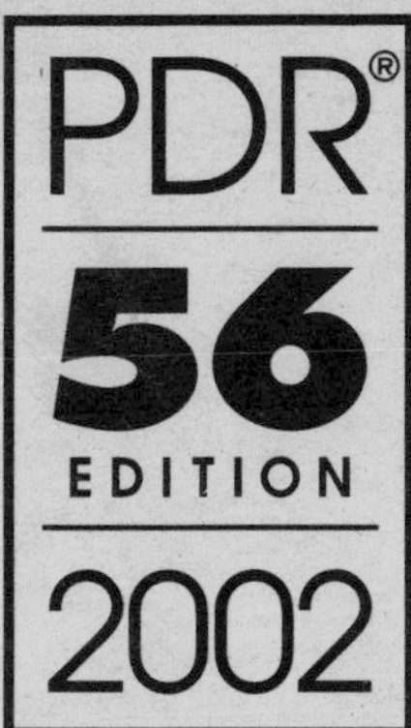

PHYSICIANS' DESK REFERENCE®

Supplement A

For important errata, turn the page.

IMPORTANT NOTICE

Supplements to PHYSICIANS' DESK REFERENCE are published twice yearly to provide readers with significant revisions of existing product listings as well as comprehensive information on new drugs and other products not included in the current annual edition. Before prescribing or administering any product described in PHYSICIANS' DESK REFERENCE, be sure to consult this supplement to determine whether revisions have occurred since the 2002 edition of PDR went to press.

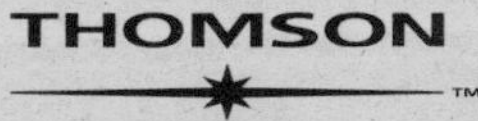

ERRATA

Paddock Laboratories, Inc.

In the list of the company's products found on page 14 of the Manufacturers' Index to the 2002 edition, an entry for **Bacitracin USP Micronized Powder** should appear under "Other Products Available."

Product Identification Guide

Under the photos of the **Ultram** 50-milligram tablet on page 330 of the 2002 edition, the generic name should be listed as "tramadol HCl tablets," not "topiramate tablets."

NEW PRODUCT LISTINGS INDEX

Listed below are new *PDR* listings first appearing in 2002 *PDR Supplement A*. These listings include comprehensive descriptions of new pharmaceutical products introduced since publication of the 2002 *PDR*, new dosage forms of products already described, and existing pharmaceutical products not described in the 2002 *PDR*.

REVISED PRODUCT INFORMATION INDEX

As new research data and clinical findings become available, the product information in *PDR* is revised accordingly. Revisions submitted since the 2002 edition went to press can be found below. To remind yourself of a revision, write "See Supplement A" next to the product's heading in the book.

Brand/Generic (Manufacturer, PDR Page No.) — **Supplement Page**

NEW PRODUCT LISTINGS

This section contains comprehensive descriptions of new pharmaceutical products introduced since publication of the 2002 *PDR*, new dosage forms of products already described, and existing pharmaceutical products not described in the 2002 *PDR*.

Actelion Pharmaceuticals US, Inc.

601 GATEWAY BLVD., SUITE 100
S. SAN FRANCISCO, CA 94080

Direct Inquiries to:
Michael Halstead
650-624-6900

TRACLEER™ ℞
[*trək' lĕr*]
(bosentan)
62.5 mg and 125 mg film-coated tablets

Use of TRACLEER™ requires attention to two significant concerns: 1) potential for serious liver injury, and 2) potential damage to a fetus.

WARNING: Potential liver injury
TRACLEER™ causes at least 3-fold (upper limit of normal; ULN) elevation of liver aminotransferases (ALT and AST) in about 11% of patients, accompanied by elevated bilirubin in a small number of cases. Because these changes are a marker for potential serious liver injury, serum aminotransferase levels must be measured prior to initiation of treatment and then monthly (see WARNINGS: Potential Liver Injury and DOSAGE AND ADMINISTRATION). To date, in a setting of close monitoring, elevations have been reversible, within a few days to 9 weeks, either spontaneously or after dose reduction or discontinuation, and without sequelae.
Elevations in aminotransferases require close attention (see DOSAGE AND ADMINISTRATION). TRACLEER™ should generally be avoided in patients with elevated aminotransferases (> 3 × ULN) at baseline because monitoring liver injury may be more difficult.
If liver aminotransferase elevations are accompanied by clinical symptoms of liver injury (such as nausea, vomiting, fever, abdominal pain, jaundice, or unusual lethargy or fatigue) or increases in bilirubin ≥ 2 × ULN, treatment should be stopped. There is no experience with the re-introduction of TRACLEER™ in these circumstances.

CONTRAINDICATION: Pregnancy
TRACLEER™ (bosentan) is very likely to produce major birth defects if used by pregnant women, as this effect has been seen consistently when it is administered to animals (see CONTRAINDICATIONS). Therefore, pregnancy must be excluded before the start of treatment with TRACLEER™ and prevented thereafter by the use of a reliable method of contraception. Hormonal contraceptives, including oral, injectable and implantable contraceptives should not be used as the sole means of contraception because these may not be effective in patients receiving TRACLEER™ (see Precautions: Drug Interactions). Monthly pregnancy tests should be obtained.
Because of potential liver injury and in an effort to make the chance of fetal exposure to TRACLEER™ (bosentan) as small as possible, TRACLEER™ may be prescribed only through the TRACLEER™ Access Program by calling 1 866 228 3546. Adverse events can also be reported directly via this number.

DESCRIPTION

Bosentan is the first of a new drug class, an endothelin receptor antagonist.

TRACLEER™ (bosentan) belongs to a class of highly substituted pyrimidine derivatives, with no chiral centers. It is designated chemically as 4-tert-butyl-N-[6-(2-hydroxy-ethoxy)-5-(2-methoxy-phenoxy)-[2,2']-bipyrimidin-4-yl]-benzenesulfonamide monohydrate and has the following structural formula:

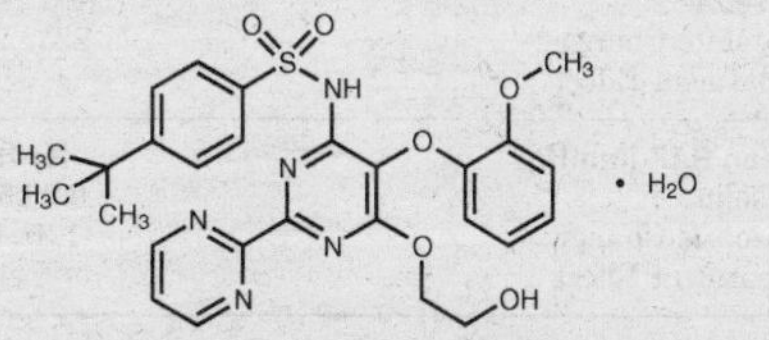

Bosentan has a molecular weight of 569.64 and a molecular formula of $C_{27}H_{29}N_5O_6S{\bullet}H_2O$. Bosentan is a white to yellowish powder. It is poorly soluble in water (1.0 mg/100 ml) and in aqueous solutions at low pH (0.1 mg/100 ml at pH 1.1 and 4.0; 0.2 mg/100 ml at pH 5.0). Solubility increases at higher pH values (43 mg/100 ml at pH 7.5). In the solid state, bosentan is very stable, is not hygroscopic and is not light sensitive.

TRACLEER™ is available as 62.5 mg and 125 mg film-coated tablets for oral administration, and contains the following excipients: corn starch, pregelatinized starch, sodium starch glycolate, povidone, glyceryl behenate, magnesium stearate, hydroxypropylmethylcellulose, triacetin, talc, titanium dioxide, iron oxide yellow, iron oxide red, and ethylcellulose. Each TRACLEER™ 62.5 mg tablet contains 64.541 mg of bosentan, equivalent to 62.5 mg of anhydrous bosentan. Each TRACLEER™ 125 mg tablet contains 129.082 mg of bosentan, equivalent to 125 mg of anhydrous bosentan.

CLINICAL PHARMACOLOGY

Mechanism of Action

Endothelin-1 (ET-1) is a neurohormone, the effects of which are mediated by binding to ET_A and ET_B receptors in the endothelium and vascular smooth muscle. ET-1 concentrations are elevated in plasma and lung tissue of patients with pulmonary arterial hypertension, suggesting a pathogenic role for ET-1 in this disease. Bosentan is a specific and competitive antagonist at endothelin receptor types ET_A and ET_B. Bosentan has a slightly higher affinity for ET_A receptors than for ET_B receptors.

Pharmacokinetics

General

After oral administration, maximum plasma concentrations of bosentan are attained within 3–5 hours and the terminal elimination half-life ($t_{1/2}$) is about 5 hours. Pharmacokinetics of bosentan was not studied in patients with pulmonary arterial hypertension, but exposure is expected to be greater in such patients because increased (30-40%) bosentan exposure was observed in patients with severe chronic heart failure.

Absorption and Distribution

The absolute bioavailability of bosentan in normal volunteers is about 50% and is unaffected by food. The volume of distribution is about 18 L. Bosentan is highly bound (> 98%) to plasma proteins, mainly albumin. Bosentan does not penetrate into erythrocytes.

Metabolism and Elimination

Bosentan has three metabolites, one of which is pharmacologically active and may contribute 10%–20% of the effect of bosentan. Bosentan is an inducer of CYP2C9 and CYP3A4 and possibly also of CYP2C19. Total clearance after a single intravenous dose is about 8 L/hr. Upon multiple dosing, plasma concentrations decrease gradually to 50–65% of those seen after single dose administration, probably the effect of auto-induction of the metabolizing liver enzymes. Steady-state is reached within 3–5 days. Bosentan is eliminated by biliary excretion following metabolism in the liver. Less than 3% of an administered oral dose is recovered in urine.

Special Populations

It is not known whether bosentan pharmacokinetics is influenced by gender, body weight, race, or age.

Liver Function Impairment

The influence of liver impairment on the pharmacokinetics of bosentan has not been evaluated, but *in vitro* and *in vivo* evidence showing extensive hepatic metabolism of bosentan suggests that liver impairment would significantly increase exposure of bosentan. Caution should be exercised during the use of TRACLEER™ in patients with mildly impaired liver function. TRACLEER™ should generally be avoided in patients with moderate or severe liver abnormalities and/or elevated aminotransferases > 3 × ULN (See **DOSAGE AND ADMINISTRATION**).

Renal Impairment

In patients with severe renal impairment (creatinine clearance 1530 ml/min), plasma concentrations of bosentan were essentially unchanged and plasma concentrations of the three metabolites were increased about 2-fold compared to people with normal renal function. These differences do not appear to be clinically important (See **DOSAGE AND ADMINISTRATION**).

Clinical Studies

Two randomized, double-blind, multi-center, placebo-controlled trials were conducted in 32 and 213 patients. The larger study (BREATHE-1) compared 2 doses (125 mg b.i.d. and 250 mg b.i.d.) of TRACLEER™ with placebo. The smaller study (Study 351) compared 125 mg b.i.d. with placebo. Patients had severe (WHO functional Class III-IV) pulmonary arterial hypertension: primary pulmonary hypertension (72%) or pulmonary hypertension secondary to scleroderma or other connective tissue diseases (21%), or to autoimmune diseases (7%). There were no patients with pulmonary hypertension secondary to other conditions such as HIV disease, or recurrent pulmonary emboli.

In both studies, TRACLEER™ or placebo was added to patients' current therapy, which could have included a combination of digoxin, anticoagulants, diuretics, and vasodilators (e.g., calcium channel blockers, ACE inhibitors), but not epoprostenol. TRACLEER™ was given at a dose of 62.5 mg b.i.d. for 4 weeks and then at 125 mg b.i.d. or 250 mg b.i.d. for either 12 (BREATHE-1) or 8 (Study 351) additional weeks. The primary study endpoint was 6-minute walk distance. In addition, symptoms and functional status were assessed. Hemodynamic measurements were made at 12 weeks in Study 351.

The mean age was about 49 years. About 80% of patients were female, and about 80% were Caucasian. Patients had been diagnosed with pulmonary hypertension for a mean of 2.4 years.

Submaximal Exercise Capacity

Results of the 6-minute walk distance at 3 months (Study 351) or 4 months (BREATHE-1) are shown in Table 1.

[See table 1 at top of next page]

Figure 1. Mean Change in 6-min Walk Distance (BREATHE-1)

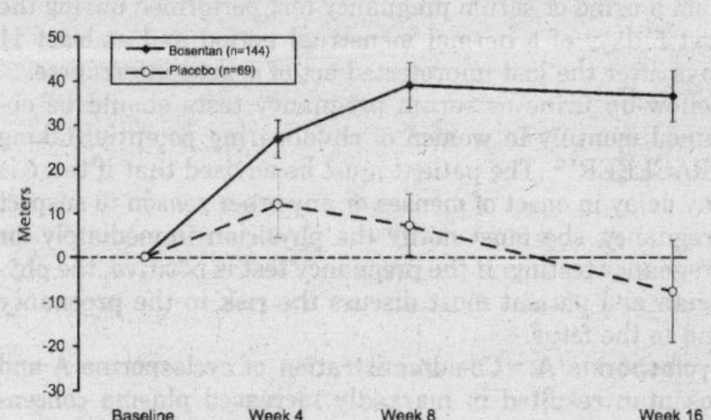

Change from baseline in 6-minute walk distance from start of therapy to week 16 in the placebo and combined bosentan (125 mg b.i.d. and 250 mg b.i.d.) groups. Values are expressed as mean ± standard error of the mean.

Continued on next page

Tracleer—Cont.

In both trials, treatment with TRACLEER™ resulted in a significant increase in exercise capacity. The improvement in walk distance was apparent after 1 month of treatment (with 62.5 mg b.i.d.) and fully developed by about 2 months of treatment (Figure 1). It was maintained for up to 7 months of double-blind treatment. Walking distance was somewhat greater with 250 mg b.i.d., but the potential for increased liver injury causes this dose not to be recommended (See **DOSAGE AND ADMINISTRATION**). There were no apparent differences in treatment effects on walk distance among subgroups analyzed by demographic factors, baseline disease severity, or disease etiology, but the studies had little power to detect such differences.

Hemodynamic Changes

Invasive hemodynamic parameters were assessed in Study 351. Treatment with TRACLEER™ led to a significant increase in cardiac index (CI) associated with a significant reduction in pulmonary artery pressure (PAP), pulmonary vascular resistance (PVR), and mean right atrial pressure (RAP) (Table 2).

Symptoms and Functional Status

Symptoms of pulmonary arterial hypertension were assessed by Borg dyspnea score, WHO functional class, and rate of "clinical worsening." Clinical worsening was assessed as the sum of death, hospitalizations for PAH, discontinuation of therapy because of PAH, and need for epoprostenol. There was a significant reduction in dyspnea during walk tests (Borg dyspnea score), and significant improvement in WHO functional class in TRACLEER™-treated patients. There was a significant reduction in the rate of clinical worsening (Table 3 and Figure 2). Figure 2 shows the Log-rank test reflecting clinical worsening over 28 weeks. The long-term effect of TRACLEER™ was further assessed in an open-label study with 29 patients receiving at least one year of treatment. Without a control group, these data must be interpreted cautiously. During this period, no patients died and one patient deteriorated, requiring treatment with epoprostenol.

[See table 2 above]
[See table 3 above]

INDICATIONS AND USAGE

TRACLEER™ is indicated for the treatment of pulmonary arterial hypertension in patients with WHO Class III or IV symptoms, to improve exercise ability and decrease the rate of clinical worsening (see **Clinical Studies**).

CONTRAINDICATIONS

See **BOX WARNING** for **CONTRAINDICATION** to use in pregnancy.

Pregnancy Category X. TRACLEER™ is expected to cause fetal harm if administered to pregnant women. Bosentan was teratogenic in rats given oral doses ≥ 60 mg/kg/day (twice the maximum recommended human oral dose of 125 mg, b.i.d., on a mg/m^2 basis). In an embryo-fetal toxicity study in rats, bosentan showed dose-dependent teratogenic effects, including malformations of the head, mouth, face and large blood vessels. Bosentan increased stillbirths and pup mortality at oral doses of 60 and 300 mg/kg/day (2 and 10 times, respectively, the maximum recommended human dose on a mg/m^2 basis). Although birth defects were not observed in rabbits given oral doses of up to 1500 mg/kg/day, plasma concentrations of bosentan in rabbits were lower than those reached in the rat. The similarity of malformations induced by bosentan and those observed in endothelin-1 knockout mice and in animals treated with other endothelin receptor antagonists indicates that teratogenicity is a class effect of these drugs. There are no data on the use of TRACLEER™ in pregnant women.

Pregnancy must be excluded before the start of treatment with TRACLEER™ and prevented thereafter by use of reliable contraception. Hormonal contraceptives, including oral, injectable, and implantable contraceptives may not be reliable in the presence of TRACLEER™ and should not be used as the sole contraceptive method in patients receiving TRACLEER™ (see **Drug Interactions**: Hormonal Contraceptives, Including Oral, Injectable, and Implantable Contraceptives). Input from a gynecologist or similar expert on adequate contraception should be sought as needed.

TRACLEER™ should be started only in patients known not to be pregnant. For female patients of childbearing potential, a prescription for TRACLEER™ should not be issued by the prescriber unless the patient assures the prescriber that she is not sexually active or provides negative results from a urine or serum pregnancy test performed during the first 5 days of a normal menstrual period and at least 11 days after the last unprotected act of sexual intercourse.

Follow-up urine or serum pregnancy tests should be obtained monthly in women of childbearing potential taking TRACLEER™. The patient must be advised that if there is any delay in onset of menses or any other reason to suspect pregnancy, she must notify the physician immediately for pregnancy testing. If the pregnancy test is positive, the physician and patient must discuss the risk to the pregnancy and to the fetus.

Cyclosporine A: Co-administration of cyclosporine A and bosentan resulted in markedly increased plasma concentrations of bosentan. Therefore, concomitant use of TRACLEER™ and cyclosporine A is contraindicated.

Glyburide: An increased risk of liver enzyme elevations was observed in patients receiving glyburide concomitantly with bosentan. Therefore co-administration of glyburide and TRACLEER™ is contraindicated.

Table 1 Effects of bosentan on 6-minute walk distance

	BREATHE-1			Study 351	
	Bosentan 125 mg b.i.d. (n = 74)	*Bosentan 250 mg b.i.d. (n = 70)*	Placebo (n = 69)	Bosentan 125 mg b.i.d. (n = 21)	Placebo (n =11)
Baseline	*326 ± 73*	*333 ± 75*	344 ± 76	360 ± 86	355 ± 82
End point	*353 ± 115*	*379 ± 101*	336 ± 129	431 ± 66	350 ± 147
Change from baseline	*27 ± 75*	*46 ± 62*	-8 ± 96	70 ± 56	-6 ± 121
Placebo - substracted	*35[(a)]*	*54[(b)]*		76[(c)]	

Distance in meters: mean ± standard deviation. Changes are to week 16 for BREATHE-1 and to week 12 for Study 351.

[(a)]p = 0.01; by Wilcoxon
[(b)]p = 0.0001 for 250 mg; by Wilcoxon
[(c)]p = 0.02 by Student's t-test.

Table 2. Change from Baseline to Week 12: Hemodynamic Parameters

	Bosentan 125 mg b.i.d.		Placebo
Mean CI (L/min/m^2)	N=20		N=10
Baseline	2.35±0.73		2.48±1.03
Absolute Change	0.50±0.46		-0.52±0.48
Treatment Effect		1.02[(a)]	
Mean PAP (mmHg)	N=20		N=10
Baseline	53.7±13.4		55.7±10.5
Absolute Change	-1.6±5.1		5.1±8.8
Treatment Effect		-6.7[(b)]	
Mean PVR (dyn•sec•cm^{-5})	N=19		N=10
Baseline	896±425		942±430
Absolute Change	-223±245		191±235
Treatment Effect		-415[(a)]	
Mean RAP (mmHg)	N=19		N=10
Baseline	9.7±5.6		9.9±4.1
Absolute Change	-1.3±4.1		4.9±4.6
Treatment Effect		-6.2[(a)]	

Values shown are means ± SD

[(a)]p≤0.001
[(b)]p<0.02

Table 3. Incidence of Clinical Worsening, Intent To Treat Population

	BREATHE-1		Study 351	
	Bonsentan 125/250 mg b.i.d. (N = 144)	Placebo (N = 69)	Bonsentan 125 mg b.i.d. (N = 21)	Placebo (N = 11)
Patients with clinical worsening [n (%)]	9 (6%)[(a)]	14 (20%)	0 (0%)[(b)]	3 (27%)
Death	1 (1%)	2 (3%)	0 (0%)	0 (0%)
Hospitalization for PAH	6 (4%)	9 (13%)	0 (0%)	3 (27%)
Discontinuation due to worsening of PAH	5 (3%)	6 (9%)	0 (0%)	3 (27%)
Receipt of epoprostenol[(c)]	4 (3%)	3 (4%)	0 (0%)	3 (27%)

Note: Patients may have had more than one reason for clinical worsening.

[(a)]p=0.0015 vs. placebo by log-rank test. There was no relevant difference between the 125 mg and 250 mg b.i.d. groups.
[(b)]p=0.033 vs. placebo by Fisher's exact test.
[(c)]Receipt of epoprostenol was always a consequence of clinical worsening.

Hypersensitivity. TRACLEER™ is also contraindicated in patients who are hypersensitive to bosentan or any component of the medication.

WARNINGS

Potential Liver Injury (see **BOX WARNING**)

Elevations in ALT or AST by more than 3 × ULN were observed in 11% of bosentan-treated patients (N = 658) compared to 2% of placebo-treated patients (N = 280). Threefold increases were seen in 12% of 95 PAH patients on 125 mg b.i.d. and 14% of 70 PAH patients on 250 mg b.i.d. Eight-fold increases were seen in 2% of PAH patients on 125 mg b.i.d. and 7% of PAH patients on 250 mg b.i.d. Bilirubin increases to ≥ 3 × ULN were associated with aminotransferase increases in 2 of 658 (0.3%) of patients treated with bosentan.

The combination of hepatocellular injury (increases in aminotransferases of > 3 × ULN) and increases in total bilirubin (≥ 3 × ULN) is a marker for potential serious liver injury.[1]

Elevations of AST and/or ALT associated with bosentan are dose-dependent, occur both early and late in treatment, usually progress slowly, are typically asymptomatic, and to date have been reversible after treatment interruption or cessation. These aminotransferase elevations may reverse spontaneously while continuing treatment with TRACLEER.™

[See figure at top of next column]

Liver aminotransferase levels must be measured prior to initiation of treatment and then monthly. If elevated aminotransferase levels are seen, changes in monitoring and

Figure 2. Time to Clinical Worsening (BREATHE-1)

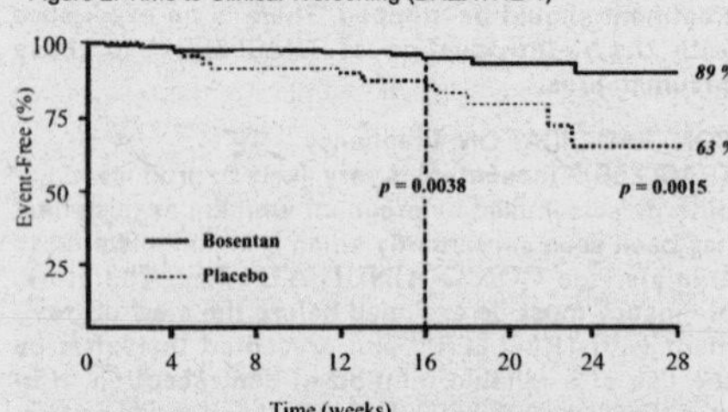

Time from randomization to clinical worsening with Kaplan-Meier estimates of the proportions of failures in BREATHE-1. All patients (N=144 in the bosentan group and N=69 in the placebo group) participated in the first 16 weeks of the study. A subset of this population (N=35 in the bosentan group and 13 in the placebo group) continued double-blind therapy for up to 28 weeks.

treatment must be initiated (see **DOSAGE AND ADMINISTRATION**). If liver aminotransferase elevations are accompanied by clinical symptoms of liver injury (such as nausea, vomiting, fever, abdominal pain, jaundice, or unusual lethargy or fatigue) or increases in bilirubin ≥ 2 × ULN, treatment should be stopped. There is no experience with the re-introduction of TRACLEER™ in these circumstances.

Pre-existing Liver Impairment

Liver aminotransferase levels must be measured prior to initiation of treatment and then monthly. TRACLEER™ should generally be avoided in patients with moderate or severe liver impairment (see **Clinical Pharmacology** and **DOSAGE AND ADMINISTRATION**). In addition, TRACLEER™ should generally be avoided in patients with elevated aminotransferases (> 3 × ULN) because monitoring liver injury in these patients may be more difficult (see **BOX WARNING**).

PRECAUTIONS

Hematologic Changes

Treatment with TRACLEER™ caused a dose-related decrease in hemoglobin and hematocrit. Hemoglobin levels should be monitored after 1 and 3 months of treatment and then every 3 months. The overall mean decrease in hemoglobin concentration for bosentan-treated patients was 0.9 g/dl (change to end of treatment). Most of this decrease of hemoglobin concentration was detected during the first few weeks of bosentan treatment and hemoglobin levels stabilized by 4–12 weeks of bosentan treatment.

In placebo-controlled studies of all uses of bosentan, marked decreases in hemoglobin (> 15% decrease from baseline resulting in values < 11 g/dl) were observed in 6% of bosentan-treated patients and 3% of placebo-treated patients. In patients with pulmonary arterial hypertension treated with doses of 125 and 250 mg b.i.d., marked decreases in hemoglobin occurred in 3% compared to 1% in placebo-treated patients.

A decrease in hemoglobin concentration by at least 1 g/dl was observed in 57% of bosentan-treated patients as compared to 29% of placebo-treated patients. In 80% of those patients whose hemoglobin decreased by at least 1 g/dl, the decrease occurred during the first 6 weeks of bosentan treatment.

During the course of treatment the hemoglobin concentration remained within normal limits in 68% of bosentan-treated patients compared to 76% of placebo patients.

The explanation for the change in hemoglobin is not known, but it does not appear to be hemorrhage or hemolysis.

It is recommended that hemoglobin concentrations be checked after 1 and 3 months, and every 3 months thereafter. If a marked decrease in hemoglobin concentration occurs, further evaluation should be undertaken to determine the cause and need for specific treatment.

Information for Patients

Patients are advised to consult the TRACLEER™ Medication Guide on the safe use of TRACLEER™.

The physician should discuss with the patient the importance of monthly monitoring of serum aminotransferases and urine or serum pregnancy testing and of avoidance of pregnancy. The physician should discuss options for effective contraception and measures to prevent pregnancy with their female patients. Input from a gynecologist or similar expert on adequate contraception should be sought as needed.

Drug Interactions

Bosentan is metabolized by CYP2C9 and CYP3A4. Inhibition of these isoenzymes may increase the plasma concentration of bosentan (see ketoconazole). Bosentan is an inducer of CYP3A4 and CYP2C9. Consequently, plasma concentrations of drugs metabolized by these two isoenzymes will be decreased when TRACLEER™ is co-administered. Bosentan had no relevant inhibitory effect on any CYP isoenzymes tested (CYP1A2, CYP2C9, CYP2C19, CYP2D6, CYP3A4). Consequently, TRACLEER™ is not expected to increase the plasma concentrations of drugs metabolized by these enzymes.

Hormonal Contraceptives, Including Oral, Injectable, and Implantable Contraceptives: Specific interaction studies have not been performed to evaluate the effect of co-administration of bosentan and hormonal contraceptives, including oral, injectable or implantable contraceptives. Since many of these drugs are metabolized by CYP3A4, there is a possibility of failure of contraception when TRACLEER™ is co-administered. Women should not rely on hormonal contraception alone when taking TRACLEER™.

Specific interaction studies have demonstrated the following:

Cyclosporine A: During the first day of concomitant administration, trough concentrations of bosentan were increased by about 30-fold. Steady-state bosentan plasma concentrations were 3- to 4-fold higher than in the absence of cyclosporine A. The concomitant administration of bosentan and cyclosporine A is contraindicated (see **CONTRAINDICATIONS**). Co-administration of bosentan decreased the plasma concentrations of cyclosporine A (a CYP3A4 substrate) by approximately 50%.

Glyburide: An increased risk of elevated liver aminotransferases was observed in patients receiving concomitant therapy with glyburide. Therefore, the concomitant administration of TRACLEER™ and glyburide is contraindicated, and alternative hypoglycemic agents should be considered (see **CONTRAINDICATIONS**).

Co-administration of bosentan decreased the plasma concentrations of glyburide by approximately 40%. The plasma concentrations of bosentan were also decreased by approximately 30%. Bosentan is also expected to reduce plasma concentrations of other oral hypoglycemic agents that are predominantly metabolized by CYP2C9 or CYP3A4. The possibility of worsened glucose control in patients using these agents should be considered.

Ketoconazole: Co-administration of bosentan 125 mg b.i.d. and ketoconazole, a potent CYP3A4 inhibitor, increased the plasma concentrations of bosentan by approximately 2-fold. No dose adjustment of bosentan is necessary, but increased effects of bosentan should be considered.

Simvastatin and Other Statins: Co-administration of bosentan decreased the plasma concentrations of simvastatin (a CYP3A4 substrate), and its active β-hydroxy acid metabolite, by approximately 50%. The plasma concentrations of bosentan were not affected. Bosentan is also expected to reduce plasma concentrations of other statins that have significant metabolism by CYP3A4, such as lovastatin and atorvastatin. The possibility of reduced statin efficacy should be considered. Patients using CYP3A4 metabolized statins should have cholesterol levels monitored after TRACLEER™ is initiated to see whether the statin dose needs adjustment.

Warfarin: Co-administration of bosentan 500 mg b.i.d. for 6 days decreased the plasma concentrations of both S-warfarin (a CYP2C9 substrate) and R-warfarin (a CYP3A4 substrate) by 29 and 38%, respectively. Clinical experience with concomitant administration of bosentan and warfarin in patients with pulmonary arterial hypertension did not show clinically relevant changes in INR or warfarin dose (baseline vs. end of the clinical studies), and the need to change the warfarin dose during the trials due to changes in INR or due to adverse events was similar among bosentan- and placebo-treated patients.

Digoxin, Nimodipine and Losartan: Bosentan has been shown to have no pharmacokinetic interactions with digoxin and nimodipine, and losartan has no effect on plasma levels of bosentan.

Carcinogenesis, Mutagenesis, Impairment of Fertility

Two years of dietary administration of bosentan to mice produced an increased incidence of hepatocellular adenomas and carcinomas in males at doses as low as 450 mg/kg/day (about 8 times the maximum recommended human dose [MRHD] of 125 mg b.i.d., on a mg/m^2 basis). In the same study, doses greater than 2000 mg/kg/day (about 32 times the MRHD) were associated with an increased incidence of colon adenomas in both males and females. In rats, dietary administration of bosentan for two years was associated with an increased incidence of brain astrocytomas in males at doses as low as 500 mg/kg/day (about 16 times the MRHD). In a comprehensive battery of *in vitro* tests (the microbial mutagenesis assay, the unscheduled DNA synthesis assay, the V-79 mammalian cell mutagenesis assay, and human lymphocyte assay) and an *in vivo* mouse micronucleus assay, there was no evidence for any mutagenic or clastogenic activity of bosentan.

Impairment of Fertility/Testicular Function

Many endothelin receptor antagonists have profound effects on the histology and function of the testes in animals. These drugs have been shown to induce atrophy of the seminiferous tubules of the testes and to reduce sperm counts and male fertility in rats when administered for longer than 10 weeks. Where studied, testicular tubular atrophy and decreases in male fertility observed with endothelin receptor antagonists appear irreversible.

In fertility studies in which male and female rats were treated with bosentan at oral doses of up to 1500 mg/kg/day (50 times the MRHD on a mg/m^2 basis) or intravenous doses up to 40 mg/kg/day, no effects on sperm count, sperm motility, mating performance or fertility were observed. An increased incidence of testicular tubular atrophy was observed in rats given bosentan orally at doses as low as 125 mg/kg/day (about 4 times the MRHD and the lowest doses tested) for two years but not at doses as high as 1500 mg/kg/day (about 50 times the MRHD) for 6 months. Effects on sperm count and motility were evaluated only in the much shorter duration fertility studies in which males had been exposed to the drug for 4-6 weeks. An increased incidence of tubular atrophy was not observed in mice treated for 2 years at doses up to 4500 mg/kg/day (about 75 times the MRHD) or in dogs treated up to 12 months at doses up to 500 mg/kg/day (about 50 times the MRHD).

There are no data on the effects of bosentan or other endothelin receptor antagonists on testicular function in man.

Pregnancy, Teratogenic Effects: Category X (See **CONTRAINDICATIONS**).

Nursing Mothers

It is not known whether this drug is excreted in human milk. Because many drugs are excreted in human milk, breastfeeding while taking TRACLEER™ is not recommended.

Pediatric Use

Safety and efficacy in pediatric patients have not been established. (see **DOSAGE AND ADMINISTRATION**).

Use in Elderly Patients

Clinical experience with TRACLEER™ in subjects aged 65 or older has not included a sufficient number of such subjects to identify a difference in response between elderly and younger patients (see **DOSAGE AND ADMINISTRATION**).

ADVERSE REACTIONS

Adverse Events

See **BOX WARNING** for discussion of liver injury and **PRECAUTIONS** for discussion of hemoglobin and hematocrit abnormalities.

Safety data on bosentan were obtained from 12 clinical studies (8 placebo-controlled and 4 open-label) in 777 patients with pulmonary arterial hypertension, and other diseases. Doses up to 8 times the currently recommended clinical dose (125 mg b.i.d.) were administered for a variety of durations. The exposure to bosentan in these trials ranged from 1 day to 4.1 years (N=89 for 1 year; N=61 for 1.5 years and N=39 for more than 2 years). Exposure of pulmonary arterial hypertension patients (N=235) to bosentan ranged from 1 day to 1.7 years (N=126 more than 6 months and N=28 more than 12 months).

Treatment discontinuations due to adverse events other than those related to pulmonary hypertension during the clinical trials in patients with pulmonary arterial hypertension were more frequent on bosentan (5%; 8/165 patients) than on placebo (3%; 2/80 patients). In this database the only cause of discontinuations > 1%, and occurring more often on bosentan was abnormal liver function.

The adverse drug reactions that occurred in ≥ 3% of the bosentan-treated patients and were more common on bosentan in placebo-controlled trials in pulmonary arterial hypertension at doses of 125 or 250 mg b.i.d. are shown in Table 4:

Table 4. Adverse events* occurring in ≥ 3% of patients treated with bosentan 125-250 mg b.i.d. and more common on bosentanin placebo-controlled studies in pulmonary arterial hypertension

Adverse Event	Bosentan N=165		Placebo N=80	
	No.	%	No.	%
Headache	36	22%	16	20%
Nasopharyngitis	18	11%	6	8%
Flushing	15	9%	4	5%
Hepatic function abnormal	14	8%	2	3%
Edema, lower limb	13	8%	4	5%
Hypotension	11	7%	3	4%
Palpitations	8	5%	1	1%
Dyspepsia	7	4%	0	0%
Edema	7	4%	2	3%
Fatigue	6	4%	1	1%
Pruritus	6	4%	0	0%

***Note: only AEs with onset from start of treatment to 1 calendar day after end of treatment are included. All reported events (at least 3%) are included except those too general to be informative, and those not reasonably associated with the use of the drug because they were associated with the condition being treated or are very common in the treated population.**

In placebo-controlled studies of bosentan in pulmonary arterial hypertension and for other diseases (primarily chronic heart failure), a total of 677 patients were treated with bosentan at daily doses ranging from 100 mg to 2000 mg and 288 patients were treated with placebo. The duration of treatment ranged from 4 weeks to 6 months. For the adverse drug reactions that occurred in ≥ 3% of bosentan-treated patients, the only ones that occurred more frequently on bosentan than on placebo (≥ 2% difference) were headache (16% vs. 13%), flushing (7% vs. 2%), abnormal hepatic function (6% vs. 2%), leg edema (5% vs. 1%), and anemia (3% vs. 1%).

Laboratory Abnormalities

Increased Liver Aminotransferases (see BOX WARNING and WARNINGS).

Decreased Hemoglobin and Hematocrit (see **PRECAUTIONS**)

OVERDOSAGE

Bosentan has been given as a single dose of up to 2400 mg in normal volunteers, or up to 2000 mg/day for 2 months in patients, without any major clinical consequences. The most common side effect was headache of mild to moderate intensity. In the cyclosporine A interaction study, in which doses of 500 and 1000 mg b.i.d. of bosentan were given concomitantly with cyclosporine A, trough plasma concentrations of bosentan increased 30-fold, resulting in severe headache, nausea, and vomiting, but no serious adverse events. Mild decreases in blood pressure and increases in heart rate were observed.

There is no specific experience of overdosage with bosentan beyond the doses described above. Massive overdosage may result in pronounced hypotension requiring active cardiovascular support.

DOSAGE AND ADMINISTRATION

General

TRACLEER™ treatment should be initiated at a dose of 62.5 mg b.i.d. for 4 weeks and then increased to the maintenance dose of 125 mg b.i.d. Doses above 125 mg b.i.d. did not appear to confer additional benefit sufficient to offset the increased risk of liver injury.

Tablets should be administered morning and evening with or without food.

Dosage Adjustment and Monitoring in Patients Developing Aminotransferase Abnormalities

ALT/AST levels	Treatment and monitoring recommendations
> 3 and ≤ 5 × ULN	Confirm by another aminotransferase test; if confirmed, reduce the daily dose or interrupt treatment, and monitor aminotransferase levels at least every 2 weeks. If the aminotransferase levels return to pre-treatment

Continued on next page

Tracleer—Cont.

	values, continue or re-introduce the treatment as appropriate (see below).
> 5 and ≤ 8 × ULN	Confirm by another aminotransferase test; if confirmed, stop treatment and monitor aminotransferase levels at least every 2 weeks. Once the aminotransferase levels return to pre-treatment values, consider re-introduction of the treatment (see below).
> 8 × ULN	Treatment should be stopped and reintroduction of TRACLEER™ should not be considered. There is no experience with re-introduction of TRACLEER™ in these circumstances.

If TRACLEER™ is re-introduced it should be at the starting dose; aminotransferase levels should be checked within 3 days and thereafter according to the recommendations above.

If liver aminotransferase elevations are accompanied by clinical symptoms of liver injury (such as nausea, vomiting, fever, abdominal pain, jaundice, or unusual lethargy or fatigue) or increases in bilirubin ≥2 x ULN, treatment should be stopped. There is no experience with the re-introduction of TRACLEER™ in these circumstances.

Use in Women of Child-bearing Potential

TRACLEER™ treatment should only be initiated in women of child-bearing potential following a negative pregnancy test and only in those who practice adequate contraception that does not rely solely upon hormonal contraceptives, including oral, injectable or implantable contraceptives (see **DRUG INTERACTIONS:** Hormonal contraceptives, Including Oral, Injectable and Implantable Contraceptives). Input from a gynecologist or similar expert on adequate contraception should be sought as needed. Urine or serum pregnancy tests should be obtained monthly in women of child-bearing potential taking TRACLEER™.

Dosage Adjustment in Renally Impaired Patients

The effect of renal impairment on the pharmacokinetics of bosentan is small and does not require dosing adjustment.

Dosage Adjustment in Geriatric Patients

Clinical studies of TRACLEER™ did not include sufficient numbers of subjects aged 65 and older to determine whether they respond differently from younger subjects. Clinical experience has not identified differences in responses between elderly and younger patients. In general, caution should be exercised in dose selection for elderly patients given the greater frequency of decreased hepatic, renal, or cardiac function, and of concomitant disease or other drug therapy in this age group.

Dosage Adjustment in Hepatically Impaired Patients

The influence of liver impairment on the pharmacokinetics of TRACLEER™ has not been evaluated. Because there is *in vivo* and *in vitro* evidence that the main route of excretion of TRACLEER™ is biliary, liver impairment would be expected to increase exposure (Cmax, AUC) to bosentan. There are no specific data to guide dosing in hepatically impaired patients (See **WARNINGS**); caution should be exercised in patients with mildly impaired liver function. TRACLEER™ should generally be avoided in patients with moderate or severe liver impairment.

Dosage Adjustment in Children

Safety and efficacy in pediatric patients have not been established.

Dosage Adjustment in Patients with Low Body Weight

In patients with a body weight below 40 kg but who are over 12 years of age the recommended initial and maintenance dose is 62.5 mg b.i.d.

Discontinuation of Treatment

There is limited experience with abrupt discontinuation of TRACLEER™. No evidence for acute rebound has been observed. Nevertheless, to avoid the potential for clinical deterioration, gradual dose reduction (62.5 mg b.i.d. for 3 to 7 days) should be considered.

HOW SUPPLIED

62.5 mg film-coated, round, biconvex, orange-white tablets, embossed with identification marking "62,5", packaged in a white high density polyethylene bottle and a white polypropylene child-resistant cap.

NDC 66215-101-06: Bottle containing 60 tablets.

125 mg film-coated, oval, biconvex, orange-white tablets, embossed with identification marking "125", packaged in a white high density polyethylene bottle and a white polypropylene child-resistant cap.

NDC 66215-102-06: Bottle containing 60 tablets.

Rx only.

STORAGE

Store at 20°C–25°C (68°F–77°F). Excursions are permitted between 15°C and 30°C (59°F and 86°F). [See USP Controlled Room Temperature].

Manufactured by:

Patheon Inc.
Mississauga, Ontario, CANADA

Marketed by:

Actelion Pharmaceuticals US, Inc.
South San Francisco, CA

REFERENCE

1. Zimmerman HJ. Hepatotoxicity—The adverse effects of drugs and other chemicals on the liver. Second ed. Philadelphia: Lippincott, 1999.

IN-5083/S REV 3

Amgen

AMGEN INC.
ONE AMGEN CENTER DRIVE
THOUSAND OAKS, CA 91320-1789

Direct Inquiries to:
Customer Service Department
(800) 282-6436
FAX: (800) 292-6436

For Medical Information Contact:
Professional Services Department
(800) 772-6436
FAX: 805-376-8550

In Emergencies:
(800) 772-6436

After Hours and Weekends:
(800) 772-6436

Sales and Ordering:
Customer Service Department
(800) 282-6436
FAX: (800) 292-6436

ARANESP™ ℞

(darbepoetin alfa)
For Injection

DESCRIPTION

Aranesp™ is an erythropoiesis stimulating protein closely related to erythropoietin that is produced in Chinese hamster ovary (CHO) cells by recombinant DNA technology. Aranesp™ is a 165-amino acid protein that differs from recombinant human erythropoietin in containing 5 N-linked oligosaccharide chains, whereas recombinant human erythropoietin contains 3.[1] The 2 additional N-glycosylation sites result from amino acid substitutions in the erythropoietin peptide backbone. The additional carbohydrate chains increase the approximate molecular weight of the glycoprotein from 30,000 to 37,000 daltons. Aranesp™ is formulated as a sterile, colorless, preservative-free protein solution for intravenous (IV) or subcutaneous (SC) administration.

Single-dose vials are available containing either 25, 40, 60, 100, or 200 mcg of Aranesp™. Two formulations contain excipients as follows:

Polysorbate solution contains 0.05 mg polysorbate 80, 2.12 mg sodium phosphate monobasic monohydrate, 0.66 mg sodium phosphate dibasic anhydrous, and 8.18 mg sodium chloride in Water for Injection, USP (per 1 mL) at pH 6.2 ± 0.2.

Albumin solution contains 2.5 mg albumin (human), 2.23 mg sodium phosphate monobasic monohydrate, 0.53 mg sodium phosphate dibasic anhydrous, and 8.18 mg sodium chloride in Water for Injection, USP (per 1 mL) at pH 6.0 ± 0.3.

CLINICAL PHARMACOLOGY

Mechanism of Action

Aranesp™ stimulates erythropoiesis by the same mechanism as endogenous erythropoietin. A primary growth factor for erythroid development, erythropoietin is produced in the kidney and released into the bloodstream in response to hypoxia. In responding to hypoxia, erythropoietin interacts with progenitor stem cells to increase red cell production. Production of endogenous erythropoietin is impaired in patients with chronic renal failure (CRF), and erythropoietin deficiency is the primary cause of their anemia. Increased hemoglobin levels are not generally observed until 2 to 6 weeks after initiating treatment with Aranesp™.

Pharmacokinetics

Aranesp™ has an approximately 3-fold longer terminal half-life than Epoetin alfa when administered by either the IV or SC route.

Following IV administration to adult CRF patients, Aranesp™ serum concentration-time profiles are biphasic, with a distribution half-life of approximately 1.4 hours and mean terminal half-life of approximately 21 hours.

Following SC administration, the absorption is slow and rate-limiting, and the terminal half-life is 49 hours (range: 27 to 89 hours), which reflects the absorption half-life. The peak concentration occurs at 34 hours (range: 24 to 72 hours) post-SC administration in adult CRF patients, and bioavailability is approximately 37% (range: 30% to 50%).

The distribution of Aranesp™ in adult CRF patients is predominantly confined to the vascular space (approximately 60 mL/kg). The pharmacokinetic parameters indicate dose-linearity over the therapeutic dose range. With once weekly dosing, steady-state serum levels are achieved within 4 weeks with < 2-fold increase in peak concentration when compared to the initial dose. Accumulation was negligible following both IV and SC dosing over 1 year of treatment.

CLINICAL STUDIES

The safety and effectiveness of Aranesp™ have been assessed in multicenter studies. Two studies evaluated the safety and efficacy of Aranesp™ for the correction of anemia in adult patients with CRF, and 2 studies assessed the ability of Aranesp™ to maintain hemoglobin concentrations in adult patients with CRF who had been receiving other recombinant erythropoietins.

De Novo Use of Aranesp™

In 2 open-label studies, Aranesp™ or Epoetin alfa were administered for the correction of anemia in CRF patients who had not been receiving prior treatment with exogenous erythropoietin. Study 1 evaluated CRF patients receiving dialysis; Study 2 evaluated patients not requiring dialysis (predialysis patients). In both studies, the starting dose of Aranesp™ was 0.45 mcg/kg administered once weekly. The starting dose of Epoetin alfa was 50 U/kg 3 times weekly in Study 1 and 50 U/kg twice weekly in Study 2. When necessary, dosage adjustments were instituted to maintain hemoglobin in the study target range of 11 to 13 g/dL. (Note: The recommended hemoglobin target is lower than the target range of these studies. See DOSAGE AND ADMINISTRATION: General for recommended clinical hemoglobin target.) The primary efficacy endpoint was the proportion of patients who experienced at least a 1.0 g/dL increase in hemoglobin concentration to a level of at least 11.0 g/dL by 20 weeks (Study 1) or 24 weeks (Study 2). The studies were designed to assess the safety and effectiveness of Aranesp™ but not to support conclusions regarding comparisons between the 2 products.

In Study 1, the hemoglobin target was achieved by 72% (95% CI: 62%, 81%) of the 90 patients treated with Aranesp™ and 84% (95% CI: 66%, 95%) of the 31 patients treated with Epoetin alfa. The mean increase in hemoglobin over the initial 4 weeks of Aranesp™ treatment was 1.10 g/dL (95% CI: 0.82 g/dL, 1.37 g/dL).

In Study 2, the primary efficacy endpoint was achieved by 93% (95% CI: 87%, 97%) of the 129 patients treated with Aranesp™ and 92% (95% CI: 78%, 98%) of the 37 patients treated with Epoetin alfa. The mean increase in hemoglobin from baseline through the initial 4 weeks of Aranesp™ treatment was 1.38 g/dL (95% CI: 1.21 g/dL, 1.55 g/dL).

Conversion From Other Recombinant Erythropoietins

Two studies (Studies 3 and 4) were conducted in adult patients with CRF who had been receiving other recombinant erythropoietins and compared the abilities of Aranesp™ and other erythropoietins to maintain hemoglobin concentrations within a study target range of 9 to 13 g/dL. (Note: The recommended hemoglobin target is lower than the target range of these studies. See DOSAGE AND ADMINISTRATION: General for recommended clinical hemoglobin target.) CRF patients who had been receiving stable doses of other recombinant erythropoietins were randomized to Aranesp™, or to continue with their prior erythropoietin at the previous dose and schedule. For patients randomized to Aranesp™, the initial weekly dose was determined on the basis of the previous total weekly dose of recombinant erythropoietin. Study 3 was a double-blind study conducted in North America, in which 169 hemodialysis patients were randomized to treatment with Aranesp™ and 338 patients continued on Epoetin alfa. Study 4 was an open-label study conducted in Europe and Australia in which 347 patients were randomized to treatment with Aranesp™ and 175 patients were randomized to continue on Epoetin alfa or Epoetin beta. Of the 347 patients randomized to Aranesp™, 92% were receiving hemodialysis and 8% were receiving peritoneal dialysis.

In Study 3, a median weekly dose of 0.53 mcg/kg Aranesp™ (25th, 75th percentiles: 0.30, 0.93 mcg/kg) was required to maintain hemoglobin in the study target range. In Study 4, a median weekly dose of 0.41 mcg/kg Aranesp™ (25th, 75th percentiles: 0.26, 0.65 mcg/kg) was required to maintain hemoglobin in the study target range.

INDICATIONS AND USAGE

Aranesp™ is indicated for the treatment of anemia associated with chronic renal failure, including patients on dialysis and patients not on dialysis.

CONTRAINDICATIONS

Aranesp™ is contraindicated in patients with:

- uncontrolled hypertension
- known hypersensitivity to the active substance or any of the excipients

WARNINGS

Cardiovascular Events, Hemoglobin, and Rate of Rise of Hemoglobin

Aranesp™ and other erythropoietic therapies may increase the risk of cardiovascular events, including death, in patients with CRF. The higher risk of cardiovascular events may be associated with higher hemoglobin and/or higher rates of rise of hemoglobin.

In a clinical trial of Epoetin alfa treatment in hemodialysis patients with clinically evident cardiac disease, patients were randomized to a target hemoglobin of either 14 ± 1 g/dL or 10 ± 1 g/dL.[2] Higher mortality (35% versus 29%) was observed in the 634 patients randomized to a target hemoglobin of 14 g/dL than in the 631 patients assigned a target hemoglobin of 10 g/dL. The reason for the increased mortality observed in this study is unknown; however, the incidence of nonfatal myocardial infarction, vascular access thrombosis, and other thrombotic events was also higher in the group randomized to a target hemoglobin of 14 g/dL.

In CRF patients the hemoglobin should be managed carefully, not to exceed a target of 12 g/dL.

In patients treated with Aranesp™ or other recombinant erythropoietins in Aranesp™ clinical trials, increases in hemoglobin greater than approximately 1.0 g/dL during any

2-week period were associated with increased incidence of cardiac arrest, neurologic events (including seizures and stroke), exacerbations of hypertension, congestive heart failure, vascular thrombosis/ischemia/infarction, acute myocardial infarction, and fluid overload/edema. It is recommended that the dose of Aranesp™ be decreased if the hemoglobin increase exceeds 1.0 g/dL in any 2-week period, because of the association of excessive rate of rise of hemoglobin with these events.

Hypertension

Patients with uncontrolled hypertension should not be treated with Aranesp™; blood pressure should be controlled adequately before initiation of therapy. Blood pressure may rise during treatment of anemia with Aranesp™ or Epoetin alfa. In Aranesp™ clinical trials, approximately 40% of patients required initiation or intensification of antihypertensive therapy during the early phase of treatment when the hemoglobin was increasing. Hypertensive encephalopathy and seizures have been observed in patients with CRF treated with Aranesp™ or Epoetin alfa.

Special care should be taken to closely monitor and control blood pressure in patients treated with Aranesp™. During Aranesp™ therapy, patients should be advised of the importance of compliance with antihypertensive therapy and dietary restrictions. If blood pressure is difficult to control by pharmacologic or dietary measures, the dose of Aranesp™ should be reduced or withheld (see DOSAGE AND ADMINISTRATION: Dose Adjustment). A clinically significant decrease in hemoglobin may not be observed for several weeks.

Seizures

Seizures have occurred in patients with CRF participating in clinical trials of Aranesp™ and Epoetin alfa. During the first several months of therapy, blood pressure and the presence of premonitory neurologic symptoms should be monitored closely. While the relationship between seizures and the rate of rise of hemoglobin is uncertain, it is recommended that the dose of Aranesp™ be decreased if the hemoglobin increase exceeds 1.0 g/dL in any 2-week period.

Albumin (Human)

Aranesp™ is supplied in 2 formulations with different excipients, one containing polysorbate 80 and another containing albumin (human), a derivative of human blood (see DESCRIPTION). Based on effective donor screening and product manufacturing processes, Aranesp™ formulated with albumin carries an extremely remote risk for transmission of viral diseases. A theoretical risk for transmission of Creutzfeldt-Jakob disease (CJD) also is considered extremely remote. No cases of transmission of viral diseases or CJD have ever been identified for albumin.

PRECAUTIONS

General

A lack of response or failure to maintain a hemoglobin response with Aranesp™ doses within the recommended dosing range should prompt a search for causative factors. Deficiencies of folic acid or vitamin B_{12} should be excluded or corrected. Intercurrent infections, inflammatory or malignant processes, osteofibrosis cystica, occult blood loss, hemolysis, severe aluminum toxicity, and bone marrow fibrosis may compromise an erythropoietic response.

The safety and efficacy of Aranesp™ therapy have not been established in patients with underlying hematologic diseases (eg, hemolytic anemia, sickle cell anemia, thalassemia, porphyria).

Hematology

Sufficient time should be allowed to determine a patient's responsiveness to a dosage of Aranesp™ before adjusting the dose. Because of the time required for erythropoiesis and the red cell half-life, an interval of 2 to 6 weeks may occur between the time of a dose adjustment (initiation, increase, decrease, or discontinuation) and a significant change in hemoglobin.

In order to prevent the hemoglobin from exceeding the recommended target (12 g/dL) or rising too rapidly (greater than 1.0 g/dL in 2 weeks), the guidelines for dose and frequency of dose adjustments should be followed (see DOSAGE AND ADMINISTRATION: Dose Adjustment).

Patients With CRF Not Requiring Dialysis

Patients with CRF not yet requiring dialysis may require lower maintenance doses of Aranesp™ than patients receiving dialysis. Though predialysis patients generally receive less frequent monitoring of blood pressure and laboratory parameters than dialysis patients, predialysis patients may be more responsive to the effects of Aranesp™, and require judicious monitoring of blood pressure and hemoglobin. Renal function and fluid and electrolyte balance should also be closely monitored.

Dialysis Management

Therapy with Aranesp™ results in an increase in red blood cells and a decrease in plasma volume, which could reduce dialysis efficiency; patients who are marginally dialyzed may require adjustments in their dialysis prescription.

Laboratory Tests

After initiation of Aranesp™ therapy, the hemoglobin should be determined weekly until it has stabilized and the maintenance dose has been established (see DOSAGE AND ADMINISTRATION). After a dose adjustment, the hemoglobin should be determined weekly for at least 4 weeks until it has been determined that the hemoglobin has stabilized in response to the dose change. The hemoglobin should then be monitored at regular intervals.

In order to ensure effective erythropoiesis, iron status should be evaluated for all patients before and during treatment, as the majority of patients will eventually require supplemental iron therapy. Supplemental iron therapy is recommended for all patients whose serum ferritin is below 100 mcg/L or whose serum transferrin saturation is below 20%.

Information for Patients

Patients should be informed of the possible side effects of Aranesp™ and be instructed to report them to the prescribing physician. Patients should be informed of the signs and symptoms of allergic drug reactions and be advised of appropriate actions. Patients should be counseled on the importance of compliance with their Aranesp™ treatment, dietary and dialysis prescriptions, and the importance of judicious monitoring of blood pressure and hemoglobin concentration should be stressed.

If it is determined that a patient can safely and effectively administer Aranesp™ at home, appropriate instruction on the proper use of Aranesp™ should be provided for patients and their caregivers, including careful review of the "Information for Patients and Caregivers" insert. Patients and caregivers should also be cautioned against the reuse of needles, syringes, or drug product, and be thoroughly instructed in their proper disposal. A puncture-resistant container for the disposal of used syringes and needles should be made available to the patient.

Drug Interactions

No formal drug interaction studies of Aranesp™ with other medications commonly used in CRF patients have been performed.

Carcinogenesis, Mutagenesis, and Impairment of Fertility

Carcinogenicity: The carcinogenic potential of Aranesp™ has not been evaluated in long-term animal studies. Aranesp™ did not alter the proliferative response of nonhematological cells in vitro or in vivo. In toxicity studies of approximately 6 months duration in rats and dogs, no tumorigenic or unexpected mitogenic responses were observed in any tissue type. Using a panel of human tissues, the in vitro tissue binding profile of Aranesp™ was identical to Epoetin alfa. Neither molecule bound to human tissues other than those expressing the erythropoietin receptor.

Mutagenicity: Aranesp™ was negative in the in vitro bacterial and CHO cell assays to detect mutagenicity and in the in vivo mouse micronucleus assay to detect clastogenicity.

Impairment of Fertility: When administered intravenously to male and female rats prior to and during mating, reproductive performance, fertility, and sperm assessment parameters were not affected at any doses evaluated (up to 10 mcg/kg/dose, administered 3 times weekly). An increase in postimplantation fetal loss was seen at doses equal to or greater than 0.5 mcg/kg/dose, administered 3 times weekly (3-fold higher than the recommended weekly starting human dose).

Pregnancy Category C

When Aranesp™ was administered intravenously to rats and rabbits during gestation, no evidence of a direct embryotoxic, fetotoxic, or teratogenic outcome was observed at doses up to 20 mcg/kg/day (40-fold higher than the recommended weekly starting human dose). The only adverse effect observed was a slight reduction in fetal weight, which occurred at doses causing exaggerated pharmacological effects in the dams (1 mcg/kg/day and higher). No deleterious effects on uterine implantation were seen in either species. No significant placental transfer of Aranesp™ was observed in rats. An increase in postimplantation fetal loss was observed in studies assessing fertility (see Carcinogenesis, Mutagenesis, and Impairment of Fertility: Impairment of Fertility).

Intravenous injection of Aranesp™ to female rats every other day from day 6 of gestation through day 23 of lactation at doses of 2.5 mcg/kg/dose and higher resulted in offspring (F1 generation) with decreased body weights, which correlated with a low incidence of deaths, as well as delayed eye opening and delayed preputial separation. No adverse effects were seen in the F2 offspring.

There are no adequate and well controlled studies in pregnant women. Aranesp™ should be used during pregnancy only if the potential benefit justifies the potential risk to the fetus.

Nursing Mothers

It is not known whether Aranesp™ is excreted in human milk. Because many drugs are excreted in human milk, caution should be exercised when Aranesp™ is administered to a nursing woman.

Pediatric Use

The safety and efficacy of Aranesp™ in pediatric patients have not been established.

Geriatric Use

Of the 1598 CRF patients in clinical studies of Aranesp™, 42% were age 65 and over, while 15% were 75 and over. No overall differences in safety or efficacy were observed between these patients and younger patients, but greater sensitivity of some older individuals cannot be ruled out.

ADVERSE REACTIONS

In all studies, the most frequently reported serious adverse reactions with Aranesp™ were vascular access thrombosis, congestive heart failure, sepsis, and cardiac arrhythmia. The most commonly reported adverse reactions were infection, hypertension, hypotension, myalgia, headache, and diarrhea (see WARNINGS: Cardiovascular Events, Hemoglobin, and Rate of Rise of Hemoglobin/Hypertension). The most frequently reported adverse reactions resulting in clinical intervention (eg, discontinuation of Aranesp™, adjustment in dosage, or the need for concomitant medication to treat an adverse reaction symptom) were hypotension, hypertension, fever, myalgia, nausea, and chest pain.

Because clinical trials are conducted under widely varying conditions, adverse reaction rates observed in the clinical trials of Aranesp™ cannot be directly compared to rates in the clinical trials of other drugs and may not reflect the rates observed in practice.

The data described below reflect exposure to Aranesp™ in 1598 CRF patients, including 675 exposed for at least 6 months, of whom 185 were exposed for greater than 1 year. Aranesp™ was evaluated in active-controlled (n = 823) and uncontrolled studies (n = 775).

The rates of adverse events and association with Aranesp™ are best assessed in the results from studies in which Aranesp™ was used to stimulate erythropoiesis in patients anemic at study baseline (n = 348), and, in particular, the subset of these patients in randomized controlled trials (n = 276). Because there were no substantive differences in the rates of adverse reactions between these subpopulations, or between these subpopulations and the entire population of patients treated with Aranesp™, data from all 1598 patients were pooled.

The population encompassed an age range from 18 to 91 years. Fifty-seven percent of the patients were male. The percentages of Caucasian, Black, Asian, and Hispanic patients were 83%, 11%, 3%, and 1%, respectively. The median weekly dose of Aranesp™ was 0.45 mcg/kg (25th, 75th percentiles: 0.29, 0.66 mcg/kg).

Some of the adverse events reported are typically associated with CRF, or recognized complications of dialysis, and may not necessarily be attributable to Aranesp™ therapy. No important differences in adverse event rates between treatment groups were observed in controlled studies in which patients received Aranesp™ or other recombinant erythropoietins.

The data in Table 1 reflect those adverse events occurring in at least 5% of patients treated with Aranesp™:

Table 1. Adverse Events Occurring in ≥ 5% of Patients

Event	Patients Treated With Aranesp™ (n = 1598)
APPLICATION SITE	
Injection Site Pain	7%
BODY AS A WHOLE	
Peripheral Edema	11%
Fatigue	9%
Fever	9%
Death	7%
Chest Pain, Unspecified	6%
Fluid Overload	6%
Access Infection	6%
Influenza-like Symptoms	6%
Access Hemorrhage	6%
Asthenia	5%
CARDIOVASCULAR	
Hypertension	23%
Hypotension	22%
Cardiac Arrhythmias/Cadiac Arrest	10%
Angina Pectoris/Cardiac Chest Pain	8%
Thrombosis Vascular Access	8%
Congestive Heart Failure	6%
CNS/PNS	
Headache	16%
Dizziness	8%
GASTROINTESTINAL	
Diarrhea	16%
Vomiting	15%
Nausea	14%
Abdominal Pain	12%
Constipation	5%
MUSCULO-SKELETAL	
Myalgia	21%
Arthralgia	11%
Limb Pain	10%
Back Pain	8%
RESISTANCE MECHANISM	
Infection[a]	27%
RESPIRATORY	
Upper Respiratory Infection	14%
Dyspnea	12%
Cough	10%
Bronchitis	6%
SKIN AND APPENDAGES	
Pruritus	8%

[a] Infection includes sepsis, bacteremia, pneumonia, peritonitis, and abscess.

The incidence rates for other clinically significant events are shown in Table 2.

Table 2. Percent Incidence of Other Clinically Significant Events

Event	Patients Treated With Aranesp™ (n = 1598)
Acute Myocardial Infarction	2%
Seizure	1%
Stroke	1%
Transient Ischemic Attack	1%

Continued on next page

Aranesp—Cont.

Thrombotic Events

Vascular access thrombosis in hemodialysis patients occurred in clinical trials at an annualized rate of 0.22 events per patient year of Aranesp™ therapy. Rates of thrombotic events (eg, vascular access thrombosis, venous thrombosis, and pulmonary emboli) with Aranesp™ therapy were similar to those observed with other recombinant erythropoietins in these trials.

Immunogenicity

As with all therapeutic proteins, there is a potential for immunogenicity. The incidence of antibody development in patients receiving Aranesp™ has not been adequately determined. Radioimmunoprecipitation and neutralizing antibody assays were performed on sera from 1534 patients treated with Aranesp™. High-titer antibodies were not detected, but assay sensitivity may be inadequate to reliably detect lower titers. Since the incidence of antibody formation is highly dependent on the sensitivity and specificity of the assay, and the observed incidence of antibody positivity in an assay may additionally be influenced by several factors including sample handling, concomitant medications, and underlying disease, comparison of the incidence of antibodies to Aranesp™ with the incidence of antibodies to other products may be misleading.

Erythrocyte aplasia, in association with antibodies to erythropoietin, has been reported on rare occasions in patients treated with other recombinant erythropoietins. Due to the close relationship of Aranesp™ to endogenous erythropoietin, such a response is a theoretical possibility with Aranesp™ treatment, but has not been observed to date.

There have been rare reports of potentially serious allergic reactions including skin rash and urticaria associated with Aranesp™. Symptoms have recurred with rechallenge, suggesting a causal relationship exists in some instances. If an anaphylactic reaction occurs, Aranesp™ should be immediately discontinued and appropriate therapy should be administered.

OVERDOSAGE

The maximum amount of Aranesp™ that can be safely administered in single or multiple doses has not been determined. Doses over 3.0 mcg/kg/week for up to 28 weeks have been administered. Excessive rise and rate of rise in hemoglobin, however, have been associated with adverse events (see WARNINGS and DOSAGE AND ADMINISTRATION: Dose Adjustment). In the event of polycythemia, Aranesp™ should be temporarily withheld (see DOSAGE AND ADMINISTRATION: Dose Adjustment). If clinically indicated, phlebotomy may be performed.

DOSAGE AND ADMINISTRATION

General

Aranesp™ is administered either IV or SC as a single weekly injection. The dose should be started and slowly adjusted as described below based on hemoglobin levels. If a patient fails to respond or maintain a response, other etiologies should be considered and evaluated (see PRECAUTIONS: General/Laboratory Tests). When Aranesp™ therapy is initiated or adjusted, the hemoglobin should be followed weekly until stabilized and monitored at least monthly thereafter.

For patients who respond to Aranesp™ with a rapid increase in hemoglobin (eg, more than 1.0 g/dL in any 2-week period), the dose of Aranesp™ should be reduced (see DOSAGE AND ADMINISTRATION: Dose Adjustment) because of the association of excessive rate of rise of hemoglobin with adverse events (see WARNINGS: Cardiovascular Events, Hemoglobin, and Rate of Rise of Hemoglobin).

The dose should be adjusted for each patient to achieve and maintain a target hemoglobin level not to exceed 12 g/dL.

Starting Dose

Correction of Anemia

The recommended starting dose of Aranesp™ for the correction of anemia in CRF patients is 0.45 mcg/kg body weight, administered as a single IV or SC injection once weekly. Because of individual variability, doses should be titrated to not exceed a target hemoglobin concentration of 12 g/dL (see Dose Adjustment). For many patients, the appropriate maintenance dose will be lower than this starting dose. Predialysis patients, in particular, may require lower maintenance doses. Also, some patients have been treated successfully with a SC dose of Aranesp™ administered once every 2 weeks.

Conversion From Epoetin alfa to Aranesp™

The starting weekly dose of Aranesp™ should be estimated on the basis of the weekly Epoetin alfa dose at the time of substitution (see Table 3). Because of individual variability, doses should then be titrated to maintain the target hemoglobin. Due to the longer serum half-life, Aranesp™ should be administered less frequently than Epoetin alfa. Aranesp™ should be administered once a week if a patient was receiving Epoetin alfa 2 to 3 times weekly. Aranesp™ should be administered once every 2 weeks if a patient was receiving Epoetin alfa once per week. The route of administration (IV or SC) should be maintained.

Table 3. Estimated Aranesp™ Starting Doses (mcg/week) Based on Previous Epoetin alfa Dose (Units/week)

Previous Weekly Epoetin alfa Dose (Units/week)	Weekly Aranesp™ Dose (mcg/week)
< 2,500	6.25
2,500 to 4,999	12.5
5,000 to 10,999	25
11,000 to 17,999	40
18,000 to 33,999	60
34,000 to 89,999	100
≥ 90,000	200

Dose Adjustment

The dose should be adjusted for each patient to achieve and maintain a target hemoglobin not to exceed 12 g/dL.

Increases in dose should not be made more frequently than once a month. If the hemoglobin is increasing and approaching 12 g/dL, the dose should be reduced by approximately 25%. If the hemoglobin continues to increase, doses should be temporarily withheld until the hemoglobin begins to decrease, at which point therapy should be reinitiated at a dose approximately 25% below the previous dose. If the hemoglobin increases by more than 1.0 g/dL in a 2-week period, the dose should be decreased by approximately 25%. If the increase in hemoglobin is less than 1 g/dL over 4 weeks and iron stores are adequate (see PRECAUTIONS: Laboratory Tests), the dose of Aranesp™ may be increased by approximately 25% of the previous dose. Further increases may be made at 4-week intervals until the specified hemoglobin is obtained.

Maintenance Dose

Aranesp™ dosage should be adjusted to maintain a target hemoglobin not to exceed 12 g/dL. If the hemoglobin exceeds 12 g/dL, the dose may be adjusted as described above. Doses must be individualized to ensure that hemoglobin is maintained at an appropriate level for each patient.

Preparation and Administration of Aranesp™

1. Do not shake Aranesp™. Vigorous shaking may denature Aranesp™, rendering it biologically inactive.
2. Parenteral drug products should be inspected visually for particulate matter and discoloration prior to administration. Do not use any vials exhibiting particulate matter or discoloration.
3. Do not dilute Aranesp™.
4. Do not administer Aranesp™ in conjunction with other drug solutions.
5. Aranesp™ is packaged in single-use vials and contains no preservative. Discard any unused portion. Do not pool unused portions.
6. See the accompanying "Information for Patients and Caregivers" leaflet for complete instructions on the preparation and administration of Aranesp™.

HOW SUPPLIED

Aranesp™ is available in 2 solutions, an albumin solution and a polysorbate solution. The words "Albumin Free" appear on the polysorbate container labels and the package main panels as well as other panels as space permits. Aranesp™ is available in the following packages:

1 mL Single-dose Vial, Polysorbate Solution

1 Vial/Pack, 4 Packs/Case	4 Vials/Pack, 10 Packs/Case
200 mcg/1 mL (NDC 55513-006-01)	25 mcg/1 mL (NDC 55513-002-04)
	40 mcg/1 mL (NDC 55513-003-04)
	60 mcg/1 mL (NDC 55513-004-04)
	100 mcg/1 mL (NDC 55513-005-04)

1 mL Single-dose Vial, Albumin Solution

1 Vial/Pack, 4 Packs/Case	4 Vials/Pack, 10 Packs/Case
200 mcg/1 mL (NDC 55513-014-01)	25 mcg/1 mL (NDC 55513-010-04)
	40 mcg/1 mL (NDC 55513-011-04)
	60 mcg/1 mL (NDC 55513-012-04)
	100 mcg/1 mL (NDC 55513-013-04)

Storage

Store at 2° to 8°C (36° to 46°F). Do not freeze or shake. Protect from light.

REFERENCES

1. Egrie JC and Browne JK. Development and characterization of novel erythropoiesis stimulating protein (NESP). *Brit J Cancer.* 2001;84(Suppl 1):3–10.
2. Besarab A, Bolton WK, Browne JK, et al. The effects of normal as compared with low hematocrit values in patients with cardiac disease who are receiving hemodialysis and epoetin. *N Engl J Med.* 1998;339:584–90.

Rx only

This product, or its use, may be covered by one or more US Patents, including US Patent No. 5,618,698, in addition to others including patents pending.

Amgen Inc., One Amgen Center Drive, Thousand Oaks, CA 91320-1799

Issue Date 09/17/2001

KINERET™ ℞

[kĭn' ĕ-rĕt]

(Anakinra)

DESCRIPTION

Kineret™ (anakinra) is a recombinant, nonglycosylated form of the human interleukin-1 receptor antagonist (IL-1Ra). Kineret™ differs from native human IL-1Ra in that it has the addition of a single methionine residue at its amino terminus. Kineret™ consists of 153 amino acids and has a molecular weight of 17.3 kilodaltons. It is produced by recombinant DNA technology using an *E. coli* bacterial expression system.

Kineret™ is supplied in single use 1 mL prefilled glass syringes with 27 gauge needles as a sterile, clear, colorless-to-white, preservative-free solution for daily subcutaneous (SC) administration. Each 1 mL prefilled glass syringe contains: 0.67 mL (100 mg) of anakinra in a solution (pH 6.5) containing sodium citrate (1.29 mg), sodium chloride (5.48 mg), disodium EDTA (0.12 mg), and polysorbate 80 (0.70 mg) in Water for Injection, USP.

CLINICAL PHARMACOLOGY

Kineret™ blocks the biologic activity of IL-1 by competitively inhibiting IL-1 binding to the interleukin-1 type I receptor (IL-1RI), which is expressed in a wide variety of tissues and organs.[1]

IL-1 production is induced in response to inflammatory stimuli and mediates various physiologic responses including inflammatory and immunological responses. IL-1 has a broad range of activities including cartilage degradation by its induction of the rapid loss of proteoglycans, as well as stimulation of bone resorption.[2] The levels of the naturally occurring IL-1Ra in synovium and synovial fluid from rheumatoid arthritis (RA) patients are not sufficient to compete with the elevated amount of locally produced IL-1.[3,4,5]

Pharmacokinetics

The absolute bioavailability of Kineret™ after a 70 mg SC bolus injection in healthy subjects (n=11) is 95%. In subjects with RA, maximum plasma concentrations of Kineret™ occurred 3 to 7 hours after SC administration of Kineret™ at clinically relevant doses (1 to 2 mg/kg; n = 18); the terminal half-life ranged from 4 to 6 hours. In RA patients, no unexpected accumulation of Kineret™ was observed after daily SC doses for up to 24 weeks.

The influence of demographic covariates on the pharmacokinetics of Kineret™ was studied using population pharmacokinetic analysis encompassing 341 patients receiving daily SC injection of Kineret™ at doses of 30, 75, and 150 mg for up to 24 weeks. The estimated Kineret™ clearance increased with increasing creatinine clearance and body weight. After adjusting for creatinine clearance and body weight, gender and age were not significant factors for mean plasma clearance.

Patients with Renal Impairment: The mean plasma clearance of Kineret™ decreased 70-75% in normal subjects with severe or end stage renal disease (defined as creatinine clearance less than 30 mL/minute, as estimated from serum creatinine levels[6]). No formal studies have been conducted examining the pharmacokinetics of Kineret™ administered subcutaneously in rheumatoid arthritis patients with renal impairment.

Patients with Hepatic Dysfunction: No formal studies have been conducted examining the pharmacokinetics of Kineret™ administered subcutaneously in rheumatoid arthritis patients with hepatic impairment.

CLINICAL STUDIES

The safety and efficacy of Kineret™ have been evaluated in three randomized, double-blind, placebo-controlled trials of 1392 patients ≥ 18 years of age with active rheumatoid arthritis (RA). An additional fourth study was conducted to assess safety. In the efficacy trials, Kineret™ was studied in combination with other disease-modifying antirheumatic drugs (DMARDs) (studies 1 and 2) or as a monotherapy (study 3).

Study 1 evaluated 501 patients with active RA who had been on a stable dose of methotrexate (MTX) (10 to 25 mg/week) for at least 8 weeks. In addition, they had at least 6 swollen/painful and 9 tender joints and either a C-reactive protein (CRP) of ≥1.5 mg/dL or an erythrocyte sedimentation rate (ESR) of ≥ 28 mm/hr. Patients were randomized to Kineret™ or placebo in addition to their stable doses of MTX.

Study 2 evaluated 419 patients with active RA who had received MTX for at least 6 months including a stable dose (15 to 25 mg/week) for at least 3 consecutive months prior to enrollment. Patients were randomized to receive placebo or one of five doses of Kineret™ SC daily for 12 to 24 weeks in addition to their stable doses of MTX.

Study 3 evaluated 472 patients with active RA and had similar inclusion criteria to Study 1 except that these patients had received no DMARD for the previous 6 weeks or during the study.[7] Patients were randomized to receive either Kineret™ or placebo. Patients were DMARD-naïve or had failed no more than 3 DMARDs.

Study 4 was a placebo-controlled, randomized trial designed to assess the safety of Kineret™ in 1414 patients receiving a variety of concurrent medications for their RA including some DMARD therapies, as well as patients who were DMARD-free. The TNF blocking agents etanercept and infliximab were specifically excluded. Concurrent DMARDs included MTX, sulfasalazine, hydrochloroquine, gold, penicillamine, leflunomide, and azathioprine. Unlike studies 1, 2 and 3, patients predisposed to infection due to a history of underlying disease such as pneumonia, asthma, controlled diabetes, and chronic obstructive pulmonary disease (COPD) were also enrolled. (See **ADVERSE REACTIONS**-Infections).

In Studies 1, 2, and 3, the improvement in signs and symptoms of RA was assessed using the American College of Rheumatology (ACR) response criteria (ACR_{20}, ACR_{50}, ACR_{70}). In all three studies, patients treated with Kineret™

were more likely to achieve an ACR_{20} or higher magnitude of response (ACR_{50} and ACR_{70}) than patients treated with placebo (Table 1). The treatment response rates did not differ based on gender or ethnic group. The results of the ACR component scores in Study 1 are shown in Table 2.

Most clinical responses, both in patients receiving placebo and patients receiving Kineret™, occurred within 12 weeks of enrollment.

[See table 1 at right]
[See table 2 at right]

Table 1. Percent of Patients with ACR Responses in Studies 1 and 3

Response	Study 1 (Patients on MTX) Placebo (n=251)	Study 1 Kineret™ 100 mg/day (n=250)	Study 3 (No DMARDs) Placebo (n=119)	Study 3 Kineret™ 75 mg/day (n=115)	Study 3 Kineret™ 150 mg/day (n=115)
ACR 20					
Month 3	24%	34%[a]	23%	33%	33%
Month 6	22%	38%[c]	27%	34%	43%[a]
ACR 50					
Month 3	6%	13%[b]	5%	10%	8%
Month 6	8%	17%[b]	8%	11%	19%[a]
ACR 70					
Month 3	0%	3%[a]	0%	0%	0%
Month 6	2%	6%[a]	1%	1%	1%

[a] $p<0.05$, Kineret™ versus placebo
[b] $p<0.01$, Kineret™ versus placebo
[c] $p<0.001$, Kineret™ versus placebo

Table 2. Effect of Kineret™ on Median ACR Component Scores in Study 1

Parameter (median)	Placebo/MTX (N = 251) Baseline	Placebo/MTX Month 6	Kineret™/MTX 100 mg/day (N = 250) Baseline	Kineret™/MTX Month 6
Patient Reported Outcomes				
Disability index[a]	1.38	1.13	1.38	1.00
Patient global assessment[b]	51.0	41.0	51.0	29.0
Pain[b]	56.0	44.0	63.0	34.0
Objective Measures				
ESR (mm/hr)	35.0	32.0	36.0	19.0
CRP (mg/dL)	2.2	1.6	2.2	0.5
Physician's Assessments				
Tender/painful joints[c]	20.0	11.0	23.0	9.0
Physician global assessment[b]	59.0	31.0	59.0	26.0
Swollen joints[d]	18.0	10.5	17.0	9.0

[a] Health assessment questionnaire; 0 = best, 3 = worst; includes eight categories: dressing and grooming, arising, eating, walking, hygiene, reach, grip, and activities.
[b] Visual analog scale; 0 = best, 100 = worst
[c] Scale 0 to 68
[d] Scale 0 to 66

INDICATIONS AND USAGE

Kineret™ is indicated for the reduction in signs and symptoms of moderately to severely active rheumatoid arthritis, in patients 18 years of age or older who have failed 1 or more disease modifying antirheumatic drugs (DMARDs). Kineret™ can be used alone or in combination with DMARDs other than Tumor Necrosis Factor (TNF) blocking agents (See **WARNINGS**).

CONTRAINDICATIONS

Kineret™ is contraindicated in patients with known hypersensitivity to *E.coli*-derived proteins, Kineret™, or any components of the product.

WARNINGS

KINERET™ HAS BEEN ASSOCIATED WITH AN INCREASED INCIDENCE OF SERIOUS INFECTIONS (2%) vs. PLACEBO (< 1%). ADMINISTRATION OF KINERET™ SHOULD BE DISCONTINUED IF A PATIENT DEVELOPS A SERIOUS INFECTION. TREATMENT WITH KINERET™ SHOULD NOT BE INITIATED IN PATIENTS WITH ACTIVE INFECTIONS. THE SAFETY AND EFFICACY OF KINERET™ IN IMMUNOSUPPRESSED PATIENTS OR IN PATIENTS WITH CHRONIC INFECTIONS HAVE NOT BEEN EVALUATED. THE SAFETY OF KINERET™ USED IN COMBINATION WITH TNF BLOCKING AGENTS HAS NOT BEEN ESTABLISHED. PRELIMINARY DATA SUGGEST A HIGHER RATE OF SERIOUS INFECTIONS (7%, 4/58) WHEN KINERET™ AND ETANERCEPT ARE USED IN COMBINATION COMPARED WITH WHEN KINERET™ IS USED ALONE. IN THIS COMBINATION STUDY NEUTROPENIA (NEUTROPHIL COUNT ≤ 1000/mm³) WAS OBSERVED IN 3% OF PATIENTS (2/58). USE OF KINERET™ WITH TNF BLOCKING AGENTS SHOULD ONLY BE DONE WITH EXTREME CAUTION AND WHEN NO SATISFACTORY ALTERNATIVES EXIST.

PRECAUTIONS

General

Hypersensitivity reactions associated with Kineret™ administration are rare. If a severe hypersensitivity reaction occurs, administration of Kineret™ should be discontinued and appropriate therapy initiated.

Immunosuppression

The impact of treatment with Kineret™ on active and/or chronic infections and the development of malignancies is not known. (See **WARNINGS, ADVERSE REACTIONS, Infections and Malignancies**).

Immunizations

No data are available on the effects of vaccination in patients receiving Kineret™. Live vaccines should not be given concurrently with Kineret™. No data are available on the secondary transmission of infection by live vaccines in patients receiving Kineret™ (See **Precautions, Immunosuppression**). Since Kineret™ interferes with normal immune response mechanisms to new antigens such as vaccines, vaccination may not be effective in patients receiving Kineret™.

Information for Patients

If a physician has determined that a patient can safely and effectively receive Kineret™ at home, patients and their caregivers should be instructed on the proper dosage and administration of Kineret™. All patients should be provided with the "Information for Patients and Caregivers" insert. While this "Information for Patients and Caregivers" insert provides information about the product and its use, it is not intended to take the place of regular discussions between the patient and healthcare provider.

Patients should be informed of the signs and symptoms of allergic and other adverse drug reactions and advised of appropriate actions. Patients and their caregivers should be thoroughly instructed in the importance of proper disposal and cautioned against the reuse of needles, syringes, and drug product. A puncture-resistant container for the disposal of used syringes should be available to the patient. The full container should be disposed of according to the directions provided by the healthcare professional.

Laboratory Tests

Patients receiving Kineret™ may experience a decrease in neutrophil counts. In the placebo-controlled studies, 8% of patients receiving Kineret™ had decreases in neutrophil counts of at least 1 World Health Organization (WHO) toxicity grade compared with 2% in the placebo control group. Six Kineret™-treated patients (0.3%) experienced neutropenia (ANC $\leq 1 \times 10^9$/L). This is discussed in more detail in the Adverse Events-Hematologic Events section. Neutrophil counts should be assessed prior to initiating Kineret™ treatment, and while receiving Kineret™, monthly for 3 months, and thereafter quarterly for a period up to 1 year.

Drug Interactions

No drug-drug interaction studies in human subjects have been conducted. Toxicologic and toxicokinetic studies in rats did not demonstrate any alterations in the clearance or toxicologic profile of either methotrexate or Kineret™ when the two agents were administered together.

Carcinogenesis, Mutagenesis, And Impairment Of Fertility

Kineret™ has not been evaluated for its carcinogenic potential in animals. Using a standard *in vivo* and *in vitro* battery of mutagenesis assays, Kineret™ did not induce gene mutations in either bacteria or mammalian cells. In rats and rabbits, Kineret™ at doses of up to 100-fold greater than the human dose had no adverse effects on male or female fertility.

Pregnancy Category B

Reproductive studies have been conducted with Kineret™ on rats and rabbits at doses up to 100 times the human dose and have revealed no evidence of impaired fertility or harm to the fetus. There are, however, no adequate and well-controlled studies in pregnant women. Because animal reproduction studies are not always predictive of human response, Kineret™ should be used during pregnancy only if clearly needed.

Nursing Mothers

It is not known whether Kineret™ is secreted in human milk. Because many drugs are secreted in human milk, caution should be exercised if Kineret™ is administered to nursing women.

Pediatric Use

The safety and efficacy of Kineret™ in patients with juvenile rheumatoid arthritis (JRA) have not been established.

Geriatric Use

A total of 653 patients ≥ 65 years of age, including 135 patients ≥ 75 years of age, were studied in clinical trials. No differences in safety or effectiveness were observed between these patients and younger patients, but greater sensitivity of some older individuals cannot be ruled out. Because there is a higher incidence of infections in the elderly population in general, caution should be used in treating the elderly. This drug is known to be substantially excreted by the kidney, and the risk of toxic reactions to this drug may be greater in patients with impaired renal function.

ADVERSE REACTIONS

The most serious adverse reactions were:

- Serious Infections - see **WARNINGS**
- Neutropenia, particularly when used in combination with TNF blocking agents – see **WARNINGS**

The most common adverse reaction with Kineret™ is injection site reactions. These reactions were the most common reason for withdrawing from studies.

Because clinical trials are conducted under widely varying and controlled conditions, adverse reaction rates observed in clinical trials of a drug cannot be directly compared to rates in the clinical trials of another drug and may not predict the rates observed in a broader patient population in clinical practice.

The data described herein reflect exposure to Kineret™ in 2606 patients, including 1812 exposed for at least 6 months and 570 exposed for at least one year. Studies 1 and 4 used the recommended dose of 100 mg per day. The patients studied were representative of the general population of patients with rheumatoid arthritis.

Injection-Site Reactions

The most common and consistently reported treatment-related adverse event associated with Kineret™ is injection-site reaction (ISR). The majority of ISRs were reported as mild. These typically lasted for 14 to 28 days and were characterized by 1 or more of the following: erythema, ecchymosis, inflammation, and pain. In Studies 1 and 4, 71% of patients developed an ISR, which was typically reported within the first 4 weeks of therapy. The development of ISRs in patients who had not previously experienced ISRs was uncommon after the first month of therapy.

Infections

In Studies 1 and 4 combined, the incidence of infection was 40% in the Kineret™-treated patients and 35% in placebo-treated patients. The incidence of serious infections in studies 1 and 4 was 1.8% in Kineret™-treated patients and 0.6% in placebo-treated patients over 6 months. These infections consisted primarily of bacterial events such as cellulitis, pneumonia, and bone and joint infections, rather than unusual, opportunistic, fungal, or viral infections. Patients with asthma appeared to be at higher risk of developing serious infections; Kineret™ 5% versus placebo <1%. Most patients continued on study drug after the infection resolved. There were no on-study deaths due to serious infectious episodes in either study.

In a study in which patients were receiving both etanercept and Kineret™ for up to 24 weeks, the incidence of serious infections was 7%. These infections consisted of bacterial pneumonia (2 cases) and cellulitis (2 cases), which recovered with antibiotic treatment.

Malignancies

Twenty-one malignancies of various types were observed in 2531 RA patients treated in clinical trials with Kineret™ for up to 50 months. The observed rates and incidences were similar to those expected for the population studied.

Hematologic Events

In placebo-controlled studies with Kineret™, treatment was associated with small reductions in the mean values for total white blood count, platelets, and absolute neutrophil blood count (ANC), and a small increase in the mean eosinophil differential percentage.

In all placebo-controlled studies, 8% of patients receiving Kineret™ had decreases in ANC of at least 1 WHO toxicity grade, compared with 2% of placebo patients. Six Kineret™-treated patients (0.3%) developed neutropenia (ANC $\leq 1 \times 10^9$/L). Additional patients treated with Kineret™ plus etanercept (2/58, 3%) developed ANC $\leq 1 \times 10^9$/L. While neutropenic, one patient developed cellulitis and the other patient developed pneumonia. Both patients recovered with antibiotic therapy.

Immunogenicity

In Study 4, 28% of patients tested positively for anti-Kineret™ antibodies at month 6 in a highly sensitive, Kineret™-binding biosensor assay. Of the 1274 subjects

Continued on next page

Kineret—Cont.

with available data, <1% (n = 9) were seropositive in a cell-based bioassay for antibodies capable of neutralizing the biologic effects of Kineret™. None of these 9 subjects were positive for neutralizing antibodies at more than 1 time point, and all of these subjects were negative for neutralizing antibodies by 9 months. No correlation between antibody development and clinical response or adverse events was observed. The long-term immunogenicity of Kineret™ is unknown.

Antibody assay results are highly dependent on the sensitivity and specificity of the assays. Additionally, the observed incidence of antibody positivity in an assay may be influenced by several factors, including sample handling, concomitant medications, and underlying disease. For these reasons, comparison of the incidence of antibodies to Kineret™ with the incidence of antibodies to other products may be misleading.

Other Adverse Events

Table 3 reflects adverse events in Studies 1 and 4, that occurred with a frequency of ≥ 5% and a higher frequency in Kineret™-treated patients.

Table 3. Percent of RA Patients Reporting Adverse Events (Studies 1 and 4)

Preferred Term	Placebo (N = 534)	Kineret™ 100 mg/day (N = 1366)
Injection Site Reaction	28 %	71 %
Infection	35 %	40 %
URI	13 %	13 %
Sinusitis	4 %	6 %
Influenza-Like Symptoms	4 %	5 %
Other	23 %	26 %
Headache	9 %	12 %
Nausea	6 %	8 %
Diarrhea	5 %	7 %
Sinusitis	6 %	7 %
Influenza-Like Symptoms	5 %	6 %
Pain Abdominal	4 %	5 %

OVERDOSAGE

There have been no cases of overdose reported with Kineret™ in clinical trials of RA. In sepsis trials no serious toxicities attributed to Kineret™ were seen when administered at mean calculated doses of up to 35 times those given patients with RA over a 72-hour treatment period.

DOSAGE AND ADMINISTRATION

The recommended dose of Kineret™ for the treatment of patients with rheumatoid arthritis is 100 mg/day administered daily by subcutaneous injection. Higher doses did not result in a higher response. The dose should be administered at approximately the same time every day. Kineret™ is provided in single-use 1 mL prefilled glass syringes. Instructions on appropriate use should be given by the health care professional to the patient or care provider. Patients or care providers should not be allowed to administer Kineret™ until he/she has demonstrated a thorough understanding of procedures and an ability to inject the product. After administration of Kineret™, it is essential to follow the proper procedure for disposal of syringes and needles. See the "Information for Patients and Caregivers" leaflet for detailed instructions on the handling and injection of Kineret™.

Visually inspect the solution for particulate matter and discoloration before administration. If particulates or discoloration are observed, the prefilled syringe should not be used. Administer only 1 dose (the entire contents of 1 prefilled glass syringe) per day. Discard any unused portions; Kineret™ contains no preservative. Do not save unused drug for later administration.

HOW SUPPLIED

Kineret™ is supplied in single-use preservative free, 1 mL prefilled glass syringes with 27 gauge needles. Each prefilled glass syringe contains 0.67 mL (100 mg) of anakinra. Kineret™ is dispensed in packs containing 7 syringes. It is also available in a 4×7 syringe dispensing pack (28 syringes). The NDC number for Kineret™ is 55513-177-07.

Storage

Do not use Kineret™ beyond the expiration date shown on the carton. Kineret™ should be stored in the refrigerator at 2° to 8°C (36° to 46°F). **DO NOT FREEZE OR SHAKE.** Protect from light.

REFERENCES

1. Hannum CH, Wilcox CJ, Arend WP, et al. Interleukin-1 receptor antagonist activity of a human interleukin-1 inhibitor. *Nature*. 1990; 343:336-40.
2. Van Lent, PLEM, Fons, AJ, Van De Loo, AEM et al. Major role for interleukin 1 but not for tumor necrosis factor in early cartilage damage in immune complex in mice. *J Rheumatol*. 1995; 22:2250-2258
3. Deleuran BW, Shu CQ, Field M, et al. Localization of interleukin-1 alpha, type 1 interleukin-1 receptor and interleukin-1 receptor antagonist in the synovial membrane and cartilage/pannus junction in rheumatoid arthritis. *Br J Rheumatol*. 1992; 31:801-809.
4. Chomarat P, Vannier E, Dechanet J, et al. Balance of IL-1 receptor antagonist/IL-1*B* in rheumatoid synovium and its regulation by IL-4 and IL-10. *J Immunol.* 1995; 1432-1439.
5. Firestein GS, Boyle DL, Yu C, et al. Synovial interleukin -1 receptor antagonist and interleukin-1 balance in rheumatoid arthritis. *Arthritis Rheum.* 1994; 37:644-652.
6. Cockcroft,.DW and Gault, HM. Prediction of creatinine clearance from serum creatinine. *Nephron* 1976; 16:31-41.
7. Bresnihan B, Alvaro-Gracia JM, Cobby M, et al. Treatment of rheumatoid arthritis with recombinant human interleukin-1 receptor antagonist. *Arthritis Rheum.* 1998; 41:2196-2204.

Amgen Inc.
One Amgen Center Drive
Thousand Oaks, CA 91320-1799

Issue Date: 11/14/2001

NEULASTA™ ℞

[*nū' läs-tă*]
(pegfilgrastim)

DESCRIPTION

Neulasta™ (pegfilgrastim) is a covalent conjugate of recombinant methionyl human G-CSF (Filgrastim) and monomethoxypolyethylene glycol. Filgrastim is a water-soluble 175 amino acid protein with a molecular weight of approximately 19 kilodaltons (kd). Filgrastim is obtained from the bacterial fermentation of a strain of *Escherichia coli* transformed with a genetically engineered plasmid containing the human G-CSF gene. To produce pegfilgrastim, a 20 kd monomethoxypolyethylene glycol molecule is covalently bound to the N-terminal methionyl residue of Filgrastim. The average molecular weight of pegfilgrastim is approximately 39 kd.

Neulasta™ is supplied in 0.6 mL prefilled syringes for subcutaneous (SC) injection. Each syringe contains 6 mg pegfilgrastim (based on protein weight), in a sterile, clear, colorless, preservative-free solution (pH 4.0) containing acetate (0.35 mg), sorbitol (30.0 mg), polysorbate 20 (0.02 mg), and sodium (0.02 mg) in water for injection, USP.

CLINICAL PHARMACOLOGY

Both Filgrastim and pegfilgrastim are Colony Stimulating Factors that act on hematopoietic cells by binding to specific cell surface receptors thereby stimulating proliferation, differentiation, commitment, and end cell functional activation.[1,2] Studies on cellular proliferation, receptor binding, and neutrophil function demonstrate that Filgrastim and pegfilgrastim have the same mechanism of action. Pegfilgrastim has reduced renal clearance and prolonged persistence in vivo as compared to Filgrastim.

Pharmacokinetics

The pharmacokinetics and pharmacodynamics of Neulasta™ were studied in 379 patients with cancer. The pharmacokinetics of Neulasta™ were nonlinear in cancer patients and clearance decreased with increases in dose. Neutrophil receptor binding is an important component of the clearance of Neulasta™, and serum clearance is directly related to the number of neutrophils. For example, the concentration of Neulasta™ declined rapidly at the onset of neutrophil recovery that followed myelosuppressive chemotherapy. In addition to numbers of neutrophils, body weight appeared to be a factor. Patients with higher body weights experienced higher systemic exposure to Neulasta™ after receiving a dose normalized for body weight. A large variability in the pharmacokinetics of Neulasta™ was observed in cancer patients. The half- life of Neulasta™ ranged from 15 to 80 hours after SC injection.

Special Populations

No gender-related differences were observed in the pharmacokinetics of Neulasta™, and no differences were observed in the pharmacokinetics of geriatric patients (≥ 65 years of age) compared to younger patients (< 65 years of age) (see PRECAUTIONS, Geriatric Use). The pharmacokinetic profile in pediatric populations or in patients with hepatic or renal insufficiency has not been assessed.

CLINICAL STUDIES

Neulasta™ was evaluated in two randomized, double-blind, active control studies, employing doxorubicin 60 mg/m^2 and docetaxel 75 mg/m^2 administered every 21 days for up to 4 cycles for the treatment of metastatic breast cancer. Study 1 investigated the utility of a fixed dose of Neulasta™. Study 2 employed a weight-adjusted dose. In the absence of growth factor support, similar chemotherapy regimens have been reported to result in a 100% incidence of severe neutropenia (absolute neutrophil count [ANC] $< 0.5 \times 10^9$/L) with a mean duration of 5–7 days, and a 30 to 40% incidence of febrile neutropenia. Based on the correlation between the duration of severe neutropenia and the incidence of febrile neutropenia found in studies with Filgrastim, duration of severe neutropenia was chosen as the primary endpoint in both studies, and the efficacy of Neulasta™ was demonstrated by establishing comparability to Filgrastim (NEUPOGEN®)-treated subjects in the mean days of severe neutropenia.

In study 1, 157 subjects were randomized to receive a single SC dose of 6 mg of Neulasta™ on day 2 of each chemotherapy cycle or Filgrastim at 5 mcg/kg/day SC beginning on day 2 of each cycle. In study 2, 310 subjects were randomized to receive a single SC injection of Neulasta™ at 100 mcg/kg on day 2 or Filgrastim at 5 mcg/kg/day SC beginning on day 2 of each cycle of chemotherapy.

Both studies met the primary objective of demonstrating that the mean days of severe neutropenia of Neulasta™-treated patients did not exceed that of Filgrastim-treated patients by more than one day in cycle 1 of chemotherapy (see Table 1). The rates of febrile neutropenia in the two studies were comparable for Neulasta™ and Filgrastim (in the range of 10 to 20%). Other secondary endpoints included days of severe neutropenia in cycles 2–4, the depth of ANC nadir in cycles 1–4, and the time to ANC recovery after nadir. In both studies, the results for the secondary endpoints were similar between the two treatment groups.

Table 1. Mean Days of Severe Neutropenia (in Cycle 1)

Study	Mean days of severe neutropenia		Difference in means (95% CI)
	Neulasta™[a]	NEUPOGEN® (5 mcg/kg/day)	
Study 1 n = 157	1.8	1.6	0.2 (−0.2, 0.6)
Study 2 n = 310	1.7	1.6	0.1 (−0.2, 0.4)

a. Study 1 dose = 6 mg × 1; study 2 dose = 100 mcg/kg × 1

INDICATIONS AND USAGE

Neulasta™ is indicated to decrease the incidence of infection, as manifested by febrile neutropenia, in patients with non-myeloid malignancies receiving myelosuppressive anti-cancer drugs associated with a clinically significant incidence of febrile neutropenia.

CONTRAINDICATIONS

Neulasta™ is contraindicated in patients with known hypersensitivity to *E coli*-derived proteins, pegfilgrastim, Filgrastim, or any other component of the product.

WARNINGS

Splenic Rupture

RARE CASES OF SPLENIC RUPTURE HAVE BEEN REPORTED FOLLOWING THE ADMINISTRATION OF THE PARENT COMPOUND OF NEULASTA™, FILGRASTIM, FOR PBPC MOBILIZATION IN BOTH HEALTHY DONORS AND PATIENTS WITH CANCER. SOME OF THESE CASES WERE FATAL. NEULASTA™ HAS NOT BEEN EVALUATED IN THIS SETTING, THEREFORE, NEULASTA™ SHOULD NOT BE USED FOR PBPC MOBILIZATION. PATIENTS RECEIVING NEULASTA™ WHO REPORT LEFT UPPER ABDOMINAL OR SHOULDER TIP PAIN SHOULD BE EVALUATED FOR AN ENLARGED SPLEEN OR SPLENIC RUPTURE.

Adult Respiratory Distress Syndrome (ARDS)

Adult respiratory distress syndrome (ARDS) has been reported in neutropenic patients with sepsis receiving Filgrastim, the parent compound of Neulasta™, and is postulated to be secondary to an influx of neutrophils to sites of inflammation in the lungs. Neutropenic patients receiving Neulasta™ who develop fever, lung infiltrates, or respiratory distress should be evaluated for the possibility of ARDS. In the event that ARDS occurs, Neulasta™ should be discontinued and/or withheld until resolution of ARDS and patients should receive appropriate medical management for this condition.

Allergic Reactions

Allergic-type reactions, including anaphylaxis, skin rash, and urticaria, occurring on initial or subsequent treatment have been reported with the parent compound of Neulasta™, Filgrastim. In some cases, symptoms have recurred with rechallenge, suggesting a causal relationship. Allergic-type reactions to Neulasta™ have not been observed in clinical trials. If a serious allergic reaction or an anaphylactic reaction occurs, appropriate therapy should be administered and further use of Neulasta™ should be discontinued.

Sickle Cell Disease

Severe sickle cell crises have been reported in patients with sickle cell disease (specifically homozygous sickle cell anemia, sickle/hemoglobin C disease, and sickle/β+ thalassemia) who received Filgrastim, the parent compound of pegfilgrastim, for PBPC mobilization or following chemotherapy. One of these cases was fatal. Pegfilgrastim should be used with caution in patients with sickle cell disease, and only after careful consideration of the potential risks and benefits. Patients with sickle cell disease who receive Neulasta™ should be kept well hydrated and monitored for the occurrence of sickle cell crises. In the event of severe sickle cell crisis supportive care should be administered, and interventions to ameliorate the underlying event, such as therapeutic red blood cell exchange transfusion, should be considered.

PRECAUTIONS

General

Use With Chemotherapy and/or Radiation Therapy

Neulasta™ should not be administered in the period between 14 days before and 24 hours after administration of cytotoxic chemotherapy (see DOSAGE AND ADMINISTRATION) because of the potential for an increase in sensitivity of rapidly dividing myeloid cells to cytotoxic chemotherapy. The use of Neulasta™ has not been studied in patients receiving chemotherapy associated with delayed myelosuppression (eg, nitrosoureas, mitomycin C).

The administration of Neulasta™ concomitantly with 5-fluorouracil or other antimetabolites has not been evaluated in patients. Administration of pegfilgrastim at 0, 1, and 3 days before 5-fluorouracil resulted in increased mortality in mice; administration of pegfilgrastim 24 hours after 5-fluorouracil did not adversely affect survival.
The use of Neulasta™ has not been studied in patients receiving radiation therapy.

Potential Effect on Malignant Cells

Pegfilgrastim is a growth factor that primarily stimulates neutrophils and neutrophil precursors; however, the G-CSF receptor through which pegfilgrastim and Filgrastim act has been found on tumor cell lines, including some myeloid, T-lymphoid, lung, head and neck, and bladder tumor cell lines. The possibility that pegfilgrastim can act as a growth factor for any tumor type cannot be excluded. Use of Neulasta™ in myeloid malignancies and myelodysplasia (MDS) has not been studied. In a randomized study comparing the effects of the parent compound of Neulasta™, Filgrastim, to placebo in patients undergoing remission induction and consolidation chemotherapy for acute myeloid leukemia, important differences in remission rate between the two arms were excluded. Disease-free survival and overall survival were comparable; however, the study was not designed to detect important differences in these endpoints.[3]

Information for Patients

Patients should be informed of the possible side effects of Neulasta™, and be instructed to report them to the prescribing physician. Patients should be informed of the signs and symptoms of allergic drug reactions and be advised of appropriate actions. Patients should be counseled on the importance of compliance with their Neulasta™ treatment, including regular monitoring of blood counts.
If it is determined that a patient or caregiver can safely and effectively administer Neulasta™ (pegfilgrastim) at home, appropriate instruction on the proper use of Neulasta™ (pegfilgrastim) should be provided for patients and their caregivers, including careful review of the "Information for Patients and Caregivers" insert. Patients and caregivers should be cautioned against the reuse of needles, syringes, or drug product, and be thoroughly instructed in their proper disposal. A puncture-resistant container for the disposal of used syringes and needles should be available.

Laboratory Monitoring

To assess a patient's hematologic status and ability to tolerate myelosuppressive chemotherapy, a complete blood count and platelet count should be obtained before chemotherapy is administered. Regular monitoring of hematocrit value and platelet count is recommended.

Drug Interaction

No formal drug interaction studies between Neulasta™ and other drugs have been performed. Drugs such as lithium may potentiate the release of neutrophils; patients receiving lithium and Neulasta™ should have more frequent monitoring of neutrophil counts.

Carcinogenesis, Mutagenesis, Impairment of Fertility

No mutagenesis studies were conducted with pegfilgrastim. The carcinogenic potential of pegfilgrastim has not been evaluated in long-term animal studies. In a toxicity study of 6 months duration in rats given once weekly subcutaneous injections of up to 1000 mcg/kg of pegfilgrastim (approximately 23-fold higher than the recommended human dose), no precancerous or cancerous lesions were noted.
When administered once weekly via subcutaneous injections to male and female rats at doses up to 1000 mcg/kg prior to, and during mating, reproductive performance, fertility and sperm assessment parameters were not affected.

Pregnancy Category C

Pegfilgrastim has been shown to have adverse effects in pregnant rabbits when administered SC every other day during gestation at doses as low as 50 mcg/kg/dose (approximately 4-fold higher than the recommended human dose). Decreased maternal food consumption, accompanied by a decreased maternal body weight gain and decreased fetal body weights were observed at 50 to 1000 mcg/kg/dose. Pegfilgrastim doses of 200 and 250 mcg/kg/dose resulted in an increased incidence of abortions. Increased post-implantation loss due to early resorptions, was observed at doses of 200 to 1000 mcg/kg/dose and decreased numbers of live rabbit fetuses were observed at pegfilgrastim doses of 200 to 1000 mcg/kg/dose, given every other day.
Subcutaneous injections of pegfilgrastim of up to 1000 mcg/kg/dose every other day during the period of organogenesis in rats were not associated with an embryotoxic or fetotoxic outcome. However, an increased incidence (compared to historical controls) of wavy ribs was observed in rat fetuses at 1000 mcg/kg/dose every other day. Very low levels (< 0.5%) of pegfilgrastim crossed the placenta when administered subcutaneously to pregnant rats every other day during gestation.
Once weekly subcutaneous injections of pegfilgrastim to female rats from day 6 of gestation through day 18 of lactation at doses up to 1000 mcg/kg/dose did not result in any adverse maternal effects. There were no deleterious effects on the growth and development of the offspring and no adverse effects were found upon assessment of fertility indices.
There are no adequate and well-controlled studies in pregnant women. Neulasta™ should be used during pregnancy only if the potential benefit to the mother justifies the potential risk to the fetus.

Nursing Mothers

It is not known whether pegfilgrastim is excreted in human milk. Because many drugs are excreted in human milk, caution should be exercised when Neulasta™ is administered to a nursing woman.

Pediatric Use

The safety and effectiveness of Neulasta™ in pediatric patients have not been established. The 6 mg fixed dose single-use syringe formulation should not be used in infants, children, and smaller adolescents weighing less than 45 kg.

Geriatric Use

Of the 465 subjects with cancer who received Neulasta™ in clinical studies, 85 (18%) were age 65 and over, and 14 (3%) were age 75 and over. No overall differences in safety or effectiveness were observed between these patients and younger patients; however, due to the small number of elderly subjects, small but clinically relevant differences cannot be excluded.

ADVERSE REACTIONS

See WARNINGS sections regarding Splenic Rupture, ARDS, Allergic Reactions, and Sickle Cell Disease.
Safety data are based upon 465 subjects with lymphoma and solid tumors (breast, lung, and thoracic tumors) enrolled in six randomized clinical studies. Subjects received Neulasta™ after nonmyeloablative cytotoxic chemotherapy. Most adverse experiences were attributed by the investigators to the underlying malignancy or cytotoxic chemotherapy and occurred at similar rates in subjects who received Neulasta™ (n = 465) or Filgrastim (n = 331). These adverse experiences occurred at rates between 72% and 15% and included: nausea, fatigue, alopecia, diarrhea, vomiting, constipation, fever, anorexia, skeletal pain, headache, taste perversion, dyspepsia, myalgia, insomnia, abdominal pain, arthralgia, generalized weakness, peripheral edema, dizziness, granulocytopenia, stomatitis, mucositis, and neutropenic fever.
The most common adverse event attributed to Neulasta™ in clinical trials was medullary bone pain, reported in 26% of subjects, which was comparable to the incidence in Filgrastim-treated patients. This bone pain was generally reported to be of mild-to-moderate severity. Approximately 12% of all subjects utilized non-narcotic analgesics and less than 6% utilized narcotic analgesics in association with bone pain. No patient withdrew from study due to bone pain.
In clinical studies, leukocytosis (WBC counts > 100×10^9/L) was observed in less than 1% of 465 subjects with non-myeloid malignancies receiving Neulasta™. Leukocytosis was not associated with any adverse effects.
In subjects receiving Neulasta™ in clinical trials, the only serious event that was not deemed attributable to underlying or concurrent disease, or to concurrent therapy was a case of hypoxia.
Reversible elevations in LDH, alkaline phosphatase, and uric acid, which did not require treatment intervention, were observed. The incidences of these changes, presented for Neulasta™ relative to Filgrastim, were: LDH (19% vs 29%), alkaline phosphatase (9% vs 16%), and uric acid (8% vs 9% [1% of reported cases for both treatment groups were classified as severe]).

Immunogenicity

As with all therapeutic proteins, there is a potential for immunogenicity. The incidence of antibody development in patients receiving Neulasta™ has not been adequately determined. While available data suggest that a small proportion of patients developed binding antibodies to Filgrastim or pegfilgrastim, the nature and specificity of these antibodies has not been adequately studied. No neutralizing antibodies have been detected using a cell-based bioassay in 46 patients who apparently developed binding antibodies. The detection of antibody formation is highly dependent on the sensitivity and specificity of the assay, and the observed incidence of antibody positivity in an assay may be influenced by several factors including sample handling, concomitant medications, and underlying disease. Therefore, comparison of the incidence of antibodies to Neulasta™ with the incidence of antibodies to other products may be misleading.
Cytopenias resulting from an antibody response to exogenous growth factors have been reported on rare occasions in patients treated with other recombinant growth factors. There is a theoretical possibility that an antibody directed against pegfilgrastim may cross-react with endogenous G-CSF, resulting in immune-mediated neutropenia, but this has not been observed in clinical studies.

OVERDOSAGE

The maximum amount of Neulasta™ that can be safely administered in single or multiple doses has not been determined. Single doses of 300 mcg/kg have been administered SC to 8 normal volunteers and 3 patients with non-small cell lung cancer without serious adverse effects. These subjects experienced a mean maximum ANC of 55×10^9/L, with a corresponding mean maximum WBC of 67×10^9/L. The absolute maximum ANC observed was 96×10^9/L with a corresponding absolute maximum WBC observed of 120×10^9/L. The duration of leukocytosis ranged from 6 to 13 days. Leukapheresis should be considered in the management of symptomatic individuals.

DOSAGE AND ADMINISTRATION

The recommended dosage of Neulasta™ is a single SC injection of 6 mg administered once per chemotherapy cycle. Neulasta™ should not be administered in the period between 14 days before and 24 hours after administration of cytotoxic chemotherapy (see PRECAUTIONS).
The 6 mg fixed dose formulation should not be used in infants, children, and smaller adolescents weighing less than 45 kg.
Neulasta™ should be visually inspected for discoloration and particulate matter before administration. Neulasta™ should not be administered if discoloration or particulates are observed.
Neulasta™ is supplied in prefilled syringes with UltraSafe® Needle Guards. Following administration of Neulasta™ from the prefilled syringe, the UltraSafe® Needle Guard should be activated to prevent accidental needle sticks. To activate the UltraSafe® Needle Guard, place your hands behind the needle, grasp the guard with one hand, and slide the guard forward until the needle is completely covered and the guard clicks into place. NOTE: If an audible click is not heard, the needle guard may not be completely activated. The prefilled syringe should be disposed of by placing the entire prefilled syringe with guard activated into an approved puncture-proof container.

Storage

Neulasta™ should be stored refrigerated at 2° to 8°C (36° to 46°F); syringes should be kept in their carton to protect from light until time of use. Shaking should be avoided. Before injection Neulasta™ may be allowed to reach room temperature for a maximum of 48 hours but should be protected from light. Neulasta™ left at room temperature for more than 48 hours should be discarded. Freezing should be avoided; however, if accidentally frozen, Neulasta™ should be allowed to thaw in the refrigerator before administration. If frozen a second time, Neulasta™ should be discarded.

HOW SUPPLIED

Neulasta™ is supplied as a preservative-free solution containing 6 mg (0.6 mL) of pegfilgrastim (10 mg/mL) in a single-dose syringe with a 27 gauge, 1/2 inch needle with an UltraSafe® Needle Guard.
Neulasta™ is provided in a dispensing pack containing one syringe (NDC 55513-190-01).

REFERENCES

1. Morstyn G, Dexter T, Foote M. *Filgrastim (r-metHuG-CSF) in clinical practice*. 2nd Edition. 1998;3:51–71.
2. Valerius T, Elsasser D, Repp R, et al. HLA Class-II antibodies recruit G-CSF activated neutrophils for treatment of B-cell malignancies. *Leukemia and Lymphoma*. 1997;26, 261–269.
3. Heil G, Hoelzer D, Sanz MA, et al. A randomized, double-blind, placebo-controlled, phase III study of Filgrastim in remission induction and consolidation therapy for adults with de novo Acute Myeloid Leukemia. *Blood*. 1997;90:4710–4718.

AMGEN®

Manufactured by: Amgen Manufacturing, Limited, a subsidiary of Amgen Inc.
One Amgen Center Drive
Thousand Oaks, California 91320-1799

Issue Date: 01/31/02

AstraZeneca LP

WILMINGTON, DE 19850-5437

For Medical Information, Adverse Drug Experiences, and Customer Service
Contact: (800) 236-9933

ENTOCORT™ EC ℞
(budesonide)
Capsules
Rx only

DESCRIPTION

Budesonide, the active ingredient of ENTOCORT™ EC capsules, is a synthetic corticosteroid. It is designated chemically as (RS)-11β,16α, 17,21-tetrahydroxypregna-1,4-diene-3,20-dione cyclic 16, 17-acetal with butyraldehyde. Budesonide is provided as a mixture of two epimers (22R and 22S). The empirical formula of budesonide is $C_{25}H_{34}O_6$ and its molecular weight is 430.5. Its structural formula is:

CH₂OH / C=O / CH₃ / HO / CH₃ / O–C–H / CH₂–CH₂–CH₃

Epimer 22R of budesonide

Epimer 22S of budesonide

Continued on next page

Entocort EC—Cont.

Budesonide is a white to off-white, tasteless, odorless powder that is practically insoluble in water and heptane, sparingly soluble in ethanol, and freely soluble in chloroform. Its partition coefficient between octanol and water at pH 5 is 1.6×10^3 ionic strength 0.01.

Each capsule contains 3 mg of micronized budesonide with the following inactive ingredients: ethylcellulose, acetyltributyl citrate, methacrylic acid copolymer type C, triethyl citrate, antifoam M, polysorbate 80, talc, and sugar spheres. The capsule shells have the following inactive ingredients: gelatin, iron oxide, and titanium dioxide.

CLINICAL PHARMACOLOGY

Budesonide has a high topical glucocorticosteroid (GCS) activity and a substantial first pass elimination. The formulation contains granules which are coated to protect dissolution in gastric juice, but which dissolve at pH >5.5, ie, normally when the granules reach the duodenum. Thereafter, a matrix of ethylcellulose with budesonide controls the release of the drug into the intestinal lumen in a time-dependent manner.

Pharmacokinetics

Absorption

The absorption of ENTOCORT EC seems to be complete, although C_{max} and T_{max} are variable. Time to peak concentration varies in individual patients between 30 and 600 minutes. Following oral administration of 9 mg of budesonide in healthy subjects, a peak plasma concentration of approximately 5 nmol/L is observed and the area under the plasma concentration time curve is approximately 30 nmol•hr/mL.

The systemic availability after a single dose is higher in patients with Crohn's disease compared to healthy volunteers, (21% vs 9%) but approaches that in healthy volunteers after repeated dosing.

Distribution

The mean volume of distribution (V_{ss}) of budesonide varies between 2.2 and 3.9 L/kg in healthy subjects and in patients. Plasma protein binding is estimated to be 85 to 90% in the concentration range 1 to 230 nmol/L, independent of gender. The erythrocyte/plasma partition ratio at clinically relevant concentrations is about 0.8.

Metabolism

Following absorption, budesonide is subject to high first pass metabolism (80–90%). *In vitro* experiments in human liver microsomes demonstrate that budesonide is rapidly and extensively biotransformed, mainly by CYP3A4, to its 2 major metabolites, 6β-hydroxy budesonide and 16α-hydroxy prednisolone. The glucocorticoid activity of these metabolites is negligible (<1/100) in relation to that of the parent compound.

In vivo investigations with intravenous doses in healthy subjects are in agreement with the *in vitro* findings and demonstrate that budesonide has a high plasma clearance, 0.9–1.8 L/min. Similarly, high plasma clearance values have been shown in patients with Crohn's disease. These high plasma clearance values approach the estimated liver blood flow, and, accordingly, suggest that budesonide is a high hepatic clearance drug.

The plasma elimination half-life, $t_{1/2}$, after administration of intravenous doses ranges between 2.0 and 3.6 hours, and does not differ between healthy adults and patients with Crohn's disease.

Excretion

Budesonide is excreted in urine and feces in the form of metabolites. After oral as well as intravenous administration of micronized [^{3}H]-budesonide, approximately 60% of the recovered radioactivity is found in urine. The major metabolites, including 6β-hydroxy budesonide and 16α-hydroxy prednisolone, are mainly renally excreted, intact or in conjugated forms. No unchanged budesonide is detected in urine.

Special Populations

No significant pharmacokinetic differences have been identified due to sex.

Hepatic Insufficiency

In patients with liver cirrhosis, systemic availability of orally administered budesonide correlates with disease severity and is, on average, 2.5-fold higher compared with healthy controls. Patients with mild liver disease are minimally affected. Patients with severe liver dysfunction were not studied. Absorption parameters are not altered, and for the intravenous dose, no significant differences in CL or V_{ss} are observed.

Renal Insufficiency

The pharmacokinetics of budesonide in patients with renal impairment has not been studied. Intact budesonide is not renally excreted, but metabolites are to a large extent, and might therefore reach higher levels in patients with impaired renal function. However, these metabolites have negligible corticosteroid activity as compared with budesonide (<1/100). Thus, patients with impaired renal function taking budesonide are not expected to have an increased risk of adverse effects.

Drug-Drug Interactions

Budesonide is metabolized via CYP3A4. Potent inhibitors of CYP3A4 can increase the plasma levels of budesonide severalfold. Co-administration of ketoconazole results in an eight-fold increase in AUC of budesonide, compared to budesonide alone. Grapefruit juice, an inhibitor of gut mucosal CYP3A, approximately doubles the systemic exposure of oral budesonide. Conversely, induction of CYP3A4 can result in the lowering of budesonide plasma levels. Oral contraceptives containing ethinyl estradiol, which are also metabolized by CYP3A4, do not affect the pharmacokinetics of budesonide. Budesonide does not affect the plasma levels of oral contraceptives (ie, ethinyl estradiol).

Since the dissolution of the coating of ENTOCORT EC is pH dependent (dissolves at pH >5.5), the release properties and uptake of the compound may be altered after treatment with drugs that change the gastrointestinal pH. However, the gastric acid inhibitory drug omeprazole, 20 mg qd, does not affect the absorption or pharmacokinetics of ENTOCORT EC. When an uncoated oral formulation of budesonide is co-administered with a daily dose of cimetidine 1g, a slight increase in the budesonide peak plasma concentration and rate of absorption occurs, resulting in significant cortisol suppression.

Food Effects

A mean delay in time to peak concentration of 2.5 hours is observed with the intake of a high-fat meal, with no significant differences in AUC.

PHARMACODYNAMICS

Budesonide has a high glucocorticoid effect and a weak mineralocorticoid effect, and the affinity of budesonide to GCS receptors, which reflects the intrinsic potency of the drug, is about 200-fold that of cortisol and 15-fold that of prednisolone.

Treatment with systemically active GCS is associated with a suppression of endogenous cortisol concentrations and an impairment of the hypothalamus-pituitary-adrenal (HPA) axis function. Markers, indirect and direct, of this are cortisol levels in plasma or urine and response to ACTH stimulation.

Plasma cortisol suppression was compared following five days' administration of ENTOCORT EC capsules and prednisolone in a crossover study in healthy volunteers. The mean decrease in the integrated 0–24 hour plasma cortisol concentration was greater (78%) with prednisolone 20 mg/day compared to 45% with ENTOCORT EC 9 mg/day.

CLINICAL STUDIES

The safety and efficacy of ENTOCORT EC were evaluated in 994 patients with mild to moderate active Crohn's disease of the ileum and/or ascending colon in 5 randomized and double-blind studies. The study patients ranged in age from 17 to 85 (mean 35), 40% were male and 97% were white. Of the 651 patients treated with ENTOCORT EC, 17 (2.6%) were ≥65 years of age and none were >74 years of age. The Crohn's Disease Activity Index (CDAI) was the main clinical assessment used for determining efficacy in these 5 studies. The CDAI is a validated index based on subjective aspects rated by the patient (frequency of liquid or very soft stools, abdominal pain rating and general well-being) and objective observations (number of extraintestinal symptoms, need for antidiarrheal drugs, presence of abdominal mass, body weight and hematocrit). Clinical improvement, defined as a CDAI score of ≤150 assessed after 8 weeks of treatment, was the primary efficacy variable in these 5 comparative efficacy studies of ENTOCORT EC capsules. Safety assessments in these studies included monitoring of adverse experiences. A checklist of potential symptoms of hypercorticism was used.

One study (Study 1) compared the safety and efficacy of ENTOCORT EC 9 mg qd in the morning to a comparator. At baseline, the median CDAI was 272. ENTOCORT EC 9 mg qd resulted in a significantly higher clinical improvement rate at Week 8 than the comparator (Table 1).

[See table above]

Table 1: Clinical Improvement Rates (CDAI ≤150) After 8 weeks of Treatment

Clinical Study	ENTOCORT EC 9 mg QD	ENTOCORT EC 4.5 mg BID	Comparator [a]	Placebo	Prednisolone
1	62/91 (69%)		37/83 (45%)		
2		31/61 (51%)		13/64 (20%)	
3	38/79 (48%)	41/78 (53%)		13/40 (33%)	
4	35/58 (60%)	25/60 (42%)			35/58 (60%)
5	45/86 (52%)				56/85 (65%)

[a] This drug is not approved for the treatment of Crohn's disease in the United States.

Two placebo-controlled clinical trials (Studies 2 and 3) were conducted. Study 2 involved 258 patients and tested the effects of grading doses of ENTOCORT EC (1.5 mg bid, 4.5 mg bid, or 7.5 mg bid) versus placebo. At baseline, the median CDAI was 290. The 3 mg per day dose level (data not shown) could not be differentiated from placebo. The 9 mg per day arm was statistically different from placebo (Table 1), while no additional benefit was seen when the daily ENTOCORT EC dose was increased to 15 mg per day (data not shown). In Study 3, the median CDAI at baseline was 263. Neither 9 mg qd nor 4.5 mg bid ENTOCORT EC dose levels was statistically different from placebo (Table 1).

Two clinical trials (Studies 4 and 5) compared ENTOCORT EC capsules with oral prednisolone (initial dose 40 mg per day). At baseline, the median CDAI was 277. Equal clinical improvement rates (60%) were seen in the ENTOCORT EC 9 mg qd and the prednisolone groups in Study 4. In Study 5, 13% fewer patients in the ENTOCORT EC group experience clinical improvement than in the prednisolone group (no statistical difference) (Table 1).

The proportion of patients with normal plasma cortisol values (≥150 nmol/L) was significantly higher in the ENTOCORT EC groups in both trials (60 to 66%) than in the prednisolone groups (26 to 28%) at Week 8.

INDICATIONS AND USAGE

ENTOCORT EC is indicated for the treatment of mild to moderate active Crohn's disease involving the ileum and/or the ascending colon.

CONTRAINDICATIONS

ENTOCORT EC is contraindicated in patients with known hypersensitivity to budesonide.

WARNINGS

Glucocorticosteroids can reduce the response of the hypothalamuspituitary-adrenal (HPA) axis to stress. In situations where patients are subject to surgery or other stress situations, supplementation with a systemic glucocorticosteroid is recommended. Since ENTOCORT EC is a glucocorticosteroid, general warnings concerning glucocorticoids should be followed.

Care is needed in patients who are transferred from glucocorticosteroid treatment with high systemic effects to corticosteroids with lower systemic availability, since symptoms attributed to withdrawal of steroid therapy, including those of acute adrenal suppression or benign intracranial hypertension, may develop. Adrenocortical function monitoring may be required in these patients and the dose of systemic steroid should be reduced cautiously.

Patients who are on drugs that suppress the immune system are more susceptible to infection than healthy individuals. Chicken pox and measles, for example, can have a more serious or even fatal course in susceptible patients or patients on immunosuppressant doses of glucocorticosteroids. In patients who have not had these diseases, particular care should be taken to avoid exposure. How the dose, route and duration of glucocorticosteroid administration affect the risk of developing a disseminated infection is not known. The contribution of the underlying disease and/or prior glucocorticosteroid treatment to the risk is also not known. If exposed, therapy with varicella zoster immune globulin (VZIG) or pooled intravenous immunoglobulin (IVIG), as appropriate, may be indicated. If exposed to measles, prophylaxis with pooled intramuscular immunoglobulin (IG) may be indicated. (See the respective package insert for complete VZIG and IG prescribing information.) If chicken pox develops, treatment with antiviral agents may be considered.

PRECAUTIONS

General

Caution should be taken in patients with tuberculosis, hypertension, diabetes mellitus, osteoporosis, peptic ulcer, glaucoma or cataracts, or with a family history of diabetes or glaucoma, or with any other condition where glucocorticosteroids may have unwanted effects.

Replacement of systemic glucocorticosteroids with ENTOCORT EC capsules may unmask allergies, eg, rhinitis and eczema, which were previously controlled by the systemic drug.

When ENTOCORT EC capsules are used chronically, systemic glucocorticosteroid effects such as hypercorticism and adrenal suppression may occur.

Reduced liver function affects the elimination of glucocorticosteroids, and increased systemic availability of oral budesonide has been demonstrated in patients with liver cirrhosis.

Information for Patients

ENTOCORT EC capsules should be swallowed whole and NOT CHEWED OR BROKEN.

Patients should be advised to avoid the consumption of grapefruit juice for the duration of their ENTOCORT EC therapy.

Patients should be given the patient package insert for additional information.

Drug Interactions

Concomitant oral administration of ketoconazole (a known inhibitor of CYP3A4 activity in the liver and in the intestinal mucosa) caused an eight-fold increase of the systemic exposure to oral budesonide. If treatment with inhibitors of CYP3A4 activity (such as ketoconazole, intraconazole, ritonavir, indinavir, saquinavir, erythromycin, etc.) is indicated, reduction of the budesonide dose should be considered. After extensive intake of grapefruit juice (which inhibits CYP3A4 activity predominantly in the intestinal mucosa), the systemic exposure for oral budesonide increased about two times. As with other drugs primarily being metabolized through CYP3A4, ingestion of grapefruit or grapefruit juice should be avoided in connection with budesonide administration.

Carcinogenesis, Mutagenesis, Impairment of Fertility

Carcinogenicity studies with budesonide were conducted in rats and mice. In a two-year study in Sprague-Dawley rats, budesonide caused a statistically significant increase in the incidence of gliomas in male rats at an oral dose of 50 mcg/kg (approximately 0.05 times the maximum recommended human dose on a body surface area basis). In addition, there were increased incidences of primary hepatocellular tumors in male rats at 25 mcg/kg (approximately 0.023 times the maximum recommended human dose on a body surface area basis) and above. No tumorigenicity was seen in female rats at oral doses up to 50 mcg/kg (approximately 0.05 times the maximum recommended human dose on a body surface area basis). In an additional two-year study in male Sprague-Dawley rats, budesonide caused no gliomas at an oral dose of 50 mcg/kg (approximately 0.05 times the maximum recommended human dose on a body surface area basis). However, it caused a statistically significant increase in the incidence of hepatocellular tumors at an oral dose of 50 mcg/kg (approximately 0.05 times the maximum recommended human dose on a body surface area basis). The concurrent reference corticosteroids (prednisolone and triamcinolone acetonide) showed similar findings. In a 91-week study in mice, budesonide caused no treatment-related carcinogenicity at oral doses up to 200 mcg/kg (approximately 0.1 times the maximum recommended human dose on a body surface area basis).

Budesonide was not genotoxic in the Ames test, the mouse lymphoma cell forward gene mutation (TK $^{+/-}$) test, the human lymphocyte chromosome aberration test, the *Drosophila melanogaster* sex-linked recessive lethality test, the rat hepatocyte UDS test and the mouse micronucleus test.

In rats, budesonide had no effect on fertility at subcutaneous doses up to 80 mcg/kg (approximately 0.07 times the maximum recommended human dose on a body surface area basis). However, it caused a decrease in prenatal viability and viability in pups at birth and during lactation, along with a decrease in maternal body-weight gain, at subcutaneous doses of 20 mcg/kg (approximately 0.02 times the maximum recommended human dose on a body surface area basis) and above. No such effects were noted at 5 mcg/kg (approximately 0.005 times the maximum recommended human dose on a body surface area basis).

Pregnancy

Teratogenic Effects: Pregnancy Category C: As with other corticosteroids, budesonide was teratogenic and embryocidal in rabbits and rats. Budesonide produced fetal loss, decreased pup weights, and skeletal abnormalities at subcutaneous doses of 25 mcg/kg in rabbits (approximately 0.05 times the maximum recommended human dose on a body surface area basis) and 500 mcg/kg in rats (approximately 0.5 times the maximum recommended human dose on a body surface area basis).

There are no adequate and well-controlled studies in pregnant women. Budesonide should be used during pregnancy only if the potential benefit justifies the potential risk to the fetus.

Nonteratogenic Effects: Hypoadrenalism may occur in infants born of mothers receiving corticosteroids during pregnancy. Such infants should be carefully observed.

Nursing Mothers

Glucocorticosteroids are secreted in human milk. Because of the potential for adverse reactions in nursing infants from any corticosteroid, a decision should be made whether to discontinue nursing or discontinue the drug, taking into account the importance of the drug to the mother. The amount of budesonide secreted in breast milk has not been determined.

Pediatric Use

Safety and effectiveness in pediatric patients have not been established.

Geriatric Use

Clinical studies of ENTOCORT EC did not include sufficient numbers of subjects aged 65 and over to determine whether they respond differently from younger subjects. Other reported clinical experience has not identified differences in responses between the elderly and younger patients. In general, dose selection for an elderly patient should be cautious, usually starting at the low end of the dosing range, reflecting the greater frequency of decreased hepatic, renal, or cardiac function, and of concomitant disease or other drug therapy.

ADVERSE REACTIONS

The safety of ENTOCORT EC was evaluated in 651 patients. They ranged in age from 17 to 74 (mean 35), 40% were male and 97% were white, 2.6% were ≥65 years of age. Five hundred and twenty patients were treated with ENTOCORT EC 9 mg (total daily dose). In general, ENTOCORT EC was well tolerated in these trials. The most common adverse events reported were headache, respiratory infection, nausea, and symptoms of hypercorticism. Clinical studies have shown that the frequency of glucocorticosteroid-associated adverse events was substantially reduced with ENTOCORT EC capsules compared with prednisolone at therapeutically equivalent doses. Adverse events occurring in ≥5% of the patients are listed in Table 2:

[See table 2 above]

Table 2: Adverse Events Occurring in ≥5% of the Patients in any Treated Group

	ENTOCORT EC 9 mg n=520	Placebo n=107	Prednisolone 40 mg n=145	Comparator* n=88
Adverse Event	**Number (%)**	**Number (%)**	**Number (%)**	**Number (%)**
Headache	107(21)	19(18)	31(21)	11(13)
Respiratory Infection	55(11)	7(7)	20(14)	5(6)
Nausea	57(11)	10(9)	18(12)	7(8)
Back Pain	36(7)	10(9)	17(12)	5(6)
Dyspepsia	31(6)	4(4)	17(12)	3(3)
Dizziness	38(7)	5(5)	18(12)	5(6)
Abdominal Pain	32(6)	18(17)	6(4)	10(11)
Flatulence	30(6)	6(6)	12(8)	5(6)
Vomiting	29(6)	6(6)	6(4)	6(7)
Fatigue	25(5)	8(7)	11(8)	0(0)
Pain	24(5)	8(7)	17(12)	2(2)

*This drug is not approved for the treatment of Crohn's disease in the United States.

Adverse events occurring in 520 patients treated with ENTOCORT EC 9 mg (total daily dose), with an incidence <5% and greater than placebo (n=107), are listed below by body system: ***Body as a Whole:*** *asthenia, C-Reactive protein increased, chest pain, dependent edema, face edema, flu-like disorder, malaise;* ***Cardiovascular:*** *hypertension;* ***Central and Peripheral Nervous System:*** *hyperkinesia, paresthesia, tremor, vertigo;* ***Gastrointestinal:*** *anus disorder, Crohn's disease aggravated, enteritis, epigastric pain, gastrointestinal fistula, glossitis, hemorrhoids, intestinal obstruction, tongue edema, tooth disorder;* ***Hearing and Vestibular:*** *Ear infection-not otherwise specified;* ***Heart Rate and Rhythm:*** *palpitation, tachycardia;* ***Metabolic and Nutritional:*** *hypokalemia, weight increase;* ***Musculoskeletal:*** *arthritis aggravated, cramps, myalgia;* ***Psychiatric:*** *agitation, appetite increased, confusion, insomnia, nervousness, sleep disorder, somnolence;* ***Resistance Mechanism:*** *moniliasis;* ***Reproductive, Female:*** *intermenstrual bleeding, menstrual disorder;* ***Respiratory:*** *bronchitis, dyspnea;* ***Skin and Appendages:*** *acne, alopecia, dermatitis, eczema, skin disorder, sweating increased;* ***Urinary:*** *dysuria, micturition frequency, nocturia;* ***Vascular:*** *flushing;* ***Vision:*** *eye abnormality, vision abnormal;* ***White Blood Cell:*** leukocytosis

Glucocorticosteroid Adverse Reactions

Table 3 displays the frequency and incidence of symptoms of hypercorticism by active questioning of patients in clinical trials.

[See table 3 above]

Table 3: Summary and Incidence of Symptoms of Hypercorticism

	ENTOCORT EC 9 mg n=427	Placebo n=107	Prednisolone Taper 40 mg n=145
Symptom	**Number (%)**	**Number (%)**	**Number (%)**
Acne	63(15)	14(13)	33(23)*
Bruising Easily	63(15)	12(11)	13(9)
Moon Face	46(11)	4(4)	53(37)*
Swollen Ankles	32(7)	6(6)	13(9)
Hirsutism[a]	22(5)	2(2)	5(3)
Buffalo Hump	6(1)	2(2)	5(3)
Skin Striae	4(1)	2(2)	0(0)

[a] Adverse event dictionary included term hair growth increased, local and hair growth increased, general.
*Statistically significantly different from ENTOCORT EC 9 mg

In addition to the symptoms in Table 3, three cases of benign intracranial hypertension have been reported in patients treated with budesonide from post-marketing surveillance. A cause and effect relationship has not been established.

CLINICAL LABORATORY TEST FINDINGS

The following potentially clinically significant laboratory changes in clinical trials, irrespective of relationship to ENTOCORT EC, were reported in ≥1% of patients: hypokalemia, leukocytosis, anemia, hematuria, pyuria, erythrocyte sedimentation rate increased, alkaline phosphatase increased, atypical neutrophils, C-reactive protein increased, and adrenal insufficiency.

OVERDOSAGE

Reports of acute toxicity and/or death following overdosage of glucocorticosteroids are rare. Treatment consists of immediate gastric lavage or emesis followed by supportive and symptomatic therapy.

If glucocorticosteroids are used at excessive doses for prolonged periods, systemic glucocorticosteroid effects such as hypercorticism and adrenal suppression may occur. For chronic overdosage in the face of severe disease requiring continuous steroid therapy, the dosage may be reduced temporarily.

Single oral doses of 200 and 400 mg/kg were lethal in female and male mice, respectively. The signs of acute toxicity were decreased motor activity, piloerection and generalized edema.

DOSAGE AND ADMINISTRATION

The recommended adult dosage for the treatment of mild to moderate active Crohn's disease involving the ileum and/or the ascending colon is 9 mg taken once daily in the morning for up to 8 weeks. Safety and efficacy of ENTOCORT EC in the treatment of active Crohn's Disease have not been established beyond 8 weeks.

For recurring episodes of active Crohn's Disease, a repeat 8 week course of ENTOCORT EC can be given.

Treatment with ENTOCORT EC capsules can be tapered to 6 mg daily for 2 weeks prior to complete cessation.

Patients with mild to moderate active Crohn's disease involving the ileum and/or ascending colon have been switched from oral prednisolone to ENTOCORT EC with no reported episodes of adrenal insufficiency. Since prednisolone should not be stopped abruptly, tapering should begin concomitantly with initiating ENTOCORT EC treatment.

Hepatic Insufficiency: Patients with moderate to severe liver disease should be monitored for increased signs and/or symptoms of hypercorticism. Reducing the dose of ENTOCORT EC capsules should be considered in these patients.

CYP3A4 inhibitors: If concomitant administration with ketoconazole, or any other CYP3A4 inhibitor, is indicated, patients should be closely monitored for increased signs and/or symptoms of hypercorticism. Reduction in the dose of ENTOCORT EC capsules should be considered.

ENTOCORT EC capsules should be swallowed whole and not chewed or broken.

HOW SUPPLIED

ENTOCORT EC 3 mg capsules are hard gelatin capsules with an opaque light grey body and an opaque pink cap, coded with CIR and 3 mg on the capsule.

They are supplied as follows:

NDC 0186-0702-10 Bottles of 100

Storage

Store at 25°C (77°F); excursions permitted to 15–30°C (59–86°F) [See USP Controlled Room Temperature].

Keep container tightly closed.

Manufactured for:
AstraZeneca LP, Wilmington, DE 19850
By: AstraZeneca AB
S-151 85 Sodertalje, Sweden
20569-00
Rev 08/01

Continued on next page

Entocort EC—Cont.

PATIENT INFORMATION

Entocort™ EC
(budesonide) Capsules

Read this information carefully before you begin treatment. Read the information you get whenever you get more medicine. There may be new information. This information does not take the place of talking with your doctor about your medical condition or your treatment. If you have any questions about ENTOCORT EC (EN-toe-cort EE-CEE), ask your health care provider (provider). Only your provider can determine if ENTOCORT EC is right for you.

What is ENTOCORT EC?

ENTOCORT EC is a medicine to treat mild to moderate Crohn's Disease in many people. However, it does not work for everyone who takes it. ENTOCORT EC is a *nonsystemic* corticosteroid, which means it works mainly in one area of the body. The medicine in ENTOCORT EC is released in the intestine. Therefore, it controls the symptoms of Crohn's disease even though 90% of the drug does not go into the bloodstream. Because of this, it causes fewer severe side effects than other corticosteroids. (See the end of this Patient Information for information about Crohn's Disease.)

Who should not take ENTOCORT EC?

Do not take ENTOCORT EC if:

- you are breast feeding. Because ENTOCORT EC is carried in human milk, it may harm the baby. Talk with your provider about whether you should stop breast feeding to take ENTOCORT EC or should use another treatment
- you have had an allergic reaction to ENTOCORT EC or any of its ingredients

To help your provider decide if ENTOCORT EC is right for you, tell your provider:

- if you had an allergic reaction to any medicine in the past
- the names of all the prescription and nonprescription medicines you now take. Be sure to tell your provider if you take ketoconazole, which can affect processing of ENTOCORT EC by the liver, steroids such as prednisone, or any other drug that suppresses your immune system
- if you are pregnant, think you may be pregnant, or plan to get pregnant. Your provider will talk about whether ENTOCORT EC is right for you
- if you ever had liver problems. Liver problems affect the amount of ENTOCORT EC that stays in your system, and dosage may need to be changed
- if you are about to have surgery for any reason. Your dosage may need to be changed
- if you have chicken pox or measles, or any other condition that suppresses the immune system
- if you or anyone in your family has had diabetes or glaucoma
- if you ever had tuberculosis, high blood pressure, osteoporosis, ulcers, or cataracts.

How should I take ENTOCORT EC?

Take ENTOCORT EC in the morning. Swallow each ENTOCORT EC capsule whole. **Do not open, chew, or crush ENTOCORT EC capsules.** Your provider will tell you how long to take ENTOCORT EC.

What should I avoid while taking ENTOCORT EC?

Patients who take medicines that suppress the immune system, such as ENTOCORT EC, are more likely to get infections. Avoid people with infections. Also, if you never had chicken pox or measles, be careful to avoid people with these conditions. These conditions can be more serious if you get them while taking ENTOCORT EC.

While you are taking ENTOCORT EC, do not drink grapefruit juice regularly. Grapefruit juice can increase the amount of ENTOCORT EC in your blood. Other juices, like orange juice or apple juice, do not have this effect.

What are the side effects of ENTOCORT EC?

The most common side effects of ENTOCORT EC are headache, infection in your air passages (respiratory infection), nausea, and symptoms of hypercorticism (too much steroids in your body).

These symptoms include an increase in the size of the face and neck, acne, and bruising. Most symptoms of too much steroids in your body occur less often with ENTOCORT EC than with other steroids.

Call your provider right away if you notice itching, skin rash, fever, swelling of your face and neck, or trouble breathing while you are taking ENTOCORT EC. These may be signs that you are allergic to the medicine and you may need emergency medical help.

Switching from a systemic medicine, like prednisone, to a nonsystemic medicine, such as ENTOCORT EC, can cause allergies controlled by the systemic medicine to come back. These allergies may include eczema (a skin disease) or rhinitis (inflammation inside the nose).

Call your provider if:

- your Crohn's disease symptoms worsen during treatment
- you notice any side effects or any other symptoms that concern you

These are not all the possible side effects of ENTOCORT EC. Ask your provider or pharmacist for a complete listing of all possible side effects of ENTOCORT EC.

What is Crohn's disease?

Crohn's disease is an inflammatory bowel disease. The inflammation caused by Crohn's disease is usually found in a part of the small intestine called the ileum and in the large intestine (colon). It may also occur in any part of the gastrointestinal tract (digestive system) from the mouth to the anus (rectum). The cause of Crohn's disease is not yet known.

There are many symptoms of Crohn's disease. These include diarrhea, crampy abdominal (stomach area) pain, fever, and sometimes bleeding from the rectum. Appetite loss followed by weight loss may occur. There may also be redness and soreness of the eyes, joint pain, and sores on the skin. These symptoms may range from mild to severe.

There is no cure yet for Crohn's disease. However, it is possible for the disease to quiet down (go into remission). During these periods of remission, there may be times when the symptoms get worse. In general, people with Crohn's disease are able to lead productive lives.

General advice about prescription medicines

Medicines are sometimes prescribed for conditions that are not mentioned in patient information leaflets. Do not use ENTOCORT EC for a condition for which it was not prescribed. Do not give ENTOCORT EC to other people, even if they have the same symptoms you have. It may harm them.

Keep ENTOCORT EC and all medicines out of the reach of children.

This leaflet summarizes the most important information about ENTOCORT EC. If you would like more information, talk with your provider. You can ask your pharmacist or provider for information about ENTOCORT EC that is written for health professionals. You can also visit the ENTOCORT EC Web site at (**www.EntocortEC.com**) or call the information center at AstraZeneca toll-free (**1-800-237-8898**).

Manufactured for:
AstraZeneca LP, Wilmington, DE 19850
By: AstraZeneca AB
S-151 85 Sodertalje, Sweden
20583-01 Rev 10/01 **AstraZeneca**

Ballay Pharmaceuticals, Inc.

P.O. BOX 1356
WIMBERLEY, TX 78676

Direct Inquiries to:
Terry Ballay, President
512-847-6458

In addition to the full labeling of the products listed below, the following products are also available from Ballay Pharmaceuticals:
Balagan® (Otic Solution)
Baltussin® HC Ⓒⅲ
Nortemp®
Pulexn® DM

ALACOL DM® SYRUP ℞

[*'alə - kōl*]
Alcohol Free–Sugar Free

DESCRIPTION

Antihistamine/Nasal Decongestant/Antitussive syrup for oral administration. An alcohol-free, sugar-free, black raspberry flavored syrup. Each teaspoonful (5 mL) contains: Dextromethorphan HBr. 10 mg; Phenylephrine HCl, 5mg; Brompheniramine Maleate, 2 mg.

INACTIVE INGREDIENTS

Propylene Glycol, Sodium Saccharin, Glycerin, Sorbitol, Purified Water, Raspberry Flavor, FD&C Red#40, and FD&C Blue#1

CLINICAL PHARMACOLOGY

Dextromethorphan Hydrobromide acts centrally to elevate the threshold for coughing. It has no analgesic or addictive properties. The onset of antitussive action occurs in 15 to 30 minutes after administration and is of long duration. Phenylephrine HCl is a sympathomimetic drug which is readily absorbed from the gastrointestinal tract and produces nasal vasoconstriction (decongestion). Phenylephrine effects its vasoconstrictor activity by releasing noradrenaline from sympathetic nerve endings and from direct stimulation of α-adreno receptors in blood vessels. Brompheniramine Maleate is a histamine antagonist, specifically an H_1-receptor blocking agent belonging to the alkylamine class of antihistamines. Antihistamines appear to compete with histamine for receptor sites on effector cells. Brompheniramine also has anticholinergic (drying) and sedative effects. Among the antihistaminic effects, it antagonizes the allergic response (vasodilatation, increased vascular permeability, increased mucous secretion) of nasal tissue. Brompheniramine is well absorbed from the gastrointestinal tract, with peak plasma concentration after a single oral dose of 4 mg reached in 5 hours: urinary excretion is the major route of elimination, mostly as products of biodegradation; the liver is assumed to be the main sight of metabolic transformation.

INDICATIONS

ALACOL DM is indicated for the relief of coughs and upper respiratory symptoms, including nasal congestion, associated with allergy or the common cold.

CONTRAINDICATIONS

Hypersensitivity to any of the ingredients. Do not use in newborns, in premature infants, in nursing mothers, in patients with severe hypertension or severe coronary artery disease, or in those receiving MAO inhibitors. Antihistamines should not be used to treat lower respiratory tract conditions including asthma.

WARNINGS

A persistent cough may be a sign of a serious condition. If cough persists for more than one week, tends to recur or is accompanied by fever, rash, or persistent headache, consult a physician. Do not take this product for persistent or chronic cough such as occurs with smoking, asthma, emphysema, or if cough is accompanied by excessive phlegm (mucus) unless directed by a physician. Especially in infants and small children, antihistamines in overdosage may cause hallucinations, convulsions, and death. Antihistamines may diminish mental alertness. In young children they may produce excitation.

PRECAUTIONS

General- Because of its antihistamine component, ALACOL DM should be used with caution in patients with a history of bronchial asthma, narrow-angle glaucoma, gastrointestinal obstruction, urinary bladder neck obstruction. Because of its sympathomimetic component, ALACOL DM should be used with caution in patients with diabetes, hypertension, heart disease, thyroid disease.

Information for Patients- Patients should be warned about engaging in activities requiring mental alertness, such as driving a car or operating dangerous machinery.

Drug Interactions: Antihistamines have additive effects with alcohol and other CNS depressants (hypnotics, sedatives, tranquilizers, antianxiety agents, etc.). MAO inhibitors prolong and intensify the anticholinergic (drying) effects of antihistamines. MAO inhibitors may enhance the effect of phenylephrine. Sympathomimetics may reduce the effects of antihypertensive drugs.

Carcinogenesis, Mutagenesis, Impairment of Fertility- Animal studies of ALACOL DM to assess carcinogenic and mutagenic potential, or the effect on fertility have not been performed.

Usage in Pregnancy-Pregnancy Category C. Teratogenic Effects- Animal reproduction studies have not been conducted with ALACOL DM. It is also not known whether ALACOL DM can cause fetal harm when administered to a pregnant woman or can affect reproduction capacity. ALACOL DM should be used during pregnancy only if the potential benefit justifies the potential risk to the fetus. Reproduction studies of brompheniramine maleate in rats and mice at doses up to 16 times the maximum human dose have revealed no evidence of impaired fertility or harm to the fetus.

Nursing Mothers- Because of the higher risk of intolerance of antihistamines in small infants generally, and in newborns and prematures in particular, ALACOL DM is contraindicated in nursing mothers.

ADVERSE REACTIONS

The most frequent adverse reactions to ALACOL DM include sedation, dryness of mouth, nose and throat, thickening of bronchial secretions, and dizziness. Other adverse reactions may include: ***Dermatologic-*** Urticaria, drug rash, photosensitivity, and pruritus. ***Cardiovascular System-*** Hypotension, hypertension, cardiac arrhythmias. ***Central Nervous System-*** disturbed coordination, tremor, irritability, insomnia, visual disturbance, weakness, nervousness, convulsions, headache, euphoria and dysphoria. ***G.U. System-*** Urinary frequency, difficult urination. ***G.I. System-*** Epigastric discomfort, anorexia, nausea, vomiting, diarrhea, or constipation. ***Respiratory System-*** Tightness of chest and wheezing, shortness of breath. ***Hematologic System-*** Hemolytic anemia, thrombocytopenia, agranulocytosis.

OVERDOSAGE

Signs and Symptoms- Dextromethorphan in toxic doses will cause drowsiness, ataxia, nystagmus, opisthotonos, and convulsive seizures. Overdosage of phenylephrine may be associated with tachycardia, hypertension, and cardiac arrhythmias. The effect on the central nervous system of an overdosage of brompheniramine may vary from depression to stimulation, especially in children. Anticholinergic effects may also occur. ***Treatment-*** Induce emesis if patient is alert and is seen by a physician prior to 6 hours following ingestion. Precautions against aspiration must be taken, especially in infants and small children. Gastric lavage may be carried out, although in some instances tracheostomy may be necessary prior to lavage. Naloxone HCl 0.005 mg/kg intravenously may be of value in reversing the CNS depression that may occur from an overdose of Dextromethorphan. CNS stimulants may counter CNS depression. Should CNS hyperactivity or convulsive seizures occur, intravenous short-acting barbiturates may be indicated. Hypertensive responses and/or tachycardia should be treated appropriately. Oxygen, intravenous fluids, and other supportive measures should be employed as indicated.

DOSAGE AND ADMINISTRATION

Adults and Children over 12 years- 2 teaspoonful (10 mL) every 4 hours. ***Children 6 to 12 years-*** 1 teaspoonful (5 mL) every 4 hours. ***Children 2 to 6 years-*** ½ teaspoonful (2.5 mL) every 4 hours. ***Children under 2 years-*** as directed by a physician. Do not exceed 6 doses during a 24 hour period.

HOW SUPPLIED

NDC 63162-507-16 16 oz (473 mL) bottles, and NDC 63162-507-20 20 mL sample bottles.
Store between 59°-86°F (15°-30°C)
Dispense in tight, light resistant containers as defined by the USP.
KEEP THIS AND ALL MEDICATIONS OUT OF THE REACH OF CHILDREN.

Rx Only
Manufactured in USA for
BALLAY PHARMACEUTICALS, INC.
Wimberley, TX 78676
By
Elge, Inc. Rosenberg, TX 77471 REV 11/01

BALAMINE DM® ORAL DROPS ℞

[bal'-ə' mīn]
For Infants

BALAMINE®-DM SYRUP ℞

[bal'-ə' mīn]
For adults and children (18 months and over)

DESCRIPTION

Antihistamine/Decongestant/Antitussive for oral use

ACTIVE INGREDIENTS

BALAMINE DM ORAL DROPS
Each dropperful (1 mL) contains:
Carbinoxamine Maleate .... 2 mg
Pseudoephedrine Hydrochloride .... 25 mg
Dextromethorphan Hydrobromide .... 3.5 mg
BALAMINE-DM SYRUP
Each teaspoonful (5 mL) contains:
Carbinoxamine Maleate .... 4 mg
Pseudoephedrine Hydrochloride .... 60 mg
Dextromethorphan Hydrobromide .... 12.5 mg

INACTIVE INGREDIENTS

BALAMINE DM ORAL DROPS
Citric acid, D&C Red No. 33, FD&C Blue No. 1, glycerin, sodium benzoate, sodium citrate, sorbitol, purified water, flavoring and other ingredients.
BALAMINE-DM SYRUP
Citric acid, D&C Red No. 33, FD&C Blue No. 1, glycerin, menthol, povidone, purified water, sodium benzoate, sodium citrate, sorbitol, and flavoring.
Carbinoxamine maleate (2-[p-Chloro-α-[2-(dimethylamino) ethoxyl] benzyl]pyridine maleate) is one of the ethanolamine class of H_1 antihistamines. Pseudoephedrine hydrochloride (Benzenemethanol,α-[1-(methylamino) ethyl]-,[S-R*,R*)]-, hydrochloride) is the hydrochloride of pseudoephedrine, a naturally occurring dextrorotatory stereoisomer of ephedrine. Dextromethorphan Hydrobromide (Morphinan, 3-methoxy-17-methyl-, (9α, 13α, 14α)-, hydrobromide, monohydrate) is the hydrobromide of d-form racemethorphan.

CLINICAL PHARMACOLOGY

Antihistaminic, decongestant and antitussive actions.
Carbinoxamine maleate possesses H_1 antihistaminic activity and mild anticholinergic and sedative effects. Serum half-life for carbinoxamine is estimated to be 10 to 20 hours. Virtually no intact drug is excreted in the urine.
Pseudoephedrine hydrochloride is an oral sympathomimetic amine that acts as a decongestant to respiratory tract mucous membranes. While its vasoconstrictor action is similar to that of ephedrine, pseudoephedrine has less pressor effect in normotensive adults. Serum half-life for pseudoephedrine is 6 to 8 hours. Acidic urine is associated with faster elimination of the drug. About one-half of the administered dose is excreted in the urine.
Dextromethorphan hydrobromide is a nonnarcotic antitussive with effectiveness equal to codeine. It acts in the medulla oblongata to elevate the cough threshold. Dextromethorphan does not produce analgesia or induce tolerance, and has no potential for addiction. At usual doses, it will not depress respiration or inhibit ciliary activity. Dextromethorphan is rapidly metabolized with trace amounts of the parent compound in blood and urine. About one-half of the administered dose is excreted in the urine as conjugated metabolites.

INDICATIONS AND USAGE

For relief of coughs and upper respiratory symptoms, including nasal congestion, associated with allergy or the common cold.

CONTRAINDICATIONS

Patients with hypersensitivity or idiosyncrasy to any of its ingredients. Sympathomimetic amines are contraindicated in patients with severe hypertension, severe coronary artery disease and patients on monoamine oxidase (MAO) inhibitor therapy. Antihistamines are contraindicated in patients with narrow-angle glaucoma, urinary retention, peptic ulcer and during an asthma attack. Dextromethorphan should not be used in patients receiving a monoamine oxidase inhibitor (MAOI) or for 2 weeks after stopping the MAOI drug.

WARNINGS

Sympathomimetic amines should be used judiciously and sparingly in patients with hypertension, diabetes, ischemic heart disease, hyperthyroidism, increased intraocular pressure or prostatic hypertrophy. See Contraindications. Sympathomimetic amines may produce CNS stimulation with convulsions or cardiovascular collapse with accompanying hypotension. The elderly (60 years and older) are more likely to exhibit adverse reactions. Antihistamines may cause excitability, especially in children. At doses higher than the recommended dose, nervousness, dizziness, or sleeplessness may occur. Do not exceed recommended dosage. Administration of dextromethorphan may be accompanied by histamine release and should be used with caution in atopic children.

AGE	DOSE*	FREQUENCY*
Balamine DM Oral Drops		
For Oral Use Only		
1-3 months	1/4 dropperful (1/4 mL)	q.i.d.
3-6 months	1/2 dropperful (1/2 mL)	q.i.d.
6-9 months	3/4 dropperful (3/4 mL)	q.i.d.
9-18 months	1 dropperful (1 mL)	q.i.d.
Balamine DM Syrup		
18 months-6 years	1/2 teaspoonful (2.5 mL)	q.i.d.
adults and children 6 years and over	1 teaspoonful (5 mL)	q.i.d.

* In mild cases or in particularly sensitive patients, less frequent or reduced doses may be adequate.

PRECAUTIONS

General
Before prescribing medication to suppress or modify cough, identify and provide therapy for the underlying cause of cough and take caution that modification of cough does not increase the risk of clinical or physiologic complications. Dextromethorphan should be used with caution in sedated or debilitated patients and in patients confined to supine positions.
Use with caution in patients with hypertension, heart disease, asthma, hyperthyroidism, increased intraocular pressure, diabetes mellitus and prostatic hypertrophy.
Information for Patients: Avoid alcohol and other CNS depressants while taking these products. Patients sensitive to antihistamines may experience moderate to severe drowsiness. Patients sensitive to sympathomimetic amines may note mild CNS stimulation. While taking these products, exercise care in driving or operating appliances, machinery, etc.
Drug Interactions: Antihistamines may enhance the effects of tricyclic antidepressants, barbiturates, alcohol, and other CNS depressants. MAO inhibitors prolong and intensify the anticholinergic effects of antihistamines.
Sympathomimetic amines may reduce the antihypertensive effects of reserpine, veratrum alkaloids, methyldopa and mecamylamine. Effects of sympathomimetics are increased with MAO inhibitors and beta-adrenergic blockers. The cough-suppressant action of dextromethorphan and narcotic antitussives are additive. Dextromethorphan is contraindicated with monoamine oxidase inhibitors (MAOI). See Contraindications section.
Pregnancy Category C: Animal reproduction studies have not been conducted with Balamine DM. It is also not known whether these products can cause fetal harm when administered to a pregnant woman or affect reproduction capacity. Give to pregnant women only if clearly needed.
Nursing Mothers: It is not known whether the drugs in Balamine DM are excreted in human milk. Because many drugs are excreted in human milk and because of the potential for serious adverse reactions in nursing infants, a decision should be made whether to discontinue nursing or discontinue the product, taking into account the importance of the drug to the mother.

ADVERSE REACTIONS

Antihistamines: Sedation, dizziness, diplopia, vomiting, diarrhea, dry mouth, headache, nervousness, nausea, anorexia, heartburn, weakness, polyuria and dysuria and, rarely, excitability in children. Urinary retention may occur in patients with prostatic hypertrophy.
Sympathomimetic Amines: Convulsions, CNS stimulation, cardiac arrhythmias, respiratory difficulty, increased heart rate or blood pressure, hallucinations, tremors, nervousness, insomnia, weakness, pallor and dysuria.
Dextromethorphan: Drowsiness, dizziness, and GI disturbance.

OVERDOSAGE

No information is available as to specific results of an overdose of these products. The signs, symptoms and treatment described below are those of H_1 antihistamine, ephedrine and dextromethorphan overdose.
Symptoms: Should antihistamine effects predominate, central action constitutes the greatest danger. In the small child, predominant symptoms are excitation, hallucination, ataxia, incoordination, tremors, flushed face and fever. Convulsions, fixed and dilated pupils, coma and death may occur in severe cases. In the adult, fever and flushing are uncommon; excitement leading to convulsions and postictal depression is often preceded by drowsiness and coma. Respiration is usually not seriously depressed; blood pressure is usually stable.
Should sympathomimetic symptoms predominate, central effects include restlessness, dizziness, tremor, hyperactive reflexes, talkativeness, irritability and insomnia. Cardiovascular and renal effects include difficulty in micturition, headache, flushing, palpitation, cardiac arrhythmias, hypertension with subsequent hypotension and circulatory collapse. Gastrointestinal effects include dry mouth, metallic taste, anorexia, nausea, vomiting, diarrhea, and abdominal cramps.
Dextromethorphan may cause respiratory depression with a large overdose.
Treatment: a) Evacuate stomach as condition warrants. Activated charcoal may be useful. b) Maintain a nonstimulating environment. c) Monitor cardiovascular status. d) Do not give stimulants. e) Reduce fever with cool sponging. f) Treat respiratory depression with naloxone if dextromethorphan toxicity is suspected. g) Use sedatives or anticonvulsants to control CNS excitation and convulsions. h) Physostigmine may reverse anticholinergic symptoms. i) Ammonium chloride may acidify the urine to increase urinary excretion of pseudoephedrine. j) Further care is symptomatic and supportive.

DOSAGE AND ADMINISTRATION

[See table above]

HOW SUPPLIED

Balamine DM Oral Drops, grape flavored, in 30 mL bottles, with calibrated droppers, **NDC** 63162-509-30.
Balamine DM Syrup, grape flavored, in 16 fl. oz. (1-pint) bottles, **NDC** 63162-508-16.
Dispense in USP tight, light-resistant container. Avoid exposure to excessive heat.
Rx ONLY
Revised 12/01
BALLY
Manufactured for: **Ballay Pharmaceutical, Inc.** Wimberley, Tx. 78676
Manufactured by: Elge, Inc. Rosenberg, Tx. 77471

BioMolecular Sciences Inc.

13701 MARINA POINT DRIVE
SUITE 346
MARINA DEL REY, CA 90292

Direct Inquiries to:
800-273-2846

SEROPRO RX™ OTC

Lactoferrin and Cysteine Delivery
(biologically active whey protein concentrate)
Powder - 300gram jar

DESCRIPTION

SeroPro RX™ is a proprietary whey protein concentrate, derived from hormone treatment free milk. It provides biologically active protein fractions that assist the body in maintaining levels of glutathione (GSH) and support the immune system. SeroPro Rx™ contains high levels of naturally occurring Lactoferrin, Immunoglobulins and Bovine Serum Albumin. Lactoferrin has been shown to have anti-microbial, anti-viral and anti-fungal effects. The protein fractions in SeroPro Rx™ contain exceptional amounts of cysteine and glutamine (glutamate), the precursors required for the production of intracellular GSH.

KEY FACTS

GSH is a tripeptide composed of the three amino acids glutamate, cysteine and glycine. SeroPro Rx™ is a primary product, not a by-product of cheese manufacturing. The full range of protein fractions are maintained in their original conformation. This process enables SeroPro Rx™ to have high levels of cysteine. Cysteine is the critical amino acid for the efficient intracellular production of GSH.
Lactoferrin is an iron binding and iron modulating protein. Lactoferrin resides in the chemical family called cytokines. SeroPro Rx™ provides naturally occurring lactoferrin in its most biologically available state.
SeroPro Rx™ can be viewed as a delivery system of both cysteine and lactoferrin.

RECOMMENDED USE

Biologically active protein supplementation may be used to address GSH deficiency, wasting, oxidative stress, iron deficiency, chemical toxicity, detoxification, protein deficiency and immune suppression. Reduced levels of GSH have been observed in: AIDS, cancer, CFIDS, catabolic cachexia, hepatitis, radiation poisoning, malnutritive states, chemotherapy and over training syndrome, and has been associated with numerous neurological disease states. These clinical pathologies have been associated with oxidative stress and have been published in peer-reviewed research.
Maintenance dose is two servings (10 grams) per day. For mild to moderate health challenges, higher doses are recommended. Observational studies with AIDS, cancer and CFIDS patients have noted consumption of 20–30 grams per day without ill effect. SeroPro Rx™ is best administered on an empty stomach or with light food consumption.
Do not use hot or acidic liquids to mix the product.

Continued on next page

Seropro RX—Cont.

SAFETY

SeroPro Rx™ is contraindicated in individuals who have known hypersensitivity to milk proteins.

Each 5 gram serving of SeroPro Rx™ contains 4 grams of protein. Patients on a protein restricted diet need to take this into account when calculating their daily protein intake. SeroPro Rx™ contains less then 6% lactose and is generally well-tolerated by lactose-intolerant individuals.

Patients undergoing immunosuppressive therapy should discuss the use of this product with their health professional.

RECOMMENDED DOSAGE

Maintenance dosage is 5gram BID. For advanced disease states, higher dosages are recommended.

HOW SUPPLIED

5 grams of milk protein concentrate powder per serving scoop.

60 servings per jar.

Storage: Cool and dry. Refrigeration is not necessary.

REFERENCES

1. The Journal of Immunology 61: 503–508, 1987, "Glutathione and Lymphosite Activation"

2. The Journal of the American College of Nutrition Volume 5, 1986, Anderson and Meister, "Intracellular Delivery of Cysteine and Glutathione Delivery Systems"

3. Immune depressed individuals have lower GSH levels when fighting disease. Lymphocytes, cells vital for immune response, depend on GSH for their proper function and replication. Immunology 61: 503–508 1987

4. Glutathione is essential in supporting the immune system, including natural killer cells (Droege et al., 1997

5. Cancer Letters 57: 91–94 1991

6. Lower GSH levels are implicated in many diseases associated with aging, including cataracts, Alzheimer's, Parkinson's, atherosclerosis and others. Journal of Clinical Epidemiology 47: 1021–28 1994

7. Whey proteins promote muscular development. Sports Medicine 21; 213–238, 1996

8. Low GSH has been demonstrated in nuerodegenerative diseases such as MS (Multiple Sclerosis), ALS (Lou Gehrig's Disease), Alzheimer's, and Parkinson's disease and others. The Lancet 344: 796–798 1994

9. GSH detoxifies many pollutants, carcinogens and poisons, including many in fuel exhaust and cigarette smoke. It retards damage from radiation such as seen with the loss of the ozone layer. Annual Review of Biochemistry 52: 711–780 1983.

10. Numerous studies have demonstrated that patients with compromised liver function due to alcohol abuse have significant reduction of GSH in the liver. (Lamestro, 1995) AIDS

11. Low GSH levels with poor survival in AIDS patients. Proc. National Acad. Science USA 94: 2967–72 1997

12. Biochemical Pharmacology 47:2113–2123 1994

13. Droege W, Holm E. Role of cysteine and GSH HIV-wasting and other diseases associated with muscle wasting and immunoglobulin function. FASEB J 1997; 11:10771089

SeroPro Rx™ is a trademark of Wellwisdom, LLC
Distributed by BioMolecular Sciences Inc.

***These statements have not been evaluated by the Food and Drug Administration. This product is not intended to diagnose, treat, cure or prevent any disease.**

Biovail Pharmaceuticals, Inc.

170 SOUTHPORT DRIVE
MORRISVILLE, NC 27560

For direct inquiries contact:
Phone: 1-866-Biovail
1-866-246-8245

ZOVIRAX® ℞

[zō-vī 'răx]
(acyclovir)
Ointment 5%

Prescribing information for this product, which appears in the GlaxoSmithKline section on pages 1707–1708 of the 2002 PDR, has been completely revised for marketing by Biovail Pharmaceuticals as follows. Please write "See Supplement A" next to the product heading.

DESCRIPTION

ZOVIRAX is the brand name for acyclovir, a synthetic nucleoside analogue active against herpes viruses. ZOVIRAX Ointment 5% is a formulation for topical administration. Each gram of ZOVIRAX Ointment 5% contains 50 mg of acyclovir in a polyethylene glycol (PEG) base.

Acyclovir is a white, crystalline powder with the molecular formula $C_8H_{11}N_5O_3$ and a molecular weight of 225. The maximum solubility in water at 37°C is 2.5 mg/mL. The pka's of acyclovir are 2.27 and 9.25.

The chemical name of acyclovir is 2-amino-1,9-dihydro-9-[(2-hydroxyethoxy)methyl]-6*H*-purin-6-one.

VIROLOGY

Mechanism of Antiviral Action: Acyclovir is a synthetic purine nucleoside analogue with in vitro and in vivo inhibitory activity against herpes simplex virus types 1 (HSV-1), 2 (HSV-2), and varicella-zoster virus (VZV).

The inhibitory activity of acyclovir is highly selective due to its affinity for the enzyme thymidine kinase (TK) encoded by HSV and VZV. This viral enzyme converts acyclovir into acyclovir monophosphate, a nucleotide analogue. The monophosphate is further converted into diphosphate by cellular guanylate kinase and into triphosphate by a number of cellular enzymes. In vitro, acyclovir triphosphate stops replication of herpes viral DNA. This is accomplished in 3 ways: 1) competitive inhibition of viral DNA polymerase, 2) incorporation into and termination of the growing viral DNA chain, and 3) inactivation of the viral DNA polymerase. The greater antiviral activity of acyclovir against HSV compared to VZV is due to its more efficient phosphorylation by the viral TK.

Antiviral Activities: The quantitative relationship between the in vitro susceptibility of herpes viruses to antivirals and the clinical response to therapy has not been established in humans, and virus sensitivity testing has not been standardized. Sensitivity testing results, expressed as the concentration of drug required to inhibit by 50% the growth of virus in cell culture (IC_{50}), vary greatly depending upon a number of factors. Using plaque-reduction assays, the IC_{50} against herpes simplex virus isolates ranges from 0.02 to 13.5 mcg/mL for HSV-1 and from 0.01 to 9.9 mcg/mL for HSV-2. The IC_{50} for acyclovir against most laboratory strains and clinical isolates of VZV ranges from 0.12 to 10.8 mcg/mL. Acyclovir also demonstrates activity against the Oka vaccine strain of VZV with a mean IC_{50} of 1.35 mcg/mL.

Drug Resistance: Resistance of HSV and VZV to acyclovir can result from qualitative and quantitative changes in the viral TK and/or DNA polymerase. Clinical isolates of HSV and VZV with reduced susceptibility to acyclovir have been recovered from immunocompromised patients, especially with advanced HIV infection. While most of the acyclovir-resistant mutants isolated thus far from immunocompromised patients have been found to be TK-deficient mutants, other mutants involving the viral TK gene (TK partial and TK altered) and DNA polymerase have been isolated. TK-negative mutants may cause severe disease in infants and immunocompromised adults. The possibility of viral resistance to acyclovir should be considered in patients who show poor clinical response during therapy.

CLINICAL PHARMACOLOGY

Two clinical pharmacology studies were performed with ZOVIRAX Ointment 5% in immunocompromised adults at risk of developing mucocutaneous Herpes simplex virus infections or with localized varicella-zoster infections. These studies were designed to evaluate the dermal tolerance, systemic toxicity, and percutaneous absorption of acyclovir.

In 1 of these studies, which included 16 inpatients, the complete ointment or its vehicle were randomly administered in a dose of 1-cm strips (25 mg acyclovir) 4 times a day for 7 days to an intact skin surface area of 4.5 square inches. No local intolerance, systemic toxicity, or contact dermatitis were observed. In addition, no drug was detected in blood and urine by radioimmunoassay (sensitivity, 0.01 mcg/mL).

The other study included 11 patients with localized varicella-zoster infections. In this uncontrolled study, acyclovir was detected in the blood of 9 patients and in the urine of all patients tested. Acyclovir levels in plasma ranged from <0.01 to 0.28 mcg/mL in 8 patients with normal renal function, and from <0.01 to 0.78 mcg/mL in 1 patient with impaired renal function. Acyclovir excreted in the urine ranged from <0.02% to 9.4% of the daily dose. Therefore, systemic absorption of acyclovir after topical application is minimal.

CLINICAL TRIALS

In clinical trials of initial genital herpes infections, ZOVIRAX Ointment 5% has shown a decrease in healing time and, in some cases, a decrease in duration of viral shedding and duration of pain. In studies in immunocompromised patients mainly with herpes labialis, there was a decrease in duration of viral shedding and a slight decrease in duration of pain.

In studies of recurrent genital herpes and of herpes labialis in nonimmunocompromised patients, there was no evidence of clinical benefit; there was some decrease in duration of viral shedding.

INDICATIONS AND USAGE

ZOVIRAX (acyclovir) Ointment 5% is indicated in the management of initial genital herpes and in limited non-life-threatening mucocutaneous Herpes simplex virus infections in immunocompromised patients.

CONTRAINDICATIONS

ZOVIRAX Ointment 5% is contraindicated in patients who develop hypersensitivity to the components of the formulation.

WARNINGS

ZOVIRAX Ointment 5% is intended for cutaneous use only and should not be used in the eye.

PRECAUTIONS:

General: The recommended dosage, frequency of applications, and length of treatment should not be exceeded (see DOSAGE AND ADMINISTRATION). There are no data to support the use of ZOVIRAX Ointment 5% to prevent transmission of infection to other persons or prevent recurrent infections when applied in the absence of signs and symptoms. ZOVIRAX Ointment 5% should not be used for the prevention of recurrent HSV infections. Although clinically significant viral resistance associated with the use of ZOVIRAX Ointment 5% has not been observed, this possibility exists.

Drug Interactions: Clinical experience has identified no interactions resulting from topical or systemic administration of other drugs concomitantly with ZOVIRAX Ointment 5%.

Carcinogenesis, Mutagenesis, Impairment of Fertility: Systemic exposure following topical administration of acyclovir is minimal. Dermal carcinogenicity studies were not conducted. Results from the studies of carcinogenesis, mutagenesis, and fertility are not included in the full prescribing information for ZOVIRAX Ointment 5% due to the minimal exposures of acyclovir that result from dermal application. Information on these studies is available in the full prescribing information for ZOVIRAX Capsules, Tablets, and Suspension and ZOVIRAX for Injection.

Pregnancy: ***Teratogenic Effects:*** Pregnancy Category B. Acyclovir was not teratogenic in the mouse, rabbit, or rat at exposures greatly in excess of human exposure. There are no adequate and well-controlled studies of systemic acyclovir in pregnant women. A prospective epidemiologic registry of acyclovir use during pregnancy was established in 1984 and completed in April 1999. There were 749 pregnancies followed in women exposed to systemic acyclovir during the first trimester of pregnancy resulting in 756 outcomes. The occurrence rate of birth defects approximates that found in the general population. However, the small size of the registry is insufficient to evaluate the risk for less common defects or to permit reliable or definitive conclusions regarding the safety of acyclovir in pregnant women and their developing fetuses. Systemic acyclovir should be used during pregnancy only if the potential benefit justifies the potential risk to the fetus.

Nursing Mothers: It is not known whether topically applied acyclovir is excreted in breast milk. Systemic exposure following topical administration is minimal. After oral administration of ZOVIRAX, acyclovir concentrations have been documented in breast milk in 2 women and ranged from 0.6 to 4.1 times the corresponding plasma levels. These concentrations would potentially expose the nursing infant to a dose of acyclovir up to 0.3 mg/kg per day. Nursing mothers who have active herpetic lesions near or on the breast should avoid nursing.

Geriatric Use: Clinical studies of ZOVIRAX Ointment did not include sufficient numbers of subjects aged 65 and over to determine whether they respond differently from younger subjects. Other reported clinical experience has not identified differences in responses between the elderly and younger patients. Systemic absorption of acyclovir after topical administration is minimal (see CLINICAL PHARMACOLOGY).

Pediatric Use: Safety and effectiveness in pediatric patients have not been established.

ADVERSE REACTIONS

In the controlled clinical trials, mild pain (including transient burning and stinging) was reported by about 30% of patients in both the active and placebo arms; treatment was discontinued in 2 of these patients. Local pruritus occurred in 4% of these patients. In all studies, there was no significant difference between the drug and placebo group in the rate or type of reported adverse reactions nor were there any differences in abnormal clinical laboratory findings.

Observed During Clinical Practice: Based on clinical practice experience in patients treated with ZOVIRAX Ointment in the US, spontaneously reported adverse events are uncommon. Data are insufficient to support an estimate of their incidence or to establish causation. These events may also occur as part of the underlying disease process. Voluntary reports of adverse events that have been received since market introduction include:

General: Edema and/or pain at the application site.

Skin: Pruritus, rash.

OVERDOSAGE

Overdosage by topical application of ZOVIRAX Ointment 5% is unlikely because of limited transcutaneous absorption (see CLINICAL PHARMACOLOGY).

DOSAGE AND ADMINISTRATION

Apply sufficient quantity to adequately cover all lesions every 3 hours, 6 times per day for 7 days. The dose size per application will vary depending upon the total lesion area but should approximate a one-half inch ribbon of ointment per 4 square inches of surface area. A finger cot or rubber glove should be used when applying ZOVIRAX to prevent autoinoculation of other body sites and transmission of infection to other persons. **Therapy should be initiated as early as possible following onset of signs and symptoms.**

HOW SUPPLIED

Each gram of ZOVIRAX Ointment 5% contains 50 mg acyclovir in a polyethylene glycol base. It is supplied as follows:

15-g tubes (NDC 64455-993-94)

3-g tubes (NDC 64455-993-41).

Store at 15° to 25°C (59° to 77°F) in a dry place.

Manufactured by GlaxoSmithKline, Research Triangle Park, NC 27709
for Biovail Pharmaceuticals, Inc., Morrisville, NC 27560

December 2001/RL-1044

Elan Pharmaceuticals
7475 LUSK BLVD.
SAN DIEGO, CA 92121

For Medical Information Contact:
(888) NEURO-05
(888) 638-7605
To Report Adverse Events Contact:
(877) ELAN GSS
(877) 352–6477
The products below are distributed by Elan Pharmaceuticals

FROVA™ ℞

[frō' va]
(frovatriptan succinate) Tablets

DESCRIPTION

FROVA* (frovatriptan succinate) tablets contain frovatriptan succinate, a selective 5-hydroxy-tryptamine$_1$ (5-HT$_{1B/1D}$) receptor subtype agonist, as the active ingredient. Frovatriptan succinate is chemically designated as R-(+) 3-methylamino-6-carboxamido-1,2,3,4-tetrahydrocarbazole monosuccinate monohydrate and it has the following structure:

[Structure: H_2N–C(=O)– carbazole ring with NHCH$_3$; N–H; $(CH_2COOH)_2$ H_2O]

The empirical formula is $C_{14}H_{17}N_3O.C_4H_6O_4.H_2O$, representing a molecular weight of 379.4.
Frovatriptan succinate is a white to off-white powder that is soluble in water. Each FROVA tablet for oral administration contains 3.91 mg frovatriptan succinate, equivalent to 2.5 mg of frovatriptan base. Each tablet also contains the inactive ingredients lactose NF, microcrystalline cellulose NF, colloidal silicon dioxide NF, sodium starch glycolate NF, magnesium stearate NF, hydroxypropylmethylcellulose USP, polyethylene glycol 3000 USP, triacetin USP, and titanium dioxide USP.

* FROVA is a trademark of Elan Pharmaceuticals, Inc.

CLINICAL PHARMACOLOGY

Mechanism of Action

Frovatriptan is a 5-HT receptor agonist that binds with high affinity for 5-HT$_{1B}$ and 5-HT$_{1D}$ receptors. Frovatriptan has no significant effects on GABA$_A$ mediated channel activity and has no significant affinity for benzodiazepine binding sites.
Frovatriptan is believed to act on extracerebral, intracranial arteries and to inhibit excessive dilation of these vessels in migraine. In anesthetized dogs and cats, intravenous administration of frovatriptan produced selective constriction of the carotid vascular bed and had no effect on blood pressure (both species) or coronary resistance (in dogs).

Pharmacokinetics

Mean maximum blood concentrations (C_{max}) in patients are achieved approximately 2 - 4 hours after administration of a single oral dose of frovatriptan 2.5 mg. The absolute bioavailability of an oral dose of frovatriptan 2.5 mg in healthy subjects is about 20% in males and 30% in females. Food has no significant effect on the bioavailability of frovatriptan, but delays t_{max} by one hour.
Binding of frovatriptan to serum proteins is low (approximately 15%). Reversible binding to blood cells at equilibrium is approximately 60%, resulting in a blood:plasma ratio of about 2:1 in both males and females. The mean steady state volume of distribution of frovatriptan following intravenous administration of 0.8 mg is 4.2 L/kg in males and 3.0 L/kg in females.
In vitro, cytochrome P450 1A2 appears to be the principal enzyme involved in the metabolism of frovatriptan. Following administration of a single oral dose of radiolabeled frovatriptan 2.5 mg to healthy male and female subjects, 32% of the dose was recovered in urine and 62% in feces. Radiolabeled compounds excreted in urine were unchanged frovatriptan, hydroxylated frovatriptan, N-acetyl desmethyl frovatriptan, hydroxylated N-acetyl desmethyl frovatriptan and desmethyl frovatriptan, together with several other minor metabolites. Desmethyl frovatriptan has lower affinity for 5-HT$_{1B/1D}$ receptors compared to the parent compound. The N-acetyl desmethyl metabolite has no significant affinity for 5-HT receptors. The activity of the other metabolites is unknown.
After an intravenous dose, mean clearance of frovatriptan was 220 and 130 mL/min in males and females, respectively. Renal clearance accounted for about 40% (82 mL/min) and 45% (60 mL/min) of total clearance in males and females, respectively. The mean terminal elimination half-life of frovatriptan in both males and females is approximately 26 hours.
The pharmacokinetics of frovatriptan are similar in migraine patients and healthy subjects.

Special Populations

Age: Mean AUC of frovatriptan was 1.5- to 2-fold higher in healthy elderly subjects (age 65 - 77 years) compared to those in healthy younger subjects (age 21 - 37 years). There was no difference in t_{max} or $t_{1/2}$ between the two populations.
Gender: There was no difference in the mean terminal elimination half-life of frovatriptan in males and females. Bioavailability was higher, and systemic exposure to frovatriptan was approximately 2-fold greater, in females than males, irrespective of age.
Renal Impairment: Since less than 10% of FROVA is excreted in urine after an oral dose, it is unlikely that the exposure to frovatriptan will be affected by renal impairment. The pharmacokinetics of frovatriptan following a single oral dose of 2.5 mg was not different in patients with renal impairment (5 males and 6 females, creatinine clearance 16 - 73 mL/min) and in subjects with normal renal function.
Hepatic Impairment: There is no clinical or pharmacokinetic experience with FROVA in patients with severe hepatic impairment. The AUC in subjects with mild (Child-Pugh 5 - 6) to moderate (Child-Pugh 7 - 9) hepatic impairment is about twice as high as the AUC in young, healthy subjects, but within the range found among normal elderly subjects.
Race: The effect of race on the pharmacokinetics of frovatriptan has not been examined.

***Drug Interactions* (see also PRECAUTIONS, *Drug Interactions*)**

Frovatriptan is not an inhibitor of human monoamine oxidase (MAO) enzymes or cytochrome P450 (isozymes 1A2, 2C9, 2C19, 2D6, 2E1, 3A4) *in vitro* at concentrations up to 250 to 500-fold higher than the highest blood concentrations observed in man at a dose of 2.5 mg. No induction of drug metabolizing enzymes was observed following multiple dosing of frovatriptan to rats or on addition to human hepatocytes *in vitro*. Although no clinical studies have been performed, it is unlikely that frovatriptan will affect the metabolism of co-administered drugs metabolized by these mechanisms.
Oral contraceptives: Retrospective analysis of pharmacokinetic data from females across trials indicated that the mean C_{max} and AUC of frovatriptan are 30% higher in those subjects taking oral contraceptives compared to those not taking oral contraceptives.
Ergotamine: The AUC and C_{max} of frovatriptan (2×2.5 mg dose) were reduced by approximately 25% when co-administered with ergotamine tartrate.
Propranolol: Propranolol increased the AUC of frovatriptan 2.5 mg in males by 60% and in females by 29%. The C_{max} of frovatriptan was increased 23% in males and 16% in females in the presence of propranolol. The t_{max} as well as half-life of frovatriptan, though slightly longer in the females, were not affected by concomitant administration of propranolol.
Moclobemide: The pharmacokinetic profile of frovatriptan was unaffected when a single oral dose of frovatriptan 2.5 mg was administered to healthy female subjects receiving the MAO-A inhibitor, moclobemide, at an oral dose of 150 mg bid for 8 days.

Clinical Trials

The efficacy of FROVA in the acute treatment of migraine headaches was demonstrated in five randomized, double-blind, placebo-controlled, outpatient trials. Two of these were dose-finding studies in which patients were randomized to receive doses of frovatriptan ranging from 0.5 - 40 mg. The three studies evaluating only one dose studied 2.5 mg. In these controlled short-term studies combined, patients were predominately female (88%) and Caucasian (94%) with a mean age of 42 years (range 18 - 69). Patients were instructed to treat a moderate to severe headache. Headache response, defined as a reduction in headache severity from moderate or severe pain to mild or no pain, was assessed for up to 24 hours after dosing. The associated symptoms nausea, vomiting, photophobia and phonophobia were also assessed. Maintenance of response was assessed for up to 24 hours post dose. In two of the trials a second dose of FROVA was provided after the initial treatment, to treat recurrence of the headache within 24 hours. Other medication, excluding other 5-HT$_1$ agonists and ergotamine containing compounds, was permitted from 2 hours after the first dose of FROVA. The frequency and time to use of additional medications were also recorded.
In all five placebo-controlled trials, the percentage of patients achieving a headache response 2 hours after treatment was significantly greater for those taking FROVA compared to those taking placebo (Table 1).
Lower doses of frovatriptan (1 mg or 0.5 mg) were not effective at 2 hours. Higher doses (5 mg to 40 mg) of frovatriptan showed no added benefit over 2.5 mg but did cause a greater incidence of adverse events.

Table 1
Percentage of Patients with Headache Response (Mild or No Headache) 2 Hours Following Treatment[a]

Trial	FROVA (frovatriptan 2.5 mg)	Placebo
1	42%* (n=90)	22% (n=91)
2	38%* (n=121)	25% (n=115)
3	39%* (n=187)	21% (n=99)
4	46%** (n=672)	27% (n=347)
5	37%** (n=438)	23% (n=225)

[a]ITT observed data, excludes patients who had missing data or were asleep; *p<0.05, **p<0.001 in comparison with placebo

Comparisons of drug performance based upon results obtained in different clinical trials are never reliable. Because trials are conducted at different times, with different samples of patients, by different investigators, employing different criteria and/or different interpretations of the same criteria, under different conditions (dose, dosing regimen, etc.), quantitative estimates of treatment response and the timing of response may be expected to vary considerably from study to study.
The estimated probability of achieving an initial headache response by 2 hours following treatment is depicted in Figure 1.

Figure 1
Estimated Probability of Achieving Initial Headache Response Within 2 Hours

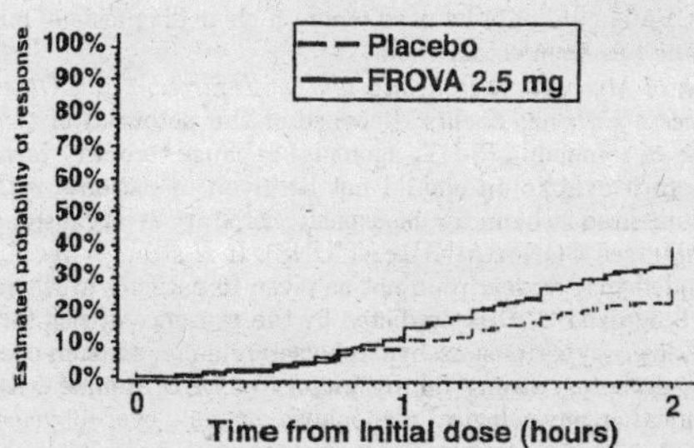

Figure 1 shows a Kaplan-Meier plot of the probability over time of obtaining headache response (no or mild pain) following treatment with frovatriptan 2.5 mg or placebo. The probabilities displayed are based on pooled data from four placebo-controlled trials described in Table 1 (Trials 1, 3, 4 and 5). Patients who did not achieve a response were censored at 24 hours.
In patients with migraine-associated nausea, photophobia and phonophobia at baseline there was a decreased incidence of these symptoms in FROVA treated patients compared to placebo. The estimated probability of patients taking a second dose or other medication for their migraine over the 24 hours following the initial dose of study treatment is summarized in Figure 2.

Figure 2
Estimated Probability of Patients Taking a Second Dose or Other Medication for Migraine Over the 24 Hours Following the Initial Dose of Study Treatment

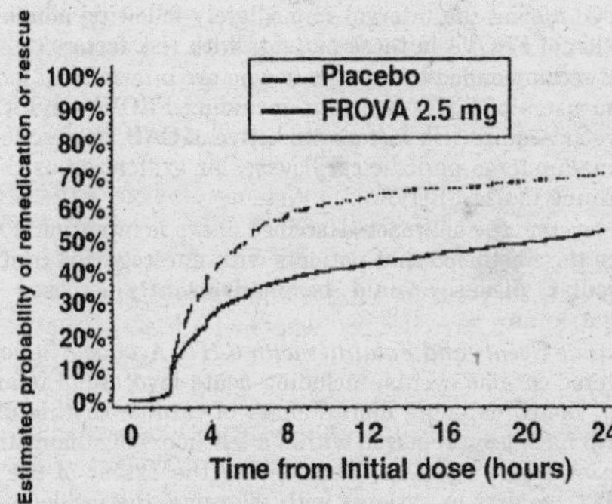

Figure 2 is a Kaplan-Meier plot showing the probability of patients taking a second dose or other medication for migraine over the 24 hours following the initial dose of study medication based on the data from four placebo-controlled trials described in Table 1 (Trials 1, 3, 4 and 5). The plot includes those patients who had a response to the initial dose and those who did not. The protocols did not permit remedication within 2 hours of the initial dose.
Efficacy was unaffected by a history of aura; gender; age, or concomitant medications commonly used by migraine patients.

INDICATIONS AND USAGE

FROVA is indicated for the acute treatment of migraine attacks with or without aura in adults.
FROVA is not intended for the prophylactic therapy of migraine or for use in the management of hemiplegic or basilar migraine (see CONTRAINDICATIONS). The safety and effectiveness of FROVA have not been established for cluster headache, which is present in an older, predominately male, population.

CONTRAINDICATIONS

FROVA should not be given to patients with ischemic heart disease (e.g. angina pectoris, history of myocardial infarction, or documented silent ischemia), or to patients who have symptoms or findings consistent with ischemic heart disease, coronary artery vasospasm, including Prinzmetal's variant angina or other significant underlying cardiovascular disease (see WARNINGS).
FROVA should not be given to patients with cerebrovascular syndromes including (but not limited to) strokes of any type as well as transient ischemic attacks.

Continued on next page

Frova—Cont.

FROVA should not be given to patients with peripheral vascular disease including (but is not limited to) ischemic bowel disease (see WARNINGS).
FROVA should not be given to patients with uncontrolled hypertension (see WARNINGS).
FROVA should not be administered to patients with hemiplegic or basilar migraine.
FROVA should not be used within 24 hours of treatment with another 5-HT_1 agonist, an ergotamine containing or ergot-type medication such as dihydroergotamine (DHE) or methysergide.
FROVA is contraindicated in patients who are hypersensitive to frovatriptan or any of the inactive ingredients in the tablets.

WARNINGS

FROVA should only be used where a clear diagnosis of migraine has been established.
Risk of Myocardial Ischemia and/or Infarction and Other Adverse Cardiac Events: Because of the potential of this class of compound (5-HT_1 agonists) to cause coronary vasospasm, frovatriptan should not be given to patients with documented ischemic or vasospastic coronary artery disease (CAD) (see CONTRAINDICATIONS). It is strongly recommended that frovatriptan not be given to patients in whom unrecognized CAD is predicted by the presence of risk factors (e.g., hypertension, hypercholesterolemia, smoker, obesity, diabetes, strong family history of CAD, female with surgical or physiological menopause, or male over 40 years of age) unless a cardiovascular evaluation provides satisfactory clinical evidence that the patient is reasonably free of coronary artery and ischemic myocardial disease or other significant underlying cardiovascular disease. The sensitivity of cardiac diagnostic procedures to detect cardiovascular disease or predisposition to coronary artery vasospasm is modest, at best. If, during the cardiovascular evaluation, the patient's medical history, electrocardiographic, or other investigations reveal findings indicative of, or consistent with, coronary artery vasospasm or myocardial ischemia, frovatriptan should not be administered (see CONTRAINDICATIONS).
For patients with risk factors predictive of CAD, who are determined to have a satisfactory cardiovascular evaluation, it is strongly recommended that administration of the first dose of frovatriptan take place in the setting of a physician's office or similar medically staffed and equipped facility unless the patient has previously received frovatriptan. Because cardiac ischemia can occur in the absence of clinical symptoms, consideration should be given to obtaining on the first occasion of use an electrocardiogram (ECG) during the interval immediately following administration of FROVA in these patients with risk factors.
It is recommended that patients who are intermittent long-term users of 5-HT_1 agonists, including FROVA, and who have or acquire risk factors predictive of CAD, as described above, undergo periodic cardiovascular evaluation as they continue to use FROVA.
The systematic approach described above is intended to reduce the likelihood that patients with unrecognized cardiovascular disease would be inadvertently exposed to frovatriptan.
Cardiac Events and Fatalities with 5-HT_1 Agonists: Serious adverse cardiac events, including acute myocardial infarction, life-threatening disturbances of cardiac rhythm and death have been reported within a few hours of administration of 5-HT_1 agonists. Considering the extent of use of 5-HT_1 agonists in patients with migraine, the incidence of these events is extremely low.
Premarketing experience with frovatriptan: Among more than 3000 patients with migraine who participated in premarketing clinical trials of FROVA, no deaths or serious cardiac events were reported which were related to the use of FROVA.
Cerebrovascular Events and Fatalities with 5-HT_1 Agonists: Cerebral hemorrhage, subarachnoid hemorrhage, stroke and other cerebrovascular events have been reported in patients treated with 5-HT_1 agonists; and some have resulted in fatalities. In a number of cases, it appears possible that the cerebrovascular events were primary, the agonist having been administered in the incorrect belief that the symptoms experienced were a consequence of migraine, when they were not. It should be noted that patients with migraine may be at increased risk of certain cerebrovascular events (e.g. stroke, hemorrhage, transient ischemic attack).
Other Vasospasm-Related Events: 5-HT_1 agonists may cause vasospastic reactions other than coronary artery spasm. Both peripheral vascular ischemia and colonic ischemia with abdominal pain and bloody diarrhea have been reported with 5-HT_1 agonists.
Effects on Blood Pressure: In young healthy subjects, there were statistically significant increases in systolic and diastolic blood pressure after single doses of 80 mg frovatriptan (32 times the clinical dose) and above. These increases were transient, resolved spontaneously and were not clinically significant. At the recommended dose of 2.5 mg, transient changes in systolic blood pressure were recorded in some elderly subjects (65 - 77 years). Any increases were generally small, resolved spontaneously, and blood pressure remained within the normal range. Frovatriptan is contraindicated in patients with uncontrolled hypertension (See CONTRAINDICATIONS).
An 18% increase in mean pulmonary artery pressure was seen following dosing with another 5-HT_1 agonist in a study evaluating subjects undergoing cardiac catheterization.

PRECAUTIONS

General: As with other 5-HT_1 agonists, sensations of pain, tightness, pressure and heaviness have been reported in the chest, throat, neck and jaw after treatment with FROVA. These events have not been associated with arrhythmias or ischemic ECG changes in clinical trials with FROVA. Because 5-HT_1 agonists may cause coronary vasospasm, patients who experience signs or symptoms suggestive of angina following dosing should be evaluated for the presence of CAD. Patients shown to have CAD and those with Prinzmetal's variant angina should not receive 5-HT_1 agonists (see CONTRAINDICATIONS). Patients who experience other symptoms or signs suggestive of decreased arterial flow, such as ischemic bowel syndrome or Raynaud's syndrome following the use of any 5-HT_1 agonist are candidates for further evaluation. If a patient has no response for the first migraine attack treated with FROVA, the diagnosis of migraine should be reconsidered before frovatriptan is administered to treat any subsequent attacks.
Hepatically Impaired Patients: There is no clinical or pharmacokinetic experience with FROVA in patients with severe hepatic impairment. The AUC of frovatriptan in patients with mild (Child-Pugh 5 - 6) to moderate (Child-Pugh 7 - 9) hepatic impairment was about twice that of young, healthy subjects, but within the range observed in healthy elderly subjects and was considerably lower than the values attained with higher doses of frovatriptan (up to 40 mg), which were not associated with any serious adverse effects. Therefore, no dosage adjustment is necessary when FROVA is given to patients with mild to moderate hepatic impairment (see CLINICAL PHARMACOLOGY, *Special Populations*).
Binding to Melanin-Containing Tissues: When pigmented rats were given a single oral dose of 5 mg/kg of radiolabeled frovatriptan, the radioactivity in the eye after 28 days was 87% of the value measured after 8 hours. This suggests that frovatriptan and/or its metabolites may bind to the melanin of the eye. Because there could be accumulation in melanin rich tissues over time, this raises the possibility that frovatriptan could cause toxicity in these tissues after extended use. However, no effects on the retina related to treatment with frovatriptan were noted in the toxicity studies. Although no systematic monitoring of ophthalmologic function was undertaken in clinical trials and no specific recommendations for ophthalmologic monitoring are made, prescribers should be aware of the possibility of long-term ophthalmologic effects.

Information for Patients

Physicians should instruct their patients to read the patient package insert before taking FROVA. See PATIENT INFORMATION at the end of this labeling for the text of the separate leaflet provided for patients.

Laboratory Tests

No specific laboratory tests are recommended for monitoring patients prior to and/or after treatment with FROVA.

Drug Interactions (see also CLINICAL PHARMACOLOGY, *Drug Interactions*)

Ergot-containing drugs have been reported to cause prolonged vasospastic reactions. Due to a theoretical risk of a pharmacodynamic interaction, use of ergotamine-containing or ergot-type medications (like dihydroergotamine or methysergide) and FROVA within 24 hours of each other should be avoided (see CONTRAINDICATIONS).
Concomitant use of other 5-$HT_{1B/1D}$ agonists within 24 hours of FROVA treatment is not recommended (see CONTRAINDICATIONS).
Selective serotonin reuptake inhibitors (SSRIs) (e.g., fluoxetine, fluvoxamine, paroxetine, sertraline) have been reported, rarely, to cause weakness, hyperreflexia, and incoordination when coadministered with 5-HT_1 agonists. If concomitant treatment with frovatriptan and an SSRI is clinically warranted, appropriate observation of the patient is advised.

Drug/Laboratory Test Interactions

FROVA is not known to interfere with commonly employed clinical laboratory tests.

Carcinogenesis, Mutagenesis, Impairment of Fertility

Carcinogenesis: The carcinogenic potential of frovatriptan was evaluated in an 84-week study in mice (4, 13, and 40 mg/kg/day), a 104-week study in rats (8.5, 27 and 85 mg/kg/day), and a 26-week study in p53(+/-) transgenic mice (20, 62.5, 200, and 400 mg/kg/day). Although the maximum tolerated dose (MTD) was not achieved in the 84-week mouse study and in female rats, exposures at the highest doses studied were many fold greater than those achieved at the maximum recommended daily human dose (MRHD) of 7.5 mg. There were no increases in tumor incidence in the 84-week mouse study at doses producing 140 times the exposure achieved at the MRHD based on blood AUC comparisons. In the rat study, there was a statistically significant increase in the incidence of pituitary adenomas in males only at 85 mg/kg/day, a dose that produced 250 times the exposure achieved at the MRHD based on AUC comparisons. In the 26-week p53(+/-) transgenic mouse study, there was an increased incidence of subcutaneous sarcomas in females dosed at 200 and 400 mg/kg/day, or 390 and 630 times the human exposure based on AUC comparisons. The incidence of sarcomas was not increased at lower doses that achieved exposures 180 and 60 times the human exposure. These sarcomas were physically associated with subcutaneously implanted animal identification transponders. There were no other increases in tumor incidence of any type in any dose group. These sarcomas are not considered to be relevant to humans.
Mutagenesis: Frovatriptan was clastogenic in human lymphocyte cultures, in the absence of metabolic activation. In the bacterial reverse mutation assay (Ames test), frovatriptan produced an equivocal response in the absence of metabolic activation. No mutagenic or clastogenic activities were seen in an *in vitro* mouse lymphoma assay, an *in vivo* mouse bone marrow micronucleus test, or an *ex vivo* assay for unscheduled DNA synthesis in rat liver.
Impairment of Fertility: Male and female rats were dosed prior to and during mating, and up to implantation, at doses of 100, 500, and 1000 mg/kg/day (equivalent to approximately 130, 650 and 1300 times the MRHD on a mg/m^2 basis). At all dose levels there was an increase in the number of females that mated on the first day of pairing compared to control animals. This occurred in conjunction with a prolongation of the estrous cycle. In addition females had a decreased mean number of corpora lutea, and consequently a lower number of live fetuses per litter, which suggested a partial impairment of ovulation. There were no other fertility-related effects.

Pregnancy: Pregnancy Category C

When pregnant rats were administered frovatriptan during the period of organogenesis at oral doses of 100, 500 and 1000 mg/kg/day (equivalent to 130, 650 and 1300 times the maximum recommended human dose [MRHD] on a mg/m^2 basis) there were dose related increases in incidences of both litters and total numbers of fetuses with dilated ureters, unilateral and bilateral pelvic cavitation, hydronephrosis, and hydroureters. A no-effect dose for renal effects was not established. This signifies a syndrome of related effects on a specific organ in the developing embryo in all treated groups, which is consistent with a slight delay in fetal maturation. This delay was also indicated by a treatment related increased incidence of incomplete ossification of the sternebrae, skull and nasal bones in all treated groups. Slightly lower fetal weights and an increased incidence of early embryonic deaths in treated rats were observed; although not statistically significant compared to control, the latter effect occurred in both the embryo-fetal developmental study and in the prenatal-postnatal developmental study. There was no evidence of this latter effect at the lowest dose level studied, 100 mg/kg/day (equivalent to 130 times the MRHD on a mg/m^2 basis). When pregnant rabbits were dosed throughout organogenesis at doses up to 80 mg/kg/day (equivalent to 210 times the MRHD on a mg/m^2 basis) no effects on fetal development were observed. There are no adequate and well-controlled studies in pregnant women; therefore, frovatriptan should be used during pregnancy only if the potential benefit justifies the potential risk to the fetus.

Nursing Mothers

It is not known whether frovatriptan is excreted in human milk. Frovatriptan and/or its metabolites are excreted in the milk of lactating rats with the maximum concentration being four-fold higher than that seen in blood. Therefore, caution should be exercised when considering the administration of FROVA to a nursing woman.

Pediatric Use

Safety and effectiveness of FROVA in pediatric patients have not been established; therefore, FROVA is not recommended for use in patients under 18 years of age. Postmarketing experience with other triptans includes a limited number of reports that describe pediatric patients who have experienced clinically serious adverse events that are similar in nature to those reported rarely in adults.

Use in the Elderly

Mean blood concentrations of frovatriptan in elderly subjects were 1.5- to 2-times higher than those seen in younger adults (see CLINICAL PHARMACOLOGY, *Special Populations*). Because migraine occurs infrequently in the elderly, clinical experience with FROVA is limited in such patients.

ADVERSE REACTIONS

Serious cardiac events, including some that have been fatal, have occurred following use of 5-HT_1 agonists. These events are extremely rare and most have been reported in patients with risk factors predictive of CAD. Events reported have included coronary artery vasospasm, transient myocardial ischemia, myocardial infarction, ventricular tachycardia and ventricular fibrillation (see CONTRAINDICATIONS, WARNINGS and PRECAUTIONS).
Incidence in Controlled Clinical Trials: Among 1554 patients treated with FROVA in four placebo-controlled trials (Trials 1, 3, 4 and 5 in Table 1), only 1% (16) patients withdrew because of treatment-emergent adverse events. In a long term, open-label study where patients were allowed to treat multiple migraine attacks with FROVA for up to 1 year, 5% (26/496) patients discontinued due to treatment-emergent adverse events.
The treatment-emergent adverse events that occurred most frequently following administration of frovatriptan 2.5 mg (*i.e.*, in at least 2% of patients), and at an incidence $\geq$1% greater than with placebo, in the four placebo-controlled trials were dizziness, paresthesia, headache, dry mouth, fatigue, flushing, hot or cold sensation and chest pain.
Table 2 lists treatment-emergent adverse events reported within 48 hours of drug administration that occurred with frovatriptan 2.5 mg at an incidence of $\geq$2% and more often than on placebo, in the first attack in four placebo-controlled trials (Trials 1, 3, 4 and 5 in Table 1). These studies involved 2392 patients (1554 frovatriptan 2.5 mg and 838 placebo). The events cited reflect experience gained un-

der closely monitored conditions of clinical trials in a highly selected patient population. In actual clinical practice or in other clinical trials, these incidence estimates may not apply, as the conditions of use, reporting behavior, and the kinds of patients treated may differ.

Table 2
Treatment-Emergent Adverse Events (Incidence ≥2% and Greater Than Placebo) of Patients in Four Placebo-Controlled Migraine Trials

Adverse events	Frovatriptan 2.5 mg (n=1554)	Placebo (n=838)
Central & peripheral nervous system		
Dizziness	8%	5%
Headache	4%	3%
Paresthesia	4%	2%
Gastrointestinal system disorders		
Mouth dry	3%	1%
Dyspepsia	2%	1%
Body as a whole — general disorders		
Fatigue	5%	2%
Hot or cold sensation	3%	2%
Chest pain	2%	1%
Musculo-skeletal		
Skeletal pain	3%	2%
Vascular		
Flushing	4%	2%

Other events that occurred at ≥2% on frovatriptan that were equally or more common in the placebo group were somnolence and nausea.

FROVA is generally well tolerated. The incidence of adverse events in clinical trials did not increase when up to 3 doses were used within 24 hours. The majority of adverse events were mild or moderate and transient. The incidence of adverse events in four placebo-controlled clinical trials was not affected by gender, age or concomitant medications commonly used by migraine patients. There were insufficient data to assess the impact of race on the incidence of adverse events.

Other Events Observed in Association with FROVA: In the paragraphs that follow, the incidence of less commonly reported adverse events in four placebo-controlled trials are presented. Variability associated with adverse event reporting, the terminology used to describe adverse events etc, limit the value of the incidence estimates provided. The incidence of each adverse event is calculated as the number of patients reporting the event at least once divided by the number of patients who used FROVA. All adverse events reported within 48 hours of drug administration in the first attack in four placebo-controlled trials involving 2392 patients (1554 frovatriptan 2.5 mg and 838 placebo) are included, except those already listed in Table 2, those too general to be informative, those not reasonably associated with the use of the drug and those which occurred at the same or a greater incidence in the placebo group. Events are further classified within body system categories and enumerated in order of decreasing frequency using the following definitions: frequent adverse events are those occurring in at least 1/100 patients, infrequent adverse events are those occurring in between 1/100 and 1/1000 patients, and rare adverse events are those occurring in fewer than 1/1000 patients.

Central and peripheral nervous system: Frequent: dysesthesia and hypoesthesia. Infrequent: tremor, hyperesthesia, migraine aggravated, involuntary muscle contractions, vertigo, ataxia, abnormal gait and speech disorder. Rare: hypertonia, hypotonia, abnormal reflexes and tongue paralysis.

Gastrointestinal: Frequent: vomiting, abdominal pain and diarrhea. Infrequent: dysphagia, flatulence, constipation, anorexia, esophagospasm and increased salivation. Rare: change in bowel habits, cheilitis, eructation, gastroesophageal reflux, hiccup, peptic ulcer, salivary gland pain, stomatitis and toothache.

Body as a whole: Frequent: pain. Infrequent: asthenia, rigors, fever, hot flushes and malaise. Rare: feeling of relaxation, leg pain and edema mouth.

Psychiatric: Frequent: insomnia and anxiety. Infrequent: confusion, nervousness, agitation, euphoria, impaired concentration, depression, emotional lability, amnesia, thinking abnormal and depersonalization. Rare: depression aggravated, abnormal dreaming and personality disorder.

Musculoskeletal: Infrequent: myalgia, back pain, arthralgia, arthrosis, leg cramps and muscle weakness.

Respiratory: Frequent: sinusitis and rhinitis. Infrequent: pharyngitis, dyspnea, hyperventilation and laryngitis.

Vision disorders: Frequent: vision abnormal. Infrequent: eye pain, conjunctivitis and abnormal lacrimation.

Skin and appendages: Frequent: sweating increased. Infrequent: pruritis, and bullous eruption.

Hearing and vestibular disorders: Frequent: tinnitus. Infrequent: ear ache, and hyperacusis.

Heart rate and rhythm: Frequent: palpitation. Infrequent: tachycardia. Rare: bradycardia.

Metabolic and nutritional disorders: Infrequent: thirst and dehydration. Rare: hypocalcemia and hypoglycemia.

Special senses, other disorders: Infrequent: taste perversion.

Urinary system disorders: Infrequent: micturition frequency and polyuria. Rare: nocturia, renal pain and abnormal urine.

Cardiovascular disorders, general: Infrequent: abnormal ECG.

Platelet, bleeding and clotting disorders: Infrequent: epistaxis. Rare: purpura.

Autonomic nervous system: Rare: syncope.

DRUG ABUSE AND DEPENDENCE

Although the abuse potential of FROVA has not been specifically assessed in clinical trials, no abuse of, tolerance to, withdrawal from, or drug-seeking behavior was observed in patients who received FROVA. The 5-HT_1 agonists, as a class, have not been associated with drug abuse.

OVERDOSAGE

There is no direct experience of any patient taking an overdose of FROVA. The maximum single dose of frovatriptan given to male and female patients with migraine was 40 mg (16 times the clinical dose) and the maximum single dose given to healthy male subjects was 100 mg (40 times the clinical dose) without significant adverse events.

As with other 5-HT_1 receptor agonists, there is no specific antidote for frovatriptan. The elimination half-life of frovatriptan is 26 hours, therefore if overdose occurs, the patient should be monitored closely for at least 48 hours and be given any necessary symptomatic treatment.

The effects of hemo- or peritoneal dialysis on blood concentrations of frovatriptan are unknown.

DOSAGE AND ADMINISTRATION

The recommended dose is a single tablet of FROVA (frovatriptan 2.5 mg) taken orally with fluids.

If the headache recurs after initial relief, a second tablet may be taken, providing there is an interval of at least 2 hours between doses. The total daily dose of frovatriptan should not exceed 3 tablets (3 × 2.5 mg per day).

There is no evidence that a second dose of frovatriptan is effective in patients who do not respond to a first dose of the drug for the same headache.

The safety of treating an average of more than 4 migraine attacks in a 30-day period has not been established.

HOW SUPPLIED

FROVA tablets, containing 2.5 mg of frovatriptan (base) as the succinate, are available as round, white, film-coated tablets with 77 on one side and the "e" logo on the other side. The tablets are available in:

Blister card of 9 tablets, 1 blister card per carton (NDC 59075-740-89)

Store at controlled room temperature, 25°C (77°F) excursions permitted to 15 - 30°C (59°F - 86°F) [see USP Controlled Room Temperature], Protect from moisture and light.

U.S. Patent Nos. 5,962,501, 5,827,871, 5,637,611 and 5,464,864 and 5,616,603.

Rx Only

Manufactured by:
Galen Limited
Craigavon, BT63 5UA, UK

Distributed by:
Elan Biopharmaceuticals
San Diego, CA 92121, USA

FROVA is a trademark of Elan Pharmaceuticals, Inc., a member of the Elan Group.

6000348 / PX422/1 Rev. 12/2001

PATIENT INFORMATION: The following wording is contained in a separate leaflet provided for patients.

Patient information about
FROVA™ (frovatriptan succinate) Tablets

Read this information before you start taking FROVA (FRO-va). Also, read the information each time you renew your prescription, in case anything has changed. This leaflet does not contain all of the information about FROVA. For further information or advice ask your doctor or pharmacist. You and your doctor should discuss FROVA before you start taking the medicine and at regular checkups.

What is FROVA?

FROVA is a prescription medicine used to treat migraine attacks in adults. It is in the class of drugs called selective serotonin receptor agonists.

FROVA should only be taken for a migraine headache. Do not use FROVA to treat headaches that might be caused by other conditions. Tell your doctor about your symptoms. Your doctor will decide if you have migraine headaches and if FROVA is for you.

There is more information about migraine at the end of this leaflet.

Who should not take FROVA?

Do not take FROVA if you:

- have uncontrolled high blood pressure
- have heart disease or a history of heart disease
- have hemiplegic or basilar migraine (if you are not sure about this, ask your doctor)
- have had a stroke
- have circulation (blood flow) problems
- have taken a similar drug (a serotonin receptor agonist) in the last 24 hours. These include sumatriptan (IMITREX®), naratriptan (AMERGE™), zolmitriptan (ZOMIG™), rizatriptan (MAXALT™), or almotriptan (AXERT™)
- have taken ergotamine type medicines in the last 24 hours. These include BELLERGAL®, CAFERGOT®, ERGOMAR®, WIGRAINE®, DHE 45®, or SANSERT®
- have any allergic reaction to the tablet

What you should tell your doctor before and during treatment with FROVA?

To help your doctor decide if FROVA is right for you, tell your doctor if you:

- are pregnant, or planning to become pregnant
- are breast-feeding or plan to breast-feed
- have any history of chest pain, shortness of breath, or palpitations
- have any risk factors for heart disease, including
  - high blood pressure
  - diabetes
  - high cholesterol
  - overweight
  - smoking
  - a family history of heart disease
  - past menopause
  - male over 40 years old
- are taking any other medicine, including prescription and non-prescription medicines, and herbal supplements
- have any past or present medical problems
- have previous allergies to any medicine

Tell your doctor if you take

- propranolol
- selective serotonin reuptake inhibitors (SSRIs) such as Prozac (fluoextine), Luvox (fluvoxamine), Paxil (paroxetine), and Zoloft (sertraline)

These medicines may affect how FROVA works, or FROVA may affect how these medicines work.

How should you take FROVA?

Take one FROVA tablet anytime after the start of your migraine headache.

If your headache comes back after your first dose, you may take a second tablet after two (2) hours. Do not take more than three (3) FROVA tablets in a 24-hour period.

If you take too much medicine, contact your doctor, hospital emergency department, or poison control center right away.

What are the common side effects of FROVA?

The most common side effects associated with use of FROVA are:

- dizziness
- fatigue (tiredness)
- headache (other than a migraine headache)
- paresthesia (feeling of tingling)
- dry mouth
- flushing (hot flashes)
- feeling hot or cold
- chest pain
- dyspepsia (indigestion)
- skeletal pain (pain in joints or bones)

Tell your doctor about any symptoms that you develop while taking FROVA. If you feel dizziness or fatigue, take extra care or avoid driving and operating machinery.

In very rare cases, patients taking this class of medicines experience serious heart problems, stroke, or increased blood pressure. If you develop pain, tightness, heaviness, or pressure in your chest, throat, neck, or jaw, contact your doctor right away.

Also contact your doctor right away if you develop a rash or itching after taking FROVA. You may be allergic to this medicine.

What is a migraine and how does it differ from other headaches?

Migraine is an intense, throbbing headache that often affects one side of the head. It often includes nausea, vomiting, and sensitivity to light and sound. The pain and symptoms from a migraine headache may be worse than the pain and symptoms of a common headache. Migraine headaches usually last for hours or longer.

Some people have problems with vision (an aura) before they get a migraine headache. These include flashing lights, wavy lines, and dark spots.

Only your doctor can determine that your headache is a migraine headache, so it is important that you discuss all of your symptoms with your doctor.

FROVA is a trademark of Elan Pharmaceuticals, Inc., a member of the Elan Group.

Gilead Sciences, Inc.

333 LAKESIDE DRIVE
FOSTER CITY, CA 94404

Direct Inquiries To:
Customer Service
(800) GILEAD5

Medical Emergency Contact:
Director, Medical Information
(800) GILEAD5
FAX: (650) 522-5477

VIREAD® ℞
[*vĕr 'ē ăd*]
(tenofovir disoproxil fumarate) Tablets
Rx Only

WARNING
LACTIC ACIDOSIS AND SEVERE HEPATOMEGALY WITH STEATOSIS, INCLUDING FATAL CASES, HAVE BEEN REPORTED WITH THE USE OF NUCLEOSIDE ANALOGS ALONE OR IN COMBINATION WITH OTHER ANTIRETROVIRALS (SEE WARNINGS).

Continued on next page

Viread—Cont.

DESCRIPTION

VIREAD is the brand name for tenofovir disoproxil fumarate (a prodrug of tenofovir) which is a fumaric acid salt of *bis*-isopropoxycarbonyloxymethyl ester derivative of tenofovir. In vivo tenofovir disoproxil fumarate is converted to tenofovir, an acyclic nucleoside phosphonate (nucleotide) analog of adenosine 5′- monophosphate. Tenofovir exhibits activity against HIV reverse transcriptase.

The chemical name of tenofovir disoproxil fumarate is 9-[(*R*)-2-[[bis[[(isopropoxycarbonyl) oxy]methoxy]phosphinyl]methoxy]propyl]adenine fumarate (1:1). It has a molecular formula of $C_{19}H_{30}N_5O_{10}P \bullet C_4H_4O_4$ and a molecular weight of 635.52. It has the following structural formula:

Tenofovir disoproxil fumarate is a white to off-white crystalline powder with a solubility of 13.4 mg/mL in distilled water at 25°C. It has an octanol/phosphate buffer (pH 6.5) partition coefficient (*log p*) of 1.25 at 25°C.

VIREAD tablets are for oral administration. Each tablet contains 300 mg of tenofovir disoproxil fumarate, which is equivalent to 245 mg of tenofovir disoproxil, and the following inactive ingredients: croscarmellose sodium, lactose monohydrate, magnesium stearate, microcrystalline cellulose, and pregelatinized starch. The tablets are coated with a blue colored film (Opadry II Y-30-10671-A) that is made of FD&C blue #2 aluminum lake, hydroxypropyl methylcellulose 2910, lactose monohydrate, titanium dioxide, and triacetin.

In this insert, all dosages are expressed in terms of tenofovir disoproxil fumarate except where otherwise noted.

CLINICAL PHARMACOLOGY

Microbiology

Mechanism of Action: Tenofovir disoproxil fumarate is an acyclic nucleoside phosphonate diester analog of adenosine monophosphate. Tenofovir disoproxil fumarate requires initial diester hydrolysis for conversion to tenofovir and subsequent phosphorylations by cellular enzymes to form tenofovir diphosphate. Tenofovir diphosphate inhibits the activity of HIV reverse transcriptase by competing with the natural substrate deoxyadenosine 5′-triphosphate and, after incorporation into DNA, by DNA chain termination. Tenofovir diphosphate is a weak inhibitor of mammalian DNA polymerases α, β, and mitochondrial DNA polymerase γ.

Antiviral Activity In Vitro: The in vitro antiviral activity of tenofovir against laboratory and clinical isolates of HIV was assessed in lymphoblastoid cell lines, primary monocyte/macrophage cells and peripheral blood lymphocytes. The IC_{50} (50% inhibitory concentrations) for tenofovir was in the range of 0.04 μM to 8.5 μM. In drug combination studies of tenofovir with nucleoside and nonnucleoside analog inhibitors of HIV reverse transcriptase, and protease inhibitors, additive to synergistic effects were observed. Most of these drug combinations have not been studied in humans.

In Vitro Resistance: HIV isolates with reduced susceptibility to tenofovir have been selected in vitro. These viruses expressed a K65R mutation in reverse transcriptase and showed a 3 - 4 fold reduction in susceptibility to tenofovir.

In Vitro Cross-resistance: Cross-resistance among certain reverse transcriptase inhibitors has been recognized. The in vitro activity of tenofovir against HIV-1 strains with zidovudine-associated mutations (M41L, D67N, K70R, L210W, T215Y/F or K219Q/E/N) was evaluated. Zidovudine-associated mutations may also confer reductions in susceptibility to other NRTIs and these mutations have been reported to emerge during combination therapy with stavudine and didanosine. In 20 samples that had multiple zidovudine-associated mutations (mean 3), a mean 3.1-fold increase of the IC_{50} of tenofovir was observed (range 0.8 to 8.4). The K65R mutation is selected both in vitro and in some HIV-infected subjects treated with didanosine, zalcitabine, or abacavir; therefore, some cross-resistance may occur in patients who develop this mutation following treatment with these drugs. Multinucleoside resistant HIV-1 with a T69S double insertion mutation in the reverse transcriptase showed reduced susceptibility to tenofovir.

Genotypic and Phenotypic Analyses of VIREAD in Patients with Previous Antiretroviral Therapy (Studies 902 and 907): See Description of Clinical Studies.

In Vivo Resistance:

Post baseline genotyping in Studies 902 and 907 showed that seven of 237 VIREAD-treated patients' HIV (3%) developed the K65R mutation, a mutation selected by VIREAD and other NRTIs in vitro. Among VIREAD-treated patients whose HIV developed NRTI-associated mutations, there was continued HIV RNA suppression through 24 weeks. The rate and extent of tenofovir-associated resistance mutations has not been characterized in antiretroviral naïve patients initiating VIREAD treatment.

Phenotypic analyses of HIV isolates after 48 weeks (Study 902, n=30) or 24 weeks (Study 907, n=35) of VIREAD therapy showed no significant changes in VIREAD susceptibility unless the K65R mutation had developed.

Table 1. Drug Interactions: Changes in Pharmacokinetic Parameters for Tenofovir[1] in the Presence of the Co-administered Drug

Co-administered Drug	Dose of Co-administered Drug (mg)	N	% Change of Tenofovir Pharmacokinetic Parameters[2] (90% CI)		
			C_{max}	AUC	C_{min}
Lamivudine	150 twice daily× 7 days	15	⇔	⇔	⇔
Didanosine[3]	250 or 400 once daily× 7 days	14	⇔	⇔	⇔
Indinavir	800 three times daily× 7 days	13	↑ 14 (↓ 3 to ↑ 33)	⇔	⇔
Lopinavir/ Ritonavir	400/100 twice daily × 14 days	21	↑ 31 (↑ 12 to ↑ 53)	↑ 34 (↑ 25 to ↑ 44)	↑ 29 (↑ 11 to ↑ 48)
Efavirenz	600 once daily× 14 days	29	⇔	⇔	⇔

1. Patients received VIREAD 300 mg once daily
2. Increase = ↑; Decrease = ↓; No Effect = ⇔
3. Buffered formulation

Table 2. Drug Interactions: Changes in Pharmacokinetic Parameters for Co-administered Drug in the Presence of VIREAD 300 mg Once Daily

Co-administered Drug	Dose of Co-administered Drug (mg)	N	% Change of Co-administered Drug Pharmacokinetic Parameters[1] (90% CI)		
			C_{max}	AUC	C_{min}
Lamivudine	150 twice daily× 7 days	15	↓ 24 (↓ 34 to ↓ 12)	⇔	⇔
Didanosine[2] (see PRECAUTIONS)	250 or 400 once daily × 7 days	14	↑ 28 (↑ 11 to ↑ 48)	↑ 44 (↑ 31 to ↑ 59)	—
Indinavir	800 three times daily× 7 days	12	↓ 11 (↓ 30 to ↑ 12)	⇔	⇔
Lopinavir	Lopinavir/Ritonavir 400/100 twice daily × 14 days	21	↓ 15 (↓ 23 to ↓ 6)	↓ 15 (↓ 22 to ↓ 7)	⇔
Ritonavir	Lopinavir/Ritonavir 400/100 twice daily × 14 days	21	↓ 28 (↓ 43 to ↓ 9)	↓ 24 (↓ 33 to ↓ 13)	↑ 7 (↓ 22 to ↑ 37)
Efavirenz	600 once daily× 14 days	30	⇔	⇔	⇔

1. Increase = ↑; Decrease = ↓; No Effect = ⇔
2. Buffered formulation

Pharmacokinetics

The pharmacokinetics of tenofovir disoproxil fumarate have been evaluated in healthy volunteers and HIV-infected individuals. Tenofovir pharmacokinetics are similar between these populations.

Absorption: VIREAD is a water soluble diester prodrug of the active ingredient tenofovir. The oral bioavailability of tenofovir from VIREAD in fasted patients is approximately 25%. Following oral administration of a single dose of VIREAD 300 mg to HIV-infected patients in the fasted state, maximum serum concentrations (C_{max}) are achieved in 1.0 ± 0.4 hours. C_{max} and AUC values are 296 ± 90 ng/mL and 2287 ± 685 ng*h/mL, respectively.

The pharmacokinetics of tenofovir are dose proportional over a VIREAD dose range of 75 to 600 mg and are not affected by repeated dosing.

Effects of Food on Oral Absorption: Administration of VIREAD following a high-fat meal (~700 to 1000 kcal containing 40 to 50% fat) increases the oral bioavailability, with an increase in tenofovir $AUC_{0-\infty}$ of approximately 40% and an increase in C_{max} of approximately 14%. Food delays the time to tenofovir C_{max} by approximately 1 hour. C_{max} and AUC of tenofovir are 326 ± 119 ng/mL and 3324 ± 1370 ng*h/mL following multiple doses of VIREAD 300 mg once daily in the fed state. VIREAD should be taken with a meal to enhance the bioavailability of tenofovir.

Distribution: In vitro binding of tenofovir to human plasma or serum proteins is less than 0.7 and 7.2%, respectively, over the tenofovir concentration range 0.01 to 25 μg/mL. The volume of distribution at steady-state is 1.3 ± 0.6 L/kg and 1.2 ± 0.4 L/kg, following intravenous administration of tenofovir 1.0 mg/kg and 3.0 mg/kg.

Metabolism and Elimination: In vitro studies indicate that neither tenofovir disoproxil nor tenofovir are substrates of CYP450 enzymes.

Following IV administration of tenofovir, approximately 70–80% of the dose is recovered in the urine as unchanged tenofovir within 72 hours of dosing. After multiple oral doses of VIREAD 300 mg once daily (under fed conditions), 32 ± 10% of the administered dose is recovered in urine over 24 hours.

Tenofovir is eliminated by a combination of glomerular filtration and active tubular secretion. There may be competition for elimination with other compounds that are also renally eliminated.

Special Populations:

There were insufficient numbers from racial and ethnic groups other than Caucasian to adequately determine potential pharmacokinetic differences among these populations.

Tenofovir pharmacokinetics are similar in male and female patients.

Pharmacokinetic studies have not been performed in children or in the elderly.

The pharmacokinetics of tenofovir have not been studied in patients with hepatic impairment; however, tenofovir and tenofovir disoproxil are not metabolized by liver enzymes, so the impact of liver impairment should be limited. (See PRECAUTIONS, Hepatic Impairment)

The pharmacokinetics of tenofovir have not been evaluated in patients with renal impairment (creatinine clearance < 60 mL/min). Because tenofovir is primarily renally eliminated, tenofovir pharmacokinetics are likely to be affected by renal impairment. (See WARNINGS, Renal Insufficiency)

Drug Interactions:

At concentrations substantially higher (~ 300-fold) than those observed in vivo, tenofovir did not inhibit in vitro drug metabolism mediated by any of the following human CYP450 isoforms: CYP3A4, CYP2D6, CYP2C9 or CYP2E1. However, a small (6%) but statistically significant reduction in metabolism of CYP1A substrate was observed. Based on the results of in vitro experiments and the known elimination pathway of tenofovir, the potential for CYP450 mediated interactions involving tenofovir with other medicinal products is low. (See Pharmacokinetics)

Tenofovir is primarily excreted by the kidneys by a combination of glomerular filtration and active tubular secretion. Co-administration of VIREAD with drugs that are eliminated by active tubular secretion may increase serum concentrations of either tenofovir or the co-administered drug, due to competition for this elimination pathway. Drugs that decrease renal function may also increase serum concentrations of tenofovir.

VIREAD has been evaluated in healthy volunteers in combination with didanosine, lamivudine, indinavir, efavirenz, and lopinavir/ritonavir. Tables 1 and 2 summarize pharmacokinetic effects of co-administered drug on tenofovir pharmacokinetics and effects of tenofovir on the pharmacokinetics of co-administered drug.

[See table 1 above]
[See table 2 above]

INDICATIONS AND USAGE

VIREAD is indicated in combination with other antiretroviral agents for the treatment of HIV-1 infection. This indication is based on analyses of plasma HIV-1 RNA levels and CD4 cell counts in a controlled study of VIREAD of 24 weeks duration and in a controlled, dose ranging study of VIREAD of 48 weeks duration. Both studies were conducted in treatment experienced adults with evidence of HIV-1 viral replication despite ongoing antiretroviral therapy. Studies in antiretroviral naïve patients are ongoing; consequently, the risk-benefit ratio for this population has yet to be determined.

Additional important information regarding the use of VIREAD for the treatment of HIV infection:

- There are no study results demonstrating the effect of VIREAD on clinical progression of HIV.
- The use of VIREAD should be considered for treating adult patients with HIV strains that are expected to be susceptible to tenofovir as assessed by laboratory testing or treatment history. (See Description of Clinical Studies)

Description of Clinical Studies: Treatment Experienced Patients

Study 907: VIREAD + Standard Background Therapy (SBT) Compared to Placebo + SBT

Study 907 was a 24 week, double-blind placebo-controlled multicenter study of VIREAD added to a stable background regimen of antiretroviral agents in 550 treatment-experienced patients. Patients had a mean baseline CD4 cell count of 426 cells/mm^3 (range 23–1385), median baseline plasma HIV RNA of 2340 (range 50–75,900) copies/mL, and mean duration of prior HIV treatment was 5.4 years. Mean age of the patients was 42 years, 85% were male and 69% were Caucasian, 17% African-American and 12% Hispanic.

Changes from baseline in $\log_{10}$ copies/mL plasma HIV RNA levels over time up to week 24 are presented below in Figure 1.

Figure 1
Mean Change from Baseline in Plasma HIV RNA ($\log_{10}$ copies/mL) Through Week 24: Study 907 (All Available Data)

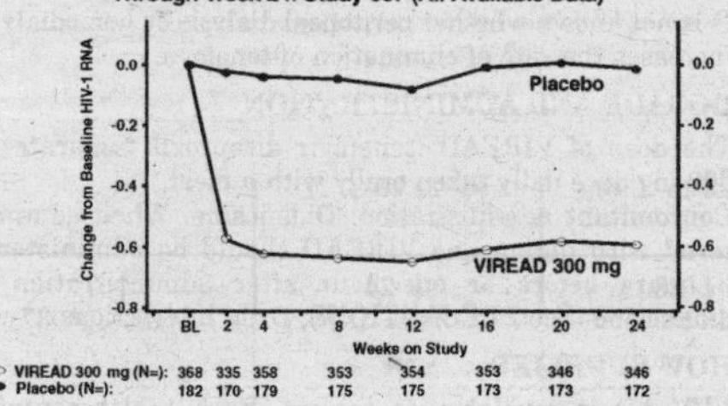

The percent of patients with HIV RNA < 400 copies/mL, < 50 copies/mL and outcomes of patients through 24 weeks are summarized in Table 3.

[See table 3 above]

Mean change in absolute CD4 counts by week 24 was +11 cells/mm^3 for the VIREAD group and -5 cells/mm^3 for the placebo group.

One patient in the VIREAD group and no patients in the placebo arm experienced a new CDC Class C event.

Study 902: VIREAD + Standard Background Therapy (SBT) Compared to Placebo + SBT

Study 902 was a double-blind placebo-controlled multicenter study evaluating treatment with VIREAD at three dose levels (75 mg QD, 150 mg QD and 300 mg QD) when added to a stable background regimen of antiretroviral agents in 186 treatment-experienced patients. Placebo patients received VIREAD 300 mg QD at week 24. All patients received open label VIREAD 300 mg QD after week 48. Patients had a mean baseline CD4 cell count of 374 cells/mm^3 (range 9–1240), median baseline plasma HIV RNA of 5010 copies/mL (range 52–575,000), and mean duration of prior HIV treatment was 4.6 years. Mean age was 42 years, 92% were male and 74% were Caucasian, 13% African-American, and 11% Hispanic. At week 24, the rate of drug discontinuation was 11% for the VIREAD group versus 25% for the placebo group.

Changes from baseline in $\log_{10}$ copies/mL plasma HIV RNA levels over time up to week 48 are presented below in Figure 2.

Figure 2
Mean Change from Baseline in Plasma HIV RNA ($\log_{10}$ copies/mL) Through Week 48: Study 902 (All Available Data)

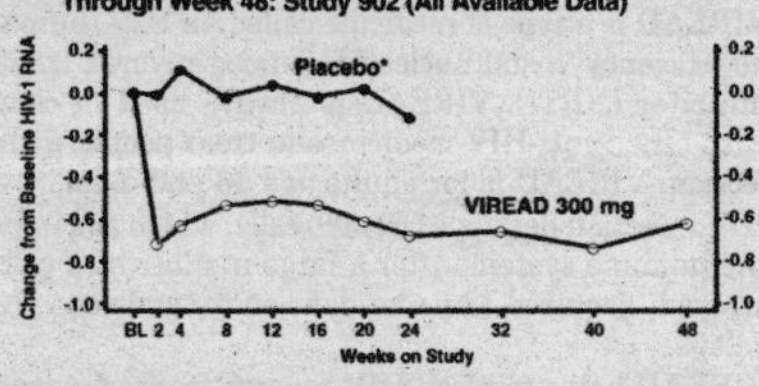

*At week 24, 21 placebo patients crossed over to receive VIREAD 300 mg once daily. At week 48 mean change from week 24 was -0.56 $\log_{10}$ copies/mL.

Through week 24 the proportion of patients achieving < 400 copies/mL was 19% VIREAD vs. 7% placebo and < 50 copies/mL was 11% VIREAD vs. 0% placebo. The differences for these secondary endpoints were not statistically significant.

Mean change in absolute CD4 counts by week 24 were -14 cells/mm^3 for the VIREAD group and +20 cells/mm^3 for the placebo group. This result was not statistically significant. Mean change in CD4 count at week 48 was +11 cells/mm^3 for the VIREAD group.

No patients experienced a new CDC Class C event through week 24.

Table 3. Outcomes of Randomized Treatment at Week 24 (Study 907)

Outcomes	VIREAD 300 mg (N=368)	Placebo (N=182)
HIV RNA < 400 copies/mL	149 (40%)	20 (11%)
HIV RNA > 400 copies/mL	189 (51%)	146 (80%)
HIV RNA < 50 copies/mL	71 (19%)	2 (1%)
HIV RNA > 50 copies/mL	267 (73%)	164 (90%)
Discontinued due to adverse reactions	11 (3%)	5 (3%)
Discontinued due to virologic failure	0	1 (1%)
Discontinued due to other reasons[1]	12 (3%)	5 (3%)
Missing HIV RNA level	7 (2%)	5 (3%)

1. Includes discontinuations due to consent withdrawn, lost to follow up, non-compliance, protocol violations, pregnancy, and other reasons.

Table 4. HIV RNA Response At Week 24 by Number of Baseline Zidovudine-Associated Mutations in Studies 902 and 907 (Intent-To-Treat)[1]

Number of baseline zidovudine-associated mutations[2]	Change in HIV RNA[3] (N)	
	VIREAD 300 mg	Placebo
None	−0.80 (68)	−0.11 (29)
Any	−0.50 (154)	0 (81)
1 – 2	−0.66 (55)	−0.04 (33)
≥ 3 including M41L or L210W	−0.21 (57)	+0.01 (29)
≥ 3 without M41L or L210W	−0.67 (42)	+0.07 (19)

1. Genotypic testing performed by Virco Laboratories and Visible Genetics TruGene™ technology
2. M41L, D67N, K70R, L210W, T215Y/F or K219Q/E/N in RT
3. Average HIV RNA change from baseline through week 24 ($DAVG_{24}$) in $\log_{10}$ copies/mL

Genotypic Analyses of VIREAD in Patients with Previous Antiretroviral Therapy (Studies 902 and 907)

The virologic response to VIREAD therapy has been evaluated with respect to baseline viral genotype (N=222) in treatment experienced patients participating in trials 902 and 907. In both of these studies, 94% of the participants evaluated had baseline HIV isolates expressing at least one NRTI mutation. These included resistance mutations associated with zidovudine (M41L, D67N, K70R, L210W, T215Y/F or K219Q/E/N), the lamivudine/abacavir-associated mutation (M184V), and others. In addition the majority of participants evaluated had mutations associated with either PI or NNRTI use. Virologic responses for patients in the genotype substudy were similar to the overall results in studies 902 and 907.

The use of resistance testing and the clinical interpretation of genotypic mutations is a complex and evolving field. Conclusions regarding the relevance of particular mutations or mutational patterns are subject to change pending additional data.

Several exploratory analyses were conducted to evaluate the effect of specific mutations and mutational patterns on virologic outcome. Descriptions of numerical differences in HIV RNA response are displayed in Table 4. Because of the large number of potential comparisons, statistical testing was not conducted.

Varying degrees of cross-resistance of VIREAD to pre-existing zidovudine-associated mutations were observed and appeared to depend on the number of specific mutations. VIREAD-treated patients whose HIV expressed 3 or more zidovudine-associated mutations that included either the M41L or L210W reverse transcriptase mutation showed reduced responses to VIREAD therapy; however, these responses were still improved compared with placebo. The presence of the D67N, K70R, T215Y/F or K219Q/E/N mutation did not appear to affect responses to VIREAD therapy. The HIV RNA responses by number and type of baseline zidovudine-associated mutations are shown in Table 4.

[See table 4 above]

In the protocol defined analyses, virologic response to VIREAD was not reduced in patients with HIV that expressed the lamivudine/abacavir-associated M184V mutation. In the absence of zidovudine-associated mutations, patients with the M184V mutation receiving VIREAD showed a -0.84 $\log_{10}$ copies/mL decrease in their HIV RNA relative to placebo. In the presence of zidovudine-associated mutations, the M184V mutation did not affect the mean HIV RNA responses to VIREAD treatment. More data are needed to determine the impact of M184V alone (in the absence of all other NRTI mutations) on subsequent virologic response in patients receiving VIREAD. There were limited data on patients expressing some primary nucleoside reverse transcriptase inhibitor mutations and multi-drug resistant mutations at baseline. However, patients expressing mutations at K65R (N=6), or L74V without zidovudine-associated mutations (N=6) appeared to have reduced virologic responses to VIREAD.

The presence of at least one HIV protease inhibitor or non nucleoside reverse transcriptase inhibitor mutation at baseline did not appear to affect the virologic response to VIREAD. Cross-resistance between VIREAD and HIV protease inhibitors is unlikely because of the different enzyme targets involved.

Phenotypic Analyses of VIREAD in Patients with Previous Antiretroviral Therapy (Studies 902 and 907)

The virologic response to VIREAD therapy has been evaluated with respect to baseline phenotype (N=100) in treatment experienced patients partcipating in trials 902 and 907. Phenotypic analysis of baseline HIV from patients in Studies 902 and 907 demonstrated a correlation between baseline susceptibility to VIREAD and response to VIREAD therapy. Table 5 summarizes the HIV RNA response by baseline VIREAD susceptibility.

Table 5. HIV RNA Response at Week 24 by Baseline VIREAD Susceptibility in Studies 902 and 907 (Intent-To-Treat)[1]

Baseline VIREAD Susceptibility[2]	Change in HIV RNA[3] (N)
≤ 1	−0.74 (35)
> 1 and ≤ 3	−0.56 (49)
> 3 and ≤ 4	−0.3 (7)
≤ 4	−0.61 (91)
> 4	−0.12 (9)

1. Tenofovir susceptibility was determined by recombinant phenotypic Antivirogram™ assay (Virco)
2. Fold change in susceptibility from wild-type
3. Average HIV RNA change from baseline through week 24 ($DAVG_{24}$) in $\log_{10}$ copies/mL

CONTRAINDICATIONS

VIREAD is contraindicated in patients with previously demonstrated hypersensitivity to any of the components of the product.

WARNINGS

Lactic Acidosis/Severe Hepatomegaly with Steatosis

Lactic acidosis and severe hepatomegaly with steatosis, including fatal cases, have been reported with the use of nucleoside analogs alone or in combination with other antiretrovirals. A majority of these cases have been in women. Obesity and prolonged nucleoside exposure may be risk factors. Particular caution should be exercised when administering nucleoside analogs to any patient with known risk factors for liver disease; however, cases have also been reported in patients with no known risk factors. Treatment with VIREAD should be suspended in any patient who develops clinical or laboratory findings suggestive of lactic ac-

Continued on next page

Viread—Cont.

idosis or pronounced hepatotoxicity (which may include hepatomegaly and steatosis even in the absence of marked transaminase elevations).

Renal Impairment
Tenofovir is principally eliminated by the kidney. VIREAD should not be administered to patients with renal insufficiency (creatinine clearance < 60 mL/min) until data become available describing the disposition of VIREAD in these patients.

PRECAUTIONS

Drug Interactions
When administered with VIREAD, C_{max} and AUC of didanosine (administered as the buffered formulation) increased by 28% and 44%, respectively. The mechanism for this interaction is unknown. Although an increased rate of didanosine–associated adverse events has not been observed in pooled clinical studies at this time, long term effects are unknown. Patients taking VIREAD and didanosine concomitantly should be monitored for long term didanosine-associated adverse events. (See CLINICAL PHARMACOLOGY, Drug Interactions and DOSAGE AND ADMINISTRATION)
Since tenofovir is primarily eliminated by the kidneys, coadministration of VIREAD with drugs that reduce renal function or compete for active tubular secretion may increase serum concentrations of tenofovir and/or increase the concentrations of other renally eliminated drugs. Some examples include, but are not limited to, cidofovir, acyclovir, valacyclovir, ganciclovir and valganciclovir.

Hepatic Impairment
The pharmacokinetics of tenofovir have not been studied in patients with hepatic impairment. As tenofovir and tenofovir disoproxil are not metabolized by liver enzymes, the impact of liver impairment should be limited. However, because tenofovir is not entirely renally excreted (70–80%), tenofovir pharmacokinetics may be altered in patients with hepatic insufficiency.

Fat Redistribution
Redistribution/accumulation of body fat including central obesity, dorsocervical fat enlargement (buffalo hump), peripheral wasting, facial wasting, breast enlargement, and "cushingoid appearance" have been observed in patients receiving antiretroviral therapy. The mechanism and long-term consequences of these events are currently unknown. A causal relationship has not been established.

Animal Toxicology
Tenofovir and tenofovir disoproxil fumarate administered in toxicology studies to rats, dogs and monkeys at exposures (based on AUCs) between 6 and 12 fold those observed in humans caused bone toxicity. In monkeys the bone toxicity was diagnosed as osteomalacia. Osteomalacia observed in monkeys appeared to be reversible upon dose reduction or discontinuation of tenofovir. In rats and dogs, the bone toxicity manifested as reduced bone mineral density. The mechanism(s) underlying bone toxicity is unknown.
Evidence of renal toxicity was noted in 4 animal species. Increases in serum creatinine, BUN, glycosuria, proteinuria, phosphaturia and/or calciuria and decreases in serum phosphate were observed to varying degrees in these animals. These toxicities were noted at exposures (based on AUCs) 2–20 times higher than those observed in humans. The relationship of the renal abnormalities, particularly the phosphaturia, to the bone toxicity is not known.

Clinical Monitoring for Bone and Renal Toxicity
It is not known if long term administration of VIREAD (> 1 year) will cause bone abnormalities. Therefore if bone abnormalities are suspected then appropriate consultation should be obtained.
Although tenofovir-associated renal toxicity has not been observed in pooled clinical studies for up to one year, long term renal effects are unknown. Consideration should be given to monitoring for changes in serum creatinine and serum phosphorus in patients at risk or with a history of renal dysfunction.

Carcinogenesis, Mutagenesis, Impairment of Fertility
Long-term carcinogenicity studies of tenofovir disoproxil fumarate in rats and mice are in progress.
Tenofovir disoproxil fumarate was mutagenic in the in vitro mouse lymphoma assay and negative in an in vitro bacterial mutagenicity test (Ames test). In an in vivo mouse micronucleus assay, tenofovir disoproxil fumarate was negative at doses up to 2000 mg/kg when administered to male mice.
There were no effects on fertility, mating performance or early embryonic development when tenofovir disoproxil fumarate was administered at 600 mg/kg/day to male rats for 28 days prior to mating and to female rats for 15 days prior to mating through day seven of gestation. There was, however, an alteration of the estrous cycle in female rats. A dose of 600 mg/kg/day is equivalent to 10 times the human dose based on body surface area comparisons.

Pregnancy
Pregnancy category B: Reproduction studies have been performed in rats and rabbits at doses up to 14 and 19 times the human dose based on body surface area comparisons and revealed no evidence of impaired fertility or harm to the fetus due to tenofovir. There are, however, no adequate and well-controlled studies in pregnant women. Because animal reproduction studies are not always predictive of human response, VIREAD should be used during pregnancy only if clearly needed.
Antiretroviral Pregnancy Registry: To monitor fetal outcomes of pregnant women exposed to VIREAD, an Antiretroviral Pregnancy Registry has been established. Healthcare providers are encouraged to register patients by calling 1-800-258-4263.

Nursing Mothers: The Centers for Disease Control and Prevention recommend that HIV-infected mothers not breast-feed their infants to avoid risking postnatal transmission of HIV. Studies in rats have demonstrated that tenofovir is secreted in milk. It is not known whether tenofovir is excreted in human milk. Because of both the potential for HIV transmission and the potential for serious adverse reactions in nursing infants, **mothers should be instructed not to breast-feed if they are receiving VIREAD.**

Pediatric Use
Safety and effectiveness in pediatric patients have not been established.

Geriatric Use
Clinical studies of VIREAD did not include sufficient numbers of subjects aged 65 and over to determine whether they respond differently from younger subjects. In general, dose selection for the elderly patient should be cautious, keeping in mind the greater frequency of decreased hepatic, renal, or cardiac function, and of concomitant disease or other drug therapy.

ADVERSE REACTIONS

More than 1000 patients have been treated with VIREAD alone or in combination with other antiretroviral medicinal products for periods of 28 days to 143 weeks in Phase I-III clinical trials and a compassionate access study.
Assessment of adverse reactions is based on two studies (902 and 907) in which 653 treatment experienced patients received double-blind treatment with VIREAD 300 mg (n=443) or placebo (n=210) for 24 weeks followed by extended treatment with VIREAD.
Treatment-Related Adverse Events: The most common adverse events that occurred in patients receiving VIREAD with other antiretroviral agents in clinical trials were mild to moderate gastrointestinal events, such as nausea, diarrhea, vomiting and flatulence. Less than 1% of patients discontinued participation in the clinical studies due to gastrointestinal adverse events.
A summary of treatment related adverse events is provided in Table 6 below.

Table 6. Treatment-Related Adverse Events (Grades 1–4) Reported in ≥ 3% of VIREAD-Treated Patients in the Pooled 902 – 907 Studies (0–24 weeks)

	VIREAD 300 mg	Placebo
Number of Patients Treated	443	210
Nausea	11%	10%
Diarrhea	9%	8%
Asthenia	8%	8%
Headache	6%	7%
Vomiting	5%	2%
Flatulence	4%	0%
Abdominal Pain	3%	3%
Anorexia	3%	1%

Laboratory Abnormalities: Laboratory abnormalities observed in these studies occurred with similar frequency in the VIREAD and placebo treated groups. A summary of Grade 3 and 4 laboratory abnormalities is provided in Table 7 below.
[See table above]

Table 7. Grade 3/4 Laboratory Abnormalities Reported in ≥ 1% of VIREAD-Treated Patients in the Pooled 902 – 907 Studies (0–24 weeks)

	VIREAD 300 mg	Placebo
Number of Patients Treated	443	210
Number of Patients with Grade 3 or 4 Laboratory Abnormalities	117 (26%)	78 (37%)
Laboratory abnormalities		
Triglyceride (> 750 mg/dL)	37 (8%)	28 (13%)
Creatine kinase (> 782 U/L)	53 (12%)	38 (18%)
Serum amylase (> 175 U/L)	21 (5%)	14 (7%)
AST (M: >180 U/L) (F: >170 U/L)	16 (4%)	6 (3%)
Urine glucose (3+ or 4+)	12 (3%)	6 (3%)
ALT elevation (M: >215 U/L) (F: >170 U/L)	10 (2%)	4 (2%)
Serum glucose (>250 mg/dL)	8 (2%)	8 (4%)
Neutrophil (<650/mm^3)	6 (1%)	3 (1%)

OVERDOSAGE

Limited clinical experience at doses higher than the therapeutic dose of VIREAD 300 mg is available. In Study 901 tenofovir disoproxil fumarate 600 mg was administered to 8 patients orally for 28 days. No severe adverse reactions were reported. The effects of higher doses are not known.
If overdose occurs the patient must be monitored for evidence of toxicity, and standard supportive treatment applied as necessary.
It is not known whether peritoneal dialysis or hemodialysis increases the rate of elimination of tenofovir.

DOSAGE AND ADMINISTRATION

The dose of VIREAD (tenofovir disoproxil fumarate) is 300 mg once daily taken orally with a meal.
Concomitant administration: Didanosine. When administered with didanosine VIREAD should be administered 2 hours before or one hour after administration of didanosine (See PRECAUTIONS, Drug Interactions).

HOW SUPPLIED

VIREAD is available as tablets. Each tablet contains 300 mg of tenofovir disoproxil fumarate, which is equivalent to 245 mg of tenofovir disoproxil. The tablets are almond-shaped, light blue film-coated, and debossed with "GILEAD" and "4331" on one side and with "300" on the other side. They are packaged as follows: Bottles of 30 tablets (NDC 61958-0401-1) containing a desiccant (silica gel canister or sachet) and closed with child-resistant closure.
Store at 25°C (77°F), excursions permitted to 15–30°C (59–86°F) (see USP Controlled Room Temperature).
Gilead Sciences, Inc.
Foster City, CA 94404
26 October 2001
VIREAD™ is a trademark of Gilead Sciences, Inc.
IN-5078/S
 RM-1351

VIREAD™
(tenofovir disoproxil fumarate) Tablets

Patient Information

VIREAD (veer ee ad)
Generic Name: tenofovir disoproxil fumarate
(te NOE' fo veer dye soe PROX il FYOU-marate)
Read this leaflet carefully before you start taking VIREAD. Also, read it each time you get your VIREAD prescription refilled, in case something has changed. This information does not take the place of talking with your doctor when you start this medicine and at check ups. You should stay under a doctor's care when taking VIREAD. Do not change or stop your medicine without first talking with your doctor. Talk to your doctor if you have any questions about VIREAD.

What is VIREAD and how does it work?
VIREAD is a type of medicine called an HIV (human immunodeficiency virus) nucleotide analog reverse transcriptase inhibitor (NRTI). VIREAD is always used in combination with other anti-HIV medicines to treat people with HIV infection. VIREAD is for adults age 18 and older.
HIV infection destroys CD4 (T) cells, which are important to the immune system. After a large number of T cells are destroyed, acquired immune deficiency syndrome (AIDS) develops.
VIREAD helps to block HIV reverse transcriptase, a chemical in your body (enzyme) that is needed for HIV to multiply. VIREAD lowers the amount of HIV in the blood (called viral load) and may help to increase the number of T cells (called CD4 cells). Lowering the amount of HIV in the blood lowers the chance of death or infections that happen when your immune system is weak (opportunistic infections).

Does VIREAD cure HIV or AIDS?
VIREAD does not cure HIV infection or AIDS. The long-term effects of VIREAD are not known at this time. People taking VIREAD may still get opportunistic infections or

other conditions that happen with HIV infection. Opportunistic infections are infections that develop because the immune system is weak. Some of these conditions are pneumonia, herpes virus infections, and *Mycobacterium avium* complex (MAC) infections.

Does VIREAD reduce the risk of passing HIV to others?
VIREAD does not reduce the risk of passing HIV to others through sexual contact or blood contamination. Continue to practice safe sex and do not use or share dirty needles.

Who should not take VIREAD?
Together with your doctor, you need to decide whether VIREAD is right for you.
Do not take VIREAD if

- you have kidney problems. VIREAD has not been studied in people with kidney problems
- you are allergic to VIREAD or any of its ingredients

What should I tell my doctor before taking VIREAD?
Tell your doctor

- *If you are pregnant or planning to become pregnant:* The effects of VIREAD on pregnant women or their unborn babies are not known.
- *If you are breast-feeding:* Do not breast-feed if you are taking VIREAD. Do not breast-feed if you have HIV. If you are a woman who has or will have a baby, talk with your doctor about the best way to feed your baby. If your baby does not already have HIV, there is a chance that the baby can get HIV through breast-feeding.
- **Tell your doctor about all your medical conditions,** especially liver and kidney problems.
- **Tell your doctor about all the medicines you take,** including prescription and non-prescription medicines and dietary supplements. VIREAD may increase the amount of Videx (didanosine) in your blood. You may need to be followed more carefully if you are taking these two drugs together.

It is a good idea to keep a complete list of all the medicines that you take. Make a new list when medicines are added or stopped. Give copies of this list to all of your healthcare providers **every** time you visit your doctor or fill a prescription.

How should I take VIREAD?

- Stay under a doctor's care when taking VIREAD. Do not change your treatment or stop treatment without first talking with your doctor.
- Take VIREAD every day exactly as your doctor prescribed it. Follow the directions from your doctor, exactly as written on the label. Set up a dosing schedule and follow it carefully.
- The usual dose of VIREAD is 1 tablet once a day, in combination with other anti-HIV medicines.
- Take VIREAD with a meal. The amount of VIREAD in your blood increases with food. Taking it with food helps it work better.
- If you are also taking didanosine you should take VIREAD two hours before or one hour after didanosine.
- When your VIREAD supply starts to run low, get more from your doctor or pharmacy. This is very important because the amount of virus in your blood may increase if the medicine is stopped for even a short time. The virus may develop resistance to VIREAD and become harder to treat.
- Only take medicine that has been prescribed specifically for you. Do not give VIREAD to others or take medicine prescribed for someone else.

What should I do if I miss a dose of VIREAD?
It is important that you do not miss any doses. If you miss a dose of VIREAD, take it as soon as possible and then take your next scheduled dose at its regular time. If it is almost time for your next dose, do not take the missed dose. Wait and take the next dose at the regular time. Do not double the next dose.

What happens if I take too much VIREAD?
If you suspect that you took more than the prescribed dose of VIREAD, contact your local poison control center or emergency room right away.
As with all medicines, VIREAD should be kept out of reach of children.

What should I avoid while taking VIREAD?

- Do not breast-feed. See "What should I tell my doctor before taking VIREAD?"

What are the possible side effects of VIREAD?

- The most common side effects of VIREAD are: diarrhea, nausea, vomiting, and flatulence (intestinal gas).
- VIREAD caused harm to the bones of animals. These effects have not been seen in persons taking VIREAD for up to one year. It is not known if the effects will be seen in persons taking VIREAD for longer periods of time.
- Changes in body fat have been seen in some patients taking anti-HIV medicine. These changes may include increased amount of fat in the upper back and neck ("buffalo hump"), breast, and around the main part of your body (trunk). Loss of fat from the legs, arms and face may also happen. The cause and long term health effects of these conditions are not known at this time.
- There have been other side effects in patients taking VIREAD. However, these side effects may have been due to other medicines that patients were taking or to the illness itself. Some of these side effects can be serious.
- This list of side effects is not complete. If you have questions about side effects, ask your doctor, nurse, or pharmacist. You should report any new or continuing symptoms to your doctor right away. Your doctor may be able to help you manage these side effects.

How do I store VIREAD?

- Keep VIREAD and all other medications out of reach of children.
- Store VIREAD at room temperature 77°F (25°C). It should remain stable until the expiration date printed on the label.
- Do not keep your medicine in places that are too hot or cold.
- Do not keep medicine that is out of date or that you no longer need. If you throw any medicines away make sure that children will not find them.

General advice about prescription medicines:
Talk to your doctor or other health care provider if you have any questions about this medicine or your condition. Medicines are sometimes prescribed for purposes other than those listed in a Patient Information Leaflet. If you have any concerns about this medicine, ask your doctor. Your doctor or pharmacist can give you information about this medicine that was written for health care professionals. Do not use this medicine for a condition for which it was not prescribed. Do not share this medicine with other people.

October 2001
RM-1351

Key Pharmaceuticals, Inc.

GALLOPING HILL ROAD
KENILWORTH, NJ 07033

For Medical Information Contact:
Generally:
Drug Information Services
(800) 526-4099
(9:00 AM to 5:00 PM EST)

After Hours and Weekends:
(908) 298-4000

PROVENTIL® HFA ℞

[*prō 'vĕn-tĭl*]
(albuterol sulfate)
Inhalation Aerosol
FOR ORAL INHALATION ONLY
Prescribing Information

DESCRIPTION

The active component of PROVENTIL HFA (albuterol sulfate) Inhalation Aerosol is albuterol sulfate, USP racemic α^1[(*tert*-Butylamino)methyl]-4-hydroxy-*m*-xylene-α,α'-diol sulfate (2:1)(salt), a relatively selective beta$_2$-adrenergic bronchodilator having the following chemical structure:

Albuterol sulfate is the official generic name in the United States. The World Health Organization recommended name for the drug is salbutamol sulfate. The molecular weight of albuterol sulfate is 576.7, and the empirical formula is $(C_{13}H_{21}NO_3)_2 \bullet H_2SO_4$. Albuterol sulfate is a white to off-white crystalline solid. It is soluble in water and slightly soluble in ethanol. PROVENTIL HFA Inhalation Aerosol is a pressurized metered-dose aerosol unit for oral inhalation. It contains a microcrystalline suspension of albuterol sulfate in propellant HFA-134a (1,1,1,2-tetrafluoroethane), ethanol, and oleic acid.

Each actuation delivers 120 mcg albuterol sulfate, USP from the valve and 108 mcg albuterol sulfate, USP from the mouthpiece (equivalent to 90 mcg of albuterol base from the mouthpiece). Each canister provides 200 inhalations. It is recommended to prime the inhaler before using for the first time and in cases where the inhaler has not been used for more than 2 weeks by releasing four "test sprays" into the air, away from the face.

This product does not contain chlorofluorocarbons (CFCs) as the propellant.

CLINICAL PHARMACOLOGY

Mechanism of Action *In vitro* studies and *in vivo* pharmacologic studies have demonstrated that albuterol has a preferential effect on beta$_2$-adrenergic receptors compared with isoproterenol. While it is recognized that beta$_2$-adrenergic receptors are the predominant receptors on bronchial smooth muscle, data indicate that there is a population of beta$_2$ receptors in the human heart existing in a concentration between 10% and 50% of cardiac beta-adrenergic receptors. The precise function of these receptors has not been established. (See **WARNINGS** for **Cardiovascular Effects.**)

Activation of beta$_2$-adrenergic receptors on airway smooth muscle leads to the activation of adenylcyclase and to an increase in the intracellular concentration of cyclic-3',5'-adenosine monophosphate (cyclic AMP). This increase of cyclic AMP leads to the activation of protein kinase A, which inhibits the phosphorylation of myosin and lowers intracellular ionic calcium concentrations, resulting in relaxation. Albuterol relaxes the smooth muscles of all airways, from the trachea to the terminal bronchioles. Albuterol acts as a functional antagonist to relax the airway irrespective of the spasmogen involved, thus protecting against all bronchoconstrictor challenges. Increased cyclic AMP concentrations are also associated with the inhibition of release of mediators from mast cells in the airway.

Albuterol has been shown in most clinical trials to have more effect on the respiratory tract, in the form of bronchial smooth muscle relaxation, than isoproterenol at comparable doses while producing fewer cardiovascular effects. Controlled clinical studies and other clinical experience have shown that inhaled albuterol, like other beta-adrenergic agonist drugs, can produce a significant cardiovascular effect in some patients, as measured by pulse rate, blood pressure, symptoms, and/or electrocardiographic changes.

Preclinical Intravenous studies in rats with albuterol sulfate have demonstrated that albuterol crosses the blood-brain barrier and reaches brain concentrations amounting to approximately 5% of the plasma concentrations. In structures outside the blood-brain barrier (pineal and pituitary glands), albuterol concentrations were found to be 100 times those in the whole brain.

Studies in laboratory animals (minipigs, rodents, and dogs) have demonstrated the occurrence of cardiac arrhythmias and sudden death (with histologic evidence of myocardial necrosis) when β-agonists and methylxanthines were administered concurrently. The clinical significance of these findings is unknown.

Propellant HFA-134a is devoid of pharmacological activity except at very high doses in animals (380–1300 times the maximum human exposure based on comparisons of AUC values), primarily producing ataxia, tremors, dyspnea, or salivation. These are similar to effects produced by the structurally related chlorofluorocarbons (CFCs), which have been used extensively in metered dose inhalers.

In animals and humans, propellant HFA-134a was found to be rapidly absorbed and rapidly eliminated, with an elimination half-life of 3 to 27 minutes in animals and 5 to 7 minutes in humans. Time to maximum plasma concentration (Tmax) and mean residence time are both extremely short leading to a transient appearance of HFA-134a in the blood with no evidence of accumulation.

Pharmacokinetics In a single-dose bioavailability study which enrolled six healthy, male volunteers, transient low albuterol levels (close to the lower limit of quantitation) were observed after administration of two puffs from both PROVENTIL HFA Inhalation Aerosol and a CFC 11/12 propelled albuterol inhaler. No formal pharmacokinetic analyses were possible for either treatment, but systemic albuterol levels appeared similar.

Clinical Trials In a 12-week, randomized, double-blind, double-dummy, active- and placebo-controlled trial, 565 patients with asthma were evaluated for the bronchodilator efficacy of PROVENTIL HFA Inhalation Aerosol (193 patients) in comparison to a CFC 11/12 propelled albuterol inhaler (186 patients) and an HFA-134a placebo inhaler (186 patients).

Serial FEV$_1$ measurements (shown below as percent change from test-day baseline) demonstrated that two inhalations of PROVENTIL HFA Inhalation Aerosol produced significantly greater improvement in pulmonary function than placebo and produced outcomes which were clinically comparable to a CFC 11/12 propelled albuterol inhaler.

The mean time to onset of a 15% increase in FEV$_1$ was 6 minutes and the mean time to peak effect was 50 to 55 minutes. The mean duration of effect as measured by a 15% increase in FEV$_1$ was 3 hours. In some patients, duration of effect was as long as 6 hours.

In another clinical study in adults, two inhalations of PROVENTIL HFA Inhalation Aerosol taken 30 minutes before exercise prevented exercise-induced bronchospasm as demonstrated by the maintenance of FEV$_1$ within 80% of baseline values in the majority of patients.

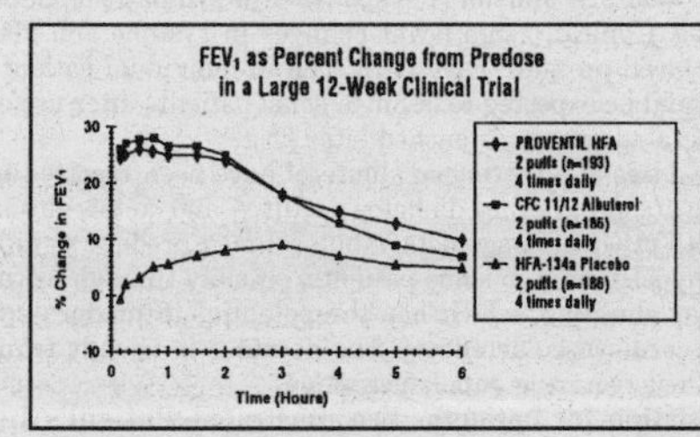

In a 4-week, randomized, open-label trial, 63 children, 4 to 11 years of age, with asthma were evaluated for the bronchodilator efficacy of PROVENTIL HFA Inhalation Aerosol (33 pediatric patients) in comparison to a CFC 11/12 propelled albuterol inhaler (30 pediatric patients).

Serial FEV$_1$ measurements as percent change from test-day baseline demonstrated that two inhalations of PROVENTIL HFA Inhalation Aerosol produced outcomes which were clinically comparable to a CFC 11/12 propelled albuterol inhaler.

The mean time to onset of a 12% increase in FEV$_1$ for PROVENTIL HFA Inhalation Aerosol was 7 minutes and the mean time to peak effect was approximately 50 minutes.

Continued on next page

Proventil HFA—Cont.

The mean duration of effect as measured by a 12% increase in FEV_1 was 2.3 hours. In some pediatric patients, duration of effect was as long as 6 hours.
In another clinical study in pediatric patients, two inhalations of PROVENTIL HFA Inhalation Aerosol taken 30 minutes before exercise provided comparable protection against exercise-induced bronchospasm as a CFC 11/12 propelled albuterol inhaler.

INDICATIONS AND USAGE

PROVENTIL HFA Inhalation Aerosol is indicated in adults and children 4 years of age and older for the treatment or prevention of bronchospasm with reversible obstructive airway disease and for the prevention of exercise-induced bronchospasm.

CONTRAINDICATIONS

PROVENTIL HFA Inhalation Aerosol is contraindicated in patients with a history of hypersensitivity to albuterol or any other PROVENTIL HFA components.

WARNINGS

1. Paradoxical Bronchospasm: Inhaled albuterol sulfate can produce paradoxical bronchospasm that may be life threatening. If paradoxical bronchospasm occurs, PROVENTIL HFA Inhalation Aerosol should be discontinued immediately and alternative therapy instituted. It should be recognized that paradoxical bronchospasm, when associated with inhaled formulations, frequently occurs with the first use of a new canister.
2. Deterioration of Asthma: Asthma may deteriorate acutely over a period of hours or chronically over several days or longer. If the patient needs more doses of PROVENTIL HFA Inhalation Aerosol than usual, this may be a marker of destabilization of asthma and requires reevaluation of the patient and treatment regimen, giving special consideration to the possible need for anti-inflammatory treatment, eg, corticosteroids.
3. Use of Anti-inflammatory Agents: The use of beta-adrenergic-agonist bronchodilators alone may not be adequate to control asthma in many patients. Early consideration should be given to adding anti-inflammatory agents, eg, corticosteroids, to the therapeutic regimen.
4. Cardiovascular Effects: PROVENTIL HFA Inhalation Aerosol, like other beta-adrenergic agonists, can produce clinically significant cardiovascular effects in some patients as measured by pulse rate, blood pressure, and/or symptoms. Although such effects are uncommon after administration of PROVENTIL HFA Inhalation Aerosol at recommended doses, if they occur, the drug may need to be discontinued. In addition, beta agonists have been reported to produce ECG changes, such as flattening of the T wave, prolongation of the QT_c interval, and ST segment depression. The clinical significance of these findings is unknown. Therefore, PROVENTIL HFA Inhalation Aerosol, like all sympathomimetic amines, should be used with caution in patients with cardiovascular disorders, especially coronary insufficiency, cardiac arrhythmias, and hypertension.
5. Do Not Exceed Recommended Dose: Fatalities have been reported in association with excessive use of inhaled sympathomimetic drugs in patients with asthma. The exact cause of death is unknown, but cardiac arrest following an unexpected development of a severe acute asthmatic crisis and subsequent hypoxia is suspected.
6. Immediate Hypersensitivity Reactions: Immediate hypersensitivity reactions may occur after administration of albuterol sulfate, as demonstrated by rare cases of urticaria, angioedema, rash, bronchospasm, anaphylaxis, and oropharyngeal edema.

PRECAUTIONS

General Albuterol sulfate, as with all sympathomimetic amines, should be used with caution in patients with cardiovascular disorders, especially coronary insufficiency, cardiac arrhythmias, and hypertension; in patients with convulsive disorders, hyperthyroidism, or diabetes mellitus; and in patients who are unusually responsive to sympathomimetic amines. Clinically significant changes in systolic and diastolic blood pressure have been seen in individual patients and could be expected to occur in some patients after use of any beta-adrenergic bronchodilator.
Large doses of intravenous albuterol have been reported to aggravate preexisting diabetes mellitus and ketoacidosis. As with other beta-agonists, albuterol may produce significant hypokalemia in some patients, possibly through intracellular shunting, which has the potential to produce adverse cardiovascular effects. The decrease is usually transient, not requiring supplementation.
Information for Patients See illustrated **Patient's Instructions for Use**. SHAKE WELL BEFORE USING. Patients should be given the following information:
It is recommended to prime the inhaler before using for the first time and in cases where the inhaler has not been used for more than 2 weeks by releasing four "test sprays" into the air, away from the face.
KEEPING THE PLASTIC MOUTHPIECE CLEAN IS VERY IMPORTANT TO PREVENT MEDICATION BUILD-UP AND BLOCKAGE. THE MOUTHPIECE SHOULD BE WASHED, SHAKEN TO REMOVE EXCESS WATER, AND AIR DRIED THOROUGHLY AT LEAST ONCE A WEEK. INHALER MAY CEASE TO DELIVER MEDICATION IF NOT PROPERLY CLEANED.
The mouthpiece should be cleaned (with the canister removed) by running warm water through the top and bottom for 30 seconds at least once a week. The mouthpiece must be shaken to remove excess water, then air dried thoroughly

Adverse Experience Incidences (% of patients) in a Large 12-week Clinical Trial*

Body System/ Adverse Event (Preferred Term)		PROVENTIL HFA Inhalation Aerosol (N = 193)	CFG 11/12 Propelled Albuterol Inhaler (N = 186)	HFA-134a Placebo Inhaler (N = 186)
Application Site Disorders	Inhalation Site Sensation	6	9	2
	Inhalation Taste Sensation	4	3	3
Body as a Whole	Allergic Reaction/Symptoms	6	4	<1
	Back Pain	4	2	3
	Fever	6	2	5
Central and Peripheral Nervous System	Tremor	7	8	2
Gastrointestinal System	Nausea	10	9	5
	Vomiting	7	2	3
Heart Rate and Rhythm Disorder	Tachycardia	7	2	<1
Psychiatric Disorders	Nervousness	7	9	3
Respiratory System Disorders	Respiratory Disorder (unspecified)	6	4	5
	Rhinitis	16	22	14
	Upper Resp Tract Infection	21	20	18
Urinary System Disorder	Urinary Tract Infection	3	4	2

*This table includes all adverse events (whether considered by the investigator drug related or unrelated to drug) which occurred at an incidence rate of at least 3.0% in the PROVENTIL HFA Inhalation Aerosol group and more frequently in the PROVENTIL HFA Inhalation Aerosol group than in the HFA-134a placebo inhaler group.

(such as overnight). Blockage from medication build-up or improper medication delivery may result from failure to thoroughly air dry the mouthpiece.
If the mouthpiece should become blocked (little or no medication coming out of the mouthpiece), the blockage may be removed by washing as described above.
If it is necessary to use the inhaler before it is completely dry, shake off excess water, replace canister, test spray twice away from face, and take the prescribed dose. After such use, the mouthpiece should be rewashed and allowed to air dry thoroughly.
The action of PROVENTIL HFA Inhalation Aerosol should last up to 4 to 6 hours. PROVENTIL HFA Inhalation Aerosol should not be used more frequently than recommended. Do not increase the dose or frequency of doses of PROVENTIL HFA Inhalation Aerosol without consulting your physician. If you find that treatment with PROVENTIL HFA Inhalation Aerosol becomes less effective for symptomatic relief, your symptoms become worse, and/or you need to use the product more frequently than usual, medical attention should be sought immediately. While you are taking PROVENTIL HFA Inhalation Aerosol, other inhaled drugs and asthma medications should be taken only as directed by your physician.
Common adverse effects of treatment with inhaled albuterol include palpitations, chest pain, rapid heart rate, tremor, or nervousness. If you are pregnant or nursing, contact your physician about use of PROVENTIL HFA Inhalation Aerosol. Effective and safe use of PROVENTIL HFA Inhalation Aerosol includes an understanding of the way that it should be administered. Use PROVENTIL HFA Inhalation Aerosol only with the actuator supplied with the product. Discard the canister after 200 sprays have been used.
In general, the technique for administering PROVENTIL HFA Inhalation Aerosol to children is similar to that for adults. Children should use PROVENTIL HFA Inhalation Aerosol under adult supervision, as instructed by the patient's physician. (See Patient's Instructions for Use).
Drug Interactions
1. Beta Blockers: Beta-adrenergic-receptor blocking agents not only block the pulmonary effect of beta agonists, such as PROVENTIL HFA Inhalation Aerosol, but may produce severe bronchospasm in asthmatic patients. Therefore, patients with asthma should not normally be treated with beta blockers. However, under certain circumstances, eg, as prophylaxis after myocardial infarction, there may be no acceptable alternatives to the use of beta-adrenergic-blocking agents in patients with asthma. In this setting, cardioselective beta blockers should be considered, although they should be administered with caution.
2. Diuretics: The ECG changes and/or hypokalemia which may result from the administration of nonpotassium sparing diuretics (such as loop or thiazide diuretics) can be acutely worsened by beta agonists, especially when the recommended dose of the beta agonist is exceeded. Although the clinical significance of these effects is not known, caution is advised in the coadministration of beta agonists with nonpotassium sparing diuretics.
3. Albuterol-Digoxin: Mean decreases of 16% and 22% in serum digoxin levels were demonstrated after single-dose intravenous and oral administration of albuterol, respectively, to normal volunteers who had received digoxin for 10 days. The clinical significance of these findings for patients with obstructive airway disease who are receiving albuterol and digoxin on a chronic basis is unclear; nevertheless, it would be prudent to carefully evaluate the serum digoxin levels in patients who are currently receiving digoxin and albuterol.
4. Monoamine Oxidase Inhibitors or Tricyclic Antidepressants: PROVENTIL HFA Inhalation Aerosol should be administered with extreme caution to patients being treated with monoamine oxidase inhibitors or tricyclic antidepressants, or within 2 weeks of discontinuation of such agents, because the action of albuterol on the cardiovascular system may be potentiated.
Carcinogenesis, Mutagenesis, and Impairment of Fertility
In a 2-year study in Sprague-Dawley rats, albuterol sulfate caused a dose-related increase in the incidence of benign leiomyomas of the mesovarium at and above dietary doses of 2 mg/kg (approximately 15 times the maximum recommended daily inhalation dose for adults on a mg/m^2 basis and approximately 6 times the maximum recommended daily inhalation dose for children on a mg/m^2 basis). In another study this effect was blocked by the coadministration of propranolol, a nonselective beta-adrenergic antagonist. In an 18-month study in CD-1 mice, albuterol sulfate showed no evidence of tumorigenicity at dietary doses of up to 500 mg/kg (approximately 1700 times the maximum recommended daily inhalation dose for adults on a mg/m^2 basis and approximately 800 times the maximum recommended daily inhalation dose for children on a mg/m^2 basis). In a 22-month study in Golden Hamsters, albuterol sulfate showed no evidence of tumorigenicity at dietary doses of up to 50 mg/kg (approximately 225 times the maximum recommended daily inhalation dose for adults on a mg/m^2 basis and approximately 110 times the maximum recommended daily inhalation dose for children on a mg/m^2 basis).
Albuterol sulfate was not mutagenic in the Ames test or a mutation test in yeast. Albuterol sulfate was not clastogenic in a human peripheral lymphocyte assay or in an AH1 strain mouse micronucleus assay.
Reproduction studies in rats demonstrated no evidence of impaired fertility at oral doses up to 50 mg/kg (approximately 340 times the maximum recommended daily inhalation dose for adults on a mg/m^2 basis).
Pregnancy: *Teratogenic Effects:* Pregnancy Category C
Albuterol sulfate has been shown to be teratogenic in mice. A study in CD-1 mice given albuterol sulfate subcutaneously showed cleft palate formation in 5 of 111 (4.5%) fetuses at 0.25 mg/kg (less than the maximum recommended daily inhalation dose for adults on a mg/m^2 basis) and in 10 of 108 (9.3%) fetuses at 2.5 mg/kg (approximately 8 times the maximum recommended daily inhalation dose for adults on a mg/m^2 basis). The drug did not induce cleft palate formation at a dose of 0.025 mg/kg (less than the maximum recommended daily inhalation dose for adults on a mg/m^2 basis). Cleft palate also occurred in 22 of 72 (30.5%) fetuses from females treated subcutaneously with 2.5 mg/kg of isoproterenol (positive control).
A reproduction study in Stride Dutch rabbits revealed cranioschisis in 7 of 19 (37%) fetuses when albuterol sulfate was administered orally at 50 mg/kg dose (approximately 680 times the maximum recommended daily inhalation dose for adults on a mg/m^2 basis).
In an inhalation reproduction study in Sprague-Dawley rats, the albuterol sulfate/HFA-134a formulation did not exhibit any teratogenic effects at 10.5 mg/kg (approximately 70 times the maximum recommended daily inhalation dose for adults on a mg/m^2 basis).
A study in which pregnant rats were dosed with radiolabeled albuterol sulfate demonstrated that drug-related material is transferred from the maternal circulation to the fetus.
There are no adequate and well-controlled studies of PROVENTIL HFA Inhalation Aerosol or albuterol sulfate in pregnant women. PROVENTIL HFA Inhalation Aerosol should be used during pregnancy only if the potential benefit justifies the potential risk to the fetus.
During worldwide marketing experience, various congenital anomalies, including cleft palate and limb defects, have been reported in the offspring of patients being treated with albuterol. Some of the mothers were taking multiple medications during their pregnancies. Because no consistent pattern of defects can be discerned, a relationship between albuterol use and congenital anomalies has not been established.

Use in Labor and Delivery
Because of the potential for beta-agonist interference with uterine contractility, use of PROVENTIL HFA Inhalation Aerosol for relief of bronchospasm during labor should be restricted to those patients in whom the benefits clearly outweigh the risk.
Tocolysis: Albuterol has not been approved for the management of preterm labor. The benefit:risk ratio when albuterol is administered for tocolysis has not been established. Serious adverse reactions, including pulmonary edema, have been reported during or following treatment of premature labor with $beta_2$-agonists, including albuterol.
Nursing Mothers
Plasma levels of albuterol sulfate and HFA-134a after inhaled therapeutic doses are very low in humans, but it is not known whether the components of PROVENTIL HFA Inhalation Aerosol are excreted in human milk.
Because of the potential for tumorigenicity shown for albuterol in animal studies and lack of experience with the use of PROVENTIL HFA Inhalation Aerosol by nursing mothers, a decision should be made whether to discontinue nursing or to discontinue the drug, taking into account the importance of the drug to the mother. Caution should be exercised when albuterol sulfate is administered to a nursing woman.
Pediatrics
The safety and effectiveness of PROVENTIL HFA Inhalation Aerosol in pediatric patients below the age of 4 years have not been established.
Geriatrics
PROVENTIL HFA Inhalation Aerosol has not been studied in a geriatric population. As with other $beta_2$-agonists, special caution should be observed when using PROVENTIL HFA Inhalation Aerosol in elderly patients who have concomitant cardiovascular disease that could be adversely affected by this class of drug.

ADVERSE REACTIONS

Adverse reaction information concerning PROVENTIL HFA Inhalation Aerosol is derived from a 12-week, double-blind, double-dummy study which compared PROVENTIL HFA Inhalation Aerosol, a CFC 11/12 propelled albuterol inhaler, and an HFA-134a placebo inhaler in 565 asthmatic patients. The following table lists the incidence of all adverse events (whether considered by the investigator drug related or unrelated to drug) from this study which occurred at a rate of 3% or greater in the PROVENTIL HFA Inhalation Aerosol treatment group and more frequently in the PROVENTIL HFA Inhalation Aerosol treatment group than in the placebo group. Overall, the incidence and nature of the adverse reactions reported for PROVENTIL HFA Inhalation Aerosol and a CFC 11/12 propelled albuterol inhaler were comparable.
[See table at top of previous page]
Adverse events reported by less than 3% of the patients receiving PROVENTIL HFA Inhalation Aerosol, and by a greater proportion of PROVENTIL HFA Inhalation Aerosol patients than placebo patients, which have the potential to be related to PROVENTIL HFA Inhalation Aerosol include: dysphonia, increased sweating, dry mouth, chest pain, edema, rigors, ataxia, leg cramps, hyperkinesia, eructation, flatulence, tinnitus, diabetes mellitus, anxiety, depression, somnolence, rash. Palpitation and dizziness have also been observed with PROVENTIL HFA Inhalation Aerosol.
Adverse events reported in a 4-week pediatric clinical trial comparing PROVENTIL HFA Inhalation Aerosol and a CFC 11/12 propelled albuterol inhaler occurred at a low incidence rate and were similar to those seen in the adult trials.
In small, cumulative dose studies, tremor, nervousness, and headache appeared to be dose related.
Rare cases of urticaria, angioedema, rash, bronchospasm, and oropharyngeal edema have been reported after the use of inhaled albuterol. In addition, albuterol, like other sympathomimetic agents, can cause adverse reactions such as hypertension, angina, vertigo, central nervous system stimulation, insomnia, headache, and drying or irritation of the oropharynx.

OVERDOSAGE

The expected symptoms with overdosage are those of excessive beta-adrenergic stimulation and/or occurrence or exaggeration of any of the symptoms listed under **ADVERSE REACTIONS**, eg, seizures, angina, hypertension or hypotension, tachycardia with rates up to 200 beats per minute, arrhythmias, nervousness, headache, tremor, dry mouth, palpitation, nausea, dizziness, fatigue, malaise, and insomnia.
Hypokalemia may also occur. As with all sympathomimetic medications, cardiac arrest and even death may be associated with abuse of PROVENTIL HFA Inhalation Aerosol. Treatment consists of discontinuation of PROVENTIL HFA Inhalation Aerosol together with appropriate symptomatic therapy. The judicious use of a cardioselective beta-receptor blocker may be considered, bearing in mind that such medication can produce bronchospasm. There is insufficient evidence to determine if dialysis is beneficial for overdosage of PROVENTIL HFA Inhalation Aerosol.
The oral median lethal dose of albuterol sulfate in mice is greater than 2000 mg/kg (approximately 6800 times the maximum recommended daily inhalation dose for adults on a mg/m^2 basis and approximately 3200 times the maximum recommended daily inhalation dose for children on a mg/m^2 basis). In mature rats, the subcutaneous median lethal dose of albuterol sulfate is approximately 450 mg/kg (approximately 3000 times the maximum recommended daily inhalation dose for adults on a mg/m^2 basis and approximately 1400 times the maximum recommended daily inhalation dose for children on a mg/m^2 basis). In young rats, the subcutaneous median lethal dose is approximately 2000 mg/kg (approximately 14,000 times the maximum recommended daily inhalation dose for adults on a mg/m^2 basis and approximately 6400 times the maximum recommended daily inhalation dose for children on a mg/m^2 basis). The inhalation median lethal dose has not been determined in animals.

DOSAGE AND ADMINISTRATION

For treatment of acute episodes of bronchospasm or prevention of asthmatic symptoms, the usual dosage for adults and children 4 years of age and older is two inhalations repeated every 4 to 6 hours. More frequent administration or a larger number of inhalations is not recommended. In some patients, one inhalation every 4 hours may be sufficient. Each actuation of PROVENTIL HFA Inhalation Aerosol delivers 108 mcg of albuterol sulfate (equivalent to 90 mcg of albuterol base) from the mouthpiece. It is recommended to prime the inhaler before using for the first time and in cases where the inhaler has not been used for more than 2 weeks by releasing four "test sprays" into the air, away from the face.
Exercise Induced Bronchospasm Prevention: The usual dosage for adults and children 4 years of age and older is two inhalations 15 to 30 minutes before exercise.
To maintain proper use of this product, it is important that the mouthpiece be washed and dried thoroughly at least once a week. The inhaler may cease to deliver medication if not properly cleaned and dried thoroughly. See **Information for Patients**. Keeping the plastic mouthpiece clean is very important to prevent medication build-up and blockage. The inhaler may cease to deliver medication if not properly cleaned and air dried thoroughly. If the mouthpiece becomes blocked, washing the mouthpiece will remove the blockage.
If a previously effective dose regimen fails to provide the usual response, this may be a marker of destabilization of asthma and requires reevaluation of the patient and the treatment regimen, giving special consideration to the possible need for anti-inflammatory treatment, eg, corticosteroids.

HOW SUPPLIED

PROVENTIL HFA (albuterol sulfate) Inhalation Aerosol is supplied as a pressurized aluminum canister with a yellow plastic actuator and orange dust cap each in boxes of one. Each actuation delivers 120 mcg of albuterol sulfate from the valve and 108 mcg of albuterol sulfate from the mouthpiece (equivalent to 90 mcg of albuterol base). Canisters with a labeled net weight of 6.7 g contain 200 inhalations (NDC 0085-1132-01).
Rx only. Store between 15° and 25°C (59° and 77°F). For best results, canister should be at room temperature before use.
SHAKE WELL BEFORE USING.
The yellow actuator supplied with PROVENTIL HFA Inhalation Aerosol should not be used with any other product canisters, and actuator from other products should not be used with a PROVENTIL HFA Inhalation Aerosol canister. The correct amount of medication in each canister cannot be assured after 200 actuations, even though the canister is not completely empty. The canister should be discarded when the labeled number of actuations have been used.
WARNING: Avoid spraying in eyes. Contents under pressure. Do not puncture or incinerate. Exposure to temperatures above 120°F may cause bursting. Keep out of reach of children.
PROVENTIL HFA Inhalation Aerosol does not contain chlorofluorocarbons (CFCs) as the propellant.
Developed and Manufactured by
3M Health Care Limited
Loughborough UK
or
3M Pharmaceuticals,
Northridge, CA 91324
for
Key Pharmaceuticals, Inc.
Kenilworth, NJ 07033 USA

B03085

 23800110T
Rev. 10/01 23549620

PROVENTIL® HFA
(albuterol sulfate)
Inhalation Aerosol
FOR ORAL INHALATION ONLY
Patient's Instructions for Use

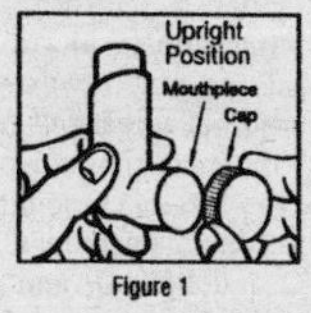

Figure 1

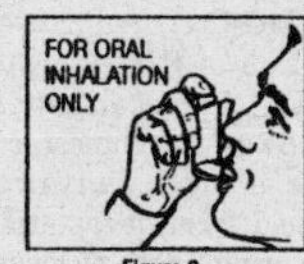

Figure 2

Before using your PROVENTIL HFA (albuterol sulfate) Inhalation Aerosol, read complete instructions carefully. Children should use PROVENTIL HFA Inhalation Aerosol under adult supervision, as instructed by the patient's doctor. Please note that (CFC-free symbol) indicates that this inhalation aerosol does not contain chlorofluorocarbons (CFCs) as the propellant.

1. SHAKE THE INHALER WELL immediately before each use. **Then remove the cap from the mouthpiece** (see Figure 1). **Check mouthpiece for foreign objects prior to use.** Make sure the canister is fully inserted into the actuator.
2. As with all aerosol medications, it is recommended to prime the inhaler before using for the first time and in cases where the inhaler has not been used for more than 2 weeks. Prime by releasing four "test sprays" into the air, away from your face.
3. BREATHE OUT FULLY THROUGH THE MOUTH, expelling as much air from your lungs as possible. Place the mouthpiece fully into the mouth holding the inhaler in its upright position (see Figure 2) and closing the lips around it.
4. WHILE BREATHING IN DEEPLY AND SLOWLY THROUGH THE MOUTH, FULLY DEPRESS THE TOP OF THE METAL CANISTER with your index finger (see Figure 2).
5. HOLD YOUR BREATH AS LONG AS POSSIBLE, up to 10 seconds. Before breathing out, remove the inhaler from your mouth and release your finger from the canister.
6. If your physician has prescribed additional puffs, wait 1 minute, shake the inhaler again, and repeat steps 2 through 4. Replace the cap after use.
7. KEEPING THE PLASTIC MOUTHPIECE CLEAN IS EXTREMELY IMPORTANT TO PREVENT MEDICATION BUILD-UP AND BLOCKAGE. THE MOUTHPIECE SHOULD BE WASHED, SHAKEN TO REMOVE EXCESS WATER, AND AIR DRIED THOROUGHLY AT LEAST ONCE A WEEK. INHALER MAY STOP SPRAYING IF NOT PROPERLY CLEANED.
   Routine cleaning instructions:
   Step 1. To clean, remove the canister and mouthpiece cap. Wash the mouthpiece through the top and bottom with warm running water for 30 seconds at least once a week (see Figure A). **Never immerse the metal canister in water.**

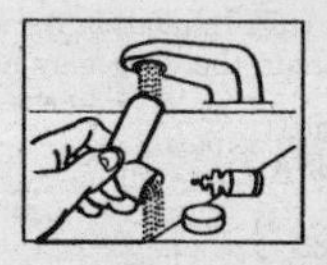
Figure A Wash mouthpiece under warm running water.

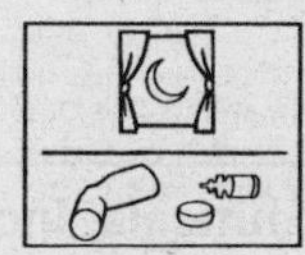
Figure B Allow mouthpiece to air dry, such as overnight.

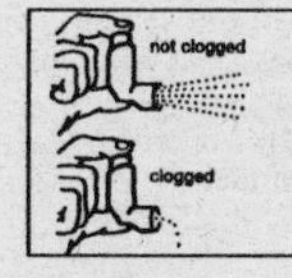

Figure C When blocked, little or no medicine comes out.

   Step 2. To dry, shake off excess water and let the mouthpiece air dry thoroughly, such as overnight (see Figure B). When the mouthpiece is dry, replace the canister and the mouthpiece cap. Blockage from medication build-up is more likely to occur if the mouthpiece is not allowed to air dry thoroughly.
   IF YOUR INHALER HAS BECOME BLOCKED (little or no medication coming out of the mouthpiece, see Figure C), wash the mouthpiece as described in Step 1 and air dry thoroughly as described in Step 2.
   IF YOU NEED TO USE YOUR INHALER BEFORE IT IS COMPLETELY DRY, SHAKE OFF EXCESS WATER, replace the canister, and test spray twice into the air, away from your face, to remove most of the water remaining in the mouthpiece. Then take your dose as prescribed. **After such use, rewash and air dry thoroughly as described in Steps 1 and 2.**
8. The correct amount of medication in each inhalation cannot be assured after 200 actuations, even though the canister is not completely empty. The canister should be discarded when the labeled number of actuations have been used. Before you reach the specific number of actuations, you should consult your physician to determine whether a refill is needed. Just as you should not take extra doses without consulting your physician, you also should not stop using PROVENTIL HFA Inhalation Aerosol without consulting your physician.

You may notice a slightly different taste or spray force than you are used to with PROVENTIL HFA Inhalation Aerosol, compared to other albuterol inhalation aerosol products.

Continued on next page

Proventil HFA—Cont.

DOSAGE:

Use only as directed by your physician.

WARNINGS:

The action of PROVENTIL HFA Inhalation Aerosol should last up to 4 to 6 hours. PROVENTIL HFA Inhalation Aerosol should not be used more frequently than recommended. Do not increase the number of puffs or frequency of doses of PROVENTIL HFA Inhalation Aerosol without consulting your physician. If you find that treatment with PROVENTIL HFA Inhalation Aerosol becomes less effective for symptomatic relief, your symptoms become worse, and/or you need to use the product more frequently than usual, medical attention should be sought immediately. While you are taking PROVENTIL HFA Inhalation Aerosol, other inhaled drugs should be taken only as directed by your physician. If you are pregnant or nursing, contact your physician about the use of PROVENTIL HFA Inhalation Aerosol.

Common adverse effects of treatment with PROVENTIL HFA Inhalation Aerosol include palpitations, chest pain, rapid heart rate, tremor, or nervousness. Effective and safe use of PROVENTIL HFA Inhalation Aerosol includes an understanding of the way that it should be administered. Use PROVENTIL HFA Inhalation Aerosol only with the yellow actuator supplied with the product. The PROVENTIL HFA Inhalation Aerosol actuator should not be used with other aerosol medications.

For best results, use at room temperature. Avoid exposing product to extreme heat and cold.

Shake well before use.

Contents Under Pressure.

Do not puncture. Do not store near heat or open flame. Exposure to temperatures above 120°F may cause bursting. Never throw container into fire or incinerator. Store between 15° and 25°C (59° and 77°F). Avoid spraying in eyes. Keep out of reach of children.

Further Information: Your PROVENTIL HFA (albuterol sulfate) Inhalation Aerosol does not contain chlorofluorocarbons (CFCs) as the propellant. Instead, the inhaler contains a hydrofluoroalkane (HFA-134a) as the propellant.

Developed and Manufactured by
3M Health Care Limited
Loughborough UK
or
3M Pharmaceuticals
Northridge, CA 91324
for
Key Pharmaceuticals, Inc.
Kenilworth, NJ 07033 USA
Rev. 10/01 23549620
U.S. Patent No. 5,225,183

Kos Pharmaceuticals, Inc.

1001 BRICKELL BAY DRIVE
25TH FLOOR
MIAMI, FL 33131

For medical information contact:

Drug Information Services
1-888-4-LIPIDS
1-888-454-7437

ADVICOR™ ℞

[ad' vĭ kor"]

(niacin extended-release and lovastatin tablets)

Rx Only

DESCRIPTION

ADVICOR contains niacin extended-release and lovastatin in combination. Niacin, a B-complex vitamin, and lovastatin, an inhibitor of 3-hydroxy-3-methylglutaryl-coenzyme A (HMG-CoA) reductase, are both lipid-altering agents.

Niacin is nicotinic acid, or 3-pyridinecarboxylic acid. Niacin is a white, nonhygroscopic crystalline powder that is very soluble in water, boiling ethanol and propylene glycol. It is insoluble in ethyl ether. The empirical formula of niacin is $C_6H_5NO_2$ and its molecular weight is 123.11. Niacin has the following structural formula:

[structural formula: pyridine ring with N and COOH]

Lovastatin is [1S -[1(alpha)(R *), 3(alpha), 7(beta), 8(beta)(2S *, 4S *), 8a(beta)]]-1,2,3, 7,8,8a-hexahydro-3,7-dimethyl-8-[2-(tetrahydro-4-hydroxy-6-oxo-2H-pyran-2-yl) ethyl]-1-naphthalenyl 2-methylbutanoate. Lovastatin is a white, nonhygroscopic crystalline powder that is insoluble in water and sparingly soluble in ethanol, methanol, and acetonitrile. The empirical formula of lovastatin is $C_{24}H_{36}O_5$ and its molecular weight is 404.55. Lovastatin has the following structural formula:

[structural formula: lovastatin, with labels HO, H, O, H_3C, H, CH_3, H_3C, H]

ADVICOR tablets contain the labeled amount of niacin and lovastatin and have the following inactive ingredients: hydroxypropyl methylcellulose, povidone, stearic acid, polyethylene glycol, titanium dioxide, polysorbate 80. The individual tablet strengths (expressed in terms of mg niacin/mg lovastatin) contain the following coloring agents:

ADVICOR 500 mg/20 mg - synthetic red and yellow iron oxides.

ADVICOR 750 mg/20 mg - FD & C Yellow # 6 Aluminum Lake.

ADVICOR 1000 mg/20 mg - synthetic red, yellow, and black iron oxides.

CLINICAL PHARMACOLOGY

A variety of clinical studies have demonstrated that elevated levels of total cholesterol (TC), low-density lipoprotein cholesterol (LDL-C), and apolipoprotein B-100 (Apo B) promote human atherosclerosis. Similarly, decreased levels of high-density lipoprotein cholesterol (HDL-C) are associated with the development of atherosclerosis. Epidemiological investigations have established that cardiovascular morbidity and mortality vary directly with the level of TC and LDL-C, and inversely with the level of HDL-C.

Cholesterol-enriched triglyceride-rich lipoproteins, including very low-density lipoproteins (VLDL), intermediate-density lipoproteins (IDL), and their remnants, can also promote atherosclerosis. Elevated plasma triglycerides (TG) are frequently found in a triad with low HDL-C levels and small LDL particles, as well as in association with non-lipid metabolic risk factors for coronary heart disease (CHD). As such, total plasma TG have not consistently been shown to be an independent risk factor for CHD.

As an adjunct to diet, the efficacy of niacin and lovastatin in improving lipid profiles (either individually, or in combination with each other, or niacin in combination with other statins) for the treatment of dyslipidemia has been well documented. The effect of combined therapy with niacin and lovastatin on cardiovascular morbidity and mortality has not been determined.

Effects on Lipids

ADVICOR

ADVICOR reduces LDL-C, TC, and TG, and increases HDL-C due to the individual actions of niacin and lovastatin. The magnitude of individual lipid and lipoprotein responses may be influenced by the severity and type of underlying lipid abnormality.

Niacin

Niacin functions in the body after conversion to nicotinamide adenine dinucleotide (NAD) in the NAD coenzyme system. Niacin (but not nicotinamide) in gram doses reduces LDL-C, Apo B, Lp(a), TG, and TC, and increases HDL-C. The increase in HDL-C is associated with an increase in apolipoprotein A-I (Apo A-I) and a shift in the distribution of HDL subfractions. These shifts include an increase in the HDL_2:HDL_3 ratio, and an elevation in lipoprotein A-I (Lp A-I, an HDL-C particle containing only Apo A-I). In addition, preliminary reports suggest that niacin causes favorable LDL particle size transformations, although the clinical relevance of this effect is not yet clear.

Lovastatin

Lovastatin has been shown to reduce both normal and elevated LDL-C concentrations. Apo B also falls substantially during treatment with lovastatin. Since each LDL-C particle contains one molecule of Apo B, and since little Apo B is found in other lipoproteins, this strongly suggests that lovastatin does not merely cause cholesterol to be lost from LDL-C, but also reduces the concentration of circulating LDL particles. In addition, lovastatin can produce increases of variable magnitude in HDL-C, and modestly reduces VLDL-C and plasma TG. The effects of lovastatin on Lp(a), fibrinogen, and certain other independent biochemical risk markers for coronary heart disease are not well characterized.

Mechanism of Action

Niacin

The mechanism by which niacin alters lipid profiles is not completely understood and may involve several actions, including partial inhibition of release of free fatty acids from adipose tissue, and increased lipoprotein lipase activity (which may increase the rate of chylomicron triglyceride removal from plasma). Niacin decreases the rate of hepatic synthesis of VLDL-C and LDL-C, and does not appear to affect fecal excretion of fats, sterols, or bile acids.

Lovastatin

Lovastatin is a specific inhibitor of 3-hydroxy-3-methylglutaryl-coenzyme A (HMG-CoA) reductase, the enzyme that catalyzes the conversion of HMG-CoA to mevalonate. The conversion of HMG-CoA to mevalonate is an early step in the biosynthetic pathway for cholesterol. Lovastatin is a prodrug and has little, if any, activity until hydrolyzed to its active beta-hydroxyacid form, lovastatin acid. The mechanism of the LDL-lowering effect of lovastatin may involve both reduction of VLDL-C concentration and induction of the LDL receptor, leading to reduced production and/or increased catabolism of LDL-C.

Pharmacokinetics

Absorption and Bioavailability

ADVICOR

In single-dose studies of ADVICOR, rate and extent of niacin and lovastatin absorption were bioequivalent under fed conditions to that from NIASPAN® and Mevacor® tablets, respectively. After administration of two ADVICOR 1000 mg/20 mg tablets, peak niacin concentrations averaged about 18 mcg/mL and occurred about 5 hours after dosing; about 72% of the niacin dose was absorbed according to the urinary excretion data. Peak lovastatin concentrations averaged about 11 ng/mL and occurred about 2 hours after dosing.

The extent of niacin absorption from ADVICOR was increased by administration with food. The administration of two ADVICOR 1000 mg/20 mg tablets under low-fat or high-fat conditions resulted in a 22 to 30% increase in niacin bioavailability relative to dosing under fasting conditions. Lovastatin bioavailability is affected by food. Lovastatin Cmax was increased 48% and 21% after a high- and a low-fat meal, respectively, but the lovastatin AUC was decreased 26% and 24% after a high- and a low-fat meal, respectively, compared to those under fasting conditions.

Niacin

Due to extensive and saturable first-pass metabolism, niacin concentrations in the general circulation are dose dependent and highly variable. Peak steady-state niacin concentrations were 0.6, 4.9, and 15.5 mcg/mL after doses of 1000, 1500, and 2000 mg NIASPAN once daily (given as two 500 mg, two 750 mg, and two 1000 mg tablets, respectively).

Lovastatin

Lovastatin appears to be incompletely absorbed after oral administration. Because of extensive hepatic extraction, the amount of lovastatin reaching the systemic circulation as active inhibitors after oral administration is low (<5%) and shows considerable inter-individual variation. Peak concentrations of active and total inhibitors occur within 2 to 4 hours after Mevacor administration.

Lovastatin absorption appears to be increased by at least 30% by grapefruit juice; however, the effect is dependent on the amount of grapefruit juice consumed and the interval between grapefruit juice and lovastatin ingestion.

With a once-a-day dosing regimen, plasma concentrations of total inhibitors over a dosing interval achieved a steady-state between the second and third days of therapy and were about 1.5 times those following a single dose of Mevacor.

Distribution

Niacin

Niacin is less than 20% bound to human serum proteins and distributes into milk. Studies using radiolabeled niacin in mice show that niacin and its metabolites concentrate in the liver, kidney, and adipose tissue.

Lovastatin

Both lovastatin and its beta-hydroxyacid metabolite are highly bound (>95%) to human plasma proteins. Distribution of lovastatin or its metabolites into human milk is unknown; however, lovastatin distributes into milk in rats. In animal studies, lovastatin concentrated in the liver, and crossed the blood-brain and placental barriers.

Metabolism

Niacin

Niacin undergoes rapid and extensive first-pass metabolism that is dose-rate specific and, at the doses used to treat dyslipidemia, saturable. In humans, one pathway is through a simple conjugation step with glycine to form nicotinuric acid (NUA). NUA is then excreted, although there may be a small amount of reversible metabolism back to niacin. The other pathway results in the formation of NAD. It is unclear whether nicotinamide is formed as a precursor to, or following the synthesis of, NAD. Nicotinamide is further metabolized to at least N-methylnicotinamide (MNA) and nicotinamide-N-oxide (NNO). MNA is further metabolized to two other compounds, N-methyl-2-pyridone-5-carboxamide (2PY) and N-methyl-4-pyridone-5-carboxamide (4PY). The formation of 2PY appears to predominate over 4PY in humans.

Lovastatin

Lovastatin undergoes extensive first-pass extraction and metabolism by cytochrome P450 3A4 in the liver, its primary site of action. The major active metabolites present in human plasma are the beta-hydroxyacid of lovastatin (lovastatin acid), its 6'-hydroxy derivative, and two additional metabolites.

Elimination

ADVICOR

Niacin is primarily excreted in urine mainly as metabolites. After a single dose of ADVICOR, at least 60% of the niacin dose was recovered in urine as unchanged niacin and its metabolites. The plasma half-life for lovastatin was about 4.5 hours in single-dose studies.

Niacin

The plasma half-life for niacin is about 20 to 48 minutes after oral administration and dependent on dose administered. Following multiple oral doses of NIASPAN, up to 12% of the dose was recovered in urine as unchanged niacin depending on dose administered. The ratio of metabolites recovered in the urine was also dependent on the dose administered.

Lovastatin

Lovastatin is excreted in urine and bile, based on studies of Mevacor. Following an oral dose of radiolabeled lovastatin in man, 10% of the dose was excreted in urine and 83% in feces. The latter represents absorbed drug equivalents excreted in bile, as well as any unabsorbed drug.

Special Populations

Hepatic

No pharmacokinetic studies have been conducted in patients with hepatic insufficiency for either niacin or lovastatin (see **WARNINGS, Liver Dysfunction**).

Renal

No information is available on the pharmacokinetics of niacin in patients with renal insufficiency.

In a study of patients with severe renal insufficiency (creatinine clearance 10 to 30 mL/min), the plasma concentrations of total inhibitors after a single dose of lovastatin were approximately two-fold higher than those in healthy volunteers.

ADVICOR should be used with caution in patients with renal disease.

Gender

Plasma concentrations of niacin and metabolites after single- or multiple-dose administration of niacin are generally higher in women than in men, with the magnitude of the difference varying with dose and metabolite. Recovery of niacin and metabolites in urine, however, is generally similar for men and women, indicating similar absorption for both genders. The gender differences observed in plasma niacin and metabolite levels may be due to gender-specific differences in metabolic rate or volume of distribution. Data from clinical trials suggest that women have a greater hypolipidemic response than men at equivalent doses of NIASPAN and ADVICOR.

In a multiple-dose study, plasma concentrations of active and total HMG-CoA reductase inhibitors were 20 to 50% higher in women than in men. In two single-dose studies with ADVICOR, lovastatin concentrations were about 30% higher in women than men, and total HMG-CoA reductase inhibitor concentrations were about 20 to 25% greater in women.

In a multi-center, randomized, double-blind, active comparator study in patients with Type IIa and IIb hyperlipidemia, ADVICOR was compared to single-agent treatment (NIASPAN and lovastatin). The treatment effects of ADVICOR compared to lovastatin and NIASPAN differed for males and females with a significantly larger treatment effect seen for females. The mean percent change from baseline at endpoint for LDL-C, TG, and HDL-C by gender are as follows (Table 1):

Table 1. Mean percent change from baseline at endpoint for LDL-C, HDL-C and TG by gender

	ADVICOR 2000 mg/40 mg		NIASPAN 2000 mg		Lovastatin 40 mg	
	Women (n=22)	Men (n=30)	Women (n=28)	Men (n=28)	Women (n=21)	Men (n-38)
LDL-C	-47%	-34%	-12%	-9%	-31%	-31%
HDL-C	+33%	+24%	+22%	+15%	+3%	+7%
TG	-48%	-35%	-25%	-15%	-15%	-23%

Clinical Studies

In a multi-center, randomized, double-blind, parallel, 28-week, active-comparator study in patients with Type IIa and IIb hyperlipidemia, ADVICOR was compared to each of its components (NIASPAN and lovastatin). Using a forced dose-escalation study design, patients received each dose for at least 4 weeks. Patients randomized to treatment with ADVICOR initially received 500 mg/20 mg. The dose was increased at 4-week intervals to a maximum of 1000 mg/20 mg in one-half of the patients and 2000 mg/40 mg in the other half. The NIASPAN monotherapy group underwent a similar titration from 500 mg to 2000 mg. The patients randomized to lovastatin monotherapy received 20 mg for 12 weeks titrated to 40 mg for up to 16 weeks. Up to a third of the patients randomized to ADVICOR or NIASPAN discontinued prior to Week 28. In this study, ADVICOR decreased LDL-C, TG and Lp(a), and increased HDL-C in a dose-dependent fashion (Tables 2, 3, 4 and 5 below). Results from this study for LDL-C mean percent change from baseline (the primary efficacy variable) showed that:

1) LDL-lowering with ADVICOR was significantly greater than that achieved with lovastatin 40 mg only after 28 weeks of titration to a dose of 2000 mg/40 mg (p<.0001)
2) ADVICOR at doses of 1000 mg/20 mg or higher achieved greater LDL-lowering than NIASPAN (p<.0001)

The LDL-C results are summarized in Table 2.

[See table 2 above]

ADVICOR achieved significantly greater HDL-raising compared to lovastatin and NIASPAN monotherapy at all doses (Table 3).

[See table 3 above]

In addition, ADVICOR achieved significantly greater TG-lowering at doses of 1000 mg/20 mg or greater compared to lovastatin and NIASPAN monotherapy (Table 4).

[See table 4 above]

The Lp(a) lowering effects of ADVICOR and NIASPAN were similar, and both were superior to lovastatin (Table 5). The independent effect of lowering Lp(a) with NIASPAN or ADVICOR on the risk of coronary and cardiovascular morbidity and mortality has not been determined.

[See table 5 above]

ADVICOR Long-Term Study

A total of 814 patients were enrolled in a long-term (52-week), open-label, single-arm study of ADVICOR. Patients were force dose-titrated to 2000 mg/40 mg over 16 weeks. After titration, patients were maintained on the maximum tolerated dose of ADVICOR for a total of 52 weeks. Five hundred-fifty (550) patients (68%) completed the study, and fifty-six percent (56%) of all patients were able to maintain a dose of 2000 mg/40 mg for the 52 weeks of treatment. The lipid-altering effects of ADVICOR peaked after 4 weeks on the maximum tolerated dose, and were maintained for the duration of treatment. These effects were comparable to what was observed in the double-blind study of ADVICOR (Tables 2-4).

Table 2. LDL-C mean percent change from baseline

Week	ADVICOR			NIASPAN			Lovastatin		
	n*	Dose (mg/mg)	LDL	n*	Dose (mg)	LDL	n*	Dose (mg)	LDL
Baseline	57	-	190.9 mg/dL	61	-	189.7 mg/dL	61	-	185.6 mg/dL
12	47	1000/20	-30%	46	1000	-3%	56	20	-29%
16	45	1000/40	-36%	44	1000	-6%	56	40	-31%
20	42	1500/40	-37%	43	1500	-12%	54	40	-34%
28	42	2000/40	-42%	41	2000	-14%	53	40	-32%

*n = number of patients remaining in the trial at each timepoint

Table 3. HDL-C mean percent change from baseline

Week	ADVICOR			NIASPAN			Lovastatin		
	n*	Dose (mg/mg)	HDL	n*	Dose (mg)	HDL	n*	Dose (mg)	HDL
Baseline	57	-	45 mg/dL	61	-	47 mg/dL	61	-	43 mg/dL
12	47	1000/20	+20%	46	1000	+14%	56	20	+3%
16	45	1000/40	+20%	44	1000	+15%	56	40	+5%
20	42	1500/40	+27%	43	1500	+22%	54	40	+6%
28	42	2000/40	+30%	41	2000	+24%	53	40	+6%

*n = number of patients remaining in the trial at each timepoint

Table 4. TG median percent change from baseline

Week	ADVICOR			NIASPAN			Lovastatin		
	n*	Dose (mg/mg)	TG	n*	Dose (mg)	TG	n*	Dose (mg)	TG
Baseline	57	-	174 mg/dL	61	-	186 mg/dL	61	-	171 mg/dL
12	47	1000/20	-32%	46	1000	-22%	56	20	-20%
16	45	1000/40	-39%	44	1000	-23%	56	40	-17%
20	42	1500/40	-44%	43	1500	-31%	54	40	-21%
28	42	2000/40	-44%	41	2000	-31%	53	40	-20%

*n = number of patients remaining in the trial at each timepoint

Table 5. Lp(a) median percent change from baseline

Week	ADVICOR			NIASPAN			Lovastatin		
	n	Dose (mg/mg)	Lp(a)	n	Dose (mg)	Lp(a)	n	Dose (mg)	Lp(a)
Baseline	57	-	34 mg/dL	61	-	41 mg/dL	60	-	42 mg/dL
12	47	1000/20	-9%	46	1000	-8%	55	20	+8%
16	45	1000/40	-9%	44	1000	-12%	55	40	+8%
20	42	1500/40	-17%	43	1500	-22%	53	40	+6%
28	42	2000/40	-22%	41	2000	-32%	52	40	0%

*n = number of patients remaining in the trial at each timepoint

INDICATIONS AND USAGE

ADVICOR is a fixed-dose combination product and is not indicated for initial therapy (see **DOSAGE AND ADMINISTRATION**). Therapy with lipid-altering agents should be only one component of multiple risk factor intervention in individuals at significantly increased risk for atherosclerotic vascular disease due to hypercholesterolemia. Initial medical therapy is indicated with a single agent as an adjunct to diet when the response to a diet restricted in saturated fat and cholesterol and other nonpharmacologic measures alone has been inadequate (see also Table 7 and the NCEP treatment guidelines[1]).

ADVICOR is indicated for the treatment of primary hypercholesterolemia (heterozygous familial and nonfamilial) and mixed dyslipidemia (Frederickson Types IIa and IIb; Table 6) in:

- Patients treated with lovastatin who require further TG-lowering or HDL-raising who may benefit from having niacin added to their regimen
- Patients treated with niacin who require further LDL-lowering who may benefit from having lovastatin added to their regimen

Table 6. Classification of Hyperlipoproteinemias

Type	Lipoproteins Elevated	Lipid Elevations	
		Major	Minor
I (rare)	Chylomicrons	TG	↑→TC
IIa	LDL	TC	-
IIb	LDL, VLDL	TC	TG
III (rare)	IDL	TC/TG	-
IV	VLDL	TG	↑→TC
V (rare)	Chylomicrons, VLDL	TG	↑→TC

TC = total cholesterol; TG = triglycerides; LDL = low-density lipoprotein; VLDL = very low-density lipoprotein; IDL = intermediate-density lipoprotein
↑→ = increased or no change

General Recommendations

Prior to initiating therapy with a lipid-lowering agent, secondary causes for hypercholesterolemia (e.g., poorly controlled diabetes mellitus, hypothyroidism, nephrotic syndrome, dysproteinemias, obstructive liver disease, other drug therapy, alcoholism) should be excluded, and a lipid profile performed to measure TC, HDL-C, and TG. For patients with TG < 400 mg/dL, LDL-C can be estimated using the following equation:

$$\text{LDL-C} = \text{TC} - [(0.20 \times \text{TG}) + \text{HDL-C}]$$

For TG levels > 400 mg/dL, this equation is less accurate and LDL-C concentrations should be determined by ultracentrifugation. Lipid determinations should be performed at intervals of no less than 4 weeks and dosage adjusted according to the patient's response to therapy. The NCEP Treatment Guidelines are summarized in Table 7.

[See table 7 at top of next page]

After the LDL-C goal has been achieved, if the TG is still ≥ 200 mg/dL, non-HDL-C (TC minus HDL-C) becomes a secondary target of therapy. Non-HDL-C goals are set 30 mg/dL higher than LDL-C goals for each risk category.

CONTRAINDICATIONS

ADVICOR is contraindicated in patients with a known hypersensitivity to niacin, lovastatin or any component of this medication, active liver disease or unexplained persistent elevations in serum transaminases (see **WARNINGS**), active peptic ulcer disease, or arterial bleeding.

Pregnancy and lactation—Atherosclerosis is a chronic process and the discontinuation of lipid-lowering drugs during pregnancy should have little impact on the outcome of long-term therapy of primary hypercholesterolemia. Moreover, cholesterol and other products of the cholesterol biosynthesis pathway are essential components for fetal development,

Continued on next page

Advicor—Cont.

including synthesis of steroids and cell membranes. Because of the ability of inhibitors of HMG-CoA reductase, such as lovastatin, to decrease the synthesis of cholesterol and possibly other products of the cholesterol biosynthesis pathway, ADVICOR is contraindicated in women who are pregnant and in lactating mothers. ADVICOR may cause fetal harm when administered to pregnant women. **ADVICOR should be administered to women of childbearing age only when such patients are highly unlikely to conceive.** If the patient becomes pregnant while taking this drug, ADVICOR should be discontinued immediately and the patient should be apprised of the potential hazard to the fetus (see **PRECAUTIONS, Pregnancy**).

WARNINGS

ADVICOR should not be substituted for equivalent doses of immediate-release (crystalline) niacin. For patients switching from immediate-release niacin to NIASPAN, therapy with NIASPAN should be initiated with low doses (i.e., 500 mg once daily at bedtime) and the NIASPAN dose should then be titrated to the desired therapeutic response (see DOSAGE AND ADMINISTRATION).

Liver Dysfunction

Cases of severe hepatic toxicity, including fulminant hepatic necrosis, have occurred in patients who have substituted sustained-release (modified-release, timed-release) niacin products for immediate-release (crystalline) niacin at equivalent doses.

ADVICOR should be used with caution in patients who consume substantial quantities of alcohol and/or have a past history of liver disease. Active liver disease or unexplained transaminase elevations are contraindications to the use of ADVICOR.

Niacin preparations and lovastatin preparations have been associated with abnormal liver tests. In studies using NIASPAN alone, 0.8% of patients were discontinued for transaminase elevations. In studies using lovastatin alone, 0.2% of patients were discontinued for transaminase elevations.[2] In three safety and efficacy studies involving titration to final daily ADVICOR doses ranging from 500 mg/10 mg to 2500 mg/40 mg, ten of 1028 patients (1.0%) experienced reversible elevations in AST/ALT to more than 3 times the upper limit of normal (ULN). Three of ten elevations occurred at doses outside the recommended dosing limit of 2000 mg/40 mg; no patient receiving 1000 mg/20 mg had 3-fold elevations in AST/ALT.

In clinical studies with ADVICOR, elevations in transaminases did not appear to be related to treatment duration; elevations in AST and ALT levels did appear to be dose related. Transaminase elevations were reversible upon discontinuation of ADVICOR.

Liver function tests should be performed on all patients during therapy with ADVICOR. Serum transaminase levels, including AST and ALT (SGOT and SGPT), should be monitored before treatment begins, every 6 to 12 weeks for the first 6 months, and periodically thereafter (e.g., at approximately 6-month intervals). Special attention should be paid to patients who develop elevated serum transaminase levels, and in these patients, measurements should be repeated promptly and, if confirmed, then performed more frequently. If the transaminase levels show evidence of progression, particularly if they rise to 3 times ULN and are persistent, or if they are associated with symptoms of nausea, fever, and/or malaise, the drug should be discontinued.

Skeletal Muscle

Lovastatin

Lovastatin and other inhibitors of HMG-CoA reductase occasionally cause myopathy, which is manifested as muscle pain or weakness associated with grossly elevated creatine kinase (> 10 times ULN).

Rhabdomyolysis, with or without acute renal failure secondary to myoglobinuria, has been reported rarely and can occur at any time. In a large, long-term, clinical safety and efficacy study (the EXCEL study)[3,4] with lovastatin, myopathy occurred in up to 0.2% of patients treated with lovastatin 20 to 80 mg for up to 2 years. When drug treatment was interrupted or discontinued in these patients, muscle symptoms and creatine kinase (CK) increases promptly resolved. The risk of myopathy is increased by concomitant therapy with certain drugs, some of which were excluded by the EXCEL study design.

The risk of myopathy appears to be increased by high levels of HMG-CoA reductase inhibitory activity in plasma. Lovastatin is metabolized by the cytochrome P450 isoform 3A4. Certain drugs which share this metabolic pathway can raise the plasma levels of lovastatin and may increase the risk of myopathy. These include cyclosporine, itraconazole, ketoconazole and other antifungal azoles, the macrolide antibiotics erythromycin and clarithromycin, HIV protease inhibitors, the antidepressant nefazodone, or large quantities of grapefruit juice (>1 quart daily).

ADVICOR

Myopathy and/or rhabdomyolysis have been reported when lovastatin is used in combination with lipid-altering doses (≥1g/day) of niacin. Physicians contemplating the use of ADVICOR, a combination of lovastatin and niacin, should weigh the potential benefits and risks, and should carefully monitor patients for any signs and symptoms of muscle pain, tenderness, or weakness, particularly during the initial month of treatment or during any period of upward dosage titration of either drug. Periodic CK determinations may be considered in such situations, but there is no assurance that such monitoring will prevent myopathy. In clinical studies, no cases of rhabdomyolysis and one suspected case of myopathy have been reported in 1079 patients who were treated with ADVICOR at doses up to 2000 mg/40 mg for periods up to 2 years.

Table 7. NCEP Treatment Guidelines: LDL-C Goals and Cutpoints for Therapeutic Lifestyle Changes and Drug Therapy in Different Risk Categories

Risk Category	LDL Goal (mg/dL)	LDL Level at Which to Initiate Therapeutic Lifestyle Changes (mg/dL)	LDL Level at Which to Consider Drug Therapy (mg/dL)
CHD[†] or CHD risk equivalents (10-year risk >20%)	<100	≥100	≥130 (100-129: drug optional)[††]
2+ Risk factors (10-year risk ≤20%)	<130	≥130	10-year risk 10%-20%:≥130 10-year risk <10%:≥160
0-1 Risk factor[†††]	<160	≥160	≥190 (160-189: LDL-lowering drug optional)

†CHD, coronary heart disease
††Some authorities recommend use of LDL-lowering drugs in this category if an LDL-C level of <100 mg/dL cannot be achieved by therapeutic lifestyle changes. Others prefer use of drugs that primarily modify triglycerides and HDL-C, e.g., nicotinic acid or fibrate. Clinical judgement also may call for deferring drug therapy in this subcategory.
†††Almost all people with 0-1 risk factor have 10-year risk <10%; thus, 10-year risk assessment in people with 0-1 risk factor is not necessary.

Patients starting therapy with ADVICOR should be advised of the risk of myopathy, and told to report promptly unexplained muscle pain, tenderness, or weakness. A CK level above 10 times ULN in a patient with unexplained muscle symptoms indicates myopathy. ADVICOR therapy should be discontinued if myopathy is diagnosed or suspected.

In patients with complicated medical histories predisposing to rhabdomyolysis, such as preexisting renal insufficiency, dose escalation requires caution. Also, as there are no known adverse consequences of brief interruption of therapy, treatment with ADVICOR should be stopped for a few days before elective major surgery and when any major acute medical or surgical condition supervenes.

Use of ADVICOR with other Drugs

The incidence and severity of myopathy may be increased by concomitant administration of ADVICOR with drugs that can cause myopathy when given alone, such as gemfibrozil and other fibrates.

The use of ADVICOR in combination with fibrates should be avoided unless the benefit of further alterations in lipid levels is likely to outweigh the increased risk of this drug combination. In patients taking concomitant cyclosporine or fibrates, the dose of ADVICOR should generally not exceed 1000 mg/20 mg (see DOSAGE AND ADMINISTRATION), as the risk of myopathy may increase at higher doses. Interruption of ADVICOR therapy during a course of treatment with a systemic antifungal azole or a macrolide antibiotic should be considered.

PRECAUTIONS

General

Before instituting therapy with a lipid-altering medication, an attempt should be made to control dyslipidemia with appropriate diet, exercise, and weight reduction in obese patients, and to treat other underlying medical problems (see **INDICATIONS AND USAGE**).

Patients with a past history of jaundice, hepatobiliary disease, or peptic ulcer should be observed closely during ADVICOR therapy. Frequent monitoring of liver function tests and blood glucose should be performed to ascertain that the drug is producing no adverse effects on these organ systems.

Diabetic patients may experience a dose-related rise in fasting blood sugar (FBS). In three clinical studies, which included 1028 patients exposed to ADVICOR (6 to 22% of whom had diabetes type II at baseline), increases in FBS above normal occurred in 46 to 65% of patients at any time during study treatment with ADVICOR. Fourteen patients (1.4%) were discontinued from study treatment: 3 patients for worsening diabetes, 10 patients for hyperglycemia and 1 patient for a new diagnosis of diabetes. In the studies in which lovastatin and NIASPAN were used as active controls, 24 to 41% of patients receiving lovastatin and 43 to 58% of patients receiving NIASPAN also had increases in FBS above normal. One patient (1.1%) receiving lovastatin was discontinued for hyperglycemia. Diabetic or potentially diabetic patients should be observed closely during treatment with ADVICOR, and adjustment of diet and/or hypoglycemic therapy may be necessary.

In one long-term study of 106 patients treated with ADVICOR, elevations in prothrombin time (PT) >3 X ULN occurred in 2 patients (2%) during study drug treatment. In a long-term study of 814 patients treated with ADVICOR, 7 patients were noted to have platelet counts <100,000 during study drug treatment. Four of these patients were discontinued, and one patient with a platelet count <100,000 had prolonged bleeding after a tooth extraction. Prior studies have shown that NIASPAN can be associated with dose-related reductions in platelet count (mean of -11% with 2000 mg) and increases of PT (mean of approximately +4%). Accordingly, patients undergoing surgery should be carefully evaluated. In controlled studies, ADVICOR has been associated with small but statistically significant dose-related reductions in phosphorus levels (mean of -10% with 2000 mg/40 mg). Phosphorus levels should be monitored periodically in patients at risk for hypophosphatemia. In clinical studies with ADVICOR, hypophosphatemia was more common in males than in females. The clinical relevance of hypophosphatemia in this population is not known.

Niacin

Caution should also be used when ADVICOR is used in patients with unstable angina or in the acute phase of MI, particularly when such patients are also receiving vasoactive drugs such as nitrates, calcium channel blockers, or adrenergic blocking agents.

Elevated uric acid levels have occurred with niacin therapy; therefore, in patients predisposed to gout, niacin therapy should be used with caution. Niacin is rapidly metabolized by the liver, and excreted through the kidneys. ADVICOR is contraindicated in patients with significant or unexplained hepatic dysfunction (see **CONTRAINDICATIONS** and **WARNINGS**) and should be used with caution in patients with renal dysfunction.

Lovastatin

Lovastatin may elevate creatine phosphokinase and transaminase levels (see **WARNINGS** and **ADVERSE REACTIONS**). This should be considered in the differential diagnosis of chest pain in a patient on therapy with lovastatin.

Endocrine function—HMG-CoA reductase inhibitors interfere with cholesterol synthesis and as such might theoretically blunt adrenal and/or gonadal steroid production. Results of clinical studies with drugs in this class have been inconsistent with regard to drug effects on basal and reserve steroid levels. However, clinical studies have shown that lovastatin does not reduce basal plasma cortisol concentration or impair adrenal reserve, and does not reduce basal plasma testosterone concentration. Another HMG-CoA reductase inhibitor has been shown to reduce the plasma testosterone response to human chorionic gonadotropin (HCG). In the same study, the mean testosterone response to HCG was slightly but not significantly reduced after treatment with lovastatin 40 mg daily for 16 weeks in 21 men. The effects of HMG-CoA reductase inhibitors on male fertility have not been studied in adequate numbers of male patients. The effects, if any, on the pituitary-gonadal axis in premenopausal women are unknown. Patients treated with lovastatin who develop clinical evidence of endocrine dysfunction should be evaluated appropriately. Caution should also be exercised if an HMG-CoA reductase inhibitor or other agent used to lower cholesterol levels is administered to patients also receiving other drugs (e.g., ketoconazole, spironolactone, cimetidine) that may decrease the levels or activity of endogenous steroid hormones.

CNS toxicity—Lovastatin produced optic nerve degeneration (Wallerian degeneration of retinogeniculate fibers) in clinically normal dogs in a dose-dependent fashion starting at 60 mg/kg/day, a dose that produced mean plasma drug levels about 30 times higher than the mean drug level in humans taking the highest recommended dose (as measured by total enzyme inhibitory activity). Vestibulocochlear Wallerian-like degeneration and retinal ganglion cell chromatolysis were also seen in dogs treated for 14 weeks at 180 mg/kg/day, a dose which resulted in a mean plasma drug level (Cmax) similar to that seen with the 60 mg/kg/day dose.

CNS vascular lesions, characterized by perivascular hemorrhage and edema, mononuclear cell infiltration of perivascular spaces, perivascular fibrin deposits and necrosis of small vessels, were seen in dogs treated with lovastatin at a dose of 180 mg/kg/day, a dose which produced plasma drug levels (Cmax) which were about 30 times higher than the mean values in humans taking 80 mg/day.

Similar optic nerve and CNS vascular lesions have been observed with other drugs of this class.

Cataracts were seen in dogs treated with lovastatin for 11 and 28 weeks at 180 mg/kg/day and 1 year at 60 mg/kg/day.

Information for Patients

Patients should be advised of the following:

— to report promptly unexplained muscle pain, tenderness, or weakness (see **WARNINGS, Skeletal Muscle**);

— to take ADVICOR at bedtime, with a low-fat snack. Administration on an empty stomach is not recommended;

— to carefully follow the prescribed dosing regimen (see **DOSAGE AND ADMINISTRATION**);
— that flushing is a common side effect of niacin therapy that usually subsides after several weeks of consistent niacin use. Flushing may last for several hours after dosing, may vary in severity, and will, by taking ADVICOR at bedtime, most likely occur during sleep. If awakened by flushing, especially if taking antihypertensives, rise slowly to minimize the potential for dizziness and/or syncope;
— that taking aspirin (up to approximately 30 minutes before taking ADVICOR) or another non-steroidal anti-inflammatory drug (e.g., ibuprofen) may minimize flushing;
— to avoid ingestion of alcohol or hot drinks around the time of ADVICOR administration, to minimize flushing;
— should not be administered with grapefruit juice;
— that if ADVICOR therapy is discontinued for an extended length of time, their physician should be contacted prior to re-starting therapy; re-titration is recommended (see **DOSAGE AND ADMINISTRATION**);
— to notify their physician if they are taking vitamins or other nutritional supplements containing niacin or related compounds such as nicotinamide (see **Drug Interactions**);
— to notify their physician if symptoms of dizziness occur;
— if diabetic, to notify their physician of changes in blood glucose;
— that ADVICOR tablets should not be broken, crushed, or chewed, but should be swallowed whole.

Drug Interactions

Niacin

Antihypertensive Therapy—Niacin may potentiate the effects of ganglionic blocking agents and vasoactive drugs resulting in postural hypotension.

Aspirin: Concomitant aspirin may decrease the metabolic clearance of niacin. The clinical relevance of this finding is unclear.

Bile Acid Sequestrants—An *in vitro* study was carried out investigating the niacin-binding capacity of colestipol and cholestyramine. About 98% of available niacin was bound to colestipol, with 10 to 30% binding to cholestyramine. These results suggest that 4 to 6 hours, or as great an interval as possible, should elapse between the ingestion of bile acid-binding resins and the administration of ADVICOR.

Other—Concomitant alcohol or hot drinks may increase the side effects of flushing and pruritus and should be avoided around the time of ADVICOR ingestion. Vitamins or other nutritional supplements containing large doses of niacin or related compounds such as nicotinamide may potentiate the adverse effects of ADVICOR.

Lovastatin

Serious skeletal muscle disorders, e.g., rhabdomyolysis, have been reported during concomitant therapy of lovastatin or other HMG-CoA reductase inhibitors with cyclosporine, itraconazole, ketoconazole, gemfibrozil, niacin, erythromycin, clarithromycin, nefazodone or HIV protease inhibitors. (See **WARNINGS, Skeletal Muscle**).

Coumarin Anticoagulants—In a small clinical study in which lovastatin was administered to warfarin-treated patients, no effect on PT was detected. However, another HMG-CoA reductase inhibitor has been found to produce a less than two seconds increase in PT in healthy volunteers receiving low doses of warfarin. Also, bleeding and/or increased PT have been reported in a few patients taking coumarin anticoagulants concomitantly with lovastatin. It is recommended that in patients taking anticoagulants, PT be determined before starting ADVICOR and frequently enough during early therapy to insure that no significant alteration of PT occurs. Once a stable PT has been documented, PT can be monitored at the intervals usually recommended for patients on coumarin anticoagulants. If the dose of ADVICOR is changed, the same procedure should be repeated.

Antipyrine—Lovastatin had no effect on the pharmacokinetics of antipyrine or its metabolites. However, since lovastatin is metabolized by the cytochrome P450 isoform 3A4 enzyme system, this does not preclude an interaction with other drugs metabolized by the same isoform.

Propranolol—In normal volunteers, there was no clinically significant pharmacokinetic or pharmacodynamic interaction with concomitant administration of single doses of lovastatin and propranolol.

Digoxin—In patients with hypercholesterolemia, concomitant administration of lovastatin and digoxin resulted in no effect on digoxin plasma concentrations.

Oral Hypoglycemic Agents—In pharmacokinetic studies of lovastatin in hypercholesterolemic, non-insulin dependent diabetic patients, there was no drug interaction with glipzide or with chlorpropamide.

Drug/Laboratory Test Interactions

Niacin may produce false elevations in some fluorometric determinations of plasma or urinary catecholamines. Niacin may also give false-positive reactions with cupric sulfate solution (Benedict's reagent) in urine glucose tests.

Carcinogenesis, Mutagenesis, Impairment of Fertility

No studies have been conducted with ADVICOR regarding carcinogenesis, mutagenesis, or impairment of fertility.

Niacin

Niacin, administered to mice for a lifetime as a 1% solution in drinking water, was not carcinogenic. The mice in this study received approximately 6 to 8 times a human dose of 3000 mg/day as determined on a mg/m^2 basis. Niacin was negative for mutagenicity in the Ames test. No studies on impairment of fertility have been performed.

Table 8. Treatment-Emergent Adverse Events in ≥ 5% of Patients
(Events Irrespective of Causality; Data from Controlled, Double-Blind Studies)

Adverse Event	ADVICOR	NIASPAN	Lovastatin
Total Number of Patients	214	92	94
Cardiovascular	**163 (76%)**	**66 (72%)**	**24 (26%)**
Flushing	152 (71%)	60 (65%)	17 (18%)
Body as a Whole	**104 (49%)**	**50 (54%)**	**42 (45%)**
Asthenia	10 (5%)	6 (7%)	5 (5%)
Flu Syndrome	12 (6%)	7 (8%)	4 (4%)
Headache	20 (9%)	12 (13%)	5 (5%)
Infection	43 (20%)	14 (15%)	19 (20%)
Pain	18 (8%)	3 (3%)	9 (10%)
Pain, Abdominal	9 (4%)	1 (1%)	6 (6%)
Pain, Back	10 (5%)	5 (5%)	5 (5%)
Digestive System	**51 (24%)**	**26 (28%)**	**16 (17%)**
Diarrhea	13 (6%)	8 (9%)	2 (2%)
Dyspepsia	6 (3%)	5 (5%)	4 (4%)
Nausea	14 (7%)	11 (12%)	2 (2%)
Vomiting	7 (3%)	5 (5%)	0
Metabolic and Nutrit. System	**37 (17%)**	**18 (20%)**	**13 (14%)**
Hyperglycemia	8 (4%)	6 (7%)	6 (6%)
Musculoskeletal System	**19 (9%)**	**9 (10%)**	**17 (18%)**
Myalgia	6 (3%)	5 (5%)	8 (9%)
Skin and Appendages	**3 (2%)**	**19 (21%)**	**11 (12%)**
Pruritus	14 (7%)	7 (8%)	3 (3%)
Rash	11 (5%)	11 (12%)	3 (3%)

Note: Percentages are calculated from the total number of patients in each column.

Lovastatin

In a 21-month carcinogenic study in mice, there was a statistically significant increase in the incidence of hepatocellular carcinomas and adenomas in both males and females at 500 mg/kg/day. This dose produced a total plasma drug exposure 3 to 4 times that of humans given the highest recommended dose of lovastatin (drug exposure was measured as total HMG-CoA reductase inhibitory activity in extracted plasma). Tumor increases were not seen at 20 and 100 mg/kg/day, doses that produced drug exposures of 0.3 to 2 times that of humans at the 80 mg/day dose. A statistically significant increase in pulmonary adenomas was seen in female mice at approximately 4 times the human drug exposure. (Although mice were given 300 times the human dose on a mg/kg body weight basis, plasma levels of total inhibitory activity were only 4 times higher in mice than in humans given 80 mg of lovastatin.)

There was an increase in incidence of papilloma in the non-glandular mucosa of the stomach of mice beginning at exposures of 1 to 2 times that of humans. The glandular mucosa was not affected. The human stomach contains only glandular mucosa.

In a 24-month carcinogenicity study in rats, there was a positive dose-response relationship for hepatocellular carcinogenicity in males at drug exposures between 2 to 7 times that of human exposure at 80 mg/day (doses in rats were 5, 30, and 180 mg/kg/day).

An increased incidence of thyroid neoplasms in rats appears to be a response that has been seen with other HMG-CoA reductase inhibitors.

A drug in this class chemically similar to lovastatin was administered to mice for 72 weeks at 25, 100, and 400 mg/kg body weight, which resulted in mean serum drug levels approximately 3, 15, and 33 times higher than the mean human serum drug concentration (as total inhibitory activity) after a 40 mg oral dose. Liver carcinomas were significantly increased in high-dose females and mid- and high-dose males, with a maximum incidence of 90 percent in males. The incidence of adenomas of the liver was significantly increased in mid- and high-dose females. Drug treatment also significantly increased the incidence of lung adenomas in mid- and high-dose males and females. Adenomas of the Harderian gland (a gland of the eye of rodents) were significantly higher in high-dose mice than in controls.

No evidence of mutagenicity was observed in a microbial mutagen test using mutant strains of *Salmonella typhimurium* with or without rat or mouse liver metabolic activation. In addition, no evidence of damage to genetic material was noted in an *in vitro* alkaline elution assay using rat or mouse hepatocytes, a V-79 mammalian cell forward mutation study, an *in vitro* chromosome aberration study in CHO cells, or an *in vivo* chromosomal aberration assay in mouse bone marrow.

Drug-related testicular atrophy, decreased spermatogenesis, spermatocytic degeneration and giant cell formation were seen in dogs starting at 20 mg/kg/day. Similar findings were seen with another drug in this class. No drug-related effects on fertility were found in studies with lovastatin in rats. However, in studies with a similar drug in this class, there was decreased fertility in male rats treated for 34 weeks at 25 mg/kg body weight, although this effect was not observed in a subsequent fertility study when this same dose was administered for 11 weeks (the entire cycle of spermatogenesis, including epididymal maturation). In rats treated with this same reductase inhibitor at 180 mg/kg/day, seminiferous tubule degeneration (necrosis and loss of spermatogenic epithelium) was observed. No microscopic changes were observed in the testes from rats of either study. The clinical significance of these findings is unclear.

Pregnancy

Pregnancy Category X—See **CONTRAINDICATIONS**.

ADVICOR should be administered to women of childbearing potential only when such patients are highly unlikely to conceive and have been informed of the potential hazard. Safety in pregnant women has not been established and there is no apparent benefit to therapy with ADVICOR during pregnancy (see **CONTRAINDICATIONS**). Treatment should be immediately discontinued as soon as pregnancy is recognized.

Niacin

Animal reproduction studies have not been conducted with niacin or with ADVICOR. It is also not known whether niacin at doses typically used for lipid disorders can cause fetal harm when administered to pregnant women or whether it can affect reproductive capacity. If a woman receiving niacin or ADVICOR for primary hypercholesterolemia (Types IIa or IIb) becomes pregnant, the drug should be discontinued.

Lovastatin

Rare reports of congenital anomalies have been received following intrauterine exposure to HMG-CoA reductase inhibitors. In a review[5] of approximately 100 prospectively followed pregnancies in women exposed to lovastatin or another structurally related HMG-CoA reductase inhibitor, the incidences of congenital anomalies, spontaneous abortions and fetal deaths/stillbirths did not exceed what would be expected in the general population. The number of cases is adequate only to exclude a 3- to 4-fold increase in congenital anomalies over the background incidence. In 89% of the prospectively followed pregnancies, drug treatment was initiated prior to pregnancy and was discontinued at some point in the first trimester when pregnancy was identified. Lovastatin has been shown to produce skeletal malformations at plasma levels 40 times the human exposure (for mouse fetus) and 80 times the human exposure (for rat fetus) based on mg/m^2 surface area (doses were 800 mg/kg/day). No drug-induced changes were seen in either species at multiples of 8 times (rat) or 4 times (mouse) based on surface area. No evidence of malformations was noted in rabbits at exposures up to 3 times the human exposure (dose of 15 mg/kg/day, highest tolerated dose).

Labor and Delivery

No studies have been conducted on the effect of ADVICOR, niacin or lovastatin on the mother or the fetus during labor or delivery, on the duration of labor or delivery, or on the growth, development, and functional maturation of the child.

Nursing Mothers

No studies have been conducted with ADVICOR in nursing mothers.

Because of the potential for serious adverse reactions in nursing infants from lipid-altering doses of niacin and lovastatin (see **CONTRAINDICATIONS**), ADVICOR should not be taken while a woman is breastfeeding.

Niacin has been reported to be excreted in human milk. It is not known whether lovastatin is excreted in human milk. A small amount of another drug in this class is excreted in human breast milk.

Pediatric use

No studies in patients under 18 years-of-age have been conducted with ADVICOR. Because pediatric patients are not

Continued on next page

Advicor—Cont.

likely to benefit from cholesterol lowering for at least a decade and because experience with this drug or its active ingredients is limited, treatment of pediatric patients with ADVICOR is not recommended at this time.

Geriatric Use

Of the 214 patients who received ADVICOR in double-blind clinical studies, 37.4% were 65 years-of-age and older, and of the 814 patients who received ADVICOR in open-label clinical studies, 36.2% were 65 years-of-age and older. Responses in LDL-C, HDL-C, and TG were similar in geriatric patients. No overall differences in the percentage of patients with adverse events were observed between older and younger patients. No overall differences were observed in selected chemistry values between the two groups except for amylase which was higher in older patients.

ADVERSE REACTIONS

Overview

In controlled clinical studies, 40/214 (19%) of patients randomized to ADVICOR discontinued therapy prior to study completion, 18/214 (8%) of discontinuations being due to flushing. In the same controlled studies, 9/94 (10%) of patients randomized to lovastatin and 19/92 (21%) of patients randomized to NIASPAN also discontinued treatment prior to study completion secondary to adverse events. Flushing episodes (i.e., warmth, redness, itching and/or tingling) were the most common treatment-emergent adverse events, and occurred in 53% to 83% of patients treated with ADVICOR. Spontaneous reports with NIASPAN and clinical studies with ADVICOR suggest that flushing may also be accompanied by symptoms of dizziness or syncope, tachycardia, palpitations, shortness of breath, sweating, chills, and/or edema.

Adverse Reactions Information

Because clinical studies are conducted under widely varying conditions, adverse reaction rates observed in clinical studies of a drug cannot be directly compared to rates in the clinical studies of another drug and may not reflect the rates observed in clinical practice. The adverse reaction information from clinical studies does, however provide a basis for identifying the adverse events that appear to be related to drug use and for approximating rates.

The data described in this section reflect the exposure to ADVICOR in two double-blind, controlled clinical studies of 400 patients. The population was 28 to 86 years-of-age, 54% male, 85% Caucasian, 9% Black, and 7% Other, and had mixed dyslipidemia (Frederickson Types IIa and IIb).

In addition to flushing, other adverse events occurring in 5% or greater of patients treated with ADVICOR are shown in Table 8 below.

[See table at top of previous page]

The following adverse events have also been reported with niacin, lovastatin, and/or other HMG-CoA reductase inhibitors, but not necessarily with ADVICOR, either during clinical studies or in routine patient management.

Body as a Whole:	chest pain; abdominal pain; edema; chills; malaise
Cardiovascular:	atrial fibrillation; tachycardia; palpitations, and other cardiac arrhythmias; orthostasis; hypotension; syncope
Eye:	toxic amblyopia; cystoid macular edema; ophthalmoplegia; eye irritation
Gastrointestinal:	activation of peptic ulcers and peptic ulceration; dyspepsia; vomiting; anorexia; constipation; flatulence, pancreatitis; hepatitis; fatty change in liver; jaundice; and rarely, cirrhosis, fulminant hepatic necrosis, and hepatoma
Metabolic:	gout
Musculoskeletal:	muscle cramps; myopathy; rhabdomyolysis; arthralgia
Nervous:	dizziness; insomnia; dry mouth; paresthesia; anxiety; tremor; vertigo; memory loss; peripheral neuropathy; psychic disturbances; dysfunction of certain cranial nerves
Skin:	hyper-pigmentation; acanthosis nigricans; urticaria; alopecia; dry skin; sweating; and a variety of skin changes (e.g., nodules, discoloration, dryness of mucous membranes, changes to hair/nails)
Respiratory:	dyspnea; rhinitis
Urogenital:	gynecomastia; loss of libido; erectile dysfunction
Hypersensitivity reactions:	An apparent hypersensitivity syndrome has been reported rarely, which has included one or more of the following features: anaphylaxis, angioedema, lupus erythematous-like syndrome, polymyalgia rheumatica, vasculitis, purpura, thrombocytopenia, leukopenia, hemolytic anemia, positive ANA, ESR increase, eosinophilia, arthritis, arthralgia, urticaria, asthenia, photosensitivity, fever, chills, flushing, malaise, dyspnea, toxic epidermal necrolysis, erythema multiforme, including Stevens-Johnson syndrome.
Other:	migraine

Clinical Laboratory Abnormalities

Chemistry

Elevations in serum transaminases (see **WARNINGS - Liver Dysfunction**), CPK and fasting glucose, and reductions in phosphorus. Niacin extended-release tablets have been associated with slight elevations in LDH, uric acid, total bilirubin, and amylase. Lovastatin and/or HMG-CoA reductase inhibitors have been associated with elevations in alkaline phosphatase, γ-glutamyl transpeptidase and bilirubin, and thyroid function abnormalities.

Hematology

Niacin extended-release tablets have been associated with slight reductions in platelet counts and prolongation in PT (see **WARNINGS**).

DRUG ABUSE AND DEPENDENCE

Neither niacin nor lovastatin is a narcotic drug. ADVICOR has no known addiction potential in humans.

OVERDOSAGE

Information on acute overdose with ADVICOR in humans is limited. Until further experience is obtained, no specific treatment of overdose with ADVICOR can be recommended. The patient should be carefully observed and given supportive treatment.

Niacin

The s.c. LD50 of niacin is 5 g/kg in rats.

The signs and symptoms of an acute overdose of niacin can be anticipated to be those of excessive pharmacologic effect: severe flushing, nausea/vomiting, diarrhea, dyspepsia, dizziness, syncope, hypotension, possibly cardiac arrhythmias and clinical laboratory abnormalities. Insufficient information is available on the potential for the dialyzability of niacin.

Lovastatin

After oral administration of lovastatin to mice the median lethal dose observed was >15 g/m^2.

Five healthy human volunteers have received up to 200 mg of lovastatin as a single dose without clinically significant adverse experiences. A few cases of accidental overdose have been reported; no patients had any specific symptoms, and all patients recovered without sequelae. The maximum dose taken was 5 to 6 g. The dialyzability of lovastatin and its metabolites in man is not known at present.

DOSAGE AND ADMINISTRATION

The usual recommended starting dose for NIASPAN is 500 mg qhs. NIASPAN must be titrated and the dose should not be increased by more than 500 mg every 4 weeks up to a maximum dose of 2000 mg a day, to reduce the incidence and severity of side effects. Patients already receiving a stable dose of NIASPAN may be switched directly to a niacin-equivalent dose of ADVICOR.

The usual recommended starting dose of lovastatin is 20 mg once a day. Dose adjustments should be made at intervals of 4 weeks or more. Patients already receiving a stable dose of lovastatin may receive concomitant dosage titration with NIASPAN, and switch to ADVICOR once a stable dose of NIASPAN has been reached.

Flushing of the skin (see **ADVERSE REACTIONS**) may be reduced in frequency or severity by pretreatment with aspirin (taken up to approximately 30 minutes prior to ADVICOR dose) or other non-steroidal anti-inflammatory drugs. Flushing, pruritus, and gastrointestinal distress are also greatly reduced by slowly increasing the dose of niacin and avoiding administration on an empty stomach.

Equivalent doses of ADVICOR may be substituted for equivalent doses of NIASPAN but should not be substituted for other modified-release (sustained-release or time-release) niacin preparations or immediate-release (crystalline) niacin preparations (see WARNINGS). Patients previously receiving niacin products other than NIASPAN should be started on NIASPAN with the recommended NIASPAN titration schedule, and the dose should subsequently be individualized based on patient response.

ADVICOR should be taken at bedtime, with a low-fat snack, and the dose should be individualized according to patient response. ADVICOR tablets should be taken whole and should not be broken, crushed, or chewed before swallowing. The dose of ADVICOR should not be increased by more than 500 mg daily (based on the NIASPAN component) every 4 weeks. The lowest dose of ADVICOR is 500 mg/20 mg. Doses of ADVICOR greater than 2000 mg/40 mg daily are not recommended. **If ADVICOR therapy is discontinued for an extended period (>7 days), reinstitution of therapy should begin with the lowest dose of ADVICOR.**

HOW SUPPLIED

ADVICOR is an unscored, capsule-shaped tablet containing either 500, 750, or 1000 mg of niacin in an extended-release formulation and 20 mg of lovastatin in an immediate-release formulation. Tablets are color-coated and debossed with "KOS" on one side and the tablet strength code on the other side. ADVICOR 500 mg/20 mg tablets are light yellow, code "502". ADVICOR 750 mg/20 mg tablets are light orange, code "752". ADVICOR 1000 mg/20 mg tablets are dark pink/light purple, code "1002". Tablets are supplied in bottles of 30, 90, or 180 tablets as shown below.

500 mg/20 mg tablets:	bottles of 30 - NDC# 60598-006-30
	bottles of 90 - NDC# 60598-006-90
	bottles of 180 - NDC# 60598-006-18
750 mg/20 mg tablets:	bottles of 30 - NDC# 60598-007-30
	bottles of 90 - NDC# 60598-007-90
	bottles of 180 - NDC# 60598-007-18
1000 mg/20 mg tablets:	bottles of 30 - NDC# 60598-008-30
	bottles of 90 - NDC# 60598-008-90
	bottles of 180 - NDC# 60598-008-18

Store at room temperature (20° to 25°C or 68° to 77°F).

Rx Only

REFERENCES

1. Executive Summary of the Third Report of the National Cholesterol Education Program (NCEP) Expert Panel on Detection, Evaluation, and Treatment of High Blood Cholesterol in Adults (Adult Treatment Panel III). *JAMA* 2001; 285:2486-2497.
2. Downs JR, et al. *JAMA* 1998; 279:1615-1622.
3. Bradford RH, et al. *Arch Intern Med* 1991;151:43-49.
4. Bradford RH, et al. *Am J Cardiol* 1994; 74:667-673.
5. Manson JM, et al. *Reprod Toxicol* 1996; 10(6): 439-446.

Mfr. by:
KOS PHARMACEUTICALS, INC.
Miami, FL 33131

400161/1101
Printed in USA

The Medicines Company

5 SYLVAN WAY
PARSIPPANY, NJ 07054

Direct Inquiries to:
(800) 264-4662

ANGIOMAX® ℞

[an-'jē-ō max]
(bivalirudin)
FOR INJECTION

DESCRIPTION

Angiomax® (bivalirudin) is a specific and reversible direct thrombin inhibitor. The active substance is a synthetic, 20 amino acid peptide. The chemical name is D-phenylalanyl-L-prolyl-L-arginyl-L-prolyl-glycyl-glycyl-glycyl-glycyl-L-asparagyl-glycyl-L-aspartyl-L-phenylalanyl-L-glutamyl-L-glutamyl-L-isoleucyl-L-prolyl-L-glutamyl-L-glutamyl-L-tyrosyl-L-leucine trifluoroacetate (salt) hydrate (Figure 1). The molecular weight of Angiomax is 2180 daltons (anhydrous free base peptide). Angiomax is supplied in single-use vials as a white lyophilized cake, which is sterile. Each vial contains 250 mg bivalirudin, 125 mg mannitol, and sodium hydroxide to adjust the pH to 5 to 6 (equivalent of approximately 12.5 mg sodium). When reconstituted with Sterile Water for Injection the product yields a clear to opalescent, colorless to slightly yellow solution, pH 5–6.

[See chemical structure at top of next page]

CLINICAL PHARMACOLOGY

General:

Angiomax directly inhibits thrombin by specifically binding both to the catalytic site and to the anion-binding exosite of circulating and clot-bound thrombin. Thrombin is a serine proteinase that plays a central role in the thrombotic process, acting to cleave fibrinogen into fibrin monomers and to activate Factor XIII to Factor XIIIa, allowing fibrin to develop a covalently cross-linked framework which stabilizes the thrombus; thrombin also activates Factors V and VIII, promoting further thrombin generation, and activates platelets, stimulating aggregation and granule release. The binding of Angiomax to thrombin is reversible as thrombin slowly cleaves the Angiomax-Arg_3-Pro_4 bond, resulting in recovery of thrombin active site functions.

In *in vitro* studies, bivalirudin inhibited both soluble (free) and clot-bound thrombin, was not neutralized by products of the platelet release reaction, and prolonged the activated partial thromboplastin time (aPTT), thrombin time (TT), and prothrombin time (PT) of normal human plasma in a concentration-dependent manner. The clinical relevance of these findings is unknown.

Pharmacokinetics:

Bivalirudin exhibits linear pharmacokinetics following intravenous (IV) administration to patients undergoing percutaneous transluminal coronary angioplasty (PTCA). In these patients, a mean steady state bivalirudin concentration of 12.3 ± 1.7 mcg/mL is achieved following an IV bolus of 1 mg/kg and a 4-hour 2.5 mg/kg/h IV infusion. Bivalirudin is cleared from plasma by a combination of renal mechanisms and proteolytic cleavage, with a half-life in patients with normal renal function of 25 minutes. The disposition of bivalirudin was studied in PTCA patients with mild and moderate renal impairment and in patients with severe renal impairment. Drug elimination was related to glomerular filtration rate (GFR). Total body clearance was similar for patients with normal renal function and with mild renal impairment (60–89mL/min). Clearance was reduced approximately 20% in patients with moderate and severe renal impairment and was reduced approximately 80% in dialysis-dependent patients. See Table 1 for pharmacokinetic parameters and dose reduction recommendations. For patients with renal impairment the activated clotting time (ACT) should be monitored. Bivalirudin is hemodialyzable. Approximately 25% is cleared by hemodialysis.

Bivalirudin does not bind to plasma proteins (other than thrombin) or to red blood cells.

[See table 1 at right]

Pharmacodynamics:

In healthy volunteers and patients (with ≥ 70% vessel occlusion undergoing routine angioplasty), bivalirudin exhibits its linear dose- and concentration-dependent anticoagulant activity as evidenced by prolongation of the ACT, aPTT, PT, and TT. Intravenous administration of Angiomax produces an immediate anticoagulant effect. Coagulation times return to baseline approximately 1 hour following cessation of Angiomax administration.

In 291 patients with ≥ 70% vessel occlusion undergoing routine angioplasty, a positive correlation was observed between the dose of Angiomax and the proportion of patients achieving ACT values of 300 sec or 350 sec. At an Angiomax dose of 1.0 mg/kg IV bolus plus 2.5 mg/kg/h IV infusion for 4 hours, followed by 0.2 mg/kg/h, all patients reached maximal ACT values > 300 sec.

Clinical Trials:

Angiomax was evaluated in patients with unstable angina undergoing PTCA in two randomized, double-blind, multicenter studies with identical protocols. Patients must have had unstable angina defined as: (1) a new onset of severe or accelerated angina or rest pain within the month prior to study entry or (2) angina or ischemic rest pain which developed between four hours and two weeks after an acute myocardial infarction (MI). Overall, 4312 patients with unstable angina, including 741 (17%) patients with post-MI angina, were treated in a 1:1 randomized fashion with Angiomax or heparin. Patients ranged in age from 29–90 (median 63) years, their weight was a median of 80 kg (39–120kg), 68% were male, and 91% were Caucasian. Twenty-three percent of patients were treated with heparin within one hour prior to randomization. All patients were administered aspirin 300–325 mg prior to PTCA and daily thereafter. Patients randomized to Angiomax were started on an intravenous infusion of Angiomax (2.5 mg/kg/h). Within 5 minutes after starting the infusion, and prior to PTCA, a 1 mg/kg loading dose was administered as an intravenous bolus. The infusion was continued for 4 hours, then the infusion was changed under double-blinded conditions to Angiomax (0.2 mg/kg/h) for up to an additional 20 hours (patients received this infusion for an average of 14 hours). The ACT was checked at 5 minutes and at 45 minutes following commencement. If on either occasion the ACT was <350 seconds, an additional double-blinded bolus of placebo was administered. The Angiomax dose was not titrated to ACT. Median ACT values were: ACT in seconds (5th percentile-95th percentile): 345 sec (240–595 seconds) at 5 min and 346 sec (range 269–583 sec) at 45 min after initiation of dosing. Patients randomized to heparin were given a loading dose (175 IU/kg) as an intravenous bolus 5-minutes before the planned procedure, with immediate commencement of an infusion of heparin (15 IU/kg/h). The infusion was continued for 4 hours. After 4-hours of infusion, the heparin infusion was changed under double-blinded conditions to heparin (15 IU/kg/hour) for up to 20 additional hours. The ACT was checked at 5 minutes and at 45 minutes following commencement. If on either occasion the ACT was <350 seconds, an additional double-blind bolus of heparin (60 IU/kg) was administered. Once the target ACT was achieved for heparin patients, no further ACT measurements were performed. All ACTs were determined with the Hemochron® device. The protocol allowed use of open-label heparin at the discretion of the investigator after discontinuation of blinded study medication, whether or not an endpoint event (procedural failure) had occurred. The use of open-label heparin was similar between Angiomax and heparin treatment groups (about 20% in both groups).

The studies were designed to demonstrate the safety and efficacy of Angiomax in patients undergoing PTCA as a treatment for unstable angina as compared with a control group of similar patients receiving heparin during and up to 24 hours after initiation of PTCA. The primary protocol endpoint was a composite endpoint called procedural failure, which included both clinical and angiographic elements measured during hospitalization. The clinical elements were: the occurrence of death, MI, or urgent revascularization, adjudicated under double-blind conditions. The angiographic elements were: impending or abrupt vessel closure. The protocol-specified safety endpoint was major hemorrhage.

The median duration of hospitalization was 4 days for both the Angiomax treatment group and the heparin treatment group. The rates of procedural failure were similar in the Angiomax and heparin treatment groups. Study outcomes are shown in Table 2.

[See table 2 above]

INDICATIONS AND USAGE

Angiomax is indicated for use as an anticoagulant in patients with unstable angina undergoing percutaneous transluminal coronary angioplasty (PTCA). Angiomax is intended for use with aspirin and has been studied only in patients receiving concomitant aspirin (see Clinical Trials and DOSAGE AND ADMINISTRATION).

The safety and effectiveness of Angiomax have not been established when used in conjunction with platelet inhibitors other than aspirin, such as glycoprotein IIb/IIIa inhibitors (see PRECAUTIONS, Drug Interactions).

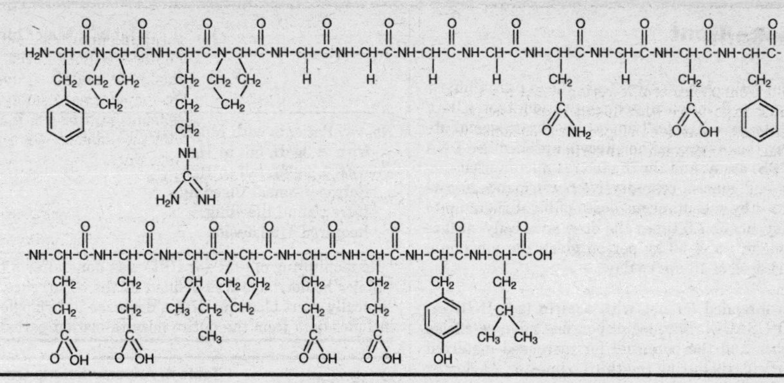

Table 1. PK parameters and dose adjustments in renal impairment*

Renal Function (GFR, mL/min)	Clearance (mL/min/kg)	Half-life (minutes)	% reduction in infusion dose
Normal renal function (≥90 mL/min)	3.4	25	0
Mild renal impairment (60–89 mL/min)	3.4	22	0
Moderate renal impairment (30–59 mL/min)	2.7	34	20
Severe renal impairment (10–29 mL/min)	2.8	57	60
Dialysis-dependent patients (off dialysis)	1.0	3.5 hours	90

* The ACT should be monitored in renally-impaired patients

Table 2. Incidences of In-hospital Clinical Endpoints In Randomized Clinical Trials Occurring within 7 Days

All Patients	ANGIOMAX® n=2161	HEPARIN n=2151
Efficacy Endpoints:		
Procedural Failure[1]	7.9%	9.3%
Death, MI, Revascularization	6.2%	7.9%
Death	0.2%	0.2%
MI[2]	3.3%	4.2%
Revascularization[3]	4.2%	5.6%
Safety Endpoint:		
Major Hemorrhage[4]	3.5%	9.3%

[1] The protocol specified primary endpoint (a composite of death or MI or clinical deterioration of cardiac origin requiring revascularization or placement of an aortic balloon pump or angiographic evidence of abrupt vessel closure).

[2] Defined as: Q-wave MI; CK-MB elevation ≥ 2×ULN, new ST- or T-wave abnormality, and chest pain ≥30 mins; OR new LBBB with chest pain ≥30 mins and/or elevated CK-MB enzymes; OR elevated CK-MB and new ST- or T-wave abnormality without chest pain; OR elevated CK-MB.

[3] Defined as: any revascularization procedure, including angioplasty, CABG, stenting, or placement of an intra-aortic balloon pump.

[4] Defined as the occurrence of any of the following: intracranial bleeding, retroperitoneal bleeding, clinically overt bleeding with a decrease in hemoglobin ≥3 g/dL or leading to a transfusion of ≥2 units of blood.

The safety and effectiveness of Angiomax have not been established in patients with unstable angina who are not undergoing PTCA or in patients with other acute coronary syndromes.

CONTRAINDICATIONS

Angiomax is contraindicated in patients with:

— active major bleeding;

— hypersensitivity to Angiomax or its components.

WARNINGS

Angiomax is not intended for intramuscular administration. Although most bleeding associated with the use of Angiomax in PTCA occurs at the site of arterial puncture, hemorrhage can occur at any site. An unexplained fall in blood pressure or hematocrit, or any unexplained symptom, should lead to serious consideration of a hemorrhagic event and cessation of Angiomax administration.

There is no known antidote to Angiomax. Angiomax is hemodialyzable (see CLINICAL PHARMACOLOGY, Pharmacokinetics).

PRECAUTIONS

General:

Clinical trials have provided limited information for use of Angiomax in patients with heparin-induced thrombocytopenia/heparin-induced thrombocytopenia-thrombosis syndrome (HIT/HITTS) undergoing PTCA. The number of HIT/HITTS patients treated is inadequate to reliably assess efficacy and safety in these patients undergoing PTCA. Angiomax was administered to a small number of patients with a history of HIT/HITTS or active HIT/HITTS and undergoing PTCA in an uncontrolled, open-label study and in an emergency treatment program and appeared to provide adequate anticoagulation in these patients. In *in vitro* studies, bivalirudin exhibited no platelet aggregation response against sera from patients with a history of HIT/HITTS.

Drug Interactions:

Bivalirudin does not exhibit binding to plasma proteins (other than thrombin) or red blood cells.

Drug-drug interaction studies have been conducted with the adenosine diphosphate (ADP) antagonist, ticlopidine, and the glycoprotein IIb/IIIa inhibitor, abciximab, and with low molecular weight heparin. Although data are limited, precluding conclusions regarding efficacy and safety in combination with these agents, the results do not suggest pharmacodynamic interactions. In patients treated with low molecular weight heparin, low molecular weight heparin was discontinued at least 8 hours prior to the procedure and administration of Angiomax.

The safety and effectiveness of Angiomax have not been established when used in conjunction with platelet inhibitors other than aspirin, such as glycoprotein IIb/IIIa inhibitors. In clinical trials in patients undergoing PTCA, co-administration of Angiomax with heparin, warfarin or thrombolytics was associated with increased risks of major bleeding events compared to patients not receiving these concomitant medications. There is no experience with co-administration of Angiomax and plasma expanders such as dextran. Angiomax should be used with caution in patients with disease states associated with an increased risk of bleeding.

Pediatric Use:

The safety and effectiveness of Angiomax in pediatric patients have not been established.

Immunogenicity/Re-exposure:

Among 494 subjects who received Angiomax in clinical trials and were tested for antibodies, 2 subjects had treatment-emergent positive bivalirudin antibody tests. Neither subject demonstrated clinical evidence of allergic or anaphylactic reactions and repeat testing was not performed. Nine additional patients who had initial positive tests were negative on repeat testing.

Carcinogenesis, mutagenesis, and impairment of fertility:

No long-term studies in animals have been performed to evaluate the carcinogenic potential of Angiomax. Bivalirudin displayed no genotoxic potential in the *in vitro* bacterial

Continued on next page

Angiomax—Cont.

cell reverse mutation assay (Ames test), the *in vitro* Chinese hamster ovary cell forward gene mutation test (CHO/HGPRT), the *in vitro* human lymphocyte chromosomal aberration assay, the *in vitro* rat hepatocyte unscheduled DNA synthesis (UDS) assay, and the *in vivo* rat micronucleus assay. Fertility and general reproductive performance in rats were unaffected by subcutaneous doses of bivalirudin up to 150 mg/kg/day, about 1.6 times the dose on a body surface area basis (mg/m^2) of a 50 kg person given the maximum recommended dose of 15 mg/kg/day.

Pregnancy:

Angiomax is intended for use with aspirin (see INDICATIONS AND USAGE). Because of possible adverse effects on the neonate and the potential for increased maternal bleeding, particularly during the third trimester, Angiomax and aspirin should be used together during pregnancy only if clearly needed.

Pregnancy Category B:

Teratogenicity studies have been performed in rats at subcutaneous doses up to 150 mg/kg/day, (1.6 times the maximum recommended human dose based on body surface area) and rabbits at subcutaneous doses up to 150 mg/kg/day (3.2 times the maximum recommended human dose based on body surface area). These studies revealed no evidence of impaired fertility or harm to the fetus attributable to bivalirudin. There are, however, no adequate and well-controlled studies in pregnant women. Because animal reproduction studies are not always predictive of human response, this drug should be used during pregnancy only if clearly needed.

Nursing mothers:

It is not known whether bivalirudin is excreted in human milk. Because many drugs are excreted in human milk, caution should be exercised when Angiomax is administered to a nursing woman.

Geriatric patients:

Of the total number of patients in clinical studies of Angiomax undergoing PTCA, 41% were ≥65 years of age, while 11% were >75 years old. A difference of ≥5% between age groups was observed for heparin-treated but not Angiomax-treated patients with regard to the percentage of patients with major bleeding events. There were no individual bleeding events which were observed with a difference of ≥5% between treatment groups, although puncture site hemorrhage and catheterization site hematoma were each observed in a higher percentage of patients ≥65 years than in patients <65 years. This difference between age groups was more pronounced for heparin-treated than Angiomax-treated patients.

ADVERSE REACTIONS

Bleeding:

In 4312 patients undergoing PTCA for treatment of unstable angina in 2 randomized, double-blind studies comparing Angiomax to heparin, Angiomax patients exhibited lower rates of major bleeding and lower requirements for blood transfusions. The incidence of major bleeding is presented in Table 3. The incidence of major bleeding was lower in the Angiomax group than in the heparin group.

[See table 3 above]

Table 3. Major bleeding and transfusions: All Patients[1]

	ANGIOMAX® n=2161	HEPARIN n=2151
No. (%) Patients with Major Hemorrhage[2]	79 (3.7)	199 (9.3)
–with ≥ 3g/dL fall in Hgb	41 (1.9)	124 (5.8)
–with ≥ 5g/dL fall in Hgb	14 (<1)	47 (2.2)
–Retroperitoneal Bleeding	5 (<1)	15 (<1)
–Intracranial Bleeding	1 (<1)	2 (<1)
–Required Transfusion	43 (2.0)	123 (5.7)

[1] No monitoring of ACT (or PTT) was done after a target ACT was achieved.
[2] Major hemorrhage was defined as the occurrence of any of the following: intracranial bleeding, retroperitoneal bleeding, clinically overt bleeding with a decrease in hemoglobin ≥3 g/dL or leading to a transfusion of ≥2 units of blood. This table includes data from the entire hospitalization period.

Other adverse events:

In the 2 randomized double-blind clinical trials of Angiomax in patients undergoing PTCA, 82% of 2161 Angiomax-treated patients and 83% of 2151 heparin-treated patients experienced at least one treatment-emergent adverse event. The most frequent treatment-emergent events were back pain (42%), pain (15%), nausea (15%), headache (12%), and hypotension (12%) in the Angiomax-treated group. Treatment-emergent adverse events other than bleeding reported for ≥5% of patients in either treatment group are shown in Table 4.

[See table 4 above]

Table 4. Adverse Events Other Than Bleeding Occurring in ≥5% Of Patients In Either Treatment Group In Randomized Clinical Trials

EVENT	Treatment Group: ANGIOMAX® (n=2161)	Treatment Group: HEPARIN (n=2151)
	Number of Patients (%)	
Cardiovascular		
Hypotension	262 (12)	371 (17)
Hypertension	135 (6)	115 (5)
Bradycardia	118 (5)	164 (8)
Gastrointestinal		
Nausea	318 (15)	347 (16)
Vomiting	138 (6)	169 (8)
Dyspepsia	100 (5)	111 (5)
Genitourinary		
Urinary retention	89 (4)	98 (5)
Miscellaneous		
Back pain	916 (42)	944 (44)
Pain	330 (15)	358 (17)
Headache	264 (12)	225 (10)
Injection site pain	174 (8)	274 (13)
Insomnia	142 (7)	139 (6)
Pelvic pain	130 (6)	169 (8)
Anxiety	127 (6)	140 (7)
Abdominal pain	103 (5)	104 (5)
Fever	103 (5)	108 (5)
Nervousness	102 (5)	87 (4)

Serious, non-bleeding adverse events were experienced in 2% of 2161 Angiomax-treated patients and 2% of 2151 heparin-treated patients. The following individual serious non-bleeding adverse events were rare (>0.1% to <1%) and similar in incidence between Angiomax and heparin-treated patients. These events are listed by body system: *Body as a Whole*: fever, infection, sepsis; *Cardiovascular*: hypotension, syncope, vascular anomaly, ventricular fibrillation; *Nervous*: cerebral ischemia, confusion, facial paralysis; *Respiratory*: lung edema; *Urogenital*: kidney failure, oliguria.

OVERDOSAGE

Discontinuation of Angiomax leads to a gradual reduction in anticoagulant effects due to metabolism of the drug. There has been no experience of overdosage in human clinical trials. In case of overdosage, Angiomax should be discontinued and the patient should be closely monitored for signs of bleeding. There is no known antidote to Angiomax. Angiomax is hemodialyzable (see CLINICAL PHARMACOLOGY, Pharmacokinetics).

DOSAGE AND ADMINISTRATION

The recommended dosage of Angiomax is intravenous (IV) bolus dose of 1.0 mg/kg followed by a 4-hour IV infusion at a rate of 2.5 mg/kg/h. After completion of the initial 4-hour infusion, an additional IV infusion of Angiomax may be initiated at a rate of 0.2 mg/kg/h for up to 20 hours, if needed. Angiomax is intended for use with aspirin (300–325 mg daily) and has been studied only in patients receiving concomitant aspirin. Treatment with Angiomax should be initiated just prior to PTCA. The dose of Angiomax may need to be reduced, and anticoagulation status monitored, in patients with renal impairment (see CLINICAL PHARMACOLOGY, Pharmacokinetics).

Table 5. Dosing Table

Weight (kg)	Using 5 mg/mL concentration: Bolus (1 mg/kg) (mL)	Using 5 mg/mL concentration: Initial 4-hour Infusion (2.5 mg/kg/hr) (mL/hr)	Using 0.5 mg/mL concentration: Subsequent Low-rate Infusion (0.2mg/kg/hr) (mL/hr)
43–47	9	22.5	18
48–52	10	25	20
53–57	11	27.5	22
58–62	12	30	24
63–67	13	32.5	26
68–72	14	35	28
73–77	15	37.5	30
78–82	16	40	32
83–87	17	42.5	34
88–92	18	45	36
93–97	19	47.5	38
98–102	20	50	40
103–107	21	52.5	42
108–112	22	55	44
113–117	23	57.5	46
118–122	24	60	48
123–127	25	62.5	50
128–132	26	65	52
133–137	27	67.5	54
138–142	28	70	56
143–147	29	72.5	58
148–152	30	75	60

Instructions for Administration:

Angiomax® (bivalirudin) is intended for intravenous injection and infusion. To each 250 mg vial add 5 mL of Sterile Water for Injection, USP. Gently swirl until all material is dissolved. Each reconstituted vial should be further diluted in 50 mL of 5% Dextrose in Water or 0.9% Sodium Chloride for Injection to yield a final concentration of 5 mg/mL (e.g., 1 vial in 50 mL; 2 vials in 100 mL; 5 vials in 250 mL). The dose to be administered is adjusted according to the patient's weight, see Table 5.

If the low-rate infusion is used after the initial infusion, a lower concentration bag should be prepared. In order to prepare this bag, reconstitute the 250 mg vial with 5 mL of Sterile Water for Injection, USP. Gently swirl until all material is dissolved. Each reconstituted vial should be further diluted in 500 mL of 5% Dextrose in Water or 0.9% Sodium Chloride for Injection to yield a final concentration of 0.5 mg/mL. The infusion rate to be administered should be selected from the right-hand column in Table 5.

[See table 5 above]

Angiomax should be administered via an intravenous line. No incompatibilities have been observed with glass bottles or polyvinyl chloride bags and administration sets. Ninety-six intravenous medications including those commonly administered to patients with coronary artery disease undergoing PTCA were tested for Y-site physical compatibility with Angiomax. Eighty-seven of the 96 test drugs were compatible with Angiomax including: abciximab, dexamethasone sodium phosphate, digoxin, diphenhydramine HCl, dobutamine HCl, dopamine HCl, epinephrine HCl, eptifibatide, esmolol, furosemide, heparin sodium, hydrocortisone sodium succinate, lidocaine HCl, meperidine HCl, methylprednisolone sodium succinate, midazolam HCl, morphine sulphate, nitroglycerin, potassium chloride, sodium bicarbonate, tirofiban HCl, and verapamil HCl.

Nine drugs related in haze formation, microparticulate formation, or gross precipitation and should not be administered in the same intravenous line with Angiomax. These nine incompatible drugs are: alteplase, amiodarone HCl, amphotericin B, chlorpromazine HCl, diazepam, prochlorperazine edisylate, reteplase, streptokinase, and vancomycin HCl.

Parenteral drug products should be inspected visually for particulate matter and discoloration prior to administration. Preparations of Angiomax containing particulate matter should not be used. Reconstituted material will be a clear to slightly opalescent, colorless to slightly yellow solution.

Storage after Reconstitution:
Do not freeze reconstituted or diluted Angiomax. Reconstituted material may be stored at 2–8°C for up to 24 hours. Diluted Angiomax with a concentration of between 0.5 mg/mL and 5 mg/mL is stable at room temperature for up to 24 hours. Discard any unused portion of reconstituted solution remaining in the vial.

HOW SUPPLIED

Angiomax® (bivalirudin) is supplied as a sterile, lyophilized product in single-use, glass vials. After reconstitution, each vial delivers 250 mg of Angiomax.
Store Angiomax dosage units at 20–25°C (68–77°F). Excursions to 15–30°C permitted. [See USP Controlled Room Temperature.]
NDC# 65293-001-01
Manufactured by:
Ben Venue Laboratories
Bedford, Ohio
Distributed by:
ICS
Louisville, KY
Marketed by:
THE MEDICINES COMPANY
Cambridge, MA 02142
For information call: (800) 264-4662
U.S. Patent 5,196,404
Rx only
Hemochron® is a registered trademark of International Technidyne Corporation, Edison, NJ.
TMC PN 1002 Rev. 1 (06/08/2001)

Merck & Co., Inc.
WEST POINT, PA 19486

For Medical Information Contact:
Generally:
Product and service information:
Call the Merck National Service Center, 8:00 AM to 7:00 PM (ET), Monday through Friday:
(800) NSC-MERCK
(800) 672-6372
FAX: (800) MERCK-68
FAX: (800) 637-2568
Adverse Drug Experiences:
Call the Merck National Service Center, 8:00 AM to 7:00 PM (ET), Monday through Friday:
(800) NSC-MERCK
(800) 672-6372
In Emergencies:
24-hour emergency information for healthcare professionals:
(800) NSC-MERCK
(800) 672-6372
Sales and Ordering:
For product orders and direct account inquiries only, call the Order Management Center,
8:00 AM to 7:00 PM (ET), Monday through Friday:
(800) MERCK RX
(800) 637-2579

INVANZ™ ℞
(ERTAPENEM FOR INJECTION)

For Intravenous or Intramuscular Use

DESCRIPTION

INVANZ* (Ertapenem for Injection) is a sterile, synthetic, parenteral, 1-β methyl-carbapenem that is structurally related to beta-lactam antibiotics.
Chemically, INVANZ is described as [4*R*-[3(3*S**,5*S**), 4α,5β,6β(*R**)]]-3-[[5-[[(3-carboxyphenyl)amino]carbonyl-3-pyrrolidinyl]thio]-6-(1-hydroxyethyl)-4-methyl-7-oxo-1-azabicyclo[3.2.0]hept-2-ene-2-carboxylic acid monosodium salt. Its molecular weight is 497.50. The empirical formula is $C_{22}H_{24}N_3O_7SNa$, and its structural formula is:

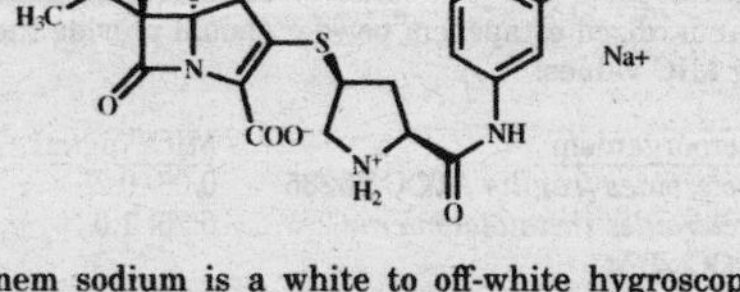

Ertapenem sodium is a white to off-white hygroscopic, weakly crystalline powder. It is soluble in water and 0.9% sodium chloride solution, practically insoluble in ethanol, and insoluble in isopropyl acetate and tetrahydrofuran.
INVANZ is supplied as sterile lyophilized powder for intravenous infusion after reconstitution with appropriate diluent (see DOSAGE AND ADMINISTRATION, PREPARATION OF SOLUTION) and transfer to 50 mL 0.9% Sodium Chloride Injection or for intramuscular injection following

Table 1
Plasma Concentrations of Ertapenem After Single Dose Administration

Dose/Route	Average Plasma Concentrations (mcg/mL) 0.5 hr	1 hr	2 hr	4 hr	6 hr	8 hr	12 hr	18 hr	24 hr
1 g IV*	155	115	83	48	31	20	9	3	1
1 g IM	33	53	67	57	40	27	13	4	2

*Infused at a constant rate over 30 minutes

Table 2
Concentrations (mcg/mL) of Ertapenem in Skin Blister Fluid at each Sampling Point on the Third Day of 1-g Once Daily IV Doses

0.5 hr	1 hr	2 hr	4 hr	8 hr	12 hr	24 hr
7	12	17	24	24	21	8

reconstitution with 1% lidocaine hydrochloride. Each vial contains 1.046 grams ertapenem sodium, equivalent to 1 gram ertapenem. The sodium content is approximately 137 mg (approximately 6.0 mEq).
Each vial of INVANZ contains the following inactive ingredients: 175 mg sodium bicarbonate and sodium hydroxide to adjust pH to 7.5.

* Trademark of MERCK & CO., Inc.

CLINICAL PHARMACOLOGY

Pharmacokinetics
Average plasma concentrations (mcg/mL) of ertapenem following a single 30-minute infusion of a 1 g intravenous (IV) dose and administration of a single 1 g intramuscular (IM) dose in healthy young adults are presented in Table 1.
[See table 1 above]
The area under the plasma concentration-time curve (AUC) of ertapenem increased less-than dose-proportional based on total ertapenem concentrations over the 0.5 to 2 g dose range, whereas the AUC increased greater-than dose proportional based on unbound ertapenem concentrations. Ertapenem exhibits non-linear pharmacokinetics due to concentration-dependent plasma protein binding at the proposed therapeutic dose. (See CLINICAL PHARMACOLOGY, *Distribution*.)
There is no accumulation of ertapenem following multiple IV or IM 1g daily doses in healthy adults.
Absorption
Ertapenem, reconstituted with 1% lidocaine HCl injection, USP (in saline without epinephrine), is almost completely absorbed following intramuscular (IM) administration at the recommended dose of 1 g. The mean bioavailability is approximately 90%. Following 1 g daily IM administration, mean peak plasma concentrations (C_{max}) are achieved in approximately 2.3 hours (T_{max}).
Distribution
Ertapenem is highly bound to human plasma proteins, primarily albumin. In healthy young adults, the protein binding of ertapenem decreases as plasma concentrations increase, from approximately 95% bound at an approximate plasma concentration of <100 micrograms (mcg)/mL to approximately 85% bound at an approximate plasma concentration of 300 mcg/mL.
The apparent volume of distribution at steady state (V_{ss}) of ertapenem is approximately 8.2 liters.
The concentrations of ertapenem achieved in suction-induced skin blister fluid at each sampling point on the third day of 1 g once daily IV doses are presented in Table 2. The ratio of AUC_{0-24} in skin blister fluid/AUC_{0-24} in plasma is 0.61.
[See table 2 above]
The concentration of ertapenem in breast milk from 5 lactating women with pelvic infections (5 to 14 days postpartum) was measured at random time points daily for 5 consecutive days following the last 1 g dose of intravenous therapy (3–10 days of therapy). The concentration of ertapenem in breast milk within 24 hours of the last dose of therapy in all 5 women ranged from <0.13 (lower limit of quantitation) to 0.38 mcg/mL; peak concentrations were not assessed. By day 5 after discontinuation of therapy, the level of ertapenem was undetectable in the breast milk of 4 women and below the lower limit of quantitation (<0.13 mcg/mL) in 1 woman.
Metabolism
In healthy young adults, after infusion of 1 g IV radiolabeled ertapenem, the plasma radioactivity consists predominantly (94%) of ertapenem. The major metabolite of ertapenem is the inactive ring-opened derivative formed by hydrolysis of the beta-lactam ring.
In vitro studies in human liver microsomes indicate that ertapenem does not inhibit metabolism mediated by any of the following cytochrome p450 (CYP) isoforms: 1A2, 2C9, 2C19, 2D6, 2E1 and 3A4. (See DRUG INTERACTIONS.)
In vitro studies indicate that ertapenem does not inhibit P-glycoprotein-mediated transport of digoxin or vinblastine and that ertapenem is not a substrate for P-glycoprotein-mediated transport. (See PRECAUTIONS, *Drug Interactions*.)
Elimination
Ertapenem is eliminated primarily by the kidneys. The mean plasma half-life in healthy young adults is approximately 4 hours and the plasma clearance is approximately 1.8 L/hour.
Following the administration of 1 g IV radiolabeled ertapenem to healthy young adults, approximately 80% is recovered in urine and 10% in feces. Of the 80% recovered in urine, approximately 38% is excreted as unchanged drug and approximately 37% as the ring-opened metabolite.
In healthy young adults given a 1 g IV dose, the mean percentage of the administered dose excreted in urine was 17.4% during 0–2 hours postdose, 5.4% during 4–6 hours postdose, and 2.4% during 12–24 hours postdose.
Special Populations
Renal Insufficiency
Total and unbound fractions of ertapenem pharmacokinetics were investigated in 26 adult subjects (31 to 80 years of age) with varying degrees of renal impairment. Following a single 1 g IV dose of ertapenem, the unbound AUC increased 1.5-fold and 2.3-fold in subjects with mild renal insufficiency (CL_{CR} 60–90 mL/min/1.73 m^2) and moderate renal insufficiency (CL_{CR} 31–59 mL/min/1.73 m^2), respectively, compared with healthy young subjects (25 to 45 years of age). No dosage adjustment is necessary in patients with CL_{CR} ≥31 mL/min/1.73 m^2. The unbound AUC increased 4.4-fold and 7.6-fold in subjects with advanced renal insufficiency (CL_{CR} 5–30 mL/min/1.73 m^2) and end-stage renal insufficiency (CL_{CR} <10 mL/min/1.73 m^2), respectively, compared with healthy young subjects. The effects of renal insufficiency on AUC of total drug were of smaller magnitude. The recommended dose of ertapenem in patients with CL_{CR} ≤30 mL/min/1.73 m^2 is 0.5 grams every 24 hours. Following a single 1 g IV dose given immediately prior to a 4 hour hemodialysis session in 5 patients with end-stage renal insufficiency, approximately 30% of the dose was recovered in the dialysate. A supplementary dose of 150 mg is recommended if ertapenem is administered within 6 hours prior to hemodialysis. (See DOSAGE AND ADMINISTRATION.)
Hepatic Insufficiency
The pharmacokinetics of ertapenem in patients with hepatic insufficiency have not been established. However, ertapenem does not appear to undergo hepatic metabolism based on *in vitro* studies and approximately 10% of an administered dose is recovered in the feces. (See PRECAUTIONS and DOSAGE AND ADMINISTRATION.)
Gender
The effect of gender on the pharmacokinetics of ertapenem was evaluated in healthy male (n=8) and healthy female (n=8) subjects. The differences observed could be attributed to body size when body weight was taken into consideration. No dose adjustment is recommended based on gender.
Geriatric Patients
The impact of age on the pharmacokinetics of ertapenem was evaluated in healthy male (n=7) and healthy female (n=7) subjects ≥65 years of age. The total and unbound AUC increased 37% and 67%, respectively, in elderly adults relative to young adults. These changes were attributed to age-related changes in creatinine clearance. No dosage adjustment is necessary for elderly patients with normal (for their age) renal function.
Pediatric Patients
The pharmacokinetics of ertapenem in pediatric patients have not been established.
Microbiology
Ertapenem has *in vitro* activity against gram-positive and gram-negative aerobic and anaerobic bacteria. The bactericidal activity of ertapenem results from the inhibition of cell wall synthesis and is mediated through ertapenem binding to penicillin binding proteins (PBPs). In *Escherichia coli*, it has strong affinity toward PBPs 1a, 1b, 2, 3, 4 and 5 with preference for PBPs 2 and 3. Ertapenem is stable against hydrolysis by a variety of beta-lactamases, including penicillinases, and cephalosporinases and extended spectrum beta-lactamases. Ertapenem is hydrolyzed by metallo-beta-lactamases.
Ertapenem has been shown to be active against most strains of the following microorganisms *in vitro* and in clinical infections. (See INDICATIONS AND USAGE):
Aerobic gram-positive microorganisms:
Staphylococcus aureus (methicillin susceptible strains only)
Streptococcus agalactiae
Streptococcus pneumoniae (penicillin susceptible strains only)
Streptococcus pyogenes
Note: Methicillin-resistant staphylococci and *Enterococcus* spp. are resistant to ertapenem.

Continued on next page

Information on the Merck & Co., Inc., products listed on these pages is from the prescribing information in use April 1, 2002.

Invanz—Cont.

Aerobic gram-negative microorganisms:
Escherichia coli
Haemophilus influenzae (Beta-lactamase negative strains only)
Klebsiella pneumoniae
Moraxella catarrhalis
Anaerobic microorganisms:
Bacteroides fragilis
Bacteroides distasonis
Bacteroides ovatus
Bacteroides thetaiotaomicron
Bacteroides uniformis
Clostridium clostridioforme
Eubacterium lentum
Peptostreptococcus species
Porphyromonas asaccharolytica
Prevotella bivia
The following *in vitro* data are available, **but their clinical significance is unknown.**
At least 90% of the following microorganisms exhibit an *in vitro* minimum inhibitory concentration (MIC) less than or equal to the susceptible breakpoint for ertapenem; however, the safety and effectiveness of ertapenem in treating clinical infections due to these microorganisms have not been established in adequate and well-controlled clinical studies:
Aerobic gram-positive microorganisms:
Streptococcus pneumoniae (penicillin-intermediate strains only)
Aerobic gram-negative microorganisms:
Citrobacter freundii
Citrobacter koseri
Enterobacter aerogenes
Enterobacter cloacae
Haemophilus influenzae (Beta-lactamase positive strains)
Haemophilus parainfluenzae
Klebsiella oxytoca (excluding ESBL producing strains)
Morganella morganii
Proteus mirabilis
Proteus vulgaris
Serratia marcescens
Anaerobic microorganisms:
Clostridium perfringens
Fusobacterium spp.
Susceptibility Tests:
When available, the results of *in vitro* susceptibility tests should be provided to the physician as periodic reports which describe the susceptibility profile of nosocomial and community-acquired pathogens. These reports should aid the physician in selecting the most effective antimicrobial.
Dilution Techniques:
Quantitative methods are used to determine antimicrobial minimum inhibitory concentrations (MICs). These MICs provide estimates of the susceptibility of bacteria to antimicrobial compounds. The MICs should be determined using a standardized procedure. Standardized procedures are based on a broth dilution method[1,4] or equivalent with standardized inoculum concentrations and standardized concentrations of ertapenem powder. The MIC values should be interpreted according to the following criteria:
For testing Enterobacteriaceae and *Staphylococcus* spp.:

MIC (μg/mL)	Interpretation
≤2.0	Susceptible (S)
4.0	Intermediate (I)
≥8.0	Resistant (R)

Note: *Staphylococcus* spp. can be considered susceptible to ertapenem if the penicillin MIC is ≤ 0.12 μg/mL. If the penicillin MIC is >0.12 μg/mL, then test oxacillin. *Staphylococcus aureus* can be considered susceptible to ertapenem if the oxacillin MIC is ≤2.0 μg/mL and resistant to ertapenem if the oxacillin MIC is ≥4.0 μg/mL. Coagulase negative staphylococci can be considered susceptible to ertapenem if the oxacillin MIC is ≤0.25 μg/mL and resistant to ertapenem if the oxacillin MIC ≥0.5 μg/mL.

For testing *Haemophilus* spp.[a]:

MIC (μg/mL)	Interpretation[b]
≤0.5	Susceptible (S)

[a]This interpretive standard is applicable only to broth microdilution susceptibility tests with *Haemophilus* spp. using *Haemophilus* Test Medium (HTM)[1] inoculated with a direct colony suspension and incubated in ambient air at 35°C for 20–24 hrs.
[b]The current absence of data in resistant strains precludes defining any results other than "Susceptible". Strains yielding MIC results suggestive of a "nonsusceptible" category should be submitted to a reference laboratory for further testing.

For testing *Streptococcus pneumoniae*[c,d]:

MIC (μg/mL)	Interpretation[b]
≤1.0	Susceptible (S)

[c]This interpretive standard is applicable only to broth microdilution susceptibility tests using cation-adjusted Mueller-Hinton broth with 2–5% lysed horse blood inoculated with direct colony suspension and incubated in ambient air at 35°C for 20–24 hrs.
[d]*Streptococcus pneumoniae* that are susceptible to penicillin (penicillin MIC ≤0.06 μg/mL) can be considered susceptible to ertapenum. Testing of ertapenem against penicillin-intermediate or penicillin-resistant isolates is not recommended since reliable interpretive criteria for ertapenem are not available.

For testing *Streptococcus* spp. other than *Streptococcus pneumoniae*[c,e]:

MIC (μg/mL)	Interpretation[b]
≤1.0	Susceptible (S)

[e]*Streptococcus* spp. that are susceptible to penicillin (MIC ≤0.12 μg/mL) can be considered susceptible to ertapenum. Testing of ertapenem against penicillin-intermediate or penicillin-resistant isolates is not recommended since reliable interpretive criteria for ertapenem are not available.

A report of "Susceptible" indicates that the pathogen is likely to be inhibited if the antimicrobial compound in blood reaches the concentrations usually achievable. A report of "Intermediate" indicates that the result should be considered equivocal, and, if the microorganism is not fully susceptible to alternative, clinically feasible drugs, the test should be repeated. This category implies possible clinical applicability in body sites where the drug is physiologically concentrated or in situations where high dosage of drug can be used. This category also provides a buffer zone which prevents small uncontrolled technical factors from causing major discrepancies in interpretation. A report of "Resistant" indicates that the pathogen is not likely to be inhibited if the antimicrobial compound in the blood reaches the concentrations usually achievable; other therapy should be selected.
Standardized susceptibility test procedures require the use of laboratory control microorganisms to control the technical aspects of the laboratory procedures. Quality control microorganisms are specific strains of organisms with intrinsic biological properties. QC strains are very stable strains which will give a standard and repeatable susceptibility pattern. The specific strains used for microbiological quality control are not clinically significant. Standard ertapenem powder should provide the following MIC values.

Microorganism	MIC Range (μg/mL)
Enterococcus faecalis ATCC 29212	4.0–16.0
Escherichia coli ATCC 25922	0.004–0.016
Haemophilus influenzae[f] ATCC 49766	0.016–0.06
Pseudomonas aeruginosa ATCC 27853	2.0–8.0
Staphylococcus aureus ATCC 29213	0.06–0.25
Streptococcus pneumoniae[g] ATCC 49619	0.03–0.25

[f]This quality control range is applicable to only *H. influenzae* ATCC 49766 tested by the broth microdilution procedure using HTM[1] inoculated with a direct colony suspension and incubated in ambient air at 35°C for 20–24 hrs.
[g]This quality control range is applicable to only *S. pneumonaie* ATCC 49619 tested by a broth microdilution procedure using cation-adjusted Mueller-Hinton broth with 2–5% lysed horse blood inoculated with a direct colony suspension and incubated in ambient air at 35°C for 20–24 hrs.

Diffusion Techniques:
Quantitative methods that require measurement of zone diameters also provide reproducible estimates of the susceptibility of bacteria to antimicrobial compounds. One such standardized procedure[2,4] requires the use of standardized inoculum concentrations. This procedure uses paper disks impregnated with 10-μg ertapenem to test the suspectibility of microorganisms to ertapenem.
Reports from the laboratory providing results of the standard single-disk susceptibility test with a 10-μg ertapenem disk should be interpreted according to the following criteria:
For testing Enterobacteriaceae and *Staphylococcus* spp.:

Zone Diameter (mm)	Interpretation
≥19	Susceptible (S)
16–18	Intermediate (I)
≤15	Resistant (R)

Note: *Staphylococcus* spp. can be considered susceptible to ertapenem if the penicillin (10 U disk) zone is ≥29 mm. If the penicillin zone is ≤28 mm, then test oxacillin by disk diffusion (1 μg disk). *Staphylococcus aureus* can be considered susceptible to ertapenem if the oxacillin (1 μg disk) zone is ≥13 mm and resistant to ertapenem if the oxacillin zone is ≤10 mm. Coagulase negative staphylococci can be considered susceptible to ertapenem if the oxacillin zone is ≥18 mm and resistant to ertapenem if the oxacillin (1 μg disk) zone is ≤17 mm.

For testing *Haemophilus* spp.[h]:

Zone Diameter (mm)	Interpretation[b]
≥19	Susceptible (S)

[h]This zone diameter standard is applicable only to tests performed by disk diffusion with *Haemophilus* spp. using HTM[2] inoculated with a direct colony suspension and incubated in 5% CO_2 at 35°C for 16–18 hrs.

For testing *Streptococcus pneumoniae*[i,j]:

Zone Diameter (mm)	Interpretation[b]
≥19	Susceptible (S)

[i]These zone diameter standards apply only to tests performed using Mueller-Hinton agar supplemented with 5% sheep blood inoculated with a direct colony suspension and incubated in 5% CO_2 at 35°C for 20–24 hrs.
[j]*Streptococcus pneumoniae* that is susceptible to penicillin (1-μg oxacillin disk zone diameter ≥20 mm), can be considered susceptible to ertapenum. Isolates with 1-μg oxacillin zone diameter ≤19 mm should be tested against ertapenem using an MIC method.

For testing *Streptococcus* spp. other than *Streptococcus pneumoniae*[k,l]:

Zone Diameter (mm)	Interpretation[b]
≥19	Susceptible (S)

[k]These zone diameter standards apply only to tests performed using Mueller-Hinton agar supplemented with 5% sheep blood inoculated with a direct colony suspension and incubated in ambient air at 35°C for 20–24 hrs.
[l]Beta-hemolytic *Streptococcus* spp. that are susceptible to penicillin (10-units penicillin disk zone diameter ≥24 mm), can be considered susceptible to ertapenum. Isolates with 10-units penicillin disk zone diameter <24 mm should be tested against ertapenem using an MIC method. Penicillin disk diffusion interpretive criteria are not available for viridans group streptococci and they should not be tested against ertapenem.

Interpretation should be as stated above for results using dilution techniques. Interpretation involves correlation of the diameter obtained in the disk test with the MIC for ertapenem.
As with standardized dilution techniques, diffusion methods require the use of laboratory control microorganisms that are used to control the technical aspects of the laboratory procedures. Quality control microorganisms are specific strains of organisms with intrinsic biological properties. QC strains are very stable strains that will give a standard and repeatable susceptibility pattern. The specific strains used for microbiological quality control are not clinically significant. For the diffusion technique, the 10-μg ertapenem disk should provide the following zone diameters in these laboratory quality control strains:

Microorganism	Zone Diameter Range (mm)
Escherichia coli ATCC 25922	29–36
Haemophilus influenzae[m] ATCC 49766	27–33
Pseudomonas aeruginosa ATCC 27853	13–21
Staphylococcus aureus ATCC 25923	24–31
Streptococcus pneumoniae[n] ATCC 49619	28–35

[m]This quality control range is applicable to *Haemophilus influenzae* ATCC 49766 tested by disk diffusion using HTM[2] agar inoculated with a direct colony suspension and incubated in 5% CO_2 at 35°C for 16–18 hrs.
[n]This quality control range is applicable to *Streptococcus pneumoniae* ATCC 49619 tested by disk diffusion using Mueller-Hinton agar supplemented with 5% sheep blood inoculated with a direct colony suspension and incubated in 5% CO_2 at 35°C for 20–24 hrs.

Anaerobic Techniques:
For anaerobic bacteria, the susceptibility to ertapenem as MICs can be determined by standardized test methods[3]. The MIC values obtained should be interpreted according to the following criteria:

MIC (μg/mL)	Interpretation
≤4.0	Susceptible (S)
8.0	Intermediate (I)
≥16.0	Resistant (R)

Interpretation is identical to that stated above for results using dilution techniques.
As with other susceptibility techniques, the use of laboratory control microorganisms is required to control the technical aspects of the laboratory standardized procedures. Standardized ertapenem powder should provide the following MIC values:

Microorganism	MIC[o] (μg/mL)
Bacteroides fragilis ATCC 25285	0.06–0.25
Bacteroides thetaiotaomicron ATCC 29741	0.25–1.0
Eubacterium lentum ATCC 43055	0.5–2.0

[o]These quality control ranges are applicable only to agar dilution using *Brucella* agar supplemented with hemin, vitamin K1 and 5% defibrinated or laked sheep blood inoculated with a direct colony suspension or a 6- to 24-hour fresh culture in enriched thioglycollate medium and incubated in an anaerobic jar or chamber at 35–37°C for 42–48 hrs.

INDICATIONS AND USAGE

INVANZ is indicated for the treatment of adult patients with the following moderate to severe infections caused by susceptible strains of the designated microorganisms. (See DOSAGE AND ADMINISTRATION):

Complicated Intra-abdominal Infections due to *Escherichia coli, Clostridium clostridioforme, Eubacterium lentum, Peptostreptococcus* species, *Bacteroides fragilis, Bacteroides distasonis, Bacteroides ovatus, Bacteroides thetaiotaomicron,* or *Bacteroides uniformis.*

Complicated Skin and Skin Structure Infections due to *Staphylococcus aureus* (methicillin susceptible strains only), *Streptococcus pyogenes, Escherichia coli,* or *Peptostreptococcus* species.

Community Acquired Pneumonia due to *Streptococcus pneumoniae* (penicillin susceptible strains only) including cases with concurrent bacteremia, *Haemophilus influenzae* (beta-lactamase negative strains only), or *Moraxella catarrhalis.*

Complicated Urinary Tract Infections including pyelonephritis due to *Escherichia coli,* including cases with concurrent bacteremia, or *Klebsiella pneumoniae.*

Acute Pelvic Infections including postpartum endomyometritis, septic abortion and post surgical gynecologic infections due to *Streptococcus agalactiae, Escherichia coli, Bacteroides fragilis, Porphyromonas asaccharolytica, Peptostreptococcus* species, or *Prevotella bivia.*

Appropriate specimens for bacteriological examination should be obtained in order to isolate and identify the causative organisms and to determine their susceptibility to ertapenem. Therapy with INVANZ (ertapenem) may be initiated empirically before results of these tests are known; once results become available, antimicrobial therapy should be adjusted accordingly.

CONTRAINDICATIONS

INVANZ is contraindicated in patients with known hypersensitivity to any component of this product or to other drugs in the same class or in patients who have demonstrated anaphylactic reactions to beta-lactams.

Due to the use of lidocaine HCl as a diluent, INVANZ administered intramuscularly is contraindicated in patients with a known hypersensitivity to local anesthetics of the amide type. (Refer to the prescribing information for lidocaine HCl.)

WARNINGS

SERIOUS AND OCCASIONALLY FATAL HYPERSENSITIVITY (ANAPHYLACTIC) REACTIONS HAVE BEEN REPORTED IN PATIENTS RECEIVING THERAPY WITH BETA-LACTAMS. THESE REACTIONS ARE MORE LIKELY TO OCCUR IN INDIVIDUALS WITH A HISTORY OF SENSITIVITY TO MULTIPLE ALLERGENS. THERE HAVE BEEN REPORTS OF INDIVIDUALS WITH A HISTORY OF PENICILLIN HYPERSENSITIVITY WHO HAVE EXPERIENCED SEVERE HYPERSENSITIVITY REACTIONS WHEN TREATED WITH ANOTHER BETA-LACTAM. BEFORE INITIATING THERAPY WITH INVANZ, CAREFUL INQUIRY SHOULD BE MADE CONCERNING PREVIOUS HYPERSENSITIVITY REACTIONS TO PENICILLINS, CEPHALOSPORINS, OTHER BETA-LACTAMS AND OTHER ALLERGENS. IF AN ALLERGIC REACTION TO INVANZ OCCURS, DISCONTINUE THE DRUG IMMEDIATELY. **SERIOUS ANAPHYLACTIC REACTIONS REQUIRE IMMEDIATE EMERGENCY TREATMENT WITH EPINEPHRINE, OXYGEN, INTRAVENOUS STEROIDS, AND AIRWAY MANAGEMENT, INCLUDING INTUBATION. OTHER THERAPY MAY ALSO BE ADMINISTERED AS INDICATED.**

Seizures and other CNS adverse experiences have been reported during treatment with INVANZ. (See PRECAUTIONS and ADVERSE REACTIONS.)

Pseudomembranous colitis has been reported with nearly all antibacterial agents, including ertapenem, and may range in severity from mild to life-threatening. Therefore, it is important to consider this diagnosis in patients who present with diarrhea subsequent to the administration of antibacterial agents.

Treatment with antibacterial agents alters the normal flora of the colon and may permit overgrowth of clostridia. Studies indicate that a toxin produced by *Clostridium difficile* is a primary cause of "antibiotic-associated colitis".

After the diagnosis of pseudomembranous colitis has been established, therapeutic measures should be initiated. Mild cases of pseudomembranous colitis usually respond to drug discontinuation alone. In moderate to severe cases, consideration should be given to management with fluids and electrolytes, protein supplementation and treatment with an antibacterial drug clinically effective against *Clostridium difficile* colitis.

Lidocaine HCl is the diluent for intramuscular administration of INVANZ. Refer to the prescribing information for lidocaine HCl.

PRECAUTIONS

General

During clinical investigations in adult patients treated with INVANZ (1 g once a day), seizures, irrespective of drug relationship, occurred in 0.5% of patients during study therapy plus 14-day follow-up period. (See ADVERSE REACTIONS.) These experiences have occurred most commonly in patients with CNS disorders (e.g., brain lesions or history of seizures) and/or comprised renal function. Close adherence to the recommended dosage regimen is urged, especially in patients with known factors that predispose to convulsive activity. Anticonvulsant therapy should be continued in patients with known seizure disorders. If focal tremors, myoclonus, or seizures occur, patients should be evaluated neurologically, placed on anticonvulsant therapy if not already instituted, and the dosage of INVANZ reexamined to determine whether it should be decreased or the antibiotic discontinued. Dosage adjustment of INVANZ is recommended in patients with reduced renal function. (See DOSAGE AND ADMINISTRATION.)

As with other antibiotics, prolonged use of INVANZ may result in overgrowth of non-suspectible organisms. Repeated evaluation of the patient's condition is essential. If superinfection occurs during therapy, appropriate measures should be taken.

Caution should be taken when administering INVANZ intramuscularly to avoid inadvertent injection into a blood vessel. (See DOSAGE AND ADMINISTRATION.)

Lidocaine HCl is the diluent for intramuscular administration of INVANZ. Refer to the prescribing information for Lidocaine HCl for additional precautions.

Laboratory Tests

While INVANZ possesses toxicity similar to the beta-lactam group of antibiotics, periodic assessment of organ system function, including renal, hepatic, and hematopoietic, is advisable during prolonged therapy.

Drug Interactions

When ertapenem is co-administered with probenecid (500 mg p.o. every 6 hours), probenecid competes for active tubular secretion and reduces the renal clearance of ertapenem. Based on total ertapenem concentrations, probenecid increased the AUC by 25% and reduced the plasma and renal clearances by 20% and 35%, respectively. The half-life increased from 4.0 to 4.8 hours. Because of the small effect on half-life, the coadministration with probenecid to extend the half-life of ertapenem is not recommended.

In vitro studies indicate that ertapenem does not inhibit P-glycoprotein-mediated transport of digoxin or vinblastine and that ertapenem is not a substrate for P-glycoprotein-mediated transport. *In vitro* studies in human liver microsomes indicate that ertapenem does not inhibit metabolism mediated by any of the following six cytochrome p450 (CYP) isoforms: 1A2, 2C9, 2C19, 2D6, 2E1 and 3A4. Drug interactions caused by inhibition of P-glycoprotein-mediated drug clearance or CYP-mediated drug clearance with the listed isoforms are unlikely. (See CLINICAL PHARMACOLOGY, *Distribution* and *Metabolism.*)

Other than with probenecid, no specific clinical drug interaction studies have been conducted.

Table 3
Incidence (%) of Adverse Experiences Reported
During Study Therapy Plus 14-Day Follow-Up in ≥1.0% of Patients
Treated With INVANZ in Clinical Studies

Adverse Events	INVANZ* 1 g daily (N=802)	Piperacillin/ Tazobactam* 3.375 g q6h (N=774)	INVANZ† 1 g daily (N=1152)	Ceftriaxone† 1 or 2 g daily (N=942)
Local:				
Extravasation	1.9	1.7	0.7	1.1
Infused vein complication	7.1	7.9	5.4	6.7
Phlebitis/thrombophlebitis	1.9	2.7	1.6	2.0
Systemic:				
Asthenia/fatigue	1.2	0.9	1.2	1.1
Death	2.5	1.6	1.3	1.6
Edema/swelling	3.4	2.5	2.9	3.3
Fever	5.0	6.6	2.3	3.4
Abdominal pain	3.6	4.8	4.3	3.9
Chest pain	1.5	1.4	1.0	2.5
Hypertension	1.6	1.4	0.7	1.0
Hypotension	2.0	1.4	1.0	1.2
Tachycardia	1.6	1.3	1.3	0.7
Acid regurgitation	1.6	0.9	1.1	0.6
Oral candidiasis	0.1	1.3	1.4	1.9
Constipation	4.0	5.4	3.3	3.1
Diarrhea	10.3	12.1	9.2	9.8
Dyspepsia	1.1	0.6	1.0	1.6
Nausea	8.5	8.7	6.4	7.4
Vomiting	3.7	5.3	4.0	4.0
Leg pain	1.1	0.5	0.4	0.3
Anxiety	1.4	1.3	0.8	1.2
Altered mental status‡	5.1	3.4	3.3	2.5
Dizziness	2.1	3.0	1.5	2.1
Headache	5.6	5.4	6.8	6.9
Insomnia	3.2	5.2	3.0	4.1
Cough	1.6	1.7	1.3	0.5
Dyspnea	2.6	1.8	1.0	2.4
Pharyngitis	0.7	1.4	1.1	0.6
Rales/rhonchi	1.1	1.0	0.5	1.0
Respiratory distress	1.0	0.4	0.2	0.2
Erythema	1.6	1.7	1.2	1.2
Pruritus	2.0	2.6	1.0	1.9
Rash	2.5	3.1	2.3	1.5
Vaginitis	1.4	1.0	3.3	3.7

* Includes Phase IIb/III Complicated intra-abdominal infections, Complicated skin and skin structure infections and Acute pelvic infections studies

† Includes Phase IIb/III Community acquired pneumonia and Complicated urinary tract infections, and Phase IIa studies

‡ Includes agitation, confusion, disorientation, decreased mental acuity, changed mental status, somnolence, stupor

Carcinogenesis, Mutagenesis, Impairment of Fertility

No long-term studies in animals have been performed to evaluate the carcinogenic potential of ertapenem.

Ertapenem was neither mutagenic nor genotoxic in the following *in vitro* assays: alkaline elution/rat hepatocyte assay, chromosomal aberration assay in Chinese hamster ovary cells, and TK6 human lymphoblastoid cell mutagenesis assay; and in the *in vivo* mouse micronucleus assay.

In mice and rats, IV doses of up to 700 mg/kg/day (for mice, approximately 3 times the recommended human dose of 1 g based on body surface area and for rats, approximately 1.2 times the human exposure at the recommended dose of 1 g based on plasma AUCs) resulted in no effects on mating performance, fecundity, fertility, or embryonic survival.

Pregnancy: Teratogenic Effects

Pregnancy Category B: In mice and rats given IV doses of up to 700 mg/kg/day (for mice, approximately 3 times the recommended human dose of 1 g based on body surface area and for rats, approximately 1.2 times the human exposure at the recommended dose of 1 g based on plasma AUCs), there was no evidence of developmental toxicity as assessed by external, visceral, and skeletal examination of the fetuses. However, in mice given 700 mg/kg/day, slight decreases in average fetal weights and an associated decrease in the average number of ossified sacrocaudal vertebrae were observed. Ertapenem crosses the placental barrier in rats.

There are, however, no adequate and well-controlled studies in pregnant women. Because animal reproduction studies are not always predictive of human response, this drug should be used during pregnancy only if clearly needed.

Nursing Mothers

Ertapenem is excreted in human breast milk. (See CLINICAL PHARMACOLOGY, *Distribution.*) Caution should be exercised when INVANZ is administered to a nursing woman. INVANZ should be administered to nursing mothers only when the expected benefit outweighs the risk.

Labor and delivery

INVANZ has not been studied for use during labor and delivery.

Pediatric Use

Safety and effectiveness in pediatric patients have not been established. Therefore, use in patients under 18 years of age is not recommended.

Continued on next page

Information on the Merck & Co., Inc., products listed on these pages is from the prescribing information in use April 1, 2002.

Invanz—Cont.

Geriatric Use

Of the 1,835 patients in Phase llb/lll studies treated with INVANZ, approximately 26 percent were 65 and over, while approximately 12 percent were 75 and over. No overall differences in safety or effectiveness were observed between these patients and younger patients. Other reported clinical experience has not identified differences in responses between the elderly and younger patients, but greater sensitivity of some older individuals cannot be ruled out.

This drug is known to be substantially excreted by the kidney, and the risk of toxic reactions to this drug may be greater in patients with impaired renal function. Because elderly patients are more likely to have decreased renal function, care should be taken in dose selection, and it may be useful to monitor renal function. (See DOSAGE AND ADMINISTRATION.)

Hepatic Insufficiency

The pharmacokinetics of ertapenem in patients with hepatic insufficiency have not been established. Of the total number of patients in clinical studies, 37 patients receiving ertapenem 1 g daily and 36 patients receiving comparator drugs were considered to have Child-Pugh Class A, B, or C liver impairment. The incidence of adverse experiences in patients with hepatic impairment was similar between the ertapenem group and the comparator groups.

ANIMAL PHARMACOLOGY

In repeat-dose studies in rats, treatment-related neutropenia occurred at every dose-level tested, including the lowest dose (2 mg/kg, 12 mg/m^2).

Studies in rabbits and Rhesus monkeys were inconclusive with regard to the effect on neutrophil counts.

ADVERSE REACTIONS

Clinical studies enrolled 1954 patients treated with ertapenem; in some of the clinical studies, parenteral therapy was followed by a switch to an appropriate oral antimicrobial. (See CLINICAL STUDIES.) Most adverse experiences reported in these clinical studies were described as mild to moderate in severity. Ertapenem was discontinued due to adverse experiences in 4.7% of patients. Table 3 shows the incidence of adverse experiences reported in ≥1.0% of patients in these studies. The most common drug-related adverse experiences in patients treated with INVANZ, including those who were switched to therapy with an oral antimicrobial, were diarrhea (5.5%), infused vein complication (3.7%), nausea (3.1%), headache (2.2%), vaginitis in females (2.1%), phlebitis/thrombophlebitis (1.3%), and vomiting (1.1%).

[See table 3 at top of previous page]

In patients treated for complicated intra-abdominal infections, death occurred in 4.7% (15/316) of patients receiving ertapenem and 2.6% (8/307) of patients receiving comparator drug. These deaths occurred in patients with significant co-morbidity and/or severe baseline infections. Deaths were considered unrelated to study drugs by investigators.

In clinical studies, seizure was reported during study therapy plus 14-day follow-up period in 0.5% of patients treated with ertapenem, 0.3% of patients treated with piperacillin/tazobactam and 0% of patients treated with ceftriaxone. (See PRECAUTIONS.)

Additional adverse experiences that were reported with INVANZ with an incidence >0.1% within each body system are listed below:

Body as a whole: abdominal distention, pain, chills, septicemia, septic shock, dehydration, gout, malaise, necrosis, candidiasis, weight loss, facial edema, injection site induration, injection site pain, flank pain, and syncope;

Cardiovascular System: heart failure, hematoma, cardiac arrest, bradycardia, arrhythmia, atrial fibrillation, heart murmur, ventricular tachycardia, asystole, and subdural hemorrhage;

Digestive System: gastrointestinal hemorrhage, anorexia, flatulence, *C. difficile* associated diarrhea, stomatitis, dysphagia, hemorrhoids, ileus, cholelithiasis, duodenitis, esophagitis, gastritis, jaundice, mouth ulcer, pancreatitis, and pyloric stenosis;

Nervous System & Psychiatric: nervousness, seizure (see WARNINGS and PRECAUTIONS), tremor, depression, hypesthesia, spasm, paresthesia, aggressive behavior, and vertigo;

Respiratory System: pleural effusion, hypoxemia, bronchoconstriction, pharyngeal discomfort, epistaxis, pleuritic pain, asthma, hemoptysis, hiccups, and voice disturbance;

Skin & Skin Appendage: sweating, dermatitis, desquamation, flushing, and urticaria;

Special Senses: taste perversion;

Urogenital System: renal insufficiency, oliguria/anuria, vaginal pruritus, hematuria, urinary retention, bladder dysfunction, vaginal candidiasis, and vulvovaginitis.

Adverse Laboratory Changes

Laboratory adverse experiences that were reported during therapy in ≥1.0% of patients treated with INVANZ in clinical studies are presented in Table 4. Drug-related laboratory adverse experiences that were reported during therapy in ≥1.0% of patients treated with INVANZ, including those who were switched to therapy with an oral antimicrobial, in clinical studies were ALT increased (6.0%), AST increased (5.2%), serum alkaline phosphatase increased (3.4%), platelet count increased (2.8%), and eosinophils increased (1.1%). Ertapenem was discontinued due to laboratory adverse experiences in 0.3% of patients.

[See table 4 above]

Additional laboratory adverse experiences that were reported during therapy in >0.1% but <1.0% of patients treated with INVANZ in clinical studies include: increases in BUN, direct and indirect serum bilirubin, serum sodium, monocytes, PTT, urine epithelial cells; decreases in serum bicarbonate.

Table 4
Incidence* (%) of Specific Laboratory Adverse Experiences Reported During Study Therapy Plus 14-Day Follow-Up in ≥1.0% of Patients Treated With INVANZ in Clinical Studies

Adverse laboratory experiences	INVANZ‡ 1 g daily (n†=766)	Piperacillin/ Tazobactam‡ 3.375 g q6h (n†=755)	INVANZ§ 1 g daily (n†=1122)	Ceftriaxone§ 1 or 2 g daily (n†=920)
ALT increased	8.8	7.3	8.3	6.9
AST increased	8.4	8.3	7.1	6.5
Serum albumin decreased	1.7	1.5	0.9	1.6
Serum alkaline phosphatase increased	6.6	7.2	4.3	2.8
Serum creatinine increased	1.1	2.7	0.9	1.2
Serum glucose increased	1.2	2.3	1.7	2.0
Serum potassium decreased	1.7	2.8	1.8	2.4
Serum potassium increased	1.3	0.5	0.5	0.7
Total serum bilirubin increased	1.7	1.4	0.6	1.1
Eosinophils increased	1.1	1.1	2.1	1.8
Hematocrit decreased	3.0	2.9	3.4	2.4
Hemoglobin decreased	4.9	4.7	4.5	3.5
Platelet count decreased	1.1	1.2	1.1	1.0
Platelet count increased	6.5	6.3	4.3	3.5
Segmented neutrophils decreased	1.0	0.3	1.5	0.8
Prothrombin time increased	1.2	2.0	0.3	0.9
WBC decreased	0.8	0.7	1.5	1.4
Urine RBCs increased	2.5	2.9	1.1	1.0
Urine WBCs increased	2.5	3.2	1.6	1.1

* Number of patients with laboratory adverse experiences/Number of patients with the laboratory test
† Number of patients with one or more laboratory tests
‡ Includes Phase IIb/III Complicated intra-abdominal infections, Complicated skin and skin structure infections and Acute pelvic infections studies
§ Includes Phase IIb/III Community acquired pneumonia and Complicated urinary tract infections, and Phase IIa studies

OVERDOSAGE

No specific information is available on the treatment of overdosage with INVANZ. Intentional overdosing of INVANZ is unlikely. Intravenous administration of INVANZ at a dose of 2 g over 30 min or 3 g over 1–2h in healthy volunteers resulted in an increased incidence of nausea. In clinical studies, inadvertent administration of three 1 g doses of INVANZ in a 24 hour period resulted in diarrhea and transient dizziness in one patient.

In the event of an overdose, INVANZ should be discontinued and general supportive treatment given until renal elimination takes place.

INVANZ can be removed by hemodialysis; the plasma clearance of the total fraction of ertapenem was increased 30% in subjects with end-stage renal insufficiency when hemodialysis (4 hour session) was performed immediately following administration. However, no information is available on the use of hemodialysis to treat overdosage.

DOSAGE AND ADMINISTRATION

The dose of INVANZ in adults is 1 gram (g) given once a day. INVANZ may be administered by intravenous infusion for up to 14 days or intramuscular injection for up to 7 days. When administered intravenously, INVANZ should be infused over a period of 30 minutes.

Intramuscular administration of INVANZ may be used as an alternative to intravenous administration in the treatment of those infections for which intramuscular therapy is appropriate.

DO NOT MIX OR CO-INFUSE INVANZ WITH OTHER MEDICATIONS. DO NOT USE DILUENTS CONTAINING DEXTROSE (α-D-GLUCOSE).

Table 5 presents dosage guidelines for INVANZ.

[See table 5 above]

Table 5
Dosage Guidelines for Adults With Normal Renal Function* and Body Weight

Infection†	Daily Dose (IV or IM)	Recommended Duration of Total Antimcirobial Treatment
Complicated intra-abdominal infections	1 g	5 to 14 days
Complicated skin and skin structure infections	1 g	7 to 14 days
Community acquired pneumonia	1 g	10 to 14 days‡
Complicated urinary tract infections, including pyelonephritis	1 g	10 to 14 days‡
Acute pelvic infections including postpartum endomyometritis, septic abortion and post surgical gynecologic infections	1 g	3 to 10 days

* defined as creatinine clearance >90 mL/min/1.73 m^2
† due to the designated pathogens (see INDICATIONS AND USAGE)
‡ duration includes a possible switch to an appropraite oral therapy, after at least 3 days of parenteral therapy, once clinical improvement has been demonstrated.

Patients with Renal Insufficiency: INVANZ may be used for the treatment of infections in patients with renal insufficiency. In patients whose creatinine clearance is >30 mL/min/1.73 m^2, no dosage adjustment is necessary. Patients with advanced renal insufficiency (creatinine clearance ≤30 mL/min/1.73 m^2) and end-stage renal insufficiency (creatinine clearance ≤10 mL/min/1.73 m^2) should receive 500 mg daily.

Patients on Hemodialysis: When patients on hemodialysis are given the recommended daily dose of 500 mg of INVANZ within 6 hours prior to hemodialysis, a supplementary dose of 150 mg is recommended following the hemodialysis session. If INVANZ is given at least 6 hours prior to hemodialysis, no supplementary dose is needed. There are no data in patients undergoing peritoneal dialysis or hemofiltration.

When only the serum creatinine is available, the following formula** may be used to estimate creatinine clearance. The serum creatinine should represent a steady state of renal function.

$$\text{Males: } \frac{(\text{weight in kg}) \times (140\text{-age in years})}{(72) \times \text{serum creatinine (mg/100 mL)}}$$

$$\text{Females: } (0.85) \times (\text{value calculated for males})$$

Patients with Hepatic Insufficiency: No dose adjustment recommendations can be made in patients with impaired hepatic function. (See CLINICAL PHARMACOLOGY, *Special Populations, Hepatic Insufficiency* and PRECAUTIONS.)

No dosage adjustment is recommended based on age or gender. (See CLINICAL PHARMACOLOGY, *Special Populations.*)

** Cockcroft and Gault equation: Cockcroft DW, Gault MH. Prediction of creatinine clearance from serum creatinine. Nephron. 1976

PREPARATION OF SOLUTION

Preparation for intravenous administration:

DO NOT MIX OR CO-INFUSE INVANZ WITH OTHER MEDICATIONS. DO NOT USE DILUENTS CONTAINING DEXTROSE (α-D-GLUCOSE).

INVANZ MUST BE RECONSTITUTED AND THEN DILUTED PRIOR TO ADMINISTRATION.

1. Reconstitute the contents of a 1 g vial of INVANZ with 10 mL of one of the following: Water for Injection, 0.9% Sodium Chloride Injection or Bacteriostatic Water for Injection.
2. Shake well to dissolve and immediately transfer contents of the reconstituted vial to 50 mL of 0.9% Sodium Chloride Injection.
3. Complete the infusion within 6 hours of reconstitution.

Preparation for intramuscular administration:

INVANZ MUST BE RECONSTITUTED PRIOR TO ADMINISTRATION.

1. Reconstitute the contents of a 1 g vial of INVANZ with 3.2 mL of 1.0% lidocaine HCl injection*** (**without epinephrine**). Shake vial thoroughly to form solution.
2. Immediately withdraw the contents of the vial and administer by deep intramuscular injection into a large muscle mass (such as the gluteal muscles or lateral part of the thigh).
3. The reconstituted IM solution should be used within 1 hour after preparation. **NOTE: THE RECONSTITUTED SOLUTION SHOULD NOT BE ADMINISTERED INTRAVENOUSLY.**

Parenteral drug products should be inspected visually for particulate matter and discoloration prior to use, whenever solution and container permit. Solutions of INVANZ range from colorless to pale yellow. Variations of color within this range do not affect the potency of the product.

***Refer to the prescribing information for lidocaine HCl.

STORAGE AND STABILITY

Before reconstitution

Do not store lyophilized powder above 25°C (77°F).

Reconstituted and infusion solutions

The reconstituted solution, immediately diluted in 0.9% Sodium Chloride Injection (see DOSAGE AND ADMINISTRATION, PREPARATION OF SOLUTION), **may be stored at room temperature (25°C) and used within 6 hours or stored for 24 hours under refrigeration (5°C) and used within 4 hours after removal from refrigeration. Solutions of INVANZ should not be frozen.**

HOW SUPPLIED

INVANZ is supplied as a sterile lyophilized powder in single dose vials containing ertapenem for intravenous infusion or for intramuscular injection as follows:

No. 3843—1 g ertapenem equivalent
NDC 0006-3843-71 in trays of 10 vials
No. 3843—1 g ertapenem equivalent
NDC 0006-3843-45 in trays of 25 vials.

CLINICAL STUDIES

Complicated Intra-Abdominal Infections

Ertapenem was evaluated in adults for the treatment of complicated intra-abdominal infections in a clinical trial. This study compared ertapenem (1 g intravenously once a day) with piperacillin/tazobactam (3.375 g intravenously every 6 hours) for 5 to 14 days and enrolled 665 patients with localized complicated appendicitis, and any other complicated intra-abdominal infection including colonic, small intestinal, and biliary infections and generalized peritonitis. The combined clinical and microbiologic success rates in the microbiologically evaluable population at 4 to 6 weeks posttherapy (test of cure) were 83.6% (163/195) for ertapenem and 80.4% (152/189) for piperacillin/tazobactam.

Complicated Skin and Skin Structure Infections

Ertapenem was evaluated in adults for the treatment of complicated skin and skin structure infections in a clinical trial. This study compared ertapenem (1 g intravenously once a day) with piperacillin/tazobactam (3.375 g intravenously every 6 hours) for 7 to 14 days and enrolled 540 patients including patients with deep soft tissue abscess, posttraumatic wound infection and cellulitis with purulent drainage. The clinical success rates at 10 to 21 days posttherapy (test of cure) were 83.9% (141/168) for ertapenem and 85.3% (145/170) for piperacillin/tazobactam.

Community Acquired Pneumonia

Ertapenem was evaluated in adults for the treatment of community acquired pneumonia in two clinical trials. Both studies compared ertapenem (1 g parenterally once a day) with ceftriaxone (1 g parenterally once a day) and enrolled a total of 866 patients. Both regimens allowed the option to switch to oral amoxicillin/clavulanate for a total of 10 to 14 days of treatment (parenteral and oral). In the first study the primary efficacy parameter was the clinical success rate in the clinically evaluable population and success rates were 92.3% (168/182) for ertapenem and 91.0% (183/201) for ceftriaxone at 7 to 14 days posttherapy (test of cure). In the second study the primary efficacy parameter was the clinical success rates in the microbiologically evaluable population and success rates were 91% (91/100) for ertapenem and 91.8% (45/49) for ceftriaxone at 7 to 14 days posttherapy (test of cure).

Complicated Urinary Tract Infections Including Pyelonephritis

Ertapenem was evaluated in adults for the treatment of complicated urinary tract infections including pyelonephritis in two clinical trials. Both studies compared ertapenem (1 g parenterally once a day) with ceftriaxone (1 g parenterally once a day) and enrolled a total of 850 patients. Both regimens allowed the option to switch to oral ciprofloxacin (500 mg twice daily) for a total of 10 to 14 days of treatment (parenteral and oral). The microbiological success rates (combined studies) at 5 to 9 days posttherapy (test of cure) were 89.5% (229/256) for ertapenem and 91.1% (204/224) for ceftriaxone.

Acute Pelvic Infections Including Endomyometritis, Septic Abortion And Post-Surgical Gynecological Infections

Ertapenem was evaluated in adults for the treatment of acute pelvic infections in a clinical trial. This study compared ertapenem (1 g intravenously once a day) with piperacillin/tazobactam (3.375 g intravenously every 6 hours) for 3 to 10 days and enrolled 412 patients including 350 patients with obstetric/postpartum infections and 45 patients with septic abortion. The clinical success rates in the clinically evaluable population at 2 to 4 weeks posttherapy (test of cure) were 93.9% (153/163) for ertapenem and 91.5% (140/153) for piperacillin/tazobactam.

REFERENCES

1. National Committee for Clinical Laboratory Standardards. Methods for Dilution Antimicrobial Susceptibility Tests for Bacteria that Grow Aerobically. Fifth Edition; Approved Standard, NCCLS Document M7-A5, Vol. 17, No. 2 NCCLS, Wayne, PA, December 2000.
2. National Committee for Clinical Laboratory Standardards. Performance Standards for Antimicrobial Disk Susceptibility Tests. Seventh Edition; Approved Standard, NCCLS Document M2-A7, Vol. 17, No. 1 NCCLS, Wayne, PA, January 2000.
3. National Committee for Clinical Laboratory Standardards. *Methods for Antimicrobial Susceptibility Testing of Anaerobic Bacteria* - Fourth Edition; Approved Standard, NCCLS Document M11-A4, Vol. 17, No. 22. NCCLS, Wayne, PA, December 1997.
4. National Committee for Clinical Laboratory Standardards. Performance Standards for Antimicrobial Susceptibility Testing - Eleventh Informational Supplement. Approved Standard, NCCLS Document M100-S11, Vol. 21, No. 1. NCCLS, Wayne, PA, January 2001.

MERCK & CO., INC., Whitehouse Station, NJ 08889, USA
9500000 Issued November 2001

Novartis Pharmaceuticals Corporation

NOVARTIS PHARMACEUTICALS CORPORATION
One Health Plaza
East Hanover, NJ 07936
(for branded products)

For Information Contact *(branded products):*

Customer Response Department
(888) NOW-NOVARTIS [888-669-6682]

Global Internet Address:
http: //www.novartis.com

ELIDEL® ℞

[ĕl'-ĭ dĕl]

(pimecrolimus) Cream 1%
FOR DERMATOLOGIC USE ONLY
NOT FOR OPHTHALMIC USE

Rx only

Prescribing Information

DESCRIPTION

Elidel® (pimecrolimus) Cream 1% contains the compound pimecrolimus, the 33-epi-chloro-derivative of the macrolactam ascomycin.

Chemically, pimecrolimus is (1R,9S,12S,13R,14S,17R, 18E,21S,23S,24R,25S,27R)-12-[(1E)-2-[(1R,3R,4S)-4-chloro-3-methoxycyclohexyl]-1- methylvinyl]- 17-ethyl-1, 14- dihydroxy-23, 25-dimethoxy-13, 19, 21, 27-tetramethyl- 11, 28-dioxa-4-aza-tricyclo[22.3.1.$0^{4,9}$]octacos-18-ene-2, 3,10, 16-tetraone.

The compound has the empirical formula $C_{43}H_{68}ClNO_{11}$ and the molecular weight of 810.47. The structural formula is

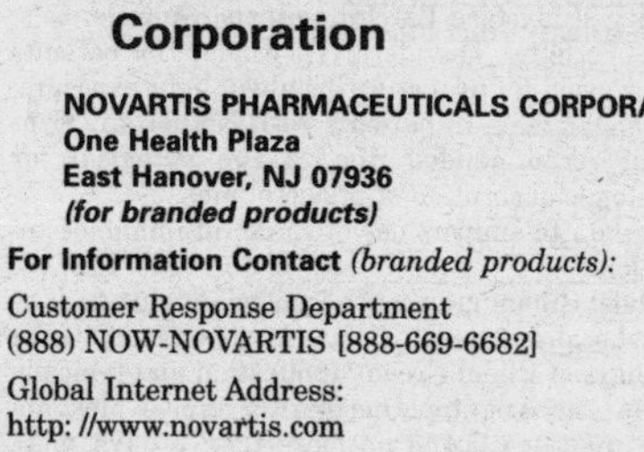

Pimecrolimus is a white to off-white fine crystalline powder. It is soluble in methanol and ethanol and insoluble in water. Each gram of Elidel Cream 1% contains 10 mg of pimecrolimus in a whitish cream base of benzyl alcohol, cetyl alcohol, citric acid, mono- and di-glycerides, oleyl alcohol, propylene glycol, sodium cetostearyl sulphate, sodium hydroxide, stearyl alcohol, triglycerides, and water.

CLINICAL PHARMACOLOGY

Mechanism of Action/Pharmacodynamics

The mechanism of action of pimecrolimus in atopic dermatitis is not known. While the following have been observed, the clinical significance of these observations in atopic dermatitis is not known. It has been demonstrated that pimecrolimus binds with high affinity to macrophilin-12 (FKBP-12) and inhibits the calcium-dependent phosphatase, calcineurin. As a consequence, it inhibits T cell activation by blocking the transcription of early cytokines. In particular, pimecrolimus inhibits at nanomolar concentrations Interleukin-2 and interferon gamma (Th1-type) and Interleukin-4 and Interleukin-10 (Th2-type) cytokine synthesis in human T cells. In addition, pimecrolimus prevents the release of inflammatory cytokines and mediators from mast cells in vitro after stimulation by antigen/IgE.

Pharmacokinetics

Absorption

In adult patients being treated for atopic dermatitis [13%-62% Body Surface Area (BSA) involvement] for periods up to a year, blood concentrations of pimecrolimus are routinely either at or below the limit of quantification of the assay (< 0.5 ng/mL). In those subjects with detectable blood levels they are routinely < 2 ng/mL and show no sign of drug accumulation with time. Because of the low systemic absorption of pimecrolimus following topical application the calculation of standard pharmacokinetic measures such as AUC, C_{max}, $T_{1/2}$, et cetera cannot be reliably done.

Distribution

In vitro studies of the protein binding of pimecrolimus indicate that it is 74%-87% bound to plasma proteins.

Metabolism

Following the administration of a single oral radiolabeled dose of pimecrolimus numerous circulating O-demethylation metabolites were seen. Studies with human liver microsomes indicate that pimecrolimus is metabolized in vitro by the CYP3A sub-family of metabolizing enzymes. No evidence of skin mediated drug metabolism was identified in vivo using the minipig or in vitro using stripped human skin.

Elimination

Based on the results of the aforementioned radiolabeled study, following a single oral dose of pimecrolimus ~81% of the administered radioactivity was recovered, primarily in the feces (78.4%) as metabolites. Less than 1% of the radioactivity found in the feces was due to unchanged pimecrolimus.

Special Populations

Pediatrics

The systemic exposure to pimecrolimus from Elidel® (pimecrolimus) Cream 1% was investigated in 26 pediatric patients with atopic dermatitis (20%-69% BSA involvement) between the ages of 2–14 yrs. Following twice daily application for three weeks, blood concentrations of pimecrolimus were consistently low (< 3 ng/mL), with the majority of the blood samples being below the limit of quantification (0.5 ng/mL). However, the children (20 children out of the total 23 children investigated) had at least one detectable blood level as compared to the adults (13 adults out of the total 25 adults investigated) over a 3-week treatment period. Due to the low and erratic nature of the blood levels observed, no correlation could be made between amount of cream, degree of BSA involvement, and blood concentrations. In general, the blood concentrations measured in adult atopic dermatitis patients were comparable to those seen in the pediatric population.

In a second group of 22 pediatric patients aged 3-23 months with 10%-92% BSA involvement, a higher proportion of detectable blood levels was seen ranging from 0.1 ng/mL to 2.6 ng/mL (limit of quantification 0.1 ng/mL). This increase in the absolute number of positive blood levels may be due to the larger surface area to body mass ratio seen in these younger subjects. In addition, a higher incidence of upper respiratory symptoms/infections was also seen relative to the older age group in the PK studies. At this time a causal relationship between these findings and Elidel use cannot be ruled out. Use of Elidel in this population is not recommended (see **Pediatric Use**).

Renal Insufficiency

The effect of renal insufficiency on the pharmacokinetics of topically administered pimecrolimus has not been evaluated. Given the very low systemic exposure of pimecrolimus via the topical route, no change in dosing is required.

Hepatic Insufficiency

The effect of hepatic insufficiency on the pharmacokinetics of topically administered pimecrolimus has not been evaluated. Given the very low systemic exposure of pimecrolimus via the topical route, no change in dosing is required.

CLINICAL STUDIES

Three randomized, double-blind, vehicle-controlled, multicenter, Phase 3 studies were conducted in 1335 pediatric patients ages 3 months-17 years old to evaluate Elidel® (pimecrolimus) Cream 1% for the treatment of mild to moderate atopic dermatitis. Two of the three trials support the use of Elidel Cream in patients 2 years and older with mild to moderate atopic dermatitis (see **Pediatric Use**). Three other trials provided additional data regarding the safety of Elidel Cream in the treatment of atopic dermatitis. Two of these other trials were vehicle-controlled with optional sequential use of a medium potency topical corticosteroid in

Continued on next page

Elidel—Cont.

pediatric patients and one trial was an active comparator trial in adult patients with atopic dermatitis (see **Pediatric Use** and **ADVERSE REACTIONS**).

Two identical 6-week, randomized, vehicle-controlled, multi-center, Phase 3 trials were conducted to evaluate Elidel Cream for the treatment of mild to moderate atopic dermatitis. A total of 403 pediatric patients 2–17 years old were included in the studies. The male/female ratio was approximately 50% and 29% of the patients were African American. At study entry, 59% of patients had moderate disease and the mean body surface area (BSA) affected was 26%. About 75% of patients had atopic dermatitis affecting the face and/or neck region. In these studies, patients applied either Elidel Cream or vehicle cream twice daily to 5% to 96% of their BSA for up to 6 weeks. At endpoint, based on the physicians global evaluation of clinical response, 35% of patients treated with Elidel Cream were clear or almost clear of signs of atopic dermatitis compared to only 18% of vehicle-treated patients. More Elidel patients (57%) had mild or no pruritus at 6 weeks compared to vehicle patients (34%). The improvement in pruritus occurred in conjunction with the improvement of the patients' atopic dermatitis.

In these two 6-week studies of Elidel, the combined efficacy results at endpoint are as follows:

	% Patients	
	Elidel® (N= 267)	Vehicle (N= 136)
Global Assessment		
Clear	28 (10%)	5 (4%)
Clear or Almost Clear	93 (35%)	25 (18%)
Clear to Mild Disease	180 (67%)	55 (40%)

In the two pediatric studies that independently support the use of Elidel Cream in mild to moderate atopic dermatitis, a significant treatment effect was seen by day 15. Of the key signs of atopic dermatitis, erythema, infiltration/papulation, lichenification, and excoriations, erythema and infiltration/papulation were reduced at day 8 when compared to vehicle.

The following graph depicts the time course of improvement in the percent body surface area affected as a result of treatment with Elidel Cream in 2–17 year olds.

Figure 1
Body Surface Area Over Time

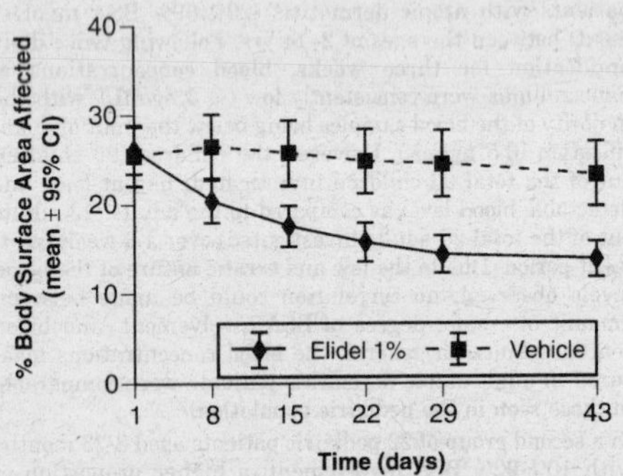

The following graph shows the time course of improvement in erythema as a result of treatment with Elidel Cream in 2–17 year olds.

Figure 2
Mean Erythema Over Time

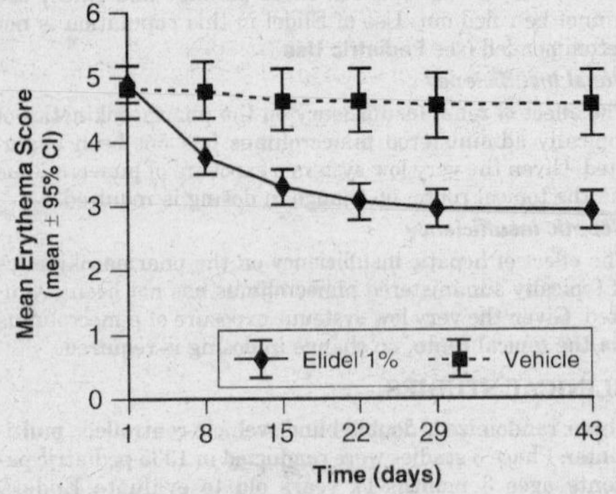

INDICATIONS AND USAGE

Elidel® (pimecrolimus) Cream 1% is indicated for short-term and intermittent long-term therapy in the treatment of *mild to moderate* atopic dermatitis in non-immunocompromised patients 2 years of age and older, in whom the use of alternative, conventional therapies is deemed inadvisable because of potential risks, or in the treatment of patients who are not adequately responsive to or intolerant of alternative, conventional therapies (see **DOSAGE AND ADMINISTRATION**).

CONTRAINDICATIONS

Elidel® (pimecrolimus) Cream 1% is contraindicated in individuals with a history of hypersensitivity to pimecrolimus or any of the components of the cream.

PRECAUTIONS

General

Elidel® (pimecrolimus) Cream 1% should not be applied to areas of active cutaneous viral infections.

Studies have not evaluated the safety and efficacy of Elidel Cream in the treatment of clinically infected atopic dermatitis. Before commencing treatment with Elidel Cream, clinical infections at treatment sites should be cleared.

While patients with atopic dermatitis are predisposed to superficial skin infections including eczema herpeticum (Kaposi's varicelliform eruption), treatment with Elidel Cream may be associated with an increased risk of varicella zoster virus infection (chicken pox or shingles), herpes simplex virus infection, or eczema herpeticum. In the presence of these skin infections, the balance of risks and benefits associated with Elidel Cream use should be evaluated.

In clinical studies, 14 cases of lymphadenopathy (0.9%) were reported while using Elidel Cream. These cases of lymphadenopathy were usually related to infections and noted to resolve upon appropriate antibiotic therapy. Of these 14 cases, the majority had either a clear etiology or were known to resolve. Patients who receive Elidel Cream and who develop lymphadenopathy should have the etiology of their lymphadenopathy investigated. In the absence of a clear etiology for the lymphadenopathy, or in the presence of acute infectious mononucleosis, discontinuation of Elidel Cream should be considered. Patients who develop lymphadenopathy should be monitored to ensure that the lymphadenopathy resolves.

In clinical studies, 15 cases of skin papilloma or warts (1%) were observed in patients using Elidel Cream. The youngest patient was age 2 and the oldest was age 12. In cases where there is worsening of skin papillomas or they do not respond to conventional therapy, discontinuation of Elidel Cream should be considered until complete resolution of the warts is achieved.

The enhancement of ultraviolet carcinogenicity is not necessarily dependent on phototoxic mechanisms. Despite the absence of observed phototoxicity in humans (see **ADVERSE REACTIONS**), Elidel Cream shortened the time to skin tumor formation in an animal photocarcinogenicity study (see **Carcinogenesis, Mutagenesis, Impairment of Fertility**). Therefore, it is prudent for patients to minimize or avoid natural or artificial sunlight exposure.

The use of Elidel Cream in patients with Netherton's Syndrome is not recommended due to the potential for increased systemic absorption of pimecrolimus.

There are no data to support use of Elidel in immunocompromised patients.

The use of Elidel Cream may cause local symptoms such as skin burning. Localized symptoms are most common during the first few days of Elidel Cream application and typically improve as the lesions of atopic dermatitis resolve. Most application site reactions lasted no more than 5 days, were mild to moderate in severity, and started within 1-5 days of treatment. (See **ADVERSE REACTIONS**.)

Information for Patients

Patients using Elidel should receive the following information and instructions:

- Patients should use Elidel Cream as directed by the physician. Elidel Cream is for external use on the skin only. As with any topical medication, patients or caregivers should wash hands after application if hands are not an area for treatment.
- Patients should minimize or avoid exposure to natural or artificial sunlight (tanning beds or UVA/B treatment) while using Elidel Cream.
- Patients should not use this medication for any disorder other than that for which it was prescribed.
- Patients should report any signs or symptoms of adverse reactions to their physician.
- Therapy should be discontinued after signs and symptoms of atopic dermatitis have resolved. Treatment with Elidel should be resumed at the first signs or symptoms of recurrence.
- Use of Elidel may cause reactions at the site of application such as a mild to moderate feeling of warmth and/or sensation of burning. Patients should see a physician if an application site reaction is severe or persists for more than 1 week.
- The patient should contact the physician if no improvement in the atopic dermatitis is seen following 6 weeks of treatment, or if at any time the condition worsens.

Drug Interactions

Potential interactions between Elidel and other drugs, including immunizations, have not been systematically evaluated. Due to the very low blood levels of pimecrolimus detected in some patients after topical application, systemic drug interactions are not expected, but cannot be ruled out. The concomitant administration of known CYP3A family of inhibitors in patients with widespread and/or erythrodermic disease should be done with caution. Some examples of such drugs are erythromycin, itraconazole, ketoconazole, fluconazole, calcium channel blockers and cimetidine.

Carcinogenesis, Mutagenesis, Impairment of Fertility

In a 2-year rat dermal carcinogenicity study using Elidel Cream, a statistically significant increase in the incidence of follicular cell adenoma of the thyroid was noted in low, mid and high dose male animals compared to vehicle and saline control male animals. Follicular cell adenoma of the thyroid was noted in the dermal rat carcinogenicity study at the lowest dose of 2 mg/kg/day [0.2% pimecrolimus cream; 1.5× the Maximum Recommended Human Dose (MRHD) based on AUC comparisons]. No increase in the incidence of follicular cell adenoma of the thyroid was noted in the oral carcinogenicity study in male rats up to 10 mg/kg/day (66× MRHD based on AUC comparisons). However, oral studies may not reflect continuous exposure or the same metabolic profile as by the dermal route. In a mouse dermal carcinogenicity study using pimecrolimus in an ethanolic solution, no increase in incidence of neoplasms was observed in the skin or other organs up to the highest dose of 4 mg/kg/day (0.32% pimecrolimus in ethanol) 27× MRHD based on AUC comparisons. However, lymphoproliferative changes (including lymphoma) were noted in a 13 week repeat dose dermal toxicity study conducted in mice using pimecrolimus in an ethanolic solution at a dose of 25 mg/kg/day (47× MRHD based on AUC comparisons). No lymphoproliferative changes were noted in this study at a dose of 10 mg/kg/day (17× MRHD based on AUC comparison). However, the latency time to lymphoma formation was shortened to 8 weeks after dermal administration of pimecrolimus dissolved in ethanol at a dose of 100 mg/kg/day (179-217× MRHD based on AUC comparisons).

In a mouse oral (gavage) carcinogenicity study, a statistically significant increase in the incidence of lymphoma was noted in high dose male and female animals compared to vehicle control male and female animals. Lymphomas were noted in the oral mouse carcinogenicity study at a dose of 45 mg/kg/day (258-340× MRHD based on AUC comparisons). No drug-related tumors were noted in the mouse oral carcinogenicity study at a dose of 15 mg/kg/day (60-133× MRHD based on AUC comparisons). In an oral (gavage) rat carcinogenicity study, a statistically significant increase in the incidence of benign thymoma was noted in 10 mg/kg/day pimecrolimus treated male and female animals compared to vehicle control treated male and female animals. In addition, a significant increase in the incidence of benign thymoma was noted in another oral (gavage) rat carcinogenicity study in 5 mg/kg/day pimecrolimus treated male animals compared to vehicle control treated male animals. No drug-related tumors were noted in the rat oral carcinogenicity study at a dose of 1 mg/kg/day male animals (1.1× MRHD based on AUC comparisons) and at a dose of 5 mg/kg/day for female animals (21× MRHD based on AUC comparisons).

In a 52-week dermal photo-carcinogenicity study, the median time to onset of skin tumor formation was decreased in hairless mice following chronic topical dosing with concurrent exposure to UV radiation (40 weeks of treatment followed by 12 weeks of observation) with the Elidel Cream vehicle alone. No additional effect on tumor development beyond the vehicle effect was noted with the addition of the active ingredient, pimecrolimus, to the vehicle cream.

A battery of in vitro genotoxicity tests, including Ames assay, mouse lymphoma L5178Y assay, and chromosome aberration test in V79 Chinese hamster cells and an in vivo mouse micronucleus test revealed no evidence for a mutagenic or clastogenic potential for the drug.

An oral fertility and embryofetal developmental study in rats revealed estrus cycle disturbances, post-implantation loss and reduction in litter size at the 45 mg/kg/day dose (38× MRHD based on AUC comparisons). No effect on fertility in female rats was noted at 10 mg/kg/day (12× MRHD based on AUC comparisons). No effect on fertility in male rats was noted at 45 mg/kg/day (23× MRHD based on AUC comparisons), which was the highest dose tested in this study.

Pregnancy

Teratogenic Effects: Pregnancy Category C

There are no adequate and well-controlled studies of topically administered pimecrolimus in pregnant women. The experience with Elidel Cream when used by pregnant women is too limited to permit assessment of the safety of its use during pregnancy.

In dermal embryofetal developmental studies, no maternal or fetal toxicity was observed up to the highest practicable doses tested, 10 mg/kg/day (1% pimecrolimus cream) in rats (0.14× MRHD based on body surface area) and 10 mg/kg/day (1% pimecrolimus cream) in rabbits (0.65× MRHD based on AUC comparisons). The 1% pimecrolimus cream was administered topically for 6 hours/day during the period of organogenesis in rats and rabbits (gestational days 6–21 in rats and gestational days 6–20 in rabbits).

A combined oral fertility and embryofetal developmental study was conducted in rats and an oral embryofetal developmental study was conducted in rabbits. Pimecrolimus was administered during the period of organogenesis (2 weeks prior to mating until gestational day 16 in rats, gestational days 6-18 in rabbits) up to dose levels of 45 mg/kg/day in rats and 20 mg/kg/day in rabbits. In the absence of maternal toxicity, indicators of embryofetal toxicity (post-implantation loss and reduction in litter size) were noted at 45 mg/kg/day (38× MRHD based on AUC comparisons) in the oral fertility and embryofetal developmental study conducted in rats. No malformations in the fetuses were noted at 45 mg/kg/day (38× MRHD based on AUC comparisons) in this study. No maternal toxicity, embryotoxicity or teratogenicity were noted in the oral rabbit embryofetal developmental toxicity study at 20 mg/kg/day (3.9× MRHD based on AUC comparisons), which was the highest dose tested in this study.

An oral peri- and post-natal developmental study was conducted in rats. Pimecrolimus was administered from gestational day 6 through lactational day 21 up to a dose level of

Treatment Emergent Adverse Events (≥ 1%) in Elidel® Treatment Groups

	Pediatric Patients* Vehicle-Controlled (6 weeks)		Pediatric Patients* Open-Label (20 weeks)	Pediatric Patients* Vehicle-Controlled (1 year)		Adult Active Comparator (1 year)
	Elidel® Cream (N=267) N (%)	Vehicle (N=136) N (%)	Elidel® Cream (N=335) N (%)	Elidel® Cream (N=272) N (%)	Vehicle (N=75) N (%)	Elidel® Cream (N=328) N (%)
At least 1 AE	182 (68.2%)	97 (71.3%)	240 (72.0%)	230 (84.6%)	56 (74.7%)	256 (78.0%)
Infections and Infestations						
Upper Respiratory Tract Infection NOS	38 (14.2%)	18 (13.2%)	65 (19.4%)	13 (4.8%)	6 (8.0%)	14 (4.3%)
Nasopharyngitis	27 (10.1%)	10 (7.4%)	32 (19.6%)	72 (26.5%)	16 (21.3%)	25 (7.6%)
Skin Infection NOS	8 (3.0%)	9 (5.1%)	18 (5.4%)	6 (2.2%)	3 (4.0%)	21 (6.4%)
Influenza	8 (3.0%)	1 (0.7%)	22 (6.6%)	36 (13.2%)	3 (4.0%)	32 (9.8%)
Ear Infection NOS	6 (2.2%)	2 (1.5%)	19 (5.7%)	9 (3.3%)	1 (1.3%)	2 (0.6%)
Otitis Media	6 (2.2%)	1 (0.7%)	10 (3.0%)	8 (2.9%)	4 (5.3%)	2 (0.6%)
Impetigo	5 (1.9%)	3 (2.2%)	12 (3.6%)	11 (4.0%)	4 (5.3%)	8 (2.4%)
Bacterial Infection	4 (1.5%)	3 (2.2%)	4 (1.2%)	3 (1.1%)	0	6 (1.8%)
Folliculitis	3 (1.1%)	1 (0.7%)	3 (0.9%)	6 (2.2%)	3 (4.0%)	20 (6.1%)
Sinusitis	3 (1.1%)	1 (0.7%)	11 (3.3%)	6 (2.2%)	1 (1.3%)	2 (0.6%)
Pneumonia NOS	3 (1.1%)	1 (0.7%)	5 (1.5%)	0	1 (1.3%)	1 (0.3%)
Pharyngitis NOS	2 (0.7%)	2 (1.5%)	3 (0.9%)	22 (8.1%)	2 (2.7%)	3 (0.9%)
Pharyngitis Streptococcal	2 (0.7%)	2 (1.5%)	10 (3.0%)	0	<1%	0
Molluscum Contagiosum	2 (0.7%)	0	4 (1.2%)	5 (1.8%)	0	0
Staphylococcal Infection	1 (0.4%)	5 (3.7%)	7 (2.1%)	0	<1%	3 (0.9%)
Bronchitis NOS	1 (0.4%)	3 (2.2%)	4 (1.2%)	29 (10.7%)	6 (8.0%)	8 (2.4%)
Herpes Simplex	1 (0.4%)	0	4 (1.2%)	9 (3.3%)	2 (2.7%)	13 (4.0%)
Tonsillitis NOS	1 (0.4%)	0	3 (0.9%)	17 (6.3%)	0	2 (0.6%)
Viral Infection NOS	2 (0.7%)	1 (0.7%)	1 (0.3%)	18 (6.6%)	1 (1.3%)	0
Gastroenteritis NOS	0	3 (2.2%)	2 (0.6%)	20 (7.4%)	2 (2.7%)	6 (1.8%)
Chickenpox	2 (0.7%)	0	3 (0.9%)	8 (2.9%)	3 (4.0%)	1 (0.3%)
Skin Papilloma	1 (0.4%)	0	2 (0.6%)	9 (3.3%)	<1%	0
Tonsillitis Acute NOS	0	0	0	7 (2.6%)	0	0
Upper Respiratory Tract Infection Viral NOS	1 (0.4%)	0	3 (0.9%)	4 (1.5%)	0	1 (0.3%)
Herpes Simplex Dermatitis	0	0	1 (0.3%)	4 (1.5%)	0	2 (0.6%)
Bronchitis Acute NOS	0	0	0	4 (1.5%)	0	0
Eye Infection NOS	0	0	0	3 (1.1%)	<1%	1 (0.3%)
General Disorders and Administration Site Conditions						
Application Site Burning	28 (10.4%)	17 (12.5%)	5 (1.5%)	23 (8.5%)	5 (6.7%)	85 (25.9%)
Pyrexia	20 (7.5%)	12 (8.8%)	41 (12.2%)	34 (12.5%)	4 (5.3%)	4 (1.2%)
Application Site Reaction NOS	8 (3.0%)	7 (5.1%)	7 (2.1%)	9 (3.3%)	2 (2.7%)	48 (14.6%)
Application Site Irritation	8 (3.0%)	8 (5.9%)	3 (0.9%)	1 (0.4%)	3 (4.0%)	21 (6.4%)
Influenza Like Illness	1 (0.4%)	0	2 (0.6%)	5 (1.8%)	2 (2.7%)	6 (1.8%)
Application Site Erythema	1 (0.4%)	0	0	6 (2.2%)	0	7 (2.1%)
Application Site Pruritus	3 (1.1%)	2 (1.5%)	2 (0.6%)	5 (1.8%)	0	18 (5.5%)
Respiratory, Thoracic and Mediastinal Disorders						
Cough	31 (11.6%)	11 (8.1%)	31 (9.3%)	43 (15.8%)	8 (10.7%)	8 (2.4%)
Nasal Congestion	7 (2.6%)	2 (1.5%)	6 (1.8%)	4 (1.5%)	1 (1.3%)	2 (0.6%)
Rhinorrhea	5 (1.9%)	1 (0.7%)	3 (0.9%)	1 (0.4%)	1 (1.3%)	0
Asthma Aggravated	4 (1.5%)	3 (2.2%)	13 (3.9%)	3 (1.1%)	1 (1.3%)	0
Sinus Congestion	3 (1.1%)	1 (0.7%)	2 (0.6%)	<1%	<1%	3 (0.9%)
Rhinitis	1 (0.4%)	0	5 (1.5%)	12 (4.4%)	5 (6.7%)	7 (2.1%)
Wheezing	1 (0.4%)	1 (0.7%)	4 (1.2%)	2 (0.7%)	<1%	0
Asthma NOS	2 (0.7%)	1 (0.7%)	11 (3.3%)	10 (3.7%)	2 (2.7%)	8 (2.4%)
Epistaxis	0	1 (0.7%)	0	9 (3.3%)	1 (1.3%)	1 (0.3%)
Dyspnea NOS	0	0	0	5 (1.8%)	1 (1.3%)	2 (0.6%)
Gastrointestinal Disorders						
Abdominal Pain Upper	11 (4.1%)	6 (4.4%)	10 (3.0%)	15 (5.5%)	5 (6.7%)	1 (0.3%)
Sore Throat	9 (3.4%)	5 (3.7%)	15 (5.4%)	22 (8.1%)	4 (5.3%)	12 (3.7%)
Vomiting NOS	8 (3.0%)	6 (4.4%)	14 (4.2%)	18 (6.6%)	6 (8.0%)	2 (0.6%)
Diarrhea NOS	3 (1.1%)	1 (0.7%)	2 (0.6%)	21 (7.7%)	4 (5.3%)	7 (2.1%)
Nausea	1 (0.4%)	3 (2.2%)	4 (1.2%)	11 (4.0%)	5 (6.7%)	6 (1.8%)
Abdominal Pain NOS	1 (0.4%)	1 (0.7%)	5 (1.5%)	12 (4.4%)	3 (4.0%)	1 (0.3%)
Toothache	1 (0.4%)	1 (0.7%)	2 (0.6%)	7 (2.6%)	1 (1.3%)	2 (0.6%)
Constipation	1 (0.4%)	0	2 (0.6%)	10 (3.7%)	<1%	0
Loose Stools	0	1 (0.7%)	4 (1.2%)	<1%	<1%	0
Reproductive System and Breast Disorders						
Dysmenorrhea	3 (1.1%)	0	5 (1.5%)	3 (1.1%)	1 (1.3%)	4 (1.2%)
Eye Disorders						
Conjunctivitis NEC	2 (0.7%)	1 (0.7%)	7 (2.1%)	6 (2.2%)	3 (4.0%)	10 (3.0%)
Skin & Subcutaneous Tissue Disorders						
Urticaria	3 (1.1%)	0	1 (0.3%)	1 (0.4%)	<1%	3 (0.9%)
Acne NOS	0	1 (0.7%)	1 (0.3%)	4 (1.5%)	<1%	6 (1.8%)
Immune System Disorders						
Hypersensitivity NOS	11 (4.1%)	6 (4.4%)	16 (4.8%)	14 (5.1%)	1 (1.3%)	11 (3.4%)
Injury and Poisoning						
Accident NOS	3 (1.1%)	1 (0.7%)	1 (0.3%)	<1%	1 (1.3%)	0
Laceration	2 (0.7%)	1 (0.7%)	5 (1.5%)	<1%	<1%	0
Musculoskeletal, Connective Tissue and Bone Disorders						
Back Pain	1 (0.4%)	2 (1.5%)	1 (0.3%)	<1%	0	6 (1.8%)
Arthralgias	0	0	1 (0.3%)	3 (1.1%)	1 (1.3%)	5 (1.5%)
Ear and Labyrinth Disorders						
Earache	2 (0.7%)	1 (0.7%)	0	8 (2.9%)	2 (2.7%)	0
Nervous System Disorders						
Headache	37 (13.9%)	12 (8.8%)	38 (11.3%)	69 (25.4%)	12 (16.0%)	23 (7.0%)

* Ages 2-17 years

40 mg/kg/day. Only 2 of 22 females delivered live pups at the highest dose of 40 mg/kg/day. Postnatal survival, development of the F1 generation, their subsequent maturation and fertility were not affected at 10 mg/kg/day (12× MRHD based on AUC comparisons), the highest dose evaluated in this study.

Pimecrolimus was transferred across the placenta in oral rat and rabbit embryofetal developmental studies.

There are, however, no adequate and well-controlled studies in pregnant women. Because animal reproduction studies are not always predictive of human response, this drug should be used only if clearly needed during pregnancy.

Nursing Mothers

It is not known whether this drug is excreted in human milk. Because of the potential for serious adverse reactions in nursing infants from pimecrolimus, a decision should be made whether to discontinue nursing or to discontinue the drug, taking into account the importance of the drug to the mother.

Pediatric Use

Elidel Cream may be used in pediatric patients 2 years of age and older. Three Phase 3 pediatric studies were conducted involving 1114 patients 2-17 years of age. Two studies were 6-week randomized vehicle-controlled studies with a 20-week open-label phase and one was a vehicle-controlled long-term (up to 1 year) safety study with the option for sequential topical corticosteroid use. Of these patients 542 (49%) were 2-6 years of age. In the short-term studies, 11% of Elidel patients did not complete these studies and 1.5% of Elidel patients discontinued due to adverse events. In the one-year study, 32% of Elidel patients did not complete this study and 3% of Elidel patients discontinued due to adverse events. Most discontinuations were due to unsatisfactory therapeutic effect.

The most common local adverse event in the short-term studies of Elidel Cream in pediatric patients ages 2-17 was application site burning (10% vs. 13% vehicle); the incidence in the long-term study was 9% Elidel vs. 7% vehicle (see **ADVERSE REACTIONS**). Adverse events that were more frequent (>5%) in patients treated with Elidel Cream compared to vehicle were headache (14% vs. 9%) in the short-term trial. Nasopharyngitis (26% vs. 21%), influenza (13% vs. 4%), pharyngitis (8% vs. 3%), viral infection (7% vs. 1%), pyrexia (13% vs. 5%), cough (16% vs. 11%), and headache (25% vs. 16%) were increased over vehicle in the 1-year safety study (see **ADVERSE REACTIONS**). In 843 patients ages 2-17 years treated with Elidel Cream, 9 (0.8%) developed eczema herpeticum (5 on Elidel Cream alone and 4 on Elidel Cream used in sequence with corticosteroids). In 211 patients on vehicle alone, there were no cases of eczema herpeticum. The majority of adverse events were mild to moderate in severity.

Elidel Cream is not recommended for use in pediatric patients below the age of 2 years. Two Phase 3 studies were conducted involving 436 infants age 3 months – 23 months. One 6-week randomized vehicle-controlled study with a 20-week open-label phase and one long term safety study were conducted. In the 6-week study, 11% of Elidel and 48% of vehicle patients did not complete this study; no patient in either group discontinued due to adverse events. Infants on Elidel Cream had an increased incidence of some adverse events compared to vehicle. In the 6-week vehicle-controlled study these adverse events included pyrexia (32% vs. 13% vehicle), URI (24% vs. 14%), nasopharyngitis (15% vs. 8%), gastroenteritis (7% vs. 3%), otitis media (4% vs. 0%), and diarrhea (8% vs. 0%). In the open-label phase of the study, for infants who switched to Elidel Cream from vehicle, the incidence of the above-cited adverse events approached or equaled the incidence of those patients who remained on Elidel Cream. In the 6 month safety data, 16% of Elidel and 35% of vehicle patients discontinued early and 1.5% of Elidel and 0% of vehicle patients discontinued due to adverse events. Infants on Elidel Cream had a greater incidence of some adverse events as compared to vehicle. These included pyrexia (30% vs. 20%), URI (21% vs. 17%), cough (15% vs. 9%), hypersensitivity (8% vs. 2%), teething (27% vs. 22%), vomiting (9% vs. 4%), rhinitis (13% vs. 9%), viral rash (4% vs. 0%), rhinorrhea (4% vs. 0%), and wheezing (4% vs. 0%).

The effects of Elidel Cream on the developing immune system in infants are unknown.

Geriatric Use

Nine (9) patients ≥ 65 years old received Elidel Cream in Phase 3 studies. Clinical studies of Elidel did not include sufficient numbers of patients aged 65 and over to assess efficacy and safety.

ADVERSE REACTIONS

In human dermal safety studies, Elidel® (pimecrolimus) Cream 1% did not induce contact sensitization, phototoxicity, or photoallergy, nor did it show any cumulative irritation.

In a one-year safety study in pediatric patients age 2-17 years old involving sequential use of Elidel Cream and a topical corticosteroid, 43% of Elidel patients and 68% of vehicle patients used corticosteroids during the study. Corticosteroids were used for more than 7 days by 34% of Elidel patients and 54% of vehicle patients. An increased incidence of impetigo, skin infection, superinfection (infected atopic dermatitis), rhinitis, and urticaria were found in the patients that had used Elidel Cream and topical corticosteroid sequentially as compared to Elidel Cream alone.

In 3 randomized, double-blind vehicle-controlled pediatric studies and one active-controlled adult study, 843 and 328 patients respectively, were treated with Elidel Cream. In these clinical trials, 48 (4%) of the 1171 Elidel patients and 13 (3%) of 408 vehicle-treated patients discontinued therapy due to adverse events. Discontinuations for AEs were primarily due to application site reactions, and cutaneous

Continued on next page

Elidel—Cont.

infections. The most common application site reaction was application site burning, which occurred in 8%-26% of patients treated with Elidel Cream.

The following table depicts the incidence of adverse events pooled across the 2 identically designed 6-week studies with their open label extensions and the 1-year safety study for pediatric patients ages 2-17. Data from the adult active-controlled study is also included in this table. Adverse events are listed regardless of relationship to study drug.

[See table at top of previous page]

OVERDOSAGE

There has been no experience of overdose with Elidel® (pimecrolimus) Cream 1%. No incidents of accidental ingestion have been reported. If oral ingestion occurs, medical advice should be sought.

DOSAGE AND ADMINISTRATION

Apply a thin layer of Elidel® (pimecrolimus) Cream 1% to the affected skin twice daily and rub in gently and completely. Elidel may be used on all skin surfaces, including the head, neck, and intertriginous areas.

Elidel should be used twice daily for as long as signs and symptoms persist. Treatment should be discontinued if resolution of disease occurs. If symptoms persist beyond 6 weeks, the patient should be re-evaluated.

The safety of Elidel Cream under occlusion, which may promote systemic exposure, has not been evaluated. **Elidel Cream should not be used with occlusive dressings.**

HOW SUPPLIED

Elidel® (pimecrolimus) Cream 1% is available in tubes of 15 grams, 30 grams, and 100 grams.

15 gram tube .... NDC 0078-0375-40
30 gram tube .... NDC 0078-0375-46
100 gram tube .... NDC 0078-0375-63

Store at 25°C (77°F); excursions permitted to 15°C-30°C (59°F-86°F). Do not freeze.

Manufactured by:
Novartis Pharma GmbH
Wehr, Germany
Distributed by:
Novartis Pharmaceuticals Corp.
East Hanover, NJ 07936

89012001
DECEMBER 2001 T2001-06
492360/1 US

FOCALIN™ Ⓒ℞

[fōk' ă-lĭn]
dexmethylphenidate hydrochloride tablets

Rx only

Prescribing Information

DESCRIPTION

Focalin™ (dexmethylphenidate hydrochloride) is the *d-threo*-enantiomer of racemic methylphenidate hydrochloride, which is a 50/50 mixture of the *d-threo* and *l-threo*-enantiomers. Focalin is a central nervous system (CNS) stimulant, available in three tablet strengths. Each tablet contains dexmethylphenidate hydrochloride 2.5, 5, or 10 mg for oral administration. Dexmethylphenidate hydrochloride is methyl α-phenyl-2-piperidineacetate hydrochloride, (R,R')-(+)-. Its empirical formula is $C_{14}H_{19}NO_2$•HCl.

Its molecular weight is 269.77 and its structural formula is

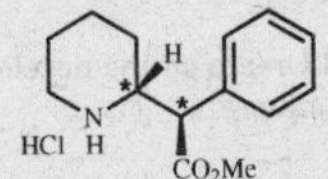

Note: * = asymmetric carbon centers

Dexmethylphenidate hydrochloride is a white to off white powder. Its solutions are acid to litmus. It is freely soluble in water and in methanol, soluble in alcohol, and slightly soluble in chloroform and in acetone.

Focalin also contains the following inert ingredients: pregelatinized starch, lactose monohydrate, sodium starch glycolate, microcrystalline cellulose, magnesium stearate, and FD&C Blue No.1 #5516 aluminum lake (2.5 mg tablets), D&C Yellow Lake #10 (5 mg tablets); the 10 mg tablet contains no dye.

CLINICAL PHARMACOLOGY

Pharmacodynamics

Dexmethylphenidate hydrochloride is a central nervous system stimulant. Focalin, the more pharmacologically active enantiomer of the *d*- and *l*-enantiomers, is thought to block the reuptake of norepinephrine and dopamine into the presynaptic neuron and increase the release of these monoamines into the extraneuronal space. The mode of therapeutic action in Attention Deficit Hyperactivity Disorder (ADHD) is not known.

Pharmacokinetics

Absorption

Dexmethylphenidate hydrochloride is readily absorbed following oral administration of Focalin. In patients with ADHD, plasma dexmethylphenidate concentrations increase rapidly, reaching a maximum in the fasted state at about 1 to 1½ hours post-dose. No differences in the pharmacokinetics of Focalin were noted following single and repeated twice daily dosing, thus indicating no significant drug accumulation in children with ADHD.

When given to children as capsules in single doses of 2.5 mg, 5 mg, and 10 mg, C_{max} and $AUC_{0\text{-}inf}$ of dexmethylphenidate were proportional to dose. In the same study, plasma dexmethylphenidate levels were comparable to those achieved following single *dl-threo*-methylphenidate HCl doses given as capsules in twice the total mg amount (equimolar with respect to Focalin).

Food Effects

In a single dose study conducted in adults, coadministration of 2 × 10 mg Focalin with a high fat breakfast resulted in a dexmethylphenidate t_{max} of 2.9 hours post-dose as compared to 1.5 hours post-dose when given in a fasting state. C_{max} and $AUC_{0\text{-}inf}$ were comparable in both the fasted and non-fasted states.

Distribution

Plasma dexmethylphenidate concentrations in children decline exponentially following oral administration of Focalin.

Metabolism and Excretion

In humans, dexmethylphenidate is metabolized primarily to *d*-α-phenylpiperidine acetic acid (also known as *d*-ritalinic acid) by de-esterification. This metabolite has little or no pharmacological activity. There is little or no *in vivo* interconversion to the *l-threo*-enantiomer, based on a finding of minute levels of *l-threo*-methylphenidate being detectable in a few samples in only 2 of 58 children and adults. After oral dosing of radiolabeled racemic methylphenidate in humans, about 90% of the radioactivity was recovered in urine. The main urinary metabolite was ritalinic acid, accountable for approximately 80% of the dose.

In vitro studies showed that dexmethylphenidate did not inhibit cytochrome P450 isoenzymes.

The mean plasma elimination half-life of dexmethylphenidate is approximately 2.2 hours.

Special Populations

Gender

Pharmacokinetic parameters were similar for boys and girls (mean age 10 years).

In a single dose study conducted in adults, the mean dexmethylphenidate $AUC_{0\text{-}inf}$ values (adjusted for body weight) following single 2 × 10 mg doses of Focalin were 25%-35% higher in adult female volunteers (n=6) compared to male volunteers (n=9). Both t_{max} and $t_{½}$ were comparable for males and females.

Race

There is insufficient experience with the use of Focalin to detect ethnic variations in pharmacokinetics.

Age

The pharmacokinetics of dexmethylphenidate after Focalin administration have not been studied in children less than 6 years of age. When single doses of Focalin were given to children between the ages of 6 to 12 years and healthy adult volunteers, C_{max} of dexmethylphenidate was similar, however, children showed somewhat lower AUCs compared to the adults.

Renal Insufficiency

There is no experience with the use of Focalin in patients with renal insufficiency. After oral administration of radiolabeled racemic methylphenidate in humans, methylphenidate was extensively metabolized and approximately 80% of the radioactivity was excreted in the urine in the form of ritalinic acid. Since very little unchanged drug is excreted in the urine, renal insufficiency is expected to have little effect on the pharmacokinetics of Focalin.

Hepatic Insufficiency

There is no experience with the use of Focalin in patients with hepatic insufficiency. (For Drug Interactions, see PRECAUTIONS.)

Clinical Studies

Focalin was evaluated in two double-blind, parallel-group, placebo-controlled trials in untreated or previously treated patients aged 6 to 17 years old with a DSM-IV diagnosis of Attention Deficit Hyperactivity Disorder (ADHD). Both studies included all three subtypes of ADHD, *i.e.*, Combined Type, Predominantly Inattentive Type, or Predominantly Hyperactive-Impulsive Type. While both children and adolescents were included, the sample was predominantly children, thus, the findings are most pertinent to this age group. In both studies, the primary comparison of interest was Focalin *versus* placebo.

Focalin (5, 10, or 20 mg/day total dose), *dl-threo*-methylphenidate HCl (10, 20, or 40 mg/day total dose), and placebo were compared in a multicenter, 4-week, parallel group study in n=132 patients. Patients took the study medication twice daily, 3.5 to 5.5 hours between doses. Treatment was initiated with the lowest dose, and doses could be doubled at weekly intervals, depending on clinical response and tolerability, up to the maximum dose. The change from baseline to week 4 of the averaged score (an average of two ratings during the week) of the teacher's version of the SNAP-ADHD Rating Scale, a scale for assessing ADHD symptoms, was the primary outcome. Patients treated with Focalin showed a statistically significant improvement in symptom scores from baseline over patients who received placebo.

[See figure at top of next column]

The other study, involving n=75 patients, was a multicenter, placebo-controlled, double-blind, 2-week treatment withdrawal study in children who were responders during a 6-week, open label initial treatment period. Children took study medication twice a day separated by a 3.5 to 5.5 hour interval. The primary outcome was proportion of treatment failures at the end of the 2-week withdrawal phase, where

Figure 1
Mean Change from Baseline in Teacher SNAP-ADHD Scores in a 4-week Double-Blind Placebo-Controlled Study of Focalin™*

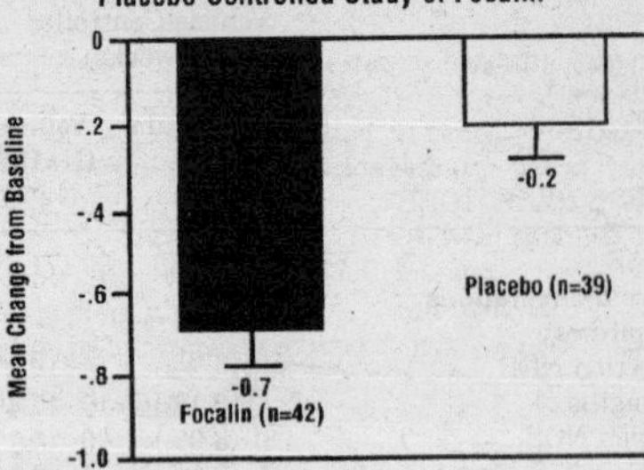

*Figure 1: Error bars represent the standard error of the mean.

treatment failure was defined as a rating of 6 (much worse) or 7 (very much worse) on the Investigator Clinical Global Impression - Improvement (CGI-I). Patients continued on Focalin showed a statistically significant lower rate of failure over patients who received placebo.

Figure 2
Percent of Treatment Failures following a 2-week Double-Blind Placebo-Controlled Withdrawal of Focalin™

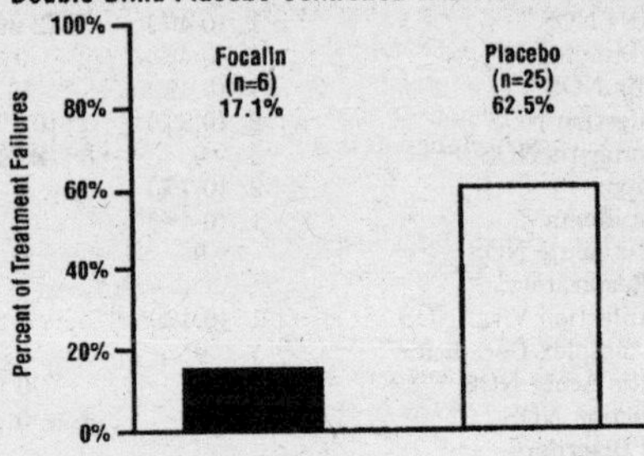

INDICATION AND USAGE

Focalin is indicated for the treatment of Attention Deficit Hyperactivity Disorder (ADHD).

The efficacy of Focalin in the treatment of ADHD was established in two controlled trials of patients aged 6 to 17 years of age who met DSM-IV criteria for ADHD (see Clinical Studies).

A diagnosis of ADHD (DSM-IV) implies the presence of hyperactive-impulsive or inattentive symptoms that cause impairment and were present before age 7 years. The symptoms must cause clinically significant impairment, *e.g.*, in social, academic, or occupational functioning; and be present in two or more settings, *e.g.*, school (or work) and at home. The symptoms must not be better accounted for by another mental disorder. For the inattentive type, at least six of the following symptoms must have persisted for at least 6 months: lack of attention to details/careless mistakes; lack of sustained attention; poor listener; failure to follow through on tasks; poor organization; avoids tasks requiring sustained mental effort; loses things; easily distracted; forgetful. For the Hyperactive-Impulsive Type, at least six of the following symptoms must have persisted for at least 6 months: fidgeting/squirming; leaving seat; inappropriate running/climbing; difficulty with quiet activities; "on the go," excessive talking; blurting answers; can't wait turn; intrusive. The Combined Type requires both inattentive and hyperactive-impulsive criteria to be met.

Special Diagnostic Considerations

Specific etiology of this syndrome is unknown, and there is no single diagnostic test. Adequate diagnosis requires the use not only of medical but of special psychological, educational, and social resources. Learning may or may not be impaired. The diagnosis must be based upon a complete history and evaluation of the child and not solely on the presence of the required number of DSM-IV characteristics.

Need for Comprehensive Treatment Program

Focalin is indicated as an integral part of a total treatment program for ADHD that may include other measures (psychological, educational, social) for patients with this syndrome. Drug treatment may not be indicated for all patients with this syndrome. Stimulants are not intended for use in the patient who exhibits symptoms secondary to environmental factors and/or other primary psychiatric disorders, including psychosis. Appropriate educational placement is essential and psychosocial intervention is often helpful. When remedial measures alone are insufficient, the decision to prescribe stimulant medication will depend upon the physician's assessment of the chronicity and severity of the patient's symptoms.

Long-term Use

The effectiveness of Focalin for long-term use, *i.e.*, for more than 6 weeks, has not been systematically evaluated in controlled trials. Therefore, the physician who elects to use Focalin for extended periods should periodically re-evaluate the long-term usefulness of the drug for the individual patient (see DOSAGE AND ADMINISTRATION).

CONTRAINDICATIONS

Agitation

Focalin is contraindicated in patients with marked anxiety, tension, and agitation, since the drug may aggravate these symptoms.

Hypersensitivity to Methylphenidate
Focalin is contraindicated in patients known to be hypersensitive to methylphenidate or other components of the product.
Glaucoma
Focalin is contraindicated in patients with glaucoma.
Tics
Focalin is contraindicated in patients with motor tics or with a family history or diagnosis of Tourette's syndrome (see ADVERSE REACTIONS).
Monoamine Oxidase Inhibitors
Focalin is contraindicated during treatment with monoamine oxidase inhibitors, and also within a minimum of 14 days following discontinuation of a monoamine oxidase inhibitor (hypertensive crises may result).

WARNINGS

Depression
Focalin should not be used to treat severe depression.
Fatigue
Focalin should not be used for the prevention or treatment of normal fatigue states.
Long-Term Suppression of Growth
Sufficient data on safety of long-term use of Focalin in children are not yet available. Although a causal relationship has not been established, suppression of growth (*i.e.*, weight gain and/or height) has been reported with the long-term use of stimulants in children. Therefore, patients requiring long-term therapy should be carefully monitored. Patients who are not growing or gaining weight as expected should have their treatment interrupted.
Psychosis
Clinical experience suggests that in psychotic children, administration of methylphenidate may exacerbate symptoms of behavior disturbance and thought disorder.
Seizures
There is some clinical evidence that methylphenidate may lower the convulsive threshold in patients with prior history of seizures, in patients with prior EEG abnormalities in the absence of a history of seizures, and, very rarely, in the absence of a history of seizures and no prior EEG evidence of seizures. In the presence of seizures, the drug should be discontinued.
Hypertension and Other Cardiovascular Conditions
Use cautiously in patients with hypertension. Blood pressure should be monitored at appropriate intervals in all patients taking Focalin, especially those with hypertension. In the placebo controlled studies, the mean pulse increase was 2-5 bpm for both Focalin and racemic methylphenidate compared to placebo, with mean increases of systolic and diastolic blood pressure of 2-3 mmHg, compared to placebo. Therefore, caution is indicated in treating patients whose underlying medical conditions might be compromised by increases in blood pressure or heart rate, *e.g.*, those with pre-existing hypertension, heart failure, recent myocardial infarction, or hyperthyroidism.
Visual Disturbance
Symptoms of visual disturbances have been encountered in rare cases following use of methylphenidate. Difficulties with accommodation and blurring of vision have been reported.
Use in Children Under 6 Years of Age
Focalin should not be used in children under 6 years, since safety and efficacy in this age group have not been established.

DRUG DEPENDENCE: Focalin should be given cautiously to patients with a history of drug dependence or alcoholism. Chronic, abusive use can lead to marked tolerance and psychological dependence with varying degrees of abnormal behavior. Frank psychotic episodes can occur, especially with parenteral abuse. Careful supervision is required during drug withdrawal from abusive use since severe depression may occur. Withdrawal following chronic therapeutic use may unmask symptoms of the underlying disorder that may require follow-up.

PRECAUTIONS

Hematologic Monitoring
Periodic CBC, differential, and platelet counts are advised during prolonged therapy.
Information for Patients
Patient information is printed at the end of this insert. To assure safe and effective use of Focalin, the information and instructions provided in the patient information section should be discussed with patients.
Drug Interactions
Methylphenidate may decrease the effectiveness of drugs used to treat hypertension. Because of possible effects on blood pressure, Focalin should be used cautiously with pressor agents.
Human pharmacologic studies have shown that racemic methylphenidate may inhibit the metabolism of coumarin anticoagulants, anticonvulsants (*e.g.*, phenobarbital, phenytoin, primidone), and some antidepressants (tricyclics and selective serotonin reuptake inhibitors). Downward dose adjustments of these drugs may be required when given concomitantly with methylphenidate. It may be necessary to adjust the dosage and monitor plasma drug concentration (or, in the case of coumarin, coagulation times), when initiating or discontinuing concomitant methylphenidate.
Serious adverse events have been reported in concomitant use with clonidine, although no causality for the combination has been established. The safety of using methylphenidate in combination with clonidine or other centrally acting alpha-2 agonists has not been systematically evaluated.
Carcinogenesis, Mutagenesis, and Impairment of Fertility
Lifetime carcinogenicity studies have not been carried out with dexmethylphenidate. In a lifetime carcinogenicity study carried out in B6C3F1 mice, racemic methylphenidate caused an increase in hepatocellular adenomas, and in males only, an increase in hepatoblastomas at a daily dose of approximately 60 mg/kg/day. Hepatoblastoma is a relatively rare rodent malignant tumor type. There was no increase in total malignant hepatic tumors. The mouse strain used is sensitive to the development of hepatic tumors, and the significance of these results to humans is unknown.
Racemic methylphenidate did not cause any increase in tumors in a lifetime carcinogenicity study carried out in F344 rats; the highest dose used was approximately 45 mg/kg/day.
In a 24-week study of racemic methylphenidate in the transgenic mouse strain p53+/-, which is sensitive to genotoxic carcinogens, there was no evidence of carcinogenicity. Mice were fed diets containing the same concentrations as in the lifetime carcinogenicity study; the high-dose group was exposed to 60-74 mg/kg/day of racemic methylphenidate.
Dexmethylphenidate was not mutagenic in the *in vitro* Ames reverse mutation assay, the *in vitro* mouse lymphoma cell forward mutation assay, or the *in vivo* mouse bone marrow micronucleus test.
Racemic methylphenidate was not mutagenic in the *in vitro* Ames reverse mutation assay or the *in vitro* mouse lymphoma cell forward mutation assay, and was negative *in vivo* in the mouse bone marrow micronucleus assay. However, sister chromatid exchanges and chromosome aberrations were increased, indicative of a weak clastogenic response, in an *in vitro* assay of racemic methylphenidate in cultured Chinese Hamster Ovary (CHO) cells.
Racemic methylphenidate did not impair fertility in male or female mice that were fed diets containing the drug in an 18-week Continuous Breeding study. The study was conducted at doses of up to 160 mg/kg/day.
Pregnancy
Pregnancy Category C
In studies conducted in rats and rabbits, dexmethylphenidate was administered orally at doses of up to 20 and 100 mg/kg/day, respectively, during the period of organogenesis. No evidence of teratogenic activity was found in either the rat or rabbit study; however, delayed fetal skeletal ossification was observed at the highest dose level in rats. When dexmethylphenidate was administered to rats throughout pregnancy and lactation at doses of up to 20 mg/kg/day, postweaning body weight gain was decreased in male offspring at the highest dose, but no other effects on postnatal development were observed. At the highest doses tested, plasma levels (AUCs) of dexmethylphenidate in pregnant rats and rabbits were approximately 5 and 1 times, respectively, those in adults dosed with the maximum recommended human dose of 20 mg/day.
Racemic methylphenidate has been shown to have teratogenic effects in rabbits when given in doses of 200 mg/kg/day throughout organogenesis.
Adequate and well-controlled studies in pregnant women have not been conducted. Focalin should be used during pregnancy only if the potential benefit justifies the potential risk to the fetus.
Nursing Mothers
It is not known whether dexmethylphenidate is excreted in human milk. Because many drugs are excreted in human milk, caution should be exercised if Focalin is administered to a nursing woman.
Pediatric Use
The safety and efficacy of Focalin in children under 6 years old have not been established. Long-term effects of Focalin in children have not been well established (see WARNINGS).

ADVERSE REACTIONS

The pre-marketing development program for Focalin included exposures in a total of 696 participants in clinical trials (684 patients, 12 healthy adult subjects). These participants received Focalin 5, 10, or 20 mg/day. The 684 ADHD patients (ages 6 to 17 years) were evaluated in two controlled clinical studies, two clinical pharmacology studies, and two uncontrolled long-term safety studies. Safety data on all patients are included in the discussion that follows. Adverse reactions were assessed by collecting adverse events, and results of physical examinations, vital sign and body weight measurements, and laboratory analyses.
Adverse events during exposure were primarily obtained by general inquiry and recorded by clinical investigators using terminology of their own choosing. Consequently, it is not possible to provide a meaningful estimate of the proportion of individuals experiencing adverse events without first grouping similar types of events into a smaller number of standardized event categories. In the tables and tabulations that follow, standard COSTART dictionary terminology has been used to classify reported adverse events.
The stated frequencies of adverse events represent the proportion of individuals who experienced, at least once, a treatment-emergent adverse event of the type listed. An event was considered treatment emergent if it occurred for the first time or worsened while receiving therapy following baseline evaluation.

Adverse Findings in Clinical Trials with Focalin
Adverse Events Associated with Discontinuation of Treatment
No Focalin-treated patients discontinued due to adverse events in two placebo-controlled trials. Overall, 50 of 684 children treated with Focalin (7.3%) experienced an adverse event that resulted in discontinuation. The most common reasons for discontinuation were twitching (described as motor or vocal tics), anorexia, insomnia, and tachycardia (approximately 1% each).
Adverse Events Occurring at an Incidence of 5% or More Among Focalin-Treated Patients
Table 1 enumerates treatment-emergent adverse events for two, placebo-controlled, parallel group trials in children with ADHD at Focalin doses of 5, 10, and 20 mg/day. The table includes only those events that occurred in 5% or more of patients treated with Focalin where the incidence in patients treated with Focalin was at least twice the incidence in placebo-treated patients. The prescriber should be aware that these figures cannot be used to predict the incidence of adverse events in the course of usual medical practice where patient characteristics and other factors differ from those which prevailed in the clinical trials. Similarly, the cited frequencies cannot be compared with figures obtained from other clinical investigations involving different treatments, uses, and investigators. The cited figures, however, do provide the prescribing physician with some basis for estimating the relative contribution of drug and non-drug factors to the adverse event incidence rate in the population studied.

Table 1
Treatment-Emergent Adverse Events[1] Occurring During Double-Blind Treatment in Clinical Trials of Focalin™

Body System	Preferred Term	Focalin (n=79)	Placebo (n=82)
Body as a Whole			
	Abdominal Pain	15%	6%
	Fever	5%	1%
Digestive System			
	Anorexia	6%	1%
	Nausea	9%	1%

[1] Events, regardless of causality, for which the incidence for patients treated with Focalin was at least 5% and twice the incidence among placebo-treated patients. Incidence has been rounded to the nearest whole number.

Adverse Events with Other Methylphenidate HCl Products
Nervousness and insomnia are the most common adverse reactions reported with other methylphenidate products. In children, loss of appetite, abdominal pain, weight loss during prolonged therapy, insomnia, and tachycardia may occur more frequently; however, any of the other adverse reactions listed below may also occur.
Other reactions include:
Cardiac: angina, arrhythmia, palpitations, pulse increased or decreased
Gastrointestinal: nausea
Immune: hypersensitivity reactions including skin rash, urticaria, fever, arthralgia, exfoliative dermatitis, erythema multiforme with histopathological findings of necrotizing vasculitis, and thrombocytopenic purpura
Nervous System: dizziness, drowsiness, dyskinesia, headache, rare reports of Tourette's syndrome, toxic psychosis
Vascular: blood pressure increased or decreased, cerebral arteritis and/or occlusion
Although a definite causal relationship has not been established, the following have been reported in patients taking methylphenidate:
Blood/lymphatic: leukopenia and/or anemia
Hepatobiliary: abnormal liver function, ranging from transaminase elevation to hepatic coma
Psychiatric: transient depressed mood
Skin/subcutaneous: scalp hair loss
Very rare reports of neuroleptic malignant syndrome (NMS) have been received, and, in most of these, patients were concurrently receiving therapies associated with NMS. In a single report, a ten year old boy who had been taking methylphenidate for approximately 18 months experienced an NMS-like event within 45 minutes of ingesting his first dose of venlafaxine. It is uncertain whether this case represented a drug-drug interaction, a response to either drug alone, or some other cause.
In children, loss of appetite, abdominal pain, weight loss during prolonged therapy, insomnia, and tachycardia may occur more frequently; however, any of the other adverse reactions listed above may also occur.

DRUG ABUSE AND DEPENDENCE

Controlled Substance Class
Focalin, like other methylphenidate products, is classified as a Schedule II controlled substance by Federal regulation.
Abuse, Dependence, and Tolerance
See WARNINGS for boxed warning containing drug abuse and dependence information.

OVERDOSAGE

Signs and Symptoms
Signs and symptoms of acute methylphenidate overdosage, resulting principally from overstimulation of the CNS and from excessive sympathomimetic effects, may include the following: vomiting, agitation, tremors, hyperreflexia, mus-

Continued on next page

Focalin—Cont.

cle twitching, convulsions (may be followed by coma), euphoria, confusion, hallucinations, delirium, sweating, flushing, headache, hyperpyrexia, tachycardia, palpitations, cardiac arrhythmias, hypertension, mydriasis, and dryness of mucous membranes.

Recommended Treatment

Treatment consists of appropriate supportive measures. The patient must be protected against self-injury and against external stimuli that would aggravate overstimulation already present. Gastric contents may be evacuated by gastric lavage as indicated. Before performing gastric lavage, control agitation and seizures if present and protect the airway. Other measures to detoxify the gut include administration of activated charcoal and a cathartic. Intensive care must be provided to maintain adequate circulation and respiratory exchange; external cooling procedures may be required for hyperpyrexia.

Efficacy of peritoneal dialysis for Focalin overdosage has not been established.

Poison Control Center

As with the management of all overdosage, the possibility of multiple drug ingestion should be considered. The physician may wish to consider contacting a poison control center for up-to-date information on the management of overdosage with methylphenidate.

DOSAGE AND ADMINISTRATION

Focalin is administered twice daily, at least 4 hours apart. Focalin may be administered with or without food.

Dosage should be individualized according to the needs and responses of the patient.

Patients New to Methylphenidate

The recommended starting dose of Focalin for patients who are not currently taking racemic methylphenidate, or for patients who are on stimulants other than methylphenidate, is 5 mg/day (2.5 mg twice daily).

Dosage may be adjusted in 2.5 to 5 mg increments to a maximum of 20 mg/day (10 mg twice daily). In general, dosage adjustments may proceed at approximately weekly intervals.

Patients Currently Using Methylphenidate

For patients currently using methylphenidate, the recommended starting dose of Focalin is half the dose of racemic methylphenidate. The maximum recommended dose is 20 mg/day (10 mg twice daily).

Maintenance/Extended Treatment

There is no body of evidence available from controlled trials to indicate how long the patient with ADHD should be treated with Focalin. It is generally agreed, however, that pharmacological treatment of ADHD may be needed for extended periods. Nevertheless, the physician who elects to use Focalin for extended periods in patients with ADHD should periodically re-evaluate the long-term usefulness of the drug for the individual patient with periods off medication to assess the patient's functioning without pharmacotherapy. Improvement may be sustained when the drug is either temporarily or permanently discontinued.

Dose Reduction and Discontinuation

If paradoxical aggravation of symptoms or other adverse events occur, the dosage should be reduced, or, if necessary, the drug should be discontinued.

If improvement is not observed after appropriate dosage adjustment over a 1-month period, the drug should be discontinued.

HOW SUPPLIED

Tablets, D-shaped, embossed "D" on upper convex face and dosage strength on lower convex face

2.5 mg Tablets - blue
Bottles of 100 .... NDC 0078-0380-05

5 mg Tablets - yellow
Bottles of 100 .... NDC 0078-0381-05

10 mg Tablets - white
Bottles of 100 .... NDC 0078-0382-05

Store at 25°C (77°F); excursions permitted 15°C-30°C (59°F-86°F).
[see USP Controlled Room Temperature]
Protect from light and moisture.

REFERENCE

American Psychiatric Association. Diagnosis and Statistical Manual of Mental Disorders. 4th ed. Washington DC: American Psychiatric Association 1994.

REV: NOVEMBER 2001 T2001-85

INFORMATION FOR PATIENTS TAKING FOCALIN™, OR FOR THEIR PARENTS OR CAREGIVERS

Focalin™ Ⓒ

dexmethylphenidate hydrochloride tablets

Rx only

This information for patients or their parents or caregivers is about Focalin, a medication intended for the treatment of Attention Deficit Hyperactivity Disorder (ADHD).

Please read this before you start taking Focalin. It is not intended to replace your doctor's instructions or advice. If you have any questions about this material or about Focalin, be sure to talk to your doctor or pharmacist.

What is Focalin?

Focalin is a central nervous system stimulant for the treatment of Attention Deficit Hyperactivity Disorder (ADHD). Dexmethylphenidate hydrochloride, the active ingredient of Focalin, is also found in methylphenidate, a central nervous system stimulant that has been used to treat ADHD for more than 30 years. Focalin is available in a D-shaped tablet form, 2.5 mg, 5 mg, and 10 mg, and is intended to be used in doses of 5 to 20 mg per day, given as divided doses, as directed by your doctor.

What is Attention Deficit Hyperactivity Disorder (ADHD)?

Attention Deficit Hyperactivity Disorder (ADHD) is a disorder characterized by symptoms of inattentiveness and/or hyperactivity-impulsivity inappropriate to the patient's age which interfere with functioning in two or more settings (*e.g.*, school and home). Symptoms of inattention may include not paying attention, making careless mistakes, not listening, not finishing tasks, not following directions, and being easily distracted. Symptoms of hyperactivity-impulsiveness may include fidgeting, talking excessively, running around at inappropriate times, and interrupting others. Some patients have more symptoms of hyperactivity and impulsiveness while others have more symptoms of inattentiveness. Some patients have both types of symptoms. Symptoms must be present for at least 6 months to be certain of the diagnosis.

How Does Focalin work?

Focalin (dexmethylphenidate hydrochloride) is rapidly absorbed into the bloodstream and acts for a period of several hours. Focalin helps to increase attention and decrease impulsiveness and hyperactivity in patients with ADHD.

Before Focalin Treatment

It is very important that ADHD be accurately diagnosed and that the need for medication be carefully assessed. It is important to remember that Focalin is only part of the overall management of ADHD. Parents, teachers, physicians and other professionals are part of a team that must work together.

Before Focalin treatment, your doctor should be made aware of any current or past physical or mental problems. Tell your doctor if there is a history of drug or alcohol abuse, depression, psychosis, epilepsy or seizure disorders, high blood pressure, glaucoma, facial tics (involuntary movements), or a family history of Tourette's syndrome.

Both your doctor and your pharmacist should also be informed of all medicines that you are taking, even if these drugs are not taken on a regular basis and are available without prescription. Your doctor will decide whether you can take Focalin with other medicines. Methylphenidate is known to interact with a number of other drugs. These include medicines to treat depression, such as monoamine oxidase inhibitors; to control seizures; and to thin blood. Sometimes these interactions may require a change in dosage, or occasionally stopping one of the drugs involved.

Tell your doctor if you are pregnant or nursing a baby.

Who Should Not Take Focalin?

You should NOT take Focalin if:

- You have significant anxiety, tension, or agitation since Focalin may make these conditions worse.
- You are allergic to methylphenidate or any of the other ingredients in Focalin.
- You have glaucoma, an eye disease.
- You have tics or Tourette's syndrome, or a family history of Tourette's syndrome.
- You are taking a monoamine oxidase inhibitor, a type of drug, or have discontinued a monoamine oxidase inhibitor in the last 14 days.

Talk to your doctor if you believe any of these conditions apply to you.

How Should I Take Focalin?

Take the dose prescribed by your doctor. Your doctor may adjust the amount of drug you take until it is right for you. From time to time, your doctor may interrupt your treatment to check your symptoms while you are not taking the drug.

What are the Possible Side Effects of Focalin?

In the clinical studies with patients using Focalin, the most common side effects were stomach pain, fever, decreased appetite, and nausea. Other side effects seen with Focalin include vomiting, dizziness, sleeplessness, nervousness, tics, allergic reactions, increased blood pressure and psychosis (abnormal thinking or hallucinations).

This is not a complete list of possible side effects. Ask your doctor about other side effects. If you develop any side effect, talk to your doctor.

What Must I Discuss with my Doctor before Taking Focalin?

Talk to your doctor ***before*** taking Focalin if you:

- Are being treated for depression or have symptoms of depression such as feelings of sadness, worthlessness, and hopelessness.
- Have motion tics (hard-to-control, repeated twitching of any parts of your body) or verbal tics (hard-to-control repeating of sounds or words).
- Have someone in your family with motion tics, verbal tics, or Tourette's syndrome.
- Have abnormal thoughts or visions, hear abnormal sounds, or have been diagnosed with psychosis.
- Have had seizures (convulsions, epilepsy) or abnormal EEGs (electroencephalograms).
- Have high blood pressure.
- Have an abnormal heart rate or rhythm.

Tell your doctor ***immediately*** if you develop any of the above conditions or symptoms while taking Focalin.

Can I Take Focalin with Other Medicines?

Tell your doctor about ***all*** medicines that you are taking. Your doctor should decide whether you can take Focalin with other medicines. These include:

- Other medicines that a doctor has prescribed.
- Medicines that you buy yourself without a prescription.
- Any herbal remedies that you may be taking.

You should not take Focalin with monoamine oxidase (MAO) inhibitors.

While on Focalin, do not start taking a new medicine or herbal remedy before checking with your doctor.

Focalin may change the way your body reacts to certain medicines. These include medicines used to treat depression, prevent seizures, or prevent blood clots (commonly called "blood thinners"). Your doctor may need to change your dose of these medicines if you are taking them with Focalin.

Other Important Safety Information

Abuse of Focalin can lead to dependence.

Tell your doctor if you have ever abused or been dependent on alcohol or drugs, or if you are now abusing or dependent on alcohol or drugs.

Before taking Focalin, tell your doctor if you are pregnant or plan on becoming pregnant. If you take Focalin, it may be in your breast milk. Tell your doctor if you are nursing a baby.

Tell your doctor if you have blurred vision when taking Focalin.

Slower growth (weight gain and/or height) has been reported with long-term use of methylphenidate in children. Your doctor will be carefully watching your height and weight. If you are not growing or gaining weight as your doctor expects, your doctor may stop your Focalin treatment.

Call your doctor ***immediately*** if you take more than the amount of Focalin prescribed by your doctor.

What Else Should I Know about Focalin?

Focalin has not been studied in children under 6 years of age.

Focalin may be a part of your overall treatment for ADHD. Your doctor may also recommend that you have counseling or other therapy.

As with all medicines, never share Focalin with anyone else and take only the number of Focalin tablets prescribed by your doctor.

Focalin may be taken at the same time as food or with no food. Focalin should be stored in a safe place at room temperature (between 59°F - 86°F). Do not store this medicine in hot, damp, or humid places.

Keep the container of Focalin in a safe place, away from high-traffic areas where other people could have accidental or unauthorized access to the medication. Keep track of the number of tablets so that you will know if any are missing. Sadly, someone who has easy access to Focalin may be able to give the tablets to others or misuse the medication.

Keep Out of the Reach of Children

REV: NOVEMBER 2001 T2001-86
Printed in U.S.A. T2001-85/T2001-86
Code 888B00 89013602

Manufactured for:
Novartis Pharmaceuticals Corporation
East Hanover, NJ 07936
By:
Mikart, Inc.
Atlanta, GA 30318

Ortho-McNeil Pharmaceutical

RARITAN, NJ 08869-0602

www.ortho-mcneil.com
For Medical Information Contact:
(800) 682-6532
In Emergencies:
(908) 218-7325
For Patient Education Materials Contact:
877-323-2200
For Customer Service (Sales and Ordering):
800-631-5273

ORTHO EVRA™

[*ōr'-thō 'ev'-rā*]

(NORELGESTROMIN / ETHINYL ESTRADIOL TRANSDERMAL SYSTEM)

Prescribing Information

Patients should be counseled that this product does not protect against HIV infection (AIDS) and other sexually transmitted diseases.

℞ only

DESCRIPTION

ORTHO EVRA™ is a combination transdermal contraceptive patch with a contact surface area of 20 cm^2. It contains 6.00 mg norelgestromin and 0.75 mg ethinyl estradiol (EE), and releases 150 micrograms of norelgestromin and 20 micrograms of EE to the bloodstream per 24 hours.

ORTHO EVRA™ is a thin, matrix-type transdermal contraceptive patch consisting of three layers. The backing layer is composed of a beige flexible film consisting of a low-density pigmented polyethylene outer layer and a polyester inner layer. It provides structural support and protects the middle adhesive layer from the environment. The middle layer contains polyisobutylene/polybutene adhesive, crospovidone, non-woven polyester fabric and lauryl lactate as inactive components. The active components in this layer are the hormones, norelgestromin and ethinyl estradiol. The third layer is the release liner, which protects the adhesive layer during storage and is removed just prior to application. It is a transparent polyethylene terephthalate (PET) film with a polydimethylsiloxane coating on the side that is in contact with the middle adhesive layer.

The outside of the backing layer is heat-stamped "ORTHO EVRA™ 150/20."

The structural formulas of the components are:

norelgestromin ethinyl estradiol

Molecular weight, norelgestromin: 327.47
Molecular weight, ethinyl estradiol: 296.41
Chemical name for norelgestromin: 18, 19-dinorpregn-4-en-20-yn-3-one, 13-ethyl- 17-hydroxy-, 3-oxime, (17α)
Chemical name for ethinyl estradiol: 19-Norpregna-1, 3, 5 (10)-trien-20-yne-3, 17-diol, (17α)

CLINICAL PHARMACOLOGY

Pharmacodynamics

Norelgestromin is the active progestin largely responsible for the progestational activity that occurs in women following application of ORTHO EVRA™. Norelgestromin is also the primary active metabolite produced following oral administration of norgestimate (NGM), the progestin component of the oral contraceptive products ORTHO-CYCLEN® and ORTHO TRI-CYCLEN®.

Combination oral contraceptives act by suppression of gonadotropins. Although the primary mechanism of this action is inhibition of ovulation, other alterations include changes in the cervical mucus (which increase the difficulty of sperm entry into the uterus) and the endometrium (which reduce the likelihood of implantation).

Receptor and human sex hormone-binding globulin (SHBG) binding studies, as well as studies in animals and humans, have shown that both norgestimate and norelgestromin exhibit high progestational activity with minimal intrinsic androgenicity[90–93]. Transdermally-administered norelgestromin, in combination with ethinyl estradiol, does not counteract the estrogen-induced increases in SHBG, resulting in lower levels of free testosterone in serum compared to baseline.

Pharmacokinetic studies with ORTHO EVRA™ demonstrated consistent elimination kinetics for norelgestromin and EE with half-life values of approximately 28 hours and 17 hours, respectively. One clinical trial assessed the return of hypothalamic-pituitary-ovarian axis function post-therapy and found that FSH, LH, and Estradiol mean values, though suppressed during therapy, returned to near baseline values during the 6 weeks post therapy.

Pharmacokinetics

Absorption

Following application of ORTHO EVRA™, both norelgestromin and EE rapidly appear in the serum, reach a plateau by approximately 48 hours, and are maintained at an approximate steady-state throughout the wear period. C^{SS} concentrations for norelgestromin and EE during one week of patch wear are approximately 0.6–0.8 ng/ml and 40–50 pg/ml, respectively, and are generally consistent from all studies and application sites. These C^{SS} concentrations are within the reference ranges for norelgestromin (0.6 to 1.2 ng/ml) and EE (25 to 75 pg/ml) established based upon the C_{ave} concentrations observed with subjects taking ORTHO-CYCLEN®.

Daily absorption of norelgestromin and EE from ORTHO EVRA™ was determined by comparison to an intravenous infusion of norelgestromin and EE. The results indicated that the average dose of norelgestromin and EE absorbed into the systemic circulation is 150 mcg/day and 20 mcg/day, respectively.

The absorption of norelgestromin and EE following application of ORTHO EVRA™ to the abdomen, buttock, upper outer arm and upper torso (excluding breast) was evaluated in a cross-over design study. The results of this study indicated that C^{SS} and AUC for the buttock, upper arm and torso for each analyte were equivalent. While C^{SS} values for the abdomen were within reference ranges for EE 35 mcg/NGM 250 mcg oral contraceptive users, exposure to the drugs was lower and strict bioequivalence requirements for AUC were not met in this study. However, in a separate parallel group multiple application pharmacokinetic study, C^{SS} and AUC for the buttock and abdomen were not statistically different. Therefore, all four sites may be considered therapeutically equivalent.

The absorption of norelgestromin and EE following application of ORTHO EVRA™ was studied under conditions encountered in a health club (sauna, whirlpool and treadmill) and in a cold water bath. The results indicated that for norelgestromin there were no significant treatment effects on C^{SS} or AUC when compared to normal wear. For EE, slight increases were observed due to sauna, whirlpool and treadmill, however, the C^{SS} values following these treatments were within the reference range. There was no significant effect of cold water on these parameters.

In multiple dose studies, C^{SS} and AUC for norelgestromin and EE were found to increase slightly over time when compared to Week 1 of Cycle 1. In a three-cycle study, these pharmacokinetic parameters reached steady-state conditions during all three weeks of Cycle 3. (See Table 1, Figures 1 and 2).

Table 1: Mean (SD) Pharmacokinetic Parameters of Norelgestromin and EE Following 3 Consecutive Cycles of ORTHO EVRA™ Wear on the Buttock

Analyte	Parameter	Cycle 1 Week 1	Cycle 3 Week 1	Cycle 3 Week 2	Cycle 3 Week 3
Norelgestromin	$C^{ss\ a}$	0.70 (0.28)	0.70 (0.29)	0.80 (0.23)	0.70 (0.32)
	$AUC_{0\text{-}168}{}^{b}$	107 (44.2)	105 (45.5)	132 (57.1)	120 (52.8)
	t ½^{c}	nc	nc	nc	32.1 (12.9)
EE	$C^{ss\ d}$	46.4 (17.9)	47.6 (17.3)	59.0 (25.1)	49.6 (27.0)
	$AUC_{0\text{-}168}{}^{e}$	6796 (2673)	7160 (2893)	10054 (4205)	8840 (5176)
	t ½^{c}	nc	nc	nc	21.0 (9.07)

[a] ng/mL
[b] ng·h/mL
[c] h
[d] pg/mL
[e] pg·h/mL
nc = not calculated

[See table above]

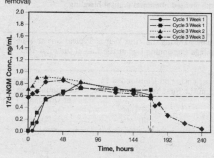

Figure 1: Mean Norelgestromin Serum Concentrations (ng/mL) in Healthy Female Volunteers Following Application of ORTHO EVRA™ on the Buttock for Three Consecutive Cycles (Dotted horizontal lines indicate the reference range. Dotted vertical arrow indicates time of patch removal)

Figure 2: Mean Ethinyl Estradiol Serum Concentrations (pg/mL) in Healthy Female Volunteers Following Application of ORTHO EVRA™ on the Buttock for Three Consecutive Cycles (Dotted horizontal lines indicate the reference range. Dotted vertical arrow indicates time of patch removal.)

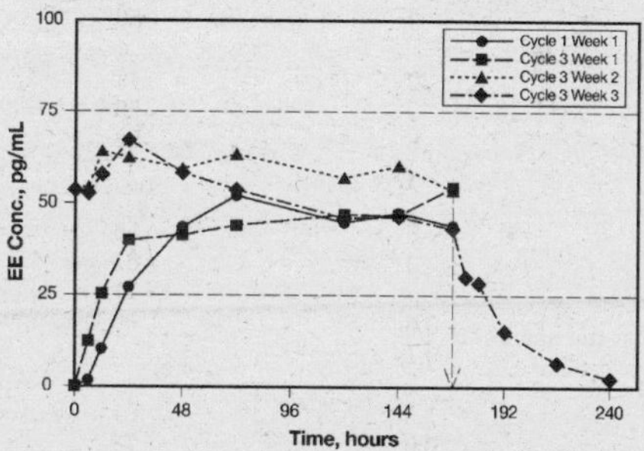

Results from a study of consecutive ORTHO EVRA™ wear for 7 days and 10 days indicated that serum concentrations of norelgestromin and EE dropped slightly during the first 6 hours after the patch replacement, still stayed within the reference range and recovered within 12 hours. Target C^{ss} of norelgestromin and EE were maintained during 2 days of extended wear of ORTHO EVRA™.

Figure 3: Mean (SD) Norelgestromin Serum Concentrations (ng/mL) Following Application of ORTHO EVRA™ to the Abdomen for 7 Days and 10 Days (Dotted horizontal lines indicate the reference range. Solid vertical arrows indicate actual time of patch removal. Dotted vertical arrow indicates theoretical time of patch removal under normal use.)

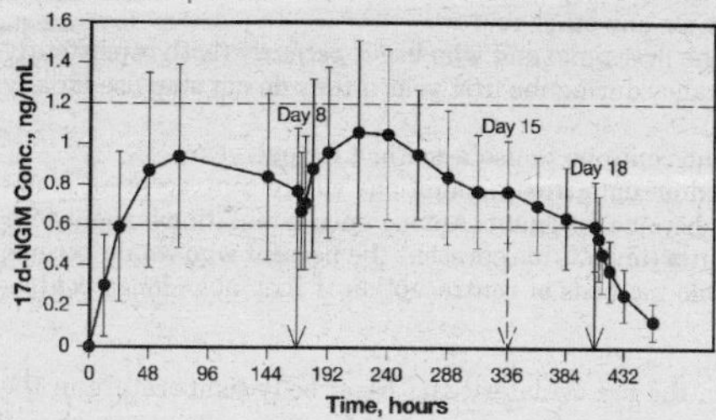

[See figure at top of next column]

Metabolism

Since ORTHO EVRA™ is applied transdermally, first-pass metabolism (via the gastrointestinal tract and/or liver) of norelgestromin and EE that would be expected with oral administration is avoided. Hepatic metabolism of norelgestromin occurs and metabolites include norgestrel, which is highly bound to SHBG, and various hydroxylated

Figure 4: Mean (SD) EE Serum Concentrations (pg/mL) Following Application of ORTHO EVRA™ to Abdomen for 7 Days and 10 Days (Dotted horizontal lines indicate reference range. Solid vertical arrows indicate actual time of patch removal. Dotted vertical arrow indicates theoretical time of patch removal under normal use.)

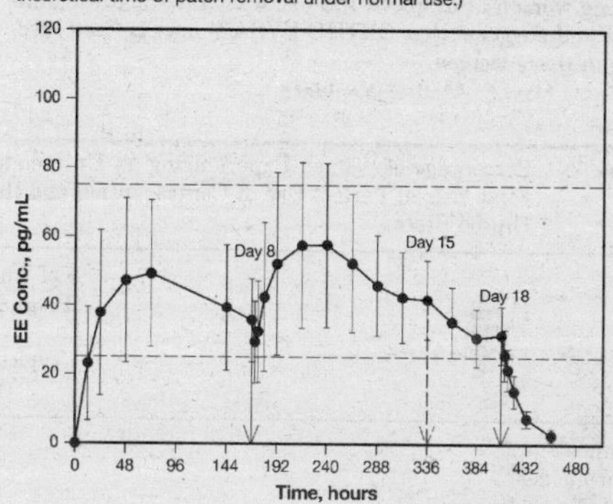

and conjugated metabolites. Ethinyl estradiol is also metabolized to various hydroxylated products and their glucuronide and sulfate conjugates.

Distribution

Norelgestromin and norgestrel (a serum metabolite of norelgestromin) are highly bound (>97%) to serum proteins. Norelgestromin is bound to albumin and not to SHBG, while norgestrel is bound primarily to SHBG, which limits its biological activity. Ethinyl estradiol is extensively bound to serum albumin.

Elimination

Following removal of patches, the elimination kinetics of norelgestromin and EE were consistent for all studies with half-life values of approximately 28 hours and 17 hours, respectively. The metabolites of norelgestromin and EE are eliminated by renal and fecal pathways.

Special Populations

Effects of Age, Body Weight, Body Surface Area and Race: The effects of age, body weight, body surface area and race on the pharmacokinetics of norelgestromin and EE were evaluated in 230 healthy women from nine pharmacokinetic studies of single 7-day applications of ORTHO EVRA™. For both norelgestromin and EE, increasing age, body weight and body surface area each were associated with slight decreases in C^{ss} and AUC values. However, only a small fraction (10–25%) of the overall variability in the pharmacokinetics of norelgestromin and EE following application of ORTHO EVRA™ may be associated with any or all of the above demographic parameters. There was no significant effect of race with respect to Caucasians, Hispanics and Blacks.

Renal and Hepatic Impairment

No formal studies were conducted with ORTHO EVRA™ to evaluate the pharmacokinetics, safety, and efficacy in women with renal or hepatic impairment. Steroid hormones may be poorly metabolized in patients with impaired liver function (see PRECAUTIONS).

Drug Interactions

The metabolism of hormonal contraceptives may be influenced by various drugs. Of potential clinical importance are drugs that cause the induction of enzymes that are responsible for the degradation of estrogens and progestins, and drugs that interrupt entero-hepatic recirculation of estrogen (e.g. certain antibiotics)[72].

The proposed mechanism of interaction of antibiotics is different from that of liver enzyme-inducing drugs. Literature suggests possible interactions with the concomitant use of hormonal contraceptives and ampicillin or tetracycline. In a pharmacokinetic drug interaction study, oral administration of tetracycline HCl, 500 mg q.i.d. for 3 days prior to and 7 days during wear of ORTHO EVRA™ did not significantly affect the pharmacokinetics of norelgestromin or EE.

Continued on next page

Ortho Evra—Cont.

The major target for enzyme inducers is the hepatic microsomal estrogen-2-hydroxylase (cytochrome P450 3A4)[99]. See also PRECAUTIONS, Drug Interactions.

Patch Adhesion

In the clinical trials with ORTHO EVRA™, approximately 2% of the cumulative number of patches completely detached. The proportion of subjects with at least 1 patch that completely detached ranged from 2% to 6%, with a reduction from Cycle 1 (6%) to Cycle 13 (2%). For instructions on how to manage detachment of patches, refer to the DOSAGE AND ADMINISTRATION section.

INDICATIONS AND USAGE

ORTHO EVRA™ is indicated for the prevention of pregnancy.

Like oral contraceptives, ORTHO EVRA™ is highly effective if used as recommended in this label.

In 3 large clinical trials in North America, Europe and South Africa, 3,330 women (ages 18–45) completed 22,155 cycles of ORTHO EVRA™ use, pregnancy rates were approximately 1 per 100 women-years of ORTHO EVRA™ use. The racial distribution was 91% Caucasian, 4.9% Black, 1.6% Asian, and 2.4% Other.

With respect to weight, 5 of the 15 pregnancies reported with ORTHO EVRA™ use were among women with a baseline body weight ≥198 lbs. (90kg), which constituted <3% of the study population. The greater proportion of pregnancies among women at or above 198 lbs. was statistically significant and suggests that ORTHO EVRA™ may be less effective in these women.

Health Care Professionals who consider ORTHO EVRA™ for women at or above 198 lbs. should discuss the patient's individual needs in choosing the most appropriate contraceptive option.

Table 2 lists the accidental pregnancy rates for users of various methods of contraception. The efficacy of these contraceptive methods, except sterilization, IUD, and Norplant depends upon the reliability with which they are used. Correct and consistent use of methods can result in lower failure rates.

[See table below]

ORTHO EVRA™ has not been studied for and is not indicated for use in emergency contraception.

CONTRAINDICATIONS

ORTHO EVRA™ should not be used in women who currently have the following conditions:

- Thrombophlebitis, thromboembolic disorders
- A past history of deep vein thrombophlebitis or thromboembolic disorders
- Cerebrovascular or coronary artery disease (current or past history)
- Valvular heart disease with complications[103]
- Severe hypertension[103]
- Diabetes with vascular involvement[103]
- Headaches with focal neurological symptoms
- Major surgery with prolonged immobilization
- Known or suspected carcinoma of the breast or personal history of breast cancer
- Carcinoma of the endometrium or other known or suspected estrogen-dependent neoplasia
- Undiagnosed abnormal genital bleeding
- Cholestatic jaundice of pregnancy or jaundice with prior hormonal contraceptive use
- Acute or chronic hepatocellular disease with abnormal liver function[103]
- Hepatic adenomas or carcinomas
- Known or suspected pregnancy
- Hypersensitivity to any component of this product

Table 2: Percentage of Women Experiencing an Unintended Pregnancy During the First Year of Typical Use and the First Year of Perfect Use of Contraception and the Percentage Continuing Use at the End of the First Year. United States.

Method (1)	% of Women Experiencing an Unintended Pregnancy within the First Year of Use: Typical Use[1] (2)	Perfect Use[2] (3)	% of Women Continuing Use at One Year[3] (4)
Chance[4]	85	85	
Spermicides[5]	26	6	40
Periodic abstinence	25		63
Calendar		9	
Ovulation Method		3	
Sympto-Thermal[6]		2	
Post-Ovulation		1	
Cap[7]			
Parous Women	40	26	42
Nulliparous Women	20	9	56
Sponge			
Parous Women	40	20	42
Nulliparous Women	20	9	56
Diaphragm[7]	20	6	56
Withdrawal	19	4	
Condom[8]			
Female (Reality)	21	5	56
Male	14	3	61
Pill	5		71
Progestin Only		0.5	
Combined		0.1	
IUD			
Progesterone T	2.0	1.5	81
Copper T380A	0.8	0.6	78
LNg 20	0.1	0.1	81
Depo-Provera	0.3	0.3	70
Norplant and Norplant-2	0.05	0.05	88
Female Sterilization	0.5	0.5	100
Male Sterilization	0.15	0.10	100

Hatcher et al, 1998, Ref. # 1.

Emergency Contraceptive Pills: Treatment initiated within 72 hours after unprotected intercourse reduces the risk of pregnancy by at least 75%.[9]

Lactational Amenorrhea Method: LAM is highly effective, *temporary* method of contraception.[10]

Source: Trussell J, Contraceptive efficacy. In Hatcher RA, Trussell J, Stewart F, Cates W, Stewart GK, Kowal D, Guest F, Contraceptive Technology: Seventeenth Revised Edition. New York NY: Irvington Publishers, 1998.

[1] Among *typical* couples who initiate use of a method (not necessarily for the first time), the percentage who experience an accidental pregnancy during the first year if they do not stop use for any other reason.

[2] Among couples who initiate use of a method (not necessarily for the first time) and who use it *perfectly* (both consistently and correctly), the percentage who experience an accidental pregnancy during the first year if they do not stop use for any other reason.

[3] Among couples attempting to avoid pregnancy, the percentage who continue to use a method for one year.

[4] The percents becoming pregnant in columns (2) and (3) are based on data from populations where contraception is not used and from women who cease using contraception in order to become pregnant. Among such populations, about 89% become pregnant within one year. This estimate was lowered slightly (to 85%) to represent the percent who would become pregnant within one year among women now relying on reversible methods of contraception if they abandoned contraception altogether.

[5] Foams, creams, gels, vaginal suppositories, and vaginal film.

[6] Cervical mucus (ovulation) method supplemented by calendar in the pre-ovulatory and basal body temperature in the post-ovulatory phases.

[7] With spermicidal cream or jelly.

[8] Without spermicides.

[9] The treatment schedule is one dose within 72 hours after unprotected intercourse, and a second dose 12 hours after the first dose. The Food and Drug Administration has declared the following brands of oral contraceptives to be safe and effective for emergency contraception: Ovral (1 dose is 2 white pills), Alesse (1 dose is 5 pink pills), Nordette or Levlen (1 dose is 2 light-orange pills), Lo/Ovral (1 dose is 4 white pills), Triphasil or Tri-Levlen (1 dose is 4 yellow pills).

[10] However, to maintain effective protection against pregnancy, another method of contraception must be used as soon as menstruation resumes, the frequency or duration of breastfeeds is reduced, bottle feeds are introduced, or the baby reaches six months of age.

WARNINGS

Cigarette smoking increases the risk of serious cardiovascular side effects from hormonal contraceptive use. This risk increases with age and with heavy smoking (15 or more cigarettes per day) and is quite marked in women over 35 years of age. Women who use hormonal contraceptives, including ORTHO EVRA, should be strongly advised not to smoke.

ORTHO EVRA™ and other contraceptives that contain both an estrogen and a progestin are called combination hormonal contraceptives. There is no epidemiologic data available to determine whether safety and efficacy with the transdermal route of administration would be different than the oral route. Practitioners prescribing ORTHO EVRA™ should be familiar with the following information relating to risks.

The use of combination hormonal contraceptives is associated with increased risks of several serious conditions including myocardial infarction, thromboembolism, stroke, hepatic neoplasia, and gallbladder disease, although the risk of serious morbidity or mortality is very small in healthy women without underlying risk factors. The risk of morbidity and mortality increases significantly in the presence of other underlying risk factors such as hypertension, hyperlipidemias, obesity and diabetes.

The information contained in this package insert is principally based on studies carried out in women who used combination oral contraceptives with higher formulations of estrogens and progestins than those in common use today. The effect of long-term use of combination hormonal contraceptives with lower doses of both estrogen and progestin administered by any route remains to be determined.

Throughout this labeling, epidemiological studies reported are of two types: retrospective or case control studies and prospective or cohort studies. Case control studies provide a measure of the relative risk of a disease, namely, a ratio of the incidence of a disease among oral contraceptive users to that among nonusers. The relative risk does not provide information on the actual clinical occurrence of a disease. Cohort studies provide a measure of attributable risk, which is the *difference* in the incidence of disease between hormonal contraceptive users and nonusers. The attributable risk does provide information about the actual occurrence of a disease in the population (adapted from refs. 2 and 3 with the author's permission). For further information, the reader is referred to a text on epidemiological methods.

1. Thromboembolic Disorders And Other Vascular Problems

a. Thromboembolism

An increased risk of thromboembolic and thrombotic disease associated with the use of hormonal contraceptives is well established. Case control studies have found the relative risk of users compared to nonusers to be 3 for the first episode of superficial venous thrombosis, 4 to 11 for deep vein thrombosis or pulmonary embolism, and 1.5 to 6 for women with predisposing conditions for venous thromboembolic disease[2,3,19–24]. Cohort studies have shown the relative risk to be somewhat lower, about 3 for new cases and about 4.5 for new cases requiring hospitalization[25]. The risk of thromboembolic disease associated with hormonal contraceptives is not related to length of use and disappears after hormonal contraceptive use is stopped[2]. A two- to four-fold increase in relative risk of post-operative thromboembolic complications has been reported with the use of hormonal contraceptives[9,26]. The relative risk of venous thrombosis in women who have predisposing conditions is twice that of women without such medical conditions[9,26]. If feasible, hormonal contraceptives should be discontinued at least four weeks prior to and for two weeks after elective surgery of a type associated with an increase in risk of thromboembolism and during and following prolonged immobilization. Since the immediate postpartum period is also associated with an increased risk of thromboembolism, hormonal contraceptives should be started no earlier than four weeks after delivery in women who elect not to breast-feed.

In the large clinical trials (N=3,330 with 1,704 women-years of exposure), one case of non-fatal pulmonary embolism occurred during ORTHO EVRA™ use, and one case of post-operative non-fatal pulmonary embolism was reported following ORTHO EVRA™ use. It is unknown if the risk of venous thromboembolism with ORTHO EVRA™ use is different than with use of combination oral contraceptives.

As with any combination hormonal contraceptives, the clinician should be alert to the earliest manifestations of thrombotic disorders (thrombophlebitis, pulmonary embolism, cerebrovascular disorders, and retinal thrombosis). Should any of these occur or be suspected, ORTHO EVRA™ should be discontinued immediately.

b. Myocardial Infarction

An increased risk of myocardial infarction has been attributed to hormonal contraceptive use. This risk is primarily in smokers or women with other underlying risk factors for coronary artery disease such as hypertension, hypercholesterolemia, morbid obesity, and diabetes. The relative risk of heart attack for current hormonal contraceptive users has been estimated to be two to six[4–10] compared to non-users. The risk is very low under the age of 30.

Smoking in combination with oral contraceptive use has been shown to contribute substantially to the incidence of myocardial infarctions in women in their mid-thirties or older with smoking accounting for the majority of excess cases[11]. Mortality rates associated with circulatory disease have been shown to increase substantially in smokers, especially in those 35 years of age and older among women who use oral contraceptives. (See Figure 5)

Figure 5: Circulatory Disease Mortality Rates Per 100,000 Women-Years by Age, Smoking Status and Oral Contraceptive Use

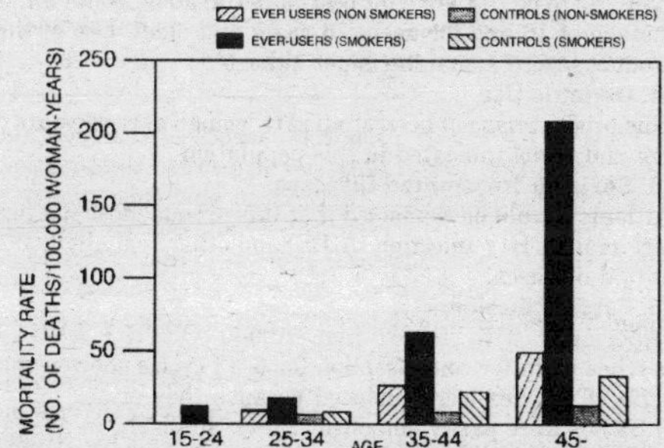

Hormonal contraceptives may compound the effects of well-known risk factors, such as hypertension, diabetes, hyperlipidemias, age and obesity[13]. In particular, some progestins are known to decrease HDL cholesterol and cause glucose intolerance, while estrogens may create a state of hyperinsulinism[14–18]. Hormonal contraceptives have been shown to increase blood pressure among some users (see Section 9 in WARNINGS). Similar effects on risk factors have been associated with an increased risk of heart disease. Hormonal contraceptives, including ORTHO EVRA™, must be used with caution in women with cardiovascular disease risk factors.

Norgestimate and norelgestromin have minimal androgenic activity (see CLINICAL PHARMACOLOGY). There is some evidence that the risk of myocardial infarction associated with hormonal contraceptives is lower when the progestin has minimal androgenic activity than when the activity is greater[97].

c. Cerebrovascular diseases

Hormonal contraceptives have been shown to increase both the relative and attributable risks of cerebrovascular events (thrombotic and hemorrhagic strokes), although, in general, the risk is greatest among older (>35 years), hypertensive women who also smoke. Hypertension was found to be a risk factor for both users and nonusers, for both types of strokes, and smoking interacted to increase the risk of stroke[27–29].

In a large study, the relative risk of thrombotic strokes has been shown to range from 3 for normotensive users to 14 for users with severe hypertension[30]. The relative risk of hemorrhagic stroke is reported to be 1.2 for non-smokers who used hormonal contraceptives, 2.6 for smokers who did not use hormonal contraceptives, 7.6 for smokers who used hormonal contraceptives, 1.8 for normotensive users and 25.7 for users with severe hypertension[30]. The attributable risk is also greater in older women[3].

d. Dose-related risk of vascular disease from hormonal contraceptives

A positive association has been observed between the amount of estrogen and progestin in hormonal contraceptives and the risk of vascular disease[31–33]. A decline in serum high-density lipoproteins (HDL) has been reported with many progestational agents[14–16]. A decline in serum high-density lipoproteins has been associated with an increased incidence of ischemic heart disease. Because estrogens increase HDL cholesterol, the net effect of a hormonal contraceptive depends on a balance achieved between doses of estrogen and progestin and the activity of the progestin used in the contraceptives. The activity and amount of both hormones should be considered in the choice of a hormonal contraceptive.

e. Persistence of risk of vascular disease

There are two studies that have shown persistence of risk of vascular disease for ever-users of combination hormonal contraceptives. In a study in the United States, the risk of developing myocardial infarction after discontinuing combination hormonal contraceptives persists for at least 9 years for women 40–49 years who had used combination hormonal contraceptives for five or more years, but this increased risk was not demonstrated in other age groups[8]. In another study in Great Britain, the risk of developing cerebrovascular disease persisted for at least 6 years after discontinuation of combination hormonal contraceptives, although excess risk was very small[34]. However, both studies were performed with combination hormonal contraceptive formulations containing 50 micrograms or higher of estrogens.

It is unknown whether ORTHO EVRA™ is distinct from other combination hormonal contraceptives with regard to the occurrence of venous and arterial thrombosis.

2. Estimates Of Mortality From Combination Hormonal Contraceptive Use

One study gathered data from a variety of sources that have estimated the mortality rate associated with different methods of contraception at different ages (Table 3). These estimates include the combined risk of death associated with contraceptive methods plus the risk attributable to pregnancy in the event of method failure. Each method of contraception has its specific benefits and risks. The study concluded that with the exception of combination oral contraceptive users 35 and older who smoke, and 40 and older who do not smoke, mortality associated with all methods of birth control is low and below that associated with childbirth.

Table 3. Annual Number of Birth-Related or Method-Related Deaths Associated With Control of Fertility Per 100,000 Non-Sterile Women, by Fertility Control Method According to Age

Method of control and outcome	15–19	20–24	25–29	30–34	35–39	40–44
No fertility control methods*	7.0	7.4	9.1	14.8	25.7	28.2
Oral contraceptives, non-smoker**	0.3	0.5	0.9	1.9	13.8	31.6
Oral contraceptives, smoker**	2.2	3.4	6.6	13.5	51.1	117.2
IUD**	0.8	0.8	1.0	1.0	1.4	1.4
Condom*	1.1	1.6	0.7	0.2	0.3	0.4
Diaphragm/spermicide*	1.9	1.2	1.2	1.3	2.2	2.8
Periodic abstinence*	2.5	1.6	1.6	1.7	2.9	3.6

*Deaths are birth-related
**Deaths are method-related
Adapted from H.W. Ory, ref. # 35.

The observation of a possible increase in risk of mortality with age for combination oral contraceptive users is based on data gathered in the 1970's but not reported until 1983[35]. Current clinical recommendation involves the use of lower estrogen dose formulations and a careful consideration of risk factors. In 1989, the Fertility and Maternal Health Drugs Advisory Committee was asked to review the use of combination hormonal contraceptives in women 40 years of age and over. The Committee concluded that although cardiovascular disease risks may be increased with combination hormonal contraceptive use after age 40 in healthy non-smoking women (even with the newer low-dose formulations), there are also greater potential health risks associated with pregnancy in older women and with the alternative surgical and medical procedures that may be necessary if such women do not have access to effective and acceptable means of contraception. The Committee recommended that the benefits of low-dose combination hormonal contraceptive use by healthy non-smoking women over 40 may outweigh the possible risks[36, 37].

Although the data are mainly obtained with oral contraceptives, this is likely to apply to ORTHO EVRA™ as well. Women of all ages who use combination hormonal contraceptives, should use the lowest possible dose formulation that is effective and meets the individual patient needs. [See table above]

3. Carcinoma Of The Reproductive Organs And Breasts

Numerous epidemiological studies give conflicting reports on the relationship between breast cancer and COC use. The risk of having breast cancer diagnosed may be slightly increased among current and recent users of combination oral contraceptives. However, this excess risk appears to decrease over time after COC discontinuation and by 10 years after cessation the increased risk disappears. Some studies report an increased risk with duration of use while other studies do not and no consistent relationships have been found with dose or type of steroid. Some studies have found a small increase in risk for women who first use COCs before age 20. Most studies show a similar pattern of risk with COC use regardless of a woman's reproductive history or her family breast cancer history.

In addition, breast cancers diagnosed in current or ever oral contraceptive users may be less clinically advanced than in never-users.

Women who currently have or have had breast cancer should not use hormonal contraceptives because breast cancer is usually a hormonally sensitive tumor.

Some studies suggest that combination oral contraceptive use has been associated with an increase in the risk of cervical intraepithelial neoplasia in some populations of women[45–48]. However, there continues to be controversy about the extent to which such findings may be due to differences in sexual behavior and other factors.

In spite of many studies of the relationship between oral contraceptive use and breast and cervical cancers, a cause-and-effect relationship has not been established. It is not known whether ORTHO EVRA™ is distinct from oral contraceptives with regard to the above statements.

4. Hepatic Neoplasia

Benign hepatic adenomas are associated with hormonal contraceptive use, although the incidence of benign tumors is rare in the United States. Indirect calculations have estimated the attributable risk to be in the range of 3.3 cases/100,000 for users, a risk that increases after four or more years of use, especially with hormonal contraceptives containing 50 micrograms or more of estrogen[49]. Rupture of benign, hepatic adenomas may cause death through intra-abdominal hemorrhage[50,51].

Studies from Britain and the US have shown an increased risk of developing hepatocellular carcinoma in long term (≥ 8 years)[52–54,96] oral contraceptive users. However, these cancers are extremely rare in the US and the attributable risk (the excess incidence) of liver cancers in oral contraceptive users approaches less than one per million users. It is unknown whether ORTHO EVRA™ is distinct from oral contraceptives in this regard.

5. Ocular Lesions

There have been clinical case reports of retinal thrombosis associated with the use of hormonal contraceptives. ORTHO EVRA™ should be discontinued if there is unexplained partial or complete loss of vision; onset of proptosis or diplopia; papilledema; or retinal vascular lesions. Appropriate diagnostic and therapeutic measures should be undertaken immediately.

6. Hormonal Contraceptive Use Before Or During Early Pregnancy

Extensive epidemiological studies have revealed no increased risk of birth defects in women who have used oral contraceptives prior to pregnancy[56,57]. Studies also do not indicate a teratogenic effect, particularly in so far as cardiac anomalies and limb reduction defects are concerned[55,56,58,59], when oral contraceptives are taken inadvertently during early pregnancy.

Combination hormonal contraceptives such as ORTHO EVRA™ should not be used to induce withdrawal bleeding as a test for pregnancy. ORTHO EVRA™ should not be used during pregnancy to treat threatened or habitual abortion.

It is recommended that for any patient who has missed two consecutive periods, pregnancy should be ruled out. If the patient has not adhered to the prescribed schedule for the use of ORTHO EVRA™ the possibility of pregnancy should be considered at the time of the first missed period. Hormonal contraceptive use should be discontinued if pregnancy is confirmed.

7. Gallbladder Disease

Earlier studies have reported an increased lifetime relative risk of gallbladder surgery in users of hormonal contraceptives and estrogens[60,61]. More recent studies, however, have shown that the relative risk of developing gallbladder disease among hormonal contraceptive users may be minimal[62–64]. The recent findings of minimal risk may be related to the use of hormonal contraceptive formulations containing lower hormonal doses of estrogens and progestins.

Combination hormonal contraceptives such as ORTHO EVRA™ may worsen existing gallbladder disease and may accelerate the development of this disease in previously asymptomatic women. Women with a history of combination hormonal contraceptive-related cholestasis are more likely to have the condition recur with subsequent combination hormonal contraceptive use.

8. Carbohydrate And Lipid Metabolic Effects

Hormonal contraceptives have been shown to cause a decrease in glucose tolerance in some users[17]. However, in the non-diabetic woman, combination hormonal contraceptives appear to have no effect on fasting blood glucose[67]. Prediabetic and diabetic women in particular should be carefully monitored while taking combination hormonal contraceptives such as ORTHO EVRA™.

In clinical trials with oral contraceptives containing ethinyl estradiol and norgestimate there were no clinically significant changes in fasting blood glucose levels. There were no clinically significant changes in glucose levels over 24 cycles of use. Moreover, glucose tolerance tests showed no clinically significant changes from baseline to cycles 3, 12 and 24. In a 6-cycle clinical trial with ORTHO EVRA™ there were no clinically significant changes in fasting blood glucose from baseline to end of treatment.

A small proportion of women will have persistent hypertriglyceridemia while taking hormonal contraceptives. As discussed earlier (see WARNINGS 1a and 1d), changes in serum triglycerides and lipoprotein levels have been reported in hormonal contraceptive users.

9. Elevated Blood Pressure

Women with significant hypertension should not be started on hormonal contraception[103]. Women with a history of hypertension or hypertension-related diseases, or renal disease[70] should be encouraged to use another method of contraception. If women elect to use ORTHO EVRA™, they should be monitored closely and if a clinically significant elevation of blood pressure occurs, ORTHO EVRA™ should be discontinued. For most women, elevated blood pressure will return to normal after stopping hormonal contraceptives, and there is no difference in the occurrence of hypertension between former and never users[68–71].

An increase in blood pressure has been reported in women taking hormonal contraceptives[68] and this increase is more likely in older hormonal contraceptive users[69] and with extended duration of use[61]. Data from the Royal College of

Continued on next page

Ortho Evra—Cont.

General Practitioners[12] and subsequent randomized trials have shown that the incidence of hypertension increases with increasing progestational activity.

10. Headache

The onset or exacerbation of migraine headache or the development of headache with a new pattern that is recurrent, persistent or severe requires discontinuation of ORTHO EVRA™ and evaluation of the cause.

11. Bleeding Irregularities

Breakthrough bleeding and spotting are sometimes encountered in women using ORTHO EVRA™. Non-hormonal causes should be considered and adequate diagnostic measures taken to rule out malignancy, other pathology, or pregnancy in the event of breakthrough bleeding, as in the case of any abnormal vaginal bleeding. If pathology has been excluded, time or a change to another contraceptive product may resolve the bleeding. In the event of amenorrhea, pregnancy should be ruled out before initiating use of ORTHO EVRA™.

Some women may encounter amenorrhea or oligomenorrhea after discontinuation of hormonal contraceptive use, especially when such a condition was pre-existent.

Bleeding Patterns:

In the clinical trials most women started their withdrawal bleeding on the fourth day of the drug-free interval, and the median duration of withdrawal bleeding was 5 to 6 days. On average 26% of women per cycle had 7 or more total days of bleeding and/or spotting (this includes both withdrawal flow and breakthrough bleeding and/or spotting).

12. Ectopic Pregnancy

Ectopic as well as intrauterine pregnancy may occur in contraceptive failures.

PRECAUTIONS

Women should be counseled that ORTHO EVRA™ does not protect against HIV infection (AIDS) and other sexually transmitted infections.

1. Body Weight ≥198 lbs. (90 kg)

Results of clinical trials suggest that ORTHO EVRA™ may be less effective in women with body weight ≥198 lbs. (90 kg) than in women with lower body weights.

2. Physical Examination And Follow-Up

It is good medical practice for women using ORTHO EVRA™, as for all women, to have annual medical evaluation and physical examinations. The physical examination, however, may be deferred until after initiation of hormonal contraceptives if requested by the woman and judged appropriate by the clinician. The physical examination should include special reference to blood pressure, breasts, abdomen and pelvic organs, including cervical cytology, and relevant laboratory tests. In case of undiagnosed, persistent or recurrent abnormal vaginal bleeding, appropriate measures should be conducted to rule out malignancy or other pathology. Women with a strong family history of breast cancer or who have breast nodules should be monitored with particular care.

3. Lipid Disorders

Women who are being treated for hyperlipidemias should be followed closely if they elect to use ORTHO EVRA™. Some progestins may elevate LDL levels and may render the control of hyperlipidemias more difficult.

4. Liver Function

If jaundice develops in any woman using ORTHO EVRA™, the medication should be discontinued. The hormones in ORTHO EVRA™ may be poorly metabolized in patients with impaired liver function.

5. Fluid Retention

Steroid hormones like those in ORTHO EVRA™ may cause some degree of fluid retention. ORTHO EVRA™ should be prescribed with caution, and only with careful monitoring, in patients with conditions which might be aggravated by fluid retention.

6. Emotional Disorders

Women who become significantly depressed while using combination hormonal contraceptives such as ORTHO EVRA™ should stop the medication and use another method of contraception in an attempt to determine whether the symptom is drug related. Women with a history of depression should be carefully observed and ORTHO EVRA™ discontinued if significant depression occurs.

7. Contact Lenses

Contact lens wearers who develop visual changes or changes in lens tolerance should be assessed by an ophthalmologist.

8. Drug Interactions

Changes in Contraceptive Effectiveness Associated with Co-Administration of Other Drugs:

Contraceptive effectiveness may be reduced when hormonal contraceptives are co-administered with some antibiotics, antifungals, anticonvulsants, and other drugs that increase metabolism of contraceptive steroids. This could result in unintended pregnancy or breakthrough bleeding. Examples include barbiturates, griseofulvin, rifampin, phenylbutazone, phenytoin, carbamazepine, felbamate, oxcarbazepine, topiramate and possibly with ampicillin.

The proposed mechanism of interaction of antibiotics is different from that of liver enzyme-inducing drugs. Literature suggests possible interactions with the concomitant use of hormonal contraceptives and ampicillin or tetracycline. In a pharmacokinetic drug interaction study, oral administration of tetracycline HCl, 500 mg q.i.d. for 3 days prior to and 7 days during wear of ORTHO EVRA™ did not significantly affect the pharmacokinetics of norelgestromin or EE.

Several of the anti-HIV protease inhibitors have been studied with co-administration of oral combination hormonal contraceptives; significant changes (increase and decrease) in the mean AUC of the estrogen and progestin have been noted in some cases. The efficacy and safety of oral contraceptive products may be affected; it is unknown whether this applies to ORTHO EVRA™. Healthcare professionals should refer to the label of the individual anti-HIV protease inhibitors for further drug-drug interaction information.

Herbal products containing St. John's Wort (hypericum perforatum) may induce hepatic enzymes (cytochrome P450) and p-glycoprotein transporter and may reduce the effectiveness of contraceptive steroids. This may also result in breakthrough bleeding.

Increase in Plasma Hormone Levels Associated with Co-Administered Drugs:

Co-administration of atorvastatin and certain oral contraceptives containing ethinyl estradiol increase AUC values for ethinyl estradiol by approximately 20%. Ascorbic acid and acetaminophen may increase plasma ethinyl estradiol levels, possibly by inhibition of conjugation. CYP 3A4 inhibitors such as itraconazole or ketoconazole may increase plasma hormone levels.

Changes in Plasma Levels of Co-Administered Drugs:

Combination hormonal contraceptives containing some synthetic estrogens (e.g., ethinyl estradiol) may inhibit the metabolism of other compounds. Increased plasma concentrations of cyclosporine, prednisolone, and theophylline have been reported with concomitant administration of oral contraceptives. In addition, oral contraceptives may induce the conjugation of other compounds. Decreased plasma concentrations of acetaminophen and increased clearance of temazepam, salicylic acid, morphine and clofibric acid have been noted when these drugs were administered with oral contraceptives.

Although norelgestromin and its metabolites inhibit a variety of P450 enzymes in human liver microsomes, the clinical consequence of such an interaction on the levels of other concomitant medications is likely to be insignificant. Under the recommended dosing regimen, the in vivo concentrations of norelgestromin and its metabolites, even at the peak serum levels, are relatively low compared to the inhibitory constant (Ki) (based on results of *in vitro* studies).

Health care professionals are advised to also refer to prescribing information of co-administered drugs for recommendations regarding management of concomitant therapy.

9. Interactions With Laboratory Tests

Certain endocrine and liver function tests and blood components may be affected by hormonal contraceptives:

a. Increased prothrombin and factors VII, VIII, IX, and X; decreased antithrombin 3; increased norepinephrine-induced platelet aggregability.

b. Increased thyroid binding globulin (TBG) leading to increased circulating total thyroid hormone, as measured by protein-bound iodine (PBI), T4 by column or by radioimmunoassay. Free T3 resin uptake is decreased, reflecting the elevated TBG, free T4 concentration is unaltered.

c. Other binding proteins may be elevated in serum.

d. Sex hormone binding globulins are increased and result in elevated levels of total circulating endogenous sex steroids and corticoids; however, free or biologically active levels either decrease or remain unchanged.

e. Triglycerides may be increased and levels of various other lipids and lipoproteins may be affected.

f. Glucose tolerance may be decreased.

g. Serum folate levels may be depressed by hormonal contraceptive therapy. This may be of clinical significance if a woman becomes pregnant shortly after discontinuing ORTHO EVRA™.

10. Carcinogenesis

No carcinogenicity studies were conducted with norelgestromin. However, bridging PK studies were conducted using doses of NGM/EE which were used previously in the 2-year rat carcinogenicity study and 10-year monkey toxicity study to support the approval of ORTHO-CYCLEN and ORTHO TRI-CYCLEN under NDAs 19-653 and 19-697, respectively. The PK studies demonstrated that rats and monkeys were exposed to 16 and 8 times the human exposure, respectively, with the proposed ORTHO EVRA™ transdermal contraceptive system.

Norelgestromin was tested in in-vitro mutagenicity assays (bacterial plate incorporation mutation assay, CHO/HGPRT mutation assay, chromosomal aberration assay using cultured human peripheral lymphocytes) and in one in-vivo test (rat micronucleus assay) and found to have no genotoxic potential.

See WARNINGS Section.

11. Pregnancy

Pregnancy Category X. See CONTRAINDICATIONS and WARNINGS Sections.

Norelgestromin was tested for its reproductive toxicity in a rabbit developmental toxicity study by the SC route of administration. Doses of 0, 1, 2, 4 and 6 mg/kg body weight, which gave systemic exposure of approximately 25 to 125 times the human exposure with ORTHO EVRA™, were administered daily on gestation days 7–19. Malformations reported were paw hyperflexion at 4 and 6 mg/kg and paw hyperextension and cleft palate at 6 mg/kg.

12. Nursing Mothers

The effects of ORTHO EVRA™ in nursing mothers have not been evaluated and are unknown. Small amounts of combination hormonal contraceptive steroids have been identified in the milk of nursing mothers and a few adverse effects on the child have been reported, including jaundice and breast enlargement. In addition, combination hormonal contraceptives given in the postpartum period may interfere with lactation by decreasing the quantity and quality of breast milk. Long-term follow-up of infants whose mothers used combination hormonal contraceptives while breast feeding has shown no deleterious effects. However, the nursing mother should be advised not to use ORTHO EVRA™ but to use other forms of contraception until she has completely weaned her child.

13. Pediatric Use

Safety and efficacy of ORTHO EVRA™ have been established in women of reproductive age. Safety and efficacy are expected to be the same for post-pubertal adolescents under the age of 16 and for users 16 years and older. Use of this product before menarche is not indicated.

14. Geriatric Use

This product has not been studied in women over 65 years of age and is not indicated in this population.

15. Sexually Transmitted Diseases

Patients should be counseled that this product does not protect against HIV infection (AIDS) and other sexually transmitted diseases.

16. Patch Adhesion

Experience with more than 70,000 ORTHO EVRA™ patches worn for contraception for 6–13 cycles showed that 4.7% of patches were replaced because they either fell off (1.8%) or were partly detached (2.9%). Similarly, in a small study of patch wear under conditions of physical exertion and variable temperature and humidity, less than 2% of patches were replaced for complete or partial detachment.

If the ORTHO EVRA™ patch becomes partially or completely detached and remains detached, insufficient drug delivery occurs. A patch should not be re-applied if it is no longer sticky, if it has become stuck to itself or another surface, if it has other material stuck to it, or if it has become loose or fallen off before. If a patch cannot be re-applied, a new patch should be applied immediately. Supplemental adhesives or wraps should not be used to hold the ORTHO EVRA™ patch in place.

If a patch is partially or completely detached for more than one day (24 hours or more) OR if the woman is not sure how long the patch has been detached, she may not be protected from pregnancy. She should stop the current contraceptive cycle and start a new cycle immediately by applying a new patch. Back-up contraception, such as condoms, spermicide, or diaphragm, must be used for the first week of the new cycle.

INFORMATION FOR THE PATIENT

See Patient Labeling printed below.

ADVERSE REACTIONS

The most common adverse events reported by 9 to 22% of women using ORTHO EVRA™ in clinical trials (N=3,330) were the following, in order of decreasing incidence: breast symptoms, headache, application site reaction, nausea, upper respiratory infection, menstrual cramps, and abdominal pain.

The most frequent adverse events leading to discontinuation in 1 to 2.4% of women using ORTHO EVRA™ in the trials included the following: nausea and/or vomiting, application site reaction, breast symptoms, headache, and emotional lability.

Listed below are adverse events that have been associated with the use of combination hormonal contraceptives. These are also likely to apply to combination transdermal hormonal contraceptives such as ORTHO EVRA™.

An increased risk of the following serious adverse reactions has been associated with the use of combination hormonal contraceptives (see WARNINGS Section).

- Thrombophlebitis and venous thrombosis with or without embolism
- Arterial thromboembolism
- Pulmonary embolism
- Myocardial infarction
- Cerebral hemorrhage
- Cerebral thrombosis
- Hypertension
- Gallbladder disease
- Hepatic adenomas or benign liver tumors

There is evidence of an association between the following conditions and the use of combination hormonal contraceptives:

- Mesenteric thrombosis
- Retinal thrombosis

The following adverse reactions have been reported in users of combination hormonal contraceptives and are believed to be drug-related:

- Nausea
- Vomiting
- Gastrointestinal symptoms (such as abdominal cramps and bloating)
- Breakthrough bleeding
- Spotting
- Change in menstrual flow
- Amenorrhea
- Temporary infertility after discontinuation of treatment
- Edema
- Melasma which may persist
- Breast changes: tenderness, enlargement, secretion
- Change in weight (increase or decrease)
- Change in cervical erosion and secretion
- Diminution in lactation when given immediately postpartum

- Cholestatic jaundice
- Migraine
- Rash (allergic)
- Mental depression
- Reduced tolerance to carbohydrates
- Vaginal candidiasis
- Change in corneal curvature (steepening)
- Intolerance to contact lenses

The following adverse reactions have been reported in users of combination hormonal contraceptives and a cause and effect association has been neither confirmed nor refuted:

- Pre-menstrual syndrome
- Cataracts
- Changes in appetite
- Cystitis-like syndrome
- Headache
- Nervousness
- Dizziness
- Hirsutism
- Loss of scalp hair
- Erythema multiforme
- Erythema nodosum
- Hemorrhagic eruption
- Vaginitis
- Porphyria
- Impaired renal function
- Hemolytic uremic syndrome
- Acne
- Changes in libido
- Colitis
- Budd-Chiari Syndrome

OVERDOSAGE

Serious ill effects have not been reported following accidental ingestion of large doses of hormonal contraceptives. Overdosage may cause nausea and vomiting, and withdrawal bleeding may occur in females. Given the nature and design of the ORTHO EVRA™ patch, it is unlikely that overdosage will occur. Serious ill effects have not been reported following acute ingestion of large doses of oral contraceptives by young children. In case of suspected overdose, all ORTHO EVRA™ patches should be removed and symptomatic treatment given.

DOSAGE AND ADMINISTRATION

To achieve maximum contraceptive effectiveness, ORTHO EVRA™ must be used exactly as directed.

Complete instructions to facilitate patient counseling on proper system usage may be found in the Detailed Patient Labeling.

Transdermal Contraceptive System Overview

This system uses a 28-day (four-week) cycle. A new patch is applied each week for three weeks (21 total days). Week Four is patch-free. Withdrawal bleeding is expected during this time.

Every new patch should be applied on the same day of the week. This day is known as the "Patch Change Day." For example, if the first patch is applied on a Monday, all subsequent patches should be applied on a Monday. Only one patch should be worn at a time.

On the day after Week Four ends a new four-week cycle is started by applying a new patch. Under no circumstances should there be more than a seven-day patch-free interval between dosing cycles.

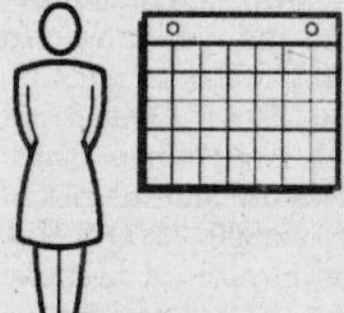

If the woman is starting ORTHO EVRA™ for the **first time**, she should **wait until the day she begins her menstrual period**. Either a First Day start or Sunday start may be chosen (see below). The day she applies her first patch will be Day 1. Her "Patch Change Day" will be on this day every week.

CHOOSE ONE OPTION:

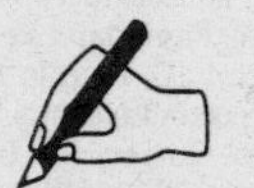

☐ First Day Start

or

☐ Sunday Start

- for **First Day Start**: the patient should apply her first patch during the first 24 hours of her menstrual period.

If therapy starts after Day 1 of the menstrual cycle, a non-hormonal back-up contraceptive (such as a condoms, spermicide, or diaphragm) should be used concurrently for the first 7 consecutive days of the first treatment cycle.

OR

- for **Sunday Start**: the woman should apply her first patch on the first Sunday after her menstrual period starts. She must use back-up contraception for the first week of her first cycle.

If the menstrual period begins on a Sunday, the first patch should be applied on that day, and no back-up contraception is needed.

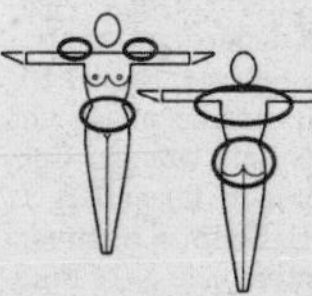

Where to apply the patch. The patch should be applied to clean, dry, intact healthy skin on the buttock, abdomen, upper outer arm or upper torso, in a place where it won't be rubbed by tight clothing. ORTHO EVRA™ should not be placed on skin that is red, irritated or cut, nor should it be placed on the breasts.

To prevent interference with the adhesive properties of ORTHO EVRA™, no make-up, creams, lotions, powders or other topical products should be applied to the skin area where the ORTHO EVRA™ patch is or will be placed.

Application of the ORTHO EVRA™ patch

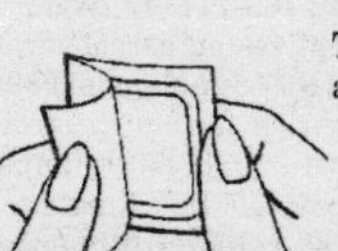

The foil pouch is opened by tearing it along the edge using the fingers.

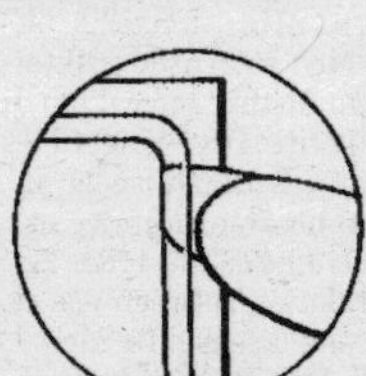

The foil pouch should be peeled apart and open flat.

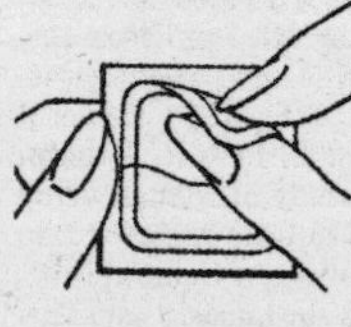

A corner of the patch is grasped firmly and it is gently removed from the foil pouch.

The woman should be instructed to use her fingernail, to lift one corner of the patch and peel the patch <u>and</u> the plastic liner off the foil liner. **Sometimes patches can stick to the inside of the pouch – the woman should be careful not to accidentally remove the clear liner as she removes the patch.**

Half of the clear protective liner is to be peeled away. (The woman should avoid touching the sticky surface of the patch).

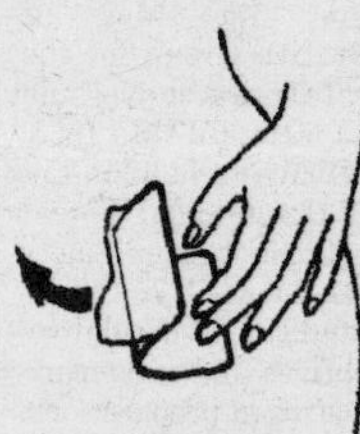

The sticky surface of the patch is applied to the skin and the other half of the liner is removed. The woman should press down firmly on the patch with the palm of her hand for 10 seconds, making sure that the edges stick well. She should check her patch every day to make sure it is sticking.

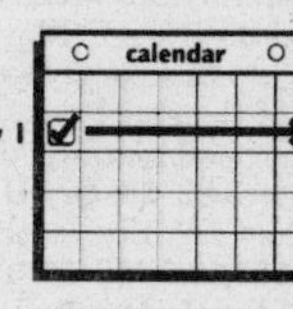

The patch is worn for seven days (one week). On the "Patch Change Day", Day 8, the used patch is removed and a new one is applied immediately. The used patch still contains some active hormones – it should be carefully folded in half so that it sticks to itself before throwing it away.

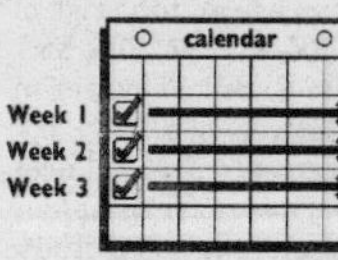

A new patch is applied for Week Two (on Day 8) and again for Week Three (on Day 15), on the usual "Patch Change Day". Patch changes may occur at any time on the Change Day. Each new ORTHO EVRA™ patch should be applied to a new spot on the skin to help avoid irritation, although they may be kept within the same anatomic area.

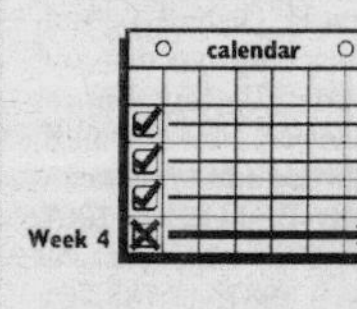

Week Four is patch-free (Day 22 through Day 28), thus completing the four-week contraceptive cycle. Bleeding is expected to begin during this time.

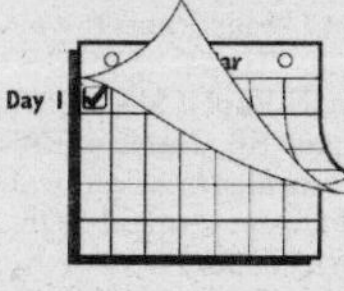

The next four-week cycle is started by applying a new patch on the usual "Patch Change Day," the day after Day 28, no matter when the menstrual period begins or ends. Under no circumstances should there be more than a seven-day patch-free interval between patch cycles.

If the ORTHO EVRA™ patch becomes partially or completely detached and remains detached, insufficient drug delivery occurs.

If a patch is partially or completely detached:

- **for less than one day** (up to 24 hours), the woman should try to reapply it to the same place or replace it with a new patch immediately. No back-up contraception is needed. The woman's "Patch Change Day" will remain the same.
- **for more than one day** (24 hours or more) **OR if the woman is not sure how long the patch has been detached**, SHE MAY NOT BE PROTECTED FROM PREGNANCY. She should stop the current contraceptive cycle and start a new cycle immediately by applying a new patch. There is now a new "Day 1" and a new "Patch Change Day." Back-up contraception, such as condoms, spermicide, or diaphragm, must be used for the first week of the new cycle.

A patch should not be re-applied if it is no longer sticky, if it has become stuck to itself or another surface, if it has other material stuck to it or if it has previously become loose or fallen off. If a patch cannot be re-applied, a new patch should be applied immediately. Supplemental adhesives or wraps should not be used to hold the ORTHO EVRA™ patch in place.

If the woman forgets to change her patch...

- **at the start of any patch cycle** (Week One /Day 1): SHE MAY NOT BE PROTECTED FROM PREGNANCY. She should apply the first patch of her new cycle as soon as she remembers. There is now a new "Patch Change Day" and a new "Day 1." The woman must use back-up contraception, such as condoms, spermicide, or diaphragm, for the first week of the new cycle.
- **in the middle of the patch cycle (Week Two/Day 8 or Week Three/Day 15),**
  - — for **one or two days** (up to 48 hours), she should apply a new patch immediately. The next patch should be applied on the usual "Patch Change Day." No back-up contraception is needed. (See Figures 3 and 4 in the Clinical Pharmacology section.)
  - — for **more than two days** (48 hours or more), SHE MAY NOT BE PROTECTED FROM PREGNANCY. She should stop the current contraceptive cycle and start a new four-week cycle immediately by putting on a new patch. There is now a new "Patch Change Day" and a new "Day 1." The woman must use back-up contraception for one week.
- **at the end of the patch cycle (Week Four/Day 22),**

Week Four (Day 22): If the woman forgets to remove her patch, she should take it off as soon as she remembers. The next cycle should be started on the usual "Patch Change Day," which is the day after Day 28. No back-up contraception is needed.

Under no circumstances should there be more than a seven-day patch-free interval between cycles. If there are more than seven patch-free days, THE WOMAN MAY NOT BE PROTECTED FROM PREGNANCY and back-up contraception, such as condoms, spermicide, or diaphragm, must be used for seven days. As with combined oral contraceptives, the risk of ovulation increases with each day beyond the recommended drug-free period. If coital exposure has occurred during such an extended patch-free interval, the possibility of fertilization should be considered.

Change Day Adjustment

If the woman wishes to change her Patch Change Day she should complete her current cycle, removing the third ORTHO EVRA™ patch on the correct day. During the patch-free week, she may select an earlier Patch Day Change by applying a new ORTHO EVRA™ patch on the desired day. In no case should there be more than 7 consecutive patch-free days.

Switching from an Oral Contraceptive

Treatment with ORTHO EVRA™ should begin on the first day of withdrawal bleeding. If there is no withdrawal bleeding within 5 days of the last active (hormone-containing) tablet, pregnancy must be ruled out. If therapy starts later than the first day of withdrawal bleeding, a non-hormonal contraceptive should be used concurrently for 7 days. If more than 7 days elapse after taking the last active oral contraceptive tablet, the possibility of ovulation and conception should be considered.

Use after Childbirth

Women who elect not to breast-feed should start contraceptive therapy with ORTHO EVRA™ no sooner than 4 weeks after childbirth. If a woman begins using ORTHO EVRA™ postpartum, and has not yet had a period, the possibility of ovulation and conception occurring prior to use of ORTHO EVRA™ should be considered, and she should be instructed to use an additional method of contraception, such as condoms, spermicide, or diaphragm, for the first seven days. (See *Precautions: Nursing Mothers, and Warnings: Thromboembolic and Other Vascular Problems.*)

Use after Abortion or Miscarriage[106]

After an abortion or miscarriage that occurs in the first trimester, ORTHO EVRA™ may be started immediately. An additional method of contraception is not needed if ORTHO EVRA™ is started immediately. If use of ORTHO EVRA™ is not started within 5 days following a first trimester abortion, the woman should follow the instructions for a woman starting ORTHO EVRA™ for the first time. In the meantime she should be advised to use a non-hormonal contraceptive method. Ovulation may occur within 10 days of an abortion or miscarriage.

ORTHO EVRA™ should be started no earlier than 4 weeks after a second trimester abortion or miscarriage. When ORTHO EVRA™ is used postpartum or postabortion, the increased risk of thromboembolic disease must be considered. (See CONTRAINDICATIONS and WARNINGS concerning thromboembolic disease. See PRECAUTIONS for "Nursing Mothers".)

Continued on next page

Ortho Evra—Cont.

Breakthrough Bleeding or Spotting

In the event of breakthrough bleeding or spotting (bleeding that occurs on the days that ORTHO EVRA™ is worn), treatment should be continued. If breakthrough bleeding persists longer than a few cycles, a cause other than ORTHO EVRA™ should be considered.

In the event of no withdrawal bleeding (bleeding that should occur during the patch-free week), treatment should be resumed on the next scheduled Change Day. If ORTHO EVRA™ has been used correctly, the absence of withdrawal bleeding is not necessarily an indication of pregnancy. Nevertheless, the possibility of pregnancy should be considered, especially if absence of withdrawal bleeding occurs in 2 consecutive cycles. ORTHO EVRA™ should be discontinued if pregnancy is confirmed.

In Case of Vomiting or Diarrhea

Given the nature of transdermal application, dose delivery should be unaffected by vomiting.

In Case of Skin Irritation

If patch use results in uncomfortable irritation, the patch may be removed and a new patch may be applied to a different location until the next Change Day. Only one patch should be worn at a time.

ADDITIONAL INSTRUCTIONS FOR DOSING

Breakthrough bleeding, spotting, and amenorrhea are frequent reasons for patients discontinuing hormonal contraceptives. In case of breakthrough bleeding, as in all cases of irregular bleeding from the vagina, non-functional causes should considered. In case of undiagnosed persistent or recurrent abnormal bleeding from the vagina, adequate diagnostic measures are indicated to rule out pregnancy or malignancy. If pathology has been excluded, time or a change to another method of contraception may solve the problem.

Use of hormonal contraceptives in the event of a missed menstrual period:

1. If the woman has not adhered to the prescribed schedule, the possibility of pregnancy should be considered at the time of the first missed period. Hormonal contraceptive use should be discontinued if pregnancy is confirmed.
2. If the woman has adhered to the prescribed regimen and misses one period, she should continue using her contraceptive patches.
3. If the woman has adhered to the prescribed regimen and misses two consecutive periods, pregnancy should be ruled out. ORTHO EVRA™ use should be discontinued if pregnancy is confirmed.

HOW SUPPLIED

Each beige ORTHO EVRA™ patch contains 6.0 mg norelgestromin and 0.75 mg EE, and releases 150 micrograms of norelgestromin and 20 micrograms of EE to the bloodstream per 24 hours. Each patch surface is heat stamped with ORTHO EVRA™ 150/20. Each patch is packaged in a protective pouch.

ORTHO EVRA™ is available in folding cartons of 1 cycle each (NDC # 0062-1920-15); each cycle contains 3 patches. ORTHO EVRA™ is also available in folding cartons containing a single patch (NDC # 0062-1920-01), intended for use as a replacement in the event that a patch is inadvertently lost or destroyed.

Special Precautions for Storage and Disposal

Store at 25°C (77°F); excursions permitted to 15–30°C (59–86°F).

Store patches in their protective pouches. Apply immediately upon removal from the protective pouch.

Do not store in the refrigerator or freezer.

Used patches still contain some active hormones. Each patch should be carefully folded in half so that it sticks to itself before throwing it away.

REFERENCES

1. Trussel J. Contraceptive efficacy. In Hatcher RA, Trussel J, Stewart F, Cates W, Stewart GK, Kowal D, Guest F. *Contraceptive Technology: Seventeenth Revised Edition.* New York NY: Irvington Publishers, 1998. **2.** Stadel BV. Oral contraceptives and cardiovascular disease. (Pt.1). N Engl J Med 1981; 305:612-618. **3.** Stadel BV. Oral contraceptives and cardiovascular disease. (Pt.2). N Engl J Med 1981; 305:672-677. **4.** Adam SA, Thorogood M. Oral contraception and myocardial infarction revisited: the effects of new preparations and prescribing patterns. Br J Obstet Gynaecol 1981; 88:838-845. **5.** Mann JI, Inman WH. Oral contraceptives and death from myocardial infarction. Br Med J 1975; 2(5965):245-248. **6.** Mann JI, Vessey MP, Thorogood M, Doll R. Myocardial infarction in young women with special reference to oral contraceptive practice. Br Med J 1975; 2(5956):241-245. **7.** Royal College of General Practitioners' Oral Contraception Study: Further analyses of mortality in oral contraceptive users. Lancet 1981; 1:541-546. **8.** Slone D, Shapiro S, Kaufman DW, Rosenberg L, Miettinen OS, Stolley PD. Risk of myocardial infarction in relation to current and discontinued use of oral contraceptives. N Engl J Med 1981:305:420-424. **9.** Vessey MP. Female hormones and vascular disease-an epidemiological overview. Br J Fam Plann 1980; 6 (Supplement): 1-12. **10.** Russell-Briefel RG, Ezzati TM, Fulwood R, Perlman JA, Murphy RS. Cardiovascular risk status and oral contraceptive use, United States, 1976-80. Prevent Med 1986; 15:352-362. **11.** Goldbaum GM, Kendrick JS, Hogelin GC, Gentry EM. The relative impact of smoking and oral contraceptive use on women in the United States. JAMA 1987; 258:1339-1342. **12.** Layde PM, Beral V. Further analyses of mortality in oral contraceptive users; Royal College of General Practitioners' Oral Contraception Study. (Table 5) Lancet 1981; 1:541-546. **13.** Knopp RH. Arteriosclerosis risk: the roles of oral contraceptives and postmenopausal estrogens. J Reprod Med 1986; 31(9) (Supplement):913-921. **14.** Krauss RM, Roy S, Mishell DR, Casagrande J, Pike MC. Effects of two low-dose oral contraceptives on serum lipids and lipoproteins: Differential changes in high-density lipoproteins subclasses. Am J Obstet 1983; 145:446-452. **15.** Wahl P, Walden C, Knopp R, Hoover J, Wallace R, Heiss G, Rifkind B. Effect of estrogen/progestin potency on lipid/lipoprotein cholesterol. N Engl J Med 1983; 308:862-867. **16.** Wynn V, Niththyananthan R. The effect of progestin in combined oral contraceptives on serum lipids with special reference to high density lipoproteins. Am J Obstet Gynecol 1982;142:766-771. **17.** Wynn V, Godsland I. Effects of oral contraceptives on carbohydrate metabolism. J Reprod Med 1986;31(9)(Supplement):892-897. **18.** LaRosa JC. Atherosclerotic risk factors in cardiovascular disease. J Reprod Med 1986;31(9)(Supplement):906-912. **19.** Inman WH, Vessey MP. Investigation of death from pulmonary, coronary, and cerebral thrombosis and embolism in women of child-bearing age. Br Med J 1968;2(5599):193-199. **20.** Maguire MG, Tonascia J, Sartwell PE, Stolley PD, Tockman MS. Increased risk of thrombosis due to oral contraceptives:a further report. Am J Epidemiol 1979; 110(2):188-195. **21.** Petitti DB, Wingerd J, Pellegrin F, Ramacharan S. Risk of vascular disease in women: smoking, oral contraceptives, noncontraceptive estrogens, and other factors. JAMA 1979;242:1150-1154. **22.** Vessey MP, Doll R. Investigation of relation between use of oral contraceptives and thromboembolic disease. Br Med J 1968;2(5599):199-205. **23.** Vessey MP, Doll R. Investigation of relation between use of oral contraceptives and thromboembolic disease. A further report. Br Med J 1969; 2(5658):651-657. **24.** Porter JB, Hunter JR, Danielson DA, Jick H, Stergachis A. Oral contraceptives and non-fatal vascular disease-recent experience. Obstet Gynecol 1982;59(3):299-302. **25.** Vessey M, Doll R, Peto R, Johnson B, Wiggins P. A long-term follow-up study of women using different methods of contraception: an interim report. J Biosocial Sci 1976;8:375-427. **26.** Royal College of General Practitioners: Oral Contraceptives, venous thrombosis, and varicose veins. J Royal Coll Gen Pract 1978; 28:393-399. **27.** Collaborative Group for the Study of Stroke in Young Women: Oral contraception and increased risk of cerebral ischemia or thrombosis. N Engl J Med 1973;288:871-878. **28.** Petitti DB, Wingerd J. Use of oral contraceptives, cigarette smoking, and risk of subarachnoid hemorrhage. Lancet 1978;2:234-236. **29.** Inman WH. Oral contraceptives and fatal subarachnoid hemorrhage. Br Med J 1979:2(6203):1468-1470. **30.** Collaborative Group for the Study of Stroke in Young Women: Oral Contraceptives and stroke in young women: associated risk factors. JAMA 1975; 231:718-722. **31.** Inman WH, Vessey MP, Westerholm B, Engelund A. Thromboembolic disease and the steroidal content of oral contraceptives. A report to the Committee on Safety of Drugs. Br Med J 1970;2:203-209. **32.** Meade TW, Greenberg G, Thompson SG. Progestogens and cardiovascular reactions associated with oral contraceptives and a comparison of the safety of 50- and 35-mcg oestrogen preparations. Br Med J 1980;280(6224):1157-1161. **33.** Kay CR. Progestogens and arterial disease-evidence from the Royal College of General Practitioners' Study. Am J Obstet Gynecol 1982;142:762-765. **34.** Royal College of General Practitioners: Incidence of arterial disease among oral contraceptive users. J Royal Coll Gen Pract 1983;33:75-82. **35.** Ory HW. Mortality associated with fertility and fertility control: 1983. Family Planning Perspectives 1983;15:50-56. **36.** The Cancer and Steroid Hormone Study of the Centers for Disease Control and the National Institute of Child Health and Human Development: Oral contraceptive use and the risk of breast cancer. N Engl J Med 1986;315:405-411. **37.** Pike MC, Henderson BE, Krailo MD, Duke A, Roy S. Breast cancer in young women and use of oral contraceptives: possible modifying effect of formulation and age at use. Lancet 1983;2:926-929. **38.** Paul C, Skegg DG, Spears GFS, Kaldor JM. Oral contraceptives and breast cancer: A national study. Br Med J 1986; 293:723-725. **39.** Miller DR, Rosenberg L, Kaufman DW, Schottenfeld D, Stolley PD, Shapiro S. Breast cancer risk in relation to early oral contraceptive use. Obstet Gynecol 1986;68:863-868. **40.** Olson H, Olson KL, Moller TR, Ranstam J, Holm P. Oral contraceptive use and breast cancer in young women in Sweden (letter). Lancet 1985; 2:748-749. **41.** McPherson K, Vessey M, Neil A, Doll R, Jones L, Roberts M. Early contraceptive use and breast cancer: Results of another case-control study. Br J Cancer 1987; 56:653-660. **42.** Huggins GR, Zucker PF. Oral contraceptives and neoplasia; 1987 update. Fertil Steril 1987; 47:733-761. **43.** McPherson K, Drife JO. The pill and breast cancer: why the uncertainty? Br Med J 1986; 293:709-710. **44.** Shapiro S. Oral contraceptives-time to take stock. N Engl J Med 1987; 315:450-451. **45.** Ory H, Naib Z, Conger SB, Hatcher RA, Tyler CW. Contraceptive choice and prevalence of cervical dysplasia and carcinoma in situ. Am J Obstet Gynecol 1976; 124:573-577. **46.** Vessey MP, Lawless M, McPherson K, Yeates D. Neoplasia of the cervix uteri and contraception: a possible adverse effect of the pill. Lancet 1983; 2:930. **47.** Brinton LA, Huggins GR, Lehman HF, Malli K, Savitz DA, Trapido E, Rosenthal J, Hoover R. Long term use of oral contraceptives and risk of invasive cervical cancer. Int J Cancer 1986; 38:339-344. **48.** WHO Collaborative Study of Neoplasia and Steroid Contraceptives: Invasive cervical cancer and combined oral contraceptives. Br Med J 1985; 290:961-965. **49.** Rooks JB, Ory HW, Ishak KG, Strauss LT, Greenspan JR, Hill AP, Tyler CW. Epidemiology of hepatocellular adenoma: the role of oral contraceptive use. JAMA 1979; 242:644-648. **50.** Bein NN, Goldsmith HS. Recurrent massive hemorrhage from benign hepatic tumors secondary to oral contraceptives. Br J Surg 1977; 64:433-435. **51.** Klatskin G. Hepatic tumors: possible relationship to use of oral contraceptives. Gastroenterology 1977; 73:386-394. **52.** Henderson BE, Preston-Martin S, Edmondson HA, Peters RL, Pike MC. Hepatocellular carcinoma and oral contraceptives. Br J Cancer 1983;48:437-440. **53.** Neuberger J, Forman D, Doll R, Williams R. Oral contraceptives and hepatocellular carcinoma. Br Med J 1986; 292:1355-1357. **54.** Forman D, Vincent TJ, Doll R. Cancer of the liver and oral contraceptives. Br Med J 1986; 292:1357-1361. **55.** Harlap S, Eldor J. Births following oral contraceptive failures. Obstet Gynecol 1980; 55:447-452. **56.** Savolainen E, Saksela E, Saxen L. Teratogenic hazards of oral contraceptives analyzed in a national malformation register. Am J Obstet Gynecol 1981: 140:521-524. **57.** Janerich DT, Piper JM, Glebatis DM. Oral contraceptives and birth defects. Am J Epidemiol 1980; 112:73-79. **58.** Ferencz C, Matanoski GM, Wilson PD, Rubin JD, Neill CA, Gutberlet R. Maternal hormone therapy and congenital heart disease. Teratology 1980; 21:225-239. **59.** Rothman KJ, Fyler DC, Goldblatt A, Kreidberg MB. Exogenous hormones and other drug exposures of children with congenital heart disease. Am J Epidemiol 1979; 109:433-439. **60.** Boston Collaborative Drug Surveillance Program: Oral contraceptives and venous thromboembolic disease, surgically confirmed gallbladder disease, and breast tumors. Lancet 1973; 1:1399-1404. **61.** Royal College of General Practitioners: Oral contraceptives and health. New York, Pittman 1974. **62.** Layde PM, Vessey MP, Yeates D. Risk of gallbladder disease: a cohort study of young women attending family planning clinics. J Epidemiol Community Health 1982; 36:274-278. **63.** Rome Group for Epidemiology and Prevention of Cholelithiasis (GREPCO): Prevalence of gallstone disease in an Italian adult female population. Am J Epidemiol 1984; 119:796-805. **64.** Strom BL, Tamragouri RT, Morse ML, Lazar EL, West SL, Stolley PD, Jones JK. Oral contraceptives and other risk factors for gallbladder disease. Clin Pharmacol Ther 1986; 39:335-341. **65.** Wynn V, Adams PW, Godsland IF, Melrose J, Niththyananthan R, Oakley NW, Seedj A. Comparison of effects of different combined oral contraceptive formulations on carbohydrate and lipid metabolism. Lancet 1979; 1:1045-1049. **66.** Wynn V. Effect of progesterone and progestins on carbohydrate metabolism. In: Progesterone and Progestin. Bardin CW, Milgrom E, Mauvis-Jarvis P. eds. New York, Raven Press 1983; pp. 395-410. **67.** Perlman JA, Roussell-Briefel RG, Ezzati TM, Lieberknecht G. Oral glucose tolerance and the potency of oral contraceptive progestogens. J Chronic Dis 1985;38:857-864. **68.** Royal College of General Practitioners' Oral Contraception Study: Effect on hypertension and benign breast disease of progestogen component in combined oral contraceptives. Lancet 1977; 1:624. **69.** Fisch IR, Frank J. Oral contraceptives and blood pressure. JAMA 1977; 237:2499-2503. **70.** Laragh AJ. Oral contraceptive induced hypertension-nine years later. Am J Obstet Gynecol 1976; 126:141-147. **71.** Ramcharan S, Peritz E, Pellegrin FA, Williams WT. Incidence of hypertension in the Walnut Creek Contraceptive Drug Study cohort: In: Pharmacology of steroid contraceptive drugs. Garattini S, Berendes HW. Eds. New York, Raven Press, 1977; pp. 277-288, (Monographs of the Mario Negri Institute for Pharmacological Research Milan.) **72.** Stockley I. Interactions with oral contraceptives. J Pharm 1976;216:140-143. **73.** The Cancer and Steroid Hormone Study of the Centers for Disease Control and the National Institute of Child Health and Human Development: Oral contraceptive use and the risk of ovarian cancer. JAMA 1983; 249:1596-1599. **74.** The Cancer and Steroid Hormone Study of the Centers for Disease Control and the National Institute of Child Health and Human Development: Combination oral contraceptive use and the risk of endometrial cancer. JAMA 1987; 257:796-800. **75.** Ory HW. Functional ovarian cysts and oral contraceptives: negative association confirmed surgically. JAMA 1974; 228:68-69. **76.** Ory HW, Cole P, MacMahon B, Hoover R. Oral contraceptives and reduced risk of benign breast disease. N Engl J Med 1976; 294:419-422. **77.** Ory HW. The noncontraceptive health benefits from oral contraceptive use. Fam Plann Perspect 1982; 14:182-184. **78.** Ory HW, Forrest JD, Lincoln R. Making choices: Evaluating the health risks and benefits of birth control methods. New York, The Alan Guttmacher Institute, 1983; p.1. **79.** Schlesselman J, Stadel BV, Murray P, Lai S. Breast cancer in relation to early use of oral contraceptives. JAMA 1988; 259:1828-1833. **80.** Hennekens CH, Speizer FE, Lipnick RJ, Rosner B, Bain C, Belanger C, Stampfer MJ, Willett W, Peto R. A case-control study of oral contraceptive use and breast cancer. JNCI 1984; 72:39-42. **81.** LaVecchia C, Decarli A, Fasoli M, Franceschi S, Gentile A, Negri E, Parazzini F, Tognoni G. Oral contraceptives and cancers of the breast and of the female genital tract. Interim results from a case-control study. Br J Cancer 1986; 54:311-317. **82.** Meirik O, Lund E, Adami H, Bergstrom R, Christoffersen T, Bergsjo P. Oral contraceptive use and breast cancer in young women. A Joint National Case-control study in Sweden and Norway. Lancet 1986; 11:650-654. **83.** Kay CR, Hannaford PC. Breast cancer and the pill-A further report from the Royal College of General Practitioners' oral contraception study. Br J Cancer 1988;58:675-680. **84.** Stadel BV, Lai S, Schlesselman JJ, Murray P. Oral contraceptives and premenopausal breast cancer in nulliparous women. Contraception 1988; 38:287-299. **85.** Miller DR, Rosenberg L, Kaufman DW, Stolley P, Warshauer ME, Shapiro S. Breast cancer before age 45 and oral contraceptive use: New Findings. Am J Epidemiol 1989; 129:269-280. **86.** The UK National Case-Control Study Group, Oral contraceptive use and breast cancer risk in young women. Lancet 1989; 1:973-982. **87.** Schlesselman JJ. Cancer of the breast and reproductive tract in relation to use of oral contraceptives. Contraception 1989; 40:1-38. **88.** Vessey MP, McPherson K, Villard-Mackintosh L, Yeates D. Oral contraceptives and breast cancer: latest findings in a large cohort study. Br J Cancer 1989; 59:613-617. **89.** Jick SS, Walker AM, Stergachis A, Jick H. Oral contraceptives and breast cancer. Br J Cancer 1989; 59:618-621. **90.** Anderson FD, Selectivity and minimal androgenicity of norgestimate in monophasic and triphasic oral contraceptives. Acta Obstet Gynecol Scand 1992; 156 (Supplement):15-21. **91.** Chapdelaine A, Desmaris J-L, Derman RJ. Clinical evidence of minimal androgenic activity of norgestimate. Int J Fertil 1989; 34(51):347-352. **92.** Phillips A, Demarest K, Hahn DW, Wong F, McGuire JL. Progestational and androgenic receptor binding affinities and in vivo activities of norgestimate and other progestins. Contraception 1989; 41(4):399-409. **93.** Phillips A, Hahn DW, Klimek S, McGuire JL. A comparison of the potencies and activities of progestogens used in contraceptives. Contraception 1987; 36(2):181-192. **94.** Janaud A, Rouffy J, Upmalis D, Dain M-P. A comparison study of lipid and androgen metabolism with triphasic oral contraceptive formulations containing norgestimate or levonorgestrel Acta Obstet Gynecol Scand 1992; 156 (Supplement):34-38. **95.** Collaborative Group on Hormonal Factors in Breast Cancer. Breast cancer and hormonal contraceptives: collaborative reanalysis of individual data on 53 297 women with breast cancer and 100 239 women without breast cancer from 54 epidemiological studies. Lancet 1996; 347:1713-1727. **96.** Palmer JR, Rosenberg L, Kaufman DW, Warshauer ME, Stolley P, Shapiro S. Oral Contraceptive Use and Liver Cancer. Am J Epidemiol 1989;130:878-882. **97.** Lewis M, Spitzer WO, Heinemann LAJ, MacRae KD, Bruppacher R, Thorogood M on behalf of Transnational Research Group on Oral Contraceptives and Health of Young Women. Third generation oral contraceptives and risk of myocardial infarction: an international case-control study. Br Med J, 1996;312:88-90. **98.** Vessey MP, Smith MA, Yeates D. Return of fertility after discontinuation of oral contraceptives: influence of age and parity. Brit J Fam Plan; 1986; 11:120-124. **99.** Back DJ, Orme M.L'E. Pharmacokinetic drug interactions with oral contraceptives. Clin Pharmacokinet 1990; 18:472-484. **100.** Rosenfeld WE, Doose DR, Walker SA, Nayak RK. Effect of topiramate on the pharmacokinetics of an oral contraceptive containing norethindrone and ethinyl estradiol in patients with epilepsy. Epilepsia 1997 Mar;38(3):317-323. **101.** Shenfield GM. Oral Contraceptives. Are drug interaction of clinical significance? Drug Saf 1993 Jul;9(1):21-37. **102.** Ouellet D, Hsu A, Qian J, Locke CS, Eason CJ, Cavanaugh JH, Leonard JM, Granneman GR. Effect of ritonavir on the pharmacokinetics of ethinyl oestradiol in healthy female volunteers. Br J Clin Pharmacol 1998;46(2):111-116. **103.** Improving access to quality care in family planning: Medical eligibility criteria for contraceptive use. Geneva, WHO, Family and Reproductive Health, 1996 (WHO/FRH/FPP/96.9). **104.** Skolnick JL, Stoler BS, Katz DG, Anderson WH. Rifampicin, oral contraceptives and pregnancy. J Am Med Assoc 1976;236-1382. **105.** Henney JE. Risk of drug interactions with St. John's Wort. JAMA 2000;283(13). **106.** Lahteennmaki P et al, Coagulation factors in women using oral contraceptives or intrauterine devices immediately after abortion. American Journal of Obstetrics and Gynecology, (1981); 141: 175-179.

DETAILED PATIENT LABELING

ORTHO EVRA™

(norelgestromin/ethinyl estradiol transdermal system)

℞ only

This product is intended to prevent pregnancy. It does not protect against HIV (AIDS) or other sexually transmitted diseases.

DESCRIPTION

The contraceptive patch ORTHO EVRA™ is a thin, beige, plastic patch that sticks to the skin. The sticky part of the patch contains the hormones norelgestromin and ethinyl estradiol, which are absorbed continuously through the skin and into the bloodstream. Each patch is sealed in a pouch that protects it until you are ready to wear it.

INTRODUCTION

Any woman who considers using the contraceptive patch ORTHO EVRA™ should understand the benefits and risks of using this form of birth control. This leaflet will give you much of the information you will need to make this decision and will also help you determine if you are at risk of developing any serious side effects. It will tell you how to use the contraceptive patch properly so that it will be as effective as possible. However, this leaflet is not a replacement for a careful discussion between you and your health care professional. You should discuss the information provided in this leaflet with him or her, both when you first start using the contraceptive patch ORTHO EVRA™ and during your revisits. You should also follow your health care professional's advice with regard to regular check-ups while you are using the contraceptive patch.

EFFECTIVENESS OF HORMONAL CONTRACEPTIVE METHODS

Hormonal contraceptives, including ORTHO EVRA™, are used to prevent pregnancy and are more effective than most other non-surgical methods of birth control. When ORTHO EVRA™ is used correctly, the chance of becoming pregnant is approximately 1% (1 pregnancy per 100 women per year of use when used correctly), which is comparable to that of the pill. The chance of becoming pregnant increases with incorrect use.

Annual Number of Birth-Related or Method-Related Deaths Associated With Control of Fertility Per 100,000 Nonsterile Women by Fertility Control Method According to Age

Method of control and outcome	15–19	20–24	25–29	30–34	35–39	40–44
No fertility control methods*	7.0	7.4	9.1	14.8	25.7	28.2
Oral contraceptives, non-smoker**	0.3	0.5	0.9	1.9	13.8	31.6
Oral contraceptives, smoker**	2.2	3.4	6.6	13.5	51.1	117.2
IUD**	0.8	0.8	1.0	1.0	11.4	1.4
Condom*	1.1	1.6	0.7	0.2	0.3	0.4
Diaphragm/spermicide*	1.9	1.2	1.2	1.3	2.2	2.8
Periodic abstinence*	2.5	1.6	1.6	1.7	2.9	3.6

*Deaths are birth-related
**Deaths are method-related
Adapted from H.W. Ory, ref. # 35.

Clinical trials suggested that ORTHO EVRA™ may be less effective in women weighing more than 198 lbs. (90 kg). If you weigh more than 198 lbs. (90 kg) you should talk to your health care professional about which method of birth control may be best for you.

Typical failure rates for other methods of birth control during the first year of use are as follows:

Implant: <1%
Injection: <1%
IUD: <1–2%
Diaphragm with spermicides: 20%
Spermicides alone: 26%
Female sterilization: <1%
Male sterilization: <1%
Cervical Cap with spermicide: 20 to 40%
Condom alone (male): 14%
Condom alone (female): 21%
Periodic abstinence: 25%
No birth control method: 85%
Withdrawal: 19%

WHO SHOULD NOT USE ORTHO EVRA™

Hormonal contraceptives include birth control pills, injectables, implants, the vaginal ring, and the contraceptive patch. The following information is derived primarily from studies of birth control pills. The contraceptive patch is expected to be associated with similar risks:

Cigarette smoking increases the risk of serious cardiovascular side effects from hormonal contraceptive use. This risk increases with age and with heavy smoking (15 or more cigarettes per day) and is quite marked in women over 35 years of age. Women who use hormonal contraceptives, including ORTHO EVRA™, are strongly advised not to smoke.

Some women should not use the ORTHO EVRA™ contraceptive patch. For example, you should not use ORTHO EVRA™ if you are pregnant or think you may be pregnant. You should also not use ORTHO EVRA™ if you have any of the following conditions:

- A history of heart attack or stroke
- Blood clots in the legs (thrombophlebitis), lungs (pulmonary embolism), or eyes
- A history of blood clots in the deep veins of your legs
- Chest pain (angina pectoris)
- Known or suspected breast cancer or cancer of the lining of the uterus, cervix or vagina.
- Unexplained vaginal bleeding (until your doctor reaches a diagnosis)
- Hepatitis or yellowing of the whites of your eyes or of the skin (jaundice) during pregnancy or during previous use of hormonal contraceptives such as ORTHO EVRA™, NORPLANT, or the birth control pill
- Liver tumor (benign or cancerous)
- Known or suspected pregnancy
- Severe high blood pressure
- Diabetes with complications of the kidneys, eyes, nerves, or blood vessels
- Headaches with neurological symptoms
- Use of oral contraceptives (birth control pills)
- Disease of heart valves with complications
- Need for a prolonged period of bed rest following major surgery
- An allergic reaction to any of the components of ORTHO EVRA™

Tell your health care professional if you have ever had any of these conditions. Your health care professional can recommend a non-hormonal method of birth control.

OTHER CONSIDERATIONS BEFORE USING ORTHO EVRA™

Talk to your health care professional about using ORTHO EVRA™ if

- you smoke
- you are recovering from the birth of a baby
- you are recovering from a second trimester miscarriage or abortion
- you are breast feeding
- you weigh 198 pounds or more
- you are taking any other medications

Also, tell your health care professional if you have or have had:

- Breast nodules, fibrocystic disease of the breast, an abnormal breast x-ray or mammogram
- A family history of breast cancer
- Diabetes
- Elevated cholesterol or triglycerides
- High blood pressure
- Migraine or other headaches or epilepsy
- Depression
- Gallbladder disease
- Liver disease
- Heart disease
- Kidney disease
- Scanty or irregular menstrual periods

If you have any of these conditions you should be checked often by your health care professional if you use the contraceptive patch.

RISKS OF USING HORMONAL CONTRACEPTIVES, INCLUDING ORTHO EVRA™

The following information is derived primarily from studies of birth control pills. Since ORTHO EVRA™ contains hormones similar to those found in birth control pills, it is expected to be associated with similar risks:

1. Risk of developing blood clots

Blood clots and blockage of blood vessels that can cause death or serious disability are some of the most serious side effects of using hormonal contraceptives, including the ORTHO EVRA™ contraceptive patch. In particular, a clot in the legs can cause thrombophlebitis, and a clot that travels to the lungs can cause sudden blocking of the vessel carrying blood to the lungs. Rarely, clots occur in the blood vessels of the eye and may cause blindness, double vision, or impaired vision.

If you use ORTHO EVRA™ and need elective surgery, need to stay in bed for a prolonged illness or injury or have recently delivered a baby, you may be at risk of developing blood clots. You should consult your doctor about stopping ORTHO EVRA™ four weeks before surgery and not using it for two weeks after surgery or during bed rest. You should also not use ORTHO EVRA™ soon after delivery of a baby. It is advisable to wait for at least four weeks after delivery if you are not breast-feeding. If you are breast-feeding, you should wait until you have weaned your child before using ORTHO EVRA™. (See also the section on Breast Feeding in General Precautions.)

2. Heart attacks and strokes

Hormonal contraceptives, including ORTHO EVRA™, may increase the risk of developing strokes (blockage or rupture of blood vessels in the brain) and angina pectoris and heart attacks (blockage of blood vessels in the heart). Any of these conditions can cause death or serious disability.

Smoking and the use of hormonal contraceptives including ORTHO EVRA™ greatly increase the chances of developing and dying of heart disease. Smoking also greatly increases the possibility of suffering heart attacks and strokes.

3. Gallbladder disease

Women who use hormonal contraceptives, including ORTHO EVRA™, probably have a greater risk than nonusers of having gallbladder disease.

4. Liver tumors

In rare cases, combination oral contraceptives can cause benign but dangerous liver tumors. Since ORTHO EVRA™ contains hormones similar to those in birth control pills, this association may also exist with ORTHO EVRA™. These benign liver tumors can rupture and cause fatal internal bleeding. In addition, some studies report an increased risk of developing liver cancer. However, liver cancers are rare.

5. Cancer of the reproductive organs and breasts

Various studies give conflicting reports on the relationship between breast cancer and hormonal contraceptive use. Combination hormonal contraceptives, including ORTHO EVRA™, may slightly increase your chance of having breast cancer diagnosed, particularly after using hormonal contraceptives at a younger age. After you stop using hormonal contraceptives, the chances of having breast cancer diagnosed begin to go back down. You should have regular breast examinations by a health care professional and examine your own breasts monthly. Tell your health care professional if you have a family history of breast cancer or if you have had breast nodules or an abnormal mammogram. Women who currently have or have had breast cancer should not use oral contraceptives because breast cancer is usually a hormone-sensitive tumor.

Some studies have found an increase in the incidence of cancer of the cervix in women who use oral contraceptives, al-

Continued on next page

Ortho Evra—Cont.

though this finding may be related to factors other than the use of oral contraceptives. However, there is insufficient evidence to rule out the possibility that oral contraceptives may cause such cancers.

ESTIMATED RISK OF DEATH FROM A BIRTH CONTROL METHOD OR PREGNANCY

All methods of birth control and pregnancy are associated with a risk of developing certain diseases that may lead to disability or death. An estimate of the number of deaths associated with different methods of birth control and pregnancy has been calculated and is shown in the following table.

ORTHO EVRA™ is expected to be associated with similar risks as oral contraceptives:

[See table at top of previous page]

In the above table, the risk of death from any birth control method is less than the risk of childbirth, except for oral contraceptive users over the age of 35 who smoke and pill users over the age of 40 even if they do not smoke. It can be seen in the table that for women aged 15 to 39, the risk of death was highest with pregnancy (7–26 deaths per 100,000 women, depending on age). Among pill users who do not smoke, the risk of death is always lower than that associated with pregnancy for any age group, although over the age of 40, the risk increases to 32 deaths per 100,000 women, compared to 28 associated with pregnancy at that age. However, for pill users who smoke and are over the age of 35, the estimated number of deaths exceeds those for other methods of birth control. If a woman is over the age of 40 and smokes, her estimated risk of death is four times higher (117/100,000 women) than the estimated risk associated with pregnancy (28/100,000 women) in that age group. In 1989 an Advisory Committee of the FDA concluded that the benefits of low-dose hormonal contraceptive use by healthy, non-smoking women over 40 years of age may outweigh the possible risks.

WARNING SIGNALS

If any of these adverse effects occur while you are using ORTHO EVRA™, call your doctor immediately:

- Sharp chest pain, coughing of blood, or sudden shortness of breath (indicating a possible clot in the lung)
- Pain in the calf (indicating a possible clot in the leg)
- Crushing chest pain or tightness in the chest (indicating a possible heart attack)
- Sudden severe headache or vomiting, dizziness or fainting, disturbances of vision or speech, weakness, or numbness in an arm or leg (indicating a possible stroke)
- Sudden partial or complete loss of vision (indicating a possible clot in the eye)
- Breast lumps (indicating possible breast cancer or fibrocystic disease of the breast; ask your doctor or health care professional to show you how to examine your breasts)
- Severe pain or tenderness in the stomach area (indicating a possibly ruptured liver tumor)
- Severe problems with sleeping, weakness, lack of energy, fatigue, or change in mood (possibly indicating severe depression)
- Jaundice or a yellowing of the skin or eyeballs accompanied frequently by fever, fatigue, loss of appetite, dark colored urine, or light colored bowel movements (indicating possible liver problems)

SIDE EFFECTS OF ORTHO EVRA™

1. Skin irritation

Skin irritation, redness or rash may occur at the site of application. If this occurs, the patch may be removed and a new patch may be applied to a new location until the next Change Day. Single replacement patches are available from pharmacies.

2. Vaginal bleeding

Irregular vaginal bleeding or spotting may occur while you are using ORTHO EVRA™. Irregular bleeding may vary from slight staining between menstrual periods to breakthrough bleeding which is a flow much like a regular period. Irregular bleeding may occur during the first few months of contraceptive patch use but may also occur after you have been using the contraceptive patch for some time. Such bleeding may be temporary and usually does not indicate any serious problems. It is important to continue using your contraceptive patches on schedule. If the bleeding occurs in more than a few cycles or lasts for more than a few days, talk to your health care professional.

3. Problems wearing contact lenses

If you wear contact lenses and notice a change in vision or an inability to wear your lenses, contact your health care professional.

4. Fluid retention or raised blood pressure

Hormonal contraceptives, including the contraceptive patch, may cause edema (fluid retention) with swelling of the fingers or ankles and may raise your blood pressure. If you experience fluid retention, contact your health care professional.

5. Melasma

A spotty darkening of the skin is possible, particularly of the face. This may persist after use of hormonal contraceptives is discontinued.

6. Other side effects

The most common side effects of ORTHO EVRA™ include nausea and vomiting, breast symptoms, headache, menstrual cramps, and abdominal pain. In addition, change in appetite, nervousness, depression, dizziness, loss of scalp hair, rash, and vaginal infections may occur.

GENERAL PRECAUTIONS

1. Weight > 198 lbs. (90 kg)

Clinical trials suggest that ORTHO EVRA™ may be less effective in women weighing more than 198 lbs. (90 kg) compared with its effectiveness in women with lower body weights. If you weigh more than 198 lbs. (90 kg) you should talk to your health care professional about which method of birth control may be best for you.

2. Missed periods and use of ORTHO EVRA™ before or during early pregnancy

There may be times when you may not menstruate regularly during your patch-free week. If you have used ORTHO EVRA™ correctly and miss one menstrual period, continue using your contraceptive patches for the next cycle but be sure to inform your health care professional before doing so. If you have not used ORTHO EVRA™ as instructed and missed a menstrual period, or if you missed two menstrual periods in a row, you could be pregnant. Check with your health care professional immediately to determine whether you are pregnant. Stop using ORTHO EVRA™ if you are pregnant.

There is no conclusive evidence that hormonal contraceptive use causes birth defects when taken accidentally during early pregnancy. Previously, a few studies had reported that oral contraceptives might be associated with birth defects, but these findings have not been seen in more recent studies. Nevertheless, hormonal contraceptives, including ORTHO EVRA™, should not be used during pregnancy. You should check with your health care professional about risks to your unborn child from any medication taken during pregnancy.

3. While breast-feeding

If you are breast-feeding, consult your health care professional before starting ORTHO EVRA™. Hormonal contraceptives are passed on to the child in the milk. A few adverse effects on the child have been reported, including yellowing of the skin (jaundice) and breast enlargement. In addition, combination hormonal contraceptives may decrease the amount and quality of your milk. If possible, do not use combination hormonal contraceptives such as ORTHO EVRA™ while breast-feeding. You should use a barrier method of contraception since breast-feeding provides only partial protection from becoming pregnant and this partial protection decreases significantly as you breastfeed for longer periods of time. You should consider starting ORTHO EVRA™ only after you have weaned your child completely.

4. Laboratory tests

If you are scheduled for any laboratory tests, tell your doctor you are using ORTHO EVRA™ since certain blood tests may be affected by hormonal contraceptives.

5. Drug interactions

Certain drugs may interact with hormonal contraceptives, including ORTHO EVRA™, to make them less effective in preventing pregnancy or cause an increase in breakthrough bleeding. Such drugs include rifampin, drugs used for epilepsy such as barbiturates (for example, phenobarbital), anticonvulsants such as topiramate (TOPAMAX), carbamazepine (Tegretol is one brand of this drug), phenytoin (Dilantin is one brand of this drug), phenylbutazone (Butazolidin is one brand), certain drugs used in the treatment of HIV or AIDS, and possibly certain antibiotics. Tetracycline has been shown not to interact with ORTHO EVRA™. Pregnancies and breakthrough bleeding have been reported by users of combined hormonal contraceptives who also used some form of St. John's Wort.

As with all prescription products, you should notify your health care professional of any other medications you are taking. You may need to use a barrier contraceptive when you take drugs that can make ORTHO EVRA™ less effective.

6. Sexually transmitted diseases

ORTHO EVRA™ is intended to prevent pregnancy. It does not protect against HIV (AIDS) or other sexually transmitted diseases such as chlamydia, genital herpes, genital warts, gonorrhea, hepatitis B, and syphilis.

HOW TO USE ORTHO EVRA ™

Instructions for Use

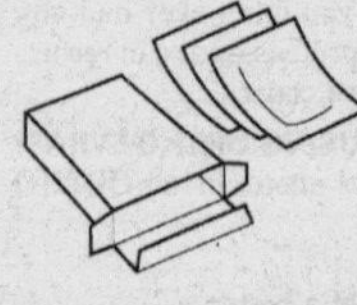

ORTHO EVRA™ keeps you from becoming pregnant by transferring hormones to your body through your skin. The patch must stick securely to your skin in order for it to work properly.

This method uses a 28 day (four week) cycle. You should apply a new patch each week for three weeks (21 total days). You should not apply a patch during the fourth week. Your menstrual period should start during this patch-free week.

Every new patch should be applied on the same day of the week. This day will be your 'Patch Change Day.' *For example, if you apply your first patch on a Monday, all of your patches should be applied on a Monday.* You should wear only one patch at a time.

On the day after week four ends, you should begin a new four week cycle by applying a new patch.

Save these instructions.

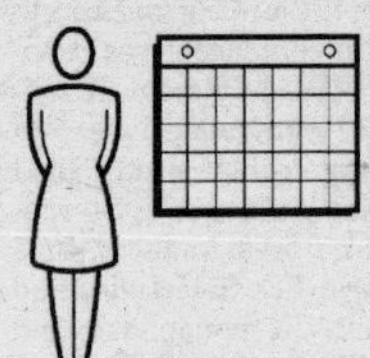

1

If this is the **first time** you are using ORTHO EVRA™, **wait until the day you get your menstrual period.** *The day you apply your first patch will be Day 1. Your 'Patch Change Day' will be on this day every week.*

CHOOSE ONE OPTION:

☐ **First Day Start**

or

☐ **Sunday Start**

2

You may choose a first day start or Sunday start

- *for **First Day** start:* apply your first patch during the first 24 hours of your menstrual period.

OR

- for ***Sunday** start:* apply your first patch on the first Sunday after your menstrual period starts. *You must use back-up contraception, such as a condom, spermicide, or diaphragm for the first week of your first cycle.*
- *The day you apply your first patch will be Day 1. Your 'Patch Change Day' will be on this day every week.*

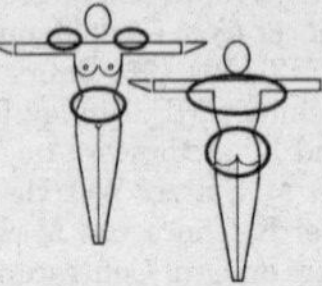

3

Choose a place on your body to put the patch. Put the patch on your buttock, abdomen, upper outer arm or upper torso, in a place where it won't be rubbed by tight clothing. *Never put the patch on your breasts. To avoid irritation, apply each new patch to a different place on your skin.*

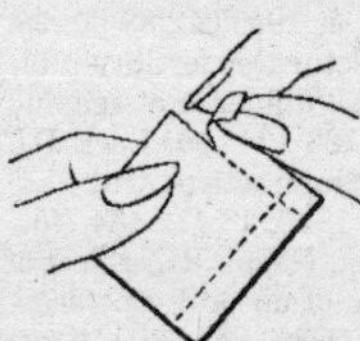

4

Open the foil pouch by tearing it along the top edge <u>**and**</u> one side edge.

Peel the foil pouch apart and open it flat.

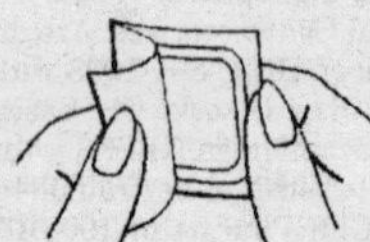

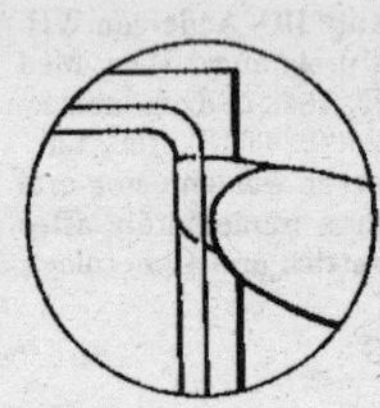

5

You will see that the patch is covered by a layer of clear plastic. It is important to remove the patch <u>**and**</u> the plastic together from the foil pouch.

Using your fingernail, lift one corner of the patch and peel the patch <u>**and**</u> the plastic off the foil liner.

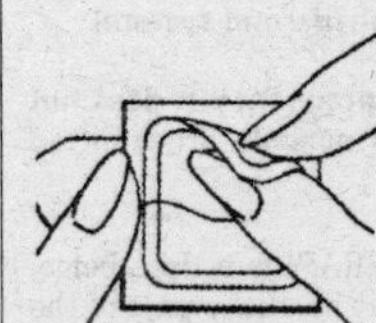

Sometimes patches can stick to the inside of the pouch – be careful not to accidentally remove the clear liner as you remove the patch.

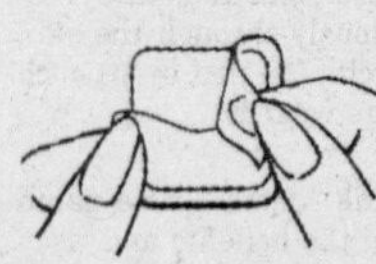

6

Peel away half of the clear plastic and **be careful** not to touch the exposed sticky surface of the patch **with your fingers.**

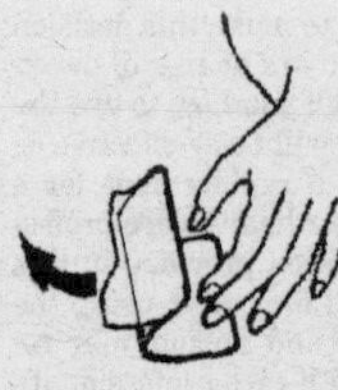

7

Apply the sticky side of the patch to the skin you've cleaned and dried, then remove the other half of the clear plastic.

Press firmly on the patch with the palm of your hand for 10 seconds, making sure the edges stick well. Run your finger around the edge of the patch to make sure it is sticking properly.

Check your patch every day to make sure all the edges are sticking.

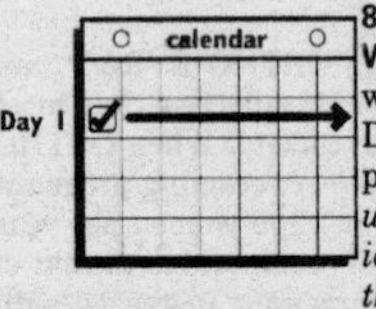

8

Wear the patch for seven days (one week). On your 'Patch Change Day,' Day 8, remove the used patch. Apply a new patch immediately. *The used patch still contains some medicine—carefully fold it in half so that it sticks to itself before throwing it away.*

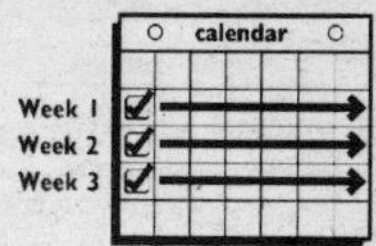

9
Apply a new patch for week two (on Day 8) and for week three (on Day 15), on your 'Patch Change Day.' *To avoid irritation, do not apply the new patch to the same exact place on your skin.*

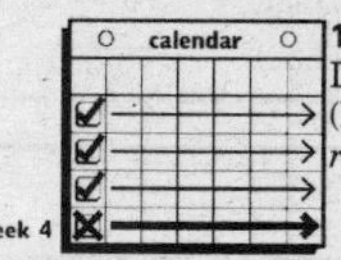

10
Do not wear a patch on week four (Day 22 through Day 28). *Your period should start during this week.*

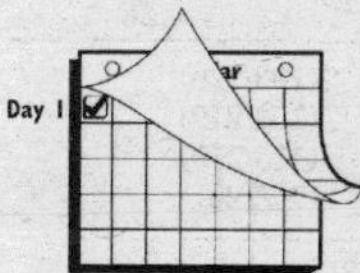

11
Begin your next four week cycle by applying a new patch on your normal 'Patch Change Day,' the day after Day 28 – *no matter when your period begins or ends.*

If your patch has become loose or has fallen off...

- **for less than one day**, try to re-apply it or apply a new patch immediately. No back-up contraception is needed. *Your 'Patch Change Day' will remain the same.*
- **for more than one day OR if you are not sure for how long**, YOU MAY BECOME PREGNANT – **Start a new four week cycle immediately** by putting on a new patch. *You now have a new Day 1 and a new 'Patch Change Day.' You must use back-up contraception, such as a condom, spermicide, or diaphragm for the first week of your new cycle.*
- do not try to re-apply a patch if it's no longer sticky, if it has become stuck to itself or another surface, if it has other material stuck to it or if it has previously become loose or fallen off. No tapes or wraps should be used to keep the patch in place. If you cannot re-apply a patch, apply a new patch immediately.

If you forget to change your patch...

- **at the start of any patch cycle,**
  Week one (Day 1): If you forget to apply your patch, YOU COULD BECOME PREGNANT – *you must use back-up contraception for one week.* Apply the first patch of your new cycle as soon as you remember. *You now have a new 'Patch Change Day' and new Day 1.*
- **in the middle of your patch cycle,**
  Week two or week three: If you forget to change your patch for **one or two days**, apply a new patch as soon as you remember. Apply your next patch on your normal 'Patch Change Day.' No back-up contraception is needed.
  Week two or week three: If you forget to change your patch for **more than two days**, YOU COULD BECOME PREGNANT – **start a new four week cycle as soon as you remember by putting on a new patch.** *You now have a different 'Patch Change Day' and a new Day 1. You must use back-up contraception for the first week of your new cycle.*
- **at the end of your patch cycle,**
  Week four: If you forget to remove your patch, take it off as soon as you remember. Start your next cycle on your normal 'Patch Change Day,' the day after Day 28. No back-up contraception is needed.
- **at the start of your next patch cycle,**
  Day 1 (week one): If you forget to apply your patch, YOU COULD BECOME PREGNANT – apply the first patch of your new cycle as soon as you remember. *You now have a new 'Patch Change Day' and new Day 1. You must use back-up contraception for the first week of your new cycle.*
- ***you should never have the patch off for more than seven days.***

Other information...

- Always apply your patch to clean, dry skin. Avoid skin that is red, irritated or cut. Do not use creams, oils, powder or makeup on your skin where you will put a patch or near a patch you are wearing. It may cause the patch to become loose.
- If patch use results in uncomfortable irritation, the patch may be removed and a new patch may be applied to a new location until the next Change Day. Only one patch should be worn at a time.
- Some medicines may change the way ORTHO EVRA™ works. If you are taking any medication, you must talk to your health care professional BEFORE you use the patch. *You may need to use back-up contraception.*
- Store at 25°C (77°F).
- Single replacement patches are available through your pharmacist.
- For further information log on to **www.orthoevra.com** or call toll free **1 877 EVRA 888**

WHEN YOU SWITCH FROM THE PILL TO ORTHO EVRA™:

If you are switching from the pill to ORTHO EVRA™, wait until you get your menstrual period. If you do not get your period within five days of taking the last active pill, check with your health care professional to be sure that you are not pregnant.

IMPORTANT POINTS TO REMEMBER

1. IT IS IMPORTANT TO USE ORTHO EVRA™ exactly as directed in this leaflet. Incorrect use increases your chances of becoming pregnant. This includes starting your contraceptive cycle late or missing your scheduled CHANGE DAYS.
2. You should wear one patch per week for three weeks, followed by one week off. **You should never have the patch off for more than seven days in a row.** If you have the patch off for more than seven days in a row and you have had sex during this time, YOU COULD BECOME PREGNANT.
3. **IF YOU ARE NOT SURE WHAT TO DO ABOUT MISTAKES WITH PATCH USE:**
   - Use a BACK-UP METHOD, *such as a condom, spermicide, or diaphragm* anytime you have sex.
   - Contact your health care professional for instructions.
4. Do not skip patches even if you do not have sex very often.
5. SOME WOMEN HAVE SPOTTING OR LIGHT BLEEDING, BREAST TENDERNESS OR MAY FEEL SICK TO THEIR STOMACH DURING ORTHO EVRA™ USE. If these symptoms occur, do not stop using the contraceptive patch. The problem will usually go away. If it doesn't go away, check with your health care professional.
6. MISTAKES IN USING YOUR PATCHES CAN ALSO CAUSE SPOTTING OR LIGHT BLEEDING.
7. If you miss TWO PERIODS IN A ROW contact your health care professional because you might be pregnant.
8. The amount of drug you get from the ORTHO EVRA™ patch should not be affected by VOMITING OR DIARRHEA.
9. IF YOU TAKE CERTAIN MEDICINES, ORTHO EVRA™ may not work as well. Use a non-hormonal back-up method (such as condoms, spermicide, or diaphragm) until you check with your health care professional.
10. IF YOU WANT TO MOVE YOUR PATCH CHANGE DAY to a different day of the week, finish your current cycle, removing your third ORTHO EVRA™ patch on the correct day. **During week four**, the "patch-free week" (Day 22 through Day 28), you may choose an earlier Patch Change Day by applying a new patch on the day you prefer. You now have a new Day 1 and a new Patch Change Day. **You should never have the patch off for more than seven days in a row.**
11. BE SURE YOU HAVE READY AT ALL TIMES:
    - A NON-HORMONAL BIRTH CONTROL method (such as condoms, spermicide, or diaphragm) to use as a back-up in case of dosing errors.
12. IF YOU HAVE TROUBLE REMEMBERING TO CHANGE YOUR CONTRACEPTIVE PATCH, talk to your health care professional about how to make patch-changing easier or about using another method of birth control.
13. Single replacement patches are available through your pharmacist.
14. For Patch replacement, see "How to use ORTHO EVRA™" section.

IF YOU HAVE ANY QUESTIONS OR ARE UNSURE ABOUT THE INFORMATION IN THIS LEAFLET, call your health care professional.

PREGNANCY DUE TO ORTHO EVRA™ FAILURE

The incidence of pregnancy from hormonal contraceptive failure is approximately one percent (i.e., one pregnancy per 100 women per year) if used correctly. The chance of becoming pregnant increases with incorrect use. If contraceptive patch failure does occur, the risk to the fetus is minimal.

PREGNANCY AFTER STOPPING ORTHO EVRA™

There may be some delay in becoming pregnant after you stop using ORTHO EVRA™, especially if you had irregular menstrual cycles before you used hormonal contraceptives. It may be best to postpone conception until you begin menstruation regularly once you have stopped using ORTHO EVRA™ and want to become pregnant.

There does not appear to be any increase in birth defects in newborn babies when pregnancy occurs soon after stopping hormonal contraceptives.

OVERDOSAGE

ORTHO EVRA™ is unlikely to cause an overdose because the patch releases a steady amount of the hormones. Do not use more than one patch at a time. Serious ill effects have not been reported when large doses of oral contraceptives were accidentally taken by young children. Overdosage may cause nausea and vomiting. Vaginal bleeding may occur in females. In case of overdosage, contact your health care professional or pharmacist.

OTHER INFORMATION

Your health care professional will take a medical and family history before prescribing ORTHO EVRA™ and will examine you. The physical examination may be delayed to another time if you request it and the health care professional believes that it is a good medical practice to postpone it. You should be reexamined at least once a year. Be sure to inform your health care professional if there is a family history of any of the conditions listed previously in this leaflet. Be sure to keep all appointments with your health care professional, because this is a time to determine if there are early signs of side effects of hormonal contraceptive use.

Do not use the drug for any condition other than the one for which it was prescribed. This drug has been prescribed specifically for you; do not give it to others who may want birth control.

If you want more information about ORTHO EVRA™, ask your health care professional or pharmacist. They have a more technical leaflet called the Prescribing Information that you may wish to read.

Special Precautions for Storage and Disposal

Store at room temperature.

Store patches in their protective pouches. Apply to the skin immediately upon removal from the protective pouch.

Do not store in the refrigerator or freezer.

Used patches still contain some active hormones. Fold each patch in half so that it sticks to itself before throwing it away.

ORTHO-McNEIL

ORTHO-McNEIL PHARMACEUTICAL, INC.
Raritan, New Jersey 08869
 ISSUED NOVEMBER 2001 631-10-660-1

Pfizer Inc.

**235 EAST 42ND STREET
NEW YORK, NY 10017–5755**

For Medical Information Contact:
(800) 438-1985
24 hours a day, seven days a week.

BEXTRA™ ℞
(valdecoxib tablets)

DESCRIPTION

Valdecoxib is chemically designated as 4-(5-methyl-3-phenyl-4-isoxazolyl) benzenesulfonamide and is a diaryl substituted isoxazole. It has the following chemical structure:

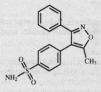

Valdecoxib

The empirical formula for valdecoxib is $C_{16}H_{14}N_2O_3S$, and the molecular weight is 314.36. Valdecoxib is a white crystalline powder that is relatively insoluble in water (10 mcg/mL) at 25°C and pH 7.0, soluble in methanol and ethanol, and freely soluble in organic solvents and alkaline (pH=12) aqueous solutions.

BEXTRA Tablets for oral administration contain either 10 mg or 20 mg of valdecoxib. Inactive ingredients include lactose monohydrate, microcrystalline cellulose, pregelatinized starch, croscarmellose sodium, magnesium stearate, hydroxypropyl methylcellulose, polyethylene glycol, polysorbate 80, and titanium dioxide.

CLINICAL PHARMACOLOGY

Mechanism of Action

Valdecoxib is a nonsteroidal anti-inflammatory drug (NSAID) that exhibits anti-inflammatory, analgesic and antipyretic properties in animal models. The mechanism of action is believed to be due to inhibition of prostaglandin synthesis primarily through inhibition of cyclooxygenase-2 (COX-2). At therapeutic plasma concentrations in humans valdecoxib does not inhibit cyclooxygenase-1 (COX-1).

Pharmacokinetics

Absorption

Valdecoxib achieves maximal plasma concentrations in approximately 3 hours. The absolute bioavailability of valdecoxib is 83% following oral administration of BEXTRA compared to intravenous infusion of valdecoxib.

Dose proportionality was demonstrated after single doses (1–400 mg) of valdecoxib. With multiple doses (up to 100 mg/day for 14 days), valdecoxib exposure as measured by the AUC, increases in a more than proportional manner at doses above 10 mg BID. Steady state plasma concentrations of valdecoxib are achieved by day 4.

The steady state pharmacokinetic parameters of valdecoxib in healthy male subjects are shown in Table 1.

[See table 1 at top of next page]

No clinically significant age or gender differences were seen in pharmacokinetic parameters that would require dosage adjustments.

Effect of Food and Antacid

BEXTRA can be taken with or without food. Food had no significant effect on either the peak plasma concentration (C_{max}) or extent of absorption (AUC) of valdecoxib when BEXTRA was taken with a high fat meal. The time to peak plasma concentration (T_{max}), however, was delayed by 1–2 hours. Administration of BEXTRA with antacid (aluminum/magnesium hydroxide) had no significant effect on either the rate or extent of absorption of valdecoxib.

Distribution

Plasma protein binding for valdecoxib is about 98% over the concentration range (21–2384 ng/mL). Steady state apparent volume of distribution (Vss/F) of valdecoxib is approximately 86 L after oral administration. Valdecoxib and its ac-

Continued on next page

Bextra—Cont.

tive metabolite preferentially partition into erythrocytes with a blood to plasma concentration ratio of about 2.5:1. This ratio remains approximately constant with time and therapeutic blood concentrations.

Metabolism

In humans, valdecoxib undergoes extensive hepatic metabolism involving both P450 isoenzymes (3A4 and 2C9) and non-P450 dependent pathways (i.e., glucuronidation). Concomitant administration of BEXTRA with known CYP 3A4 and 2C9 inhibitors (e.g., fluconazole and ketoconazole) can result in increased plasma exposure of valdecoxib (see PRECAUTIONS—Drug Interactions).

One active metabolite of valdecoxib has been identified in human plasma at approximately 10% the concentration of valdecoxib. This metabolite, which is a less potent COX-2 specific inhibitor than the parent, also undergoes extensive metabolism and constitutes less than 2% of the valdecoxib dose excreted in the urine and feces. Due to its low concentration in the systemic circulation, it is not likely to contribute significantly to the efficacy profile of BEXTRA.

Excretion

Valdecoxib is eliminated predominantly via hepatic metabolism with less than 5% of the dose excreted unchanged in the urine and feces. About 70% of the dose is excreted in the urine as metabolites, and about 20% as valdecoxib N-glucuronide. The apparent oral clearance (CL/F) of valdecoxib is about 6 L/hr. The elimination half-life ($T_{1/2}$) is approximately 8–11 hours.

Special Populations

Geriatric

In elderly subjects (>65 years), weight-adjusted steady state plasma concentrations ($AUC_{(0-12hr)}$) are about 30% higher than in young subjects. No dose adjustment is needed based on age.

Pediatric

BEXTRA has not been investigated in pediatric patients below 18 years of age.

Race

Pharmacokinetic differences due to race have not been identified in clinical and pharmacokinetic studies conducted to date.

Hepatic Insufficiency

Valdecoxib plasma concentrations are significantly increased (130%) in patients with moderate (Child-Pugh Class B) hepatic impairment. In clinical trials, doses of BEXTRA above those recommended have been associated with fluid retention. Hence, treatment with BEXTRA should be initiated with caution in patients with mild to moderate hepatic impairment and fluid retention. The use of BEXTRA in patients with severe hepatic impairment (Child-Pugh Class C) is not recommended.

Renal Insufficiency

The pharmacokinetics of valdecoxib have been studied in patients with varying degrees of renal impairment. Because renal elimination of valdecoxib is not important to its disposition, no clinically significant changes in valdecoxib clearance were found even in patients with severe renal impairment or in patients undergoing renal dialysis. In patients undergoing hemodialysis the plasma clearance (CL/F) of valdecoxib was similar to the CL/F found in healthy elderly subjects (CL/F about 6 to 7 L/hr.) with normal renal function (based on creatinine clearance).

NSAIDs have been associated with worsening renal function and use in advanced renal disease is not recommended (see PRECAUTIONS—Renal Effects).

Drug Interactions

Also see **PRECAUTIONS—Drug Interactions.**

General

Valdecoxib undergoes both P450 (CYP) dependent and non-P450 dependent (glucuronidation) metabolism. In vitro studies indicate that valdecoxib is not a significant inhibitor of CYP 1A2, 3A4, or 2D6 and is only a weak inhibitor of CYP 2C9 and 2C19 at therapeutic concentrations. The P450-mediated metabolic pathway of valdecoxib predominantly involves the 3A4 and 2C9 isozymes. Using prototype inhibitors and substrates of these isozymes, the following results were obtained. Coadministration of a known inhibitor of CYP 2C9/3A4 (fluconazole) and a CYP 3A4 (ketoconazole) inhibitor enhanced the total plasma exposure (AUC) of valdecoxib. Coadministration of valdecoxib with warfarin caused a small, but statistically significant increase in plasma exposures of R-warfarin and S-warfarin, and also in the pharmacodynamic effects (International Normalized Ratio - INR) of warfarin. (See PRECAUTIONS—Drug Interactions.)

Coadministration of valdecoxib, or its injectable prodrug, with substrates of CYP 2C9 (propofol) and CYP 3A4 (midazolam, alfentanil, fentanyl) did not inhibit the metabolism of either substrate.

Coadministration of valdecoxib with a CYP 3A4 substrate (glyburide) or a CYP 2D6 substrate (dextromethorphan) did not result in clinically important inhibition in the metabolism of these agents.

CLINICAL STUDIES

The efficacy and clinical utility of BEXTRA Tablets have been demonstrated in osteoarthritis (OA), rheumatoid arthritis (RA) and in the treatment of primary dysmenorrhea.

Osteoarthritis

BEXTRA was evaluated for treatment of the signs and symptoms of osteoarthritis of the knee or hip, in five double-blind, randomized, controlled trials in which 3918 patients were treated for 3 to 6 months. BEXTRA was shown to be superior to placebo in improvement in three domains of OA symptoms: (1) the WOMAC (Western Ontario and McMaster Universities) osteoarthritis index, a composite of pain, stiffness and functional measures in OA, (2) the overall patient assessment of pain, and (3) the overall patient global assessment. The two 3-month pivotal trials in OA generally showed changes statistically significantly different from placebo, and comparable to the naproxen control, in measures of these domains for the 10 mg/day dose. No additional benefit was seen with a valdecoxib 20 mg daily dose.

Rheumatoid Arthritis

BEXTRA demonstrated significant reduction compared to placebo in the signs and symptoms of RA, as measured by the ACR (American College of Rheumatology) 20 improvement, a composite defined as both improvement of 20% in the number of tender and number of swollen joints, and a 20% improvement in three of the following five: patient global, physician global, patient pain, patient function assessment, and the erythrocyte sedimentation rate (ESR). BEXTRA was evaluated for treatment of the signs and symptoms of rheumatoid arthritis in four double-blind, randomized, controlled studies in which 3444 patients were treated for 3 to 6 months. The two 3-month pivotal trials compared valdecoxib to naproxen and placebo. The results for the ACR20 responses in these trials are shown below (Table 2). Trials of BEXTRA in rheumatoid arthritis allowed concomitant use of corticosteroids and/or disease-modifying anti-rheumatic drugs (DMARDs), such as methotrexate, gold salts, and hydroxychloroquine. No additional benefit was seen with a valdecoxib 20 mg daily dose.

[See table 2 above]

Table 1

Mean (SD) Steady State Pharmacokinetic Parameters

Steady State Pharmacokinetic Parameters after Valdecoxib 10 mg Once Daily for 14 Days	Healthy Male Subjects (n=8, 20 to 42 yr.)
AUC(0–24hr) (hr · ng/mL)	1479.0 (291.9)
C_{max} (ng/mL)	161.1 (48.1)
T_{max} (hr)	2.25 (0.71)
C_{min} (ng/mL)	21.9 (7.68)
Terminal Half-life (hr)	8.11 (1.32)

Table 2

ACR20 Response Rate (%) in Rheumatoid Arthritis

	Study 1		Study 2	
BEXTRA 10 mg/day	49%**	(103/209)	46%**	(103/226)
BEXTRA 20 mg/day	48%**	(102/212)	47%*	(103/219)
Naproxen 500 mg BID	44%*	(100/225)	53%**	(115/219)
Placebo	32%	(70/222)	32%	(71/220)

* p<0.01;
** p<0.001 compared to placebo

Figure 1

Incidence of Endoscopically Observed Gastroduodenal Ulcers in OA Patients

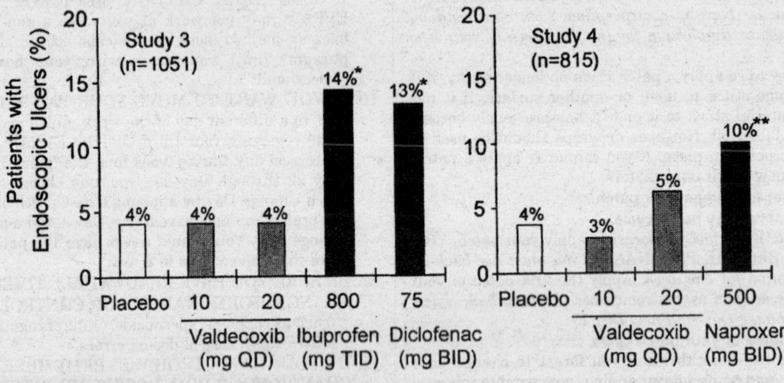

* Significantly different vs placebo and both valdecoxib treatment groups; p<0.05
** Significantly different vs placebo and valdecoxib 10 mg; p<0.05

Primary Dysmenorrhea

BEXTRA was compared to naproxen sodium 550 mg in two placebo-controlled studies of women with moderate to severe primary dysmenorrhea. The onset of analgesia was within 60 minutes for BEXTRA 20 mg. The onset, magnitude, and duration of analgesic effect with BEXTRA 20 mg were comparable to naproxen sodium 550 mg.

Safety Studies

Gastrointestinal (GI) Endoscopy Studies with Therapeutic Doses: Scheduled upper GI endoscopic evaluations were performed with BEXTRA at doses of 10 and 20 mg daily in over 800 OA patients who were enrolled into two randomized 3-month studies using active comparators and placebo controls (Study 3 and Study 4). These studies enrolled patients free of endoscopic ulcers at baseline and compared rates of endoscopic ulcers, defined as any gastroduodenal ulcer seen endoscopically provided it was of "unequivocal depth" and at least 3 mm in diameter.

In both studies, BEXTRA 10 mg daily was associated with a statistically significant lower incidence of endoscopic gastroduodenal ulcers over the study period compared to the active comparators. Figure 1 summarizes the incidence of gastroduodenal ulcers in Studies 3 and 4 for the placebo, valdecoxib, and active control arms.

[See figure 1 above]

Safety Study with Supratherapeutic Doses: Scheduled upper GI endoscopic evaluations were performed in a randomized 6-month study of 1217 patients with OA and RA comparing valdecoxib 20 mg BID (40 mg daily) and 40 mg BID (80 mg daily) (4 to 8 times the recommended therapeutic dose) to naproxen 500 mg BID (Study 5). This study also formally assessed renal events as a primary outcome with supratherapeutic doses of BEXTRA. The renal endpoint was defined as any of the following: new/increase in edema, new/increase in congestive heart failure, increase in blood pressure (BP; >20 mm Hg systolic, >10 mm Hg diastolic), new/increase in BP treatment, new/increase in diuretic therapy, creatinine increase over 30% (or >1.2 mg/dL if baseline <0.9 mg/dL), BUN increase over 200% or >50 mg/dL, 24-hr urinary protein increase to >500 mg (if baseline 0–150 mg or >750 if baseline 151–300 or >1000 if baseline 301–500), serum potassium increase to >6 mEq/L, or serum sodium decrease to <130 mEq/L.

Figure 2 summarizes the incidence rates of gastroduodenal ulcers and renal events that were seen in Study 5. BEXTRA 40 mg daily and 80 mg daily were associated with a statistically significant lower incidence of endoscopic gastroduodenal ulcers over the study period compared to naproxen. The incidence of renal events was significantly different between the BEXTRA 80 mg daily group and naproxen. The clinical relevance of renal events observed with supratherapeutic doses (4 to 8 times the recommended therapeutic dose) of BEXTRA is not known (see PRECAUTIONS—Renal Effects).

[See figure 2 at top of next page]

Renal Safety at the Therapeutic Chronic Dose: The renal effects of valdecoxib compared with placebo and conventional NSAIDs were also assessed by prospectively designed pooled analyses of renal events data (see definition above—Supratherapeutic Doses) from five placebo- and active-controlled 12-week arthritis trials that included 995 OA or RA patients given valdecoxib 10 mg daily. The incidence of renal events observed in this analysis with valdecoxib 10 mg daily (3%), ibuprofen 800 mg TID (7%), naproxen 500 mg BID (2%) and diclofenac 75 mg BID (4%) were significantly higher than placebo-treated patients (1%). In all treatment groups, the majority of renal events were either due to the occurrence of edema or worsening BP.

Gastrointestinal Ulcers in High-Risk Patients: Subset analyses were performed of patients with risk factors (age, concomitant low-dose aspirin use, history of prior ulcer disease) enrolled in four upper GI endoscopic studies. Table 3 summarizes the trends seen.

[See table above]

The correlation between findings of endoscopic studies, and the incidence of clinically significant serious upper GI events has not been established.

Platelets: In four clinical studies with young and elderly (≥65 years) subjects, single and multiple doses up to 7 days of BEXTRA 10 to 40 mg BID had no effect on platelet aggregation.

INDICATIONS AND USAGE

BEXTRA Tablets are indicated:

- For relief of the signs and symptoms of osteoarthritis and adult rheumatoid arthritis.
- For the treatment of primary dysmenorrhea.

CONTRAINDICATIONS

BEXTRA Tablets are contraindicated in patients with known hypersensitivity to valdecoxib. BEXTRA should not be given to patients who have experienced asthma, urticaria, or allergic-type reactions after taking aspirin or NSAIDs. Severe, rarely fatal, anaphylactic-like reactions to NSAIDs are possible in such patients (see WARNINGS—Anaphylactoid Reactions, and PRECAUTIONS—Pre-existing Asthma).

WARNINGS

Gastrointestinal (GI) Effects—Risk of GI Ulceration, Bleeding, and Perforation

Serious gastrointestinal toxicity such as bleeding, ulceration and perforation of the stomach, small intestine or large intestine can occur at any time with or without warning symptoms in patients treated with nonsteroidal anti-inflammatory drugs (NSAIDs). Minor gastrointestinal problems such as dyspepsia are common and may also occur at any time during NSAID therapy. Therefore, physicians and patients should remain alert for ulceration and bleeding even in the absence of previous GI tract symptoms. Patients should be informed about the signs and symptoms of serious GI toxicity and the steps to take if they occur. The utility of periodic laboratory monitoring has not been demonstrated, nor has it been adequately assessed. Only one in five patients who develop a serious upper GI adverse event on NSAID therapy is symptomatic. It has been demonstrated that upper GI ulcers, gross bleeding or perforation caused by NSAIDs appear to occur in approximately 1% of patients treated for 3 to 6 months and 2–4% of patients treated for one year. These trends continue, thus increasing the likelihood of developing a serious GI event at some time during the course of therapy. However, even short-term therapy is not without risk.

NSAIDs should be prescribed with extreme caution in patients with a prior history of ulcer disease or gastrointestinal bleeding. Most spontaneous reports of fatal GI events are in elderly or debilitated patients and therefore special care should be taken in treating this population. For high risk patients, alternate therapies that do not involve NSAIDs should be considered.

Studies have shown that patients with a *prior history of peptic ulcer disease and/or gastrointestinal bleeding* and who use NSAIDs, have a greater than 10-fold higher risk for developing a GI bleed than patients with neither of these risk factors. In addition to a past history of ulcer disease, pharmacoepidemiological studies have identified several other co-therapies or co-morbid conditions that may increase the risk for GI bleeding such as: treatment with oral corticosteroids, treatment with anticoagulants, longer duration of NSAID therapy, smoking, alcoholism, older age, and poor general health status. (See CLINICAL STUDIES—Safety Studies.)

Anaphylactoid Reactions

Anaphylactoid reactions were not reported in patients receiving BEXTRA in clinical trials. However, as with NSAIDs in general, anaphylactoid reactions may occur in patients without known prior exposure to BEXTRA. BEXTRA should not be given to patients with the aspirin triad. This symptom complex typically occurs in asthmatic patients who experience rhinitis with or without nasal polyps, or who exhibit severe, potentially fatal bronchospasm after taking aspirin or other NSAIDs (see CONTRAINDICATIONS and PRECAUTIONS—Pre-existing Asthma). Emergency help should be sought in cases where an anaphylactoid reaction occurs.

Advanced Renal Disease

No information is available regarding the safe use of BEXTRA Tablets in patients with advanced kidney disease. Therefore, treatment with BEXTRA is not recommended in these patients. If therapy with BEXTRA must be initiated, close monitoring of the patient's kidney function is advisable (see PRECAUTIONS—Renal Effects).

Pregnancy

In late pregnancy, BEXTRA should be avoided because it may cause premature closure of the ductus arteriosus.

PRECAUTIONS

General

BEXTRA Tablets cannot be expected to substitute for corticosteroids or to treat corticosteroid insufficiency. Abrupt discontinuation of corticosteroids may lead to exacerbation of corticosteroid-responsive illness. Patients on prolonged corticosteroid therapy should have their therapy tapered slowly if a decision is made to discontinue corticosteroids.

Figure 2
Incidence of Endoscopic Gastroduodenal Ulcers and Renal Events in the High-Dose Safety Study

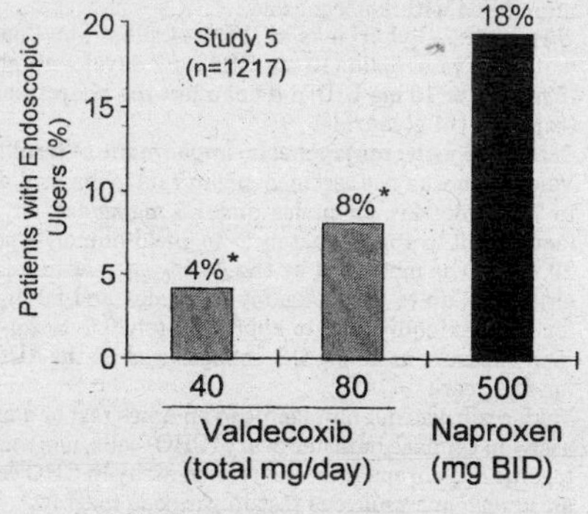

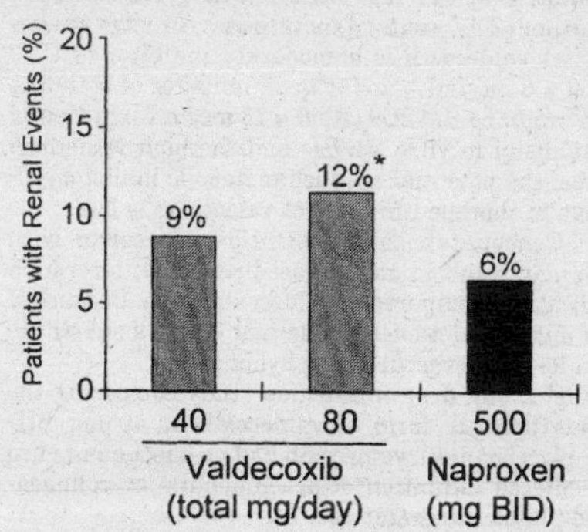

* Significantly different vs naproxen, p<0.05

Table 3
Incidence of Endoscopic Gastroduodenal Ulcers in Patients With and Without Selected Risk Factors

	Placebo-controlled Studies		Active-Controlled Studies			
Risk Factor	Placebo	Valdecoxib (10–20 mg daily)	Valdecoxib (10–80 mg daily)	Ibuprofen 800 mg TID	Naproxen 500 mg BID	Diclofenac 75 mg BID
Age						
<65 yrs	3.7% (8/219)	3.5% (17/484)	3.7% (48/1306)	8.2% (9/110)	12.8% (51/397)	13.2% (34/258)
≥65 yrs	5.8% (8/137)	4.6% (12/262)	7.6% (43/568)	21.6% (16/74)	22.0% (33/150)	18.2% (25/137)
Concomitant Low Dose Aspirin Use						
no	4.4% (13/298)	3.2% (21/650)	3.8% (64/1671)	9.8% (15/153)	16.0% (75/468)	12.8% (45/351)
yes	5.2% (3/58)	8.3% (8/96)	13.3% (27/203)	32.3% (10/31)	11.4% (9/79)	31.8% (14/44)
History of Ulcer Disease						
no	4.4% (14/317)	3.4% (22/647)	4.1% (681/1666)	13.8% (22/160)	13.3% (63/475)	14.7% (52/354)
yes	5.1% (2/39)	7.1% (7/99)	11.1% (23/208)	12.5% (3/24)	29.2% (21/72)	17.1% (7/41)

No statistical conclusions can be drawn from these comparisons.

The pharmacological activity of valdecoxib in reducing fever and inflammation may diminish the utility of these diagnostic signs in detecting complications of presumed noninfectious, painful conditions.

Hepatic Effects

Borderline elevations of one or more liver tests may occur in up to 15% of patients taking NSAIDs. Notable elevations of ALT or AST (approximately three or more times the upper limit of normal) have been reported in approximately 1% of patients in clinical trials with NSAIDs. These laboratory abnormalities may progress, may remain unchanged, or may remain transient with continuing therapy. Rare cases of severe hepatic reactions, including jaundice and fatal fulminant hepatitis, liver necrosis and hepatic failure (some with fatal outcome) have been reported with NSAIDs. In controlled clinical trials of valdecoxib, the incidence of borderline (defined as 1.2- to 3.0-fold) elevations of liver tests was 8.0% for valdecoxib and 8.4% for placebo, while approximately 0.3% of patients taking valdecoxib, and 0.2% of patients taking placebo, had notable (defined as greater than 3-fold) elevations of ALT or AST.

A patient with symptoms and/or signs suggesting liver dysfunction, or in whom an abnormal liver test has occurred, should be monitored carefully for evidence of the development of a more severe hepatic reaction while on therapy with BEXTRA. If clinical signs and symptoms consistent with liver disease develop, or if systemic manifestations occur (e.g., eosinophilia, rash), BEXTRA should be discontinued.

Renal Effects

Long-term administration of NSAIDs has resulted in renal papillary necrosis and other renal injury. Renal toxicity has also been seen in patients in whom renal prostaglandins have a compensatory role in the maintenance of renal perfusion. In these patients, administration of a nonsteroidal anti-inflammatory drug may cause a dose-dependent reduction in prostaglandin formation and, secondarily, in renal blood flow, which may precipitate overt renal decompensation. Patients at greatest risk of this reaction are those with impaired renal function, heart failure, liver dysfunction, those taking diuretics and Angiotensin Converting Enzyme (ACE) inhibitors, and the elderly. Discontinuation of NSAID therapy is usually followed by recovery to the pretreatment state.

Caution should be used when initiating treatment with BEXTRA in patients with considerable dehydration. It is advisable to rehydrate patients first and then start therapy with BEXTRA. Caution is also recommended in patients with pre-existing kidney disease. (See WARNINGS—Advanced Renal Disease.)

Hematological Effects

Anemia is sometimes seen in patients receiving BEXTRA. Patients on long-term treatment with BEXTRA should have their hemoglobin or hematocrit checked if they exhibit any signs or symptoms of anemia.

BEXTRA does not generally affect platelet counts, prothrombin time (PT), or partial prothrombin time (PTT), and does not appear to inhibit platelet aggregation at indicated dosages (See CLINICAL STUDIES—Safety Studies—Platelets).

Fluid Retention and Edema

Fluid retention and edema have been observed in some patients taking BEXTRA (see ADVERSE REACTIONS). Therefore, BEXTRA should be used with caution in patients with fluid retention, hypertension, or heart failure.

Preexisting Asthma

Patients with asthma may have aspirin-sensitive asthma. The use of aspirin in patients with aspirin-sensitive asthma has been associated with severe bronchospasm, which can be fatal. Since cross reactivity, including bronchospasm, between aspirin and other nonsteroidal anti-inflammatory drugs has been reported in such aspirin-sensitive patients, BEXTRA should not be administered to patients with this form of aspirin sensitivity and should be used with caution in patients with preexisting asthma.

Information for Patients

BEXTRA can cause GI discomfort and, rarely, more serious GI side effects, which may result in hospitalization and even fatal outcomes. Although serious GI tract ulcerations and bleeding can occur without warning symptoms, patients should be alert for the signs and symptoms of ulcerations and bleeding, and should ask for medical advice when observing any indicative sign or symptoms. Patients should be apprised of the importance of this follow-up (see WARNINGS—Gastrointestinal (GI) Effects—Risk of GI Ulceration, Bleeding, and Perforation).

Patients should report to their physicians, signs or symptoms of gastrointestinal ulceration or bleeding, skin rash, weight gain, or edema.

Patients should be informed of the warning signs and symptoms of hepatotoxicity (e.g., nausea, fatigue, lethargy, pruritus, jaundice, right upper quadrant tenderness, and flu-like symptoms). If these occur, patients should be instructed to stop therapy and seek immediate medical attention.

Patients should also be instructed to seek immediate emergency help in the case of an anaphylactoid reaction (see WARNINGS—Anaphylactoid Reactions).

In late pregnancy, BEXTRA should be avoided because it may cause premature closure of the ductus arteriosus.

Laboratory Tests

Because serious GI tract ulcerations and bleeding can occur without warning symptoms, physicians should monitor for signs and symptoms of GI bleeding.

Drug Interactions

The drug interaction studies with valdecoxib were performed both with valdecoxib and a rapidly hydrolyzed intravenous prodrug form. The results from trials using the intravenous prodrug are reported in this section as they relate to the role of valdecoxib in drug interactions.

Continued on next page

Bextra—Cont.

General: In humans, valdecoxib metabolism is predominantly mediated via CYP 3A4 and 2C9 with glucuronidation being a further (20%) route of metabolism. In vitro studies indicate that valdecoxib is a moderate inhibitor of CYP 2C19 (IC50 = 6 mcg/mL), and a weak inhibitor of both 3A4 (IC50 = 44 mcg/mL) and 2C9 (IC50 = 13 mcg/mL). In view of the limitations of in vitro studies and the high valdecoxib IC50 values, the potential for such metabolic inhibitory effects in vivo at therapeutic doses of valdecoxib is low.

Aspirin: Concomitant administration of aspirin with valdecoxib may result in an increased risk of GI ulceration and complications compared to valdecoxib alone. Because of its lack of anti-platelet effect valdecoxib is not a substitute for aspirin for cardiovascular prophylaxis.

In a parallel group drug interaction study comparing the intravenous prodrug form of valdecoxib at 40 mg BID (n=10) vs. placebo (n=9), valdecoxib had no effect on in vitro aspirin-mediated inhibition of arachidonate- or collagen-stimulated platelet aggregation.

Methotrexate: Valdecoxib 10 mg BID did not show a significant effect on the plasma exposure or renal clearance of methotrexate.

ACE-inhibitors: Reports suggest that NSAIDs may diminish the antihypertensive effect of ACE-inhibitors. This interaction should be given consideration in patients taking BEXTRA concomitantly with ACE-inhibitors.

Furosemide: Clinical studies, as well as post-marketing observations, have shown that NSAIDs can reduce the natriuretic effect of furosemide and thiazides in some patients. This response has been attributed to inhibition of renal prostaglandin synthesis.

Anticonvulsants: Anticonvulsant drug interaction studies with valdecoxib have not been conducted. As with other drugs, routine monitoring should be performed when therapy with BEXTRA is either initiated or discontinued in patients on anticonvulsant therapy.

Dextromethorphan: Dextromethorphan is primarily metabolized by CYP 2D6 and to a lesser extent by 3A4. Coadministration with valdecoxib (40 mg BID for 7 days) resulted in a significant increase in dextromethorphan plasma levels suggesting that, at these doses, valdecoxib is a weak inhibitor of 2D6. Dextromethorphan plasma concentrations in the presence of high doses of valdecoxib were almost 5-fold lower than those seen in CYP 2D6 poor metabolizers.

Lithium: Valdecoxib 40 mg BID for 7 days produced significant decreases in lithium serum clearance (25%) and renal clearance (30%) with a 34% higher serum exposure compared to lithium alone. Lithium serum concentrations should be monitored closely when initiating or changing therapy with BEXTRA in patients receiving lithium. Lithium carbonate (450 mg BID for 7 days) had no effect on valdecoxib pharmacokinetics.

Warfarin: The effect of valdecoxib on the anticoagulant effect of warfarin (1–8 mg/day) was studied in healthy subjects by coadministration of BEXTRA 40 mg BID for 7 days. Valdecoxib caused a statistically significant increase in plasma exposures of R-warfarin and S-warfarin (12% and 15%, respectively), and in the pharmacodynamic effects (prothrombin time, measured as INR) of warfarin. While mean INR values were only slightly increased with coadministration of valdecoxib, the day-to-day variability in individual INR values was increased. Anticoagulant therapy should be monitored, particularly during the first few weeks, after initiating therapy with BEXTRA in patients receiving warfarin or similar agents.

Fluconazole and Ketoconazole: Ketoconazole and fluconazole are predominantly CYP 3A4 and 2C9 inhibitors, respectively. Concomitant single dose administration of valdecoxib 20 mg with multiple doses of ketoconazole and fluconazole produced a significant increase in exposure of valdecoxib. Plasma exposure (AUC) to valdecoxib was increased 62% when coadministered with fluconazole and 38% when coadministered with ketoconazole.

Glyburide: Glyburide is a CYP 3A4 substrate. Coadministration of valdecoxib (10 mg BID for 7 days) with glyburide (5 mg QD or 10 mg BID) did not affect the pharmacokinetics (exposure) of glyburide.

Carcinogenesis, mutagenesis, impairment of fertility

Valdecoxib was not carcinogenic in rats given oral doses up to 7.5 mg/kg/day for males and 1.5 mg/kg/day for females (equivalent to approximately 2- to 6-fold human exposure at 20 mg QD as measured by the $AUC_{(0-24hr)}$) or in mice given oral doses up to 25 mg/kg/day for males and 50 mg/kg/day for females (equivalent to approximately 0.6- to 2.4-fold human exposure at 20 mg QD as measured by the $AUC_{(0-24hr)}$) for two years.

Valdecoxib was not mutagenic in an Ames test or a mutation assay in Chinese hamster ovary (CHO) cells, nor was it clastogenic in a chromosome aberration assay in CHO cells or in an *in vivo* micronucleus test in rat bone marrow.

Valdecoxib did not impair male rat fertility at oral doses up to 9.0 mg/kg/day (equivalent to approximately 3- to 6-fold human exposure at 20 mg QD as measured by the $AUC_{(0-24hr)}$). In female rats, a decrease in ovulation with increased pre- and post-implantation loss resulted in decreased live embryos/fetuses at doses ≥2 mg/kg/day (equivalent to approximately 2-fold human exposure at 20 mg QD as measured by the $AUC_{(0-24hr)}$ for valdecoxib). The effects on female fertility were reversible. This effect is expected with inhibition of prostaglandin synthesis and is not the result of irreversible alteration of female reproductive function.

Pregnancy

Teratogenic Effects: Pregnancy Category C.

The incidence of fetuses with skeletal anomalies such as semi-bipartite thoracic vertebra centra and fused sternebrae was slightly higher in rabbits at an oral dose of 40 mg/kg/day (equivalent to approximately 72-fold human exposures at 20 mg QD as measured by the $AUC_{(0-24hr)}$) throughout organogenesis.

Valdecoxib was not teratogenic in rabbits up to an oral dose of 10 mg/kg/day (equivalent to approximately 8-fold human exposures at 20 mg QD as measured by the $AUC_{(0-24hr)}$).

Valdecoxib was not teratogenic in rats up to an oral dose of 10 mg/kg/day (equivalent to approximately 19-fold human exposure at 20 mg QD as measured by the $AUC_{(0-24hr)}$). There are no studies in pregnant women. However, valdecoxib crosses the placenta in rats and rabbits. BEXTRA should be used during pregnancy only if the potential benefit justifies the potential risk to the fetus.

Non-Teratogenic Effects: Valdecoxib caused increased pre- and post-implantation loss with reduced live fetuses at oral doses ≥10 mg/kg/day (equivalent to approximately 19-fold human exposure at 20 mg QD as measured by the $AUC_{(0-24hr)}$) in rats and an oral dose of 40 mg/kg/day (equivalent to approximately 72-fold human exposure at 20 mg QD as measured by the $AUC_{(0-24hr)}$) in rabbits throughout organogenesis. In addition, reduced neonatal survival and decreased neonatal body weight when rats were treated with valdecoxib at oral doses ≥6 mg/kg/day (equivalent to approximately 7-fold human exposure at 20 mg QD as measured by the $AUC_{(0-24hr)}$) throughout organogenesis and lactation period. No studies have been conducted to evaluate the effect of valdecoxib on the closure of the ductus arteriosus in humans. Therefore, as with other drugs known to inhibit prostaglandin synthesis, use of BEXTRA during the third trimester of pregnancy should be avoided.

Labor and Delivery

Valdecoxib produced no evidence of delayed labor or parturition at oral doses up to 10 mg/kg/day in rats (equivalent to approximately 19-fold human exposure at 20 mg QD as measured by the $AUC_{(0-24hr)}$). The effects of BEXTRA on labor and delivery in pregnant women are unknown.

Nursing Mothers

Valdecoxib and its active metabolite are excreted in the milk of lactating rats. It is not known whether this drug is excreted in human milk. Because many drugs are excreted in human milk, and because of the potential for adverse reactions in nursing infants from BEXTRA, a decision should be made whether to discontinue nursing or to discontinue the drug, taking into account the importance of the drug to the mother and the importance of nursing to the infant.

Pediatric Use

Safety and effectiveness of BEXTRA in pediatric patients below the age of 18 years have not been evaluated.

Geriatric Use

Of the patients who received BEXTRA in arthritis clinical trials of three months duration, or greater, approximately 2100 were 65 years of age or older, including 570 patients who were 75 years or older. No overall differences in effectiveness were observed between these patients and younger patients.

ADVERSE REACTIONS

Of the patients treated with BEXTRA Tablets in controlled arthritis trials, 2665 were patients with OA, and 2684 were patients with RA. More than 4000 patients have received a chronic total daily dose of BEXTRA 10 mg or more. More than 2800 patients have received BEXTRA 10 mg/day, or more, for at least 6 months and 988 of these have received BEXTRA for at least 1 year.

Osteoarthritis and Rheumatoid Arthritis

Table 4 lists all adverse events, regardless of causality, that occurred in ≥2.0% of patients receiving BEXTRA 10 and 20 mg/day in studies of three months or longer from 7 controlled studies conducted in patients with OA or RA that included a placebo and/or a positive control group.

[See table below]

Table 4
Adverse Events with Incidence ≥2.0% in Valdecoxib Treatment Groups: Controlled Arthritis Trials of Three Months or Longer

		(Total Daily Dose)				
		Valdecoxib		Diclofenac	Ibuprofen	Naproxen
Adverse Event	**Placebo**	**10 mg**	**20 mg**	**150 mg**	**2400 mg**	**1000 mg**
Number Treated	973	1214	1358	711	207	766
Autonomic Nervous System Disorders						
Hypertension	0.6	1.6	2.1	2.5	2.4	1.7
Body as a Whole						
Back pain	1.6	1.6	2.7	2.8	1.4	1.0
Edema peripheral	0.7	2.4	3.0	3.2	2.9	2.1
Influenza-like symptoms	2.2	2.0	2.2	3.1	2.9	2.0
Injury accidental	2.8	4.0	3.7	3.9	3.9	3.0
Central and Peripheral Nervous System Disorders						
Dizziness	2.1	2.6	2.7	4.2	3.4	2.7
Headache	7.1	4.8	8.5	6.6	4.3	5.5
Gastrointestinal System Disorders						
Abdominal fullness	2.0	2.1	1.9	3.0	2.9	2.5
Abdominal pain	6.3	7.0	8.2	17.0	8.2	10.1
Diarrhea	4.2	5.4	6.0	10.8	3.9	4.7
Dyspepsia	6.3	7.9	8.7	13.4	15.0	12.9
Flatulence	4.1	2.9	3.5	3.1	7.7	5.4
Nausea	5.9	7.0	6.3	8.4	7.7	8.7
Musculoskeletal System Disorders						
Myalgia	1.6	2.0	1.9	2.4	2.4	1.4
Respiratory System Disorders						
Sinusitis	2.2	2.6	1.8	1.1	3.4	3.4
Upper Respiratory Tract Infection	6.0	6.7	5.7	6.3	4.3	6.4
Skin and Appendages disorders						
Rash	1.0	1.4	2.1	1.5	0.5	1.4

In these placebo- and active-controlled clinical trials, the discontinuation rate due to adverse events was 7.5% for arthritis patients receiving valdecoxib 10 mg daily, 7.9% for arthritis patients receiving valdecoxib 20 mg daily and 6.0% for patients receiving placebo.

In the seven controlled OA and RA studies, the following adverse events occurred in 0.1–1.9% of patients treated with BEXTRA 10–20 mg daily, regardless of causality.

Application site disorders: Cellulitis, dermatitis contact

Cardiovascular: Aggravated hypertension, aneurysm, angina pectoris, arrhythmia, cardiomyopathy, congestive heart failure, coronary artery disorder, heart murmur, hypotension

Central, peripheral nervous system: Cerebrovascular disorder, hypertonia, hypoesthesia, migraine, neuralgia, neuropathy, paresthesia, tremor, twitching, vertigo

Endocrine: Goiter

Female reproductive: Amenorrhea, dysmenorrhea, leukorrhea, mastitis, menstrual disorder, menorrhagia, menstrual bloating, vaginal hemorrhage

Gastrointestinal: Abnormal stools, constipation, diverticulosis, dry mouth, duodenal ulcer, duodenitis, eructation, esophagitis, fecal incontinence, gastric ulcer, gastritis, gastroenteritis, gastroesophageal reflux, hematemesis, hematochezia, hemorrhoids, hemorrhoids bleeding, hiatal hernia, melena, stomatitis, stool frequency increased, tenesmus, tooth disorder, vomiting

General: Allergy aggravated, allergic reaction, asthenia, chest pain, chills, cyst NOS, edema generalized, face edema, fatigue, fever, hot flushes, halitosis, malaise, pain, periorbital swelling, peripheral pain

Hearing and vestibular: Ear abnormality, earache, tinnitus

Heart rate and rhythm: Bradycardia, palpitation, tachycardia

Hemic: Anemia

Liver and biliary system: Hepatic function abnormal, hepatitis, ALT increased, AST increased

Male reproductive: Impotence, prostatic disorder

Metabolic and nutritional: Alkaline phosphatase increased, BUN increased, CPK increased, creatinine increased, diabetes mellitus, glycosuria, gout, hypercholesterolemia, hyperglycemia, hyperkalemia, hyperlipemia, hyperuricemia, hypocalcemia, hypokalemia, LDH increased, thirst increased, weight decrease, weight increase, xerophthalmia

Musculoskeletal: Arthralgia, fracture accidental, neck stiffness, osteoporosis, synovitis, tendonitis

Neoplasm: Breast neoplasm, lipoma, malignant ovarian cyst

Platelets (bleeding or clotting): Ecchymosis, epistaxis, hematoma NOS, thrombocytopenia

Psychiatric: Anorexia, anxiety, appetite increased, confusion, depression, depression aggravated, insomnia, nervousness, morbid dreaming, somnolence

Resistance mechanism disorders: Herpes simplex, herpes zoster, infection fungal, infection soft tissue, infection viral, moniliasis, moniliasis genital, otitis media

Respiratory: Abnormal breath sounds, bronchitis, bronchospasm, coughing, dyspnea, emphysema, laryngitis, pneumonia, pharyngitis, pleurisy, rhinitis

Skin and appendages: Acne, alopecia, dermatitis, dermatitis fungal, eczema, photosensitivity allergic reaction, pruritus, rash erythematous, rash maculopapular, rash psoriaform, skin dry, skin hypertrophy, skin ulceration, sweating increased, urticaria

Special senses: Taste perversion

Urinary system: Albuminuria, cystitis, dysuria, hematuria, micturition frequency increased, pyuria, urinary incontinence, urinary tract infection

Vascular: Claudication intermittent, hemangioma acquired, varicose vein

Vision: Blurred vision, cataract, conjunctival hemorrhage, conjunctivitis, eye pain, keratitis, vision abnormal

White Cell and RES Disorders: Eosinophilia, leukopenia, leukocytosis, lymphadenopathy, lymphangitis, lymphopenia

Other serious adverse events that were reported rarely (estimated <0.1%) in clinical trials, regardless of causality, in patients taking BEXTRA:

Autonomic nervous system disorders: Hypertensive encephalopathy, vasospasm

Cardiovascular: Abnormal ECG, aortic stenosis, atrial fibrillation, carotid stenosis, coronary thrombosis, heart block, heart valve disorders, mitral insufficiency, myocardial infarction, myocardial ischemia, pericarditis, syncope, thrombophlebitis, unstable angina, ventricular fibrillation

Central, peripheral nervous system: Convulsions

Endocrine: Hyperparathyroidism

Female reproductive: Cervical dysplasia

Gastrointestinal: Appendicitis, colitis with bleeding, dysphagia, esophageal perforation, gastrointestinal bleeding, ileus, intestinal obstruction, peritonitis

Hemic: Lymphoma-like disorder, pancytopenia

Liver and biliary system: Cholelithiasis

Metabolic: Dehydration

Musculoskeletal: Pathological fracture, osteomyelitis

Neoplasm: Benign brain neoplasm, bladder carcinoma, carcinoma, gastric carcinoma, prostate carcinoma, pulmonary carcinoma

Platelets (bleeding or clotting): Embolism, pulmonary embolism, thrombosis

Psychiatric: Manic reaction, psychosis

Renal: Acute renal failure

Resistance mechanism disorders: Sepsis

Respiratory: Apnea, pleural effusion, pulmonary edema, pulmonary fibrosis, pulmonary infarction, pulmonary hemorrhage, respiratory insufficiency

Skin: Basal cell carcinoma, malignant melanoma

Urinary system: Pyelonephritis, renal calculus

Vision: Retinal detachment

OVERDOSAGE

Symptoms following acute NSAID overdoses are usually limited to lethargy, drowsiness, nausea, vomiting, and epigastric pain, which are generally reversible with supportive care. Gastrointestinal bleeding can occur. Hypertension, acute renal failure, respiratory depression and coma may occur, but are rare.

Anaphylactoid reactions have been reported with therapeutic ingestion of NSAIDs, and may occur following an overdose.

Patients should be managed by symptomatic and supportive care following an NSAID overdose. There are no specific antidotes. Hemodialysis removed only about 2% of administered valdecoxib from the systemic circulation of 8 patients with end-stage renal disease and, based on its degree of plasma protein binding (>98%), dialysis is unlikely to be useful in overdose. Forced diuresis, alkalinization of urine, or hemoperfusion also may not be useful due to high protein binding.

DOSAGE AND ADMINISTRATION

Osteoarthritis and Adult Rheumatoid Arthritis

The recommended dose of BEXTRA Tablets for the relief of the signs and symptoms of arthritis is 10 mg once daily.

Primary Dysmenorrhea

The recommended dose of BEXTRA Tablets for treatment of primary dysmenorrhea is 20 mg twice daily, as needed.

HOW SUPPLIED

BEXTRA Tablets 10 mg are white, film-coated, and capsule-shaped, debossed "10" on one side with a four pointed star shape on the other, supplied as:

NDC Number	Size
0025-1975-31	Bottle of 100
0025-1975-51	Bottle of 500
0025-1975-34	Carton of 100 unit dose

BEXTRA Tablets 20 mg are white, film-coated, and capsule-shaped, debossed "20" on one side with a four pointed star shape on the other, supplied as:

NDC Number	Size
0025-1980-31	Bottle of 100
0025-1980-51	Bottle of 500
0025-1980-34	Carton of 100 unit dose

Store at 25°C (77°F); excursions permitted to 15°–30°C (59°–86°F). [See USP Controlled Room Temperature]

Rx only

November 2001

Manufactured for:
G.D. Searle LLC
A subsidiary of Pharmacia Corporation
Chicago, IL 60680 USA
Pfizer Inc
New York, NY 10017, USA
by: Searle Ltd.
Caguas, PR 00725

818 763 000 P04001 / PS4001

Pharmacia & Upjohn

100 ROUTE 206 NORTH
PEAPACK, NEW JERSEY 07977

Direct Inquiries to:
1-888-768-5501

For Medical and Pharmaceutical Information, Including Emergencies, Contact:
800-323-4204 or www.MEDINFO@pharmacia.com

CAMPTOSAR® ℞

irinotecan hydrochloride injection
For Intravenous Use Only

WARNINGS

CAMPTOSAR Injection should be administered only under the supervision of a physician who is experienced in the use of cancer chemotherapeutic agents. Appropriate management of complications is possible only when adequate diagnostic and treatment facilities are readily available.

CAMPTOSAR can induce both early and late forms of diarrhea that appear to be mediated by different mechanisms. Both forms of diarrhea may be severe. Early diarrhea (occurring during or shortly after infusion of CAMPTOSAR) may be accompanied by cholinergic symptoms of rhinitis, increased salivation, miosis, lacrimation, diaphoresis, flushing, and intestinal hyperperistalsis that can cause abdominal cramping. Early diarrhea and other cholinergic symptoms may be prevented or ameliorated by atropine (see PRECAUTIONS, General). Late diarrhea (generally occurring more than 24 hours after administration of CAMPTOSAR) can be life threatening since it may be prolonged and may lead to dehydration, electrolyte imbalance, or sepsis. Late diarrhea should be treated promptly with loperamide. Patients with diarrhea should be carefully monitored and given fluid and electrolyte replacement if they become dehydrated or antibiotic therapy if they develop ileus, fever, or severe neutropenia (see WARNINGS). Administration of CAMPTOSAR should be interrupted and subsequent doses reduced if severe diarrhea occurs (see DOSAGE AND ADMINISTRATION).

Severe myelosuppression may occur (see WARNINGS).

DESCRIPTION

CAMPTOSAR Injection (irinotecan hydrochloride injection) is an antineoplastic agent of the topoisomerase I inhibitor class. Irinotecan hydrochloride was clinically investigated as CPT-11.

CAMPTOSAR is supplied as a sterile, pale yellow, clear, aqueous solution. It is available in two single-dose sizes: 2 mL-fill vials contain 40 mg irinotecan hydrochloride and 5 mL-fill vials contain 100 mg irinotecan hydrochloride. Each milliliter of solution contains 20 mg of irinotecan hydrochloride (on the basis of the trihydrate salt), 45 mg of sorbitol NF powder, and 0.9 mg of lactic acid, USP. The pH of the solution has been adjusted to 3.5 (range, 3.0 to 3.8) with sodium hydroxide or hydrochloric acid. CAMPTOSAR is intended for dilution with 5% Dextrose Injection, USP (D5W), or 0.9% Sodium Chloride Injection, USP, prior to intravenous infusion. The preferred diluent is 5% Dextrose Injection, USP.

Irinotecan hydrochloride is a semisynthetic derivative of camptothecin, an alkaloid extract from plants such as *Camptotheca acuminata*. The chemical name is ***(S)***-4,11-diethyl-3,4,12,14-tetrahydro-4-hydroxy-3,14-dioxo-1***H***-pyrano[3′,4′:6,7]-indolizino[1,2-b]quinolin-9-yl-[1,4′-bipiperidine]-1′-carboxylate, monohydrochloride, trihydrate. Its structural formula is as follows:

Irinotecan Hydrochloride

Irinotecan hydrochloride is a pale yellow to yellow crystalline powder, with the empirical formula $C_{33}H_{38}N_4O_6 \bullet HCl \bullet 3\ H_2O$ and a molecular weight of 677.19. It is slightly soluble in water and organic solvents.

CLINICAL PHARMACOLOGY

Irinotecan is a derivative of camptothecin. Camptothecins interact specifically with the enzyme topoisomerase I which relieves torsional strain in DNA by inducing reversible single-strand breaks. Irinotecan and its active metabolite SN-38 bind to the topoisomerase I-DNA complex and prevent religation of these single-strand breaks. Current research suggests that the cytotoxicity of irinotecan is due to double-strand DNA damage produced during DNA synthesis when replication enzymes interact with the ternary complex formed by topoisomerase I, DNA, and either irinotecan or SN-38. Mammalian cells cannot efficiently repair these double-strand breaks.

Irinotecan serves as a water-soluble precursor of the lipophilic metabolite SN-38. SN-38 is formed from irinotecan by carboxylesterase-mediated cleavage of the carbamate bond between the camptothecin moiety and the dipiperidino side chain. SN-38 is approximately 1000 times as potent as irinotecan as an inhibitor of topoisomerase I purified from human and rodent tumor cell lines. In vitro cytotoxicity assays show that the potency of SN-38 relative to irinotecan varies from 2- to 2000-fold. However, the plasma area under the concentration versus time curve (AUC) values for SN-38 are 2% to 8% of irinotecan and SN-38 is 95% bound to plasma proteins compared to approximately 50% bound to plasma proteins for irinotecan (see Pharmacokinetics). The precise contribution of SN-38 to the activity of CAMPTOSAR is thus unknown. Both irinotecan and SN-38 exist in an active lactone form and an inactive hydroxy acid anion form. A pH-dependent equilibrium exists between the two forms such that an acid pH promotes the formation of the lactone, while a more basic pH favors the hydroxy acid anion form.

Administration of irinotecan has resulted in antitumor activity in mice bearing cancers of rodent origin and in human carcinoma xenografts of various histological types.

Pharmacokinetics

After intravenous infusion of irinotecan in humans, irinotecan plasma concentrations decline in a multiexponential manner, with a mean terminal elimination half-life of about 6 to 12 hours. The mean terminal elimination half-life of the active metabolite SN-38 is about 10 to 20 hours. The half-lives of the lactone (active) forms of irinotecan and SN-38 are similar to those of total irinotecan and SN-38, as the lactone and hydroxy acid forms are in equilibrium.

Over the recommended dose range of 50 to 350 mg/m^2, the AUC of irinotecan increases linearly with dose; the AUC of SN-38 increases less than proportionally with dose. Maximum concentrations of the active metabolite SN-38 are generally seen within 1 hour following the end of a 90-minute infusion of irinotecan. Pharmacokinetic parameters for irinotecan and SN-38 following a 90-minute infusion of irinotecan at dose levels of 125 and 340 mg/m^2 determined in two clinical studies in patients with solid tumors are summarized in Table 1:

[See table 1 at top of next page]

Irinotecan exhibits moderate plasma protein binding (30% to 68% bound). SN-38 is highly bound to human plasma proteins (approximately 95% bound). The plasma protein to which irinotecan and SN-38 predominantly binds is albumin.

Metabolism and Excretion: The metabolic conversion of irinotecan to the active metabolite SN-38 is mediated by carboxylesterase enzymes and primarily occurs in the liver. SN-38 subsequently undergoes conjugation to form a glucuronide metabolite. SN-38 glucuronide had 1/50 to 1/100 the activity of SN-38 in cytotoxicity assays using two cell lines in vitro. The disposition of irinotecan has not been fully elucidated in humans. The urinary excretion of irinotecan is 11% to 20%; SN-38, <1%; and SN-38 glucuronide, 3%. The cumulative biliary and urinary excretion of irinotecan and its metabolites (SN-38 and SN-38 glucuronide) over a period of 48 hours following administration of irinotecan in two patients ranged from approximately 25% (100 mg/m^2) to 50% (300 mg/m^2).

Pharmacokinetics in Special Populations

Geriatric: In studies using the weekly schedule, the terminal half-life of irinotecan was 6.0 hours in patients who were 65 years or older and 5.5 hours in patients younger than 65 years. Dose-normalized AUC_{0-24} for SN-38 in patients who were at least 65 years of age was 11% higher than in patients younger than 65 years. No change in the starting dose is recommended for geriatric patients receiving the weekly dosage schedule of irinotecan. The pharmacokinetics of irinotecan given once every 3 weeks has not been studied in the geriatric population; a lower starting dose is recommended in patients 70 years or older based on clinical toxicity experience with this schedule (see DOSAGE AND ADMINISTRATION).

Pediatric: Information regarding the pharmacokinetics of irinotecan is not available.

Gender: The pharmacokinetics of irinotecan do not appear to be influenced by gender.

Race: The influence of race on the pharmacokinetics of irinotecan has not been evaluated.

Hepatic Insufficiency: The influence of hepatic insufficiency on the pharmacokinetic characteristics of irinotecan and its metabolites has not been formally studied. Among patients with known hepatic tumor involvement (a majority of patients), irinotecan and SN-38 AUC values were somewhat higher than values for patients without liver metastases (see PRECAUTIONS).

Renal Insufficiency: The influence of renal insufficiency on the pharmacokinetics of irinotecan has not been evaluated.

Drug-Drug Interactions

In a phase 1 clinical study involving irinotecan, 5-fluorouracil (5-FU), and leucovorin (LV) in 26 patients with solid tumors, the disposition of irinotecan was not substantially altered when the drugs were co-administered. Although the C_{max} and AUC_{0-24} of SN-38, the active metabolite, were reduced (by 14% and 8%, respectively) when irinotecan was followed by 5-FU and LV administration compared with when irinotecan was given alone, this sequence of administration was used in the combination trials and is recommended (see DOSAGE AND ADMINISTRATION). Formal in vivo or in vitro drug interaction studies to evaluate the influence of irinotecan on the disposition of 5-FU and LV have not been conducted.

Continued on next page

Camptosar—Cont.

Possible pharmacokinetic interactions of CAMPTOSAR with other concomitantly administered medications have not been formally investigated.

CLINICAL STUDIES

Irinotecan has been studied in clinical trials in combination with 5-fluorouracil (5-FU) and leucovorin (LV) and as a single agent (see DOSAGE AND ADMINISTRATION). When given as a component of combination-agent treatment, irinotecan was either given with a weekly schedule of bolus 5-FU/LV or with an every-2-week schedule of infusional 5-FU/LV. Weekly and a once-every-3-week dosage schedules were used for the single-agent irinotecan studies. Clinical studies of combination and single-agent use are described below.

First-Line Therapy in Combination with 5-FU/LV for the Treatment of Metastatic Colorectal Cancer

Two phase 3, randomized, controlled, multinational clinical trials support the use of CAMPTOSAR Injection as first-line treatment of patients with metastatic carcinoma of the colon or rectum. In each study, combinations of irinotecan with 5-FU and LV were compared with 5-FU and LV alone. Study 1 compared combination irinotecan/bolus 5-FU/LV therapy given weekly with a standard bolus regimen of 5-FU/LV alone given daily for 5 days every 4 weeks; an irinotecan-alone treatment arm given on a weekly schedule was also included. Study 2 evaluated two different methods of administering infusional 5-FU/LV, with or without irinotecan. In both studies, concomitant medications such as antiemetics, atropine, and loperamide were given to patients for prophylaxis and/or management of symptoms from treatment. In Study 2, a 7-day course of fluoroquinolone antibiotic prophylaxis was given in patients whose diarrhea persisted for greater than 24 hours despite loperamide or if they developed a fever in addition to diarrhea. Treatment with oral fluoroquinolone was also initiated in patients who developed an absolute neutrophil count (ANC) $<500/mm^3$, even in the absence of fever or diarrhea. Patients in both studies also received treatment with intravenous antibiotics if they had persistent diarrhea or fever or if ileus developed.

In both studies, the combination of irinotecan/5-FU/LV therapy resulted in significant improvements in objective tumor response rates, time to tumor progression, and survival when compared with 5-FU/LV alone. These differences in survival were observed in spite of second-line therapy in a majority of patients on both arms, including crossover to irinotecan-containing regimens in the control arm. Patient characteristics and major efficacy results are shown in Table 2.

[See table 2 at right]

Improvement was noted with irinotecan-based combination therapy relative to 5-FU/LV when response rates and time to tumor progression were examined across the following demographic and disease-related subgroups (age, gender, ethnic origin, performance status, extent of organ involvement with cancer, time from diagnosis of cancer, prior adjuvant therapy, and baseline laboratory abnormalities). Figures 1 and 2 illustrate the Kaplan-Meier survival curves for the comparison of irinotecan/5-FU/LV versus 5-FU/LV in Studies 1 and 2, respectively.

Figure 1. Survival First-Line Irinotecan/5-FU/LV vs 5-FU/LV Study 1

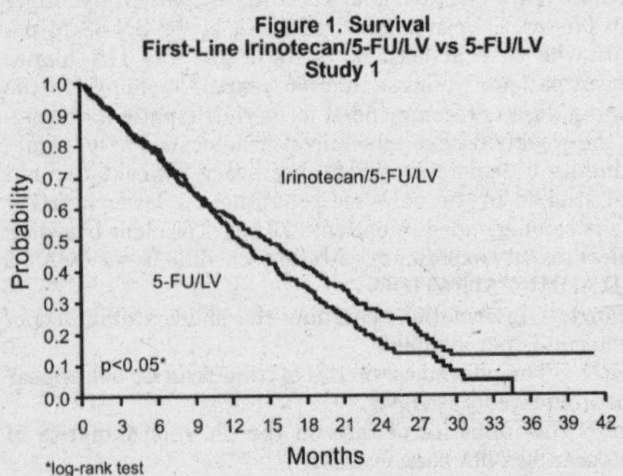

Figure 2. Survival First-Line Irinotecan/5-FU/LV vs 5-FU/LV Study 2

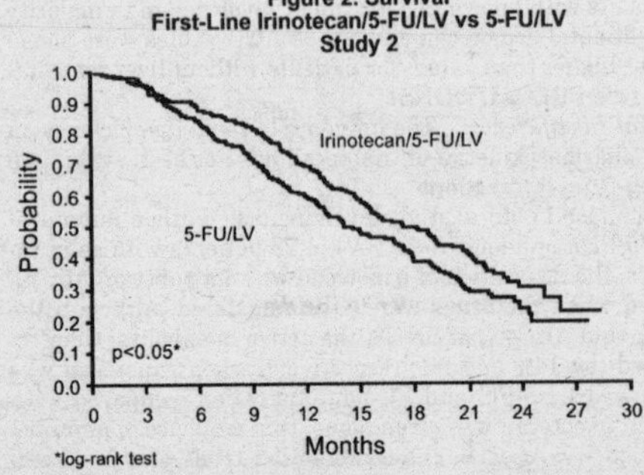

Second-Line Treatment for Recurrent or Progressive Metastatic Colorectal Cancer After 5-FU-Based Treatment

Weekly Dosage Schedule

Data from three open-label, single-agent, clinical studies, involving a total of 304 patients in 59 centers, support the use of CAMPTOSAR in the treatment of patients with metastatic cancer of the colon or rectum that has recurred or progressed following treatment with 5-FU-based therapy. These studies were designed to evaluate tumor response rate and do not provide information on actual clinical benefit, such as effects on survival and disease-related symptoms. In each study, CAMPTOSAR was administered in repeated 6-week cycles consisting of a 90-minute intravenous infusion once weekly for 4 weeks, followed by a 2-week rest period. Starting doses of CAMPTOSAR in these trials were 100, 125, or 150 mg/m^2, but the 150-mg/m^2 dose was poorly tolerated (due to unacceptably high rates of grade 4 late diarrhea and febrile neutropenia). Study 1 enrolled 48 patients and was conducted by a single investigator at several regional hospitals. Study 2 was a multicenter study conducted by the North Central Cancer Treatment Group. All 90 patients enrolled in Study 2 received a starting dose of 125 mg/m^2. Study 3 was a multicenter study that enrolled 166 patients from 30 institutions. The initial dose in Study 3 was 125 mg/m^2 but was reduced to 100 mg/m^2 because the toxicity seen at the 125-mg/m^2 dose was perceived to be greater than that seen in previous studies. All patients in these studies had metastatic colorectal cancer, and the majority had disease that recurred or progressed following a 5-FU-based regimen administered for metastatic disease. The results of the individual studies are shown in Table 3.

[See table 3 at bottom of next page]

In the intent-to-treat analysis of the pooled data across all three studies, 193 of the 304 patients began therapy at the recommended starting dose of 125 mg/m^2. Among these 193 patients, 2 complete and 27 partial responses were observed, for an overall response rate of 15.0% (95% Confidence Interval [CI], 10.0% to 20.1%) at this starting dose. A considerably lower response rate was seen with a starting dose of 100 mg/m^2. The majority of responses were observed within the first two cycles of therapy, but responses did occur in later cycles of treatment (one response was observed after the eighth cycle). The median response duration for patients beginning therapy at 125 mg/m^2 was 5.8 months (range, 2.6 to 15.1 months). Of the 304 patients treated in

Table 1. Summary of Mean (± Standard Deviation) Irinotecan and SN-38 Pharmacokinetic Parameters in Patients with Solid Tumors

Dose (mg/m^2)	Irinotecan					SN-38		
	C_{max} (ng/mL)	AUC_{0-24} (ng·h/mL)	$t_{1/2}$ (h)	V_z (L/m^2)	CL ($L/h/m^2$)	C_{max} (ng/mL)	AUC_{0-24} (ng·h/mL)	$t_{1/2}$ (h)
125 (N=64)	1,660 ±797	10,200 ±3,270	5.8[a] ±0.7	110 ±48.5	13.3 ±6.01	26.3 ±11.9	229 ±108	10.4[a] ±3.1
340 (N=6)	3,392 ±874	20,604 ±6,027	11.7[b] ±1.0	234 ±69.6	13.9 ±4.0	56.0 ±28.2	474 ±245	21.0[b] ±4.3

C_{max} - Maximum plasma concentration
AUC_{0-24} - Area under the plasma concentration-time curve from time 0 to 24 hours after the end of the 90-minute infusion
$t_{1/2}$ - Terminal elimination half-life
V_z - Volume of distribution of terminal elimination phase
CL - Total systemic clearance
[a] Plasma specimens collected for 24 hours following the end of the 90-minute infusion.
[b] Plasma specimens collected for 48 hours following the end of the 90-minute infusion. Because of the longer collection period, these values provide a more accurate reflection of the terminal elimination half-lives of irinotecan and SN-38.

Table 2. Combination Dosage Schedule: Study Results

	Study 1			Study 2	
	Irinotecan + Bolus 5-FU/LV weekly× 4 q 6 weeks	Bolus 5-FU/LV daily× 5 q 4 weeks	Irinotecan weekly× 4 q 6 weeks	Irinotecan + Infusional 5-FU/LV	Infusional 5-FU/LV
Number of Patients	231	226	226	198	187
Demographics and Treatment Administration					
Female/Male (%)	34/65	45/54	35/64	33/67	47/53
Median Age in years (range)	62 (25–85)	61 (19–85)	61 (30–87)	62 (27–75)	59 (24–75)
Performance Status (%)					
0	39	41	46	51	51
1	46	45	46	42	41
2	15	13	8	7	8
Primary Tumor (%)					
Colon	81	85	84	55	65
Rectum	17	14	15	45	35
Median Time from Diagnosis to Randomization (months, range)	1.9 (0–161)	1.7 (0–203)	1.8 (0.1–185)	4.5 (0–88)	2.7 (0–104)
Prior Adjuvant 5-FU Therapy (%)					
No	89	92	90	74	76
Yes	11	8	10	26	24
Median Duration of Study Treatment[a] (months)	5.5	4.1	3.9	5.6	4.5
Median Relative Dose Intensity (%)[a]					
Irinotecan	72	—	75	87	—
5-FU	71	86	—	86	93
Efficacy Results					
Confirmed Objective Tumor Response Rate[b] (%)	39	21 ($p<0.0001$)[c]	18	35	22 ($p<0.005$)[c]
Median Time to Tumor Progression[d] (months)	7.0	4.3 ($p=0.004$)[d]	4.2	6.7	4.4 ($p<0.001$)[d]
Median Survival (months)	14.8	12.6 ($p<0.05$)[d]	12.0	17.4	14.1 ($p<0.05$)[d]

[a] Study 1: N=225 (irinotecan/5-FU/LV), N=219 (5-FU/LV), N=223 (irinotecan)
Study 2: N=199 (irinotecan/5-FU/LV), N=186 (5-FU/LV)
[b] Confirmed ≥4 to 6 weeks after first evidence of objective response
[c] Chi-square test
[d] Log-rank test

the three studies, response rates to CAMPTOSAR were similar in males and females and among patients older and younger than 65 years. Rates were also similar in patients with cancer of the colon or cancer of the rectum and in patients with single and multiple metastatic sites. The response rate was 18.5% in patients with a performance status of 0 and 8.2% in patients with a performance status of 1 or 2. Patients with a performance status of 3 or 4 have not been studied. Over half of the patients responding to CAMPTOSAR had not responded to prior 5-FU. Patients who had received previous irradiation to the pelvis responded to CAMPTOSAR at approximately the same rate as those who had not previously received irradiation.

Once-Every-3-Week Dosage Schedule

Single-Arm Studies: Data from an open-label, single-agent, single-arm, multicenter, clinical study involving a total of 132 patients support a once every-3-week dosage schedule of irinotecan in the treatment of patients with metastatic cancer of the colon or rectum that recurred or progressed following treatment with 5-FU. Patients received a starting dose of 350 mg/m^2 given by 30-minute intravenous infusion once every 3 weeks. Among the 132 previously treated patients in this trial, the intent-to-treat response rate was 12.1% (95% CI, 7.0% to 18.1%).

Randomized Trials: Two multicenter, randomized, clinical studies further support the use of irinotecan given by the once-every-3-week dosage schedule in patients with metastatic colorectal cancer whose disease has recurred or progressed following prior 5-FU therapy. In the first study, second-line irinotecan therapy plus best supportive care was compared with best supportive care alone. In the second study, second-line irinotecan therapy was compared with infusional 5-FU-based therapy. In both studies, irinotecan was administered intravenously at a starting dose of 350 mg/m^2 over 90 minutes once every 3 weeks. The starting dose was 300 mg/m^2 for patients who were 70 years and older or who had a performance status of 2. The highest total dose permitted was 700 mg. Dose reductions and/or administration delays were permitted in the event of severe hematologic and/or nonhematologic toxicities while on treatment. Best supportive care was provided to patients in both arms of Study 1 and included antibiotics, analgesics, corticosteroids, transfusions, psychotherapy, or any other symptomatic therapy as clinically indicated. In both studies, concomitant medications such as antiemetics, atropine, and loperamide were given to patients for prophylaxis and/or management of symptoms from treatment. If late diarrhea persisted for greater than 24 hours despite loperamide, a 7-day course of fluoroquinolone antibiotic prophylaxis was given. Patients in the control arm of the second study received one of the following 5-FU regimens: (1) LV, 200 mg/m^2 IV over 2 hours; followed by 5-FU, 400 mg/m^2 IV bolus; followed by 5-FU, 600 mg/m^2 continuous IV infusion over 22 hours on days 1 and 2 every 2 weeks; (2) 5-FU, 250 to 300 mg/m^2/day protracted continuous IV infusion until toxicity; (3) 5-FU, 2.6 to 3 g/m^2 IV over 24 hours every week for 6 weeks with or without LV, 20 to 500 mg/m^2/day every week IV for 6 weeks with 2-week rest between cycles. Patients were to be followed every 3 to 6 weeks for 1 year. A total of 535 patients were randomized in the two studies at 94 centers. The primary endpoint in both studies was survival. The studies demonstrated a significant overall survival advantage for irinotecan compared with best supportive care (p=0.0001) and infusional 5-FU-based therapy (p=0.035) as shown in Figures 3 and 4. In Study 1, median survival for patients treated with irinotecan was 9.2 months compared with 6.5 months for patients receiving best supportive care. In Study 2, median survival for patients treated with irinotecan was 10.8 months compared with 8.5 months for patients receiving infusional 5-FU-based therapy. Multiple regression analyses determined that patients' baseline characteristics also had a significant effect on survival. When adjusted for performance status and other baseline prognostic factors, survival among patients treated with irinotecan remained significantly longer than in the control populations (p=0.001 for Study 1 and p=0.017 for Study 2). Measurements of pain, performance status, and weight loss were collected prospectively in the two studies; however, the plan for the analysis of these data was defined retrospectively. When comparing irinotecan with best supportive care in Study 1, this analysis showed a statistically significant advantage for irinotecan, with longer time to development of pain (6.9 months versus 2.0 months), time to performance status deterioration (5.7 months versus 3.3 months), and time to > 5% weight loss (6.4 months versus 4.2 months). Additionally, 33.3% (33/99) of patients with a baseline performance status of 1 or 2 showed an improvement in performance status when treated with irinotecan versus 11.3% (7/62) of patients receiving best supportive care (p=0.002). Because of the inclusion of patients with non-measurable disease, intent-to-treat response rates could not be assessed.

Figure 3. Survival
Second-Line Irinotecan vs Best Supportive Care (BSC)
Study 1

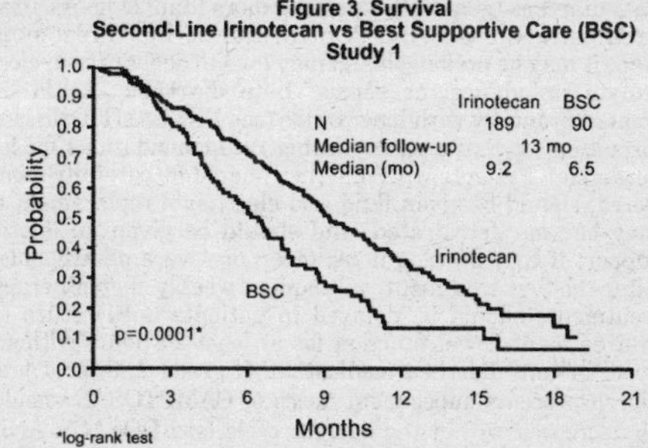

Figure 4. Survival
Second-Line Irinotecan vs Infusional 5-FU
Study 2

Irinotecan 5-FU
N 127 129
Median follow-up 15 mo
Median (mo) 10.8 8.5
p=0.035*
Months
*log-rank test

In the two randomized studies, the EORTC QLQ-C30 instrument was utilized. At the start of each cycle of therapy, patients completed a questionnaire consisting of 30 questions, such as "Did pain interfere with daily activities?" (1 = Not at All, to 4 = Very Much) and "Do you have any trouble taking a long walk?" (Yes or No). The answers from the 30 questions were converted into 15 subscales, that were scored from 0 to 100, and the global health status subscale that was derived from two questions about the patient's sense of general well being in the past week. In addition to the global health status subscale, there were five functional (i.e., cognitive, emotional, social, physical, role) and nine symptom (i.e., fatigue, appetite loss, pain assessment, insomnia, constipation, dyspnea, nausea/vomiting, financial impact, diarrhea) subscales. The results as summarized in Table 5 are based on patients' worst post-baseline scores. In Study 1, a multivariate analysis and univariate analyses of the individual subscales were performed and corrected for multivariate testing. Patients receiving irinotecan reported significantly better results for the global health status, on two of five functional subscales, and on four of nine symptom subscales. As expected, patients receiving irinotecan noted significantly more diarrhea than those receiving best supportive care. In Study 2, the multivariate analysis on all 15 subscales did not indicate a statistically significant difference between irinotecan and infusional 5-FU.

[See table 4 at top of next page]
[See table 5 at top of next page]

INDICATIONS AND USAGE

CAMPTOSAR Injection is indicated as a component of first-line therapy in combination with 5-fluorouracil and leucovorin for patients with metastatic carcinoma of the colon or rectum. CAMPTOSAR is also indicated for patients with metastatic carcinoma of the colon or rectum whose disease has recurred or progressed following initial fluorouracil-based therapy.

CONTRAINDICATIONS

CAMPTOSAR Injection is contraindicated in patients with a known hypersensitivity to the drug.

WARNINGS

General

Outside of a well-designed clinical study, CAMPTOSAR Injection should not be used in combination with the "Mayo Clinic" regimen of 5-FU/LV (administration for 4–5 consecutive days every 4 weeks) because of reports of increased toxicity, including toxic deaths. CAMPTOSAR should be used as recommended (see DOSAGE AND ADMINISTRATION, Table 10).

Table 3. Weekly Dosage Schedule: Study Results

	Study			
	1	2	3	
Number of Patients	48	90	64	102
Starting Dose (mg/m^2/wk × 4)	125[a]	125	125	100
Demographics and Treatment Administration				
Female/Male (%)	46/54	36/64	50/50	51/49
Median Age in years (range)	63 (29–78)	63 (32–81)	61 (42–84)	64 (25–84)
Ethnic Origin (%)				
White	79	96	81	91
African American	12	4	11	5
Hispanic	8	0	8	2
Oriental/Asian	0	0	0	2
Performance Status (%)				
0	60	38	59	44
1	38	48	33	51
2	2	14	8	5
Primary Tumor (%)				
Colon	100	71	89	87
Rectum	0	29	11	8
Unknown	0	0	0	5
Prior 5-FU Therapy (%)				
For Metastatic Disease	81	66	73	68
≤6 months after Adjuvant	15	7	27	28
>6 months after Adjuvant	2	16	0	2
Classification Unknown	2	12	0	3
Prior Pelvic/Abdominal Irradiation (%)				
Yes	3	29	0	0
Other	0	9	2	4
None	97	62	98	96
Duration of Treatment with CAMPTOSAR (median, months)	5	4	4	3
Relative Dose Intensity[b] (median %)	74	67	73	81
Efficacy				
Confirmed Objective Response Rate (%)[c] (95% CI)	21 (9.3–32.3)	13 (6.3–20.4)	14 (5.5–22.6)	9 (3.3–14.3)
Time to Response (median, months)	2.6	1.5	2.8	2.8
Response Duration (median, months)	6.4	5.9	5.6	6.4
Survival (median, months)	10.4	8.1	10.7	9.3
1-Year Survival (%)	46	31	45	43

[a] Nine patients received 150 mg/m^2 as a starting dose; two (22.2%) responded to CAMPTOSAR.
[b] Relative dose intensity for CAMPTOSAR based on planned dose intensity of 100, 83.3, and 66.7 mg/m^2/wk corresponding with 150, 125, and 100 mg/m^2 starting doses, respectively.
[c] Confirmed ≥ 4 to 6 weeks after first evidence of objective response.

Continued on next page

Camptosar—Cont.

In patients receiving either irinotecan/5-FU/LV or 5-FU/LV in the clinical trials, higher rates of hospitalization, neutropenic fever, thromboembolism, first-cycle treatment discontinuation, and early deaths were observed in patients with a baseline performance status of 2 than in patients with a baseline performance status of 0 or 1.

Diarrhea

CAMPTOSAR can induce both early and late forms of diarrhea that appear to be mediated by different mechanisms. Early diarrhea (occurring during or shortly after infusion of CAMPTOSAR) is cholinergic in nature. It is usually transient and only infrequently is severe. It may be accompanied by symptoms of rhinitis, increased salivation, miosis, lacrimation, diaphoresis, flushing, and intestinal hyperperistalsis that can cause abdominal cramping. Early diarrhea and other cholinergic symptoms may be prevented or ameliorated by administration of atropine (see PRECAUTIONS, General, for dosing recommendations for atropine). Late diarrhea (generally occurring more than 24 hours after administration of CAMPTOSAR) can be life threatening since it may be prolonged and may lead to dehydration, electrolyte imbalance, or sepsis. Late diarrhea should be treated promptly with loperamide (see PRECAUTIONS, Information for Patients, for dosing recommendations for loperamide). Patients with diarrhea should be carefully monitored, should be given fluid and electrolyte replacement if they become dehydrated, and should be given antibiotic support if they develop ileus, fever, or severe neutropenia. After the first treatment, subsequent weekly chemotherapy treatments should be delayed in patients until return of pretreatment bowel function for at least 24 hours without need for anti-diarrhea medication. If grade 2, 3, or 4 late diarrhea occurs subsequent doses of CAMPTOSAR should be decreased within the current cycle (see DOSAGE AND ADMINISTRATION).

Neutropenia

Deaths due to sepsis following severe neutropenia have been reported in patients treated with CAMPTOSAR. Neutropenic complications should be managed promptly with antibiotic support (see PRECAUTIONS). Therapy with CAMPTOSAR should be temporarily omitted during a cycle of therapy if neutropenic fever occurs or if the absolute neutrophil count drops $<1000/mm^3$. After the patient recovers to an absolute neutrophil count $\geq 1000/mm^3$, subsequent doses of CAMPTOSAR should be reduced depending upon the level of neutropenia observed (see DOSAGE AND ADMINISTRATION).

Routine administration of a colony-stimulating factor (CSF) is not necessary, but physicians may wish to consider CSF use in individual patients experiencing significant neutropenia.

Hypersensitivity

Hypersensitivity reactions including severe anaphylactic or anaphylactoid reactions have been observed.

Colitis/Ileus

Cases of colitis complicated by ulceration, bleeding, ileus, and infection have been observed. Patients experiencing ileus should receive prompt antibiotic support (see PRECAUTIONS).

Renal Impairment/Renal Failure

Rare cases of renal impairment and acute renal failure have been identified, usually in patients who became volume depleted from severe vomiting and/or diarrhea.

Thromboembolism

Thromboembolic events have been observed in patients receiving irinotecan-containing regimens; the specific cause of these events has not been determined.

Pregnancy

CAMPTOSAR may cause fetal harm when administered to a pregnant woman. Radioactivity related to ^{14}C-irinotecan crosses the placenta of rats following intravenous administration of 10 mg/kg (which in separate studies produced an irinotecan C_{max} and AUC about 3 and 0.5 times, respectively, the corresponding values in patients administered 125 mg/m^2). Administration of 6 mg/kg/day intravenous irinotecan to rats (which in separate studies produced an irinotecan C_{max} and AUC about 2 and 0.2 times, respectively, the corresponding values in patients administered 125 mg/m^2) and rabbits (about one-half the recommended human weekly starting dose on a mg/m^2 basis) during the period of organogenesis, is embryotoxic as characterized by increased post-implantation loss and decreased numbers of live fetuses. Irinotecan was teratogenic in rats at doses greater than 1.2 mg/kg/day (which in separate studies produced an irinotecan C_{max} and AUC about 2/3 and 1/40th, respectively, of the corresponding values in patients administered 125 mg/m^2) and in rabbits at 6.0 mg/kg/day (about one-half the recommended human weekly starting dose on a mg/m^2 basis). Teratogenic effects included a variety of external, visceral, and skeletal abnormalities. Irinotecan administered to rat dams for the period following organogenesis through weaning at doses of 6 mg/kg/day caused decreased learning ability and decreased female body weights in the offspring. There are no adequate and well-controlled studies of irinotecan in pregnant women. If the drug is used during pregnancy, or if the patient becomes pregnant while receiving this drug, the patient should be apprised of the potential hazard to the fetus. Women of childbearing potential should be advised to avoid becoming pregnant while receiving treatment with CAMPTOSAR.

PRECAUTIONS

General

Care of Intravenous Site: CAMPTOSAR Injection is administered by intravenous infusion. Care should be taken to avoid extravasation, and the infusion site should be monitored for signs of inflammation. Should extravasation occur, flushing the site with sterile water and applications of ice are recommended.

Premedication with Antiemetics: Irinotecan is emetigenic. It is recommended that patients receive premedication with antiemetic agents. In clinical studies of the weekly dosage schedule, the majority of patients received 10 mg of dexamethasone given in conjunction with another type of antiemetic agent, such as a 5-HT^3 blocker (e.g., ondansetron or granisetron). Antiemetic agents should be given on the day of treatment, starting at least 30 minutes before administration of CAMPTOSAR. Physicians should also consider providing patients with an antiemetic regimen (e.g., prochlorperazine) for subsequent use as needed.

Treatment of Cholinergic Symptoms: Prophylactic or therapeutic administration of 0.25 to 1 mg of intravenous or subcutaneous atropine should be considered (unless clinically contraindicated) in patients experiencing rhinitis, increased salivation, miosis, lacrimation, diaphoresis, flushing, abdominal cramping, or diarrhea (occurring during or shortly after infusion of CAMPTOSAR). These symptoms are expected to occur more frequently with higher irinotecan doses.

Patients at Particular Risk: In patients receiving either irinotecan/5-FU/LV or 5-FU/LV in the clinical trials, higher rates of hospitalization, neutropenic fever, thromboembolism, first-cycle treatment discontinuation, and early deaths were observed in patients with a baseline performance status of 2 than in patients with a baseline performance status of 0 or 1. Patients who had previously received pelvic/abdominal radiation and elderly patients with comorbid conditions should be closely monitored.

The use of CAMPTOSAR in patients with significant hepatic dysfunction has not been established. In clinical trials of either dosing schedule, irinotecan was not administered to patients with serum bilirubin >2.0 mg/dL, or transaminase >3 times the upper limit of normal if no liver metasta-

Table 4. Once-Every-3-Week Dosage Schedule: Study Results

	Study 1		Study 2	
	Irinotecan	BSC[a]	Irinotecan	5-FU
Number of Patients	189	90	127	129
Demographics and Treatment Administration				
Female/Male (%)	32/68	42/58	43/57	35/65
Median Age in years (range)	59 (22–75)	62 (34–75)	58 (30–75)	58 (25–75)
Performance Status (%)				
0	47	31	58	54
1	39	46	35	43
2	14	23	8	3
Primary Tumor (%)				
Colon	55	52	57	62
Rectum	45	48	43	38
Prior 5-FU Therapy (%)				
For Metastatic Disease	70	63	58	68
As Adjuvant Treatment	30	37	42	32
Prior Irradiation (%)	26	27	18	20
Duration of Study Treatment (median, months) (Log-rank test)	4.1	—	4.2 (p=0.02)	2.8
Relative Dose Intensity (median %)[b]	94	—	95	81–99
Survival				
Survival (median, months) (Log-rank test)	9.2 (p=0.0001)	6.5	10.8 (p=0.035)	8.5

[a] BSC = best supportive care

[b] Relative dose intensity for irinotecan based on planned dose intensity of 116.7 and 100 mg/m^2/wk corresponding with 350 and 300 mg/m^2 starting doses, respectively.

Table 5. EORTC QLQ-C30: Mean Worst Post-Baseline Score[a]

QLQ-C30 Subscale	Study 1			Study 2		
	Irinotecan	BSC	p-value	Irinotecan	5-FU	p-value
Global Health Status	47	37	0.03	53	52	0.9
Functional Scales						
Cognitive	77	68	0.07	79	83	0.9
Emotional	68	64	0.4	64	68	0.9
Social	58	47	0.06	65	67	0.9
Physical	60	40	0.0003	66	66	0.9
Role	53	35	0.02	54	57	0.9
Symptom Scales						
Fatigue	51	63	0.03	47	46	0.9
Appetite Loss	37	57	0.0007	35	38	0.9
Pain Assessment	41	56	0.009	38	34	0.9
Insomnia	39	47	0.3	39	33	0.9
Constipation	28	41	0.03	25	19	0.9
Dyspnea	31	40	0.2	25	24	0.9
Nausea/Vomiting	27	29	0.5	25	16	0.09
Financial Impact	22	26	0.5	24	15	0.3
Diarrhea	32	19	0.01	32	22	0.2

[a] For the five functional subscales and global health status subscale, higher scores imply better functioning, whereas, on the nine symptom subscales, higher scores imply more severe symptoms. The subscale scores of each patient were collected at each visit until the patient dropped out of the study.

sis, or transaminase >5 times the upper limit of normal with liver metastasis. However in clinical trials of the weekly dosage schedule, it has been noted that patients with modestly elevated baseline serum total bilirubin levels (1.0 to 2.0 mg/dL) have had a significantly greater likelihood of experiencing first-cycle grade 3 or 4 neutropenia than those with bilirubin levels that were less than 1.0 mg/dL (50.0% [19/38] versus 17.7% [47/226]; $p<0.001$). Patients with abnormal glucuronidation of bilirubin, such as those with Gilbert's syndrome, may also be at greater risk of myelosuppression when receiving therapy with CAMPTOSAR. An association between baseline bilirubin elevations and an increased risk of late diarrhea has not been observed in studies of the weekly dosage schedule.

Information for Patients

Patients and patients' caregivers should be informed of the expected toxic effects of CAMPTOSAR, particularly of its gastrointestinal complications, such as nausea, vomiting, abdominal cramping, diarrhea, and infection. Each patient should be instructed to have loperamide readily available and to begin treatment for late diarrhea (generally occurring more than 24 hours after administration of CAMPTOSAR) at the first episode of poorly formed or loose stools or the earliest onset of bowel movements more frequent than normally expected for the patient. One dosage regimen for loperamide used in clinical trials consisted of the following (Note: This dosage regimen exceeds the usual dosage recommendations for loperamide.): 4 mg at the first onset of late diarrhea and then 2 mg every 2 hours until the patient is diarrhea-free for at least 12 hours. During the night, the patient may take 4 mg of loperamide every 4 hours. Premedication with loperamide is not recommended. The use of drugs with laxative properties should be avoided because of the potential for exacerbation of diarrhea. Patients should be advised to contact their physician to discuss any laxative use.

Patients should be instructed to contact their physician or nurse if any of the following occur: diarrhea for the first time during treatment; black or bloody stools; symptoms of dehydration such as lightheadedness, dizziness, or faintness; inability to take fluids by mouth due to nausea or vomiting; inability to get diarrhea under control within 24 hours; or fever or evidence of infection.

Patients should be alerted to the possibility of alopecia.

Laboratory Tests

Careful monitoring of the white blood cell count with differential, hemoglobin, and platelet count is recommended before each dose of CAMPTOSAR.

Drug Interactions

The adverse effects of CAMPTOSAR, such as myelosuppression and diarrhea, would be expected to be exacerbated by other antineoplastic agents having similar adverse effects. Patients who have previously received pelvic/abdominal irradiation are at increased risk of severe myelosuppression following the administration of CAMPTOSAR. The concurrent administration of CAMPTOSAR with irradiation has not been adequately studied and is not recommended.

Lymphocytopenia has been reported in patients receiving CAMPTOSAR, and it is possible that the administration of dexamethasone as antiemetic prophylaxis may have enhanced the likelihood of this effect. However, serious opportunistic infections have not been observed, and no complications have specifically been attributed to lymphocytopenia.

Hyperglycemia has also been reported in patients receiving CAMPTOSAR. Usually, this has been observed in patients with a history of diabetes mellitus or evidence of glucose intolerance prior to administration of CAMPTOSAR. It is probable that dexamethasone, given as antiemetic prophylaxis, contributed to hyperglycemia in some patients.

The incidence of akathisia in clinical trials of the weekly dosage schedule was greater (8.5%, 4/47 patients) when prochlorperazine was administered on the same day as CAMPTOSAR than when these drugs were given on separate days (1.3%, 1/80 patients). The 8.5% incidence of akathisia, however, is within the range reported for use of prochlorperazine when given as a premedication for other chemotherapies.

It would be expected that laxative use during therapy with CAMPTOSAR would worsen the incidence or severity of diarrhea, but this has not been studied.

In view of the potential risk of dehydration secondary to vomiting and/or diarrhea induced by CAMPTOSAR, the physician may wish to withhold diuretics during dosing with CAMPTOSAR and, certainly, during periods of active vomiting or diarrhea.

Drug-Laboratory Test Interactions

There are no known interactions between CAMPTOSAR and laboratory tests.

Carcinogenesis, Mutagenesis & Impairment of Fertility

Long-term carcinogenicity studies with irinotecan were not conducted. Rats were, however, administered intravenous doses of 2 mg/kg or 25 mg/kg irinotecan once per week for 13 weeks (in separate studies, the 25 mg/kg dose produced an irinotecan C_{max} and AUC that were about 7.0 times and 1.3 times the respective values in patients administered 125 mg/m^2 weekly) and were then allowed to recover for 91 weeks. Under these conditions, there was a significant linear trend with dose for the incidence of combined uterine horn endometrial stromal polyps and endometrial stromal sarcomas. Neither irinotecan nor SN-38 was mutagenic in the in vitro Ames assay. Irinotecan was clastogenic both in vitro (chromosome aberrations in Chinese hamster ovary cells) and in vivo (micronucleus test in mice). No significant adverse effects on fertility and general reproductive performance were observed after intravenous administration of irinotecan in doses of up to 6 mg/kg/day to rats and rabbits. However, atrophy of male reproductive organs was observed after multiple daily irinotecan doses both in rodents at 20 mg/kg (which in separate studies produced an irinotecan C_{max} and AUC about 5 and 1 times, respectively, the corresponding values in patients administered 125 mg/m^2 weekly) and dogs at 0.4 mg/kg (which in separate studies produced an irinotecan C_{max} and AUC about one-half and 1/15th, respectively, the corresponding values in patients administered 125 mg/m^2 weekly).

Table 6. Study 1: Percent (%) of Patients Experiencing Clinically Relevant Adverse Events in Combination Therapies[a]

Adverse Event	Study 1: Irinotecan + Bolus 5-FU/LV weekly × 4 q 6 weeks N=225		Bolus 5-FU/LV daily × 5 q 4 weeks N=219		Irinotecan weekly × 4 q 6 weeks N=223	
	Grade 1–4	Grade 3&4	Grade 1–4	Grade 3&4	Grade 1–4	Grade 3&4
TOTAL Adverse Events	100	53.3	100	45.7	99.6	45.7
GASTROINTESTINAL						
Diarrhea						
late	84.9	22.7	69.4	13.2	83.0	31.0
grade 3	—	15.1	—	5.9	—	18.4
grade 4	—	7.6	—	7.3	—	12.6
early	45.8	4.9	31.5	1.4	43.0	6.7
Nausea	79.1	15.6	67.6	8.2	81.6	16.1
Abdominal pain	63.1	14.6	50.2	11.5	67.7	13.0
Vomiting	60.4	9.7	46.1	4.1	62.8	12.1
Anorexia	34.2	5.8	42.0	3.7	43.9	7.2
Constipation	41.3	3.1	31.5	1.8	32.3	0.4
Mucositis	32.4	2.2	76.3	16.9	29.6	2.2
HEMATOLOGIC						
Neutropenia	96.9	53.8	98.6	66.7	96.4	31.4
grade 3	—	29.8	—	23.7	—	19.3
grade 4	—	24.0	—	42.5	—	12.1
Leukopenia	96.9	37.8	98.6	23.3	96.4	21.5
Anemia	96.9	8.4	98.6	5.5	96.9	4.5
Neutropenic fever	—	7.1	—	14.6	—	5.8
Thrombocytopenia	96.0	2.6	98.6	2.7	96.0	1.7
Neutropenic infection	—	1.8	—	0	—	2.2
BODY AS A WHOLE						
Asthenia	70.2	19.5	64.4	11.9	69.1	13.9
Pain	30.7	3.1	26.9	3.6	22.9	2.2
Fever	42.2	1.7	32.4	3.6	43.5	0.4
Infection	22.2	0	16.0	1.4	13.9	0.4
METABOLIC & NUTRITIONAL						
↑ Bilirubin	87.6	7.1	92.2	8.2	83.9	7.2
DERMATOLOGIC						
Exfoliative dermatitis	0.9	0	3.2	0.5	0	0
Rash	19.1	0	26.5	0.9	14.3	0.4
Alopecia[b]	43.1	—	26.5	—	46.1	—
RESPIRATORY						
Dyspnea	27.6	6.3	16.0	0.5	22.0	2.2
Cough	26.7	1.3	18.3	0	20.2	0.4
Pneumonia	6.2	2.7	1.4	1.0	3.6	1.3
NEUROLOGIC						
Dizziness	23.1	1.3	16.4	0	21.1	1.8
Somnolence	12.4	1.8	4.6	1.8	9.4	1.3
Confusion	7.1	1.8	4.1	0	2.7	0
CARDIOVASCULAR						
Vasodilation	9.3	0.9	5.0	0	9.0	0
Hypotension	5.8	1.3	2.3	0.5	5.8	1.7
Thromboembolic events[c]	9.3	—	11.4	—	5.4	—

[a] Severity of adverse events based on NCI CTC (version 1.0)

[b] Complete hair loss = Grade 2

[c] Includes angina pectoris, arterial thrombosis, cerebral infarct, cerebrovascular accident, deep thrombophlebitis, embolus lower extremity, heart arrest, myocardial infarct, myocardial ischemia, peripheral vascular disorder, pulmonary embolus, sudden death, thrombophlebitis, thrombosis, vascular disorder.

Pregnancy

Pregnancy Category D—see WARNINGS.

Nursing Mothers

Radioactivity appeared in rat milk within 5 minutes of intravenous administration of radiolabeled irinotecan and was concentrated up to 65-fold at 4 hours after administration relative to plasma concentrations. Because many drugs are excreted in human milk and because of the potential for serious adverse reactions in nursing infants, it is recommended that nursing be discontinued when receiving therapy with CAMPTOSAR.

Pediatric Use

The safety and effectiveness of CAMPTOSAR in pediatric patients have not been established.

Geriatric Use

Patients greater than 65 years of age should be closely monitored because of a greater risk of late diarrhea in this population (see CLINICAL PHARMACOLOGY, Pharmacokinetics in Special Populations and ADVERSE REACTIONS, Overview of Adverse Events). The starting dose of CAMPTOSAR in patients 70 years and older for the once-every-3-week-dosage schedule should be 300 mg/m^2 (see DOSAGE AND ADMINISTRATION).

ADVERSE REACTIONS

First-Line Combination Therapy

A total of 955 patients with metastatic colorectal cancer received the recommended regimens of irinotecan in combination with 5-FU/LV, 5-FU/LV alone, or irinotecan alone. In the two phase 3 studies, 370 patients received irinotecan in combination with 5-FU/LV, 362 patients received 5-FU/LV alone, and 223 patients received irinotecan alone. (See Table 10 in DOSAGE AND ADMINISTRATION for recommended combination-agent regimens.)

In Study 1, 49 (7.3%) patients died within 30 days of last study treatment: 21 (9.3%) received irinotecan in combination with 5-FU/LV, 15 (6.8%) received 5-FU/LV alone, and 13 (5.8%) received irinotecan alone. Deaths potentially related to treatment occurred in 2 (0.9%) patients who received irinotecan in combination with 5-FU/LV (2 neutropenic fever/sepsis), 3 (1.4%) patients who received 5-FU/LV alone (1 neutropenic fever/sepsis, 1 CNS bleeding during thrombocytopenia, 1 unknown) and 2 (0.9%) patients who received irinotecan alone (2 neutropenic fever). Deaths from any cause within 60 days of first study treatment were reported for 15 (6.7%) patients who received irinotecan in combination with 5-FU/LV, 16 (7.3%) patients who received 5-FU/LV alone, and 15 (6.7%) patients who received irinotecan alone. Discontinuations due to adverse events were reported for 17 (7.6%) patients who received irinotecan in combination with 5-FU/LV, 14 (6.4%) patients who received 5-FU/LV alone, and 26 (11.7%) patients who received irinotecan alone.

In Study 2, 10 (3.5%) patients died within 30 days of last study treatment: 6 (4.1%) received irinotecan in combination with 5-FU/LV and 4 (2.8%) received 5-FU/LV alone. There was one potentially treatment-related death, which

Continued on next page

Camptosar—Cont.

occurred in a patient who received irinotecan in combination with 5-FU/LV (0.7%, neutropenic sepsis). Deaths from any cause within 60 days of first study treatment were reported for 3 (2.1%) patients who received irinotecan in combination with 5-FU/LV and 2 (1.4%) patients who received 5-FU/LV alone. Discontinuations due to adverse events were reported for 9 (6.2%) patients who received irinotecan in combination with 5-FU/LV and 1 (0.7%) patient who received 5-FU/LV alone.

The most clinically significant adverse events for patients receiving irinotecan-based therapy were diarrhea, nausea, vomiting, neutropenia, and alopecia. The most clinically significant adverse events for patients receiving 5-FU/LV therapy were diarrhea, neutropenia, neutropenic fever, and mucositis. In Study 1, grade 4 neutropenia, neutropenic fever (defined as grade 2 fever and grade 4 neutropenia), and mucositis were observed less often with weekly irinotecan/5-FU/LV than with monthly administration of 5-FU/LV.

Tables 6 and 7 list the clinically relevant adverse events reported in Studies 1 and 2, respectively.

[See table at top of previous page]

[See table 7 below]

Second-Line Single-Agent Therapy

Weekly Dosage Schedule

In three clinical studies evaluating the weekly dosage schedule, 304 patients with metastatic carcinoma of the colon or rectum that had recurred or progressed following 5-FU-based therapy were treated with CAMPTOSAR. Seventeen of the patients died within 30 days of the administration of CAMPTOSAR; in five cases (1.6%, 5/304), the deaths were potentially drug-related. These five patients experienced a constellation of medical events that included known effects of CAMPTOSAR. One of these patients died of neutropenic sepsis without fever. Neutropenic fever occurred in nine (3.0%) other patients; these patients recovered with supportive care.

One hundred nineteen (39.1%) of the 304 patients were hospitalized a total of 156 times because of adverse events; 81 (26.6%) patients were hospitalized for events judged to be related to administration of CAMPTOSAR. The primary reasons for drug-related hospitalization were diarrhea, with or without nausea and/or vomiting (18.4%); neutropenia/leukopenia, with or without diarrhea and/or fever (8.2%); and nausea and/or vomiting (4.9%).

Table 8. Adverse Events Occurring in >10% of 304 Previously Treated Patients with Metastatic Carcinoma of the Colon or Rectum[a]

Body System & Event	% of Patients Reporting	
	NCI Grades 1–4	NCI Grades 3 & 4
GASTROINTESTINAL		
Diarrhea (late)[b]	88	31
7–9 stools/day (grade 3)	—	(16)
≥10 stools/day (grade 4)	—	(14)
Nausea	86	17
Vomiting	67	12
Anorexia	55	6
Diarrhea (early)[c]	51	8
Constipation	30	2
Flatulence	12	0
Stomatitis	12	1
Dyspepsia	10	0
HEMATOLOGIC		
Leukopenia	63	28
Anemia	60	7
Neutropenia	54	26
500 to <1000/mm^3 (grade 3)	—	(15)
<500/mm^3 (grade 4)	—	(12)
BODY AS A WHOLE		
Asthenia	76	12
Abdominal cramping/pain	57	16
Fever	45	1
Pain	24	2
Headache	17	1
Back pain	14	2
Chills	14	0
Minor infection[d]	14	0
Edema	10	1
Abdominal Enlargement	10	0
METABOLIC & NUTRITIONAL		
↓ Body weight	30	1
Dehydration	15	4
↑ Alkaline phosphatase	13	4
↑ SGOT	10	1
DERMATOLOGIC		
Alopecia	60	NA[e]
Sweating	16	0
Rash	13	1
RESPIRATORY		
Dyspnea	22	4
↑ Coughing	17	0
Rhinitis	16	0
NEUROLOGIC		
Insomnia	19	0
Dizziness	15	0
CARDIOVASCULAR		
Vasodilation (flushing)	11	0

[a] Severity of adverse events based on NCI CTC (version 1.0)
[b] Occurring >24 hours after administration of CAMPTOSAR
[c] Occurring ≤24 hours after administration of CAMPTOSAR
[d] Primarily upper respiratory infections
[e] Not applicable; complete hair loss = NCI grade 2

Table 7. Study 2: Percent (%) of Patients Experiencing Clinically Relevant Adverse Events in Combination Therapies[a]

Adverse Event	Study 2			
	Irinotecan + 5-FU/LV Infusional d 1&2 q 2 weeks N=145		5-FU/LV Infusional d 1&2 q 2 weeks N=143	
	Grade 1–4	Grade 3&4	Grade 1–4	Grade 3&4
TOTAL Adverse Events	100	72.4	100	39.2
GASTROINTESTINAL				
Diarrhea				
late	72.4	14.4	44.8	6.3
grade 3	—	10.3	—	4.2
grade 4	—	4.1	—	2.1
Cholinergic syndrome[b]	28.3	1.4	0.7	0
Nausea	66.9	2.1	55.2	3.5
Abdominal pain	17.2	2.1	16.8	0.7
Vomiting	44.8	3.5	32.2	2.8
Anorexia	35.2	2.1	18.9	0.7
Constipation	30.3	0.7	25.2	1.4
Mucositis	40.0	4.1	28.7	2.8
HEMATOLOGIC				
Neutropenia	82.5	46.2	47.9	13.4
grade 3	—	36.4	—	12.7
grade 4	—	9.8	—	0.7
Leukopenia	81.3	17.4	42.0	3.5
Anemia	97.2	2.1	90.9	2.1
Neutropenic fever	—	3.4	—	0.7
Thrombocytopenia	32.6	0	32.2	0
Neutropenic infection	—	2.1	—	0
BODY AS A WHOLE				
Asthenia	57.9	9.0	48.3	4.2
Pain	64.1	9.7	61.5	8.4
Fever	22.1	0.7	25.9	0.7
Infection	35.9	7.6	33.6	3.5
METABOLIC & NUTRITIONAL				
↑ Bilirubin	19.1	3.5	35.9	10.6
DERMATOLOGIC				
Hand & foot syndrome	10.3	0.7	12.6	0.7
Cutaneous signs	17.2	0.7	20.3	0
Alopecia[c]	56.6	—	16.8	—
RESPIRATORY				
Dyspnea	9.7	1.4	4.9	0
CARDIOVASCULAR				
Hypotension	3.4	1.4	0.7	0
Thromboembolic events[d]	11.7	—	5.6	—

[a] Severity of adverse events based on NCI CTC (version 1.0)
[b] Includes rhinitis, increased salivation, miosis, lacrimation, diaphoresis, flushing, abdominal cramping or diarrhea (occurring during or shortly after infusion of irinotecan)
[c] Complete hair loss = Grade 2
[d] Includes angina pectoris, arterial thrombosis, cerebral infarct, cerebrovascular accident, deep thrombophlebitis, embolus lower extremity, heart arrest, myocardial infarct, myocardial ischemia, peripheral vascular disorder, pulmonary embolus, sudden death, thrombophlebitis, thrombosis, vascular disorder.

Table 9. Percent of Patients Experiencing Grade 3 & 4 Adverse Events in Comparative Studies of Once-Every-3-Week Irinotecan Therapy[a]

Adverse Event	Study 1		Study 2	
	Irinotecan N=189	BSC[b] N=90	Irinotecan N=127	5-FU N=129
TOTAL Grade 3/4 Adverse Events	79	67	69	54
GASTROINTESTINAL				
Diarrhea	22	6	22	11
Vomiting	14	8	14	5
Nausea	14	3	11	4
Abdominal pain	14	16	9	8
Constipation	10	8	8	6
Anorexia	5	7	6	4
Mucositis	2	1	2	5
HEMATOLOGIC				
Leukopenia/ Neutropenia	22	0	14	2
Anemia	7	6	6	3
Hemorrhage	5	3	1	3
Thrombocytopenia	1	0	4	2
Infection				
without grade 3/4 neutropenia	8	3	1	4
with grade 3/4 neutropenia	1	0	2	0
Fever				
without grade 3/4 neutropenia	2	1	2	0
with grade 3/4 neutropenia	2	0	4	2
BODY AS A WHOLE				
Pain	19	22	17	13
Asthenia	15	19	13	12
METABOLIC & NUTRITIONAL				
Hepatic[c]	9	7	9	6
DERMATOLOGIC				
Hand & foot syndrome	0	0	0	5
Cutaneous signs[d]	2	0	1	3
RESPIRATORY[e]	10	8	5	7
NEUROLOGIC[f]	12	13	9	4
CARDIOVASCULAR[g]	9	3	4	2
OTHER[h]	32	28	12	14

[a] Severity of adverse events based on NCI CTC (version 1.0)
[b] BSC = best supportive care
[c] Hepatic includes events such as ascites and jaundice

[d] Cutaneous signs include events such as rash
[e] Respiratory includes events such as dyspnea and cough
[f] Neurologic includes events such as somnolence
[g] Cardiovascular includes events such as dysrhythmias, ischemia, and mechanical cardiac dysfunction
[h] Other includes events such as accidental injury, hepatomegaly, syncope, vertigo, and weight loss

Adjustments in the dose of CAMPTOSAR were made during the cycle of treatment and for subsequent cycles based on individual patient tolerance. The first dose of at least one cycle of CAMPTOSAR was reduced for 67% of patients who began the studies at the 125-mg/m^2 starting dose. Within-cycle dose reductions were required for 32% of the cycles initiated at the 125-mg/m^2 dose level. The most common reasons for dose reduction were late diarrhea, neutropenia, and leukopenia. Thirteen (4.3%) patients discontinued treatment with CAMPTOSAR because of adverse events. The adverse events in Table 8 are based on the experience of the 304 patients enrolled in the three studies described in the CLINICAL STUDIES, Studies Evaluating the Weekly Dosage Schedule, section.

Once-Every-3-Week Dosage Schedule

A total of 535 patients with metastatic colorectal cancer whose disease had recurred or progressed following prior 5-FU therapy participated in the two phase 3 studies: 316 received irinotecan, 129 received 5-FU, and 90 received best supportive care. Eleven (3.5%) patients treated with irinotecan died within 30 days of treatment. In three cases (1%, 3/316), the deaths were potentially related to irinotecan treatment and were attributed to neutropenic infection, grade 4 diarrhea, and asthenia, respectively. One (0.8%, 1/129) patient treated with 5-FU died within 30 days of treatment; this death was attributed to grade 4 diarrhea. Hospitalizations due to serious adverse events (whether or not related to study treatment) occurred at least once in 60% (188/316) of patients who received irinotecan, 63% (57/90) who received best supportive care, and 39% (50/129) who received 5-FU-based therapy. Eight percent of patients treated with irinotecan and 7% treated with 5-FU-based therapy discontinued treatment due to adverse events.

Of the 316 patients treated with irinotecan, the most clinically significant adverse events (all grades, 1–4) were diarrhea (84%), alopecia (72%), nausea (70%), vomiting (62%), cholinergic symptoms (47%), and neutropenia (30%). Table 9 lists the grade 3 and 4 adverse events reported in the patients enrolled to all treatment arms of the two studies described in the CLINICAL STUDIES, Studies Evaluating the Once-Every-3-Week Dosage Schedule, section.

Overview of Adverse Events

Gastrointestinal: Nausea, vomiting, and diarrhea are common adverse events following treatment with CAMPTOSAR and can be severe. When observed, nausea and vomiting usually occur during or shortly after infusion of CAMPTOSAR. In the clinical studies testing the every 3-week-dosage schedule, the median time to the onset of late diarrhea was 5 days after irinotecan infusion. In the clinical studies evaluating the weekly dosage schedule, the median time to onset of late diarrhea was 11 days following administration of CAMPTOSAR. For patients starting treatment at the 125-mg/m^2 weekly dose, the median duration of any grade of late diarrhea was 3 days. Among those patients treated at the 125-mg/m^2 weekly dose who experienced grade 3 or 4 late diarrhea, the median duration of the entire episode of diarrhea was 7 days. The frequency of grade 3 or 4 late diarrhea was somewhat greater in patients starting treatment at 125 mg/m^2 than in patients given a 100-mg/m^2 weekly starting dose (34% [65/193] versus 23% [24/102]; p=0.08). The frequency of grade 3 and 4 late diarrhea by age was significantly greater in patients ≥65 years than in patients <65 years (40% [53/133] versus 23% [40/171]; p=0.002). In one study of the weekly dosage treatment, the frequency of grade 3 and 4 late diarrhea was significantly greater in male than in female patients (43% [25/58] versus 16% [5/32]; p=0.01), but there were no gender differences in the frequency of grade 3 and 4 late diarrhea in the other two studies of the weekly dosage treatment schedule. Colonic ulceration, sometimes with gastrointestinal bleeding, has been observed in association with administration of CAMPTOSAR.

Hematology: CAMPTOSAR commonly causes neutropenia, leukopenia (including lymphocytopenia), and anemia. Serious thrombocytopenia is uncommon. When evaluated in the trials of weekly administration, the frequency of grade 3 and 4 neutropenia was significantly higher in patients who received previous pelvic/abdominal irradiation than in those who had not received such irradiation (48% [13/27] versus 24% [67/277]; p=0.04). In these same studies, patients with baseline serum total bilirubin levels of 1.0 mg/dL or more also had a significantly greater likelihood of experiencing first-cycle grade 3 or 4 neutropenia than those with bilirubin levels that were less than 1.0 mg/dL (50% [19/38] versus 18% [47/266]; p<0.001). There were no significant differences in the frequency of grade 3 and 4 neutropenia by age or gender. In the clinical studies evaluating the weekly dosage schedule, neutropenic fever (concurrent NCI grade 4 neutropenia and fever of grade 2 or greater) occurred in 3% of the patients; 6% of patients received G-CSF for the treatment of neutropenia. NCI grade 3 or 4 anemia was noted in 7% of the patients receiving weekly treatment; blood transfusions were given to 10% of the patients in these trials.

Body as a Whole: Asthenia, fever, and abdominal pain are generally the most common events of this type.

Cholinergic Symptoms: Patients may have cholinergic symptoms of rhinitis, increased salivation, miosis, lacrimation, diaphoresis, flushing, and intestinal hyperperistalsis that can cause abdominal cramping and early diarrhea. If these symptoms occur, they manifest during or shortly after drug infusion. They are thought to be related to the anticholinesterase activity of the irinotecan parent compound and are expected to occur more frequently with higher irinotecan doses.

Table 10. Combination-Agent Dosage Regimens & Dose Modifications[a]

Regimen	Agent	Dose		
Regimen 1 6-wk cycle with bolus 5-FU/LV (next cycle begins on day 43)	CAMPTOSAR LV 5-FU	125 mg/m^2 IV over 90 min, d 1,8,15,22 20 mg/m^2 IV bolus, d 1,8,15,22 500 mg/m^2 IV bolus, d 1,8,15,22		
		Starting Dose & Modified Dose Levels (mg/m^2)		
		Starting Dose	Dose Level -1	Dose Level -2
	CAMPTOSAR LV 5-FU	125 20 500	100 20 400	75 20 300
Regimen 2 6-wk cycle with infusional 5-FU/LV (next cycle begins on day 43)	CAMPTOSAR LV 5-FU Bolus 5-FU Infusion[b]	180 mg/m^2 IV over 90 min, d 1,15,29 200 mg/m^2 IV over 2 h, d 1,2,15,16,29,30 400 mg/m^2 IV bolus, d 1,2,15,16,29,30 600 mg/m^{2}IV over 22 h, d 1,2,15,16,29,30		
		Starting Dose & Modified Dose Levels (mg/m^2)		
		Starting Dose	Dose Level −1	Dose Level −2
	CAMPTOSAR LV 5-FU Bolus 5-FU Infusion[b]	180 200 400 600	150 200 320 480	120 200 240 360

[a] Dose reductions beyond dose level −2 by decrements of ≈20% may be warranted for patients continuing to experience toxicity. Provided intolerable toxicity does not develop, treatment with additional cycles may be continued indefinitely as long as patients continue to experience clinical benefit.
[b] Infusion follows bolus administration.

Table 11. Recommended Dose Modifications for CAMPTOSAR/5-Fluorouracil (5-FU)/Leucovorin (LV) Combination Schedules

Patients should return to pre-treatment bowel function without requiring antidiarrhea medications for at least 24 hours before the next chemotherapy administration. A new cycle of therapy should not begin until the granulocyte count has recovered to ≥1500/mm^3, and the platelet count has recovered to ≥100,000/mm^3, and treatment-related diarrhea is fully resolved. Treatment should be delayed 1 to 2 weeks to allow for recovery from treatment-related toxicities. If the patient has not recovered after a 2-week delay, consideration should be given to discontinuing therapy.

Toxicity NCI CTC Grade[a] (Value)	During a Cycle of Therapy	At the Start of Subsequent Cycles of Therapy[b]
No toxicity	Maintain dose level	Maintain dose level
Neutropenia		
1 (1500 to 1999/mm^3)	Maintain dose level	Maintain dose level
2 (1000 to 1499/mm^3)	↓ 1 dose level	Maintain dose level
3 (500 to 999/mm^3)	Omit dose until resolved to ≤ grade 2, then ↓ 1 dose level	↓ 1 dose level
4 (<500/mm^3)	Omit dose until resolved to ≤ grade 2, then ↓ 2 dose levels	↓ 2 dose levels
Neutropenic fever	Omit dose until resolved, then ↓ 2 dose levels	
Other hematologic toxicities	Dose modifications for leukopenia or thrombocytopenia during a cycle of therapy and at the start of subsequent cycles of therapy are also based on NCI toxicity criteria and are the same as recommended for neutropenia above.	
Diarrhea		
1 (2–3 stools/day > pretx[c])	Delay dose until resolved to baseline, then give same dose	Maintain dose level
2 (4–6 stools/day > pretx)	Omit dose until resolved to baseline, then ↓ 1 dose level	Maintain dose level
3 (7–9 stools/day > pretx)	Omit dose until resolved to baseline, then ↓ 1 dose level	↓ 1 dose level
4 (≥10 stools/day > pretx)	Omit dose until resolved to baseline, then ↓ 2 dose levels	↓ 2 dose levels
Other nonhematologic toxicities[d]		
1	Maintain dose level	Maintain dose level
2	Omit dose until resolved to ≤ grade 1, then ↓ 1 dose level	Maintain dose level
3	Omit dose until resolved to ≤ grade 2, then ↓ 1 dose level	↓ 1 dose level
4	Omit dose until resolved to ≤ grade 2, then ↓ 2 dose levels	↓ 2 dose levels
	For mucositis / stomatitis decrease only 5-FU, not CAMPTOSAR	*For mucositis / stomatitis decrease only 5-FU, not CAMPTOSAR*

[a] National Cancer Institute Common Toxicity Criteria (version 1.0)
[b] Relative to the starting dose used in the previous cycle
[c] Pretreatment
[d] Excludes alopecia, anorexia, asthenia

Hepatic: In the clinical studies evaluating the weekly dosage schedule, NCI grade 3 or 4 liver enzyme abnormalities were observed in fewer than 10% of patients. These events typically occur in patients with known hepatic metastases.

Dermatologic: Alopecia has been reported during treatment with CAMPTOSAR. Rashes have also been reported but did not result in discontinuation of treatment.

Respiratory: Severe pulmonary events are infrequent. In the clinical studies evaluating the weekly dosage schedule, NCI grade 3 or 4 dyspnea was reported in 4% of patients. Over half the patients with dyspnea had lung metastases; the extent to which malignant pulmonary involvement or other preexisting lung disease may have contributed to dyspnea in these patients is unknown.

Neurologic: Insomnia and dizziness can occur, but are not usually considered to be directly related to the administration of CAMPTOSAR. Dizziness may sometimes represent symptomatic evidence of orthostatic hypotension in patients with dehydration.

Cardiovascular: Vasodilation (flushing) may occur during administration of CAMPTOSAR. Bradycardia may also occur, but has not required intervention. These effects have been attributed to the cholinergic syndrome sometimes observed during or shortly after infusion of CAMPTOSAR. Thromboembolic events have been observed in patients receiving CAMPTOSAR; the specific cause of these events has not been determined.

Other Non-U.S. Clinical Trials

Irinotecan has been studied in over 1100 patients in Japan. Patients in these studies had a variety of tumor types, including cancer of the colon or rectum, and were treated with several different doses and schedules. In general, the types

Continued on next page

Camptosar—Cont.

of toxicities observed were similar to those seen in U.S. trials with CAMPTOSAR. There is some information from Japanese trials that patients with considerable ascites or pleural effusions were at increased risk for neutropenia or diarrhea. A potentially life-threatening pulmonary syndrome, consisting of dyspnea, fever, and a reticulonodular pattern on chest x-ray, was observed in a small percentage of patients in early Japanese studies. The contribution of irinotecan to these preliminary events was difficult to assess because these patients also had lung tumors and some had preexisting nonmalignant pulmonary disease. As a result of these observations, however, clinical studies in the United States have enrolled few patients with compromised pulmonary function, significant ascites, or pleural effusions.

Post-Marketing Experience

The following events have been identified during postmarketing use of CAMPTOSAR in clinical practice. Cases of colitis complicated by ulceration, bleeding, ileus, or infection have been observed. There have been rare cases of renal impairment and acute renal failure, generally in patients who became infected and/or volume depleted from severe gastrointestinal toxicities (see WARNINGS).

Hypersensitivity reactions including severe anaphylactic or anaphylactoid reactions have also been observed (see WARNINGS).

OVERDOSAGE

In U.S. phase 1 trials, single doses of up to 345 mg/m^2 of irinotecan were administered to patients with various cancers. Single doses of up to 750 mg/m^2 of irinotecan have been given in non-U.S. trials. The adverse events in these patients were similar to those reported with the recommended dosage and regimen. There is no known antidote for overdosage of CAMPTOSAR. Maximum supportive care should be instituted to prevent dehydration due to diarrhea and to treat any infectious complications.

DOSAGE AND ADMINISTRATION

Combination-Agent Dosage

Dosage Regimens

CAMPTOSAR Injection in Combination with 5-Fluorouracil (5-FU) and Leucovorin (LV)

CAMPTOSAR should be administered as an intravenous infusion over 90 minutes (see Preparation of Infusion Solution). For all regimens, the dose of LV should be administered immediately after CAMPTOSAR, with the administration of 5-FU to occur immediately after receipt of LV. CAMPTOSAR should be used as recommended; the currently recommended regimens are shown in Table 10.

Dosing for patients with bilirubin >2 mg/dL cannot be recommended since such patients were not included in clinical studies. It is recommended that patients receive premedication with antiemetic agents. Prophylactic or therapeutic administration of atropine should be considered in patients experiencing cholinergic symptoms. See PRECAUTIONS, General.

Dose Modifications

Patients should be carefully monitored for toxicity and assessed prior to each treatment. Doses of CAMPTOSAR and 5-FU should be modified as necessary to accommodate individual patient tolerance to treatment. Based on the recommended dose-levels described in Table 10, Combination-Agent Dosage Regimens & Dose Modifications, subsequent doses should be adjusted as suggested in Table 11, Recommended Dose Modifications for Combination Schedules. All dose modifications should be based on the worst preceding toxicity. After the first treatment, patients with active diarrhea should return to pre-treatment bowel function without requiring antidiarrhea medications for at least 24 hours before the next chemotherapy administration.

A new cycle of therapy should not begin until the toxicity has recovered to NCI grade 1 or less. Treatment may be delayed 1 to 2 weeks to allow for recovery from treatment-related toxicity. If the patient has not recovered, consideration should be given to discontinuing therapy. Provided intolerable toxicity does not develop, treatment with additional cycles of CAMPTOSAR/5-FU/LV may be continued indefinitely as long as patients continue to experience clinical benefit.

[See table 10 at top of previous page]
[See table 11 at top of previous page]

Single-Agent Dosage Schedules

Dosage Regimens

CAMPTOSAR should be administered as an intravenous infusion over 90 minutes for both the weekly and once-every-3-week dosage schedules (see Preparation of Infusion Solution). Single-agent dosage regimens are shown in Table 12.

A reduction in the starting dose by one dose level of CAMPTOSAR may be considered for patients with any of the following conditions: age ≥65 years, prior pelvic/abdominal radiotherapy, performance status of 2, or increased bilirubin levels. Dosing for patients with bilirubin >2 mg/dL cannot be recommended since such patients were not included in clinical studies.

It is recommended that patients receive premedication with antiemetic agents. Prophylactic or therapeutic administration of atropine should be considered in patients experiencing cholinergic symptoms. See PRECAUTIONS, General.

Dose Modifications

Patients should be carefully monitored for toxicity and doses of CAMPTOSAR should be modified as necessary to accommodate individual patient tolerance to treatment. Based on recommended dose-levels described in Table 12, Single-Agent Regimens of CAMPTOSAR and Dose Modifications, subsequent doses should be adjusted as suggested in Table 13, Recommended Dose Modifications for Single-Agent Schedules. All dose modifications should be based on the worst preceding toxicity.

Table 13. Recommended Dose Modifications for Single-Agent Schedules[a]

A new cycle of therapy should not begin until the granulocyte count has recovered to ≥1500/mm^3, and the platelet count has recovered to ≥100,000/mm^3, and treatment-related diarrhea is fully resolved. Treatment should be delayed 1 to 2 weeks to allow for recovery from treatment-related toxicities. If the patient has not recovered after a 2-week delay, consideration should be given to discontinuing CAMPTOSAR.

Worst Toxicity NCI Grade[b] (Value)	During a Cycle of Therapy	At the Start of the Next Cycles of Therapy (After Adequate Recovery), Compared with the Starting Dose in the Previous Cycle[a]	
	Weekly	Weekly	Once Every 3 Weeks
No toxicity	Maintain dose level	↑ 25 mg/m^2 up to a maximum dose of 150 mg/m^2	Maintain dose level
Neutropenia			
1 (1500 to 1999/mm^3)	Maintain dose level	Maintain dose level	Maintain dose level
2 (1000 to 1499/mm^3)	↓ 25 mg/m^2	Maintain dose level	Maintain dose level
3 (500 to 999/mm^3)	Omit dose until resolved to ≤ grade 2, then ↓ 25 mg/m^2	↓ 25 mg/m^2	↓ 50 mg/m^2
4 (<500/mm^3)	Omit dose until resolved to ≤ grade 2, then ↓ 50 mg/m^2	↓ 50 mg/m^2	↓ 50 mg/m^2
Neutropenic fever	Omit dose until resolved, then ↓ 50 mg/m^2 when resolved	↓ 50 mg/m^2	↓ 50 mg/m^2
Other hematologic toxicities	Dose modifications for leukopenia, thrombocytopenia, and anemia during a cycle of therapy and at the start of subsequent cycles of therapy are also based on NCI toxicity criteria and are the same as recommended for neutropenia above.		
Diarrhea			
1 (2–3 stools/day > pretx[c])	Maintain dose level	Maintain dose level	Maintain dose level
2 (4–6 stools/day > pretx)	↓ 25 mg/m^2	Maintain dose level	Maintain dose level
3 (7–9 stools/day > pretx)	Omit dose until resolved to ≤ grade 2, then ↓ 25 mg/m^2	↓ 25 mg/m^2	↓ 50 mg/m^2
4 (≥ 10 stools/day > pretx)	Omit dose until resolved to ≤ grade 2, then ↓ 50 mg/m^2	↓ 50 mg/m^2	↓ 50 mg/m^2
Other nonhematologic toxicities[d]			
1	Maintain dose level	Maintain dose level	Maintain dose level
2	↓ 25 mg/m^2	↓ 25 mg/m^2	↓ 50 mg/m^2
3	Omit dose until resolved to ≤ grade 2, then ↓ 25 mg/m^2	↓ 25 mg/m^2	↓ 50 mg/m^2
4	Omit dose until resolved to ≤ grade 2, then ↓ 50 mg/m^2	↓ 50 mg/m^2	↓ 50 mg/m^2

[a] All dose modifications should be based on the worst preceding toxicity
[b] National Cancer Institute Common Toxicity Criteria (version 1.0)
[c] Pretreatment
[d] Excludes alopecia, anorexia, asthenia

A new cycle of therapy should not begin until the toxicity has recovered to NCI grade 1 or less. Treatment may be delayed 1 to 2 weeks to allow for recovery from treatment-related toxicity. If the patient has not recovered, consideration should be given to discontinuing this combination therapy. Provided intolerable toxicity does not develop, treatment with additional cycles of CAMPTOSAR may be continued indefinitely as long as patients continue to experience clinical benefit.

Table 12. Single-Agent Regimens of CAMPTOSAR and Dose Modifications

Weekly Regimen[a]	125 mg/m^2 IV over 90 min, d 1,8,15,22 then 2-wk rest		
	Starting Dose & Modified Dose Levels[c] (mg/m^2)		
	Starting Dose	Dose Level −1	Dose Level −2
	125	100	75
Once-Every-3-Week Regimen[b]	350 mg/m^2 IV over 90 min, once every 3 wks[c]		
	Starting Dose & Modified Dose Levels (mg/m^2)		
	Starting Dose	Dose Level −1	Dose Level −2
	350	300	250

[a] Subsequent doses may be adjusted as high as 150 mg/m^2 or to as low as 50 mg/m^2 in 25 to 50 mg/m^2 decrements depending upon individual patient tolerance.
[b] Subsequent doses may be adjusted as low as 200 mg/m^2 in 50 mg/m^2 decrements depending upon individual patient tolerance.
[c] Provided intolerable toxicity does not develop, treatment with additional cycles may be continued indefinitely as long as patients continue to experience clinical benefit.

[See table above]

Preparation & Administration Precautions

As with other potentially toxic anticancer agents, care should be exercised in the handling and preparation of infusion solutions prepared from CAMPTOSAR Injection. The use of gloves is recommended. If a solution of CAMPTOSAR contacts the skin, wash the skin immediately and thoroughly with soap and water. If CAMPTOSAR contacts the mucous membranes, flush thoroughly with water. Several published guidelines for handling and disposal of anticancer agents are available.[1–7]

Preparation of Infusion Solution

Inspect vial contents for particulate matter and repeat inspection when drug product is withdrawn from vial into syringe.

CAMPTOSAR Injection must be diluted prior to infusion. CAMPTOSAR should be diluted in 5% Dextrose Injection, USP, (preferred) or 0.9% Sodium Chloride Injection, USP, to a final concentration range of 0.12 to 2.8 mg/mL. In most clinical trials, CAMPTOSAR was administered in 250 mL to 500 mL of 5% Dextrose Injection, USP.

The solution is physically and chemically stable for up to 24 hours at room temperature (approximately 25°C) and in ambient fluorescent lighting. Solutions diluted in 5% Dextrose Injection, USP, and stored at refrigerated temperatures (approximately 2° to 8°C), and protected from light are physically and chemically stable for 48 hours. Refrigeration of admixtures using 0.9% Sodium Chloride Injection, USP, is not recommended due to a low and sporadic incidence of visible particulates. Freezing CAMPTOSAR and admixtures of CAMPTOSAR may result in precipitation of the drug and should be avoided. Because of possible microbial contamination during dilution, it is advisable to use the admixture prepared with 5% Dextrose Injection, USP, within 24 hours if refrigerated (2° to 8°C, 36° to 46°F). In the case of admixtures prepared with 5% Dextrose Injection, USP, or Sodium Chloride Injection, USP, the solutions should be used within 6 hours if kept at room temperature (15° to 30°C, 59° to 86°F).

Other drugs should not be added to the infusion solution. Parenteral drug products should be inspected visually for particulate matter and discoloration prior to administration whenever solution and container permit.

HOW SUPPLIED

Each mL of CAMPTOSAR Injection contains 20 mg irinotecan (on the basis of the trihydrate salt); 45 mg sorbitol; and 0.9 mg lactic acid. When necessary, pH has been adjusted to 3.5 (range, 3.0 to 3.8) with sodium hydroxide or hydrochloric acid.

CAMPTOSAR Injection is available in single-dose amber glass vials in the following package sizes:

2 mL	NDC 0009-7529-02
5 mL	NDC 0009-7529-01

This is packaged in a backing/plastic blister to protect against inadvertent breakage and leakage. The vial should be inspected for damage and visible signs of leaks before removing the backing/plastic blister. If damaged, incinerate the unopened package.

Store at controlled room temperature 15° to 30°C (59° to 86°F). Protect from light. It is recommended that the vial (and backing/plastic blister) should remain in the carton until the time of use.

Rx only

REFERENCES

1. Recommendations for the Safe Handling of Parenteral Antineoplastic Drugs. NIH Publication No. 83-2621. For sale by the Superintendent of Documents, U.S. Government Printing Office, Washington, DC 20402.
2. AMA Council Report. Guidelines for handling parenteral antineoplastics. JAMA 1985;253(11): 1590–2.
3. National Study Commission on Cytotoxic Exposure. Recommendations for handling cytotoxic agents. Available from Louis P. Jeffrey, ScD, Chairman, National Study Commission on Cytotoxic Exposure, Massachusetts College of Pharmacy and Allied Health Sciences, 179 Longwood Avenue, Boston, MA 02115.
4. Clinical Oncological Society of Australia. Guidelines and recommendations for safe handling of antineoplastic agents. Med J Australia 1983;1:426–8.
5. Jones RB, et. al. Safe handling of chemotherapeutic agents: a report from the Mount Sinai Medical Center. CA-A Cancer J for Clinicians, 1983;Sept./Oct., 258–63.
6. American Society of Hospital Pharmacists Technical Assistance Bulletin on handling cytotoxic and hazardous drugs. Am J Hosp Pharm 1990;47:1033–49.
7. Controlling Occupational Exposure to Hazardous Drugs (OSHA Work-Practice Guidelines). Am J Health-Syst Pharm 1996;53:1669–85.

Manufactured by Pharmacia & Upjohn Company
A subsidiary of Pharmacia Corporation
Kalamazoo, Michigan 49001, USA
Licensed from Yakult Honsha Co., LTD, Japan, and Daiichi Pharmaceutical Co., LTD, Japan
Revised May 2002 816 907 112
692839

Pharmanex, LLC

75 WEST CENTER STREET
PROVO, UT 84601

For Technical Information and Product Support:
1-800-487-1000
www.pharmanex.com

Founded in 1994, Pharmanex is a science-based developer and marketer of natural, preventive healthcare products. Pharmanex products are researched and developed by an internal staff of 50 scientists and Ph.D.s, as well as through an advisory network of professionals from institutions across the United States and around the world. All Pharmanex products are subjected to a stringent, scientific analysis known as the Pharmanex 6S Quality Manufacturing Process™. Pharmanex products are distributed through independent sales representatives. For more information about Pharmanex product availability, visit the company Web site at www.pharmanex.com.

BIOGINKGO™ Extra Strength OTC

[*bī 'ō-gĭng 'ko*]
Standardized *Ginkgo biloba* leaf Extract
60 mg tablets
Dietary Supplement

DESCRIPTION

BioGinkgo [patent #6,174,531] is an all-natural, standardized extract of the leaves of *Ginkgo biloba* trees for use as a dietary supplement to improve blood circulation to the brain and extremities, improve cognitive function and conserve mental sharpness, and protect the body from oxidative cellular damage caused by free radicals.* *Ginkgo biloba* extract is primarily used to affect the age-related, relatively slow decline in cognitive function.* There have been several controlled clinical trials designed to test the effectiveness of *Ginkgo biloba* extract (GBE) in mitigating symptoms such as: difficulties of concentration and memory, absent mindedness, confusion, lack of energy, tiredness and decreased physical performance.

Ginkgo biloba is one of the most widely used botanicals in the world and the focus of extensive scientific research, including over 300 published studies and reports to its credit. Twenty years of research led to the development of a standardized, concentrated extract from the leaves—with a scientifically supported composition of 22 to 27% flavonoid glycoside content and 5 to 7% terpene lactone content as specified by European health authority standards for phytomedicines.

INGREDIENTS

BioGinkgo 27/7 is a standardized 50:1 extract of *Ginkgo biloba* leaf supplied in 60 mg tablets. Each tablet contains 60 mg *Ginkgo biloba* leaf extract. Each capsule is scientifically standardized to contain 27% Ginkgo flavone glycosides (kaempferol, quercetin and isorhamnetin) and 7% terpene lactones (ginkgolide A, B, C, and bilobalide).

SCIENTIFIC SUPPORT

In a bioavailability study in rabbits published in *Planta Medica* (Li CL and Wong YY, Dec 1997) comparing BioGinkgo 27/7 to another commercially available GBE, BioGinkgo 27/7 reached higher levels of plasma concentration of anti-Platelet Activating Factor (PAF) components, and manifested a faster onset and longer duration of action of anti-PAF activity over a 12-hour period.

<u>GBE promotes healthy blood flow:</u> A meta-analysis of several controlled clinical studies shows that GBE helps to maintain normal blood circulation in the body, including the brain and the extremities (arms, legs, eyes, inner ear, etc.) without a "borrowing" effect on adjacent areas of normal flow. GBE promotes efficient circulation by helping to maintain the elasticity of arteries and capillaries. Terpene lactones specific to GBE inhibit PAF, which may contribute to circulation blockage. Ginkgolide B is the most potent PAF antaganist and binds to PAF receptors.*

<u>GBE improves memory and enhances cognitive function:</u> GBE increases the rate at which information is transmitted between nerve cells by increasing blood flow to the brain and the Central Nervous System (CNS). Also, by inhibiting PAF-induced platelet aggregation and reducing the resulting viscosity or "stickiness" of the blood, the ginkgolides increase cerebral blood flow and contribute to the improvement in cognitive function seen after GBE treatment.*

<u>GBE promotes eye health:</u> The macular area of the retina is responsible for fine reading, and is particularly sensitive to damage by lipid free radicals. GBE may promote eye health in the elderly through its protective antioxidant properties.*

For additional clinical results, please see the following reference:

- Ernst E, Pittler MH. Ginkgo biloba for dementia: A systematic review of double-blind, placebo-controlled trails. Clinical Drug Investigation 1999;4:301-308.

RECOMMENDED USE

As a dietary supplement, take one 60 mg tablet bid. Allow from 2 weeks up to 12 weeks for optimum benefits.

SAFETY

GBE appears to be well tolerated at prescribed doses. Adverse reactions include mild gastrointestinal discomfort, and rare reports of allergic skin reactions. Some people may experience a mild, transient headache for the first two or three days of use.

WARNINGS

BioGinkgo has not been evaluated in children and should only be used by adults. Pregnant or breast feeding mothers should consult a physician prior to use. Consult a physician if using concurrently with anticoagulant or NSAID medications.

HOW SUPPLIED

BioGinkgo 27/7 tablets of 60 mg each are supplied in 60 count packages, and can be purchased from independent distributors and pharmacies.

STORAGE/SHELF LIFE

For all Pharmanex dietary supplements:

Storage: Store in a dry, cool place. Avoid excessive heat. Protect from light.

Shelf Life: Expiration date is imprinted on box and bottle.

EDUCATIONAL MATERIALS

For more information, including scientific references and scientific support papers for Pharmanex Healthcare Products: Call toll free 1-800-487-1000, Monday - Friday, 8 am to 5 pm, MST. Website: www.pharmanex.com

***These statements have not been evaluated by the Food and Drug Administration. This product is not intended to diagnose, treat, cure or prevent any disease.**

CORDYMAX Cs-4™ OTC

***Cordyceps sinensis* mushroom mycelia**
[*kord 'ə-măk sē ēs fŏr, kord' ə-seps sĭ-nĕn-sĭs*]
525 mg capsules
Dietary Supplement

DESCRIPTION

CordyMax Cs-4 (Patent Pending) is a dietary supplement used to reduce symptoms of fatigue, and to promote vitality and overall well-being.* It is an exclusive fermentation product derived from the mycelia of the principal fungal strain (*Paecilomyces hepiali* Chen Cs-4) isolated from the renowned *Cordyceps sinensis* mushroom. CordyMax has been profiled extensively by chemical and pharmacological methods, and is recognized as having activity most similar to wild *Cordyceps sinensis*. For over two-thousand years, *Cordyceps sinensis* has remained the premier agent in the pharmacopoeia of traditional Chinese medicine to restore vitality and energy, and to serve as a potent tonic conducive to general health and normal aging concerns.*

SCIENTIFIC SUPPORT

In humans and animals, CordyMax substantially increases the serum levels of the enzyme superoxide dismutase (SOD). This enhancement of the enzyme's proven ability to scavenge the free radicals associated with age-related oxidative cellular damage may explain the traditional use of the mushroom as a dietary supplement to improve vitality, energy, and quality of life. Scientific studies also indicate that supplementation with CordyMax may (1) Reduce oxidative stress by scavenging oxygen-free radicals in mitochondria; (2) Promote efficient utilization of oxygen, increase VO_2Max, and enhance lung function; (3) Elevate energy states (ATP) in organs; (3) Redistribute blood flow to essential organs; (4) Maintain normal liver and kidney functions; (5) Improve exercise capacity and resistance to fatigue.*

For additional clinical results, please see the following references:

- Zhu JS, et al. The Scientific Rediscovery of an Ancient Chinese Herbal Medicine: Cordyceps sinensis Part I and II. J Alt Comp Med 1998;4(3):289-303 and 1998;4(4):429-457.
- Nicodemus KJ, et al. Supplementation with Cordyceps Cs-4 fermentation product promotes fat metabolism during prolonged exercise. Med Sci Sport Exercise 2001;33:S164.
- Xiao, Y., et al. "Increased Aerobic Capacity in Healthy Elderly Humans Given a Fermentation Product of Cordyceps Cs-4". Med Sci Sport Exercise 1999;31(5):S120.

INGREDIENTS

Each capsule of CordyMax CS-4 contains 525 mg of the fermentation product of mycelia (*Paecilomyces hepiali* Chen, Cs-4) isolated from the mushroom *Cordyceps sinensis* (Berk.) Sacc., and is scientifically standardized to contain a minimum of 0.14% adenosine and 5% mannitol (an indicatory of pholysaccharide content).

RECOMMENDED USE

As a dietary supplement, take two 525 mg capsules bid or tid with water or food. Optimal results typically take 3 to 6 weeks.

SAFETY

With the exception of one case of allergic skin reaction, no other adverse reactions have been reported. During clinical trails in China, some subjects noted a mild sensation of thirst, and one subject noted slight nausea. All subjects considered these effects quite tolerable. No cases of CNS effects have been reported. No contraindications were identified based on Chinese human studies. CordyMax is non-mutagenic and non-teratogenic.

WARNINGS

CordyMax has not been evaluated in children and should only be used by adults. Pregnant and breast feeding mothers should consult a physician prior to use. Consult a physician prior to use if using anticoagulants, MAO inhibitors, or any other prescription medication.

HOW SUPPLIED

CordyMax capsules of 525 mg each are supplied in 120 count packages, and can be purchased from independent distributors and pharmacies.

STORAGE/SHELF LIFE

For all Pharmanex dietary supplements:

Storage: Store in a dry, cool place. Avoid excessive heat. Protect from light.

Shelf Life: Expiration date is imprinted on box and bottle.

EDUCATIONAL MATERIALS

For more information, including scientific references and scientific support papers for Pharmanex Healthcare Products: Call toll free 1-800-487-1000, Monday - Friday, 8 am to 5 pm, MST. Website: www.pharmanex.com

***These statements have not been evaluated by the Food and Drug Administration. This product is not intended to diagnose, treat, cure or prevent any disease.**

LIFEPAK® OTC

Multivitamin/mineral/phytonutrient supplement
Multinutrient capsules in packets
Dietary Supplement

DESCRIPTION

LifePak is a comprehensive wellness program, delivering the optimum types and amounts of vitamins, minerals, trace elements, antioxidants, and phytonutrients for general health and well-being.* LifePak addresses all common nutrient deficiencies, such as vitamins A, E, B6, the bone nutrients calcium and magnesium, and the minerals iron and zinc; provides the key anti-aging nutrients such as alpha-lipoic acid, vitamins C, E, and B12, folic acid, flavonoids, and mixed carotenoids that promote cellular protection and regeneration; and supports cardiovascular health, bone metabolism, and normal immune function.* The amounts of vitamins and minerals included in LifePak were chosen not only to prevent vitamin and mineral deficiencies, but also to correct any pre-existing deficiencies with regular use.* LifePak is intended for the general adult

Continued on next page

Life Pak—Cont.

population. Pharmanex also offers LifePak Women for premenopausal women, LifePak PreNatal for pregnant and lactating women, and LifePak Prime for men over age 40 and postmenopausal women.

SCIENTIFIC SUPPORT

LifePak's antioxidant and cardiovascular benefits are supported by two double-blind clinical studies. In a completely randomized crossover study, 25 subjects received LifePak, and 25 received placebo for 6 weeks. After a six-week washout period, the treatments were reversed. The results showed that LifePak significantly improved antioxidant status as evidenced by increased serum concentrations of ascorbic acid, α-carotene, β-carotene, and vitamin E, with no changes in placebo treatment. Most important, LifePak significantly decreased LDL oxidizability, as the lag time was prolonged by 17 % and oxidation rate was reduced, with no changes in placebo treatment. Results also confirmed the assumption that a complex antioxidant nutrient combination can be efficacious in the presence of a full spectrum of non-antioxidant nutrients in a nutritionally complete vitamin/mineral/phytonutrient supplement.

A second LifePak clinical study confirmed the results obtained from the crossover study in essentially all measurements. Thus, the antioxidant and cardiovascular benefits of LifePak are supported by two independent well-designed, double-blind clinical studies.*

For additional clinical results, please refer to the following references:

- Smidt CR, Seidehamel RJ, Devaraj S, Jialal I. The Effects of a Nutritionally Complete Dietary Supplement (LifePak®) on Antioxidant Status and LDL-Oxidation in Healthy Non-Smokers. FASEB Journal 1999;13(4):A546.
- Over 1,000 clinical studies support the benefits of the ingredients in LifePak. For a complete list of references, please contact Pharmanex at 1-800-487-1000.

INGREDIENTS

LifePak provides 39 vitamins, minerals, trace elements, antioxidants, and phytonutrients, which are provided in two daily packets. For a detailed ingredient list call Pharmanex at 1-800-487-1000.

RECOMMENDED USE

As a dietary supplement, take the contents of one LifePak packet bid with water or food.

SAFETY

All individual nutrient levels in LifePak are documented to be safe and clinical studies showed no adverse effects due to LifePak supplementation. The daily amounts of all vitamins and minerals are well below the No-Observed Adverse Effect Levels (NOAEL) established by the Council for Responsible Nutrition (CRN) in 1997 and the Upper Limits (UL) established by the Food and Nutrition Board of the National Research Council. The other nutrients in LifePak, including the phytonutrients, are added in amounts that can be obtained from diets high in fruits and vegetables (5-10 servings/day) or other commonly consumed foods and beverages.

WARNINGS

Keep this product out of reach of children. Accidental overdose of iron-containing products is a leading cause of fatal poisoning in children under six years of age. In case of accidental overdose, call a doctor or poison control center immediately. Consult a physician prior to use of taking a prescription medication. Discontinue use of this product 2 weeks prior to and after surgery.

HOW SUPPLIED

Each box provides 60 individual packets, or the equivalent of a one-month supply, and can be purchased from independent distributors and pharmacies.

STORAGE/SHELF LIFE

For all Pharmanex dietary supplements:

Storage: Store in a dry, cool place. Avoid excessive heat. Protect from light.

Shelf Life: Expiration date is imprinted on box and bottle.

EDUCATIONAL MATERIALS

For more information, including scientific references and scientific support papers for Pharmanex Healthcare Products: Call toll free 1-800-487-1000, Monday - Friday, 8 am to 5 pm, MST. Website: www.pharmanex.com

***These statements have not been evaluated by the Food and Drug Administration. This product is not intended to diagnose, treat, cure or prevent any disease.**

REISHIMAX™ OTC

Standardized Reishi Mushroom Extract
500 mg capsules
Dietary Supplement

DESCRIPTION

ReishiMax is a proprietary, standardized extract of Reishi (*Ganoderma lucidum*) mushroom. ReishiMax™ supports healthy immune system function by stimulating cell-mediated immunity with a proprietary standardized Reishi formula. ReishiMax is intended for adults who wish to maintain a healthy immune system; who smoke or who are frequently exposed to environmental pollutants; who do not get enough sleep; or who are under constant stress.*

In China, Reishi is a TCM herb of choice as a general tonic for promoting longevity, vitality and endurance, and for health preservation. As recorded in New Compilation of Materia Medica (y. 1757), Reishi "benefits heart and lung, nourishes the essence and vital energy, prevents from illness, and acts for millennia as a longevity-promoting herbal tonic."*

INGREDIENTS

ReishiMax is composed of Reishi fruiting bodies and cracked spores. The key active constituents found in Reishi include polysaccharides (beta-1,3-glucans) and triterpenes (ganoderic acids and others). Other ingredients naturally found in Reishi include nucleosides, fatty acids (oleic acid), and amino acids. The active ingredients in ReishiMax are standardized to 6% triterpenes and 13.5% polysaccharides. ReishiMax also contains a 1% extract of 100% cracked spores.

SCIENTIFIC SUPPORT

According to the results of animal and *in vitro* studies, ReishiMax has been demonstrated to stimulate the formation of antibodies, stimulate the ability of proliferation of immune cells, and modulate the functions of T cells. Ample amounts of data from animal and *in vitro* studies strongly support that Reishi extracts can enhance cell-mediated immunity by influencing lymphocytes, natural killer (NK) cells, tumor necrosis factor (TNF) and other cytokines, macrophages, and histamine release from mast cells, thus resulting in improved health benefits.*

An unpublished comparative study recently conducted by the Medical Institute at National Taiwan University found that ReishiMax enhanced immune function in mice compared to placebo and the leading Reishi competitor in Taiwan (Chiang 2002, manuscript in preparation). After six weeks, ReishiMax increased serum immunoglobulins (IgG, IgM, IgA), increased proliferation of lymphocytes, and increased secretion of cytokines (IL-2, IL-5, IL-6) and IFNγ.*

In clinical studies, Reishi extracts have been shown to increase levels of T-cell counts, CD4/CD8 ratio, cytokine IL-2, complement C3 and immunoglobulin G, lower levels of T-suppressor cell counts, improve vigor and appetite, and shorten recovery time (Kupin 1992, Yang 1996).*

For additional clinical results, please see the following references:

- Kupin, V. (1992). A new biological response modifier—*Ganoderma lucidum*—and its application in oncology, in: *The 4th International Symposium on Ganoderma lucidum*, Hyatt Regency hotel, June 10, 1992, Seoul, Korea, Program and Abstracts, pp. 36-39.
- Yang QY, Wang, M. M. (1996). The anti-aging effects of *Ganoderma* essence, in: *1996 Teipei International Ganoderma Research Conference*, Taipei International Convention Center (TICC), August 15-15, 1996, Abstracts, Special Lecture.

SAFETY

ReishiMax is safe and well tolerated at the recommended dosage. In animal studies, Reishi has been shown to be non-carcinogenic, has not produced hepatic toxicity, and has not impaired growth or development. In high doses (1.5 to 1.9 grams/day), some people have experienced temporary symptoms of sleepiness, thirst, rashes, bloating, frequent urination, abnormal sweating, and loose stools.

WARNINGS

Keep out of reach of children. If you are pregnant or nursing, or taking a prescription medication, consult a physician before using this product. Consult a physician if you are concurrently using anticoagulants, receiving immunosuppressive therapies or have an immune disorder. Individuals with known fungal allergies should be cautious when taking Reishi. Discontinue use of this product 2 weeks prior to and after surgery.

RECOMMENDED USE

Take one to two capsules of ReishiMax with liquid at your morning and evening meals. For optimal health benefits, take one (1) capsule twice daily for health maintenance, and two (2) capsules twice daily for immune modulation.

HOW SUPPLIED

ReishiMax is supplied in a 15-30 day supply of 60 capsules. Each capsule contains 495 mg of standardized Reishi mushroom extract and 5 mg of Reishi cracked spores.

STORAGE/SHELF LIFE

For all Pharmanex dietary supplements:

Storage: Store in a dry, cool place. Avoid excessive heat. Protect from light.

Shelf Life: Expiration date is imprinted on box and bottle.

EDUCATIONAL MATERIALS

For more information, including scientific references and scientific support papers for Pharmanex Healthcare Products: Call toll free 1-800-487-1000, Monday - Friday, 8 am to 5 pm, MST. Website: www.pharmanex.com

***These statements have not been evaluated by the Food and Drug Administration. This product is not intended to diagnose, treat, cure or prevent any disease.**

TĒGREEN 97™ OTC

[*tē ' grēn 97*]

Standardized Green Tea Polyphenol Extract
250 mg capsules
Dietary Supplement

DESCRIPTION

Tēgreen 97 is a standardized, caffeine-free polyphenol extract of the fresh leaves of the tea plant *Camellia sinensis*. The major components of Tēgreen are polyphenols, which have proven free radical scavenging and antioxidant properties. The polyphenols with the most active antioxidant activity are the catechins, specifically epigallocatechin gallate (EGCg) and epigallocatechin (EGC).*

INGREDIENTS

Each 250 mg capsule of proprietary Tēgreen 97 contains a 20:1 extract of green tea leaves (*Camellia sinensis*) standardized to a minimum 97% pure polyphenols including 162 mg catechins, of which 95 mg is EGCg, 37 mg is ECG, and 15 mg is EGC. Tegreen 97 is decaffeinated (<0.5 mg).

SCIENTIFIC SUPPORT

The ingestion of green tea polyphenols promotes general well-being by affecting a very broad spectrum of functions. In large-scale epidemiological studies in Asia (totaling more than 100,000 people for study periods up to 10 years), daily consumption of 4 or more cups of a green tea beverage was associated with significant overall health benefits (*Mitscher et al., Medicinal Res Rev 1997; 17: 327-365*). Even after adjustments were made for potential confounding factors including age, tobacco and alcohol use, and body weight such benefits were still evident.*

In addition to providing direct protection from the oxidative effects of potentially toxic free radicals, green tea polyphenols may also enhance the body's natural resistance to environmental toxins and stresses by increasing the activity of certain antioxidant and detoxifying enzymes, including glutathione peroxidase, glutathione reductase, glutathione S-transferase, catalase, and quinone reductase in some cells and tissues. Supplementation with green tea polyphenols (especially the catechin EGCg) may help: (1) block the formation of toxic compounds, including nitrosamines (2) suppress the activation of free radicals (3) detoxify or trap free radicals (4) inhibit spontaneous and photo-enhanced lipid peroxidation (5) inhibit the enzyme urokinase.*

For additional clinical results, refer to the following references:

- Mitscher L, et al. Chemoprotection: A review of the potential therapeutic antioxidant properties of green tea (*Camillia sinensis*) and certain of its constituents. Medicinal Research Reviews 1997;17(4):327-365.
- Mitscher L, et al. Naturally occurring antimutagens and cytoprotective agents, biologically active natural products: agrochemicals and pharmaceuticals. CRC Press [In Press].
- Pillai S, et al (1999) "Antimutagenic/Antioxidant activity of green tea components and related compounds". Journal of Environmental Pathology, Toxicology and Oncology 1999;18(3):lead article.

RECOMMENDED USE

As a dietary supplement, take one 250 mg capsule qd with food. Each capsule provides the green tea polyphenols typically found in approximately 7 cups of high-quality brewed green tea.

SAFETY

Not known to be associated with any significant side effects or toxicity. Since Tēgreen contains only trace amounts of caffeine (approximately 1-1.3 mg/capsule), it should not produce the stimulant caused by the consumption of caffeine-containing beverages.

WARNINGS

Tēgreen has not been evaluated in children and should only be used by adults. Pregnant or breast feeding mothers should consult a physician prior to use. Consult a physician prior to use if taking anticoagulants, or other prescription medications. Discontinue use of this product 2 weeks prior to and after surgery.

HOW SUPPLIED

Tēgreen capsules are supplied in 30 count packages, and can be purchased from independent distributors and pharmacies.

STORAGE/SHELF LIFE

For all Pharmanex dietary supplements:

Storage: Store in a dry, cool place. Avoid excessive heat. Protect from light.

Shelf Life: Expiration date is imprinted on box and bottle.

EDUCATIONAL MATERIALS

For more information, including scientific references and scientific support papers for Pharmanex Healthcare Products: Call toll free 1-800-487-1000, Monday - Friday, 8 am to 5 pm, MST. Website: www.pharmanex.com

***These statements have not been evaluated by the Food and Drug Administration. This product is not intended to diagnose, treat, cure or prevent any disease.**

Sankyo Pharma Inc.

TWO HILTON COURT
PARISPPANY, NJ 07054

Direct Inquiries to:
1-877-4SANKYO
www.sankyopharma.com

BENICAR™ Tablets ℞
(OLMESARTAN MEDOXOMIL)

> **USE IN PREGNANCY**
> **When used in pregnancy during the second and third trimesters, drugs that act directly on the renin-angiotensin system can cause injury and even death to the developing fetus.** When pregnancy is detected, BENICAR™ should be discontinued as soon as possible. See **WARNINGS, Fetal/Neonatal Morbidity and Mortality.**

DESCRIPTION

BENICAR™ (olmesartan medoxomil), a prodrug, is hydrolyzed to olmesartan during absorption from the gastrointestinal tract. Olmesartan is a selective AT_1 subtype angiotensin II receptor antagonist.

Olmesartan medoxomil is described chemically as 2,3-dihydroxy-2-butenyl 4-(1-hydroxy-1-methylethyl)-2-propyl-1-[*p*-(*o*-1H-tetrazol-5-ylphenyl)benzyl]imidazole-5-carboxylate, cyclic 2,3-carbonate.

Its empirical formula is $C_{29}H_{30}N_6O_6$ and its structural formula is:

Olmesartan medoxomil is a white to light yellowish-white powder or crystalline powder with a molecular weight of 558.59. It is practically insoluble in water and sparingly soluble in methanol. BENICAR™ is available for oral use as film-coated tablets containing 5 mg, 20 mg, or 40 mg of olmesartan medoxomil and the following inactive ingredients: hydroxypropylcellulose, lactose, low-substituted hydroxypropylcellulose, magnesium stearate, microcrystalline cellulose, talc, titanium dioxide, and (5 mg only) yellow iron oxide.

CLINICAL PHARMACOLOGY

Mechanism of Action

Angiotensin II is formed from angiotensin I in a reaction catalyzed by angiotensin converting enzyme (ACE, kininase II). Angiotensin II is the principal pressor agent of the renin-angiotensin system, with effects that include vasoconstriction, stimulation of synthesis and release of aldosterone, cardiac stimulation and renal reabsorption of sodium. Olmesartan blocks the vasoconstrictor effects of angiotensin II by selectively blocking the binding of angiotensin II to the AT_1 receptor in vascular smooth muscle. Its action is, therefore, independent of the pathways for angiotensin II synthesis.

An AT_2 receptor is found also in many tissues, but this receptor is not known to be associated with cardiovascular homeostasis. Olmesartan has more than a 12,500-fold greater affinity for the AT_1 receptor than for the AT_2 receptor.

Blockade of the renin-angiotensin system with ACE inhibitors, which inhibit the biosynthesis of angiotensin II from angiotensin I, is a mechanism of many drugs used to treat hypertension. ACE inhibitors also inhibit the degradation of bradykinin, a reaction also catalyzed by ACE. Because olmesartan medoxomil does not inhibit ACE (kininase II), it does not affect the response to bradykinin. Whether this difference has clinical relevance is not yet known.

Blockade of the angiotensin II receptor inhibits the negative regulatory feedback of angiotensin II on renin secretion, but the resulting increased plasma renin activity and circulating angiotensin II levels do not overcome the effect of olmesartan on blood pressure.

Pharmacokinetics

General

Olmesartan medoxomil is rapidly and completely bioactivated by ester hydrolysis to olmesartan during absorption from the gastrointestinal tract. Olmesartan appears to be eliminated in a biphasic manner with a terminal elimination half-life of approximately 13 hours. Olmesartan shows linear pharmacokinetics following single oral doses of up to 320 mg and multiple oral doses of up to 80 mg. Steady-state levels of olmesartan are achieved within 3 to 5 days and no accumulation in plasma occurs with once-daily dosing.

The absolute bioavailability of olmesartan is approximately 26%. After oral administration, the peak plasma concentration (C_{max}) of olmesartan is reached after 1 to 2 hours. Food does not affect the bioavailability of olmesartan.

Metabolism and Excretion

Following the rapid and complete conversion of olmesartan medoxomil to olmesartan during absorption, there is virtually no further metabolism of olmesartan. Total plasma clearance of olmesartan is 1.3 L/h, with a renal clearance of 0.6 L/h. Approximately 35% to 50% of the absorbed dose is recovered in urine while the remainder is eliminated in feces via the bile.

Distribution

The volume of distribution of olmesartan is approximately 17 L. Olmesartan is highly bound to plasma proteins (99%) and does not penetrate red blood cells. The protein binding is constant at plasma olmesartan concentrations well above the range achieved with recommended doses.

In rats, olmesartan crossed the blood-brain barrier poorly, if at all. Olmesartan passed across the placental barrier in rats and was distributed to the fetus. Olmesartan was distributed to milk at low levels in rats.

Special Populations

Pediatric: The pharmacokinetics of olmesartan have not been investigated in patients <18 years of age.

Geriatrics: The pharmacokinetics of olmesartan were studied in the elderly (≥65 years). Overall, maximum plasma concentrations of olmesartan were similar in young adults and the elderly. Modest accumulation of olmesartan was observed in the elderly with repeated dosing; $AUC_{ss,\tau}$ was 33% higher in elderly patients, corresponding to an approximate 30% reduction in CL_R.

Gender: Minor differences were observed in the pharmacokinetics of olmesartan in women compared to men. AUC and C_{max} were 10-15% higher in women than in men.

Renal Insufficiency: In patients with renal insufficiency, serum concentrations of olmesartan were elevated compared to subjects with normal renal function. After repeated dosing, the AUC was approximately tripled in patients with severe renal impairment (creatinine clearance <20 mL/min). The pharmacokinetics of olmesartan in patients undergoing hemodialysis has not been studied.

Hepatic Insufficiency: Increases in $AUC_{0-\infty}$ and C_{max} were observed in patients with moderate hepatic impairment compared to those in matched controls, with an increase in AUC of about 60%.

Drug Interactions: See PRECAUTIONS, Drug Interactions.

Pharmacodynamics

Olmesartan medoxomil doses of 2.5 to 40 mg inhibit the pressor effects of angiotensin I infusion. The duration of the inhibitory effect was related to dose, with doses of olmesartan medoxomil >40 mg giving >90% inhibition at 24 hours.

Plasma concentrations of angiotensin I and angiotensin II and plasma renin activity (PRA) increase after single and repeated administration of olmesartan medoxomil to healthy subjects and hypertensive patients. Repeated administration of up to 80 mg olmesartan medoxomil had minimal influence on aldosterone levels and no effect on serum potassium.

Clinical Trials

The antihypertensive effects of BENICAR™ have been demonstrated in seven placebo-controlled studies at doses ranging from 2.5 to 80 mg for 6 to 12 weeks, each showing statistically significant reductions in peak and trough blood pressure. A total of 2693 patients (2145 BENICAR™; 548 placebo) with essential hypertension were studied. BENICAR™ once daily (QD) lowered diastolic and systolic blood pressure. The response was dose-related, as shown in the following graph. An olmesartan medoxomil dose of 20 mg daily produces a trough sitting BP reduction over placebo of about 10/6 mm Hg and a dose of 40 mg daily produces a trough sitting BP reduction over placebo of about 12/7 mm Hg. Olmesartan medoxomil doses greater than 40 mg had little additional effect. The onset of the antihypertensive effect occurred within 1 week and was largely manifest after 2 weeks.

BENICAR™ Dose Response Placebo-Adjusted Reduction in Blood Pressure (mm Hg)

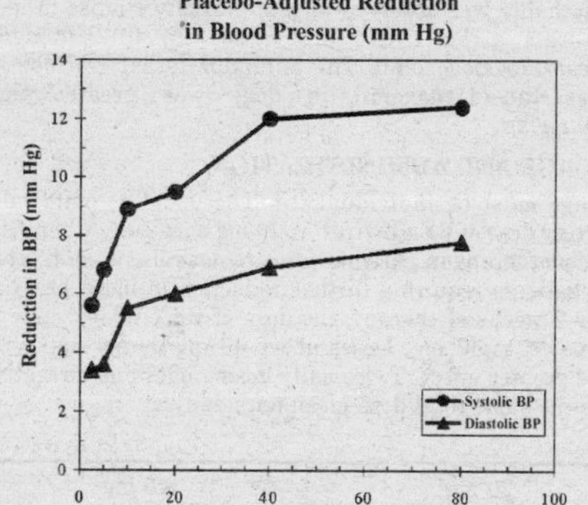

Data above are from seven placebo-controlled studies (2145 BENICAR™ patients, 548 placebo patients).

The blood pressure lowering effect was maintained throughout the 24-hour period with BENICAR™ once daily, with trough-to-peak ratios for systolic and diastolic response between 60 and 80%.

The blood pressure lowering effect of BENICAR™, with and without hydrochlorothiazide, was maintained in patients treated for up to 1 year. There was no evidence of tachyphylaxis during long-term treatment with BENICAR™ or rebound effect following abrupt withdrawal of olmesartan medoxomil after 1 year of treatment.

The antihypertensive effect of BENICAR™ was similar in men and women and in patients older and younger than 65 years. The effect was smaller in black patients (usually a low-renin population), as has been seen with other ACE inhibitors, angiotensin receptor blockers and beta-blockers. BENICAR™ had an additional blood pressure lowering effect when added to hydrochlorothiazide.

INDICATIONS AND USAGE

BENICAR™ is indicated for the treatment of hypertension. It may be used alone or in combination with other antihypertensive agents.

CONTRAINDICATIONS

BENICAR™ is contraindicated in patients who are hypersensitive to any component of this product.

WARNINGS

Fetal/Neonatal Morbidity and Mortality

Drugs that act directly on the renin-angiotensin system can cause fetal and neonatal morbidity and death when administered to pregnant women. Several dozen cases have been reported in the world literature of patients who were taking angiotensin converting enzyme inhibitors. When pregnancy is detected, BENICAR™ should be discontinued as soon as possible.

The use of drugs that act directly on the renin-angiotensin system during the second and third trimesters of pregnancy has been associated with fetal and neonatal injury, including hypotension, neonatal skull hypoplasia, anuria, reversible or irreversible renal failure and death. Oligohydramnios has also been reported, presumably resulting from decreased fetal function; oligohydramnios in this setting has been associated with fetal limb contractures, craniofacial deformation and hypoplastic lung development. Prematurity, intrauterine growth retardation and patent ductus arteriosus have also been reported, although it is not clear whether these occurrences were due to exposure to the drug.

These adverse effects do not appear to have resulted from intrauterine drug exposure that has been limited to the first trimester. Mothers whose embryos and fetuses are exposed to an angiotensin II receptor antagonist only during the first trimester should be so informed. Nonetheless, when patients become pregnant, physicians should have the patient discontinue the use of BENICAR™ as soon as possible. Rarely (probably less often than once in every thousand pregnancies), no alternative to a drug acting on the renin-angiotensin system will be found. In these rare cases, the mothers should be apprised of the potential hazards to their fetuses and serial ultrasound examinations should be performed to assess the intra-amniotic environment.

If oligohydramnios is observed, BENICAR™ should be discontinued unless it is considered life-saving for the mother. Contraction stress testing (CST), a nonstress test (NST) or biophysical profiling (BPP) may be appropriate, depending upon the week of pregnancy. Patients and physicians should be aware, however, that oligohydramnios may not appear until after the fetus has sustained irreversible injury.

Infants with histories of *in utero* exposure to an angiotensin II receptor antagonist should be closely observed for hypotension, oliguria and hyperkalemia. If oliguria occurs, attention should be directed toward support of blood pressure and renal perfusion. Exchange transfusion or dialysis may be required as means of reversing hypotension and/or substituting for disordered renal function.

There is no clinical experience with the use of BENICAR™ in pregnant women. No teratogenic effects were observed when olmesartan medoxomil was administered to pregnant rats at oral doses up to 1000 mg/kg/day (240 times the maximum recommended human dose [MRHD] of olmesartan medoxomil on a mg/m^2 basis) or pregnant rabbits at oral doses up to 1 mg/kg/day (half the MRHD on a mg/m^2 basis; higher doses could not be evaluated for effects on fetal development as they were lethal to the does). In rats, significant decreases in pup birth weight and weight gain were observed at doses ≥1.6 mg/kg/day, and delays in developmental milestones and dose-dependent increases in the incidence of dilation of the renal pelvis were observed at doses ≥8 mg/kg/day. The no observed effect dose for developmental toxicity in rats is 0.3 mg/kg/day, about one-tenth the MRHD of 40 mg/day.

Hypotension in Volume- or Salt-Depleted Patients

In patients with an activated renin-angiotensin system, such as volume- and/or salt-depleted patients (e.g., those being treated with high doses of diuretics), symptomatic hypotension may occur after initiation of treatment with BENICAR™. Treatment should start under close medical supervision. If hypotension does occur, the patient should be placed in the supine position and, if necessary, given an intravenous infusion of normal saline (See **DOSAGE AND ADMINISTRATION**). A transient hypotensive response is not a contraindication to further treatment, which usually can be continued without difficulty once the blood pressure has stabilized.

Continued on next page

Benicar—Cont.

PRECAUTIONS

General

Impaired Renal Function: As a consequence of inhibiting the renin-angiotensin-aldosterone system, changes in renal function may be anticipated in susceptible individuals treated with olmesartan medoxomil. In patients whose renal function may depend upon the activity of the renin-angiotensin-aldosterone system (e.g. patients with severe congestive heart failure), treatment with angiotensin converting enzyme inhibitors and angiotensin receptor antagonists has been associated with oliguria and/or progressive azotemia and (rarely) with acute renal failure and/or death. Similar results may be anticipated in patients treated with olmesartan medoxomil. (See **CLINICAL PHARMACOLOGY, Special Populations.**)

In studies of ACE inhibitors in patients with unilateral or bilateral renal artery stenosis, increases in serum creatinine or blood urea nitrogen (BUN) have been reported. There has been no long-term use of olmesartan medoxomil in patients with unilateral or bilateral renal artery stenosis, but similar results may be expected.

Information for Patients

Pregnancy: Female patients of childbearing age should be told about the consequences of second and third trimester exposure to drugs that act on the renin-angiotensin system and they should be told also that these consequences do not appear to have resulted from intrauterine drug exposure that has been limited to the first trimester. These patients should be asked to report pregnancies to their physicians as soon as possible.

Drug Interactions

No significant drug interactions were reported in studies in which olmesartan medoxomil was co-administered with digoxin or warfarin in healthy volunteers. The bioavailability of olmesartan was not significantly altered by the co-administration of antacids [$Al(OH)_3$/$Mg(OH)_2$]. Olmesartan medoxomil is not metabolized by the cytochrome P450 system and has no effects on P450 enzymes; thus, interactions with drugs that inhibit, induce or are metabolized by those enzymes are not expected.

Carcinogenesis, Mutagenesis, Impairment of Fertility

Olmesartan medoxomil was not carcinogenic when administered by dietary administration to rats for up to 2 years. The highest dose tested (2000 mg/kg/day) was, on a mg/m^2 basis, about 480 times the maximum recommended human dose (MRHD) of 40 mg/day. Two carcinogenicity studies conducted in mice, a 6-month gavage study in the p53 knockout mouse and a 6-month dietary administration study in the Hras2 transgenic mouse, at doses of up to 1000 mg/kg/day (about 120 times the MRHD), revealed no evidence of a carcinogenic effect of olmesartan medoxomil.

Both olmesartan medoxomil and olmesartan tested negative in the *in vitro* Syrian hamster embryo cell transformation assay and showed no evidence of genetic toxicity in the Ames (bacterial mutagenicity) test. However, both were shown to induce chromosomal aberrations in cultured cells *in vitro* (Chinese hamster lung). Olmesartan medoxomil also tested positive for thymidine kinase mutations in the *in vitro* mouse lymphoma assay (olmesartan not tested). Olmesartan medoxomil tested negative *in vivo* for mutations in the MutaMouse intestine and kidney, for DNA damage in the rat kidney (comet assay) and for clastogenicity in mouse bone marrow (micronucleus test) at oral doses of up to 2000 mg/kg (olmesartan not tested).

Fertility of rats was unaffected by administration of olmesartan medoxomil at dose levels as high as 1000 mg/kg/day (240 times the MRHD) in a study in which dosing was begun 2 (female) or 9 (male) weeks prior to mating.

Pregnancy

Pregnancy Categories C (first trimester) and D (second and third trimesters). See **WARNINGS, Fetal/Neonatal Morbidity and Mortality.**

Nursing Mothers

It is not known whether olmesartan is excreted in human milk, but olmesartan is secreted at low concentration in the milk of lactating rats. Because of the potential for adverse effects on the nursing infant, a decision should be made whether to discontinue nursing or discontinue the drug, taking into account the importance of the drug to the mother.

Pediatric Use

Safety and effectiveness in pediatric patients have not been established.

Geriatric Use

Of the total number of hypertensive patients receiving BENICAR™ in clinical studies, more than 20% were 65 years of age and over, while more than 5% were 75 years of age and older. No overall differences in effectiveness or safety were observed between elderly patients and younger patients. Other reported clinical experience has not identified differences in responses between the elderly and younger patients, but greater sensitivity of some older individuals cannot be ruled out.

ADVERSE REACTIONS

BENICAR™ has been evaluated for safety in more than 3825 patients/subjects, including more than 3275 patients treated for hypertension in controlled trials. This experience included about 900 patients treated for at least 6 months and more than 525 for at least 1 year. Treatment with BENICAR™ was well tolerated, with an incidence of adverse events similar to placebo. Events generally were mild, transient and had no relationship to the dose of olmesartan medoxomil.

The overall frequency of adverse events was not dose-related. Analysis of gender, age and race groups demonstrated no differences between olmesartan medoxomil and placebo-treated patients. The rate of withdrawals due to adverse events in all trials of hypertensive patients was 2.4% (i.e. 79/3278) of patients treated with olmesartan medoxomil and 2.7% (i.e. 32/1179) of control patients. In placebo-controlled trials, the only adverse event that occurred in more than 1% of patients treated with olmesartan medoxomil and at a higher incidence versus placebo was dizziness (3% vs. 1%).

The following adverse events occurred in placebo-controlled clinical trials at an incidence of more than 1% of patients treated with olmesartan medoxomil, but also occurred at about the same or greater incidence in patients receiving placebo: back pain, bronchitis, creatine phosphokinase increased, diarrhea, headache, hematuria, hyperglycemia, hypertriglyceridemia, inflicted injury, influenza-like symptoms, pharyngitis, rhinitis, sinusitis and upper respiratory tract infection.

The incidence of cough was similar in placebo (0.7%) and BENICAR™ (0.9%) patients.

Other (potentially important) adverse events that have been reported with an incidence of greater than 0.5%, whether or not attributed to treatment, in the more than 3100 hypertensive patients treated with olmesartan medoxomil monotherapy in controlled or open-label trials are listed below.

Body as a Whole: chest pain, fatigue, pain, peripheral edema
Central and Peripheral Nervous System: vertigo
Gastrointestinal: abdominal pain, dyspepsia, gastroenteritis, nausea
Heart Rate and Rhythm Disorders: tachycardia
Metabolic and Nutritional Disorders: hypercholesterolemia, hyperlipemia, hyperuricemia
Musculoskeletal: arthralgia, arthritis, myalgia, skeletal pain
Psychiatric Disorders: insomnia
Skin and Appendages: rash
Urinary System: urinary tract infection

Facial edema was reported in 5 patients receiving olmesartan medoxomil. Angioedema has been reported with other angiotensin II antagonists.

Laboratory Test Findings: In controlled clinical trials, clinically important changes in standard laboratory parameters were rarely associated with administration of olmesartan medoxomil.

Hemoglobin and Hematocrit: Small decreases in hemoglobin and hematocrit (mean decreases of approximately 0.3 g/dL and 0.3 volume percent, respectively) were observed.

Liver Function Tests: Elevations of liver enzymes and/or serum bilirubin were observed infrequently. Five patients (0.1%) assigned to olmesartan medoxomil and one patient (0.2%) assigned to placebo in clinical trials were withdrawn because of abnormal liver chemistries (transaminases or total bilirubin). Of the five olmesartan medoxomil patients, three had elevated transaminases, which were attributed to alcohol use, and one had a single elevated bilirubin value, which normalized while treatment continued.

OVERDOSAGE

Limited data are available related to overdosage in humans. The most likely manifestations of overdosage would be hypotension and tachycardia; bradycardia could be encountered if parasympathetic (vagal) stimulation occurs. If symptomatic hypotension should occur, supportive treatment should be initiated. The dialyzability of olmesartan is unknown.

No lethality was observed in acute toxicity studies in mice and rats given single oral doses up to 2000mg/kg olmesartan medoxomil. The minimum lethal oral dose of olmesartan medoxomil in dogs was greater than 1500 mg/kg.

DOSAGE AND ADMINISTRATION

Dosage must be individualized. The usual recommended starting dose of BENICAR™ is 20 mg once daily when used as monotherapy in patients who are not volume-contracted. For patients requiring further reduction in blood pressure after 2 weeks of therapy, the dose of BENICAR™ may be increased to 40 mg. Doses above 40 mg do not appear to have greater effect. Twice-daily dosing offers no advantage over the same total dose given once daily.

No initial dosage adjustment is recommended for elderly patients, for patients with moderate to marked renal impairment (creatinine clearance <40mL/min) or with moderate to marked hepatic dysfunction (see CLINICAL PHARMACOLOGY, Special Populations). For patients with possible depletion of intravascular volume (e.g., patients treated with diuretics, particularly those with impaired renal function), BENICAR™ should be initiated under close medical supervision and consideration should be given to use of a lower starting dose (see WARNINGS, Hypotension in Volume- and Salt-Depleted Patients).

BENICAR™ may be administered with or without food.

If blood pressure is not controlled by BENICAR™ alone, a diuretic may be added. BENICAR™ may be administered with other antihypertensive agents.

HOW SUPPLIED

BENICAR™ is supplied as yellow, round, film-coated tablets containing 5 mg of olmesartan medoxomil, as white, round, film-coated tablets containing 20 mg of olmesartan medoxomil, and as white, oval-shaped, film-coated tablets containing 40 mg of olmesartan medoxomil. Tablets are debossed with Sankyo on one side and C12, C14, or C15 on the other side of the 5, 20, and 40 mg tablets, respectively.

Tablets are supplied as follows:

[See table below]

	5 mg	20 mg	40 mg
Bottle of 30	NDC 65597-101-30	NDC 65597-103-30	NDC 65597-104-30
Bottle of 90	Not available	NDC 65597-103-90	NDC 65597-104-90
Blister 10 cards X 10		NDC 65597-103-10	NDC 65597-104-10

Storage

Store at 20-25°C (68-77°F) [See USP Controlled Room Temperature].

Manufactured by Sankyo Pharma GmbH, Munich, Germany

Manufactured for Sankyo Pharma Inc., New York, NY 10017

Rx Only

P1800601

Sanofi-Synthelabo Inc.

90 PARK AVENUE
NEW YORK, NY 10016

Direct Inquiries to:
(212) 551-4000

For Medical Information Contact:
Product Information Services
(800) 446-6267

Sales and Ordering:
East Coast: (800) 223-1062
West Coast: (800) 223-5511

AMBIEN® Ⓒ℞

[am' bē-ĕn]
(zolpidem tartrate)

DESCRIPTION

Ambien (zolpidem tartrate), is a non-benzodiazepine hypnotic of the imidazopyridine class and is available in 5-mg and 10-mg strength tablets for oral administration.

Chemically, zolpidem is N,N,6-trimethyl-2-p-tolylimidazo[1,2-a] pyridine-3-acetamide L-(+)-tartrate (2:1). It has the following structure:

Zolpidem tartrate is a white to off-white crystalline powder that is sparingly soluble in water, alcohol, and propylene glycol. It has a molecular weight of 764.88.

Each Ambien tablet includes the following inactive ingredients: hydroxypropyl methylcellulose, lactose, magnesium stearate, microcrystalline cellulose, polyethylene glycol, sodium starch glycolate, and titanium dioxide; the 5-mg tablet also contains FD&C Red No. 40, iron oxide colorant, and polysorbate 80.

CLINICAL PHARMACOLOGY

Pharmacodynamics: Subunit modulation of the $GABA_A$ receptor chloride channel macromolecular complex is hypothesized to be responsible for sedative, anticonvulsant, anxiolytic, and myorelaxant drug properties. The major modulatory site of the $GABA_A$ receptor complex is located on its alpha (α) subunit and is referred to as the benzodiazepine (BZ) or omega (ω) receptor. At least three subtypes of the (ω) receptor have been identified.

While zolpidem is a hypnotic agent with a chemical structure unrelated to benzodiazepines, barbiturates, or other drugs with known hypnotic properties, it interacts with a GABA-BZ receptor complex and shares some of the pharmacological properties of the benzodiazepines. In contrast to the benzodiazepines, which nonselectively bind to and activate all omega receptor subtypes, zolpidem in vitro binds the (ω_1) receptor preferentially with a high affinity ratio of the alpha$_1$/alpha$_5$ subunits. The (ω_1) receptor is found primarily on the Lamina IV of the sensorimotor cortical regions, substantia nigra (parsreticulata), cerebellum molecular layer, olfactory bulb, ventral thalamic complex, pons, inferior colliculus, and globus pallidus. This selective binding of zolpidem on the (ω_1) receptor is not absolute, but it may explain the relative absence of myorelaxant and anticonvulsant effects in animal studies as well as the preservation of deep sleep (stages 3 and 4) in human studies of zolpidem at hypnotic doses.

Pharmacokinetics: The pharmacokinetic profile of Ambien is characterized by rapid absorption from the GI tract and a short elimination half-life ($T_{1/2}$) in healthy subjects. In a single-dose crossover study in 45 healthy subjects administered 5- and 10-mg zolpidem tartrate tablets, the mean peak concentrations (C_{max}) were 59 (range: 29 to 113) and 121 (range: 58 to 272) ng/mL, respectively, occurring at a mean time (T_{max}) of 1.6 hours for both. The mean Ambien elimination half-life was 2.6 (range: 1.4 to 4.5) and 2.5 (range: 1.4 to 3.8) hours, for the 5- and 10-mg tablets, respectively. Ambien is converted to inactive metabolites that are eliminated primarily by renal excretion. Ambien demonstrated linear kinetics in the dose range of 5 to 20 mg. Total protein binding was found to be 92.5 ± 0.1% and remained constant, independent of concentration between 40 and 790 ng/mL. Zolpidem did not accumulate in young adults following nightly dosing with 20-mg zolpidem tartrate tablets for 2 weeks.

A food-effect study in 30 healthy male volunteers compared the pharmacokinetics of Ambien 10 mg when administered while fasting or 20 minutes after a meal. Results demonstrated that with food, mean AUC and C_{max} were decreased by 15% and 25%, respectively, while mean T_{max} was prolonged by 60% (from 1.4 to 2.2 hr). The half-life remained unchanged. These results suggest that, for faster sleep onset, Ambien should not be administered with or immediately after a meal.

In the elderly, the dose for Ambien should be 5 mg (see *Precautions and Dosage and Administration*). This recommendation is based on several studies in which the mean C_{max}, $T_{1/2}$, and AUC were significantly increased when compared to results in young adults. In one study of eight elderly subjects (>70 years), the means for C_{max}, $T_{1/2}$, and AUC significantly increased by 50% (255 vs 384 ng/mL), 32% (2.2 vs 2.9 hr), and 64% (955 vs 1,562 ng hr/mL), respectively, as compared to younger adults (20 to 40 years) following a single 20-mg oral zolpidem dose. Ambien did not accumulate in elderly subjects following nightly oral dosing of 10 mg for 1 week.

The pharmacokinetics of Ambien in eight patients with chronic hepatic insufficiency were compared to results in healthy subjects. Following a single 20-mg oral zolpidem dose, mean C_{max} and AUC were found to be two times (250 vs 499 ng/mL) and five times (788 vs 4,203 ng hr/mL) higher, respectively, in hepatically compromised patients. T_{max} did not change. The mean half-life in cirrhotic patients of 9.9 hr (range: 4.1 to 25.8 hr) was greater than that observed in normals of 2.2 hr (range: 1.6 to 2.4 hr). Dosing should be modified accordingly in patients with hepatic insufficiency (see *Precautions and Dosage and Administration*).

The pharmacokinetics of zolpidem tartrate were studied in 11 patients with end-stage renal failure (mean Cl_{Cr} = 6.5 ± 1.5 mL/min) undergoing hemodialysis three times a week, who were dosed with zolpidem 10 mg orally each day for 14 or 21 days. No statistically significant differences were observed for C_{max}, T_{max}, half-life, and AUC between the first and last day of drug administration when baseline concentration adjustments were made. On day 1, C_{max} was 172 ± 29 ng/mL (range: 46 to 344 ng/mL). After repeated dosing for 14 or 21 days, C_{max} was 203 ± 32 ng/mL (range: 28 to 316 ng/mL). On day 1, T_{max} was 1.7 ± 0.3 hr (range: 0.5 to 3.0 hr); after repeated dosing T_{max} was 0.8 ± 0.2 hr (range: 0.5 to 2.0 hr). This variation is accounted for by noting that last-day serum sampling began 10 hours after the previous dose, rather than after 24 hours. This resulted in residual drug concentration and a shorter period to reach maximal serum concentration. On day 1, $T_{1/2}$ was 2.4 ± 0.4 hr (range: 0.4 to 5.1 hr). After repeated dosing, $T_{1/2}$ was 2.5 ± 0.4 hr (range: 0.7 to 4.2 hr). AUC was 796 ± 159 ng hr/mL after the first dose and 818 ± 170 ng• hr/mL after repeated dosing. Zolpidem was not hemodialyzable. No accumulation of unchanged drug appeared after 14 or 21 days. Ambien (zolpidem tartrate) pharmacokinetics were not significantly different in renally impaired patients. No dosage adjustment is necessary in patients with compromised renal function. As a general precaution, these patients should be closely monitored.

Postulated relationship between elimination rate of hypnotics and their profile of common untoward effects: The type and duration of hypnotic effects and the profile of unwanted effects during administration of hypnotic drugs may be influenced by the biologic half-life of administered drug and any active metabolites formed. When half-lives are long, drug or metabolites may accumulate during periods of nightly administration and be associated with impairment of cognitive and/or motor performance during waking hours; the possibility of interaction with other psychoactive drugs or alcohol will be enhanced. In contrast, if half-lives, including half-lives of active metabolites, are short, drug and metabolites will be cleared before the next dose is ingested, and carryover effects related to excessive sedation or CNS depression should be minimal or absent. Ambien has a short half-life and no active metabolites. During nightly use for an extended period, pharmacodynamic tolerance or adaptation to some effects of hypnotics may develop. If the drug has a short elimination half-life, it is possible that a relative deficiency of the drug or its active metabolites (ie, in relationship to the receptor site) may occur at some point in the interval between each night's use. This sequence of events may account for two clinical findings reported to occur after several weeks of nightly use of other rapidly eliminated hypnotics, namely, increased wakefulness during the last third of the night, and the appearance of increased signs of daytime anxiety. Increased wakefulness during the last third of the night as measured by polysomnography has not been observed in clinical trials with Ambien.

Controlled trials supporting safety and efficacy

Transient insomnia: Normal adults experiencing transient insomnia (n=462) during the first night in a sleep laboratory were evaluated in a double-blind, parallel group, single-night trial comparing two doses of zolpidem (7.5 and 10 mg) and placebo. Both zolpidem doses were superior to placebo on objective (polysomnographic) measures of sleep latency, sleep duration, and number of awakenings.

Normal elderly adults (mean age 68) experiencing transient insomnia (n=35) during the first two nights in a sleep laboratory were evaluated in a double-blind, crossover, 2-night trial comparing four doses of zolpidem (5, 10, 15 and 20 mg) and placebo. All zolpidem doses were superior to placebo on the two primary PSG parameters (sleep latency and efficiency) and all four subjective outcome measures (sleep duration, sleep latency, number of awakenings, and sleep quality).

Chronic insomnia: Zolpidem was evaluated in two controlled studies for the treatment of patients with chronic insomnia (most closely resembling primary insomnia, as defined in the APA Diagnostic and Statistical Manual of Mental Disorders, DSM-IV™). Adult outpatients with chronic insomnia (n=75) were evaluated in a double-blind, parallel group, 5-week trial comparing two doses of zolpidem tartrate (10 and 15 mg) and placebo. On objective (polysomnographic) measures of sleep latency and sleep efficiency, zolpidem 15 mg was superior to placebo for all 5 weeks; zolpidem 10 mg was superior to placebo on sleep latency for the first 4 weeks and on sleep efficiency for weeks 2 and 4. Zolpidem was comparable to placebo on number of awakenings at both doses studied.

Adult outpatients (n=141) with chronic insomnia were also evaluated in a double-blind, parallel group, 4-week trial comparing two doses of zolpidem (10 and 15 mg) and placebo. Zolpidem 10 mg was superior to placebo on a subjective measure of sleep latency for all 4 weeks, and on subjective measures of total sleep time, number of awakenings, and sleep quality for the first treatment week. Zolpidem 15 mg was superior to placebo on a subjective measure of total sleep latency for the first 3 weeks, on a subjective measure of total sleep time for the first week, and on number of awakenings and sleep quality for the first 2 weeks.

Next-day residual effects: Next-day residual effects of Ambien were evaluated in seven studies involving normal volunteers. In three studies in adults (including one study in a phase advance model of transient insomnia) and in one study in elderly subjects, a small but statistically significant decrease in performance was observed in the Digit Symbol Substitution Test (DSST) when compared to placebo. Studies of Ambien in non-elderly patients with insomnia did not detect evidence of next-day residual effects using the DSST, the Multiple Sleep Latency Test (MSLT), and patient ratings of alertness.

Rebound effects: There was no objective (polysomnographic) evidence of rebound insomnia at recommended doses seen in studies evaluating sleep on the nights following discontinuation of Ambien (zolpidem tartrate). There was subjective evidence of impaired sleep in the elderly on the first post-treatment night at doses above the recommended elderly dose of 5 mg.

Memory impairment: Controlled studies in adults utilizing objective measures of memory yielded no consistent evidence of next-day memory impairment following the administration of Ambien. However, in one study involving zolpidem doses of 10 and 20 mg, there was a significant decrease in next-morning recall of information presented to subjects during peak drug effect (90 minutes post-dose), ie, these subjects experienced anterograde amnesia. There was also subjective evidence from adverse event data for anterograde amnesia occurring in association with the administration of Ambien, predominantly at doses above 10 mg.

Effects on sleep stages: In studies that measured the percentage of sleep time spent in each sleep stage, Ambien has generally been shown to preserve sleep stages. Sleep time spent in stages 3 and 4 (deep sleep) was found comparable to placebo with only inconsistent, minor changes in REM (paradoxical) sleep at the recommended dose.

INDICATIONS AND USAGE

Ambien (zolpidem tartrate) is indicated for the short-term treatment of insomnia. Ambien has been shown to decrease sleep latency and increase the duration of sleep for up to 35 days in controlled clinical studies (see *Clinical Pharmacology: Controlled trials supporting safety and efficacy*).

Hypnotics should generally be limited to 7 to 10 days of use, and reevaluation of the patient is recommended if they are to be taken for more than 2 to 3 weeks. Ambien should not be prescribed in quantities exceeding a 1-month supply (see *Warnings*).

CONTRAINDICATIONS

None known.

WARNINGS

Since sleep disturbances may be the presenting manifestation of a physical and/or psychiatric disorder, symptomatic treatment of insomnia should be initiated only after a careful evaluation of the patient. The failure of insomnia to remit after 7 to 10 days of treatment may indicate the presence of a primary psychiatric and/or medical illness which should be evaluated. Worsening of insomnia or the emergence of new thinking or behavior abnormalities may be the consequence of an unrecognized psychiatric or physical disorder. Such findings have emerged during the course of treatment with sedative/hypnotic drugs, including Ambien. Because some of the important adverse effects of Ambien appear to be dose related (see *Precautions* and *Dosage and Administration*), it is important to use the smallest possible effective dose, especially in the elderly.

A variety of abnormal thinking and behavior changes have been reported to occur in association with the use of sedative/hypnotics. Some of these changes may be characterized by decreased inhibition (eg, aggressiveness and extroversion that seemed out of character), similar to effects produced by alcohol and other CNS depressants. Other reported behavioral changes have included bizarre behavior, agitation, hallucinations, and depersonalization. Amnesia and other neuro-psychiatric symptoms may occur unpredictably. In primarily depressed patients, worsening of depression, including suicidal thinking, has been reported in association with the use of sedative/hypnotics.

It can rarely be determined with certainty whether a particular instance of the abnormal behaviors listed above is drug induced, spontaneous in origin, or a result of an underlying psychiatric or physical disorder. Nonetheless, the emergence of any new behavioral sign or symptom of concern requires careful and immediate evaluation.

Following the rapid dose decrease or abrupt discontinuation of sedative/hypnotics, there have been reports of signs and symptoms similar to those associated with withdrawal from other CNS-depressant drugs (see *Drug Abuse* and *Dependence*).

Ambien, like other sedative/hypnotic drugs, has CNS-depressant effects. Due to the rapid onset of action, Ambien should only be ingested immediately prior to going to bed. Patients should be cautioned against engaging in hazardous occupations requiring complete mental alertness or motor coordination such as operating machinery or driving a motor vehicle after ingesting the drug, including potential impairment of the performance of such activities that may occur the day following ingestion of Ambien. Ambien showed additive effects when combined with alcohol and should not be taken with alcohol. Patients should also be cautioned about possible combined effects with other CNS-depressant drugs. Dosage adjustments may be necessary when Ambien is administered with such agents because of the potentially additive effects.

PRECAUTIONS

General

Use in the elderly and/or debilitated patients: Impaired motor and/or cognitive performance after repeated exposure or unusual sensitivity to sedative/hypnotic drugs is a concern in the treatment of elderly and/or debilitated patients. Therefore, the recommended Ambien dosage is 5 mg in such patients (see *Dosage and Administration*) to decrease the possibility of side effects. These patients should be closely monitored.

Use in patients with concomitant illness: Clinical experience with Ambien (zolpidem tartrate) in patients with concomitant systemic illness is limited. Caution is advisable in using Ambien in patients with diseases or conditions that could affect metabolism or hemodynamic responses. Although studies did not reveal respiratory depressant effects at hypnotic doses of Ambien in normals or in patients with mild to moderate chronic obstructive pulmonary disease (COPD), a reduction in the Total Arousal Index together with a reduction in lowest oxygen saturation and increase in the times of oxygen desaturation below 80% and 90% was observed in patients with mild-to-moderate sleep apnea when treated with Ambien (10 mg) when compared to placebo. However, precautions should be observed if Ambien is prescribed to patients with compromised respiratory function, since sedative/hypnotics have the capacity to depress respiratory drive. Post-marketing reports of respiratory insufficiency, most of which involved patients with preexisting respiratory impairment, have been received. Data in end-stage renal failure patients repeatedly treated with Ambien did not demonstrate drug accumulation or alterations in pharmacokinetic parameters. No dosage adjustment in renally impaired patients is required; however, these patients should be closely monitored (see *Pharmacokinetics*). A study in subjects with hepatic impairment did reveal prolonged elimination in this group; therefore, treatment should be initiated with 5 mg in patients with hepatic compromise, and they should be closely monitored.

Use in depression: As with other sedative/hypnotic drugs, Ambien should be administered with caution to patients exhibiting signs or symptoms of depression. Suicidal tendencies may be present in such patients and protective measures may be required. Intentional over-dosage is more common in this group of patients; therefore, the least amount of drug that is feasible should be prescribed for the patient at any one time.

Information for patients: Patient information is printed at the end of this insert. To assure safe and effective use of

Continued on next page

Ambien—Cont.

Ambien, this information and instructions provided in the patient information section should be discussed with patients.

Laboratory tests: There are no specific laboratory tests recommended.

Drug interactions

CNS-active drugs: Ambien was evaluated in healthy volunteers in single-dose interaction studies for several CNS drugs. A study involving haloperidol and zolpidem revealed no effect of haloperidol on the pharmacokinetics or pharmacodynamics of zolpidem. Imipramine in combination with zolpidem produced no pharmacokinetic interaction other than a 20% decrease in peak levels of imipramine, but there was an additive effect of decreased alertness. Similarly, chlorpromazine in combination with zolpidem produced no pharmacokinetic interaction, but there was an additive effect of decreased alertness and psychomotor performance. The lack of a drug interaction following single-dose administration does not predict a lack following chronic administration.

An additive effect on psychomotor performance between alcohol and zolpidem was demonstrated.

A single-dose interaction study with zolpidem 10 mg and fluoxetine 20 mg at steady-state levels in male volunteers did not demonstrate any clinically significant pharmacokinetic or pharmacodynamic interactions. When multiple doses of zolpidem and fluoxetine at steady-state concentrations were evaluated in healthy females, the only significant change was a 17% increase in the zolpidem half-life. There was no evidence of an additive effect in psychomotor performance.

Following five consecutive nightly doses of zolpidem 10 mg in the presence of sertraline 50 mg (17 consecutive daily doses, at 7:00 am, in healthy female volunteers), zolpidem C_{max} was significantly higher (43%) and T_{max} was significantly decreased (53%). Pharmacokinetics of sertraline and N-desmethylsertraline were unaffected by zolpidem.

Since the systematic evaluations of Ambien (zolpidem tartrate) in combination with other CNS-active drugs have been limited, careful consideration should be given to the pharmacology of any CNS-active drug to be used with zolpidem. Any drug with CNS-depressant effects could potentially enhance the CNS-depressant effects of zolpidem.

Drugs that affect drug metabolism via cytochrome P450: A randomized, double-blind, crossover interaction study in ten healthy volunteers between itraconazole (200 mg once daily for 4 days) and a single dose of zolpidem (10 mg) given 5 hours after the last dose of itraconazole resulted in a 34% increase in $AUC_{0-\infty}$ of zolpidem. There were no significant pharmacodynamic effects of zolpidem on subjective drowsiness, postural sway, or psychomotor performance.

A randomized, placebo-controlled, crossover interaction study in eight healthy female volunteers between 5 consecutive daily doses of rifampin (600 mg) and a single dose of zolpidem (20 mg) given 17 hours after the last dose of rifampin showed significant reductions of the AUC (−73%), C_{max} (−58%), and $T_{1/2}$ (−36%) of zolpidem together with significant reductions in the pharmacodynamic effects of zolpidem.

Other drugs: A study involving cimetidine/zolpidem and ranitidine/zolpidem combinations revealed no effect of either drug on the pharmacokinetics or pharmacodynamics of zolpidem. Zolpidem had no effect on digoxin kinetics and did not affect prothrombin time when given with warfarin in normal subjects. Zolpidem's sedative/hypnotic effect was reversed by flumazenil; however, no significant alterations in zolpidem pharmacokinetics were found.

Drug/Laboratory test interactions: Zolpidem is not known to interfere with commonly employed clinical laboratory tests. In addition, clinical data indicate that zolpidem does not cross-react with benzodiazepines, opiates, barbiturates, cocaine, cannabinoids, or amphetamines in two standard urine drug screens.

Carcinogenesis, mutagenesis, impairment of fertility

Carcinogenesis: Zolpidem was administered to rats and mice for 2 years at dietary dosages of 4, 18, and 80 mg/kg/day. In mice, these dosages are 26 to 520 times or 2 to 35 times the maximum 10-mg human dose on a mg/kg or mg/m^2 basis, respectively. In rats these doses are 43 to 876 times or 6 to 115 times the maximum 10-mg human dose on a mg/kg or mg/m^2 basis, respectively. No evidence of carcinogenic potential was observed in mice. Renal liposarcomas were seen in 4/100 rats (3 males, 1 female) receiving 80 mg/kg/day and a renal lipoma was observed in one male rat at the 18 mg/kg/ day dose. Incidence rates of lipoma and liposarcoma for zolpidem were comparable to those seen in historical controls and the tumor findings are thought to be a spontaneous occurrence.

Mutagenesis: Zolpidem did not have mutagenic activity in several tests including the Ames test, genotoxicity in mouse lymphoma cells in vitro, chromosomal aberrations in cultured human lymphocytes, unscheduled DNA synthesis in rat hepatocytes in vitro, and the micronucleus test in mice.

Impairment of fertility: In a rat reproduction study, the high dose (100 mg base/kg) of zolpidem resulted in irregular estrus cycles and prolonged precoital intervals, but there was no effect on male or female fertility after daily oral doses of 4 to 100 mg base/kg or 5 to 130 times the recommended human dose in mg/m^2. No effects on any other fertility parameters were noted.

Pregnancy

Teratogenic effects: Pregnancy Category B. Studies to assess the effects of zolpidem on human reproduction and development have not been conducted.

Teratology studies were conducted in rats and rabbits.

In rats, adverse maternal and fetal effects occurred at 20 and 100 mg base/kg and included dose-related maternal lethargy and ataxia and a dose-related trend to incomplete ossification of fetal skull bones. Underossification of various fetal bones indicates a delay in maturation and is often seen in rats treated with sedative/hypnotic drugs. There were no teratogenic effects after zolpidem administration. The no-effect dose for maternal or fetal toxicity was 4 mg base/kg or 5 times the maximum human dose on a mg/m^2 basis.

In rabbits, dose-related maternal sedation and decreased weight gain occurred at all doses tested. At the high dose, 16 mg base/kg, there was an increase in postimplantation fetal loss and underossification of sternebrae in viable fetuses. These fetal findings in rabbits are often secondary to reductions in maternal weight gain. There were no frank teratogenic effects. The no-effect dose for fetal toxicity was 4 mg base/kg or 7 times the maximum human dose on a mg/m^2 basis.

Because animal reproduction studies are not always predictive of human response, this drug should be used during pregnancy only if clearly needed.

Nonteratogenic effects: Studies to assess the effects on children whose mothers took zolpidem during pregnancy have not been conducted. However, children born of mothers taking sedative/hypnotic drugs may be at some risk for withdrawal symptoms from the drug during the postnatal period. In addition, neonatal flaccidity has been reported in infants born of mothers who received sedative/hypnotic drugs during pregnancy.

Labor and delivery: Ambien (zolpidem tartrate) has no established use in labor and delivery.

Nursing mothers: Studies in lactating mothers indicate that the half-life of zolpidem is similar to that in young normal volunteers (2.6 ± 0.3 hr). Between 0.004 and 0.019% of the total administered dose is excreted into milk, but the effect of zolpidem on the infant is unknown.

In addition, in a rat study, zolpidem inhibited the secretion of milk. The no-effect dose was 4 mg base/kg or 6 times the recommended human dose in mg/m^2.

The use of Ambien in nursing mothers is not recommended.

Pediatric use: Safety and effectiveness in pediatric patients below the age of 18 have not been established.

Geriatric use: A total of 154 patients in U.S. controlled clinical trials and 897 patients in non-U.S. clinical trials who received zolpidem were ≥60 years of age. For a pool of U.S. patients receiving zolpidem at doses of ≤10 mg or placebo, there were three adverse events occurring at an incidence of at least 3% for zolpidem and for which the zolpidem incidence was at least twice the placebo incidence (ie, they could be considered drug related).

Adverse Event	Zolpidem	Placebo
Dizziness	3%	0%
Drowsiness	5%	2%
Diarrhea	3%	1%

A total of 30/1,959 (1.5%) non-U.S. patients receiving zolpidem reported falls, including 28/30 (93%) who were ≥70 years of age. Of these 28 patients, 23 (82%) were receiving zolpidem doses >10 mg. A total of 24/1,959 (1.2%) non-U.S. patients receiving zolpidem reported confusion, including 18/24 (75%) who were ≥70 years of age. Of these 18 patients, 14 (78%) were receiving zolpidem doses >10 mg.

ADVERSE REACTIONS

Associated with discontinuation of treatment: Approximately 4% of 1,701 patients who received zolpidem at all doses (1.25 to 90 mg) in U.S. premarketing clinical trials discontinued treatment because of an adverse clinical event. Events most commonly associated with discontinuation from U.S. trials were daytime drowsiness (0.5%), dizziness (0.4%), headache (0.5%), nausea (0.6%), and vomiting (0.5%).

Approximately 4% of 1,959 patients who received zolpidem at all doses (1 to 50 mg) in similar foreign trials discontinued treatment because of an adverse event. Events most commonly associated with discontinuation from these trials were daytime drowsiness (1.1%), dizziness/vertigo (0.8%), amnesia (0.5%), nausea (0.5%), headache (0.4%), and falls (0.4%).

Data from a clinical study in which selective serotonin reuptake inhibitor- (SSRI) treated patients were given zolpidem revealed that four of the seven discontinuations during double-blind treatment with zolpidem (n=95) were associated with impaired concentration, continuing or aggravated depression, and manic reaction; one patient treated with placebo (n=97) was discontinued after an attempted suicide.

Incidence in controlled clinical trials

Most commonly observed adverse events in controlled trials: During short-term treatment (up to 10 nights) with Ambien at doses up to 10 mg, the most commonly observed adverse events associated with the use of zolpidem and seen at statistically significant differences from placebo-treated patients were drowsiness (reported by 2% of zolpidem patients), dizziness (1%), and diarrhea (1%). During longer-term treatment (28 to 35 nights) with zolpidem at doses up to 10 mg, the most commonly observed adverse events associated with the use of zolpidem and seen at statistically significant differences from placebo-treated patients were dizziness (5%) and drugged feelings (3%).

Adverse events observed at an incidence of ≥1% in controlled trials: The following tables enumerate treatment-emergent adverse event frequencies that were observed at an incidence equal to 1% or greater among patients with insomnia who received Ambien in U.S. placebo-controlled trials. Events reported by investigators were classified utilizing a modified World Health Organization (WHO) dictionary of preferred terms for the purpose of establishing event frequencies. The prescriber should be aware that these figures cannot be used to predict the incidence of side effects in the course of usual medical practice, in which patient characteristics and other factors differ from those that prevailed in these clinical trials. Similarly, the cited frequencies cannot be compared with figures obtained from other clinical investigators involving related drug products and uses, since each group of drug trials is conducted under a different set of conditions. However, the cited figures provide the physician with a basis for estimating the relative contribution of drug and nondrug factors to the incidence of side effects in the population studied.

The following table was derived from a pool of 11 placebo-controlled short-term U.S. efficacy trials involving zolpidem in doses ranging from 1.25 to 20 mg. The table is limited to data from doses up to and including 10 mg, the highest dose recommended for use.

[See table below]

The following table was derived from a pool of three placebo-controlled long-term efficacy trials involving Ambien (zolpidem tartrate). These trials involved patients with chronic insomnia who were treated for 28 to 35 nights with zolpidem at doses of 5, 10, or 15 mg. The table is limited to data from doses up to and including 10 mg, the highest dose recommended for use. The table includes only adverse events occurring at an incidence of at least 1% for zolpidem patients.

[See table at bottom of next page]

Dose relationship for adverse events: There is evidence from dose comparison trials suggesting a dose relationship for many of the adverse events associated with zolpidem use, particularly for certain CNS and gastrointestinal adverse events.

Adverse event incidence across the entire preapproval database: Ambien (zolpidem tartrate) was administered to 3,660 subjects in clinical trials throughout the U.S., Canada, and Europe. Treatment-emergent adverse events associated with clinical trial participation were recorded by clinical investigators using terminology of their own choosing. To provide a meaningful estimate of the proportion of individuals experiencing treatment-emergent adverse events, similar types of untoward events were grouped into a smaller number of standardized event categories and classified utilizing a modified World Health Organization (WHO) dictionary of preferred terms. The frequencies presented, therefore, represent the proportions of the 3,660 individuals exposed to zolpidem, at all doses, who experienced an event of the type cited on at least one occasion while receiving zolpidem. All reported treatment-emergent adverse events are included, except those already listed in the table above of adverse events in placebo-controlled studies, those coding terms that are so general as to be uninformative, and those events where a drug cause was remote. It is important to emphasize that, although the events reported did occur during treatment with Ambien, they were not necessarily caused by it.

Incidence of Treatment-Emergent Adverse Experiences in Short-term Placebo-Controlled Clinical Trials
(Percentage of patients reporting)

Body System/ Adverse Event*	Zolpidem (≤10 mg) (N=685)	Placebo (N=473)
Central and Peripheral Nervous System		
Headache	7	6
Drowsiness	2	–
Dizziness	1	–
Gastrointestinal System		
Nausea	2	3
Diarrhea	1	–
Musculoskeletal System		
Myalgia	1	2

*Events reported by at least 1% of Ambien patients are included.

Adverse events are further classified within body system categories and enumerated in order of decreasing frequency using the following definitions: frequent adverse events are defined as those occurring in greater than 1/100 subjects; infrequent adverse events are those occurring in 1/100 to 1/1,000 patients; rare events are those occurring in less than 1/1,000 patients.

Autonomic nervous system: Infrequent: increased sweating, pallor, postural hypotension, syncope. Rare: abnormal accommodation, altered saliva, flushing, glaucoma, hypotension, impotence, increased saliva, tenesmus.

Body as a whole: Frequent: asthenia. Infrequent: edema, falling, fever, malaise, trauma. Rare: allergic reaction, allergy aggravated, abdominal body sensation, anaphylactic shock, face edema, hot flashes, increased ESR, pain, restless legs, rigors, tolerance increased, weight decrease.

Cardiovascular system: Infrequent: cerebrovascular disorder, hypertension, tachycardia. Rare: angina pectoris, arrhythmia, arteritis, circulatory failure, extrasystoles, hypertension aggravated, myocardial infarction, phlebitis, pulmonary embolism, pulmonary edema, varicose veins, ventricular tachycardia.

Central and peripheral nervous system: Frequent: ataxia, confusion, euphoria, insomnia, vertigo. Infrequent: agitation, decreased cognition, detached, difficulty concentrating, dysarthria, emotional lability, hallucination, hypoesthesia, illusion, leg cramps, migraine, paresthesia, sleeping (after daytime dosing), speech disorder, stupor, tremor. Rare: abnormal gait, abnormal thinking, aggressive reaction, apathy, appetite increased, decreased libido, delusion, dementia, depersonalization, dysphasia, feeling strange, hypokinesia, hypotonia, hysteria, intoxicated feeling, manic reaction, neuralgia, neuritis, neuropathy, neurosis, panic attacks, paresis, personality disorder, somnambulism, suicide attempts, tetany, yawning.

Gastrointestinal system: Frequent: hiccup. Infrequent: constipation, dysphagia, flatulence, gastroenteritis. Rare: enteritis, eructation, esophagospasm, gastritis, hemorrhoids, intestinal obstruction, rectal hemorrhage, tooth caries.

Hematologic and lymphatic system: Rare: anemia, hyperhemoglobinemia, leukopenia, lymphadenopathy, macrocytic anemia, purpura, thrombosis.

Immunologic system: Rare: abscess, herpes simplex, herpes zoster, otitis externa, otitis media.

Liver and biliary system: Infrequent: abnormal hepatic function, increased SGPT. Rare: bilirubinemia, increased SGOT.

Metabolic and nutritional: Infrequent: hyperglycemia, thirst. Rare: gout, hypercholesteremia, hyperlipidemia, increased alkaline phosphatase, increased BUN, periorbital edema.

Musculoskeletal system: Infrequent: arthritis. Rare: arthrosis, muscle weakness, sciatica, tendinitis.

Reproductive system: Infrequent: menstrual disorder, vaginitis. Rare: breast fibroadenosis, breast neoplasm, breast pain.

Respiratory system: Infrequent: bronchitis, coughing, dyspnea. Rare: bronchospasm, epistaxis, hypoxia, laryngitis, pneumonia.

Skin and appendages: Infrequent: pruritus. Rare: acne, bullous eruption, dermatitis, furunculosis, injection-site inflammation, photosensitivity reaction, urticaria.

Special senses: Frequent: diplopia, vision abnormal. Infrequent: eye irritation, eye pain, scleritis, taste perversion, tinnitus. Rare: conjunctivitis, corneal ulceration, lacrimation abnormal, parosmia, photopsia.

Urogenital system: Infrequent: cystitis, urinary incontinence. Rare: acute renal failure, dysuria, micturition frequency, nocturia, polyuria, pyelonephritis, renal pain, urinary retention.

DRUG ABUSE AND DEPENDENCE

Controlled substance: Zolpidem tartrate is classified as a Schedule IV controlled substance by federal regulation.

Abuse and dependence: Studies of abuse potential in former drug abusers found that the effects of single doses of Ambien (zolpidem tartrate) 40 mg were similar, but not identical, to diazepam 20 mg, while zolpidem tartrate 10 mg was difficult to distinguish from placebo.

Sedative/hypnotics have produced withdrawal signs and symptoms following abrupt discontinuation. These reported symptoms range from mild dysphoria and insomnia to a withdrawal syndrome that may include abdominal and muscle cramps, vomiting, sweating, tremors, and convulsions. The U.S. clinical trial experience from zolpidem does not reveal any clear evidence for withdrawal syndrome. Nevertheless, the following adverse events included in DSM-III-R criteria for uncomplicated sedative/hypnotic withdrawal were reported during U.S. clinical trials following placebo substitution occurring within 48 hours following last zolpidem treatment: fatigue, nausea, flushing, lightheadedness, uncontrolled crying, emesis, stomach cramps, panic attack, nervousness, and abdominal discomfort. These reported adverse events occurred at an incidence of 1% or less. However, available data cannot provide a reliable estimate of the incidence, if any, of dependence during treatment at recommended doses. Rare post-marketing reports of abuse, dependence and withdrawal have been received.

Because persons with a history of addiction to, or abuse of, drugs or alcohol are at increased risk of habituation and dependence, they should be under careful surveillance when receiving zolpidem or any other hypnotic.

Incidence of Treatment-Emergent Adverse Experiences in Long-term Placebo-Controlled Clinical Trials
(Percentage of patients reporting)

Body System/ Adverse Event*	Zolpidem (≤10 mg) (N=152)	Placebo (N=161)
Autonomic Nervous System		
Dry mouth	3	1
Body as a Whole		
Allergy	4	1
Back pain	3	2
Influenza-like symptoms	2	–
Chest pain	1	–
Fatigue	1	2
Cardiovascular System		
Palpitation	2	–
Central and Peripheral Nervous System		
Headache	19	22
Drowsiness	8	5
Dizziness	5	1
Lethargy	3	1
Drugged feeling	3	–
Lightheadedness	2	1
Depression	2	1
Abnormal dreams	1	–
Amnesia	1	–
Anxiety	1	1
Nervousness	1	3
Sleep disorder	1	–
Gastrointestinal System		
Nausea	6	6
Dyspepsia	5	6
Diarrhea	3	2
Abdominal pain	2	2
Constipation	2	1
Anorexia	1	1
Vomiting	1	1
Immunologic System		
Infection	1	1
Musculoskeletal System		
Myalgia	7	7
Arthralgia	4	4
Respiratory System		
Upper respiratory infection	5	6
Sinusitis	4	2
Pharyngitis	3	1
Rhinitis	1	3
Skin and Appendages		
Rash	2	1
Urogenital System		
Urinary tract infection	2	2

*Events reported by at least 1% of patients treated with Ambien.

OVERDOSAGE

Signs and symptoms: In European postmarketing reports of overdose with zolpidem alone, impairment of consciousness has ranged from somnolence to light coma. There was one case each of cardiovascular and respiratory compromise. Individuals have fully recovered from zolpidem tartrate overdoses up to 400 mg (40 times the maximum recommended dose). Overdose cases involving multiple CNS-depressant agents, including zolpidem, have resulted in more severe symptomatology, including fatal outcomes.

Recommended treatment: General symptomatic and supportive measures should be used along with immediate gastric lavage where appropriate. Intravenous fluids should be administered as needed. Flumazenil may be useful. As in all cases of drug overdose, respiration, pulse, blood pressure, and other appropriate signs should be monitored and general supportive measures employed. Hypotension and CNS depression should be monitored and treated by appropriate medical intervention. Sedating drugs should be withheld following zolpidem overdosage, even if excitation occurs. The value of dialysis in the treatment of overdosage has not been determined, although hemodialysis studies in patients with renal failure receiving therapeutic doses have demonstrated that zolpidem is not dialyzable.

Poison control center: As with the management of all overdosage, the possibility of multiple drug ingestion should be considered. The physician may wish to consider contacting a poison control center for up-to-date information on the management of hypnotic drug product overdosage.

DOSAGE AND ADMINISTRATION

The dose of Ambien should be individualized.

The recommended dose for adults is 10 mg immediately before bedtime.

Downward dosage adjustment may be necessary when Ambien is administered with agents having known CNS-depressant effects because of the potentially additive effects. Elderly or debilitated patients may be especially sensitive to the effects of Ambien (zolpidem tartrate). Patients with hepatic insufficiency do not clear the drug as rapidly as normals. An initial 5-mg dose is recommended in these patients (see *Precautions*).

The total Ambien dose should not exceed 10 mg.

HOW SUPPLIED

Ambien 5-mg tablets are capsule-shaped, pink, film coated, with, AMB 5 debossed on one side and 5401 on the other and supplied as:

NDC Number	Size
0024-5401-31	bottle of 100
0024-5401-34	carton of 100 unit dose

Ambien 10-mg tablets are capsule-shaped, white, film coated, with AMB 10 debossed on one side and 5421 on the other and supplied as:

NDC Number	Size
0024-5421-31	bottle of 100
0024-5421-34	carton of 100 unit dose

Store at controlled room temperature 20°–25° C (68°–77°F).

Rx only

INFORMATION FOR PATIENTS TAKING AMBIEN

Your doctor has prescribed Ambien to help you sleep. The following information is intended to guide you in the safe use of this medicine.

It is not meant to take the place of your doctor's instructions. If you have any questions about Ambien tablets be sure to ask your doctor or pharmacist.

Ambien is used to treat different types of sleep problems, such as:

- trouble falling asleep
- waking up too early in the morning
- waking up often during the night

Some people may have more than one of these problems.

Ambien belongs to a group of medicines known as the "sedative/hypnotics," or simply, sleep medicines. There are many different sleep medicines available to help people sleep better. Sleep problems are usually temporary, requiring treatment for only a short time, usually 1 or 2 days up to 1 or 2 weeks. Some people have chronic sleep problems that may require more prolonged use of sleep medicine. However, you should not use these medicines for long periods without talking with your doctor about the risks and benefits of prolonged use.

SIDE EFFECTS

Most common side effects: All medicines have side effects. Most common side effects of sleep medicines include:

- drowsiness
- dizziness
- lightheadedness
- difficulty with coordination

You may find that these medicines make you sleepy during the day. How drowsy you feel depends upon how your body reacts to the medicine, which sleep medicine you are taking, and how large a dose your doctor has prescribed. Daytime drowsiness is best avoided by taking the lowest dose possi-

Continued on next page

Ambien—Cont.

ble that will still help you sleep at night. Your doctor will work with you to find the dose of Ambien that is best for you.

To manage these side effects while you are taking this medicine:

- When you first start taking Ambien or any other sleep medicine until you know whether the medicine will still have some carryover effect in you the next day, use extreme care while doing anything that requires complete alertness, such as driving a car, operating machinery, or piloting an aircraft.
- NEVER drink alcohol while you are being treated with Ambien or any sleep medicine. Alcohol can increase the side effects of Ambien or any other sleep medicine.
- Do not take any other medicines without asking your doctor first. This includes medicines you can buy without a prescription. Some medicines can cause drowsiness and are best avoided while taking Ambien.
- Always take the exact dose of Ambien prescribed by your doctor. Never change your dose without talking to your doctor first.

SPECIAL CONCERNS

There are some special problems that may occur while taking sleep medicines.

Memory problems: Sleep medicines may cause a special type of memory loss or "amnesia." When this occurs, a person may not remember what has happened for several hours after taking the medicine. This is usually not a problem since most people fall asleep after taking the medicine. Memory loss can be a problem, however, when sleep medicines are taken while traveling, such as during an airplane flight and the person wakes up before the effect of the medicine is gone. This has been called "traveler's amnesia."

Memory problems are not common while taking Ambien. In most instances memory problems can be avoided if you take Ambien only when you are able to get a full night's sleep (7 to 8 hours) before you need to be active again. Be sure to talk to your doctor if you think you are having memory problems.

Tolerance: When sleep medicines are used every night for more than a few weeks, they may lose their effectiveness to help you sleep. This is known as "tolerance." Sleep medicines should, in most cases, be used only for short periods of time, such as 1 or 2 days and generally no longer than 1 or 2 weeks. If your sleep problems continue, consult your doctor, who will determine whether other measures are needed to overcome your sleep problems.

Dependence: Sleep medicines can cause dependence, especially when these medicines are used regularly for longer than a few weeks or at high doses. Some people develop a need to continue taking their medicines. This is known as dependence or "addiction."

When people develop dependence, they may have difficulty stopping the sleep medicine. If the medicine is suddenly stopped, the body is not able to function normally and unpleasant symptoms (see *Withdrawal*) may occur. They may find they have to keep taking the medicine either at the prescribed dose or at increasing doses just to avoid withdrawal symptoms.

All people taking sleep medicines have some risk of becoming dependent on the medicine. However, people who have been dependent on alcohol or other drugs in the past may have a higher chance of becoming addicted to sleep medicines. This possibility must be considered before using these medicines for more than a few weeks.

If you have been addicted to alcohol or drugs in the past, it is important to tell your doctor before starting Ambien or any sleep medicine.

Withdrawal: Withdrawal symptoms may occur when sleep medicines are stopped suddenly after being used daily for a long time. In some cases, these symptoms can occur even if the medicine has been used for only a week or two.

In mild cases, withdrawal symptoms may include unpleasant feelings. In more severe cases, abdominal and muscle cramps, vomiting, sweating, shakiness, and rarely, seizures may occur. These more severe withdrawal symptoms are very uncommon.

Another problem that may occur when sleep medicines are stopped is known as "rebound insomnia." This means that a person may have more trouble sleeping the first few nights after the medicine is stopped than before starting the medicine. If you should experience rebound insomnia, do not get discouraged. This problem usually goes away on its own after 1 or 2 nights.

If you have been taking Ambien or any other sleep medicine for more than 1 or 2 weeks, do not stop taking it on your own. Always follow your doctor's directions.

Changes in behavior and thinking: Some people using sleep medicines have experienced unusual changes in their thinking and/or behavior. These effects are not common. However, they have included:

- more outgoing or aggressive behavior than normal
- loss of personal identity
- confusion
- strange behavior
- agitation
- hallucinations
- worsening of depression
- suicidal thoughts

How often these effects occur depends on several factors, such as a person's general health, the use of other medicines, and which sleep medicine is being used. Clinical experience with Ambien suggests that it is uncommonly associated with these behavior changes.

It is also important to realize that it is rarely clear whether these behavior changes are caused by the medicine, an illness, or occur on their own. In fact, sleep problems that do not improve may be due to illnesses that were present before the medicine was used. If you or your family notice any changes in your behavior, or if you have any unusual or disturbing thoughts, call your doctor immediately.

Pregnancy: Sleep medicines may cause sedation of the unborn baby when used during the last weeks of pregnancy. Be sure to tell your doctor if you are pregnant, if you are planning to become pregnant, or if you become pregnant while taking Ambien.

SAFE USE OF SLEEPING MEDICINES

To ensure the safe and effective use of Ambien or any other sleep medicine, you should observe the following cautions:

1. Ambien is a prescription medicine and should be used ONLY as directed by your doctor. Follow your doctor's instructions about how to take, when to take, and how long to take Ambien.
2. Never use Ambien or any other sleep medicine for longer than directed by your doctor.
3. If you notice any unusual and/or disturbing thoughts or behavior during treatment with Ambien or any other sleep medicine, contact your doctor.
4. Tell your doctor about any medicines you may be taking, including medicines you may buy without a prescription. You should also tell your doctor if you drink alcohol. DO NOT use alcohol while taking Ambien or any other sleep medicine.
5. Do not take Ambien unless you are able to get a full night's sleep before you must be active again. For example, Ambien should not be taken on an overnight airplane flight of less than 7 to 8 hours since "traveler's amnesia" may occur.
6. Do not increase the prescribed dose of Ambien or any other sleep medicine unless instructed by your doctor.
7. When you first start taking Ambien or any other sleep medicine until you know whether the medicine will still have some carryover effect in you the next day, use extreme care while doing anything that requires complete alertness, such as driving a car, operating machinery, or piloting an aircraft.
8. Be aware that you may have more sleeping problems the first night or two after stopping Ambien or any other sleep medicine.
9. Be sure to tell your doctor if you are pregnant, if you are planning to become pregnant, or if you become pregnant while taking Ambien.
10. As with all prescription medicines, never share Ambien or any other sleep medicine with anyone else. Always store Ambien or any other sleep medicine in the original container out of reach of children.
11. Ambien works very quickly. You should only take Ambien right before going to bed and are ready to go to sleep.

sanofi~synthelabo

Distributed by:
Sanofi-Synthelabo Inc.
New York, NY 10016

Ambien® Ⓒ
(zolpidem tartrate)

Printed in USA Revised February 2002

ZSS-5

ELIGARD™ 7.5 mg ℞

[*ĕl'-ə gärd*]

(leuprolide acetate for injectable suspension)

DESCRIPTION

ELIGARD™ 7.5 mg is a sterile polymeric matrix formulation of leuprolide acetate for subcutaneous injection. It is designed to deliver 7.5 mg of leuprolide acetate at a controlled rate over a one month therapeutic period.

Leuprolide acetate is a synthetic nonapeptide analog of naturally occurring gonadotropin releasing hormone (GnRH or LH-RH) that, when given continuously, inhibits pituitary gonadotropin secretion and suppresses testicular and ovarian steroidogenesis. The analog possesses greater potency than the natural hormone. The chemical name is 5-oxo-L-prolyl-L-histidyl-L-tryptophyl-L-seryl-L-tyrosyl-D-leucyl-L-leucyl-L-arginyl-N-ethyl-L-prolinamide acetate (salt) with the following structural formula:

ELIGARD™ 7.5 mg is prefilled and supplied in two separate, sterile syringes whose contents are mixed immediately prior to administration. The two syringes are joined and the single dose product is mixed until it is homogenous. ELIGARD™ 7.5 mg is administered subcutaneously where it forms a solid drug delivery depot.

One syringe contains the ATRIGEL® Delivery System and the other contains leuprolide acetate. The ATRIGEL® Delivery System is a polymeric (non-gelatin containing) delivery system consisting of a biodegradable poly(DL-lactide-co-glycolide) (PLGH) polymer formulation dissolved in a biocompatible solvent, *N*-methyl-2-pyrrolidone (NMP). PLGH is a co-polymer with a 50:50 molar ratio of DL-lactide to glycolide containing carboxyl end groups. The second syringe contains leuprolide acetate and the constituted product is designed to deliver 7.5 mg of leuprolide acetate at the time of subcutaneous injection.

ELIGARD™ 7.5 mg delivers 7.5 mg of leuprolide acetate (equivalent to approximately 7.0 mg leuprolide free base) dissolved in 160 mg *N*-methyl-2-pyrrolidone and 82.5 mg poly(DL-lactide-co-glycolide). The approximate weight of the administered formulation is 250 mg.

CLINICAL PHARMACOLOGY

Leuprolide acetate, an LH-RH agonist, acts as a potent inhibitor of gonadotropin secretion when given continuously in therapeutic doses. Animal and human studies indicate that after an initial stimulation, chronic administration of leuprolide acetate results in suppression of ovarian and testicular steroidogenesis. This effect is reversible upon discontinuation of drug therapy.

In humans, administration of leuprolide acetate results in an initial increase in circulating levels of luteinizing hormone (LH) and follicle stimulating hormone (FSH), leading to a transient increase in levels of the gonadal steroids (testosterone and dihydrotestosterone in males, and estrone and estradiol in premenopausal females). However, continuous administration of leuprolide acetate results in decreased levels of LH and FSH. In males, testosterone is reduced to below castrate threshold (≤ 50 ng/dL). These decreases occur within two to four weeks after initiation of treatment. Long-term studies have shown that continuation of therapy with leuprolide acetate maintains testosterone below the castrate level for up to seven years.

PHARMACODYNAMICS

Following the first dose of ELIGARD™ 7.5 mg, mean serum testosterone concentrations transiently increased, then fell to below castrate threshold (≤ 50 ng/dL) within three weeks (Figure 1). Continued monthly treatment maintained castrate testosterone suppression throughout the study. No breakthrough of testosterone concentrations above castrate threshold (> 50 ng/dL) occurred at any time during the study once castrate suppression was achieved.

Leuprolide acetate is not active when given orally.

PHARMACOKINETICS

Absorption: The pharmacokinetics/pharmacodynamics observed during three once monthly injections (ELIGARD™ 7.5 mg) in 20 patients with advanced carcinoma of the prostate is shown in Figure 1. Mean serum leuprolide concentrations following the initial injection rose to 25.3 ng/mL (C_{max}) at approximately 5 hours after injection. After the initial increase following each injection, serum concentrations remained relatively constant (0.28 – 2.00 ng/mL). There was no evidence of significant accumulation during repeated dosing. Nondetectable leuprolide plasma concentrations have been observed during chronic ELIGARD™ 7.5 mg administration, but testosterone levels were maintained at castrate levels.

Figure 1-Pharmacokinetic/Pharmacodynamic Response (N=20) to ELIGARD™ 7.5 mg - Patients dosed initially and at Months 1 and 2

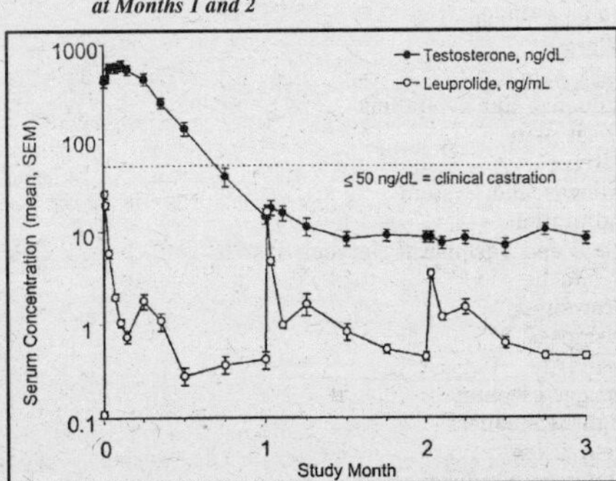

A reduced number of sampling timepoints resulted in the apparent decrease in C_{max} values with the second and third doses of ELIGARD™ 7.5 mg (Figure 1).

Distribution: The mean steady-state volume of distribution of leuprolide following intravenous bolus administration to healthy male volunteers was 27 L.[1] *In vitro* binding to human plasma proteins ranged from 43% to 49%.

Metabolism: In healthy male volunteers, a 1 mg bolus of leuprolide administered intravenously revealed that the mean systemic clearance was 8.34 L/h, with a terminal elimination half-life of approximately 3 hours based on a two compartment model.[1]

No drug metabolism study was conducted with ELIGARD™ 7.5 mg. Upon administration with different leuprolide acetate formulations, the major metabolite of leuprolide acetate is a pentapeptide (M-1) metabolite.

Excretion: No drug excretion study was conducted with ELIGARD™ 7.5 mg.

Special Populations:

Geriatrics: The majority (70%) of the 128 patients studied in these clinical trials were age 70 and older.

Pediatrics: The safety and effectiveness of ELIGARD™ 7.5 mg in pediatric patients have not been established (see **CONTRAINDICATIONS**).

Race: In patients studied (26 White, 2 Hispanic), mean serum leuprolide concentrations were similar.

Renal and Hepatic Insufficiency: The pharmacokinetics of ELIGARD™ 7.5 mg in hepatically and renally impaired patients have not been determined.

Drug-Drug Interactions: No pharmacokinetic drug-drug interaction studies were conducted with ELIGARD™ 7.5 mg.

CLINICAL STUDIES

In one open-label, multicenter study (AGL9904), 120 patients with advanced prostate cancer were treated with six monthly injections of ELIGARD™ 7.5 mg. Eighty-nine patients had stage C disease and 31 patients had stage D disease. This study evaluated the achievement and maintenance of serum testosterone suppression over six months of therapy.

The mean testosterone concentration increased from 361.3 ng/dL at Baseline to 574.6 ng/dL at Day 3 following the initial subcutaneous injection. The mean serum testosterone concentration then decreased to below Baseline by Day 10 and was 21.8 ng/dL on Day 28. At the conclusion of the study (Month 6), mean testosterone concentration was 6.1 ng/dL (Figure 2).

Serum testosterone was suppressed to below the castrate threshold (≤ 50 ng/dL) by Day 28 (Week 4) in 112 of 119 (94.1%) patients remaining in the study. The remaining seven patients all attained the castrate threshold by Day 42. Once testosterone suppression at or below serum concentrations of 50 ng/dL was achieved, no patients (0%) demonstrated breakthrough (concentration above 50 ng/dL) at any time in the study. All 117 evaluable patients in the study at Month 6 (two patients withdrew for reasons unrelated to drug) had testosterone concentrations of ≤ 50 ng/dL.

Figure 2. ELIGARD™ 7.5 mg Mean Serum Testosterone Concentrations (n=117)

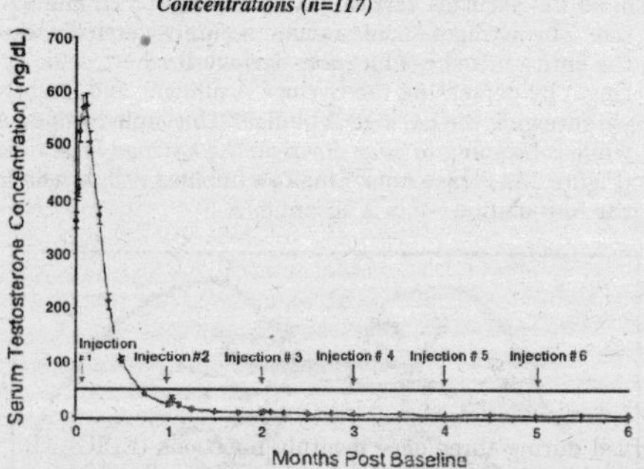

Serum PSA decreased in all patients whose Baseline values were elevated above the normal limit. Mean values were reduced 94% from Baseline to Month 6. At Month 6, PSA levels had decreased to within normal limits in 94% of patients who presented with elevated levels at Baseline.

Other secondary efficacy endpoints evaluated included WHO performance status, bone pain, urinary pain and urinary signs and symptoms. At Baseline, 88% of patients were classified as "fully active" by the WHO performance status scale (Status=0) and 11% as "restricted in strenuous activity but ambulatory and able to carry out work of a light or sedentary nature" (Status=1). These percentages were unchanged at Month 6. At Baseline, patients experienced little bone pain, with a mean score of 1.22 (range 1–9) on a scale of 1 (no pain) to 10 (worst pain possible). At Month 6, the mean bone pain score was essentially unchanged at 1.26 (range 1–7). Urinary pain, scored on the same scale, was similarly low, with a mean of 1.12 at Baseline (range 1–5) and 1.07 at Month 6 (range 1–8). Urinary signs and symptoms were similarly low at Baseline and decreased modestly at Month 6. In addition, there was a reduction in patients with prostate abnormalities detected during physical exam from 102 (85%) at Screening to 77 (64%) at Month 6.

INDICATIONS AND USAGE

ELIGARD™ 7.5 mg is indicated for the palliative treatment of advanced prostate cancer.

CONTRAINDICATIONS

1. ELIGARD™ 7.5 mg is contraindicated in patients with hypersensitivity to GnRH, GnRH agonist analogs or any of the components of ELIGARD™ 7.5 mg. Anaphylactic reactions to synthetic GnRH or GnRH agonist analogs have been reported in the literature.[2]
2. ELIGARD™ 7.5 mg is contraindicated in women and in pediatric patients and was not studied in women or children. Moreover, leuprolide acetate can cause fetal harm when administered to a pregnant woman. Major fetal abnormalities were observed in rabbits but not in rats after administration of leuprolide acetate throughout gestation. There were increased fetal mortality and decreased fetal weights in rats and rabbits. The effects on fetal mortality are expected consequences of the alterations in hormonal levels brought about by this drug. The possibility exists that spontaneous abortion may occur.

WARNINGS

ELIGARD™ 7.5 mg, like other LH-RH agonists, causes a transient increase in serum concentrations of testosterone during the first week of treatment. Patients may experience worsening of symptoms or onset of new signs and symptoms during the first few weeks of treatment, including bone pain, neuropathy, hematuria, or bladder outlet obstruction. Isolated cases of ureteral obstruction and/or spinal cord compression, which may contribute to paralysis with or without fatal complications, have been observed in the palliative treatment of advanced prostate cancer using LH-RH agonists. (see **PRECAUTIONS**).

If spinal cord compression or renal impairment develops, standard treatment of these complications should be instituted.

Table 1: Incidence (%) of Possibly or Probably Related Systemic Adverse Events Reported by ≥ 2% of Patients (n = 120) Treated with ELIGARD™ 7.5 mg for up to Six Months in Study AGL9904

Body System	Adverse Event	Number	Percent
Body as a Whole	Malaise and Fatigue	21	17.5%
	Dizziness	4	3.3%
Cardiovascular	Hot flashes/sweats*	68	56.7%
Genitourinary	Atrophy of Testes*	6	5.0%
Digestive	Gastroenteritis/Colitis	3	2.5%

Table 2: Incidence (%) of Possibly or Probably-Related Systemic Adverse Events Reported by ≥ 2% of Surgically Castrated Patients (n = 8) Treated with a Single-Dose of ELIGARD™ 7.5 mg in Study AGL9802

Body System	Adverse Event	Number	Percent
Cardiovascular	Hot flashes/sweats*	2	25.0%

PRECAUTIONS

General: Patients with metastatic vertebral lesions and/or with urinary tract obstruction should be closely observed during the first few weeks of therapy (see **WARNINGS** section).

Laboratory tests: Response to ELIGARD™ 7.5 mg should be monitored by measuring serum concentrations of testosterone and prostate-specific antigen periodically.

In the majority of patients, testosterone levels increased above Baseline during the first week, declining thereafter to Baseline levels or below by the end of the second week. Castrate levels were generally reached within two to four weeks and once achieved were maintained for the duration of treatment. No increases to above the castrate level occurred in any of the patients.

Results of testosterone determinations are dependent on assay methodology. It is advisable to be aware of the type and precision of the assay methodology to make appropriate clinical and therapeutic decisions.

Drug Interactions: See **PHARMACOKINETICS**

Drug/Laboratory Test Interactions: Therapy with leuprolide results in suppression of the pituitary-gonadal system. Results of diagnostic tests of pituitary gonadotropic and gonadal functions conducted during and after leuprolide therapy may be affected.

Carcinogenesis, Mutagenesis, Impairment of Fertility: Two-year carcinogenicity studies were conducted with leuprolide acetate in rats and mice. In rats, a dose-related increase of benign pituitary hyperplasia and benign pituitary adenomas was noted at 24 months when the drug was administered subcutaneously at high daily doses (0.6 to 4 mg/kg). There was a significant but not dose-related increase of pancreatic islet-cell adenomas in females and of testicular interstitial cell adenomas in males (highest incidence in the low dose group). In mice, no leuprolide acetate-induced tumors or pituitary abnormalities were observed at a dose as high as 60 mg/kg for two years. Patients have been treated with leuprolide acetate for up to three years with doses as high as 10 mg/day and for two years with doses as high as 20 mg/day without demonstrable pituitary abnormalities. No carcinogenicity studies have been conducted with ELIGARD™ 7.5 mg.

Mutagenicity studies have been performed with leuprolide acetate using bacterial and mammalian systems and with ELIGARD™ 7.5 mg in bacterial systems. These studies provided no evidence of a mutagenic potential.

Pregnancy, Teratogenic Effects: Pregnancy category X. (See **CONTRAINDICATIONS**).

Pediatric Use: ELIGARD 7.5 mg is contraindicated in pediatric patients and was not studied in children (see **CONTRAINDICATIONS**).

ADVERSE REACTIONS

The safety of ELIGARD™ 7.5 mg was evaluated in eight surgically castrated males and 120 patients with advanced prostate cancer in two clinical trials. ELIGARD™ 7.5 mg, like other LH-RH analogs, caused a transient increase in serum testosterone concentrations during the first week of treatment. Therefore, potential exacerbations of signs and symptoms of the disease during the first few weeks of treatment are of concern in patients with vertebral metastases and/or urinary obstruction or hematuria. If these conditions are aggravated, it may lead to neurological problems such as weakness and/or paresthesia of the lower limbs or worsening of urinary symptoms (see **WARNINGS** and **PRECAUTIONS**).

In Study AGL9904, 120 patients were dosed with ELIGARD™ 7.5 mg for up to six months and injection sites were closely monitored. In all, 716 injections of ELIGARD™ 7.5 mg were administered. Transient burning/stinging was reported following 248 (34.6%) injections, with the majority (84%) of these events reported as mild. Pain was reported following 4.3% of study injections (18.3% of patients) and was generally reported as brief in duration and mild in intensity.

Erythema was reported following 2.6% of injections (12.5% of patients). These events were all reported as mild and generally resolved within a few days post-injection. Mild bruising was reported following 2.5% of injections (11.7% of patients). Pruritis, induration, and ulceration was reported following 1.4% (11 patients), 0.4% (3 patients), and 0.1% (1 patient) of study injections, respectively.

These localized adverse events were non-recurrent over time. No patient discontinued therapy due to an injection site adverse event.

The following possibly or probably related systemic adverse events occurred during clinical trials of up to six months of treatment with ELIGARD™ 7.5 mg, and were reported in ≥ 2% of patients (Tables 1 and 2). Often, causality is difficult to assess in patients with metastatic prostate cancer. Reactions considered not drug-related are excluded.

[See table 1 above]

[See table 2 above]

In addition, the following possibly or probably related systemic adverse events were reported by < 2% of the patients using ELIGARD™ 7.5 mg in clinical studies.

General: Sweating, insomnia, syncope

Gastrointestinal: Flatulence, constipation

Hematologic: Decreased red blood cell count, hematocrit and hemoglobin

Metabolic: Weight gain

Musculoskeletal: Tremor, backache, joint pain

Nervous: Disturbance of smell and taste, depression, vertigo

Skin: Alopecia

Urogenital: Testicular soreness, impotence*, decreased libido*, gynecomastia, breast soreness

*Expected pharmacological consequences of testosterone suppression. In the patient populations studied, a total of 86 hot flash/sweats adverse events were reported in 70 patients. Of these, 71 events (83%) were mild; 14 (16%) were moderate; 1 (1%) was severe.

Changes in Bone Density: Decreased bone density has been reported in the medical literature in men who have had orchiectomy or who have been treated with an LH-RH agonist analog.[3] It can be anticipated that long periods of medical castration in men will have effects on bone density.

OVERDOSAGE

In clinical trials using daily subcutaneous leuprolide acetate in patients with prostate cancer, doses as high as 20 mg/day for up to two years caused no adverse effects differing from those observed with the 1 mg/day dose.

DOSAGE AND ADMINISTRATION

The recommended dose of ELIGARD™ 7.5 mg is one injection every month. The injection delivers 7.5 mg of leuprolide acetate, incorporated in a polymer formulation. It is administered subcutaneously and provides continuous release of leuprolide for one month.

Once mixed, ELIGARD 7.5 mg should be discarded if not administered within 30 minutes.

As with other drugs administered by subcutaneous injection, the injection site should vary periodically.

Mixing Procedure

IMPORTANT: Allow the product to reach room temperature before using. **Once mixed, the product must be administered within 30 minutes.**

Follow the instructions as directed to ensure proper preparation of ELIGARD™ 7.5 mg prior to administration:

ELIGARD™ 7.5 mg is packaged in a pouch that contains two smaller pouches (Figure 3), a needle cartridge and a desiccant pack (Figure 4). Syringe A pouch contains the sterile Syringe A pre-filled with the ATRIGEL® polymer system and a long white replacement plunger rod (Figure 5). Syringe B pouch contains the sterile Syringe B pre-filled with leuprolide acetate powder (Figure 6).

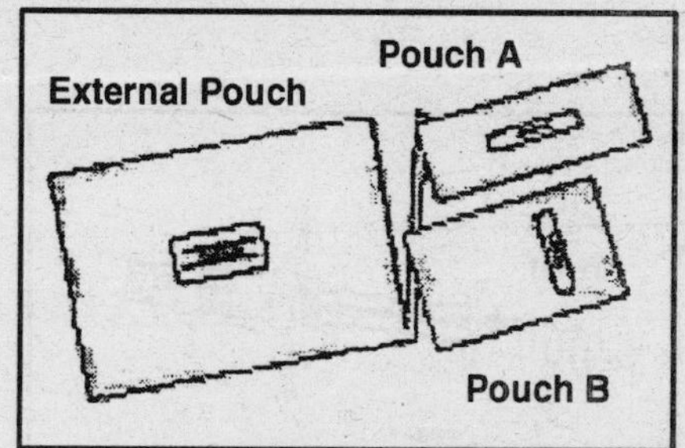

Figure 3

Continued on next page

Eligard—Cont.

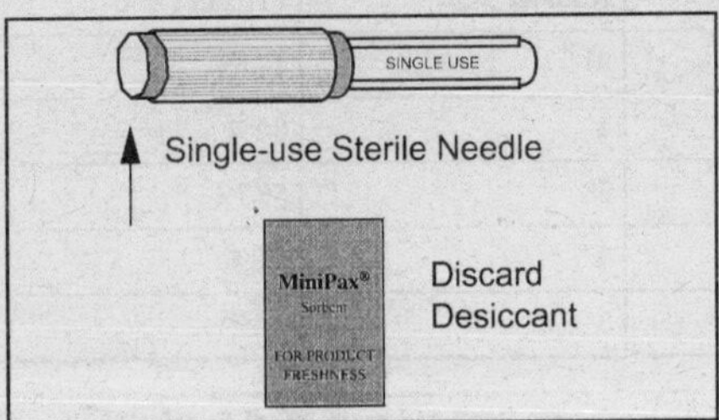

Figure 4

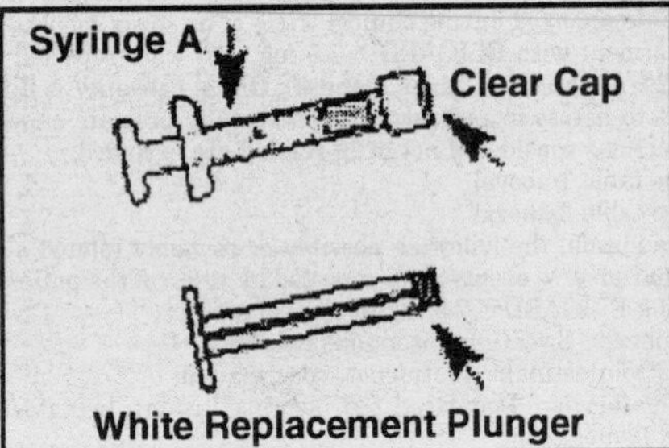

Figure 5

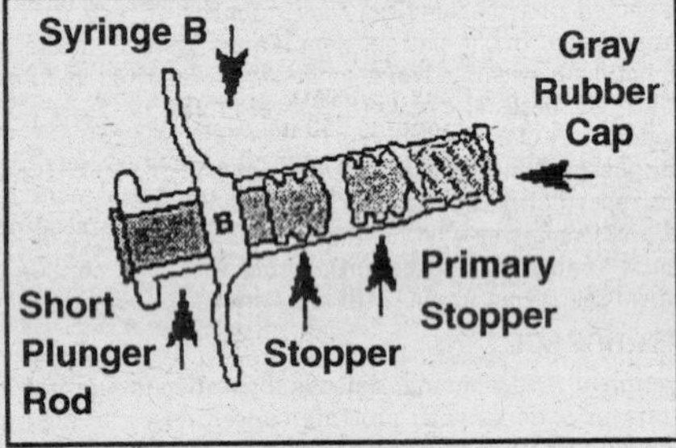

Figure 6

1. On a clean field, open all of the pouches and remove the contents. Discard the desiccant pack.

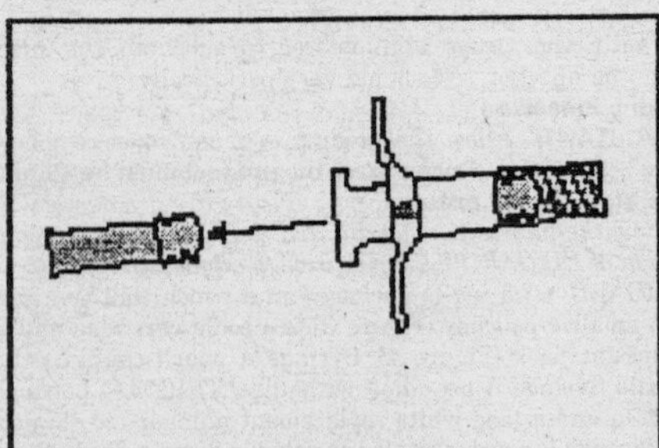

Figure 7

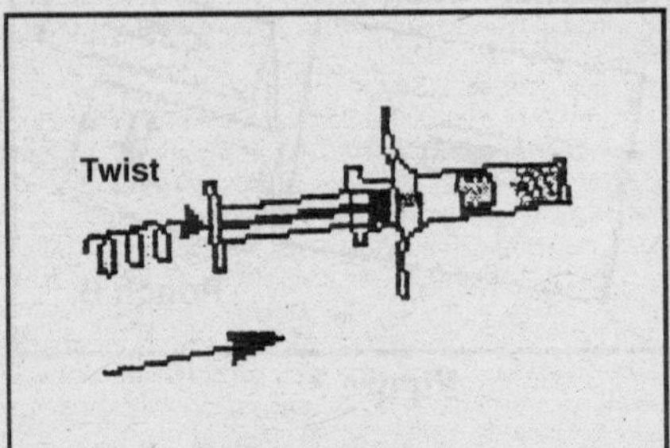

Figure 8

2. Pull out the blue-tipped short plunger rod and attached stopper from Syringe B and discard (Figure 7). Gently insert the long, white replacement plunger rod into the gray primary stopper remaining in Syringe B by twisting it in place (Figure 8).

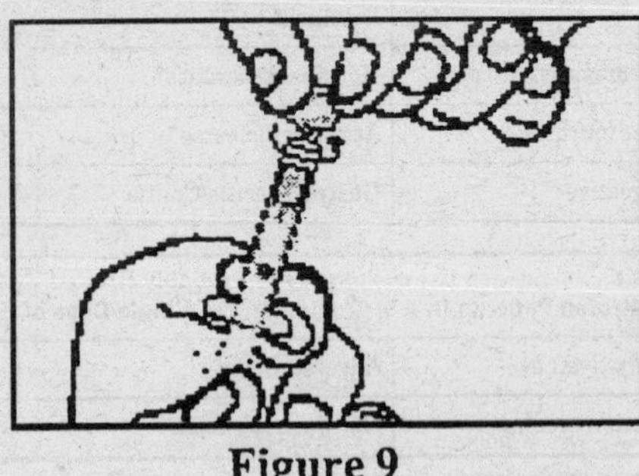

Figure 9

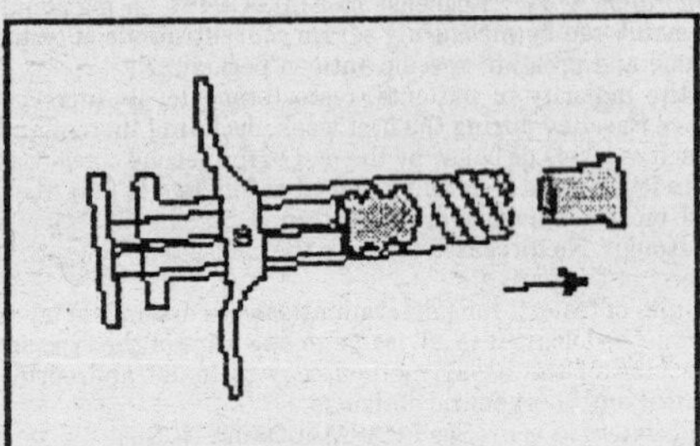

Figure 10

3. Unscrew the clear cap from Syringe A (Figure 9). Remove the gray rubber cap from Syringe B (Figure 10).

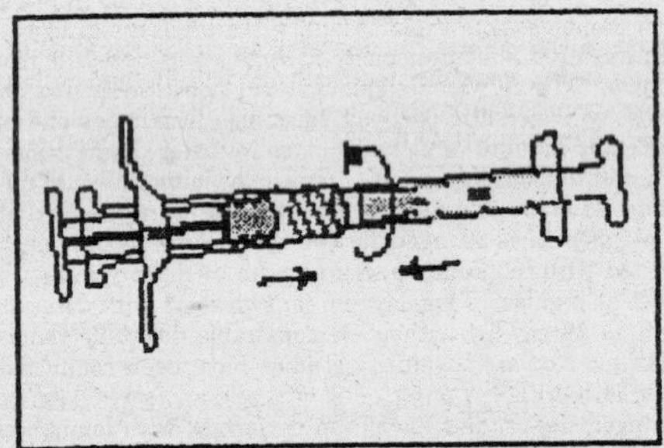

Figure 11

4. Join the two syringes together by pushing in and twisting until secure (Figure 11).

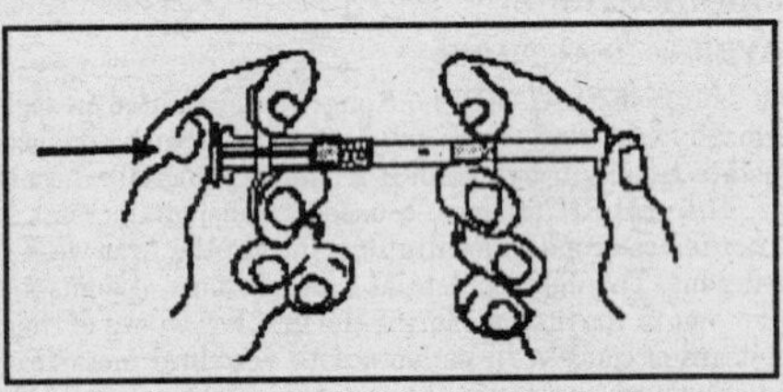

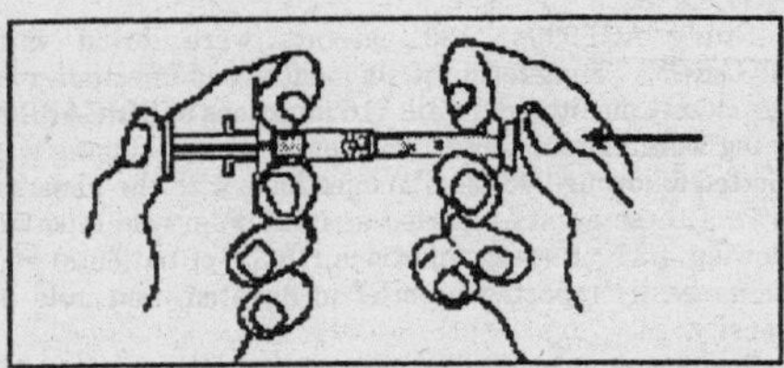

Figure 12

5. Thoroughly mix the product by pushing the contents of both syringes back and forth between syringes (approximately 45 seconds) to obtain a uniform suspension (Figure 12). When thoroughly mixed, the suspension will appear a light tan to tan color. **Please note: Product must be mixed as described; shaking will not provide adequate mixing of the product.**

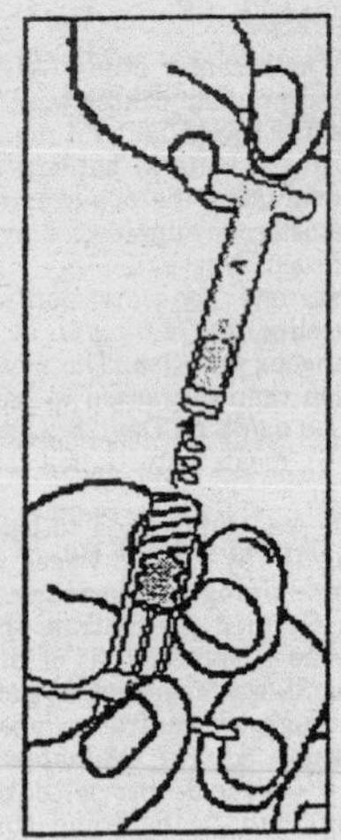

Figure 13

6. Hold the syringes vertically with Syringe B on the bottom. The syringes should remain securely coupled. Draw the entire mixed product into Syringe B (short, wide syringe) by depressing the Syringe A plunger and slightly withdrawing the Syringe B plunger. Uncouple Syringe A while continuing to push down on the Syringe A plunger (Figure 13). **Please note: Small air bubbles will remain in the formulation—this is acceptable.**

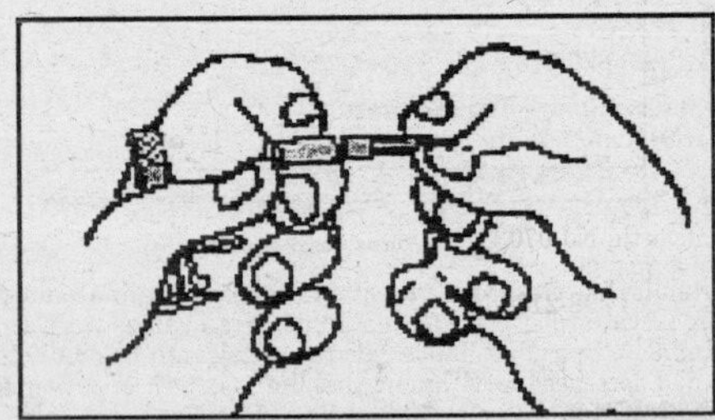

Figure 14

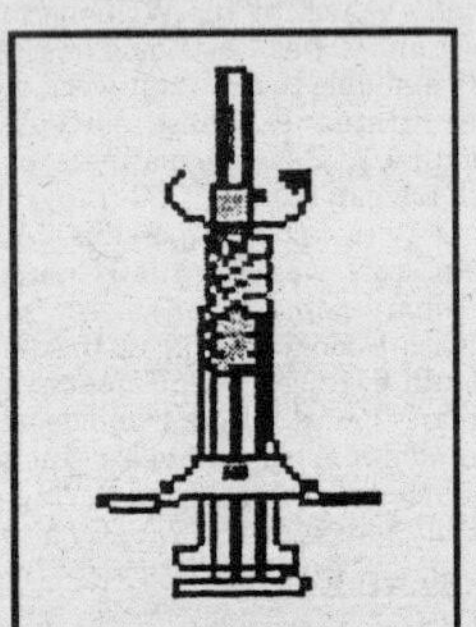

Figure 15

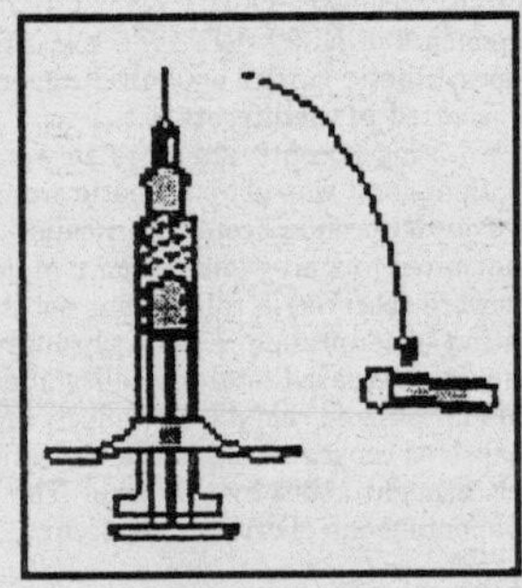

Figure 16

7. Hold Syringe B upright. Remove the pink cap on the bottom of the sterile needle cartridge by twisting it (Figure 14). Attach the needle cartridge to the end of Syringe B (Figure 15) by pushing in and turning the needle until it is firmly seated. Do not twist the needle onto the syringe until it is stripped. Pull off the clear needle cartridge cover prior to administration (Figure 16). After administration discard all components safely in an appropriate biohazard container.

HOW SUPPLIED

ELIGARD™ 7.5 mg is available in a single use kit. The kit consists of a two-syringe mixing system, a 20-gauge half-

inch needle, a silicone desiccant pouch to control moisture uptake, and package insert for constitution and administration procedures. Each syringe is individually packaged. One contains the ATRIGEL® Delivery System and the other contains leuprolide acetate. When constituted, ELIGARD™ 7.5 mg is administered as a single dose.
(NDC 0024-05970-07)
Rx only
Store at 2–8 °C (36–46 °F)
Sanofi-Synthelabo
Manufactured for Sanofi-Synthelabo Inc.
New York, NY 10016
by Atrix Laboratories, Inc.
Fort Collins, CO 80525

1. Sennello LT et al. Single-dose pharmacokinetics of leuprolide in humans following intravenous and subcutaneous administration. J Pharm Sci 1986; 75(2): 158–160.
2. MacLeod TL et. al. Anaphylactic reaction to synthetic luteinizing hormone releasing hormone. Fertil Steril 1987 Sept; 48(3): 500–502.
3. Hatano T et. al. Incidence of bone fracture in patients receiving luteinizing hormone-releasing hormone agonists for prostate cancer. BJU International 2000 86: 449–452.
04295 Rev 1 4/02 Revised April 2002

Schering Corporation

a wholly-owned subsidiary of Schering-Plough Corporation
GALLOPING HILL ROAD
KENILWORTH, NJ 07033

Direct Inquiries to:
(908) 298-4000
CUSTOMER SERVICE:
(800) 222-7579
FAX: (908) 820-6400

For Medical Information Contact:
Schering Laboratories
Drug Information Services
2000 Galloping Hill Road
Kenilworth, NJ 07033
(800) 526-4099
FAX: (908) 298-2188

CLARINEX® ℞

[klar'-ə-neks"]
(desloratadine)
TABLETS

DESCRIPTION

CLARINEX (desloratadine) Tablets are light blue, round, film coated tablets containing 5 mg desloratadine, an antihistamine, to be administered orally. It also contains the following excipients: dibasic calcium phosphate dihydrate USP, microcrystalline cellulose NF, corn starch NF, talc USP, carnauba wax NF, white wax NF, coating material consisting of lactose monohydrate, hydroxypropyl methylcellulose, titanium dioxide, polyethylene glycol, and FD&C Blue # 2 Aluminum Lake.

Desloratadine is a white to off-white powder that is slightly soluble in water, but very soluble in ethanol and propylene glycol. It has an empirical formula: $C_{19}H_{19}ClN_2$ and a molecular weight of 310.8. The chemical name is 8-chloro-6,11-dihydro-11-(4-piperdinylidene)-5*H*-benzo[5,6]cyclo-hepta [1,2-*b*]pyridine and has the following structure:

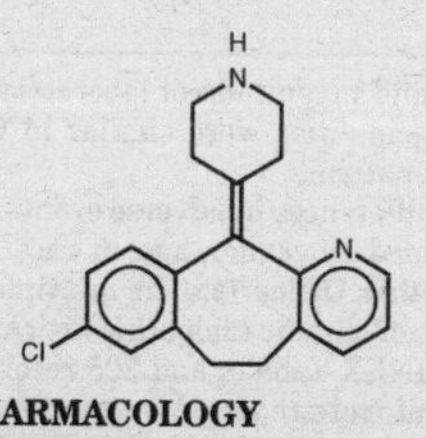

CLINICAL PHARMACOLOGY

Mechanism of Action: Desloratadine is a long-acting tricyclic histamine antagonist with selective H_1-receptor histamine antagonist activity. Receptor binding data indicates that at a concentration of 2-3 ng/mL (7 nanomolar), desloratadine shows significant interaction with the human histamine H_1 receptor. Desloratadine inhibited histamine release from human mast cells *in vitro*.

Results of a radiolabeled tissue distribution study in rats and a radioligand H_1-receptor binding study in guinea pigs showed that desloratadine did not readily cross the blood brain barrier.

Pharmacokinetics: Absorption: Following oral administration of desloratadine 5 mg once daily for 10 days to normal healthy volunteers, the mean time to maximum plasma concentrations (T_{max}) occurred at approximately 3 hours post dose and mean steady state peak plasma concentrations (C_{max}) and area under the concentration-time curve (AUC) of 4 ng/mL and 56.9 ng•hr/mL were observed, respectively. Neither food nor grapefruit juice had an effect on the bioavailability (C_{max} and AUC) of desloratadine.

Distribution: Desloratadine and 3-hydroxydesloratadine are approximately 82% to 87% and 85% to 89%, bound to plasma proteins, respectively. Protein binding of desloratadine and 3-hydroxydesloratadine was unaltered in subjects with impaired renal function.

Table 1

Changes in Desloratadine and 3-Hydroxydesloratadine Pharmacokinetics in Healthy Male and Female Volunteers

	Desloratadine C_{max}	Desloratadine AUC 0–24 hrs	3-Hydroxydesloratadine C_{max}	3-Hydroxydesloratadine AUC 0–24 hrs
Erythromycin (500 mg Q8h)	+24%	+14%	+43%	+40%
Ketoconazole (200 mg Q12h)	+45%	+39%	+43%	+72%
Azithromycin (500 mg day 1,250 mg QD × 4 days)	+15%	+5%	+15%	+4%
Fluoxetine (20 mg QD)	+15%	+0%	+17%	+13%
Cimetidine (600 mg Q12h)	+12%	+19%	-11%	-3%

Metabolism: Desloratadine (a major metabolite of loratadine) is extensively metabolized to 3-hydroxydesloratadine, an active metabolite, which is subsequently glucuronidated. The enzyme(s) responsible for the formation of 3-hydroxydesloratadine have not been identified. Data from clinical trials indicate that a subset of the general patient population has a decreased ability to form 3-hydroxydesloratadine, and are slow metabolizers of desloratadine. In pharmacokinetic studies (n=1087), approximately 7% of subjects were slow metabolizers of desloratadine (defined as a subject with an AUC ratio of 3-hydroxydesloratadine to desloratadine less than 0.1, or a subject with a desloratadine half-life exceeding 50 hours). The frequency of slow metabolizers is higher in Blacks (approximately 20% of Blacks were slow metabolizers in pharmacokinetic studies, n=276). The median exposure (AUC) to desloratadine in the slow metabolizers was approximately 6-fold greater than the subjects who are not slow metabolizers. Subjects who are slow metabolizers of desloratadine cannot be prospectively identified and will be exposed to higher levels of desloratadine following dosing with the recommended dose of desloratadine. Although not seen in these pharmacokinetic studies, patients who are slow metabolizers may be more susceptible to dose-related adverse events.

Elimination: The mean elimination half-life of desloratadine was 27 hours. C_{max} and AUC values increased in a dose proportional manner following single oral doses between 5 and 20 mg. The degree of accumulation after 14 days of dosing was consistent with the half-life and dosing frequency. A human mass balance study documented a recovery of approximately 87% of the ^{14}C-desloratadine dose, which was equally distributed in urine and feces as metabolic products. Analysis of plasma 3-hydroxydesloratadine showed similar T_{max} and half-life values compared to desloratadine.

Special Populations: Geriatric: In older subjects (≥ 65 years old; n=17) following multiple-dose administration of CLARINEX Tablets, the mean C_{max} and AUC values for desloratadine were 20% greater than in younger subjects (< 65 years old). The oral total body clearance (CL/F) when normalized for body weight was similar between the two age groups. The mean plasma elimination half-life of desloratadine was 33.7 hr in subjects ≥ 65 years old. The pharmacokinetics for 3-hydroxydesloratadine appeared unchanged in older versus younger subjects. These age-related differences are unlikely to be clinically relevant and no dosage adjustment is recommended in elderly subjects.

Renally Impaired: Desloratadine pharmacokinetics following a single dose of 7.5 mg were characterized in patients with mild (n=7; creatinine clearance 51-69 mL/min/1.73 m^2), moderate (n=6; creatinine clearance 34-43 mL/min/1.73 m^2), and severe (n=6; creatinine clearance 5–29 mL/min/1.73 m^2) renal impairment or hemodialysis dependent (n=6) patients. In patients with mild and moderate renal impairment, median C_{max} and AUC values increased by approximately 1.2- and 1.9-fold, respectively, relative to subjects with normal renal function. In patients with severe renal impairment or who were hemodialysis dependent, C_{max} and AUC values increased by approximately 1.7- and 2.5-fold, respectively. Minimal changes in 3-hydroxydesloratadine concentrations were observed. Desloratadine and 3-hydroxydesloratadine were poorly removed by hemodialysis. Plasma protein binding of desloratadine and 3-hydroxydesloratadine was unaltered by renal impairment. Dosage adjustment for patients with renal impairment is recommended (see **DOSAGE AND ADMINISTRATION** section).

Hepatically Impaired: Desloratadine pharmacokinetics were characterized following a single oral dose in patients with mild (n=4), moderate (n=4), and severe (n=4) hepatic impairment as defined by the Child-Pugh classification of hepatic function and 8 subjects with normal hepatic function. Patients with hepatic impairment, regardless of severity, had approximately a 2.4-fold increase in AUC as compared with normal subjects. The apparent oral clearance of desloratadine in patients with mild, moderate, and severe hepatic impairment was 37%, 36%, and 28% of that in normal subjects, respectively. An increase in the mean elimination half-life of desloratadine in patients with hepatic impairment was observed. For 3-hydroxydesloratadine, the mean C_{max} and AUC values for patients with hepatic impairment were not statistically significantly different from subjects with normal hepatic function. Dosage adjustment for patients with hepatic impairment is recommended (see **DOSAGE AND ADMINISTRATION** section).

Gender: Female subjects treated for 14 days with CLARINEX Tablets had 10% and 3% higher desloratadine C_{max} and AUC values, respectively, compared with male subjects. The 3-hydroxydesloratadine C_{max} and AUC values were also increased by 45% and 48%, respectively, in females compared with males. However, these apparent differences are not likely to be clinically relevant and therefore no dosage adjustment is recommended.

Race: Following 14 days of treatment with CLARINEX Tablets, the C_{max} and AUC values for desloratadine were 18% and 32% higher, respectively, in Blacks compared with Caucasians. For 3-hydroxydesloratadine there was a corresponding 10% reduction in C_{max} and AUC values in Blacks compared to Caucasians. These differences are not likely to be clinically relevant and therefore no dose adjustment is recommended.

Drug Interactions: In two controlled crossover clinical pharmacology studies in healthy male (n=12 in each study) and female (n=12 in each study) volunteers, desloratadine 7.5 mg (1.5 times the daily dose) once daily was coadministered with erythromycin 500 mg every 8 hours or ketoconazole 200 mg every 12 hours for 10 days. In 3 separate controlled, parallel group clinical pharmacology studies, desloratadine at the clinical dose of 5 mg has been coadministered with azithromycin 500 mg followed by 250 mg once daily for 4 days (n=18) or with fluoxetine 20 mg once daily for 7 days after a 23 day pretreatment period with fluoxetine (n=18) or with cimetidine 600 mg every 12 hours for 14 days (n=18) under steady state conditions to normal healthy male and female volunteers. Although increased plasma concentrations (C_{max} and AUC 0-24 hrs) of desloratadine and 3-hydroxydesloratadine were observed (see Table 1), there were no clinically relevant changes in the safety profile of desloratadine, as assessed by electrocardiographic parameters (including the corrected QT interval), clinical laboratory tests, vital signs, and adverse events.
[See table above]

Pharmacodynamics: Wheal and Flare: Human histamine skin wheal studies following single and repeated 5 mg doses of desloratadine have shown that the drug exhibits an antihistaminic effect by 1 hour; this activity may persist for as long as 24 hours. There was no evidence of histamine-induced skin wheal tachyphylaxis within the desloratadine 5 mg group over the 28 day treatment period. The clinical relevance of histamine wheal skin testing is unknown.

Effects on QT_c: Single dose administration of desloratadine did not alter the corrected QT interval (QT_c) in rats (up to 12 mg/kg, oral), or guinea pigs (25 mg/kg, intravenous). Repeated oral administration at doses up to 24 mg/kg for durations up to 3 months in monkeys did not alter the QT_c at an estimated desloratadine exposure (AUC) that was approximately 955 times the mean AUC in humans at the recommended daily oral dose. See **OVERDOSAGE** section for information on human QT_c experience.

Clinical Trials: Seasonal Allergic Rhinitis: The clinical efficacy and safety of CLARINEX Tablets were evaluated in over 2,300 patients 12 to 75 years of age with seasonal allergic rhinitis. A total of 1,838 patients received 2.5-20 mg/day of CLARINEX in 4 double-blind, randomized, placebo-controlled clinical trials of 2- to 4- weeks duration conducted in the United States. The results of these studies demonstrated the efficacy and safety of CLARINEX 5 mg in the treatment of adult and adolescent patients with seasonal allergic rhinitis. In a dose ranging trial, CLARINEX 2.5-20 mg/day was studied. Doses of 5, 7.5, 10, and 20 mg/day were superior to placebo; and no additional benefit was seen at doses above 5.0 mg. In the same study, an increase in the incidence of somnolence was observed at doses of 10 mg/day and 20 mg/day (5.2% and 7.6%, respectively), compared to placebo (2.3%).

In 2 four-week studies of 924 patients (aged 15 to 75 years) with seasonal allergic rhinitis and concomitant asthma, CLARINEX Tablets 5 mg once daily improved rhinitis symptoms, with no decrease in pulmonary function. This supports the safety of administering CLARINEX Tablets to adult patients with seasonal allergic rhinitis with mild to moderate asthma.

CLARINEX Tablets 5 mg once daily significantly reduced the Total Symptom Scores (the sum of individual scores of nasal and non-nasal symptoms) in patients with seasonal allergic rhinitis. See Table 2.

Continued on next page

Clarinex—Cont.

[See table 2 above]
There were no significant differences in the effectiveness of CLARINEX Tablets 5 mg across subgroups of patients defined by gender, age, or race.

Perennial Allergic Rhinitis: The clinical efficacy and safety of CLARINEX Tablets 5 mg were evaluated in over 1,300 patients 12 to 80 years of age with perennial allergic rhinitis. A total of 685 patients received 5 mg/day of CLARINEX in 2 double blind, randomized, placebo controlled clinical trials of 4 weeks duration conducted in the United States and internationally. In one of these studies CLARINEX Tablets 5 mg once daily was shown to significantly reduce symptoms of perennial allergic rhinitis (Table 3).
[See table 3 at right]

Chronic Idiopathic Urticaria: The efficacy and safety of CLARINEX Tablets 5 mg once daily was studied in 416 chronic idiopathic urticaria patients 12 to 84 years of age, of whom 211 received CLARINEX. In two double-blind, placebo-controlled, randomized clinical trials of six weeks duration, at the pre-specified one-week primary time point evaluation, CLARINEX Tablets significantly reduced the severity of pruritus when compared to placebo (Table 4). Secondary endpoints were also evaluated and during the first week of therapy CLARINEX Tablets 5 mg reduced the secondary endpoints, "Number of Hives" and the "Size of the Largest Hive," when compared to placebo.
[See table 4 at right]

INDICATIONS AND USAGE

Allergic Rhinitis: CLARINEX Tablets 5 mg are indicated for the relief of the nasal and non-nasal symptoms of allergic rhinitis (seasonal and perennial) in patients 12 years of age and older.

Chronic Idiopathic Urticaria: CLARINEX Tablets are indicated for the symptomatic relief of pruritus, reduction in the number of hives, and size of hives, in patients with chronic idiopathic urticaria 12 years of age and older.

CONTRAINDICATIONS

CLARINEX Tablets 5 mg are contraindicated in patients who are hypersensitive to this medication or to any of its ingredients, or to loratadine.

PRECAUTIONS

Carcinogenesis, Mutagenesis, Impairment of Fertility: The carcinogenic potential of desloratadine was assessed using loratadine studies. In an 18-month study in mice and a 2-year study in rats, loratadine was administered in the diet at doses up to 40 mg/kg/day in mice (estimated desloratadine and desloratadine metabolite exposures were approximately 3 times the AUC in humans at the recommended daily oral dose) and 25 mg/kg/day in rats (estimated desloratadine and desloratadine metabolite exposures were approximately 30 times the AUC in humans at the recommended daily oral dose). Male mice given 40 mg/kg/day loratadine had a significantly higher incidence of hepatocellular tumors (combined adenomas and carcinomas) than concurrent controls. In rats, a significantly higher incidence of hepatocellular tumors (combined adenomas and carcinomas) was observed in males given 10 mg/kg/day and in males and females given 25 mg/kg/day. The estimated desloratadine and desloratadine metabolite exposures of rats given 10 mg/kg of loratadine were approximately 7 times the AUC in humans at the recommended daily oral dose. The clinical significance of these findings during long-term use of desloratadine is not known.

In genotoxicity studies with desloratadine, there was no evidence of genotoxic potential in a reverse mutation assay (*Salmonella/E. coli* mammalian microsome bacterial mutagenicity assay) or in two assays for chromosomal aberrations (human peripheral blood lymphocyte clastogenicity assay and mouse bone marrow micronucleus assay).

There was no effect on female fertility in rats at desloratadine doses up to 24 mg/kg/day (estimated desloratadine and desloratadine metabolite exposures were approximately 130 times the AUC in humans at the recommended daily oral dose). A male specific decrease in fertility, demonstrated by reduced female conception rates, decreased sperm numbers and motility, and histopathologic testicular changes, occurred at an oral desloratadine dose of 12 mg/kg in rats (estimated desloratadine exposures were approximately 45 times the AUC in humans at the recommended daily oral dose). Desloratadine had no effect on fertility in rats at an oral dose of 3 mg/kg/day (estimated desloratadine and desloratadine metabolite exposures were approximately 8 times the AUC in humans at the recommended daily oral dose).

Pregnancy Category C: Desloratadine was not teratogenic in rats at doses up to 48 mg/kg/day (estimated desloratadine and desloratadine metabolite exposures were approximately 210 times the AUC in humans at the recommended daily oral dose) or in rabbits at doses up to 60 mg/kg/day (estimated desloratadine exposures were approximately 230 times the AUC in humans at the recommended daily oral dose). In a separate study, an increase in pre-implantation loss and a decreased number of implantations and fetuses were noted in female rats at 24 mg/kg (estimated desloratadine and desloratadine metabolite exposures were approximately 120 times the AUC in humans at the recommended daily oral dose). Reduced body weight and slow righting reflex were reported in pups at doses of 9 mg/kg/day or greater (estimated desloratadine and desloratadine metabolite exposures were approximately 50 times or greater than the AUC in humans at the recommended daily oral dose).

Table 2

TOTAL SYMPTOM SCORE (TSS)
Changes in a 2 Week Clinical Trial in Patients with Seasonal Allergic Rhinitis

Treatment Group (n)	Mean Baseline* (sem)	Change from Baseline** (sem)	Placebo Comparison (P-value)
CLARINEX 5.0 mg (171)	14.2 (0.3)	-4.3 (0.3)	P=<0.01
Placebo (173)	13.7 (0.3)	-2.5 (0.3)	

* At baseline, a total nasal symptom score (sum of 4 individual symptoms) of least 6 and a total non-nasal symptom score (sum of 4 individual symptoms) of at least 5 (each symptom scored 0 to 3 where 0=no symptom and 3=severe symptoms) was required for trial eligibility. TSS ranges from 0=no symptoms to 24=maximal symptoms.
**Mean reduction in TSS averaged over the 2-week treatment period.

Table 3

TOTAL SYMPTOM SCORE (TSS)
Changes in a 4 Week Clinical Trial in Patients with Perennial Allergic Rhinitis

Treatment Group (n)	Mean Baseline* (sem)	Change from Baseline** (sem)	Placebo Comparison (P-value)
CLARINEX 5.0 mg (337)	12.37 (0.18)	-4.06 (0.21)	P=0.01
Placebo (337)	12.30 (0.18)	-3.27 (0.21)	

* At baseline, a total nasal symptom score (sum of 5 individual nasal symptoms and 3 non-nasal symptoms, each symptom scored 0 to 3 where 0=no symptom and 3=severe symptoms) of at least 10 was required for trial eligibility. TSS ranges from 0=no symptoms to 24=maximal symptoms.
**Mean reduction in TSS averaged over the 4-week treatment period.

Table 4

PRURITUS SYMPTOM SCORE
Changes in the First Week of a Clinical Trial in Patients with Chronic Idiopathic Urticaria

Treatment Group (n)	Mean Baseline (sem)	Change from Baseline* (sem)	Placebo Comparison (P-value)
CLARINEX 5.0 mg (115)	2.19 (0.04)	-1.05 (0.07)	P=<0.01
Placebo (110)	2.21 (0.04)	-0.52 (0.07)	

Pruritus scored 0 to 3 where 0=no symptom to 3=maximal symptom
*Mean reduction in pruritus averaged over the first week of treatment.

Desloratadine had no effect on pup development at an oral dose of 3 mg/kg/day (estimated desloratadine and desloratadine metabolite exposures were approximately 7 times the AUC in humans at the recommended daily oral dose). There are, however, no adequate and well-controlled studies in pregnant women. Because animal reproduction studies are not always predictive of human response, desloratadine should be used during pregnancy only if clearly needed.

Nursing Mothers: Desloratadine passes into breast milk, therefore a decision should be made whether to discontinue nursing or to discontinue desloratadine, taking into account the importance of the drug to the mother.

Pediatric Use: The safety and effectiveness of CLARINEX Tablets in pediatric patients under 12 years of age have not been established.

Geriatric Use: Clinical studies of desloratadine did not include sufficient numbers of subjects aged 65 and over to determine whether they respond differently from younger subjects. Other reported clinical experience has not identified differences between the elderly and younger patients. In general, dose selection for an elderly patient should be cautious, reflecting the greater frequency of decreased hepatic, renal, or cardiac function, and of concomitant disease or other drug therapy. (see **CLINICAL PHARMACOLOGY—Special Populations**).

Information for Patients: Patients should be instructed to use CLARINEX Tablets as directed. As there are no food effects on bioavailability, patients can be instructed that CLARINEX Tablets may be taken without regard to meals. Patients should be advised not to increase the dose or dosing frequency as studies have not demonstrated increased effectiveness at higher doses and somnolence may occur.

ADVERSE REACTIONS

Allergic Rhinitis: In multiple-dose placebo-controlled trials, 2,834 patients received CLARINEX Tablets at doses of 2.5 mg to 20 mg daily, of whom 1,655 patients received the recommended daily dose of 5 mg. In patients receiving 5 mg daily, the rate of adverse events was similar between CLARINEX and placebo-treated patients. The percent of patients who withdrew prematurely due to adverse events was 2.4% in the CLARINEX group and 2.6% in the placebo group. There were no serious adverse events in these trials in patients receiving desloratadine. All adverse events that were reported by greater than or equal to 2% of patients who received the recommended daily dose of CLARINEX Tablets (5.0 mg once-daily), and that were more common with CLARINEX Tablet than placebo, are listed in Table 5.

Table 5

Incidence of Adverse Events Reported by ≥ 2% of Allergic Rhinitis Patients in Placebo-Controlled, Multiple-Dose Clinical Trials

Adverse Experience	CLARINEX Tablets 5 mg (n=1,655)	Placebo (n=1,652)
Pharyngitis	4.1%	2.0%
Dry Mouth	3.0%	1.9%
Myalgia	2.1%	1.8%
Fatigue	2.1%	1.2%
Somnolence	2.1%	1.8%
Dysmenorrhea	2.1%	1.6%

The frequency and magnitude of laboratory and electrocardiographic abnormalities were similar in CLARINEX and placebo-treated patients.

There were no differences in adverse events for subgroups of patients as defined by gender, age, or race.

Chronic Idiopathic Urticaria: In multiple-dose, placebo-controlled trials of chronic idiopathic urticaria, 211 patients received CLARINEX Tablets and 205 received placebo. Adverse events that were reported by greater than or equal to 2% of patients who received CLARINEX Tablets and that were more common with CLARINEX Tablets than placebo were (rates for CLARINEX and placebo, respectively): headache (14%, 13%), nausea (5%, 2%), fatigue (5%, 1%), dizziness (4%, 3%), pharyngitis (3%, 2%), dyspepsia (3%, 1%), and myalgia (3%, 1%).

The following spontaneous adverse events have been reported during the marketing of desloratadine: tachycardia, and rarely hypersensitivity reactions (such as rash, pruritus, urticaria, edema, dyspnea, and anaphylaxis), and elevated liver enzymes including bilirubin.

DRUG ABUSE AND DEPENDENCE

There is no information to indicate that abuse or dependency occurs with CLARINEX Tablets.

OVERDOSAGE

Information regarding acute overdosage is limited to experience from clinical trials conducted during the development of the CLARINEX product. In a dose ranging trial, at doses of 10 mg and 20 mg/day somnolence was reported.

Single daily doses of 45 mg were given to normal male and female volunteers for 10 days. All ECGs obtained in this study were manually read in a blinded fashion by a cardiologist. In CLARINEX-treated subjects, there was an increase in mean heart rate of 9.2 bpm relative to placebo. The QT interval was corrected for heart rate (QT_c) by both the Bazett and Fridericia methods. Using the QT_c (Bazett) there was a mean increase of 8.1 msec in CLARINEX-treated subjects relative to placebo. Using QT_c (Fridericia) there was a mean increase of 0.4 msec in CLARINEX-treated subjects relative to placebo. No clinically relevant adverse events were reported.

In the event of overdose, consider standard measures to remove any unabsorbed drug. Symptomatic and supportive treatment is recommended. Desloratadine and 3-hydroxydesloratadine are not eliminated by hemodialysis.

Lethality occurred in rats at oral doses of 250 mg/kg or greater (estimated desloratadine and desloratadine metabolite exposures were approximately 120 times the AUC in humans at the recommended daily oral dose). The oral median lethal dose in mice was 353 mg/kg (estimated desloratadine exposures were approximately 290 times the human daily oral dose on a mg/m^2 basis). No deaths occurred at oral doses up to 250 mg/kg in monkeys (estimated desloratadine exposures were approximately 810 times the human daily oral dose on a mg/m^2 basis).

DOSAGE AND ADMINISTRATION

In adults and children 12 years of age and over; the recommended dose of CLARINEX Tablets is 5 mg once daily. In patients with liver or renal impairment, a starting dose of one 5 mg tablet every other day is recommended based on pharmacokinetic data.

HOW SUPPLIED

CLARINEX Tablets: Embossed "C5", light blue film coated tablets; that are packaged in high-density polyethylene plastic bottles of 100 (NDC 0085-1264-01) and 500 (NDC 0085-1264-02). Also available, CLARINEX Unit-of-Use package of 30 tablets (3 × 10; 10 blisters per card) (NDC 0085-1264-04); and Unit Dose-Hospital Pack of 100 Tablets (10 × 10; 10 blisters per card) (NDC 0085-1264-03).

Protect Unit-of-Use packaging and Unit Dose-Hospital Pack from excessive moisture.

Store between 2° and 25°C (36° and 77°F).

Heat sensitive. Avoid exposure at or above 30°C (86°F).

Schering®
Schering Corporation
Kenilworth, NJ 07033 USA

2/02 **23882116T**

U.S. Patent Nos. 4,659,716; 4,863,931; 4,804,666; 5,595,997; and 6,100,274.

MIRADON® ℞

brand of anisindione
[*mīr' a-don*]
Tablets

DESCRIPTION

MIRADON Tablets contain a synthetic anticoagulant, anisindione, an indanedione derivative. Each tablet contains 50 mg anisindione. They also contain: corn starch, FD&C Red No. 3, gelatin, lactose, and hydrogenated cottonseed oil.

ACTIONS

Like phenindione, to which it is related chemically, anisindione exercises its therapeutic action by reducing the prothrombin activity of the blood.

INDICATIONS

Anisindione is indicated for the prophylaxis and treatment of venous thrombosis and its extension, the treatment of atrial fibrillation with embolization, the prophylaxis and treatment of pulmonary embolism, and as an adjunct in the treatment of coronary occlusion.

CONTRAINDICATIONS

All contraindications to oral anticoagulant therapy are relative rather than absolute. Contraindications should be evaluated for each patient, giving consideration to the need for and the benefits to be achieved by anticoagulant therapy, the potential dangers of hemorrhage, the expected duration of therapy, and the quality of patient monitoring and compliance.

Hemorrhagic Tendencies or Blood Dyscrasias: In general, oral anticoagulants are contraindicated in patients who are bleeding or who have hemorrhagic blood dyscrasias or hemorrhagic tendencies (eg, hemophilia, polycythemia vera, purpura, leukemia) or a history of bleeding diathesis. They are contraindicated in patients with recent cerebral hemorrhage, active ulceration of the gastrointestinal tract, including ulcerative colitis, or open ulcerative, traumatic, or surgical wounds. Oral anticoagulants may be contraindicated in patients with recent or contemplated brain, eye, or spinal cord surgery or prostatectomy, and in those undergoing regional or lumbar block anesthesia or continuous tube drainage of the small intestine. Oral anticoagulants may be contraindicated in patients who have severe renal or hepatic disease, subacute bacterial endocarditis, pericarditis, polyarthritis, diverticulitis, visceral carcinoma, or aneurysm. Other conditions in which the oral anticoagulants may be contraindicated include severe or malignant hypertension, eclampsia or preeclampsia, threatened abortion, emaciation, malnutrition, and vitamin C or K deficiencies. Since a high degree of patient cooperation is required for the outpatient use of oral anticoagulants, a lack of such cooperation is a relative contraindication to their use.

Pregnancy: Anisindione is contraindicated in pregnancy because the drug crosses the placental barrier. Oral anticoagulants may cause fetal damage when administered to pregnant women. Fetal or neonatal hemorrhage and intrauterine fetal death have occurred even when maternal prothrombin times were within the therapeutically accepted range. Maternal use of warfarin and anisindione during the first trimester of pregnancy has been reported to cause hypoplastic nasal structures or other signs of the Conradi-Hunermann syndrome in the offspring. These patients received other drugs in addition to anticoagulants and a positive causal relationship has not been established. If oral anticoagulants must be used during pregnancy, or if the patient becomes pregnant while taking one of these drugs, the patient should be apprised of the potential hazard to the fetus. The possibility of termination of the pregnancy should be considered in light of these risks.

As an alternative to the use of oral anticoagulants in pregnant patients, the use of heparin, which does not cross the placenta, should be considered.

WARNINGS

Anisindione should be reserved for patients who cannot tolerate the coumarins.

Oral anticoagulants are potent drugs with prolonged and cumulative effects. Treatment must be individualized according to patient response, and the benefit expected from anticoagulant therapy should be weighed against the possible hazards associated with the use of these drugs.

Oral anticoagulants should not be used in the treatment of acute completed strokes due to the risk of fatal cerebral hemorrhage (see **INDICATIONS**).

Because agranulocytosis and hepatitis have been associated with the use of anisindione, liver function and blood studies should be performed periodically. Patients should be instructed to report to the physician symptoms such as marked fatigue, chills, fever, or sore throat; the drug should be discontinued promptly since these symptoms may signal the onset of severe toxicity. If leukopenia or evidence of hypersensitivity occurs, the drug should be discontinued. Because of the possibility of renal damage associated with the use of phenindione, the urine should be tested periodically for albumin whenever phenindione or any indanedione anticoagulant is used.

Relatively minor bleeding episodes and hemorrhage occur in 2% to 10% of patients treated with oral anticoagulants. Bleeding will vary in intensity, and may be related to the quality of patient monitoring, compliance on the part of the patient, the incidence of potentially hemorrhagic lesions, or the extent of anticoagulation induced. Severe and moderate hypertension, severe to moderate hepatic and renal insufficiency, and infectious diseases or disturbances of intestinal flora as in sprue, or with antibiotic therapy may increase the risks associated with anticoagulant therapy.

Occasionally, fatal hemorrhages can occur. Massive hemorrhage from organ systems may involve cerebral, pericardial, pulmonary, adrenal, hepatic, spinal, gastrointestinal, or genitourinary sites. Gastrointestinal hemorrhage may be secondary to peptic ulceration or silent neoplasm and is responsible for 25% of all deaths due to oral anticoagulant therapy. Bleeding complications in the genitourinary tract may range in severity from microscopic hematuria to gross hematuria to extensive uterine hemorrhage.

Hemorrhagic necrosis and/or gangrene of the skin and subcutaneous tissue, petechial and purpuric hemorrhage, ecchymosis, epistaxis, hematemesis, or hemoptysis, may also occur. Hemorrhage and necrosis have in some cases been reported to result in death or permanent disability. Necrosis appears to be associated with local thrombosis and usually appears within a few days of the start of anticoagulant therapy. In severe cases of necrosis, treatment through debridement or amputation of the affected tissue, limb, breast, or penis has been reported. Careful diagnosis is required to determine whether necrosis is caused by an underlying disease. MIRADON therapy should be discontinued when anisindione is suspected to be the cause of developing necrosis and heparin therapy may be considered for anticoagulation. Although various treatments have been attempted, no treatment for necrosis has been considered uniformly effective. (See below for information on predisposing conditions.)

The risks of anticoagulant therapy may be increased in patients with known or suspected hereditary, familial, or clinical deficiency in protein C. This condition, which should be suspected if there is a history of recurrent episodes of thromboembolic disorders in the patient or in the family, has been associated with an increased risk of developing necrosis following warfarin administration, and may be expected following anisindione therapy. Skin necrosis may occur in the absence of protein C deficiency. It has been reported that initiation of anticoagulation therapy with heparin for 4 to 5 days before initiation of therapy with anisindione may minimize the incidence of this reaction. Anisindione therapy should be discontinued when it is suspected to be the cause of developing necrosis and heparin therapy may be considered for anticoagulation.

Concurrent use of anticoagulants with streptokinase, urokinase, or alteplase (recombinant tissue plasminogen activator) is not recommended and may be hazardous. (Consult the product information accompanying those preparations.)

Abrupt cessation of anticoagulant therapy is not generally recommended; if possible, taper the dose gradually over 3 to 4 weeks.

PRECAUTIONS

General: Periodic determination of prothrombin time or other suitable coagulation test is essential. The availability of suitable laboratory facilities to monitor therapy accurately with oral anticoagulants is mandatory, both to assure adequate anticoagulation and to avoid toxicity due to overdosage. The dosage of oral anticoagulants depends on the clinical response as monitored by prothrombin time determinations (see **DOSAGE AND ADMINISTRATION**).

Since heparin prolongs the one-stage prothrombin time, a period of at least 5 hours should elapse after the last intravenous dose and after the last subcutaneous dose of heparin before drawing blood to determine the prothrombin time when heparin and anisindione have been given together. In addition to adequate laboratory facilities, a supply of oral or parenteral phytonadione (vitamin K_1) and a source of whole blood or plasma should be available when emergency treatment of acute overdosage is required (see **OVERDOSAGE**).

A number of factors including environmental, mental, medical, and nutritional states may affect an individual's response to anticoagulant therapy. Factors which increase sensitivity to the drug and lengthen prothrombin time include: initial hypoprothrombinemia, increased age, poor nutritional status, vitamin K deficiency or malabsorption, congestive heart failure or vascular damage, hepatic disorders including hepatitis or obstructive jaundice, biliary fistula, febrile states, hyperthyroidism, preparatory bowel sterilization, recent surgery, and X-ray therapy.

Factors which may decrease the response to oral anticoagulants and shorten the prothrombin time include: pregnancy, diabetes mellitus, hyperlipidemia, hypothyroidism, hypercholesterolemia, and hereditary or acquired resistance.

Information for Patients: The physician should instruct patients:

- To follow carefully the physician's directions for taking this drug and not to alter these directions without authorization.
- To follow carefully the physician's directions for the periodic blood test (prothrombin time) required to assure that the correct dose of the drug is being used.
- To discuss with the physician any other medication (prescription or nonprescription) to be used.
- To report to the physician any abnormal bleeding, such as blood in the urine, blood in the stool (a black, tarry appearance); bleeding from the gums or nose; patches of discoloration or bruises on the arms, legs, or toes; or excessive bleeding following minor cuts (eg, while shaving).
- To discuss with the physician any plan to become pregnant or to report any pregnancy promptly.

Laboratory Tests: The need for careful control of the degree of anticoagulation, as determined by changes in prothrombin activity, cannot be overemphasized. It should be noted, however, that bleeding during anticoagulant therapy may not always correlate with prothrombin activity.

The stool guaiac test should be used to detect occult gastrointestinal bleeding.

In long-term therapy with anticoagulants, periodic laboratory evaluation of organ systems, including hematopoietic, renal, and hepatic studies, should be performed (see **WARNINGS**).

Drug Interactions: Addition or deletion of any drug from the therapeutic regimen of patients receiving oral anticoagulants may affect patient response to the anticoagulant. Frequent determination of prothrombin time and close monitoring of the patient is essential to ascertain when adjustment of dosage of anticoagulant may be needed.

Because of the variability of individual patient response, multiple interacting mechanisms with some drugs, the dependency of the extent of the interaction on the dosage and duration of therapy, and the possible administration of several interacting drugs simultaneously, it is difficult to predict the direction and degree of the ultimate effect of concomitant medications on anticoagulant response. For example, since cholestyramine may reduce the gastrointestinal absorption of both the oral anticoagulants and vitamin K, the net effects are unpredictable. Chloral hydrate may cause an increased prothrombin response by displacing the anticoagulant from protein binding sites or a diminished prothrombin response through increased metabolism of the unbound drug by hepatic enzyme induction, thus leading to inter-patient variation in ultimate prothrombin effect. An interacting drug which leads to a decrease in prothrombin time necessitating an increased dose of oral anticoagulant to maintain an adequate degree of anticoagulation may, if abruptly discontinued, increase the risk of subsequent bleeding.

Drugs that have been reported to diminish oral anticoagulant response, ie, decreased prothrombin time response, in man significantly include: adrenocortical steroids; alcohol*; antacids; antihistamines; barbiturates; carbamazepine; chloral hydrate*; chlordiazepoxide; cholestyramine; diet high in vitamin K; diuretics*; ethchlorvynol; glutethimide; griseofulvin; haloperidol; meprobamate; oral contraceptives; paraldehyde; primidone; ranitidine*; rifampin; unreliable prothrombin time determinations; vitamin C; warfarin sodium underdosage.

Drugs that reportedly may increase oral anticoagulant response, ie, increased prothrombin response, in man include: alcohol*; allopurinol; aminosalicylic acid; amiodarone; anabolic steroids; antibiotics; bromelains; chloral hydrate*; chlorpropamide; chymotrypsin; cimetidine; cinchophen; clofibrate; dextran; dextrothyroxine; diazoxide; dietary deficiencies; diflunisal; diuretics*; disulfiram; drugs affecting blood elements; ethacrynic acid; fenoprofen; glucagon; hepatotoxic drugs; ibuprofen; indomethacin; influenza virus

Continued on next page

Miradon—Cont.

vaccine; inhalation anesthetics; mefenamic acid; methyldopa; methylphenidate; metronidazole; miconazole; monoamine oxidase inhibitors; nalidixic acid; naproxen; oxolinic acid; oxyphenbutazone; pentoxifylline; phenylbutazone; phenyramidol; phenytoin; prolonged hot weather; prolonged narcotics; pyrazolones; quinidine; quinine; ranitidine*; salicylates; sulfinpyrazone; sulfonamides, long acting; sulindac; thyroid drugs; tolbutamide; triclofos sodium; trimethoprim/sulfamethoxazole; unreliable prothrombin time determinations; warfarin sodium overdosage.

Oral anticoagulants may potentiate the hypoglycemic action of hypoglycemic agents, eg, tolbutamide and chlorpropamide, by inhibiting their metabolism in the liver. Because oral anticoagulants may interfere with the hepatic metabolism of phenytoin, toxic levels of the anticonvulsant may occur when an oral anticoagulant and phenytoin are administered concurrently.

Drugs that reduce the number of blood platelets by causing bone marrow depression (such as antineoplastic agents) or drugs which inhibit platelet function (eg, aspirin and other nonsteroidal anti-inflammatory drugs, dipyridamole, hydrochloroquine, clofibrate, dextran) may increase the bleeding tendency produced by anticoagulants without altering prothrombin time determinations. The beneficial effects on arterial thrombus formation from combined therapy with antiplatelet and anticoagulant medication must be weighed against an increased risk of inducing hemorrhage.

*Increased and decreased prothrombin time responses have been reported.

Drug/Laboratory Test Interferences: Dicumarol and indanedione anticoagulants, including anisindione, or their metabolites may color alkaline urine red-orange, which may interfere with spectrophotometrically determined urinary laboratory tests. The color reverses when the test sample is acidified *in vitro* to a pH below 4.

Carcinogenesis, Mutagenesis, Impairment of Fertility: Long-term dosing studies to determine the carcinogenic potential of oral anticoagulants, including anisindione, have not been done. Information on mutagenesis is unknown.

Pregnancy: Teratogenic and other effects—Pregnancy Category X: (See **CONTRAINDICATIONS**.)

Labor and Delivery: Anisindione is contraindicated in pregnancy. If oral anticoagulants are used in pregnant women, they should not be administered during the first trimester, and should be discontinued prior to labor and delivery.

Some clinicians suggest the replacement of oral anticoagulants with heparin therapy before term. Heparin is withheld during early labor and reinstituted 6 hours postpartum. After 5 to 7 days, therapy with oral anticoagulants may be resumed if indicated.

See **CONTRAINDICATIONS** for the use of oral anticoagulants in pregnancy.

Nursing Mothers: Oral anticoagulants or their metabolites are excreted in the milk of nursing mothers, possibly in amounts sufficient to cause a prothrombopenic state and bleeding in the newborn. As a general rule, nursing should not be undertaken while a patient is receiving an oral anticoagulant.

Pediatric Use: The use of oral anticoagulants in pediatric patients is not well documented. However, they may be beneficial in pediatric patients with rare thromboembolic disorder secondary to other disease states such as the nephrotic syndrome or congenital heart lesions. Heparin is probably the initial anticoagulant of choice because of its immediate onset of action.

ADVERSE REACTIONS

Multisystem adverse reactions have been reported, and some may be serious enough to warrant hospital admission. In general, they may be divided into 2 categories: those which involve abnormal bleeding and other effects which do not. Hemorrhage and/or necrosis are among the hazards of treatment with any anticoagulant and are the main serious complications of therapy. For additional discussion of possible hemorrhagic complications following oral anticoagulant therapy see **WARNINGS**. Although most of the adverse reactions for oral anticoagulant drugs have been reported for warfarin, dicumarol, and phenindione, all the drugs within this class have similar pharmacologic and clinical properties, and require the same degree of caution in monitoring adverse reactions regardless of the drug administered.

Some indanediones (phenindione) have been associated with undesirable reactions which have not been reported with the coumarins and are not counterbalanced by advantages, thus perhaps favoring the use of the coumarin-type anticoagulants. Changing from one chemical type of oral anticoagulant to the other may eliminate an adverse reaction, such as rash or diarrhea. Dermatitis is the only untoward reaction consistently associated with anisindione therapy.

Adverse reactions reported following therapy with either coumarin or indanedione anticoagulants include: nausea, diarrhea, pyrexia, dermatitis or exfoliative dermatitis, urticaria, alopecia, and sore mouth or mouth ulcers.

Side effects which have additionally been reported for coumarin derivatives include: vomiting, abdominal cramps, anorexia, priapism, erythema and necrosis of the skin and other tissues, manifesting as purple toes and cutaneous gangrene. There is no reason to expect that some or all of these adverse reactions might not occur in patients receiving anisindione.

Additional side effects attributed to the indanedione anticoagulants include: headache, sore throat, blurred vision, paralysis of accommodation, steatorrhea, hepatitis, jaundice, liver damage, renal tubular necrosis, albuminuria, anuria, myeloid immaturity, agranulocytosis, leukocyte agglutinins, red cell aplasia, atypical mononuclear cells, leukopenia, leukocytosis, anemia, thrombocytopenia, and eosinophilia.

Phenprocoumon-induced delayed callus formation following bone fracture has been reported.

DOSAGE AND ADMINISTRATION

Initial dosage of MIRADON Tablets is 300 mg the first day, 200 mg the second day, and 100 mg the third day. With initiation of treatment, prothrombin activity decreases rapidly to 50 percent of baseline values within 6 hours; thereafter it decreases slowly until it reaches 15 to 30 percent of baseline values in 48 to 72 hours. *Maintenance dosage* is established from daily prothrombin-time determinations for each patient, although with MIRADON Tablets, the uniform, predictable action of the drug makes it possible to reduce the frequency of prothrombin-time determinations in some cases. Maintenance dosage will vary between 25 to 250 mg a day and should be set to keep the prothrombin time one and one-half to two times the normal value. The dose may be repeated for many days; anisindione does not accumulate in the body.

Prothrombin activity returns to normal within 24 to 72 hours after treatment when the drug is discontinued. Some studies suggest that gradual reduction of dosage over a 2-week period may decrease the frequency of recurrence of thromboembolic disease by preventing a rapid rise in prothrombin activity.

OVERDOSAGE

Vitamin K_1 is a specific antidote for anticoagulants, such as anisindione, which reduce prothrombin activity in the blood. Vitamin K_1 may be administered orally or by injection, if the patient is not bleeding or if bleeding is slight. A few hours after administration of vitamin K_1 preparations, such as phytonadione, prothrombin activity increases and clotting time decreases. In the presence of more active hemorrhage, however, transfusions of whole blood or plasma are required until the desired level of prothrombin activity is achieved. Treatment with vitamin K_1 preparations is only adjunctive in such cases.

HOW SUPPLIED

MIRADON Tablets, 50 mg, pink, scored, compressed tablets impressed with the Schering trademark and product identification numbers 795; bottle of 100 (NDC 0085-0795-05).

Store at Controlled Room Temperature 20°–25°C (68°–77°F) [See USP].

MIRADON®
brand of anisindione
Tablets

Schering Corporation
Kenilworth, NJ 07033 USA

Rev. 7/01 B-16099775

REBETOL® ℞

[rē' bə-tōl]
(ribavirin, USP)
Capsules

- **REBETOL monotherapy is not effective for the treatment of chronic hepatitis C virus infection and should not be used alone for this indication. (See WARNINGS).**
- **The primary toxicity of ribavirin is hemolytic anemia. The anemia associated with REBETOL therapy may result in worsening of cardiac disease that has lead to fatal and nonfatal myocardial infarctions. Patients with a history of significant or unstable cardiac disease should not be treated with REBETOL. (See WARNINGS, ADVERSE REACTIONS and DOSAGE AND ADMINISTRATION).**
- **Significant teratogenic and/or embryocidal effects have been demonstrated in all animal species exposed to ribavirin. In addition, ribavirin has a multiple dose half-life of 12 days, and so it may persist in non plasma compartments for as long as six months. Therefore, REBETOL therapy is contraindicated in women who are pregnant and in the male partners of women who are pregnant. Extreme care must be taken to avoid pregnancy during therapy and for 6 months after completion of treatment in both female patients and in female partners of male patients who are taking REBETOL therapy. At least two reliable forms of effective contraception must be utilized during treatment and during the 6-month posttreatment follow-up period. (See CONTRAINDICATIONS, WARNINGS, PRECAUTIONS-Information for Patients and Pregnancy Category X).**

DESCRIPTION

REBETOL®

REBETOL is Schering Corporation's brand name for ribavirin, a nucleoside analog. The chemical name of ribavirin is 1-β-D-ribofuranosyl-1*H*-1,2,4-triazole-3-carboxamide and has the following structural formula:

Ribavirin is a white, crystalline powder. It is freely soluble in water and slightly soluble in anhydrous alcohol. The empirical formula is $C_8H_{12}N_4O_5$ and the molecular weight is 244.21.

REBETOL Capsules consist of a white powder in a white, opaque, gelatin capsule. Each capsule contains 200 mg ribavirin and the inactive ingredients microcrystalline cellulose, lactose monohydrate, croscarmellose sodium, and magnesium stearate. The capsule shell consists of gelatin, sodium lauryl sulfate, silicon dioxide, and titanium dioxide. The capsule is printed with edible blue pharmaceutical ink which is made of shellac, anhydrous ethyl alcohol, isopropyl alcohol, n-butyl alcohol, propylene glycol, ammonium hydroxide, and FD&C Blue #2 aluminum lake.

Mechanism of Action

Ribavirin/Interferon alfa-2b, recombinant. The mechanism of inhibition of hepatitis C virus (HCV) RNA by combination therapy with REBETOL and INTRON A has not been established.

CLINICAL PHARMACOLOGY

Pharmacokinetics

Ribavirin Single- and multiple-dose pharmacokinetic properties in adults with chronic hepatitis C are summarized in **TABLE 1**. Ribavirin was rapidly and extensively absorbed following oral administration. However, due to first-pass metabolism, the absolute bioavailability averaged 64% (44%). There was a linear relationship between dose and AUC_{tf} (AUC from time zero to last measurable concentration) following single doses of 200–1200 mg ribavirin. The relationship between dose and C_{max} was curvilinear, tending to asymptote above single doses of 400–600 mg.

Upon multiple oral dosing, based on $AUC12_{hr}$, a sixfold accumulation of ribavirin was observed in plasma. Following oral dosing with 600 mg BID, steady-state was reached by approximately 4 weeks, with mean steady-state plasma concentrations of 2200 (37%) ng/mL. Upon discontinuation of dosing, the mean half-life was 298 (30%) hours, which probably reflects slow elimination from nonplasma compartments.

Effect of Food on Absorption of Ribavirin Both AUC_{tf} and C_{max} increased by 70% when REBETOL Capsules were administered with a high-fat meal (841 kcal, 53.8 g fat, 31.6 g protein, and 57.4 g carbohydrate) in a single-dose pharmacokinetic study. There are insufficient data to address the clinical relevance of these results. Clinical efficacy studies were conducted without instructions with respect to food consumption. (See **DOSAGE AND ADMINISTRATION**.)

Effect of Antacid on Absorption of Ribavirin Coadministration with an antacid containing magnesium, aluminum, and simethicone (Mylanta®[1]) resulted in a 14% decrease in mean ribavirin AUC_{tf}. The clinical relevance of results from this single-dose study is unknown.

TABLE 1. Mean (% CV) Pharmacokinetic Parameters for REBETOL When Administered Individually to Adults with Chronic Hepatitis C

Parameter	REBETOL (N=12)	
	Single Dose 600 mg	Multiple Dose 600 mg BID
T_{max} (hr)	1.7 (46)***	3 (60)
C_{max}*	782 (37)	3680 (85)
AUC_{tf}**	13400 (48)	228000 (25)
$T_{½}$ (hr)	43.6 (47)	298 (30)
Apparent Volume of Distribution (L)	2825 (9)†	
Apparent Clearance (L/hr)	38.2 (40)	
Absolute Bioavailability	64% (44)† †	

* ng/mL
** ng.hr/mL
*** N=11
† data obtained from a single-dose pharmacokinetic study using ^{14}C labeled ribavirin; N=5
† † N=6

Ribavirin transport into nonplasma compartments has been most extensively studied in red blood cells, and has been identified to be primarily via an e_s-type equilibrative nucleoside transporter. This type of transporter is present on virtually all cell types and may account for the extensive volume of distribution. Ribavirin does not bind to plasma proteins.

Ribavirin has two pathways of metabolism: (i) a reversible phosphorylation pathway in nucleated cells; and (ii) a degradative pathway involving deribosylation and amide hydrolysis to yield a triazole carboxylic acid metabolite. Ribavirin and its triazole carboxamide and triazole carboxylic acid metabolites are excreted renally. After oral administration of 600 mg of ^{14}C-ribavirin, approximately 61% and

12% of the radioactivity was eliminated in the urine and feces, respectively, in 336 hours. Unchanged ribavirin accounted for 17% of the administered dose.
Results of *in vitro* studies using both human and rat liver microsome preparations indicated little or no cytochrome P450 enzyme-mediated metabolism of ribavirin, with minimal potential for P450 enzyme-based drug interactions.
No pharmacokinetic interactions were noted between INTRON A Injection and REBETOL Capsules in a multiple-dose pharmacokinetic study.

[1]Trademark of Johnson & Johnson-Merck Consumer Pharmaceuticals Co.

Special Populations

Renal Dysfunction The pharmacokinetics of ribavirin were assessed after administration of a single oral dose (400 mg) of ribavirin to non HCV-infected subjects with varying degrees of renal dysfunction. The mean AUC_{tf} value was threefold greater in subjects with creatinine clearance values between 10 to 30 mL/min when compared to control subjects (creatinine clearance >90 mL/min). In subjects with creatinine clearance values between 30 to 60 mL/min, AUC_{tf} was twofold greater when compared to control subjects. The increased AUC_{tf} appears to be due to reduction of renal and non-renal clearance in these patients. Phase III efficacy trials included subjects with creatinine clearance values > 50 mL/min. The multiple dose pharmacokinetics of ribavirin cannot be accurately predicted in patients with renal dysfunction. Ribavirin is not effectively removed by hemodialysis. Patients with creatinine clearance <50 mL/min should not be treated with REBETOL (See **WARNINGS**.)
Hepatic Dysfunction The effect of hepatic dysfunction was assessed after a single oral dose of ribavirin (600 mg). The mean AUC_{tf} values were not significantly different in subjects with mild, moderate, or severe hepatic dysfunction (Child-Pugh Classification A, B, or C), when compared to control subjects. However, the mean C_{max} values increased with severity of hepatic dysfunction and was twofold greater in subjects with severe hepatic dysfunction when compared to control subjects.
Pediatric Patients Pharmacokinetic evaluations in pediatric subjects have not been performed.
Elderly Patients Pharmacokinetic evaluations in elderly subjects have not been performed.
Gender There were no clinically significant pharmacokinetic differences noted in a single-dose study of eighteen male and eighteen female subjects.
****In this section of the label, numbers in parenthesis indicate % coefficient of variation.***

INDICATIONS AND USAGE

REBETOL (ribavirin, USP) Capsules are indicated only in combination with INTRON A (interferon alfa-2b, recombinant) Injection for the treatment of chronic hepatitis C in patients with compensated liver disease previously untreated with alpha interferon or who have relapsed following alpha interferon therapy.
The safety and efficacy of REBETOL Capsules with interferons other than INTRON A have not been established.

Description of Clinical Studies

Previously Untreated Patients Adults with compensated chronic hepatitis C and detectable HCV RNA (assessed by a central laboratory using a research-based RT-PCR assay) who were previously untreated with alpha interferon therapy were enrolled into two multicenter, double-blind trials (US and International) and randomized to receive REBETOL Capsules 1200 mg/day (1000 mg/day for patients weighing ≤75 kg) plus INTRON A Injection 3 MIU TIW or INTRON A Injection plus placebo for 24 or 48 weeks followed by 24 weeks of off-therapy follow-up. The International study did not contain a 24-week INTRON A plus placebo treatment arm. The US study enrolled 912 patients who, at baseline, were 67% male, 89% Caucasian with a mean Knodell HAI score (I+II+III) of 7.5, and 72% genotype 1. The International study, conducted in Europe, Israel, Canada, and Australia, enrolled 799 patients (65% male, 95% Caucasian, mean Knodell score 6.8, and 58% genotype 1).
Study results are summarized in **TABLE 2**.
[See table 2 above]
Of patients who had not achieved HCV RNA below the limit of detection of the research based assay by week 24 of REBETOL/INTRON A treatment, less than 5% responded to an additional 24 weeks of combination treatment.
Among patients with HCV genotype 1 treated with REBETOL/INTRON A therapy who achieved HCV RNA below the detection limit of the research-based assay by 24 weeks, those randomized to 48 weeks of treatment had higher virologic responses compared to those in the 24 week treatment group. There was no observed increase in response rates for patients with HCV non-genotype 1 randomized to REBETOL/INTRON A therapy for 48 weeks compared to 24 weeks.
Relapse Patients Patients with compensated chronic hepatitis C and detectable HCV RNA (assessed by a central laboratory using a research-based RT-PCR assay) who had relapsed following one or two courses of interferon therapy (defined as abnormal serum ALT levels) were enrolled into two multicenter, double-blind trials (US and International) and randomized to receive REBETOL 1200 mg/day (1000 mg/day for patients weighing ≤75 kg) plus INTRON A 3 MIU TIW or INTRON A plus placebo for 24 weeks followed by 24 weeks of off-therapy follow-up. The US study enrolled 153 patients who, at baseline, were 67% male, 92% Caucasian with a mean Knodell HAI score (I+II+III) of 6.8, and 58% genotype 1. The International study, conducted in Europe, Israel, Canada, and Australia, enrolled 192 patients (64% male, 95% Caucasian, mean Knodell score 6.6, and 56% genotype 1).
Study results are summarized in **TABLE 3**.
[See table 3 above]
Virologic and histologic responses were similar among male and female patients in both the previously untreated and relapse studies.

TABLE 2. Virologic and Histologic Responses: Previously Untreated Patients*

	US Study			
	24 weeks of treatment		48 weeks of treatment	
	INTRON A plus REBETOL (N=228)	INTRON A plus Placebo (N=231)	INTRON A plus REBETOL (N=228)	INTRON A plus Placebo (N=225)
Virologic Response				
-Responder[1]	65 (29)	13 (6)	85 (37)	27 (12)
-Nonresponder	147 (64)	194 (84)	110 (48)	168 (75)
-Missing data	16 (7)	24 (10)	33 (14)	30 (13)
Histologic Response				
-Improvement[2]	102 (45)	77 (33)	96 (42)	65 (29)
-No improvement	77 (34)	99 (43)	61 (27)	93 (41)
-Missing data	49 (21)	55 (24)	71 (31)	67 (30)

	International Study		
	24 weeks of treatment	48 weeks of treatment	
	INTRON A plus REBETOL (N=265)	INTRON A plus REBETOL (N=268)	INTRON A plus Placebo (N=266)
Virologic Response			
-Responder[1]	86 (32)	113 (42)	46 (17)
-Nonresponder	158 (60)	120 (45)	196 (74)
-Missing data	21 (8)	35 (13)	24 (9)
Histologic Response			
-Improvement[2]	103 (39)	102 (38)	69 (26)
-No improvement	85 (32)	58 (22)	111 (41)
-Missing data	77 (29)	108 (40)	86 (32)

* Number (%) of patients.
[1] Defined as HCV RNA below limit of detection using a research based RT-PCR assay at end of treatment and during follow-up period.
[2] Defined as posttreatment (end of follow-up) minus pretreatment liver biopsy Knodell HAI score (I+II+III) improvement of ≥2 points.

TABLE 3. Virologic and Histologic Responses: Relapse Patients*

	US Study		International Study	
	INTRON A plus REBETOL (N=77)	INTRON A plus Placebo (N=76)	INTRON A plus REBETOL (N=96)	INTRON A plus Placebo (N=96)
Virologic Responses				
-Responder[1]	33 (43)	3 (4)	46 (48)	5 (5)
-Nonresponder	36 (47)	66 (87)	45 (47)	91 (95)
-Missing data	8 (10)	7 (9)	5 (5)	0 (0)
Histologic Response				
-Improvement[2]	38 (49)	27 (36)	49 (51)	30 (31)
-No improvement	23 (30)	37 (49)	29 (30)	44 (46)
-Missing data	16 (21)	12 (16)	18 (19)	22 (23)

* Number (%) of Patients.
[1] Defined as HCV RNA below limit of detection using a research based RT-PCR assay at end of treatment and during follow-up period.
[2] Defined as posttreatment (end of follow-up) minus pretreatment liver biopsy Knodell HAI score (I+II+III) improvement of ≥2 points.

CONTRAINDICATIONS

Pregnancy

REBETOL may cause birth defects and/or death of the exposed fetus. REBETOL therapy is contraindicated for use in women who are pregnant or in men whose female partners are pregnant. (See **WARNINGS, PRECAUTIONS-Information for Patients and Pregnancy Category X**).
REBETOL Capsules are contraindicated in patients with a history of hypersensitivity to ribavirin or any component of the capsule.
Patients with autoimmune hepatitis must not be treated with combination REBETOL/INTRON A therapy because using these medicines can make the hepatitis worse.

WARNINGS

Based on results of clinical trials ribavirin monotherapy is not effective for the treatment of chronic hepatitis C virus infection; therefore, REBETOL Capsules must not be used alone. The safety and efficacy of REBETOL Capsules have only been established when used together with INTRON A (interferon alfa-2b, recombinant) as REBETRON Combination Therapy.
There are significant adverse events caused by REBETOL/INTRON A, including severe depression and suicidal ideation, hemolytic anemia, suppression of bone marrow function, pulmonary dysfunction, pancreatitis, and diabetes. The REBETRON Combination Therapy package insert should be reviewed in its entirety prior to initiation of combination treatment for additional safety information.
The safety and efficacy of oral ribavirin for the treatment of HIV infection, adenovirus, RSV, parainfluenza, or influenza infections have not been established. REBETOL Capsules should not be used for these indications. Ribavirin for inhalation has a separate package insert, which should be consulted if ribavirin inhalation therapy is being considered.
The safety and efficacy of REBETOL/INTRON A therapy has not been established in liver or other organ transplant patients, patients with decompensated liver disease due to hepatitis C infection, patients who are nonresponders to interferon therapy, or patients coinfected with HBV or HIV.

Pregnancy

REBETOL may cause birth defects and/or death of the exposed fetus. Extreme care must be taken to avoid pregnancy in female patients and in female partners of male patients. REBETOL has demonstrated significant teratogenic and/or embryocidal effects in all animal species in which adequate studies have been conducted. These effects occurred at doses as low as one twentieth of the recommended human dose of ribavirin. REBETOL THERAPY SHOULD NOT BE STARTED UNTIL A REPORT OF A NEGATIVE PREGNANCY TEST HAS BEEN OBTAINED IMMEDIATELY PRIOR TO PLANNED INITIATION OF THERAPY. Patients should be instructed to use at least two forms of effective contraception during treatment and during the six month period after treatment has been stopped based on multiple dose half-life of ribavirin of 12 days. Pregnancy testing should occur monthly during REBETOL therapy and for six months after therapy has stopped (see CONTRAINDICATIONS and PRECAUTIONS: Information for Patients and Pregnancy Category X).

Continued on next page

Rebetol—Cont.

Anemia

THE PRIMARY TOXICITY OF RIBAVIRIN IS HEMOLYTIC ANEMIA, WHICH WAS OBSERVED IN APPROXIMATELY 10% OF REBETOL/INTRON A-TREATED PATIENTS IN CLINICAL TRIALS. (SEE ADVERSE REACTIONS LABORATORY VALUES – *HEMOGLOBIN*). THE ANEMIA ASSOCIATED WITH REBETOL CAPSULES OCCURS WITHIN 1–2 WEEKS OF INITIATION OF THERAPY. BECAUSE THE INITIAL DROP IN HEMOGLOBIN MAY BE SIGNIFICANT, IT IS ADVISED THAT HEMOGLOBIN OR HEMATOCRIT BE OBTAINED PRETREATMENT AND AT WEEK 2 AND WEEK 4 OF THERAPY, OR MORE FREQUENTLY IF CLINICALLY INDICATED. PATIENTS SHOULD THEN BE FOLLOWED AS CLINICALLY APPROPRIATE.

Fatal and nonfatal myocardial infarctions have been reported in patients with anemia caused by REBETOL. Patients should be assessed for underlying cardiac disease before initiation of ribavirin therapy and should be appropriately monitored during therapy. If there is any deterioration of cardiovascular status, therapy should be suspended or discontinued. (See DOSAGE AND ADMINISTRATION: Guidelines for Dose Modification.) Because cardiac disease may be worsened by drug induced anemia, patients with a history of significant or unstable cardiac disease should not use REBETOL. (See ADVERSE REACTIONS.)

Patients with hemoglobinopathies (e.g., thalassemia major, sickle-cell anemia) should not be treated with REBETOL.

REBETOL therapy should be suspended in patients with signs and symptoms of pancreatitis and discontinued in patients with confirmed pancreatitis.

REBETOL should not be used in patients with creatinine clearance <50 mL/min. (**See Clinical Pharmacology, Special populations.**)

PRECAUTIONS

Information for Patients Patients must be informed that REBETOL may cause birth defects and/or death of the exposed fetus. REBETOL must not be used by women who are pregnant or by men whose female partners are pregnant. Extreme care must be taken to avoid pregnancy in female patients and in female partners of male patients taking REBETOL. REBETOL should not be initiated until a report of a negative pregnancy test has been obtained immediately prior to initiation of therapy. Patients must perform a pregnancy test monthly during therapy and for 6 months post therapy. Women of childbearing potential must be counseled about use of effective contraception (two reliable forms) prior to initiating therapy. Patients (male and female) must be advised of the teratogenic/embryocidal risks and must be instructed to practice effective contraception during REBETOL and for 6 months post therapy. Patients (male and female) should be advised to notify the physician immediately in the event of a pregnancy. (See **CONTRAINDICATIONS and WARNINGS.**)

If pregnancy does occur during treatment or during 6 months posttherapy, the patient must be advised of the teratogenic risk of REBETOL therapy to the fetus. Patients, or partners of patients, should immediately report any pregnancy that occurs during treatment or within 6 months after treatment cessation to their physician. Physicians should report such cases by calling 1-800-727-7064.

Patients receiving REBETOL should be informed of the benefits and risks associated with treatment, directed in its appropriate use, and referred to the patient **MEDICATION GUIDE**. Patients should be informed that the effect of treatment of hepatitis C infection on transmission is not known, and that appropriate precautions to prevent transmission of the hepatitis C virus should be taken.

The most common adverse experience occurring with REBETOL is anemia, which may be severe. (See **ADVERSE REACTIONS.**) Patients should be advised that laboratory evaluations are required prior to starting therapy and periodically thereafter. (See **Laboratory Tests.**) It is advised that patients be well hydrated, especially during the initial stages of treatment.

Laboratory Tests The following laboratory tests are recommended for all patients treated with REBETOL, prior to beginning treatment and then periodically thereafter.

- Standard hematologic tests - including hemoglobin (pretreatment, week 2 and week 4 of therapy, and as clinically appropriate [see **WARNINGS**]), complete and differential white blood cell counts, and platelet count.
- Blood chemistries - liver function tests and TSH.
- Pregnancy - including monthly monitoring for women of childbearing potential.

Carcinogenesis and Mutagenesis Adequate studies to assess the carcinogenic potential of ribavirin in animals have not been conducted. However, ribavirin is a nucleoside analog that has produced positive findings in multiple *in vitro* and animal *in vivo* genotoxicity assays, and should be considered a potential carcinogen. Further studies to assess the carcinogenic potential of ribavirin in animals are ongoing.

Ribavirin demonstrated increased incidences of mutation and cell transformation in multiple genotoxicity assays. Ribavirin was active in the Balb/3T3 *In Vitro* Cell Transformation Assay. Mutagenic activity was observed in the mouse lymphoma assay, and at doses of 20–200 mg/kg (estimated human equivalent of 1.67–16.7 mg/kg, based on body surface area adjustment for a 60 kg adult; 0.1–1 X the maximum recommended human 24-hour dose of ribavirin) in a mouse micronucleus assay. A dominant lethal assay in rats was negative, indicating that if mutations occurred in rats they were not transmitted through male gametes.

TABLE 4. Selected Treatment-Emergent Adverse Events: Previously Untreated and Relapse Patients

	Percentage of Patients					
	US Previously Untreated Study				US Relapse Study	
	24 weeks of treatment		48 weeks of treatment		24 weeks of treatment	
Patients Reporting Adverse Events*	**INTRON A plus REBETOL (N=228)**	**INTRON A plus Placebo (N=231)**	**INTRON A plus REBETOL (N=228)**	**INTRON A plus Placebo (N=225)**	**INTRON A plus REBETOL (N=77)**	**INTRON A plus Placebo (N=76)**
Application Site Disorders						
injection site inflammation	13	10	12	14	6	8
injection site reaction	7	9	8	9	5	3
Body as a Whole-General Disorders						
Headache	63	63	66	67	66	68
Fatigue	68	62	70	72	60	53
Rigors	40	32	42	39	43	37
Fever	37	35	41	40	32	36
influenza-like symptoms	14	18	18	20	13	13
Asthenia	9	4	9	9	10	4
chest pain	5	4	9	8	6	7
Central & Peripheral Nervous System Disorders						
Dizziness	17	15	23	19	26	21
Gastrointestinal System Disorders						
Nausea	38	35	46	33	47	33
Anorexia	27	16	25	19	21	14
Dyspepsia	14	6	16	9	16	9
Vomiting	11	10	9	13	12	8
Musculoskeletal System Disorders						
Myalgia	61	57	64	63	61	58
Arthralgia	30	27	33	36	29	29
musculoskeletal pain	20	26	28	32	22	28
Psychiatric Disorders						
Insomnia	39	27	39	30	26	25
Irritability	23	19	32	27	25	20
Depression	32	25	36	37	23	14
emotional lability	7	6	11	8	12	8
concentration impaired	11	14	14	14	10	12
nervousness	4	2	4	4	5	4
Respiratory System Disorders						
Dyspnea	19	9	18	10	17	12
Sinusitis	9	7	10	14	12	7
Skin and Appendages Disorders						
Alopecia	28	27	32	28	27	26
Rash	20	9	28	8	21	5
Pruritus	21	9	19	8	13	4
Special Senses, Other Disorders						
taste perversion	7	4	8	4	6	5

* Patients reporting one or more adverse events. A patient may have reported more than one adverse event within a body system/organ class category.

Impairment of Fertility Ribavirin demonstrated significant embryocidal and/or teratogenic effects at doses well below the recommended human dose in all animal species in which adequate studies have been conducted.

Fertile women and partners of fertile women should not receive REBETOL unless the patient and his/her partner are using effective contraception (two reliable forms). Based on a multiple dose half-life ($t_{1/2}$) of ribavirin of 12 days, effective contraception must be utilized for 6 months post therapy (e.g., 15 half-lives of clearance for ribavirin).

REBETOL should be used with caution in fertile men. In studies in mice to evaluate the time course and reversibility of ribavirin-induced testicular degeneration at doses of 15 to 150 mg/kg/day (estimated human equivalent of 1.25–12.5 mg/kg/day, based on body surface area adjustment for a 60 kg adult; 0.1–0.8 X the maximum human 24-hour dose of ribavirin) administered for 3 or 6 months, abnormalities in sperm occurred. Upon cessation of treatment, essentially total recovery from ribavirin-induced testicular toxicity was apparent within 1 or 2 spermatogenesis cycles.

Animal Toxicology Long-term studies in the mouse and rat (18–24 months; doses of 20–75 and 10–40 mg/kg/day, respectively [estimated human equivalent doses of 1.67–6.25 and 1.43–5.71 mg/kg/day, respectively, based on body surface area adjustment for a 60 kg adult; approximately 0.1–0.4 X the maximum human 24-hour dose of ribavirin]) have demonstrated a relationship between chronic ribavirin exposure and increased incidences of vascular lesions (microscopic hemorrhages) in mice. In rats, retinal degeneration occurred in controls, but the incidence was increased in ribavirin-treated rats.

Pregnancy Category X (see CONTRAINDICATIONS) Ribavirin produced significant embryocidal and/or teratogenic effects in all animal species in which adequate studies have been conducted. Malformations of the skull, palate, eye, jaw, limbs, skeleton, and gastrointestinal tract were noted. The incidence and severity of teratogenic effects increased with escalation of the drug dose. Survival of fetuses and offspring was reduced. In conventional embryotoxicity/teratogenicity studies in rats and rabbits, observed no effect dose levels were well below those for proposed clinical use (0.3 mg/kg/day for both the rat and rabbit; approximately 0.06 X the recommended human 24-hour dose of ribavirin). No maternal toxicity or effects on offspring were observed in a peri/postnatal toxicity study in rats dosed orally at up to 1 mg/kg/day (estimated human equivalent dose of 0.17 mg/kg based on body surface area adjustment for a 60 kg adult; approximately 0.01 X the maximum recommended human 24-hour dose of ribavirin).

Treatment and Posttreatment: Potential Risk to the Fetus Ribavirin is known to accumulate in intracellular components from where it is cleared very slowly. It is not known whether ribavirin contained in sperm will exert a potential teratogenic effect upon fertilization of the ova. In a study in rats, it was concluded that dominant lethality was not induced by ribavirin at doses up to 200 mg/kg for 5 days (estimated human equivalent doses of 7.14–28.6 mg/kg, based on body surface area adjustment for a 60 kg adult; up to 1.7 X the maximum recommended human dose of ribavirin). However, because of the potential human teratogenic effects of ribavirin, male patients should be advised to take every precaution to avoid risk of pregnancy for their female partners.

Women of childbearing potential should not receive REBETOL unless they are using effective contraception (two reliable forms) during the therapy period. In addition, effective contraception should be utilized for 6 months posttherapy based on a multiple dose half-life ($t_{1/2}$) of ribavirin of 12 days.

Male patients and their female partners must practice effective contraception (two reliable forms) during treatment with REBETOL and for the 6-month post therapy period (e.g., 15 half-lives for ribavirin clearance from the body).

TABLE 5. Selected Hematologic Values During Treatment with REBETOL plus INTRON A: Previously Untreated and Relapse Patients

	Percentage of Patients					
	US Previously Untreated Study				US Relapse Study	
	24 weeks of treatment		48 weeks of treatment		24 weeks of treatment	
	INTRON A plus REBETOL (N=228)	**INTRON A plus Placebo (N=231)**	**INTRON A plus REBETOL (N=228)**	**INTRON A plus Placebo (N=225)**	**INTRON A plus REBETOL (N=77)**	**INTRON A plus Placebo (N=76)**
Hemoglobin (g/dL)						
9.5-10.9	24	1	32	1	21	3
8.0-9.4	5	0	4	0	4	0
6.5-7.9	0	0	0	0.4	0	0
<6.5	0	0	0	0	0	0
Leukocytes (× 10^9/L)						
2.0-2.9	40	20	38	23	45	26
1.5-1.9	4	1	9	2	5	3
1.0-1.4	0.9	0	2	0	0	0
<1.0	0	0	0	0	0	0
Neutrophils (× 10^9/L)						
1.0-1.49	30	32	31	44	42	34
0.75-0.99	14	15	14	11	16	18
0.5-0.74	9	9	14	7	8	4
<0.5	11	8	11	5	5	8
Platelets (× 10^9/L)						
70-99	9	11	11	14	6	12
50-69	2	3	2	3	0	5
30-49	0	0.4	0	0.4	0	0
<30	0.9	0	1	0.9	0	0
Total Bilirubin (mg/dL)						
1.5-3.0	27	13	32	13	21	7
3.1-6.0	0.9	0.4	2	0	3	0
6.1-12.0	0	0	0.4	0	0	0
>12.0	0	0	0	0	0	0

If pregnancy occurs in a patient or partner of a patient during treatment or during the 6 months after treatment cessation, physicians should report such cases by calling 1-800-727-7064.

Nursing Mothers It is not known whether REBETOL is excreted in human milk. Because of the potential for serious adverse reactions from the drug in nursing infants, a decision should be made whether to discontinue nursing or to delay or discontinue REBETOL.

Geriatric Use Clinical studies of REBETOL/INTRON A therapy did not include sufficient numbers of subjects aged 65 and over to determine if they respond differently from younger subjects. In clinical trials, elderly subjects had a higher frequency of anemia (67%) than did younger patients (28%) (See **WARNINGS**).

In general, REBETOL Capsules should be administered to elderly patients cautiously, starting at the lower end of the dosing range, reflecting the greater frequency of decreased hepatic and/or cardiac function, and of concomitant disease or other drug therapy.

REBETOL is known to be substantially excreted by the kidney, and the risk of toxic reactions to this drug may be greater in patients with impaired renal function. Because elderly patients often have decreased renal function, care should be taken in dose selection. Renal function should be monitored and dosage adjustments should be made accordingly. REBETOL should not be used in elderly patients with creatinine clearance <50 mL/min (See **WARNINGS**).

Pediatric Use Safety and effectiveness in pediatric patients have not been established.

ADVERSE REACTIONS

The primary toxicity of ribavirin is hemolytic anemia. Reductions in hemoglobin levels occurred within the first 1–2 weeks of oral therapy. (See WARNINGS.) Cardiac and pulmonary events associated with anemia occurred in approximately 10% of patients. (See WARNINGS.)

In clinical trials, 19% and 6% of previously untreated and relapse patients, respectively, discontinued therapy due to adverse events in the combination arms compared to 13% and 3% in the interferon arms. Selected treatment-emergent adverse events that occurred in the US studies with 5% incidence are provided in **TABLE 4** by treatment group. In general, the selected treatment-emergent adverse events reported with lower incidence in the international studies as compared to the US studies with the exception of asthenia, influenza-like symptoms, nervousness, and pruritus.

[See table at top of previous page]

In addition, the following spontaneous adverse events have been reported during the marketing surveillance of REBETOL/INTRON A therapy: hearing disorder and vertigo.

Laboratory Values

Changes in selected hematologic values (hemoglobin, white blood cells, neutrophils, and platelets) during REBETOL are described below. (See **TABLE 5.**)

Hemoglobin Hemoglobin decreases among patients receiving REBETOL therapy began at Week 1, with stabilization by Week 4. In previously untreated patients treated for 48 weeks the mean maximum decrease from baseline was 3.1 g/dL in the US study and 2.9 g/dL in the International study. In relapse patients the mean maximum decrease from baseline was 2.8 g/dL in the US study and 2.6 g/dL in the International study. Hemoglobin values returned to pretreatment levels within 4–8 weeks of cessation of therapy in most patients.

Bilirubin and Uric Acid Increases in both bilirubin and uric acid, associated with hemolysis, were noted in clinical trials. Most were moderate biochemical changes and were reversed within 4 weeks after treatment discontinuation. This observation occurs most frequently in patients with a previous diagnosis of Gilbert's syndrome. This has not been associated with hepatic dysfunction or clinical morbidity.

[See table above]

OVERDOSAGE

In combination REBETOL/INTRON A clinical trials, the maximum overdose reported was a dose of 39 million units of INTRON A (13 subcutaneous injections of 3 million IU each) taken with 10 g of REBETOL (fifty 200-mg capsules) in an investigator-initiated trial. The patient was observed for 2 days in the emergency room during which time no adverse event from the overdose was noted.

DOSAGE AND ADMINISTRATION

(See **CLINICAL PHARMACOLOGY, Special populations**; See **WARNINGS**).

The recommended dose of REBETOL Capsules depends on the patient's body weight. The recommended doses of REBETOL is provided in **TABLE 6.**

The recommended duration of treatment for patients previously untreated with interferon is 24 to 48 weeks. The duration of treatment should be individualized to the patient depending on baseline disease characteristics, response to therapy, and tolerability of the regimen (see *Description of Clinical Studies* and **ADVERSE REACTIONS**). After 24 weeks of treatment virologic response should be assessed. Treatment discontinuation should be considered in any patient who has not achieved an HCV-RNA below the limit of detection of the assay by 24 weeks. There are no safety and efficacy data on treatment for longer than 48 weeks in the previously untreated patient population.

In patients who relapse following interferon therapy, the recommended duration of treatment is 24 weeks. There are no safety and efficacy data on treatment for longer than 24 weeks in the relapse patient population.

TABLE 6. Recommended Dosing

Body weight	REBETOL Capsules
≤75 kg	2 × 200-mg capsules AM, 3 × 200-mg capsules PM daily p.o.
>75 kg	3 × 200 mg capsules AM, 3 × 200 mg capsules PM daily p.o.

REBETOL may be administered without regard to food, but should be administered in a consistent manner with respect to food intake. (See **CLINICAL PHARMACOLOGY.**)

***Dose Modifications* (TABLE 7)**

In clinical trials, approximately 26% of patients required modification of their dose of REBETOL Capsules, INTRON A Injection, or both agents. If severe adverse reactions or laboratory abnormalities develop during combination REBETOL/INTRON A therapy, the dose should be modified, or discontinued if appropriate, until the adverse reactions abate. If intolerance persists after dose adjustment, REBETOL/INTRON A therapy should be discontinued.

REBETOL should not be used in patients with creatinine clearance <50 mL/min. (**See Warnings** and **Clinical Pharmacology, Special populations.**)

REBETOL should be administered with caution to patients with pre-existing cardiac disease. Patients should be assessed before commencement of therapy and should be appropriately monitored during therapy. If there is any deterioration of cardiovascular status, therapy should be stopped. (See **WARNINGS.**)

For patients with a history of stable cardiovascular disease, a permanent dose reduction is required if the hemoglobin decreases by ≥2 g/dL during any 4-week period. In addition, for these cardiac history patients, if the hemoglobin remains <12 g/dL after 4 weeks on a reduced dose, the patient should discontinue combination REBETOL/INTRON A therapy.

It is recommended that a patient whose hemoglobin level falls below 10 g/dL have his/her REBETOL dose reduced to 600 mg daily (1 × 200-mg capsule AM, 2 × 200 mg capsules PM). A patient whose hemoglobin level falls below 8.5 g/dL should be permanently discontinued from REBETOL therapy. (See **WARNINGS.**)

TABLE 7. Guidelines for Dose Modifications and Discontinuation for Anemia

	Dose Reduction* REBETOL – 600 mg daily	Permanent Discontinuation of REBETOL Treatment
Hemoglobin		
No Cardiac History	**<10 g/dL**	**<8.5 g/dL**
Cardiac History Patients	**≥2 g/dL decrease during any 4-week period during treatment**	**<12 g/dL after 4 weeks of dose reduction**

HOW SUPPLIED

REBETOL 200-mg Capsules are white, opaque capsules with REBETOL, 200 mg, and the Schering Corporation logo imprinted on the capsule shell; the capsules are packaged in a bottle containing 42 capsules (NDC 0085-1327-04), 56 capsules (NDC 0085-1351-05), 70 capsules (NDC 0085-1385-07), and 84 capsules (NDC 0085-1194-03).

Storage Conditions

The bottle of REBETOL Capsules should be stored-at 25°C (77°F); excursions are permitted between 15° and 30°C (59° and 86°F).

Schering Corporation
Kenilworth, NJ 07033 USA
U.S. Patents 4,530,901 & 4,211,771

B-24819612 Rev. 8/01

TAP Pharmaceuticals Inc.
LAKE FOREST, IL 60045

For Medical Information Contact:
Medical Department
(800) 622-2011 (LUPRON)
(800) 478-9526 (PREVACID)
In Emergencies:
(800) 622-2011 (LUPRON)
(800) 478-9526 (PREVACID)

SPECTRACEF™ Tablets ℞
(cefditoren pivoxil)
[spek' trə-sĕf]
Rx ONLY

DESCRIPTION

SPECTRACEF tablets contain cefditoren pivoxil, a semi-synthetic cephalosporin antibiotic for oral administration. It is a prodrug which is hydrolyzed by esterases during absorption, and the drug is distributed in the circulating blood as active cefditoren.

Chemically, cefditoren pivoxil is (-)-(6R,7R)-2,2-dimethylpropionyloxymethyl 7-[(Z)-2-(2-aminothiazol-4-yl)-2-methoxyiminoacetamido]-3-[(Z)-2-(4-methylthiazol-5-yl)ethenyl]-8-oxo-5-thia-1-azabicyclo[4.2.0]oct-2-ene-2-carboxylate. The empirical formula is $C_{25}H_{28}N_6O_7S_3$ and the molecular weight is 620.73. The structural formula of cefditoren pivoxil is shown below:

[See chemical structure at top of next page]

Continued on next page

Spectracef—Cont.

cefditoren pivoxil

The amorphous form of cefditoren pivoxil developed for clinical use is a light yellow powder. It is freely soluble in dilute hydrochloric acid and soluble at levels equal to 6.06 mg/mL in ethanol and <0.1 mg/mL in water.

SPECTRACEF tablets contain 200 mg of cefditoren as cefditoren pivoxil and the following inactive ingredients: croscarmellose sodium, sodium caseinate (a milk protein), D-mannitol, magnesium stearate, sodium tripolyphosphate, hydroxypropyl methylcellulose, and hydroxypropyl cellulose. The tablet coating contains hydroxypropyl methylcellulose, titanium dioxide, polyethylene glycol, and carnauba wax. Tablets are printed with ink containing FD&C Blue No. 1, D&C Red No. 27, shellac, and propylene glycol.

CLINICAL PHARMACOLOGY

Pharmacokinetics

Absorption

Oral Bioavailability

Following oral administration, cefditoren pivoxil is absorbed from the gastrointestinal tract and hydrolyzed to cefditoren by esterases. Maximal plasma concentrations (C_{max}) of cefditoren under fasting conditions average 1.8 ± 0.6 µg/mL following a single 200 mg dose and occur 1.5 to 3 hours following dosing. Less than dose-proportional increases in C_{max} and area under the concentration-time curve (AUC) were observed at doses of 400 mg and above. Cefditoren does not accumulate in plasma following twice daily administration to subjects with normal renal function. Under fasting conditions, the estimated absolute bioavailability of cefditoren pivoxil is approximately 14%. The absolute bioavailability of cefditoren pivoxil administered with a low fat meal (693 cal, 14 g fat, 122 g carb, 23 g protein) is 16.1 ± 3.0%.

Food Effect

Administration of cefditoren pivoxil following a high fat meal (858 cal, 64 g fat, 43 g carb, 31 g protein) resulted in a 70% increase in mean AUC and a 50% increase in mean C_{max} compared to administration of cefditoren pivoxil in the fasted state. After a high fat meal, the C_{max} averaged 3.1 ± 1.0 µg/mL following a single 200 mg dose of cefditoren pivoxil and 4.4 ± 0.9 µg/mL following a 400 mg dose. Cefditoren AUC and C_{max} values from studies conducted with a moderate fat meal (648 cal, 27 g fat, 73 g carb, 29 g protein) are similar to those obtained following a high fat meal.

Distribution

The mean volume of distribution at steady state (V_{ss}) of cefditoren is 9.3 ± 1.6 L. Binding of cefditoren to plasma proteins averages 88% from *in vitro* determinations, and is concentration-independent at cefditoren concentrations ranging from 0.05 to 10 µg/mL. Cefditoren is primarily bound to human serum albumin and its binding is decreased when serum albumin concentrations are reduced. Binding to α-1-acid glycoprotein ranges from 3.3 to 8.1%. Penetration into red blood cells is negligible.

Skin blister fluid

Maximal concentrations of cefditoren in suction-induced blister fluid were observed 4 to 6 hours following administration of a 400 mg dose of cefditoren pivoxil with a mean of 1.1 ± 0.42 µg/mL. Mean blister fluid AUC values were 56 ± 15% of corresponding plasma concentrations.

Tonsil tissue

In fasted patients undergoing elective tonsillectomy, the mean concentration of cefditoren in tonsil tissue 2 to 4 hours following administration of a 200 mg dose of cefditoren pivoxil was 0.18 ± 0.07 µg/g. Mean tonsil tissue concentrations of cefditoren were 12 ± 3% of the corresponding serum concentrations.

Cerebrospinal Fluid (CSF)

Data on the penetration of cefditoren into human cerebrospinal fluid are not available.

Metabolism and Excretion

Cefditoren is eliminated from the plasma, with a mean terminal elimination half-life ($t_{1/2}$) of 1.6 ± 0.4 hours in young healthy adults. Cefditoren is not appreciably metabolized. After absorption, cefditoren is mainly eliminated by excretion into the urine, with a renal clearance of approximately 4-5 L/h. Studies with the renal tubular transport blocking agent probenecid indicate that tubular secretion, along with glomerular filtration is involved in the renal elimination of cefditoren. Cefditoren renal clearance is reduced in patients with renal insufficiency. (See Special Populations, *Renal Insufficiency and Hemodialysis.*)

Hydrolysis of cefditoren pivoxil to its active component, cefditoren, results in the formation of pivalate. Following multiple doses of cefditoren pivoxil, greater than 70% of the pivalate is absorbed. Pivalate is mainly eliminated (>99%) through renal excretion, nearly exclusively as pivaloylcarnitine. Following a 200 mg BID regimen for 10 days, the mean decrease in plasma concentrations of total carnitine was 18.1 ± 7.2 nmole/mL, representing a 39% decrease in plasma carnitine concentrations. Following a 400 mg BID regimen for 14 days, the mean decrease in plasma concentrations of carnitine was 33.3 ± 9.7 nmole/mL, representing a 63% decrease in plasma carnitine concentrations. Plasma concentrations of carnitine returned to the normal control range within 7 to 10 days after discontinuation of cefditoren pivoxil. (See **PRECAUTIONS, General and CONTRAINDICATIONS.**)

Special Populations

Geriatric

The effect of age on the pharmacokinetics of cefditoren was evaluated in 48 male and female subjects aged 25 to 75 years given 400 mg cefditoren pivoxil BID for 7 days. Physiological changes related to increasing age increased the extent of cefditoren exposure in plasma, as evidenced by a 26% higher C_{max} and a 33% higher AUC for subjects aged ≥ 65 years compared with younger subjects. The rate of elimination of cefditoren from plasma was lower in subjects aged ≥ 65 years, with $t_{1/2}$ values 16–26% longer than for younger subjects. Renal clearance of cefditoren in subjects aged ≥ 65 years was 20–24% lower than in younger subjects. These changes could be attributed to age-related changes in creatinine clearance. No dose adjustments are necessary for elderly patients with normal (for their age) renal function.

Gender

The effect of gender on the pharmacokinetics of cefditoren was evaluated in 24 male and 24 female subjects given 400 mg cefditoren pivoxil BID for 7 days. The extent of exposure in plasma was greater in females than in males, as evidenced by a 14% higher C_{max} and a 16% higher AUC for females compared to males. Renal clearance of cefditoren in females was 13% lower than in males. These differences could be attributed to gender-related differences in lean body mass. No dose adjustments are necessary for gender.

Renal Insufficiency

Cefditoren pharmacokinetics were investigated in 24 adult subjects with varying degrees of renal function following administration of cefditoren pivoxil 400 mg BID for 7 days. Decreased creatinine clearance (CL_{cr}) was associated with an increase in the fraction of unbound cefditoren in plasma and a decrease in the cefditoren elimination rate, resulting in greater systemic exposure in subjects with renal impairment. The unbound C_{max} and AUC were similar in subjects with mild renal impairment (CL_{cr}: 50-80 mL/min/1.73 m^2) compared to subjects with normal renal function (CL_{cr}: >80 mL/min/1.73 m^2). Moderate (CL_{cr}: 30-49 mL/min/1.73 m^2) or severe (CL_{cr}: <30 mL/min/1.73 m^2) renal impairment increased the extent of exposure in plasma, as evidenced by mean unbound C_{max} values 90% and 114% higher and AUC values 232% and 324% higher than that for subjects with normal renal function. The rate of elimination from plasma was lower in subjects with moderate or severe renal impairment, with respective mean $t_{1/2}$ values of 2.7 and 4.7 hours. No dose adjustment is necessary for patients with mild renal impairment (CL_{cr}: 50-80 mL/min/1.73 m^2). It is recommended that not more than 200 mg BID be administered to patients with moderate renal impairment (CL_{cr}: 30-49 mL/min/1.73 m^2) and 200 mg QD be administered to patients with severe renal impairment (CL_{cr}: <30 mL/min/1.73 m^2). (See **DOSAGE AND ADMINISTRATION.**)

Hemodialysis

Cefditoren pharmacokinetics investigated in six adult subjects with end-stage renal disease (ESRD) undergoing hemodialysis given a single 400 mg dose of cefditoren pivoxil were highly variable. The mean $t_{1/2}$ was 4.7 hours and ranged from 1.5 to 15 hours. Hemodialysis (4 hours duration) removed approximately 30% of cefditoren from systemic circulation but did not change the apparent terminal elimination half-life. The appropriate dose for ESRD patients has not been determined. (See **DOSAGE AND ADMINISTRATION.**)

Hepatic Disease

Cefditoren pharmacokinetics were evaluated in six adult subjects with mild hepatic impairment (Child-Pugh Class A) and six with moderate hepatic impairment (Child-Pugh Class B). Following administration of cefditoren pivoxil 400 mg BID for 7 days in these subjects, mean C_{max} and AUC values were slightly (<15%) greater than those observed in normal subjects. No dose adjustments are necessary for patients with mild or moderate hepatic impairment (Child-Pugh Class A or B). The pharmacokinetics of cefditoren in subjects with severe hepatic impairment (Child-Pugh Class C) have not been studied.

Microbiology

Cefditoren is a cephalosporin with antibacterial activity against gram-positive and gram-negative pathogens. The bactericidal activity of cefditoren results from the inhibition of cell wall synthesis via affinity for penicillin-binding proteins (PBPs). Cefditoren is stable in the presence of a variety of β-lactamases, including penicillinases and some cephalosporinases.

Cefditoren has been shown to be active against most strains of the following bacteria, both *in vitro* and in clinical infections, as described in the **INDICATIONS AND USAGE** section.

Aerobic Gram-Positive Microorganisms

Staphylococcus aureus (methicillin-susceptible strains, including β-lactamase-producing strains)

Note: Cefditoren is inactive against methicillin-resistant *Staphylococcus aureus*

Streptococcus pneumoniae (penicillin-susceptible strains only)

Streptococcus pyogenes

Aerobic Gram-Negative Microorganisms

Haemophilus influenzae (including β-lactamase-producing strains)

Haemophilus parainfluenzae (including β-lactamase-producing strains)

Moraxella catarrhalis (including β-lactamase-producing strains)

The following *in vitro* data are available, **but their clinical significance is unknown.** Cefditoren exhibits *in vitro* minimum inhibitory concentrations (MICs) of ≤0.125 µg/mL against most (≥90%) strains of the following bacteria; however, the safety and effectiveness of cefditoren in treating clinical infections due to these bacteria have not been established in adequate and well-controlled clinical trials.

Aerobic Gram-Positive Microorganisms

Streptococcus agalactiae

Streptococcus Groups C and G

Streptococcus, viridans group (penicillin-susceptible and -intermediate strains)

Susceptibility Tests

Dilution Techniques

Quantitative methods that are used to determine MICs provide reproducible estimates of the susceptibility of bacteria to antimicrobial compounds. The MICs should be determined using a standardized procedure. Standardized procedures are based on dilution methods[1] (broth) or equivalent with standardized inoculum concentrations and standardized concentrations of cefditoren powder. The MIC values obtained should be interpreted according to the following criteria:

For testing *Haemophilus* spp.[a] and *Streptococcus* spp. including *S. pneumoniae*[b]:

Clinical Isolates	MIC (µg/mL)	Interpretation
S. pneumoniae	≤0.125 0.250 ≥0.50	Susceptible (S) Intermediate (I) Resistant (R)
Haemophilus spp.	≤0.125 0.250 ≥0.50	Susceptible (S) Intermediate (I) Resistant (R)
S. pyogenes	≤0.125	Susceptible (S)

[a] This interpretive standard is applicable only to broth microdilution susceptibility tests with *Haemophilus* spp. using *Haemophilus* Test Medium (HTM).[1]

[b] These interpretive standards are applicable only to broth microdilution susceptibility tests with *Streptococcus* spp. using cation-adjusted Mueller-Hinton broth with 2–5% lysed horse blood.[1]

Susceptibility test criteria cannot be established for *S. aureus.*

A report of "Susceptible" indicates that the pathogen is likely to be inhibited if the antimicrobial compound in the blood reaches the concentration usually achievable. A report of "Intermediate" indicates that the result should be considered equivocal, and, if the microorganism is not fully susceptible to alternative, clinically feasible drugs, the test should be repeated. This category implies possible clinical applicability in body sites where the drug is physiologically concentrated or in situations where high dosage of drug can be used. This category also provides a buffer zone that prevents small, uncontrolled technical factors from causing major discrepancies in interpretation. A report of "Resistant" indicates that the pathogen is not likely to be inhibited if the antimicrobial compound in the blood reaches the concentration usually achievable and that other therapy should be selected.

Standardized susceptibility test procedures require the use of laboratory control bacterial strains to control the technical aspects of the laboratory procedures. Standard cefditoren powder should provide the following MICs with these quality control strains:

Microorganisms	MIC Ranges (µg/mL)
Streptococcus pneumoniae[a] ATCC 49619	0.016–0.12
Haemophilus influenzae[b] ATCC 49766	0.004–0.016
Haemophilus influenzae[b] ATCC 49247	0.06–0.25

[a] This quality control range is applicable to only *S. pneumoniae* ATCC 49619 tested by a microdilution procedure using cation-adjusted Mueller-Hinton broth with 2–5% lysed horse blood.[1]

[b] This quality control range is applicable to only *H. influenzae* ATCC 49247 and ATCC 49766 tested by a microdilution procedure using HTM.[1]

INDICATIONS AND USAGE

SPECTRACEF is indicated for the treatment of mild to moderate infections in adults and adolescents (12 years of age or older) which are caused by susceptible strains of the designated microorganisms in the conditions listed below.

Acute Bacterial Exacerbation of Chronic Bronchitis caused by *Haemophilus influenzae* (including β-lactamase-producing strains), *Haemophilus parainfluenzae* (including β-lactamase-producing strains), *Streptococcus pneumoniae* (penicillin-susceptible strains only), or *Moraxella catarrhalis* (including β-lactamase-producing strains).

Pharyngitis/Tonsillitis caused by *Streptococcus pyogenes*. NOTE: SPECTRACEF is effective in the eradication of *Streptococcus pyogenes* from the oropharynx.

SPECTRACEF has not been studied for the prevention of rheumatic fever following *Streptococcus pyogenes* pharyngitis/tonsillitis. Only intramuscular penicillin has been demonstrated to be effective for the prevention of rheumatic fever.

Uncomplicated Skin and Skin-Structure Infections caused by *Staphylococcus aureus* (including β-lactamase-producing strains) or *Streptococcus pyogenes*.

CONTRAINDICATIONS

SPECTRACEF is contraindicated in patients with known allergy to the cephalosporin class of antibiotics or any of its components.

SPECTRACEF is contraindicated in patients with carnitine deficiency or inborn errors of metabolism that may result in clinically significant carnitine deficiency, because use of SPECTRACEF causes renal excretion of carnitine. (See **PRECAUTIONS, General.**)

SPECTRACEF tablets contain sodium caseinate, a milk protein. Patients with milk protein hypersensitivity (not lactose intolerance) should not be administered SPECTRACEF.

WARNINGS

BEFORE THERAPY WITH SPECTRACEF (CEFDITOREN PIVOXIL) IS INSTITUTED, CAREFUL INQUIRY SHOULD BE MADE TO DETERMINE WHETHER THE PATIENT HAS HAD PREVIOUS HYPERSENSITIVITY REACTIONS TO CEFDITOREN PIVOXIL, OTHER CEPHALOSPORINS, PENICILLINS, OR OTHER DRUGS. IF CEFDITOREN PIVOXIL IS TO BE GIVEN TO PENICILLIN-SENSITIVE PATIENTS, CAUTION SHOULD BE EXERCISED BECAUSE CROSS-HYPERSENSITIVITY AMONG β-LACTAM ANTIBIOTICS HAS BEEN CLEARLY DOCUMENTED AND MAY OCCUR IN UP TO 10% OF PATIENTS WITH A HISTORY OF PENICILLIN ALLERGY. IF AN ALLERGIC REACTION TO CEFDITOREN PIVOXIL OCCURS, THE DRUG SHOULD BE DISCONTINUED. SERIOUS ACUTE HYPERSENSITIVITY REACTIONS MAY REQUIRE TREATMENT WITH EPINEPHRINE AND OTHER EMERGENCY MEASURES, INCLUDING OXYGEN, INTRAVENOUS FLUIDS, INTRAVENOUS ANTIHISTAMINES, CORTICOSTEROIDS, PRESSOR AMINES, AND AIRWAY MANAGEMENT, AS CLINICALLY INDICATED.

Pseudomembranous colitis has been reported with nearly all antibacterial agents, including cefditoren pivoxil, and may range in severity from mild to life-threatening. Therefore, it is important to consider this diagnosis in patients who present with diarrhea subsequent to the administration of antibacterial agents.

Treatment with antibacterial agents alters normal flora of the colon and may permit overgrowth of clostridia. Studies indicate that a toxin produced by *Clostridium difficile (C. difficile)* is a primary cause of antibiotic-associated colitis.

After the diagnosis of pseudomembranous colitis has been established, appropriate therapeutic measures should be initiated. Mild cases of pseudomembranous colitis usually respond to drug discontinuation alone. In moderate to severe cases, consideration should be given to management with fluids and electrolytes, protein supplementation, and treatment with an antibacterial drug clinically effective against *C. difficile* colitis.

PRECAUTIONS

General

SPECTRACEF is not recommended when prolonged antibiotic treatment is necessary, since other pivalate-containing compounds have caused clinical manifestations of carnitine deficiency when used over a period of months. No clinical effects of carnitine decrease have been associated with short-term treatment. The effects on carnitine concentrations of repeat short-term courses of SPECTRACEF are not known.

In healthy volunteers (mean age 32.5 ± 7.6 years) given a 200 mg BID regimen for 10 days, the mean decrease in plasma concentrations of total carnitine was 18.1 ± 7.2 nmole/mL, representing a 39% decrease in plasma carnitine concentrations. In healthy volunteers (mean age 34.7 ± 7.2 years) given a 400 mg BID regimen for 14 days, the mean decrease in plasma concentrations of carnitine was 33.3 ± 9.7 nmole/mL, representing a 63% decrease in plasma carnitine concentrations. Plasma concentrations of carnitine returned to the normal control range within 7 to 10 days after discontinuation of cefditoren pivoxil. (See **CLINICAL PHARMACOLOGY.**) Neither measurement of serum carnitine nor concomitant administration of supplemental

carnitine is recommended as a general measure for patients receiving short-term treatment with cefditoren pivoxil.

As with other antibiotics, prolonged treatment may result in the possible emergence and overgrowth of resistant organisms. Careful observation of the patient is essential. If superinfection occurs during therapy, appropriate alternative therapy should be administered.

Cephalosporins may be associated with a fall in prothrombin activity. Those at risk include patients with renal or hepatic impairment, or poor nutritional state, as well as patients receiving a protracted course of antimicrobial therapy, and patients previously stabilized on anticoagulant therapy. Prothrombin time should be monitored in patients at risk and exogenous vitamin K administered as indicated. In clinical trials, there was no difference between cefditoren and comparator cephalosporins in the incidence of increased prothrombin time.

Treatment-Related Adverse Events in Trials in Adult and Adolescent Patients ≥12 Years

		SPECTRACEF 200 mg BID (N=2409)	SPECTRACEF 400 mg BID (N=1890)	COMPARATORS[a] (N=2381)
Incidence ≥ 1%	Diarrhea	11%	14%	7%
	Nausea	4%	6%	5%
	Headache	2%	2%	2%
	Abdominal Pain	2%	2%	1%
	Vaginal Moniliasis	3%[b]	6%[c]	5%[d]
	Dyspepsia	1%	2%	2%
	Vomiting	1%	1%	1%

[a] includes amoxicillin/clavulanate, cefadroxil monohydrate, cefuroxime axetil, cefpodoxime proxetil, clarithromycin, and penicillin
[b] 1296 females
[c] 1010 females
[d] 1320 females

SPECTRACEF Dosage and Administration* Adults and Adolescents (≥12 Years)

Type of Infection	Dosage	Duration (days)
Acute Bacterial Exacerbation of Chronic Bronchitis	400 mg BID	10
Pharyngitis/Tonsilitis	200 mg BID	10
Uncomplicated Skin and Skin Structure Infections	200 mg BID	10

*Should be taken with meals

Information for Patients

SPECTRACEF should be taken with meals to enhance absorption.

SPECTRACEF may be taken concomitantly with oral contraceptives.

It is not recommended that SPECTRACEF be taken concomitantly with antacids or other drugs taken to reduce stomach acids. (See **PRECAUTIONS, Drug Interactions.**)

SPECTRACEF tablets contain sodium caseinate, a milk protein. Patients with milk protein hypersensitivity (not lactose intolerance) should not be administered SPECTRACEF.

Drug Interactions

Oral Contraceptives

Multiple doses of cefditoren pivoxil had no effect on the pharmacokinetics of ethinyl estradiol, the estrogenic component in most oral contraceptives.

Antacids

Co-administration of a single dose of an antacid which contained both magnesium (800 mg) and aluminum (900 mg) hydroxides reduced the oral absorption of a single 400 mg dose of cefditoren pivoxil administered following a meal, as evidenced by a 14% decrease in mean C_{max} and an 11% decrease in mean AUC. Although the clinical significance is not known, it is not recommended that cefditoren pivoxil be taken concomitantly with antacids.

H_2-Receptor Antagonists

Co-administration of a single dose of intravenously administered famotidine (20 mg) reduced the oral absorption of a single 400 mg dose of cefditoren pivoxil administered following a meal, as evidenced by a 27% decrease in mean C_{max} and a 22% decrease in mean AUC. Although the clinical significance is not known, it is not recommended that cefditoren pivoxil be taken concomitantly with H_2 receptor antagonists.

Probenecid

As with other β-lactam antibiotics, co-administration of probenecid with cefditoren pivoxil resulted in an increase in the plasma exposure of cefditoren, with a 49% increase in mean C_{max}, a 122% increase in mean AUC, and a 53% increase in $t_{1/2}$.

Drug/Laboratory Test Interactions

Cephalosporins are known to occasionally induce a positive direct Coombs' test. A false-positive reaction for glucose in the urine may occur with copper reduction tests (Benedict's or Fehling's solution or with CLINITEST® tablets), but not with enzyme-based tests for glycosuria (e.g., CLINISTIX®, TES-TAPE®). As a false-negative result may occur in the ferricyanide test, it is recommended that either the glucose oxidase or hexokinase method be used to determine blood/plasma glucose levels in patients receiving cefditoren pivoxil.

Carcinogenesis, Mutagenesis, Impairment of Fertility

No long-term animal carcinogenicity studies have been conducted with cefditoren pivoxil. Cefditoren pivoxil was not mutagenic in the Ames bacterial reverse mutation assay, or in the mouse lymphoma mutation assay at the hypoxanthine-guanine phosphoribosyltransferase locus. In Chinese hamster lung cells, chromosomal aberrations were produced by cefditoren pivoxil, but not by cefditoren. Subsequent studies showed that the chromosome aberrations were due to the release of formaldehyde from the pivoxil ester moiety in the *in vitro* assay system. Neither cefditoren nor cefditoren pivoxil produced chromosomal aberrations when tested in an *in vitro* human peripheral blood lymphocyte assay, or in the *in vivo* mouse micronucleus assay. Cefditoren pivoxil did not induce unscheduled DNA synthesis when tested.

In rats, fertility and reproduction were not affected by cefditoren pivoxil at oral doses up to 1000 mg/kg/day, approximately 24 times a human dose of 200 mg BID based on mg/m^2/day.

Pregnancy - Teratogenic Effects

Pregnancy Category B

Cefditoren pivoxil was not teratogenic up to the highest doses tested in rats and rabbits. In rats, this dose was 1000 mg/kg/day, which is approximately 24 times a human dose of 200 mg BID based on mg/m^2/day. In rabbits, the highest dose tested was 90 mg/kg/day, which is approximately four times a human dose of 200 mg BID based on mg/m^2/day. This dose produced severe maternal toxicity and resulted in fetal toxicity and abortions.

In a postnatal development study in rats, cefditoren pivoxil produced no adverse effects on postnatal survival, physical and behavioral development, learning abilities, and reproductive capability at sexual maturity when tested at doses of up to 750 mg/kg/day, the highest dose tested. This is approximately 18 times a human dose of 200 mg BID based on mg/m^2/day.

There are however, no adequate and well-controlled studies in pregnant women. Because animal reproductive studies are not always predictive of human response, this drug should be used during pregnancy only if clearly needed.

Labor and Delivery

Cefditoren pivoxil has not been studied for use during labor and delivery.

Nursing Mothers

Cefditoren was detected in the breast milk of lactating rats. Because many drugs are excreted in human breast milk, caution should be exercised when cefditoren pivoxil is administered to nursing women.

Pediatric Use

Safety and efficacy of cefditoren pivoxil tablets in pediatric patients less than 12 years of age have not been established.

Geriatric Use

Of the 2409 patients in clinical studies who received cefditoren pivoxil 200 mg BID, 244 (10%) were >65 years of age. Of the 1890 patients in clinical studies who received cefditoren pivoxil 400 mg BID, 242 (13%) were >65 years of age. No clinically significant differences in effectiveness or safety were observed between older and younger patients. No dose adjustments are necessary in geriatric patients with normal (for their age) renal function. This drug is known to be substantially excreted by the kidney, and the risk of toxic reactions to this drug may be greater in patients with impaired renal function. Because elderly patients are more likely to have decreased renal function, care should be taken in dose selection, and it may be useful to monitor renal function. (See **DOSAGE AND ADMINISTRATION.**)

ADVERSE EVENTS

Clinical Trials – SPECTRACEF Tablets (Adults and Adolescent Patients ≥12 Years of Age)

In clinical trials, 4299 adult and adolescent patients have been treated with the recommended doses of cefditoren pivoxil tablets (200 mg or 400 mg BID). Most adverse events were mild and self-limiting. No deaths or permanent disabilities have been attributed to cefditoren.

The following adverse events were thought by the investigators to be possibly, probably, or definitely related to cefditoren tablets in multiple-dose clinical trials:

[See first table above]

Continued on next page

Spectracef—Cont.

The overall incidence of adverse events, and in particular diarrhea, increased with the higher recommended dose of SPECTRACEF.
Treatment related adverse events experienced by <1% but >0.1% of patients who received 200 mg or 400 mg BID of cefditoren pivoxil were abnormal dreams, allergic reaction, anorexia, asthenia, coagulation time increased, constipation, dizziness, dry mouth, eructation, fever, flatulence, fungal infection, gastritis, gastrointestinal disorder, hyperglycemia, increased appetite, insomnia, leukopenia, leukorrhea, liver function test abnormal, mouth ulceration, myalgia, nervousness, oral moniliasis, pain, peripheral edema, pharyngitis, pseudomembranous colitis, pruritus, rash, rhinitis, sinusitis, somnolence, stomatitis, sweating, taste perversion, thrombocythemia, urinary frequency, urticaria, vaginitis, and weight loss. Pseudomembranous colitis symptoms may begin during or after antibiotic treatment. (See **WARNINGS**.)
Fifty-three of 2409 (2%) patients who received 200 mg BID and 64 of 1890 (3%) patients who received 400 mg BID of cefditoren pivoxil discontinued medication due to adverse events thought by the investigators to be possibly, probably, or definitely associated with cefditoren therapy. The discontinuations were primarily for gastrointestinal disturbances, usually diarrhea or nausea. Diarrhea was the primary reason for discontinuation in 18 of 2409 (0.7%) patients who received 200 mg BID and in 26 of 1890 (1.4%) patients who received 400 mg BID of cefditoren pivoxil.
Changes in laboratory parameters of possible clinical significance, without regard to drug relationship and which occurred in ≥ 1% of patients who received cefditoren pivoxil 200 mg or 400 mg BID, were hematuria (2.9% and 3.2%), increased urine white blood cells (2.3% and 2.5%), decreased hematocrit (1.7% and 2.2%), and increased glucose (1.6% and 0.8%). Those events which occurred in < 1% but > 0.1% of patients included the following: increased/decreased white blood cells, increased eosinophils, decreased neutrophils, increased lymphocytes, increased platelet count, decreased hemoglobin, increased potassium, decreased chloride, decreased inorganic phosphorus, decreased calcium, increased SGPT, increased SGOT, increased cholesterol, decreased albumin, proteinuria, and increased BUN. It is not known if these abnormalities were caused by the drug or the underlying condition being treated.

Cephalosporin Class Adverse Reactions

In addition to the adverse reactions listed above which have been observed in patients treated with cefditoren pivoxil the following adverse reactions and altered laboratory test results have been reported for cephalosporin class antibiotics:
Adverse Reactions: Allergic reactions, anaphylaxis, drug fever, Stevens-Johnson syndrome, serum sickness-like reaction, erythema multiforme, toxic epidermal necrolysis, colitis, renal dysfunction, toxic nephropathy, reversible hyperactivity, hypertonia, hepatic dysfunction including cholestasis, aplastic anemia, hemolytic anemia, hemorrhage, and superinfection.
Altered Laboratory Tests: Prolonged prothrombin time, positive direct Coombs' test, false-positive test for urinary glucose, elevated alkaline phosphatase, elevated bilirubin, elevated LDH, increased creatinine, pancytopenia, neutropenia, and agranulocytosis.
Several cephalosporins have been implicated in triggering seizures, particularly in patients with renal impairment when the dosage was not reduced. (See **DOSAGE AND ADMINISTRATION**.) If seizures associated with drug therapy occur, the drug should be discontinued. Anticonvulsant therapy can be given if clinically indicated.

OVERDOSAGE

Information on cefditoren pivoxil overdosage in humans is not available. However, with other β-lactam antibiotics, adverse effects following overdosage have included nausea, vomiting, epigastric distress, diarrhea, and convulsions. Hemodialysis may aid in the removal of cefditoren from the body, particularly if renal function is compromised (30% reduction of plasma concentrations following 4 hours of hemodialysis). Treat overdosage symptomatically and institute supportive measures as required.
In acute animal toxicity studies, cefditoren pivoxil when tested at the limit oral doses of 5100 mg/kg in rats and up to 2000 mg/kg in dogs did not exhibit any health effects of concern. Certain effects, such as diarrhea and soft stool lasting for a few days were observed in some animals as expected with most oral antibiotics due to inhibition of intestinal microflora.

DOSAGE AND ADMINISTRATION

(See **INDICATIONS AND USAGE** for Indicated Pathogens.)
[See second table at top of previous page]

Patients with Renal Insufficiency

No dose adjustment is necessary for patients with mild renal impairment (CL_{cr}: 50-80 mL/min/1.73 m^2). It is recommended that not more than 200 mg BID be administered to patients with moderate renal impairment (CL_{cr}: 30–49 mL/min/1.73 m^2) and 200 mg QD be administered to patients with severe renal impairment (CL_{cr}: <30 mL/min/1.73 m^2). The appropriate dose in patients with end-stage renal disease has not been determined.

Patients with Hepatic Disease

No dose adjustments are necessary for patients with mild or moderate hepatic impairment (Child-Pugh Class A or B). The pharmacokinetics of cefditoren have not been studied in patients with severe hepatic impairment (Child-Pugh Class C).

HOW SUPPLIED

SPECTRACEF tablets containing cefditoren pivoxil equivalent to 200 mg of cefditoren are available as white, elliptical, film-coated tablets imprinted with TAP 200 mg in blue. These tablets are available in multi-dose tamper-evident containers as follows:
NDC 0300-7535-20 Bottles of 20
NDC 0300-7535-60 Bottles of 60
Store at 25°C (77°F); excursions permitted to 15–30°C (59–86°F). [See USP Controlled Room Temperature.] Protect from light and moisture. Dispense in a tight, light resistant container.

REFERENCES

1. National Committee for Clinical Laboratory Standards. *Methods for Dilution Antimicrobial Susceptibility Tests for Bacteria That Grow Aerobically – Fifth Edition*; Approved Standard, NCCLS Document M7-A5, Vol. 20, No. 2, NCCLS, Wayne, PA, January, 2000.

U.S. Patent Nos. 4,839,350; 4,918,068; and 5,958,915
Other patents pending.
Manufactured for
TAP Pharmaceuticals Inc.
Lake Forest, Illinois, 60045
™ –Trademark
® –Registered Trademark
(No. 7535)
750-01233-R1; Revised: August 2001

REVISED INFORMATION

As new research data and clinical findings become available, the product information in *PDR* is revised accordingly. Revisions submitted since the 2002 edition went to press can be found below. To remind yourself of a revision, write "See Supplement A" next to the product's heading in the book.

Abbott Laboratories Inc.

Pharmaceutical Products Division
NORTH CHICAGO, IL 60064, U.S.A.

Pharmaceutical Products Division—
Direct Inquiries to:
Customer Service:
(800) 255-5162
Technical Services:
(800) 441-4987
For Medical Information Contact:
Generally:
(800) 633-9110
Adverse Drug Experiences:
(800) 633-9110
Sales and Ordering:
(800) 255-5162

Hospital Products Division—
Direct Inquiries to:
Customer Service
(800) 222-6883
For Medical Information Contact:
(800) 615-0187
Sales and Ordering:
(800) 222-6883

HYTRIN® ℞
(terazosin hydrochloride)
Capsules

Prescribing information for this product, which appears on pages 464–467 of the 2002 PDR, has been completely revised as follows. Please write "See Supplement A" next to the product heading.

DESCRIPTION

HYTRIN (terazosin hydrochloride), an alpha-1-selective adrenoceptor blocking agent, is a quinazoline derivative represented by the following chemical name and structural formula: (RS)-Piperazine, 1-(4-amino-6,7-dimethoxy-2-quinazolinyl)-4-[(tetra-hydro-2-furanyl)carbonyl]-, monohydrochloride, dihydrate.

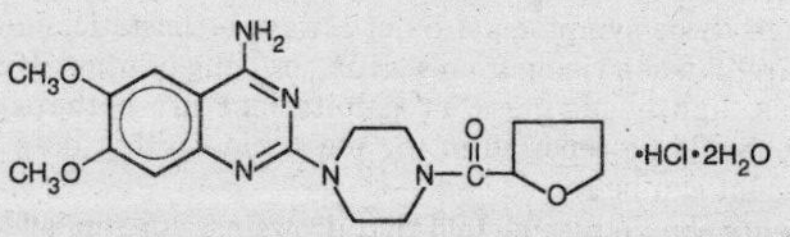

$\cdot HCl \cdot 2H_2O$

Terazosin hydrochloride is a white, crystalline substance, freely soluble in water and isotonic saline and has a molecular weight of 459.93. HYTRIN capsules (terazosin hydrochloride capsules) for oral ingestion are supplied in four dosage strengths containing terazosin hydrochloride equivalent to 1 mg, 2 mg, 5 mg, or 10 mg of terazosin.

Inactive Ingredients:

1 mg capsules: gelatin, glycerin, iron oxide, methylparaben, mineral oil, polyethylene glycol, povidone, propylparaben, titanium dioxide, and vanillin.

2 mg capsules: D&C yellow No. 10, gelatin, glycerin, methylparaben, mineral oil, polyethylene glycol, povidone, propylparaben, titanium dioxide, and vanillin.

5 mg capsules: D&C red No. 28, FD&C red No. 40, gelatin, glycerin, methylparaben, mineral oil, polyethylene glycol, povidone, propylparaben, titanium dioxide, and vanillin.

10 mg capsules: FD&C blue No. 1, gelatin, glycerin, methylparaben, mineral oil, polyethylene glycol, povidone, propylparaben, titanium dioxide, and vanillin.

CLINICAL PHARMACOLOGY

Pharmacodynamics:

A. Benign Prostatic Hyperplasia (BPH)

The symptoms associated with BPH are related to bladder outlet obstruction, which is comprised of two underlying components: a static component and a dynamic component. The static component is a consequence of an increase in prostate size. Over time, the prostate will continue to enlarge. However, clinical studies have demonstrated that the size of the prostate does not correlate with the severity of BPH symptoms or the degree of urinary obstruction. The dynamic component is a function of an increase in smooth muscle tone in the prostate and bladder neck, leading to constriction of the bladder outlet. Smooth muscle tone is mediated by sympathetic nervous stimulation of alpha-1 adrenoceptors, which are abundant in the prostate, prostatic capsule and bladder neck. The reduction in symptoms and improvement in urine flow rates following administration of terazosin is related to relaxation of smooth muscle produced by blockade of alpha-1 adrenoceptors in the bladder neck and prostate. Because there are relatively few alpha-1 adrenoceptors in the bladder body, terazosin is able to reduce the bladder outlet obstruction without affecting bladder contractility.

Terazosin has been studied in 1222 men with symptomatic BPH. In three placebo-controlled studies, symptom evaluation and uroflowmetric measurements were performed approximately 24 hours following dosing. Symptoms were quantified using the Boyarsky Index. The questionnaire evaluated both obstructive (hesitancy, intermittency, terminal dribbling, impairment of size and force of stream, sensation of incomplete bladder emptying) and irritative (nocturia, daytime frequency, urgency, dysuria) symptoms by rating each of the 9 symptoms from 0-3, for a total score of 27 points. Results from these studies indicated that terazosin statistically significantly improved symptoms and peak urine flow rates over placebo as follows:

[See table at bottom of next page]

In all three studies, both symptom scores and peak urine flow rates showed statistically significant improvement from baseline in patients treated with terazosin from week 2 (or the first clinic visit) and throughout the study duration.

Analysis of the effect of terazosin on individual urinary symptoms demonstrated that compared to placebo, terazosin significantly improved the symptoms of hesitancy, intermittency, impairment in size and force of urinary stream, sensation of incomplete emptying, terminal dribbling, daytime frequency and nocturia.

Global assessments of overall urinary function and symptoms were also performed by investigators who were blinded to patient treatment assignment. In studies 1 and 3, patients treated with terazosin had a significantly ($p \leq 0.001$) greater overall improvement compared to placebo treated patients.

In a short term study (Study 1), patients were randomized to either 2, 5 or 10 mg of terazosin or placebo. Patients randomized to the 10 mg group achieved a statistically significant response in both symptoms and peak flow rate compared to placebo (Figure 1).

[See figure 1 at top of next column]

+ for baseline values see above table
* $p \leq 0.05$, compared to placebo group

In a long-term, open-label, non-placebo controlled clinical trial, 181 men were followed for 2 years and 58 of these men were followed for 30 months. The effect of terazosin on urinary symptom scores and peak flow rates was maintained throughout the study duration (Figures 2 and 3):

[See figure 2 at top of next column]
[See figure 3 at top of next column]

In this long-term trial, both symptom scores and peak urinary flow rates showed statistically significant improvement suggesting a relaxation of smooth muscle cells.

Figure 1
Study 1

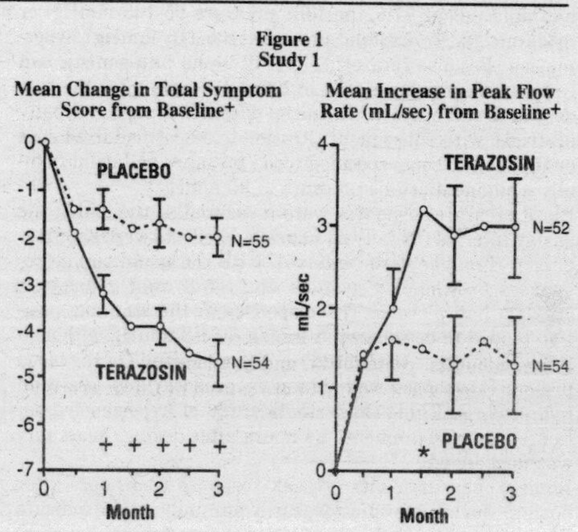

Figure 2
Mean Change in Total Symptom Score from Baseline
Long-Term, Open-Label, Non-Placebo Controlled Study
(N=494)

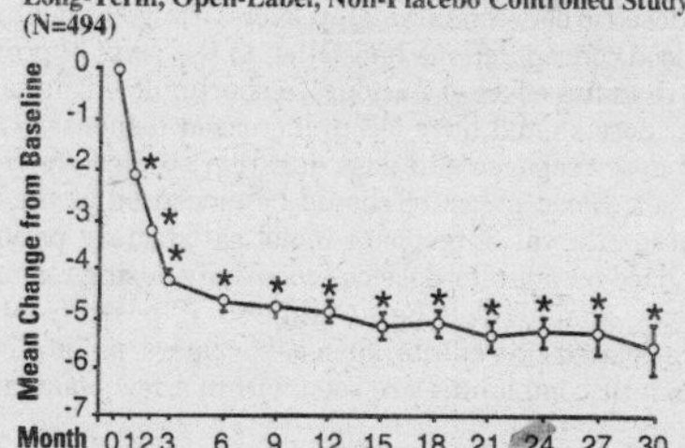

* $p \leq 0.05$ vs. baseline
mean baseline = 10.7

Figure 3
Mean Change in Peak Flow Rate from Baseline
Long-Term, Open-Label, Non-Placebo Controlled Study
(N=494)

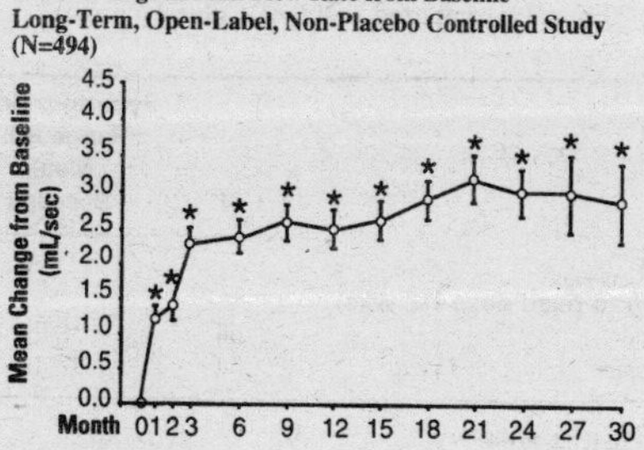

* $p \leq 0.05$ vs. baseline
mean baseline = 9.9

Although blockade of alpha-1 adrenoceptors also lowers blood pressure in hypertensive patients with increased peripheral vascular resistance, terazosin treatment of normotensive men with BPH did not result in a clinically significant blood pressure lowering effect:

Continued on next page

Hytrin—Cont.

Mean Changes in Blood Pressure from Baseline to Final Visit in all Double-Blind, Placebo-Controlled Studies

		Normotensive Patients DBP ≤ 90 mm Hg		Hypertensive Patients DBP > 90 mm Hg	
	Group	N	Mean Change	N	Mean Change
SBP (mm Hg)	Placebo	293	-0.1	45	-5.8
	Terazosin	519	-3.3*	65	-14.4*
DBP (mm Hg)	Placebo	293	+0.4	45	-7.1
	Terazosin	519	-2.2*	65	-15.1*

*p ≤ 0.05 vs. placebo

B. Hypertension

In animals, terazosin causes a decrease in blood pressure by decreasing total peripheral vascular resistance. The vasodilatory hypotensive action of terazosin appears to be produced mainly by blockade of alpha-1 adrenoceptors. Terazosin decreases blood pressure gradually within 15 minutes following oral administration.

Patients in clinical trials of terazosin were administered once daily (the great majority) and twice daily regimens with total doses usually in the range of 5-20 mg/day, and had mild (about 77%, diastolic pressure 95-105 mmHg) or moderate (23%, diastolic pressure 105-115 mmHg) hypertension. Because terazosin, like all alpha antagonists, can cause unusually large falls in blood pressure after the first dose or first few doses, the initial dose was 1 mg in virtually all trials, with subsequent titration to a specified fixed dose or titration to some specified blood pressure end point (usually a supine diastolic pressure of 90 mmHg).

Blood pressure responses were measured at the end of the dosing interval (usually 24 hours) and effects were shown to persist throughout the interval, with the usual supine responses 5-10 mmHg systolic and 3.5-8 mmHg diastolic greater than placebo. The responses in the standing position tended to be somewhat larger, by 1-3 mmHg, although this was not true in all studies. The magnitude of the blood pressure responses was similar to prazosin and less than hydrochlorothiazide (in a single study of hypertensive patients). In measurements 24 hours after dosing, heart rate was unchanged.

Limited measurements of peak response (2-3 hours after dosing) during chronic terazosin administration indicate that it is greater than about twice the trough (24 hour) response, suggesting some attenuation of response at 24 hours, presumably due to a fall in blood terazosin concentrations at the end of the dose interval. This explanation is not established with certainty, however, and is not consistent with the similarity of blood pressure response to once daily and twice daily dosing and with the absence of an observed dose-response relationship over a range of 5-20 mg, i.e., if blood concentrations had fallen to the point of providing less than full effect at 24 hours, a shorter dosing interval or larger dose should have led to increased response.

Further dose response and dose duration studies are being carried out. Blood pressure should be measured at the end of the dose interval; if response is not satisfactory, patients may be tried on a larger dose or twice daily dosing regimen. The latter should also be considered if possibly blood pressure-related side effects, such as dizziness, palpitations, or orthostatic complaints, are seen within a few hours after dosing.

The greater blood pressure effect associated with peak plasma concentrations (first few hours after dosing) appears somewhat more position-dependent (greater in the erect position) than the effect of terazosin at 24 hours and in the erect position there is also a 6-10 beat per minute increase in heart rate in the first few hours after dosing. During the first 3 hours after dosing 12.5% of patients had a systolic pressure fall of 30 mmHg or more from supine to standing, or standing systolic pressure below 90 mmHg with a fall of at least 20 mmHg, compared to 4% of a placebo group.

There was a tendency for patients to gain weight during terazosin therapy. In placebo-controlled monotherapy trials, male and female patients receiving terazosin gained a mean of 1.7 and 2.2 pounds respectively, compared to losses of 0.2 and 1.2 pounds respectively in the placebo group. Both differences were statistically significant.

During controlled clinical trials, patients receiving terazosin monotherapy had a small but statistically significant decrease (a 3% fall) compared to placebo in total cholesterol and the combined low-density and very-low-density lipoprotein fractions. No significant changes were observed in high-density lipoprotein fraction and triglycerides compared to placebo.

Analysis of clinical laboratory data following administration of terazosin suggested the possibility of hemodilution based on decreases in hematocrit, hemoglobin, white blood cells, total protein and albumin. Decreases in hematocrit and total protein have been observed with alpha-blockade and are attributed to hemodilution.

Pharmacokinetics:

Terazosin hydrochloride administered as HYTRIN capsules is essentially completely absorbed in man. Administration of capsules immediately after meals had a minimal effect on the extent of absorption. The time to reach peak plasma concentration however, was delayed by about 40 minutes. Terazosin has been shown to undergo minimal hepatic first-pass metabolism and nearly all of the circulating dose is in the form of parent drug. The plasma levels peak about one hour after dosing, and then decline with a half-life of approximately 12 hours. In a study that evaluated the effect of age on terazosin pharmacokinetics, the mean plasma half-lives were 14.0 and 11.4 hours for the age group ≥70 years and the age group of 20-39 years, respectively. After oral administration the plasma clearance was decreased by 31.7% in patients 70 years of age or older compared to that in patients 20-39 years of age.

The drug is 90-94% bound to plasma proteins and binding is constant over the clinically observed concentration range. Approximately 10% of an orally administered dose is excreted as parent drug in the urine and approximately 20% is excreted in the feces. The remainder is eliminated as metabolites. Impaired renal function had no significant effect on the elimination of terazosin, and dosage adjustment of terazosin to compensate for the drug removal during hemodialysis (approximately 10%) does not appear to be necessary. Overall, approximately 40% of the administered dose is excreted in the urine and approximately 60% in the feces. The disposition of the compound in animals is qualitatively similar to that in man.

INDICATIONS AND USAGE

HYTRIN (terazosin hydrochloride) is indicated for the treatment of symptomatic benign prostatic hyperplasia (BPH). There is a rapid response, with approximately 70% of patients experiencing an increase in urinary flow and improvement in symptoms of BPH when treated with HYTRIN. The long-term effects of HYTRIN on the incidence of surgery, acute urinary obstruction or other complications of BPH are yet to be determined.

HYTRIN is also indicated for the treatment of hypertension. It can be used alone or in combination with other antihypertensive agents such as diuretics or beta-adrenergic blocking agents.

CONTRAINDICATIONS

HYTRIN capsules are contraindicated in patients known to be hypersensitive to terazosin hydrochloride.

WARNINGS

Syncope and "First-dose" Effect:

HYTRIN capsules, like other alpha-adrenergic blocking agents, can cause marked lowering of blood pressure, especially postural hypotension, and syncope in association with the first dose or first few days of therapy. A similar effect can be anticipated if therapy is interrupted for several days and then restarted. Syncope has also been reported with other alpha-adrenergic blocking agents in association with rapid dosage increases or the introduction of another antihypertensive drug. Syncope is believed to be due to an excessive postural hypotensive effect, although occasionally the syncopal episode has been preceded by about of severe supraventricular tachycardia with heart rates of 120-160 beats per minute. Additionally, the possibility of the contribution of hemodilution to the symptoms of postural hypotension should be considered.

To decrease the likelihood of syncope or excessive hypotension, treatment should always be initiated with a 1 mg dose of terazosin, given at bedtime. The 2 mg, 5 mg and 10 mg capsules are not indicated as initial therapy. Dosage should then be increased slowly, according to recommendations in the Dosage and Administration section and additional antihypertensive agents should be added with caution. The patient should be cautioned to avoid situations, such as driving or hazardous tasks, where injury could result should syncope occur during initiation of therapy.

In early investigational studies, where increasing single doses up to 7.5 mg were given at 3 day intervals, tolerance to the first dose phenomenon did not necessarily develop and the "first-dose" effect could be observed at all doses. Syncopal episodes occurred in 3 of the 14 subjects given terazosin at doses of 2.5, 5 and 7.5 mg, which are higher than the recommended initial dose; in addition, severe orthostatic hypotension (blood pressure falling to 50/0 mmHg) was seen in two others and dizziness, tachycardia, and lightheadedness occurred in most subjects. These adverse effects all occurred within 90 minutes of dosing.

In three placebo-controlled BPH studies 1, 2, and 3 (see CLINICAL PHARMACOLOGY), the incidence of postural hypotension in the terazosin treated patients was 5.1%, 5.2%, and 3.7% respectively.

In multiple dose clinical trials involving nearly 2000 hypertensive patients treated with terazosin, syncope was reported in about 1% of patients. Syncope was not necessarily associated only with the first dose.

If syncope occurs, the patient should be placed in a recumbent position and treated supportively as necessary. There is evidence that the orthostatic effect of terazosin is greater, even in chronic use, shortly after dosing. The risk of the events is greatest during the initial seven days of treatment, but continues at all time intervals.

Priapism:

Rarely, (probably less than once in every several thousand patients) terazosin and other α_1-antagonists have been associated with priapism (painful penile erection, sustained for hours and unrelieved by sexual intercourse or masturbation). Two or three dozen cases have been reported. Because this condition can lead to permanent impotence if not promptly treated, patients must be advised about the seriousness of the condition (see **PRECAUTIONS: Information for Patients**).

PRECAUTIONS

General:

Prostatic Cancer

Carcinoma of the prostate and BPH cause many of the same symptoms. These two diseases frequently co-exist. Therefore, patients thought to have BPH should be examined prior to starting HYTRIN therapy to rule out the presence of carcinoma of the prostate.

Orthostatic Hypotension

While syncope is the most severe orthostatic effect of terazosin (see Warnings), other symptoms of lowered blood pressure, such as dizziness, lightheadedness and palpitations, were more common and occurred in some 28% of patients in clinical trials of hypertension. In BPH clinical trials, 21% of the patients experienced one or more of the following: dizziness, hypotension, postural hypotension, syncope, and vertigo. Patients with occupations in which such events represent potential problems should be treated with particular caution.

Information for Patients (see Patient Package Insert):

Patients should be made aware of the possibility of syncopal and orthostatic symptoms, especially at the initiation of therapy, and to avoid driving or hazardous tasks for 12 hours after the first dose, after a dosage increase and after interruption of therapy when treatment is resumed. They should be cautioned to avoid situations where injury could result should syncope occur during initiation of terazosin therapy. They should also be advised of the need to sit or lie down when symptoms of lowered blood pressure occur, although these symptoms are not always orthostatic, and to be careful when rising from a sitting or lying position. If dizziness, lightheadedness, or palpitations are bothersome they should be reported to the physician, so that dose adjustment can be considered.

Patients should also be told that drowsiness or somnolence can occur with terazosin, requiring caution in people who must drive or operate heavy machinery.

Patients should be advised about the possibility of priapism as a result of treatment with HYTRIN and other similar medications. Patients should know that this reaction to HYTRIN is extremely rare, but that if it is not brought to immediate medical attention, it can lead to permanent erectile dysfunction (impotence).

Laboratory Tests:

Small but statistically significant decreases in hematocrit, hemoglobin, white blood cells, total protein and albumin were observed in controlled clinical trials. These laboratory findings suggested the possibility of hemodilution. Treatment with terazosin for up to 24 months had no significant effect on prostate specific antigen (PSA) levels.

Drug Interactions:

In controlled trials, terazosin has been added to diuretics, and several beta-adrenergic blockers; no unexpected interactions were observed. Terazosin has also been used in patients on a variety of concomitant therapies; while these

	Symptom Score (Range 0-27)			Peak Flow Rate (mL/sec)		
	N	Mean Baseline	Mean Change (%)	N	Mean Baseline	Mean Change (%)
Study 1 (10 mg)[a]						
Titration to fixed dose (12 wks)						
Placebo	55	9.7	-2.3 (24)	54	10.1	+1.0 (10)
Terazosin	54	10.1	-4.5 (45)*	52	8.8	+3.0 (34)*
Study 2 (2, 5, 10, 20 mg)[b]						
Titration to response (24 wks)						
Placebo	89	12.5	-3.8 (30)	88	8.8	+1.4 (16)
Terazosin	85	12.2	-5.3 (43)*	84	8.4	+2.9 (35)*
Study 3 (1, 2, 5, 10 mg)[c]						
Titration to response (24 wks)						
Placebo	74	10.4	-1.1 (11)	74	8.8	+1.2 (14)
Terazosin	73	10.9	-4.6 (42)*	73	8.6	+2.6 (30)*

[a] Highest dose 10 mg shown.
[b] 23% of patients on 10 mg, 41% of patients on 20 mg.
[c] 67% of patients on 10 mg.
* Significantly (p ≤ 0.05) more improvement than placebo.

were not formal interaction studies, no interactions were observed. Terazosin has been used concomitantly in at least 50 patients on the following drugs or drug classes: 1) analgesic/anti-inflammatory (e.g., acetaminophen, aspirin, codeine, ibuprofen, indomethacin); 2) antibiotics (e.g., erythromycin, trimethoprim and sulfamethoxazole); 3) anticholinergic/sympathomimetics (e.g., phenylephrine hydrochloride, phenylpropanolamine hydrochloride, pseudoephedrine hydrochloride); 4) antigout (e.g., allopurinol); 5) antihistamines (e.g., chlorpheniramine); 6) cardiovascular agents (e.g., atenolol, hydrochlorothiazide, methyclothiazide, propranolol); 7) corticosteroids; 8) gastrointestinal agents (e.g., antacids); 9) hypoglycemics; 10) sedatives and tranquilizers (e.g., diazepam).

Use with Other Drugs:
In a study (n=24) where terazosin and verapamil were administered concomitantly, terazosin's mean AUC_{0-24} increased 11% after the first verapamil dose and after 3 weeks of verapamil treatment it increased by 24% with associated increases in C_{max} (25%) and C_{min} (32%) means. Terazosin mean T_{max} decreased from 1.3 hours to 0.8 hours after 3 weeks of verapamil treatment. Statistically significant differences were not found in the verapamil level with and without terazosin. In a study (n=6) where terazosin and captopril were administered concomitantly, plasma disposition of captopril was not influenced by concomitant administration of terazosin and terazosin maximum plasma concentrations increased linearly with dose at steady-state after administration of terazosin plus captopril (see Dosage and Administration).

Carcinogenesis, Mutagenesis, Impairment of Fertility:
Terazosin was devoid of mutagenic potential when evaluated *in vivo* and *in vitro* (the Ames test, *in vivo* cytogenetics, the dominant lethal test in mice, *in vivo* Chinese hamster chromosome aberration test and V79 forward mutation assay).
Terazosin, administered in the feed to rats at doses of 8, 40, and 250 mg/kg/day (70, 350, and 2100 mg/M²/day), for two years, was associated with a statistically significant increase in benign adrenal medullary tumors of male rats exposed to the 250 mg/kg dose. This dose is 175 times the maximum recommended human dose of 20 mg (12 mg/M²). Female rats were unaffected. Terazosin was not oncogenic in mice when administered in feed for 2 years at a maximum tolerated dose of 32 mg/kg/day (110 mg/M²; 9 times the maximum recommended human dose). The absence of mutagenicity in a battery of tests, of tumorigenicity of any cell type in the mouse carcinogenicity assay, of increased total tumor incidence in either species, and of proliferative adrenal lesions in female rats, suggests a male rat species-specific event. Numerous other diverse pharmaceutical and chemical compounds have also been associated with benign adrenal medullary tumors in male rats without supporting evidence for carcinogenicity in man.
The effect of terazosin on fertility was assessed in a standard fertility/reproductive performance study in which male and female rats were administered oral doses of 8, 30 and 120 mg/kg/day. Four of 20 male rats given 30 mg/kg (240 mg/M²; 20 times the maximum recommended human dose) and five of 19 male rats given 120 mg/kg (960 mg/M²; 80 times the maximum recommended human dose) failed to sire a litter. Testicular weights and morphology were unaffected by treatment. Vaginal smears at 30 and 120 mg/kg/day, however, appeared to contain less sperm than smears from control matings and good correlation was reported between sperm count and subsequent pregnancy.
Oral administration of terazosin for one or two years elicited a statistically significant increase in the incidence of testicular atrophy in rats exposed to 40 and 250 mg/kg/day (29 and 175 times the maximum recommended human dose), but not in rats exposed to 8 mg/kg/day (> 6 times the maximum recommended human dose). Testicular atrophy was also observed in dogs dosed with 300 mg/kg/day (> 500 times the maximum recommended human dose) for three months but not after one year when dosed with 20 mg/kg/day (38 times the maximum recommended human dose). This lesion has also been seen with Minipress®, another (marketed) selective-alpha-1 blocking agent.

Pregnancy:
Teratogenic effects: Pregnancy Category C. Terazosin was not teratogenic in either rats or rabbits when administered at oral doses up to 280 and 60 times, respectively, the maximum recommended human dose. Fetal resorptions occurred in rats dosed with 480 mg/kg/day, approximately 280 times the maximum recommended human dose. Increased fetal resorptions, decreased fetal weight and an increased number of supernumerary ribs were observed in offspring of rabbits dosed with 60 times the maximum recommended human dose. These findings (in both species) were most likely secondary to maternal toxicity. There are no adequate and well-controlled studies in pregnant women and the safety of terazosin in pregnancy has not been established. HYTRIN is not recommended during pregnancy unless the potential benefit justifies the potential risk to the mother and fetus.
Nonteratogenic effects: In a peri- and post-natal development study in rats, significantly more pups died in the group dosed with 120 mg/kg/day (> 75 times the maximum recommended human dose) than in the control group during the three-week postpartum period.

Nursing Mothers:
It is not known whether terazosin is excreted in breast milk. Because many drugs are excreted in breast milk, caution should be exercised when terazosin is administered to a nursing woman.

Pediatric Use:
Safety and effectiveness in children have not been determined.

ADVERSE REACTIONS

Benign Prostatic Hyperplasia

The incidence of treatment-emergent adverse events has been ascertained from clinical trials conducted worldwide. All adverse events reported during these trials were recorded as adverse reactions. The incidence rates presented below are based on combined data from six placebo-controlled trials involving once-a-day administration of terazosin at doses ranging from 1 to 20 mg. Table 1 summarizes those adverse events reported for patients in these trials when the incidence rate in the terazosin group was at least 1% and was greater than that for the placebo group, or where the reaction is of clinical interest. Asthenia, postural hypotension, dizziness, somnolence, nasal congestion/rhinitis, and impotence were the only events that were significantly ($p \leq 0.05$) more common in patients receiving terazosin than in patients receiving placebo. The incidence of urinary tract infection was significantly lower in the patients receiving terazosin than in patients receiving placebo. An analysis of the incidence rate of hypotensive adverse events (see PRECAUTIONS) adjusted for the length of drug treatment has shown that the risk of the events is greatest during the initial seven days of treatment, but continues at all time intervals.

TABLE 1
ADVERSE REACTIONS DURING PLACEBO-CONTROLLED TRIALS BENIGN PROSTATIC HYPERPLASIA

Body System	Terazosin (N=636)	Placebo (N=360)
BODY AS A WHOLE		
†Asthenia	7.4%*	3.3%
Flu Syndrome	2.4%	1.7%
Headache	4.9%	5.8%
CARDIOVASCULAR SYSTEM		
Hypotension	0.6%	0.6%
Palpitations	0.9%	1.1%
Postural Hypotension	3.9%*	0.8%
Syncope	0.6%	0.0%
DIGESTIVE SYSTEM		
Nausea	1.7%	1.1%
METABOLIC AND NUTRITIONAL DISORDERS		
Peripheral Edema	0.9%	0.3%
Weight Gain	0.5%	0.0%
NERVOUS SYSTEM		
Dizziness	9.1%*	4.2%
Somnolence	3.6%*	1.9%
Vertigo	1.4%	0.3%
RESPIRATORY SYSTEM		
Dyspnea	1.7%	0.8%
Nasal Congestion/Rhinitis	1.9%*	0.0%
SPECIAL SENSES		
Blurred Vision/Amblyopia	1.3%	0.6%
UROGENITAL SYSTEM		
Impotence	1.6%*	0.6%
Urinary Tract Infection	1.3%	3.9%*

† Includes weakness, tiredness, lassitude and fatigue.
* $p \leq 0.05$ comparison between groups.

Additional adverse events have been reported, but these are, in general, not distinguishable from symptoms that might have occurred in the absence of exposure to terazosin. The safety profile of patients treated in the long-term open-label study was similar to that observed in the controlled studies.
The adverse events were usually transient and mild or moderate in intensity, but sometimes were serious enough to interrupt treatment. In the placebo-controlled clinical trials, the rates of premature termination due to adverse events were not statistically different between the placebo and terazosin groups. The adverse events that were bothersome, as judged by their being reported as reasons for discontinuation of therapy by at least 0.5% of the terazosin group and being reported more often than in the placebo group, are shown in Table 2.

TABLE 2
DISCONTINUATION DURING PLACEBO-CONTROLLED TRIALS BENIGN PROSTATIC HYPERPLASIA

Body System	Terazosin (N=636)	Placebo (N=360)
BODY AS A WHOLE		
Fever	0.5%	0.0%
Headache	1.1%	0.8%
CARDIOVASCULAR SYSTEM		
Postural Hypotension	0.5%	0.0%
Syncope	0.5%	0.0%
DIGESTIVE SYSTEM		
Nausea	0.5%	0.3%
NERVOUS SYSTEM		
Dizziness	2.0%	1.1%
Vertigo	0.5%	0.0%
RESPIRATORY SYSTEM		
Dyspnea	0.5%	0.3%
SPECIAL SENSES		
Blurred Vision/Amblyopia	0.6%	0.0%
UROGENITAL SYSTEM		
Urinary Tract Infection	0.5%	0.3%

Hypertension

The prevalence of adverse reactions has been ascertained from clinical trials conducted primarily in the United States. All adverse experiences (events) reported during these trials were recorded as adverse reactions. The prevalence rates presented below are based on combined data from fourteen placebo-controlled trials involving once-a-day administration of terazosin, as monotherapy or in combination with other antihypertensive agents, at doses ranging from 1 to 40 mg. Table 3 summarizes those adverse experiences reported for patients in these trials where the prevalence rate in the terazosin group was at least 5%, where the prevalence rate for the terazosin group was at least 2% and was greater than the prevalence rate for the placebo group, or where the reaction is of particular interest. Asthenia, blurred vision, dizziness, nasal congestion, nausea, peripheral edema, palpitations and somnolence were the only symptoms that were significantly ($p < 0.05$) more common in patients receiving terazosin than in patients receiving placebo. Similar adverse reaction rates were observed in placebo-controlled monotherapy trials.

TABLE 3
ADVERSE REACTIONS DURING PLACEBO-CONTROLLED TRIALS HYPERTENSION

Body System	Terazosin (N=859)	Placebo (N=506)
BODY AS A WHOLE		
†Asthenia	11.3%*	4.3%
Back Pain	2.4%	1.2%
Headache	16.2%	15.8%
CARDIOVASCULAR SYSTEM		
Palpitations	4.3%*	1.2%
Postural Hypotension	1.3%	0.4%
Tachycardia	1.9%	1.2%
DIGESTIVE SYSTEM		
Nausea	4.4%*	1.4%
METABOLIC AND NUTRITIONAL DISORDERS		
Edema	0.9%	0.6%
Peripheral Edema	5.5%*	2.4%
Weight Gain	0.5%	0.2%
MUSCULOSKELETAL SYSTEM		
Pain–Extremities	3.5%	3.0%
NERVOUS SYSTEM		
Depression	0.3%	0.2%
Dizziness	19.3%*	7.5%
Libido Decreased	0.6%	0.2%
Nervousness	2.3%	1.8%
Paresthesia	2.9%	1.4%
Somnolence	5.4%*	2.6%
RESPIRATORY SYSTEM		
Dyspnea	3.1%	2.4%
Nasal Congestion	5.9%*	3.4%
Sinusitis	2.6%	1.4%
SPECIAL SENSES		
Blurred Vision	1.6%*	0.0%
UROGENITAL SYSTEM		
Impotence	1.2%	1.4%

† Includes weakness, tiredness, lassitude and fatigue.
* Statistically significant at p=0.05 level.

Additional adverse reactions have been reported, but these are, in general, not distinguishable from symptoms that might have occurred in the absence of exposure to terazosin. The following additional adverse reactions were reported by at least 1% of 1987 patients who received terazosin in controlled or open, short- or long-term clinical trials or have been reported during marketing experience: *Body as a Whole:* chest pain, facial edema, fever, abdominal pain, neck pain, shoulder pain; *Cardiovascular System:* arrhythmia, vasodilation; *Digestive System:* constipation, diarrhea, dry mouth, dyspepsia, flatulence, vomiting; *Metabolic/Nutritional Disorders:* gout; *Musculoskeletal System:* arthralgia, arthritis, joint disorder, myalgia; *Nervous System:* anxiety, insomnia; *Respiratory System:* bronchitis, cold symptoms,

Continued on next page

Hytrin—Cont.

epistaxis, flu symptoms, increased cough, pharyngitis, rhinitis; *Skin and Appendages:* pruritus, rash, sweating; *Special Senses:* abnormal vision, conjunctivitis, tinnitus; *Urogenital System:* urinary frequency, urinary incontinence primarily reported in postmenopausal women, urinary tract infection.
The adverse reactions were usually mild or moderate in intensity but sometimes were serious enough to interrupt treatment. The adverse reactions that were most bothersome, as judged by their being reported as reasons for discontinuation of therapy by at least 0.5% of the terazosin group and being reported more often than in the placebo group, are shown in Table 4.

TABLE 4
DISCONTINUATIONS DURING PLACEBO-CONTROLLED TRIALS HYPERTENSION

Body System	Terazosin (N=859)	Placebo (N=506)
BODY AS A WHOLE		
Asthenia	1.6%	0.0%
Headache	1.3%	1.0%
CARDIOVASCULAR SYSTEM		
Palpitations	1.4%	0.2%
Postural Hypotension	0.5%	0.0%
Syncope	0.5%	0.2%
Tachycardia	0.6%	0.0%
DIGESTIVE SYSTEM		
Nausea	0.8%	0.0%
METABOLIC AND NUTRITIONAL DISORDERS		
Peripheral Edema	0.6%	0.0%
NERVOUS SYSTEM		
Dizziness	3.1%	0.4%
Paresthesia	0.8%	0.2%
Somnolence	0.6%	0.2%
RESPIRATORY SYSTEM		
Dyspnea	0.9%	0.6%
Nasal Congestion	0.6%	0.0%
SPECIAL SENSES		
Blurred Vision	0.6%	0.0%

Post-marketing Experience
Post-marketing experience indicates that in rare instances patients may develop allergic reactions, including anaphylaxis, following administration of terazosin hydrochloride. There have been reports of priapism and thrombocytopenia during post-marketing surveillance. Atrial fibrillation has been reported.

OVERDOSAGE

Should overdosage of HYTRIN lead to hypotension, support of the cardiovascular system is of first importance. Restoration of blood pressure and normalization of heart rate may be accomplished by keeping the patient in the supine position. If this measure is inadequate, shock should first be treated with volume expanders. If necessary, vasopressors should then be used and renal function should be monitored and supported as needed. Laboratory data indicate that terazosin is 90-94% protein bound; therefore, dialysis may not be of benefit.

DOSAGE AND ADMINISTRATION

If HYTRIN administration is discontinued for several days, therapy should be reinstituted using the initial dosing regimen.
Benign Prostatic Hyperplasia:
Initial Dose:
1 mg at bedtime is the starting dose for all patients, and this dose should not be exceeded as an initial dose. Patients should be closely followed during initial administration in order to minimize the risk of severe hypotensive response.
Subsequent Doses:
The dose should be increased in a stepwise fashion to 2 mg, 5 mg, or 10 mg once daily to achieve the desired improvement of symptoms and/or flow rates. Doses of 10 mg once daily are generally required for the clinical response. Therefore, treatment with 10 mg for a minimum of 4–6 weeks may be required to assess whether a beneficial response has been achieved. Some patients may not achieve a clinical response despite appropriate titration. Although some additional patients responded at a 20 mg daily dose, there was an insufficient number of patients studied to draw definitive conclusions about this dose. There are insufficient data to support the use of higher doses for those patients who show inadequate or no response to 20 mg daily. **If terazosin administration is discontinued for several days or longer, therapy should be reinstituted using the initial dosing regimen.**
Use with Other Drugs:
Caution should be observed when HYTRIN is administered concomitantly with other antihypertensive agents, especially the calcium channel blocker verapamil, to avoid the possibility of developing significant hypotension. When using HYTRIN and other antihypertensive agents concomitantly, dosage reduction and retitration of either agent may be necessary (see Precautions).
Hypertension:
The dose of HYTRIN and the dose interval (12 or 24 hours) should be adjusted according to the patient's individual blood pressure response. The following is a guide to its administration:
Initial Dose:
1 mg at bedtime is the starting dose for all patients, and this dose should not be exceeded. This initial dosing regimen should be strictly observed to minimize the potential for severe hypotensive effects.
Subsequent Doses:
The dose may be slowly increased to achieve the desired blood pressure response. The usual recommended dose range is 1 mg to 5 mg administered once a day; however, some patients may benefit from doses as high as 20 mg per day. Doses over 20 mg do not appear to provide further blood pressure effect and doses over 40 mg have not been studied. Blood pressure should be monitored at the end of the dosing interval to be sure control is maintained throughout the interval. It may also be helpful to measure blood pressure 2-3 hours after dosing to see if the maximum and minimum responses are similar, and to evaluate symptoms such as dizziness or palpitations which can result from excessive hypotensive response. If response is substantially diminished at 24 hours an increased dose or use of a twice daily regimen can be considered. **If terazosin administration is discontinued for several days or longer, therapy should be reinstituted using the initial dosing regimen.** In clinical trials, except for the initial dose, the dose was given in the morning.
Use With Other Drugs: (see above)

HOW SUPPLIED

HYTRIN capsules (terazosin hydrochloride capsules) are available in four dosage strengths:
1 mg grey capsules (imprinted with and the Abbo-Code HH):
Bottles of 100 .... (**NDC** 0074-3805-13),
Abbo-Pac® unit dose strip packages
of 100 capsules .... (**NDC** 0074-3805-11).
2 mg yellow capsules (imprinted with and the Abbo-Code HY):
Bottles of 100 .... (**NDC** 0074-3806-13),
Abbo-Pac® unit dose strip packages
of 100 capsules .... (**NDC** 0074-3806-11).
5 mg red capsules (imprinted with and the Abbo-Code HK):
Bottles of 100 .... (**NDC** 0074-3807-13),
Abbo-Pac® unit dose strip packages
of 100 capsules .... (**NDC** 0074-3807-11).
10 mg blue capsules (imprinted with and the Abbo-Code HN):
Bottles of 100 .... (**NDC** 0074-3808-13),
Abbo-Pac® unit dose strip packages
of 100 capsules .... (**NDC** 0074-3808-11).
Recommended storage: Store at controlled room temperature between 20-25°C (68-77°F). See USP. Protect from light and moisture.
Revised: February, 2001
Ref.: 03-5105
ABBOTT LABORATORIES
NORTH CHICAGO, IL 60064, U.S.A. 01G-501-0118-1
MASTER

KALETRA™ ℞

[*kuh-LEE-tra*]
(lopinavir/ritonavir) capsules
(lopinavir/ritonavir) oral solution
Rx only

Prescribing information for this product, which appears on pages 471–478 of the 2002 PDR, has been completely revised as follows. Please write "See Supplement A" next to the product heading.

DESCRIPTION

KALETRA (lopinavir/ritonavir) is a co-formulation of lopinavir and ritonavir. Lopinavir is an inhibitor of the HIV protease. As co-formulated in KALETRA, ritonavir inhibits the CYP3A-mediated metabolism of lopinavir, thereby providing increased plasma levels of lopinavir.
Lopinavir is chemically designated as [1S-[1R*, (R*), 3R*, 4R*]]-N-[4-[[(2,6-dimethylphenoxy)acetyl]amino]-3-hydroxy-5-phenyl-1-(phenylmethyl)pentyl]tetrahydro-alpha-(1-methylethyl)-2-oxo-1(2H)-pyrimidineacetamide. Its molecular formula is $C_{37}H_{48}N_4O_5$, and its molecular weight is 628.80. Lopinavir has the following structural formula:

Ritonavir is chemically designated as 10-Hydroxy-2-methyl-5-(1-methylethyl)-1- [2-(1-methylethyl)-4-thiazolyl]-3,6-dioxo-8,11-bis(phenylmethyl)-2,4,7,12-tetraazatridecan-13-oic acid, 5-thiazolylmethyl ester, [5S-(5R*,8R*,10R*,11R*)]. Its molecular formula is $C_{37}H_{48}N_6O_5S_2$, and its molecular weight is 720.95. Ritonavir has the following structural formula:

Lopinavir is a white to light tan powder. It is freely soluble in methanol and ethanol, soluble in isopropanol and practically insoluble in water.
KALETRA capsules are available for oral administration in a strength of 133.3 mg lopinavir and 33.3 mg ritonavir with the following inactive ingredients: FD&C Yellow No. 6, gelatin, glycerin, oleic acid, polyoxyl 35 castor oil, propylene glycol, sorbitol special, titanium dioxide, and water.
KALETRA oral solution is available for oral administration as 80 mg lopinavir and 20 mg ritonavir per milliliter with the following inactive ingredients: Acesulfame potassium, alcohol, artificial cotton candy flavor, citric acid, glycerin, high fructose corn syrup, Magnasweet-110 flavor, menthol, natural & artificial vanilla flavor, peppermint oil, polyoxyl 40 hydrogenated castor oil, povidone, propylene glycol, saccharin sodium, sodium chloride, sodium citrate, and water.
KALETRA oral solution contains 42.4% alcohol (v/v).

CLINICAL PHARMACOLOGY

Microbiology
Mechanism of action: Lopinavir, an inhibitor of the HIV protease, prevents cleavage of the Gag-Pol polyprotein, resulting in the production of immature, non-infectious viral particles.
Antiviral activity in vitro: The *in vitro* antiviral activity of lopinavir against laboratory HIV strains and clinical HIV isolates was evaluated in acutely infected lymphoblastic cell lines and peripheral blood lymphocytes, respectively. In the absence of human serum, the mean 50% effective concentration (EC_{50}) of lopinavir against five different HIV-1 laboratory strains ranged from 10-27 nM (0.006 - 0.017 μg/mL, 1 μg/mL = 1.6 μM) and ranged from 4-11 nM (0.003 - 0.007 μg/mL) against several HIV-1 clinical isolates (n=6). In the presence of 50% human serum, the mean EC_{50} of lopinavir against these five laboratory strains ranged from 65 - 289 nM (0.04 - 0.18 μg/mL), representing a 7- to 11-fold attenuation. Combination drug activity studies with lopinavir and other protease inhibitors or reverse transcriptase inhibitors have not been completed.
Resistance: HIV-1 isolates with reduced susceptibility to lopinavir have been selected *in vitro*. The presence of ritonavir does not appear to influence the selection of lopinavir-resistant viruses *in vitro*.
The selection of resistance to KALETRA in antiretroviral treatment naive patients has not yet been characterized. In a Phase III study of 653 antiretroviral treatment naive patients (Study 863), plasma viral isolates from each patient on treatment with plasma HIV >400 copies/mL at Week 24, 32, 40 and/or 48 were analyzed. No evidence of resistance to KALETRA was observed in 37 evaluable KALETRA-treated patients (0%). Evidence of genotypic resistance to nelfinavir, defined as the presence of the D30N and/or L90M mutation in HIV protease, was observed in 25/76 (33%) of evaluable nelfinavir-treated patients. The selection of resistance to KALETRA in antiretroviral treatment naive pediatric patients (Study 940) appears to be consistent with that seen in adult patients (Study 863).
Resistance to KALETRA has been noted to emerge in patients treated with other protease inhibitors prior to KALETRA therapy. In Phase II studies of 227 antiretroviral treatment naive and protease inhibitor experienced patients, isolates from 4 of 23 patients with quantifiable (>400 copies/mL) viral RNA following treatment with KALETRA for 12 to 100 weeks displayed significantly reduced susceptibility to lopinavir compared to the corresponding baseline viral isolates. Three of these patients had previously received treatment with a single protease inhibitor (nelfinavir, indinavir, or saquinavir) and one patient had received treatment with multiple protease inhibitors (indinavir, saquinavir and ritonavir). All four of these patients had at least 4 mutations associated with protease inhibitor resistance immediately prior to KALETRA therapy. Following viral rebound, isolates from these patients all contained additional mutations, some of which are recognized to be associated with protease inhibitor resistance. However, there are insufficient data at this time to identify lopinavir-associated mutational patterns in isolates from patients on KALETRA therapy. The assessment of these mutational patterns is under study.
Cross-resistance – Preclinical Studies: Varying degrees of cross-resistance have been observed among HIV protease inhibitors. Little information is available on the cross-resistance of viruses that developed decreased susceptibility to lopinavir during KALETRA therapy.
The *in vitro* activity of lopinavir against clinical isolates from patients previously treated with a single protease inhibitor was determined. Isolates that displayed >4-fold reduced susceptibility to nelfinavir (n=13) and saquinavir (n=4), displayed <4-fold reduced susceptibility to lopinavir. Isolates with >4-fold reduced susceptibility to indinavir (n=16) and ritonavir (n=3) displayed a mean of 5.7- and 8.3-fold reduced susceptibility to lopinavir, respectively. Isolates

from patients previously treated with two or more protease inhibitors showed greater reductions in susceptibility to lopinavir, as described in the following paragraph.

Clinical Studies – Antiviral activity of KALETRA in patients with previous protease inhibitor therapies: The clinical relevance of reduced *in vitro* susceptibility to lopinavir has been examined by assessing the virologic response to KALETRA therapy, with respect to baseline viral genotype and phenotype, in 56 NNRTI-naive patients with HIV RNA >1000 copies/mL despite previous therapy with at least two protease inhibitors selected from nelfinavir, indinavir, saquinavir and ritonavir (Study 957). In this study, patients were initially randomized to receive one of two doses of KALETRA in combination with efavirenz and nucleoside reverse transcriptase inhibitors. The EC_{50} values of lopinavir against the 56 baseline viral isolates ranged from 0.5- to 96-fold higher than the wild-type EC_{50}. Fifty-five percent (31/56) of these baseline isolates displayed a >4-fold reduced susceptibility to lopinavir. These 31 isolates had a mean reduction in lopinavir susceptibility of 27.9-fold. Table 1 shows the 48 week virologic response (HIV RNA <400 and <50 copies) according to susceptibility and number of genotypic mutations at baseline in 50 evaluable patients enrolled in the study (957) described above. Because this was a select patient population and the sample size was small, the data depicted in Table 1 do not constitute definitive clinical susceptibility breakpoints. Additional data are needed to determine clinically significant breakpoints for KALETRA.

Table 1: HIV RNA Response at Week 48 by baseline KALETRA susceptibility and by number of protease inhibitor-associated mutations[1]

Lopinavir susceptibility[2] at baseline	HIV RNA < 400 copies/mL (%)	HIV RNA < 50 copies/mL (%)
<10 fold	25/27 (93%)	22/27 (81%)
>10 and <40 fold	11/15 (73%)	9/15 (60%)
≥40 fold	2/8 (25%)	2/8 (25%)
Number of protease inhibitor mutations at baseline		
Up to 5	21/23 (91%)[3]	19/23 (83%)
>5	17/27 (63%)	14/27 (52%)

[1] Lopinavir susceptibility was determined by recombinant phenotypic technology performed by virologic; genotype also performed by virologic

[2] Fold change in susceptibility from wild type

[3] Thirteen of the 23 patient isolates contained PI mutations at positions 82, 84, and/or 90

There are insufficient data at this time to identify lopinavir-associated mutational patterns in isolates from patients on KALETRA therapy. Further studies are needed to assess the association between specific mutational patterns and virologic response rates.

Pharmacokinetics

The pharmacokinetic properties of lopinavir co-administered with ritonavir have been evaluated in healthy adult volunteers and in HIV-infected patients; no substantial differences were observed between the two groups. Lopinavir is essentially completely metabolized by CYP3A. Ritonavir inhibits the metabolism of lopinavir, thereby increasing the plasma levels of lopinavir. Across studies, administration of KALETRA 400/100 mg BID yields mean steady-state lopinavir plasma concentrations 15- to 20-fold higher than those of ritonavir in HIV-infected patients. The plasma levels of ritonavir are less than 7% of those obtained after the ritonavir dose of 600 mg BID. The *in vitro* antiviral EC_{50} of lopinavir is approximately 10-fold lower than that of ritonavir. Therefore, the antiviral activity of KALETRA is due to lopinavir.

Figure 1 displays the mean steady-state plasma concentrations of lopinavir and ritonavir after KALETRA 400/100 mg BID for 3-4 weeks from a pharmacokinetic study in HIV-infected adult subjects (n=21).

Figure 1: Mean Steady-State Plasma Concentrations with 95% Confidence Intervals (CI) for HIV-Infected Adult Subjects (N=21)

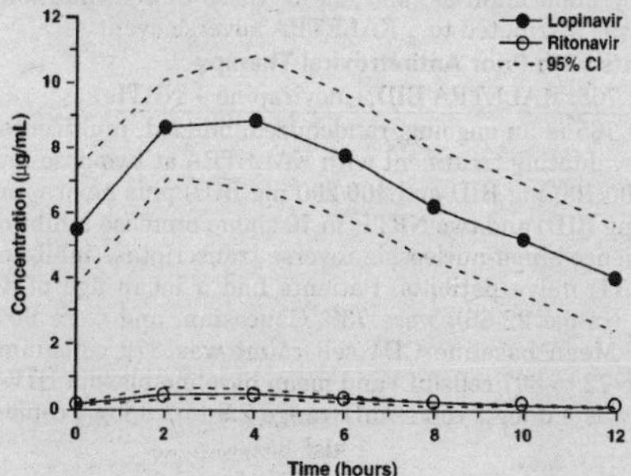

Table 2: Drug Interactions: Pharmacokinetic Parameters for Lopinavir in the Presence of the Co-administered Drug (See Precautions, Table 8 for Recommended Alterations in Dose or Regimen)

Co-administered Drug	Dose of Co-administered Drug (mg)	Dose of KALETRA (mg)	n	Ratio (with/without co-administered drug) of Lopinavir Pharmacokinetic Parameters (90% CI); No Effect = 1.00		
				C_{max}	AUC	C_{min}
Amprenavir[1]	450 BID, 5 d 750 BID, 5 d	400/100 BID, 22 d	12 10	0.89 (0.83, 0.95)	0.85 (0.81, 0.90)	0.81 (0.74, 0.89)
Atorvastatin	20 QD, 4 d	400/100 BID, 14 d	12	0.90 (0.78, 1.06)	0.90 (0.79, 1.02)	0.92 (0.78, 1.10)
Efavirenz[2]	600 QHS, 9 d	400/100 BID, 9 d	11, 7*	0.97 (0.78, 1.22)	0.81 (0.64, 1.03)	0.61 (0.38, 0.97)
Ketoconazole	200 single dose	400/100 BID, 16 d	12	0.89 (0.80, 0.99)	0.87 (0.75, 1.00)	0.75 (0.55, 1.00)
Nevirapine	200 QD, 14 days; BID, 6 days	400/100 BID, 20 d	5, 9*	0.95 (0.73, 1.25)	0.99 (0.74, 1.32)	1.02 (0.68, 1.53)
	7 mg/kg or 4 mg/kg QD, 2 wk; BID 1 wk[3]	300/75 mg/m² BID, 3 wk	12, 15*	0.86 (0.64, 1.16)	0.78 (0.56, 1.09)	0.45 (0.25, 0.81)
Pravastatin	20 QD, 4 d	400/100 BID, 14 d	12	0.98 (0.89, 1.08)	0.95 (0.85, 1.05)	0.88 (0.77, 1.02)
Rifabutin	150 QD, 10 d	400/100 BID, 20 d	14	1.08 (0.97, 1.19)	1.17 (1.04, 1.31)	1.20 (0.96, 1.65)
Rifampin	600 QD, 10 d	400/100 BID, 20 d	22	0.45 (0.40, 0.51)	0.25 (0.21, 0.29)	0.01 (0.01, 0.02)
Ritonavir[4]	100 BID, 3-4 wk	400/100 BID, 3-4 wk	8, 21*	1.28 (0.94, 1.76)	1.46 (1.04, 2.06)	2.16 (1.29, 3.62)

All interaction studies conducted in healthy, HIV-negative subjects unless otherwise indicated.

[1] Composite effect of amprenavir 450 and 750 mg Q12h regimens on lopinavir pharmacokinetics.

[2] The pharmacokinetics of ritonavir are unaffected by concurrent efavirenz.

[3] Study conducted in HIV-positive pediatric subjects ranging in age from 6 months to 12 years.

[4] Study conducted in HIV-positive adult subjects.

* Parallel group design; n for KALETRA + co-administered drug, n for KALETRA alone.

Absorption: In a pharmacokinetic study in HIV-positive subjects (n=21) without meal restrictions, multiple dosing with 400/100 mg KALETRA BID for 3 to 4 weeks produced a mean ± SD lopinavir peak plasma concentration (C_{max}) of 9.6 ± 4.4 µg/mL, occurring approximately 4 hours after administration. The mean steady-state trough concentration prior to the morning dose was 5.5 ± 4.0 µg/mL. Lopinavir AUC over a 12 hour dosing interval averaged 82.8 ± 44.5 µg•h/mL. The absolute bioavailability of lopinavir co-formulated with ritonavir in humans has not been established. Under nonfasting conditions (500 kcal, 25% from fat), lopinavir concentrations were similar following administration of KALETRA co-formulated capsules and liquid. When administered under fasting conditions, both the mean AUC and C_{max} of lopinavir were 22% lower for the KALETRA liquid relative to the capsule formulation.

Effects of Food on Oral Absorption: Administration of a single 400/100 mg dose of KALETRA capsules with a moderate fat meal (500-682 kcal, 23 to 25% calories from fat) was associated with a mean increase of 48 and 23% in lopinavir AUC and C_{max}, respectively, relative to fasting. For KALETRA oral solution, the corresponding increases in lopinavir AUC and C_{max} were 80 and 54%, respectively. Relative to fasting, administration of KALETRA with a high fat meal (872 kcal, 56% from fat) increased lopinavir AUC and C_{max} by 97 and 43%, respectively, for capsules, and 130 and 56%, respectively, for oral solution. To enhance bioavailability and minimize pharmacokinetic variability KALETRA should be taken with food.

Distribution: At steady state, lopinavir is approximately 98-99% bound to plasma proteins. Lopinavir binds to both alpha-1-acid glycoprotein (AAG) and albumin; however, it has a higher affinity for AAG. At steady state, lopinavir protein binding remains constant over the range of observed concentrations after 400/100 mg KALETRA BID, and is similar between healthy volunteers and HIV-positive patients.

Metabolism: *In vitro* experiments with human hepatic microsomes indicate that lopinavir primarily undergoes oxidative metabolism. Lopinavir is extensively metabolized by the hepatic cytochrome P450 system, almost exclusively by the CYP3A isozyme. Ritonavir is a potent CYP3A inhibitor which inhibits the metabolism of lopinavir, and therefore increases plasma levels of lopinavir. A ^{14}C-lopinavir study in humans showed that 89% of the plasma radioactivity after a single 400/100 mg KALETRA dose was due to parent drug. At least 13 lopinavir oxidative metabolites have been identified in man. Ritonavir has been shown to induce metabolic enzymes, resulting in the induction of its own metabolism. Pre-dose lopinavir concentrations decline with time during multiple dosing, stabilizing after approximately 10 to 16 days.

Elimination: Following a 400/100 mg ^{14}C-lopinavir/ritonavir dose, approximately 10.4 ± 2.3% and 82.6 ± 2.5% of an administered dose of ^{14}C-lopinavir can be accounted for in urine and feces, respectively, after 8 days. Unchanged lopinavir accounted for approximately 2.2 and 19.8% of the administered dose in urine and feces, respectively. After multiple dosing, less than 3% of the lopinavir dose is excreted unchanged in the urine. The half-life of lopinavir over a 12 hour dosing interval averaged 5-6 hours, and the apparent oral clearance (CL/F) of lopinavir is 6 to 7 L/h.

Special Populations:

Gender, Race and Age: Lopinavir pharmacokinetics have not been studied in elderly patients. No gender related pharmacokinetic differences have been observed in adult patients. No clinically important pharmacokinetic differences due to race have been identified.

Pediatric Patients: The pharmacokinetics of KALETRA 300/75 mg/m² BID and 230/57.5 mg/m² BID have been studied in a total of 53 pediatric patients, ranging in age from 6 months to 12 years. The 230/57.5 mg/m² BID regimen without nevirapine and the 300/75 mg/m² BID regimen with nevirapine provided lopinavir plasma concentrations similar to those obtained in adult patients receiving the 400/100 mg BID regimen (without nevirapine).

The mean steady-state lopinavir AUC, C_{max}, and C_{min} were 72.6 ± 31.1 µg•h/mL, 8.2 ± 2.9 and 3.4 ± 2.1 µg/mL, respectively after KALETRA 230/57.5 mg/m² BID without nevirapine (n=12), and were 85.8 ± 36.9 µg•h/mL, 10.0 ± 3.3 and 3.6 ± 3.5 µg/mL, respectively, after 300/75 mg/m² BID with nevirapine (n=12). The nevirapine regimen was 7 mg/kg BID (6 months to 8 years) or 4 mg/kg BID (>8 years).

Renal Insufficiency: Lopinavir pharmacokinetics have not been studied in patients with renal insufficiency; however, since the renal clearance of lopinavir is negligible, a decrease in total body clearance is not expected in patients with renal insufficiency.

Hepatic Impairment: Lopinavir is principally metabolized and eliminated by the liver. Although KALETRA has not been studied in patients with hepatic impairment, lopinavir concentrations may be increased in these patients (see **PRECAUTIONS**).

Drug-Drug Interactions: See also **CONTRAINDICATIONS, WARNINGS and PRECAUTIONS: Drug Interactions.**

KALETRA is an inhibitor of the P450 isoform CYP3A *in vitro*. Co-administration of KALETRA and drugs primarily metabolized by CYP3A may result in increased plasma concentrations of the other drug, which could increase or prolong its therapeutic and adverse effects (see **CONTRAINDICATIONS**).

KALETRA inhibits CYP2D6 *in vitro*, but to a lesser extent than CYP3A. Clinically significant drug interactions with drugs metabolized by CYP2D6 are possible with KALETRA at the recommended dose, but the magnitude is not known. KALETRA does not inhibit CYP2C9, CYP2C19, CYP2E1, CYP2B6 or CYP1A2 at clinically relevant concentrations.

KALETRA has been shown *in vivo* to induce its own metabolism and to increase the biotransformation of some drugs metabolized by cytochrome P450 enzymes and by glucuronidation.

KALETRA is metabolized by CYP3A. Drugs that induce CYP3A activity would be expected to increase the clearance of lopinavir, resulting in lowered plasma concentrations of lopinavir. Although not noted with concurrent ketoconazole, co-administration of KALETRA and other drugs that inhibit CYP3A may increase lopinavir plasma concentrations.

Continued on next page

Kaletra—Cont.

Drug interaction studies were performed with KALETRA and other drugs likely to be coadministered and some drugs commonly used as probes for pharmacokinetic interactions. The effects of co-administration of KALETRA on the AUC, C_{max} and C_{min} are summarized in Table 2 (effect of other drugs on lopinavir) and Table 3 (effect of KALETRA on other drugs). The effects of other drugs on ritonavir are not shown since they generally correlate with those observed with lopinavir (if lopinavir concentrations are decreased, ritonavir concentrations are decreased) unless otherwise indicated in the table footnotes. For information regarding clinical recommendations, see Table 8 in **PRECAUTIONS**.

[See table at top of previous page]

[See table 3 above]

Effect of KALETRA on other Protease Inhibitors (PIs): The pharmacokinetics of single-dose indinavir and saquinavir, and multiple-dose amprenavir obtained in healthy subjects after at least 10 days of KALETRA 400/100 mg BID were compared to historical data in HIV-infected subjects (refer to Table 3 for information on study design and doses). Because of the limitations in the study design and the use of comparisons between healthy and HIV infected subjects, it is not possible to recommend definitive dosing recommendations. However, based on these comparisons, amprenavir 750 mg BID and indinavir 600 mg BID, when co-administered with KALETRA 400/100 mg BID, may produce a similar AUC, lower C_{max}, and higher C_{min} compared to their respective established clinical dosing regimens. Saquinavir 800 mg BID, when co-administered with KALETRA 400/100 mg BID, may produce a similar AUC and higher C_{min} to its respective established clinical dosing regimen (no comparative information regarding C_{max}). The clinical significance of the lower C_{max} and higher C_{min} is unknown. Appropriate doses of amprenavir, indinavir and saquinavir in combination with KALETRA with respect to safety and efficacy have not been established (see **PRECAUTIONS** – Table 8).

INDICATIONS AND USAGE

KALETRA is indicated in combination with other antiretroviral agents for the treatment of HIV-infection. This indication is based on analyses of plasma HIV RNA levels and CD4 cell counts in a controlled study of KALETRA of 48 weeks duration and in smaller uncontrolled dose-ranging studies of KALETRA of 72 weeks duration. At present, there are no results from controlled trials evaluating the effect of KALETRA on clinical progression of HIV.

Description of Clinical Studies

Patients Without Prior Antiretroviral Therapy

Study 863: KALETRA BID + stavudine + lamivudine compared to nelfinavir TID + stavudine + lamivudine

Study 863 is an ongoing, randomized, double-blind, multicenter trial comparing treatment with KALETRA (400/100 mg BID) plus stavudine and lamivudine versus nelfinavir (750 mg TID) plus stavudine and lamivudine in 653 antiretroviral treatment naive patients. Patients had a mean age of 38 years (range: 19 to 84), 57% were Caucasian, and 80% were male. Mean baseline CD4 cell count was 259 cells/mm³ (range: 2 to 949 cells/mm³) and mean baseline plasma HIV-1 RNA was 4.9 log_{10} copies/mL (range: 2.6 to 6.8 log_{10} copies/mL).

Treatment response and outcomes of randomized treatment are presented in Figure 2 and Table 4, respectively.

Figure 2: Virologic Response Through Week 48, Study 863*†

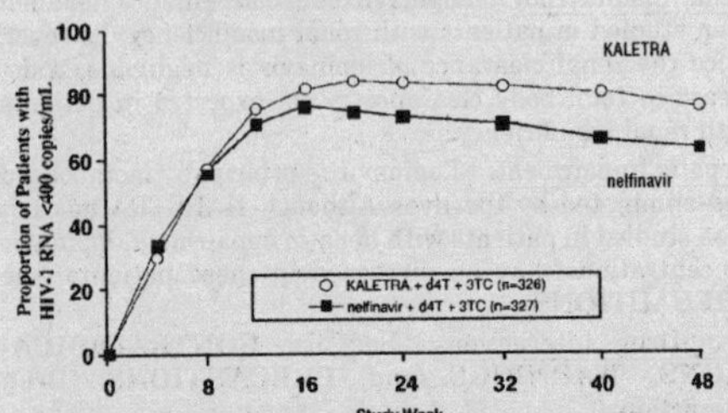

* Roche AMPLICOR HIV-1 MONITOR Assay.
† Responders at each visit are patients who had achieved and maintained HIV-1 RNA <400 copies/mL without discontinuation by that visit.

Table 3: Drug Interactions: Pharmacokinetic Parameters for Co-administered Drug in the Presence of KALETRA (See Precautions, Table 8 for Recommended Alterations in Dose or Regimen)

Co-administered Drug	Dose of Co-administered Drug (mg)	Dose of KALETRA (mg)	n	Ratio (with/without KALETRA) of Co-administered Drug Pharmacokinetic Parameters (90% CI); No Effect = 1.00		
				C_{max}	AUC	C_{min}
Amprenavir	450 BID, 5 d 750 BID, 5 d	400/100 BID, 22 d	12 10	See text below for discussion of interaction.		
Atorvastatin	20 QD, 4 d	400/100 BID, 14 d	12	4.67 (3.35, 6.51)	5.88 (4.69, 7.37)	2.28 (1.91, 2.71)
Efavirenz	600 QHS, 9 d	400/100 BID, 9 d	11, 12*	0.91 (0.72, 1.15)	0.84 (0.62, 1.15)	0.84 (0.58, 1.20)
Ethinyl Estradiol	35 µg QD, 21 d (Ortho Novum®)	400/100 BID, 14 d	12	0.59 (0.52, 0.66)	0.58 (0.54, 0.62)	0.42 (0.36, 0.49)
Indinavir	600 single dose	400/100 BID, 10 d	11	See text below for discussion of interaction.		
Ketoconazole	200 single dose	400/100 BID, 16 d	12	1.13 (0.91, 1.40)	3.04 (2.44, 3.79)	N/A
Methadone	5 single dose	400/100 BID, 10 d	11	0.55 (0.48, 0.64)	0.47 (0.42, 0.53)	N/A
Nevirapine	200 QD, 14 d; BID, 6 d	400/100 BID, 20 d	5, 6*	1.05 (0.72, 1.52)	1.08 (0.72, 1.64)	1.15 (0.71, 1.86)
Norethindrone	1 QD, 21 d (Ortho Novum®)	400/100 BID, 14 d	12	0.84 (0.75, 0.94)	0.83 (0.73, 0.94)	0.68 (0.54, 0.85)
Pravastatin	20 QD, 4 d	400/100 BID, 14 d	12	1.26 (0.87, 1.83)	1.33 (0.91, 1.94)	N/A
Rifabutin	300 QD, 10 d; 150 QD, 10 d	400/100 BID, 10 d	12	2.12 (1.89, 2.38)	3.03 (2.79, 3.30)	4.90 (3.18, 5.76)
25-*O*-des-acetyl rifabutin				23.6 (13.7, 25.3)	47.5 (29.3, 51.8)	94.9 (74.0, 122)
Rifampin + 25-*O*-des-acetyl rifabutin[1]				3.46 (3.07, 3.91)	5.73 (5.08, 6.46)	9.53 (7.56, 12.01)
Saquinavir	800 single dose	400/100 BID, 10 d	11	See text below for discussion of interaction.		

All interaction studies conducted in healthy, HIV-negative subjects unless otherwise indicated.
[1] Effect on the dose-normalized sum of rifabutin parent and 25-O-desacetyl rifabutin active metabolite.
*Parallel group design; n for KALETRA + co-administered drug, n for co-administered drug alone.
N/A=not available.

Table 5: Proportion of Responders Through Week 48 by Baseline Viral Load (Study 863)

Baseline Viral Load (HIV-1 RNA copies/mL)	KALETRA +d4T + 3TC			Nelfinavir +d4T+ 3TC		
	<400 copies/mL[1]	<50 copies/mL[2]	n	<400 copies/mL[1]	<50 copies/mL[2]	n
<30,000	74%	71%	82	79%	72%	87
≥30,000 to <100,000	81%	73%	79	67%	54%	79
≥100,000 to <250,000	75%	64%	83	60%	47%	72
≥250,000	72%	60%	82	44%	33%	89

[1] Patients achieved and maintained confirmed HIV RNA <400 copies/mL through Week 48.
[2] Patients achieved HIV RNA <50 copies/mL at Week 48.

Table 4: Outcomes of Randomized Treatment Through Week 48 (Study 863)

Outcome	KALETRA +d4T + 3TC (N=326)	Nelfinavir +d4T + 3TC (N=327)
Responder* [1]	75%	62%
Virologic failure[2]	9%	25%
Rebound	7%	15%
Never suppressed through Week 48	2%	9%
Death	2%	1%
Discontinued due to adverse event	4%	4%
Discontinued for other reasons[3]	10%	8%

*Corresponds to rates at Week 48 in Figure 2.
[1] Patients achieved and maintained confirmed HIV RNA <400 copies/mL through Week 48.
[2] Includes confirmed viral rebound and failure to achieve confirmed <400 copies/mL through Week 48.
[3] Includes lost to follow-up, patient's withdrawl, non-compliance, protocol violation and other reasons.

Through 48 weeks of therapy, there was a statistically significantly higher proportion of patients in the KALETRA arm compared to the nelfinavir arm with HIV RNA <400 copies/mL (75% vs. 62%, respectively) and HIV RNA <50 copies/mL (67% vs. 52%, respectively). Treatment response by baseline HIV RNA level subgroups is presented in Table 5.

[See table 5 above]

Through 48 weeks of therapy, the mean increase from baseline in CD4 cell count was 207 cells/mm³ for the KALETRA arm and 195 cells/mm³ for the nelfinavir arm.

Study 720: KALETRA BID + stavudine + lamivudine

Study 720 is an ongoing, randomized, blinded, multicenter trial evaluating treatment with KALETRA at three dose levels (Group I: 200/100 mg BID and 400/100 mg BID; Group II: 400/100 mg BID and 400/200 mg BID) plus lamivudine (150 mg BID) and stavudine (40 mg BID) in 100 patients. All patients were converted to open-label KALETRA at the 400/100 mg BID dose between weeks 48 and 72 of the study. Patients had a mean age of 35 years (range: 21 to 59), 70% were Caucasian, and 96% were male. Mean baseline CD4 cell count was 338 cells/mm³ (range: 3 to 918 cells/mm³) and mean baseline plasma HIV-1 RNA was 4.9 log_{10} copies/mL (range: 3.3 to 6.3 log_{10} copies/mL).

Through 72 weeks of treatment, the proportion of patients with HIV RNA < 400 (<50) copies/mL was 80% (78%) and the mean increase from baseline in CD4 cell count was 256 cells/mm³ for the 51 patients originally randomized to the 400/100 mg dose of KALETRA. At 72 weeks, 13 patients (13%) had discontinued the study for any reason. Four discontinuations (4%) were secondary to adverse events or laboratory abnormalities, and one of these discontinuations (1%) was attributed to a KALETRA adverse event.

Patients with Prior Antiretroviral Therapy

Study 765: KALETRA BID + nevirapine + NRTIs

Study 765 is an ongoing, randomized, blinded, multicenter trial evaluating treatment with KALETRA at two dose levels (400/100 mg BID and 400/200 mg BID) plus nevirapine (200 mg BID) and two NRTIs in 70 single protease inhibitor experienced, non-nucleoside reverse transcriptase inhibitor (NNRTI) naive patients. Patients had a mean age of 40 years (range 22-66), were 73% Caucasian, and were 90% male. Mean baseline CD4 cell count was 372 cells/mm³ (range 72 to 807 cells/µL) and mean baseline plasma HIV-1 RNA was 4.0 log_{10} copies/mL (range 2.9 to 5.8 log_{10} copies/mL).

Through 72 weeks of treatment, the proportion of patients with HIV RNA < 400 (<50) copies/mL was 75% (58%) and the mean increase from baseline in CD4 cell count was 174 cells/mm^3 for the 36 patients receiving the 400/100 mg dose of KALETRA. At 72 weeks, 13 patients (19%) had discontinued the study for any reason. Six discontinuations (9%) were secondary to adverse events or laboratory abnormalities, and three of these discontinuations (4%) were attributed to KALETRA adverse events.

CONTRAINDICATIONS

KALETRA is contraindicated in patients with known hypersensitivity to any of its ingredients, including ritonavir.

Co-administration of KALETRA is contraindicated with drugs that are highly dependent on CYP3A or CYP2D6 for clearance and for which elevated plasma concentrations are associated with serious and/or life-threatening events. These drugs are listed in Table 6.

Table 6: Drugs That Are Contraindicated With KALETRA

Drug Class	Drugs Within Class That Are Contraindicated With KALETRA
Antiarrhythmics	Flecainide, Propafenone
Antihistamines	Astemizole, Terfenadine
Ergot Derivatives	Dihydroergotamine, Ergonovine, Ergotamine, Methylergonovine
GI motility agent	Cisapride
Neuroleptic	Pimozide
Sedative/hypnotics	Midazolam, Triazolam

WARNINGS

ALERT: Find out about medicines that should NOT be taken with KALETRA. This statement is included on the product's bottle label.

Drug Interactions

KALETRA is an inhibitor of the P450 isoform CYP3A. Co-administration of KALETRA and drugs primarily metabolized by CYP3A or CYP2D6 may result in increased plasma concentrations of the other drug that could increase or prolong its therapeutic and adverse effects (see **Pharmacokinetics: Drug-Drug Interactions, CONTRAINDICATIONS – Table 6: Drugs That Are Contraindicated With KALETRA, PRECAUTIONS – Table 7: Drugs That Should Not Be Co-administered With KALETRA** and **Table 8: Established and Other Potentially Significant Drug Interactions**).

Particular caution should be used when prescribing sildenafil in patients receiving KALETRA. Co-administration of KALETRA with sildenafil is expected to substantially increase sildenafil concentrations and may result in an increase in sildenafil-associated adverse events including hypotension, syncope, visual changes and prolonged erection (see **PRECAUTIONS: Drug Interactions** and the complete prescribing information for sildenafil).

Concomitant use of KALETRA with lovastatin or simvastatin is not recommended. Caution should be exercised if HIV protease inhibitors, including KALETRA, are used concurrently with other HMG-CoA reductase inhibitors that are also metabolized by the CYP3A4 pathway (e.g., atorvastatin). The risk of myopathy, including rhabdomyolysis may be increased when HIV protease inhibitors, including KALETRA, are used in combination with these drugs.

Concomitant use of KALETRA and St. John's wort (hypericum perforatum), or products containing St. John's wort, is not recommended. Co-administration of protease inhibitors, including KALETRA, with St. John's wort is expected to substantially decrease protease inhibitor concentrations and may result in sub-optimal levels of lopinavir and lead to loss of virologic response and possible resistance to lopinavir or to the class of protease inhibitors.

Pancreatitis

Pancreatitis has been observed in patients receiving KALETRA therapy, including those who developed marked triglyceride elevations. In some cases, fatalities have been observed. Although a causal relationship to KALETRA has not been established, marked triglyceride elevations is a risk factor for development of pancreatitis (see **PRECAUTIONS - Lipid Elevations**). Patients with advanced HIV disease may be at increased risk of elevated triglycerides and pancreatitis, and patients with a history of pancreatitis may be at increased risk of recurrence during KALETRA therapy.

Pancreatitis should be considered if clinical symptoms (nausea, vomiting, abdominal pain) or abnormalities in laboratory values (such as increased serum lipase or amylase values) suggestive of pancreatitis should occur. Patients who exhibit these signs or symptoms should be evaluated and KALETRA and/or other antiretroviral therapy should be suspended as clinically appropriate.

Diabetes Mellitus/Hyperglycemia

New onset diabetes mellitus, exacerbation of pre-existing diabetes mellitus, and hyperglycemia have been reported during postmarketing surveillance in HIV-infected patients receiving protease inhibitor therapy. Some patients required either initiation or dose adjustments of insulin or oral hypoglycemic agents for treatment of these events. In some cases, diabetic ketoacidosis has occurred. In those patients who discontinued protease inhibitor therapy, hyperglycemia persisted in some cases. Because these events have been reported voluntarily during clinical practice, estimates of frequency cannot be made and a causal relationship between protease inhibitor therapy and these events has not been established.

PRECAUTIONS

Hepatic Impairment and Toxicity

KALETRA is principally metabolized by the liver; therefore, caution should be exercised when administering this drug to patients with hepatic impairment, because lopinavir concentrations may be increased. Patients with underlying hepatitis B or C or marked elevations in transaminases prior to treatment may be at increased risk for developing further transaminase elevations or hepatic decompensation. There have been postmarketing reports of hepatic dysfunction, including some fatalities. These have generally occurred in patients with advanced HIV disease taking multiple concomitant medications in the setting of underlying chronic hepatitis or cirrhosis. A causal relationship with KALETRA therapy has not been established. Increased AST/ALT monitoring should be considered in these patients, especially during the first several months of KALETRA treatment.

Resistance/Cross-resistance

Various degrees of cross-resistance among protease inhibitors have been observed. The effect of KALETRA therapy on the efficacy of subsequently administered protease inhibitors is under investigation (see **MICROBIOLOGY**).

Hemophilia

There have been reports of increased bleeding, including spontaneous skin hematomas and hemarthrosis, in patients with hemophilia type A and B treated with protease inhibitors. In some patients additional factor VIII was given. In more than half of the reported cases, treatment with protease inhibitors was continued or reintroduced. A causal relationship between protease inhibitor therapy and these events has not been established.

Fat Redistribution

Redistribution/accumulation of body fat including central obesity, dorsocervical fat enlargement (buffalo hump), peripheral wasting, facial wasting, breast enlargement, and "cushingoid appearance" have been observed in patients receiving antiretroviral therapy. The mechanism and long-term consequences of these events are currently unknown. A causal relationship has not been established.

Lipid Elevations

Treatment with KALETRA has resulted in large increases in the concentration of total cholesterol and triglycerides (see **ADVERSE REACTIONS** – Table 10). Triglyceride and cholesterol testing should be performed prior to initiating KALETRA therapy and at periodic intervals during therapy. Lipid disorders should be managed as clinically appropriate. See **PRECAUTIONS Table 8: Established and Other Potentially Significant Drug Interactions** for additional information on potential drug interactions with KALETRA and HMG-CoA reductase inhibitors.

Information for Patients

A statement to patients and health care providers is included on the product's bottle label: **"ALERT: Find out about medicines that should NOT be taken with KALETRA."** A Patient Package Insert (PPI) for KALETRA is available for patient information.

Patients should be told that sustained decreases in plasma HIV RNA have been associated with a reduced risk of progression to AIDS and death. Patients should remain under the care of a physician while using KALETRA. Patients should be advised to take KALETRA and other concomitant antiretroviral therapy every day as prescribed. KALETRA must always be used in combination with other antiretroviral drugs. Patients should not alter the dose or discontinue therapy without consulting with their doctor. If a dose of KALETRA is missed patients should take the dose as soon as possible and then return to their normal schedule. However, if a dose is skipped the patient should not double the next dose.

Patients should be informed that KALETRA is not a cure for HIV infection and that they may continue to develop opportunistic infections and other complications associated with HIV disease. The long-term effects of KALETRA are unknown at this time. Patients should be told that there are currently no data demonstrating that therapy with KALETRA can reduce the risk of transmitting HIV to others through sexual contact.

KALETRA may interact with some drugs; therefore, patients should be advised to report to their doctor the use of any other prescription, non-prescription medication or herbal products, particularly St. John's wort.

Patients taking didanosine should take didanosine one hour before or two hours after KALETRA.

Patients receiving sildenafil should be advised that they may be at an increased risk of sildenafil-associated adverse events including hypotension, visual changes, and sustained erection, and should promptly report any symptoms to their doctor.

Patients receiving estrogen-based hormonal contraceptives should be instructed that additional or alternate contraceptive measures should be used during therapy with KALETRA.

KALETRA should be taken with food to enhance absorption.

Patients should be informed that redistribution or accumulation of body fat may occur in patients receiving antiretroviral therapy and that the cause and long term health effects of these conditions are not known at this time.

Drug Interactions

KALETRA is an inhibitor of CYP3A (cytochrome P450 3A) both *in vitro* and *in vivo*. Co-administration of KALETRA and drugs primarily metabolized by CYP3A (e.g., dihydropyridine calcium channel blockers, HMG-CoA reductase inhibitors, immunosuppressants and sildenafil) may result in increased plasma concentrations of the other drugs that could increase or prolong their therapeutic and adverse effects (see **Table 8: Established and Other Potentially Significant Drug Interactions**). Agents that are extensively metabolized by CYP3A and have high first pass metabolism appear to be the most susceptible to large increases in AUC (>3-fold) when co-administered with KALETRA.

KALETRA inhibits CYP2D6 *in vitro*, but to a lesser extent than CYP3A. Clinically significant drug interactions with drugs metabolized by CYP2D6 are possible with KALETRA at the recommended dose, but the magnitude is not known.

KALETRA does not inhibit CYP2C9, CYP2C19, CYP2E1, CYP2B6 or CYP1A2 at clinically relevant concentrations.

KALETRA has been shown *in vivo* to induce its own metabolism and to increase the biotransformation of some drugs metabolized by cytochrome P450 enzymes and by glucuronidation.

KALETRA is metabolized by CYP3A. Co-administration of KALETRA and drugs that induce CYP3A may decrease lopinavir plasma concentrations and reduce its therapeutic effect (see **Table 8: Established and Other Potentially Significant Drug Interactions**). Although not noted with concurrent ketoconazole, co-administration of KALETRA and other drugs that inhibit CYP3A may increase lopinavir plasma concentrations.

Drugs that are contraindicated and not recommended for co-administration with KALETRA are included in **Table 7: Drugs That Should Not be Co-administered With KALETRA.** These recommendations are based on either drug interaction studies or predicted interactions due to the expected magnitude of interaction and potential for serious events or loss of efficacy.

[See table 7 at top of next page]

[See table 8 on pages 88 and 89]

Other Drugs:

Drug interaction studies reveal no clinically significant interaction between KALETRA and pravastatin, stavudine or lamivudine.

Based on known metabolic profiles, clinically significant drug interactions are not expected between KALETRA and fluvastatin, dapsone, trimethoprim/sulfamethoxazole, azithromycin, erythromycin, or fluconazole.

Zidovudine and Abacavir: KALETRA induces glucuronidation; therefore, KALETRA has the potential to reduce zidovudine and abacavir plasma concentrations. The clinical significance of this potential interaction is unknown.

Carcinogenesis, Mutagenesis and Impairment of Fertility

Long-term carcinogenicity studies of KALETRA in animal systems have not been completed.

Carcinogenicity studies in mice and rats have been carried out on ritonavir. In male mice, at levels of 50, 100 or 200 mg/kg/day, there was a dose dependent increase in the incidence of both adenomas and combined adenomas and carcinomas in the liver. Based on AUC measurements, the exposure at the high dose was approximately 4-fold for males that of the exposure in humans with the recommended therapeutic dose (400/100 mg KALETRA BID). There were no carcinogenic effects seen in females at the dosages tested. The exposure at the high dose was approximately 9-fold for the females that of the exposure in humans. In rats dosed at levels of 7, 15 or 30 mg/kg/day there were no carcinogenic effects. In this study, the exposure at the high dose was approximately 0.7-fold that of the exposure in humans with the 400/100 mg KALETRA BID regimen. Based on the exposures achieved in the animal studies, the significance of the observed effects is not known. However, neither lopinavir nor ritonavir was found to be mutagenic or clastogenic in a battery of *in vitro* and *in vivo* assays including the Ames bacterial reverse mutation assay using *S. typhimurium* and *E. coli*, the mouse lymphoma assay, the mouse micronucleus test and chromosomal aberration assays in human lymphocytes.

Lopinavir in combination with ritonavir at a 2:1 ratio produced no effects on fertility in male and female rats at levels of 10/5, 30/15 or 100/50 mg/kg/day. Based on AUC measurements, the exposures in rats at the high doses were approximately 0.7-fold for lopinavir and 1.8-fold for ritonavir of the exposures in humans at the recommended therapeutic dose (400/100 mg BID).

Pregnancy

Pregnancy Category C: No treatment-related malformations were observed when lopinavir in combination with ritonavir was administered to pregnant rats or rabbits. Embryonic and fetal developmental toxicities (early resorption, decreased fetal viability, decreased fetal body weight, increased incidence of skeletal variations and skeletal ossification delays) occurred in rats at a maternally toxic dosage (100/50 mg/kg/day). Based on AUC measurements, the drug exposures in rats at 100/50 mg/kg/day were approximately 0.7-fold for lopinavir and 1.8-fold for ritonavir for males and females that of the exposures in humans at the recommended therapeutic dose (400/100 mg BID). In a peri- and postnatal study in rats, a developmental toxicity (a decrease in survival in pups between birth and postnatal day 21) occurred at 40/20 mg/kg/day and greater.

Continued on next page

Kaletra—Cont.

No embryonic and fetal developmental toxicities were observed in rabbits at a maternally toxic dosage (80/40 mg/kg/day). Based on AUC measurements, the drug exposures in rabbits at 80/40 mg/kg/day were approximately 0.6-fold for lopinavir and 1.0-fold for ritonavir that of the exposures in humans at the recommended therapeutic dose (400/100 mg BID). There are, however, no adequate and well-controlled studies in pregnant women. KALETRA should be used during pregnancy only if the potential benefit justifies the potential risk to the fetus.

Antiretroviral Pregnancy Registry: To monitor maternal-fetal outcomes of pregnant women exposed to KALETRA, an Antiretroviral Pregnancy Registry has been established. Physicians are encouraged to register patients by calling 1-800-258-4263.

Nursing Mothers: The Centers for Disease Control and Prevention recommend that HIV-infected mothers not breast-feed their infants to avoid risking postnatal transmission of HIV. Studies in rats have demonstrated that lopinavir is secreted in milk. It is not known whether lopinavir is secreted in human milk. Because of both the potential for HIV transmission and the potential for serious adverse reactions in nursing infants, mothers should be instructed **not to breast-feed if they are receiving KALETRA.**

Geriatric Use

Clinical studies of KALETRA did not include sufficient numbers of subjects aged 65 and over to determine whether they respond differently from younger subjects. In general, appropriate caution should be exercised in the administration and monitoring of KALETRA in elderly patients reflecting the greater frequency of decreased hepatic, renal, or cardiac function, and of concomitant disease or other drug therapy.

Pediatric Use

The safety and pharmacokinetic profiles of KALETRA in pediatric patients below the age of 6 months have not been established. In HIV-infected patients age 6 months to 12 years, the adverse event profile seen during a clinical trial was similar to that for adult patients. The evaluation of the antiviral activity of KALETRA in pediatric patients in clinical trials is ongoing.

Study 940 is an ongoing open-label, multicenter trial evaluating the pharmacokinetic profile, tolerability, safety and efficacy of KALETRA oral solution containing lopinavir 80 mg/mL and ritonavir 20 mg/mL in 100 antiretroviral naive (44%) and experienced (56%) pediatric patients. All patients were non-nucleoside reverse transcriptase inhibitor naive. Patients were randomized to either 230 mg lopinavir/57.5 mg ritonavir per m^2 or 300 mg lopinavir/75 mg ritonavir per m^2. Naive patients also received lamivudine and stavudine. Experienced patients received nevirapine plus up to two nucleoside reverse transcriptase inhibitors. Safety, efficacy and pharmacokinetic profiles of the two dose regimens were assessed after three weeks of therapy in each patient. After analysis of these data, all patients were continued on the 300 mg lopinavir/75 mg ritonavir per m^2 dose. Patients had a mean age of 5 years (range 6 months to 12 years) with 14% less than 2 years. Mean baseline CD4 cell count was 838 cells/mm^3 and mean baseline plasma HIV-1 RNA was 4.7 log_{10} copies/mL.

Through 48 weeks of therapy, the proportion of patients who achieved and sustained an HIV RNA < 400 copies/mL was 80% for antiretroviral naive patients and 71% for antiretroviral experienced patients. The mean increase from baseline in CD4 cell count was 404 cells/mm^3 for antiretroviral naive and 284 cells/mm^3 for antiretroviral experienced patients treated through 48 weeks. At 48 weeks, two patients (2%) had prematurely discontinued the study. One antiretroviral naive patient prematurely discontinued secondary to an adverse event attributed to KALETRA, while one antiretroviral experienced patient prematurely discontinued secondary to an HIV-related event.

Dose selection for patients 6 months to 12 years of age was based on the following results. The 230/57.5 mg/m^2 BID regimen without nevirapine and the 300/75 mg/m^2 BID regimen with nevirapine provided lopinavir plasma concentrations similar to those obtained in adult patients receiving the 400/100 mg BID regimen (without nevirapine).

ADVERSE REACTIONS

Adults:

Treatment-Emergent Adverse Events: KALETRA has been studied in 612 patients as combination therapy in Phase I/II and Phase III clinical trials. The most common adverse event associated with KALETRA therapy was diarrhea, which was generally of mild to moderate severity. Rates of discontinuation of randomized therapy due to adverse events were 5.8% in KALETRA-treated and 4.9% in nelfinavir-treated patients in Study 863.

Drug related clinical adverse events of moderate or severe intensity in ≥ 2% of patients treated with combination therapy including KALETRA for up to 48 weeks (Phase III) and for up to 72 weeks (Phase I/II) are presented in Table 9. For other information regarding observed or potentially serious adverse events, please see **WARNINGS** and **PRECAUTIONS**.

[See table 9 at top of page 90]

Treatment-emergent adverse events occurring in less than 2% of adult patients receiving KALETRA in all phase II/III clinical trials and considered at least possibly related or of unknown relationship to treatment with KALETRA and of at least moderate intensity are listed below by body system.

Table 7: Drugs That Should Not Be Co-administered With KALETRA

Drug Class: Drug Name	Clinical Comment
Antiarrhythmics: flecainide, propafenone	CONTRAINDICATED due to potential for serious and/or life-threatening reactions such as cardiac arrhythmias.
Antihistamines: astemizole, terfenadine	CONTRAINDICATED due to potential for serious and/or life-threatening reactions such as cardiac arrhythmias.
Antimycobacterial: rifampin	May lead to loss of virologic response and possible resistance to KALETRA or to the class of protease inhibitors or other co-administered antiretroviral agents.
Ergot Derivatives: dihydroergotamine, ergonovine, ergotamine, methylergonovine	CONTRAINDICATED due to potential for serious and/or life-threatening reactions such as acute ergot toxicity characterized by peripheral vasospasm and ischemia of the extremities and other tissues.
GI Motility Agent: cisapride	CONTRAINDICATED due to potential for serious and/or life-threatening reactions such as cardiac arrhythmias.
Herbal Products: St. John's wort (hypericum perforatum)	May lead to loss of virologic response and possible resistance to KALETRA or to the class of protease inhibitors.
HMG-CoA Reductase Inhibitors: lovastatin, simvastatin	Potential for serious reactions such as risk of myopathy including rhabdomyolysis.
Neuroleptic: pimozide	CONTRAINDICATED due to the potential for serious and/or life-threatening reactions such as cardiac arrhythmias.
Sedative/Hypnotics: midazolam, triazolam	CONTRAINDICATED due to potential for serious and/or life-threatening reactions such as prolonged or increased sedation or respiratory depression.

Table 8: Established and Other Potentially Significant Drug Interactions: Alteration in Dose or Regimen May Be Recommended Based on Drug Interaction Studies or Predicted Interaction (See CLINICAL PHARMACOLOGY for Magnitude of Interaction, Tables 2 and 3)

Concomitant Drug Class: Drug Name	Effect on Concentration of lopinavir or Concomitant Drug	Clinical Comment
	HIV-Antiviral Agents	
Non-nucleoside Reverse Transcriptase Inhibitors: efavirenz*, nevirapine*	↓ Lopinavir	A dose increase of KALETRA to 533/133 mg (4 capsules or 6.5 mL) twice daily taken with food should be considered when used in combination with efavirenz or nevirapine in patients where reduced susceptibility to lopinavir is clinically suspected (by treatment history or laboratory evidence) (see **DOSAGE AND ADMINISTRATION**). NOTE: Efavirenz and nevirapine induce the activity of CYP3A and thus have the potential to decrease plasma concentrations of other protease inhibitors when used in combination with KALETRA.
Non-nucleoside Reverse Transcriptase Inhibitor: delavirdine	↑ Lopinavir	Appropriate doses of the combination with respect to safety and efficacy have not been established.
Nucleoside Reverse Transcriptase Inhibitor: didanosine		It is recommended that didanosine be administered on an empty stomach; therefore, didanosine should be given one hour before or two hours after KALETRA (given with food).
HIV-Protease Inhibitors: amprenavir*, indinavir*, saquinavir*	When co-administered with reduced doses of concomitant protease inhibitors: ↑ Amprenavir (Similar AUC, ↓ C_{max}, ↑ C_{min}) ↑ Indinavir (Similar AUC, ↓ C_{max} ↑ C_{min}) ↑ Saquinavir (Similar AUC, ↑ C_{min})	Alterations in concentrations (e.g., AUC, C_{max} and C_{min}) are noted when reduced doses of concomitant protease inhibitors are co-administered with KALETRA. Appropriate doses of the combination with respect to safety and efficacy have not been established (see **CLINICAL PHARMACOLOGY**: Table 3 and Effect of KALETRA on other Protease Inhibitors (PIs)).
HIV-Protease Inhibitor: ritonavir*	↑ Lopinavir	Appropriate doses of additional ritonavir in combination with KALETRA with respect to safety and efficacy have not been established.

(Table continued on next page)

Body as a Whole: Abdomen enlarged, back pain, chest pain, chest pain substernal, chills, cyst, drug interaction, drug level increased, face edema, fever, flu syndrome, hypertrophy, infection bacterial, malaise, and viral infection.

Cardiovascular System: Deep vein thrombosis, hypertension, migraine, palpitation, thrombophlebitis, varicose vein, and vasculitis.

Digestive System: Anorexia, cholecystitis, constipation, dry mouth, dysphagia, enterocolitis, eructation, esophagitis, fecal incontinence, flatulence, gastritis, gastroenteritis, gastrointestinal disorder, hemorrhagic colitis, increased appetite, mouth ulceration, pancreatitis, sialadenitis, stomatitis, and ulcerative stomatitis.

Endocrine System: Cushing's syndrome, diabetes mellitus, and hypothyroidism.

Hemic and Lymphatic System: Anemia, leukopenia, and lymphadenopathy.

Metabolic and Nutritional Disorders: Avitaminosis, dehydration, edema, glucose tolerance decreased, lactic acidosis, obesity, peripheral edema, weight gain, and weight loss.

Musculoskeletal System: Arthralgia, arthrosis and myalgia.

Nervous System: Abnormal dreams, agitation, amnesia, anxiety, ataxia, confusion, depression, dizziness, dyskinesia, emotional lability, encephalopathy, facial paralysis, hypertonia, libido decreased, nervousness, neuropathy, paresthesia, peripheral neuritis, somnolence, thinking abnormal, and tremor.

Respiratory System: Bronchitis, dyspnea, lung edema, rhinitis, and sinusitis.

Skin and Appendages: Acne, alopecia, dry skin, eczema, exfoliative dermatitis, furunculosis, maculopapular rash, nail disorder, pruritis, seborrhea, skin benign neoplasm, skin discoloration, skin ulcer, and sweating.

Special Senses: Abnormal vision, eye disorder, otitis media, taste perversion, and tinnitus.

Urogenital System: Abnormal ejaculation, gynecomastia, hypogonadism male, kidney calculus, and urine abnormality.

Post-Marketing Experience: Redistribution/accumulation of body fat has been reported (see **PRECAUTIONS, Fat Redistribution**).

Laboratory Abnormalities: The percentages of adult patients treated with combination therapy including KALETRA with Grade 3-4 laboratory abnormalities are presented in Table 10.

[See table 10 at top of next page]

Pediatrics:

Treatment-Emergent Adverse Events: KALETRA has been studied in 100 pediatric patients 6 months to 12 years of age. The adverse event profile seen during a clinical trial was similar to that for adult patients.

Taste aversion, vomiting, and diarrhea were the most commonly reported drug related adverse events of any severity in pediatric patients treated with combination therapy including KALETRA for up to 48 weeks in Study 940. A total of 8 children experienced moderate or severe adverse events at least possibly related to KALETRA. Rash (reported in 3%) was the only drug-related clinical adverse event of moderate to severe intensity observed in ≥ 2% of children enrolled.

Laboratory Abnormalities: The percentages of pediatric patients treated with combination therapy including KALETRA with Grade 3-4 laboratory abnormalities are presented in Table 11.

[See table 11 at top of page 91]

OVERDOSAGE

KALETRA oral solution contains 42.4% alcohol (v/v). Accidental ingestion of the product by a young child could result in significant alcohol-related toxicity and could approach the potential lethal dose of alcohol.

Human experience of acute overdosage with KALETRA is limited. Treatment of overdose with KALETRA should consist of general supportive measures including monitoring of vital signs and observation of the clinical status of the patient. There is no specific antidote for overdose with KALETRA. If indicated, elimination of unabsorbed drug should be achieved by emesis or gastric lavage. Administration of activated charcoal may also be used to aid in removal of unabsorbed drug. Since KALETRA is highly protein bound, dialysis is unlikely to be beneficial in significant removal of the drug.

Table 8: Established and Other Potentially Significant Drug Interactions: Alteration in Dose or Regimen May Be Recommended Based on Drug Interaction Studies or Predicted Interaction (See CLINICAL PHARMACOLOGY for Magnitude of Interaction, Tables 2 and 3) — *(cont.)*

Concomitant Drug Class: Drug Name	Effect on Concentration of lopinavir or Concomitant Drug	Clinical Comment
Other Agents		
Antiarrhythmics: amiodarone, bepridil, lidocaine (systemic), and quinidine	↑ Antiarrhythmics	Caution is warranted and therapeutic concentration monitoring is recommended for antiarrhythmics when co-administered with KALETRA, if available.
Anticoagulant: warfarin		Concentrations of warfarin may be affected. It is recommended that INR (international normalized ratio) be monitored.
Anticonvulsants: carbamazepine, phenobarbital, phenytoin	↓ Lopinavir	Use with caution. KALETRA may be less effective due to decreased lopinavir plasma concentrations in patients taking these agents concomitantly.
Anti-infective: clarithromycin	↑ Clarithromycin	For patients with renal impairment, the following dosage adjustments should be considered: •For patients with CL_{CR} 30 to 60 mL/min the dose of clarithromycin should be reduced by 50%. •For patients with CL_{CR} <30 mL/min the dose of clarithromycin should be decreased by 75%. No dose adjustment for patients with normal renal function is necessary.
Antifungals: ketoconazole*, itraconazole	↑ Ketoconazole ↑ Itraconazole	High doses of ketoconazole or itraconazole (>200 mg/day) are not recommended.
Antimycobacterial: rifabutin*	↑ Rifabutin and rifabutin metabolite	Dosage reduction of rifabutin by at least 75% of the usual dose of 300 mg/day is recommended (i.e., a maximum dose of 150 mg every other day or three times per week). Increased monitoring for adverse events is warranted in patients receiving the combination. Further dosage reduction of rifabutin may be necessary.
Antiparasitic: atovaquone	↓ Atovaquone	Clinical significance is unknown; however, increase in atovaquone doses may be needed.
Calcium Channel Blockers, Dihydropyridine: e.g, felodipine, nifedipine, nicardipine	↑ Dihydropyridine calcium channel blockers	Caution is warranted and clinical monitoring of patients is recommended.
Corticosteroid: Dexamethasone	↓ Lopinavir	Use with caution. KALETRA may be less effective due to decreased lopinavir plasma concentrations in patients taking these agents concomitantly.
Disulfiram/metronidazole		KALETRA oral solution contains alcohol, which can produce disulfiram-like reactions when co-administered with disulfiram or other drugs that produce this reaction (e.g., metronidazole).
Erectile Dysfunction Agent: sidenafil	↑ Sidenafil	Use with caution at reduced doses of 25 mg every 48 hours with increased monitoring for adverse events.
HMG-CoA Reductase Inhibitors: atorvastatin*	↑ Atorvastatin	Use lowest possible dose of atorvastatin with careful monitoring, or consider other HMG-CoA reductase inhibitors such as pravastatin or fluvastatin in combination with KALETRA.
Immunosuppressants: cyclosporine, tacrolimus, rapamycin	↑ Immuno-suppressants	Therapeutic concentration monitoring is recommended for immunosuppressant agents when co-administered with KALETRA.
Nacrotic Analgesic: Methadone*	↓ Methadone	Dosage of methadone may need to be increased when co-administered with KALETRA.
Oral Contraceptive: ethinyl estradiol*	↓ Ethinyl estradiol	Alternative or additional contraceptive measures should be used when estrogen-based oral contraceptives and KALETRA are co-administered.

* See **CLINICAL PHARMACOLOGY** for Magnitude of Interaction, Tables 2 and 3

DOSAGE AND ADMINISTRATION

Adults

The recommended dosage of KALETRA is 400/100 mg (3 capsules or 5.0 mL) twice daily taken with food.

Concomitant therapy: Efavirenz or nevirapine: A dose increase of KALETRA to 533/133 mg (4 capsules or 6.5 mL) twice daily taken with food should be considered when used in combination with efavirenz or nevirapine in treatment experienced patients where reduced susceptibility to lopinavir is clinically suspected (by treatment history or laboratory evidence) (see **CLINICAL PHARMACOLOGY – Drug Interactions** and/or **PRECAUTIONS** – Table 8).

Pediatric Patients

In children 6 months to 12 years of age, the recommended dosage of KALETRA oral solution is 12/3 mg/kg for those 7 to <15 kg and 10/2.5 mg/kg for those 15 to 40 kg (approximately equivalent to 230/57.5 mg/m²) twice daily taken with food, up to a maximum dose of 400/100 mg in children >40 kg (5.0 mL or 3 capsules) twice daily. **It is preferred that the prescriber calculate the appropriate milligram dose for each individual child ≤12 years old and determine the corresponding volume of solution or number of capsules.** However, as an alternative, the following table contains dosing guidelines for KALETRA oral solution based on body weight. When possible, dose should be administered using a calibrated dosing syringe.

[See second table at top of page 91]

Note: Use adult dosage recommendation for children >12 years of age.

Concomitant therapy: Efavirenz or nevirapine: A dose increase of KALETRA oral solution to 13/3.25 mg/kg for those 7 to <15 kg and 11/2.75 mg/kg for those 15 to 45 kg (approximately equivalent to 300/75 mg/m²) twice daily taken with food, up to a maximum dose of 533/133 mg in children >45 kg twice daily should be considered when used in combination with efavirenz or nevirapine in treatment experienced children 6 months to 12 years of age in which reduced susceptibility to lopinavir is clinically suspected (by treatment history or laboratory evidence). The following table contains dosing guidelines for KALETRA oral solution based on body weight, when used in combination with efavirenz or nevirapine in children (see **CLINICAL PHARMACOLOGY- Drug Interactions** and/or **PRECAUTIONS** – Table 8).

[See third table at top of page 91]

Note: Use adult dosage recommendation for children >12 years of age.

HOW SUPPLIED

KALETRA (lopinavir/ritonavir) capsules are orange soft gelatin capsules imprinted with the corporate logo and the Abbo-Code PK. KALETRA is available as 133.3 mg lopinavir/33.3 mg ritonavir capsules in the following package sizes:

Bottles of 180 capsules each .... (**NDC** 0074-3959-77)

Recommended storage: Store KALETRA soft gelatin capsules at 36°F - 46°F (2°C - 8°C) until dispensed. Avoid exposure to excessive heat. For patient use, refrigerated KALETRA capsules remain stable until the expiration date printed on the label. If stored at room temperature up to 77°F (25°C), capsules should be used within 2 months.

KALETRA (lopinavir/ritonavir) oral solution is a light yellow to orange colored liquid supplied in amber-colored multiple-dose bottles containing 400 mg lopinavir/100 mg ritonavir per 5 mL (80 mg lopinavir/20 mg ritonavir per mL) packaged with a marked dosing cup in the following size:

160 mL bottle .... (**NDC** 0074-3956-46)

Recommended storage: Store KALETRA oral solution at 36°F - 46°F (2°C - 8°C) until dispensed. Avoid exposure to excessive heat. For patient use, refrigerated KALETRA oral solution remains stable until the expiration date printed on the label. If stored at room temperature up to 77°F (25°C), oral solution should be used within 2 months.

Ref.: 03-5177-R6-Rev. January, 2002

ABBOTT LABORATORIES
NORTH CHICAGO IL, 60064, U.S.A.

02B-036-2780-1 **MASTER**
PRINTED IN U.S.A.

KALETRA™
(lopinavir/ritonavir) capsules
(lopinavir/ritonavir) oral solution

ALERT: Find out about medicines that should NOT be taken with KALETRA.

Please also read the section "MEDICINES YOU SHOULD NOT TAKE WITH KALETRA."

Patient Information
KALETRA™
(kuh-LEE-tra)

Generic Name: lopinavir/ritonavir
(lop-IN-uh-veer/rit-ON-uh-veer)

Read this leaflet carefully before you start taking KALETRA. Also, read it each time you get your KALETRA prescription refilled, in case something has changed. This information does not take the place of talking

Continued on next page

Kaletra—Cont.

with your doctor when you start this medicine and at check ups. Ask your doctor if you have any questions about KALETRA.

What is KALETRA and how does it work?

KALETRA is a combination of two medicines. They are lopinavir and ritonavir. KALETRA is a type of medicine called an HIV (human immunodeficiency virus) protease (PRO-tee-ase) inhibitor. KALETRA is always used in combination with other anti-HIV medicines to treat people with human immunodeficiency virus (HIV) infection. KALETRA is for adults and for children age 6 months and older.

HIV infection destroys CD4 (T) cells, which are important to the immune system. After a large number of T cells are destroyed, acquired immune deficiency syndrome (AIDS) develops.

KALETRA blocks HIV protease, a chemical which is needed for HIV to multiply. KALETRA reduces the amount of HIV in your blood and increases the number of T cells. Reducing the amount of HIV in the blood reduces the chance of death or infections that happen when your immune system is weak (opportunistic infections).

Does KALETRA cure HIV or AIDS?

KALETRA does not cure HIV infection or AIDS. The long-term effects of KALETRA are not known at this time. People taking KALETRA may still get opportunistic infections or other conditions that happen with HIV infection. Some of these conditions are pneumonia, herpes virus infections, and *Mycobacterium avium* complex (MAC) infections.

Does KALETRA reduce the risk of passing HIV to others?

KALETRA does not reduce the risk of passing HIV to others through sexual contact or blood contamination. Continue to practice safe sex and do not use or share dirty needles.

How should I take KALETRA?

- You should stay under a doctor's care when taking KALETRA. Do not change your treatment or stop treatment without first talking with your doctor.
- You must take KALETRA every day exactly as your doctor prescribed it. The dose of KALETRA may be different for you than for other patients. Follow the directions from your doctor, exactly as written on the label.
- Dosing in adults (including children 12 years of age and older): The usual dose for adults is 3 capsules (400/100 mg) or 5.0 mL of the oral solution twice a day (morning and night), in combination with other anti-HIV medicines.
- Dosing in children from 6 months to 12 years of age: Children from 6 months to 12 years of age can also take KALETRA. The child's doctor will decide the right dose based on the child's weight.
- Take KALETRA with food to help it work better.
- Do not change your dose or stop taking KALETRA without first talking with your doctor.
- When your KALETRA supply starts to run low, get more from your doctor or pharmacy. This is very important because the amount of virus in your blood may increase if the medicine is stopped for even a short time. The virus may develop resistance to KALETRA and become harder to treat.
- Be sure to set up a schedule and follow it carefully.
- Only take medicine that has been prescribed specifically for you. Do not give KALETRA to others or take medicine prescribed for someone else.

What should I do if I miss a dose of KALETRA?

It is important that you do not miss any doses. If you miss a dose of KALETRA, take it as soon as possible and then take your next scheduled dose at its regular time. If it is almost time for your next dose, do not take the missed dose. Wait and take the next dose at the regular time. Do not double the next dose.

What happens if I take too much KALETRA?

If you suspect that you took more than the prescribed dose of this medicine, contact your local poison control center or emergency room immediately.

As with all prescription medicines, KALETRA should be kept out of the reach of young children. KALETRA liquid contains a large amount of alcohol. If a toddler or young child accidentally drinks more than the recommended dose of KALETRA, it could make him/her sick from too much alcohol. Contact your local poison control center or emergency room immediately if this happens.

Who should not take KALETRA?

Together with your doctor, you need to decide whether KALETRA is right for you.

- Do not take KALETRA if you are taking certain medicines. These could cause serious side effects that could cause death. Before you take KALETRA, you must tell your doctor about all the medicines you are taking or are planning to take. These include other prescription and nonprescription medicines and herbal supplements.

For more information about medicines you should not take with KALETRA, please read the section titled "MEDICINES YOU SHOULD NOT TAKE WITH KALETRA."

- Do not take KALETRA if you have an allergy to KALETRA or any of its ingredients, including ritonavir or lopinavir.

Can I take KALETRA with other medications?*

KALETRA may interact with other medicines, including those you take without a prescription. You must tell your doctor about all the medicines you are taking or planning to take before you take KALETRA.

Table 9: Percentage of Patients with Treatment-Emergent[1] Adverse Events of Moderate or Severe Intensity Reported in ≥ 2% of Adult Patients

	Antiretroviral Naive Patients			Protease Inhibitor Experienced Patients
	Study 863 (48 Weeks)		Study 720 (72 Weeks)	Phase I/II and Phase III
	KALETRA 400/100 mg BID + d4T + 3TC (N=326)	Nelfinavir 750 mg TID + d4T + 3TC (N=327)	KALETRA BID[2] + d4T + 3TC (N=84)	KALETRA BID[3] + NNRTI + NRTIs (N=186)
Body as a Whole				
Abdominal Pain	4.0%	3.1%	4.8%	1.6%
Asthenia	4.0%	3.4%	7.1%	5.4%
Headache	2.5%	1.8%	7.1%	1.6%
Pain	0.6%	0.0%	2.4%	1.6%
Digestive System				
Abnormal Stools	0.0%	0.3%	6.0%	1.6%
Diarrhea	15.6%	17.1%	23.8%	15.6%
Dyspepsia	2.1%	0.3%	1.2%	0.5%
Nausea	6.7%	4.6%	15.5%	2.7%
Vomiting	2.5%	2.4%	4.8%	1.6%
Nervous System				
Insomnia	1.5%	1.2%	2.4%	1.1%
Skin and Appendages				
Rash	0.6%	1.5%	3.6%	2.0%

[1] Includes adverse events of possible, probable or unknown relationship to study drug.

[2] Includes adverse event data from dose group I (400/100 mg BID only [N=16]) and dose group II (400/100 mg BID [N=35]) and 400/200 mg BID [N=33]). Within dosing groups, moderate to severe nausea of probable/possible relationship to KALETRA occurred at a higher rate in the 400/200 mg dose arm compared to the 400/100 mg dose arm in group II.

[3] Includes adverse event data from patients receiving 400/100 mg BID, 400/200 mg BID, and 533/133 mg BID for 16-72 weeks. All 186 patients received KALETRA in combination with NRTIs and either nevirapine or efavirenz.

Table 10: Grade 3-4 Laboratory Abnormalities Reported in ≥ 2% of Adult Patients

Variable	Limit[1]	Antiretroviral Naive Patients			Antiretroviral Experienced Patients
		Study 863 (48 Weeks)		Study 720 (72 Weeks)	Phase I/II and Phase III
		KALETRA 400/100 mg BID + d4T + 3TC (N=326)	Nelfinavir 750 mg TID + d4T + 3TC (N=327)	KALETRA BID[2] + d4T + 3TC (N=84)	KALETRA BID[3] + NNRTI + NRTIs (N=186)
Chemistry	High				
Glucose	>250 mg/dL	2.2%	1.6%	2.4%	4.4%
Uric Acid	>12 mg/dL	2.2%	1.6%	3.6%	0.5%
SGOT/AST	>180 U/L	2.2%	4.1%	9.5%	5.5%
SGPT/ALT	>215 U/L	3.8%	3.8%	8.3%	7.1%
GGT	>300 U/L	N/A	N/A	3.6%	24.6%[4]
Total Cholesterol	>300 mg/dL	9.0%	5.0%	14.3%	28.4%
Triglycerides	>750 mg/dL	9.3%	1.3%	10.7%	28.4%
Amylase	>2 × ULN	3.2%	2.2%	4.8%	4.9%
Chemistry	Low				
Inorganic Phosphorus	<1.5 mg/dL	0.0%	0.0%	0.0%	2.2%
Hematology	Low				
Neutrophils	0.75×10^9/L	0.6%	2.5%	2.4%	2.7%

[1] ULN = upper limit of the normal range; N/A = Not Applicable.

[2] Includes clinical laboratory data from dose group I (400/100 mg BID only [N=16]) and dose group II (400/100 mg BID [N=35] and 400/200 mg BID [N=33]).

[3] Includes clinical laboratory data from patients receiving 400/100 mg BID, 400/200 mg BID, and 533/133 mg BID for 16-72 weeks. All 186 patients received KALETRA in combination with NRTIs and either nevirapine or efavirenz.

[4] GGT was only measured in 69 patients receiving 400/100 mg BID or 400/200 mg BID in combination with nevirapine.

MEDICINES YOU SHOULD NOT TAKE WITH KALETRA:

- Do not take the following medicines with KALETRA because they can cause serious problems or death if taken with KALETRA.
  - — Dihydroergotamine, ergonovine, ergotamine and methylergonovine such as Cafergot®, Migranal®, D.H.E. 45®, Ergotrate Maleate, Methergine, and others
  - — Halcion® (triazolam)
  - — Hismanal® (astemizole)
  - — Orap® (pimozide)
  - — Propulsid® (cisapride)
  - — Rythmol® (propafenone)
  - — Seldane® (terfenadine)
  - — Tambocor™ (flecainide)
  - — Versed® (midazolam)
- Do not take KALETRA with rifampin, also known as Rimactane®, Rifadin®, Rifater®, or Rifamate®. Rifampin may lower the amount of KALETRA in your blood and make it less effective.
- Do not take KALETRA with St. John's wort (hypericum perforatum), an herbal product sold as a dietary supplement, or products containing St. John's wort. Talk with your doctor if you are taking or planning to take St. John's wort. Taking St. John's wort may decrease KALETRA levels and lead to increased viral load and possible resistance to KALETRA or cross-resistance to other anti-HIV medicines.
- Do not take KALETRA with the cholesterol-lowering medicines Mevacor® (lovastatin) or Zocor® (simvastatin) because of possible serious reactions. There is also an increased risk of drug interactions between KALETRA and Lipitor® (atorvastatin); talk to your doctor before you take any of these cholesterol-reducing medicines with KALETRA.

Medicines that require dosage adjustments:

It is possible that your doctor may need to increase or decrease the dose of other medicines when you are also taking KALETRA. Remember to tell your doctor all medicines you are taking or plan to take.

Before you take Viagra® (sildenafil) with KALETRA, talk to your doctor about problems these two medicines can cause when taken together. You may get increased side effects of VIAGRA, such as low blood pressure, vision changes, and penis erection lasting more than 4 hours. If an erection lasts longer than 4 hours, get medical help right away to avoid permanent damage to your penis. Your doctor can explain these symptoms to you.

Table 11: Grade 3-4 Laboratory Abnormalities Reported in ≥ 2% of Pediatric Patients

Variable	Limit[1]	KALETRA BID + RTIs (N=100)
Chemistry	High	
Sodium	>149 mEq/L	3.0%
Total bilirubin	≥3.0 × ULN	3.0%
SGOT/AST	>180 U/L	8.0%
SGPT/ALT	>215 U/L	7.0%
Total cholesterol	>300 mg/dL	3.0%
Amylase	>2.5 × ULN	7.0%[2]
Chemistry	Low	
Sodium	<130 mEq/L	3.0%
Hematology	Low	
Platelet Count	< 50 × 10^9/L	4.0%
Neutrophils	< 0.40 × 10^9/L	2.0%

[1] ULN = upper limit of the normal range.
[2] Subjects with Grade 3-4 amylase confirmed by elevations in pancreatic amylase.

Weight (kg)	Dose (mg/kg)*	Volume of oral solution BID (80 mg lopinavir/ 20 mg ritonavir per mL)
Without nevirapine or efavirenz		
7 to <15 kg	12 mg/kg BID	
7 to 10 kg		1.25 mL
>10 to <15 kg		1.75 mL
15 to 40 kg	10 mg/kg BID	
15 to 20 kg		2.25 mL
>20 to 25 kg		2.75 mL
>25 to 30 kg		3.5 mL
>30 to 35 kg		4.0 mL
>35 to 40 kg		4.75 mL
>40 kg	Adult dose	5 mL (or 3 capsules)

* Dosing based on the lopinavir component of lopinavir/ritonavir solution (80 mg/20 mg per mL).

Weight (kg)	Dose (mg/kg)*	Volume of oral solution BID (80 mg lopinavir/ 20 mg ritonavir per mL)
Without nevirapine or efavirenz		
7 to <15 kg	13 mg/kg BID	
7 to 10 kg		1.5 mL
>10 to <15 kg		2.0 mL
15 to 45 kg	11 mg/kg BID	
15 to 20 kg		2.5 mL
>20 to 25 kg		3.25 mL
>25 to 30 kg		4.0 mL
>30 to 35 kg		4.5 mL
>35 to 40 kg		5.0 mL (or 3 capsules)
>40 to 45 kg		5.75 mL
>45 kg	Adult dose	6.5 mL (or 4 capsules)

* Dosing based on the lopinavir component of lopinavir/ritonavir solution (80 mg/20 mg per mL).

- If you are taking oral contraceptives ("the pill") to prevent pregnancy, you should use an additional or different type of contraception since KALETRA may reduce the effectiveness of oral contraceptives.
- Efavirenz (Sustiva™) or nevirapine (Viramune®) may lower the amount of KALETRA in your blood. Your doctor may increase your dose of KALETRA if you are also taking efavirenz or nevirapine.
- If you are taking Mycobutin® (rifabutin), your doctor will lower the dose of Mycobutin.
- **A change in therapy should be considered if you are taking KALETRA with:**
  Phenobarbital
  Phenytoin (Dilantin® and others)
  Carbamazepine (Tegretol® and others)

These medicines may lower the amount of KALETRA in your blood and make it less effective.

- **Other Special Considerations:**
  KALETRA oral solution contains alcohol. Talk with your doctor if you are taking or planning to take metronidazole or disulfiram. Severe nausea and vomiting can occur.
- **If you are taking both didanosine (Videx®) and KALETRA:**
  Didanosine (Videx®) should be taken one hour before or two hours after KALETRA.

What are the possible side effects of KALETRA?

- This list of side effects is **not** complete. If you have questions about side effects, ask your doctor, nurse, or pharmacist. You should report any new or continuing symptoms to your doctor right away. Your doctor may be able to help you manage these side effects.
- The most commonly reported side effects of moderate severity that are thought to be drug related are: abnormal stools (bowel movements), diarrhea, feeling weak/tired, headache, and nausea. Children taking KALETRA may sometimes get a skin rash.
- Blood tests in patients taking KALETRA may show possible liver problems. People with liver disease such as Hepatitis B and Hepatitis C who take KALETRA may have worsening liver disease. Liver problems including death have occurred in patients taking KALETRA. In studies, it is unclear if KALETRA caused these liver problems because some patients had other illnesses or were taking other medicines.
- Some patients taking KALETRA can develop serious problems with their pancreas (pancreatitis), which may cause death. You have a higher chance of having pancreatitis if you have had it before. Tell your doctor if you have nausea, vomiting, or abdominal pain. These may be signs of pancreatitis.
- Some patients have large increases in triglycerides and cholesterol. The long-term chance of getting complications such as heart attacks or stroke due to increases in triglycerides and cholesterol caused by protease inhibitors is not known at this time.
- Diabetes and high blood sugar (hyperglycemia) occur in patients taking protease inhibitors such as KALETRA. Some patients had diabetes before starting protease inhibitors, others did not. Some patients need changes in their diabetes medicine. Others needed new diabetes medicine.
- Changes in body fat have been seen in some patients taking antiretroviral therapy. These changes may include increased amount of fat in the upper back and neck ("buffalo hump"), breast, and around the trunk. Loss of fat from the legs, arms and face may also happen. The cause and long term health effects of these conditions are not known at this time.
- Some patients with hemophilia have increased bleeding with protease inhibitors.
- There have been other side effects in patients taking KALETRA. However, these side effects may have been due to other medicines that patients were taking or to the illness itself. Some of these side effects can be serious.

What should I tell my doctor before taking KALETRA?

- *If you are pregnant or planning to become pregnant:* The effects of KALETRA on pregnant women or their unborn babies are not known.
- *If you are breast-feeding:* Do not breast-feed if you are taking KALETRA. You should not breast-feed if you have HIV. If you are a woman who has or will have a baby, talk with your doctor about the best way to feed your baby. You should be aware that if your baby does not already have HIV, there is a chance that HIV can be transmitted through breast-feeding.
- *If you have liver problems:* If you have liver problems or are infected with Hepatitis B or Hepatitis C, you should tell your doctor before taking KALETRA.
- *If you have diabetes:* Some people taking protease inhibitors develop new or more serious diabetes or high blood sugar. Tell your doctor if you have diabetes or an increase in thirst or frequent urination.
- *If you have hemophilia:* Patients taking KALETRA may have increased bleeding.

How do I store KALETRA?

- Keep KALETRA and all other medicines out of the reach of children.
- Refrigerated KALETRA capsules and oral solution remain stable until the expiration date printed on the label. If stored at room temperature up to 77°F (25°C), KALETRA capsules and oral solution should be used within 2 months.
- Avoid exposure to excessive heat.

Do not keep medicine that is out of date or that you no longer need. Be sure that if you throw any medicine away, it is out of the reach of children.

General advice about prescription medicines:

Talk to your doctor or other health care provider if you have any questions about this medicine or your condition. Medicines are sometimes prescribed for purposes other than those listed in a Patient Information Leaflet. If you have any concerns about this medicine, ask your doctor. Your doctor or pharmacist can give you information about this medicine that was written for health care professionals. Do not use this medicine for a condition for which it was not prescribed. Do not share this medicine with other people.

*** The brands listed are trademarks of their respective owners and are not trademarks of Abbott Laboratories. The makers of these brands are not affiliated with and do not endorse Abbott Laboratories or its products.**

Ref.: 03-5177-R6
Revised: January, 2002
ABBOTT LABORATORIES
NORTH CHICAGO, IL 60064 U.S.A.

PRINTED IN U.S.A.

MERIDIA® Ⓒ℞

[mĕr-ĭdĭa]
(sibutramine hydrochloride monohydrate)
Capsules
℞ only

DESCRIPTION

MERIDIA® (sibutramine hydrochloride monohydrate) is an orally administered agent for the treatment of obesity. Chemically, the active ingredient is a racemic mixture of the (+) and (−) enantiomers of cyclobutanemethanamine, 1-(4-chlorophenyl)-*N*,*N*-dimethyl-α-(2-methylpropyl)-, hydrochloride, monohydrate, and has an empirical formula of $C_{17}H_{29}Cl_2NO$. Its molecular weight is 334.33.

The structural formula is shown below:

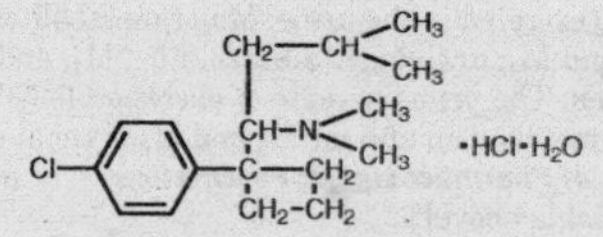

Sibutramine hydrochloride monohydrate is a white to cream crystalline powder with a solubility of 2.9 mg/mL in pH 5.2 water. Its octanol:water partition coefficient is 30.9 at pH 5.0.

Each MERIDIA capsule contains 5 mg, 10 mg, and 15 mg of sibutramine hydrochloride monohydrate. It also contains as inactive ingredients: lactose monohydrate, NF; microcrystalline cellulose, NF; colloidal silicon dioxide, NF; and magnesium stearate, NF in a hard-gelatin capsule [which contains titanium dioxide, USP; gelatin; FD&C Blue No. 2 (5- and 10-mg capsules only); D&C Yellow No. 10 (5- and 15-mg capsules only), and other inactive ingredients].

CLINICAL PHARMACOLOGY

Mode of Action

Sibutramine produces its therapeutic effects by norepinephrine, serotonin and dopamine reuptake inhibition. Sibutramine and its major pharmacologically active metabolites (M_1 and M_2) do not act via release of monoamines.

Pharmacodynamics

Sibutramine exerts its pharmacological actions predominantly via its secondary (M_1) and primary (M_2) amine metabolites. The parent compound, sibutramine, is a potent inhibitor of serotonin (5-hydroxytryptamine, 5-HT) and norepinephrine reuptake *in vivo*, but not *in vitro*. However, metabolites M_1 and M_2 inhibit the reuptake of these neurotransmitters both *in vitro* and *in vivo*.

In human brain tissue, M_1 and M_2 also inhibit dopamine reuptake *in vitro*, but with ~3-fold lower potency than for the reuptake inhibition of serotonin or norepinephrine.

Potencies of Sibutramine, M_1 and M_2 as *In Vitro* Inhibitors of Monoamine Reuptake in Human Brain

Potency to Inhibit Monoamine Reuptake (K_i; nM)

	Serotonin	Norepinephrine	Dopamine
Sibutramine	298	5451	943
M_1	15	20	49
M_2	20	15	45

A study using plasma samples taken from sibutramine-treated volunteers showed monoamine reuptake inhibition of norepinephrine > serotonin > dopamine; maximum inhibitions were norepinephrine = 73%, serotonin = 54% and dopamine = 16%.

Continued on next page

Meridia—Cont.

Sibutramine and its metabolites (M_1 and M_2) are not serotonin, norepinephrine or dopamine releasing agents. Following chronic administration of sibutramine to rats, no depletion of brain monoamines has been observed.
Sibutramine, M_1 and M_2 exhibit no evidence of anticholinergic or antihistaminergic actions. In addition, receptor binding profiles show that sibutramine, M_1 and M_2 have low affinity for serotonin (5-HT_1, 5-HT_{1A}, 5-HT_{1B}, 5-HT_{2A}, 5-HT_{2C}), norepinephrine (β, $β_1$, $β_3$, $α_1$ and $α_2$), dopamine (D_1 and D_2), benzodiazepine, and glutamate (NMDA) receptors. These compounds also lack monoamine oxidase inhibitory activity *in vitro* and *in vivo*.

Pharmacokinetics

Absorption

Sibutramine is rapidly absorbed from the GI tract (T_{max} of 1.2 hours) following oral administration and undergoes extensive first-pass metabolism in the liver (oral clearance of 1750 L/h and half-life of 1.1 h) to form the pharmacologically active mono- and di-desmethyl metabolites M_1 and M_2. Peak plasma concentrations of M_1 and M_2 are reached within 3 to 4 hours. On the basis of mass balance studies, on average, at least 77% of a single oral dose of sibutramine is absorbed. The absolute bioavailability of sibutramine has not been determined.

Distribution

Radiolabeled studies in animals indicated rapid and extensive distribution into tissues: highest concentrations of radiolabeled material were found in the eliminating organs, liver and kidney. *In vitro*, sibutramine, M_1 and M_2 are extensively bound (97%, 94% and 94%, respectively) to human plasma proteins at plasma concentrations seen following therapeutic doses.

Metabolism

Sibutramine is metabolized in the liver principally by the cytochrome P450($3A_4$) isoenzyme, to desmethyl metabolites, M_1 and M_2. These active metabolites are further metabolized by hydroxylation and conjugation to pharmacologically inactive metabolites, M_5 and M_6. Following oral administration of radiolabeled sibutramine, essentially all of the peak radiolabeled material in plasma was accounted for by unchanged sibutramine (3%), M_1 (6%), M_2 (12%), M_5 (52%), and M_6 (27%).
M_1 and M_2 plasma concentrations reached steady-state within four days of dosing and were approximately two-fold higher than following a single dose. The elimination half-lives of M_1 and M_2, 14 and 16 hours, respectively, were unchanged following repeated dosing.

Excretion

Approximately 85% (range 68–95%) of a single orally administered radiolabeled dose was excreted in urine and feces over a 15-day collection period with the majority of the dose (77%) excreted in the urine. Major metabolites in urine were M_5 and M_6; unchanged sibutramine, M_1, and M_2 were not detected. The primary route of excretion for M_1 and M_2 is hepatic metabolism and for M_5 and M_6 is renal excretion.

Summary of Pharmacokinetic Parameters

[See first table above]

Effect of Food

Administration of a single 20 mg dose of sibutramine with a standard breakfast resulted in reduced peak M1 and M2 concentrations (by 27% and 32%, respectively) and delayed the time to peak by approximately three hours. However, the AUC's of M_1 and M_2 were not significantly altered.

Special Populations

Geriatric: Plasma concentrations of M_1 and M_2 were similar between elderly (ages 61 to 77 yr) and young (ages 19 to 30 yr) subjects following a single 15-mg oral sibutramine dose. Plasma concentrations of the inactive metabolites M_5 and M_6 were higher in the elderly; these differences are not likely to be of clinical significance. In general, dose selection for an elderly patient should be cautious, reflecting the greater frequency of decreased hepatic, renal, or cardiac function, and of concomitant disease or other drug therapy.
Pediatric: The safety and effectiveness of MERIDIA in pediatric patients under 16 years old have not been established.
Gender: Pooled pharmacokinetic parameters from 54 young, healthy volunteers (37 males and 17 females) receiving a 15-mg oral dose of sibutramine showed the mean C_{max} and AUC of M_1 and M_2 to be slightly (≤19% and ≤36%, respectively) higher in females than males. Somewhat higher steady-state trough plasma levels were observed in female obese patients from a large clinical efficacy trial. However, these differences are not likely to be of clinical significance. Dosage adjustment based upon the gender of a patient is not necessary (see "**DOSAGE AND ADMINISTRATION**").
Race: The relationship between race and steady-state trough M_1 and M_2 plasma concentrations was examined in a clinical trial in obese patients. A trend towards higher concentrations in Black patients over Caucasian patients was noted for M_1 and M_2. However, these differences are not considered to be of clinical significance.
Renal Insufficiency: The effect of renal disease has not been studied. However, since sibutramine and its active metabolites M_1 and M_2 are eliminated by hepatic metabolism, renal disease is unlikely to have a significant effect on their disposition. Elimination of the inactive metabolites M_5 and M_6, which are renally excreted, may be affected in this population. MERIDIA should not be used in patients with severe renal impairment.
Hepatic Insufficiency: In 12 patients with moderate hepatic impairment receiving a single 15-mg oral dose of sibutramine, the combined AUC's of M_1 and M_2 were increased by 24% compared to healthy subjects while M_5 and M_6 plasma concentrations were unchanged. The observed differences in M_1 and M_2 concentrations do not warrant dosage adjustment in patients with mild to moderate hepatic impairment. MERIDIA should not be used in patients with severe hepatic dysfunction.

Mean (% CV) and 95% Confidence Intervals of Pharmacokinetic Parameters (Dose = 15 mg)

Study Population	C_{max} (ng/mL)	T_{max} (h)	AUC† (ng*h/mL)	T½ (h)
Metabolite M_1				
Target Population:				
Obese Subjects	4.0 (42)	3.6 (28)	25.5 (63)	--
(n=18)	3.2–4.8	3.1–4.1	18.1–32.9	
Special Population:				
Moderate Hepatic	2.2 (36)	3.3 (33)	18.7 (65)	--
Impairment (n=12)	1.8–2.7	2.7–3.9	11.9–25.5	
Metabolite M_2				
Target Population:				
Obese Subjects	6.4 (28)	3.5 (17)	92.1 (26)	17.2 (58)
(n=18)	5.6–7.2	3.2–3.8	81.2–103	12.5–21.8
Special Population:				
Moderate Hepatic	4.3 (37)	3.8 (34)	90.5 (27)	22.7 (30)
Impairment (n=12)	3.4–5.2	3.1–4.5	76.9–104	18.9–26.5

† Calculated only up to 24 hr for M_1

Mean Weight Loss (lbs) in the Six-Month and One-Year Trials

Study/Patient Group	Placebo (n)	MERIDIA (mg) 5 (n)	10 (n)	15 (n)	20 (n)
Study 1					
All patients*	2.0	6.6	9.7	12.1	13.6
	(142)	(148)	(148)	(150)	(145)
Completers**	2.9	8.1	12.1	15.4	18.0
	(84)	(103)	(95)	(94)	(89)
Early responders***	8.5	13.0	16.0	18.2	20.1
	(17)	(60)	(64)	(73)	(76)
Study 2					
All patients*	3.5		9.8	14.0	
	(157)		(154)	(152)	
Completers**	4.8		13.6	15.2	
	(76)		(80)	(93)	
Early responders***	10.7		18.2	18.8	
	(24)		(57)	(76)	
Study 3******					
All patients*	15.2		28.4		
	(78)		(81)		
Completers**	16.7		29.7		
	(48)		(60)		
Early responders***	21.5		33.0		
	(22)		(46)		

* Data for all patients who received study drug and who had any post-baseline measurement (last observation carried forward analysis).
** Data for all patients who completed the entire 6-month (Study 1) or one-year period of dosing and have data recorded for the month 6 (Study 1) or month 12 visit.
*** Data for patients who lost at least 4 lbs in the first 4 weeks of treatment and completed the study.
**** Weight loss data shown describe changes in weight from the pre-VLCD; mean weight loss during the 4-week VLCD was 16.9 lbs for sibutramine and 16.3 lbs for placebo.

CLINICAL STUDIES

Observational epidemiologic studies have established a relationship between obesity and the risks for cardiovascular disease, non-insulin dependent diabetes mellitus (NIDDM), certain forms of cancer, gallstones, certain respiratory disorders, and an increase in overall mortality. These studies suggest that weight loss, if maintained, may produce health benefits for some patients with chronic obesity who may also be at risk for other diseases.
The long-term effects of MERIDIA on the morbidity and mortality associated with obesity have not been established. Weight loss was examined in 11 double-blind, placebo-controlled obesity trials (BMI range across all studies 27–43) with study durations of 12 to 52 weeks and doses ranging from 1 to 30 mg once daily. Weight was significantly reduced in a dose-related manner in sibutramine-treated patients compared to placebo over the dose range of 5 to 20 mg once daily. In two 12-month studies, maximal weight loss was achieved by 6 months and statistically significant weight loss was maintained over 12 months. The amount of placebo-subtracted weight loss achieved on MERIDIA was consistent across studies.
Analysis of the data in three long-term (≥6 months) obesity trials indicates that patients who lose at least 4 pounds in the first 4 weeks of therapy with a given dose of MERIDIA are most likely to achieve significant long-term weight loss on that dose of MERIDIA. Approximately 60% of such patients went on to achieve a placebo-subtracted weight loss of ≥5% of their initial body weight by month 6. Conversely, of those patients on a given dose of MERIDIA who did not lose at least 4 pounds in the first 4 weeks of therapy, approximately 80% did not go on to achieve a placebo-subtracted weight loss of ≥5% of their initial body weight on that dose by month 6.
Significant dose-related reductions in waist circumference, an indicator of intra-abdominal fat, have also been observed over 6 and 12 months in placebo-controlled clinical trials. In a 12-week placebo-controlled study of non-insulin dependent diabetes mellitus patients randomized to placebo or 15 mg per day of MERIDIA, Dual Energy X-Ray Absorptiometry (DEXA) assessment of changes in body composition showed that total body fat mass decreased by 1.8 kg in the MERIDIA group versus 0.2 kg in the placebo group ($p<0.001$). Similarly, truncal (android) fat mass decreased by 0.6 kg in the MERIDIA group versus 0.1 kg in the placebo group ($p<0.01$). The changes in lean mass, fasting blood sugar, and HbA_1 were not statistically significantly different between the two groups.
Eleven double-blind, placebo-controlled obesity trials with study durations of 12 to 52 weeks have provided evidence that MERIDIA does not adversely affect glycemia, serum lipid profiles, or serum uric acid in obese patients. Treatment with MERIDIA (5 to 20 mg once daily) is associated with mean increases in blood pressure of 1 to 3 mm Hg and with mean increases in pulse rate of 4 to 5 beats per minute relative to placebo. These findings are similar in normotensives and in patients with hypertension controlled with medication. Those patients who lose significant (≥ 5% weight loss) amounts of weight on MERIDIA tend to have smaller increases in blood pressure and pulse rate (see "**WARNINGS**").
In Study 1, a 6-month, double-blind, placebo-controlled study in obese patients, Study 2, a 1-year, double-blind, placebo-controlled study in obese patients, and Study 3, a 1-year, double-blind, placebo-controlled study in obese patients who lost at least 6 kg on a 4-week very low calorie diet (VLCD), MERIDIA produced significant reductions in weight, as shown below. In the two 1-year studies, maximal weight loss was achieved by 6 months and statistically significant weight loss was maintained over 12 months.
[See second table above]
Maintenance of weight loss with sibutramine was examined in a 2-year, double-blind, placebo-controlled trial. After a 6-month run-in phase in which all patients received sibutramine 10 mg (mean weight loss, 26 lbs.), patients were randomized to sibutramine (10 to 20 mg, 352 patients) or placebo (115 patients). The mean weight loss from initial body weight to endpoint was 21 lbs. and 12 lbs. for sibutramine and placebo patients, respectively. A statistically significantly ($p<0.001$) greater proportion of sibutramine treated patients, 75%, 62%, and 43%, maintained at least 80% of their initial weight loss at 12, 18, and 24 months,

Combined Analysis (11 Studies) of Percentage Change in Serum Lipids (N)—LOCF

Category	TG	CHOL	LDL-C	HDL-C
All Placebo	0.53 (475)	−1.53 (475)	−0.09 (233)	−0.56 (248)
<5% Weight Loss	4.52 (382)	−0.42 (382)	−0.70 (205)	−0.71 (217)
≥5% Weight Loss	−15.30 (92)	−6.23 (92)	−6.19 (27)	0.94 (30)
All Sibutramine	−8.75 (1164)	−2.21 (1165)	−1.85 (642)	4.13 (664)
<5% Weight Loss	−0.54 (547)	0.17 (548)	−0.37 (320)	3.19 (331)
≥5% Weight Loss	−16.59 (612)	−4.87 (612)	−4.56 (317)	4.68 (328)

Baseline mean values:
Placebo: TG 187 mg/dL; CHOL 221 mg/dL; LDL-C 140 mg/dL; HDL-C 47 mg/dL
Sibutramine: TG 172 mg/dL; CHOL 215 mg/dL; LDL-C 140 mg/dL; HDL-C 47 mg/dL

Parameter	Systolic			Diastolic		
mm Hg	Placebo n=12	Sibutramine		Placebo	Sibutramine	
		15 mg n=14	20 mg n=16		15 mg n=12	20 mg n=16
Daytime	0.2	3.9	4.4	0.5	5.0	5.7
Nightime	−0.3	4.1	6.4	−1.0	4.3	5.4
Early am	−0.9	9.4	5.3	−3.0	6.7	5.8
24-hour mean	−0.1	4.0	4.7	0.1	5.0	5.6

Normal diurnal variation of blood pressure was maintained.

respectively, compared with the placebo group (38%, 23%, and 16%). Also 67%, 37%, 17%, and 9% of sibutramine treated patients compared with 49%, 19%, 5%, and 3% of placebo patients lost ≥5%, ≥10%, ≥15%, and ≥20%, respectively, of their initial body weight at endpoint. From endpoint to the post-study follow-up visit (about 1 month), weight regain was approximately 4 lbs for the sibutramine patients and approximately 2 lbs for the placebo patients.
MERIDIA induced weight loss has been accompanied by beneficial changes in serum lipids that are similar to those seen with nonpharmacologically-mediated weight loss. A combined, weighted analysis of the changes in serum lipids in 11 placebo-controlled obesity studies ranging in length from 12 to 52 weeks is shown below for the last observation carried forward (LOCF) analysis.
[See first table above]
MERIDIA induced weight loss has been accompanied by reductions in serum uric acid.
Certain centrally-acting weight loss agents that cause release of serotonin from nerve terminals have been associated with cardiac valve dysfunction. The possible occurrence of cardiac valve disease was specifically investigated in two studies. In one study 2-D and color Doppler echocardiography were performed on 210 patients (mean age, 54 years) receiving MERIDIA 15 mg or placebo daily for periods of 2 weeks to 16 months (mean duration of treatment, 7.6 months). In patients without a prior history of valvular heart disease, the incidence of valvular heart disease was 3/132 (2.3%) in the sibutramine treatment group (all three cases were mild aortic insufficiency) and 2/77 (2.6%) in the placebo treatment group (one case of mild aortic insufficiency and one case of severe aortic insufficiency). In another study, 25 patients underwent 2-D and color Doppler echocardiography before treatment with MERIDIA and again after treatment with MERIDIA 5 to 30 mg daily for three months; there were no cases of valvular heart disease.
The effect of sibutramine 15 mg once daily on measures of 24-hour blood pressure was evaluated in a 12-week placebo-controlled study. Twenty-six male and female, primarily Caucasian individuals with an average BMI of 34 kg/m^2 and an average age of 39 years underwent 24-hour ambulatory blood pressure monitoring (ABPM). The mean changes from baseline to Week 12 in various measures of ABPM are shown in the following table.
[See second table above]

INDICATIONS AND USAGE

MERIDIA is indicated for the management of obesity, including weight loss and maintenance of weight loss, and should be used in conjunction with a reduced calorie diet. MERIDIA is recommended for obese patients with an initial body mass index ≥30 kg/m^2, or ≥27 kg/m^2 in the presence of other risk factors (e.g., hypertension, diabetes, dyslipidemia).
Below is a chart of Body Mass Index (BMI) based on various heights and weights.
BMI is calculated by taking the patient's weight, in kg, and dividing by the patient's height, in meters, squared. Metric conversions are as follows: pounds ÷ 2.2 = kg; inches × 0.0254 = meters.

BMI		25	26	27	28	29	30	31	32	33	34	35	40
		WEIGHT (lbs)											
	4'10"	119	124	129	134	138	143	149	153	158	163	167	191
	4'11"	124	128	133	138	143	148	154	158	164	169	173	198
	5'	128	133	138	143	148	153	159	164	169	175	179	204
	5'1"	132	137	143	148	153	158	165	169	175	180	185	211
	5'2"	136	142	147	153	158	164	170	175	181	186	191	218
H	5'3"	141	146	152	158	163	169	175	181	187	192	197	225
	5'4"	145	151	157	163	169	174	181	187	193	199	204	232
E	5'5"	150	156	162	168	174	180	187	193	199	205	210	240
	5'6"	155	161	167	173	179	186	192	199	205	211	216	247
I	5'7"	159	166	172	178	185	191	198	205	211	218	223	255
	5'8"	164	171	177	184	190	197	204	211	218	224	230	262
G	5'9"	169	176	182	189	196	203	210	217	224	231	236	270
	5'10"	174	181	188	195	202	207	216	223	230	237	243	278
H	5'11"	179	186	193	200	208	215	222	230	237	244	250	286
	6'	184	191	199	206	213	221	228	236	244	251	258	294
T	6'1"	189	197	204	212	219	227	236	243	251	258	265	302
	6'2"	194	202	210	218	225	233	241	250	258	265	272	311
	6'3"	200	208	216	224	232	240	248	256	264	272	279	319

CONTRAINDICATIONS

MERIDIA is contraindicated in patients receiving monoamine oxidase inhibitors (MAOIs) (see "**WARNINGS**").
MERIDIA is contraindicated in patients with hypersensitivity to sibutramine or any of the inactive ingredients of MERIDIA.
MERIDIA is contraindicated in patients who have anorexia nervosa.
MERIDIA is contraindicated in patients taking other centrally acting appetite suppressant drugs.

WARNINGS

Blood Pressure and Pulse

MERIDIA SUBSTANTIALLY INCREASES BLOOD PRESSURE IN SOME PATIENTS. REGULAR MONITORING OF BLOOD PRESSURE IS REQUIRED WHEN PRESCRIBING MERIDIA.
In placebo-controlled obesity studies, MERIDIA 5 to 20 mg once daily was associated with mean increases in systolic and diastolic blood pressure of approximately 1 to 3 mm Hg relative to placebo, and with mean increases in pulse rate relative to placebo of approximately 4 to 5 beats per minute. Larger increases were seen in some patients, particularly when therapy with MERIDIA was initiated at the higher doses (see table below). In pre-marketing placebo-controlled obesity studies, 0.4% of patients treated with MERIDIA were discontinued for hypertension (SBP ≥ 160 mm Hg or DBP ≥ 95 mm Hg), compared with 0.4% in the placebo group, and 0.4% of patients with MERIDIA were discontinued for tachycardia (pulse rate ≥ 100 bpm), compared with 0.1% in the placebo group. Blood pressure and pulse should be measured prior to starting therapy with MERIDIA and should be monitored at regular intervals thereafter. For patients who experience a sustained increase in blood pressure or pulse rate while receiving MERIDIA, either dose reduction or discontinuation should be considered. MERIDIA should be given with caution to those patients with a history of hypertension (see "**DOSAGE AND ADMINISTRATION**"), and should not be given to patients with uncontrolled or poorly controlled hypertension.

Percent Outliers in Studies 1 and 2

Dose (mg)	%Outliers* SBP	DBP	Pulse
Placebo	9	7	12
5	6	20	16
10	12	15	28
15	13	17	24
20	14	22	37

*Outlier defined as increase from baseline of ≥15 mm Hg for three consecutive visits (SBP), ≥10 mm Hg for three consecutive visits (DBP), or pulse ≥10 bpm for three consecutive visits.

Potential Interaction With Monoamine Oxidase Inhibitors

MERIDIA is a norepinephrine, serotonin and dopamine reuptake inhibitor and should not be used concomitantly with MAOIs (see "**PRECAUTIONS**", Drug Interactions subsection). There should be at least a 2-week interval after stopping MAOIs before commencing treatment with MERIDIA. Similarly, there should be at least a 2-week interval after stopping MERIDIA before starting treatment with MAOIs.

Concomitant Cardiovascular Disease

Treatment with MERIDIA has been associated with increases in heart rate and/or blood pressure. Therefore, MERIDIA should not be used in patients with a history of coronary artery disease, congestive heart failure, arrhythmias, or stroke.

Glaucoma

Because MERIDIA can cause mydriasis, it should be used with caution in patients with narrow angle glaucoma.

Miscellaneous

Organic causes of obesity (e.g., untreated hypothyroidism) should be excluded before prescribing MERIDIA.

PRECAUTIONS

Pulmonary Hypertension

Certain centrally-acting weight loss agents that cause release of serotonin from nerve terminals have been associated with pulmonary hypertension (PPH), a rare but lethal disease. In pre-marketing clinical studies, no cases of PPH have been reported with MERIDIA® (sibutramine hydrochloride monohydrate) Capsules. Because of the low incidence of this disease in the underlying population, however, it is not known whether or not MERIDIA may cause this disease.

Seizures

During premarketing testing, seizures were reported in <0.1% of MERIDIA treated patients. MERIDIA should be used cautiously in patients with a history of seizures. It should be discontinued in any patient who develops seizures.

Gallstones

Weight loss can precipitate or exacerbate gallstone formation.

Renal/Hepatic Dysfunction

Patients with severe renal impairment or severe hepatic dysfunction have not been systematically studied; MERIDIA should therefore not be used in such patients.

Interference With Cognitive and Motor Performance

Although sibutramine did not affect psychomotor or cognitive performance in healthy volunteers, any CNS active drug has the potential to impair judgment, thinking or motor skills.

Information For Patients

Physicians should instruct their patients to read the patient package insert before starting therapy with MERIDIA and to reread it each time the prescription is renewed.
Physicians should also discuss with their patients any part of the package insert that is relevant to them. In particular, the importance of keeping appointments for follow-up visits should be emphasized.
Patients should be advised to notify their physician if they develop a rash, hives, or other allergic reactions.
Patients should be advised to inform their physicians if they are taking, or plan to take, any prescription or over-the-counter drugs, especially weight-reducing agents, decongestants, antidepressants, cough suppressants, lithium, dihydroergotamine, sumatriptan (Imitrex®), or tryptophan, since there is a potential for interactions.
Patients should be reminded of the importance of having their blood pressure and pulse monitored at regular intervals.

Drug Interactions

CNS Active Drugs: The use of MERIDIA in combination with other CNS-active drugs, particularly serotonergic agents, has not been systematically evaluated. Consequently, caution is advised if the concomitant administration of MERIDIA with other centrally-acting drugs is indicated (see "**CONTRAINDICATIONS**" and "**WARNINGS**").
In patients receiving monoamine oxidase inhibitors (MAOIs) (e.g., phenelzine, selegiline) in combination with serotonergic agents (e.g., fluoxetine, fluvoxamine, paroxetine, sertraline, venlafaxine), there have been reports of serious, sometimes fatal, reactions ("serotonin syndrome;" see below). Because MERIDIA inhibits serotonin reuptake, MERIDIA should not be used concomitantly with a MAOI (see "**CONTRAINDICATIONS**"). At least 2 weeks should elapse between discontinuation of a MAOI and initiation of treatment with MERIDIA. Similarly, at least 2 weeks should elapse between discontinuation of MERIDIA and initiation of treatment with a MAOI.
The rare, but serious, constellation of symptoms termed "serotonin syndrome" has also been reported with the concomitant use of selective serotonin reuptake inhibitors and agents for migraine therapy, such as Imitrex® (sumatriptan succinate) and dihydroergotamine, certain opioids, such as dextromethorphan, meperidine, pentazocine and fentanyl, lithium, or tryptophan. Serotonin syndrome has also been reported with the concomitant use of two serotonin reuptake inhibitors. The syndrome requires immediate medical attention and may include one or more of the following symptoms: excitement, hypomania, restlessness, loss of consciousness, confusion, disorientation, anxiety, agitation, motor weakness, myoclonus, tremor, hemiballismus, hyperreflexia, ataxia, dysarthria, incoordination, hyperthermia, shivering, pupillary dilation, diaphoresis, emesis, and tachycardia.
Because MERIDIA inhibits serotonin reuptake, in general, it should not be administered with other serotonergic agents such as those listed above. However, if such a combination is clinically indicated, appropriate observation of the patient is warranted.
Drugs That May Raise Blood Pressure and/or Heart Rate: Concomitant use of MERIDIA and other agents that may raise blood pressure or heart rate have not been evaluated.

Continued on next page

Meridia—Cont.

These include certain decongestants, cough, cold, and allergy medications that contain agents such as ephedrine, or pseudoephedrine. Caution should be used when prescribing MERIDIA to patients who use these medications.

Drugs That Inhibit Cytochrome P450($3A_4$) Metabolism: *In vitro* studies indicated that the cytochrome P450($3A_4$)-mediated metabolism of sibutramine was inhibited by ketoconazole and to a lesser extent by erythromycin. Clinical interaction trials were conducted on these substrates. The potential for such interactions is described below.

Ketoconazole: Concomitant administration of 200 mg doses of ketoconazole twice daily and 20 mg sibutramine once daily for 7 days in 12 uncomplicated obese subjects resulted in moderate increases in AUC and C_{max} of 58% and 36% for M_1 and of 20% and 19% for M_2, respectively.

Erythromycin: The steady-state pharmacokinetics of sibutramine and metabolites M_1 and M_2 were evaluated in 12 uncomplicated obese subjects following concomitant administration of 500 mg of erythromycin three times daily and 20 mg of sibutramine once daily for 7 days. Concomitant erythromycin resulted in small increases in the AUC (less than 14%) for M_1 and M_2. A small reduction in C_{max} for M_1 (11%) and a slight increase in C_{max} for M_2 (10%) were observed.

Cimetidine: Concomitant administration of cimetidine 400 mg twice daily and sibutramine 15 mg once daily for 7 days in 12 volunteers resulted in small increases in combined (M_1 and M_2) plasma C_{max} (3.4%) and AUC (7.3%); these differences are unlikely to be of clinical significance.

Alcohol: In a double-blind, placebo-controlled, crossover study in 19 volunteers, administration of a single dose of ethanol (0.5 mL/kg) together with 20 mg of sibutramine resulted in no psychomotor interactions of clinical significance between alcohol and sibutramine. However, the concomitant use of MERIDIA and excess alcohol is not recommended.

Oral Contraceptives: The suppression of ovulation by oral contraceptives was not inhibited by MERIDIA. In a crossover study, 12 healthy female volunteers on oral steroid contraceptives received placebo in one period and 15 mg sibutramine in another period over the course of 8 weeks. No clinically significant systemic interaction was observed; therefore, no requirement for alternative contraceptive precautions are needed when patients taking oral contraceptives are concurrently prescribed sibutramine.

Drugs Highly Bound to Plasma Proteins: Although sibutramine and its active metabolites M_1 and M_2 are extensively bound to plasma proteins (≥94%), the low therapeutic concentrations and basic characteristics of these compounds make them unlikely to result in clinically significant protein binding interactions with other highly protein bound drugs such as warfarin and phenytoin. *In vitro* protein binding interaction studies have not been conducted.

Carcinogenesis, Mutagenesis, Impairment of Fertility

Carcinogenicity

Sibutramine was administered in the diet to mice (1.25, 5 or 20 mg/kg/day) and rats (1, 3, or 9 mg/kg/day) for two years generating combined maximum plasma AUC's of the two major active metabolites equivalent to 0.375 and 15.75 times, respectively, those following a daily human dose of 15 mg. There was no evidence of carcinogenicity in mice or in female rats. In male rats there was a higher incidence of benign tumors of the testicular interstitial cells; such tumors are commonly seen in rats and are hormonally mediated. The relevance of these tumors to humans is not known.

Mutagenicity

Sibutramine was not mutagenic in the Ames test, *in vitro* Chinese hamster V79 cell mutation assay, *in vitro* clastogenicity assay in human lymphocytes or micronucleus assay in mice. Its two major active metabolites were found to have equivocal bacterial mutagenic activity in the Ames test. However, both metabolites gave consistently negative results in the *in vitro* Chinese hamster V79 cell mutation assay, *in vitro* clastogenicity assay in human lymphocytes, *in vitro* DNA-repair assay in HeLa cells, micronucleus assay in mice and *in vivo* unscheduled DNA-synthesis assay in rat hepatocytes.

Impairment of Fertility

In rats, there were no effects on fertility at doses generating combined plasma AUC's of the two major active metabolites up to 32.25 times those following a human dose of 15 mg. At 13 times the human combined AUC, there was maternal toxicity, and the dam's nest-building behavior was impaired, leading to a higher incidence of perinatal mortality; there was no effect at approximately 4 times the human combined AUC.

Pregnancy

Teratogenic Effects-Pregnancy Category C

Radiolabeled studies in animals indicated that tissue distribution was unaffected by pregnancy, with relatively low transfer to the fetus. In rats, there was no evidence of teratogenicity at doses of 1, 3, or 10 mg/kg/day generating combined plasma AUC's of the two major active metabolites up to approximately 32.25 times those following the human dose of 15 mg. In rabbits dosed at 3, 15, or 75 mg/kg/day, plasma AUC's greater than approximately 5 times those following the human dose of 15 mg caused maternal toxicity. At markedly toxic doses, Dutch Belted rabbits had a slightly higher than control incidence of pups with a broad short snout, short rounded pinnae, short tail and, in some, shorter thickened long bones in the limbs; at comparably high doses in New Zealand White rabbits, one study showed a slightly higher than control incidence of pups with cardiovascular anomalies while a second study showed a lower incidence than in the control group.

No adequate and well controlled studies with MERIDIA have been conducted in pregnant women. The use of MERIDIA during pregnancy is not recommended. Women of childbearing potential should employ adequate contraception while taking MERIDIA. Patients should be advised to notify their physician if they become pregnant or intend to become pregnant during therapy.

Nursing Mothers

It is not known whether sibutramine or its metabolites are excreted in human milk. MERIDIA is not recommended for use in nursing mothers. Patients should be advised to notify their physician if they are breast-feeding.

Pediatric Use

The safety and effectiveness of MERIDIA in pediatric patients under 16 years of age have not been established.

Geriatric Use

Clinical studies of MERIDIA did not include sufficient numbers of patients aged 65 and over to determine whether they respond differently from younger patients. In general, dose selection for an elderly patient should be cautious, reflecting the greater frequency of decreased hepatic, renal, or cardiac function, and of concomitant disease or other drug therapy. Pharmacokinetics in elderly patients are discussed in **"CLINICAL PHARMACOLOGY"**.

ADVERSE REACTIONS

In placebo-controlled studies, 9% of patients treated with MERIDIA (n=2068) and 7% of patients treated with placebo (n=884) withdrew for adverse events.

In placebo-controlled studies, the most common events were dry mouth, anorexia, insomnia, constipation and headache. Adverse events in these studies occurring in ≥1% of MERIDIA treated patients and more frequently than in the placebo group are shown in the following table.

[See table below]

The following additional adverse events were reported in ≥ 1% of all patients who received MERIDIA in controlled and uncontrolled pre-marketing studies.

Body as a Whole: fever.

Digestive System: diarrhea, flatulence, gastroenteritis, tooth disorder.

Metabolic and Nutritional: peripheral edema.

Musculoskeletal System: arthritis.

Nervous System: agitation, leg cramps, hypertonia, thinking abnormal.

Respiratory System: bronchitis, dyspnea.

Skin and Appendages: pruritus.

Special Senses: amblyopia.

Urogenital System: menstrual disorder.

Postmarketing Reports

Voluntary reports of adverse events temporally associated with the use of MERIDIA are listed below. It is important to emphasize that although these events occurred during treatment with MERIDIA, they may have no causal relationship with the drug. Obesity itself, concurrent disease states/risk factors, or weight reduction may be associated with an increased risk for some of these events.

abnormal dreams, abnormal ejaculation, abnormal gait, abnormal vision, alopecia, amnesia, anaphylactic shock, ana-

BODY SYSTEM Adverse Event	Obese Patients in Placebo-Controlled Studies MERIDIA® (n = 2068) %Incidence	 Placebo (n = 884) %Incidence
BODY AS A WHOLE:		
Headache	30.3	18.6
Back pain	8.2	5.5
Flu syndrome	8.2	5.8
Injury accident	5.9	4.1
Asthenia	5.9	5.3
Abdominal pain	4.5	3.6
Chest pain	1.8	1.2
Neck pain	1.6	1.1
Allergic reaction	1.5	0.8
CARDIOVASCULAR SYSTEM		
Tachycardia	2.6	0.6
Vasodilation	2.4	0.9
Migraine	2.4	2.0
Hypertension/increased blood pressure	2.1	0.9
Palpitation	2.0	0.8
DIGESTIVE SYSTEM		
Anorexia	13.0	3.5
Constipation	11.5	6.0
Increased appetite	8.7	2.7
Nausea	5.9	2.8
Dyspepsia	5.0	2.6
Gastritis	1.7	1.2
Vomiting	1.5	1.4
Rectal disorder	1.2	0.5
METABOLIC & NUTRITIONAL		
Thirst	1.7	0.9
Generalized edema	1.2	0.8
MUSCULOSKELETAL SYSTEM		
Arthralgia	5.9	5.0
Myalgia	1.9	1.1
Tenosynovitis	1.2	0.5
Joint disorder	1.1	0.6
NERVOUS SYSTEM		
Dry mouth	17.2	4.2
Insomnia	10.7	4.5
Dizziness	7.0	3.4
Nervousness	5.2	2.9
Anxiety	4.5	3.4
Depression	4.3	2.5
Paresthesia	2.0	0.5
Somnolence	1.7	0.9
CNS stimulation	1.5	0.5
Emotional lability	1.3	0.6
RESPIRATORY SYSTEM		
Rhinitis	10.2	7.1
Pharyngitis	10.0	8.4
Sinusitis	5.0	2.6
Cough increase	3.8	3.3
Laryngitis	1.3	0.9
SKIN & APPENDAGES		
Rash	3.8	2.5
Sweating	2.5	0.9
Herpes simplex	1.3	1.0
Acne	1.0	0.8
SPECIAL SENSES		
Taste perversion	2.2	0.8
Ear disorder	1.7	0.9
Ear pain	1.1	0.7
UROGENITAL SYSTEM		
Dysmenorrhea	3.5	1.4
Urinary tract infection	2.3	2.0
Vaginal monilia	1.2	0.5
Metrorrhagia	1.0	0.8

phylactoid reaction, anemia, anger, angina pectoris, arthrosis, atrial fibrillation, blurred vision, bursitis, cerebrovascular accident, chest pressure, chest tightness, cholecystitis, cholelithiasis, concentration impaired, confusion, congestive heart failure, depression aggravated, dermatitis, dry eye, duodenal ulcer, epistaxis, eructation, eye pain, facial edema, gastrointestinal hemorrhage, Gilles de la Tourette's syndrome, goiter, heart arrest, heart rate decreased, hematuria, hyperglycemia, hyperthyroidism, hypesthesia, hypoglycemia, hypothyroidism, impotence, increased intraocular pressure, increased salivation, increased urinary frequency, intestinal obstruction, leukopenia, libido decreased, libido increased, limb pain, lymphadenopathy, manic reaction, micturition difficulty, mood changes, mouth ulcer, myocardial infarction, nasal congestion, nightmares, otitis externa, otitis media, petechiae, photosensitivity (eyes), photosensitivity (skin), respiratory disorder, serotonin syndrome, short term memory loss, speech disorder, stomach ulcer, sudden unexplained death, supraventricular tachycardia, syncope, thrombocytopenia, tinnitus, tongue edema, torsade de pointes, transient ischemic attack, tremor, twitch, urticaria, vascular headache, ventricular tachycardia, ventricular extrasystoles, ventricular fibrillation, vertigo, yawn.

Other Notable Adverse Events

Seizures: Convulsions were reported as an adverse event in three of 2068 (0.1%) MERIDIA treated patients and in none of 884 placebo-treated patients in placebo-controlled premarketing obesity studies. Two of the three patients with seizures had potentially predisposing factors (one had a prior history of epilepsy; one had a subsequent diagnosis of brain tumor). The incidence in all subjects who received MERIDIA (three of 4,588 subjects) was less than 0.1%.

Ecchymosis/Bleeding Disorders: Ecchymosis (bruising) was observed in 0.7% of MERIDIA treated patients and in 0.2% of placebo-treated patients in pre-marketing placebo-controlled obesity studies. One patient had prolonged bleeding of a small amount which occurred during minor facial surgery. MERIDIA may have an effect on platelet function due to its effect on serotonin uptake.

Interstitial Nephritis: Acute interstitial nephritis (confirmed by biopsy) was reported in one obese patient receiving MERIDIA during pre-marketing studies. After discontinuation of the medication, dialysis and oral corticosteroids were administered; renal function normalized. The patient made a full recovery.

Altered Laboratory Findings: Abnormal liver function tests, including increases in AST, ALT, GGT, LDH, alkaline phosphatase and bilirubin, were reported as adverse events in 1.6% of MERIDIA-treated obese patients in placebo-controlled trials compared with 0.8% of placebo patients. In these studies, potentially clinically significant values (total bilirubin ≥ 2 mg/dL; ALT, AST, GGT, LDH, or alkaline phosphatase ≥ 3x upper limit of normal) occurred in 0% (alkaline phosphatase) to 0.6% (ALT) of the MERIDIA treated patients and in none of the placebo-treated patients. Abnormal values tended to be sporadic, often diminished with continued treatment, and did not show a clear dose-response relationship.

DRUG ABUSE AND DEPENDENCE

Controlled Substance

MERIDIA is controlled in Schedule IV of the Controlled Substances Act (CSA).

Abuse and Physical and Psychological Dependence

Physicians should carefully evaluate patients for history of drug abuse and follow such patients closely, observing them for signs of misuse or abuse (e.g., drug development of tolerance, incrementation of doses, drug seeking behavior).

OVERDOSAGE

Human Experience

Three cases of overdose have been reported with MERIDIA. The first was in a 2-year-old child of one patient who ingested up to eight 10 mg capsules. No complications were observed during the overnight hospitalization, and the child was discharged the following day with no sequela. The second report was in a 30-year-old male in a depression study who ingested approximately 100 mg of sibutramine in an attempt to commit suicide. The patient suffered no adverse effects or ECG abnormalities post-ingestion. The third report was in the 45-year-old husband of a patient in an obese dyslipidemic study. He ingested 400 mg of his wife's drug supply and was hospitalized for observation; a heart rate of 120 bpm was noted. He was discharged the next day with no apparent sequelae.

Overdose Management

There is no specific antidote to MERIDIA. Treatment should consist of general measures employed in the management of overdosage: an airway should be established; cardiac and vital sign monitoring is recommended; general symptomatic and supportive measures should be instituted. Cautious use of β-blockers may be indicated to control elevated blood pressure or tachycardia. The benefits of forced diuresis and hemodialysis are unknown.

DOSAGE AND ADMINISTRATION

The recommended starting dose of MERIDIA is 10 mg administered once daily with or without food. If there is inadequate weight loss, the dose may be titrated after four weeks to a total of 15 mg once daily. The 5 mg dose should be reserved for patients who do not tolerate the 10 mg dose. Blood pressure and heart rate changes should be taken into account when making decisions regarding dose titration (see "**PRECAUTIONS**").

Doses above 15 mg daily are not recommended. In most of the clinical trials, MERIDIA was given in the morning.

Analysis of numerous variables has indicated that approximately 60% of patients who lose at least 4 pounds in the first 4 weeks of treatment with a given dose of MERIDIA in combination with a reduced-calorie diet lose at least 5% (placebo-subtracted) of their initial body weight by the end of 6 months to 1 year of treatment on that dose of MERIDIA. Conversely, approximately, 80% of patients who do not lose at least 4 pounds in the first 4 weeks of treatment with a given dose of MERIDIA do not lose at least 5% (placebo-subtracted) of their initial body weight by the end of 6 months to 1 year of treatment on that dose. If a patient has not lost at least 4 pounds in the first 4 weeks of treatment, the physician should consider reevaluation of therapy which may include increasing the dose or discontinuation of MERIDIA.

The safety and effectiveness of MERIDIA, as demonstrated in double-blind, placebo-controlled trials, have not been determined beyond 2 years at this time.

HOW SUPPLIED

MERIDIA® (sibutramine hydrochloride monohydrate) Capsules contain 5 mg, 10 mg, or 15 mg sibutramine hydrochloride monohydrate and are supplied as follows:

5 mg, NDC 0074-2456-13, blue/yellow capsules imprinted with "MERIDIA" on the cap and "-5-" on the body, in bottles of 100 capsules.

10 mg, NDC 0074-2457-13, blue/white capsules imprinted with "MERIDIA" on the cap and "-10-" on the body, in bottles of 100 capsules.

15 mg, NDC 0074-2458-13, yellow/white capsules imprinted with "MERIDIA" on the cap and "-15-" on the body, in bottles of 100 capsules.

Storage: Store at 25°C (77°F); excursions permitted to 15°–30°C (59°–86°F) [see USP controlled room temperature]. Protect capsules from heat and moisture. Dispense in a tight, light-resistant container as defined in USP.

Manufactured for Abbott Laboratories, North Chicago, IL 60064, U.S.A. by BASF Corporation, Mount Olive, NJ 07828, U.S.A.

IMITREX is a registered trademark of Glaxo Group Limited.

Sibutramine is covered by US Patent Nos. 4,746,680; 4,929,629; and 5,436,272.

Printed in USA
Revised: Aug., 2001
03-5139-R2

ABBOTT LABORATORIES
NORTH CHICAGO, IL60064, U.S.A.

MERIDIA® ℂ

(sibutramine hydrochloride monohydrate) Capsules

PATIENT INFORMATION

IMPORTANT PATIENT INFORMATION. READ THIS PATIENT INFORMATION CAREFULLY AND COMPLETELY BEFORE YOU START TAKING MERIDIA AND REREAD IT EACH TIME THE PRESCRIPTION IS RENEWED. CONTACT YOUR DOCTOR IMMEDIATELY IF YOU HAVE ANY QUESTIONS OR CONCERNS. SAVE THIS PATIENT INFORMATION SHEET FOR FUTURE REFERENCE.

Patient information about MERIDIA® (sibutramine hydrochloride monohydrate) Capsules.

MERIDIA capsules come in three strengths: 5 mg, 10 mg, and 15 mg.

What is MERIDIA?

MERIDIA is an oral prescription medication used for the medical management of obesity, including weight loss and the maintenance of weight loss. MERIDIA can only be prescribed by a medical doctor.

MERIDIA comes in three different strength capsules (5 mg, 10 mg, and 15 mg). The recommended initial starting dose of MERIDIA is one 10 mg capsule per day. Your doctor will determine the starting dose that is best for you.

How does MERIDIA work?

MERIDIA works by affecting appetite control centers in the brain.

In medical studies in overweight people, MERIDIA, along with a reduced calorie diet, produced significant reductions in body weight.

MERIDIA should be used as part of a comprehensive weight-loss program, supervised by your doctor, that includes a reduced calorie diet and appropriate physical activity.

How long does it take for MERIDIA to work?

Every person will respond differently to MERIDIA when used as part of a comprehensive weight-loss program. You may be able to lose 4 or more pounds of body weight in the first month you take MERIDIA. If you find that you do not lose at least 4 pounds during the first month, you should notify your doctor so he or she can re-evaluate your situation. Your doctor may wish to change your dose of MERIDIA.

Most people who lose weight on MERIDIA lose it in the first 6 months of treatment. Scientific studies that lasted two years have shown that many people who lost weight and remained on MERIDIA therapy maintained their weight loss.

Who should take MERIDIA?

A weight-loss program that includes a reduced calorie diet and appropriate physical activity may be adequate in some patients. You should discuss with your doctor whether MERIDIA should be added to such a program.

MERIDIA is recommended for overweight people with an initial body mass index (BMI) of 30 or higher, or for overweight people with a BMI of 27 or higher if they have medical risk factors such as high blood pressure, diabetes, or high cholesterol. Your doctor can determine your BMI and will decide if you meet these criteria.

How and when should I take MERIDIA?

Follow your doctors instructions on how and when to take MERIDIA.

Your doctor will recommend that you take one (1) MERIDIA capsule a day.

You can take MERIDIA on an empty stomach or after a meal.

What if I miss a dose?

If you forget to take a dose of MERIDIA, do not take an extra capsule to "make up" for the dose you forgot.

How long should I take MERIDIA?

Your doctor will determine how long you should take MERIDIA. Follow your doctor's advice.

The safety and effectiveness of MERIDIA have not been determined beyond two (2) years at this time.

Who should not take MERIDIA?

MERIDIA should not be taken by people who:

1. **HAVE UNCONTROLLED OR POORLY CONTROLLED HIGH BLOOD PRESSURE BECAUSE MERIDIA SUBSTANTIALLY INCREASES BLOOD PRESSURE IN SOME PATIENTS.**
2. Are taking prescription medicines called monoamine oxidase inhibitors (MAOIs) for depression, Parkinson's Disease, or any other disorder (for example: Eldepryl®, Parnate®, Nardil®).
3. Are taking other weight loss medications that act on the brain (for example: phentermine). This includes prescription and over-the-counter medications and herbal products.
4. Have had prior allergic reactions to MERIDIA or sibutramine.
5. Have a diagnosis of coronary artery disease and/or who have angina pectoris (heart-related chest pain).
6. Have arrhythmias (irregular heart beats).
7. Have had a prior heart attack.
8. Have a diagnosis of congestive heart failure.
9. Have severe liver or kidney disease.
10. Have had a stroke or symptoms of a stroke (transient ischemic attacks [TIAs]).
11. Are pregnant or planning to become pregnant.
12. Are breast-feeding their infants.
13. Are suffering from anorexia nervosa.
14. Are taking prescription medications for depression.
15. Have had seizures (epilepsy or convulsions).
16. Have an eye disorder called narrow angle glaucoma.
17. Are under 16 years of age.
18. Are taking other medications that regulate the neurotransmitter serotonin in the brain (for example: Prozac®, Zoloft®, Effexor®, Luvox®, Paxil® or Zyban®).

If you have any concerns or questions about whether or not you should take MERIDIA, talk to your doctor.

IMPORTANT: It is very important that you make sure that your primary care doctor and all your other health care providers know what medications you take and what medical conditions and allergies you have.

What medical conditions or information should I tell my doctor?

It is important that you tell your doctor all about your medical history, whether you are taking or have taken weight loss drugs in the past, current medical problems, current symptoms, what other medications you take or have taken (prescription and over-the-counter medicines and herbal products) and any prior allergies to medicines.

It is important to make sure your doctor knows if you have heart disease of any kind, high blood pressure, migraine headaches, glaucoma, seizures, depression, Parkinson's Disease, prior strokes, prior transient ischemic attacks (TIAs), thyroid disorders, osteoporosis, gallstones, liver disease, kidney disease, history of a major eating disorder (anorexia nervosa or bulimia nervosa) or any other medical problem.

What about physician follow-up visits?

You should make sure you see your doctor as directed for regular follow-up visits, during which your doctor can follow your body weight, and carefully monitor your overall health as you try to lose weight and maintain weight loss.

What medications can cause problems if taken at the same time I take MERIDIA?

You cannot take MERIDIA if you are taking prescription medicines called monoamine oxidase inhibitors (MAOIs). It is especially important to make sure you tell your doctor if you are taking MAOIs which are sometimes used to treat depression or Parkinson's Disease (for example: Eldepryl®, Nardil®, Parnate®). This is very important because serious, sometimes even fatal, reactions can occur if MERIDIA is taken at the same time MAOIs are taken.

If you are currently taking an MAOI, your doctor will want you to stop taking it for at least two (2) full weeks before starting you on MERIDIA.

If you are currently taking MERIDIA, your doctor will want you to stop taking it for at least two (2) full weeks before starting you on an MAOI.

MERIDIA should not be taken if you are taking other weight-loss medications that act on the brain (for example: phentermine). This includes both prescription and over-the-counter medications and herbal products.

In addition to the above, a rare, but serious, medical syndrome called the "serotonin syndrome" has been reported in patients when medications like MERIDIA are taken along with other drugs that may alter serotonin activity such as:

Continued on next page

Meridia—Cont.

drugs for depression (for example: Desyrel®, Effexor®, Eldepryl®, Remeron®, Serzone®, Wellbutrin®, Nardil®, Parnate®, Paxil®, Prozac®, Zoloft®, Ludiomil®, Adapin®, Asendin®, Elavil®, Etrafon®, Limbitrol®, Norpramin®, Pamelor®, Sinequan®, Surmontil®, Tofranil®, Triavil®, Vivactil®, Luvox®, Anafranil®), drugs for migraine headache therapy (Imitrex® [sumatriptan succinate]) and dihydroergotamine, certain pain medications such as Demerol® (meperidine), Duragesic® (fentanyl), and Talwin® (pentazocine); the cough suppressant dextromethorphan found in many cough medicines; lithium; and the amino acid tryptophan. The syndrome requires immediate medical attention and may include one or more of the following symptoms: restlessness, loss of consciousness, confusion, disorientation, anxiety, agitation, weakness, tremor, incoordination, fever, shivering, sweating, vomiting and increased heart rate.

The metabolism of MERIDIA may be inhibited by ketoconazole (an anti-fungal medicine) and to a lesser degree erythromycin (an antibiotic medicine). You need to make sure your doctor knows you are taking these medicines before you take MERIDIA. If, while taking MERIDIA, your doctor decides to put you on ketoconazole or erythromycin, you should remind him or her that you are also on MERIDIA.

Many over-the-counter cough and cold remedies, as well as certain allergy products and decongestants, contain medicines such as phenylpropanolamine, ephedrine, or pseudoephedrine that may increase blood pressure or heart rate. Before taking these medications on your own, you should check with your doctor to make sure it is all right to take these medicines if you are already taking MERIDIA. Your doctor may advise you to take a certain type of cough, cold, decongestant or allergy medicine that will not interact with MERIDIA.

When should I call my doctor?

It is important that you call your doctor immediately if you experience any symptoms or feelings that make you concerned about your health or a possible drug side effect. Let your doctor advise you on your concerns. If you experience any of the following symptoms, stop taking MERIDIA and notify your doctor immediately: trouble breathing, shortness of breath, chest pain, angina, rapid heart beats over 100 beats a minute, pounding or irregular heart beats, restlessness, lightheadedness, blackout spells, disorientation, depression, mental confusion, anxiety, nervousness, tremors, loss of muscle coordination, muscle stiffness or muscle rigidity, high fever, pain in the eyes, dilated pupils, shivering, sweating, abdominal pain, nausea or vomiting, or other symptoms that concern you.

Is MERIDIA a controlled substance?

Yes, MERIDIA is a controlled substance in Schedule IV of the Controlled Substances Act (CSA).

What weight-loss results have been observed with MERIDIA?

Patients treated with MERIDIA while on a reduced calorie diet, showed a significant weight-loss during the first 6 months of treatment, and significant weight loss was maintained for one year. In one 12-month study, the average weight loss in patients taking MERIDIA, 10 mg daily, was about 10 lbs. and in those taking 15 mg daily was about 14 lbs. The average weight loss in persons on only a reduced calorie diet was 3½ lbs.

What are some of the more common side effects of MERIDIA?

MERIDIA, like all medications, may cause side effects. In studies the most common side effects were: dry mouth, constipation, and insomnia (inability to fall asleep). Other side effects that may occur include: headache, increased sweating, an increase in blood pressure, and an increase in heart rate. These side effects are generally mild, and have usually not caused people to stop taking MERIDIA. If you develop a symptom that you think might be a side effect, stop taking MERIDIA and notify your doctor immediately so he or she can advise you on what to do.

Can MERIDIA affect blood pressure or heart rate?

MERIDIA SUBSTANTIALLY INCREASES BLOOD PRESSURE IN SOME PATIENTS. REGULAR MONITORING OF BLOOD PRESSURE IS REQUIRED WHEN TAKING MERIDIA.

On average, small increases in blood pressure and small increases in heart rate were seen in overweight people who took MERIDIA in scientifically controlled studies. You should make sure you see your doctor as directed for regular follow-up visits. Your blood pressure and pulse should be measured prior to starting therapy with MERIDIA and should be monitored at regular intervals thereafter. If you experience an increase in blood pressure or heart rate while taking MERIDIA, your doctor may decide to decrease the dose or discontinue MERIDIA.

If you have high blood pressure that is controlled by medication or diet, your doctor may choose to prescribe MERIDIA for you as part of a comprehensive weight-management program. MERIDIA should not be taken by people who have uncontrolled or poorly controlled high blood pressure.

Are there any severe side effects?

Certain weight-loss drugs have been associated with pulmonary hypertension (PPH), a rare but sometimes fatal disease. In clinical studies, no cases of PPH have been reported with MERIDIA. Because this disease is so rare, however, it is not known whether or not MERIDIA may cause this disease.

The first symptom of PPH is usually shortness of breath. If you experience new or worsening shortness of breath, or if you experience chest pain, fainting, or swelling of your feet, ankles, or legs, stop taking MERIDIA, and notify your doctor immediately.

Does MERIDIA cause damage to the heart valves?

Certain weight-loss drugs have been associated with cardiac valve dysfunction (heart valve disease). Patients in two studies were examined by doctors who used cardiac ultrasound testing to carefully look at heart valve structure and function. In one study, 25 patients were examined before treatment with MERIDIA and again after three months of treatment. None of the patients had heart valve disease. In another study, patients who had received either MERIDIA or placebo (sugar pills) for periods of two weeks to 16 months were examined. Three out of 132 patients (2.3%) who had taken MERIDIA and two out of 77 patients (2.6%) who had taken placebo were found to have heart valve disease. You should discuss this further with your doctor.

Will MERIDIA change the way I need to take my nutritional supplements?

Non-drug nutritional supplements, like vitamins, minerals and amino acids (with the exception of tryptophan) can be used along with MERIDIA. You should make sure your doctor knows what nutritional supplements you are taking and why you are taking them. You should not take MERIDIA if you are taking tryptophan. You should not use herbal or over-the-counter weight-loss products while taking MERIDIA.

What about drinking alcoholic beverages?

MERIDIA may increase the sedative effects of alcohol. It is important that you let your doctor know how often, and what type of alcoholic beverages you drink. Your doctor can advise you best as to whether you should drink alcoholic beverages while on MERIDIA.

What about drinking coffee, tea and caffeinated beverages?

MERIDIA can be safely taken with moderate use of coffee, tea or caffeinated beverages. You should check with your doctor to make sure that you do not have a medical condition that can be aggravated by these beverages independent of being on MERIDIA. You should check with your doctor if you consume a great deal of caffeinated beverages or use over-the-counter pills that contain caffeine.

What if I develop allergic reactions?

Stop taking MERIDIA and notify your doctor immediately if you develop a skin rash, hives or other allergic reactions.

What if I am pregnant or nursing?

MERIDIA should not be used by pregnant women or nursing mothers. You should notify your doctor immediately if you become pregnant or plan to become pregnant.

What about sexual activity and potential pregnancy?

Women of child bearing potential should use an effective birth control method while taking MERIDIA. Check with your doctor to make sure you are on a medically safe and effective birth control method while taking MERIDIA.

Will MERIDIA affect the effectiveness of birth control pills?

No.

What about driving a car or dangerous work activities?

MERIDIA should not interfere with your ability to drive your car. However, you should be on the alert for any signs of fatigue, sedation, or lack of alertness. You should be very careful about using alcohol before you drive as MERIDIA may increase the sedative effects of alcohol.

MERIDIA was studied in healthy people and did not affect their coordination or impair their judgment. However, MERIDIA has the potential to impair judgment, thinking, coordination or motor skills. You should check with your doctor if you have any questions with regard to your work and the use of MERIDIA.

How should I keep and use MERIDIA?

MERIDIA should be stored at normal room temperature (about 60 to 85°F). Never leave MERIDIA in hot or moist places.

It is important to keep MERIDIA in a safe area where children cannot get it.

If your child swallows MERIDIA, immediately speak with your doctor and/or take your child to the emergency room for immediate medical attention. If you are unable to reach a doctor or emergency room, call the poison control center at 1-800-764-7661.

Never take more MERIDIA than prescribed by your doctor. You should never share MERIDIA with a friend.

SAVE THIS PATIENT INFORMATION SHEET ON MERIDIA. YOU SHOULD KEEP THIS SHEET TO REFER BACK TO FROM TIME TO TIME. KEEP IT IN A SAFE PLACE WHERE YOU CAN FIND IT. YOU MAY WISH TO BRING THIS SHEET WITH YOU EVERY TIME YOU VISIT YOUR DOCTOR. IT MAY HELP YOU WITH YOUR DISCUSSIONS WITH YOUR DOCTOR.

The brands listed, with the exception of MERIDIA are trademarks of their respective owners and are not trademarks of Abbott Laboratories. The makers of these brands are not affiliated with and do not endorse Abbott Laboratories or its products.

Sibutramine is covered by US Patent Nos 4,746,680; 4,929,629; and 5,436,272.

This patient information sheet is intended for information only. It is not a substitute for your doctor's instructions. Notify your doctor immediately of any questions or concerns. Never take extra doses of MERIDIA.

For additional information on MERIDIA and weight management, please talk with your doctor, nurse, pharmacist, other health care professional or call 1-800-633-9110.

Revised: Aug., 2001
03-5139-R2
Manufactured for Abbott Laboratories,
North Chicago, IL 60064, U.S.A.
by BASF Corporation,
Mount Olive, NJ 07828, U.S.A.
ABBOTT LABORATORIES
NORTH CHICAGO, IL60064, U.S.A.

TRICOR® ℞

[tri cŏr]
(fenofibrate tablets)

DESCRIPTION

TRICOR (fenofibrate tablets), is a lipid regulating agent available as tablets for oral administration. Each tablet contains 54 mg or 160 mg of fenofibrate. The chemical name for fenofibrate is 2-[4-(4-chlorobenzoyl) phenoxy]-2-methyl-propanoic acid, 1-methylethyl ester with the following structural formula:

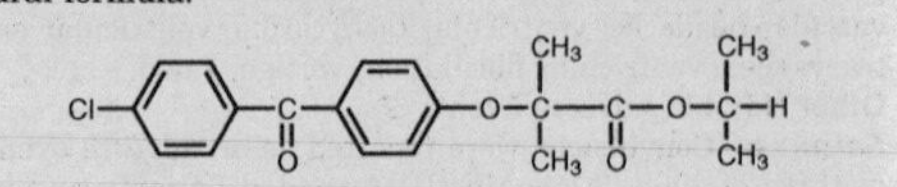

The empirical formula is $C_{20}H_{21}O_4Cl$ and the molecular weight is 360.83; fenofibrate is insoluble in water. The melting point is 79–82°C. Fenofibrate is a white solid which is stable under ordinary conditions.

Inactive Ingredients: Each tablet contains colloidal silicon dioxide, crospovidone, lactose monohydrate, lecithin, microcrystalline cellulose, polyvinyl alcohol, povidone, sodium lauryl sulfate, sodium stearyl fumarate, talc, titanium dioxide, and xanthan gum. In addition, individual tablets contain:

54 mg tablets: D&C Yellow No. 10, FD&C Yellow No. 6, FD&C Blue No. 2.

CLINICAL PHARMACOLOGY

A variety of clinical studies have demonstrated that elevated levels of total cholesterol (total-C), low density lipoprotein cholesterol (LDL-C), and apolipoprotein B (apo B), an LDL membrane complex, are associated with human atherosclerosis. Similarly, decreased levels of high density lipoprotein cholesterol (HDL-C) and its transport complex, apolipoprotein A (apo AI and apo AII) are associated with the development of atherosclerosis. Epidemiologic investigations have established that cardiovascular morbidity and mortality vary directly with the level of total-C, LDL-C, and triglycerides, and inversely with the level of HDL-C. The independent effect of raising HDL-C or lowering triglycerides (TG) on the risk of cardiovascular morbidity and mortality has not been determined.

Fenofibric acid, the active metabolite of fenofibrate, produces reductions in total cholesterol, LDL cholesterol, apolipoprotein B, total triglycerides and triglyceride rich lipoprotein (VLDL) in treated patients. In addition, treatment with fenofibrate results in increases in high density lipoprotein (HDL) and apoproteins apoAI and apoAII.

The effects of fenofibric acid seen in clinical practice have been explained *in vivo* in transgenic mice and *in vitro* in human hepatocyte cultures by the activation of peroxisome proliferator activated receptor α (PPARα). Through this mechanism, fenofibrate increases lipolysis and elimination of triglyceride-rich particles from plasma by activating lipoprotein lipase and reducing production of apoprotein C-III (an inhibitor of lipoprotein lipase activity). The resulting fall in triglycerides produces an alteration in the size and composition of LDL from small, dense particles (which are thought to be atherogenic due to their susceptibility to oxidation), to large buoyant particles. These larger particles have a greater affinity for cholesterol receptors and are catabolized rapidly. Activation of PPARα also induces an increase in the synthesis of apoproteins A-I, A-II and HDL-cholesterol.

Fenofibrate also reduces serum uric acid levels in hyperuricemic and normal individuals by increasing the urinary excretion of uric acid.

Pharmacokinetics/Metabolism

Plasma concentrations of fenofibric acid after administration of 54 mg and 160 mg tablets are equivalent under fed conditions to 67 and 200 mg capsules, respectively.

Absorption

The absolute bioavailability of fenofibrate cannot be determined as the compound is virtually insoluble in aqueous media suitable for injection. However, fenofibrate is well absorbed from the gastrointestinal tract. Following oral administration in healthy volunteers, approximately 60% of a single dose of radiolabelled fenofibrate appeared in urine, primarily as fenofibric acid and its glucuronate conjugate, and 25% was excreted in the feces. Peak plasma levels of fenofibric acid occur within 6 to 8 hours after administration.

The absorption of fenofibrate is increased when administered with food. With fenofibrate tablets, the extent of absorption is increased by approximately 35% under fed as compared to fasting conditions.

Distribution

In healthy volunteers, steady-state plasma levels of fenofibric acid were shown to be achieved within 5 days of dosing and did not demonstrate accumulation across time following multiple dose administration. Serum protein binding was approximately 99% in normal and hyperlipidemic subjects.

Metabolism

Following oral administration, fenofibrate is rapidly hydrolyzed by esterases to the active metabolite, fenofibric acid; no unchanged fenofibrate is detected in plasma.

Fenofibric acid is primarily conjugated with glucuronic acid and then excreted in urine. A small amount of fenofibric acid is reduced at the carbonyl moiety to a benzhydrol metabolite which is, in turn, conjugated with glucuronic acid and excreted in urine.

In vivo metabolism data indicate that neither fenofibrate nor fenofibric acid undergo oxidative metabolism (e.g., cytochrome P450) to a significant extent.

Excretion

After absorption, fenofibrate is mainly excreted in the urine in the form of metabolites, primarily fenofibric acid and fenofibric acid glucuronide. After administration of radiolabelled fenofibrate, approximately 60% of the dose appeared in the urine and 25% was excreted in the feces.

Fenofibric acid is eliminated with a half-life of 20 hours, allowing once daily administration in a clinical setting.

Special Populations

Geriatrics

In elderly volunteers 77–87 years of age, the oral clearance of fenofibric acid following a single oral dose of fenofibrate was 1.2 L/h, which compares to 1.1 L/h in young adults. This indicates that a similar dosage regimen can be used in the elderly, without increasing accumulation of the drug or metabolites.

Pediatrics

TRICOR has not been investigated in adequate and well-controlled trials in pediatric patients.

Gender

No pharmacokinetic difference between males and females has been observed for fenofibrate.

Race

The influence of race on the pharmacokinetics of fenofibrate has not been studied, however fenofibrate is not metabolized by enzymes known for exhibiting inter-ethnic variability. Therefore, inter-ethnic pharmacokinetic differences are very unlikely.

Renal insufficiency

In a study in patients with severe renal impairment (creatinine clearance <50 mL/min), the rate of clearance of fenofibric acid was greatly reduced, and the compound accumulated during chronic dosage. However, in patients having moderate renal impairment (creatinine clearance of 50 to 90 mL/min), the oral clearance and the oral volume of distribution of fenofibric acid are increased compared to healthy adults (2.1 L/h and 95 L versus 1.1 L/h and 30 L, respectively). Therefore, the dosage of TRICOR should be minimized in patients who have severe renal impairment, while no modification of dosage is required in patients having moderate renal impairment.

Hepatic insufficiency

No pharmacokinetic studies have been conducted in patients having hepatic insufficiency.

Drug-drug interactions

In vitro studies using human liver microsomes indicate that fenofibrate and fenofibric acid are not inhibitors of cytochrome (CYP) P450 isoforms CYP3A4, CYP2D6, CYP2E1, or CYP1A2. They are weak inhibitors of CYP2C19 and CYP2A6, and mild-to-moderate inhibitors of CYP2C9 at therapeutic concentrations.

Potentiation of coumarin-type anticoagulants has been observed with prolongation of the prothrombin time/INR.

Bile acid sequestrants have been shown to bind other drugs given concurrently. Therefore, fenofibrate should be taken at least 1 hour before or 4–6 hours after a bile acid binding resin to avoid impeding its absorption (see WARNINGS and PRECAUTIONS).

Clinical Trials

Hypercholesterolemia (Heterozygous Familial and Nonfamilial) and Mixed Dyslipidemia (Fredrickson Types IIa and IIb)

The effects of fenofibrate at a dose equivalent to 160 mg TRICOR per day were assessed from four randomized, placebo-controlled, double-blind, parallel-group studies including patients with the following mean baseline lipid values: total-C 306.9 mg/dL; LDL-C 213.8 mg/dL; HDL-C 52.3 mg/dL; and triglycerides 191.0 mg/dL. TRICOR therapy lowered LDL-C, Total-C, and the LDL-C/HDL-C ratio. TRICOR therapy also lowered triglycerides and raised HDL-C (see Table 1).

[See table 1 above]

In a subset of the subjects, measurements of apo B were conducted. TRICOR treatment significantly reduced apo B from baseline to endpoint as compared with placebo (−25.1% vs. 2.4%, p<0.0001, n=213 and 143 respectively).

Hypertriglyceridemia (Fredrickson Type IV and V)

The effects of fenofibrate on serum triglycerides were studied in two randomized, double-blind, placebo-controlled clinical trials[1] of 147 hypertriglyceridemic patients (Fredrickson Types IV and V). Patients were treated for eight weeks under protocols that differed only in that one entered patients with baseline triglyceride (TG) levels of 500 to 1500 mg/dL, and the other TG levels of 350 to 500 mg/dL. In patients with hypertriglyceridemia and normal cholesterolemia with or without hyperchylomicronemia (Type IV/V hyperlipidemia), treatment with fenofibrate at dosages equivalent to 160 mg TRICOR per day decreased primarily very low density lipoprotein (VLDL) triglycerides and VLDL cholesterol. Treatment of patients with Type IV hyperlipoproteinemia and elevated triglycerides often results in an increase of low density lipoprotein (LDL) cholesterol (see Table 2).

Table 1
Mean Percent Change in Lipid Parameters at End of Treatment[†]

Treatment Group	Total-C	LDL-C	HDL-C	TG
Pooled Cohort				
Mean baseline lipid values (n=646)	306.9 mg/dL	213.8 mg/dL	52.3 mg/dL	191.0 mg/dL
All FEN (n=361)	−18.7%*	−20.6%*	+11.0%*	−28.9%*
Placebo (n=285)	−0.4%	−2.2%	+0.7%	+7.7%
Baseline LDL-C > 160 mg/dL and TG < 150 mg/dL (Type IIa)				
Mean baseline lipid values (n=334)	307.7 mg/dL	227.7 mg/dL	58.1 mg/dL	101.7 mg/dL
All FEN (n=193)	−22.4%*	−31.4%*	+9.8%*	−23.5%*
Placebo (n=141)	+0.2%	−2.2%	+2.6%	+11.7%
Baseline LDL-C > 160 mg/dL and TG ≥ 150 mg/dL (Type IIb)				
Mean baseline lipid values (n=242)	312.8 mg/dL	219.8 mg/dL	46.7 mg/dL	231.9 mg/dL
All FEN (n=126)	−16.8%*	−20.1%*	+14.6%*	−35.9%*
Placebo (n=116)	−3.0%	−6.6%	+2.3%	+0.9%

[†]Duration of study treatment was 3 to 6 months.
*p= <0.05 vs. Placebo

Table 2
Effects of TRICOR in Patients With Fredrickson Type IV/V Hyperlipidemia

Study 1	Placebo				TRICOR			
Baseline TG levels 350 to 499 mg/dL	**N**	**Baseline (Mean)**	**Endpoint (Mean)**	**% Change (Mean)**	**N**	**Baseline (Mean)**	**Endpoint (Mean)**	**% Change (Mean)**
Triglycerides	28	449	450	−0.5	27	432	223	−46.2*
VLDL Triglycerides	19	367	350	2.7	19	350	178	−44.1*
Total Cholesterol	28	255	261	2.8	27	252	227	−9.1*
HDL Cholesterol	28	35	36	4	27	34	40	19.6*
LDL Cholesterol	28	120	129	12	27	128	137	14.5
VLDL Cholesterol	27	99	99	5.8	27	92	46	−44.7*
Study 2	**Placebo**				**TRICOR**			
Baseline TG levels 500 to 1500 mg/dL	**N**	**Baseline (Mean)**	**Endpoint (Mean)**	**% Change (Mean)**	**N**	**Baseline (Mean)**	**Endpoint (Mean)**	**% Change (Mean)**
Triglycerides	44	710	750	7.2	48	726	308	−54.5*
VLDL Triglycerides	29	537	571	18.7	33	543	205	−50.6*
Total Cholesterol	44	272	271	0.4	48	261	223	−13.8*
HDL Cholesterol	44	27	28	5.0	48	30	36	22.9*
LDL Cholesterol	42	100	90	−4.2	45	103	131	45.0*
VLDL Cholesterol	42	137	142	11.0	45	126	54	−49.4*

* = p<0.05 vs. Placebo

[See table 2 above]

The effect of TRICOR on cardiovascular morbidity and mortality has not been determined.

INDICATIONS AND USAGE

Treatment of Hypercholesterolemia

TRICOR is indicated as adjunctive therapy to diet to reduce elevated LDL-C, Total-C, Triglycerides and Apo B, and to increase HDL-C in adult patients with primary hypercholesterolemia or mixed dyslipidemia (Fredrickson Types IIa and IIb). Lipid-altering agents should be used in addition to a diet restricted in saturated fat and cholesterol when response to diet and non-pharmacological interventions alone has been inadequate (see National Cholesterol Education Program [NCEP] Treatment Guidelines, below).

Treatment of Hypertriglyceridemia

TRICOR is also indicated as adjunctive therapy to diet for treatment of adult patients with hypertriglyceridemia (Fredrickson Types IV and V hyperlipidemia). Improving glycemic control in diabetic patients showing fasting chylomicronemia will usually reduce fasting triglycerides and eliminate chylomicronemia thereby obviating the need for pharmacologic intervention.

Markedly elevated levels of serum triglycerides (e.g. > 2,000 mg/dL) may increase the risk of developing pancreatitis. The effect of TRICOR therapy on reducing this risk has not been adequately studied.

Drug therapy is not indicated for patients with Type I hyperlipoproteinemia, who have elevations of chylomicrons and plasma triglycerides, but who have normal levels of very low density lipoprotein (VLDL). Inspection of plasma refrigerated for 14 hours is helpful in distinguishing Types I, IV and V hyperlipoproteinemia[2].

The initial treatment for dyslipidemia is dietary therapy specific for the type of lipoprotein abnormality. Excess body weight and excess alcoholic intake may be important factors in hypertriglyceridemia and should be addressed prior to any drug therapy. Physical exercise can be an important ancillary measure. Diseases contributory to hyperlipidemia, such as hypothyroidism or diabetes mellitus should be looked for and adequately treated. Estrogen therapy, thiazide diuretics and beta-blockers, are sometimes associated with massive rises in plasma triglycerides, especially in subjects with familial hypertriglyceridemia. In such cases, discontinuation of the specific etiologic agent may obviate the need for specific drug therapy of hypertriglyceridemia. The use of drugs should be considered only when reasonable attempts have been made to obtain satisfactory results with non-drug methods. If the decision is made to use drugs, the patient should be instructed that this does not reduce the importance of adhering to diet. (See WARNINGS and PRECAUTIONS).

Fredrickson Classification of Hyperlipoproteinemias

Type	Lipoprotein Elevated	Lipid Elevation Major	Lipid Elevation Minor
I (rare)	chylomicrons	TG	↑↔ C
IIa	LDL	C	–
IIb	LDL, VLDL	C	TG
III (rare)	IDL	C, TG	–
IV	VLDL	TG	↑↔ C
V (rare)	chylomicrons, VLDL	TG	↑↔

C=cholesterol
TG=triglycerides
LDL=low density lipoprotein
VLDL=very low density lipoprotein
IDL=intermediate density lipoprotein

[See table at top of next page]

After the LDL-C goal has been achieved, if the TG is still >200 mg/dL, non HDL-C (total-C minus HDL-C) becomes a secondary target of therapy. Non-HDL-C goals are set 30 mg/dL higher than LDL-C goals for each risk category.

CONTRAINDICATIONS

TRICOR is contraindicated in patients who exhibit hypersensitivity to fenofibrate.

TRICOR is contraindicated in patients with hepatic or severe renal dysfunction, including primary biliary cirrhosis, and patients with unexplained persistent liver function abnormality.

TRICOR is contraindicated in patients with preexisting gallbladder disease (see WARNINGS).

WARNINGS

Liver Function: Fenofibrate at doses equivalent to 107 mg to 160 mg TRICOR per day has been associated with increases in serum transaminases [AST (SGOT) or ALT (SGPT)]. In a pooled analysis of 10 placebo-controlled trials, increases to > 3 times the upper limit of normal occurred in 5.3% of patients taking fenofibrate versus 1.1% of patients treated with placebo.

When transaminase determinations were followed either after discontinuation of treatment or during continued treat-

Continued on next page

Tricor—Cont.

ment, a return to normal limits was usually observed. The incidence of increases in transaminases related to fenofibrate therapy appear to be dose related. In an 8-week dose-ranging study, the incidence of ALT or AST elevations to at least three times the upper limit of normal was 13% in patients receiving dosages equivalent to 107 mg to 160 mg TRICOR per day and was 0% in those receiving dosages equivalent to 54 mg or less TRICOR per day, or placebo. Hepatocellular, chronic active and cholestatic hepatitis associated with fenofibrate therapy have been reported after exposures of weeks to several years. In extremely rare cases, cirrhosis has been reported in association with chronic active hepatitis.

Regular periodic monitoring of liver function, including serum ALT (SGPT) should be performed for the duration of therapy with TRICOR, and therapy discontinued if enzyme levels persist above three times the normal limit.

Cholelithiasis: Fenofibrate, like clofibrate and gemfibrozil, may increase cholesterol excretion into the bile, leading to cholelithiasis. If cholelithiasis is suspected, gallbladder studies are indicated. TRICOR therapy should be discontinued if gallstones are found.

Concomitant Oral Anticoagulants: Caution should be exercised when anticoagulants are given in conjunction with TRICOR because of the potentiation of coumarin-type anticoagulants in prolonging the prothrombin time/INR. The dosage of the anticoagulant should be reduced to maintain the prothrombin time/INR at the desired level to prevent bleeding complications. Frequent prothrombin time/INR determinations are advisable until it has been definitely determined that the prothrombin time/INR has stabilized.

Concomitant HMG-CoA Reductase Inhibitors: The combined use of TRICOR and HMG-CoA reductase inhibitors should be avoided unless the benefit of further alterations in lipid levels is likely to outweigh the increased risk of this drug combination.

In a single-dose drug interaction study in 23 healthy adults the concomitant administration of TRICOR and pravastatin resulted in no clinically important difference in the pharmacokinetics of fenofibric acid, pravastatin or its active metabolite 3a-hydroxy iso-pravastatin when compared to either drug given alone.

The combined use of fibric acid derivatives and HMG-CoA reductase inhibitors has been associated, in the absence of a marked pharmacokinetic interaction, in numerous case reports, with rhabdomyolysis, markedly elevated creatine kinase (CK) levels and myoglobinuria, leading in a high proportion of cases to acute renal failure.

The use of fibrates alone, including TRICOR, may occasionally be associated with myositis, myopathy, or rhabdomyolysis. Patients receiving TRICOR and complaining of muscle pain, tenderness, or weakness should have prompt medical evaluation for myopathy, including serum creatine kinase level determination. If myopathy/myositis is suspected or diagnosed, TRICOR therapy should be stopped.

Mortality: The effect of TRICOR on coronary heart disease morbidity and mortality and non-cardiovascular mortality has not been established.

Other Considerations: In the Coronary Drug Project, a large study of post myocardial infarction of patients treated for 5 years with clofibrate, there was no difference in mortality seen between the clofibrate group and the placebo group. There was however, a difference in the rate of cholelithiasis and cholecystitis requiring surgery between the two groups (3.0% vs. 1.8%).

Because of chemical, pharmacological, and clinical similarities between TRICOR (fenofibrate tablets), Atromid-S (clofibrate), and Lopid (gemfibrozil), the adverse findings in 4 large randomized, placebo-controlled clinical studies with these other fibrate drugs may also apply to TRICOR.

In a study conducted by the World Health Organization (WHO), 5000 subjects without known coronary artery disease were treated with placebo or clofibrate for 5 years and followed for an additional one year. There was a statistically significant, higher age-adjusted all-cause mortality in the clofibrate group compared with the placebo group (5.70% vs. 3.96%, p=<0.01). Excess mortality was due to a 33% increase in non-cardiovascular causes, including malignancy, post-cholecystectomy complications, and pancreatitis. This appeared to confirm the higher risk of gallbladder disease seen in clofibrate-treated patients studied in the Coronary Drug Project.

The Helsinki Heart Study was a large (n=4081) study of middle-aged men without a history of coronary artery disease. Subjects received either placebo or gemfibrozil for 5 years, with a 3.5 year open extension afterward. Total mortality was numerically higher in the gemfibrozil randomization group but did not achieve statistical significance (p=0.19, 95% confidence interval for relative risk G:P=.91–1.64). Although cancer deaths trended higher in the gemfibrozil group (p=0.11), cancers (excluding basal cell carcinoma) were diagnosed with equal frequency in both study groups. Due to the limited size of the study, the relative risk of death from any cause was not shown to be different than that seen in the 9 year follow-up data from World Health Organization study (RR=1.29). Similarly, the numerical excess of gallbladder surgeries in the gemfibrozil group did not differ statistically from that observed in the WHO study.

A secondary prevention component of the Helsinki Heart Study enrolled middle-aged men excluded from the primary prevention study because of known or suspected coronary heart disease. Subjects received gemfibrozil or placebo for 5 years. Although cardiac deaths trended higher in the gemfibrozil group, this was not statistically significant (hazard ratio 2.2, 95% confidence interval: 0.94–5.05). The rate of gallbladder surgery was not statistically significant between study groups, but did trend higher in the gemfibrozil group, (1.9% vs. 0.3%, p=0.07). There was a statistically significant difference in the number of appendectomies in the gemfibrozil group (6/311 vs. 0/317, p=0.029).

NCEP Treatment Guidelines: LDL-C Goals and Cutpoints for Therapeutic Lifestyle Changes and Drug Therapy in Different Risk Categories

Risk Category	LDL Goal (mg/dL)	LDL Level at Which to Initiate Therapeutic Lifestyle Changes (mg/dL)	LDL Level at which to Consider Drug Thereapy (mg/dL)
CHD† or CHD risk equivalents (10-years risk >20%)	<100	≥100	≥130 (100–129:drug optional)††
2+ Risk Factors 10-year risk ≤20%)	<130	≥130	10-year risk 10%–20%:≥130 10-Year risk <10%: ≥160
0–1 Risk Factor †††	<160	≥160	≥190 (160–189: LDL-lowering drug optional)

† CHD = coronary heart disease

†† Some authorities recommend use of LDL-lowering drugs in this category if an LDL-C level of <100 mg/dL cannot be achieved by therapeutic lifestyle changes. Others prefer use of drugs that primarily modify triglycerides and HDL-C, e.g., nicotinic acid or fibrate. Clinical judgement also may call for deferring drug therapy in this subcategory.

††† Almost all people with 0–1 risk factor have 10-year risk <10%; thus, 10-year risk assessment in people with 0–1 risk factor is not necessary.

PRECAUTIONS

Initial therapy: Laboratory studies should be done to ascertain that the lipid levels are consistently abnormal before instituting TRICOR therapy. Every attempt should be made to control serum lipids with appropriate diet, exercise, weight loss in obese patients, and control of any medical problems such as diabetes mellitus and hypothyroidism that are contributing to the lipid abnormalities. Medications known to exacerbate hypertriglyceridemia (beta-blockers, thiazides, estrogens) should be discontinued or changed if possible prior to consideration of triglyceride-lowering drug therapy.

Continued therapy: Periodic determination of serum lipids should be obtained during initial therapy in order to establish the lowest effective dose of TRICOR. Therapy should be withdrawn in patients who do not have an adequate response after two months of treatment with the maximum recommended dose of 160 mg per day.

Pancreatitis: Pancreatitis has been reported in patients taking fenofibrate, gemfibrozil, and clofibrate. This occurrence may represent a failure of efficacy in patients with severe hypertriglyceridemia, a direct drug effect, or a secondary phenomenon mediated through biliary tract stone or sludge formation with obstruction of the common bile duct.

Hypersensitivity Reactions: Acute hypersensitivity reactions including severe skin rashes requiring patient hospitalization and treatment with steroids have occurred very rarely during treatment with fenofibrate, including rare spontaneous reports of Stevens-Johnson syndrome, and toxic epidermal necrolysis. Urticaria was seen in 1.1 vs 0%, and rash in 1.4 vs 0.8% of fenofibrate and placebo patients respectively in controlled trials.

Hematologic Changes: Mild to moderate hemoglobin, hematocrit, and white blood cell decreases have been observed in patients following initiation of fenofibrate therapy. However, these levels stabilize during long-term administration. Extremely rare spontaneous reports of thrombocytopenia and agranulocytosis have been received during post-marketing surveillance outside of the U.S. Periodic blood counts are recommended during the first 12 months of TRICOR administration.

Skeletal muscle: The use of fibrates alone, including TRICOR, may occasionally be associated with myopathy. Treatment with drugs of the fibrate class has been associated on rare occasions with rhabdomyolysis, usually in patients with impaired renal function. Myopathy should be considered in any patient with diffuse myalgias, muscle tenderness or weakness, and/or marked elevations of creatine phosphokinase levels.

Patients should be advised to report promptly unexplained muscle pain, tenderness or weakness, particularly if accompanied by malaise or fever. CPK levels should be assessed in patients reporting these symptoms, and fenofibrate therapy should be discontinued if markedly elevated CPK levels occur or myopathy is diagnosed.

Drug Interactions

Oral Anticoagulants: **CAUTION SHOULD BE EXERCISED WHEN COUMARIN ANTICOAGULANTS ARE GIVEN IN CONJUNCTION WITH TRICOR. THE DOSAGE OF THE ANTICOAGULANTS SHOULD BE REDUCED TO MAINTAIN THE PROTHROMBIN TIME/INR AT THE DESIRED LEVEL TO PREVENT BLEEDING COMPLICATIONS. FREQUENT PROTHROMBIN TIME/INR DETERMINATIONS ARE ADVISABLE UNTIL IT HAS BEEN DEFINITELY DETERMINED THAT THE PROTHROMBIN TIME/INR HAS STABILIZED.**

HMG-CoA reductase inhibitors: The combined use of TRICOR and HMG-CoA reductase inhibitors should be avoided unless the benefit of further alterations in lipid levels is likely to outweigh the increased risk of this drug combination (see WARNINGS).

Resins: Since bile acid sequestrants may bind other drugs given concurrently, patients should take TRICOR at least 1 hour before or 4–6 hours after a bile acid binding resin to avoid impeding its absorption.

Cyclosporine: Because cyclosporine can produce nephrotoxicity with decreases in creatinine clearance and rises in serum creatinine, and because renal excretion is the primary elimination route of fibrate drugs including TRICOR, there is a risk that an interaction will lead to deterioration. The benefits and risks of using TRICOR with immunosuppressants and other potentially nephrotoxic agents should be carefully considered, and the lowest effective dose employed.

Carcinogenesis, Mutagenesis, Impairment of Fertility: In a 24-month study in rats (10, 45, and 200 mg/kg; 0.3, 1, and 6 times the maximum recommended human dose on the basis of mg/meter^2 of surface area), the incidence of liver carcinoma was significantly increased at 6 times the maximum recommended human dose in males and females. A statistically significant increase in pancreatic carcinomas occurred in males at 1 and 6 times the maximum recommended human dose; there were also increases in pancreatic adenomas and benign testicular interstitial cell tumors at 6 times the maximum recommended human dose in males. In a second 24-month study in a different strain of rats (doses of 10 and 60 mg/kg; 0.3 and 2 times the maximum recommended human dose based on mg/meter^2 surface area), there were significant increases in the incidence of pancreatic acinar adenomas in both sexes and increases in interstitial cell tumors of the testes at 2 times the maximum recommended human dose.

A comparative carcinogenicity study was done in rats comparing three drugs: fenofibrate (10 and 70 mg/kg; 0.3 and 1.6 times the maximum recommended human dose), clofibrate (400 mg/kg; 1.6 times the human dose), and gemfibrozil (250 mg/kg; 1.7 times the human dose) (multiples based on mg/meter^2 surface area). Pancreatic acinar adenomas were increased in males and females on fenofibrate; hepatocellular carcinoma and pancreatic acinar adenomas were increased in males and hepatic neoplastic nodules in females treated with clofibrate; hepatic neoplastic nodules were increased in males and females treated with gemfibrozil while testicular interstitial cell tumors were increased in males on all three drugs.

In a 21-month study in mice at doses of 10, 45, and 200 mg/kg (approximately 0.2, 0.7 and 3 times the maximum recommended human dose on the basis of mg/meter^2 surface area), there were statistically significant increases in liver carcinoma at 3 times the maximum recommended human dose in both males and females. In a second 18-month study at the same doses, there was a significant increase in liver carcinoma in male mice and liver adenoma in female mice at 3 times the maximum recommended human dose.

Electron microscopy studies have demonstrated peroxisomal proliferation following fenofibrate administration to the rat. An adequate study to test for peroxisome proliferation in humans has not been done, but changes in peroxisome morphology and numbers have been observed in humans after treatment with other members of the fibrate class when liver biopsies were compared before and after treatment in the same individual.

Fenofibrate has been demonstrated to be devoid of mutagenic potential in the following tests: Ames, mouse lymphoma, chromosomal aberration and unscheduled DNA synthesis.

Pregnancy Category C: Fenofibrate has been shown to be embryocidal and teratogenic in rats when given in doses 7 to

BODY SYSTEM Adverse Event	Fenofibrate* (N=439)	Placebo (N=365)
BODY AS A WHOLE		
Abdominal Pain	4.6%	4.4%
Back Pain	3.4%	2.5%
Headache	3.2%	2.7%
Asthenia	2.1%	3.0%
Flu Syndrome	2.1%	2.7%
DIGESTIVE		
Liver Function Tests Abnormal	7.5%**	1.4%
Diarrhea	2.3%	4.1%
Nausea	2.3%	1.9%
Constipation	2.1%	1.4%
METABOLIC AND NUTRITIONAL DISORDERS		
SGPT Increased	3.0%	1.6%
Creatine Phosphokinase Increased	3.0%	1.4%
SGOT Increased	3.4%**	0.5%
RESPIRATORY		
Respiratory Disorder	6.2%	5.5%
Rhinitis	2.3%	1.1%

* Dosage equivalent to 200 mg TRICOR
**Significantly different from Placebo

10 times the maximum recommended human dose and embryocidal in rabbits when given at 9 times the maximum recommended human dose (on the basis of mg/meter^2 surface area). There are no adequate and well-controlled studies in pregnant women. Fenofibrate should be used during pregnancy only if the potential benefit justifies the potential risk to the fetus.

Administration of 9 times the maximum recommended human dose of fenofibrate to female rats before and throughout gestation caused 100% of dams to delay delivery and resulted in a 60% increase in post-implantation loss, a decrease in litter size, a decrease in birth weight, a 40% survival of pups at birth, a 4% survival of pups as neonates, and a 0% survival of pups to weaning, and an increase in spina bifida.

Administration of 10 times the maximum recommended human dose to female rats on days 6–15 of gestation caused an increase in gross, visceral and skeletal findings in fetuses (domed head/hunched shoulders/rounded body/abnormal chest, kyphosis, stunted fetuses, elongated sternal ribs, malformed sternebrae, extra foramen in palatine, misshapen vertebrae, supernumerary ribs).

Administration of 7 times the maximum recommended human dose to female rats from day 15 of gestation through weaning caused a delay in delivery, a 40% decrease in live births, a 75% decrease in neonatal survival, and decreases in pup weight, at birth as well as on days 4 and 21 postpartum.

Administration of 9 and 18 times the maximum recommended human dose to female rabbits caused abortions in 10% of dams at 9 times and 25% of dams at 18 times the maximum recommended human dose and death of 7% of fetuses at 18 times the maximum recommended human dose.

Nursing mothers: Fenofibrate should not be used in nursing mothers. Because of the potential for tumorigenicity seen in animal studies, a decision should be made whether to discontinue nursing or to discontinue the drug.

Pediatric Use: Safety and efficacy in pediatric patients have not been established.

Geriatric Use: Fenofibric acid is known to be substantially excreted by the kidney, and the risk of adverse reactions to this drug may be greater in patients with impaired renal function. Because elderly patients are more likely to have decreased renal function, care should be taken in dose selection.

ADVERSE REACTIONS

CLINICAL: Adverse events reported by 2% or more of patients treated with fenofibrate during the double-blind, placebo-controlled trials, regardless of causality, are listed in the table above. Adverse events led to discontinuation of treatment in 5.0% of patients treated with fenofibrate and in 3.0% treated with placebo. Increases in liver function tests were the most frequent events, causing discontinuation of fenofibrate treatment in 1.6% of patients in double-blind trials.

[See table above]

Additional adverse events reported by three or more patients in placebo-controlled trials or reported in other controlled or open trials, regardless of causality are listed below.

BODY AS A WHOLE: Chest pain, pain (unspecified), infection, malaise, allergic reaction, cyst, hernia, fever, photosensitivity reaction, and accidental injury.

CARDIOVASCULAR SYSTEM: Angina pectoris, hypertension, vasodilatation, coronary artery disorder, electrocardiogram abnormal, ventricular extrasystoles, myocardial infarct, peripheral vascular disorder, migraine, varicose vein, cardiovascular disorder, hypotension, palpitation, vascular disorder, arrhythmia, phlebitis, tachycardia, extrasystoles, and atrial fibrillation.

DIGESTIVE SYSTEM: Dyspepsia, flatulence, nausea, increased appetite, gastroenteritis, cholelithiasis, rectal disorder, esophagitis, gastritis, colitis, tooth disorder, vomiting, anorexia, gastrointestinal disorder, duodenal ulcer, nausea and vomiting, peptic ulcer, rectal hemorrhage, liver fatty deposit, cholecystitis, eructation, gamma glutamyl transpeptidase, and diarrhea.

ENDOCRINE SYSTEM: Diabetes mellitus

HEMIC AND LYMPHATIC SYSTEM: Anemia, leukopenia, ecchymosis, eosinophilia, lymphadenopathy, and thrombocytopenia.

METABOLIC AND NUTRITIONAL DISORDERS: Creatinine increased, weight gain, hypoglycemia, gout, weight loss, edema, hyperuricemia, and peripheral edema.

MUSCULOSKELETAL SYSTEM: Myositis, myalgia, arthralgia, arthritis, tenosynovitis, joint disorder, arthrosis, leg cramps, bursitis, and myasthenia.

NERVOUS SYSTEM: Dizziness, insomnia, depression, vertigo, libido decreased, anxiety, paresthesia, dry mouth, hypertonia, nervousness, neuralgia, and somnolence.

RESPIRATORY SYSTEM: Pharyngitis, bronchitis, cough increased, dyspnea, asthma, pneumonia, laryngitis, and sinusitis.

SKIN AND APPENDAGES: Rash, pruritus, eczema, herpes zoster, urticaria, acne, sweating, fungal dermatitis, skin disorder, alopecia, contact dermatitis, herpes simplex, maculopapular rash, nail disorder, and skin ulcer.

SPECIAL SENSES: Conjunctivitis, eye disorder, amblyopia, ear pain, otitis media, abnormal vision, cataract specified, and refraction disorder.

UROGENITAL SYSTEM: Urinary frequency, prostatic disorder, dysuria, kidney function abnormal, urolithiasis, gynecomastia, unintended pregnancy, vaginal moniliasis, and cystitis.

OVERDOSAGE

There is no specific treatment for overdose with TRICOR. General supportive care of the patient is indicated, including monitoring of vital signs and observation of clinical status, should an overdose occur. If indicated, elimination of unabsorbed drug should be achieved by emesis or gastric lavage; usual precautions should be observed to maintain the airway. Because fenofibrate is highly bound to plasma proteins, hemodialysis should not be considered.

DOSAGE AND ADMINISTRATION

Patients should be placed on an appropriate lipid-lowering diet before receiving TRICOR, and should continue this diet during treatment with TRICOR. TRICOR tablets should be given with meals, thereby optimizing the bioavailability of the medication.

For the treatment of adult patients with primary hypercholesterolemia or mixed hyperlipidemia, the initial dose of TRICOR is 160 mg per day.

For adult patients with hypertriglyceridemia, the initial dose is 54 to 160 mg per day. Dosage should be individualized according to patient response, and should be adjusted if necessary following repeat lipid determinations at 4 to 8 week intervals. The maximum dose is 160 mg per day.

Treatment with TRICOR should be initiated at a dose of 54 mg/day in patients having impaired renal function, and increased only after evaluation of the effects on renal function and lipid levels at this dose. In the elderly, the initial dose should likewise be limited to 54 mg/day.

Lipid levels should be monitored periodically and consideration should be given to reducing the dosage of TRICOR if lipid levels fall significantly below the targeted range.

HOW SUPPLIED

TRICOR® (fenofibrate tablets) is available in two strengths:
54 mg yellow tablets, imprinted with ᗡ and Abbo-Code identification letters "TA", available in bottles of 90 (**NDC** 0074-4009-90).
160 mg white tablets, imprinted with ᗡ and Abbo-Code identification letters "TC", available in bottles of 90 (**NDC** 0074-4013-90).

Storage

Store at controlled room temperature, 15–30°C (59–86°F). Keep out of the reach of children. Protect from moisture.
Manufactured for Abbott Laboratories, North Chicago, IL 60064, U.S.A. by Laboratoires Fournier, S.A., 21300 Chenôve, France
Made in France

REFERENCES

1. GOLDBERG AC, *et al.* Fenofibrate for the Treatment of Type IV and V Hyperlipoproteinemias: A Double-Blind, Placebo-Controlled Multicenter US Study. *Clinical Therapeutics,* 11, pp. 69–83, 1989.
2. NIKKILA EA. Familial Lipoprotein Lipase Deficiency and Related Disorders of Chylomicron Metabolism. In Stanbury J.B., *et al.* (eds.): *The Metabolic Basis of Inherited Disease,* 5th edition, McGraw-Hill, 1983, Chap. 30, pp. 622–642.
3. BROWN WV, *et al.* Effects of Fenofibrate on Plasma Lipids: Double-Blind, Multicenter Study In Patients with Type IIA or IIB Hyperlipidemia. *Arteriosclerosis.* 6, pp. 670–678, 1986.

Revised: August, 2001
Ref.: 03-5034-R1
ABBOTT LABORATORIES
NORTH CHICAGO, IL 60064, USA

AstraZeneca LP
WILMINGTON, DE 19850-5437

For Medical Information, Adverse Drug Experiences, and Customer Service Contact: (800) 236-9933

ATACAND® ℞
[*ăt ′ă-kănd*]
(candesartan cilexetil)
TABLETS

Prescribing information for this product, which appears on page 595 of the 2002 PDR, has been completely revised as follows. Please write "See Supplement A" next to the product heading.

> **USE IN PREGNANCY**
> **When used in pregnancy during the second and third trimesters, drugs that act directly on the renin-angiotensin system can cause injury and even death to the developing fetus.** When pregnancy is detected, ATACAND should be discontinued as soon as possible. See WARNINGS, Fetal/Neonatal Morbidity and Mortality.

DESCRIPTION

ATACAND (candesartan cilexetil), a prodrug, is hydrolyzed to candesartan during absorption from the gastrointestinal tract. Candesartan is a selective AT_1 subtype angiotensin II receptor antagonist.

Candesartan cilexetil, a nonpeptide, is chemically described as (±)-1-[[(cyclohexyloxy)carbonyl]oxy]ethyl 2-ethoxy-1-[[2′-(1H- tetrazol-5-yl) [1,1′-biphenyl]-4-yl]methyl]-1H-benzimidazole-7-carboxylate.

Its empirical formula is $C_{33}H_{34}N_6O_6$, and its structural formula is

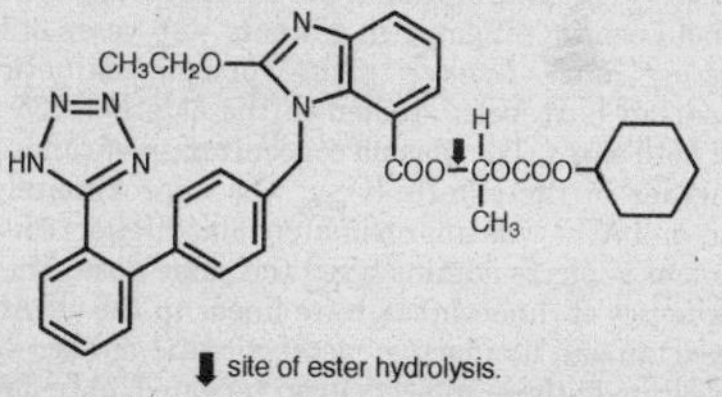
CH3CH2O
N
N=N
HN
N
COO
COCOO
H
CH3
site of ester hydrolysis.

Candesartan cilexetil is a white to off-white powder with a molecular weight of 610.67. It is practically insoluble in water and sparingly soluble in methanol. Candesartan cilexetil is a racemic mixture containing one chiral center at the cyclohexyloxycarbonyloxy ethyl ester group. Following oral administration, candesartan cilexetil undergoes hydrolysis at the ester link to form the active drug, candesartan, which is achiral.

ATACAND is available for oral use as tablets containing either 4 mg, 8 mg, 16 mg, or 32 mg of candesartan cilexetil and the following inactive ingredients: hydroxypropyl cellulose, polyethylene glycol, lactose, corn starch, carboxymethylcellulose calcium, and magnesium stearate. Ferric oxide (reddish brown) is added to the 8-mg, 16-mg, and 32-mg tablets as a colorant.

CLINICAL PHARMACOLOGY

Mechanism of Action

Angiotensin II is formed from angiotensin I in a reaction catalyzed by angiotensin-converting enzyme (ACE, kininase II). Angiotensin II is the principal pressor agent of the renin-angiotensin system, with effects that include vasoconstriction, stimulation of synthesis and release of aldosterone, cardiac stimulation, and renal reabsorption of sodium. Candesartan blocks the vasoconstrictor and aldosterone-secreting effects of angiotensin II by selectively blocking the binding of angiotensin II to the AT_1 receptor in many tissues, such as vascular smooth muscle and the adrenal gland. Its action is, therefore, independent of the pathways for angiotensin II synthesis.

There is also an AT_2 receptor found in many tissues, but AT_2 is not known to be associated with cardiovascular homeostasis. Candesartan has much greater affinity (>10,000-fold) for the AT_1 receptor than for the AT_2 receptor.

Continued on next page

Atacand—Cont.

Blockade of the renin-angiotensin system with ACE inhibitors, which inhibit the biosynthesis of angiotensin II from angiotensin I, is widely used in the treatment of hypertension. ACE inhibitors also inhibit the degradation of bradykinin, a reaction also catalyzed by ACE. Because candesartan does not inhibit ACE (kininase II), it does not affect the response to bradykinin. Whether this difference has clinical relevance is not yet known. Candesartan does not bind to or block other hormone receptors or ion channels known to be important in cardiovascular regulation.
Blockade of the angiotensin II receptor inhibits the negative regulatory feedback of angiotensin II on renin secretion, but the resulting increased plasma renin activity and angiotensin II circulating levels do not overcome the effect of candesartan on blood pressure.

Pharmacokinetics

General

Candesartan cilexetil is rapidly and completely bioactivated by ester hydrolysis during absorption from the gastrointestinal tract to candesartan, a selective AT_1 subtype angiotensin II receptor antagonist. Candesartan is mainly excreted unchanged in urine and feces (via bile). It undergoes minor hepatic metabolism by O-deethylation to an inactive metabolite. The elimination half-life of candesartan is approximately 9 hours. After single and repeated administration, the pharmacokinetics of candesartan are linear for oral doses up to 32 mg of candesartan cilexetil. Candesartan and its inactive metabolite do not accumulate in serum upon repeated once-daily dosing.
Following administration of candesartan cilexetil, the absolute bioavailability of candesartan was estimated to be 15%. After tablet ingestion, the peak serum concentration (C_{max}) is reached after 3 to 4 hours. Food with a high fat content does not affect the bioavailability of candesartan after candesartan cilexetil administration.

Metabolism and Excretion

Total plasma clearance of candesartan is 0.37 mL/min/kg, with a renal clearance of 0.19 mL/min/kg. When candesartan is administered orally, about 26% of the dose is excreted unchanged in urine. Following an oral dose of ^{14}C-labeled candesartan cilexetil, approximately 33% of radioactivity is recovered in urine and approximately 67% in feces. Following an intravenous dose of ^{14}C-labeled candesartan, approximately 59% of radioactivity is recovered in urine and approximately 36% in feces. Biliary excretion contributes to the elimination of candesartan.

Distribution

The volume of distribution of candesartan is 0.13 L/kg. Candesartan is highly bound to plasma proteins (>99%) and does not penetrate red blood cells. The protein binding is constant at candesartan plasma concentrations well above the range achieved with recommended doses. In rats, it has been demonstrated that candesartan crosses the blood-brain barrier poorly, if at all. It has also been demonstrated in rats that candesartan passes across the placental barrier and is distributed in the fetus.

Special Populations

Pediatric: The pharmacokinetics of candesartan cilexetil have not been investigated in patients <18 years of age.
Geriatric and Gender: The pharmacokinetics of candesartan have been studied in the elderly (≥65 years) and in both sexes. The plasma concentration of candesartan was higher in the elderly (C_{max} was approximately 50% higher, and AUC was approximately 80% higher) compared to younger subjects administered the same dose. The pharmacokinetics of candesartan were linear in the elderly, and candesartan and its inactive metabolite did not accumulate in the serum of these subjects upon repeated, once-daily administration. No initial dosage adjustment is necessary. (See DOSAGE AND ADMINISTRATION.) There is no difference in the pharmacokinetics of candesartan between male and female subjects.
Renal Insufficiency: In hypertensive patients with renal insufficiency, serum concentrations of candesartan were elevated. After repeated dosing, the AUC and C_{max} were approximately doubled in patients with severe renal impairment (creatinine clearance <30 mL/min/1.73m^2) compared to patients with normal kidney function. The pharmacokinetics of candesartan in hypertensive patients undergoing hemodialysis are similar to those in hypertensive patients with severe renal impairment. Candesartan cannot be removed by hemodialysis. No initial dosage adjustment is necessary in patients with renal insufficiency. (See DOSAGE AND ADMINISTRATION.)
Hepatic Insufficiency: No differences in the pharmacokinetics of candesartan were observed in patients with mild to moderate chronic liver disease. The pharmacokinetics after candesartan cilexetil administration have not been investigated in patients with severe hepatic insufficiency. No initial dosage adjustment is necessary in patients with mild hepatic disease. (See DOSAGE AND ADMINISTRATION.)

Drug Interactions

See PRECAUTIONS, Drug Interactions.

Pharmacodynamics

Candesartan inhibits the pressor effects of angiotensin II infusion in a dose-dependent manner. After 1 week of once-daily dosing with 8 mg of candesartan cilexetil, the pressor effect was inhibited by approximately 90% at peak with approximately 50% inhibition persisting for 24 hours.
Plasma concentrations of angiotensin I and angiotensin II, and plasma renin activity (PRA), increased in a dose-dependent manner after single and repeated administration of candesartan cilexetil to healthy subjects and hypertensive patients. ACE activity was not altered in healthy subjects after repeated candesartan cilexetil administration. The once-daily administration of up to 16 mg of candesartan cilexetil to healthy subjects did not influence plasma aldosterone concentrations, but a decrease in the plasma concentration of aldosterone was observed when 32 mg of candesartan cilexetil was administered to hypertensive patients. In spite of the effect of candesartan cilexetil on aldosterone secretion, very little effect on serum potassium was observed.
In multiple-dose studies with hypertensive patients, there were no clinically significant changes in metabolic function, including serum levels of total cholesterol, triglycerides, glucose, or uric acid. In a 12-week study of 161 patients with non-insulin-dependent (type 2) diabetes mellitus and hypertension, there was no change in the level of HbA_{1c}.

Clinical Trials

The antihypertensive effects of ATACAND were examined in 14 placebo-controlled trials of 4- to 12-weeks duration, primarily at daily doses of 2 to 32 mg per day in patients with baseline diastolic blood pressures of 95 to 114 mm Hg. Most of the trials were of candesartan cilexetil as a single agent, but it was also studied as add-on to hydrochlorothiazide and amlodipine. These studies included a total of 2350 patients randomized to one of several doses of candesartan cilexetil and 1027 to placebo. Except for a study in diabetics, all studies showed significant effects, generally dose related, of 2 to 32 mg on trough (24 hour) systolic and diastolic pressures compared to placebo, with doses of 8 to 32 mg giving effects of about 8-12/4-8 mm Hg. There were no exaggerated first-dose effects in these patients. Most of the antihypertensive effect was seen within 2 weeks of initial dosing, and the full effect in 4 weeks. With once-daily dosing, blood pressure effect was maintained over 24 hours, with trough to peak ratios of blood pressure effect generally over 80%. Candesartan cilexetil had an additional blood pressure lowering effect when added to hydrochlorothiazide.
The antihypertensive effect was similar in men and women and in patients older and younger than 65. Candesartan was effective in reducing blood pressure regardless of race, although the effect was somewhat less in blacks (usually a low-renin population). This has been generally true for angiotensin II antagonists and ACE inhibitors.
In long-term studies of up to 1 year, the antihypertensive effectiveness of candesartan cilexetil was maintained, and there was no rebound after abrupt withdrawal.
There were no changes in the heart rate of patients treated with candesartan cilexetil in controlled trials.

INDICATIONS AND USAGE

ATACAND is indicated for the treatment of hypertension. It may be used alone or in combination with other antihypertensive agents.

CONTRAINDICATIONS

ATACAND is contraindicated in patients who are hypersensitive to any component of this product.

WARNINGS

Fetal/Neonatal Morbidity and Mortality

Drugs that act directly on the renin-angiotensin system can cause fetal and neonatal morbidity and death when administered to pregnant women. Several dozen cases have been reported in the world literature in patients who were taking angiotensin-converting enzyme inhibitors. When pregnancy is detected, ATACAND should be discontinued as soon as possible.
The use of drugs that act directly on the renin-angiotensin system during the second and third trimesters of pregnancy has been associated with fetal and neonatal injury, including hypotension, neonatal skull hypoplasia, anuria, reversible or irreversible renal failure, and death. Oligohydramnios has also been reported, presumably resulting from decreased fetal renal function; oligohydramnios in this setting has been associated with fetal limb contractures, craniofacial deformation, and hypoplastic lung development. Prematurity, intrauterine growth retardation, and patent ductus arteriosus have also been reported, although it is not clear whether these occurrences were due to exposure to the drug.
These adverse effects do not appear to have resulted from intrauterine drug exposure that has been limited to the first trimester. Mothers whose embryos and fetuses are exposed to an angiotensin II receptor antagonist only during the first trimester should be so informed. Nonetheless, when patients become pregnant, physicians should have the patient discontinue the use of ATACAND as soon as possible.
Rarely (probably less often than once in every thousand pregnancies), no alternative to a drug acting on the renin-angiotensin system will be found. In these rare cases, the mothers should be apprised of the potential hazards to their fetuses, and serial ultrasound examinations should be performed to assess the intra-amniotic environment.
If oligohydramnios is observed, ATACAND should be discontinued unless it is considered life saving for the mother. Contraction stress testing (CST), a nonstress test (NST), or biophysical profiling (BPP) may be appropriate, depending upon the week of pregnancy. Patients and physicians should be aware, however, that oligohydramnios may not appear until after the fetus has sustained irreversible injury.
Infants with histories of *in utero* exposure to an angiotensin II receptor antagonist should be closely observed for hypotension, oliguria, and hyperkalemia. If oliguria occurs, attention should be directed toward support of blood pressure and renal perfusion. Exchange transfusion or dialysis may be required as means of reversing hypotension and/or substituting for disordered renal function.
There is no clinical experience with the use of ATACAND in pregnant women. Oral doses ≥10 mg of candesartan cilexetil/kg/day administered to pregnant rats during late gestation and continued through lactation were associated with reduced survival and an increased incidence of hydronephrosis in the offspring. The 10-mg/kg/day dose in rats is approximately 2.8 times the maximum recommended daily human dose (MRHD) of 32 mg on a mg/m^2 basis (comparison assumes human body weight of 50 kg). Candesartan cilexetil given to pregnant rabbits at an oral dose of 3 mg/kg/day (approximately 1.7 times the MRHD on a mg/m^2 basis) caused maternal toxicity (decreased body weight and death) but, in surviving dams, had no adverse effects on fetal survival, fetal weight, or external, visceral, or skeletal development. No maternal toxicity or adverse effects on fetal development were observed when oral doses up to 1000 mg of candesartan cilexetil/kg/day (approximately 138 times the MRHD on a mg/m^2 basis) were administered to pregnant mice.

Hypotension in Volume- and Salt-Depleted Patients

In patients with an activated renin-angiotensin system, such as volume- and/or salt-depleted patients (eg, those being treated with diuretics), symptomatic hypotension may occur. These conditions should be corrected prior to administration of ATACAND, or the treatment should start under close medical supervision (see DOSAGE AND ADMINISTRATION).
If hypotension occurs, the patients should be placed in the supine position and, if necessary, given an intravenous infusion of normal saline. A transient hypotensive response is not a contraindication to further treatment which usually can be continued without difficulty once the blood pressure has stabilized.

PRECAUTIONS

General

Impaired Renal Function: As a consequence of inhibiting the renin-angiotensin-aldosterone system, changes in renal function may be anticipated in susceptible individuals treated with ATACAND. In patients whose renal function may depend upon the activity of the renin-angiotensin-aldosterone system (eg, patients with severe congestive heart failure), treatment with angiotensin-converting enzyme inhibitors and angiotensin receptor antagonists has been associated with oliguria and/or progressive azotemia and (rarely) with acute renal failure and/or death. Similar results may be anticipated in patients treated with ATACAND. (See CLINICAL PHARMACOLOGY, Special Populations.)
In studies of ACE inhibitors in patients with unilateral or bilateral renal artery stenosis, increases in serum creatinine or blood urea nitrogen (BUN) have been reported. There has been no long-term use of ATACAND in patients with unilateral or bilateral renal artery stenosis, but similar results may be expected.

Information for Patients

Pregnancy: Female patients of childbearing age should be told about the consequences of second- and third-trimester exposure to drugs that act on the renin-angiotensin system, and they should also be told that these consequences do not appear to have resulted from intrauterine drug exposure that has been limited to the first trimester. These patients should be asked to report pregnancies to their physicians as soon as possible.

Drug Interactions

No significant drug interactions have been reported in studies of candesartan cilexetil given with other drugs such as glyburide, nifedipine, digoxin, warfarin, hydrochlorothiazide, and oral contraceptives in healthy volunteers. Because candesartan is not significantly metabolized by the cytochrome P450 system and at therapeutic concentrations has no effects on P450 enzymes, interactions with drugs that inhibit or are metabolized by those enzymes would not be expected.

Carcinogenesis, Mutagenesis, Impairment of Fertility

There was no evidence of carcinogenicity when candesartan cilexetil was orally administered to mice and rats for up to 104 weeks at doses up to 100 and 1000 mg/kg/day, respectively. Rats received the drug by gavage, whereas mice received the drug by dietary administration. These (maximally-tolerated) doses of candesartan cilexetil provided systemic exposures to candesartan (AUCs) that were, in mice, approximately 7 times and, in rats, more than 70 times the exposure in man at the maximum recommended daily human dose (32 mg).
Candesartan cilexetil was not genotoxic in the microbial mutagenesis and mammalian cell mutagenesis assays and in the *in vivo* chromosomal aberration and rat unscheduled DNA synthesis assays. In addition, candesartan was not genotoxic in the microbial mutagenesis, mammalian cell mutagenesis, and *in vitro* and *in vivo* chromosome aberration assays.
Fertility and reproductive performance were not affected in studies with male and female rats given oral doses of up to 300 mg/kg/day (83 times the maximum daily human dose of 32 mg on a body surface area basis).

Pregnancy

Pregnancy Categories C (first trimester) *and D* (second and third trimesters). See WARNINGS, Fetal/Neonatal Morbidity and Mortality.

Nursing Mothers

It is not known whether candesartan is excreted in human milk, but candesartan has been shown to be present in rat milk. Because of the potential for adverse effects on the nursing infant, a decision should be made whether to discontinue nursing or discontinue the drug, taking into account the importance of the drug to the mother.

Pediatric Use

Safety and effectiveness in pediatric patients have not been established.

Geriatric Use

Of the total number of subjects in clinical studies of ATACAND, 21% were 65 and over, while 3% were 75 and over. No overall differences in safety or effectiveness were observed between these subjects and younger subjects, and other reported clinical experience has not identified differences in responses between the elderly and younger patients, but greater sensitivity of some older individuals cannot be ruled out. In a placebo-controlled trial of about 200 elderly hypertensive patients (ages 65 to 87 years), administration of candesartan cilexetil was well tolerated and lowered blood pressure by about 12/6 mm Hg more than placebo.

ADVERSE REACTIONS

ATACAND has been evaluated for safety in more than 3600 patients/subjects, including more than 3200 patients treated for hypertension. About 600 of these patients were studied for at least 6 months and about 200 for at least 1 year. In general, treatment with ATACAND was well tolerated. The overall incidence of adverse events reported with ATACAND was similar to placebo.

The rate of withdrawals due to adverse events in all trials in patients (7510 total) was 3.3% (ie, 108 of 3260) of patients treated with candesartan cilexetil as monotherapy and 3.5% (ie, 39 of 1106) of patients treated with placebo. In placebo-controlled trials, discontinuation of therapy due to clinical adverse events occurred in 2.4% (ie, 57 of 2350) of patients treated with ATACAND and 3.4% (ie, 35 of 1027) of patients treated with placebo.

The most common reasons for discontinuation of therapy with ATACAND were headache (0.6%) and dizziness (0.3%).

The adverse events that occurred in placebo-controlled clinical trials in at least 1% of patients treated with ATACAND and at a higher incidence in candesartan cilexetil (n=2350) than placebo (n=1027) patients included back pain (3% vs 2%), dizziness (4% vs 3%), upper respiratory tract infection (6% vs 4%), pharyngitis (2% vs 1%), and rhinitis (2% vs 1%).

The following adverse events occurred in placebo-controlled clinical trials at a more than 1% rate but at about the same or greater incidence in patients receiving placebo compared to candesartan cilexetil: fatigue, peripheral edema, chest pain, headache, bronchitis, coughing, sinusitis, nausea, abdominal pain, diarrhea, vomiting, arthralgia, albuminuria.

Other potentially important adverse events that have been reported, whether or not attributed to treatment, with an incidence of 0.5% or greater from the more than 3200 patients worldwide treated with ATACAND are listed below. It cannot be determined whether these events were causally related to ATACAND. **Body as a Whole:** asthenia, fever; **Central and Peripheral Nervous System:** paresthesia, vertigo; **Gastrointestinal System Disorder:** dyspepsia, gastroenteritis; **Heart Rate and Rhythm Disorders:** tachycardia, palpitation; **Metabolic and Nutritional Disorders:** creatine phosphokinase increased, hyperglycemia, hypertriglyceridemia, hyperuricemia; **Musculoskeletal System Disorders:** myalgia; **Platelet/Bleeding-Clotting Disorders:** epistaxis; **Psychiatric Disorders:** anxiety, depression, somnolence; **Respiratory System Disorders:** dyspnea; **Skin and Appendages Disorders:** rash, sweating increased; **Urinary System Disorders:** hematuria.

Other reported events seen less frequently included angina pectoris, myocardial infarction, and angioedema.

Adverse events occurred at about the same rates in men and women, older and younger patients, and black and nonblack patients.

Post-Marketing Experience

The following have been very rarely reported in post-marketing experience:

Digestive: Abnormal hepatic function and hepatitis.

Hematologic: Neutropenia, leukopenia, and agranulocytosis.

Skin and Appendages Disorders: Pruritis and urticaria.

Laboratory Test Findings

In controlled clinical trials, clinically important changes in standard laboratory parameters were rarely associated with the administration of ATACAND.

Creatinine, Blood Urea Nitrogen: Minor increases in blood urea nitrogen (BUN) and serum creatinine were observed infrequently.

Hyperuricemia: Hyperuricemia was rarely found (19 or 0.6% of 3260 patients treated with candesartan cilexetil and 5 or 0.5% of 1106 patients treated with placebo).

Hemoglobin and Hematocrit: Small decreases in hemoglobin and hematocrit (mean decreases of approximately 0.2 grams/dL and 0.5 volume percent, respectively) were observed in patients treated with ATACAND alone but were rarely of clinical importance. Anemia, leukopenia, and thrombocytopenia were associated with withdrawal of one patient each from clinical trials.

Potassium: A small increase (mean increase of 0.1 mEq/L) was observed in patients treated with ATACAND alone but was rarely of clinical importance. One patient from a congestive heart failure trial was withdrawn for hyperkalemia (serum potassium = 7.5 mEq/L). This patient was also receiving spironolactone.

Liver Function Tests: Elevations of liver enzymes and/or serum bilirubin were observed infrequently. Five patients assigned to candesartan cilexetil in clinical trials were withdrawn because of abnormal liver chemistries. All had elevated transaminases. Two had mildly elevated total bilirubin, but one of these patients was diagnosed with Hepatitis A.

OVERDOSAGE

No lethality was observed in acute toxicity studies in mice, rats, and dogs given single oral doses of up to 2000 mg/kg of candesartan cilexetil. In mice given single oral doses of the primary metabolite, candesartan, the minimum lethal dose was greater than 1000 mg/kg but less than 2000 mg/kg.

Limited data are available in regard to overdosage in humans. In one recorded case of an intentional overdose, a 43-year-old female patient (Body Mass Index of 31 kg/m^2) ingested an estimated 160 mg of candesartan cilexetil in conjunction with multiple other pharmaceutical agents (ibuprofen, naproxen sodium, diphenhydramine hydrochloride, and ketoprofen). Gastric lavage was performed; the patient was monitored in hospital for several days and was discharged without sequelae.

Candesartan cannot be removed by hemodialysis.

Treatment: To obtain up-to-date information about the treatment of overdose, consult your Regional Poison Control Center. Telephone numbers of certified poison control centers are listed in the *Physicians' Desk Reference (PDR)*. In managing overdose, consider the possibilities of multiple-drug overdoses, drug-drug interactions, and altered pharmacokinetics in your patient.

The most likely manifestation of overdosage with ATACAND would be hypotension, dizziness, and tachycardia; bradycardia could occur from parasympathetic (vagal) stimulation. If symptomatic hypotension should occur, supportive treatment should be instituted.

DOSAGE AND ADMINISTRATION

Dosage must be individualized. Blood pressure response is dose related over the range of 2 to 32 mg. The usual recommended starting dose of ATACAND is 16 mg once daily when it is used as monotherapy in patients who are not volume depleted. ATACAND can be administered once or twice daily with total daily doses ranging from 8 mg to 32 mg. Larger doses do not appear to have a greater effect, and there is relatively little experience with such doses. Most of the antihypertensive effect is present within 2 weeks, and maximal blood pressure reduction is generally obtained within 4 to 6 weeks of treatment with ATACAND.

No initial dosage adjustment is necessary for elderly patients, for patients with mildly impaired renal function, or for patients with mildly impaired hepatic function (see CLINICAL PHARMACOLOGY, Special Populations). For patients with possible depletion of intravascular volume (eg, patients treated with diuretics, particularly those with impaired renal function), ATACAND should be initiated under close medical supervision and consideration should be given to administration of a lower dose (see WARNINGS, Hypotension in Volume- and Salt-Depleted Patients).

ATACAND may be administered with or without food.

If blood pressure is not controlled by ATACAND alone, a diuretic may be added. ATACAND may be administered with other antihypertensive agents.

HOW SUPPLIED

No. 3782 — Tablets ATACAND, 4 mg, are white to off-white, circular/biconvex-shaped, non-film-coated tablets, coded ACF on one side and 004 on the other. They are supplied as follows:

NDC 0186-0004-31 unit of use bottles of 30.

No. 3780 — Tablets ATACAND, 8 mg, are light pink, circular/biconvex-shaped, non-film-coated tablets, coded ACG on one side and 008 on the other. They are supplied as follows:

NDC 0186-0008-31 unit of use bottles of 30.

No. 3781 — Tablets ATACAND, 16 mg, are pink, circular/biconvex-shaped, non-film-coated tablets, coded ACH on one side and 016 on the other. They are supplied as follows:

NDC 0186-0016-31 unit of use bottles of 30

NDC 0186-0016-54 unit of use bottles of 90

NDC 0186-0016-28 unit dose packages of 100.

No. 3791 — Tablets ATACAND, 32 mg, are pink, circular/biconvex-shaped, non-film-coated tablets, coded ACL on one side and 032 on the other. They are supplied as follows:

NDC 0186-0032-31 unit of use bottles of 30

NDC 0186-0032-54 unit of use bottles of 90

NDC 0186-0032-28 unit dose packages of 100.

Storage

Store at 25°C (77°F); excursions permitted to 15–30°C (59–86°F) [see USP Controlled Room Temperature]. Keep container tightly closed.

ATACAND is a trademark of the AstraZeneca group

Manufactured under the license from Takeda Chemical Industries, Ltd.

by: AstraZeneca AB, S-151 85 Södertälje, Sweden

for: AstraZeneca LP, Wilmington, DE 19850

Made in Sweden

9174307

610002-07 Rev. 09/01

ATACAND HCT™ 16–12.5 ℞

[ăt' ă-kănd]

(Candesartan Cilexetil-Hydrochlorothiazide)

ATACAND HCT™ 32–12.5

(Candesartan Cilexetil-Hydrochlorothiazide)

TABLETS

Prescribing information for this product, which appears on page 597 of the 2002 PDR, has been completely revised as follows. Please write "See Supplement A" next to the product heading.

USE IN PREGNANCY

When used in pregnancy during the second and third trimesters, drugs that act directly on the renin-angiotensin system can cause injury and even death to the developing fetus. When pregnancy is detected, ATACAND HCT should be discontinued as soon as possible. See WARNINGS, Fetal/Neonatal Morbidity and Mortality.

DESCRIPTION

ATACAND HCT (candesartan cilexetil-hydrochlorothiazide) combines an angiotensin II receptor (type AT_1) antagonist and a diuretic, hydrochlorothiazide.

Candesartan cilexetil, a nonpeptide, is chemically described as (±)-1-[[(cyclohexyloxy)carbonyl]oxy]ethyl 2-ethoxy-1-[[2'-(1H-tetrazol-5-yl)[1,1'-biphenyl]-4-yl]methyl]-1H-benzimidazole-7-carboxylate.

Its empirical formula is $C_{33}H_{34}N_6O_6$, and its structural formula is

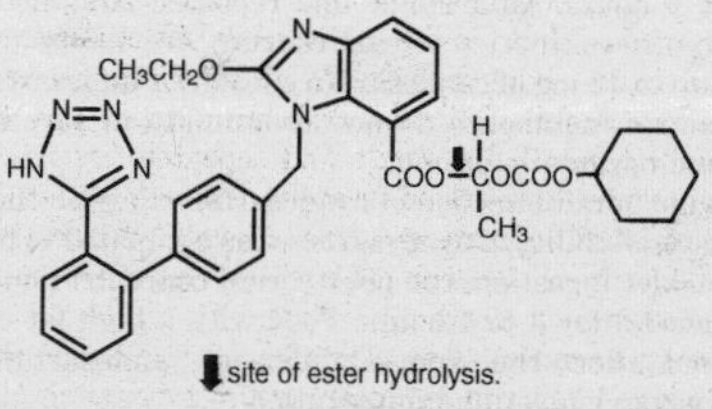

↓ site of ester hydrolysis.

Candesartan cilexetil is a white to off-white powder with a molecular weight of 610.67. It is practically insoluble in water and sparingly soluble in methanol. Candesartan cilexetil is a racemic mixture containing one chiral center at the cyclohexyloxycarbonyloxy ethyl ester group. Following oral administration, candesartan cilexetil undergoes hydrolysis at the ester link to form the active drug, candesartan, which is achiral.

Hydrochlorothiazide is 6-chloro-3,4-dihydro-*2H*-1,2,4-benzothiadiazine-7-sulfonamide 1,1-dioxide. Its empirical formula is $C_7H_8ClN_3O_4S_2$ and its structural formula is

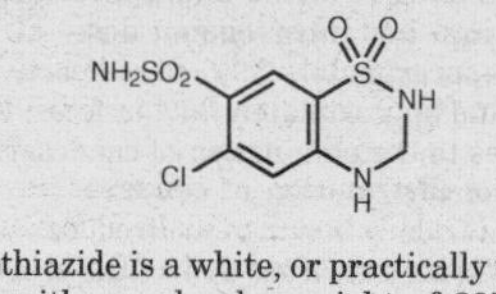

Hydrochlorothiazide is a white, or practically white, crystalline powder with a molecular weight of 297.72, which is slightly soluble in water, but freely soluble in sodium hydroxide solution.

ATACAND HCT is available for oral administration in two tablet strengths of candesartan cilexetil and hydrochlorothiazide.

ATACAND HCT 16-12.5 contains 16 mg of candesartan cilexetil and 12.5 mg of hydrochlorothiazide. ATACAND HCT 32-12.5 contains 32 mg of candesartan cilexetil and 12.5 mg of hydrochlorothiazide. The inactive ingredients of the tablets are calcium carboxymethylcellulose, hydroxypropyl cellulose, lactose monohydrate, magnesium stearate, corn starch, polyethylene glycol 8000, and ferric oxide (yellow). Ferric oxide (reddish brown) is also added to the 16-12.5 mg tablet as colorant.

CLINICAL PHARMACOLOGY

Mechanism of Action

Angiotensin II is formed from angiotensin I in a reaction catalyzed by angiotensin-converting enzyme (ACE, kininase II). Angiotensin II is the principal pressor agent of the renin-angiotensin system, with effects that include vasoconstriction, stimulation of synthesis and release of aldosterone, cardiac stimulation, and renal reabsorption of sodium. Candesartan blocks the vasoconstrictor and aldosterone-secreting effects of angiotensin II by selectively blocking the binding of angiotensin II to the AT_1 receptor in many tissues, such as vascular smooth muscle and the adrenal gland. Its action is, therefore, independent of the pathways for angiotensin II synthesis.

There is also an AT_2 receptor found in many tissues, but AT_2 is not known to be associated with cardiovascular homeostasis. Candesartan has much greater affinity (>10,000-fold) for the AT_1 receptor than for the AT_2 receptor.

Blockade of the renin-angiotensin system with ACE inhibitors, which inhibit the biosynthesis of angiotensin II from angiotensin I, is widely used in the treatment of hypertension. ACE inhibitors also inhibit the degradation of bradykinin, a reaction also catalyzed by ACE. Because candesartan does not inhibit ACE (kininase II), it does not affect the response to bradykinin. Whether this difference has clinical relevance is not yet known. Candesartan does not bind to or block other hormone receptors or ion channels known to be important in cardiovascular regulation.

Blockade of the angiotensin II receptor inhibits the negative regulatory feedback of angiotensin II on renin secretion, but the resulting increased plasma renin activity and angiotensin II circulating levels do not overcome the effect of candesartan on blood pressure.

Hydrochlorothiazide is a thiazide diuretic. Thiazides affect the renal tubular mechanisms of electrolyte reabsorption, directly increasing excretion of sodium and chloride in ap-

Continued on next page

Atacand HCT—Cont.

proximately equivalent amounts. Indirectly, the diuretic action of hydrochlorothiazide reduces plasma volume, with consequent increases in plasma renin activity, increases in aldosterone secretion, increases in urinary potassium loss, and decreases in serum potassium. The renin-aldosterone link is mediated by angiotensin II, so coadministration of an angiotensin II receptor antagonist tends to reverse the potassium loss associated with these diuretics.
The mechanism of the antihypertensive effect of thiazides is unknown.

Pharmacokinetics

General

Candesartan Cilexetil

Candesartan cilexetil is rapidly and completely bioactivated by ester hydrolysis during absorption from the gastrointestinal tract to candesartan, a selective AT_1 subtype angiotensin II receptor antagonist. Candesartan is mainly excreted unchanged in urine and feces (via bile). It undergoes minor hepatic metabolism by O-deethylation to an inactive metabolite. The elimination half-life of candesartan is approximately 9 hours. After single and repeated administration, the pharmacokinetics of candesartan are linear for oral doses up to 32 mg of candesartan cilexetil. Candesartan and its inactive metabolite do not accumulate in serum upon repeated once-daily dosing.
Following administration of candesartan cilexetil, the absolute bioavailability of candesartan was estimated to be 15%. After tablet ingestion, the peak serum concentration (C_{max}) is reached after 3 to 4 hours. Food with a high fat content does not affect the bioavailability of candesartan after candesartan cilexetil administration.

Hydrochlorothiazide

When plasma levels have been followed for at least 24 hours, the plasma half-life has been observed to vary between 5.6 and 14.8 hours.

Metabolism and Excretion

Candesartan Cilexetil

Total plasma clearance of candesartan is 0.37 mL/min/kg, with a renal clearance of 0.19 mL/min/kg. When candesartan is administered orally, about 26% of the dose is excreted unchanged in urine. Following an oral dose of ^{14}C-labeled candesartan cilexetil, approximately 33% of radioactivity is recovered in urine and approximately 67% in feces. Following an intravenous dose of ^{14}C-labeled candesartan, approximately 59% of radioactivity is recovered in urine and approximately 36% in feces. Biliary excretion contributes to the elimination of candesartan.

Hydrochlorothiazide

Hydrochlorothiazide is not metabolized but is eliminated rapidly by the kidney. At least 61% of the oral dose is eliminated unchanged within 24 hours.

Distribution

Candesartan Cilexetil

The volume of distribution of candesartan is 0.13 L/kg. Candesartan is highly bound to plasma proteins (>99%) and does not penetrate red blood cells. The protein binding is constant at candesartan plasma concentrations well above the range achieved with recommended doses. In rats, it has been demonstrated that candesartan crosses the blood-brain barrier poorly, if at all. It has also been demonstrated in rats that candesartan passes across the placental barrier and is distributed in the fetus.

Hydrochlorothiazide

Hydrochlorothiazide crosses the placental but not the blood-brain barrier and is excreted in breast milk.

Special Populations

Pediatric

The pharmacokinetics of candesartan cilexetil have not been investigated in patients <18 years of age.

Geriatric

The pharmacokinetics of candesartan have been studied in the elderly (≥65 years). The plasma concentration of candesartan was higher in the elderly (C_{max} was approximately 50% higher, and AUC was approximately 80% higher) compared to younger subjects administered the same dose. The pharmacokinetics of candesartan were linear in the elderly, and candesartan and its inactive metabolite did not accumulate in the serum of these subjects upon repeated, once-daily administration. No initial dosage adjustment is necessary. (See DOSAGE AND ADMINISTRATION.)

Gender

There is no difference in the pharmacokinetics of candesartan between male and female subjects.

Renal Insufficiency

In hypertensive patients with renal insufficiency, serum concentrations of candesartan were elevated. After repeated dosing, the AUC and C_{max} were approximately doubled in patients with severe renal impairment (creatinine clearance <30 mL/min/1.73m^2) compared to patients with normal kidney function. The pharmacokinetics of candesartan in hypertensive patients undergoing hemodialysis are similar to those in hypertensive patients with severe renal impairment. Candesartan cannot be removed by hemodialysis. No initial dosage adjustment is necessary in patients with renal insufficiency.
Thiazide diuretics are eliminated by the kidney, with a terminal half-life of 5-15 hours. In a study of patients with impaired renal function (mean creatinine clearance of 19 mL/min), the half-life of hydrochlorothiazide elimination was lengthened to 21 hours. (See DOSAGE AND ADMINISTRATION.)

Hepatic Insufficiency

No differences in the pharmacokinetics of candesartan were observed in patients with mild to moderate chronic liver disease. Thiazide diuretics should be used with caution in patients with hepatic impairment. (See DOSAGE AND ADMINISTRATION.)

Pharmacodynamics

Candesartan Cilexetil

Candesartan inhibits the pressor effects of angiotensin II infusion in a dose-dependent manner. After 1 week of once-daily dosing with 8 mg of candesartan cilexetil, the pressor effect was inhibited by approximately 90% at peak with approximately 50% inhibition persisting for 24 hours.
Plasma concentrations of angiotensin I and angiotensin II, and plasma renin activity (PRA), increased in a dose-dependent manner after single and repeated administration of candesartan cilexetil to healthy subjects and hypertensive patients. ACE activity was not altered in healthy subjects after repeated candesartan cilexetil administration. The once-daily administration of up to 16 mg of candesartan cilexetil to healthy subjects did not influence plasma aldosterone concentrations, but a decrease in the plasma concentration of aldosterone was observed when 32 mg of candesartan cilexetil was administered to hypertensive patients. In spite of the effect of candesartan cilexetil on aldosterone secretion, very little effect on serum potassium was observed.
In multiple-dose studies with hypertensive patients, there were no clinically significant changes in metabolic function including serum levels of total cholesterol, triglycerides, glucose, or uric acid. In a 12-week study of 161 patients with noninsulin-dependent (type 2) diabetes mellitus and hypertension, there was no change in the level of HbA_{1c}.

Hydrochlorothiazide

After oral administration of hydrochlorothiazide, diuresis begins within 2 hours, peaks in about 4 hours and lasts about 6 to 12 hours.

Clinical Trials

Candesartan Cilexetil—Hydrochlorothiazide

Of 12 controlled clinical trials involving 4588 patients, 5 were double-blind, placebo controlled and evaluated the antihypertensive effects of single entities vs the combination. These 5 trials, of 8 to 12 weeks duration, randomized 3037 hypertensive patients. Doses ranged from 2 to 32 mg candesartan cilexetil and from 6.25 to 25 mg hydrochlorothiazide administered once daily in various combinations.
The combination of candesartan cilexetil-hydrochlorothiazide resulted in placebo-adjusted decreases in sitting systolic and diastolic blood pressures of 14-18/8-11 mm Hg at doses of 16-12.5 mg and 32-12.5 mg. The combination of candesartan cilexetil and hydrochlorothiazide 32-25 mg resulted in placebo-adjusted decreases in sitting systolic and diastolic blood pressures of 16-19/9-11 mm Hg. The placebo corrected trough to peak ratio was evaluated in a study of candesartan cilexetil-hydrochlorothiazide 32-12.5 mg and was 88%.
Most of the antihypertensive effect of the combination of candesartan cilexetil and hydrochlorothiazide was seen in 1 to 2 weeks with the full effect observed within 4 weeks. In long-term studies of up to 1 year, the blood pressure lowering effect of the combination was maintained. The antihypertensive effect was similar regardless of age or gender, and overall response to the combination was similar in black and non-black patients. No appreciable changes in heart rate were observed with combination therapy in controlled trials.

INDICATIONS AND USAGE

ATACAND HCT is indicated for the treatment of hypertension. This fixed dose combination is not indicated for initial therapy (see DOSAGE AND ADMINISTRATION).

CONTRAINDICATIONS

ATACAND HCT is contraindicated in patients who are hypersensitive to any component of this product.
Because of the hydrochlorothiazide component, this product is contraindicated in patients with anuria or hypersensitivity to other sulfonamide-derived drugs.

WARNINGS

Fetal/Neonatal Morbidity and Mortality

Drugs that act directly on the renin-angiotensin system can cause fetal and neonatal morbidity and death when administered to pregnant women. Several dozen cases have been reported in the world literature in patients who were taking angiotensin-converting enzyme inhibitors. When pregnancy is detected, ATACAND HCT should be discontinued as soon as possible.
The use of drugs that act directly on the renin-angiotensin system during the second and third trimesters of pregnancy has been associated with fetal and neonatal injury, including hypotension, neonatal skull hypoplasia, anuria, reversible or irreversible renal failure, and death. Oligohydramnios has also been reported, presumably resulting from decreased fetal renal function; oligohydramnios in this setting has been associated with fetal limb contractures, craniofacial deformation, and hypoplastic lung development. Prematurity, intrauterine growth retardation, and patent ductus arteriosus have also been reported, although it is not clear whether these occurences were due to exposure to the drug.
These adverse effects do not appear to have resulted from intrauterine drug exposure that has been limited to the first trimester. Mothers whose embryos and fetuses are exposed to an angiotensin II receptor antagonist only during the first trimester should be so informed. Nonetheless, when patients become pregnant, physicians should have the patient discontinue the use of ATACAND HCT as soon as possible.
Rarely (probably less often than once in every thousand pregnancies), no alternative to a drug acting on the renin-angiotensin system will be found. In these rare cases, the mothers should be apprised of the potential hazards to their fetuses, and serial ultrasound examinations should be performed to assess the intra-amniotic environment.
If oligohydramnios is observed, ATACAND HCT should be discontinued unless it is considered life saving for the mother. Contraction stress testing (CST), a nonstress test (NST), or biophysical profiling (BPP) may be appropriate, depending upon the week of pregnancy. Patients and physicians should be aware, however, that oligohydramnios may not appear until after the fetus has sustained irreversible injury.
Infants with histories of *in utero* exposure to an angiotensin II receptor antagonist should be closely observed for hypotension, oliguria, and hyperkalemia. If oliguria occurs, attention should be directed toward support of blood pressure and renal perfusion. Exchange transfusion or dialysis may be required as means of reversing hypotension and/or substituting for disordered renal funtion.

Candesartan Cilexetil—Hydrochlorothiazide

There was no evidence of teratogenicity or other adverse effects on embryo-fetal development when pregnant mice, rats or rabbits were treated orally with candesartan cilexetil alone or in combination with hydrochlorothiazide. For mice, the maximum dose of candesartan cilexetil was 1000 mg/kg/day (about 150 times the maximum recommended daily human dose [MRHD]*). For rats, the maximum dose of candesartan cilexetil was 100 mg/kg/day (about 31 times the MRHD*). For rabbits, the maximum dose of candesartan cilexetil was 1 mg/kg/day (a maternally toxic dose that is about half the MRHD*). In each of these studies, hydrochlorothiazide was tested at the same dose level (10 mg/kg/day, about 4, 8, and 15 times the MRHD* in mouse, rats, and rabbit, respectively). There was no evidence of harm to the rat or mouse fetus or embryo in studies in which hydrochlorothiazide was administered alone to the pregnant rat or mouse at doses of up to 1000 and 3000 mg/kg/day, respectively.
Thiazides cross the placental barrier and appear in cord blood. There is a risk of fetal or neonatal jaundice, thrombocytopenia, and possibly other adverse reactions that have occurred in adults.

*Doses compared on the basis of body surface area. MRHD considered to be 32 mg for candesartan cilexetil and 12.5 mg for hydrochlorothiazide.

Hypotension in Volume- and Salt-Depleted Patients

Based on adverse events reported from all clinical trials of ATACAND HCT, excessive reduction of blood pressure was rarely seen in patients with uncomplicated hypertension treated with candesartan cilexetil and hydrochlorothiazide (0.4%). Initiation of antihypertensive therapy may cause symptomatic hypotension in patients with intravascular volume- or sodium-depletion, eg, in patients treated vigorously with diuretics or in patients on dialysis. These conditions should be corrected prior to administration of ATACAND HCT, or the treatment should start under close medical supervision (see DOSAGE AND ADMINISTRATION).
If hypotension occurs, the patients should be placed in the supine position and, if necessary, given an intravenous infusion of normal saline. A transient hypotensive response is not a contraindication to further treatment which usually can be continued without difficulty once the blood pressure has stabilized.

Hydrochlorothiazide

Impaired Hepatic Function

Thiazide diuretics should be used with caution in patients with impaired hepatic function or progressive liver disease, since minor alterations of fluid and electrolyte balance may precipitate hepatic coma.

Hypersensitivity Reaction

Hypersensitivity reactions to hydrochlorothiazide may occur in patients with or without a history of allergy or bronchial asthma, but are more likely in patients with such a history.

Systemic Lupus Erythematosus

Thiazide diuretics have been reported to cause exacerbation or activation of systemic lupus erythematosus.

Lithium Interaction

Lithium generally should not be given with thiazides (see PRECAUTIONS, Drug Interactions, Hydrochlorothiazide, Lithium).

PRECAUTIONS

General

Candesartan Cilexetil—Hydrochlorothiazide

In clinical trials of various doses of candesartan cilexetil and hydrochlorothiazide, the incidence of hypertensive patients who developed hypokalemia (serum potassium <3.5 mEq/L) was 2.5% versus 2.1% for placebo; the incidence of hyperkalemia (serum potassium >5.7 mEq/L) was 0.4% versus 1.0% for placebo. No patient receiving ATACAND HCT 16-12.5 mg or 32-12.5 mg was discontinued due to increases or decreases in serum potassium. Overall, the combination of candesartan cilexetil and hydrochlorothiazide had no clinically significant effect on serum potassium.

Hydrochlorothiazide
Periodic determination of serum electrolytes to detect possible electrolyte imbalance should be performed at appropriate intervals.
All patients receiving thiazide therapy should be observed for clinical signs of fluid or electrolyte imbalance: namely, hyponatremia, hypochloremic alkalosis, and hypokalemia. Serum and urine electrolyte determinations are particularly important when the patient is vomiting excessively or receiving parenteral fluids. Warning signs or symptoms of fluid and electrolyte imbalance, irrespective of cause, include dryness of mouth, thirst, weakness, lethargy, drowsiness, restlessness, confusion, seizures, muscle pains or cramps, muscular fatigue, hypotension, oliguria, tachycardia, and gastrointestinal disturbances such as nausea and vomiting.
Hypokalemia may develop, especially with brisk diuresis, when severe cirrhosis is present, or after prolonged therapy. Interference with adequate oral electrolyte intake will also contribute to hypokalemia. Hypokalemia may cause cardiac arrhythmia and may also sensitize or exaggerate the response of the heart to the toxic effects of digitalis (eg, increased ventricular irritability).
Although any chloride deficit is generally mild and usually does not require specific treatment, except under extraordinary circumstances (as in liver disease or renal disease), chloride replacement may be required in the treatment of metabolic alkalosis.
Dilutional hyponatremia may occur in edematous patients in hot weather; appropriate therapy is water restriction, rather than administration of salt, except in rare instances when the hyponatremia is life-threatening. In actual salt depletion, appropriate replacement is the therapy of choice.
Hyperuricemia may occur or acute gout may be precipitated in certain patients receiving thiazide therapy.
In diabetic patients dosage adjustments of insulin or oral hypoglycemic agents may be required. Hyperglycemia may occur with thiazide diuretics. Thus latent diabetes mellitus may become manifest during thiazide therapy.
The antihypertensive effects of the drug may be enhanced in the post-sympathectomy patient.
If progressive renal impairment becomes evident, consider withholding or discontinuing diuretic therapy.
Thiazides have been shown to increase the urinary excretion of magnesium; this may result in hypomagnesemia.
Thiazides may decrease urinary calcium excretion. Thiazides may cause intermittent and slight elevation of serum calcium in the absence of known disorders of calcium metabolism. Marked hypercalcemia may be evidence of hidden hyperparathyroidism. Thiazides should be discontinued before carrying out tests for parathyroid function.
Increases in cholesterol and triglyceride levels may be associated with thiazide diuretic therapy.

Impaired Renal Function
Candesartan Cilexetil
As a consequence of inhibiting the renin-angiotensin-aldosterone system, changes in renal function may be anticipated in susceptible individuals treated with candesartan cilexetil. In patients whose renal function may depend upon the activity of the renin-angiotensin-aldosterone system (eg, patients with severe congestive heart failure), treatment with angiotensin-converting enzyme inhibitors and angiotensin receptor antagonists has been associated with oliguria and/or progressive azotemia and (rarely) with acute renal failure and/or death. Similar results may be anticipated in patients treated with candesartan cilexetil. (See CLINICAL PHARMACOLOGY, Special Populations.)
In studies of ACE inhibitors in patients with unilateral or bilateral renal artery stenosis, increases in serum creatinine or blood urea nitrogen (BUN) have been reported. There has been no long-term use of candesartan cilexetil in patients with unilateral or bilateral renal artery stenosis, but similar results may be expected.
Hydrochlorothiazide
Thiazides should be used with caution in severe renal disease. In patients with renal disease, thiazides may precipitate azotemia. Cumulative effects of the drug may develop in patients with impaired renal function.

Information for Patients
Pregnancy
Female patients of childbearing age should be told about the consequences of second- and third-trimester exposure to drugs that act on the renin-angiotensin system, and they should also be told that these consequences do not appear to have resulted from intrauterine drug exposure that has been limited to the first trimester. These patients should be asked to report pregnancies to their physicians as soon as possible.
Symptomatic Hypotension
A patient receiving ATACAND HCT should be cautioned that lightheadedness can occur, especially during the first days of therapy, and that it should be reported to the prescribing physician. The patients should be told that if syncope occurs, ATACAND HCT should be discontinued until the physician has been consulted.
All patients should be cautioned that inadequate fluid intake, excessive perspiration, diarrhea, or vomiting can lead to an excessive fall in blood pressure, with the same consequences of lightheadedness and possible syncope.
Potassium Supplements
A patient receiving ATACAND HCT should be told not to use potassium supplements or salt substitutes containing potassium without consulting the prescribing physician.

Drug Interactions
Candesartan Cilexetil
No significant drug interactions have been reported in studies of candesartan cilexetil given with other drugs such as glyburide, nifedipine, digoxin, warfarin, hydrochlorothiazide, and oral contraceptives in healthy volunteers. Because candesartan is not significantly metabolized by the cytochrome P450 system and at therapeutic concentrations has no effects on P450 enzymes, interactions with drugs that inhibit or are metabolized by those enzymes would not be expected.
Hydrochlorothiazide
When administered concurrently the following drugs may interact with thiazide diuretics:
Alcohol, barbiturates, or narcotics—Potentiation of orthostatic hypotension may occur.
Antidiabetic drugs (oral agents and insulin)—Dosage adjustment of the antidiabetic drug may be required.
Other antihypertensive drugs—Additive effect or potentiation.
Cholestyramine and colestipol resins—Absorption of hydrochlorothiazide is impaired in the presence of anionic exchange resins. Single doses of either cholestyramine or colestipol resins bind the hydrochlorothiazide and reduce its absorption from the gastrointestinal tract by up to 85 and 43 percent, respectively.
Corticosteroids, ACTH—Intensified electrolyte depletion, particularly hypokalemia.
Pressor amines (eg, norepinephrine)—Possible decreased response to pressor amines but not sufficient to preclude their use.
Skeletal muscle relaxants, nondepolarizing (eg, tubocurarine)—Possible increased responsiveness to the muscle relaxant.
Lithium—Generally should not be given with diuretics. Diuretic agents reduce the renal clearance of lithium and add a high risk of lithium toxicity. Refer to the package insert for lithium preparations before use of such preparations with ATACAND HCT.
Non-steroidal Anti-inflammatory Drugs—In some patients, the administration of a non-steroidal anti-inflammatory agent can reduce the diuretic, natriuretic, and antihypertensive effects of loop, potassium-sparing and thiazide diuretics. Therefore, when ATACAND HCT and non-steroidal anti-inflammatory agents are used concomitantly, the patient should be observed closely to determine if the desired effect of the diuretic is obtained.

Carcinogenesis, Mutagenesis, Impairment of Fertility
Candesartan Cilexetil—Hydrochlorothiazide
No carcinogenicity studies have been conducted with the combination of candesartan cilexetil and hydrochlorothiazide. There was no evidence of carcinogenicity when candesartan cilexetil was orally administered to mice and rats for up to 104 weeks at doses up to 100 and 1000 mg/kg/day, respectively. Rats received the drug by gavage whereas mice received the drug by dietary administration. These (maximally-tolerated) doses of candesartan cilexetil provided systemic exposures to candesartan (AUCs) that were, in mice, approximately 7 times and, in rats, more than 70 times the exposure in man at the maximum recommended daily human dose (32 mg). Two-year feeding studies in mice and rats conducted under the auspices of the National Toxicology Program (NTP) uncovered no evidence of a carcinogenic potential of hydrochlorothiazide in female mice (at doses of up to approximately 600 mg/kg/day) or in male and female rats (at doses of up to approximately 100 mg/kg/day). The NTP, however, found equivocal evidence for hepatocarcinogenicity in male mice. Candesartan cilexetil, alone or in combination with hydrochlorothiazide, tested negative for mutagenicity in bacteria (Ames test), for unscheduled DNA synthesis in rat liver, for chromosomal aberrations in rat bone marrow and for micronuclei in mouse bone marrow. In addition, candesartan (the active metabolite) was not genotoxic in the microbial mutagenesis, mammalian cell mutagenesis, and *in vitro* and *in vivo* chromosome aberration assays. In the *in vitro* Chinese hamster lung cell chromosomal aberration and mouse lymphoma assays, mutagenic effects were detected when hydrochlorothiazide was tested in the presence of candesartan. Hydrochlorothiazide was not genotoxic *in vitro* in the Ames test for point mutations and the Chinese Hamster Ovary (CHO) test for chromosomal aberrations, or *in vivo* in assays using mouse germinal cell chromosomes, Chinese hamster bone marrow chromosomes, and the *Drosophila* sex-linked recessive lethal trait gene. Positive test results were obtained for hydrochlorothiazide in the *in vitro* CHO Sister Chromatid Exchange (clastogenicity) and in the Mouse Lymphoma Cell (mutagenicity) assays and in the *Aspergillus nidulans* nondisjunction assay.
No fertility studies have been conducted with the combination of candesartan cilexetil and hydrochlorothiazide. Fertility and reproductive performance were not affected in studies with male and female rats given oral doses of up to 300 mg candesartan cilexetil/kg/day (83 times the maximum daily human dose of 32 mg on a body surface area basis). Hydrochlorothiazide had no adverse effects on the fertility of mice and rats of either sex in studies wherein these species were exposed, via their diet, to doses of up to 100 and 4 mg/kg, respectively, prior to conception and throughout gestation.

Pregnancy
Pregnancy Categories C (first trimester) *and D* (second and third trimesters). See WARNINGS, Fetal/Neonatal Morbidity and Mortality.

Nursing Mothers
It is not known whether candesartan is excreted in human milk, but candesartan has been shown to be present in rat milk. Thiazides appear in human milk. Because of the potential for adverse effects on the nursing infant, a decision should be made whether to discontinue nursing or discontinue the drug, taking into account the importance of the drug to the mother.

Pediatric Use
Safety and effectiveness in pediatric patients have not been established.

Geriatric Use
Of the total number of subjects in all clinical studies of ATACAND HCT (2831), 611 (22%) were 65 and over, while 94 (3%) were 75 and over. No overall differences in safety or effectiveness were observed between these subjects and younger subjects. Other reported clinical experience has not identified differences in responses between the elderly and younger patients, but greater sensitivity of some older individuals cannot be ruled out.

ADVERSE REACTIONS
Candesartan Cilexetil—Hydrochlorothiazide
ATACAND HCT has been evaluated for safety in more than 2800 patients treated for hypertension. More than 750 of these patients were studied for at least six months and more than 500 patients were treated for at least one year. Adverse experiences have generally been mild and transient in nature and have only infrequently required discontinuation of therapy. The overall incidence of adverse events reported with ATACAND HCT was comparable to placebo. The overall frequency of adverse experiences was not related to dose, age, gender, or race.
In placebo-controlled trials that included 1089 patients treated with various combinations of candesartan cilexetil (doses of 2-32 mg) and hydrochlorothiazide (doses of 6.25-25 mg) and 592 patients treated with placebo, adverse events, whether or not attributed to treatment, occurring in greater than 2% of patients treated with ATACAND HCT and that were more frequent for ATACAND HCT than placebo were: ***Respiratory System Disorder:*** upper respiratory tract infection (3.6% vs 3.0%); ***Body as a Whole:*** back pain (3.3% vs 2.4%); influenza-like symptoms (2.5% vs 1.9%); ***Central/Peripheral Nervous System:*** dizziness (2.9% vs 1.2%).
The frequency of headache was greater than 2% (2.9%) in patients treated with ATACAND HCT but was less frequent than the rate in patients treated with placebo (5.2%).
Other adverse events that have been reported, whether or not attributed to treatment, with an incidence of 0.5% or greater from the more than 2800 patients worldwide treated with ATACAND HCT included: ***Body as a Whole:*** inflicted injury, fatigue, pain, chest pain, peripheral edema, asthenia; ***Central and Peripheral Nervous System:*** vertigo, paresthesia, hypesthesia; ***Respiratory System Disorders:*** bronchitis, sinusitis, pharyngitis, coughing, rhinitis, dyspnea; ***Musculoskeletal System Disorders:*** arthralgia, myalgia, arthrosis, arthritis, leg cramps, sciatica; ***Gastrointestinal System Disorders:*** nausea, abdominal pain, diarrhea, dyspepsia, gastritis, gastroenteritis, vomiting; ***Metabolic and Nutritional Disorders:*** hyperuricemia, hyperglycemia, hypokalemia, increased BUN, creatine phosphokinase increased; ***Urinary System Disorders:*** urinary tract infection, hematuria, cystitis; ***Liver/Biliary System Disorders:*** hepatic function abnormal, increased transaminase levels; ***Heart Rate and Rhythm Disorders:*** tachycardia, palpitation, extrasystoles, bradycardia; ***Psychiatric Disorders:*** depression, insomnia, anxiety; ***Cardiovascular Disorders:*** ECG abnormal; ***Skin and Appendages Disorders:*** eczema, sweating increased, pruritus, dermatitis, rash; ***Platelet/Bleeding Clotting Disorders:*** epistaxis; ***Resistance Mechanism Disorders:*** infection, viral infection; ***Vision Disorders:*** conjunctivitis; ***Hearing and Vestibular Disorders:*** tinnitus.
Reported events seen less frequently than 0.5% included angina pectoris, myocardial infarction and angioedema.
Candesartan Cilexetil
Other adverse experiences that have been reported with candesartan cilexetil, without regard to causality, were: ***Body as a Whole:*** fever; ***Metabolic and Nutritional Disorders:*** hypertriglyceridemia; ***Psychiatric Disorders:*** somnolence; ***Urinary System Disorders:*** albuminuria.

Post-Marketing Experience
The following have been very rarely reported in post-marketing experience with candesartan cilexetil:
Digestive: Abnormal hepatic function and hepatitis.
Hematologic: Neutropenia, leukopenia, and agranulocytosis.
Skin and Appendages Disorders: Pruritis and urticaria.
Hydrochlorothiazide
Other adverse experiences that have been reported with hydrochlorothiazide, without regard to causality, are listed below:
Body As A Whole: weakness; ***Cardiovascular:*** hypotension including orthostatic hypotension (may be aggravated by alcohol, barbiturates, narcotics or antihypertensive drugs); ***Digestive:*** pancreatitis, jaundice (intrahepatic cholestatic jaundice), sialadenitis, cramping, constipation, gastric irritation, anorexia; ***Hematologic:*** aplastic anemia, agranulocytosis, leukopenia, hemolytic anemia, thrombocytopenia; ***Hypersensitivity:*** anaphylactic reactions, necrotizing angiitis (vasculitis and cutaneous vasculitis), respiratory distress including pneumonitis and pulmonary edema, photosensitivity, urticaria, purpura; ***Metabolic:*** electrolyte imbalance, glycosuria; ***Musculoskeletal:*** muscle spasm; ***Nervous System/Psychiatric:*** restlessness; ***Renal:*** renal failure, renal dysfunction, interstitial nephritis; ***Skin:*** erythema multi-

Continued on next page

Atacand HCT—Cont.

forme including Stevens-Johnson syndrome, exfoliative dermatitis including toxic epidermal necrolysis, alopecia; ***Special Senses:*** transient blurred vision, xanthopsia; ***Urogenital:*** impotence.

Laboratory Test Findings

In controlled clinical trials, clinically important changes in standard laboratory parameters were rarely associated with the administration of ATACAND HCT.

Creatinine, Blood Urea Nitrogen—Minor increases in blood urea nitrogen (BUN) and serum creatinine were observed infrequently. One patient was discontinued from ATACAND HCT due to increased BUN. No patient was discontinued due to an increase in serum creatinine.

Hemoglobin and Hematocrit—Small decreases in hemoglobin and hematocrit (mean decreases of approximately 0.2 g/dL and 0.4 volume percent, respectively) were observed in patients treated with ATACAND HCT, but were rarely of clinical importance.

Potassium—A small decrease (mean decrease of 0.1 mEq/L) was observed in patients treated with ATACAND HCT. In placebo-controlled trials, hypokalemia was reported in 0.4% of patients treated with ATACAND HCT as compared to 1.0% of patients treated with hydrochlorothiazide or 0.2% of patients treated with placebo.

Liver Function Tests—Occasional elevations of liver enzymes and/or serum bilirubin have occurred.

OVERDOSAGE

Candesartan Cilexetil—Hydrochlorothiazide

No lethality was observed in acute toxicity studies in mice, rats and dogs given single oral doses of up to 2000 mg/kg of candesartan cilexetil or in rats given single oral doses of up to 2000 mg/kg of candesartan cilexetil in combination with 1000 mg/kg of hydrochlorothiazide. In mice given single oral doses of the primary metabolite, candesartan, the minimum lethal dose was greater than 1000 mg/kg but less than 2000 mg/kg.

Limited data are available in regard to overdosage with candesartan cilexetil in humans. The most likely manifestations of overdosage with candesartan cilexetil would be hypotension, dizziness, and tachycardia; bradycardia could occur from parasympathetic (vagal) stimulation. If symptomatic hypotension should occur, supportive treatment should be initiated. For hydrochlorothiazide, the most common signs and symptoms observed are those caused by electrolyte depletion (hypokalemia, hypochloremia, hyponatremia) and dehydration resulting from excessive diuresis. If digitalis has also been administered, hypokalemia may accentuate cardiac arrhythmias.

Candesartan cannot be removed by hemodialysis. The degree to which hydrochlorothiazide is removed by hemodialysis has not been established.

Treatment

To obtain up-to-date information about the treatment of overdose, consult your Regional Poison Control Center. Telephone numbers of certified poison control centers are listed in the *Physicians' Desk Reference (PDR)*. In managing overdose, consider the possibilities of multiple-drug overdoses, drug-drug interactions, and altered pharmacokinetics in your patient.

DOSAGE AND ADMINISTRATION

The usual recommended starting dose of candesartan cilexetil is 16 mg once daily when it is used as monotherapy in patients who are not volume depleted. ATACAND HCT can be administered once or twice daily with total daily doses ranging from 8 mg to 32 mg. Patients requiring further reduction in blood pressure should be titrated to 32 mg. Doses larger than 32 mg do not appear to have a greater blood pressure lowering effect.

Hydrochlorothiazide is effective in doses of 12.5 to 50 mg once daily.

To minimize dose-independent side effects, it is usually appropriate to begin combination therapy only after a patient has failed to achieve the desired effect with monotherapy.

The side effects (See WARNINGS) of candesartan cilexetil are generally rare and apparently independent of dose; those of hydrochlorothiazide are a mixture of dose-dependent phenomena (primarily hypokalemia) and dose-independent phenomena (eg, pancreatitis), the former much more common than the latter.

Therapy with any combination of candesartan cilexetil and hydrochlorothiazide will be associated with both sets of dose-independent side effects.

Replacement Therapy: The combination may be substituted for the titrated components.

Dose Titration by Clinical Effect: A patient whose blood pressure is not controlled on 25 mg of hydrochlorothiazide once daily can expect an incremental effect from ATACAND HCT 16-12.5 mg. A patient whose blood pressure is controlled on 25 mg of hydrochlorothiazide but is experiencing decreases in serum potassium can expect the same or incremental blood pressure effects from ATACAND HCT 16-12.5 mg and serum potassium may improve.

A patient whose blood pressure is not controlled on 32 mg of ATACAND HCT can expect incremental blood pressure effects from ATACAND HCT 32-12.5 mg and then 32-25 mg. The maximal antihypertensive effect of any dose of ATACAND HCT can be expected within 4 weeks of initiating that dose.

Patients with Renal Impairment: The usual regimens of therapy with ATACAND HCT may be followed as long as the patient's creatinine clearance is >30 mL/min. In patients with more severe renal impairment, loop diuretics are preferred to thiazides, so ATACAND HCT is not recommended.

Patients with Hepatic Impairment: Thiazide diuretics should be used with caution in patients with hepatic impairment; therefore, care should be exercised with dosing of ATACAND HCT.

ATACAND HCT may be administered with other antihypertensive agents.

ATACAND HCT may be administered with or without food.

HOW SUPPLIED

No. 3825—Tablets ATACAND HCT 16-12.5, are peach, oval, biconvex, non-film-coated tablets, coded ACS on one side and 162 on the other. They are supplied as follows:

NDC 0186-0162-28 unit dose packages of 100.

NDC 0186-0162-54 unit of use bottles of 90.

No. 3826—Tablets ATACAND HCT 32-12.5, are yellow, oval, biconvex, non-film-coated tablets, coded ACJ on one side and 322 on the other. They are supplied as follows:

NDC 0186-0322-28 unit dose packages of 100.

NDC 0186-0322-54 unit of use bottles of 90.

Storage

Store at 25°C (77°F); excursions permitted to 15-30°C (59-86°F) [see USP Controlled Room Temperature]. Keep container tightly closed.

ATACAND HCT is a trademark of the AstraZeneca group

Manufactured under the license
from Takeda Chemical Industries, Ltd.
by: AstraZeneca AB, S-151 85 Södertälje, Sweden
for: AstraZeneca LP, Wilmington, DE 19850
Made in Sweden
9329101
610517-01 Rev.09/01

NAROPIN® ℞

[nă-rōpin]

(ropivacaine HCl) Injection

Rx only

Prescribing information for this product, which appears on page 612 of the 2002 PDR, has been completely revised as follows. Please write "See Supplement A" next to the product heading.

DESCRIPTION

NAROPIN® Injection contains ropivacaine HCl which is a member of the amino amide class of local anesthetics. NAROPIN injection is a sterile, isotonic solution that contains the enantiomerically pure drug substance, sodium chloride for isotonicity and Water for Injection. Sodium hydroxide and/or hydrochloric acid may be used for pH adjustment. It is administered parenterally.

Ropivacaine HCl is chemically described as S-(-)-1-propyl-2′,6′-pipecoloxylidide hydrochloride monohydrate. The drug substance is a white crystalline powder, with a chemical formula of $C_{17}H_{26}N_2O \bullet HCl \bullet H_2O$, molecular weight of 328.89 and the following structural formula:

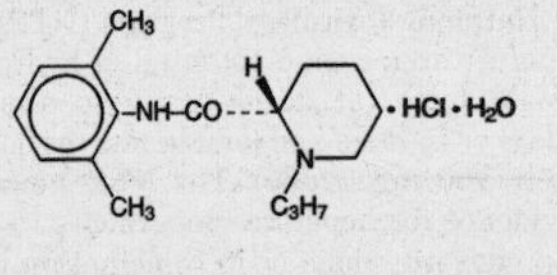

At 25°C ropivacaine HCl has a solubility of 53.8 mg/mL in water, a distribution ratio between n-octanol and phosphate buffer at pH 7.4 of 14.1 and a pKa of 8.07 in 0.1 M KCl solution. The pKa of ropivacaine is approximately the same as bupivacaine (8.1) and is similar to that of mepivacaine (7.7). However, ropivacaine has an intermediate degree of lipid solubility compared to bupivacaine and mepivacaine.

NAROPIN Injection is preservative-free and is available in single dose containers in 2.0 (0.2%), 5.0 (0.5%), 7.5 (0.75%) and 10.0 mg/mL (1.0%) concentrations. The specific gravity of NAROPIN Injection solutions range from 1.002 to 1.005 at 25°C.

CLINICAL PHARMACOLOGY

Mechanism of Action

Ropivacaine is a member of the amino amide class of local anesthetics and is supplied as the pure S-(-)-enantiomer. Local anesthetics block the generation and the conduction of nerve impulses, presumably by increasing the threshold for electrical excitation in the nerve, by slowing the propagation of the nerve impulse, and by reducing the rate of rise of the action potential. In general, the progression of anesthesia is related to the diameter, myelination and conduction velocity of affected nerve fibers. Clinically, the order of loss of nerve function is as follows: (1) pain, (2) temperature, (3) touch, (4) proprioception, and (5) skeletal muscle tone.

PHARMACOKINETICS

Absorption

The systemic concentration of ropivacaine is dependent on the total dose and concentration of drug administered, the route of administration, the patient's hemodynamic/circulatory condition, and the vascularity of the administration site.

From the epidural space, ropivacaine shows complete and biphasic absorption. The half-lives of the 2 phases, (mean ± SD) are 14 ± 7 minutes and 4.2 ± 0.9 h, respectively. The slow absorption is the rate limiting factor in the elimination of ropivacaine which explains why the terminal half-life is longer after epidural than after intravenous administration.

Ropivacaine shows dose-proportionality up to the highest intravenous dose studied, 80 mg, corresponding to a mean ± SD peak plasma concentration of 1.9 ± 0.3 µg/mL.

[See table below]

In some patients after a 300 mg dose for brachial plexus block, free plasma concentrations of ropivacaine may approach the threshold for CNS toxicity. (See PRECAUTIONS.) At a dose of greater than 300 mg, for local infiltration, the terminal half-life may be longer (>30 hours).

Distribution

After intravascular infusion, ropivacaine has a steady state volume of distribution of 41 ± 7 liters. Ropivacaine is 94% protein bound, mainly to α_1-acid glycoprotein. An increase in total plasma concentrations during continuous epidural infusion has been observed, related to a postoperative increase of α_1-acid glycoprotein. Variations in unbound, ie, pharmacologically active, concentrations have been less than in total plasma concentration. Ropivacaine readily crosses the placenta and equilibrium in regard to unbound concentration will be rapidly reached. (See PRECAUTIONS, Labor and Delivery.)

Metabolism

Ropivacaine is extensively metabolized in the liver, predominantly by aromatic hydroxylation mediated by cytochrome P4501A to 3-hydroxy ropivacaine. After a single IV dose approximately 37% of the total dose is excreted in the urine as both free and conjugated 3-hydroxy ropivacaine. Low concentrations of 3-hydroxy ropivacaine have been found in the plasma. Urinary excretion of the 4-hydroxy ropivacaine, and both the 3-hydroxy N-de-alkylated (3-OH-PPX) and 4-hydroxy N-de-alkylated (4-OH-PPX) metabolites account for less than 3% of the dose. An additional metabolite, 2-hydroxy-methyl-ropivacaine, has been identified but not quantified in the urine. The N-de-alkylated metabolite of ropivacaine (PPX) and 3-OH-ropivacaine are the major metabolites excreted in the urine during epidural infusion. Total PPX concentration in the plasma was about half as that of total ropivacaine; however, mean unbound concentrations

Table 1

Pharmacokinetic (plasma concentration-time) data from clinical trials

Route	Epidural Infusion[a]		Epidural Infusion[a]	Epidural Block[b]	Epidural Block[b]	Plexus Block[c]	IV Infusion[d]
Dose (mg)	1493±10	2075±206	1217±277	150	187.5	300	40
N	12	12	11	8	8	10	12
C_{max} (mg/L)	2.4±1[e]	2.8±0.5[e]	2.3±1.1[e]	1.1±0.2	1.6±0.6	2.3±0.8	1.2±0.2[f]
T_{max} (min)	n/a[h]	n/a	n/a	43±14	34±9	54±22	n/a
AUC_0-(mg.h/L)	135.5±50	145±34	161±90	7.2±2	11.3±4	13±3.3	1.8±0.6
CL (L/h)	11.03	13.7	n/a	5.5±2	5±2.6	n/a	21.2±7
$t_{1/2}$ (hr)[g]	5±2.5	5.7±3	6.0±3	5.7±2	7.1±3	6.8±3.2	1.9±0.5

[a] Continuous 72 hour epidural infusion after an epidural block with 5 or 10 mg/mL.
[b] Epidural anesthesia with 7.5 mg/mL (0.75%) for cesarean delivery.
[c] Brachial plexus block with 7.5 mg/mL (0.75%) ropivacaine.
[d] 20 minute IV infusion to volunteers (40 mg).
[e] C_{max} measured at the end of infusion (ie, at 72 hr).
[f] C_{max} measured at the end of infusion (ie, at 20 minutes).
[g] $t_{1/2}$ is the true terminal elimination half-life. On the other hand, $t_{1/2}$ follows absorption-dependent elimination (flip-flop) after non-intravenous administration.
[h] n/a=not applicable

of PPX were about 7 to 9 times higher than that of unbound ropivacaine following continuous epidural infusion up to 72 hours. Unbound PPX, 3-hydroxy and 4-hydroxy ropivacaine, have a pharmacological activity in animal models less than that of ropivacaine. There is no evidence of *in vivo* racemization in urine of ropivacaine.

Elimination

The kidney is the main excretory organ for most local anesthetic metabolites. In total, 86% of the ropivacaine dose is excreted in the urine after intravenous administration of which only 1% relates to unchanged drug. Ropivacaine has a mean ± SD total plasma clearance of 387 ± 107 mL/min, an unbound plasma clearance of 7.2 ± 1.6 L/min, and a renal clearance of 1 mL/min. The mean ± SD terminal half-life is 1.8 ± 0.7 h after intravascular administration and 4.2 ± 1.0 h after epidural administration (see PHARMACOKINETICS, Absorption.)

Pharmacodynamics

Studies in humans have demonstrated that, unlike most other local anesthetics, the presence of epinephrine has no major effect on either the time of onset or the duration of action of ropivacaine. Likewise, addition of epinephrine to ropivacaine has no effect on limiting systemic absorption of ropivacaine.

Systemic absorption of local anesthetics can produce effects on the central nervous and cardiovascular systems. At blood concentrations achieved with therapeutic doses, changes in cardiac conduction, excitability, refractoriness, contractility, and peripheral vascular resistance have been reported. Toxic blood concentrations depress cardiac conduction and excitability, which may lead to atrioventricular block, ventricular arrhythmias and to cardiac arrest, sometimes resulting in fatalities. In addition, myocardial contractility is depressed and peripheral vasodilation occurs, leading to decreased cardiac output and arterial blood pressure.

Following systemic absorption, local anesthetics can produce central nervous system stimulation, depression or both. Apparent central stimulation is usually manifested as restlessness, tremors and shivering, progressing to convulsions, followed by depression and coma, progressing ultimately to respiratory arrest. However, the local anesthetics have a primary depressant effect on the medulla and on higher centers. The depressed stage may occur without a prior excited stage.

In 2 clinical pharmacology studies (total n=24) ropivacaine and bupivacaine were infused (10 mg/min) in human volunteers until the appearance of CNS symptoms, eg, visual or hearing disturbances, perioral numbness, tingling and others. Similar symptoms were seen with both drugs. In 1 study, the mean ± SD maximum tolerated intravenous dose of ropivacaine infused (124 ± 38 mg) was significantly higher than that of bupivacaine (99 ± 30 mg) while in the other study the doses were not different (115 ± 29 mg of ropivacaine and 103 ± 30 mg of bupivacaine). In the latter study, the number of subjects reporting each symptom was similar for both drugs with the exception of muscle twitching which was reported by more subjects with bupivacaine than ropivacaine at comparable intravenous doses. At the end of the infusion, ropivacaine in both studies caused significantly less depression of cardiac conductivity (less QRS widening) than bupivacaine. Ropivacaine and bupivacaine caused evidence of depression of cardiac contractility, but there were no changes in cardiac output.

Clinical data in one published article indicate that differences in various pharmacodynamic measures were observed with increasing age. In one study, the upper level of analgesia increased with age, the maximum decrease of mean arterial pressure (MAP) declined with age during the first hour after epidural administration, and the intensity of motor blockade increased with age. However, no pharmacokinetic differences were observed between elderly and younger patients.

In non-clinical pharmacology studies comparing ropivacaine and bupivacaine in several animal species, the cardiac toxicity of ropivacaine was less than that of bupivacaine, although both were considerably more toxic than lidocaine. Arrhythmogenic and cardio-depressant effects were seen in animals at significantly higher doses of ropivacaine than bupivacaine. The incidence of successful resuscitation was not significantly different between the ropivacaine and bupivacaine groups.

Clinical Trials

Ropivacaine was studied as a local anesthetic both for surgical anesthesia and for acute pain management. (See DOSAGE AND ADMINISTRATION.)

The onset, depth and duration of sensory block are, in general, similar to bupivacaine. However, the depth and duration of motor block, in general, are less than that with bupivacaine.

Epidural Administration In Surgery

There were 25 clinical studies performed in 900 patients to evaluate NAROPIN epidural injection for general surgery. NAROPIN was used in doses ranging from 75 to 250 mg. In doses of 100–200 mg, the median (1st–3rd quartile) onset time to achieve a T10 sensory block was 10 (5–13) minutes and the median (1st–3rd quartile) duration at the T10 level was 4 (3–5) hours. (See DOSAGE AND ADMINISTRATION.) Higher doses produced a more profound block with a greater duration of effect.

Epidural Administration In Cesarean Section

A total of 12 studies were performed with epidural administration of NAROPIN for cesarean section. Eight of these studies involved 218 patients using the concentration of 5 mg/mL (0.5%) in doses up to 150 mg. Median onset measured at T6 ranged from 11 to 26 minutes. Median duration of sensory block at T6 ranged from 1.7 to 3.2 h, and duration of motor block ranged from 1.4 to 2.9 h. NAROPIN provided adequate muscle relaxation for surgery in all cases.

In addition, 4 active controlled studies for cesarean section were performed in 264 patients at a concentration of 7.5 mg/mL (0.75%) in doses up to 187.5 mg. Median onset measured at T6 ranged from 4 to 15 minutes. Seventy-seven to 96% of NAROPIN-exposed patients reported no pain at delivery. Some patients received other anesthetic, analgesic, or sedative modalities during the course of the operative procedure.

Epidural Administration In Labor And Delivery

A total of 9 double-blind clinical studies, involving 240 patients were performed to evaluate NAROPIN for epidural block for management of labor pain. When administered in doses up to 278 mg as intermittent injections or as a continuous infusion, NAROPIN produced adequate pain relief.

A prospective meta-analysis on 6 of these studies provided detailed evaluation of the delivered newborns and showed no difference in clinical outcomes compared to bupivacaine. There were significantly fewer instrumental deliveries in mothers receiving ropivacaine as compared to bupivacaine.

Table 2
LABOR AND DELIVERY META-ANALYSIS: MODE OF DELIVERY

Delivery Mode	NAROPIN n=199		Bupivacaine n=188	
	n	%	n	%
Spontaneous Vertex	116	58	92	49
Vacuum Extractor	26		33	
		}27*		}40
Forceps	28		42	
Cesarean Section	29	15	21	11

*p=0.004 versus bupivacaine

Epidural Administration In Postoperative Pain Management

There were 8 clinical studies performed in 382 patients to evaluate NAROPIN 2 mg/mL (0.2%) for postoperative pain management after upper and lower abdominal surgery and after orthopedic surgery. The studies utilized intravascular morphine via PCA as a rescue medication and quantified as an efficacy variable.

Epidural anesthesia with NAROPIN 5 mg/mL (0.5%) was used intraoperatively for each of these procedures prior to initiation of postoperative NAROPIN. The incidence and intensity of the motor block were dependent on the dose rate of NAROPIN and the site of injection. Cumulative doses of up to 770 mg of ropivacaine were administered over 24 hours (intraoperative block plus postoperative continuous infusion). The overall quality of pain relief, as judged by the patients, in the ropivacaine groups was rated as good or excellent (73% to 100%). The frequency of motor block was greatest at 4 hours and decreased during the infusion period in all groups. At least 80% of patients in the upper and lower abdominal studies and 42% in the orthopedic studies had no motor block at the end of the 21-hour infusion period. Sensory block was also dose rate-dependent and a decrease in spread was observed during the infusion period.

A double blind, randomized, clinical trial compared lumbar epidural infusion of NAROPIN (n=26) and bupivacaine (n=26) at 2 mg/mL (8 mL/h), for 24 hours after knee replacement. In this study, the pain scores were higher in the NAROPIN group, but the incidence and the intensity of motor block were lower.

Continuous epidural infusion of NAROPIN 2 mg/mL (0.2%) during up to 72 hours for postoperative pain management after major abdominal surgery was studied in 2 multicenter, double-blind studies. A total of 391 patients received a low thoracic epidural catheter, and NAROPIN 7.5 mg/L (0.75%) was given for surgery, in combination with GA. Postoperatively, NAROPIN 2 mg/mL (0.2%), 4–14 mL/h, alone or with fentanyl 1, 2, or 4 μg/mL was infused through the epidural catheter and adjusted according to the patient's needs. These studies support the use of NAROPIN 2 mg/mL (0.2%) for epidural infusion at 6–14 mL/h (12–28 mg) for up to 72 hours and demonstrated adequate analgesia with only slight and nonprogressive motor block in cases of moderate to severe postoperative pain.

Clinical studies with 2 mg/mL (0.2%) NAROPIN have demonstrated that infusion rates of 6–14 mL (12–28 mg) per hour provide adequate analgesia with nonprogressive motor block in cases of moderate to severe postoperative pain. In these studies, this technique resulted in a significant reduction in patients' morphine rescue dose requirement. Clinical experience supports the use of NAROPIN epidural infusions for up to 72 hours.

Peripheral Nerve Block

NAROPIN, 5 mg/mL, (0.5%), was evaluated for its ability to provide anesthesia for surgery using the techniques of Peripheral Nerve Block. There were 13 studies performed including a series of 4 pharmacodynamic and pharmacokinetic studies performed on minor nerve blocks. From these, 235 NAROPIN treated patients were evaluable for efficacy. NAROPIN was used in doses up to 275 mg. When used for brachial plexus block, onset depended on technique used. Supraclavicular blocks were consistently more successful than axillary blocks. The median onset of sensory block (anesthesia) produced by ropivacaine 0.5% via axillary block ranged from 10 minutes (medial brachial cutaneous nerve) to 45 minutes (musculocutaneous nerve). Median duration ranged from 3.7 hours (medial brachial cutaneous nerve) to 8.7 hours (ulnar nerve). The 5 mg/mL (0.5%) NAROPIN solution gave success rates from 56% to 86% for axillary blocks, compared with 92% for supraclavicular blocks.

In addition, NAROPIN, 7.5 mg/mL (0.75%), was evaluated in 99 NAROPIN treated patients, in 2 double-blind studies, performed to provide anesthesia for surgery using the techniques of Brachial Plexus Block. NAROPIN 7.5 mg/mL was compared to bupivacaine 5 mg/mL. In 1 study, patients underwent axillary brachial plexus block using injections of 40 mL (300 mg) of NAROPIN, 7.5 mg/mL (0.75%) or 40 mL injections of bupivacaine, 5 mg/mL (200 mg). In a second study, patients underwent subclavian perivascular brachial plexus block using 30 mL (225 mg) of NAROPIN, 7.5 mg/mL (0.75%) or 30 mL of bupivacaine 5 mg/mL (150 mg). There was no significant difference between the NAROPIN and bupivacaine groups in either study with regard to onset of anesthesia, duration of sensory blockade, or duration of anesthesia.

The median duration of anesthesia varied between 11.4 and 14.4 hours with both techniques. In one study, using the axillary technique, the quality of analgesia and muscle relaxation in the NAROPIN group was judged to be significantly superior to bupivacaine by both investigator and surgeon. However, using the subclavian perivascular technique, no statistically significant difference was found in the quality of analgesia and muscle relaxation as judged by both the investigator and surgeon. The use of NAROPIN 7.5 mg/mL for block of the brachial plexus via either the subclavian perivascular approach using 30 mL (225 mg) or via the axillary approach using 40 mL (300 mg) both provided effective and reliable anesthesia.

Local Infiltration

A total of 7 clinical studies were performed to evaluate the local infiltration of NAROPIN to produce anesthesia for surgery and analgesia in postoperative pain management. In these studies 297 patients who received NAROPIN in doses up to 200 mg (concentrations up to 5 mg/mL, 0.5%) were evaluable for efficacy. With infiltration of 100–200 mg NAROPIN, the time to first request for analgesic was 2–6 hours. When compared to placebo, NAROPIN produced lower pain scores and a reduction of analgesic consumption.

INDICATIONS AND USAGE

NAROPIN is indicated for the production of local or regional anesthesia for surgery and for acute pain management.

Surgical Anesthesia:	epidural block for surgery including cesarean section; major nerve block; local infiltration
Acute Pain Management:	epidural continuous infusion or intermittent bolus, eg, postoperative or labor; local infiltration

CONTRAINDICATIONS

NAROPIN is contraindicated in patients with a known hypersensitivity to ropivacaine or to any local anesthetic agent of the amide type.

WARNINGS

IN PERFORMING NAROPIN BLOCKS, UNINTENDED INTRAVENOUS INJECTION IS POSSIBLE AND MAY RESULT IN CARDIAC ARRHYTHMIA OR CARDIAC ARREST. THE POTENTIAL FOR SUCCESSFUL RESUSCITATION HAS NOT BEEN STUDIED IN HUMANS. NAROPIN SHOULD BE ADMINISTERED IN INCREMENTAL DOSES. IT IS NOT RECOMMENDED FOR EMERGENCY SITUATIONS, WHERE A FAST ONSET OF SURGICAL ANESTHESIA IS NECESSARY. HISTORICALLY, PREGNANT PATIENTS WERE REPORTED TO HAVE A HIGH RISK FOR CARDIAC ARRHYTHMIAS, CARDIAC/CIRCULATORY ARREST AND DEATH WHEN 0.75% BUPIVACAINE (ANOTHER MEMBER OF THE AMINO AMIDE CLASS OF LOCAL ANESTHETICS) WAS INADVERTENTLY RAPIDLY INJECTED INTRAVENOUSLY.

LOCAL ANESTHETICS SHOULD ONLY BE EMPLOYED BY CLINICIANS WHO ARE WELL VERSED IN THE DIAGNOSIS AND MANAGEMENT OF DOSE-RELATED TOXICITY AND OTHER ACUTE EMERGENCIES WHICH MIGHT ARISE FROM THE BLOCK TO BE EMPLOYED, AND THEN ONLY AFTER INSURING THE **IMMEDIATE (WITHOUT DELAY)** AVAILABILITY OF OXYGEN, OTHER RESUSCITATIVE DRUGS, CARDIOPULMONARY RESUSCITATIVE EQUIPMENT, AND THE PERSONNEL RESOURCES NEEDED FOR PROPER MANAGEMENT OF TOXIC REACTIONS AND RELATED EMERGENCIES (See also ADVERSE REACTIONS and PRECAUTIONS). DELAY IN PROPER MANAGEMENT OF DOSE-RELATED TOXICITY, UNDERVENTILATION FROM ANY CAUSE AND/OR ALTERED SENSITIVITY MAY LEAD TO THE DEVELOPMENT OF ACIDOSIS, CARDIAC ARREST AND, POSSIBLY, DEATH. SOLUTIONS OF NAROPIN SHOULD NOT BE USED FOR THE PRODUCTION OF OBSTETRICAL PARACERVICAL BLOCK ANESTHESIA, RETROBULBAR BLOCK, OR SPINAL ANESTHESIA (SUBARACHNOID BLOCK) DUE TO INSUFFICIENT DATA TO SUPPORT SUCH USE. INTRAVENOUS REGIONAL ANESTHESIA (BIER BLOCK) SHOULD NOT BE PERFORMED DUE TO A LACK OF CLINICAL EXPERIENCE AND THE RISK OF ATTAINING TOXIC BLOOD LEVELS OF ROPIVACAINE.

It is essential that aspiration for blood, or cerebrospinal fluid (where applicable), be done prior to injecting any local

Continued on next page

Naropin—Cont.

anesthetic, both the original dose and all subsequent doses, to avoid intravascular or subarachnoid injection. However, a negative aspiration does *not* ensure against an intravascular or subarachnoid injection.
A well-known risk of epidural anesthesia may be an unintentional subarachnoid injection of local anesthetic. Two clinical studies have been performed to verify the safety of NAROPIN at a volume of 3 mL injected into the subarachnoid space since this dose represents an incremental epidural volume that could be unintentionally injected. The 15 and 22.5 mg doses injected resulted in sensory levels as high as T5 and T4, respectively. Analgesia to pinprick started in the sacral dermatomes in 2–3 minutes, extended to the T10 level in 10–13 minutes and lasted for approximately 2 hours. The results of these two clinical studies showed that a 3 mL dose did not produce any serious adverse events when spinal anesthesia blockade was achieved.
NAROPIN should be used with caution in patients receiving other local anesthetics or agents structurally related to amide-type local anesthetics, since the toxic effects of these drugs are additive.

Table 3A
Adverse Events Reported in ≥1% of Adult Patients Receiving Regional or Local Anesthesia (Surgery, Labor, Cesarean Section, Post-Operative Pain Management, Peripheral Nerve Block and Local Infiltration)

Adverse Reaction	NAROPIN total N = 1661		Bupivacaine total N = 1443	
	N	(%)	N	(%)
Hypotension	536	(32.3)	408	(28.5)
Nausea	283	(17.0)	207	(14.4)
Vomiting	117	(7.0)	88	(6.1)
Bradycardia	96	(5.8)	73	(5.1)
Headache	84	(5.1)	68	(4.7)
Paresthesia	82	(4.9)	57	(4.0)
Back pain	73	(4.4)	75	(5.2)
Pain	71	(4.3)	71	(5.0)
Pruritus	63	(3.8)	40	(2.8)
Fever	61	(3.7)	37	(2.6)
Dizziness	42	(2.5)	23	(1.6)
Rigors (Chills)	42	(2.5)	24	(1.7)
Postoperative complications	41	(2.5)	44	(3.1)
Hypoesthesia	27	(1.6)	24	(1.7)
Urinary retention	23	(1.4)	20	(1.4)
Progression of labor poor/failed	23	(1.4)	22	(1.5)
Anxiety	21	(1.3)	11	(0.8)
Breast disorder, breast-feeding	21	(1.3)	12	(0.8)
Rhinitis	18	(1.1)	13	(0.9)

PRECAUTIONS

General

The safe and effective use of local anesthetics depends on proper dosage, correct technique, adequate precautions and readiness for emergencies.
Resuscitative equipment, oxygen and other resuscitative drugs should be available for immediate use. (See WARNINGS and ADVERSE REACTIONS.) The lowest dosage that results in effective anesthesia should be used to avoid high plasma levels and serious adverse events. Injections should be made slowly and incrementally, with frequent aspirations before and during the injection to avoid intravascular injection. When a continuous catheter technique is used, syringe aspirations should also be performed before and during each supplemental injection. During the administration of epidural anesthesia, it is recommended that a test dose of a local anesthetic with a fast onset be administered initially and that the patient be monitored for central nervous system and cardiovascular toxicity, as well as for signs of unintended intrathecal administration before proceeding. When clinical conditions permit, consideration should be given to employing local anesthetic solutions, which contain epinephrine for the test dose because circulatory changes compatible with epinephrine may also serve as a warning sign of unintended intravascular injection. An intravascular injection is still possible even if aspirations for blood are negative. Administration of higher than recommended doses of NAROPIN to achieve greater motor blockade or increased duration of sensory blockade may result in cardiovascular depression, particularly in the event of inadvertent intravascular injection. Tolerance to elevated blood levels varies with the physical condition of the patient. Debilitated, elderly patients and acutely ill patients should be given reduced doses commensurate with their age and physical condition. Local anesthetics should also be used with caution in patients with hypotension, hypovolemia or heart block.
Careful and constant monitoring of cardiovascular and respiratory vital signs (adequacy of ventilation) and the patient's state of consciousness should be performed after each local anesthetic injection. It should be kept in mind at such times that restlessness, anxiety, incoherent speech, lightheadedness, numbness and tingling of the mouth and lips, metallic taste, tinnitus, dizziness, blurred vision, tremors, twitching, depression, or drowsiness may be early warning signs of central nervous system toxicity. Because amide-type local anesthetics such as ropivacaine are metabolized by the liver, these drugs, especially repeat doses, should be used cautiously in patients with hepatic disease. Patients with severe hepatic disease, because of their inability to metabolize local anesthetics normally, are at a greater risk of developing toxic plasma concentrations. Local anesthetics should also be used with caution in patients with impaired cardiovascular function because they may be less able to compensate for functional changes associated with the prolongation of A-V conduction produced by these drugs.
Many drugs used during the conduct of anesthesia are considered potential triggering agents for malignant hyperthermia (MH). Amide-type local anesthetics are not known to trigger this reaction. However, since the need for supplemental general anesthesia cannot be predicted in advance, it is suggested that a standard protocol for management should be available.

Epidural Anesthesia

During epidural administration, NAROPIN should be administered in incremental doses of 3 to 5 mL with sufficient time between doses to detect toxic manifestations of unintentional intravascular or intrathecal injection. Syringe aspirations should also be performed before and during each supplemental injection in continuous (intermittent) catheter techniques. An intravascular injection is still possible even if aspirations for blood are negative. During the administration of epidural anesthesia, it is recommended that a test dose be administered initially and the effects monitored before the full dose is given. When clinical conditions permit, the test dose should contain an appropriate dose of epinephrine to serve as a warning of unintentional intravascular injection. If injected into a blood vessel, this amount of epinephrine is likely to produce a transient "epinephrine response" within 45 seconds, consisting of an increase in heart rate and systolic blood pressure, circumoral pallor, palpitations and nervousness in the unsedated patient. The sedated patient may exhibit only a pulse rate increase of 20 or more beats per minute for 15 or more seconds. Therefore, following the test dose, the heart should be continuously monitored for a heart rate increase. Patients on beta-blockers may not manifest changes in heart rate, but blood pressure monitoring can detect a rise in systolic blood pressure. A test dose of a short-acting amide anesthetic such as lidocaine is recommended to detect an unintentional intrathecal administration. This will be manifested within a few minutes by signs of spinal block (eg, decreased sensation of the buttocks, paresis of the legs, or, in the sedated patient, absent knee jerk). An intravascular or subarachnoid injection is still possible even if results of the test dose are negative. The test dose itself may produce a systemic toxic reaction, high spinal or epinephrine-induced cardiovascular effects.

Use in Brachial Plexus Block

Ropivacaine plasma concentrations may approach the threshold for central nervous system toxicity after the administration of 300 mg of ropivacaine for brachial plexus block. Caution should be exercised when using the 300 mg dose. (See OVERDOSAGE.)

Use in Head and Neck Area

Small doses of local anesthetics injected into the head and neck area may produce adverse reactions similar to systemic toxicity seen with unintentional intravascular injections of larger doses. The injection procedures require the utmost care. Confusion, convulsions, respiratory depression, and/or respiratory arrest, and cardiovascular stimulation or depression have been reported. These reactions may be due to intra-arterial injection of the local anesthetic with retrograde flow to the cerebral circulation. Patients receiving these blocks should have their circulation and respiration monitored and be constantly observed. Resuscitative equipment and personnel for treating adverse reactions should be immediately available. Dosage recommendations should not be exceeded. (See DOSAGE AND ADMINISTRATION.)

Use in Ophthalmic Surgery

The use of NAROPIN in retrobulbar blocks for ophthalmic surgery has not been studied. Until appropriate experience is gained, the use of NAROPIN for such surgery is not recommended.

Information for Patients

When appropriate, patients should be informed in advance that they may experience temporary loss of sensation and motor activity in the anesthetized part of the body following proper administration of lumbar epidural anesthesia. Also, when appropriate, the physician should discuss other information including adverse reactions in the NAROPIN package insert.

Drug Interactions

NAROPIN should be used with caution in patients receiving other local anesthetics or agents structurally related to amide-type local anesthetics, since the toxic effects of these drugs are additive. Cytochrome P4501A2 is involved in the formation of 3-hydroxy ropivacaine, the major metabolite. *In vivo*, the plasma clearance of ropivacaine was reduced by 70% during coadministration of fluvoxamine (25 mg bid for 2 days), a selective and potent CYP1A2 inhibitor. Thus strong inhibitors of cytochrome P4501A2, such as fluvoxamine, given concomitantly during administration of NAROPIN, can interact with NAROPIN leading to increased ropivacaine plasma levels. Caution should be exercised when CYP1A2 inhibitors are coadministered. Possible interactions with drugs known to be metabolized by CYP1A2 via competitive inhibition such as theophylline and imipramine may also occur. Coadministration of a selective and potent inhibitor of CYP3A4, ketoconazole (100 mg bid for 2 days with ropivacaine infusion administered 1 hour after ketoconazole) caused a 15% reduction in *in-vivo* plasma clearance of ropivacaine.

Carcinogenesis, Mutagenesis, Impairment of Fertility

Long term studies in animals of most local anesthetics, including ropivacaine, to evaluate the carcinogenic potential have not been conducted.
Weak mutagenic activity was seen in the mouse lymphoma test. Mutagenicity was not noted in the other assays, demonstrating that the weak signs of *in vitro* activity in the mouse lymphoma test were not manifest under diverse *in vivo* conditions.
Studies performed with ropivacaine in rats did not demonstrate an effect on fertility or general reproductive performance over 2 generations.

Pregnancy Category B

Reproduction toxicity studies have been performed in pregnant New Zealand white rabbits and Sprague-Dawley rats. During gestation days 6–18, rabbits received 1.3, 4.2, or 13 mg/kg/day subcutaneously. In rats, subcutaneous doses of 5.3, 11 and 26 mg/kg/day were administered during gestation days 6–15. No teratogenic effects were observed in rats and rabbits at the highest doses tested. The highest doses of 13 mg/kg/day (rabbits) and 26 mg/kg/day (rats) are approximately 1/3 of the maximum recommended human dose (epidural, 770 mg/24 hours) based on a mg/m^2 basis. In 2 prenatal and postnatal studies, the female rats were dosed daily from day 15 of gestation to day 20 postpartum. The doses were 5.3, 11 and 26 mg/kg/day subcutaneously. There were no treatment-related effects on late fetal development, parturition, lactation, neonatal viability, or growth of the offspring.
In another study with rats, the males were dosed daily for 9 weeks before mating and during mating. The females were dosed daily for 2 weeks before mating and then during the mating, pregnancy, and lactation, up to day 42 post coitus. At 23 mg/kg/day, an increased loss of pups was observed during the first 3 days postpartum. The effect was considered secondary to impaired maternal care due to maternal toxicity.
There are no adequate or well-controlled studies in pregnant women of the effects of NAROPIN on the developing fetus. NAROPIN should only be used during pregnancy if the benefits outweigh the risk.
Teratogenicity studies in rats and rabbits did not show evidence of any adverse effects on organogenesis or early fetal development in rats (26 mg/kg sc) or rabbits (13 mg/kg). The doses used were approximately equal to total daily dose based on body surface area. There were no treatment-related effects on late fetal development, parturition, lactation, neonatal viability, or growth of the offspring in 2 perinatal and postnatal studies in rats, at dose levels equivalent to the maximum recommended human dose based on body surface area. In another study at 23 mg/kg, an increased pup loss was seen during the first 3 days postpartum, which was considered secondary to impaired maternal care due to maternal toxicity.

Labor and Delivery

Local anesthetics, including ropivacaine, rapidly cross the placenta, and when used for epidural block can cause varying degrees of maternal, fetal and neonatal toxicity (see CLINICAL PHARMACOLOGY AND PHARMACOKINETICS). The incidence and degree of toxicity depend upon the procedure performed, the type and amount of drug used, and the technique of drug administration. Adverse reactions in the parturient, fetus and neonate involve alterations of the central nervous system, peripheral vascular tone and cardiac function.
Maternal hypotension has resulted from regional anesthesia with NAROPIN for obstetrical pain relief. Local anesthetics produce vasodilation by blocking sympathetic nerves. Elevating the patient's legs and positioning her on her left side will help prevent decreases in blood pressure. The fetal heart rate also should be monitored continuously, and electronic fetal monitoring is highly advisable. Epidural anesthesia has been reported to prolong the second stage of labor by removing the patient's reflex urge to bear down or

by interfering with motor function. Spontaneous vertex delivery occurred more frequently in patients receiving NAROPIN than in those receiving bupivacaine.

Nursing Mothers

Some local anesthetic drugs are excreted in human milk and caution should be exercised when they are administered to a nursing woman. The excretion of ropivacaine or its metabolites in human milk has not been studied. Based on the milk/plasma concentration ratio in rats, the estimated daily dose to a pup will be about 4% of the dose given to the mother. Assuming that the milk/plasma concentration in humans is of the same order, the total NAROPIN dose to which the baby is exposed by breast-feeding is far lower than by exposure *in utero* in pregnant women at term (See PRECAUTIONS, Pregnancy Category B.)

Pediatric Use

The safety and efficacy of NAROPIN in pediatric patients have not been established.

Geriatric Use

Of the 2,978 subjects that were administered NAROPIN Injection in 71 controlled and uncontrolled clinical studies, 803 patients (27%) were 65 years of age or older which includes 127 patients (4%) 75 years of age and over. NAROPIN Injection was found to be safe and effective in the patients in these studies. Clinical data in one published article indicate that differences in various pharmacodynamic measures were observed with increasing age. In one study, the upper level of analgesia increased with age, the maximum decrease of mean arterial pressure (MAP) declined with age during the first hour after epidural administration, and the intensity of motor blockade increased with age.

This drug and its metabolites are known to be excreted by the kidney, and the risk of toxic reactions to this drug may be greater in patients with impaired renal function. Elderly patients are more likely to have decreased hepatic, renal, or cardiac function, as well as concomitant disease. Therefore, care should be taken in dose selection, starting at the low end of the dosage range, and it may be useful to monitor renal function. (See PHARMACOKINETICS, Elimination.)

ADVERSE REACTIONS

Reactions to ropivacaine are characteristic of those associated with other amide-type local anesthetics. A major cause of adverse reactions to this group of drugs may be associated with excessive plasma levels, which may be due to overdosage, unintentional intravascular injection or slow metabolic degradation.

The reported adverse events are derived from clinical studies conducted in the U.S. and other countries. The reference drug was usually bupivacaine. The studies used a variety of premedications, sedatives, and surgical procedures of varying length. A total of 3988 patients have been exposed to NAROPIN at concentrations up to 1.0% in clinical trials. Each patient was counted once for each type of adverse event.

Incidence ≥5%

For the indications of epidural administration in surgery, cesarean section, post-operative pain management, peripheral nerve block, and local infiltration, the following treatment-emergent adverse events were reported with an incidence of ≥5% in all clinical studies (N=3988): hypotension (37.0%), nausea (24.8%), vomiting (11.6%), bradycardia (9.3%), fever (9.2%), pain (8.0%), postoperative complications (7.1%), anemia (6.1%), paresthesia (5.6%), headache (5.1%), pruritus (5.1%), and back pain (5.0%).

Incidence 1–5%

Urinary retention, dizziness, rigors, hypertension, tachycardia, anxiety, oliguria, hypoesthesia, chest pain, hypokalemia, dyspnea, cramps, and urinary tract infection.

Incidence in Controlled Clinical Trials

The reported adverse events are derived from controlled clinical studies with NAROPIN (concentrations ranged from 0.125% to 1.0% for NAROPIN and 0.25% to 0.75% for bupivacaine) in the U.S. and other countries involving 3094 patients. Table 3A and 3B list adverse events (number and percentage) that occurred in at least 1% of NAROPIN-treated patients in these studies. The majority of patients receiving concentrations higher than 5.0 mg/mL (0.5%) were treated with NAROPIN.

[See table at top of previous page]

[See table 3B above]

Incidence <1%

The following adverse events were reported during the NAROPIN clinical program in more than one patient (N=3988), occurred at an overall incidence of <1%, and were considered relevant:

Application Site Reactions—injection site pain

Cardiovascular System—vasovagal reaction, syncope, postural hypotension, non-specific ECG abnormalities

Female Reproductive—poor progression of labor, uterine atony

Gastrointestinal System—fecal incontinence, tenesmus, neonatal vomiting

General and Other Disorders—hypothermia, malaise, asthenia, accident and/or injury

Hearing and Vestibular—tinnitus, hearing abnormalities

Heart Rate and Rhythm—extrasystoles, non-specific arrhythmias, atrial fibrillation

Liver and Biliary System—jaundice

Metabolic Disorders—hypomagnesemia

Musculoskeletal System—myalgia

Myo/Endo/Pericardium—ST segment changes, myocardial infarction

Table 3B.
Adverse Events Reported in ≥1% of Fetuses or Neonates of Mothers Who Received Regional Anesthesia (Cesarean Section and Labor Studies)

Adverse Reaction	NAROPIN total N = 639 N	(%)	Bupivacaine total N = 573 N	(%)
Fetal bradycardia	77	(12.1)	68	(11.9)
Neonatal jaundice	49	(7.7)	47	(8.2)
Neonatal complication-NOS	42	(6.6)	38	(6.6)
Apgar score low	18	(2.8)	14	(2.4)
Neonatal respiratory disorder	17	(2.7)	18	(3.1)
Neonatal tachypnea	14	(2.2)	15	(2.6)
Neonatal fever	13	(2.0)	14	(2.4)
Fetal tachycardia	13	(2.0)	12	(2.1)
Fetal distress	11	(1.7)	10	(1.7)
Neonatal infection	10	(1.6)	8	(1.4)
Neonatal hypoglycemia	8	(1.3)	16	(2.8)

Table 4.
Common Events (Epidural Administration)

Adverse Reaction	NAROPIN						Bupivacaine			
	5 mg/mL total N=256		7.5 mg/mL total N=297		10 mg/mL total N=207		5 mg/mL total N=236		7.5 mg/mL total N=174	
	N	(%)	N	(%)	N	(%)	N	(%)	N	(%)
hypotension	99	(38.7)	146	(49.2)	113	(54.6)	91	(38.6)	89	(51.1)
nausea	34	(13.3)	68	(22.9)			41	(17.4)	36	(20.7)
bradycardia	29	(11.3)	58	(19.5)	40	(19.3)	32	(13.6)	25	(14.4)
back pain	18	(7.0)	23	(7.7)	34	(16.4)	21	(8.9)	23	(13.2)
vomiting	18	(7.0)	33	(11.1)	23	(11.1)	19	(8.1)	14	(8.0)
headache	12	(4.7)	20	(6.7)	16	(7.7)	13	(5.5)	9	(5.2)
fever	8	(3.1)	5	(1.7)	18	(8.7)	11	(4.7)		
chills	6	(2.3)	7	(2.4)	6	(2.9)	4	(1.7)	3	(1.7)
urinary retention	5	(2.0)	8	(2.7)	10	(4.8)	10	(4.2)		
paresthesia	5	(2.0)	10	(3.4)	5	(2.4)	7	(3.0)		
pruritus			14	(4.7)	3	(1.4)			7	(4.0)

Table 5
Effects of Age on Hypotension (Epidural Administration)
Total N: NAROPIN = 760, bupivacaine = 410

AGE	NAROPIN						Bupivacaine			
	5 mg/mL		7.5 mg/mL		10 mg/mL		5 mg/mL		7.5 mg/mL	
	N	(%)	N	(%)	N	(%)	N	(%)	N	(%)
<65	68	(32.2)	99	(43.2)	87	(51.5)	64	(33.5)	73	(48.3)
≥65	31	(68.9)	47	(69.1)	26	(68.4)	27	(60.0)	16	(69.6)

Table 6
Most Common Adverse Events by Gender (Epidural Administration)
Total N: Females = 405, Males = 355

Adverse Reaction	Female N	(%)	Male N	(%)
hypotension	220	(54.3)	138	(38.9)
nausea	119	(29.4)	23	(6.5)
bradycardia	65	(16.0)	56	(15.8)
vomiting	59	(14.6)	8	(2.3)
back pain	41	(10.1)	23	(6.5)
headache	33	(8.1)	17	(4.8)
chills	18	(4.4)	5	(1.4)
fever	16	(4.0)	3	(0.8)
pruritus	16	(4.0)	1	(0.3)
pain	12	(3.0)	4	(1.1)
urinary retention	11	(2.7)	7	(2.0)
dizziness	9	(2.2)	4	(1.1)
hypoesthesia	8	(2.0)	2	(0.6)
paresthesia	8	(2.0)	10	(2.8)

Nervous System—tremor, Horner's syndrome, paresis, dyskinesia, neuropathy, vertigo, coma, convulsion, hypokinesia, hypotonia, ptosis, stupor

Psychiatric Disorders—agitation, confusion, somnolence, nervousness, amnesia, hallucination, emotional lability, insomnia, nightmares

Respiratory System—bronchospasm, coughing

Skin Disorders—rash, urticaria

Urinary System Disorders—urinary incontinence, micturition disorder

Vascular—deep vein thrombosis, phlebitis, pulmonary embolism

Vision—vision abnormalities

For the indication epidural anesthesia for surgery, the 15 most common adverse events were compared between different concentrations of NAROPIN and bupivacaine. Table 4 is based on data from trials in the U.S. and other countries where NAROPIN was administered as an epidural anesthetic for surgery.

[See table 4 above]

Using data from the same studies, the number (%) of patients experiencing hypotension is displayed by patient age, drug and concentration in Table 5. In Table 6, the adverse events for NAROPIN are broken down by gender.

[See table 5 above]

[See table 6 above]

Systemic Reactions

The most commonly encountered acute adverse experiences that demand immediate countermeasures are related to the central nervous system and the cardiovascular system.

Continued on next page

Naropin—Cont.

These adverse experiences are generally dose-related and due to high plasma levels which may result from overdosage, rapid absorption from the injection site, diminished tolerance or from unintentional intravascular injection of the local anesthetic solution. In addition to systemic dose-related toxicity, unintentional subarachnoid injection of drug during the intended performance of lumbar epidural block or nerve blocks near the vertebral column (especially in the head and neck region) may result in underventilation or apnea ("Total or High Spinal"). Also, hypotension due to loss of sympathetic tone and respiratory paralysis or underventilation due to cephalad extension of the motor level of anesthesia may occur. This may lead to secondary cardiac arrest if untreated. Factors influencing plasma protein binding, such as acidosis, systemic diseases that alter protein production or competition with other drugs for protein binding sites, may diminish individual tolerance.

Epidural administration of NAROPIN has, in some cases, as with other local anesthetics, been associated with transient increases in temperature to >38.5°C. This occurred more frequently at doses of NAROPIN >16 mg/h.

Neurologic Reactions

These are characterized by excitation and/or depression. Restlessness, anxiety, dizziness, tinnitus, blurred vision or tremors may occur, possibly proceeding to convulsions. However, excitement may be transient or absent, with depression being the first manifestation of an adverse reaction. This may quickly be followed by drowsiness merging into unconsciousness and respiratory arrest. Other central nervous system effects may be nausea, vomiting, chills, and constriction of the pupils.

The incidence of convulsions associated with the use of local anesthetics varies with the route of administration and the total dose administered. In a survey of studies of epidural anesthesia, overt toxicity progressing to convulsions occurred in approximately 0.1% of local anesthetic administrations.

The incidence of adverse neurological reactions associated with the use of local anesthetics may be related to the total dose and concentration of local anesthetic administered and are also dependent upon the particular drug used, the route of administration, and the physical status of the patient. Many of these observations may be related to local anesthetic techniques, with or without a contribution from the drug. During lumbar epidural block, occasional unintentional penetration of the subarachnoid space by the catheter or needle may occur. Subsequent adverse effects may depend partially on the amount of drug administered intrathecally as well as the physiological and physical effects of a dural puncture. These observations may include spinal block of varying magnitude (including high or total spinal block), hypotension secondary to spinal block, urinary retention, loss of bladder and bowel control (fecal and urinary incontinence), and loss of perineal sensation and sexual function. Signs and symptoms of subarachnoid block typically start within 2–3 minutes of injection. Doses of 15 and 22.5 mg of NAROPIN resulted in sensory levels as high as T5 and T4, respectively. Analgesia started in the sacral dermatomes in 2–3 minutes and extended to the T10 level in 10–13 minutes and lasted for approximately 2 hours. Other neurological effects following unintentional subarachnoid administration during epidural anesthesia may include persistent anesthesia, paresthesia, weakness, paralysis of the lower extremities, and loss of sphincter control; all of which may have slow, incomplete or no recovery. Headache, septic meningitis, meningismus, slowing of labor, increased incidence of forceps delivery, or cranial nerve palsies due to traction on nerves from loss of cerebrospinal fluid have been reported (see DOSAGE AND ADMINISTRATION discussion of Lumbar Epidural Block). A high spinal is characterized by paralysis of the arms, loss of consciousness, respiratory paralysis and bradycardia.

Cardiovascular System Reactions

High doses or unintentional intravascular injection may lead to high plasma levels and related depression of the myocardium, decreased cardiac output, heart block, hypotension, bradycardia, ventricular arrhythmias, including ventricular tachycardia and ventricular fibrillation, and possibly cardiac arrest. (See WARNINGS, PRECAUTIONS, and OVERDOSAGE sections.)

Allergic Reactions

Allergic type reactions are rare and may occur as a result of sensitivity to the local anesthetic (see WARNINGS). These reactions are characterized by signs such as urticaria, pruritus, erythema, angioneurotic edema (including laryngeal edema), tachycardia, sneezing, nausea, vomiting, dizziness, syncope, excessive sweating, elevated temperature, and possibly, anaphylactoid symptomatology (including severe hypotension). Cross sensitivity among members of the amide-type local anesthetic group has been reported. The usefulness of screening for sensitivity has not been definitively established.

OVERDOSAGE

Acute emergencies from local anesthetics are generally related to high plasma levels encountered, or large doses administered, during therapeutic use of local anesthetics or to unintended subarachnoid or intravascular injection of local anesthetic solution. (See ADVERSE REACTIONS, WARNINGS, and PRECAUTIONS.)

MANAGEMENT OF LOCAL ANESTHETIC EMERGENCIES

Therapy with NAROPIN should be discontinued at the first sign of toxicity. No specific information is available for the treatment of toxicity with NAROPIN; therefore, treatment should be symptomatic and supportive. The first consideration is prevention, best accomplished by incremental injection of NAROPIN, careful and constant monitoring of cardiovascular and respiratory vital signs and the patient's state of consciousness after each local anesthetic injection and during continuous infusion. At the first sign of change in mental status, oxygen should be administered.

The first step in the management of systemic toxic reactions, as well as underventilation or apnea due to unintentional subarachnoid injection of drug solution, consists of immediate attention to the establishment and maintenance of a patent airway and effective assisted or controlled ventilation with 100% oxygen with a delivery system capable of permitting immediate positive airway pressure by mask. Circulation should be assisted as necessary. This may prevent convulsions if they have not already occurred.

If necessary, use drugs to control convulsions. Intravenous barbiturates, anticonvulsant agents, or muscle relaxants should only be administered by those familiar with their use. Immediately after the institution of these ventilatory measures, the adequacy of the circulation should be evalu-

Table 7
Dosage Recommendations

	Conc. mg/mL	(%)	Volume mL	Dose mg	Onset min	Duration hours
SURGICAL ANESTHESIA						
Lumbar Epidural	5.0	(0.5%)	15–30	75–150	15–30	2–4
Administration	7.5	(0.75%)	15–25	113–188	10–20	3–5
Surgery	10.0	(1.0%)	15–20	150–200	10–20	4–6
Lumbar Epidural	5.0	(0.5%)	20–30	100–150	15–25	2–4
Administration	7.5	(0.75%)	15–20	113–150	10–20	3–5
Cesarean Section						
Thoracic Epidural	5.0	(0.5%)	5–15	25–75	10–20	n/a[1]
Administration	7.5	(0.75%)	5–15	38–113	10–20	n/a[1]
Surgery						
Major Nerve Block	5.0	(0.5%)	35–50	175–250	15–30	5–8
(eg, brachial plexus block)	7.5	(0.75%)	10–40	75–300	10–25	6–10
Field Block	5.0	(0.5%)	1–40	5–200	1–15	2–6
(eg, minor nerve blocks and infiltration)						
LABOR PAIN MANAGEMENT						
Lumbar Epidural Administration						
Initial Dose	2.0	(0.2%)	10–20	20–40	10–15	0.5–1.5
Continuous infusion[2]	2.0	(0.2%)	6–14 mL/h	12–28 mg/h	n/a[1]	n/a[1]
Incremental injections (top-up)[2]	2.0	(0.2%)	10–15 mL/h	20–30 mg/h	n/a[1]	n/a[1]
POSTOPERATIVE PAIN MANAGEMENT						
Lumbar Epidural Administration						
Continuous infusion[3]	2.0	(0.2%)	6–14 mL/h	12–28 mg/h	n/a[1]	n/a[1]
Thoracic Epidural Administration	2.0	(0.2%)	6–14 mL/h	12–28 mg/h	n/a[1]	n/a[1]
Continuous infusion[3]						
Infiltration	2.0	(0.2%)	1–100	2–200	1–5	2–6
(eg, minor nerve block)	5.0	(0.5%)	1–40	5–200	1–5	2–6

[1] = Not Applicable

[2] = Median dose of 21 mg per hour was administered by continuous infusion or by incremental injections (top-ups) over a median delivery time of 5.5 hours.

[3] = Cumulative doses up to 770 mg of NAROPIN over 24 hours (intraoperative block plus postoperative infusion); Continuous epidural infusion at rates up to 28 mg per hour for 72 hours have been well tolerated in adults, ie, 2016 mg plus surgical dose of approximately 100–150 mg as top-up.

2.0 mg/mL (0.2%)	10 mL	NDC 0186-0859-47 Product No. 0186-0859-44
2.0 mg/mL (0.2%)	20 mL	NDC 0186-0859-57 Product No. 0186-0859-54
5.0 mg/mL (0.5%)	10 mL	NDC 0186-0863-47 Product No. 0186-0863-44
5.0 mg/mL (0.5%)	20 mL	NDC 0186-0863-57 Product No. 0186-0863-54
7.5 mg/mL (0.75%)	10 mL	NDC 0186-0867-47 Product No. 0186-0867-44
7.5 mg/mL (0.75%)	20 mL	NDC 0186-0867-57 Product No. 0186-0867-54
10.0 mg/mL (1.0%)	10 mL	NDC 0186-0868-47 Product No. 0186-0868-44
10.0 mg/mL (1.0%)	20 mL	NDC 0186-0868-57 Product No. 0186-0868-54
NAROPIN® Single Dose Vials:		
2.0 mg/mL (0.2%)	20 mL	NDC 0186-0859-51
5.0 mg/mL (0.5%)	30 mL	NDC 0186-0863-61
7.5 mg/mL (0.75%)	20 mL	NDC 0186-0867-51
10.0 mg/mL (1.0%)	20 mL	NDC 0186-0868-51
NAROPIN® E-Z OFF® Single Dose Vials:		
7.5 mg/mL (0.75%)	10 mL	NDC 0186-0867-41
10.0 mg/mL (1.0%)	10 mL	NDC 0186-0868-41
NAROPIN® Single Dose Ampules:		
2.0 mg/mL (0.2%)	20 mL	NDC 0186-0859-52
5.0 mg/mL (0.5%)	30 mL	NDC 0186-0863-62
7.5 mg/mL (0.75%)	20 mL	NDC 0186-0867-52
10.0 mg/mL (1.0%)	20 mL	NDC 0186-0868-52
NAROPIN® Single Dose Infusion Bottles:		
2.0 mg/mL (0.2%)	100 mL	NDC 0186-0859-81
2.0 mg/mL (0.2%)	200 mL	NDC 0186-0859-91
NAROPIN® Sterile-Pak Single Dose Vials: Boxes of 5		
2.0 mg/mL (0.2%)	20 mL	NDC 0186-0859-51 Product No: 0186-0859-59
5.0 mg/mL (0.5%)	30 mL	NDC 0186-0863-61 Product No: 0186-0863-69
7.5 mg/mL (0.75%)	20 mL	NDC 0186-0867-51 Product No: 0186-0867-59
10.0 mg/mL (1.0%)	20 mL	NDC 0186-0868-51 Product No: 0186-0868-59

ated. Supportive treatment of circulatory depression may require administration of intravenous fluids, and, when appropriate, a vasopressor dictated by the clinical situation (such as ephedrine or epinephrine to enhance myocardial contractile force).
The mean dosages of ropivacaine producing seizures, after intravenous infusion in dogs, nonpregnant and pregnant sheep were 4.9, 6.1 and 5.9 mg/kg, respectively. These doses were associated with peak arterial total plasma concentrations of 11.4, 4.3 and 5.0 µg/mL, respectively.
In human volunteers given intravenous NAROPIN, the mean maximum tolerated total and free arterial plasma concentrations were 4.3 and 0.6 µg/mL respectively, at which time moderate CNS symptoms (muscle twitching) were noted.
Clinical data from patients experiencing local anesthetic induced convulsions demonstrated rapid development of hypoxia, hypercarbia and acidosis within a minute of the onset of convulsions. These observations suggest that oxygen consumption and carbon dioxide production are greatly increased during local anesthetic convulsions and emphasize the importance of immediate and effective ventilation with oxygen which may avoid cardiac arrest.
If difficulty is encountered in the maintenance of a patent airway or if prolonged ventilatory support (assisted or controlled) is indicated, endotracheal intubation, employing drugs and techniques familiar to the clinician, may be indicated after initial administration of oxygen by mask.
The supine position is dangerous in pregnant women at term because of aortocaval compression by the gravid uterus. Therefore, during treatment of systemic toxicity, maternal hypotension or fetal bradycardia following regional block, the parturient should be maintained in the left lateral decubitus position if possible, or manual displacement of the uterus off the great vessels should be accomplished. Resuscitation of obstetrical patients may take longer than resuscitation of nonpregnant patients and closed-chest cardiac compression may be ineffective. Rapid delivery of the fetus may improve the response to resuscitative efforts.

DOSAGE AND ADMINISTRATION

The rapid injection of a large volume of local anesthetic solution should be avoided and fractional (incremental) doses should always be used. The smallest dose and concentration required to produce the desired result should be administered.
The dose of any local anesthetic administered varies with the anesthetic procedure, the area to be anesthetized, the vascularity of the tissues, the number of neuronal segments to be blocked, the depth of anesthesia and degree of muscle relaxation required, the duration of anesthesia desired, individual tolerance, and the physical condition of the patient. Patients in poor general condition due to aging or other compromising factors such as partial or complete heart conduction block, advanced liver disease or severe renal dysfunction require special attention although regional anesthesia is frequently indicated in these patients. To reduce the risk of potentially serious adverse reactions, attempts should be made to optimize the patient's condition before major blocks are performed, and the dosage should be adjusted accordingly.
Use an adequate test dose (3–5 mL of a short acting local anesthetic solution containing epinephrine) prior to induction of complete block. This test dose should be repeated if the patient is moved in such a fashion as to have displaced the epidural catheter. Allow adequate time for onset of anesthesia following administration of each test dose.
Parenteral drug products should be inspected visually for particulate matter and discoloration prior to administration, whenever solution and container permit. Solutions which are discolored or which contain particulate matter should not be administered.
[See table 7 at top of previous page]
The doses in the table are those considered to be necessary to produce a successful block and should be regarded as guidelines for use in adults. Individual variations in onset and duration occur. The figures reflect the expected average dose range needed. For other local anesthetic techniques standard current textbooks should be consulted.
When prolonged blocks are used, either through continuous infusion or through repeated bolus administration, the risks of reaching a toxic plasma concentration or inducing local neural injury must be considered. Experience to date indicates that a cumulative dose of up to 770 mg NAROPIN administered over 24 hours is well tolerated in adults when used for postoperative pain management: ie, 2016 mg. Caution should be exercised when administering NAROPIN for prolonged periods of time, eg, >70 hours in debilitated patients.
For treatment of postoperative pain, the following technique can be recommended: If regional anesthesia was not used intraoperatively, then an initial epidural block with 5–7 mL NAROPIN is induced via an epidural catheter. Analgesia is maintained with an infusion of NAROPIN, 2 mg/mL (0.2%). Clinical studies have demonstrated that infusion rates of 6–14 mL (12–28 mg) per hour provide adequate analgesia with nonprogressive motor block. With this technique a significant reduction in the need for opioids was demonstrated. Clinical experience supports the use of NAROPIN epidural infusions for up to 72 hours.

HOW SUPPLIED

NAROPIN® Polyamp DuoFit™ Sterile Pak:
Boxes of 5
polypropylene ampules fitting both Luer-lock and Luer-slip (tapered) syringes
[See second table at top of previous page]
The solubility of ropivacaine is limited at pH above 6. Thus care must be taken as precipitation may occur if NAROPIN is mixed with alkaline solutions.
Disinfecting agents containing heavy metals, which cause release of respective ions (mercury, zinc, copper, etc.) should not be used for skin or mucous membrane disinfection since they have been related to incidents of swelling and edema. When chemical disinfection of the container surface is desired, either isopropyl alcohol (91%) or ethyl alcohol (70%) is recommended. It is recommended that chemical disinfection be accomplished by wiping the ampule or vial stopper thoroughly with cotton or gauze that has been moistened with the recommended alcohol just prior to use. When a container is required to have a sterile outside, a Sterile-Pak should be chosen. Glass containers may, as an alternative, be autoclaved once. Stability has been demonstrated using a targeted F_0 of 7 minutes at 121°C.
Solutions should be stored at controlled room temperature 20°–25°C (68°–77°F) [see USP].
These products are intended for single use and are free from preservatives. Any solution remaining from an opened container should be discarded promptly. In addition, continuous infusion bottles should not be left in place for more than 24 hours.

AstraZeneca LP, Wilmington, DE 19850
721697-04
Rev 03/01 201808 3/01

NEXIUM™ ℞

(esomeprazole magnesium)
[*nex' ē-ŭm*]
DELAYED-RELEASE CAPSULES
Rx only

Prescribing information for this product, which appears on pages 619–623 of the 2002 PDR, has been revised as follows. Please write "See Supplement A" next to the product heading.

In the **HOW SUPPLIED** *section, the following has been added under the 40 mg strength:*
NDC 0186-5040-54 bottles of 90
Also in the **HOW SUPPLIED** *section, the following have been deleted:*
NDC 0186-5020-68 bottles of 100
NDC 0186-5040-68 bottles of 100
620514-01 Rev 4/01.

PRILOSEC® ℞

(omeprazole)
[*prī' lō-sĕc*]
DELAYED-RELEASE CAPSULES

Prescribing information for this product, which appears on page 628 of the 2002 PDR, has been completely revised as follows. Please write "See Supplement A" next to the product heading.

DESCRIPTION

The active ingredient in PRILOSEC (omeprazole) Delayed-Release Capsules is a substituted benzimidazole, 5-methoxy-2-[[(4-methoxy-3, 5-dimethyl-2-pyridinyl) methyl] sulfinyl]-1*H*-benzimidazole, a compound that inhibits gastric acid secretion. Its empirical formula is $C_{17}H_{19}N_3O_3S$, with a molecular weight of 345.42. The structural formula is:

[Structural formula: H, N, O, S, CH_2, N, H_3CO, N, H_3C, CH_3, OCH_3]

Omeprazole is a white to off-white crystalline powder which melts with decomposition at about 155°C. It is a weak base, freely soluble in ethanol and methanol, and slightly soluble in acetone and isopropanol and very slightly soluble in water. The stability of omeprazole is a function of pH; it is rapidly degraded in acid media, but has acceptable stability under alkaline conditions.
PRILOSEC is supplied as delayed-release capsules for oral administration. Each delayed-release capsule contains either 10 mg, 20 mg or 40 mg of omeprazole in the form of enteric-coated granules with the following inactive ingredients: cellulose, disodium hydrogen phosphate, hydroxypropyl cellulose, hydroxypropyl methylcellulose, lactose, mannitol, sodium lauryl sulfate and other ingredients. The capsule shells have the following inactive ingredients: gelatin-NF, FD&C Blue #1, FD&C Red #40, D&C Red #28, titanium dioxide, synthetic black iron oxide, isopropanol, butyl alcohol, FD&C Blue #2, D&C Red #7 Calcium Lake, and, in addition, the 10 mg and 40 mg capsule shells also contain D&C Yellow #10.

CLINICAL PHARMACOLOGY

Pharmacokinetics and Metabolism: Omeprazole
PRILOSEC Delayed-Release Capsules contain an enteric-coated granule formulation of omeprazole (because omeprazole is acid-labile), so that absorption of omeprazole begins only after the granules leave the stomach. Absorption is rapid, with peak plasma levels of omeprazole occurring within 0.5 to 3.5 hours. Peak plasma concentrations of omeprazole and AUC are approximately proportional to doses up to 40 mg, but because of a saturable first-pass effect, a greater than linear response in peak plasma concentration and AUC occurs with doses greater than 40 mg. Absolute bioavailability (compared to intravenous administration) is about 30–40% at doses of 20–40 mg, due in large part to presystemic metabolism. In healthy subjects the plasma half-life is 0.5 to 1 hour, and the total body clearance is 500–600 mL/min. Protein binding is approximately 95%.
The bioavailability of omeprazole increases slightly upon repeated administration of PRILOSEC Delayed-Release Capsules.
Following single dose oral administration of a buffered solution of omeprazole, little if any unchanged drug was excreted in urine. The majority of the dose (about 77%) was eliminated in urine as at least six metabolites. Two were identified as hydroxyomeprazole and the corresponding carboxylic acid. The remainder of the dose was recoverable in feces. This implies a significant biliary excretion of the metabolites of omeprazole. Three metabolites have been identified in plasma — the sulfide and sulfone derivatives of omeprazole, and hydroxyomeprazole. These metabolites have very little or no antisecretory activity.
In patients with chronic hepatic disease, the bioavailability increased to approximately 100% compared to an I.V. dose, reflecting decreased first-pass effect, and the plasma half-life of the drug increased to nearly 3 hours compared to the half-life in normals of 0.5–1 hour. Plasma clearance averaged 70 mL/min, compared to a value of 500–600 mL/min in normal subjects.
In patients with chronic renal impairment, whose creatinine clearance ranged between 10 and 62 mL/min/1.73 m^2, the disposition of omeprazole was very similar to that in healthy volunteers, although there was a slight increase in bioavailability. Because urinary excretion is a primary route of excretion of omeprazole metabolites, their elimination slowed in proportion to the decreased creatinine clearance.
The elimination rate of omeprazole was somewhat decreased in the elderly, and bioavailability was increased. Omeprazole was 76% bioavailable when a single 40 mg oral dose of omeprazole (buffered solution) was administered to healthy elderly volunteers, versus 58% in young volunteers given the same dose. Nearly 70% of the dose was recovered in urine as metabolites of omeprazole and no unchanged drug was detected. The plasma clearance of omeprazole was 250 mL/min (about half that of young volunteers) and its plasma half-life averaged one hour, about twice that of young healthy volunteers.
In pharmacokinetic studies of single 20 mg omeprazole doses, an increase in AUC of approximately four-fold was noted in Asian subjects compared to Caucasians.
Dose adjustment, particularly where maintenance of healing of erosive esophagitis is indicated, for the hepatically impaired and Asian subjects should be considered.
PRILOSEC Delayed-Release Capsule 40 mg was bioequivalent when administered with and without applesauce. However, PRILOSEC Delayed-Release Capsule 20 mg was not bioequivalent when administered with and without applesauce. When administered with applesauce, a mean 25% reduction in C_{max} was observed without a significant change in AUC for PRILOSEC Delayed-Release Capsule 20 mg. The clinical relevance of this finding is unknown.

Pharmacokinetics: Combination Therapy with Antimicrobials
Omeprazole 40 mg daily was given in combination with clarithromycin 500 mg every 8 hours to healthy adult male subjects. The steady state plasma concentrations of omeprazole were increased (C_{max}, AUC_{0-24}, and $T_{1/2}$ increases of 30%, 89% and 34% respectively) by the concomitant administration of clarithromycin. The observed increases in omeprazole plasma concentration were associated with the following pharmacological effects. The mean 24-hour gastric pH value was 5.2 when omeprazole was administered alone and 5.7 when co-administered with clarithromycin.
The plasma levels of clarithromycin and 14-hydroxy-clarithromycin were increased by the concomitant administration of omeprazole. For clarithromycin, the mean C_{max} was 10% greater, the mean C_{min} was 27% greater, and the mean AUC_{0-8} was 15% greater when clarithromycin was administered with omeprazole than when clarithromycin was administered alone. Similar results were seen for 14-hydroxy-clarithromycin, the mean C_{max} was 45% greater, the mean C_{min} was 57% greater, and the mean AUC_{0-8} was 45% greater. Clarithromycin concentrations in the gastric tissue and mucus were also increased by concomitant administration of omeprazole.

Clarithromycin Tissue Concentrations 2 hours after Dose[1]

Tissue	Clarithromycin	Clarithromycin+ Omeprazole
Antrum	10.48 ± 2.01 (n = 5)	19.96 ± 4.71 (n = 5)
Fundus	20.81 ± 7.64 (n = 5)	24.25 ± 6.37 (n = 5)
Mucus	4.15 ± 7.74 (n = 4)	39.29 ± 32.79 (n = 4)

[1]Mean ± SD (µg/g)

Continued on next page

Prilosec—Cont.

For information on clarithromycin pharmacokinetics and microbiology, consult the clarithromycin package insert, CLINICAL PHARMACOLOGY section.
The pharmacokinetics of omeprazole, clarithromycin, and amoxicillin have not been adequately studied when all three drugs are administered concomitantly.
For information on amoxicillin pharmacokinetics and microbiology, see the amoxicillin package insert, ACTIONS, PHARMACOLOGY and MICROBIOLOGY sections.

Pharmacodynamics

Mechanism of Action

Omeprazole belongs to a new class of antisecretory compounds, the substituted benzimidazoles, that do not exhibit anticholinergic or H_2 histamine antagonistic properties, but that suppress gastric acid secretion by specific inhibition of the H^+/K^+ ATPase enzyme system at the secretory surface of the gastric parietal cell. Because this enzyme system is regarded as the acid (proton) pump within the gastric mucosa, omeprazole has been characterized as a gastric acid-pump inhibitor, in that it blocks the final step of acid production. This effect is dose-related and leads to inhibition of both basal and stimulated acid secretion irrespective of the stimulus. Animal studies indicate that after rapid disappearance from plasma, omeprazole can be found within the gastric mucosa for a day or more.

Antisecretory Activity

After oral administration, the onset of the antisecretory effect of omeprazole occurs within one hour, with the maximum effect occurring within two hours. Inhibition of secretion is about 50% of maximum at 24 hours and the duration of inhibition lasts up to 72 hours. The antisecretory effect thus lasts far longer than would be expected from the very short (less than one hour) plasma half-life, apparently due to prolonged binding to the parietal H^+/K^+ ATPase enzyme. When the drug is discontinued, secretory activity returns gradually, over 3 to 5 days. The inhibitory effect of omeprazole on acid secretion increases with repeated once-daily dosing, reaching a plateau after four days.
Results from numerous studies of the antisecretory effect of multiple doses of 20 mg and 40 mg of omeprazole in normal volunteers and patients are shown below. The "max" value represents determinations at a time of maximum effect (2–6 hours after dosing), while "min" values are those 24 hours after the last dose of omeprazole.

Range of Mean Values from Multiple Studies of the Mean Antisecretory Effects of Omeprazole After Multiple Daily Dosing

Parameter	Omeprazole 20 mg		Omeprazole 40 mg	
	Max	Min	Max	Min
% Decrease in Basal Acid Output	78*	58–80	94*	80–93
% Decrease in Peak Acid Output	79*	50–59	88*	62–68
% Decrease in 24-hr. Intragastric Acidity		80–97		92–94

*Single Studies

Single daily oral doses of omeprazole ranging from a dose of 10 mg to 40 mg have produced 100% inhibition of 24-hour intragastric acidity in some patients.

Enterochromaffin-like (ECL) Cell Effects

In 24-month carcinogenicity studies in rats, a dose-related significant increase in gastric carcinoid tumors and ECL cell hyperplasia was observed in both male and female animals. (See PRECAUTIONS, Carcinogenesis, Mutagenesis, Impairment of Fertility.) Carcinoid tumors have also been observed in rats subjected to fundectomy or long-term treatment with other proton pump inhibitors or high doses of H_2-receptor antagonists.
Human gastric biopsy specimens have been obtained from more than 3000 patients treated with omeprazole in long-term clinical trials. The incidence of ECL cell hyperplasia in these studies increased with time; however, no case of ECL cell carcinoids, dysplasia, or neoplasia has been found in these patients. (See also CLINICAL PHARMACOLOGY, Pathological Hypersecretory Conditions.)

Serum Gastrin Effects

In studies involving more than 200 patients, serum gastrin levels increased during the first 1 to 2 weeks of once-daily administration of therapeutic doses of omeprazole in parallel with inhibition of acid secretion. No further increase in serum gastrin occurred with continued treatment. In comparison with histamine H_2-receptor antagonists, the median increases produced by 20 mg doses of omeprazole were higher (1.3 to 3.6 fold vs. 1.1 to 1.8 fold increase). Gastrin values returned to pretreatment levels, usually within 1 to 2 weeks after discontinuation of therapy.

Other Effects

Systemic effects of omeprazole in the CNS, cardiovascular and respiratory systems have not been found to date. Omeprazole, given in oral doses of 30 or 40 mg for 2 to 4 weeks, had no effect on thyroid function, carbohydrate me-

Per-Protocol and Intent-to-Treat *H. pylori* Eradication Rates
% of Patients Cured [95% Confidence Interval]

	PRILOSEC +clarithromycin +amoxicillin		Clarithromycin +amoxicillin	
	Per-Protocol†	Intent-to-Treat‡	Per-Protocol†	Intent-to-Treat‡
Study 126	*77 [64, 86] (n = 64)	*69 [57, 79] (n = 80)	43 [31, 56] (n = 67)	37 [27, 48] (n = 84)
Study 127	*78 [67, 88] (n = 65)	*73 [61, 82] (n = 77)	41 [29, 54] (n = 68)	36 [26, 47] (n = 83)
Study M96–446	*90 [80, 96] (n = 69)	*83 [74, 91] (n = 84)	33 [24, 44] (n = 93)	32 [23, 42] (n = 99)

† Patients were included in the analysis if they had confirmed duodenal ulcer disease (active ulcer, studies 126 and 127; history of ulcer within 5 years, study M96–446) and *H. pylori* infection at baseline defined as at least two of three positive endoscopic tests from CLOtest®, histology, and/or culture. Patients were included in the analysis if they completed the study. Additionally, if patients dropped out of the study due to an adverse event related to the study drug, they were included in the analysis as failures of therapy. The impact of eradication on ulcer recurrence has not been assessed in patients with a past history of ulcer.
‡ Patients were included in the analysis if they had documented *H. pylori* infection at baseline and had confirmed duodenal ulcer disease. All dropouts were included as failures of therapy.
*($p < 0.05$) versus clarithromycin plus amoxicillin.

H. pylori Eradication Rates (Per-Protocol Analysis at 4 to 6 Weeks)
% of Patients Cured [95% Confidence Interval]

	PRILOSEC + Clarithromycin	PRILOSEC	Clarithromycin
U.S. Studies			
Study M93–067	74 [60, 85]†‡ (n = 53)	0 [0, 7] (n = 54)	31 [18, 47] (n = 42)
Study M93–100	64 [51, 76]†‡ (n = 61)	0 [0, 6] (n = 59)	39 [24, 55] (n = 44)
Non U.S. Studies			
Study M92–812b	83 [71, 92]‡ (n = 60)	1 [0, 7] (n = 74)	N/A
Study M93–058	74 [64, 83]‡ (n = 86)	1 [0, 6] (n = 90)	N/A

† Statistically significantly higher than clarithromycin monotherapy ($p < 0.05$)
‡ Statistically significantly higher than omeprazole monotherapy ($p < 0.05$)

tabolism, or circulating levels of parathyroid hormone, cortisol, estradiol, testosterone, prolactin, cholecystokinin or secretin.
No effect on gastric emptying of the solid and liquid components of a test meal was demonstrated after a single dose of omeprazole 90 mg. In healthy subjects, a single I.V. dose of omeprazole (0.35 mg/kg) had no effect on intrinsic factor secretion. No systematic dose-dependent effect has been observed on basal or stimulated pepsin output in humans. However, when intragastric pH is maintained at 4.0 or above, basal pepsin output is low, and pepsin activity is decreased.
As do other agents that elevate intragastric pH, omeprazole administered for 14 days in healthy subjects produced a significant increase in the intragastric concentrations of viable bacteria. The pattern of the bacterial species was unchanged from that commonly found in saliva. All changes resolved within three days of stopping treatment.

Clinical Studies

Duodenal Ulcer Disease

Active Duodenal Ulcer—In a multicenter, double-blind, placebo-controlled study of 147 patients with endoscopically documented duodenal ulcer, the percentage of patients healed (per protocol) at 2 and 4 weeks was significantly higher with PRILOSEC 20 mg once a day than with placebo ($p \leq 0.01$).

Treatment of Active Duodenal Ulcer
% of Patients Healed

	PRILOSEC 20 mg a.m. (n = 99)	Placebo a.m. (n = 48)
Week 2	*41	13
Week 4	*75	27

*($p \leq 0.01$)

Complete daytime and nighttime pain relief occurred significantly faster ($p \leq 0.01$) in patients treated with PRILOSEC 20 mg than in patients treated with placebo. At the end of the study, significantly more patients who had received PRILOSEC had complete relief of daytime pain ($p \leq 0.05$) and nighttime pain ($p \leq 0.01$).
In a multicenter, double-blind study of 293 patients with endoscopically documented duodenal ulcer, the percentage of patients healed (per protocol) at 4 weeks was significantly higher with PRILOSEC 20 mg once a day than with ranitidine 150 mg b.i.d. ($p < 0.01$).

Treatment of Active Duodenal Ulcer
% of Patients Healed

	PRILOSEC 20 mg a.m. (n = 145)	Ranitidine 150 mg b.i.d (n = 148)
Week 2	42	34
Week 4	*82	63

*($p < 0.01$)

Healing occurred significantly faster in patients treated with PRILOSEC than in those treated with ranitidine 150 mg b.i.d. ($p < 0.01$).

In a foreign multinational randomized, double-blind study of 105 patients with endoscopically documented duodenal ulcer, 20 mg and 40 mg of PRILOSEC were compared to 150 mg b.i.d. of ranitidine at 2, 4 and 8 weeks. At 2 and 4 weeks both doses of PRILOSEC were statistically superior (per protocol) to ranitidine, but 40 mg was not superior to 20 mg of PRILOSEC, and at 8 weeks there was no significant difference between any of the active drugs.

Treatment of Active Duodenal Ulcer
% of Patients Healed

	PRILOSEC 20 mg (n = 34)	PRILOSEC 40 mg (n = 36)	Ranitidine 150 mg b.i.d (n = 35)
Week 2	* 83	*83	53
Week 4	* 97	*100	82
Week 8	100	100	94

*($p \leq 0.01$)

H. pylori Eradication in Patients with Duodenal Ulcer Disease

Triple Therapy (PRILOSEC/clarithromycin/amoxicillin)—Three U.S., randomized, double-blind clinical studies in patients with *H. pylori* infection and duodenal ulcer disease (n = 558) compared PRILOSEC plus clarithromycin plus amoxicillin to clarithromycin plus amoxicillin. Two studies (126 and 127) were conducted in patients with an active duodenal ulcer, and the other study (M96–446) was conducted in patients with a history of a duodenal ulcer in the past 5 years but without an ulcer present at the time of enrollment. The dose regimen in the studies was PRILOSEC 20 mg b.i.d. plus clarithromycin 500 mg b.i.d. plus amoxicillin 1 g b.i.d. for 10 days; or clarithromycin 500 mg b.i.d. plus amoxicillin 1 g b.i.d. for 10 days. In studies 126 and 127, patients who took the omeprazole regimen also received an additional 18 days of PRILOSEC 20 mg q.d. Endpoints studied were eradication of *H. pylori* and duodenal ulcer healing (studies 126 and 127 only). *H. pylori* status was determined by CLOtest®, histology and culture in all three studies. For a given patient, *H. pylori* was considered eradicated if at least two of these tests were negative, and none was positive.
The combination of omeprazole plus clarithromycin plus amoxicillin was effective in eradicating *H. pylori.*
[See first table above]

Dual Therapy (PRILOSEC/clarithromycin)—Four randomized, double-blind, multicenter studies (M93–067, M93–100, M92–812b, and M93–058) evaluated PRILOSEC 40 mg q.d. plus clarithromycin 500 mg t.i.d. for 14 days, followed by PRILOSEC 20 mg q.d. (M93–067, M93–100, M93–058) or by PRILOSEC 40 mg q.d. (M92–812b) for an additional 14 days in patients with active duodenal ulcer associated with *H. pylori.* Studies M93–067 and M93–100 were conducted in the U.S. and Canada and enrolled 242 and 256 patients, respectively. *H. pylori* infection and duodenal ulcer were confirmed in 219 patients in Study M93–067 and 228 patients in Study M93–100. These studies compared the combination regimen to PRILOSEC and clarithromycin monotherapies. Studies M92–812b and M93–058 were conducted in Europe and enrolled 154 and 215 patients, respectively. *H. pylori* infection and duodenal ulcer were confirmed in 148 patients in study M92–812b and 208 patients in Study M93–058. These studies compared the combination regimen to omeprazole monotherapy. The results for the efficacy analyses for these studies are described below. *H. pylori* eradication was defined as no positive test (culture or histology) at 4 weeks following the end of treatment, and two negative tests were required to be considered eradicated of *H. pylori*. In the per-protocol analysis, the following patients were excluded: dropouts, patients with missing *H. pylori* tests post-treatment, and patients that were not assessed for *H. pylori* eradication because they were found to have an ulcer at the end of treatment.

The combination of omeprazole and clarithromycin was effective in eradicating *H. pylori*.

[See second table at top of previous page]

Ulcer healing was not significantly different when clarithromycin was added to omeprazole therapy compared to omeprazole therapy alone.

The combination of omeprazole and clarithromycin was effective in eradicating *H. pylori* and reduced duodenal ulcer recurrence.

[See table above]

Duodenal Ulcer Recurrence Rates by *H. pylori* Eradication Status
% of Patients with Ulcer Recurrence

	H. pylori eradicated[§]	*H. pylori* not eradicated[§]
U.S. Studies[†]		
6 months post-treatment		
Study M93–067	*35 (n = 49)	60 (n = 88)
Study M93–100	*8 (n = 53)	60 (n = 106)
Non U.S. Studies[‡]		
6 months post-treatment		
Study M92–812b	*5 (n = 43)	46 (n = 78)
Study M93–058	*6 (n = 53)	43 (n = 107)
12 months post-treatment		
Study M92–812b	*5 (n = 39)	68 (n = 71)

[§] *H. pylori* eradication status assessed at same timepoint as ulcer recurrence
[†] Combined results for PRILOSEC + clarithromycin, PRILOSEC, and clarithromycin treatment arms
[‡] Combined results for PRILOSEC + clarithromycin and PRILOSEC treatment arms
*($p \leq 0.01$) versus proportion with duodenal ulcer recurrence who were not *H. pylori* eradicated

Gastric Ulcer

In a U.S. multicenter, double-blind, study of omeprazole 40 mg once a day, 20 mg once a day, and placebo in 520 patients with endoscopically diagnosed gastric ulcer, the following results were obtained.

Treatment of Gastric Ulcer
% of Patients Healed
(All Patients Treated)

	PRILOSEC 20 mg q.d. (n = 202)	PRILOSEC 40 mg q.d. (n = 214)	Placebo (n = 104)
Week 4	47.5**	55.6**	30.8
Week 8	74.8**	82.7**,+	48.1

**($p < 0.01$) PRILOSEC 40 mg or 20 mg versus placebo
+($p < 0.05$) PRILOSEC 40 mg versus 20 mg

For the stratified groups of patients with ulcer size less than or equal to 1 cm, no difference in healing rates between 40 mg and 20 mg was detected at either 4 or 8 weeks. For patients with ulcer size greater than 1 cm, 40 mg was significantly more effective than 20 mg at 8 weeks.

In a foreign, multinational, double-blind study of 602 patients with endoscopically diagnosed gastric ulcer, omeprazole 40 mg once a day, 20 mg once a day, and ranitidine 150 mg twice a day were evaluated.

Treatment of Gastric Ulcer
% of Patients Healed
(All Patients Treated)

	PRILOSEC 20 mg q.d. (n = 200)	PRILOSEC 40 mg q.d. (n = 187)	Ranitidine 150 mg b.i.d. (n = 199)
Week 4	63.5	78.1**,++	56.3
Week 8	81.5	91.4**,++	78.4

**($p < 0.01$) PRILOSEC 40 mg versus ranitidine
++($p < 0.01$) PRILOSEC 40 mg versus 20 mg

Gastroesophageal Reflux Disease (GERD)
Symptomatic GERD

A placebo controlled study was conducted in Scandinavia to compare the efficacy of omeprazole 20 mg or 10 mg once daily for up to 4 weeks in the treatment of heartburn and other symptoms in GERD patients without erosive esophagitis. Results are shown below.

% Successful Symptomatic Outcome[a]

	PRILOSEC 20 mg a.m.	PRILOSEC 10 mg a.m.	Placebo a.m.
All patients	46*,† (n = 205)	31† (n = 199)	13 (n = 105)
Patients with confirmed GERD	56*,† (n = 115)	36† (n = 109)	14 (n = 59)

[a] Defined as complete resolution of heartburn
* ($p < 0.005$) versus 10 mg
† ($p < 0.005$) versus placebo

Erosive Esophagitis

In a U.S. multicenter double-blind placebo controlled study of 20 mg or 40 mg of PRILOSEC Delayed-Release Capsules in patients with symptoms of GERD and endoscopically diagnosed erosive esophagitis of grade 2 or above, the percentage healing rates (per protocol) were as follows:

Week	20 mg PRILOSEC (n = 83)	40 mg PRILOSEC (n = 87)	Placebo (n = 43)
4	39**	45**	7
8	74**	75**	14

**($p < 0.01$) PRILOSEC versus placebo.

In this study, the 40 mg dose was not superior to the 20 mg dose of PRILOSEC in the percentage healing rate. Other controlled clinical trials have also shown that PRILOSEC is effective in severe GERD. In comparisons with histamine H_2-receptor antagonists in patients with erosive esophagitis, grade 2 or above, PRILOSEC in a dose of 20 mg was significantly more effective than the active controls. Complete daytime and nighttime heartburn relief occurred significantly faster ($p < 0.01$) in patients treated with PRILOSEC than in those taking placebo or histamine H_2-receptor antagonists.

In this and five other controlled GERD studies, significantly more patients taking 20 mg omeprazole (84%) reported complete relief of GERD symptoms than patients receiving placebo (12%).

Long Term Maintenance Treatment of Erosive Esophagitis

In a U.S. double-blind, randomized, multicenter, placebo controlled study, two dose regimens of PRILOSEC were studied in patients with endoscopically confirmed healed esophagitis. Results to determine maintenance of healing of erosive esophagitis are shown below.

Life Table Analysis

	PRILOSEC 20 mg q.d. (n = 138)	PRILOSEC 20 mg 3 days per week (n = 137)	Placebo (n = 131)
Percent in endoscopic remission at 6 months	*70	34	11

*($p < 0.01$) PRILOSEC 20 mg q.d. versus PRILOSEC 20 mg 3 consecutive days per week or placebo.

In an international multicenter double-blind study, PRILOSEC 20 mg daily and 10 mg daily were compared to ranitidine 150 mg twice daily in patients with endoscopically confirmed healed esophagitis. The table below provides the results of this study for maintenance of healing of erosive esophagitis.

Life Table Analysis

	PRILOSEC 20 mg q.d. (n = 131)	PRILOSEC 10 mg q.d. (n = 133)	Ranitidine 150 mg b.i.d. (n = 128)
Percent in endoscopic remission at 12 months	*77	‡58	46

*($p = 0.01$) PRILOSEC 20 mg q.d. versus PRILOSEC 10 mg q.d. or Ranitidine.
‡($p = 0.03$) PRILOSEC 10 mg q.d. versus Ranitidine.

In patients who initially had grades 3 or 4 erosive esophagitis, for maintenance after healing 20 mg daily of PRILOSEC was effective, while 10 mg did not demonstrate effectiveness.

Pathological Hypersecretory Conditions

In open studies of 136 patients with pathological hypersecretory conditions, such as Zollinger-Ellison (ZE) syndrome with or without multiple endocrine adenomas, PRILOSEC Delayed-Release Capsules significantly inhibited gastric acid secretion and controlled associated symptoms of diarrhea, anorexia, and pain. Doses ranging from 20 mg every other day to 360 mg per day maintained basal acid secretion below 10 mEq/hr in patients without prior gastric surgery, and below 5 mEq/hr in patients with prior gastric surgery. Initial doses were titrated to the individual patient need, and adjustments were necessary with time in some patients (see DOSAGE AND ADMINISTRATION). PRILOSEC was well tolerated at these high dose levels for prolonged periods (> 5 years in some patients). In most ZE patients, serum gastrin levels were not modified by PRILOSEC. However, in some patients serum gastrin increased to levels greater than those present prior to initiation of omeprazole therapy. At least 11 patients with ZE syndrome on long-term treatment with PRILOSEC developed gastric carcinoids. These findings are believed to be a manifestation of the underlying condition, which is known to be associated with such tumors, rather than the result of the administration of PRILOSEC. (See ADVERSE REACTIONS.)

Microbiology

Omeprazole and clarithromycin dual therapy and omeprazole, clarithromycin and amoxicillin triple therapy have been shown to be active against most strains of *Helicobacter pylori in vitro* and in clinical infections as described in the INDICATIONS AND USAGE section.

Helicobacter
Helicobacter pylori

Pretreatment Resistance

Clarithromycin pretreatment resistance rates were 3.5% (4/113) in the omeprazole/clarithromycin dual therapy studies (M93–067, M93–100) and 9.3% (41/439) in omeprazole/clarithromycin/amoxicillin triple therapy studies (126, 127, M96–446).

Amoxicillin pretreatment susceptible isolates (≤ 0.25 μg/mL) were found in 99.3% (436/439) of the patients in the omeprazole/clarithromycin/amoxicillin triple therapy studies (126, 127, M96–446). Amoxicillin pretreatment minimum inhibitory concentrations (MICs) > 0.25 μg/mL occurred in 0.7% (3/439) of the patients, all of whom were in the clarithromycin and amoxicillin study arm. One patient had an unconfirmed pretreatment amoxicillin minimum inhibitory concentration (MIC) of > 256 μg/mL by Etest®.

[See table at top of next page]

Patients not eradicated of *H. pylori* following omeprazole/clarithromycin/amoxicillin triple therapy or omeprazole/clarithromycin dual therapy will likely have clarithromycin resistant *H. pylori* isolates. Therefore, clarithromycin susceptibility testing should be done, if possible. Patients with clarithromycin resistant *H. pylori* should not be treated with any of the following: omeprazole/clarithromycin dual therapy, omeprazole/clarithromycin/amoxicillin triple therapy, or other regimens which include clarithromycin as the sole antimicrobial agent.

Amoxicillin Susceptibility Test Results and Clinical/Bacteriological Outcomes

In the triple therapy clinical trials, 84.9% (157/185) of the patients in the omeprazole/clarithromycin/amoxicillin treatment group who had pretreatment amoxicillin susceptible MICs (≤ 0.25 μg/mL) were eradicated of *H. pylori* and 15.1% (28/185) failed therapy. Of the 28 patients who failed triple therapy, 11 had no post-treatment susceptibility test results and 17 had post-treatment *H. pylori* isolates with amoxicillin susceptible MICs. Eleven of the patients who failed triple therapy also had post-treatment *H. pylori* isolates with clarithromycin resistant MICs.

Susceptibility Test for *Helicobacter pylori*

The reference methodology for susceptibility testing of *H. pylori* is agar dilution MICs[1]. One to three microliters of an inoculum equivalent to a No. 2 McFarland standard ($1 \times 10^7 - 1 \times 10^8$ CFU/mL for *H. pylori*) are inoculated directly onto freshly prepared antimicrobial containing Mueller-Hinton agar plates with 5% aged defibrinated sheep blood (≥ 2 weeks old). The agar dilution plates are incubated at 35°C in a microaerobic environment produced by a gas generating system suitable for campylobacters. After 3 days of incubation, the MICs are recorded as the lowest concentration of antimicrobial agent required to inhibit growth of the organism. The clarithromycin and amoxicillin MIC values should be interpreted according to the following criteria:

Clarithromycin MIC (μg/mL) [a]	Interpretation	
≤ 0.25	Susceptible	(S)
0.5 – 1.0	Intermediate	(I)
≥ 2.0	Resistant	(R)
Amoxicillin MIC (μg/mL) [a,b]	**Interpretation**	
≤ 0.25	Susceptible	(S)

[a] These are tentative breakpoints for the agar dilution methodology and they should not be used to interpret results obtained using alternative methods.

Continued on next page

Prilosec—Cont.

[b] There were not enough organisms with MICs > 0.25 µg/mL to determine a resistance breakpoint.

Standardized susceptibility test procedures require the use of laboratory control microorganisms to control the technical aspects of the laboratory procedures. Standard clarithromycin and amoxicillin powders should provide the following MIC values:

Microorganism	Antimicrobial Agent	MIC (µg/mL)[a]
H. pylori ATCC 43504	Clarithromycin	0.016 – 0.12 (µg/mL)
H. pylori ATCC 43504	Amoxicillin	0.016 – 0.12 (µg/mL)

[a] These are quality control ranges for the agar dilution methodology and they should not be used to control test results obtained using alternative methods.

INDICATIONS AND USAGE

Duodenal Ulcer

PRILOSEC Delayed-Release Capsules are indicated for short-term treatment of active duodenal ulcer. Most patients heal within four weeks. Some patients may require an additional four weeks of therapy.

PRILOSEC Delayed-Release Capsules, in combination with clarithromycin and amoxicillin, are indicated for treatment of patients with *H. pylori* infection and duodenal ulcer disease (active or up to 1-year history) to eradicate *H. pylori*.

PRILOSEC Delayed-Release Capsules, in combination with clarithromycin, are indicated for treatment of patients with *H. pylori* infection and duodenal ulcer disease to eradicate *H. pylori*.

Eradication of *H. pylori* has been shown to reduce the risk of duodenal ulcer recurrence. (See CLINICAL PHARMACOLOGY, Clinical Studies and DOSAGE AND ADMINISTRATION.)

[1] National Committee for Clinical Laboratory Standards. Summary Minutes, Subcommittee on Antimicrobial Susceptibility Testing, Tampa FL, January 11–13, 1998.

Among patients who fail therapy, PRILOSEC with clarithromycin is more likely to be associated with the development of clarithromycin resistance as compared with triple therapy. In patients who fail therapy, susceptibility testing should be done. If resistance to clarithromycin is demonstrated or susceptibility testing is not possible, alternative antimicrobial therapy should be instituted. (See Microbiology section, and the clarithromycin package insert, MICROBIOLOGY section.)

Gastric Ulcer

PRILOSEC Delayed-Release Capsules are indicated for short-term treatment (4–8 weeks) of active benign gastric ulcer. (See CLINICAL PHARMACOLOGY, Clinical Studies, Gastric Ulcer.)

Treatment of Gastroesophageal Reflux Disease (GERD)

Symptomatic GERD

PRILOSEC Delayed-Release Capsules are indicated for the treatment of heartburn and other symptoms associated with GERD.

Erosive Esophagitis

PRILOSEC Delayed-Release Capsules are indicated for the short-term treatment (4–8 weeks) of erosive esophagitis which has been diagnosed by endoscopy. (See CLINICAL PHARMACOLOGY, Clinical Studies.)

The efficacy of PRILOSEC used for longer than 8 weeks in these patients has not been established. In the rare instance of a patient not responding to 8 weeks of treatment, it may be helpful to give up to an additional 4 weeks of treatment. If there is recurrence of erosive esophagitis or GERD symptoms (eg, heartburn), additional 4–8 week courses of omeprazole may be considered.

Maintenance of Healing of Erosive Esophagitis

PRILOSEC Delayed-Release Capsules are indicated to maintain healing of erosive esophagitis.

Controlled studies do not extend beyond 12 months.

Pathological Hypersecretory Conditions

PRILOSEC Delayed-Release Capsules are indicated for the long-term treatment of pathological hypersecretory conditions (eg, Zollinger-Ellison syndrome, multiple endocrine adenomas and systemic mastocytosis).

CONTRAINDICATIONS

Omeprazole

PRILOSEC Delayed-Release Capsules are contraindicated in patients with known hypersensitivity to any component of the formulation.

Clarithromycin

Clarithromycin is contraindicated in patients with a known hypersensitivity to any macrolide antibiotic.

Concomitant administration of clarithromycin with cisapride, pimozide, or terfenadine is contraindicated. There have been post-marketing reports of drug interactions when clarithromycin and/or erythromycin are co-administered with cisapride, pimozide, or terfenadine resulting in cardiac arrhythmias (QT prolongation, ventricular tachycardia, ventricular fibrillation, and torsades de pointes) most likely due to inhibition of hepatic metabolism of these drugs by erythromycin and clarithromycin. Fatalities have been reported. (Please refer to full prescribing information for clarithromycin before prescribing.)

Clarithromycin Susceptibility Test Results and Clinical/Bacteriological Outcomes

Clarithromycin Susceptibility Test Results and Clinical/Bacteriological Outcomes[a]

Clarithromycin Pretreatment Results		Clarithromycin Post-treatment Results				
		H. pylori negative - eradicated	*H. pylori* positive - not eradicated Post-treatment susceptibility results			
			S[b]	I[b]	R[b]	No MIC
Dual Therapy - (omeprazole 40 mg q.d./clarithromycin 500 mg t.i.d. for 14 days followed by omeprazole 20 mg q.d. for another 14 days) (Studies M93–067, M93–100)						
Susceptible[b]	108	72	1		26	9
Intermediate[b]	1				1	
Resistant[b]	4				4	
Triple Therapy - (omeprazole 20 mg b.i.d./clarithromycin 500 mg b.i.d./amoxicillin 1 g b.i.d. for 10 days - Studies 126, 127, M96–446; followed by omeprazole 20 mg q.d. for another 18 days- Studies 126, 127)						
Susceptible[b]	171	153	7		3	8
Intermediate[b]						
Resistant[b]	14	4	1		6	3

[a]Includes only patients with pretreatment clarithromycin susceptibility test results

[b]Susceptible (S) MIC ≤ 0.25 µg/mL, Intermediate (I) MIC 0.5 – 1.0 µg/mL, Resistant (R) MIC ≥ 2 µg/mL

Amoxicillin

Amoxicillin is contraindicated in patients with a history of allergic reaction to any of the penicillins. (Please refer to full prescribing information for amoxicillin before prescribing.)

WARNINGS

Clarithromycin

CLARITHROMYCIN SHOULD NOT BE USED IN PREGNANT WOMEN EXCEPT IN CLINICAL CIRCUMSTANCES WHERE NO ALTERNATIVE THERAPY IS APPROPRIATE. IF PREGNANCY OCCURS WHILE TAKING CLARITHROMYCIN, THE PATIENT SHOULD BE APPRISED OF THE POTENTIAL HAZARD TO THE FETUS. (See WARNINGS in prescribing information for clarithromycin.)

Amoxicillin

SERIOUS AND OCCASIONALLY FATAL HYPERSENSITIVITY (anaphylactic) REACTIONS HAVE BEEN REPORTED IN PATIENTS ON PENICILLIN THERAPY. THESE REACTIONS ARE MORE LIKELY TO OCCUR IN INDIVIDUALS WITH A HISTORY OF PENICILLIN HYPERSENSITIVITY AND/OR A HISTORY OF SENSITIVITY TO MULTIPLE ALLERGENS. BEFORE INITIATING THERAPY WITH AMOXICILLIN, CAREFUL INQUIRY SHOULD BE MADE CONCERNING PREVIOUS HYPERSENSITIVITY REACTIONS TO PENICILLINS, CEPHALOSPORINS OR OTHER ALLERGENS. IF AN ALLERGIC REACTION OCCURS, AMOXICILLIN SHOULD BE DISCONTINUED AND APPROPRIATE THERAPY INSTITUTED. **SERIOUS ANAPHYLACTIC REACTIONS REQUIRE IMMEDIATE EMERGENCY TREATMENT WITH EPINEPHRINE. OXYGEN, INTRAVENOUS STEROIDS AND AIRWAY MANAGEMENT, INCLUDING INTUBATION, SHOULD ALSO BE ADMINISTERED AS INDICATED.** (See WARNINGS in prescribing information for amoxicillin.)

Antimicrobials

Pseudomembranous colitis has been reported with nearly all antibacterial agents and may range in severity from mild to life-threatening. Therefore, it is important to consider this diagnosis in patients who present with diarrhea subsequent to the administration of antibacterial agents. (See WARNINGS in prescribing information for clarithromycin and amoxicillin.)

Treatment with antibacterial agents alters the normal flora of the colon and may permit overgrowth of clostridia. Studies indicate that a toxin produced by *Clostridium difficile* is a primary cause of "antibiotic-associated colitis."

After the diagnosis of pseudomembranous colitis has been established, therapeutic measures should be initiated. Mild cases of pseudomembranous colitis usually respond to discontinuation of the drug alone. In moderate to severe cases, consideration should be given to management with fluids and electrolytes, protein supplementation, and treatment with an antibacterial drug clinically effective against *Clostridium difficile* colitis.

PRECAUTIONS

General

Symptomatic response to therapy with omeprazole does not preclude the presence of gastric malignancy.

Atrophic gastritis has been noted occasionally in gastric corpus biopsies from patients treated long-term with omeprazole.

Information for Patients

PRILOSEC Delayed-Release Capsules should be taken before eating. Patients should be cautioned that the PRILOSEC Delayed-Release Capsule should not be opened, chewed or crushed, and should be swallowed whole.

For patients who have difficulty swallowing capsules, the contents of a PRILOSEC Delayed-Release Capsule can be added to applesauce. One tablespoon of applesauce should be added to an empty bowl and the capsule should be opened. All of the pellets inside the capsule should be carefully emptied on the applesauce. The pellets should be mixed with the applesauce and then swallowed immediately with a glass of cool water to ensure complete swallowing of the pellets. The applesauce used should not be hot and should be soft enough to be swallowed without chewing. The pellets should not be chewed or crushed. The pellets/applesauce mixture should not be stored for future use.

Drug Interactions

Other

Omeprazole can prolong the elimination of diazepam, warfarin and phenytoin, drugs that are metabolized by oxidation in the liver. Although in normal subjects no interaction with theophylline or propranolol was found, there have been clinical reports of interaction with other drugs metabolized via the cytochrome P450 system (eg, cyclosporine, disulfiram, benzodiazepines). Patients should be monitored to determine if it is necessary to adjust the dosage of these drugs when taken concomitantly with PRILOSEC.

Because of its profound and long lasting inhibition of gastric acid secretion, it is theoretically possible that omeprazole may interfere with absorption of drugs where gastric pH is an important determinant of their bioavailability (eg, ketoconazole, ampicillin esters, and iron salts). In the clinical trials, antacids were used concomitantly with the administration of PRILOSEC.

Combination Therapy with Clarithromycin

Co-administration of omeprazole and clarithromycin have resulted in increases in plasma levels of omeprazole, clarithromycin, and 14-hydroxyclarithromycin. (See also CLINICAL PHARMACOLOGY, Pharmacokinetics: Combination Therapy with Antimicrobials.)

Concomitant administration of clarithromycin with cisapride, pimozide, or terfenadine is contraindicated.

There have been reports of an interaction between erythromycin and astemizole resulting in QT prolongation and torsades de pointes. Concomitant administration of erythromycin and astemizole is contraindicated. Because clarithromycin is also metabolized by cytochrome P450, concomitant administration of clarithromycin with astemizole is not recommended. (See also CONTRAINDICATIONS, Clarithromycin, above. Please refer to full prescribing information for clarithromycin before prescribing.)

Carcinogenesis, Mutagenesis, Impairment of Fertility

In two 24-month carcinogenicity studies in rats, omeprazole at daily doses of 1.7, 3.4, 13.8, 44.0 and 140.8 mg/kg/day (approximately 4 to 352 times the human dose, based on a patient weight of 50 kg and a human dose of 20 mg) produced gastric ECL cell carcinoids in a dose-related manner in both male and female rats; the incidence of this effect was markedly higher in female rats, which had higher blood levels of omeprazole. Gastric carcinoids seldom occur in the untreated rat. In addition, ECL cell hyperplasia was present in all treated groups of both sexes. In one of these studies, female rats were treated with 13.8 mg omeprazole/kg/day (approximately 35 times the human dose) for one year, then followed for an additional year without the drug. No carcinoids were seen in these rats. An increased incidence of treatment-related ECL cell hyperplasia was observed at the end of one year (94% treated vs 10% controls). By the second year the difference between treated and control rats was much smaller (46% vs 26%) but still showed more hyperplasia in the treated group. An unusual primary malignant tumor in the stomach was seen in one rat (2%). No similar tumor was seen in male or female rats treated for two years. For this strain of rat no similar tumor has been noted historically, but a finding involving only one tumor is difficult to interpret. A 78-week mouse carcinogenicity study of omeprazole did not show increased tumor occurrence, but the study was not conclusive.

Omeprazole was not mutagenic in an *in vitro* Ames *Salmonella typhimurium* assay, an *in vitro* mouse lymphoma cell assay and an *in vivo* rat liver DNA damage assay. A mouse micronucleus test at 625 and 6250 times the human dose gave a borderline result, as did an *in vivo* bone marrow chromosome aberration test. A second mouse micronucleus study at 2000 times the human dose, but with different (suboptimal) sampling times, was negative.

In a rat fertility and general reproductive performance test, omeprazole in a dose range of 13.8 to 138.0 mg/kg/day (approximately 35 to 345 times the human dose) was not toxic or deleterious to the reproductive performance of parental animals.

Pregnancy

Omeprazole

Pregnancy Category C

Teratology studies conducted in pregnant rats at doses up to 138 mg/kg/day (approximately 345 times the human dose) and in pregnant rabbits at doses up to 69 mg/kg/day (approximately 172 times the human dose) did not disclose any evidence for a teratogenic potential of omeprazole.

In rabbits, omeprazole in a dose range of 6.9 to 69.1 mg/kg/day (approximately 17 to 172 times the human dose) produced dose-related increases in embryo-lethality, fetal resorptions and pregnancy disruptions. In rats, dose-related embryo/fetal toxicity and postnatal developmental toxicity were observed in offspring resulting from parents treated with omeprazole 13.8 to 138.0 mg/kg/day (approximately 35 to 345 times the human dose). There are no adequate or well-controlled studies in pregnant women. Sporadic reports have been received of congenital abnormalities occurring in infants born to women who have received omeprazole during pregnancy. Omeprazole should be used during pregnancy only if the potential benefit justifies the potential risk to the fetus.

Clarithromycin

Pregnancy Category C. See WARNINGS (above) and full prescribing information for clarithromycin before using in pregnant women.

Nursing Mothers

It is not known whether omeprazole is excreted in human milk. In rats, omeprazole administration during late gestation and lactation at doses of 13.8 to 138 mg/kg/day (35 to 345 times the human dose) resulted in decreased weight gain in pups. Because many drugs are excreted in human milk, because of the potential for serious adverse reactions in nursing infants from omeprazole, and because of the potential for tumorigenicity shown for omeprazole in rat carcinogenicity studies, a decision should be made whether to discontinue nursing or to discontinue the drug, taking into account the importance of the drug to the mother.

Pediatric Use

Safety and effectiveness in pediatric patients have not been established.

Geriatric Use

Omeprazole was administered to over 2000 elderly individuals (≥ 65 years of age) in clinical trials in the US and Europe. There were no differences in safety and effectiveness between the elderly and younger subjects. Other reported clinical experience has not identified differences in response between the elderly and younger subjects, but greater sensitivity of some older individuals cannot be ruled out.

Pharmacokinetic studies have shown the elimination rate was somewhat decreased in the elderly and bioavailability was increased. The plasma clearance of omeprazole was 250 mL/min (about half that of young volunteers) and its plasma half-life averaged one hour, about twice that of young healthy volunteers. However, no dosage adjustment is necessary in the elderly. (See CLINICAL PHARMACOLOGY.)

ADVERSE REACTIONS

PRILOSEC Delayed-Release Capsules were generally well tolerated during domestic and international clinical trials in 3096 patients.

In the U.S. clinical trial population of 465 patients (including duodenal ulcer, Zollinger-Ellison syndrome and resistant ulcer patients), the following adverse experiences were reported to occur in 1% or more of patients on therapy with PRILOSEC. Numbers in parentheses indicate percentages of the adverse experiences considered by investigators as possibly, probably or definitely related to the drug:

	Omeprazole (n = 465)	Placebo (n = 64)	Ranitidine (n = 195)
Headache	6.9 (2.4)	6.3	7.7 (2.6)
Diarrhea	3.0 (1.9)	3.1 (1.6)	2.1 (0.5)
Abdominal Pain	2.4 (0.4)	3.1	2.1
Nausea	2.2 (0.9)	3.1	4.1 (0.5)
URI	1.9	1.6	2.6
Dizziness	1.5 (0.6)	0.0	2.6 (1.0)
Vomiting	1.5 (0.4)	4.7	1.5 (0.5)
Rash	1.5 (1.1)	0.0	0.0
Constipation	1.1 (0.9)	0.0	0.0
Cough	1.1	0.0	1.5
Asthenia	1.1 (0.2)	1.6 (1.6)	1.5 (1.0)
Back Pain	1.1	0.0	0.5

The following adverse reactions which occurred in 1% or more of omeprazole-treated patients have been reported in international double-blind, and open-label, clinical trials in which 2,631 patients and subjects received omeprazole.

Incidence of Adverse Experiences ≥ 1%
Causal Relationship not Assessed

	Omeprazole (n = 2631)	Placebo (n = 120)
Body as a Whole, site unspecified		
Abdominal pain	5.2	3.3
Asthenia	1.3	0.8
Digestive System		
Constipation	1.5	0.8
Diarrhea	3.7	2.5
Flatulence	2.7	5.8
Nausea	4.0	6.7
Vomiting	3.2	10.0
Acid regurgitation	1.9	3.3
Nervous System / Psychiatric		
Headache	2.9	2.5

Additional adverse experiences occurring in < 1% of patients or subjects in domestic and/or international trials, or occurring since the drug was marketed, are shown below within each body system. In many instances, the relationship to PRILOSEC was unclear.

Body As a Whole: Allergic reactions, including, rarely, anaphylaxis (see also *Skin* below), fever, pain, fatigue, malaise, abdominal swelling

Cardiovascular: Chest pain or angina, tachycardia, bradycardia, palpitation, elevated blood pressure, peripheral edema

Gastrointestinal: Pancreatitis (some fatal), anorexia, irritable colon, flatulence, fecal discoloration, esophageal candidiasis, mucosal atrophy of the tongue, dry mouth. During treatment with omeprazole, gastric fundic gland polyps have been noted rarely. These polyps are benign and appear to be reversible when treatment is discontinued.

Gastro-duodenal carcinoids have been reported in patients with ZE syndrome on long-term treatment with PRILOSEC. This finding is believed to be a manifestation of the underlying condition, which is known to be associated with such tumors.

Hepatic: Mild and, rarely, marked elevations of liver function tests [ALT (SGPT), AST (SGOT), γ-glutamyl transpeptidase, alkaline phosphatase, and bilirubin (jaundice)]. In rare instances, overt liver disease has occurred, including hepatocellular, cholestatic, or mixed hepatitis, liver necrosis (some fatal), hepatic failure (some fatal), and hepatic encephalopathy.

Metabolic / Nutritional: Hyponatremia, hypoglycemia, weight gain

Musculoskeletal: Muscle cramps, myalgia, muscle weakness, joint pain, leg pain

Nervous System / Psychiatric: Psychic disturbances including depression, aggression, hallucinations, confusion, insomnia, nervousness, tremors, apathy, somnolence, anxiety, dream abnormalities; vertigo; paresthesia; hemifacial dysesthesia

Respiratory: Epistaxis, pharyngeal pain

Skin: Rash and, rarely, cases of severe generalized skin reactions including toxic epidermal necrolysis (TEN; some fatal), Stevens-Johnson syndrome, and erythema multiforme (some severe); purpura and/or petechiae (some with rechallenge); skin inflammation, urticaria, angioedema, pruritus, alopecia, dry skin, hyperhidrosis

Special Senses: Tinnitus, taste perversion

Urogenital: Interstitial nephritis (some with positive rechallenge), urinary tract infection, microscopic pyuria, urinary frequency, elevated serum creatinine, proteinuria, hematuria, glycosuria, testicular pain, gynecomastia

Hematologic: Rare instances of pancytopenia, agranulocytosis (some fatal), thrombocytopenia, neutropenia, anemia, leucocytosis, and hemolytic anemia have been reported.

The incidence of clinical adverse experiences in patients greater than 65 years of age was similar to that in patients 65 years of age or less.

Combination Therapy for *H. pylori* Eradication

In clinical trials using either dual therapy with PRILOSEC and clarithromycin, or triple therapy with PRILOSEC, clarithromycin, and amoxicillin, no adverse experiences peculiar to these drug combinations have been observed. Adverse experiences that have occurred have been limited to those that have been previously reported with omeprazole, clarithromycin, or amoxicillin.

Triple Therapy (PRILOSEC / clarithromycin / amoxicillin)—The most frequent adverse experiences observed in clinical trials using combination therapy with PRILOSEC, clarithromycin, and amoxicillin (n = 274) were diarrhea (14%), taste perversion (10%), and headache (7%). None of these occurred at a higher frequency than that reported by patients taking the antimicrobial drugs alone.

For more information on clarithromycin or amoxicillin, refer to the respective package inserts, ADVERSE REACTIONS sections.

Dual Therapy (PRILOSEC / clarithromycin)—Adverse experiences observed in controlled clinical trials using combination therapy with PRILOSEC and clarithromycin (n = 346) which differed from those previously described for omeprazole alone were: Taste perversion (15%), tongue discoloration (2%), rhinitis (2%), pharyngitis (1%) and flu syndrome (1%).

For more information on clarithromycin, refer to the clarithromycin package insert, ADVERSE REACTIONS section.

OVERDOSAGE

Reports have been received of overdosage with omeprazole in humans. Doses ranged up to 2400 mg (120 times the usual recommended clinical dose). Manifestations were variable, but included confusion, drowsiness, blurred vision, tachycardia, nausea, vomiting, diaphoresis, flushing, headache, dry mouth, and other adverse reactions similar to those seen in normal clinical experience. (See ADVERSE REACTIONS.) Symptoms were transient, and no serious clinical outcome has been reported when PRILOSEC was taken alone. No specific antidote for omeprazole overdosage is known. Omeprazole is extensively protein bound and is, therefore, not readily dialyzable. In the event of overdosage, treatment should be symptomatic and supportive.

As with the management of any overdose, the possibility of multiple drug ingestion should be considered. For current information on treatment of any drug overdose, a certified Regional Poison Control Center should be contacted. Telephone numbers are listed in the Physicians' Desk Reference (PDR) or local telephone book.

Single oral doses of omeprazole at 1350, 1339, and 1200 mg/kg were lethal to mice, rats, and dogs, respectively. Animals given these doses showed sedation, ptosis, tremors, convulsions, and decreased activity, body temperature, and respiratory rate and increased depth of respiration.

DOSAGE AND ADMINISTRATION

Short-Term Treatment of Active Duodenal Ulcer

The recommended adult oral dose of PRILOSEC is 20 mg once daily. Most patients heal within four weeks. Some patients may require an additional four weeks of therapy. (See INDICATIONS AND USAGE.)

***H. pylori* Eradication for the Reduction of the Risk of Duodenal Ulcer Recurrence**

Triple Therapy (PRILOSEC / clarithromycin / amoxicillin)—The recommended adult oral regimen is PRILOSEC 20 mg plus clarithromycin 500 mg plus amoxicillin 1000 mg each given twice daily for 10 days. In patients with an ulcer present at the time of initiation of therapy, an additional 18 days of PRILOSEC 20 mg once daily is recommended for ulcer healing and symptom relief.

Dual Therapy (PRILOSEC / clarithromycin)—The recommended adult oral regimen is PRILOSEC 40 mg once daily plus clarithromycin 500 mg t.i.d. for 14 days. In patients with an ulcer present at the time of initiation of therapy, an additional 14 days of PRILOSEC 20 mg once daily is recommended for ulcer healing and symptom relief.

Please refer to clarithromycin full prescribing information for CONTRAINDICATIONS and WARNINGS, and for information regarding dosing in elderly and renally impaired patients (PRECAUTIONS: General, PRECAUTIONS: Geriatric Use and PRECAUTIONS: Drug Interactions).

Please refer to amoxicillin full prescribing information for CONTRAINDICATIONS and WARNINGS.

Gastric Ulcer

The recommended adult oral dose is 40 mg once a day for 4–8 weeks. (See CLINICAL PHARMACOLOGY, Clinical Studies, Gastric Ulcer, and INDICATIONS AND USAGE, Gastric Ulcer.)

Gastroesophageal Reflux Disease (GERD)

The recommended adult oral dose for the treatment of patients with symptomatic GERD and no esophageal lesions is 20 mg daily for up to 4 weeks. The recommended adult oral dose for the treatment of patients with erosive esophagitis and accompanying symptoms due to GERD is 20 mg daily for 4 to 8 weeks. (See INDICATIONS AND USAGE.)

Maintenance of Healing of Erosive Esophagitis

The recommended adult oral dose is 20 mg daily. (See CLINICAL PHARMACOLOGY, Clinical Studies.)

Pathological Hypersecretory Conditions

The dosage of PRILOSEC in patients with pathological hypersecretory conditions varies with the individual patient. The recommended adult oral starting dose is 60 mg once a day. Doses should be adjusted to individual patient needs and should continue for as long as clinically indicated. Doses up to 120 mg t.i.d. have been administered. Daily dosages of greater than 80 mg should be administered in divided doses. Some patients with Zollinger-Ellison syndrome have been treated continuously with PRILOSEC for more than 5 years.

No dosage adjustment is necessary for patients with renal impairment or for the elderly.

PRILOSEC Delayed-Release Capsules should be taken before eating. In the clinical trials, antacids were used concomitantly with PRILOSEC.

Patients should be cautioned that the PRILOSEC Delayed-Release Capsule should not be opened, chewed or crushed, and should be swallowed whole.

For patients who have difficulty swallowing capsules, the contents of a PRILOSEC Delayed-Release Capsule can be added to applesauce. One tablespoon of applesauce should be added to an empty bowl and the capsule should be opened. All of the pellets inside the capsule should be carefully emptied on the applesauce. The pellets should be mixed with the applesauce and then swallowed immediately with a glass of cool water to ensure complete swallowing of the pellets. The applesauce used should not be hot and should be soft enough to be swallowed without chewing. The pellets should not be chewed or crushed. The pellets/applesauce mixture should not be stored for future use.

HOW SUPPLIED

No. 3426—PRILOSEC Delayed-Release Capsules, 10 mg, are opaque, hard gelatin, apricot and amethyst colored capsules, coded 606 on cap and PRILOSEC 10 on the body. They are supplied as follows:

NDC 0186-0606-31 unit of use bottles of 30
NDC 0186-0606-68 bottles of 100
NDC 0186-0606-28 unit dose packages of 100
NDC 0186-0606-82 bottles of 1000.

No. 3440—PRILOSEC Delayed-Release Capsules, 20 mg, are opaque, hard gelatin, amethyst colored capsules, coded 742 on cap and PRILOSEC 20 on the body. They are supplied as follows:

NDC 0186-0742-31 unit of use bottles of 30

Continued on next page

Prilosec—Cont.

NDC 0186-0742-28 unit dose packages of 100
NDC 0186-0742-82 bottles of 1000.
No. 3428—PRILOSEC Delayed-Release Capsules, 40 mg, are opaque, hard gelatin, apricot and amethyst colored capsules, coded 743 on cap and PRILOSEC 40 on the body. They are supplied as follows:
NDC 0186-0743-31 unit of use bottles of 30
NDC 0186-0743-68 bottles of 100
NDC 0186-0743-28 unit dose packages of 100
NDC 0186-0743-82 bottles of 1000.

Storage
Store PRILOSEC Delayed-Release Capsules in a tight container protected from light and moisture. Store between 15°C and 30°C (59°F and 86°F).

Manufactured for: AstraZeneca LP, Wilmington, DE 19850
By: Merck & Co., Inc., Whitehouse Station, NJ 08889, USA
9194134
640004-34
Rev. 11/01

PULMICORT TURBUHALER® 200 mcg ℞

[*pull'mĭ-cōrt*]
(budesonide inhalation powder)
For Oral Inhalation Only.
Rx only

DESCRIPTION

Budesonide, the active component of PULMICORT TURBUHALER 200 mcg, is a corticosteroid designated chemically as (RS)-11β,16α,17,21-Tetrahydroxypregna-1,4-diene-3,20-dione cyclic 16,17-acetal with butyraldehyde. Budesonide is provided as a mixture of two epimers (22R and 22S). The empirical formula of budesonide is $C_{25}H_{34}O_6$ and its molecular weight is 430.5. Its structural formula is:

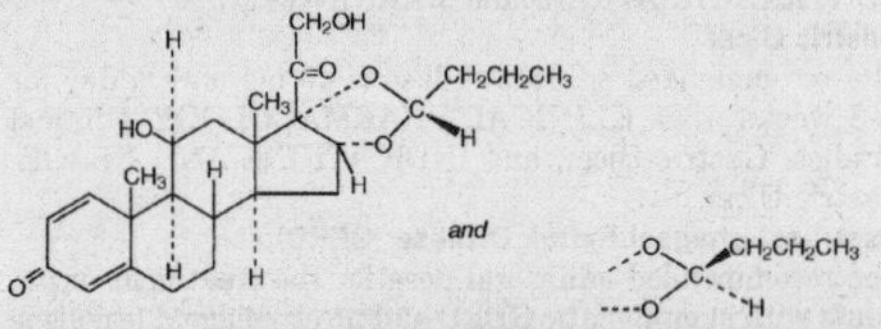

Budesonide is a white to off-white, tasteless, odorless powder that is practically insoluble in water and in heptane, sparingly soluble in ethanol, and freely soluble in chloroform. Its partition coefficient between octanol and water at pH 7.4 is 1.6×10^3.

PULMICORT TURBUHALER is an inhalation-driven multi-dose dry powder inhaler which contains only micronized budesonide. Each actuation of PULMICORT TURBUHALER provides 200 mcg budesonide per metered dose, which delivers approximately 160 mcg budesonide from the mouthpiece (based on *in vitro* testing at 60 L/min for 2 sec).

In vitro testing has shown that the dose delivery for PULMICORT TURBUHALER is substantially dependent on airflow through the device. Patient factors such as inspiratory flow rates will also affect the dose delivered to the lungs of patients in actual use (see *Patient's Instructions for Use*). In adult patients with asthma (mean FEV_1 2.9 L [0.8 – 5.1 L]) mean peak inspiratory flow (PIF) through PULMICORT TURBUHALER was 78 (40 – 111) L/min. Similar results (mean PIF 82 [43 – 125] L/min) were obtained in asthmatic children (6 to 15 years, mean FEV_1 2.1 L [0.9 – 5.4 L]). Patients should be carefully instructed on the use of this drug product to assure optimal dose delivery.

CLINICAL PHARMACOLOGY

Budesonide is an anti-inflammatory corticosteroid that exhibits potent glucocorticoid activity and weak mineralocorticoid activity. In standard *in vitro* and animal models, budesonide has approximately a 200-fold higher affinity for the glucocorticoid receptor and a 1000-fold higher topical anti-inflammatory potency than cortisol (rat croton oil ear edema assay). As a measure of systemic activity, budesonide is 40 times more potent than cortisol when administered subcutaneously and 25 times more potent when administered orally in the rat thymus involution assay.

The precise mechanism of corticosteroid actions on inflammation in asthma is not known. Corticosteroids have been shown to have a wide range of inhibitory activities against multiple cell types (eg, mast cells, eosinophils, neutrophils, macrophages, and lymphocytes) and mediators (eg, histamine, eicosanoids, leukotrienes, and cytokines) involved in allergic and non-allergic-mediated inflammation. These anti-inflammatory actions of corticosteroids may contribute to their efficacy in asthma.

Studies in asthmatic patients have shown a favorable ratio between topical anti-inflammatory activity and systemic corticosteroid effects over a wide range of doses from PULMICORT TURBUHALER. This is explained by a combination of a relatively high local anti-inflammatory effect, extensive first pass hepatic degradation of orally absorbed drug (85-95%), and the low potency of formed metabolites (see below).

Pharmacokinetics
The activity of PULMICORT TURBUHALER is due to the parent drug, budesonide. In glucocorticoid receptor affinity studies, the 22R form was two times as active as the 22S epimer. *In vitro* studies indicated that the two forms of budesonide do not interconvert. The 22R form was preferentially cleared by the liver with systemic clearance of 1.4 L/min vs. 1.0 L/min for the 22S form. The terminal half-life, 2 to 3 hours, was the same for both epimers and was independent of dose. In asthmatic patients, budesonide showed a linear increase in AUC and C_{max} with increasing dose after both a single dose and repeated dosing from PULMICORT TURBUHALER.

Absorption: After oral administration of budesonide, peak plasma concentration was achieved in about 1 to 2 hours and the absolute systemic availability was 6–13%. In contrast, most of budesonide delivered to the lungs is systemically absorbed. In healthy subjects, 34% of the metered dose was deposited in the lungs (as assessed by plasma concentration method) with an absolute systemic availability of 39% of the metered dose. Pharmacokinetics of budesonide do not differ significantly in healthy volunteers and asthmatic patients. Peak plasma concentrations of budesonide occurred within 30 minutes of inhalation from PULMICORT TURBUHALER.

Distribution: The volume of distribution of budesonide was approximately 3 L/kg. It was 85–90% bound to plasma proteins. Protein binding was constant over the concentration range (1–100 nmol/L) achieved with, and exceeding, recommended doses of PULMICORT TURBUHALER. Budesonide showed little or no binding to corticosteroid binding globulin. Budesonide rapidly equilibrated with red blood cells in a concentration independent manner with a blood/plasma ratio of about 0.8.

Metabolism: *In vitro* studies with human liver homogenates have shown that budesonide is rapidly and extensively metabolized. Two major metabolites formed via cytochrome P450 3A catalyzed biotransformation have been isolated and identified as 16α-hydroxyprednisolone and 6β-hydroxybudesonide. The corticosteroid activity of each of these two metabolites is less than 1% of that of the parent compound. No qualitative differences between the *in vitro* and *in vivo* metabolic patterns have been detected. Negligible metabolic inactivation was observed in human lung and serum preparations.

Excretion: Budesonide was excreted in urine and feces in the form of metabolites. Approximately 60% of an intravenous radiolabelled dose was recovered in the urine. No unchanged budesonide was detected in the urine.

Special Populations: No pharmacokinetic differences have been identified due to race, gender or advanced age.

Pediatric: Following intravenous dosing in pediatric patients age 10–14 years, plasma half-life was shorter than in adults (1.5 hours vs. 2.0 hours in adults). In the same population following inhalation of budesonide via a pressurized metered-dose inhaler, absolute systemic availability was similar to that in adults.

Hepatic Insufficiency: Reduced liver function may affect the elimination of corticosteroids. The pharmacokinetics of budesonide were affected by compromised liver function as evidenced by a doubled systemic availability after oral ingestion. The intravenous pharmacokinetics of budesonide were, however, similar in cirrhotic patients and in healthy subjects.

Drug-drug Interactions: Ketoconazole, a potent inhibitor of cytochrome P450 3A, the main metabolic enzyme for corticosteroids, increased plasma levels of orally ingested budesonide. At recommended doses, cimetidine had a slight but clinically insignificant effect on the pharmacokinetics of oral budesonide.

Pharmacodynamics
To confirm that systemic absorption is not a significant factor in the clinical efficacy of inhaled budesonide, a clinical study in patients with asthma was performed comparing 400 mcg budesonide administered via a pressurized metered-dose inhaler with a tube spacer to 1400 mcg of oral budesonide and placebo. The study demonstrated the efficacy of inhaled budesonide but not orally ingested budesonide despite comparable systemic levels. Thus, the therapeutic effect of conventional doses of orally inhaled budesonide are largely explained by its direct action on the respiratory tract.

Generally, PULMICORT TURBUHALER has a relatively rapid onset of action for an inhaled corticosteroid. Improvement in asthma control following inhalation of PULMICORT TURBUHALER can occur within 24 hours of beginning treatment although maximum benefit may not be achieved for 1 to 2 weeks, or longer. PULMICORT TURBUHALER has been shown to decrease airway reactivity to various challenge models, including histamine, methacholine, sodium metabisulfite, and adenosine monophosphate in hyperreactive patients. The clinical relevance of these models is not certain.

Pretreatment with PULMICORT TURBUHALER 1600 mcg daily (800 mcg twice daily) for 2 weeks reduced the acute (early-phase reaction) and delayed (late-phase reaction) decrease in FEV_1 following inhaled allergen challenge.

The effects of PULMICORT TURBUHALER on the hypothalamic-pituitary-adrenal (HPA) axis were studied in 905 adults and 404 pediatric patients with asthma. For most patients, the ability to increase cortisol production in response to stress, as assessed by cosyntropin (ACTH) stimulation test, remained intact with PULMICORT TURBUHALER treatment at recommended doses. For adult patients treated with 100, 200, 400, or 800 mcg twice daily for 12 weeks, 4%, 2%, 6%, and 13% respectively, had an abnormal stimulated cortisol response (peak cortisol <14.5 mcg/dL assessed by liquid chromatography following short-cosyntropin test) as compared to 8% of patients treated with placebo. Similar results were obtained in pediatric patients. In another study in adults, doses of 400, 800 and 1600 mcg budesonide twice daily via PULMICORT TURBUHALER for 6 weeks were examined; 1600 mcg twice daily (twice the maximum recommended dose) resulted in a 27% reduction in stimulated cortisol (6-hour ACTH infusion) while 10 mg prednisone resulted in a 35% reduction. In this study, no patient on Pulmicort Turbuhaler at doses of 400 and 800 mcg twice daily met the criterion for an abnormal stimulated cortisol response (peak cortisol <14.5 mcg/dL assessed by liquid chromatography) following ACTH infusion. An open-label, long-term follow-up of 1133 patients for up to 52 weeks confirmed the minimal effect on the HPA axis (both basal and stimulated plasma cortisol) of PULMICORT TURBUHALER when administered at recommended doses. In patients who had previously been oral steroid-dependent, use of PULMICORT TURBUHALER in recommended doses was associated with higher stimulated cortisol response compared to baseline following 1 year of therapy.

The administration of budesonide via PULMICORT TURBUHALER in doses up to 800 mcg/day (mean daily dose 445 mcg/day) or via a pressurized metered-dose inhaler in doses up to 1200 mcg/day (mean daily dose 620 mcg/day) to 216 pediatric patients (age 3 to 11 years) for 2 to 6 years had no significant effect on statural growth compared with non-corticosteroid therapy in 62 matched control patients. However, the long-term effect of PULMICORT TURBUHALER on growth is not fully known.

CLINICAL TRIALS

The therapeutic efficacy of PULMICORT TURBUHALER has been evaluated in controlled clinical trials involving more than 1300 patients (6 years and older) with asthma of varying disease duration (<1 year to >20 years) and severity.

Double-blind, parallel, placebo-controlled clinical trials of 12 weeks duration and longer have shown that, compared with placebo, PULMICORT TURBUHALER significantly improved lung function (measured by PEF and FEV_1), significantly decreased morning and evening symptoms of asthma, and significantly reduced the need for as-needed inhaled β_2-agonist use at doses of 400 mcg to 1600 mcg per day (200 mcg to 800 mcg twice daily) in adults and 400 mcg to 800 mcg per day (200 mcg to 400 mcg twice daily) in pediatric patients 6 years of age and older.

Improved lung function (morning PEF) was observed within 24 hours of initiating treatment in both adult and pediatric patients 6 years of age and older, although maximum benefit was not achieved for 1 to 2 weeks, or longer, after starting treatment. Improved lung function was maintained throughout the 12 weeks of the double-blind portion of the trials.

Patients Not Receiving Corticosteroid Therapy
In a 12-week clinical trial in 273 patients with mild to moderate asthma (mean baseline FEV_1 2.27 L) who were not well controlled by bronchodilators alone, PULMICORT TURBUHALER was evaluated at doses of 200 mcg twice daily and 400 mcg twice daily versus placebo. The FEV_1 results from this trial are shown in the figure below. Pulmonary function improved significantly on both doses of PULMICORT TURBUHALER compared with placebo.

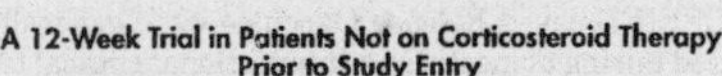
A 12-Week Trial in Patients Not on Corticosteroid Therapy Prior to Study Entry

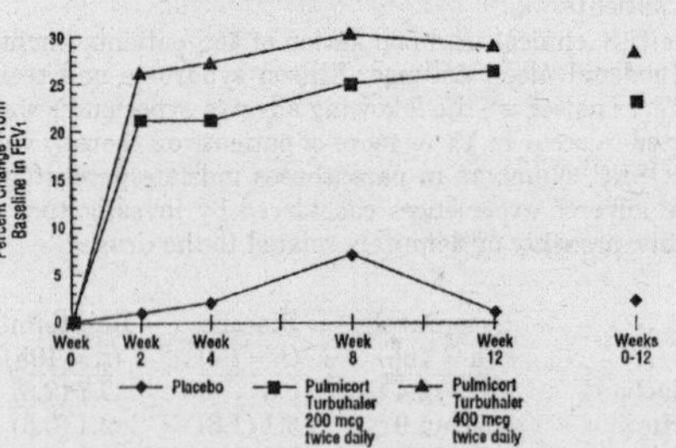

In a 12-month controlled trial in 75 patients not previously receiving corticosteroids, PULMICORT TURBUHALER at 200 mcg twice daily resulted in improved lung function (measured by PEF) and reduced bronchial hyperreactivity compared to placebo.

Patients Previously Maintained on Inhaled Corticosteroids
The safety and efficacy of PULMICORT TURBUHALER was also evaluated in adult and pediatric patients (age 6 to 18 years) previously maintained on inhaled corticosteroids (adults: N=473, mean baseline FEV_1 2.04 L, baseline doses of beclomethasone dipropionate 126-1008 mcg/day; pediatrics: N=404, mean baseline FEV_1 2.09 L, baseline doses of beclomethasone dipropionate 126-672 mcg/day or triamcinolone acetonide 300-1800 mcg/day). The FEV_1 results of these two trials, both 12 weeks in duration, are presented in the following figures. Pulmonary function improved significantly with all doses of PULMICORT TURBUHALER compared to placebo in both trials.

[See first figure at top of next column]
[See second figure at top of next column]

Patients Receiving PULMICORT TURBUHALER Once Daily
The efficacy and safety of once-daily administration of PULMICORT TURBUHALER 200 mcg and 400 mcg and

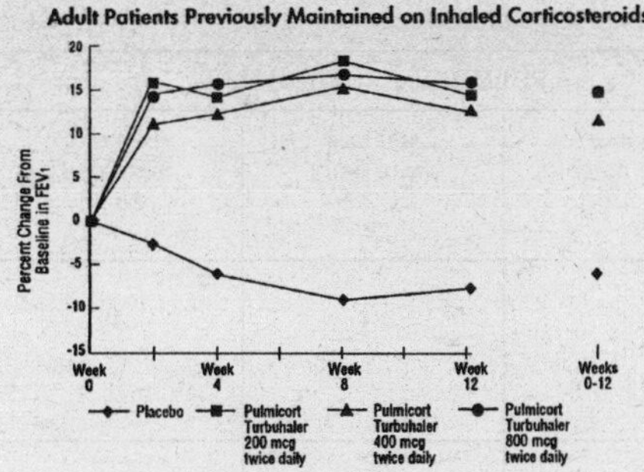

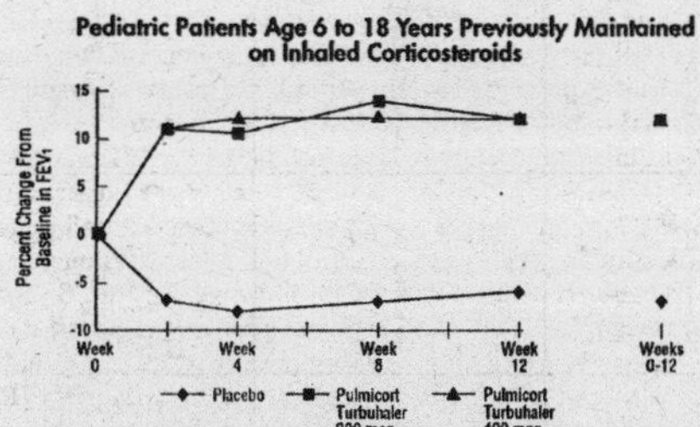

placebo were also evaluated in 309 adult asthmatic patients (mean baseline FEV_1 2.7 L) in an 18-week study. Compared with placebo, patients receiving Pulmicort 200 or 400 mcg once daily showed significantly better asthma stability as assessed by PEF and FEV_1 over an initial 6-week treatment period, which was maintained with a 200 mcg daily dose over the subsequent 12 weeks. Although the study population included both patients previously treated with inhaled corticosteroids, as well as patients not previously receiving corticosteroid therapy, the results showed that once-daily dosing was most clearly effective for those patients previously maintained on orally inhaled corticosteroids (see DOSAGE AND ADMINISTRATION).

Patients Previously Maintained on Oral Corticosteroids

In a clinical trial in 159 severe asthmatic patients requiring chronic oral prednisone therapy (mean baseline prednisone dose 19.3 mg/day) PULMICORT TURBUHALER at doses of 400 mcg twice daily and 800 mcg twice daily was compared to placebo over a 20-week period. Approximately two-thirds (68% on 400 mcg twice daily and 64% on 800 mcg twice daily) of PULMICORT TURBUHALER-treated patients were able to achieve sustained (at least 2 weeks) oral corticosteroid cessation (compared with 8% of placebo-treated patients) and improved asthma control. The average oral corticosteroid dose was reduced by 83% on 400 mcg twice daily and 79% on 800 mcg twice daily for PULMICORT TURBUHALER-treated patients vs. 27% for placebo. Additionally, 58 out of 64 patients (91%) who completely eliminated oral corticosteroids during the double-blind phase of the trial remained off oral corticosteroids for an additional 12 months while receiving PULMICORT TURBUHALER.

INDICATIONS AND USAGE

PULMICORT TURBUHALER is indicated for the maintenance treatment of asthma as prophylactic therapy in adult and pediatric patients six years of age or older. It is also indicated for patients requiring oral corticosteroid therapy for asthma. Many of those patients may be able to reduce or eliminate their requirement for oral corticosteroids over time.

PULMICORT TURBUHALER is NOT indicated for the relief of acute bronchospasm.

CONTRAINDICATIONS

PULMICORT TURBUHALER is contraindicated in the primary treatment of status asthmaticus or other acute episodes of asthma where intensive measures are required.

Hypersensitivity to budesonide contraindicates the use of PULMICORT TURBUHALER.

WARNINGS

Particular care is needed for patients who are transferred from systemically active corticosteroids to PULMICORT TURBUHALER because deaths due to adrenal insufficiency have occurred in asthmatic patients during and after transfer from systemic corticosteroids to less systemically available inhaled corticosteroids. After withdrawal from systemic corticosteroids, a number of months are required for recovery of HPA function.

Patients who have been previously maintained on 20 mg or more per day of prednisone (or its equivalent) may be most susceptible, particularly when their systemic corticosteroids have been almost completely withdrawn. During this period of HPA suppression, patients may exhibit signs and symptoms of adrenal insufficiency when exposed to trauma, surgery, or infection (particularly gastroenteritis) or other conditions associated with severe electrolyte loss. Although PULMICORT TURBUHALER may provide control of asthma symptoms during these episodes, in recommended doses it supplies less than normal physiological amounts of glucocorticoid systemically and does NOT provide the mineralocorticoid activity that is necessary for coping with these emergencies.

During periods of stress or a severe asthma attack, patients who have been withdrawn from systemic corticosteroids should be instructed to resume oral corticosteroids (in large doses) immediately and to contact their physicians for further instruction. These patients should also be instructed to carry a medical identification card indicating that they may need supplementary systemic corticosteroids during periods of stress or a severe asthma attack.

Transfer of patients from systemic corticosteroid therapy to PULMICORT TURBUHALER may unmask allergic conditions previously suppressed by the systemic corticosteroid therapy, eg, rhinitis, conjunctivitis, and eczema (see DOSAGE AND ADMINISTRATION).

Patients who are on drugs which suppress the immune system are more susceptible to infection than healthy individuals. Chicken pox and measles, for example, can have a more serious or even fatal course in susceptible pediatric patients or adults on immunosuppressant doses of corticosteroids. In pediatric or adult patients who have not had these diseases, particular care should be taken to avoid exposure. How the dose, route, and duration of corticosteroid administration affects the risk of developing a disseminated infection is not known. The contribution of the underlying disease and/or prior corticosteroid treatment to the risk is also not known. If exposed, therapy with varicella zoster immune globulin (VZIG) or pooled intravenous immunoglobulin (IVIG), as appropriate, may be indicated. If exposed to measles, prophylaxis with pooled intramuscular immunoglobulin (IG) may be indicated. (See the respective package inserts for complete VZIG and IG prescribing information.) If chicken pox develops, treatment with antiviral agents may be considered.

PULMICORT TURBUHALER is not a bronchodilator and is not indicated for rapid relief of bronchospasm or other acute episodes of asthma.

As with other inhaled asthma medications, bronchospasm, with an immediate increase in wheezing, may occur after dosing. If bronchospasm occurs following dosing with PULMICORT TURBUHALER, it should be treated immediately with a fast-acting inhaled bronchodilator. Treatment with PULMICORT TURBUHALER should be discontinued and alternate therapy instituted.

Patients should be instructed to contact their physician immediately when episodes of asthma not responsive to their usual doses of bronchodilators occur during treatment with PULMICORT TURBUHALER. During such episodes, patients may require therapy with oral corticosteroids.

PRECAUTIONS

General: During withdrawal from oral corticosteroids, some patients may experience symptoms of systemically active corticosteroid withdrawal, eg, joint and/or muscular pain, lassitude, and depression, despite maintenance or even improvement of respiratory function.

PULMICORT TURBUHALER will often permit control of asthma symptoms with less suppression of HPA function than therapeutically equivalent oral doses of prednisone. Since budesonide is absorbed into the circulation and can be systemically active at higher doses, the full beneficial effects of PULMICORT TURBUHALER in minimizing HPA dysfunction may be expected only when recommended dosages are not exceeded and individual patients are titrated to the lowest effective dose. Since individual sensitivity to effects on cortisol production exists, physicians should consider this information when prescribing PULMICORT TURBUHALER.

Because of the possibility of systemic absorption of inhaled corticosteroids, patients treated with these drugs should be observed carefully for any evidence of systemic corticosteroid effects. Particular care should be taken in observing patients postoperatively or during periods of stress for evidence of inadequate adrenal response.

It is possible that systemic corticosteroid effects such as hypercorticism and adrenal suppression may appear in a small number of patients, particularly at higher doses. If such changes occur, PULMICORT TURBUHALER should be reduced slowly, consistent with accepted procedures for management of asthma symptoms and for tapering of systemic steroids.

A reduction of growth velocity in children or teenagers may occur as a result of inadequate control of chronic diseases such as asthma or from use of corticosteroids for treatment. Physicians should closely follow the growth of all pediatric patients taking corticosteroids by any route and weigh the benefits of corticosteroid therapy and asthma control against the possibility of growth suppression (see PRECAUTIONS, Pediatric Use).

Although patients in clinical trials have received PULMICORT TURBUHALER on a continuous basis for periods of 1 to 2 years, the long-term local and systemic effects of PULMICORT TURBUHALER in human subjects are not completely known. In particular, the effects resulting from chronic use of PULMICORT TURBUHALER on developmental or immunological processes in the mouth, pharynx, trachea, and lung are unknown.

In clinical trials with PULMICORT TURBUHALER, localized infections with *Candida albicans* occurred in the mouth and pharynx in some patients. If oropharyngeal candidiasis develops, it should be treated with appropriate local or systemic (ie, oral) antifungal therapy while still continuing with PULMICORT TURBUHALER therapy, but at times therapy with PULMICORT TURBUHALER may need to be temporarily interrupted under close medical supervision.

Inhaled corticosteroids should be used with caution, if at all, in patients with active or quiescent tuberculosis infection of the respiratory tract, untreated systemic fungal, bacterial, viral or parasitic infections; or ocular herpes simplex.

Rare instances of glaucoma, increased intraocular pressure, and cataracts have been reported following the inhaled administration of corticosteroids.

Information for Patients: For proper use of PULMICORT TURBUHALER and to attain maximum improvement, the patient should read and follow the accompanying *Patient's Instructions for Use* carefully. In addition, patients being treated with PULMICORT TURBUHALER should receive the following information and instructions. This information is intended to aid the patient in the safe and effective use of the medication. It is not a disclosure of all possible adverse or intended effects.

- Patients should use PULMICORT TURBUHALER at regular intervals as directed since its effectiveness depends on regular use. The patient should not alter the prescribed dosage unless advised to do so by the physician.
- PULMICORT TURBUHALER is not a bronchodilator and is not intended to treat acute or life-threatening episodes of asthma.
- PULMICORT TURBUHALER must be in the upright position (mouthpiece on top) during loading in order to provide the correct dose. PULMICORT TURBUHALER must be primed when the unit is used for the very first time. To prime the unit, hold the unit in an upright position and turn the brown grip fully to the right, then fully to the left until it clicks. Repeat. The unit is now primed and ready to load the first dose by turning the grip fully to the right and fully to the left until it clicks.
  On subsequent uses, it is not necessary to prime the unit. However, it must be loaded in the upright position immediately prior to use. Turn the brown grip fully to the right, then fully to the left until it clicks. During inhalation, PULMICORT TURBUHALER must be held in the upright (mouthpiece up) or horizontal position. Do not shake the inhaler. Place the mouthpiece between lips and inhale forcefully and deeply. The powder is then delivered to the lungs.
- Patients should not exhale through PULMICORT TURBUHALER.
- Due to the small volume of powder, the patient may not taste or sense the presence of any medication entering the lungs when inhaling from TURBUHALER. This lack of "sensation" does not indicate that the patient is not receiving benefit from PULMICORT TURBUHALER.
- Rinsing the mouth with water without swallowing after each dosing may decrease the risk of the development of oral candidiasis.
- When there are 20 doses remaining in PULMICORT TURBUHALER, a red mark will appear in the indicator window.
- PULMICORT TURBUHALER should not be used with a spacer.
- The mouthpiece should not be bitten or chewed.
- The cover should be replaced securely after each opening.
- Keep PULMICORT TURBUHALER clean and dry at all times.
- Improvement in asthma control following inhalation of PULMICORT TURBUHALER can occur within 24 hours of beginning treatment although maximum benefit may not be achieved for 1 to 2 weeks, or longer. If symptoms do not improve in that time frame, or if the condition worsens, the patient should be instructed to contact the physician.
- Patients should be warned to avoid exposure to chicken pox or measles and if they are exposed, to consult their physicians without delay.
- For proper use of PULMICORT TURBUHALER and to attain maximum improvement, the patient should read and follow the accompanying *Patient's Instructions for Use*.

Drug Interactions: In clinical studies, concurrent administration of budesonide and other drugs commonly used in the treatment of asthma has not resulted in an increased frequency of adverse events. Ketoconazole, a potent inhibitor of cytochrome P450 3A, may increase plasma levels of budesonide during concomitant dosing. The clinical significance of concomitant administration of ketoconazole with PULMICORT TURBUHALER is not known, but caution may be warranted.

Carcinogenesis, Mutagenesis, Impairment of Fertility: Long-term studies were conducted in mice and rats using oral administration to evaluate the carcinogenic potential of budesonide.

There was no evidence of a carcinogenic effect when budesonide was administered orally for 91 weeks to mice at doses up to 200 mcg/kg/day (approximately $^1/_2$ the maximum recommended daily inhalation dose in adults and children on a mcg/m^2 basis).

In a 104-week oral study in Sprague-Dawley rats, a statistically significant increase in the incidence of gliomas was observed in male rats receiving an oral dose of 50 mcg/kg/day (approximately $^1/_4$ the maximum recommended daily inhalation dose on a mcg/m^2 basis); no such changes were seen in male rats receiving oral doses of 10 and 25 mcg/kg/day (approximately $^1/_{20}$ and $^1/_8$ the maximum recommended

Continued on next page

Pulmicort Turbuhaler—Cont.

daily inhalation dose on a mcg/m^2 basis) or in female rats at oral doses up to 50 mcg/kg/day (approximately 1/4 the maximum recommended human daily inhalation dose on a mcg/m^2 basis).

Two additional 104-week carcinogenicity studies have been performed with oral budesonide at doses of 50 mcg/kg/day (approximately 1/3 the maximum recommended daily inhalation dose in adults and children on a mcg/m^2 basis) in male Sprague-Dawley and Fischer rats. These studies did not demonstrate an increased glioma incidence in budesonide-treated animals as compared with concurrent controls or reference corticosteroid-treated groups (prednisolone and triamcinolone acetonide). Compared with concurrent controls, a statistically significant increase in the incidence of hepatocellular tumors was observed in all three steroid groups (budesonide, prednisolone, triamcinolone acetonide) in these studies.

The mutagenic potential of budesonide was evaluated in six different test systems; *Ames Salmonella*/microsome plate test, mouse micronucleus test, mouse lymphoma test, chromosome aberration test in human lymphocytes, sex-linked recessive lethal test in *Drosophila melanogaster*, and DNA repair analysis in rat hepatocyte culture. Budesonide was not mutagenic or clastogenic in any of these tests.

The effect of subcutaneous budesonide on fertility and general reproductive performance was studied in rats. At 20 mcg/kg/day (approximately 1/8 the maximum recommended daily inhalation dose in adults on a mcg/m^2 basis), decreases in maternal body weight gain, prenatal viability, and viability of the young at birth and during lactation were observed. No such effects were noted at 5 mcg/kg (approximately 1/32 the maximum recommended daily inhalation dose in adults on a mcg/m^2 basis).

Pregnancy: Teratogenic Effects: Pregnancy Category B: As with other glucocorticoids, budesonide produced fetal loss, decreased pup weight, and skeletal abnormalities at subcutaneous doses of 25 mcg/kg/day in rabbits (approximately 1/3 the maximum recommended daily inhalation dose in adults on a mcg/m^2 basis) and 500 mcg/kg/day in rats (approximately 3 times the maximum recommended daily inhalation dose in adults on a mcg/m^2 basis).

No teratogenic or embryocidal effects were observed in rats when budesonide was administered by inhalation at doses up to 250 mcg/kg/day (approximately 2 times the maximum recommended daily inhalation dose in adults on a mcg/m^2 basis).

Experience with oral corticosteroids since their introduction in pharmacologic as opposed to physiologic doses suggests that rodents are more prone to teratogenic effects from corticosteroids than humans.

Studies of pregnant women, however, have not shown that PULMICORT TURBUHALER increases the risk of abnormalities when administered during pregnancy. The results from a large population-based prospective cohort epidemiological study reviewing data from three Swedish registries covering approximately 99% of the pregnancies from 1995–1997 (i.e., Swedish Medical Birth Registry; Registry of Congenital Malformations; Child Cardiology Registry) indicate no increased risk for congenital malformations from the use of inhaled budesonide during early pregnancy. Congenital malformations were studied in 2,014 infants born to mothers reporting the use of inhaled budesonide for asthma in early pregnancy (usually 10–12 weeks after the last menstrual period), the period when most major organ malformations occur. The rate of recorded congenital malformations was similar compared to the general population rate (3.8% vs. 3.5%, respectively). In addition, after exposure to inhaled budesonide, the number of infants born with orofacial clefts was similar to the expected number in the normal population (4 children vs. 3.3, respectively).

These same data were utilized in a second study bringing the total to 2,534 infants whose mothers were exposed to inhaled budesonide. In this study, the rate of congenital malformations among infants whose mothers were exposed to inhaled budesonide during early pregnancy was not different from the rate for all newborn babies during the same period (3.6%).

Despite the animal findings, it would appear that the possibility of fetal harm is remote if the drug is used during pregnancy. Nevertheless, because the studies in humans cannot rule out the possibility of harm, PULMICORT TURBUHALER should be used during pregnancy only if clearly needed.

Nonteratogenic Effects: Hypoadrenalism may occur in infants born of mothers receiving corticosteroids during pregnancy. Such infants should be carefully observed.

Nursing Mothers: Corticosteroids are secreted in human milk. Because of the potential for adverse reactions in nursing infants from any corticosteroid, a decision should be made whether to discontinue nursing or discontinue the drug, taking into account the importance of the drug to the mother. Actual data for budesonide are lacking.

Pediatric Use: Safety and effectiveness of PULMICORT TURBUHALER in pediatric patients below 6 years of age have not been established.

In pediatric asthma patients the frequency of adverse events observed with PULMICORT TURBUHALER was similar between the 6- to 12-year age group (N=172) compared with the 13- to 17-year age group (N=124).

Oral corticosteroids have been shown to cause growth suppression in pediatric and adolescent patients, particularly with higher doses over extended periods. If a pediatric or adolescent patient on any corticosteroid appears to have growth suppression, the possibility that they are particularly sensitive to this effect of corticosteroids should be considered (see PRECAUTIONS).

Geriatric Use: One hundred patients 65 years or older were included in the US and non-US controlled clinical trials of PULMICORT TURBUHALER. There were no differences in the safety and efficacy of the drug compared to those seen in younger patients.

ADVERSE REACTIONS

The following adverse reactions were reported in patients treated with PULMICORT TURBUHALER.

The incidence of common adverse events is based upon double-blind, placebo-controlled US clinical trials in which 1,116 adult and pediatric patients age 6–70 years (472 females and 644 males) were treated with PULMICORT TURBUHALER (200 to 800 mcg twice daily for 12 to 20 weeks) or placebo.

The following table shows the incidence of adverse events in patients previously receiving bronchodilators and/or inhaled corticosteroids in US controlled clinical trials. This population included 232 male and 62 female pediatric patients (age 6 to 17 years) and 332 male and 331 female adult patients (age 18 years and greater).

[See table above]

Adverse Events with ≥ 3% Incidence reported by Patients on PULMICORT TURBUHALER

Adverse Event	Placebo N=284 %	PULMICORT TURBUHALER 200 mcg twice daily N=286 %	PULMICORT TURBUHALER 400 mcg twice daily N=289 %	PULMICORT TURBUHALER 800 mcg twice daily N=98 %
Respiratory System				
Respiratory infection	17	20	24	19
Pharyngitis	9	10	9	5
Sinusitis	7	11	7	2
Voice alteration	0	1	2	6
Body As A Whole				
Headache	7	14	13	14
Flu syndrome	6	6	6	14
Pain	2	5	5	5
Back pain	1	2	3	6
Fever	2	2	4	0
Digestive System				
Oral candidiasis	2	2	4	4
Dyspepsia	2	1	2	4
Gastroenteritis	1	1	2	3
Nausea	2	2	1	3
Average Duration of Exposure (days)	59	79	80	80

The table above includes all events (whether considered drug-related or non drug-related by the investigators) that occurred at a rate of ≥3% in any one PULMICORT TURBUHALER group and were more common than in the placebo group. In considering these data, the increased average duration of exposure for PULMICORT TURBUHALER patients should be taken into account.

The following other adverse events occurred in these clinical trials using PULMICORT TURBUHALER with an incidence of 1 to 3% and were more common on PULMICORT TURBUHALER than on placebo.

Body As A Whole: neck pain
Cardiovascular: syncope
Digestive: abdominal pain, dry mouth, vomiting
Metabolic and Nutritional: weight gain
Musculoskeletal: fracture, myalgia
Nervous: hypertonia, migraine
Platelet, Bleeding and Clotting: ecchymosis
Psychiatric: insomnia
Resistance Mechanisms: infection
Special Senses: taste perversion

In a 20-week trial in adult asthmatics who previously required oral corticosteroids, the effects of PULMICORT TURBUHALER 400 mcg twice daily (N=53) and 800 mcg twice daily (N=53) were compared with placebo (N=53) on the frequency of reported adverse events. Adverse events, whether considered drug-related or non drug-related by the investigators, reported in more than five patients in the PULMICORT TURBUHALER group and which occurred more frequently with PULMICORT TURBUHALER than placebo are shown below (% PULMICORT TURBUHALER and % placebo). In considering these data, the increased average duration of exposure for PULMICORT TURBUHALER patients (78 days for PULMICORT TURBUHALER vs. 41 days for placebo) should be taken into account.

Body As A Whole:	asthenia (9% and 2%)
	headache (12% and 2%)
	pain (10% and 2%)
Digestive:	dyspepsia (8% and 0%)
	nausea (6% and 0%)
	oral candidiasis (10% and 0%)
Musculoskeletal:	arthralgia (6% and 0%)
Respiratory:	cough increased (6% and 2%)
	respiratory infection (32% and 13%)
	rhinitis (6% and 2%)
	sinusitis (16% and 11%)

Patient Receiving PULMICORT TURBUHALER Once Daily

The adverse event profile of once-daily administration of PULMICORT TURBUHALER 200 mcg and 400 mcg, and placebo, was evaluated in 309 adult asthmatic patients in an 18-week study. The study population included both patients previously treated with inhaled corticosteroids, and patients not previously receiving corticosteroid therapy. There was no clinically relevant difference in the pattern of adverse events following once-daily administration of PULMICORT TURBUHALER when compared to twice-daily dosing.

Pediatric Studies: In a 12-week placebo-controlled trial in 404 pediatric patients 6 to 18 years of age previously maintained on inhaled corticosteroids, the frequency of adverse events for each age category (6 to 12 years, 13 to 18 years) was comparable for PULMICORT TURBUHALER (at 100, 200 and 400 mcg twice daily) and placebo. There were no clinically relevant differences in the pattern or severity of adverse events in children compared with those reported in adults.

Adverse Event Reports From Other Sources: Rare adverse events reported in the published literature or from marketing experience include: immediate and delayed hypersensitivity reactions including rash, contact dermatitis, urticaria, angioedema and bronchospasm; symptoms of hypocorticism and hypercorticism; psychiatric symptoms including depression, aggressive reactions, irritability, anxiety and psychosis.

OVERDOSAGE

The potential for acute toxic effects following overdose of Pulmicort Turbuhaler is low. If used at excessive doses for prolonged periods, systemic corticosteroid effects such as hypercorticism may occur (see PRECAUTIONS). PULMICORT TURBUHALER at twice the highest recommended dose (3200 mcg daily) administered for 6 weeks caused a significant reduction (27%) in the plasma cortisol response to a 6-hour infusion of ACTH compared with placebo (+1%). The corresponding effect of 10 mg prednisone daily was a 35% reduction in the plasma cortisol response to ACTH.

The minimal inhalation lethal dose in mice was 100 mg/kg (approximately 320 times the maximum recommended daily inhalation dose in adults and approximately 380 times the maximum recommended daily inhalation dose in children on a mcg/m^2 basis). There were no deaths following the administration of an inhalation dose of 68 mg/kg in rats (approximately 430 times the maximum recommended daily inhalation dose in adults and approximately 510 times the maximum recommended daily inhalation dose in children on a mcg/m2 basis). The minimal oral lethal dose was 200 mg/kg in mice (approximately 630 times the maximum recommended daily inhalation dose in adults and approximately 750 times the maximum recommended daily inhalation dose in children on a mcg/m^2 basis) and less than 100 mg/kg in rats (approximately 630 times the maximum recommended daily inhalation dose in adults and approximately 750 times the maximum recommended daily inhalation dose in children based on a mcg/m^2 basis).

DOSAGE AND ADMINISTRATION

PULMICORT TURBUHALER should be administered by the orally inhaled route in asthmatic patients age 6 years and older. Individual patients will experience a variable onset and degree of symptom relief. Generally, PULMICORT TURBUHALER has a relatively rapid onset of action for an inhaled corticosteroid. Improvement in asthma control following inhaled administration of PULMICORT TURBUHALER can occur within 24 hours of initiation of treatment, although maximum benefit may not be achieved for 1 to 2 weeks, or longer. The safety and efficacy of PULMICORT TURBUHALER when administered in excess of recommended doses have not been established.

The recommended starting dose and the highest recommended dose of PULMICORT TURBUHALER, based on prior asthma therapy, are listed in the following table.

[See table at top of next page]

If the once-daily treatment with PULMICORT TURBUHALER does not provide adequate control of asthma symptoms, the total daily dose should be increased and/or administered as a divided dose.

	Previous Therapy	Recommended Starting Dose	Highest Recommended Dose
Adults:	Bronchodilators alone	200 to 400 mcg twice daily	400 mcg twice daily
	Inhaled Corticosteroids*	200 to 400 mcg twice daily	800 mcg twice daily
	Oral Corticosteroids	400 to 800 mcg twice daily	800 mcg twice daily
Children:	Bronchodilators alone	200 mcg twice daily	400 mcg twice daily
	Inhaled Corticosteroids*	200 mcg twice daily	400 mcg twice daily
	Oral Corticosteroids	The highest recommended dose in children is 400 mcg twice daily	

*In patients with mild to moderate asthma who are well controlled on inhaled corticosteroids, dosing with PULMICORT TURBUHALER 200 mcg or 400 mcg once daily may be considered. PULMICORT TURBUHALER can be administered once daily either in the morning or in the evening.

Patients Maintained on Chronic Oral Corticosteroids
Initially, PULMICORT TURBUHALER should be used concurrently with the patient's usual maintenance dose of systemic corticosteroid. After approximately one week, gradual withdrawal of the systemic corticosteroid is started by reducing the daily or alternate daily dose. The next reduction is made after an interval of one or two weeks, depending on the response of the patient. Generally, these decrements should not exceed 2.5 mg of prednisone or its equivalent. A slow rate of withdrawal is strongly recommended. During reduction of oral corticosteroids, patients should be carefully monitored for asthma instability, including objective measures of airway function, and for adrenal insufficiency (see WARNINGS). During withdrawal, some patients may experience symptoms of systemic corticosteroid withdrawal, eg, joint and/or muscular pain, lassitude and depression, despite maintenance or even improvement in pulmonary function. Such patients should be encouraged to continue with PULMICORT TURBUHALER but should be monitored for objective signs of adrenal insufficiency. If evidence of adrenal insufficiency occurs, the systemic corticosteroid doses should be increased temporarily and thereafter withdrawal should continue more slowly. During periods of stress or a severe asthma attack, transfer patients may require supplementary treatment with systemic corticosteroids.

NOTE: In all patients it is desirable to titrate to the lowest effective dose once asthma stability is achieved.

Patients should be instructed to prime PULMICORT TURBUHALER prior to its initial use, and instructed to inhale deeply and forcefully each time the unit is used. Rinsing the mouth after inhalation is also recommended.

Directions for Use: Illustrated *Patient's Instructions for Use* accompany each package of PULMICORT TURBUHALER.

HOW SUPPLIED

PULMICORT TURBUHALER consists of a number of assembled plastic details, the main parts being the dosing mechanism, the storage unit for drug substance and the mouthpiece. The inhaler is protected by a white outer tubular cover screwed onto the inhaler. The body of the inhaler is white and the turning grip is brown. The following wording is printed on the grip in raised lettering, "Pulmicort™ 200 mcg". The TURBUHALER inhaler cannot be refilled and should be discarded when empty.

PULMICORT TURBUHALER is available as 200 mcg/dose, 200 doses (NDC 0186-0915-42) and has a target fill weight of 104 mg.

When there are 20 doses remaining in PULMICORT TURBUHALER, a red mark will appear in the indicator window. If the unit is used beyond the point at which the red mark appears at the bottom of the window, the correct amount of medication may not be obtained. The unit should be discarded.

Store with the cover tightened in a dry place at controlled room temperature 20–25°C (68–77°F) [see USP]. Keep out of the reach of children.

All trademarks are the property of the AstraZeneca group

Manufactured for: AstraZeneca LP, Wilmington, DE 19850
By: AstraZeneca AB, Södertälje, Sweden
808179–01 Rev. 12/01

Patient's Instructions for Use

Pulmicort Turbuhaler® 200 mcg
(budesonide inhalation powder)

Please read this leaflet carefully before you start to take your medicine. It provides a summary of information on your medicine.

FOR FURTHER INFORMATION ASK YOUR DOCTOR OR PHARMACIST.

WHAT YOU SHOULD KNOW ABOUT PULMICORT TURBUHALER®

Your doctor has prescribed PULMICORT TURBUHALER 200 mcg. It contains a medication called budesonide, which is a synthetic corticosteroid. Corticosteroids are natural substances found in the body that help fight inflammation. They are used to treat asthma because they reduce the swelling and irritation in the walls of the small air passages in the lungs and ease breathing problems. When inhaled regularly, corticosteroids also help to prevent attacks of asthma.

PULMICORT TURBUHALER treats the inflammation—the "quiet part" of asthma that you cannot hear, see, or feel. When inflammation is left untreated, your asthma symptoms and attacks can increase. PULMICORT TURBUHALER works to prevent and reduce your asthma symptoms and attacks.

IMPORTANT POINTS TO REMEMBER ABOUT PULMICORT TURBUHALER

1. MAKE SURE that this medicine is suitable for you (see "BEFORE USING YOUR PULMICORT TURBUHALER").
2. It is important that you inhale each dose as your doctor has advised.
3. Use your Turbuhaler as directed by your doctor. **DO NOT STOP TREATMENT OR REDUCE YOUR DOSE EVEN IF YOU FEEL BETTER,** unless told to do so by your doctor.
4. **DO NOT** inhale more doses or use your Turbuhaler more often than instructed by your doctor.
5. This medicine is **NOT** intended to provide rapid relief of your breathing difficulties during an asthma attack. It must be taken at regular intervals as recommended by your doctor, and not as an emergency measure.
6. Your doctor may prescribe additional medication (such as bronchodilators) for emergency relief if an acute asthma attack occurs. Please contact your doctor if:
   - an asthma attack does not respond to the additional medication,
   - you require more of the additional medication than usual.
7. If you also use another medicine by inhalation, you should consult your doctor for instructions on when to use it in relation to using your PULMICORT TURBUHALER.

BEFORE USING YOUR PULMICORT TURBUHALER

TELL YOUR DOCTOR BEFORE STARTING TO TAKE THIS MEDICINE:

- if you are pregnant (or intending to become pregnant),
- if you are breast-feeding a baby,
- if you are allergic to budesonide or any other orally inhaled corticosteroid.

In some circumstances, this medicine may not be suitable and your doctor may wish to give you a different medicine. Make sure that your doctor knows what other medicines you are taking.

USING YOUR PULMICORT TURBUHALER

- Follow the instructions shown in the section "HOW TO USE YOUR PULMICORT TURBUHALER". If you have any problems, tell your doctor or pharmacist.
- It is important that you inhale each dose as directed by your doctor. The pharmacy label will usually tell you what dose to take and how often. If it doesn't, or you are not sure, ask your doctor or pharmacist.

DOSAGE

- Use as directed by your doctor.
- It is **VERY IMPORTANT** that you follow your doctor's instructions as to how many inhalations to take and how often to use your PULMICORT TURBUHALER.
- **DO NOT** inhale more doses or use your PULMICORT TURBUHALER more often than your doctor advises.
- It may take 1 to 2 weeks or longer before you feel maximum improvement, so **IT IS VERY IMPORTANT THAT YOU USE PULMICORT TURBUHALER REGULARLY. DO NOT STOP TREATMENT OR REDUCE YOUR DOSE EVEN IF YOU ARE FEELING BETTER,** unless told to do so by your doctor.
- If you miss a dose, just take your regularly scheduled next dose when it is due. **DO NOT DOUBLE** the dose.

HOW TO USE YOUR PULMICORT TURBUHALER

Read the complete instructions carefully and use only as directed.

PRIMING INSTRUCTIONS:

Before you use a new PULMICORT TURBUHALER for the first time, you should prime it. To do this, turn the cover and lift off. Hold PULMICORT TURBUHALER upright (with mouthpiece up), then twist the brown grip fully to the right and back again to the left. Repeat. Now you are ready to take your first dose (see instructions for "TAKING A DOSE"). **You do not have to prime it any other time after this, even if you put it aside for a prolonged period of time.**

TAKING A DOSE:

1 LOADING A DOSE

- Twist the cover and lift off.
- In order to provide the correct dose, **PULMICORT TURBUHALER must be held in the upright position (mouthpiece up) whenever a dose of medication is being loaded.**
- Twist the brown grip fully to the right as far as it will go. Twist it back again fully to the left.
- You will hear a click.

2 INHALING THE DOSE

- When you are inhaling, PULMICORT TURBUHALER must be held in the upright (mouthpiece up) or horizontal position.
- Turn your head away from the inhaler and breathe out. **Do not shake the inhaler after loading it.**
- Place the mouthpiece between your lips and inhale deeply and forcefully. You may not taste or feel the medication.
- Do not chew or bite on the mouthpiece.
- Remove the inhaler from your mouth and exhale. Do not blow or exhale into the mouthpiece.
- If more than one dose is required, just repeat the steps above.
- **When you are finished, place the cover back on** the inhaler and twist shut. **Rinse your mouth with water. Do not swallow.**
- **Keep your PULMICORT TURBUHALER clean and dry at all times.**
- Do not use PULMICORT TURBUHALER if it has been damaged or if the mouthpiece has become detached.

STORING YOUR PULMICORT TURBUHALER

- After each use, place the white cover back on and twist it firmly into place.
- Keep PULMICORT TURBUHALER in a dry place at controlled room temperature, 68–77°F (20–25°C).
- Keep your PULMICORT TURBUHALER out of the **reach of young children.**
- **DO NOT** use after the date shown on the body of your Turbuhaler.

HOW TO KNOW WHEN YOUR PULMICORT TURBUHALER IS EMPTY

The label on the box or cover will tell you how many doses are in your PULMICORT TURBUHALER.

Your PULMICORT TURBUHALER has a convenient dose indicator window just below the mouthpiece.

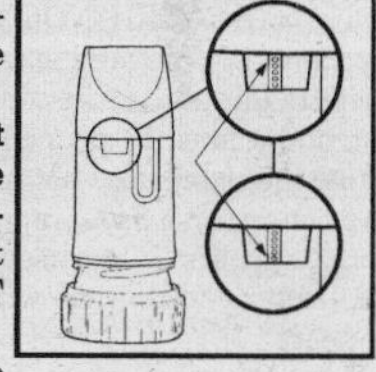

- **When a red mark appears at the top of the window, there are 20 doses of medicine remaining.** Now is the time to get your next PULMICORT TURBUHALER.
- **When the red mark reaches the bottom of the window, your inhaler should be discarded as it may no longer deliver the correct amount of medication.** (You may still hear a sound if you shake it—this sound is not the medicine. This sound is produced by the drying agent inside the Turbuhaler.)
- **Do not immerse it in water to find out if it is empty. Simply check your dose indicator window.**

FURTHER INFORMATION ABOUT PULMICORT TURBUHALER

- PULMICORT TURBUHALER delivers your medicine as a very fine powder **that you may not taste, smell, or feel.** By following the instructions for use in this leaflet, you can be confident that you have received the correct dose.
- PULMICORT TURBUHALER should not be used with a spacer.
- PULMICORT TURBUHALER contains only budesonide and does not contain any inactive ingredients.
- PULMICORT TURBUHALER is specially designed to deliver only one dose at a time, no matter how often you click the brown grip. If you accidentally blow into your inhaler after loading a dose, simply follow the instructions for loading a new dose.

This leaflet does not contain the complete information about your medicine. If you have any questions, or are not sure about something, then you should ask your doctor or pharmacist.

You may want to read this leaflet again. Please DO NOT THROW IT AWAY until you have finished your medicine.

REMEMBER: This medicine has been prescribed for you by your doctor. DO NOT give this medicine to anyone else.

USE THIS PRODUCT AS DIRECTED, UNLESS INSTRUCTED TO DO OTHERWISE BY YOUR DOCTOR. If you have further questions about the use of PULMICORT TURBUHALER, call: 1-800-237-8898

Extended Text™ INCIRC™ U.K. Pat. App. Nos. 9019032.3 & 9400832.3, Euro Pat. App. Nos. 91915912.9 & 94200154.6, U.S. Pat. No. 5399403.

PULMICORT TURBUHALER is a trademark of the AstraZeneca group

 808259-01 Rev. 12/01

RHINOCORT AQUA™ ℞

[*rhīnō-cōrt aquă*]
(budesonide)
NASAL SPRAY 32 mcg
For Intranasal Use Only.
Rx only

Prescribing information for this product, which appears on pages 642–643 of the 2002 PDR, has been completely revised as follows. Please write "See Supplement A" next to the product heading.

Continued on next page

Rhinocort Aqua—Cont.

DESCRIPTION

Budesonide, the active ingredient of RHINOCORT AQUA™ Nasal Spray, is an anti-inflammatory synthetic corticosteroid.

It is designated chemically as (RS)-11-beta, 16-alpha, 17, 21-tetrahydroxypregna-1, 4-diene-3,20-dione cyclic 16, 17-acetal with butyraldehyde.

Budesonide is provided as the mixture of two epimers (22R and 22S).

The empirical formula of budesonide is $C_{25}H_{34}O_6$ and its molecular weight is 430.5.

Its structural formula is:

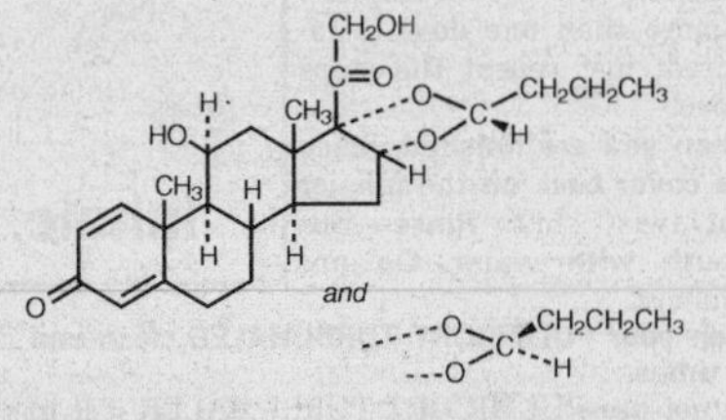

Budesonide is a white to off-white, odorless powder that is practically insoluble in water and in heptane, sparingly soluble in ethanol, and freely soluble in chloroform.

Its partition coefficient between octanol and water at pH 5 is 1.6×10^3.

RHINOCORT AQUA is an unscented, metered-dose, manual-pump spray formulation containing a micronized suspension of budesonide in an aqueous medium. Microcrystalline cellulose and carboxymethyl cellulose sodium, dextrose anhydrous, polysorbate 80, disodium edetate, potassium sorbate, and purified water are contained in this medium; hydrochloric acid is added to adjust the pH to a target of 4.5. RHINOCORT AQUA Nasal Spray delivers 32 mcg of budesonide per spray.

Each bottle of RHINOCORT AQUA Nasal Spray 32 mcg contains 120 metered sprays after initial priming.

Prior to initial use, the container must be shaken gently and the pump must be primed by actuating eight times. If used daily, the pump does not need to be reprimed. If not used for two consecutive days, reprime with one spray or until a fine spray appears. If not used for more than 14 days, rinse the applicator and reprime with two sprays or until a fine spray appears.

CLINICAL PHARMACOLOGY

Budesonide is a synthetic corticosteroid having potent glucocorticoid activity and weak mineralocorticoid activity. In standard *in vitro* and animal models, budesonide has approximately a 200-fold higher affinity for the glucocorticoid receptor and a 1000-fold higher topical anti-inflammatory potency than cortisol (rat croton oil ear edema assay). As a measure of systemic activity, budesonide is 40 times more potent than cortisol when administered subcutaneously and 25 times more potent when administered orally in the rat thymus involution assay. In glucocorticoid receptor affinity studies, the 22R form was twice as active as the 22S epimer. The precise mechanism of corticosteroid actions in seasonal and perennial allergic rhinitis is not known. Corticosteroids have been shown to have a wide range of inhibitory activities against multiple cell types (eg, mast cells, eosinophils, neutrophils, macrophages, and lymphocytes) and mediators (eg, histamine, eicosanoids, leukotrienes, and cytokines) involved in allergic mediated inflammation.

Corticosteroids affect the delayed (6 hour) response to an allergen challenge more than the histamine-associated immediate response (20 minute). The clinical significance of these findings is unknown.

Pharmacokinetics

The pharmacokinetics of budesonide have been studied following nasal, oral, and intravenous administration. Budesonide is relatively well absorbed after both inhalation and oral administration, and is rapidly metabolized into metabolites with low corticosteroid potency. The clinical activity of RHINOCORT AQUA Nasal Spray is therefore believed to be due to the parent drug, budesonide. *In vitro* studies indicate that the two epimeric forms of budesonide do not interconvert.

Absorption

Following intranasal administration of RHINOCORT AQUA, the mean peak plasma concentration occurs at approximately 0.7 hours. Compared to an intravenous dose, approximately 34% of the delivered intranasal dose reaches the systemic circulation, most of which is absorbed through the nasal mucosa. While budesonide is well absorbed from the GI tract, the oral bioavailability of budesonide is low (~10%) primarily due to extensive first pass metabolism in the liver.

Distribution

Budesonide has a volume of distribution of approximately 2–3 L/kg. The volume of distribution for the 22R epimer is almost twice that of the 22S epimer. Protein binding of budesonide *in vitro* is constant (85–90%) over a concentration range (1–100 nmol/L) which exceeded that achieved after administration of recommended doses. Budesonide shows little to no binding to glucocorticosteroid binding globulin. It rapidly equilibrates with red blood cells in a concentration independent manner with a blood/plasma ratio of about 0.8.

Metabolism

Budesonide is rapidly and extensively metabolized in humans by the liver. Two major metabolites (16α-hydroxyprednisolone and 6β-hydroxybudesonide) are formed via cytochrome P450 3A isoenzyme-catalyzed biotransformation. Known metabolic inhibitors of cytochrome P450 3A (eg, ketoconazole), or significant hepatic impairment, may increase the systemic exposure of unmetabolized budesonide (see WARNINGS and PRECAUTIONS). *In vitro* studies on the binding of the two primary metabolites to the glucocorticoid receptor indicate that they have less than 1% of the affinity for the receptor as the parent compound budesonide. *In vitro* studies have evaluated sites of metabolism and showed negligible metabolism in skin, lung, and serum. No qualitative difference between the *in vitro* and *in vivo* metabolic patterns could be detected.

Elimination

Budesonide is excreted in the urine and feces in the form of metabolites. After intranasal administration of a radiolabeled dose, 2/3 of the radioactivity was found in the urine and the remainder in the feces. The main metabolites of budesonide in the 0–24 hour urine sample following IV administration are 16α-hydroxyprednisolone (24%) and 6β-hydroxybudesonide (5%). An additional 34% of the radioactivity recovered in the urine was identified as conjugates.

The 22R form was preferentially cleared with clearance value of 1.4 L/min vs. 1.0 L/min for the 22S form. The terminal half-life, 2 to 3 hours, was similar for both epimers and it appeared to be independent of dose.

Special Populations

Geriatric: No specific pharmacokinetic study has been undertaken in subjects >65 years of age.

Pediatric: After administration of RHINOCORT AQUA Nasal Spray, the time to reach peak drug concentrations and plasma half-life were similar in children and in adults. Children had plasma concentrations approximately twice those observed in adults due primarily to differences in weight between children and adults.

Gender: No specific pharmacokinetic study has been conducted to evaluate the effect of gender on budesonide pharmacokinetics. However, following administration of 400 mcg RHINOCORT AQUA Nasal Spray to 7 male and 8 female volunteers in a pharmacokinetic study, no major gender differences in the pharmacokinetic parameters were found.

Race: No specific study has been undertaken to evaluate the effect of race on budesonide pharmacokinetics.

Renal Insufficiency: The pharmacokinetics of budesonide have not been investigated in patients with renal insufficiency.

Hepatic Insufficiency: Reduced liver function may affect the elimination of corticosteroids. The pharmacokinetics of orally administered budesonide were affected by compromised liver function as evidenced by a doubled systemic availability. The relevance of this finding to intranasally administered budesonide has not been established.

Pharmacodynamics

A 3-week clinical study in seasonal rhinitis, comparing RHINOCORT Nasal Inhaler, orally ingested budesonide, and placebo in 98 patients with allergic rhinitis due to birch pollen, demonstrated that the therapeutic effect of RHINOCORT Nasal Inhaler can be attributed to the topical effects of budesonide.

The effects of RHINOCORT AQUA Nasal Spray on adrenal function have been evaluated in several clinical trials. In a four-week clinical trial, 61 adult patients who received 256 mcg daily of RHINOCORT AQUA Nasal Spray demonstrated no significant differences from patients receiving placebo in plasma cortisol levels measured before and 60 minutes after 0.25 mg intramuscular cosyntropin. There were no consistent differences in 24-hour urinary cortisol measurements in patients receiving up to 400 mcg daily. Similar results were seen in a study of 150 children and adolescents aged 6 to 17 with perennial rhinitis who were treated with 256 mcg daily for up to 12 months.

After treatment with the recommended maximal daily dose of RHINOCORT AQUA (256 mcg) for seven days, there was a small, but statistically significant decrease in the area under the plasma cortisol-time curve over 24 hours (AUC_{0-24h}) in healthy adult volunteers.

A dose-related suppression of 24-hour urinary cortisol excretion was observed after administration of RHINOCORT AQUA doses ranging from 100–800 mcg daily for up to four days in 78 healthy adult volunteers. The clinical relevance of these results is unknown.

Clinical Trials

The therapeutic efficacy of RHINOCORT AQUA Nasal Spray has been evaluated in placebo-controlled clinical trials of seasonal and perennial allergic rhinitis of 3–6 weeks duration.

The number of patients treated with budesonide in these studies was 90 males and 51 females aged 6–12 years and 691 males and 694 females 12 years and above. The patients were predominantly Caucasian.

Overall, the results of these clinical trials showed that RHINOCORT AQUA Nasal Spray administered once daily provides statistically significant reduction in the severity of nasal symptoms of seasonal and perennial allergic rhinitis including runny nose, sneezing, and nasal congestion.

An improvement in nasal symptoms may be noted in patients within 10 hours of first using RHINOCORT AQUA Nasal Spray. This time to onset is supported by an environmental exposure unit study in seasonal allergic rhinitis patients which demonstrated that RHINOCORT AQUA Nasal Spray led to a statistically significant improvement in nasal symptoms compared to placebo by 10 hours. Further support comes from a clinical study of patients with perennial allergic rhinitis which demonstrated a statistically significant improvement in nasal symptoms for both RHINOCORT AQUA Nasal Spray and for the active comparator (mometasone furoate) compared to placebo by 8 hours. Onset was also assessed in this study with peak nasal inspiratory flow rate and this endpoint failed to show efficacy for either active treatment. Although statistically significant improvements in nasal symptoms compared to placebo were noted within 8–10 hours in these studies, about one half to two thirds of the ultimate clinical improvement with RHINOCORT AQUA Nasal Spray occurs over the first 1–2 days, and maximum benefit may not be achieved until approximately 2 weeks after initiation of treatment.

INDICATIONS AND USAGE

RHINOCORT AQUA Nasal Spray is indicated for the management of nasal symptoms of seasonal or perennial allergic rhinitis in adults and children six years of age and older.

CONTRAINDICATIONS

Hypersensitivity to any of the ingredients in this preparation contraindicates the use of RHINOCORT AQUA Nasal Spray.

WARNINGS

The replacement of a systemic corticosteroid with a topical corticosteroid can be accompanied by signs of adrenal insufficiency, and in addition some patients may experience symptoms of corticosteroid withdrawal, eg, joint and/or muscular pain, lassitude, and depression. Patients previously treated for prolonged periods with systemic corticosteroids and transferred to topical corticosteroids should be carefully monitored for acute adrenal insufficiency in response to stress. In those patients who have asthma or other clinical conditions requiring long-term systemic corticosteroid treatment, too rapid a decrease in systemic corticosteroids may cause a severe exacerbation of their symptoms.

Patients who are on drugs which suppress the immune system are more susceptible to infections than healthy individuals. Chicken pox and measles, for example, can have a more serious or even fatal course in non-immune children or adults on immunosuppressant doses of corticosteroids. In such children or adults who have not had these diseases, particular care should be taken to avoid exposure. How the dose, route, and duration of corticosteroid administration affects the risk of developing a disseminated infection is not known. The contribution of the underlying disease and/or prior corticosteroid treatment to the risk is also not known. If exposed to chicken pox, prophylaxis with varicella zoster immune globulin (VZIG) may be indicated. If exposed to measles, prophylaxis with pooled intramuscular immunoglobulin (IG) may be indicated. (See the respective package inserts for complete VZIG and IG prescribing information). If chicken pox develops, treatment with antiviral agents may be considered.

PRECAUTIONS

General

Intranasal corticosteroids may cause a reduction in growth velocity when administered to pediatric patients (see PRECAUTIONS, Pediatric Use).

Rarely, immediate and/or delayed hypersensitivity reactions may occur after the intranasal administration of budesonide. Rare instances of wheezing, nasal septum perforation, and increased intraocular pressure have been reported following the intranasal application of corticosteroids, including budesonide.

Although systemic effects have been minimal with recommended doses of RHINOCORT AQUA Nasal Spray, any such effect is dose dependent. Therefore, larger than recommended doses of RHINOCORT AQUA Nasal Spray should be avoided and the minimal effective dose for the patient should be used (see DOSAGE AND ADMINISTRATION). When used at larger doses, systemic corticosteroid effects such as hypercorticism and adrenal suppression may appear. If such changes occur, the dosage of RHINOCORT AQUA Nasal Spray should be discontinued slowly, consistent with accepted procedures for discontinuing oral corticosteroid therapy.

In clinical studies with budesonide administered intranasally, the development of localized infections of the nose and pharynx with *Candida albicans* has occurred only rarely. When such an infection develops, it may require treatment with appropriate local or systemic therapy and discontinuation of treatment with RHINOCORT AQUA Nasal Spray. Patients using RHINOCORT AQUA Nasal Spray over several months or longer should be examined periodically for evidence of *Candida* infection or other signs of adverse effects on the nasal mucosa.

RHINOCORT AQUA Nasal Spray should be used with caution, if at all, in patients with active or quiescent tuberculous infection, untreated fungal, bacterial, or systemic viral infections, or ocular herpes simplex.

Because of the inhibitory effect of corticosteroids on wound healing, patients who have experienced recent nasal septal ulcers, nasal surgery, or nasal trauma should not use a nasal corticosteroid until healing has occurred.

Hepatic dysfunction influences the pharmacokinetics of budesonide, similar to the effect on other corticosteroids, with a reduced elimination rate and increased systemic availability (see CLINICAL PHARMACOLOGY, Special Populations).

Information for Patients

Patients being treated with RHINOCORT AQUA Nasal Spray should receive the following information and instructions. Patients who are on immunosuppressant doses of corticosteroids should be warned to avoid exposure to chicken pox or measles and, if exposed, to obtain medical advice.

Patients should use RHINOCORT AQUA Nasal Spray at regular intervals since its effectiveness depends on its regular use (see DOSAGE AND ADMINISTRATION).

An improvement in nasal symptoms may be noted in patients within 10 hours of first using RHINOCORT AQUA Nasal Spray. This time to onset is supported by an environmental exposure unit study in seasonal allergic rhinitis patients which demonstrated that RHINOCORT AQUA Nasal Spray led to a statistically significant improvement in nasal symptoms compared to placebo by 10 hours. Further support comes from a clinical study of patients with perennial allergic rhinitis which demonstrated a statistically significant improvement in nasal symptoms for both RHINOCORT AQUA Nasal Spray and for the active comparator (mometasone furoate) compared to placebo by 8 hours. Onset was also assessed in this study with peak nasal inspiratory flow rate and this endpoint failed to show efficacy for either active treatment. Although statistically significant improvements in nasal symptoms compared to placebo were noted within 8–10 hours in these studies, about one half to two thirds of the ultimate clinical improvement with RHINOCORT AQUA Nasal Spray occurs over the first 1–2 days, and maximum benefit may not be achieved until approximately 2 weeks after initiation of treatment. Initial assessment for response should be made during this time frame and periodically until the patient's symptoms are stabilized.

The patient should take the medication as directed and should not exceed the prescribed dosage. The patient should contact the physician if symptoms do not improve after two weeks, or if the condition worsens. Patients who experience recurrent episodes of epistaxis (nosebleeds) or nasal septum discomfort while taking this medication should contact their physician. For proper use of this unit and to attain maximum improvement, the patient should read and follow the accompanying patient instructions carefully.

It is important to shake the bottle well before each use. The RHINOCORT AQUA Nasal Spray 32 mcg bottle has been filled with an excess to accommodate the priming activity. The bottle should be discarded after 120 sprays following initial priming, since the amount of budesonide delivered per spray thereafter may be substantially less than the labeled dose. Do not transfer any remaining suspension to another bottle.

Drug Interactions

The main route of metabolism of budesonide, as well as other corticosteroids, is via cytochrome P450 3A (CYP3A). After oral administration of ketoconazole, a potent inhibitor of cytochrome P450 3A, the mean plasma concentration of orally administered budesonide increased by more than seven-fold. Concomitant administration of other known inhibitors of CYP3A (eg, itraconazole, clarithromycin, erythromycin, etc.) may inhibit the metabolism of, and increase the systemic exposure to, budesonide (see WARNINGS and PRECAUTIONS, General).

Omeprazole, an inhibitor of cytochrome P450 2C19, did not have effects on the pharmacokinetics of oral budesonide, while cimetidine, primarily an inhibitor of cytochrome P450 1A2, caused a slight decrease in budesonide clearance and corresponding increase in its oral bioavailability.

Carcinogenesis, Mutagenesis, Impairment of Fertility

In a two-year study in Sprague-Dawley rats, budesonide caused a statistically significant increase in the incidence of gliomas in the male rats receiving an oral dose of 50 mcg/kg (approximately twice the maximum recommended daily intranasal dose in adults and children on a mcg/m^2 basis). No tumorigenicity was seen in male and female rats at respective oral doses up to 25 and 50 mcg/kg (approximately equal to and two times the maximum recommended daily intranasal dose in adults and children on a mcg/m^2 basis, respectively). In two additional two-year studies in male Fischer and Sprague-Dawley rats, budesonide caused no gliomas at an oral dose of 50 mcg/kg (approximately twice the maximum recommended daily intranasal dose in adults and children on a mcg/m^2 basis). However, in male Sprague-Dawley rats, budesonide caused a statistically significant increase in the incidence of hepatocellular tumors at an oral dose of 50 mcg/kg (approximately twice the maximum recommended daily intranasal dose in adults and children on a mcg/m^2 basis). The concurrent reference corticosteroids (prednisolone and triamcinolone acetonide) in these two studies showed similar findings.

In a 91-week study in mice, budesonide caused no treatment-related carcinogenicity at oral doses up to 200 mcg/kg (approximately 3 times the maximum recommended daily intranasal dose in adults and children on a mcg/m^2 basis).

Budesonide was not mutagenic or clastogenic in six different test systems: Ames *Salmonella*/microsome plate test, mouse micronucleus test, mouse lymphoma test, chromosome aberration test in human lymphocytes, sex-linked recessive lethal test in *Drosophila melanogaster*, and DNA repair analysis in rat hematocyte culture.

In rats, budesonide caused a decrease in prenatal viability and viability of the pups at birth and during lactation, along with a decrease in maternal body-weight gain, at subcutaneous doses of 20 mcg/kg and above (less than the maximum recommended daily intranasal dose in adults on a mcg/m^2 basis). No such effects were noted at 5 mcg/kg (less than the maximum recommended daily intranasal dose in adults on a mcg/m^2 basis).

Pregnancy

Teratogenic Effects: Pregnancy Category C: Budesonide was teratogenic and embryocidal in rabbits and rats. Budesonide produced fetal loss, decreased pup weights, and skeletal abnormalities at subcutaneous doses of 25 mcg/kg in rabbits and 500 mcg/kg in rats (approximately 2 and 16 times the maximum recommended daily intranasal dose in adults on a mcg/m^2 basis). In another study in rats, no teratogenic or embryocidal effects were seen at inhalation doses up to 250 mcg/kg (approximately 8 times the maximum recommended daily intranasal dose in adults on a mcg/m^2 basis).

There are no adequate and well-controlled studies in pregnant women. RHINOCORT AQUA Nasal Spray should be used during pregnancy only if the potential benefit justifies the potential risk to the fetus.

Experience with oral corticosteroids since their introduction in pharmacologic, as opposed to physiologic, doses suggests that rodents are more prone to teratogenic effects from corticosteroids than humans. In addition, because there is a natural increase in corticosteroid production during pregnancy, most women will require a lower exogenous corticosteroid dose and many will not need corticosteroid treatment during pregnancy.

Nonteratogenic Effects: Hypoadrenalism may occur in infants born of mothers receiving corticosteroids during pregnancy. Such infants should be carefully observed.

Nursing Mothers

It is not known whether budesonide is excreted in human milk. Because other corticosteroids are excreted in human milk, caution should be exercised when RHINOCORT AQUA Nasal Spray is administered to nursing women.

Pediatric Use

Safety and effectiveness in pediatric patients below 6 years of age have not been established.

Controlled clinical studies have shown that intranasal corticosteroids may cause a reduction in growth velocity in pediatric patients. This effect has been observed in the absence of laboratory evidence of hypothalamic-pituitary-adrenal (HPA) axis suppression, suggesting that growth velocity is a more sensitive indicator of systemic corticosteroid exposure in pediatric patients than some commonly used tests of HPA axis function. The long-term effects of this reduction in growth velocity associated with intranasal corticosteroids, including the impact on final adult height, are unknown. The potential for "catch-up" growth following discontinuation of treatment with intranasal corticosteroids has not been adequately studied. The growth of pediatric patients receiving intranasal corticosteroids, including RHINOCORT AQUA Nasal Spray, should be monitored routinely (eg, via stadiometry). The potential growth effects of prolonged treatment should be weighed against clinical benefits obtained and the availability of safe and effective noncorticosteroid treatment alternatives. To minimize the systemic effects of intranasal corticosteroids, including RHINOCORT AQUA Nasal Spray, each patient should be titrated to the lowest dose that effectively controls his/her symptoms.

Geriatric Use

Of the 2,461 patients in clinical studies of RHINOCORT AQUA Nasal Spray, 5% were 60 years of age and over. No overall differences in safety or effectiveness were observed between these subjects and younger subjects, except for an adverse event reporting frequency of epistaxis which increased with age. Further, other reported clinical experience has not identified any other differences in responses between elderly and younger patients, but greater sensitivity of some older individuals cannot be ruled out.

ADVERSE REACTIONS

The incidence of common adverse reactions is based upon two U.S. and five non-U.S. controlled clinical trials in 1,526 patients [110 females and 239 males less than 18 years of age, and 635 females and 542 males 18 years of age and older] treated with RHINOCORT AQUA Nasal Spray at doses up to 400 mcg once daily for 3–6 weeks. The table below describes adverse events occurring at an incidence of 2% or greater and more common among RHINOCORT AQUA Nasal Spray-treated patients than in placebo-treated patients in controlled clinical trials. The overall incidence of adverse events was similar between RHINOCORT AQUA and placebo.

Adverse Event	RHINOCORT AQUA	Placebo Vehicle
Epistaxis	8%	5%
Pharyngitis	4%	3%
Bronchospasm	2%	1%
Coughing	2%	<1%
Nasal Irritation	2%	<1%

A similar adverse event profile was observed in the subgroup of pediatric patients 6 to 12 years of age.

Two to three percent (2–3%) of patients in clinical trials discontinued because of adverse events. Systemic corticosteroid side effects were not reported during controlled clinical studies with RHINOCORT AQUA Nasal Spray.

If recommended doses are exceeded, however, or if individuals are particularly sensitive, symptoms of hypercorticism, ie, Cushing's Syndrome, could occur.

Rare adverse events reported from post-marketing experience include: nasal septum perforation, pharynx disorders (throat irritation, throat pain, swollen throat, burning throat, and itchy throat), angioedema, anosmia, and palpitations.

Cases of growth suppression have been reported for intranasal corticosteroids including RHINOCORT AQUA Nasal Spray (see PRECAUTIONS, Pediatric Use).

OVERDOSAGE

Acute overdosage with this dosage form is unlikely since one 120 spray bottle of RHINOCORT AQUA Nasal Spray 32 mcg only contains approximately 5.4 mg of budesonide. Chronic overdosage may result in signs/symptoms of hypercorticism (see WARNINGS and PRECAUTIONS).

DOSAGE AND ADMINISTRATION

The recommended starting dose for adults and children 6 years of age and older is 64 mcg per day administered as one spray per nostril of RHINOCORT AQUA Nasal Spray 32 mcg once daily. The maximum recommended dose for adults (12 years of age and older) is 256 mcg per day administered as four sprays per nostril once daily of RHINOCORT AQUA Nasal Spray 32 mcg and the maximum recommended dose for pediatric patients (<12 years of age) is 128 mcg per day administered as two sprays per nostril once daily

of RHINOCORT AQUA Nasal Spray 32 mcg (see HOW SUPPLIED).

Prior to initial use, the container must be shaken gently and the pump must be primed by actuating eight times. If used daily, the pump does not need to be reprimed. If not used for two consecutive days, reprime with one spray or until a fine spray appears. If not used for more than 14 days, rinse the applicator and reprime with two sprays or until a fine spray appears.

Individualization of Dosage

It is always desirable to titrate an individual patient to the minimum effective dose to reduce the possibility of side effects. In adults and children 6 years of age and older, the recommended starting dose is 64 mcg daily administered as one spray per nostril of RHINOCORT AQUA Nasal Spray 32 mcg, once daily. Some patients who do not achieve symptom control at the recommended starting dose may benefit from an increased dose. The maximum daily dose is 256 mcg for adults and 128 mcg for pediatric patients (<12 years of age). When the maximum benefit has been achieved and symptoms have been controlled, reducing the dose may be effective in maintaining control of the allergic rhinitis symptoms in patients who were initially controlled on higher doses.

An improvement in nasal symptoms may be noted in patients within 10 hours of first using RHINOCORT AQUA Nasal Spray. This time to onset is supported by an environmental exposure unit study in seasonal allergic rhinitis patients which demonstrated that RHINOCORT AQUA Nasal Spray led to a statistically significant improvement in nasal symptoms compared to placebo by 10 hours. Further support comes from a clinical study of patients with perennial allergic rhinitis which demonstrated a statistically significant improvement in nasal symptoms for both RHINOCORT AQUA Nasal Spray and for the active comparator (mometasone furoate) compared to placebo by 8 hours. Onset was also assessed in this study with peak nasal inspiratory flow rate and this endpoint failed to show efficacy for either active treatment. Although statistically significant improvements in nasal symptoms compared to placebo were noted within 8–10 hours in these studies, about one half to two thirds of the ultimate clinical improvement with RHINOCORT AQUA Nasal Spray occurs over the first 1–2 days, and maximum benefit may not be achieved until approximately 2 weeks after initiation of treatment. Initial assessment for response should be made during this time frame and periodically until the patient's symptoms are stabilized.

Directions for Use

Illustrated *Patient's Instructions for Use* accompany each package of RHINOCORT AQUA Nasal Spray 32 mcg.

HOW SUPPLIED

RHINOCORT AQUA Nasal Spray 32 mcg is available in a green coated glass bottle with a metered-dose pump spray and a green protection cap. RHINOCORT AQUA Nasal Spray 32 mcg provides 120 metered sprays after initial priming; net fill weight 8.6 g. The RHINOCORT AQUA Nasal Spray 32 mcg bottle has been filled with an excess to accommodate the priming activity. The bottle should be discarded after 120 sprays following initial priming, since the amount of budesonide delivered per spray thereafter may be substantially less than the labeled dose. Each spray delivers 32 mcg of budesonide to the patient.

NDC 0186-1070-08

RHINOCORT AQUA Nasal Spray

32 mcg, 120 metered sprays; net fill weight 8.6 g

Continued on next page

Rhinocort Aqua—Cont.

RHINOCORT AQUA Nasal Spray should be stored at controlled room temperature, 20 to 25°C (68 to 77°F) with the valve up. Do not freeze. Protect from light. **Shake gently before use.** Do not spray in eyes.

Rev. 10/01 808201-04

Distributed by:
AstraZeneca LP, Wilmington, DE 19850

TOPROL-XL® ℞

(metoprolol succinate)
[tō' prōl]
Extended-Release Tablets
Tablets: 25 mg, 50 mg, 100 mg, and 200 mg

Prescribing information for this product, which appears on page 651 of the 2002 PDR, has been completely revised as follows. Please write "See Supplement A" next to the product heading.

DESCRIPTION

Toprol-XL, metoprolol succinate, is a beta$_1$-selective (cardioselective) adrenoceptor blocking agent, for oral administration, available as extended release tablets. Toprol-XL has been formulated to provide a controlled and predictable release of metoprolol for once-daily administration. The tablets comprise a multiple unit system containing metoprolol succinate in a multitude of controlled release pellets. Each pellet acts as a separate drug delivery unit and is designed to deliver metoprolol continuously over the dosage interval. The tablets contain 23.75, 47.5, 95 and 190 mg of metoprolol succinate equivalent to 25, 50, 100 and 200 mg of metoprolol tartrate, USP, respectively. Its chemical name is (±)1-(isopropylamino)-3-[p-(2- methoxyethyl) phenoxy]-2-propanol succinate (2:1) (salt). Its structural formula is:

Metoprolol succinate is a white crystalline powder with a molecular weight of 652.8. It is freely soluble in water; soluble in methanol; sparingly soluble in ethanol; slightly soluble in dichloromethane and 2-propanol; practically insoluble in ethyl-acetate, acetone, diethylether and heptane. Inactive ingredients: silicon dioxide, cellulose compounds, sodium stearyl fumarate, polyethylene glycol, titanium dioxide, paraffin.

CLINICAL PHARMACOLOGY

General

Metoprolol is a beta$_1$-selective (cardioselective) adrenergic receptor blocking agent. This preferential effect is not absolute, however, and at higher plasma concentrations, metoprolol also inhibits beta$_2$-adrenoreceptors, chiefly located in the bronchial and vascular musculature. Metoprolol has no intrinsic sympathomimetic activity, and membrane-stabilizing activity is detectable only at plasma concentrations much greater than required for beta-blockade. Animal and human experiments indicate that metoprolol slows the sinus rate and decreases AV nodal conduction.

Clinical pharmacology studies have confirmed the beta-blocking activity of metoprolol in man, as shown by (1) reduction in heart rate and cardiac output at rest and upon exercise, (2) reduction of systolic blood pressure upon exercise, (3) inhibition of isoproterenol-induced tachycardia, and (4) reduction of reflex orthostatic tachycardia.

The relative beta$_1$-selectivity of metoprolol has been confirmed by the following: (1) In normal subjects, metoprolol is unable to reverse the beta$_2$-mediated vasodilating effects of epinephrine. This contrasts with the effect of nonselective beta-blockers, which completely reverse the vasodilating effects of epinephrine. (2) In asthmatic patients, metoprolol reduces FEV_1 and FVC significantly less than a nonselective beta-blocker, propranolol, at equivalent beta$_1$-receptor blocking doses.

In five controlled studies in normal healthy subjects, the same daily doses of Toprol-XL and immediate release metoprolol were compared in terms of the extent and duration of beta$_1$-blockade produced. Both formulations were given in a dose range equivalent to 100–400 mg of immediate release metoprolol per day. In these studies, Toprol-XL was administered once a day and immediate release metoprolol was administered once to four times a day. A sixth controlled study compared the beta$_1$-blocking effects of a 50 mg daily dose of the two formulations. In each study, beta$_1$-blockade was expressed as the percent change from baseline in exercise heart rate following standardized submaximal exercise tolerance tests at steady state. Toprol-XL administered once a day, and immediate release metoprolol administered once to four times a day, provided comparable total beta$_1$-blockade over 24 hours (area under the beta$_1$-blockade versus time curve) in the dose range 100–400 mg.

Clinical Endpoints in the MERIT-HF Study

Clinical Endpoint	Number of Patients: Placebo n=2001	Number of Patients: Toprol-XL n=1990	Relative Risk (95% Cl)	Risk Reduction with Toprol-XL	Nominal P-value
All-cause mortality plus all-cause hospitalization†	767	641	0.81 (0.73-0.90)	19%	0.00012
All-cause mortality	217	145	0.66 (0.53-0.81)	34%	0.00009
All-cause mortality plus heart failure hospitalization†	439	311	0.69 (0.60-0.80)	31%	0.0000008
Cardiovascular mortality	203	128	0.62 (0.50-0.78)	38%	0.000022
Sudden death	132	79	0.59 (0.45-0.78)	41%	0.0002
Death due to worsening heart failure	58	30	0.51 (0.33-0.79)	49%	0.0023
Hospitalizations due to worsening heart failure‡	451	317	N/A	N/A	0.0000076
Cardiovascular hospitalization‡	773	649	N/A	N/A	0.00028

† Time to first event
‡ Comparison of treatment groups examines the number of hospitalizations (Wilcoxon test); relative risk and risk reduction are not applicable.

At a dosage of 50 mg once daily, Toprol-XL produced significantly higher total beta$_1$-blockade over 24 hours than immediate release metoprolol. For Toprol-XL, the percent reduction in exercise heart rate was relatively stable throughout the entire dosage interval and the level of beta$_1$-blockade increased with increasing doses from 50 to 300 mg daily. The effects at peak/trough (ie, at 24-hours post-dosing) were: 14/9, 16/10, 24/14, 27/22 and 27/20% reduction in exercise heart rate for doses of 50, 100, 200, 300 and 400 mg Toprol-XL once a day, respectively. In contrast to Toprol-XL, immediate release metoprolol given at a dose of 50–100 mg once a day produced a significantly larger peak effect on exercise tachycardia, but the effect was not evident at 24 hours. To match the peak to trough ratio obtained with Toprol-XL over the dosing range of 200 to 400 mg, a t.i.d. to q.i.d. divided dosing regimen was required for immediate release metoprolol. A controlled crossover study in heart failure patients compared the plasma concentrations and beta$_1$-blocking effects of 50 mg immediate release metoprolol administered t.i.d., 100 mg and 200 mg Toprol-XL once daily. A 50 mg dose of immediate release metoprolol t.i.d. produced a peak plasma level of metoprolol similar to the peak level observed with 200 mg of Toprol-XL. A 200 mg dose of Toprol-XL produced a larger effect on suppression of exercise-induced and Holter-monitored heart rate over 24 hours compared to 50 mg t.i.d. of immediate release metoprolol.

The relationship between plasma metoprolol levels and reduction in exercise heart rate is independent of the pharmaceutical formulation. Using the E_{max} model, the maximal beta$_1$-blocking effect has been estimated to produce a 30% reduction in exercise heart rate. Beta$_1$-blocking effects in the range of 30–80% of the maximal effect (corresponding to approximately 8–23% reduction in exercise heart rate) are expected to occur at metoprolol plasma concentrations ranging from 30–540 nmol/L. The concentration-effect curve begins reaching a plateau between 200–300 nmol/L, and higher plasma levels produce little additional beta$_1$-blocking effect. The relative beta$_1$-selectivity of metoprolol diminishes and blockade of beta$_2$-adrenoceptors increases at higher plasma concentrations.

Although beta-adrenergic receptor blockade is useful in the treatment of angina, hypertension, and heart failure there are situations in which sympathetic stimulation is vital. In patients with severely damaged hearts, adequate ventricular function may depend on sympathetic drive. In the presence of AV block, beta-blockade may prevent the necessary facilitating effect of sympathetic activity on conduction. Beta$_2$-adrenergic blockade results in passive bronchial constriction by interfering with endogenous adrenergic bronchodilator activity in patients subject to bronchospasm and may also interfere with exogenous bronchodilators in such patients.

In other studies, treatment with Toprol-XL produced an improvement in left ventricular ejection fraction. Toprol-XL was also shown to delay the increase in left ventricular end-systolic and end-diastolic volumes after 6 months of treatment.

Hypertension

The mechanism of the antihypertensive effects of beta-blocking agents has not been elucidated. However, several possible mechanisms have been proposed: (1) competitive antagonism of catecholamines at peripheral (especially cardiac) adrenergic neuron sites, leading to decreased cardiac output; (2) a central effect leading to reduced sympathetic outflow to the periphery; and (3) suppression of renin activity.

Clinical Trials

In controlled clinical studies, an immediate release dosage form of metoprolol has been shown to be an effective antihypertensive agent when used alone or as concomitant therapy with thiazide-type diuretics at dosages of 100–450 mg daily. Toprol-XL, in dosages of 100 to 400 mg once daily, has been shown to possess comparable β_1-blockade as conventional metoprolol tablets administered two to four times daily. In addition, Toprol-XL administered at a dose of 50 mg once daily has been shown to lower blood pressure 24-hours post-dosing in placebo-controlled studies. In controlled, comparative, clinical studies, immediate release metoprolol appeared comparable as an antihypertensive agent to propranolol, methyldopa, and thiazide-type diuretics, and affected both supine and standing blood pressure. Because of variable plasma levels attained with a given dose and lack of a consistent relationship of antihypertensive activity to drug plasma concentration, selection of proper dosage requires individual titration.

Angina Pectoris

By blocking catecholamine-induced increases in heart rate, in velocity and extent of myocardial contraction, and in blood pressure, metoprolol reduces the oxygen requirements of the heart at any given level of effort, thus making it useful in the long-term management of angina pectoris.

Clinical Trials

In controlled clinical trials, an immediate release formulation of metoprolol has been shown to be an effective antianginal agent, reducing the number of angina attacks and increasing exercise tolerance. The dosage used in these studies ranged from 100 to 400 mg daily. Toprol-XL, in dosages of 100 to 400 mg once daily, has been shown to possess beta-blockade similar to conventional metoprolol tablets administered two to four times daily.

Heart Failure

The precise mechanism for the beneficial effects of beta-blockers in heart failure has not been elucidated.

Clinical Trials

MERIT-HF was a double-blind, placebo-controlled study of Toprol-XL conducted in 14 countries including the US. It randomized 3991 patients (1990 to Toprol-XL) with ejection fraction ≤ 0.40 and NYHA Class II-IV heart failure attributable to ischemia, hypertension, or cardiomyopathy. The protocol excluded patients with contraindications to beta-blocker use, those expected to undergo heart surgery, and those within 28 days of myocardial infarction or unstable angina. The primary endpoints of the trial were (1) all-cause mortality plus all-cause hospitalization (time to first event) and (2) all-cause mortality. Patients were stabilized on optimal concomitant therapy for heart failure, including diuretics, ACE inhibitors, cardiac glycosides, and nitrates. At randomization, 41% of patients were NYHA Class II, 55% NYHA Class III; 65% of patients had heart failure attributed to ischemic heart disease; 44% had a history of hypertension; 25% had diabetes mellitus; 48% had a history of myocardial infarction. Among patients in the trial, 90% were on diuretics, 89% were on ACE inhibitors, 64% were on digitalis, 27% were on a lipid-lowering agent, 37% were on an oral anticoagulant, and the mean ejection fraction was 0.28. The mean duration of follow-up was one year. At the end of the study, the mean daily dose of Toprol-XL was 159 mg.

Results for Subgroups in MERIT-HF

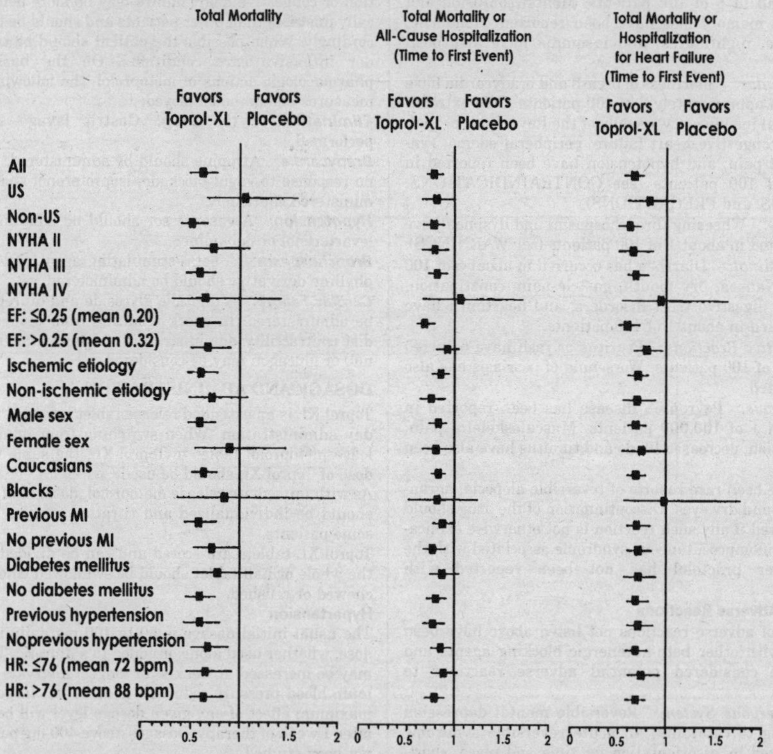

Relative risk and 95% confidence interval

US = United States; NYHA = New York Heart Association; EF = ejection fraction; MI = myocardial infarction; HR = heart rate.

Tablet	Shape	Engraving	Bottle of 100 NDC 0186-	Unit Dose Packages of 100 NDC 0186-
25 mg*	Oval	A β	1088-05	1088-39
50 mg	Round	A mo	1090-05	1090-39
100 mg	Round	A ms	1092-05	1092-39
200 mg	Oval	A my	1094-05	N/A

* The 25 mg tablet is scored on both sides.

The trial was terminated early for a statistically significant reduction in all-cause mortality (34%, nominal p= 0.00009). The risk of all-cause mortality plus all-cause hospitalization was reduced by 19% (p= 0.00012). The trial also showed improvements in heart failure-related mortality and heart failure-related hospitalizations, and NYHA functional class.

The table below shows the principal results for the overall study population. The figure below illustrates principal results for a wide variety of subgroup comparisons, including US vs. non-US populations (the latter of which was not prespecified). The combined endpoints of all-cause mortality plus all-cause hospitalization and of mortality plus heart failure hospitalization showed consistent effects in the overall study population and the subgroups, including women and the US population. However, in the US subgroup (n=1071) and women (n=898), overall mortality and cardiovascular mortality appeared less affected. Analyses of female and US patients were carried out because they each represented about 25% of the overall population. Nonetheless, subgroup analyses can be difficult to interpret and it is not known whether these represent true differences or chance effects.

[See table at top of previous page]

Pharmacokinetics

[See figure above]

In man, absorption of metoprolol is rapid and complete. Plasma levels following oral administration of conventional metoprolol tablets, however, approximate 50% of levels following intravenous administration, indicating about 50% first-pass metabolism. Metoprolol crosses the blood-brain barrier and has been reported in the CSF in a concentration 78% of the simultaneous plasma concentration.

Plasma levels achieved are highly variable after oral administration. Only a small fraction of the drug (about 12%) is bound to human serum albumin. Metoprolol is a racemic mixture of R- and S- enantiomers, and is primarily metabolized by CYP2D6. When administered orally, it exhibits stereoselective metabolism that is dependent on oxidation phenotype. Elimination is mainly by biotransformation in the liver, and the plasma half-life ranges from approximately 3 to 7 hours. Less than 5% of an oral dose of metoprolol is recovered unchanged in the urine; the rest is excreted by the kidneys as metabolites that appear to have no beta-blocking activity. Following intravenous administration of metoprolol, the urinary recovery of unchanged drug is approximately 10%. The systemic availability and half-life of metoprolol in patients with renal failure do not differ to a clinically significant degree from those in normal subjects. Consequently, no reduction in dosage is usually needed in patients with chronic renal failure.

Metoprolol is metabolized predominantly by CYP2D6, an enzyme that is absent in about 8% of Caucasians (poor metabolizers) and about 2% of most other populations. CYP2D6 can be inhibited by a number of drugs. Concomitant use of inhibiting drugs in poor metabolizers will increase blood levels of metoprolol several-fold, decreasing metoprolol's cardioselectivity. (See PRECAUTIONS, Drug Interactions.)

In comparison to conventional metoprolol, the plasma metoprolol levels following administration of Toprol-XL are characterized by lower peaks, longer time to peak and significantly lower peak to trough variation. The peak plasma levels following once-daily administration of Toprol-XL average one-fourth to one-half the peak plasma levels obtained following a corresponding dose of conventional metoprolol, administered once daily or in divided doses. At steady state the average bioavailability of metoprolol following administration of Toprol-XL, across the dosage range of 50 to 400 mg once daily, was 77% relative to the corresponding single or divided doses of conventional metoprolol. Nevertheless, over the 24-hour dosing interval, β_1-blockade is comparable and dose-related (see CLINICAL PHARMACOLOGY). The bioavailability of metoprolol shows a dose-related, although not directly proportional, increase with dose and is not significantly affected by food following Toprol-XL administration.

INDICATIONS AND USAGE

Hypertension

Toprol-XL is indicated for the treatment of hypertension. It may be used alone or in combination with other antihypertensive agents.

Angina Pectoris

Toprol-XL is indicated in the long-term treatment of angina pectoris.

Heart Failure

Toprol-XL is indicated for the treatment of stable, symptomatic (NYHA Class II or III) heart failure of ischemic, hypertensive, or cardiomyopathic origin. It was studied in patients already receiving ACE inhibitors, diuretics, and, in the majority of cases, digitalis. In this population, Toprol-XL decreased the rate of mortality plus hospitalization, largely through a reduction in cardiovascular mortality and hospitalizations for heart failure.

CONTRAINDICATIONS

Toprol-XL is contraindicated in severe bradycardia, heart block greater than first degree, cardiogenic shock, decompensated cardiac failure, and sick sinus syndrome (unless a permanent pacemaker is in place) (see WARNINGS).

WARNINGS

Ischemic Heart Disease: Following abrupt cessation of therapy with certain beta-blocking agents, exacerbations of angina pectoris and, in some cases, myocardial infarction have occurred. When discontinuing chronically administered Toprol-XL, particularly in patients with ischemic heart disease, the dosage should be gradually reduced over a period of 1–2 weeks and the patient should be carefully monitored. If angina markedly worsens or acute coronary insufficiency develops, Toprol-XL administration should be reinstated promptly, at least temporarily, and other measures appropriate for the management of unstable angina should be taken. Patients should be warned against interruption or discontinuation of therapy without the physician's advice. Because coronary artery disease is common and may be unrecognized, it may be prudent not to discontinue Toprol-XL therapy abruptly even in patients treated only for hypertension.

Bronchospastic Diseases: PATIENTS WITH BRONCHOSPASTIC DISEASES SHOULD, IN GENERAL, NOT RECEIVE BETA-BLOCKERS. Because of its relative $beta_1$-selectivity, however, Toprol-XL may be used with caution in patients with bronchospastic disease who do not respond to, or cannot tolerate, other antihypertensive treatment. Since $beta_1$-selectivity is not absolute, a $beta_2$-stimulating agent should be administered concomitantly, and the lowest possible dose of Toprol-XL should be used (see DOSAGE AND ADMINISTRATION).

Major Surgery: The necessity or desirability of withdrawing beta-blocking therapy prior to major surgery is controversial; the impaired ability of the heart to respond to reflex adrenergic stimuli may augment the risks of general anesthesia and surgical procedures.

Toprol-XL, like other beta-blockers, is a competitive inhibitor of beta-receptor agonists, and its effects can be reversed by administration of such agents, eg, dobutamine or isoproterenol. However, such patients may be subject to protracted severe hypotension. Difficulty in restarting and maintaining the heart beat has also been reported with beta-blockers.

Diabetes and Hypoglycemia: Toprol-XL should be used with caution in diabetic patients if a beta-blocking agent is required. Beta-blockers may mask tachycardia occurring with hypoglycemia, but other manifestations such as dizziness and sweating may not be significantly affected.

Thyrotoxicosis: Beta-adrenergic blockade may mask certain clinical signs (eg, tachycardia) of hyperthyroidism. Patients suspected of developing thyrotoxicosis should be managed carefully to avoid abrupt withdrawal of beta-blockade, which might precipitate a thyroid storm.

PRECAUTIONS

General

Toprol-XL should be used with caution in patients with impaired hepatic function.

Worsening cardiac failure may occur during up-titration of Toprol-XL. If such symptoms occur, diuretics should be increased and the dose of Toprol-XL should not be advanced until clinical stability is restored (see DOSAGE AND ADMINISTRATION). It may be necessary to lower the dose of Toprol-XL or temporarily discontinue it. Such episodes do not preclude subsequent successful titration of Toprol-XL.

Information for Patients

Patients should be advised to take Toprol-XL regularly and continuously, as directed, preferably with or immediately following meals. If a dose should be missed, the patient should take only the next scheduled dose (without doubling it). Patients should not interrupt or discontinue Toprol-XL without consulting the physician.

Patients should be advised (1) to avoid operating automobiles and machinery or engaging in other tasks requiring alertness until the patient's response to therapy with Toprol-XL has been determined; (2) to contact the physician if any difficulty in breathing occurs; (3) to inform the physician or dentist before any type of surgery that he or she is taking Toprol-XL.

Heart failure patients should be advised to consult their physician if they experience signs or symptoms of worsening heart failure such as weight gain or increasing shortness of breath.

Laboratory Tests

Clinical laboratory findings may include elevated levels of serum transaminase, alkaline phosphatase, and lactate dehydrogenase.

Continued on next page

Toprol-XL—Cont.

Drug Interactions

Catecholamine-depleting drugs (eg, reserpine) may have an additive effect when given with beta-blocking agents. Patients treated with Toprol-XL plus a catecholamine depletor should therefore be closely observed for evidence of hypotension or marked bradycardia, which may produce vertigo, syncope, or postural hypotension.

Drugs that inhibit CYP2D6 such as quinidine, fluoxetine, paroxetine, and propafenone are likely to increase metoprolol concentration. In healthy subjects with CYP2D6 extensive metabolizer phenotype, coadministration of quinidine 100 mg and immediate release metoprolol 200 mg tripled the concentration of S-metoprolol and doubled the metoprolol elimination half-life. In four patients with cardiovascular disease, coadministration of propafenone 150 mg t.i.d. with immediate release metoprolol 50 mg t.i.d. resulted in two- to five-fold increases in the steady-state concentration of metoprolol. These increases in plasma concentration would decrease the cardioselectivity of metoprolol.

Carcinogenesis, Mutagenesis, Impairment of Fertility

Long-term studies in animals have been conducted to evaluate the carcinogenic potential of metoprolol tartrate. In 2-year studies in rats at three oral dosage levels of up to 800 mg/kg/day (41 times, on a mg/m^2 basis, the daily dose of 200 mg for a 60-kg patient), there was no increase in the development of spontaneously occurring benign or malignant neoplasms of any type. The only histologic changes that appeared to be drug related were an increased incidence of generally mild focal accumulation of foamy macrophages in pulmonary alveoli and a slight increase in biliary hyperplasia. In a 21-month study in Swiss albino mice at three oral dosage levels of up to 750 mg/kg/day (18 times, on a mg/m^2 basis, the daily dose of 200 mg for 60-kg patient), benign lung tumors (small adenomas) occurred more frequently in female mice receiving the highest dose than in untreated control animals. There was no increase in malignant or total (benign plus malignant) lung tumors, nor in the overall incidence of tumors or malignant tumors. This 21-month study was repeated in CD-1 mice, and no statistically or biologically significant differences were observed between treated and control mice of either sex for any type of tumor.

All genotoxicity tests performed on metoprolol tartrate (a dominant lethal study in mice, chromosome studies in somatic cells, a *Salmonella*/mammalian-microsome mutagenicity test, and a nucleus anomaly test in somatic interphase nuclei) and metoprolol succinate (a *Salmonella*/mammalian-microsome mutagenicity test) were negative.

No evidence of impaired fertility due to metoprolol tartrate was observed in a study performed in rats at doses up to 22 times, on a mg/m^2 basis, the daily dose of 200 mg in a 60-kg patient.

Pregnancy Category C

Metoprolol tartrate has been shown to increase post-implantation loss and decrease neonatal survival in rats at doses up to 22 times, on a mg/m^2 basis, the daily dose of 200 mg in a 60-kg patient. Distribution studies in mice confirm exposure of the fetus when metoprolol tartrate is administered to the pregnant animal. These studies have revealed no evidence of impaired fertility or teratogenicity. There are no adequate and well-controlled studies in pregnant women. Because animal reproduction studies are not always predictive of human response, this drug should be used during pregnancy only if clearly needed.

Nursing Mothers

Metoprolol is excreted in breast milk in very small quantities. An infant consuming 1 liter of breast milk daily would receive a dose of less than 1 mg of the drug. Caution should be exercised when Toprol-XL is administered to a nursing woman.

Pediatric Use

Safety and effectiveness in pediatric patients have not been established.

Geriatric Use

Clinical studies of Toprol-XL in hypertension did not include sufficient numbers of subjects aged 65 and over to determine whether they respond differently from younger subjects. Other reported clinical experience in hypertensive patients has not identified differences in responses between elderly and younger patients.

Of the 1,990 patients with heart failure randomized to Toprol-XL in the MERIT-HF trial, 50% (990) were 65 years of age and older and 12% (238) were 75 years of age and older. There were no notable differences in efficacy or the rate of adverse events between older and younger patients.

In general, dose selection for an elderly patient should be cautious, usually starting at the low end of the dosing range, reflecting greater frequency of decreased hepatic, renal, or cardiac function, and of concomitant disease or other drug therapy.

Risk of Anaphylactic Reactions

While taking beta-blockers, patients with a history of severe anaphylactic reactions to a variety of allergens may be more reactive to repeated challenge, either accidental, diagnostic, or therapeutic. Such patients may be unresponsive to the usual doses of epinephrine used to treat allergic reaction.

ADVERSE REACTIONS

Hypertension and Angina

Most adverse effects have been mild and transient. The following adverse reactions have been reported for metoprolol tartrate.

Central Nervous System: Tiredness and dizziness have occurred in about 10 of 100 patients. Depression has been reported in about 5 of 100 patients. Mental confusion and short-term memory loss have been reported. Headache, somnolence, nightmares, and insomnia have also been reported.

Cardiovascular: Shortness of breath and bradycardia have occurred in approximately 3 of 100 patients. Cold extremities; arterial insufficiency, usually of the Raynaud type; palpitations; congestive heart failure; peripheral edema; syncope; chest pain; and hypotension have been reported in about 1 of 100 patients (see CONTRAINDICATIONS, WARNINGS, and PRECAUTIONS).

Respiratory: Wheezing (bronchospasm) and dyspnea have been reported in about 1 of 100 patients (see WARNINGS).

Gastrointestinal: Diarrhea has occurred in about 5 of 100 patients. Nausea, dry mouth, gastric pain, constipation, flatulence, digestive tract disorders, and heartburn have been reported in about 1 of 100 patients.

Hypersensitive Reactions: Pruritus or rash have occurred in about 5 of 100 patients. Worsening of psoriasis has also been reported.

Miscellaneous: Peyronie's disease has been reported in fewer than 1 of 100,000 patients. Musculoskeletal pain, blurred vision, decreased libido and tinnitus have also been reported.

There have been rare reports of reversible alopecia, agranulocytosis, and dry eyes. Discontinuation of the drug should be considered if any such reaction is not otherwise explicable. The oculomucocutaneous syndrome associated with the beta-blocker practolol has not been reported with metoprolol.

Potential Adverse Reactions

A variety of adverse reactions not listed above have been reported with other beta-adrenergic blocking agents and should be considered potential adverse reactions to Toprol-XL.

Central Nervous System: Reversible mental depression progressing to catatonia; an acute reversible syndrome characterized by disorientation for time and place, short-term memory loss, emotional lability, slightly clouded sensorium, and decreased performance on neuropsychometrics.

Cardiovascular: Intensification of AV block (see CONTRAINDICATIONS).

Hematologic: Agranulocytosis, nonthrombocytopenic purpura, thrombocytopenic purpura.

Hypersensitive Reactions: Fever combined with aching and sore throat, laryngospasm, and respiratory distress.

Heart Failure

In the MERIT-HF study, serious adverse events and adverse events leading to discontinuation of study medication were systematically collected. In the MERIT-HF study comparing Toprol-XL in daily doses up to 200 mg (mean dose 159 mg once-daily) (n=1990) to placebo (n=2001), 10.3% of Toprol-XL patients discontinued for adverse events vs. 12.2% of placebo patients.

The table below lists adverse events in the MERIT-HF study that occurred at an incidence of equal to or greater than 1% in the Toprol-XL group and greater than placebo by more than 0.5%, regardless of the assessment of causality.

Adverse Events Occurring in the MERIT-HF Study at an Incidence ≥ 1% in the Toprol-XL Group and Greater Than Placebo by More Than 0.5%

	Toprol-XL N=1990 % of patients	Placebo N=2001 % of patients
Dizziness/vertigo	1.8	1.0
Bradycardia	1.5	0.4
Accident and/or injury	1.4	0.8

Other adverse events with an incidence of > 1% on Toprol-XL and as common on placebo (within 0.5%) included myocardial infarction, pneumonia, cerebrovascular disorder, chest pain, dyspnea/dyspnea aggravated, syncope, coronary artery disorder, ventricular tachycardia/arrhythmia aggravated, hypotension, diabetes mellitus/diabetes mellitus aggravated, abdominal pain, and fatigue.

Post-Marketing Experience

The following adverse reactions have been reported in post-marketing use:

Gastrointestinal: hepatitis.

Musculoskeletal: arthralgia.

OVERDOSAGE

Acute Toxicity

There have been a few reports of overdosage with Toprol-XL and no specific overdosage information was obtained with this drug, with the exception of animal toxicology data. However, since Toprol-XL (metoprolol succinate salt) contains the same active moiety, metoprolol, as conventional metoprolol tablets (metoprolol tartrate salt), the recommendations on overdosage for metoprolol conventional tablets are applicable to Toprol-XL.

Signs and Symptoms

Overdosage of Toprol-XL may lead to severe hypotension, sinus bradycardia, atrioventricular block, heart failure, cardiogenic shock, cardiac arrest, bronchospasm, impairment of consciousness/coma, nausea, vomiting, and cyanosis.

Treatment

In general, patients with acute or recent myocardial infarction or congestive heart failure may be more hemodynamically unstable than other patients and should be treated accordingly. When possible the patient should be treated under intensive care conditions. On the basis of the pharmacologic actions of metoprolol, the following general measures should be employed:

Elimination of the Drug: Gastric lavage should be performed.

Bradycardia: Atropine should be administered. If there is no response to vagal blockade, isoproterenol should be administered cautiously.

Hypotension: A vasopressor should be administered, eg, levarterenol or dopamine.

Bronchospasm: A beta$_2$-stimulating agent and/or a theophylline derivative should be administered.

Cardiac Failure: A digitalis glycoside and diuretics should be administered. In shock resulting from inadequate cardiac contractility, administration of dobutamine, isoproterenol, or glucagon may be considered.

DOSAGE AND ADMINISTRATION

Toprol-XL is an extended release tablet intended for once-a-day administration. When switching from immediate release metoprolol tablet to Toprol-XL, the same total daily dose of Toprol-XL should be used.

As with immediate release metoprolol, dosages of Toprol-XL should be individualized and titration may be needed in some patients.

Toprol-XL tablets are scored and can be divided; however, the whole or half tablet should be swallowed whole and not chewed or crushed.

Hypertension

The usual initial dosage is 50 to 100 mg daily in a single dose, whether used alone or added to a diuretic. The dosage may be increased at weekly (or longer) intervals until optimum blood pressure reduction is achieved. In general, the maximum effect of any given dosage level will be apparent after 1 week of therapy. Dosages above 400 mg per day have not been studied.

Angina Pectoris

The dosage of Toprol-XL should be individualized. The usual initial dosage is 100 mg daily, given in a single dose. The dosage may be gradually increased at weekly intervals until optimum clinical response has been obtained or there is a pronounced slowing of the heart rate. Dosages above 400 mg per day have not been studied. If treatment is to be discontinued, the dosage should be reduced gradually over a period of 1–2 weeks (see WARNINGS).

Heart Failure

Dosage must be individualized and closely monitored during up-titration. Prior to initiation of Toprol-XL, the dosing of diuretics, ACE inhibitors, and digitalis (if used) should be stabilized. The recommended starting dose of Toprol-XL is 25 mg once daily for two weeks in patients with NYHA class II heart failure and 12.5 mg once daily in patients with more severe heart failure. The dose should then be doubled every two weeks to the highest dosage level tolerated by the patient or up to 200 mg of Toprol-XL. If transient worsening of heart failure occurs, it may be treated with increased doses of diuretics, and it may also be necessary to lower the dose of Toprol-XL or temporarily discontinue it. The dose of Toprol-XL should not be increased until symptoms of worsening heart failure have been stabilized. Initial difficulty with titration should not preclude later attempts to introduce Toprol-XL. If heart failure patients experience symptomatic bradycardia, the dose of Toprol-XL should be reduced.

HOW SUPPLIED

Tablets containing metoprolol succinate equivalent to the indicated weight of metoprolol tartrate, USP, are white, biconvex, film-coated, and scored.

[See table at top of previous page]

Store at 25°C (77°F). Excursions permitted to 15-30°C (59-86°F). (See USP Controlled Room Temperature.)

Manufactured for: AstraZeneca LP
Wilmington, DE 19850
By: AstraZeneca AB
S-151 85 Södertälje, Sweden
Made in Sweden
64193-00
Rev. 10/01

XYLOCAINE® ℞

(lidocaine HCl Injection, USP)

[*zī 'lo-caine*]

XYLOCAINE®

(lidocaine HCl and epinephrine injection, USP)
For Infiltration and Nerve Block

Prescribing information for this product, which appears on pages 653–656 of the 2002 PDR, has been revised as follows. Please write "See Supplement A" next to the product heading.

The table in the **HOW SUPPLIED** *section has been revised as follows:*

							Xylocaine-MPF								Xylocaine		
		Ampules (mL)					Polyamp DuoFit™ (mL)		Single Dose Vials (mL)						Multiple Dose Vials (mL)		
Xylocaine (lidocaine HCl) Concentration	Epinephrine Dilution (if present)	2	5	10	20	30	10	20	2	5	10	20	30	50	10	20	50
0.5%														X			X
0.5%	1:200,000																X
1%		X	X			X	X	X	X	X	X		X		X	X	X
1%	1:100,000														X	X	X
1%	1:200,000					X				X	X		X				
1.5%					X		X	X		X	X						
1.5%	1:200,000		X			X				X	X		X				
2%		X		X			X		X	X	X				X	X	X
2%	1:100,000														X	X	X
2%	1:200,000				X					X	X	X					

HOW SUPPLIED

[See table above]

721566-02, Rev 09/01.

AstraZeneca Pharmaceuticals LP

1800 CONCORD PIKE
WILMINGTON, DE 19850-5437 USA

For Product and Business Information, and Adverse Drug Experiences:
Information Center
1-800-236-9933

For Product Ordering:
Trade Customer Service
1-800-842-9920

Internet: www.astrazeneca-us.com

ACCOLATE® Tablets ℞

[ac-cō 'late]
zafirlukast

DESCRIPTION

Zafirlukast is a synthetic, selective peptide leukotriene receptor antagonist (LTRA), with the chemical name 4-(5-cyclopentyloxy-carbonylamino-1-methyl-indol-3-ylmethyl)-3-methoxy-N-o-tolylsulfonylbenzamide. The molecular weight of zafirlukast is 575.7 and the structural formula is: The empirical formula is: $C_{31}H_{33}N_3O_6S$

Zafirlukast, a fine white to pale yellow amorphous powder, is practically insoluble in water. It is slightly soluble in methanol and freely soluble in tetrahydrofuran, dimethylsulfoxide, and acetone.

ACCOLATE is supplied as 10 and 20 mg tablets for oral administration.

Inactive Ingredients: Film-coated tablets containing croscarmellose sodium, lactose, magnesium stearate, microcrystalline cellulose, povidone, hydroxypropylmethylcellulose, and titanium dioxide.

CLINICAL PHARMACOLOGY

Mechanism of Action

Zafirlukast is a selective and competitive receptor antagonist of leukotriene D_4 and E_4 (LTD_4 and LTE_4), components of slow-reacting substance of anaphylaxis (SRSA). Cysteinyl leukotriene production and receptor occupation have been correlated with the pathophysiology of asthma, including airway edema, smooth muscle constriction, and altered cellular activity associated with the inflammatory process, which contribute to the signs and symptoms of asthma. Patients with asthma were found in one study to be 25-100 times more sensitive to the bronchoconstricting activity of inhaled LTD_4 than nonasthmatic subjects.

In vitro studies demonstrated that zafirlukast antagonized the contractile activity of three leukotrienes (LTC_4, LTD_4 and LTE_4) in conducting airway smooth muscle from laboratory animals and humans. Zafirlukast prevented intradermal LTD_4-induced increases in cutaneous vascular permeability and inhibited inhaled LTD_4-induced influx of eosinophils into animal lungs. Inhalational challenge studies in sensitized sheep showed that zafirlukast suppressed the airway responses to antigen; this included both the early- and late-phase response and the nonspecific hyperresponsiveness.

In humans, zafirlukast inhibited bronchoconstriction caused by several kinds of inhalational challenges. Pretreatment with single oral doses of zafirlukast inhibited the bronchoconstriction caused by sulfur dioxide and cold air in patients with asthma. Pretreatment with single doses of zafirlukast attenuated the early- and late-phase reaction caused by inhalation of various antigens such as grass, cat dander, ragweed, and mixed antigens in patients with asthma. Zafirlukast also attenuated the increase in bronchial hyperresponsiveness to inhaled histamine that followed inhaled allergen challenge.

Clinical Pharmacokinetics and Bioavailability

Absorption: Zafirlukast is rapidly absorbed following oral administration. Peak plasma concentrations are generally achieved 3 hours after oral administration. The absolute bioavailability of zafirlukast is unknown. In two separate studies, one using a high fat and the other a high protein meal, administration of zafirlukast with food reduced the mean bioavailability by approximately 40%.

Distribution: Zafirlukast is more than 99% bound to plasma proteins, predominantly albumin. The degree of binding was independent of concentration in the clinically relevant range. The apparent steady-state volume of distribution (V_{SS}/F) is approximately 70 L, suggesting moderate distribution into tissues. Studies in rats using radiolabeled zafirlukast indicate minimal distribution across the blood-brain barrier.

Metabolism: Zafirlukast is extensively metabolized. The most common metabolic products are hydroxylated metabolites which are excreted in the feces. The metabolites of zafirlukast identified in plasma are at least 90 times less potent as LTD_4 receptor antagonists than zafirlukast in a standard in vitro test of activity. *In vitro* studies using human liver microsomes showed that the hydroxylated metabolites of zafirlukast excreted in the feces are formed through the cytochrome P450 2C9 (CYP2C9) pathway. Additional *in vitro* studies utilizing human liver microsomes show that zafirlukast inhibits the cytochrome P450 CYP3A4 and CYP2C9 isoenzymes at concentrations close to the clinically achieved total plasma concentrations (see Drug Interactions).

Excretion: The apparent oral clearance (CL/f) of zafirlukast is approximately 20 L/h. Studies in the rat and dog suggest that biliary excretion is the primary route of excretion. Following oral administration of radiolabeled zafirlukast to volunteers, urinary excretion accounts for approximately 10% of the dose and the remainder is excreted in feces. Zafirlukast is not detected in urine.

In the pivotal bioequivalence study, the mean terminal half-life of zafirlukast is approximately 10 hours in both normal adult subjects and patients with asthma. In other studies, the mean plasma half-life of zafirlukast ranged from approximately 8 to 16 hours in both normal subjects and patients with asthma. The pharmacokinetics of zafirlukast are approximately linear over the range from 5 mg to 80 mg. Steady-state plasma concentrations of zafirlukast are proportional to the dose and predictable from single-dose pharmacokinetic data. Accumulation of zafirlukast in the plasma following twice-daily dosing is approximately 45%.

The pharmacokinetic parameters of zafirlukast 20 mg administered as a single dose to 36 male volunteers are shown with the table below.

Mean (% Coefficient of Variation) pharmacokinetic parameters of zafirlukast following single 20 mg oral dose administration to male volunteers (n=36)

C_{max} ng/ml	t_{max}[1] h	AUC ng•h/mL	$t_{1/2}$ h	CL/f L/h
326 (31.0)	2 (0.5-5.0)	1137 (34)	13.3 (75.6)	19.4 (32)

[1]Median and range

Special Populations: Gender: The pharmacokinetics of zafirlukast are similar in males and females. Weight-adjusted apparent oral clearance does not differ due to gender.

Race: No differences in the pharmacokinetics of zafirlukast due to race have been observed.

Elderly: The apparent oral clearance of zafirlukast decreases with age. In patients above 65 years of age, there is an approximately 2-3 fold greater C_{max} and AUC compared to young adult patients.

Children: Following administration of a single 20 mg dose of zafirlukast to 20 boys and girls between 7 and 11 years of age, and in a second study, to 29 boys and girls between 5 and 6 years of age, the following pharmacokinetic parameters were obtained:

Parameter	Children age 5-6 years Mean (% Coefficient of Variation)	Children age 7-11 years Mean (% Coefficient of Variation)
C_{max} (ng/mL)	756 (39%)	601 (45%)
AUC (ng•h/mL)	2458 (34%)	2027 (38%)
t_{max} (h)	2.1 (61%)	2.5 (55%)
CL/f (L/h)	9.2 (37%)	11.4 (42%)

Weight unadjusted apparent clearance was 11.4 L/h (42%) in the 7-11 year old children and 9.2 L/h (37%) in the 5-6 year old children, which resulted in greater systemic drug exposures than that obtained in adults for an identical dose. To maintain similar exposure levels in children compared to adults, a dose of 10 mg twice daily is recommended in children 5-11 years of age (see DOSAGE AND ADMINISTRATION).

Zafirlukast disposition was unchanged after multiple dosing (20 mg twice daily) in children and the degree of accumulation in plasma was similar to that observed in adults.

Hepatic Insufficiency: In a study of patients with hepatic impairment (biopsy-proven cirrhosis), there was a reduced clearance of zafirlukast resulting in a 50-60% greater C_{max} and AUC compared to normal subjects.

Renal Insufficiency: Based on a cross-study comparison, there are no apparent differences in the pharmacokinetics of zafirlukast between renally-impaired patients and normal subjects.

Drug Interactions

The following drug interaction studies have been conducted with zafirlukast (see PRECAUTIONS, Drug Interactions).

- Coadministration of multiple doses of zafirlukast (160 mg/day) to steady-state with a single 25 mg dose of warfarin (a substrate of CYP2C9) resulted in a significant increase in the mean AUC (+63%) and half-life (+36%) of S-warfarin. The mean prothrombin time increased by approximately 35%. The pharmacokinetics of zafirlukast were unaffected by coadministration with warfarin.
- Coadministration of zafirlukast (80 mg/day) at steady-state with a single dose of a liquid theophylline preparation (6 mg/kg) in 13 asthmatic patients, 18 to 44 years of age, resulted in decreased mean plasma concentrations of zafirlukast by approximately 30%, but no effect on plasma theophylline concentrations was observed.
- Coadministration of zafirlukast (20 mg/day) or placebo at steady-state with a single dose of sustained release theophylline preparation (16 mg/kg) in 16 healthy boys and girls (6 through 11 years of age) resulted in no significant differences in the pharmacokinetic parameters of theophylline.
- Coadministration of zafirlukast dosed at 40 mg twice daily in a single-blind, parallel-group, 3-week study in 39 healthy female subjects taking oral contraceptives, resulted in no significant effect on ethinyl estradiol plasma concentrations or contraceptive efficacy.
- Coadministration of zafirlukast (40 mg/day) with aspirin (650 mg four times daily) resulted in mean increased plasma concentrations of zafirlukast by approximately 45%.
- Coadministration of a single dose of zafirlukast (40 mg) with erythromycin (500 mg three times daily for 5 days) to steady-state in 11 asthmatic patients resulted in decreased mean plasma concentrations of zafirlukast by approximately 40% due to a decrease in zafirlukast bioavailability.

Clinical Studies

Three U.S. double-blind, randomized, placebo-controlled, 13-week clinical trials in 1380 adults and children 12 years of age and older with mild-to-moderate asthma demonstrated that ACCOLATE improved daytime asthma symptoms, nighttime awakenings, mornings with asthma symptoms, rescue $beta_2$-agonist use, FEV_1, and morning peak expiratory flow rate. In these studies, the patients had a mean baseline FEV_1 of approximately 75% of predicted normal

Continued on next page

Accolate—Cont.

and a mean baseline beta$_2$-agonist requirement of approximately 4-5 puffs of albuterol per day. The results of the largest of the trials are shown in the table below.

Mean Change from Baseline at Study End Point

	ACCOLATE 20 mg twice daily N=514	Placebo N=248
Daytime Asthma symptom score (0-3 scale)	-0.44*	-0.25
Nighttime Awakenings (number per week)	-1.27*	-0.43
Mornings with Asthma Symptoms (days per week)	-1.32*	-0.75
Rescue β_2-agonist use (puffs per day)	-1.15*	-0.24
FEV_1 (L)	+0.15*	+0.05
Morning PEFR (L/min)	+22.06*	+7.63
Evening PEFR (L/min)	+13.12	+10.14

*$p<0.05$, compared to placebo

In a second and smaller study, the effect of ACCOLATE on most efficacy parameters was comparable to the active control (inhaled cromolyn sodium 1600 mcg four times per day) and superior to placebo at end point for decreasing rescue beta$_2$-agonist use (figure below).

Mean β_2 - agonist use (puffs/day)

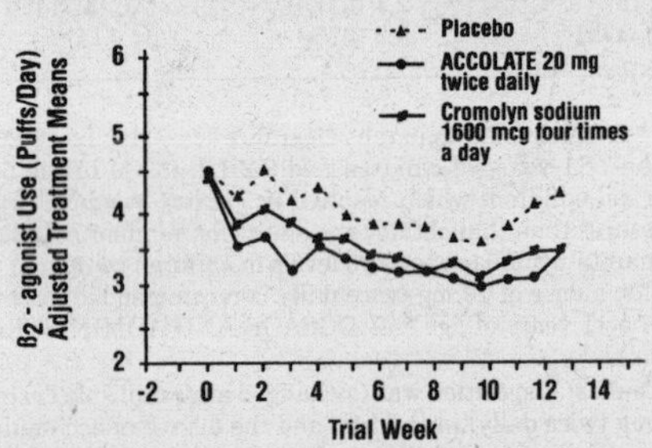

In these trials, improvement in asthma symptoms occurred within one week of initiating treatment with ACCOLATE. The role of ACCOLATE in the management of patients with more severe asthma, patients receiving antiasthma therapy other than as-needed, inhaled beta$_2$-agonists, or as an oral or inhaled corticosteroid-sparing agent remains to be fully characterized.

INDICATIONS AND USAGE

ACCOLATE is indicated for the prophylaxis and chronic treatment of asthma in adults and children 5 years of age and older.

CONTRAINDICATIONS

ACCOLATE is contraindicated in patients who are hypersensitive to zafirlukast or any of its inactive ingredients.

WARNINGS

ACCOLATE is not indicated for use in the reversal of bronchospasm in acute asthma attacks, including status asthmaticus. Therapy with ACCOLATE can be continued during acute exacerbations of asthma.

Coadministration of zafirlukast with warfarin results in a clinically significant increase in prothrombin time (PT). Patients on oral warfarin anticoagulant therapy and ACCOLATE should have their prothrombin times monitored closely and anticoagulant dose adjusted accordingly (see PRECAUTIONS, Drug Interactions).

PRECAUTIONS

Information for Patients

ACCOLATE is indicated for the chronic treatment of asthma and should be taken regularly as prescribed, even during symptom-free periods. ACCOLATE is not a bronchodilator and should not be used to treat acute episodes of asthma. Patients receiving ACCOLATE should be instructed not to decrease the dose or stop taking any other antiasthma medications unless instructed by a physician. Women who are breast-feeding should be instructed not to take ACCOLATE (see PRECAUTIONS, Nursing Mothers). Alternative antiasthma medication should be considered in such patients.

The bioavailability of ACCOLATE may be decreased when taken with food. Patients should be instructed to take ACCOLATE at least 1 hour before or 2 hours after meals.

Patients should be told that a rare side effect of ACCOLATE is hepatic dysfunction, and to contact their physician immediately if they experience symptoms of hepatic dysfunction (eg, right upper quadrant abdominal pain, nausea, fatigue, lethargy, pruritus, jaundice, flu-like symptoms, and anorexia).

Hepatic

Rarely, elevations of one or more liver enzymes have occurred in patients receiving ACCOLATE in controlled clinical trials. In clinical trials, most of these have been observed at doses four times higher than the recommended dose. The following hepatic events (which have occurred predominantly in females) have been reported from postmarketing adverse event surveillance of patients who have received the recommended dose of ACCOLATE (40 mg/day): cases of symptomatic hepatitis (with or without hyperbilirubinemia) without other attributable cause; and rarely, hyperbilirubinemia without other elevated liver function tests. In most, but not all postmarketing reports, the patient's symptoms abated and the liver enzymes returned to normal or near normal after stopping ACCOLATE. In rare cases, patients have progressed to hepatic failure.

If liver dysfunction is suspected based upon clinical signs or symptoms (eg, right upper quadrant abdominal pain, nausea, fatigue, lethargy, pruritus, jaundice, flu-like symptoms, anorexia, and enlarged liver), ACCOLATE should be discontinued. Liver function tests, in particular serum ALT, should be measured immediately and the patient managed accordingly. If liver function tests are consistent with hepatic dysfunction, ACCOLATE therapy should not be resumed. Patients in whom ACCOLATE was withdrawn because of hepatic dysfunction where no other attributable cause is identified should not be re-exposed to ACCOLATE (see PRECAUTIONS, Information for Patients and ADVERSE REACTIONS).

Eosinophilic Conditions

In rare cases, patients on ACCOLATE therapy may present with systemic eosinophilia, sometimes presenting with clinical features of vasculitis consistent with Churg-Strauss syndrome, a condition which is often treated with systemic steroid therapy. These events usually, but not always, have been associated with the reduction of oral steroid therapy. Physicians should be alert to eosinophilia, vasculitic rash, worsening pulmonary symptoms, cardiac complications, and/or neuropathy presenting in their patients. A causal association between ACCOLATE and these underlying conditions has not been established (see ADVERSE REACTIONS).

Drug Interactions

In a drug interaction study in 16 healthy male volunteers, coadministration of multiple doses of zafirlukast (160 mg/day) to steady-state with a single 25 mg dose of warfarin resulted in a significant increase in the mean AUC (+63%) and half-life (+36%) of S-warfarin. The mean prothrombin time (PT) increased by approximately 35%. This interaction is probably due to an inhibition by zafirlukast of the cytochrome P450 2C9 isoenzyme system. Patients on oral warfarin anticoagulant therapy and ACCOLATE should have their prothrombin times monitored closely and anticoagulant dose adjusted accordingly (see WARNINGS). No formal drug-drug interaction studies with ACCOLATE and other drugs known to be metabolized by the cytochrome P450 2C9 isoenzyme (eg, tolbutamide, phenytoin, carbamazepine) have been conducted; however, care should be exercised when ACCOLATE is coadministered with these drugs.

In a drug interaction study in 11 asthmatic patients, coadministration of a single dose of zafirlukast (40 mg) with erythromycin (500 mg three times daily for 5 days) to steady-state resulted in decreased mean plasma levels of zafirlukast by approximately 40% due to a decrease in zafirlukast bioavailability.

Coadministration of zafirlukast (20 mg/day) or placebo at steady-state with a single dose of sustained release theophylline preparation (16 mg/kg) in 16 healthy boys and girls (6 through 11 years of age) resulted in no significant differences in the pharmacokinetic parameters of theophylline.

Coadministration of zafirlukast (80 mg/day) at steady-state with a single dose of a liquid theophylline preparation (6 mg/kg) in 13 asthmatic patients, 18 to 44 years of age, resulted in decreased mean plasma levels of zafirlukast by approximately 30%, but no effect on plasma theophylline levels was observed.

Rare cases of patients experiencing increased theophylline levels with or without clinical signs or symptoms of theophylline toxicity after the addition of ACCOLATE to an existing theophylline regimen have been reported. The mechanism of the interaction between ACCOLATE and theophylline in these patients is unknown (see ADVERSE REACTIONS).

Coadministration of zafirlukast (40 mg/day) with aspirin (650 mg four times daily) resulted in mean increased plasma levels of zafirlukast by approximately 45%.

In a single-blind, parallel-group, 3-week study in 39 healthy female subjects taking oral contraceptives, 40 mg twice daily of zafirlukast had no significant effect on ethinyl estradiol plasma concentrations or contraceptive efficacy.

No formal drug-drug interaction studies between ACCOLATE and marketed drugs known to be metabolized by the P450 3A4 (CYP3A4) isoenzyme (eg, dihydropyridine calcium-channel blockers, cyclosporin, cisapride) have been conducted. As ACCOLATE is known to be an inhibitor of CYP3A4 *in vitro*, it is reasonable to employ appropriate clinical monitoring when these drugs are coadministered with ACCOLATE.

Carcinogenesis, Mutagenesis, Impairment of Fertility

In two-year carcinogenicity studies, zafirlukast was administered at dietary doses of 10, 100, and 300 mg/kg to mice and 40, 400, and 2000 mg/kg to rats. Male mice at an oral dose of 300 mg/kg/day (approximately 30 times the maximum recommended daily oral dose in adults and in children on a mg/m^2 basis) showed an increased incidence of hepatocellular adenomas; female mice at this dose showed a greater incidence of whole body histocytic sarcomas. Male and female rats at an oral dose of 2000 mg/kg/day (resulting in approximately 160 times the exposure to drug plus metabolites from the maximum recommended daily oral dose in adults and in children based on a comparison of the plasma area-under the curve [AUC] values) of zafirlukast showed an increased incidence of urinary bladder transitional cell papillomas. Zafirlukast was not tumorigenic at oral doses up to 100 mg/kg (approximately 10 times the maximum recommended daily oral dose in adults and in children on a mg/m^2 basis) in mice and at oral doses up to 400 mg/kg (resulting in approximately 140 times the exposure to drug plus metabolites from the maximum recommended daily oral dose in adults and in children based on a comparison of the plasma AUC values) in rats. The clinical significance of these findings for the long-term use of ACCOLATE is unknown.

Zafirlukast showed no evidence of mutagenic potential in the reverse microbial assay, in 2 forward point mutation (CHO-HGPRT and mouse lymphoma) assays or in two assays for chromosomal aberrations (the *in vitro* human peripheral blood lymphocyte clastogenic assay and the *in vivo* rat bone marrow micronucleus assay).

No evidence of impairment of fertility and reproduction was seen in male and female rats treated with zafirlukast at oral doses up to 2000 mg/kg (approximately 410 times the maximum recommended daily oral dose in adults on a mg/m^2 basis).

Pregnancy Category B

No teratogenicity was observed at oral doses up to 1600 mg/kg/day in mice (approximately 160 times the maximum recommended daily oral dose in adults on a mg/m^2 basis), up to 2000 mg/kg/day in rats (approximately 410 times the maximum recommended daily oral dose in adults on a mg/m^2 basis) and up to 2000 mg/kg/day in cynomolgus monkeys (which resulted in approximately 20 times the exposure to drug plus metabolites compared to that from the maximum recommended daily oral dose in adults based on comparison of the AUC values). At an oral dose of 2000 mg/kg/day in rats, maternal toxicity and deaths were seen with increased incidence of early fetal resorption. Spontaneous abortions occurred in cynomolgus monkeys at the maternally toxic oral dose of 2000 mg/kg/day. There are no adequate and well-controlled trials in pregnant women. Because animal reproductive studies are not always predictive of human response, ACCOLATE should be used during pregnancy only if clearly needed.

Nursing Mothers

Zafirlukast is excreted in breast milk. Following repeated 40 mg twice-a-day dosing in healthy women, average steady-state concentrations of zafirlukast in breast milk were 50 ng/mL compared to 255 ng/mL in plasma. Because of the potential for tumorigenicity shown for zafirlukast in mouse and rat studies and the enhanced sensitivity of neonatal rats and dogs to the adverse effects of zafirlukast, ACCOLATE should not be administered to mothers who are breast-feeding.

Pediatric Use

The safety of ACCOLATE at doses of 10 mg twice daily has been demonstrated in 205 pediatric patients 5 through 11 years of age in placebo-controlled trials lasting up to six weeks and with 179 patients in this age range participating in 52 weeks of treatment in an open label extension.

The effectiveness of ACCOLATE for the prophylaxis and chronic treatment of asthma in pediatric patients 5 through 11 years of age is based on an extrapolation of the demonstrated efficacy of ACCOLATE in adults with asthma and the likelihood that the disease course, and pathophysiology and the drug's effect are substantially similar between the two populations. The recommended dose for the patients 5 through 11 years of age is based upon a cross-study comparison of the pharmacokinetics of zafirlukast in adults and pediatric subjects, and on the safety profile of zafirlukast in both adult and pediatric patients at doses equal to or higher than the recommended dose.

The safety and effectiveness of zafirlukast for pediatric patients less than 5 years of age has not been established.

Geriatric Use

Based on cross-study comparison, the clearance of zafirlukast is reduced in patients 65 years of age and older such that C_{max} and AUC are approximately 2- to 3-fold greater than those of younger patients (see DOSAGE AND ADMINISTRATION and CLINICAL PHARMACOLOGY).

A total of 8094 patients were exposed to zafirlukast in North American and European short-term placebo-controlled clinical trials. Of these, 243 patients were elderly (age 65 years and older). No overall difference in adverse events was seen in the elderly patients, except for an increase in the frequency of infections among zafirlukast-treated elderly patients compared to placebo-treated elderly patients (7.0% vs. 2.9%). The infections were not severe, occurred mostly in the lower respiratory tract, and did not necessitate withdrawal of therapy.

An open-label, uncontrolled, 4-week trial of 3759 asthma patients compared the safety and efficacy of ACCOLATE 20 mg given twice daily in three patient age groups, adolescents (12-17 years), adults (18-65 years), and elderly (greater than 65 years). A higher percentage of elderly patients (n=384) reported adverse events when compared to adults and adolescents. These elderly patients showed less improvement in efficacy measures. In the elderly patients, adverse events occurring in greater than 1% of the population included headache (4.7%), diarrhea and nausea (1.8%), and pharyngitis (1.3%). The elderly reported the lowest percentage of infections of all three age groups in this study.

ADVERSE REACTIONS

Adults and Children 12 years of age and older

The safety database for ACCOLATE consists of more than 4000 healthy volunteers and patients who received ACCOLATE, of which 1723 were asthmatics enrolled in trials of 13 weeks duration or longer. A total of 671 patients

received ACCOLATE for 1 year or longer. The majority of the patients were 18 years of age or older; however, 222 patients between the age of 12 and 18 years received ACCOLATE.
A comparison of adverse events reported by ≥ 1% of zafirlukast-treated patients, and at rates numerically greater than in placebo-treated patients, is shown for all trials in the table below.

Adverse Event	ACCOLATE N=4058	PLACEBO N=2032
Headache	12.9%	11.7%
Infection	3.5%	3.4%
Nausea	3.1%	2.0%
Diarrhea	2.8%	2.1%
Pain (generalized)	1.9%	1.7%
Asthenia	1.8%	1.6%
Abdominal Pain	1.8%	1.1%
Accidental Injury	1.6%	1.5%
Dizziness	1.6%	1.5%
Myalgia	1.6%	1.5%
Fever	1.6%	1.1%
Back Pain	1.5%	1.2%
Vomiting	1.5%	1.1%
SGPT Elevation	1.5%	1.1%
Dyspepsia	1.3%	1.2%

The frequency of less common adverse events was comparable between ACCOLATE and placebo.
Rarely, elevations of one or more liver enzymes have occurred in patients receiving ACCOLATE in controlled clinical trials. In clinical trials, most of these have been observed at doses four times higher than the recommended dose. The following hepatic events (which have occurred predominantly in females) have been reported from postmarketing adverse event surveillance of patients who have received the recommended dose of ACCOLATE (40 mg/day): cases of symptomatic hepatitis (with or without hyperbilirubinemia) without other attributable cause; and rarely, hyperbilirubinemia without other elevated liver function tests. In most, but not all postmarketing reports, the patient's symptoms abated and the liver enzymes returned to normal or near normal after stopping ACCOLATE. In rare cases, patients have progressed to hepatic failure.
In clinical trials, an increased proportion of zafirlukast patients over the age of 55 years reported infections as compared to placebo-treated patients. A similar finding was not observed in other age groups studied. These infections were mostly mild or moderate in intensity and predominantly affected the respiratory tract. Infections occurred equally in both sexes, were dose-proportional to total milligrams of zafirlukast exposure, and were associated with coadministration of inhaled corticosteroids. The clinical significance of this finding is unknown.
In rare cases, patients on ACCOLATE therapy may present with systemic eosinophilia, sometimes presenting with clinical features of vasculitis consistent with Churg-Strauss syndrome, a condition which is often treated with systemic steroid therapy. These events usually, but not always, have been associated with the reduction of oral steroid therapy. Physicians should be alert to eosinophilia, vasculitic rash, worsening pulmonary symptoms, cardiac complications, and/or neuropathy presenting in their patients. A causal association between ACCOLATE and these underlying conditions has not been established (see PRECAUTIONS, Eosinophilic Conditions).
Hypersensitivity reactions, including urticaria, angioedema and rashes, with or without blistering, have been reported in association with ACCOLATE therapy. Additionally, there have been reports of patients experiencing agranulocytosis, bleeding, bruising, or edema, arthralgia, and myalgia in association with ACCOLATE therapy.
Rare cases of patients experiencing increased theophylline levels with or without clinical signs or symptoms of theophylline toxicity after the addition of ACCOLATE to an existing theophylline regimen have been reported. The mechanism of the interaction between ACCOLATE and theophylline in these patients is unknown and not predicted by available *in vitro* metabolism data and the results of two clinical drug interaction studies (see CLINICAL PHARMACOLOGY and PRECAUTIONS, Drug Interactions).

Pediatric Patients 5 through 11 years of age
ACCOLATE has been evaluated for safety in 788 pediatric patients 5 through 11 years of age. Cumulatively, 313 pediatric patients were treated with ACCOLATE 10 mg twice daily or higher for at least 6 months, and 113 of them were treated for one year or longer in clinical trials. The safety profile of ACCOLATE 10 mg twice daily versus placebo in the 4- and 6-week double-blind trials was generally similar to that observed in the adult clinical trials with ACCOLATE 20 mg twice daily.
In pediatric patients receiving ACCOLATE in multi-dose clinical trials, the following events occurred with a frequency of ≥2% and more frequently than in pediatric patients who received placebo, regardless of causality assessment: headache (4.5 vs. 4.2%) and abdominal pain (2.8 vs. 2.3%).

OVERDOSAGE
No deaths occurred at oral zafirlukast doses of 2000 mg/kg in mice (approximately 210 times the maximum recommended daily oral dose in adults and children on a mg/m^2 basis), 2000 mg/kg in rats (approximately 420 times the maximum recommended daily oral dose in adults and children on a mg/m^2 basis), and 500 mg/kg in dogs (approximately 350 times the maximum recommended daily oral dose in adults and children on a mg/m^2 basis).
Overdosage with ACCOLATE has been reported in four patients surviving reported doses as high as 200 mg. The predominant symptoms reported following ACCOLATE overdose were rash and upset stomach. There were no acute toxic effects in humans that could be consistently ascribed to the administration of ACCOLATE. It is reasonable to employ the usual supportive measures in the event of an overdose; eg, remove unabsorbed material from the gastrointestinal tract, employ clinical monitoring, and institute supportive therapy, if required.

DOSAGE AND ADMINISTRATION
Because food can reduce the bioavailability of zafirlukast, ACCOLATE should be taken at least 1 hour before or 2 hours after meals.
Adults and Children 12 years of age and older
The recommended dose of ACCOLATE in adults and children 12 years and older is 20 mg twice daily.
Pediatric Patients 5 through 11 years of age
The recommended dose of ACCOLATE in children 5 through 11 years of age is 10 mg twice daily.
Elderly Patients: Based on cross-study comparisons, the clearance of zafirlukast is reduced in elderly patients (65 years of age and older), such that C_{max} and AUC are approximately twice those of younger adults. In clinical trials, a dose of 20 mg twice daily was not associated with an increase in the overall incidence of adverse events or withdrawals because of adverse events in elderly patients.
Patients with Hepatic Impairment: The clearance of zafirlukast is reduced in patients with stable alcoholic cirrhosis such that the C_{max} and AUC are approximately 50 - 60% greater than those of normal adults. ACCOLATE has not been evaluated in patients with hepatitis or in long-term studies of patients with cirrhosis.
Patients with Renal Impairment: Dosage adjustment is not required for patients with renal impairment.

HOW SUPPLIED
ACCOLATE 10 mg Tablets, (NDC 0310-0401) white, unflavored, round, biconvex, film-coated, mini-tablets identified with "ACCOLATE 10" debossed on one side are supplied in opaque HDPE bottles of 60 tablets and Hospital Unit Dose blister packages of 100 tablets.
ACCOLATE 20 mg Tablets, (NDC 0310-0402) white, round, biconvex, coated tablets identified with "ACCOLATE 20" debossed on one side are supplied in opaque HDPE bottles of 60 tablets and Hospital Unit Dose blister packages of 100 tablets.
Store at controlled room temperature, 20-25°C (68-77°F) [see USP]. Protect from light and moisture. Dispense in the original air-tight container.
All trademarks are the property of the AstraZeneca group

Manufactured for:
AstraZeneca Pharmaceuticals LP
Wilmington, DE 19850
By: IPR Pharmaceuticals, Inc.
Carolina, PR 00984
64198-00 Rev 4/01
203597 8/01

ZOMIG® ℞
[*zō-mĭg*]
(zolmitriptan)
Tablets
ZOMIG-ZMT™ ℞
(zolmitriptan)
Orally Disintegrating Tablets

Prescribing information for this product, which appears on pages 708–711 of the 2002 PDR, has been revised as follows. Please write "See Supplement A" next to the product heading.

The 3rd paragraph under **DESCRIPTIONS** *section was revised to read:*
ZOMIG-ZMT™ Orally Disintegrating Tablets are available as 2.5 mg and 5.0 mg white uncoated tablets for oral administration. The orally disintegrating tablets contain mannitol USP, microcrystalline cellulose NF, crospovidone NF, aspartame NF, sodium bicarbonate USP, citric acid anhydrous USP, colloidal silicon dioxide NF, magnesium stearate NF and orange flavor SN 027512.
Under **PRECAUTIONS,** *subsection* **Phenylketonurics,** *the paragraph was revised to read:*
Phenylketonuric patients should be informed that ZOMIG-ZMT Tablets contain phenylalanine (a component of aspartame). Each 2.5 mg orally disintegrating tablet contains 2.81 mg phenylalanine. Each 5 mg orally disintegrating tablet contains 5.62 mg phenylalanine.
The following new 4th paragraph was added under the **HOW SUPPLIED** *section:*
5 mg Orally Disintegrating Tablets - White, flat faced, round, uncoated, bevelled tablet containing 5.0 mg of zolmitriptan identified with a debossed "Z" and "5" on one side and plain on the other are supplied in cartons containing a blister pack of 3 tablets (NDC 0310-0213-21).
64192-01, Rev 10/01.

Aventis Pharmaceuticals
300 SOMERSET CORPORATE BOULEVARD
BRIDGEWATER, NJ 08807-2854

Direct Inquiries to:
Customer Service
300 Somerset Corporate Boulevard
Bridgewater, NJ 08807-2854
(800) 207-8049

For Medical Information Contact:
Generally:
Medical Informatics
300 Somerset Corporate Boulevard
Bridgewater, NJ 08807-2854
(800) 633-1610
For information on the following products which are not described, contact the Customer Information Center at (800) 552-3656:
Bentyl® (dicyclomine hydrochloride USP) Capsules, Tablets, Injection, Syrup
Cantil® (mepenzolate bromide USP) Tablets
Cephulac® (lactulose solution)
Chronulac® (lactulose solution)
DDAVP® Rhinal Tube 2.5 mL (desmopressin acetate)
Hiprex® (methenamine hippurate)
Tenuate® (diethylpropion hydrochloride USP) Tablets/Dospan

AMARYL® ℞
[*am'ə ril*]
(glimepiride tablets)
1, 2, and 4 mg
Rx Only
Prescribing Information as of July 2001

Prescribing information for this product, which appears on pages 717–719 of the 2002 PDR, has been completely revised as follows. Please write "See Supplement A" next to the product heading.

DESCRIPTION
AMARYL® (glimepiride tablets) is an oral blood-glucose-lowering drug of the sulfonylurea class. Glimepiride is a white to yellowish-white, crystalline, odorless to practically odorless powder formulated into tablets of 1-mg, 2-mg, and 4-mg strengths for oral administration. AMARYL tablets contain the active ingredient glimepiride and the following inactive ingredients: lactose (hydrous), sodium starch glycolate, povidone, microcrystalline cellulose, and magnesium stearate. In addition, AMARYL 1-mg tablets contain Ferric Oxide Red, AMARYL 2-mg tablets contain Ferric Oxide Yellow and FD&C Blue #2 Aluminum Lake, and AMARYL 4-mg tablets contain FD&C Blue #2 Aluminum Lake.
Chemically, glimepiride is identified as 1-[[p-[2-(3-ethyl-4-methyl-2-oxo-3-pyrroline-1-carboxamido) ethyl]phenyl]sulfonyl]-3-(trans-4-methylcyclohexyl)urea.
The CAS Registry Number is 93479-97-1
The structural formula is:

Molecular Formula: $C_{24}H_{34}N_4O_5S$
Molecular Weight: 490.62
Glimepiride is practically insoluble in water.

CLINICAL PHARMACOLOGY
Mechanism Of Action
The primary mechanism of action of glimepiride in lowering blood glucose appears to be dependent on stimulating the release of insulin from functioning pancreatic beta cells. In addition, extrapancreatic effects may also play a role in the activity of sulfonylureas such as glimepiride. This is supported by both preclinical and clinical studies demonstrating that glimepiride administration can lead to increased sensitivity of peripheral tissues to insulin. These findings are consistent with the results of a long-term, randomized, placebo-controlled trial in which AMARYL therapy improved postprandial insulin/C-peptide responses and overall glycemic control without producing clinically meaningful increases in fasting insulin/C-peptide levels. However, as with other sulfonylureas, the mechanism by which glimepiride lowers blood glucose during long-term administration has not been clearly established.
AMARYL is effective as initial drug therapy. In patients where monotherapy with AMARYL or metformin has not produced adequate glycemic control, the combination of AMARYL and metformin may have a synergistic effect, since both agents act to improve glucose tolerance by different primary mechanisms of action. This complementary effect has been observed with metformin and other sulfonylureas, in multiple studies.
Pharmacodynamics
A mild glucose-lowering effect first appeared following single oral doses as low as 0.5–0.6 mg in healthy subjects. The time required to reach the maximum effect (i.e., minimum blood glucose level [T_{min}]) was about 2 to 3 hours. In noninsulin-dependent (Type II) diabetes mellitus (NIDDM) pa-

Continued on next page

Amaryl—Cont.

tients, both fasting and 2-hour postprandial glucose levels were significantly lower with glimepiride (1, 2, 4, and 8 mg once daily) than with placebo after 14 days of oral dosing. The glucose-lowering effect in all active treatment groups was maintained over 24 hours.

In larger dose-ranging studies, blood glucose and HbA_{1c} were found to respond in a dose-dependent manner over the range of 1 to 4 mg/day of AMARYL. Some patients, particularly those with higher fasting plasma glucose (FPG) levels, may benefit from doses of AMARYL up to 8 mg once daily. No difference in response was found when AMARYL was administered once or twice daily.

In two 14-week, placebo-controlled studies in 720 subjects, the average net reduction in HbA_{1c} for AMARYL (glimepiride tablets) -patients treated with 8 mg once daily was 2.0% in absolute units compared with placebo-treated patients. In a long-term, randomized, placebo-controlled study of NIDDM patients unresponsive to dietary management, AMARYL therapy improved postprandial insulin/C-peptide responses, and 75% of patients achieved and maintained control of blood glucose and HbA_{1c}. Efficacy results were not affected by age, gender, weight, or race.

In long-term extension trials with previously-treated patients, no meaningful deterioration in mean fasting blood glucose (FBG) or HbA_{1c} levels was seen after 2 1/2 years of AMARYL therapy.

Combination therapy with AMARYL and insulin (70% NPH/30% regular) was compared to placebo/insulin in secondary failure patients whose body weight was >130% of their ideal body weight. Initially, 5–10 units of insulin were administered with the main evening meal and titrated upward weekly to achieve predefined FPG values. Both groups in this double-blind study achieved similar reductions in FPG levels but the AMARYL/insulin therapy group used approximately 38% less insulin.

AMARYL therapy is effective in controlling blood glucose without deleterious changes in the plasma lipoprotein profiles of patients treated for NIDDM.

Pharmacokinetics

Absorption. After oral administration, glimepiride is completely (100%) absorbed from the GI tract. Studies with single oral doses in normal subjects and with multiple oral doses in patients with NIDDM have shown significant absorption of glimepiride within 1 hour after administration and peak drug levels (C_{max}) at 2 to 3 hours. When glimepiride was given with meals, the mean T_{max} (time to reach C_{max}) was slightly increased (12%) and the mean C_{max} and AUC (area under the curve) were slightly decreased (8% and 9%, respectively).

Distribution. After intravenous (IV) dosing in normal subjects, the volume of distribution (Vd) was 8.8 L (113 mL/kg), and the total body clearance (CL) was 47.8 mL/min. Protein binding was greater than 99.5%.

Metabolism. Glimepiride is completely metabolized by oxidative biotransformation after either an IV or oral dose. The major metabolites are the cyclohexyl hydroxy methyl derivative (M1) and the carboxyl derivative (M2). Cytochrome P450 II C9 has been shown to be involved in the biotransformation of glimepiride to M1. M1 is further metabolized to M2 by one or several cytosolic enzymes. M1, but not M2, possesses about 1/3 of the pharmacological activity as compared to its parent in an animal model; however, whether the glucose-lowering effect of M1 is clinically meaningful is not clear.

Excretion. When ^{14}C-glimepiride was given orally, approximately 60% of the total radioactivity was recovered in the urine in 7 days and M1 (predominant) and M2 accounted for 80–90% of that recovered in the urine. Approximately 40% of the total radioactivity was recovered in feces and M1 and M2 (predominant) accounted for about 70% of that recovered in feces. No parent drug was recovered from urine or feces. After IV dosing in patients, no significant biliary excretion of glimepiride or its M1 metabolite has been observed.

Pharmacokinetic Parameters. The pharmacokinetic parameters of glimepiride obtained from a single-dose, crossover, dose-proportionality (1, 2, 4, and 8 mg) study in normal subjects and from a single- and multiple-dose, parallel, dose-proportionality (4 and 8 mg) study in patients with NIDDM are summarized below:

[See table below]

These data indicate that glimepiride did not accumulate in serum, and the pharmacokinetics of glimepiride were not different in healthy volunteers and in NIDDM patients. Oral clearance of glimepiride did not change over the 1–8-mg dose range, indicating linear pharmacokinetics.

Variability. In normal healthy volunteers, the intra-individual variabilities of C_{max}, AUC, and CL/f for glimepiride were 23%, 17%, and 15%, respectively, and the inter-individual variabilities were 25%, 29%, and 24%, respectively.

Special Populations

Geriatric. Comparison of glimepiride pharmacokinetics in NIDDM patients ≤65 years and those >65 years was performed in a study using a dosing regimen of 6 mg daily. There were no significant differences in glimepiride pharmacokinetics between the two age groups. The mean AUC at steady state for the older patients was about 13% lower than that for the younger patients; the mean weight-adjusted clearance for the older patients was about 11% higher than that for the younger patients.

Pediatric. No studies were performed in pediatric patients.

Gender. There were no differences between males and females in the pharmacokinetics of glimepiride when adjustment was made for differences in body weight.

Race. No pharmacokinetic studies to assess the effects of race have been performed, but in placebo-controlled studies of AMARYL (glimepiride tablets) in patients with NIDDM, the antihyperglycemic effect was comparable in whites (n = 536), blacks (n = 63), and Hispanics (n = 63).

Renal Insufficiency. A single-dose, open-label study was conducted in 15 patients with renal impairment. AMARYL (3 mg) was administered to 3 groups of patients with different levels of mean creatinine clearance (CLcr); (Group I, CLcr = 77.7 mL/min, n = 5), (Group II, CLcr = 27.7 mL/min, n = 3), and (Group III, CLcr = 9.4 mL/min, n = 7). AMARYL was found to be well tolerated in all 3 groups. The results showed that glimepiride serum levels decreased as renal function decreased. However, M1 and M2 serum levels (mean AUC values) increased 2.3 and 8.6 times from Group I to Group III. The apparent terminal half-life ($T_{1/2}$) for glimepiride did not change, while the half-lives for M1 and M2 increased as renal function decreased. Mean urinary excretion of M1 plus M2 as percent of dose, however, decreased (44.4%, 21.9%, and 9.3% for Groups I to III).

A multiple-dose titration study was also conducted in 16 NIDDM patients with renal impairment using doses ranging from 1–8 mg daily for 3 months. The results were consistent with those observed after single doses. All patients with a CLcr less than 22 mL/min had adequate control of their glucose levels with a dosage regimen of only 1 mg daily. The results from this study suggested that a starting dose of 1 mg AMARYL may be given to NIDDM patients with kidney disease, and the dose may be titrated based on fasting blood glucose levels.

Hepatic Insufficiency. No studies were performed in patients with hepatic insufficiency.

Other Populations. There were no important differences in glimepiride metabolism in subjects identified as phenotypically different drug-metabolizers by their metabolism of sparteine.

The pharmacokinetics of glimepiride in morbidly obese patients were similar to those in the normal weight group, except for a lower C_{max} and AUC. However, since neither C_{max} nor AUC values were normalized for body surface area, the lower values of C_{max} and AUC for the obese patients were likely the result of their excess weight and not due to a difference in the kinetics of glimepiride.

Drug Interactions. The hypoglycemic action of sulfonylureas may be potentiated by certain drugs, including nonsteroidal anti-inflammatory drugs and other drugs that are highly protein bound, such as salicylates, sulfonamides, chloramphenicol, coumarins, probenecid, monoamine oxidase inhibitors, and beta adrenergic blocking agents. When these drugs are administered to a patient receiving AMARYL, the patient should be observed closely for hypoglycemia. When these drugs are withdrawn from a patient receiving AMARYL, the patient should be observed closely for loss of glycemic control.

Certain drugs tend to produce hyperglycemia and may lead to loss of control. These drugs include the thiazides and other diuretics, corticosteroids, phenothiazines, thyroid products, estrogens, oral contraceptives, phenytoin, nicotinic acid, sympathomimetics, and isoniazid. When these drugs are administered to a patient receiving AMARYL, the patient should be closely observed for loss of control. When these drugs are withdrawn from a patient receiving AMARYL, the patient should be observed closely for hypoglycemia.

Coadministration of aspirin (1 g tid) and AMARYL led to a 34% decrease in the mean glimepiride AUC and, therefore, a 34% increase in the mean CL/f. The mean C_{max} had a decrease of 4%. Blood glucose and serum C-peptide concentrations were unaffected and no hypoglycemic symptoms were reported. Pooled data from clinical trials showed no evidence of clinically significant adverse interactions with uncontrolled concurrent administration of aspirin and other salicylates.

Coadministration of either cimetidine (800 mg once daily) or ranitidine (150 mg bid) with a single 4-mg oral dose of AMARYL did not significantly alter the absorption and disposition of glimepiride, and no differences were seen in hypoglycemic symptomatology. Pooled data from clinical trials showed no evidence of clinically significant adverse interactions with uncontrolled concurrent administration of H2-receptor antagonists.

Concomitant administration of propranolol (40 mg tid) and AMARYL significantly increased C_{max}, AUC, and $T_{1/2}$ of glimepiride by 23%, 22%, and 15%, respectively, and it decreased CL/f by 18%. The recovery of M1 and M2 from urine, however, did not change. The pharmacodynamic responses to glimepiride were nearly identical in normal subjects receiving propranolol and placebo. Pooled data from clinical trials in patients with NIDDM showed no evidence of clinically significant adverse interactions with uncontrolled concurrent administration of beta-blockers. However, if beta-blockers are used, caution should be exercised and patients should be warned about the potential for hypoglycemia.

Concomitant administration of AMARYL (glimepiride tablets) (4 mg once daily) did not alter the pharmacokinetic characteristics of R- and S-warfarin enantiomers following administration of a single dose (25 mg) of racemic warfarin to healthy subjects. No changes were observed in warfarin plasma protein binding. AMARYL treatment did result in a slight, but statistically significant, decrease in the pharmacodynamic response to warfarin. The reductions in mean area under the prothrombin time (PT) curve and maximum PT values during AMARYL treatment were very small (3.3% and 9.9%, respectively) and are unlikely to be clinically important.

The responses of serum glucose, insulin, C-peptide, and plasma glucagon to 2 mg AMARYL were unaffected by coadministration of ramipril (an ACE inhibitor) 5 mg once daily in normal subjects. No hypoglycemic symptoms were reported. Pooled data from clinical trials in patients with NIDDM showed no evidence of clinically significant adverse interactions with uncontrolled concurrent administration of ACE inhibitors.

A potential interaction between oral miconazole and oral hypoglycemic agents leading to severe hypoglycemia has been reported. Whether this interaction also occurs with the intravenous, topical, or vaginal preparations of miconazole is not known. Potential interactions of glimepiride with other drugs metabolized by cytochrome P450 II C9 also include phenytoin, diclofenac, ibuprofen, naproxen, and mefenamic acid.

Although no specific interaction studies were performed, pooled data from clinical trials showed no evidence of clinically significant adverse interactions with uncontrolled concurrent administration of calcium-channel blockers, estrogens, fibrates, NSAIDS, HMG CoA reductase inhibitors, sulfonamides, or thyroid hormone.

INDICATIONS AND USAGE

AMARYL is indicated as an adjunct to diet and exercise to lower the blood glucose in patients with noninsulin-dependent (Type II) diabetes mellitus (NIDDM) whose hyperglycemia cannot be controlled by diet and exercise alone.

AMARYL may be used concomitantly with metformin when diet, exercise, and AMARYL or metformin alone do not result in adequate glycemic control.

AMARYL is also indicated for use in combination with insulin to lower blood glucose in patients whose hyperglycemia cannot be controlled by diet and exercise in conjunction with an oral hypoglycemic agent. Combined use of glimepiride and insulin may increase the potential for hypoglycemia.

In initiating treatment for noninsulin-dependent diabetes, diet and exercise should be emphasized as the primary form of treatment. Caloric restriction, weight loss, and exercise are essential in the obese diabetic patient. Proper dietary management and exercise alone may be effective in controlling the blood glucose and symptoms of hyperglycemia. In addition to regular physical activity, cardiovascular risk factors should be identified and corrective measures taken where possible.

If this treatment program fails to reduce symptoms and/or blood glucose, the use of an oral sulfonylurea or insulin should be considered. Use of AMARYL must be viewed by both the physician and patient as a treatment in addition to diet and exercise and not as a substitute for diet and exercise or as a convenient mechanism for avoiding dietary restraint. Furthermore, loss of blood glucose control on diet and exercise alone may be transient, thus requiring only short-term administration of AMARYL.

During maintenance programs, AMARYL monotherapy should be discontinued if satisfactory lowering of blood glucose is no longer achieved. Judgments should be based on regular clinical and laboratory evaluations. Secondary failures to AMARYL monotherapy can be treated with AMARYL-insulin combination therapy. In considering the use of AMARYL in asymptomatic patients, it should be recognized that blood glucose control in NIDDM has not defi-

	Volunteers Single Dose Mean±SD	Patients with NIDDM Single Dose (Day 1) Mean±SD	Multiple Dose (Day 10) Mean±SD
C_{max} (ng/mL)			
1 mg	103 ± 34 (12)	—	—
2 mg	177 ± 44 (12)	—	—
4 mg	308 ± 69 (12)	352 ± 222 (12)	309 ± 134 (12)
8 mg	557 ± 152 (12)	591 ± 232 (14)	578 ± 265 (11)
T_{max} (h)	2.4 ± 0.8 (48)	2.5 ± 1.2 (26)	2.8 ± 2.2 (23)
CL/f (mL/min)	52.1 ± 16.0 (48)	48.5 ± 29.3 (26)	52.7 ± 40.3 (23)
Vd/f (L)	21.8 ± 13.9 (48)	19.8 ± 12.7 (26)	37.1 ± 18.2 (23)
T1/2 (h)	5.3 ± 4.1 (48)	5.0 ± 2.5 (26)	9.2 ± 3.6 (23)

( ) = No. of subjects
CL/f = Total body clearance after oral dosing
Vd/f = Volume of distribution calculated after oral dosing

nitely been established to be effective in preventing the long-term cardiovascular and neural complications of diabetes. However, the Diabetes Control and Complications Trial (DCCT) demonstrated that control of HbA_{1c} and glucose was associated with a decrease in retinopathy, neuropathy, and nephropathy for insulin-dependent diabetic (IDDM) patients.

CONTRAINDICATIONS

AMARYL is contraindicated in patients with

1. Known hypersensitivity to the drug.
2. Diabetic ketoacidosis, with or without coma. This condition should be treated with insulin.

WARNINGS

SPECIAL WARNING ON INCREASED RISK OF CARDIOVASCULAR MORTALITY

The administration of oral hypoglycemic drugs has been reported to be associated with increased cardiovascular mortality as compared to treatment with diet alone or diet plus insulin. This warning is based on the study conducted by the University Group Diabetes Program (UGDP), a long-term, prospective clinical trial designed to evaluate the effectiveness of glucose-lowering drugs in preventing or delaying vascular complications in patients with non-insulin-dependent diabetes. The study involved 823 patients who were randomly assigned to one of four treatment groups (Diabetes, 19 supp. 2: 747–830, 1970).

UGDP reported that patients treated for 5 to 8 years with diet plus a fixed dose of tolbutamide (1.5 grams per day) had a rate of cardiovascular mortality approximately 2-1/2 times that of patients treated with diet alone. A significant increase in total mortality was not observed, but the use of tolbutamide was discontinued based on the increase in cardiovascular mortality, thus limiting the opportunity for the study to show an increase in overall mortality. Despite controversy regarding the interpretation of these results, the findings of the UGDP study provide an adequate basis for this warning. The patient should be informed of the potential risks and advantages of AMARYL (glimepiride tablets) and of alternative modes of therapy.

Although only one drug in the sulfonylurea class (tolbutamide) was included in this study, it is prudent from a safety standpoint to consider that this warning may also apply to other oral hypoglycemic drugs in this class, in view of their close similarities in mode of action and chemical structure.

PRECAUTIONS

General

Hypoglycemia: All sulfonylurea drugs are capable of producing severe hypoglycemia. Proper patient selection, dosage, and instructions are important to avoid hypoglycemic episodes. Patients with impaired renal function may be more sensitive to the glucose-lowering effect of AMARYL. A starting dose of 1 mg once daily followed by appropriate dose titration is recommended in those patients. Debilitated or malnourished patients, and those with adrenal, pituitary, or hepatic insufficiency are particularly susceptible to the hypoglycemic action of glucose-lowering drugs. Hypoglycemia may be difficult to recognize in the elderly and in people who are taking beta-adrenergic blocking drugs or other sympatholytic agents. Hypoglycemia is more likely to occur when caloric intake is deficient, after severe or prolonged exercise, when alcohol is ingested, or when more than one glucose-lowering drug is used. Combined use of glimepiride with insulin or metformin may increase the potential for hypoglycemia.

Loss of control of blood glucose: When a patient stabilized on any diabetic regimen is exposed to stress such as fever, trauma, infection, or surgery, a loss of control may occur. At such times, it may be necessary to add insulin in combination with AMARYL or even use insulin monotherapy. The effectiveness of any oral hypoglycemic drug, including AMARYL, in lowering blood glucose to a desired level decreases in many patients over a period of time, which may be due to progression of the severity of the diabetes or to diminished responsiveness to the drug. This phenomenon is known as secondary failure, to distinguish it from primary failure in which the drug is ineffective in an individual patient when first given. Should secondary failure occur with AMARYL or metformin monotherapy, combined therapy with AMARYL and metformin or AMARYL and insulin may result in a response. Should secondary failure occur with combined AMARYL/metformin therapy, it may be necessary to initiate insulin therapy.

Information for Patients

Patients should be informed of the potential risks and advantages of AMARYL and of alternative modes of therapy. They should also be informed about the importance of adherence to dietary instructions, of a regular exercise program, and of regular testing of blood glucose.

The risks of hypoglycemia, its symptoms and treatment, and conditions that predispose to its development should be explained to patients and responsible family members. The potential for primary and secondary failure should also be explained.

Laboratory Tests

Fasting blood glucose should be monitored periodically to determine therapeutic response. Glycosylated hemoglobin should also be monitored, usually every 3 to 6 months, to more precisely assess long-term glycemic control.

Drug Interactions

(See CLINICAL PHARMACOLOGY, Drug Interactions.)

Carcinogenesis, Mutagenesis, and Impairment of Fertility

Studies in rats at doses of up to 5000 ppm in complete feed (approximately 340 times the maximum recommended human dose, based on surface area) for 30 months showed no evidence of carcinogenesis. In mice, administration of glimepiride for 24 months resulted in an increase in benign pancreatic adenoma formation which was dose related and is thought to be the result of chronic pancreatic stimulation. The no-effect dose for adenoma formation in mice in this study was 320 ppm in complete feed, or 46–54 mg/kg body weight/day. This is about 35 times the maximum human recommended dose of 8 mg once daily based on surface area. Glimepiride was non-mutagenic in a battery of *in vitro* and *in vivo* mutagenicity studies (Ames test, somatic cell mutation, chromosomal aberration, unscheduled DNA synthesis, mouse micronucleus test).

There was no effect of glimepiride on male mouse fertility in animals exposed up to 2500 mg/kg body weight (>1,700 times the maximum recommended human dose based on surface area). Glimepiride had no effect on the fertility of male and female rats administered up to 4000 mg/kg body weight (approximately 4,000 times the maximum recommended human dose based on surface area).

Pregnancy

Teratogenic Effects. Pregnancy Category C. Glimepiride did not produce teratogenic effects in rats exposed orally up to 4000 mg/kg body weight (approximately 4,000 times the maximum recommended human dose based on surface area) or in rabbits exposed up to 32 mg/kg body weight (approximately 60 times the maximum recommended human dose based on surface area). Glimepiride has been shown to be associated with intrauterine fetal death in rats when given in doses as low as 50 times the human dose based on surface area and in rabbits when given in doses as low as 0.1 times the human dose based on surface area. This fetotoxicity, observed only at doses inducing maternal hypoglycemia, has been similarly noted with other sulfonylureas, and is believed to be directly related to the pharmacologic (hypoglycemic) action of glimepiride.

There are no adequate and well-controlled studies in pregnant women. On the basis of results from animal studies, AMARYL (glimepiride tablets) should not be used during pregnancy. Because recent information suggests that abnormal blood glucose levels during pregnancy are associated with a higher incidence of congenital abnormalities, many experts recommend that insulin be used during pregnancy to maintain glucose levels as close to normal as possible.

Nonteratogenic Effects. In some studies in rats, offspring of dams exposed to high levels of glimepiride during pregnancy and lactation developed skeletal deformities consisting of shortening, thickening, and bending of the humerus during the postnatal period. Significant concentrations of glimepiride were observed in the serum and breast milk of the dams as well as in the serum of the pups. These skeletal deformations were determined to be the result of nursing from mothers exposed to glimepiride.

Prolonged severe hypoglycemia (4 to 10 days) has been reported in neonates born to mothers who were receiving a sulfonylurea drug at the time of delivery. This has been reported more frequently with the use of agents with prolonged half-lives. Patients who are planning a pregnancy should consult their physician, and it is recommended that they change over to insulin for the entire course of pregnancy and lactation.

Nursing Mothers

In rat reproduction studies, significant concentrations of glimepiride were observed in the serum and breast milk of the dams, as well as in the serum of the pups. Although it is not known whether AMARYL is excreted in human milk, other sulfonylureas are excreted in human milk. Because the potential for hypoglycemia in nursing infants may exist, and because of the effects on nursing animals, AMARYL should be discontinued in nursing mothers. If AMARYL is discontinued, and if diet and exercise alone are inadequate for controlling blood glucose, insulin therapy should be considered. (See above Pregnancy, Nonteratogenic Effects.)

Pediatric Use

Safety and effectiveness in pediatric patients have not been established.

Geriatric Use

In US clinical studies of AMARYL, 608 of 1986 patients were 65 and over. No overall differences in safety or effectiveness were observed between these subjects and younger subjects, but greater sensitivity of some older individuals cannot be ruled out.

Comparison of glimepiride pharmacokinetics in NIDDM patients ≤65 years (n=49) and those >65 years (n=42) was performed in a study using a dosing regimen of 6 mg daily. There were no significant differences in glimepiride pharmacokinetics between the two age groups (see CLINICAL PHARMACOLOGY, Special Populations, Geriatric).

The drug is known to be substantially excreted by the kidney, and the risk of toxic reactions to this drug may be greater in patients with impaired renal function. Because elderly patients are more likely to have decreased renal function, care should be taken in dose selection, and it may be useful to monitor renal function.

Elderly patients are particularly susceptible to hypoglycemic action of glucose-lowering drugs. In elderly, debilitated, or malnourished patients, or in patients with renal and hepatic insufficiency, the initial dosing, dose increments, and maintenance dosage should be conservative based upon blood glucose levels prior to and after initiation of treatment to avoid hypoglycemic reactions. Hypoglycemia may be difficult to recognize in the elderly and in people who are taking beta-adrenergic blocking drugs or other sympatholytic agents (see CLINICAL PHARMACOLOGY, Special Populations, Renal Insufficiency; PRECAUTIONS, General; and DOSING AND ADMINISTRATION, Special Patient Population).

ADVERSE REACTIONS

The incidence of hypoglycemia with AMARYL, as documented by blood glucose values <60 mg/dL, ranged from 0.9–1.7% in two large, well-controlled, 1-year studies. (See WARNINGS and PRECAUTIONS.)

AMARYL has been evaluated for safety in 2,013 patients in US controlled trials, and in 1,551 patients in foreign controlled trials. More than 1,650 of these patients were treated for at least 1 year.

Adverse events, other than hypoglycemia, considered to be possibly or probably related to study drug that occurred in US placebo-controlled trials in more than 1% of patients treated with AMARYL are shown below.

Adverse Events Occurring in <1% AMARYL Patients

	AMARYL		Placebo	
	No.	%	No.	%
Total Treated	746	100	294	100
Dizziness	13	1.7	1	0.3
Asthenia	12	1.6	3	1.0
Headache	11	1.5	4	1.4
Nausea	8	1.1	0	0.0

Gastrointestinal Reactions

Vomiting, gastrointestinal pain, and diarrhea have been reported, but the incidence in placebo-controlled trials was less than 1%. In rare cases, there may be an elevation of liver enzyme levels. In isolated instances, impairment of liver function (e.g. with cholestasis and jaundice), as well as hepatitis, which may also lead to liver failure have been reported with sulfonylureas, including AMARYL.

Dermatologic Reactions

Allergic skin reactions, e.g., pruritus, erythema, urticaria, and morbilliform or maculopapular eruptions, occur in less than 1% of treated patients. These may be transient and may disappear despite continued use of AMARYL. If those hypersensitivity reactions persist or worsen, the drug should be discontinued. Porphyria cutanea tarda, photosensitivity reactions, and allergic vasculitis have been reported with sulfonylureas.

Hematologic Reactions

Leukopenia, agranulocytosis, thrombocytopenia, hemolytic anemia, aplastic anemia, and pancytopenia have been reported with sulfonylureas.

Metabolic Reactions

Hepatic porphyria reactions and disulfiram-like reactions have been reported with sulfonylureas; however, no cases have yet been reported with AMARYL (glimepiride tablets). Cases of hyponatremia have been reported with glimepiride and all other sulfonylureas, most often in patients who are on other medications or have medical conditions known to cause hyponatremia or increase release of antidiuretic hormone. The syndrome of inappropriate antidiuretic hormone (SIADH) secretion has been reported with certain other sulfonylureas, and it has been suggested that these sulfonylureas may augment the peripheral (antidiuretic) action of ADH and/or increase release of ADH.

Other Reactions

Changes in accommodation and/or blurred vision may occur with the use of AMARYL. This is thought to be due to changes in blood glucose, and may be more pronounced when treatment is initiated. This condition is also seen in untreated diabetic patients, and may actually be reduced by treatment. In placebo-controlled trials of AMARYL, the incidence of blurred vision was placebo, 0.7%, and AMARYL, 0.4%.

OVERDOSAGE

Overdosage of sulfonylureas, including AMARYL, can produce hypoglycemia. Mild hypoglycemic symptoms without loss of consciousness or neurologic findings should be treated aggressively with oral glucose and adjustments in drug dosage and/or meal patterns. Close monitoring should continue until the physician is assured that the patient is out of danger. Severe hypoglycemic reactions with coma, seizure, or other neurological impairment occur infrequently, but constitute medical emergencies requiring immediate hospitalization. If hypoglycemic coma is diagnosed or suspected, the patient should be given a rapid intravenous injection of concentrated (50%) glucose solution. This should be followed by a continuous infusion of a more dilute (10%) glucose solution at a rate that will maintain the blood glucose at a level above 100 mg/dL. Patients should be closely monitored for a minimum of 24 to 48 hours, because hypoglycemia may recur after apparent clinical recovery.

DOSAGE AND ADMINISTRATION

There is no fixed dosage regimen for the management of diabetes mellitus with AMARYL or any other hypoglycemic agent. The patient's fasting blood glucose and HbA_{1c} must be measured periodically to determine the minimum effective dose for the patient; to detect primary failure, i.e., inadequate lowering of blood glucose at the maximum recommended dose of medication; and to detect secondary failure, i.e., loss of adequate blood glucose lowering response after an initial period of effectiveness. Glycosylated hemoglobin levels should be performed to monitor the patient's response to therapy.

Continued on next page

Amaryl—Cont.

Short-term administration of AMARYL may be sufficient during periods of transient loss of control in patients usually controlled well on diet and exercise.

Usual Starting Dose

The usual starting dose of AMARYL as initial therapy is 1–2 mg once daily, administered with breakfast or the first main meal. Those patients who may be more sensitive to hypoglycemic drugs should be started at 1 mg once daily, and should be titrated carefully. (See PRECAUTIONS Section for patients at increased risk.)

No exact dosage relationship exists between AMARYL and the other oral hypoglycemic agents. The maximum starting dose of AMARYL should be no more than 2 mg.

Failure to follow an appropriate dosage regimen may precipitate hypoglycemia. Patients who do not adhere to their prescribed dietary and drug regimen are more prone to exhibit unsatisfactory response to therapy.

Usual Maintenance Dose

The usual maintenance dose is 1 to 4 mg once daily. The maximum recommended dose is 8 mg once daily. After reaching a dose of 2 mg, dosage increases should be made in increments of no more than 2 mg at 1–2 week intervals based upon the patient's blood glucose response. Long-term efficacy should be monitored by measurement of HbA_{1c} levels, for example, every 3 to 6 months.

AMARYL-Metformin Combination Therapy

If patients do not respond adequately to the maximal dose of AMARYL monotherapy, addition of metformin may be considered. Published clinical information exists for the use of other sulfonylureas including glyburide, glipizide, chlorpropamide, and tolbutamide in combination with metformin.

With concomitant AMARYL and metformin therapy, the desired control of blood glucose may be obtained by adjusting the dose of each drug. However, attempts should be made to identify the minimum effective dose of each drug to achieve this goal. With concomitant AMARYL and metformin therapy, the risk of hypoglycemia associated with AMARYL therapy continues and may be increased. Appropriate precautions should be taken.

AMARYL-Insulin Combination Therapy

Combination therapy with AMARYL and insulin may also be used in secondary failure patients. The fasting glucose level for instituting combination therapy is in the range of >150 mg/dL in plasma or serum depending on the patient. The recommended AMARYL dose is 8 mg once daily administered with the first main meal. After starting with low-dose insulin, upward adjustments of insulin can be done approximately weekly as guided by frequent measurements of fasting blood glucose. Once stable, combination-therapy patients should monitor their capillary blood glucose on an ongoing basis, preferably daily. Periodic adjustments of insulin may also be necessary during maintenance as guided by glucose and HbA_{1c} levels.

Specific Patient Populations

AMARYL (glimepiride tablets) is not recommended for use in pregnancy, nursing mothers, or children. In elderly, debilitated, or malnourished patients, or in patients with renal or hepatic insufficiency, the initial dosing, dose increments, and maintenance dosage should be conservative to avoid hypoglycemic reactions (See CLINICAL PHARMACOLOGY, Special Populations and PRECAUTIONS, General).

Patients Receiving Other Oral Hypoglycemic Agents

As with other sulfonylurea hypoglycemic agents, no transition period is necessary when transferring patients to AMARYL. Patients should be observed carefully (1–2 weeks) for hypoglycemia when being transferred from longer half-life sulfonylureas (e.g., chlorpropamide) to AMARYL due to potential overlapping of drug effect.

HOW SUPPLIED

AMARYL tablets are available in the following strengths and package sizes:

1 mg (pink, flat-faced, oblong with notched sides at double bisect, imprinted with "AMA RYL" on one side and the Hoechst logo on both sides of the bisect on the other side)

Bottles of 100 (NDC 0039-0221-10)

2 mg (green, flat-faced, oblong with notched sides at double bisect, imprinted with "AMA RYL" on one side and the Hoechst logo on both sides of the bisect on the other side)

Bottles of 100 (NDC 0039-0222-10)

Unit Dose Cartons (100) (NDC 0039-0222-11)

4 mg (blue, flat-faced, oblong with notched sides at double bisect, imprinted with "AMA RYL" on one side and the Hoechst logo on both sides of the bisect on the other side)

Bottles of 100 (NDC 0039-0223-10)

Unit Dose Cartons (100) (NDC 0039-0223-11)

Store between 59 and 86° F (15 and 30° C).

Dispense in well-closed containers with safety closures.

AMARYL® REG TM HOECHST AG

*US Patent 4,379,785

ANIMAL TOXICOLOGY

Reduced serum glucose values and degranulation of the pancreatic beta cells were observed in beagle dogs exposed to 320 mg glimepiride/kg/day for 12 months (approximately 1,000 times the recommended human dose based on surface area). No evidence of tumor formation was observed in any organ. One female and one male dog developed bilateral subcapsular cataracts. Non-GLP studies indicated that glimepiride was unlikely to exacerbate cataract formation. Evaluation of the co-cataractogenic potential of glimepiride in several diabetic and cataract rat models was negative and there was no adverse effect of glimepiride on bovine ocular lens metabolism in organ culture.

HUMAN OPHTHALMOLOGY DATA

Ophthalmic examinations were carried out in over 500 subjects during long-term studies using the methodology of Taylor and West and Laties et al. No significant differences were seen between AMARYL and glyburide in the number of subjects with clinically important changes in visual acuity, intra-ocular tension, or in any of the five lens-related variables examined.

Ophthalmic examinations were carried out during long-term studies using the method of Chylack et al. No significant or clinically meaningful differences were seen between AMARYL and glipizide with respect to cataract progression by subjective LOCS II grading and objective image analysis systems, visual acuity, intraocular pressure, and general ophthalmic examination.

Prescribing Information as of July 2001

Hoechst-Roussel Pharmaceuticals

Division of Aventis Pharmaceuticals Inc.

Kansas City, MO 64137 USA

www.aventispharma-us.com

amap701p

LOVENOX® ℞

(enoxaparin sodium) Injection

Rx only

Prescribing information for this product, which appears on pages 746–750 of the 2002 PDR, has been completely revised as follows. Please write "See Supplement A" next to the product heading.

SPINAL / EPIDURAL HEMATOMAS

When neuraxial anesthesia (epidural/spinal anesthesia) or spinal puncture is employed, patients anticoagulated or scheduled to be anticoagulated with low molecular weight heparins or heparinoids for prevention of thromboembolic complications are at risk of developing an epidural or spinal hematoma which can result in long-term or permanent paralysis.

The risk of these events is increased by the use of indwelling epidural catheters for administration of analgesia or by the concomitant use of drugs affecting hemostasis such as non steroidal anti-inflammatory drugs (NSAIDs), platelet inhibitors, or other anticoagulants. The risk also appears to be increased by traumatic or repeated epidural or spinal puncture.

Patients should be frequently monitored for signs and symptoms of neurological impairment. If neurologic compromise is noted, urgent treatment is necessary.

The physician should consider the potential benefit versus risk before neuraxial intervention in patients anticoagulated or to be anticoagulated for thromboprophylaxis (see also **WARNINGS, Hemorrhage,** and **PRECAUTIONS, Drug Interactions**).

DESCRIPTION

Lovenox Injection is a sterile solution containing enoxaparin sodium, a low molecular weight heparin.

Lovenox Injection is available in two concentrations:

1 100mg per mL of Water for Injection

-Prefilled Syringes 30 mg / 0.3 mL, 40 mg / 0.4 mL

-Graduated Prefilled Syringes 60 mg / 0.6 mL, 80 mg / 0.8 mL, 100 mg / 1 mL

-Ampules 30 mg / 0.3 mL

Lovenox Injection 100 mg/mL Concentration contains 10 mg enoxaparin sodium (or approximate anti-Factor Xa activity of 1000 IU [with reference to the W.H.O. First International Low Molecular Weight Heparin Reference Standard]) per 0.1 mL Water for Injection.

2 150 mg per mL of Water for Injection

-Graduated Prefilled Syringes 120 mg / 0.8 mL, 150 mg / 1 mL

Lovenox Injection 150 mg/mL Concentration contains 15 mg enoxaparin sodium (or appropriate anti-Factor Xa activity of 1500 IU [with reference to the W.H.O. First International Low Molecular Weight Heparin Reference Standard]) per 0.1 mL Water for Injection.

The solutions are preservative-free and intended for use only as a single-dose injection. (See **DOSAGE AND ADMINISTRATION** and **HOW SUPPLIED** for dosage unit descriptions.) The pH of the injection is 5.5 to 7.5. Nitrogen is used in the headspace to inhibit oxidation.

Enoxaparin is obtained by alkaline degradation of heparin benzyl ester derived from porcine intestinal mucosa. Its structure is characterized by a 2-O-sulfo-4-enepyranosuronic acid group at the non-reducing end and a 2-N,6-O-disulfo-D-glucosamine at the reducing end of the chain. The substance is the sodium salt. The average molecular weight is about 4500 daltons. The molecular weight distribution is:

<2000 daltons	≤20%
2000 to 8000 daltons	≥68%
>8000 daltons	≤18%

STRUCTURAL FORMULA

R	R′	n
–H or –SO_3Na	–SO_3Na or –C(=O)–CH_3	3 to 20

CLINICAL PHARMACOLOGY

Enoxaparin is a low molecular weight heparin which has antithrombotic properties. In humans, enoxaparin given at a dose of 1.5 mg/kg subcutaneously (SC) is characterized by a higher ratio of anti-Factor Xa to anti-Factor IIa activity (mean±SD, 14.0±3.1) (based on areas under anti-Factor activity versus time curves) compared to the ratios observed for heparin (mean±SD, 1.22±0.13). Increases of up to 1.8 times the control values were seen in the thrombin time (TT) and the activated partial thromboplastin time (aPTT). Enoxaparin at a 1 mg/kg dose (100 mg / mL concentration), administered SC every 12 hours to patients in a large clinical trial resulted in aPTT values of 45 seconds or less in the majority of patients (n = 1607).

Pharmacodynamics (conducted using 100 mg/mL concentration): Maximum anti-Factor Xa and anti-thrombin (anti-Factor IIa) activities occur 3 to 5 hours after SC injection of enoxaparin. Mean peak anti-Factor Xa activity was 0.16 IU/mL (1.58 μg/mL) and 0.38 IU/mL (3.83 μg/mL) after the 20 mg and the 40 mg clinically tested SC doses, respectively. Mean (n = 46) peak anti-Factor Xa activity was 1.1 IU/mL at steady state in patients with unstable angina receiving 1mg/kg SC every 12 hours for 14 days. Mean absolute bioavailability of enoxaparin, given SC, based on anti-Factor Xa activity is 92% in healthy volunteers. The volume of distribution of anti-Factor Xa activity is about 6 L. Following intravenous (i.v.) dosing, the total body clearance of enoxaparin is 26 mL/min. After i.v. dosing of enoxaparin labeled with the gamma-emitter, ^{99m}Tc, 40% of radioactivity and 8 to 20% of anti-Factor Xa activity were recovered in urine in 24 hours. Elimination half-life based on anti-Factor Xa activity was 4.5 hours after SC administration. Following a 40 mg SC once a day dose, significant anti-Factor Xa activity persists in plasma for about 12 hours.

Following SC dosing, the apparent clearance (CL/F) of enoxaparin is approximately 15 mL/min. Apparent clearance and A_{max} derived from anti-Factor Xa values following single SC dosing (40 mg and 60 mg) were slightly higher in males than in females. The source of the gender difference in these parameters has not been conclusively identified, however, body weight may be a contributing factor.

Apparent clearance and A_{max} derived from anti-Factor Xa values following single and multiple SC dosing in elderly

Pharmacokinetic Parameters* After 5 Days of 1.5 mg/kg SC Once Daily Doses of Enoxaparin Sodium Using 100 mg/mL *or* 200 mg/mL Concentrations

	Concentration	Anti-Xa	Anti-IIa	Heptest	aPTT
Amax (IU/mL or Δ sec)	100 mg/mL	1.37 (±0.23)	0.23 (±0.05)	104.5 (±16.6)	19.3 (±4.7)
	200 mg/mL	1.45 (±0.22)	0.26 (±0.05)	110.9 (±17.1)	22 (±6.7)
	90% CI	102–110%		102–111%	
tmax** (h)	100 mg/mL	3 (2–6)	4 (2–5)	2.5 (2–4.5)	3 (2–4.5)
	200 mg/mL	3.5 (2–6)	4.5 (2.5–6)	3.3 (2–5)	3 (2–5)
AUC (ss) (h*IU/mL or h* Δ sec)	100 mg/mL	14.26 (±2.93)	1.54 (±0.61)	1321 (±219)	
	200 mg/mL	15.43 (±2.96)	177 (±0.67)	1401 (±227)	
	90% CI	105–112%		103–109%	

*Means ± SD at Day 5 and 90% Confidence Interval (CI) of the ratio

**Median (range)

subjects were close to those observed in young subjects. Following once a day SC dosing of 40 mg enoxaparin, the Day 10 mean area under anti-Factor Xa activity versus time curve (AUC) was approximately 15% greater than the mean Day 1 AUC value. In subjects with moderate renal impairment (creatinine clearance 30 to 80 mL/min), anti-Factor Xa CL/F values were similar to those in healthy subjects. However, mean CL/F values of subjects with severe renal impairment (creatinine clearance <30 mL/min), were approximately 30% lower than the mean CL/F value of control group subjects. (See **PRECAUTIONS.**)

Although not studied clinically, the 150 mg/mL concentration of enoxaparin sodium is projected to result in anticoagulant activities similar to those of 100 mg/mL and 200 mg/mL concentrations at the same enoxaparin dose. When a daily 1.5 mg/kg SC injection of enoxaparin sodium was given to 25 healthy male and female subjects using a 100 mg/mL or a 200 mg/mL concentration the following pharmacokinetic profiles were obtained (see table below):

[See table at bottom of previous page]

CLINICAL TRIALS

Prophylaxis of Deep Vein Thrombosis Following Abdominal Surgery in Patients at Risk for Thromboembolic Complications: Abdominal surgery patients at risk include those who are over 40 years of age, obese, undergoing surgery under general anesthesia lasting longer than 30 minutes or who have additional risk factors such as malignancy or a history of deep vein thrombosis or pulmonary embolism.

In a double-blind, parallel group study of patients undergoing elective cancer surgery of the gastrointestinal, urological, or gynecological tract, a total of 1116 patients were enrolled in the study, and 1115 patients were treated. Patients ranged in age from 32 to 97 years (mean age 67 years) with 52.7% men and 47.3% women. Patients were 98% Caucasian, 1.1% Black, 0.4% Oriental, and 0.4% others. Lovenox Injection 40 mg SC, administered once a day, beginning 2 hours prior to surgery and continuing for a maximum of 12 days after surgery, was comparable to heparin 5000 U every 8 hours SC in reducing the risk of deep vein thrombosis (DVT). The efficacy data are provided below.

Efficacy of Lovenox Injection in the Prophylaxis of Deep Vein Thrombosis Following Abdominal Surgery

	Dosing Regimen	
Indication	**Lovenox Inj.** 40 mg q.d. SC n (%)	**Heparin** 5000 U q8h SC n (%)
All Treated Abdominal Surgery Patients	555 (100)	560 (100)
Treatment Failures Total VTE[1] (%)	56 (10.1) (95% CI[2]: 8 to 13)	63 (11.3) (95% CI: 9 to 14)
DVT Only (%)	54 (9.7) (95% CI: 7 to 12)	61 (10.9) (95% CI: 8 to 13)

[1] VTE=Venous thromboembolic events which included DVT, PE, and death considered to be thromboembolic in origin.
[2] CI=Confidence Interval

In a second double-blind, parallel group study, Lovenox Injection 40 mg SC once a day was compared to heparin 5000 U every 8 hours SC in patients undergoing colorectal surgery (one-third with cancer). A total of 1347 patients were randomized in the study and all patients were treated. Patients ranged in age from 18 to 92 years (mean age 50.1 years) with 54.2% men and 45.8% women. Treatment was initiated approximately 2 hours prior to surgery and continued for approximately 7 to 10 days after surgery. The efficacy data are provided below.

Efficacy of Lovenox Injection in the Prophylaxis of Deep Vein Thrombosis Following Colorectal Surgery

	Dosing Regimen	
Indication	**Lovenox Inj.** 40 mg q.d. SC n (%)	**Heparin** 5000 U q8h SC n (%)
All Treated Colorectal Surgery Patients	673 (100)	674 (100)
Treatment Failures Total VTE[1] (%)	48 (7.1) (95% CI[2]: 5 to 9)	45 (6.7) (95% CI: 5 to 9)
DVT Only (%)	47 (7.0) (95% CI: 5 to 9)	44 (6.5) (95% CI: 5 to 8)

[1] VTE=Venous thromboembolic events which included DVT, PE, and death considered to be thromboembolic in origin.
[2] CI=Confidence Interval

Prophylaxis of Deep Vein Thrombosis Following Hip or Knee Replacement Surgery: Lovenox Injection has been shown to reduce the risk of post-operative deep vein thrombosis (DVT) following hip or knee replacement surgery.

In a double-blind study, Lovenox Injection 30 mg every 12 hours SC was compared to placebo in patients with hip replacement. A total of 100 patients were randomized in the study and all patients were treated. Patients ranged in age from 41 to 84 years (mean age 67.1 years) with 45% men and 55% women. After hemostasis was established, treatment was initiated 12 to 24 hours after surgery and was continued for 10 to 14 days after surgery. The efficacy data are provided below.

Efficacy of Lovenox Injection in the Prophylaxis of Deep Vein Thrombosis Following Hip Replacement Surgery

	Dosing Regimen	
Indication	**Lovenox Inj.** 30 mg q12h SC n (%)	**Placebo** q12h SC n (%)
All Treated Hip Replacement Patients	50 (100)	50 (100)
Treatment Failures Total DVT (%)	5 (10)[1]	23 (46)
Proximal DVT (%)	1 (2)[2]	11 (22)

[1] p value versus placebo = 0.0002
[2] p value versus placebo = 0.0134

A double-blind, multicenter study compared three dosing regimens of Lovenox Injection in patients with hip replacement. A total of 572 patients were randomized in the study and 568 patients were treated. Patients ranged in age from 31 to 88 years (mean age 64.7 years) with 63% men and 37% women. Patients were 93% Caucasian, 6% Black, <1% Oriental, and 1% others. Treatment was initiated within two days after surgery and was continued for 7 to 11 days after surgery. The efficacy data are provided below.

[See table above]

Efficacy of Lovenox Injection in the Prophylaxis of Deep Vein Thrombosis Following Hip Replacement Surgery

	Dosing Regimen		
Indication	**10 mg q.d. SC** n (%)	**30 mg q12h SC** n (%)	**40 mg q.d. SC** n (%)
All Treated Hip Replacement Patients	161 (100)	208 (100)	199 (100)
Treatment Failures Total DVT (%)	40 (25)	22 (11)[1]	27 (14)
Proximal DVT (%)	17 (11)	8 (4)[2]	9 (5)

[1] p value versus Lovenox 10 mg once a day = 0.0008
[2] p value versus Lovenox 10 mg once a day = 0.0168

There was no significant difference between the 30 mg every 12 hours and 40 mg once a day regimens. In a double-blind study, Lovenox Injection 30 mg every 12 hours SC was compared to placebo in patients undergoing knee replacement surgery. A total of 132 patients were randomized in the study and 131 patients were treated, of which 99 had total knee replacement and 32 had either unicompartmental knee replacement or tibial osteotomy. The 99 patients with total knee replacement ranged in age from 42 to 85 years (mean age 70.2 years) with 36.4% men and 63.6% women. After hemostasis was established, treatment was initiated 12 to 24 hours after surgery and was continued up to 15 days after surgery. The incidence of proximal and total DVT after surgery was significantly lower for Lovenox Injection compared to placebo. The efficacy data are provided below.

Efficacy of Lovenox Injection in the Prophylaxis of Deep Vein Thrombosis Following Total Knee Replacement Therapy

	Dosing Regimen	
Indication	**Lovenox Inj.** 30 mg q12h SC n (%)	**Placebo** q12h SC n (%)
All Treated Total Knee Replacement Patients	47 (100)	52 (100)
Treatment Failures Total DVT (%)	5 (11)[1] (95% CI[2]: 1 to 21)	32 (62) (95% CI: 47 to 76)
Proximal DVT (%)	0 (0)[3] (95% Upper CL[4]: 5	7 (13) (95% CI: 3 to 24)

[1] p value versus placebo = 0.0001
[2] CI = Confidence Interval
[3] p value versus placebo = 0.013
[4] CL = Confidence Limit

Additionally, in an open-label, parallel group, randomized clinical study, Lovenox Injection 30 mg every 12 hours SC in patients undergoing elective knee replacement surgery was compared to heparin 5000 U every 8 hours SC. A total of 453 patients were randomized in the study and all were treated. Patients ranged in age from 38 to 90 years (mean age 68.5 years) with 43.7% men and 56.3% women. Patients were 92.5% Caucasian, 5.3% Black, 0.2% Oriental, and 0.4% others. Treatment was initiated after surgery and continued up to 14 days. The incidence of deep vein thrombosis was significantly lower for Lovenox Injection compared to heparin.

Extended Prophylaxis of Deep Vein Thrombosis Following Hip Replacement Surgery: In a study of extended prophylaxis for patients undergoing hip replacement surgery, patients were treated, while hospitalized, with Lovenox Injection 40 mg SC, initiated up to 12 hours prior to surgery for the prophylaxis of post-operative DVT. At the end of the perioperative period, all patients underwent bilateral venography. In a double-blind design, those patients with no venous thromboembolic disease were randomized to a post-discharge regimen of either Lovenox Injection 40 mg (n = 90) once a day SC or to placebo (n = 89) for 3 weeks. A total of 179 patients were randomized in the double-blind phase of the study and all patients were treated. Patients ranged in age from 47 to 87 years (mean age 69.4 years) with 57% men and 43% women. In this population of patients, the incidence of DVT during extended prophylaxis was significantly lower for Lovenox Injection compared to placebo. The efficacy data are provided below.

Efficacy of Lovenox Injection in the Extended Prophylaxis of Deep Vein Thrombosis Following Hip Replacement Therapy

	Post-Discharge Dosing Regimen	
Indication (Post-Discharge)	**Lovenox Inj.** 40 mg q.d. SC n (%)	**Placebo** q.d. SC n (%)
All Treated Extended Prophylaxis Patients	90 (100)	89 (100)
Treatment Failures Total DVT (%)	6 (7)[1] (95% CI[2]: 3 to 14)	18 (20) (95% CI: 12 to 30)
Proximal DVT (%)	5 (6)[3] (95% CI: 2 to 13)	7 (8) (95% CI: 3 to 16)

[1] p value versus placebo = 0.008
[2] CI = Confidence Interval
[3] p value versus placebo = 0.537

In a second study, patients undergoing hip replacement surgery were treated, while hospitalized, with Lovenox Injection 40 mg SC, initiated up to 12 hours prior to surgery. All patients were examined for clinical signs and symptoms of venous thromboembolic (VTE) disease. In a double-blind design, patients without clinical signs and symptoms of VTE disease were randomized to a post-discharge regimen of either Lovenox Injection 40 mg (n = 131) once a day SC or to placebo (n = 131) for 3 weeks. A total of 262 patients were randomized in the study double-blind phase and all patients were treated. Patients ranged in age from 44 to 87 years (mean age 68.5 years) with 43.1% men and 56.9% women. Similar to the first study the incidence of DVT during extended prophylaxis was significantly lower for Lovenox Injection compared to placebo, with a statistically significant difference in both total DVT (Lovenox Injection 21 [16%] versus placebo 45 [34%]; p = 0.001) and proximal DVT (Lovenox Injection 8 [6%] versus placebo 28 [21%]; p = <0.001).

Prophylaxis of Deep Vein Thrombosis (DVT) In Medical Patients with Severely Restricted Mobility During Acute Illness: In a double blind multicenter, parallel group study, Lovenox Injection 20 mg or 40 mg once a day SC was compared to placebo in the prophylaxis of DVT in medical patients with severely restricted mobility during acute illness (defined as walking distance of <10 meters for ≤3 days). This study included patients with heart failure (NYHA Class III or IV); acute respiratory failure or complicated chronic respiratory insufficiency (not requiring ventilatory support): acute infection (excluding septic shock); or acute rheumatic disorder [acute lumbar or sciatic pain, vertebral compression (due to osteoporosis or tumor), acute arthritic episodes of the lower extremities]. A total of 1102 patients were enrolled in the study, and 1073 patients were treated. Patients ranged in age from 40 to 97 years (mean

Continued on next page

Lovenox—Cont.

age 73 years) with equal proportions of men and women. Treatment continued for a maximum of 14 days (median duration 7 days). When given at a dose of 40 mg once a day SC, Lovenox Injection significantly reduced the incidence of DVT as compared to placebo. The efficacy data are provided below.

[See first table above]

At approximately 3 months following enrollment, the incidence of venous thromboembolism remained significantly lower in the Lovenox Injection 40 mg treatment group versus the placebo treatment group.

Prophylaxis of Ischemic Complications in Unstable Angina and Non-Q-Wave Myocardial Infarction: In a multicenter, double-blind, parallel group study, patients who recently experienced unstable angina or non-Q-wave myocardial infarction were randomized to either Lovenox Injection 1 mg/kg every 12 hours SC or heparin i.v. bolus (5000 U) followed by a continuous infusion (adjusted to achieve an aPTT of 55 to 85 seconds). A total of 3171 patients were enrolled in the study, and 3107 patients were treated. Patients ranged in age from 25–94 years (median age 64 years), with 33.4% of patients female and 66.6% male. Race was distributed as follows: 89.8% Caucasian, 4.8% Black, 2.0% Oriental, and 3.5% other. **All** patients were also treated with aspirin 100 to 325 mg per day. Treatment was initiated within 24 hours of the event and continued until clinical stabilization, revascularization procedures, or hospital discharge, with a maximal duration of 8 days of therapy. The combined incidence of the triple endpoint of death, myocardial infarction, or recurrent angina was lower for Lovenox Injection compared with heparin therapy at 14 days after initiation of treatment. The lower incidence of the triple endpoint was sustained up to 30 days after initiation of treatment. These results were observed in an analysis of both all-randomized and all-treated patients. The efficacy data are provided below.

[See second table above]

The combined incidence of death or myocardial infarction at all time points was lower for Lovenox Injection compared to standard heparin therapy, but did not achieve statistical significance. The efficacy data are provided below.

[See third table above]

In a survey one year following treatment, with information available for 92% of enrolled patients, the combined incidence of death, myocardial infarction, or recurrent angina remained lower for Lovenox Injection versus heparin (32.0% vs 35.7%). Urgent revascularization procedures were performed less frequently in the Lovenox Injection group as compared to the heparin group, 6.3% compared to 8.2% at 30 days (p = 0.047).

Treatment of Deep Vein Thrombosis (DVT) with or without Pulmonary Embolism (PE): In a multicenter, parallel group study, 900 patients with acute lower extremity DVT with or without PE were randomized to an inpatient (hospital) treatment of either (i) Lovenox Injection 1.5 mg/kg once a day SC, (ii) Lovenox Injection 1 mg/kg every 12 hours SC, or (iii) heparin i.v. bolus (5000 IU) followed by a continuous infusion (administered to achieve an aPTT of 55 to 85 seconds). A total of 900 patients were randomized in the study and all patients were treated. Patients ranged in age from 18 to 92 years (mean age 60.7 years) with 54.7% men and 45.3% women. All patients also received warfarin sodium (dose adjusted according to PT to achieve an International Normalization Ratio [INR] of 2.0 to 3.0), commencing within 72 hours of initiation of Lovenox Injection or standard heparin therapy, and continuing for 90 days. Lovenox Injection or standard heparin therapy was administered for a minimum of 5 days and until the targeted warfarin sodium INR was achieved. Both Lovenox Injection regimens were equivalent to standard heparin therapy in reducing the risk of recurrent venous thromboembolism (DVT and/or PE). The efficacy data are provided below.

[See first table at top of next page]

Similarly, in a multicenter, open-label, parallel group study, patients with acute proximal DVT were randomized to Lovenox Injection or heparin. Patients who could not receive outpatient therapy were excluded from entering the study. Outpatient exclusion criteria included the following: inability to receive outpatient heparin therapy because of associated co-morbid conditions or potential for non-compliance and inability to attend follow-up visits as an outpatient because of geographic inaccessibility. Eligible patients could be treated in the hospital, but ONLY Lovenox Injection patients were permitted to go home on therapy (72%). A total of 501 patients were randomized in the study and all patients were treated. Patients ranged in age from 19 to 96 years (mean age 57.8 years) with 60.5% men and 39.5% women. Patients were randomized to either Lovenox Injection 1 mg/kg every 12 hours SC or heparin i.v. bolus (5000 IU) followed by a continuous infusion administered to achieve an aPTT of 60 to 85 seconds (in-patient treatment). All patients also received warfarin sodium as described in the previous study. Lovenox Injection or standard heparin therapy was administered for a minimum of 5 days. Lovenox Injection was equivalent to standard heparin therapy in reducing the risk of recurrent venous thromboembolism. The efficacy data are provided below.

Efficacy of Lovenox Injection in the Prophylaxis of Deep Vein Thrombosis in Medical Patients With Severely Restricted Mobility During Acute Illness

	Dosing Regimen		
Indication	Lovenox Inj. 20 mg q.d. SC n (%)	Lovenox Inj. 40 mg q.d. SC n (%)	Placebo n (%)
All Treated Medical Patients During Acute Illness	351 (100)	360 (100)	362 (100)
Treatment Failure[1] Total VTE[2] (%)	43 (12.3)	16 (4.4)	43 (11.9)
Total DVT (%)	43 (12.3) (95% CI[3] 8.8 to 15.7)	16 (4.4) (95% CI[3] 2.3 to 6.6)	41 (11.3) (95% CI[3] 8.1 to 14.6)
Proximal DVT (%)	13 (3.7)	5 (1.4)	14 (3.9)

[1] Treatment failures during therapy, between Days 1 and 14.
[2] VTE = Venous thromboembolic events which included DVT, PE, and death considered to be thromboembolic in origin.
[3] CI = Confidence Interval

Efficacy of Lovenox Injection in the Prophylaxis of Ischemic Complications in Unstable Angina and Non-Q-Wave Myocardial Infarction (Combined Endpoint of Death, Myocardial Infarction, or Recurrent Angina)

	Dosing Regimen[1]			
Indication	Lovenox Inj. 1 mg/kg q12h SC n (%)	Heparin aPTT Adjusted i.v. Therapy n (%)	Reduction (%)	p Value
All Treated Unstable Angina and Non-Q-Wave MI Patients	1578 (100)	1529 (100)		
Timepoint[2] 48 Hours	96 (6.1)	112 (7.3)	1.2	0.120
14 Days	261 (16.5)	303 (19.8)	3.3	0.017
30 Days	313 (19.8)	358 (23.4)	3.6	0.014

[1] All patients were also treated with aspirin 100 to 325 mg per day.
[2] Evaluation timepoints are after initiation of treatment. Therapy continued for up to 8 days (median duration of 2.6 days).

Efficacy of Lovenox Injection in the Prophylaxis of Ischemic Complications in Unstable Angina and Non-Q-Wave Myocardial Infarction (Combined Endpoint of Death or Myocardial Infarction)

	Dosing Regimen[1]			
Indication	Lovenox Inj. 1 mg/kg q12h SC n (%)	Heparin aPTT Adjusted i.v. Therapy n (%)	Reduction (%)	p Value
All Treated Unstable Angina and Non-Q-Wave MI Patients	1578 (100)	1529 (100)		
Timepoint[2] 48 Hours	16 (1.0)	20 (1.3)	0.3	0.126
14 Days	76 (4.8)	93 (6.1)	1.3	0.115
30 Days	96 (6.1)	118 (7.7)	1.6	0.069

[1] All patients were also treated with aspirin 100 to 325 mg per day.
[2] Evaluation timepoints are after initiation of treatment. Therapy continued for up to 8 days (median duration of 2.6 days).

Efficacy of Lovenox Injection in Treatment of Deep Vein Thrombosis

	Dosing Regimen[1]	
Indication	Lovenox Inj. 1 mg/kg q12h SC n (%)	Heparin aPTT Adjusted i.v. Therapy n (%)
All Treated DVT Patients	247 (100)	254 (100)
Patient Outcome Total VTE[2] (%)	13 (5.3)[3]	17 (6.7)
DVT Only (%)	11 (4.5)	14 (5.5)
Proximal DVT (%)	10 (4.0)	12 (4.7)
PE (%)	2 (0.8)	3 (1.2)

[1] All patients were also treated with warfarin sodium commencing on the evening of the second day of Lovenox Injection or standard heparin therapy.
[2] VTE = venous thromboembolic event (deep vein thrombosis [DVT] and/or pulmonary embolism [PE]).
[3] The 95% Confidence Intervals for the treatment difference for total VTE was: Lovenox Injection versus heparin (−5.6 to 2.7).

INDICATIONS AND USAGE

- Lovenox Injection is indicated for the prophylaxis of deep vein thrombosis, which may lead to pulmonary embolism:
  - in patients undergoing abdominal surgery who are at risk for thromboembolic complications;
  - in patients undergoing hip replacement surgery, during and following hospitalization;
  - in patients undergoing knee replacement surgery;
  - in medical patients who are at risk for thromboembolic complications due to severely restricted mobility during acute illness.
- Lovenox Injection is indicated for the prophylaxis of ischemic complications of unstable angina and non-Q-wave myocardial infarction, when concurrently administered with aspirin.
- Lovenox Injection is indicated for:
  - the **inpatient treatment** of acute deep vein thrombosis **with or without pulmonary embolism**, when administered in conjunction with warfarin sodium;
  - the **outpatient treatment** of acute deep vein thrombosis **without pulmonary embolism** when administered in conjunction with warfarin sodium.

See **DOSAGE AND ADMINISTRATION: Adult Dosage** for appropriate dosage regimens.

CONTRAINDICATIONS

Lovenox Injection is contraindicated in patients with active major bleeding, in patients with thrombocytopenia associated with a positive *in vitro* test for anti-platelet antibody in the presence of enoxaparin sodium, or in patients with hypersensitivity to enoxaparin sodium.

Patients with known hypersensitivity to heparin or pork products should not be treated with Lovenox Injection.

WARNINGS

Lovenox Injection is not intended for intramuscular administration.

Lovenox Injection cannot be used interchangeably (unit for unit) with heparin or other low molecular weight heparins as they differ in manufacturing process, molecular weight distribution, anti-Xa and anti-IIa activities, units, and dosage. Each of these medicines has its own instructions for use.

Lovenox Injection should be used with extreme caution in patients with a history of heparin-induced thrombocytopenia.

Hemorrhage: Lovenox Injection, like other anticoagulants, should be used with extreme caution in conditions with increased risk of hemorrhage, such as bacterial endocarditis, congenital or acquired bleeding disorders, active ulcerative and angiodysplastic gastrointestinal disease, hemorrhagic stroke, or shortly after brain, spinal, or ophthalmological surgery, or in patients treated concomitantly with platelet inhibitors.

Cases of epidural or spinal hematomas have been reported with the associated use of Lovenox Injection and spinal/epidural anesthesia or spinal puncture resulting in long-term or permanent paralysis. The risk of these events is higher with the use of post-operative indwelling epidural catheters or by the concomitant use of additional drugs affecting hemostasis such as NSAIDs (see boxed WARNING; ADVERSE REACTIONS, Ongoing Safety Surveillance; and PRECAUTIONS, Drug Interactions).

Major hemorrhages including retroperitoneal and intracranial bleeding have been reported. Some of these cases have been fatal.

Bleeding can occur at any site during therapy with Lovenox Injection. An unexplained fall in hematocrit or blood pressure should lead to a search for a bleeding site.

Thrombocytopenia: Thrombocytopenia can occur with the administration of Lovenox Injection.

Moderate thrombocytopenia (platelet counts between 100,000/mm^3 and 50,000/mm^3) occurred at a rate of 1.3% in patients given Lovenox Injection, 1.2% in patients given heparin, and 0.7% in patients given placebo in clinical trials.

Platelet counts less than 50,000/mm^3 occurred at a rate of 0.1% in patients given Lovenox Injection, in 0.2% of patients given heparin, and 0.4% of patients given placebo in the same trials.

Thrombocytopenia of any degree should be monitored closely. If the platelet count falls below 100,000/mm^3, Lovenox Injection should be discontinued. Cases of heparin-induced thrombocytopenia with thrombosis have also been observed in clinical practice. Some of these cases were complicated by organ infarction, limb ischemia, or death.

Prosthetic Heart Valves: The use of Lovenox Injection is not recommended for thromboprophylaxis in patients with prosthetic heart valves. Cases of prosthetic heart valve thrombosis have been reported in patients with prosthetic valves who have received enoxaparin for thromboprophylaxis. Some of these cases were pregnant women in whom thrombosis led to maternal deaths and fetal deaths. Pregnant women with prosthetic heart valves may be at higher risk for thromboembolism **(see PRECAUTIONS: Pregnancy)**.

PRECAUTIONS

General: Lovenox Injection should not be mixed with other injections or infusions.

Lovenox Injection should be used with care in patients with a bleeding diathesis, uncontrolled arterial hypertension or a history of recent gastrointestinal ulceration, diabetic retinopathy, and hemorrhage. Elderly patients and patients with renal insufficiency may show delayed elimination of enoxaparin. Lovenox Injection should be used with care in these patients. Adjustment of enoxaparin sodium dose may be considered for low weight (<45 kg) patients and/or for patients with severe renal impairment (creatinine clearance <30 mL/min).

If thromboembolic events occur despite Lovenox Injection prophylaxis, appropriate therapy should be initiated.

Laboratory Tests: Periodic complete blood counts, including platelet count, and stool occult blood tests are recommended during the course of treatment with Lovenox Injection. When administered at recommended prophylaxis doses, routine coagulation tests such as Prothrombin Time (PT) and Activated Partial Thromboplastin Time (aPTT) are relatively insensitive measures of Lovenox Injection activity and, therefore, unsuitable for monitoring. Anti-Factor Xa may be used to monitor the anticoagulant effect of Lovenox Injection in patients with significant renal impairment. If during Lovenox Injection therapy abnormal coagulation parameters or bleeding should occur, anti-Factor Xa levels may be used to monitor the anticoagulant effects of Lovenox Injection (see **CLINICAL PHARMACOLOGY: Pharmacodynamics**).

Drug Interactions: Unless really needed, agents which may enhance the risk of hemorrhage should be discontinued prior to initiation of Lovenox Injection therapy. These agents include medications such as: anticoagulants, platelet inhibitors including acetylsalicylic acid, salicylates, NSAIDs (including ketorolac tromethamine), dipyridamole, or sulfinpyrazone. If co-administration is essential, conduct close clinical and laboratory monitoring (see **PRECAUTIONS: Laboratory Tests**).

Carcinogenesis, Mutagenesis, Impairment of Fertility: No long-term studies in animals have been performed to evaluate the carcinogenic potential of enoxaparin. Enoxaparin was not mutagenic in *in vitro* tests, including the Ames test, mouse lymphoma cell forward mutation test, and human lymphocyte chromosomal aberration test, and the *in vivo* rat bone marrow chromosomal aberration test. Enoxaparin was found to have no effect on fertility or reproductive performance of male and female rats at SC doses up to 20 mg/kg/day or 141 mg/m^2/day. The maximum human dose in clinical trials was 2.0 mg/kg/day or 78 mg/m^2/day (for an average body weight of 70 kg, height of 170 cm, and body surface area of 1.8 m^2).

Efficacy of Lovenox Injection in Treatment of Deep Vein Thrombosis With or Without Pulmonary Embolism

	Dosing Regimen[1]		
Indication	**Lovenox Inj.** 1.5 mg/kg q.d. SC n (%)	**Lovenox Inj.** 1 mg/kg q12h SC n (%)	**Heparin** aPTT Adjusted i.v. Therapy n (%)
All Treated DVT Patients with or without PE	298 (100)	312 (100)	290 (100)
Patient Outcome Total VTE[2] (%)	13 (4.4)[3]	9 (2.9)[3]	12 (4.1)
DVT Only (%)	11 (3.7)	7 (2.2)	8 (2.8)
Proximal DVT (%)	9 (3.0)	6 (1.9)	7 (2.4)
PE (%)	2 (0.7)	2 (0.6)	4 (1.4)

[1] All patients were also treated with warfarin sodium commencing within 72 hours of Lovenox Injection or standard heparin therapy.

[2] VTE = venous thromboembolic event (DVT and/or PE).

[3] The 95% Confidence Intervals for the treatment differences for total VTE were:
Lovenox Injection once a day versus heparin (−3.0 to 3.5)
Lovenox Injection every 12 hours versus heparin (−4.2 to 1.7).

Major Bleeding Episodes Following Hip or Knee Replacement Surgery[1]

	Dosing Regimen		
Indications	**Lovenox Inj.** 40 mg q.d. SC	**Lovenox Inj.** 30 mg q12h SC	**Heparin** 15,000 U/24h SC
Hip Replacement Surgery Without Extended Prophylaxis[2]		n = 786 31 (4%)	n = 541 32 (6%)
Hip Replacement Surgery With Extended Prophylaxis			
Peri-operative Period[3]	n = 288 4 (2%)		
Extended Prophylaxis Period[4]	n = 221 0 (0%)		
Knee Replacement Surgery Without Extended Prophylaxis[2]		n = 294 3 (1%)	n = 225 3 (1%)

[1] Bleeding complications were considered major: (1) if the hemorrhage caused a significant clinical event, or (2) if accompanied by a hemoglobin decrease ≥ 2 g/dL or transfusion of 2 or more units of blood products. Retroperitoneal and intracranial hemorrhages were always considered major. In the knee replacement surgery trials, intraocular hemorrhages were also considered major hemorrhages.

[2] Lovenox Injection 30 mg every 12 hours SC initiated 12 to 24 hours after surgery and continued for up to 14 days after surgery.

[3] Lovenox Injection 40 mg SC once a day initiated up to 12 hours prior to surgery and continued for up to 7 days after surgery.

[4] Lovenox Injection 40 mg SC once a day for up to 21 days after discharge.

NOTE: At no time point were the 40 mg once a day pre-operative and the 30 mg every 12 hours post-operative hip replacement surgery prophylactic regimens compared in clinical trials.

Adverse Events Occurring at ≥2% Incidence in Lovenox Injection Treated Patients[1] Undergoing Abdominal or Colorectal Surgery

	Dosing Regimen			
	Lovenox Inj. 40 mg q.d. SC n = 1228		**Heparin** 5000 U q8h SC n = 1234	
Adverse Event	**Severe**	**Total**	**Severe**	**Total**
Hemorrhage	<1%	7%	<1%	6%
Anemia	<1%	3%	<1%	3%
Ecchymosis	0%	3%	0%	3%

[1] Excluding unrelated adverse events.

Pregnancy: *Teratogenic Effects:* Pregnancy Category B: Teratology studies have been conducted in pregnant rats and rabbits at SC doses of enoxaparin up to 30 mg/kg/day or 211 mg/m^2/day and 410 mg/m^2/day, respectively. There was no evidence of teratogenic effects or fetotoxicity due to enoxaparin. There are, however, no adequate and well-controlled studies in pregnant women. Because animal reproduction studies are not always predictive of human response, this drug should be used during pregnancy only if clearly needed.

There have been reports of congenital anomalies in infants born to women who received enoxaparin during pregnancy including cerebral anomalies, limb anomalies, hypospadias, peripheral vascular malformation, fibrotic dysplasia, and cardiac defect. A cause and effect relationship has not been established nor has the incidence been shown to be higher than in the general population.

Non-teratogenic Effects: There have been post-marketing reports of fetal death when pregnant women received Lovenox Injection. Causality for these cases has not been determined. Pregnant women receiving anti-coagulants, including enoxaparin, are at increased risk for bleeding. Hemorrhage can occur at any site and may lead to death of mother and/or fetus. Pregnant women receiving enoxaparin should be carefully monitored. Pregnant women and women of child-bearing potential should be apprised of the potential hazard to the fetus and the mother if enoxaparin is administered during pregnancy.

In a clinical study of pregnant women with prosthetic heart valves given enoxaparin (1 mg/kg bid) to reduce the risk of thromboembolism, 2 of 7 women developed clots resulting in blockage of the valve and leading to maternal and fetal death. There are postmarketing reports of prosthetic valve thrombosis in pregnant women with prosthetic heart valves while receiving enoxaparin for thromboprophylaxis. These events resulted in maternal death or surgical interventions. The use of Lovenox Injection is not recommended for thromboprophylaxis in pregnant women with prosthetic heart valves (see **WARNINGS: Prosthetic Heart Valves**).

Nursing Mothers: It is not known whether this drug is excreted in human milk. Because many drugs are excreted in human milk, caution should be exercised when Lovenox Injection is administered to nursing women.

Pediatric Use: Safety and effectiveness of Lovenox Injection in pediatric patients have not been established.

Geriatric Use: Over 2800 patients, 65 years and older, have received Lovenox Injection in pivotal clinical trials. The efficacy of Lovenox Injection in the elderly (≥65 years) was similar to that seen in younger patients (<65 years).

Continued on next page

Lovenox—Cont.

The incidence of bleeding complications was similar between elderly and younger patients when 30 mg every 12 hours or 40 mg once a day doses of Lovenox Injection were employed. The incidence of bleeding complications was higher in elderly patients as compared to younger patients when Lovenox Injection was administered at doses of 1.5 mg/kg once a day or 1 mg/kg every 12 hours. The risk of Lovenox Injection-associated bleeding increased with age. Serious adverse events increased with age for patients receiving Lovenox Injection. Other clinical experience (including postmarketing surveillance and literature reports) has not revealed additional differences in the safety of Lovenox Injection between elderly and younger patients. Careful attention to dosing intervals and concomitant medications (especially antiplatelet medications) is advised. Monitoring of geriatric patients with low body weight (<45 kg) and those predisposed to decreased renal function should be considered. (see **CLINICAL PHARMACOLOGY** and **General** and **Laboratory Tests** subsections of **PRECAUTIONS**)

ADVERSE REACTIONS

Hemorrhage: The incidence of major hemorrhagic complications during Lovenox Injection treatment has been low. The following rates of major bleeding events have been reported during clinical trials with Lovenox Injection.

Major Bleeding Episodes Following Abdominal and Colorectal Surgery[1]

Indications	Dosing Regimen: Lovenox Inj. 40 mg q.d. SC	Heparin 5000 U q8h SC
Abdominal Surgery	n = 555 23 (4%)	n = 560 16 (3%)
Colorectal Surgery	n = 673 28 (4%)	n = 674 21 (3%)

[1] Bleeding complications were considered major: (1) if the hemorrhage caused a significant clinical event, or (2) if accompanied by a hemoglobin decrease ≥2 g/dL or transfusion of 2 or more units of blood products. Retroperitoneal, intraocular, and intracranial hemorrhages were always considered major.

[See second table at top of previous page]

Injection site hematomas during the extended prophylaxis period after hip replacement surgery occurred in 9% of the Lovenox Injection patients versus 1.8% of the placebo patients.

Major Bleeding Episodes in Medical Patients With Severely Restricted Mobility During Acute Illness[1]

Indications	Dosing Regimen: Lovenox Inj.[2] 20 mg q.d. SC	Lovenox Inj.[2] 40 mg q.d. SC	Placebo[2]
Medical Patients During Acute Illness	n = 351 1 (<1%)	n = 360 3 (<1%)	n = 362 2 (<1%)

[1] Bleeding complications were considered major: (1) if the hemorrhage caused a significant clinical event, (2) if the hemorrhage caused a decrease in hemoglobin of ≥ 2 g/dL or transfusion of 2 or more units of blood products. Retroperitoneal and intracranial hemorrhages were always considered major although none were reported during the trial.

[2] The rates represent major bleeding on study medication up to 24 hours after last dose.

Major Bleeding Episodes in Unstable Angina and Non-Q-Wave Myocardial Infarction

Indication	Dosing Regimen: Lovenox Inj.[1] 1 mg/kg q12h SC	Heparin[1] aPTT Adjusted i.v. Therapy
Unstable Angina and Non-Q-Wave MI[2,3]	n = 1578 17 (1%)	n = 1529 18 (1%)

[1] The rates represent major bleeding on study medication up to 12 hours after dose.

[2] Aspirin therapy was administered concurrently (100 to 325 mg per day).

[3] Bleeding complications were considered major: (1) if the hemorrhage caused a significant clinical event, or (2) if accompanied by a hemoglobin decrease by ≥ 3 g/dL or transfusion of 2 or more units of blood products. Intraocular, retroperitoncal, and intracranial hemorrhages were always considered major.

Adverse Events Occurring at ≥2% Incidence in Lovenox Injection Treated Patients[1] Undergoing Hip or Knee Replacement Surgery

Adverse Event	Lovenox Inj. 40 mg q.d. SC, Peri-operative Period n = 288[2] Severe	Total	Lovenox Inj. 40 mg q.d. SC, Extended Prophylaxis Period n = 131[3] Severe	Total	Lovenox Inj. 30 mg q12h SC n = 1080 Severe	Total	Heparin 15,000 U/24h SC n = 766 Severe	Total	Placebo q12h SC n = 115 Severe	Total
Fever	0%	8%	0%	0%	<1%	5%	<1%	4%	0%	3%
Hemorrhage	<1%	13%	0%	5%	<1%	4%	1%	4%	0%	3%
Nausea					<1%	3%	<1%	2%	0%	2%
Anemia	0%	16%	0%	<2%	<1%	2%	2%	5%	<1%	7%
Edema					<1%	2%	<1%	2%	0%	2%
Peripheral edema	0%	6%	0%	0%	<1%	3%	<1%	4%	0%	3%

[1] Excluding unrelated adverse events.

[2] Data represents Lovenox Injection 40 mg SC once a day initiated up to 12 hours prior to surgery in 288 hip replacement surgery patients who received Lovenox Injection peri-operatively in an unblinded fashion in one clinical trial.

[3] Data represents Lovenox Injection 40 mg SC once a day given in a blinded fashion as extended prophylaxis at the end of the peri-operative period in 131 of the original 288 hip replacement surgery patients for up to 21 days in one clinical trial.

Major Bleeding Episodes in Deep Vein Thrombosis With or Without Pulmonary Embolism Treatment[1]

Indication	Dosing Regimen[2]: Lovenox Inj. 1.5 mg/kg q.d. SC	Lovenox Inj. 1 mg/kg q12h SC	Heparin aPTT Adjusted i.v. Therapy
Treatment of DVT and PE	n = 298 5 (2%)	n = 559 9 (2%)	n = 554 9 (2%)

[1] Bleeding complications were considered major: (1) if the hemorrhage caused a significant clinical event, or (2) if accompanied by a hemoglobin decrease ≥2 g/dL or transfusion of 2 or more units of blood products. Retroperitoneal, intraocular, and intracranial hemorrhages were always considered major.

[2] All patients also received warfarin sodium (dose-adjusted according to PT to achieve an INR of 2.0 to 3.0) commencing within 72 hours of Lovenox Injection or standard heparin therapy and continuing for up to 90 days.

Thrombocytopenia: see **WARNINGS: Thrombocytopenia.**
Elevations of Serum Aminotransferases: Asymptomatic increases in aspartate (AST [SGOT]) and alanine (ALT [SGPT]) aminotransferase levels greater than three times the upper limit of normal of the laboratory reference range have been reported in up to 6.1% and 5.9% of patients, respectively, during treatment with Lovenox Injection. Similar significant increases in aminotransferase levels have also been observed in patients and healthy volunteers treated with heparin and other low molecular weight heparins. Such elevations are fully reversible and are rarely associated with increases in bilirubin. Since aminotransferase determinations are important in the differential diagnosis of myocardial infarction, liver disease, and pulmonary emboli, elevations that might be caused by drugs like Lovenox Injection should be interpreted with caution.
Local Reactions: Mild local irritation, pain, hematoma, ecchymosis, and erythema may follow SC injection of Lovenox Injection.
Other: Other adverse effects that were thought to be possibly or probably related to treatment with Lovenox Injection, heparin, or placebo in clinical trials with patients undergoing hip or knee replacement surgery, abdominal or colorectal surgery, or treatment for DVT and that occurred at a rate of at least 2% in the Lovenox Injection group, are provided below.

[See third table at top of previous page]
[See table above]

Adverse Events Occurring at ≥2% Incidence in Lovenox Injection Treated Medical Patients[1] With Severely Restricted Mobility During Acute Illness

Adverse Event	Dosing Regimen: Lovenox Inj. 40 mg q.d. SC n = 360 (%)	Placebo q.d. SC n = 362 (%)
Dyspnea	3.3	5.2
Thrombocytopenia	2.8	2.8
Confusion	2.2	1.1
Diarrhea	2.2	1.7
Nausea	2.5	1.7

[1] Excluding unrelated and unlikely adverse events.

Adverse Events in Lovenox Injection Treated Patients With Unstable Angina or Non-Q-Wave Myocardial Infarction: Non-hemorrhagic clinical events reported to be related to Lovenox Injection therapy occurred at an incidence of ≤1%. Non-major hemorrhagic episodes, primarily injection site ecchymoses and hematomas, were more frequently reported in patients treated with SC Lovenox Injection than in patients treated with i.v. heparin.
Serious adverse events with Lovenox Injection or heparin in a clinical trial in patients with unstable angina or non-Q-wave myocardial infarction that occurred at a rate of at least 0.5% in the Lovenox Injection group, are provided below (irrespective of relationship to drug therapy).

Serious Adverse Events Occurring at ≥0.5% Incidence in Lovenox Injection Treated Patients With Unstable Angina or Non-Q-Wave Myocardial Infarction

Adverse Event	Dosing Regimen: Lovenox Inj. 1 mg/kg q12h SC n = 1578 n (%)	Heparin aPTT Adjusted i.v. Therapy n = 1529 n (%)
Atrial fibrillation	11 (0.70)	3 (0.20)
Heart failure	15 (0.95)	11 (0.72)
Lung edema	11 (0.70)	11 (0.72)
Pneumonia	13 (0.82)	9 (0.59)

[See first table at top of next page]

Ongoing Safety Surveillance: Since 1993, there have been over 80 reports of epidural or spinal hematoma formation with concurrent use of Lovenox Injection and spinal/epidural anesthesia or spinal puncture. The majority of patients had a post-operative indwelling epidural catheter placed for analgesia or received additional drugs affecting hemostasis such as NSAIDs. Many of the epidural or spinal hematomas caused neurologic injury, including long-term or permanent paralysis. Because these events were reported voluntarily from a population of unknown size, estimates of frequency cannot be made.
Other Ongoing Safety Surveillance Reports: Local reactions at the injection site (i.e., skin necrosis, nodules, inflammation, oozing), systemic allergic reactions (i.e., pruritus, urticaria, anaphylactoid reactions), vesiculobullous rash, purpura, thrombocytosis, and thrombocytopenia with thrombosis (see **WARNINGS, Thrombocytopenia**). Very rare cases of hyperlipidemia have been reported, with one case of hyperlipidemia, with marked hypertriglyceridemia, reported in a diabetic pregnant woman; causality has not been determined.

OVERDOSAGE

Symptoms/Treatment: Accidental overdosage following administration of Lovenox Injection may lead to hemorrhagic complications. Injected Lovenox Injection may be largely neutralized by the slow i.v. injection of protamine sulfate (1% solution). The dose of protamine sulfate should be equal to the dose of Lovenox Injection injected: 1 mg protamine sulfate should be administered to neutralize 1 mg Lovenox Injection. A second infusion of 0.5 mg protamine sulfate per 1 mg of Lovenox Injection may be administered if the aPTT measured 2 to 4 hours after the first infusion remains prolonged. However, even with higher doses of protamine, the aPTT may remain more prolonged than under normal conditions found following administration of heparin. In all cases, the anti-Factor Xa activity is never completely neutralized (maximum about 60%). Particular care should be taken to avoid overdosage with protamine sulfate. Administration of protamine sulfate can cause severe hypo-

Adverse Events Occurring at ≥2% Incidence in Lovenox Injection Treated Patients[1] Undergoing Treatment of Deep Vein Thrombosis With or Without Pulmonary Embolism

	Dosing Regimen					
	Lovenox Inj. 1.5 mg/kg q.d. SC n = 298		Lovenox Inj. 1 mg/kg q12h SC n = 559		Heparin aPTT Adjusted i.v. Therapy n = 544	
Adverse Event	**Severe**	**Total**	**Severe**	**Total**	**Severe**	**Total**
Injection Site Hemorrhage	0%	5%	0%	3%	<1%	<1%
Injection Site Pain	0%	2%	0%	2%	0%	0%
Hematuria	0%	2%	0%	<1%	<1%	2%

[1] Excluding unrelated adverse events.

100 mg/mL Concentration

Dosage Unit/Strength[1]	Anti-Xa Activity[2]	Package Size (per carton)	Syringe Label Color	NDC # 0075-
Ampules				
30 mg/0.3 mL	3000 IU	10 ampules	Medium Blue	0624-03
Prefilled Syringes[3]				
30 mg/0.3 mL	3000 IU	10 syringes	Medium Blue	0624-30
40 mg/0.4 mL	4000 IU	10 syringes	Yellow	0620-40
Graduated Prefilled Syringes[3]				
60 mg/0.6 mL	6000 IU	10 syringes	Orange	0621-60
80 mg/0.8 mL	8000 IU	10 syringes	Brown	0622-80
100 mg/1 mL	10,000 IU	10 syringes	Black	0623-00

[1] Strength represents the number of milligrams of enoxaparin sodium in Water for Injection. **Lovenox Injection** ampules, 30 and 40 mg prefilled syringes, and 60, 80, and 100 mg graduated prefilled syringes each contain **10 mg enoxaparin sodium per 0.1 mL Water for Injection.**

[2] Approximate anti-Factor Xa activity based on reference to the W.H.O. First International Low Molecular Weight Heparin Reference Standard.

[3] Each **Lovenox Injection** syringe is affixed with a 27 gauge × 1/2 inch needle.

150 mg/mL Concentration

Dosage Unit/Strength[1]	Anti-Xa Activity[2]	Package Size (per carton)	Syringe Label Color	NDC # 0075-
Graduated Prefilled Syringes[3]				
120 mg/0.8 mL	12,000 IU	10 syringes	Purple	2912-01
150 mg/1 mL	15,000 IU	10 syringes	Navy Blue	2915-01

[1] Strength represents the number of milligrams of enoxaparin sodium in Water for Injection. **Lovenox Injection** 120 and 150 mg graduated prefilled syringes contain **150 mg enoxaparin sodium per 0.1 mL** Water for Injection.

[2] Approximate anti-Factor Xa activity based on reference to the W.H.O. First International Low Molecular Weight Heparin Reference Standard.

[3] Each **Lovenox Injection** graduated prefilled syringe is affixed with a 27 gauge × 1/2 inch needle.

tensive and anaphylactoid reactions. Because fatal reactions, often resembling anaphylaxis, have been reported with protamine sulfate, it should be given only when resuscitation techniques and treatment of anaphylactic shock are readily available. For additional information consult the labeling of Protamine Sulfate Injection, USP, products.

A single SC dose of 46.4 mg/kg enoxaparin was lethal to rats. The symptoms of acute toxicity were ataxia, decreased motility, dyspnea, cyanosis, and coma.

DOSAGE AND ADMINISTRATION

All patients should be evaluated for a bleeding disorder before administration of Lovenox Injection, unless the medication is needed urgently. Since coagulation parameters are unsuitable for monitoring Lovenox Injection activity, routine monitoring of coagulation parameters is not required (see **PRECAUTIONS, Laboratory Tests**).

Note: Lovenox Injection is available in two concentrations:

1 100 mg/mL Concentration: 30 mg / 0.3 mL ampules, 30 mg / 0.3 mL and 40 mg / 0.4 mL prefilled single-dose syringes, 60 mg / 0.6 mL, 80 mg / 0.8 mL, and 100 mg / 1 mL prefilled, graduated, single-dose syringes.

2 150 mg/mL Concentration: 120 mg / 0.8 mL and 150 mg / 1 mL prefilled, graduated, single-dose syringes.

Adult Dosage:

Abdominal Surgery: In patients undergoing abdominal surgery who are at risk for thromboembolic complications, the recommended dose of Lovenox Injection is **40 mg once a day** administered by SC injection with the initial dose given 2 hours prior to surgery. The usual duration of administration is 7 to 10 days; up to 12 days administration has been well tolerated in clinical trials.

Hip or Knee Replacement Surgery: In patients undergoing hip or knee replacement surgery, the recommended dose of Lovenox Injection is **30 mg every 12 hours** administered by SC injection. Provided that hemostasis has been established, the initial dose should be given 12 to 24 hours after surgery. For hip replacement surgery, a dose of **40 mg once a day** SC, given initially 12 (±3) hours prior to surgery, may be considered. Following the initial phase of thromboprophylaxis in hip replacement surgery patients, continued prophylaxis with Lovenox Injection 40 mg once a day administered by SC injection for 3 weeks is recommended. The usual duration of administration is 7 to 10 days; up to 14 days administration has been well tolerated in clinical trials.

Medical Patients During Acute Illness: In medical patients at risk for thromboembolic complications due to severely restricted mobility during acute illness, the recommended dose of Lovenox Injection is **40 mg once a day** administered by SC injection. The usual duration of administration is 6 to 11 days; up to 14 days of Lovenox Injection has been well tolerated in the controlled clinical trial.

Unstable Angina and Non-Q-Wave Myocardial Infarction: In patients with unstable angina or non-Q-wave myocardial infarction, the recommended dose of Lovenox Injection is **1 mg/kg** administered SC **every 12 hours** in conjunction with oral aspirin therapy (100 to 325 mg once daily). Treatment with Lovenox Injection should be prescribed for a minimum of 2 days and continued until clinical stabilization. To minimize the risk of bleeding following vascular instrumentation during the treatment of unstable angina, adhere precisely to the intervals recommended between Lovenox Injection doses. The vascular access sheath for instrumentation should remain in place for 6 to 8 hours following a dose of Lovenox Injection. The next scheduled dose should be given no sooner than 6 to 8 hours after sheath removal. The site of the procedure should be observed for signs of bleeding or hematoma formation. The usual duration of treatment is 2 to 8 days; up to 12.5 days of Lovenox Injection has been well tolerated in clinical trials.

Treatment of Deep Vein Thrombosis With or Without Pulmonary Embolism: In **outpatient treatment**, patients with acute deep vein thrombosis without pulmonary embolism who can be treated at home, the recommended dose of Lovenox Injection is **1 mg/kg every 12 hours** administered SC. In **inpatient (hospital) treatment**, patients with acute deep vein thrombosis with pulmonary embolism or patients with acute deep vein thrombosis without pulmonary embolism (who are not candidates for outpatient treatment), the recommended dose of Lovenox Injection is **1 mg/kg every 12 hours** administered SC **or 1.5 mg/kg once a day** administered SC at the same time every day. In both outpatient and inpatient (hospital) treatments, warfarin sodium therapy should be initiated when appropriate (usually within 72 hours of Lovenox Injection). Lovenox Injection should be continued for a minimum of 5 days and until a therapeutic oral anticoagulant effect has been achieved (International Normalization Ratio 2.0 to 3.0). The average duration of administration is 7 days; up to 17 days of Lovenox Injection administration has been well tolerated in controlled clinical trials.

Administration: Lovenox Injection is a clear, colorless to pale yellow sterile solution, and as with other parenteral drug products, should be inspected visually for particulate matter and discoloration prior to administration.

When using Lovenox Injection ampules, to assure withdrawal of the appropriate volume of drug, the use of a tuberculin syringe or equivalent is recommended.

Lovenox Injection is administered by SC injection. It must not be administered by intramuscular injection. Lovenox Injection is intended for use under the guidance of a physician. Patients may self-inject only if their physician determines that it is appropriate and with medical follow-up, as necessary. Proper training in subcutaneous injection technique (with or without the assistance of an injection device) should be provided.

Subcutaneous Injection Technique: Patients should be lying down and Lovenox Injection administered by deep SC injection. To avoid the loss of drug when using the 30 and 40 mg prefilled syringes, do not expel the air bubble from the syringe before the injection. Administration should be alternated between the left and right anterolateral and left and right posterolateral abdominal wall. The whole length of the needle should be introduced into a skin fold held between the thumb and forefinger; the skin fold should be held throughout the injection. To minimize bruising, do not rub the injection site after completion of the injection. An automatic injector, Lovenox EasyInjector™, is available for patients to administer Lovenox Injection packaged in 30 mg and 40 mg prefilled syringes. Please see directions accompanying the Lovenox EasyInjector™ automatic injection device.

HOW SUPPLIED

Lovenox® (enoxaparin sodium) Injection is available in two concentrations:

[See second table above]

[See third table above]

Store at Controlled Room Temperature, 15–25°C (59–77°F) [see USP].

Keep out of the reach of children.

Lovenox Injection prefilled and graduated prefilled syringes manufactured in France.

Lovenox Injection ampules manufactured in England.

Aventis Pharmaceuticals Products Inc.
BRIDGEWATER, NJ 08807

Prescribing information as of July 2001.

PRIFTIN® ℞

[*prĭf-tĭn*]

(rifapentine)

150 mg Tablets

Prescribing information for this product, which appears on pages 758–761 of the 2002 PDR, has been completely revised as follows. Please write "See Supplement A" next to the product heading.

Prescribing Information as of February 2002

DESCRIPTION

PRIFTIN® (rifapentine) for oral administration contains 150 mg of the active ingredient rifapentine per tablet.

The 150 mg tablets also contain, as inactive ingredients: calcium stearate, disodium EDTA, FD&C Blue No. 2 aluminum lake, hydroxypropyl cellulose, hydroxypropyl methylcellulose, microcrystalline cellulose, polyethylene glycol, pregelatinized starch, propylene glycol, sodium ascorbate, sodium lauryl sulfate, sodium starch glycolate, synthetic red iron oxide, and titanium dioxide.

Rifapentine is a rifamycin derivative antibiotic and has a similar profile of microbiological activity to rifampin (rifampicin).

The molecular weight is 877.04.

The molecular formula is $C_{47}H_{64}N_4O_{12}$.

The chemical name for rifapentine is rifamycin, 3-[[(4-cyclopentyl-1-piperazinyl)imino]methyl]-

or

3-[N-(4-Cyclopentyl - 1-piperazinyl)formimidoyl] rifamycin or 5,6,9,17,19, 21-hexahydroxy-23-methoxy-2,4,12,16,18,20, 22-heptamethyl-8-[N-(4-cyclopentyl-l-piperazinyl)-formimidoyl]-2,7-(epoxypenta-deca[1,11,13]trienimino)naphtho [2,1-b]furan-1,11(2H)-dione 21-acetate. It has the following structure:

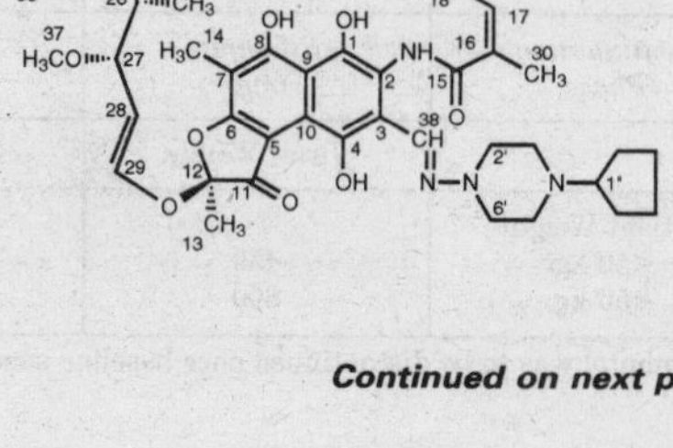

Continued on next page

Priftin—Cont.

ACTIONS/CLINICAL PHARMACOLOGY

Pharmacokinetics

Absorption

The absolute bioavailability of rifapentine has not been determined. The relative bioavailability (with an oral solution as a reference) of rifapentine after a single 600 mg dose to healthy adult volunteers was 70%. The maximum concentrations were achieved from 5 to 6 hours after administration of the 600 mg rifapentine dose. Food (850 total calories: 33 g protein, 55 g fat and 58 g carbohydrate) increased AUC(0-∞) and C_{max} by 43% and 44%, respectively over that observed when administered under fasting conditions. When oral doses of rifapentine were administered once daily or once every 72 hours to healthy volunteers for 10 days, single dose AUC(0-∞) value of rifapentine was similar to its steady-state AUC_{ss} (0–24h) or AUC_{ss} (0–72h) values, suggesting no significant auto-induction effect on steady-state pharmacokinetics of rifapentine. Steady-state conditions were achieved by day 10 following daily administration of rifapentine 600 mg. The pharmacokinetic characteristics of rifapentine and 25-desacetyl rifapentine (active metabolite) on day 10 following oral administration of 600 mg rifapentine every 72 hours to healthy volunteers are contained in the following table.

Table 1. Pharmacokinetics and rifapentine and 25-desacetyl rifapentine in healthy volunteers

Parameter	Rifapentine	25-desacetyl Rifapentine
	Mean ± SD (n=12)	
C_{max} (µg/mL)	15.05 ± 4.62	6.26 ± 2.06
AUC (0–72h)(µg*h/mL)	319.54 ± 91.52	215.88 ± 85.96
$T_{½}$(h)	13.19 ± 1.38	13.35 ± 2.67
T_{max} (h)	4.83 ± 1.80	11.25 ± 2.73
Clpo (L/h)	2.03 ± 0.60	—

Distribution

In a population pharmacokinetic analysis in 351 tuberculosis patients who received 600 mg rifapentine in combination with isoniazid, pyrazinamide and ethambutol, the estimated apparent volume of distribution was 70.2 ± 9.1 L. In healthy volunteers, rifapentine and 25-desacetyl rifapentine were 97.7% and 93.2% bound to plasma proteins, respectively. Rifapentine was mainly bound to albumin. Similar extent of protein binding was observed in healthy volunteers, asymptomatic HIV-infected subjects and hepatically impaired subjects.

Metabolism/Excretion

Following a single 600 mg oral dose of radiolabelled rifapentine to healthy volunteers (n=4), 87% of the total ^{14}C rifapentine was recovered in the urine (17%) and feces (70%). Greater than 80% of the total ^{14}C rifapentine dose was excreted from the body within 7 days. Rifapentine was hydrolyzed by an esterase enzyme to form a microbiologically active 25-desacetyl rifapentine. Rifapentine and 25-desacetyl rifapentine accounted for 99% of the total radioactivity in plasma. Plasma AUC (0-∞) and C_{max} values of the 25-desacetyl rifapentine metabolite were one-half and one-third those of the rifapentine, respectively. Based upon relative in vitro activities and AUC(0-∞) values, rifapentine and 25-desacetyl rifapentine potentially contributes 62% and 38% to the clinical activities against *M. tuberculosis*, respectively.

Special Populations

Gender: In a population pharmacokinetics analysis of sparse blood samples obtained from 351 tuberculosis patients who received 600 mg rifapentine in combination with isoniazid, pyrazinamide and ethambutol, the estimated apparent oral clearance of rifapentine for males and females was 2.51 ± 0.14 L/h and 1.69 ± 0.41 L/h, respectively. The clinical significance of the difference in the estimated apparent oral clearance is not known.

Elderly: Following oral administration of a single 600 mg dose of rifapentine to elderly (≥65 years) male healthy volunteers (n=14), the pharmacokinetics of rifapentine and 25-desacetyl metabolite were similar to that observed for young (18 to 45 years) healthy male volunteers (n=20).

Pediatric (Adolescents): In a pharmacokinetics study of rifapentine in healthy adolescents (age 12 to 15), 600 mg rifapentine was administered to those weighing ≥45 kg (n=10) and 450 mg was administered to those weighing <45 kg (n=2). The pharmacokinetics of rifapentine were similar to those observed in healthy adults.

Renal Impaired Patients: The pharmacokinetics of rifapentine have not been evaluated in renal impaired patients. Although only about 17% of an administered dose is excreted via the kidneys, the clinical significance of impaired renal function on the disposition of rifapentine and its 25-desacetyl metabolite is not known.

Hepatic Impaired Patients: Following oral administration of a single 600 mg dose of rifapentine to mild to severe hepatic impaired patients (n=15), the pharmacokinetics of rifapentine and 25-desacetyl metabolite were similar in patients with various degrees of hepatic impairment and to that observed in another study for healthy volunteers (n=12). Since the elimination of these agents are primarily via the liver, the clinical significance of impaired hepatic function on the disposition of rifapentine and its 25-desacetyl metabolite is not known.

Asymptomatic HIV-Infected Volunteers: Following oral administration of a single 600 mg dose of rifapentine to asymptomatic HIV-infected volunteers (n=15) under fasting conditions, mean C_{max} and AUC(0-∞) of rifapentine were lower (20–32%) than that observed in other studies in healthy volunteers (n=55). In a cross-study comparison, mean C_{max} and AUC values of the 25-desacetyl metabolite of rifapentine, when compared to healthy volunteers were higher (6–21%) in one study (n=20), but lower (15–16%) in a different study (n=40). The clinical significance of this observation is not known. Food (850 total calories: 33 g protein, 55 g fat, and 58 g carbohydrate) increases the mean AUC and C_{max} of rifapentine observed under fasting conditions in asymptomatic HIV-infected volunteers by about 51% and 53%, respectively.

Microbiology

Mechanism of Action

Rifapentine, a cyclopentyl rifamycin, inhibits DNA-dependent RNA polymerase in susceptible strains of *Mycobacterium tuberculosis* but not in mammalian cells. At therapeutic levels, rifapentine exhibits bactericidal activity against both intracellular and extracellular *M. tuberculosis* organisms. Both rifapentine and the 25-desacetyl metabolite accumulate in human monocyte-derived macrophages with intracellular/extracellular ratios of approximately 24:1 and 7:1, respectively.

Resistance Development

In the treatment of tuberculosis (see INDICATIONS AND USAGE), a small number of resistant cells present within large populations of susceptible cells can rapidly become predominant. Rifapentine resistance development in *M. tuberculosis* strains is principally due to one of several single point mutations that occur in the rpoB portion of the gene coding for the beta subunit of the DNA-dependent RNA polymerase. The incidence of rifapentine resistant mutants in an otherwise susceptible population of *M. tuberculosis* strains is approximately one in 10^7 to 10^8 bacilli. Due to the potential for resistance development to rifapentine, appropriate susceptibility tests should be performed in the event of persistently positive cultures.

M. tuberculosis organisms resistant to other rifamycins are likely to be resistant to rifapentine. A high level of cross-resistance between rifampin and rifapentine has been demonstrated with *M. tuberculosis* strains. Cross-resistance does not appear between rifapentine and non-rifamycin antimycobacterial agents such as isoniazid and streptomycin.

In Vitro Activity of Rifapentine against *M. tuberculosis*

Rifapentine and its 25-desacetyl metabolite have demonstrated in vitro activity against rifamycin-susceptible strains of *Mycobacterium tuberculosis* including cidal activity against phagocytized *M. tuberculosis* organisms grown in activated human macrophages.

In vitro results indicate that rifapentine MIC values for *M. tuberculosis* organisms are influenced by study conditions. Rifapentine MIC values were substantially increased employing egg-based medium compared to liquid or agar-based solid media. The addition of Tween 80 in these assays has been shown to lower MIC values for rifamycin compounds.

In mouse infection studies a therapeutic effect, in terms of enhanced survival time or reduction of organ bioburden, has been observed in *M. tuberculosis*-infected animals treated with various intermittent rifapentine-containing regimens. Animal studies have shown that the activity of rifapentine is influenced by dose and frequency of administration.

Susceptibility testing for *Mycobacterium tuberculosis*

Breakpoints to determine whether clinical isolates of *M. tuberculosis* are susceptible or resistant to rifapentine have not been established. The clinical relevance of rifapentine in vitro susceptibility test results for other mycobacterial species has not been determined.

CLINICAL TRIALS

A total of 722 patients were enrolled in Clinical Study 008, an open label, prospective, randomized, parallel group, active controlled trial, for the treatment of pulmonary tuberculosis. This population was mostly comprised of Black (>60%) or Multiracial (>31%) patients and the mean ± standard deviation age was 37 ± 11 years. Treatment groups were comparable with respect to age and race. The percentage of male patients was higher in the rifapentine combination group (80%) than in the rifampin combination group (73%). The study was divided into two phases on the basis of dosing frequency. For the first phase, designated as the Intensive Phase, 361 patients were randomized to receive rifapentine, isoniazid, pyrazinamide, and ethambutol for 60 days and 361 patients were randomized to receive rifampin, isoniazid, pyrazinamide, and ethambutol for 60 days. (Ethambutol was to be discontinued once baseline susceptibility test results were available.) Rifapentine and isoniazid were each administered at a fixed dose regardless of body weight. Rifampin, pyrazinamide, and ethambutol were administered based on body weight according to Table 2-1. **Note:** All drugs were administered ***daily*** in the Intensive Phase **except for rifapentine** which was administered twice weekly. During the second phase, designated as the Continuation Phase, 321 patients who had received rifapentine in the Intensive Phase continued to receive rifapentine and isoniazid once weekly for up to 120 days. Three hundred seven patients who had received rifampin in the Intensive Phase continued to receive rifampin and isoniazid during the Continuation Phase twice weekly for up to 120 days. Rifampin and isoniazid were administered based on body weight according to Table 2-1.

Patients in either treatment group were scheduled to receive study drug over a 180-day period with a subsequent 24-month follow-up. Additionally, both treatment groups received pyridoxine (Vitamin B_6) over the 180-day treatment period.

[See table 2-1 below]

Table 2-2 presents clinical outcome in Study 008.

[See table 2-2 at bottom of next page]

Risk of relapse was higher in the rifapentine regimen. During the Intensive Phase of treatment the rate of noncompliance with companion medications was somewhat higher for the rifapentine regimen than for the rifampin regimen. Most of the relapses occurred among those with poor compliance with these companion medications and this group also had the largest risk of relapse for the rifapentine regimen relative to the rifampin regimen. This factor appears to explain most, but not all, of the higher relapse rate observed in the rifapentine arm. Failure to convert sputum after two months of treatment (ie, end of Intensive Phase) was associated with a greater risk of relapse for both treatment regi-

Table 2-1. Dose of Rifapentine, Rifampin, Isoniazid, Pyrazinamide, and Ethambutol

Rifapentine Combination Treatment

Intensive Phase	*Rifapentine (mg)*	*Isoniazid (mg)*	*Pyrazinamide (mg)*	*Ethambutol* (mg)*
	Twice Weekly	*Daily*	*Daily*	*Daily*
Patient Weight				
<50 kg	600	300	1500	800
≥50 kg	600	300	2000	1200
Continuation Phase	*Rifapentine (mg)*	*Isoniazid (mg)*		
	Once Weekly	*Once Weekly*		
Patient Weight				
<50 kg	600	600		
≥50 kg	600	900		

Rifampin Combination Treatment

Intensive Phase	*Rifampin (mg)*	*Isoniazid (mg)*	*Pyrazinamide (mg)*	*Ethambutol (mg)*
	Daily	*Daily*	*Daily*	*Daily*
Patient Weight				
<50 kg	450	300	1500	800
≥50 kg	600	300	2000	1200
Continuation Phase	*Rifampin (mg)*	*Isoniazid (mg)*		
	Twice Weekly	*Twice Weekly*		
Patient Weight				
<50 kg	450	600		
≥50 kg	600	900		

***Ethambutol was to be discontinued once baseline susceptibility test results were available**

mens. Relapse rates were also higher for males in both regimens. Relapse in the rifapentine group was not associated with development of mono-resistance to rifampin.

In vitro susceptibility testing was conducted against *M. tuberculosis* isolates recovered from 620 patients enrolled in the study. Rifapentine and rifampin MIC values were determined employing the radiometric susceptibility testing method utilizing 7H12 broth at pH 6.8 (NCCLS procedure M24-T). Six hundred and twelve patients had *M. tuberculosis* isolates that were susceptible to rifampin (MIC < 0.5 µg/ml). Of these patients, six hundred and ten had *M. tuberculosis* isolates (99.7%) with rifapentine MICs of < 0.125 µg/ml. The other two patients that had rifampin susceptible *M. tuberculosis* isolates had rifapentine MICs of 0.25 µg/ml. The remaining eight patients had *M. tuberculosis* isolates that were resistant to rifampin (MIC > 8.0 µg/ml). These *M. tuberculosis* isolates had rifapentine MICs of > 8.0 µg/ml. In this study high rifampin and rifapentine MICs were associated with multi-drug resistant *M. tuberculosis* (MDRTB) isolates. Rifamycin mono-resistance was not observed in either treatment arm. This information is provided for comparative purposes only as rifapentine breakpoints have not been established.

INDICATIONS AND USAGE

PRIFTIN is indicated for the treatment of pulmonary tuberculosis. PRIFTIN must always be used in conjunction with at least one other antituberculosis drug to which the isolate is susceptible. In the intensive phase of the short-course treatment of pulmonary tuberculosis, **PRIFTIN should be administered twice weekly for two months,** with an interval of no less than 3 days (72 hours) between doses, as part of an appropriate regimen which includes daily companion drugs (Table 2-1). It may also be necessary to add either streptomycin or ethambutol until the results of susceptibility testing are known. ***Compliance with all drugs in the Intensive Phase (ie, PRIFTIN, isoniazid, pyrazinamide, ethambutol or streptomycin) is imperative to assure early sputum conversion and protection against relapse.*** Following the intensive phase, Continuation Phase treatment should be continued with PRIFTIN for 4 months. **During this phase, PRIFTIN should be administered on a once-weekly basis** in combination with an appropriate antituberculous agent for susceptible organisms (Table 2-1) (see DOSAGE AND ADMINISTRATION section).

In the treatment of tuberculosis, the small number of resistant cells present within large populations of susceptible cells can rapidly become the predominant type. Consequently, clinical samples for mycobacterial culture and susceptibility testing should be obtained prior to the initiation of therapy, as well as during treatment to monitor therapeutic response. The susceptibility of *M. tuberculosis* organisms to isoniazid, rifampin, pyrazinamide, ethambutol, rifapentine and other appropriate agents should be measured. If test results show resistance to any of these drugs and the patient is not responding to therapy, the drug regimen should be modified.

CONTRAINDICATIONS

This product is contraindicated in patients with a history of hypersensitivity to any of the rifamycins (eg, rifampin and rifabutin).

WARNINGS

Poor compliance with the dosage regimen, particularly the daily administered non-rifamycin drugs in the Intensive Phase, was associated with late sputum conversion and a high relapse rate in the rifapentine arm of Clinical Study 008. Therefore, compliance with the full course of therapy must be emphasized, and the importance of not missing any doses must be stressed. (See PRECAUTIONS and DOSAGE AND ADMINISTRATION.)

Since antituberculous multidrug treatments, including the rifamycin class, are associated with serious hepatic events, patients with abnormal liver tests and/or liver disease should only be given rifapentine in cases of necessity and then with caution and under strict medical supervision. In these patients, careful monitoring of liver tests (especially serum transaminases) should be carried out prior to therapy and then every 2 to 4 weeks during therapy. If signs of liver disease occur or worsen, rifapentine should be discontinued. Hepatotoxicity of other antituberculosis drugs (eg, isoniazid, pyrazinamide) used in combination with rifapentine should also be taken into account.

Hyperbilirubinemia resulting from competition for excretory pathways between rifapentine and bilirubin cannot be excluded since competition between the related drug rifampin and bilirubin can occur. An isolated report showing a moderate rise in bilirubin and/or transaminase level is not in itself an indication for interrupting treatment; rather, the decision should be made after repeating the tests, noting trends in the levels and considering them in conjunction with the patient's clinical condition. Pseudomembranous colitis has been reported to occur with various antibiotics, including other rifamycins. Diarrhea, particularly if severe and/or persistent, occurring during treatment or in the initial weeks following treatment may be symptomatic of *Clostridium difficile*-associated disease, the most severe form of which is pseudomembranous colitis. If pseudomembranous colitis is suspected, rifapentine should be stopped immediately and the patient should be treated with supportive and specific treatment without delay (eg, oral vancomycin). Products inhibiting peristalsis are contraindicated in this clinical situation.

Experience in HIV-infected patients is limited. In an ongoing CDC TB trial, five out of 30 HIV-infected patients randomized to once weekly rifapentine (plus INH) in the Continuation Phase who completed treatment, relapsed. Four of these patients developed rifampin mono-resistant (RMR) TB. Each RMR patient had late-stage HIV infection, low CD4 counts and extrapulmonary disease, and documented co-administration of antifungal azoles (See Reference 1). These findings are consistent with the literature in which an emergence of RMR TB in HIV-infected TB patients has been reported in recent years. Further study in this subpopulation is warranted. As with other antituberculous treatments, when rifapentine is used in HIV-infected patients, a more aggressive regimen should be employed (eg, more frequent dosing). Based on results to date of the CDC trial (see above), once weekly dosing during the Continuation Phase of treatment is not recommended at this time.

Because rifapentine has been shown to increase indinavir metabolism (see DRUG INTERACTIONS), it should be used with extreme caution, if at all, in patients who are also taking protease inhibitors.

PRECAUTIONS

General

Rifapentine may produce a predominately red-orange discoloration of body tissues and/or fluids (eg, skin, teeth, tongue, urine, feces, saliva, sputum, tears, sweat, and cerebrospinal fluid).

Contact lenses or dentures may become permanently stained.

Rifapentine should not be used in patients with porphyria. Rifampin has enzyme-inducing properties, including induction of delta amino levulinic acid synthetase. Isolated reports have associated porphyria exacerbation with rifampin administration. Based on these isolated reports with rifampin, it may be assumed that rifapentine has a similar effect.

Information for Patients

The patient should be told that PRIFTIN may produce a reddish coloration of the urine, sweat, sputum, tears, and breast milk and the patient should be forewarned that contact lenses or dentures may be permanently stained. The patient should be advised that the reliability of oral or other systemic hormonal contraceptives may be affected; consideration should be given to using alternative contraceptive measures. For those patients with a propensity to nausea, vomiting, or gastrointestinal upset, administration of PRIFTIN with food may be useful. Patients should be instructed to notify their physician promptly if they experience any of the following: fever, loss of appetite, malaise, nausea and vomiting, darkened urine, yellowish discoloration of the skin and eyes, and pain or swelling of the joints. Compliance with the full course of therapy must be emphasized, and the importance of not missing any doses of the daily administered companion medications in the Intensive Phase must be stressed. (See DOSAGE AND ADMINISTRATION and WARNINGS).

Laboratory Tests

Adults treated for tuberculosis with rifapentine should have baseline measurements of hepatic enzymes, bilirubin, a complete blood count, and a platelet count (or estimate).

Patients should be seen at least monthly during therapy and should be specifically questioned concerning symptoms associated with adverse reactions. All patients with abnormalities should have follow-up, including laboratory testing, if necessary. Routine laboratory monitoring for toxicity in people with normal baseline measurements is generally not necessary.

Therapeutic concentrations of rifampin have been shown to inhibit standard microbiological assays for serum folate and Vitamin B_{12}. Similar drug-laboratory interactions should be considered for rifapentine; thus, alternative assay methods should be considered.

Drug Interaction

Rifapentine-Indinavir Interaction: In a study in which 600 mg rifapentine was administered twice weekly for 14 days followed by rifapentine twice weekly plus 800 mg indinavir 3 times a day for an additional 14 days, indinavir C_{max} decreased by 55% while AUC reduced by 70%. Clearance of indinavir increased by 3-fold in the presence of rifapentine while half-life did not change. But when indinavir was administered for 14 days followed by coadministration with rifapentine for an additional 14 days, indinavir did not affect the pharmacokinetics of rifapentine. **Rifapentine should be used with extreme caution, if at all, in patients who are also taking protease inhibitors.** (See WARNINGS and DOSAGE AND ADMINISTRATION.)

Rifapentine is an inducer of cytochromes P4503A4 and P4502C8/9. Therefore, rifapentine may increase the metabolism of other coadministered drugs that are metabolized by these enzymes. Induction of enzyme activities by rifapentine occurred within 4 days after the first dose. Enzyme activities returned to baseline levels 14 days after discontinuing rifapentine. In addition, the magnitude of enzyme induction by rifapentine was dose and dosing frequency dependent; less enzyme induction occurred when 600 mg oral doses of rifapentine were given once every 72 hours versus daily. In vitro and in vivo enzyme induction studies have suggested rifapentine induction potential may be less than rifampin but more potent than rifabutin.

Rifampin has been reported to accelerate the metabolism and may reduce the activity of the following drugs; hence, rifapentine may also increase the metabolism and decrease the activity of these drugs. Dosage adjustments of the following drugs or of drugs metabolized by cytochrome P4503A4 or P4502C8/9 may be necessary if they are given concurrently with rifapentine. Patients using oral or other systemic hormonal contraceptives should be advised to change to nonhormonal methods of birth control.

Anticonvulsants: eg, phenytoin
Antiarrhythmics: eg, disopyramide, mexiletine, quinidine, tocainide
Antibiotics: eg, chloramphenicol, clarithromycin, dapsone, doxycycline, fluoroquinolones (such as ciprofloxacin)
Oral anticoagulants: eg, warfarin
Antifungals: eg, fluconazole, itraconazole, ketoconazole
Barbiturates
Benzodiazepines: eg, diazepam
Beta-blockers, calcium channel blockers: eg, diltiazem, nifedipine, verapamil
Corticosteroids
Cardiac glycoside preparations
Clofibrate
Oral or other systemic hormonal contraceptives
Haloperidol
HIV protease inhibitors: eg, indinavir, ritonavir, nelfinavir, saquinavir (see Rifapentine-Indinavir Interaction above)
Oral hypoglycemic agents: eg, sulfonylureas
Immunosuppressants: eg, cyclosporine, tacrolimus
Levothyroxine
Narcotic analgesics: eg, methadone
Progestins
Quinine
Reverse transcriptase inhibitors: eg, delavirdine, zidovudine
Sildenafil
Theophylline
Tricyclic antidepressants: eg, amitriptyline, nortriptyline

The conversion of rifapentine to 25-desacetyl rifapentine is mediated by an esterase enzyme. There is minimal potential for rifapentine metabolism to be inhibited or induced by another drug, or for rifapentine to inhibit the metabolism of another drug based upon the characteristics of the esterase enzymes. Rifapentine does not induce its own metabolism. Since rifapentine is highly bound to albumin, drug displacement interactions may also occur.

In Clinical Study 008 patients were advised to take rifapentine at least 1 hour before or 2 hours after ingestion of antacids.

Carcinogenesis, Mutagenesis, Impairment of Fertility

Carcinogenicity studies with rifapentine have not been completed. Rifapentine was negative in the following genotoxicity tests: in vitro gene mutation assay in bacteria (Ames test); in vitro point mutation test in *Aspergillus nidulans*; in vitro gene conversion assay in *Saccharomyces cerevisiae*; host-mediated (mouse) gene conversion assay with *Saccharomyces cerevisiae*; in vitro Chinese hamster ovary cell/hypoxanthine-guanine-phosphoribosyl transferase (CHO/HGPRT) forward mutation assay; in vitro chromosomal aberration assay utilizing rat lymphocytes; and in vivo mouse bone marrow micronucleus assay. The 25-desacetyl metabolite of rifapentine was also negative in the in vitro gene mutation assay in bacteria (Ames test), the in vitro Chinese hamster ovary cell/hypoxanthine-guanine-phosphoribosyl transferase (CHO/HGPRT) forward mutation assay, and the in vivo mouse bone marrow micronucleus assay. This metabolite did induce chromosomal aberrations in an in vitro chromosomal aberration assay. Fertility and reproductive performance were not affected by oral administration of rifapentine to male and female rats at doses of up to one-third of the human dose (based on body surface area conversions).

Pregnancy Category C

Teratogenic Effects

Rifapentine has been shown to be teratogenic in rats and rabbits. In rats, when given in doses 0.6 times the human dose (based on body surface area comparisons) during the period of organogenesis, pups showed cleft palates, right aortic arch and increased incidence of delayed ossification and increased number of ribs. Rabbits treated with drug at doses between 0.3 and 1.3 times the human dose (based on

Table 2-2. Clinical Outcome in Study 008*

	Rifapentine Combination	Rifampin Combination
Status of End of Treatment		
Converted	87% (248/286)	80% (226/283)
Not Converted	1% (4/286)	3% (8/283)
Lost to Follow-up	12% (34/286)	17% (49/283)
Status Through 24 Month Follow-up:		
Relapsed	12% (29/248)	7% (15/226)
Sputum Negative	57% (142/248)	64% (145/226)
Lost to Follow-up	31% (77/248)	29% (66/226)

***All data for patients with confirmed susceptible MTB (rifapentine combination, n=286; rifampin combination, n=283).**

Continued on next page

Priftin—Cont.

body surface area comparison) displayed major malformations including ovarian agenesis, pes varus, arhinia, microphthalmia and irregularities of the ossified facial tissues (4 of 321 examined fetuses).

Nonteratogenic Effects

In rats, rifapentine administration was associated with increased resorption rate and post implantation loss, decreased mean fetus weight, increased number of stillborn pups and slightly increased mortality during lactation. Rabbits given 1.3 times the human dose (based on body surface area comparisons) showed higher post-implantation losses and an increased incidence of stillborn pups.

When rifapentine was administered at 0.3 times the human dose (based on body surface area comparisons) to mated female rats late in gestation (from day 15 of gestation to day 21 postpartum), pup weights and gestational survival (live pups born/pups born) were reduced compared to controls.

Pregnancy–Human Experience

There are no adequate and well-controlled studies in pregnant women. In Clinical Study 008, six patients randomized to rifapentine became pregnant; two had normal deliveries; two had first trimester spontaneous abortions, one had an elective abortion and one patient was lost to follow-up. Of the two patients who spontaneously aborted, co-morbid conditions of ethanol abuse in one and HIV infection in the other were noted.

When administered during the last few weeks of pregnancy, rifampin can cause postnatal hemorrhages in the mother and infant for which treatment with Vitamin K may be indicated. Thus, patients and infants who receive rifapentine during the last few weeks of pregnancy should have appropriate clotting parameters evaluated.

Rifapentine should be used during pregnancy only if the potential benefit justifies the potential risk to the fetus.

Nursing Mothers

It is not known whether rifapentine is excreted in human milk. Because many drugs are excreted in human milk and because of the potential for serious adverse reactions in nursing infants, a decision should be made whether to discontinue nursing or discontinue the drug, taking into account the importance of the drug to the mother. Since rifapentine may produce a red-orange discoloration of body fluids, there is a potential for discoloration of breast milk.

Pediatric Use

The safety and effectiveness of rifapentine in pediatric patients under the age of 12 have not been established. A pharmacokinetic study was conducted in 12- to 15-year-old healthy volunteers. (See ACTIONS/CLINICAL PHARMACOLOGY Special Populations for pharmacokinetic information).

Geriatric Use

Clinical studies of PRIFTIN did not include sufficient numbers of subjects aged 65 and over to determine whether they respond differently from younger subjects. Other reported clinical experience has not identified differences in responses between the elderly and younger patients. In general, dose selection for an elderly patient should be cautious, usually starting at the low end of the dosing range, reflecting the greater frequency of decreased hepatic, renal, or cardiac function and of concomitant disease or other drug therapy. (See ACTIONS/CLINICAL PHARMACOLOGY, Pharmacokinetics, Special Populations-Elderly).

Table 2-3. Treatment-Related Adverse Events Occurring in ≥1% of the Patients in Study 008

	Intensive Phase[1]		*Continuation Phase*[2]		*Total*	
Preferred Term	*Rifapentine Combination (N=361) N (%)*	*Rifampin Combination (N=361) N (%)*	*Rifapentine Combination (N=321) N (%)*	*Rifampin Combination (N=307) N (%)*	*Rifapentine Combination (N=361) N (%)*	*Rifampin Combination (N=361) N (%)*
Hyperuricemia	78 (21.6)	55 (15.2)	0	0	78 (21.6)	55 (15.2)
ALT increased	12 (3.3)	17 (4.7)	6 (1.9)	7 (2.3)	18 (5.0)	24 (6.6)
AST increased	11 (3.0)	16 (4.4)	5 (1.6)	7 (2.3)	15 (4.2)	23 (6.4)
Neutropenia	7 (1.9)	9 (2.5)	12 (3.7)	9 (2.9)	18 (5.0)	18 (5.0)
Pyuria	11 (3.0)	10 (2.8)	6 (1.9)	3 (1.0)	14 (3.9)	12 (3.3)
Proteinuria	15 (4.2)	10 (2.8)	2 (0.6)	1 (0.3)	17 (4.7)	11 (3.0)
Hematuria	10 (2.8)	12 (3.3)	4 (1.2)	4 (1.3)	13 (3.6)	15 (4.2)
Lymphopenia	14 (3.9)	13 (3.6)	3 (0.9)	1 (0.3)	16 (4.4)	14 (3.9)
Urinary casts	11 (3.0)	3 (0.8)	4 (1.2)	0	14 (3.9)	3 (0.8)
Rash	9 (2.5)	19 (5.3)	4 (1.2)	3 (1.0)	13 (3.6)	21 (5.8)
Pruritus	8 (2.2)	15 (4.2)	1 (0.3)	1 (0.3)	9 (2.5)	16 (4.4)
Acne	5 (1.4)	3 (0.8)	2 (0.6)	1 (0.3)	7 (1.9)	4 (1.1)
Anorexia	6 (1.7)	8 (2.2)	3 (0.9)	4 (1.3)	8 (2.2)	10 (2.8)
Anemia	7 (1.9)	9 (2.5)	2 (0.6)	1 (0.3)	9 (2.5)	10 (2.8)
Leukopenia	4 (1.1)	4 (1.1)	3 (0.9)	5 (1.6)	7 (1.9)	8 (2.2)
Arthralgia	9 (2.5)	7 (1.9)	0	0	9 (2.5)	7 (1.9)
Pain	7 (1.9)	5 (1.4)	0	1 (0.3)	7 (1.9)	6 (1.7)
Nausea	7 (1.9)	2 (0.6)	0	1 (0.3)	7 (1.9)	3 (0.8)
Vomiting	4 (1.1)	6 (1.7)	1 (0.3)	1 (0.3)	5 (1.4)	7 (1.9)
Headache	3 (0.8)	4 (1.1)	1 (0.3)	3 (1.0)	4 (1.1)	7 (1.9)
Dyspepsia	3 (0.8)	5 (1.4)	2 (0.6)	3 (1.0)	4 (1.1)	8 (2.2)
Hypertension	3 (0.8)	0 (0.0)	1 (0.3)	1 (0.3)	4 (1.1)	1 (0.3)
Dizziness	4 (1.1)	0	0	1 (0.3)	4 (1.1)	1 (0.3)
Thrombocytosis	4 (1.1)	2 (0.6)	0	0	4 (1.1)	2 (0.6)
Diarrhea	4 (1.1)	0	0	0	4 (1.1)	0
Rash maculopapular	4 (1.1)	3 (0.8)	0	0	4 (1.1)	3 (0.8)
Hemoptysis	2 (0.6)	0	2 (0.6)	0	4 (1.1)	0

Note: ≥1% refers to rifapentine in the TOTAL column.

Note: A patient may have experienced the same adverse event more than once during the course of the study, therefore, patient counts across the columns may not equal the patient counts in the TOTAL column.

[1] Intensive Phase consisted of therapy with either rifapentine or rifampin combined with isoniazid, pyrazinamide, and ethambutol administered daily (rifapentine twice weekly) for 60 days.

[2] Continuation Phase consisted of therapy with either rifapentine or rifampin combined with isoniazid for 120 days. Rifapentine patients were dosed once weekly; rifampin patients were dosed twice weekly. Events recorded in this phase includes those reported up to 3 months after Continuation Phase therapy was completed.

ADVERSE REACTIONS

The investigators in the tuberculosis treatment clinical trial (Study 008) assessed the causality of adverse events as definitely, probably, possibly, unlikely or not related to one of the two drug regimens tested. The following table (Table 2-3) presents treatment-related adverse events deemed by the investigators to be at least possibly related to any of the four drugs in the regimens (rifapentine/rifampin, isoniazid, pyrazinamide, or ethambutol) which occurred in ≥1% of patients. Hyperuricemia was the most frequently reported event that was assessed as treatment related and was most likely related to the pyrazinamide since no cases were reported in the Continuation Phase when this drug was no longer included in the treatment regimen.

[See table below]

Treatment-related adverse events of moderate or severe intensity in <1% of the rifapentine combination therapy patients in Study 008 are presented below by body system.

Hepatic & Biliary: bilirubinemia, hepatitis

Dermatologic: urticaria, skin discoloration

Hematologic: thrombocytopenia, neutrophilia, leukocytosis, purpura, hematoma

Metabolic & Nutritional: hyperkalemia, hypovolemia, alkaline phosphatase increased, LDH increased

Body as a Whole - General: peripheral edema, fatigue

Gastrointestinal: constipation, esophagitis, gastritis, pancreatitis

Musculoskeletal: gout, arthrosis

Psychiatric: aggressive reaction

Three patients (two rifampin combination therapy patients and one rifapentine combination therapy patient) were discontinued in the Intensive Phase as a result of hepatitis with increased liver function tests (ALT, AST, LDH, and bilirubin). Concomitant medications for all three patients included isoniazid, pyrazinamide, ethambutol, and pyridoxine. The two rifampin patients and one rifapentine patient recovered without sequelae.

Twenty-two deaths occurred in Study 008 (eleven in the rifampin combination therapy group and eleven in the rifapentine combination therapy group). None of the deaths were attributed to study medication. In the study, 18/361 (5.0%) rifampin combination therapy patients discontinued the study due to an adverse event compared to 11/361 (3.0%) rifapentine combination therapy patients.

The overall occurrence rate of treatment-related adverse events was higher in males with the rifapentine combination regimen (50%) versus the rifampin combination regimen (43%), while in females the overall rate was greater in the rifampin combination group (68%) compared to the rifapentine combination group (59%). However, there were higher frequencies of treatment-related hematuria and ALT increases for female patients in both treatment groups compared to those for male patients.

Adverse events associated with rifampin may occur with rifapentine: effects of enzyme induction to increase metabolism resulting in decreased concentration of endogenous substrates, including adrenal hormones, thyroid hormones, and vitamin D.

OVERDOSAGE

There is no experience with the treatment of acute overdose with rifapentine at doses exceeding 1200 mg per dose. In a pharmacokinetic study involving healthy volunteers (n=9), single oral doses up to 1200 mg have been administered without serious adverse events. The only adverse events reported with the 1200 mg dose were heartburn (3/8), headache (2/8) and increased urinary frequency (1/8). In clinical trials, tuberculosis patients ranging in age from 20 to 74 years accidentally received continuous daily doses of rifapentine 600 mg. Some patients received continuous daily dosing for up to 20 days without evidence of serious adverse effects. One patient experienced a transient elevation in SGPT and glucose (the latter attributed to pre-existing diabetes); a second patient experienced slight pruritus. While there is no experience with the treatment of acute overdose with rifapentine, clinical experience with rifamycins suggests that gastric lavage to evacuate gastric contents (within a few hours of overdose), followed by instillation of an activated charcoal slurry into the stomach, may help adsorb any remaining drug from the gastrointestinal tract.

Rifapentine and 25-desacetyl rifapentine are 97.7% and 93.2% plasma protein bound, respectively. Rifapentine and related compounds excreted in urine account for only 17% of the administered dose, therefore, neither hemodialysis nor forced diuresis is expected to enhance the systemic elimination of unchanged rifapentine from the body of a patient with PRIFTIN overdose.

DOSAGE AND ADMINISTRATION

PRIFTIN should not be used alone, in initial treatment or in retreatment of pulmonary tuberculosis. In the intensive phase of short-course therapy which is to continue for 2 months, 600 mg **(four 150 mg tablets)** of PRIFTIN should be given twice weekly with an interval of not less than 3 days (72 hours) between doses. For those patients with propensity to nausea, vomiting or gastrointestinal upset, administration of PRIFTIN with food may be useful. In the Intensive Phase, PRIFTIN must be administered in combination as part of an appropriate regimen which includes daily companion drugs. *Compliance with all drugs in the Intensive Phase (ie, PRIFTIN, isoniazid, pyrazinamide, ethambutol, or streptomycin), especially on days when rifapentine is not administered, is imperative to assure early sputum conversion and protection against relapse.* The Advisory Council for the Elimination of Tuberculosis, the American Thoracic Society and the Centers for Disease Control and Prevention also recommend that either streptomycin or ethambutol be added to the regimen unless the likelihood of isoniazid resistance is very low. The need for streptomycin or ethambutol should be reassessed when the results of susceptibility testing are known. An initial treatment regimen with less than four drugs may be considered if there is little possibility of drug resistance (that is, less than 4% primary resistance to isoniazid in the community, and the patient has had no previous treatment with antituberculosis medications, is not from a country with a high prevalence of drug resistance, and has no known exposure to a drug-resistant case) (see Reference 2).

Following the intensive phase, treatment should be continued with PRIFTIN once weekly for 4 months in combination with isoniazid or an appropriate agent for susceptible organisms. If the patient is still sputum smear or culture positive, if resistant organisms are present, or if the patient is HIV positive, follow the ATS/CDC treatment guidelines (see Reference 2).

Concomitant administration of pyridoxine (Vitamin B_6) is recommended in the malnourished, in those predisposed to neuropathy (eg, alcoholics and diabetics), and in adolescents.

The above recommendations apply to patients with drug-susceptible organisms. Patients with drug-resistant organisms may require longer duration treatment with other drug regimens.

HOW SUPPLIED

PRIFTIN (rifapentine) 150 mg round normal convex dark-pink film-coated tablets debossed "Priftin" on top and "150" on the bottom, are packaged in aluminum formable foil blister strips placed in cartons of 32 tablets (4 strips of 8). Each strip of 8 tablets is inserted into an aluminum foil laminated pouch. (NDC 0088-2100-03).

Store at 25°C (77°F); excursions permitted 15–30°C (59–86°F) (see USP Controlled Room Temperature). Protect from excessive heat and humidity.

Prescribing Information as of February 2002

Manufactured by:
Gruppo Lepetit S.p.A.
20020 Lainate, Italy
Manufactured for:
Aventis Pharmaceuticals Inc.
Kansas City, MO 64137 USA
MADE IN ITALY

REFERENCES

1. Vernon A, et al. Acquired rifamycin monoresistance in patients with HIV-related tuberculosis treated with once-weekly rifapentine and isoniazid. The Lancet 1999; 353: 1843–1847.
2. American Thoracic Society, CDC. Treatment of tuberculosis and tuberculosis infection in adults and children. Am J Respir Crit Care Med. 149:1359–1374, 1994.

TAXOTERE® ℞

[*tax-ō-tĕr*]
(docetaxel)
for Injection Concentrate

Prescribing Information as of January 2002

Prescribing information for this product, which appears on pages 778–784 of the 2002 PDR, has been completely revised as follows. Please write "See Supplement A" next to the product heading.

WARNING

TAXOTERE® (docetaxel) for Injection Concentrate should be administered under the supervision of a qualified physician experienced in the use of antineoplastic agents. Appropriate management of complications is possible only when adequate diagnostic and treatment facilities are readily available.

The incidence of treatment-related mortality associated with TAXOTERE therapy is increased in patients with abnormal liver function, in patients receiving higher doses, and in patients with non-small cell lung carcinoma and a history of prior treatment with platinum-based chemotherapy who receive TAXOTERE at a dose of 100 mg/m² (see WARNINGS).

TAXOTERE should generally not be given to patients with bilirubin > upper limit of normal (ULN), or to patients with SGOT and/or SGPT >1.5 × ULN concomitant with alkaline phosphatase > 2.5 × ULN. Patients with elevations of bilirubin or abnormalities of transaminase concurrent with alkaline phosphatase are at increased risk for the development of grade 4 neutropenia, febrile neutropenia, infections, severe thrombocytopenia, severe stomatitis, severe skin toxicity, and toxic death. Patients with isolated elevations of transaminase > 1.5 × ULN also had a higher rate of febrile neutropenia grade 4 but did not have an increased incidence of toxic death. Bilirubin, SGOT or SGPT, and alkaline phosphatase values should be obtained prior to each cycle of TAXOTERE therapy and reviewed by the treating physician.

TAXOTERE therapy should not be given to patients with neutrophil counts of < 1500 cells/mm³. In order to monitor the occurrence of neutropenia, which may be severe and result in infection, frequent blood cell counts should be performed on all patients receiving TAXOTERE.

Severe hypersensitivity reactions characterized by hypotension and/or bronchospasm, or generalized rash/erythema occurred in 2.2% (2/92) of patients who received the recommended 3-day dexamethasone premedication. Hypersensitivity reactions requiring discontinuation of the TAXOTERE infusion were reported in five patients who did not receive premedication. These reactions resolved after discontinuation of the infusion and the administration of appropriate therapy. TAXOTERE must not be given to patients who have a history of severe hypersensitivity reactions to TAXOTERE or to other drugs formulated with polysorbate 80 (see WARNINGS).

Severe fluid retention occurred in 6.5% (6/92) of patients despite use of a 3-day dexamethasone premedication regimen. It was characterized by one or more of the following events: poorly tolerated peripheral edema, generalized edema, pleural effusion requiring urgent drainage, dyspnea at rest, cardiac tamponade, or pronounced abdominal distention (due to ascites) (see PRECAUTIONS).

DESCRIPTION

Docetaxel is an antineoplastic agent belonging to the taxoid family. It is prepared by semisynthesis beginning with a precursor extracted from the renewable needle biomass of yew plants. The chemical name for docetaxel is (2R,3S)-N-carboxy-3-phenylisoserine,N-*tert*-butyl ester, 13-ester with 5β-20-epoxy-1,2α,4,7β,10β,13α-hexahydroxytax-11-en-9-one 4-acetate 2- benzoate, trihydrate. Docetaxel has the following structural formula:

Docetaxel is a white to almost-white powder with an empirical formula of $C_{43}H_{53}NO_{14} \cdot 3H_2O$, and a molecular weight of 861.9. It is highly lipophilic and practically insoluble in water. TAXOTERE (docetaxel) for Injection Concentrate is a clear yellow to brownish-yellow viscous solution. TAXOTERE is sterile, non-pyrogenic, and is available in single-dose vials containing 20 mg (0.5 mL) or 80 mg (2.0 mL) docetaxel (anhydrous). Each mL contains 40 mg docetaxel (anhydrous) and 1040 mg polysorbate 80.

TAXOTERE for Injection Concentrate requires dilution prior to use. A sterile, non-pyrogenic, single-dose diluent is supplied for that purpose. The diluent for TAXOTERE contains 13% ethanol in Water for Injection, and is supplied in 1.5 mL (to be used with 20 mg TAXOTERE for Injection Concentrate) and 6.0 mL (to be used with 80 mg TAXOTERE for Injection Concentrate) vials.

CLINICAL PHARMACOLOGY

Docetaxel is an antineoplastic agent that acts by disrupting the microtubular network in cells that is essential for mitotic and interphase cellular functions. Docetaxel binds to free tubulin and promotes the assembly of tubulin into stable microtubules while simultaneously inhibiting their disassembly. This leads to the production of microtubule bundles without normal function and to the stabilization of microtubules, which results in the inhibition of mitosis in cells. Docetaxel's binding to microtubules does not alter the number of protofilaments in the bound microtubules, a feature which differs from most spindle poisons currently in clinical use.

HUMAN PHARMACOKINETICS

The pharmacokinetics of docetaxel have been evaluated in cancer patients after administration of 20–115 mg/m² in phase I studies. The area under the curve (AUC) was dose proportional following doses of 70–115 mg/m² with infusion times of 1 to 2 hours. Docetaxel's pharmacokinetic profile is consistent with a three-compartment pharmacokinetic model, with half-lives for the α, β, and γ phases of 4 min, 36 min, and 11.1 hr, respectively. The initial rapid decline represents distribution to the peripheral compartments and the late (terminal) phase is due, in part, to a relatively slow efflux of docetaxel from the peripheral compartment. Mean values for total body clearance and steady state volume of distribution were 21 L/h/m² and 113 L, respectively. Mean total body clearance for Japanese patients dosed at the range of 10–90 mg/m² was similar to that of European/American populations dosed at 100 mg/m², suggesting no significant difference in the elimination of docetaxel in the two populations.

A study of ^{14}C-docetaxel was conducted in three cancer patients. Docetaxel was eliminated in both the urine and feces following oxidative metabolism of the *tert*-butyl ester group, but fecal excretion was the main elimination route. Within 7 days, urinary and fecal excretion accounted for approximately 6% and 75% of the administered radioactivity, respectively. About 80% of the radioactivity recovered in feces is excreted during the first 48 hours as 1 major and 3 minor metabolites with very small amounts (less than 8%) of unchanged drug.

A population pharmacokinetic analysis was carried out after TAXOTERE treatment of 535 patients dosed at 100 mg/m². Pharmacokinetic parameters estimated by this analysis were very close to those estimated from phase I studies. The pharmacokinetics of docetaxel were not influenced by age or gender and docetaxel total body clearance was not modified by pretreatment with dexamethasone. In patients with clinical chemistry data suggestive of mild to moderate liver function impairment (SGOT and/or SGPT >1.5 times the upper limit of normal [ULN] concomitant with alkaline phosphatase >2.5 times ULN), total body clearance was lowered by an average of 27%, resulting in a 38% increase in systemic exposure (AUC). This average, however, includes a substantial range and there is, at present, no measurement that would allow recommendation for dose adjustment in such patients. Patients with combined abnormalities of transaminase and alkaline phosphatase should, in general, not be treated with TAXOTERE.

In vitro studies showed that docetaxel is about 94% protein bound, mainly to α_1-acid glycoprotein, albumin, and lipoproteins. In three cancer patients, the *in vitro* binding to plasma proteins was found to be approximately 97%. Dexamethasone does not affect the protein binding of docetaxel.

In vitro drug interaction studies revealed that docetaxel is metabolized by the CYP3A4 isoenzyme, and its metabolism can be inhibited by CYP3A4 inhibitors, such as ketoconazole, erythromycin, troleandomycin, and nifedipine. Based on *in vitro* findings, it is likely that CYP3A4 inhibitors and/or substrates may lead to substantial increases in docetaxel blood concentrations. No clinical studies have been performed to evaluate this finding (see **PRECAUTIONS**).

CLINICAL STUDIES

Breast Cancer: The efficacy and safety of TAXOTERE have been evaluated in locally advanced or metastatic breast cancer after failure of previous chemotherapy (alkylating agent-containing regimens or anthracycline-containing regimens), primarily at a dose of 100 mg/m² given as a 1-hour infusion every 3 weeks, but with some experience at 60 mg/m², in two large randomized trials and a number of smaller single arm studies.

Randomized Trials: In one randomized trial, patients with a history of prior treatment with an anthracycline-containing regimen were assigned to treatment with TAXOTERE or the combination of mitomycin (12 mg/m² every 6 weeks) and vinblastine (6 mg/m² every 3 weeks). 203 patients were randomized to TAXOTERE and 189 to the comparator arm. Most patients had received prior chemotherapy for metastatic disease; only 27 patients on the

Efficacy of TAXOTERE in the Treatment of Breast Cancer Patients Previously Treated with an Anthracycline-Containing Regimen (Intent-to-Treat Analysis)

Efficacy Parameter	Docetaxel (n=203)	Mitomycin/ Vinblastine (n=189)	p-value
Median Survival	11.4 months	8.7 months	
Risk Ratio*, Mortality (Docetaxel: Control)	0.73		p=0.01 Log Rank
95% CI (Risk Ratio)	0.58–0.93		
Median Time to Progression	4.3 months	2.5 months	
Risk Ratio*, Progression (Docetaxel: Control)	0.75		p=0.01 Log Rank
95% CI (Risk Ratio)	0.61–0.94		
Overall Response Rate	28.1%	9.5%	p<0.0001 Chi Square
Complete Response Rate	3.4%	1.6%	

*For the risk ratio, a value less than 1.00 favors docetaxel.

Continued on next page

Taxotere—Cont.

TAXOTERE arm and 33 patients on the comparator arm entered the study following relapse after adjuvant therapy. Three-quarters of patients had measurable, visceral metastases. The primary endpoint was time to progression. The following table summarizes the study results:

[See table at top of previous page]

In a second randomized trial, patients previously treated with an alkylating-containing regimen were assigned to treatment with TAXOTERE or doxorubicin (75 mg/m^2 every 3 weeks). 161 patients were randomized to TAXOTERE and 165 patients to doxorubicin. Approximately one-half of patients had received prior chemotherapy for metastatic disease, and one-half entered the study following relapse after adjuvant therapy. Three-quarters of patients had measurable, visceral metastases. The primary endpoint was time to progression. The study results are summarized below:

[See first table below]

Single Arm Studies: TAXOTERE at a dose of 100 mg/m^2 was studied in six single arm studies involving a total of 309 patients with metastatic breast cancer in whom previous chemotherapy had failed. Among these, 190 patients had anthracycline-resistant breast cancer, defined as progression during an anthracycline-containing chemotherapy regimen for metastatic disease, or relapse during an anthracycline-containing adjuvant regimen. In anthracycline-resistant patients, the overall response rate was 37.9% (72/190; 95% C.I.: 31.0–44.8) and the complete response rate was 2.1%.

TAXOTERE was also studied in three single arm Japanese studies at a dose of 60 mg/m^2, in 174 patients who had received prior chemotherapy for locally advanced or metastatic breast cancer. Among 26 patients whose best response to an anthracycline had been progression, the response rate was 34.6% (95% C.I.: 17.2–55.7), similar to the response rate in single arm studies of 100 mg/m^2.

Hematologic and Other Toxicity: Relation to dose and baseline liver chemistry abnormalities. Hematologic and other toxicity is increased at higher doses and in patients with elevated baseline liver function tests (LFTs). In the following tables, adverse drug reactions are compared for three populations: 730 patients with normal LFTs given TAXOTERE at 100 mg/m^2 in the randomized and single arm studies of metastatic breast cancer after failure of previous chemotherapy; 18 patients in these studies who had abnormal baseline LFTs (defined as SGOT and/or SGPT > 1.5 times ULN concurrent with alkaline phosphatase > 2.5 times ULN); and 174 patients in Japanese studies given TAXOTERE at 60 mg/m^2 who had normal LFTs.

[See second table below]

[See first table at bottom of next page]

Non-Small Cell Lung Cancer (NSCLC): The efficacy and safety of TAXOTERE in non-small cell lung cancer have been evaluated in patients with locally advanced or metastatic disease and a history of prior treatment with a platinum-based chemotherapy regimen. Two randomized, controlled trials established that a TAXOTERE dose of 75 mg/m^2 was tolerable and yielded a favorable outcome (see below). TAXOTERE at a dose of 100 mg/m^2, however, was associated with unacceptable hematologic toxicity, infections, and treatment-related mortality and this dose should not be used (see **BOXED WARNING, WARNINGS,** and **DOSAGE AND ADMINISTRATION** sections).

One trial (TAX317), randomized patients with locally advanced or metastatic non-small cell lung cancer, a history of prior platinum-based chemotherapy, no history of taxane exposure, and an ECOG performance status ≤2 to TAXOTERE or best supportive care. The primary endpoint of the study was survival. Patients were initially randomized to TAXOTERE 100 mg/m^2 or best supportive care, but early toxic deaths at this dose led to a dose reduction to TAXOTERE 75 mg/m^2. A total of 104 patients were randomized in this amended study to either TAXOTERE 75 mg/m^2 or best supportive care.

In a second randomized trial (TAX320), 373 patients with locally advanced or metastatic non-small cell lung cancer, a history of prior platinum-based chemotherapy, and an ECOG performance status ≤2 were randomized to TAXOTERE 75 mg/m^2, TAXOTERE 100 mg/m^2 and a treatment in which the investigator chose either vinorelbine 30 mg/m^2 days 1, 8, and 15 repeated every 3 weeks <u>or</u> ifosfamide 2 g/m^2 days 1–3 repeated every 3 weeks. Forty percent of the patients in this study had a history of prior paclitaxel exposure. The primary endpoint was survival in both trials. The efficacy data for the TAXOTERE 75 mg/m^2 arm and the comparator arms are summarized in the table below and in figures 1 and 2 showing the survival curves for the two studies.

[See second table at bottom of next page]

Only one of the two trials (TAX317) showed a clear effect on survival, the primary endpoint; that trial also showed an increased rate of survival to one year. In the second study (TAX320) the rate of survival at one year favored TAXOTERE 75 mg/m^2.

TAX317 Survival K-M Curves - Docetaxel 75 mg/m^2 vs. Best Supportive Care

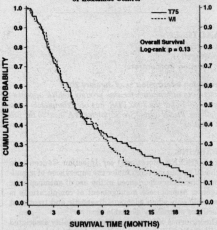

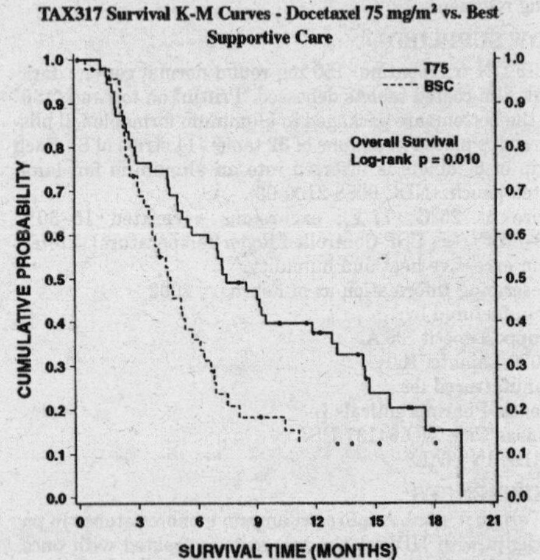

TAX320 Survival K-M Curves - Docetaxel 75 mg/m^2 vs. Vinorelbine or Ifosfamide Control

T75
V/I
Overall Survival
Log-rank p = 0.13
CUMULATIVE PROBABILITY
SURVIVAL TIME (MONTHS)

Patients treated with TAXOTERE at a dose of 75 mg/m^2 experienced no deterioration in performance status and body weight relative to the comparator arms used in these trials.

INDICATIONS AND USAGE

Breast Cancer: TAXOTERE is indicated for the treatment of patients with locally advanced or metastatic breast cancer after failure of prior chemotherapy.

Non-Small Cell Lung Cancer: TAXOTERE is indicated for the treatment of patients with locally advanced or metastatic non-small cell lung cancer after failure of prior platinum-based chemotherapy.

CONTRAINDICATIONS

TAXOTERE is contraindicated in patients who have a history of severe hypersensitivity reactions to docetaxel or to other drugs formulated with polysorbate 80.

TAXOTERE should not be used in patients with neutrophil counts of <1500 cells/mm^3.

WARNINGS

TAXOTERE should be administered under the supervision of a qualified physician experienced in the use of antineoplastic agents. Appropriate management of complications is possible only when adequate diagnostic and treatment facilities are readily available.

Efficacy of TAXOTERE in the Treatment of Breast Cancer Patients Previously Treated with an Alkylating-Containing Regimen (Intent-to-Treat Analysis)

Efficacy Parameter	Docetaxel (n=161)	Doxorubicin (n=165)	p-value
Median Survival	14.7 months	14.3 months	
Risk Ratio*, Mortality (Docetaxel: Control)	0.89		p=0.39 Log Rank
95% CI (Risk Ratio)	0.68–1.16		
Median Time to Progression	6.5 months	5.3 months	
Risk Ratio*, Progression (Docetaxel: Control)	0.93		p=0.45 Log Rank
95% CI (Risk Ratio)	0.71–1.16		
Overall Response Rate Complete Response Rate	45.3% 6.8%	29.7% 4.2%	p=0.004 Chi Square

*For the risk ratio, a value less than 1.00 favors docetaxel.

Hematologic Adverse Events in Breast Cancer Patients Previously Treated with Chemotherapy Treated at TAXOTERE 100 mg/m^2 with Normal or Elevated Liver Function Tests or 60 mg/m^2 with Normal Liver Function Tests

		TAXOTERE 100 mg/m^2		TAXOTERE 60 mg/m^2
Adverse Event		**Normal LFTs* n=730 %**	**Elevated LFTs** n=18 %**	**Normal LFTs* n=174 %**
Neutropenia				
Any	<2000 cells/mm^3	98.4	100	95.4
Grade 4	<500 cells/mm^3	84.4	93.8	74.9
Thrombocytopenia				
Any	<100,000 cells/mm^3	10.8	44.4	14.4
Grade 4	<20,000 cells/mm^3	0.6	16.7	1.1
Anemia	<11 g/dL	94.6	94.4	64.9
Infection***				
Any		22.5	38.9	1.1
Grade 3 and 4		7.1	33.3	0
Febrile Neutropenia****				
By Patient		11.8	33.3	0
By Course		2.4	8.6	0
Septic Death		1.5	5.6	1.1
Non-Septic Death		1.1	11.1	0

*Normal Baseline LFTs: Transaminases ≤ 1.5 times ULN or alkaline phosphatase ≤ 2.5 times ULN or isolated elevations of transaminases or alkaline phosphatase up to 5 times ULN

**Elevated Baseline LFTs: SGOT and/or SGPT >1.5 times ULN concurrent with alkaline phosphatase >2.5 times ULN

***Incidence of infection requiring hospitalization and/or intravenous antibiotics was 8.5% (n=62) among the 730 patients with normal LFTs at baseline; 7 patients had concurrent grade 3 neutropenia, and 46 patients had grade 4 neutropenia.

****Febrile Neutropenia: For 100 mg/m^2, ANC grade 4 and fever > 38°C with IV antibiotics and/or hospitalization; for 60 mg/m^2, ANC grade 3/4 and fever > 38.1°C

Toxic Deaths

Breast Cancer: TAXOTERE administered at 100 mg/m^2 was associated with deaths considered possibly or probably related to treatment in 2.0% (19/965) of metastatic breast cancer patients, both previously treated and untreated, with normal baseline liver function and in 11.5% (7/61) of patients with various tumor types who had abnormal baseline liver function (SGOT and/or SGPT > 1.5 times ULN together with AP > 2.5 times ULN). Among patients dosed at 60 mg/m^2, mortality related to treatment occurred in 0.6% (3/481) of patients with normal liver function, and in 3 of 7 patients with abnormal liver function. Approximately half of these deaths occurred during the first cycle. Sepsis accounted for the majority of the deaths.

Non-Small Cell Lung Cancer: TAXOTERE administered at a dose of 100 mg/m^2 in patients with locally advanced or metastatic non-small cell lung cancer who had a history of prior platinum-based chemotherapy was associated with increased treatment-related mortality (14% and 5% in two randomized, controlled studies). There were 2.8% treatment-related deaths among the 176 patients treated at the 75 mg/m^2 dose in the randomized trials. Among patients who experienced treatment-related mortality at the 75 mg/m^2 dose level, 3 of 5 patients had a PS of 2 at study entry (see **BOXED WARNING, CLINICAL STUDIES,** and **DOSAGE AND ADMINISTRATION** sections).

Non-Hematologic Adverse Events in Breast Cancer Patients Previously Treated with Chemotherapy Treated at TAXOTERE 100 mg/m^2 with Normal or Elevated Liver Function Tests or 60 mg/m^2 with Normal Liver Function Tests

Adverse Event	TAXOTERE 100 mg/m^2 Normal LFTs* n=730 %	TAXOTERE 100 mg/m^2 Elevated LFTs** n=18 %	TAXOTERE 60 mg/m^2 Normal LFTs* n=174 %
Acute Hypersensitivity Reaction Regardless of Premedication			
Any	13.0	5.6	0.6
Severe	1.2	0	0
Fluid Retention* Regardless of Premedication**			
Any	56.2	61.1	12.6
Severe	7.9	16.7	0
Neurosensory			
Any	56.8	50	19.5
Severe	5.8	0	0
Myalgia	22.7	33.3	3.4
Cutaneous			
Any	44.8	61.1	30.5
Severe	4.8	16.7	0
Asthenia			
Any	65.2	44.4	65.5
Severe	16.6	22.2	0
Diarrhea			
Any	42.2	27.8	NA
Severe	6.3	11.1	
Stomatitis			
Any	53.3	66.7	19.0
Severe	7.8	38.9	0.6

***Normal Baseline LFTs: Transaminases ≤ 1.5 times ULN or alkaline phosphatase ≤ 2.5 times ULN or isolated elevations of transaminases or alkaline phosphatase up to 5 times ULN**
****Elevated Baseline Liver Function: SGOT and/or SGPT >1.5 times ULN concurrent with alkaline phosphatase >2.5 times ULN**
*****Fluid Retention includes (by COSTART): edema (peripheral, localized, generalized, lymphedema, pulmonary edema, and edema otherwise not specified) and effusion (pleural, pericardial, and ascites); no premedication given with the 60 mg/m^2 dose**
NA = not available

Efficacy of TAXOTERE in the Treatment of Non-Small Cell Lung Cancer Patients Previously Treated with a Platinum-Based Chemotherapy Regimen (Intent-to-Treat Analysis)

	TAX317		TAX320	
	Docetaxel 75 mg/m^2 n=55	Best Supportive Care/75 n=49	Docetaxel 75 mg/m^2 n=125	Control (V/I) n=123
Overall Survival Log-rank Test	p=0.01		p=0.13	
Risk Ratio[††], Mortality (Docetaxel: Control)	0.56		0.82	
95% CI (Risk Ratio)	(0.35, 0.88)		(0.63, 1.06)	
Median Survival	7.5 months*	4.6 months	5.7 months	5.6 months
95% CI	(5.5, 12.8)	(3.7, 6.1)	(5.1, 7.1)	(4.4, 7.9)
% 1-year Survival	37%*[†]	12%	30%*[†]	20%
95% CI	(24, 50)	(2, 23)	(22, 39)	(13, 27)
Time to Progression	12.3 weeks*	7.0 weeks	8.3 weeks	7.6 weeks
95% CI	(9.0, 18.3)	(6.0, 9.3)	(7.0, 11.7)	(6.7, 10.1)
Response Rate	5.5%	Not Applicable	5.7%	0.8%
95% CI	(1.1, 15.1)		(2.3, 11.3)	(0.0, 4.5)

* p≤0.05; [†] uncorrected for multiple comparisons; [††] a value less than 1.00 favors docetaxel.

Premedication Regimen: All patients should be premedicated with oral corticosteroids such as dexamethasone 16 mg per day (*e.g.*, 8 mg BID) for 3 days starting 1 day prior to TAXOTERE to reduce the severity of fluid retention and hypersensitivity reactions (see **DOSAGE AND ADMINISTRATION** section). This regimen was evaluated in 92 patients with metastatic breast cancer previously treated with chemotherapy given TAXOTERE at a dose of 100 mg/m^2 every 3 weeks.

Hypersensitivity Reactions: Patients should be observed closely for hypersensitivity reactions, especially during the first and second infusions. Severe hypersensitivity reactions characterized by hypotension and/or bronchospasm, or generalized rash/erythema occurred in 2.2% of the 92 patients premedicated with 3-day corticosteroids. Hypersensitivity reactions requiring discontinuation of the TAXOTERE infusion were reported in 5 out of 1260 patients with various tumor types who did not receive premedication, but in 0/92 patients premedicated with 3-day corticosteroids. Patients with a history of severe hypersensitivity reactions should not be rechallenged with TAXOTERE.

Hematologic Effects: Neutropenia (< 2000 neutrophils/mm^3) occurs in virtually all patients given 60–100 mg/m^2 of TAXOTERE and grade 4 neutropenia (< 500 cells/mm^3) occurs in 85% of patients given 100 mg/m^2 and 75% of patients given 60 mg/m^2. Frequent monitoring of blood counts is, therefore, essential so that dose can be adjusted. TAXOTERE should not be administered to patients with neutrophils < 1500 cells/mm^3.

Febrile neutropenia occurred in about 12% of patients given 100 mg/m^2 but was very uncommon in patients given 60 mg/m^2. Hematologic responses, febrile reactions and infections, and rates of septic death for different regimens are dose related and are described in **CLINICAL STUDIES.**

Three breast cancer patients with severe liver impairment (bilirubin > 1.7 times ULN) developed fatal gastrointestinal bleeding associated with severe drug-induced thrombocytopenia.

Hepatic Impairment: (see **BOXED WARNING**).

Fluid Retention: (see **BOXED WARNING**).

Pregnancy: TAXOTERE can cause fetal harm when administered to pregnant women. Studies in both rats and rabbits at doses ≥ 0.3 and 0.03 mg/kg/day, respectively (about 1/50 and 1/300 the daily maximum recommended human dose on a mg/m^2 basis), administered during the period of organogenesis, have shown that TAXOTERE is embryotoxic and fetotoxic (characterized by intrauterine mortality, increased resorption, reduced fetal weight, and fetal ossification delay). The doses indicated above also caused maternal toxicity.

There are no adequate and well-controlled studies in pregnant women using TAXOTERE. If TAXOTERE is used during pregnancy, or if the patient becomes pregnant while receiving this drug, the patient should be apprised of the potential hazard to the fetus or potential risk for loss of the pregnancy. Women of childbearing potential should be advised to avoid becoming pregnant during therapy with TAXOTERE.

PRECAUTIONS

General: Responding patients may not experience an improvement in performance status on therapy and may experience worsening. The relationship between changes in performance status, response to therapy, and treatment-related side effects has not been established.

Hematologic Effects: In order to monitor the occurrence of myelotoxicity, it is recommended that frequent peripheral blood cell counts be performed on all patients receiving TAXOTERE. Patients should not be retreated with subsequent cycles of TAXOTERE until neutrophils recover to a level > 1500 cells/mm^3 and platelets recover to a level > 100,000 cells/mm^3.

A 25% reduction in the dose of TAXOTERE® (docetaxel) for Injection Concentrate is recommended during subsequent cycles following severe neutropenia (< 500 cells/mm^3) lasting 7 days or more, febrile neutropenia, or a grade 4 infection in a TAXOTERE cycle (see **DOSAGE AND ADMINISTRATION** section).

Hypersensitivity Reactions: Hypersensitivity reactions may occur within a few minutes following initiation of a TAXOTERE infusion. If minor reactions such as flushing or localized skin reactions occur, interruption of therapy is not required. More severe reactions, however, require the immediate discontinuation of TAXOTERE and aggressive therapy. All patients should be premedicated with an oral corticosteroid prior to the initiation of the infusion of TAXOTERE (see **BOXED WARNING** and **WARNINGS: Premedication Regimen**).

Cutaneous: Localized erythema of the extremities with edema followed by desquamation has been observed. In case of severe skin toxicity, an adjustment in dosage is recommended (see **DOSAGE AND ADMINISTRATION** section). The discontinuation rate due to skin toxicity was 1.6% (15/965) for metastatic breast cancer patients. Among 92 breast cancer patients premedicated with 3-day corticosteroids, there were no cases of severe skin toxicity reported and no patient discontinued TAXOTERE due to skin toxicity.

Fluid Retention: Severe fluid retention has been reported following TAXOTERE therapy (see **BOXED WARNING** and **WARNINGS: Premedication Regimen**). Patients should be premedicated with oral corticosteroids prior to

Continued on next page

Taxotere—Cont.

each TAXOTERE administration to reduce the incidence and severity of fluid retention (see **DOSAGE AND ADMINISTRATION** section). Patients with pre-existing effusions should be closely monitored from the first dose for the possible exacerbation of the effusions.

When fluid retention occurs, peripheral edema usually starts in the lower extremities and may become generalized with a median weight gain of 2 kg.

Among 92 breast cancer patients premedicated with 3-day corticosteroids, moderate fluid retention occurred in 27.2% and severe fluid retention in 6.5%. The median cumulative dose to onset of moderate or severe fluid retention was 819 mg/m^2. 9.8% (9/92) of patients discontinued treatment due to fluid retention: 4 patients discontinued with severe fluid retention; the remaining 5 had mild or moderate fluid retention. The median cumulative dose to treatment discontinuation due to fluid retention was 1021 mg/m^2. Fluid retention was completely, but sometimes slowly, reversible with a median of 16 weeks from the last infusion of TAXOTERE to resolution (range: 0 to 42+ weeks). Patients developing peripheral edema may be treated with standard measures, *e.g.*, salt restriction, oral diuretic(s).

Neurologic: Severe neurosensory symptoms (paresthesia, dysesthesia, pain) were observed in 5.5% (53/965) of metastatic breast cancer patients, and resulted in treatment discontinuation in 6.1%. When these symptoms occur, dosage must be adjusted. If symptoms persist, treatment should be discontinued (see **DOSAGE AND ADMINISTRATION** section). Patients who experienced neurotoxicity in clinical trials and for whom follow-up information on the complete resolution of the event was available had spontaneous reversal of symptoms with a median of 9 weeks from onset (range: 0 to 106 weeks). Severe peripheral motor neuropathy mainly manifested as distal extremity weakness occurred in 4.4% (42/965).

Asthenia: Severe asthenia has been reported in 14.9% (144/965) of metastatic breast cancer patients but has led to treatment discontinuation in only 1.8%. Symptoms of fatigue and weakness may last a few days up to several weeks and may be associated with deterioration of performance status in patients with progressive disease.

Information for Patients: For additional information, see the accompanying Patient Information Leaflet.

Drug Interactions: There have been no formal clinical studies to evaluate the drug interactions of TAXOTERE with other medications. *In vitro* studies have shown that the metabolism of docetaxel may be modified by the concomitant administration of compounds that induce, inhibit, or are metabolized by cytochrome P450 3A4, such as cyclosporine, terfenadine, ketoconazole, erythromycin, and troleandomycin. Caution should be exercised with these drugs when treating patients receiving TAXOTERE as there is a potential for a significant interaction.

Carcinogenicity, Mutagenicity, Impairment of Fertility: No studies have been conducted to assess the carcinogenic potential of TAXOTERE. TAXOTERE has been shown to be clastogenic in the *in vitro* chromosome aberration test in CHO-K_1 cells and in the *in vivo* micronucleus test in the mouse, but it did not induce mutagenicity in the Ames test or the CHO/HGPRT gene mutation assays. TAXOTERE produced no impairment of fertility in rats when administered in multiple IV doses of up to 0.3 mg/kg (about 1/50 the recommended human dose on a mg/m^2 basis), but decreased testicular weights were reported. This correlates with findings of a 10-cycle toxicity study (dosing once every 21 days for 6 months) in rats and dogs in which testicular atrophy or degeneration was observed at IV doses of 5 mg/kg in rats and 0.375 mg/kg in dogs (about 1/3 and 1/15 the recommended human dose on a mg/m^2 basis, respectively). An increased frequency of dosing in rats produced similar effects at lower dose levels.

Pregnancy: Pregnancy Category D (see **WARNINGS** section).

Nursing Mothers: It is not known whether TAXOTERE is excreted in human milk. Because many drugs are excreted in human milk, and because of the potential for serious adverse reactions in nursing infants from TAXOTERE, mothers should discontinue nursing prior to taking the drug.

Pediatric Use: The safety and effectiveness of TAXOTERE in pediatric patients have not been established.

ADVERSE REACTIONS

The adverse reactions are described separately for TAXOTERE 100 mg/m^2, the maximum dose approved for breast cancer, and 75 mg/m^2, the dose approved for advanced non-small cell lung carcinoma after prior platinum-based chemotherapy.

TAXOTERE 100 mg/m^2: Adverse drug reactions occurring in at least 5% of patients are compared for three populations who received TAXOTERE administered at 100 mg/m^2 as a 1-hour infusion every 3 weeks: 2045 patients with various tumor types and normal baseline liver function tests; the subset of 965 patients with locally advanced or metastatic breast cancer, both previously treated and untreated with chemotherapy, who had normal baseline liver function tests; and an additional 61 patients with various tumor types who had abnormal liver function tests at baseline. These reactions were described using COSTART terms and were considered possibly or probably related to TAXOTERE. At least 95% of these patients did not receive hematopoietic support. The safety profile is generally similar in patients receiving TAXOTERE for the treatment of breast cancer and in patients with other tumor types.

[See table below]

Summary of Adverse Events in Patients Receiving TAXOTERE at 100 mg/m^2

Adverse Event	All Tumor Types Normal LFTs* n=2045 %	All Tumor Types Elevated LFTs** n=61 %	Breast Cancer Normal LFTs* n=965 %
Hematologic			
Neutropenia			
<2000 cells/mm^3	95.5	96.4	98.5
<500 cells/mm^3	75.4	87.5	85.9
Leukopenia			
<4000 cells/mm^3	95.6	98.3	98.6
<1000 cells/mm^3	31.6	46.6	43.7
Thrombocytopenia			
<100,000 cells/mm^3	8.0	24.6	9.2
Anemia			
<11 g/dL	90.4	91.8	93.6
<8 g/dL	8.8	31.1	7.7
Febrile Neutropenia***	11.0	26.2	12.3
Septic Death	1.6	4.9	1.4
Non-Septic Death	0.6	6.6	0.6
Infections			
Any	21.6	32.8	22.2
Severe	6.1	16.4	6.4
Fever in Absence of Infection			
Any	31.2	41.0	35.1
Severe	2.1	8.2	2.2
Hypersensitivity Reactions			
Regardless of Premedication			
Any	21.0	19.7	17.6
Severe	4.2	9.8	2.6
With 3-day Premedication	n=92	n=3	n=92
Any	15.2	33.3	15.2
Severe	2.2	0	2.2
Fluid Retention			
Regardless of Premedication			
Any	47.0	39.3	59.7
Severe	6.9	8.2	8.9
With 3-day Premedication	n=92	n=3	n=92
Any	64.1	66.7	64.1
Severe	6.5	33.3	6.5
Neurosensory			
Any	49.3	34.4	58.3
Severe	4.3	0	5.5
Cutaneous			
Any	47.6	54.1	47.0
Severe	4.8	9.8	5.2
Nail Changes			
Any	30.6	23.0	40.5
Severe	2.5	4.9	3.7
Gastrointestinal			
Nausea	38.8	37.7	42.1
Vomiting	22.3	23.0	23.4
Diarrhea	38.7	32.8	42.6
Severe	4.7	4.9	5.5
Stomatitis			
Any	41.7	49.2	51.7
Severe	5.5	13.0	7.4
Alopecia	75.8	62.3	74.2
Asthenia			
Any	61.8	52.5	66.3
Severe	12.8	24.6	14.9
Myalgia			
Any	18.9	16.4	21.1
Severe	1.5	1.6	1.8
Arthralgia	9.2	6.6	8.2
Infusion Site Reactions	4.4	3.3	4.0

*Normal Baseline LFTs: Transaminases ≤ 1.5 times ULN or alkaline phosphatase ≤ 2.5 times ULN or isolated elevations of transaminases or alkaline phosphatase up to 5 times ULN

**Elevated Baseline LFTs: SGOT and/or SGPT >1.5 times ULN concurrent with alkaline phosphatase >2.5 times ULN

***Febrile Neutropenia: ANC grade 4 with fever > 38°C with IV antibiotics and/or hospitalization

Hematologic: (see **WARNINGS**). Reversible marrow suppression was the major dose-limiting toxicity of TAXOTERE. The median time to nadir was 7 days, while the median duration of severe neutropenia (<500 cells/mm^3) was 7 days. Among 2045 patients with solid tumors and normal baseline LFTs, severe neutropenia occurred in 75.4% and lasted for more than 7 days in 2.9% of cycles.

Febrile neutropenia (<500 cells/mm^3 with fever > 38°C with IV antibiotics and/or hospitalization) occurred in 11% of patients with solid tumors, in 12.3% of patients with metastatic breast cancer, and in 9.8% of 92 breast cancer patients premedicated with 3-day corticosteroids.

Severe infectious episodes occurred in 6.1% of patients with solid tumors, in 6.4% of patients with metastatic breast cancer, and in 5.4% of 92 breast cancer patients premedicated with 3-day corticosteroids.

Thrombocytopenia (<100,000 cells/mm^3) associated with fatal gastrointestinal hemorrhage has been reported.

Hypersensitivity Reactions: Severe hypersensitivity reactions are discussed in the **BOXED WARNING, WARNINGS,** and **PRECAUTIONS** sections. Minor events, including flushing, rash with or without pruritus, chest tightness, back pain, dyspnea, drug fever, or chills, have been reported and resolved after discontinuing the infusion and appropriate therapy.

Fluid Retention: (see **BOXED WARNING, WARNINGS: Premedication Regimen,** and **PRECAUTIONS** sections).

Cutaneous: Severe skin toxicity is discussed in **PRECAUTIONS**. Reversible cutaneous reactions characterized by a rash including localized eruptions, mainly on the feet and/or hands, but also on the arms, face, or thorax, usually associated with pruritus, have been observed. Eruptions generally occurred within 1 week after TAXOTERE infusion, recovered before the next infusion, and were not disabling.

Severe nail disorders were characterized by hypo- or hyperpigmentation, and occasionally by onycholysis (in 0.8% of patients with solid tumors) and pain.

Neurologic: (see **PRECAUTIONS**).

Gastrointestinal: Gastrointestinal reactions (nausea and/or vomiting and/or diarrhea) were generally mild to moderate. Severe reactions occurred in 3–5% of patients with solid tumors and to a similar extent among metastatic breast cancer patients. The incidence of severe reactions was 1% or less for the 92 breast cancer patients premedicated with 3-day corticosteroids.

Severe stomatitis occurred in 5.5% of patients with solid tumors, in 7.4% of patients with metastatic breast cancer, and in 1.1% of the 92 breast cancer patients premedicated with 3-day corticosteroids.

Cardiovascular: Hypotension occurred in 2.8% of patients with solid tumors; 1.2% required treatment. Clinically meaningful events such as heart failure, sinus tachycardia, atrial flutter, dysrhythmia, unstable angina, pulmonary edema, and hypertension occurred rarely. 8.1% (7/86) of metastatic breast cancer patients receiving TAXOTERE 100 mg/m^2 in a randomized trial and who had serial left ventricular ejection fractions assessed developed deterioration of LVEF by ≥ 10% associated with a drop below the institutional lower limit of normal.

Infusion Site Reactions: Infusion site reactions were generally mild and consisted of hyperpigmentation, inflammation, redness or dryness of the skin, phlebitis, extravasation, or swelling of the vein.

Hepatic: In patients with normal LFTs at baseline, bilirubin values greater than the ULN occurred in 8.9% of patients. Increases in SGOT or SGPT > 1.5 times the ULN, or alkaline phosphatase > 2.5 times ULN, were observed in 18.9% and 7.3% of patients, respectively. While on TAXOTERE, increases in SGOT and/or SGPT > 1.5 times ULN concomitant with alkaline phosphatase > 2.5 times ULN occurred in 4.3% of patients with normal LFTs at baseline. (Whether these changes were related to the drug or underlying disease has not been established.) TAXOTERE 75 mg/m^2: Treatment emergent adverse drug reactions are shown below. Included in this table are safety data for a total of 176 patients with non-small cell lung carcinoma and a history of prior treatment with platinum-based chemotherapy who were treated in two randomized, controlled trials. These reactions were described using NCI Common Toxicity Criteria regardless of relationship to study treatment, except for the hematologic toxicities or otherwise noted.

[See table at top of next page]

Post-marketing Experiences

The following adverse events have been identified from clinical trials and/or post-marketing surveillance. Because they are reported from a population of unknown size, precise estimates of frequency cannot be made.

Body as a whole: diffuse pain, chest pain, radiation recall phenomenon

Cardiovascular: atrial fibrillation, deep vein thrombosis, ECG abnormalities, thrombophlebitis, pulmonary embolism, syncope, tachycardia, myocardial infarction

Cutaneous: rare cases of bullous eruption such as erythema multiforme or Stevens-Johnson syndrome. Multiple factors may have contributed to the development of these effects.

Gastrointestinal: abdominal pain, anorexia, constipation, duodenal ulcer, esophagitis, gastrointestinal hemorrhage. Rare occurrences of dehydration as a consequence to gastrointestinal events, gastrointestinal perforation, ischemic colitis, colitis, intestinal obstruction, ileus, and neutropenic enterocolitis have been reported.

Hematologic: bleeding episodes

Hepatic: rare cases of hepatitis have been reported.

Neurologic: confusion, rare cases of seizures or transient loss of consciousness have been observed, sometimes appearing during the infusion of the drug.

Ophthalmologic: conjunctivitis, lacrimation or lacrimation with or without conjunctivitis. Rare cases of lacrimal duct obstruction resulting in excessive tearing have been reported primarily in patients receiving other anti-tumor agents concomitantly.

Respiratory: dyspnea, acute pulmonary edema, acute respiratory distress syndrome, interstitial pneumonia

Urogenital: renal insufficiency

OVERDOSAGE

There is no known antidote for TAXOTERE overdosage. In case of overdosage, the patient should be kept in a specialized unit where vital functions can be closely monitored. Anticipated complications of overdosage include: bone marrow suppression, peripheral neurotoxicity, and mucositis. Patients should receive therapeutic G-CSF as soon as possible after discovery of overdose. Other appropriate symptomatic measures should be taken, as needed.

In two reports of overdose, one patient received 150 mg/m^2 and the other received 200 mg/m^2 as 1-hour infusions. Both patients experienced severe neutropenia, mild asthenia, cutaneous reactions, and mild paresthesia, and recovered without incident.

In mice, lethality was observed following single IV doses that were ≥154 mg/kg (about 4.5 times the recommended human dose on a mg/m^2 basis); neurotoxicity associated with paralysis, nonextension of hind limbs, and myelin degeneration was observed in mice at 48 mg/kg (about 1.5 times the recommended human dose on a mg/m^2 basis). In male and female rats, lethality was observed at a dose of 20 mg/kg (comparable to the recommended human dose on a mg/m^2 basis) and was associated with abnormal mitosis and necrosis of multiple organs.

DOSAGE AND ADMINISTRATION

Breast Cancer: The recommended dose of TAXOTERE is 60–100 mg/m^2 administered intravenously over 1 hour every 3 weeks.

Non-Small Cell Lung Cancer: The recommended dose of TAXOTERE is 75 mg/m^2 administered intravenously over 1 hour every 3 weeks. A dose of 100 mg/m^2 in patients previously treated with chemotherapy was associated with increased hematologic toxicity, infection, and treatment-related mortality in randomized, controlled trials (see **BOXED WARNING, WARNINGS** and **CLINICAL STUDIES** sections).

Premedication Regimen: All patients should be premedicated with oral corticosteroids such as dexamethasone 16 mg per day (*e.g.*, 8 mg BID) for 3 days starting 1 day prior to TAXOTERE administration in order to reduce the incidence and severity of fluid retention as well as the severity of hypersensitivity reactions (see **BOXED WARNING, WARNINGS**, and **PRECAUTIONS** sections).

Dosage Adjustments During Treatment

Breast Cancer: Patients who are dosed initially at 100 mg/m^2 and who experience either febrile neutropenia, neutrophils < 500 cells/mm^3 for more than 1 week, or severe or cumulative cutaneous reactions during TAXOTERE therapy should have the dosage adjusted from 100 mg/m^2 to 75 mg/m^2. If the patient continues to experience these reactions, the dosage should either be decreased from 75 mg/m^2 to 55 mg/m^2 or the treatment should be discontinued. Conversely, patients who are dosed initially at 60 mg/m^2 and who do not experience febrile neutropenia, neutrophils <500 cells/mm^3 for more than 1 week, severe or cumulative cutaneous reactions, or severe peripheral neuropathy during TAXOTERE therapy may tolerate higher doses. Patients who develop ≥ grade 3 peripheral neuropathy should have TAXOTERE treatment discontinued entirely.

Non-Small Cell Lung Cancer: Patients who are dosed initially at 75 mg/m^2 and who experience either febrile neutropenia, neutrophils <500 cells/mm^3 for more than one week, severe or cumulative cutaneous reactions, or other grade 3/4 non-hematological toxicities during TAXOTERE treatment should have treatment withheld until resolution of the toxicity and then resumed at 55 mg/m^2. Patients who develop ≥ grade 3 peripheral neuropathy should have TAXOTERE treatment discontinued entirely.

Special Populations:

Hepatic Impairment: Patients with bilirubin > ULN should generally not receive TAXOTERE. Also, patients with SGOT and/or SGPT > 1.5 × ULN concomitant with alkaline phosphatase > 2.5 × ULN should generally not receive TAXOTERE.

Children: The safety and effectiveness of docetaxel in pediatric patients below the age of 16 years have not been established.

Elderly: No dosage adjustments are required for use in elderly.

PREPARATION AND ADMINISTRATION PRECAUTIONS

TAXOTERE is a cytotoxic anticancer drug and, as with other potentially toxic compounds, caution should be exercised when handling and preparing TAXOTERE solutions. The use of gloves is recommended. Please refer to **Handling and Disposal** section.

If TAXOTERE concentrate, initial diluted solution, or final dilution for infusion should come into contact with the skin, immediately and thoroughly wash with soap and water. If TAXOTERE concentrate, initial diluted solution, or final dilution for infusion should come into contact with mucosa, immediately and thoroughly wash with water.

TAXOTERE for Injection Concentrate requires two dilutions prior to administration. Please follow the preparation instructions provided below. **Note:** Both the TAXOTERE for Injection Concentrate and the diluent vials contain an overfill.

A. Preparation of the Initial Diluted Solution

1. Remove the appropriate number of vials of TAXOTERE for Injection Concentrate and diluent (13% Ethanol in Water for Injection) from the refrigerator. Allow the vials to stand at room temperature for approximately 5 minutes.
2. Aseptically withdraw the contents of the appropriate diluent vial into a syringe and transfer it to the appropriate vial of TAXOTERE for Injection Concentrate. **If the procedure is followed as described, an initial diluted solution of 10mg docetaxel/mL will result.**
3. Gently rotate the initial diluted solution for approximately 15 seconds to assure full mixture of the concentrate and diluent.
4. The initial diluted TAXOTERE solution (10 mg docetaxel/mL) should be clear; however, there may be some foam on top of the solution due to the polysorbate 80. Allow the solution to stand for a few minutes to allow any foam to dissipate. It is not required that all foam dissipate prior to continuing the preparation process.
   The initial diluted solution may be used immediately or stored either in the refrigerator or at room temperature for a maximum of 8 hours.

B. Preparation of the Final Dilution for Infusion

1. Aseptically withdraw the required amount of initial diluted TAXOTERE solution (10 mg docetaxel/mL) with a calibrated syringe and inject into a 250 mL infusion bag or bottle of either 0.9% Sodium Chloride solution or 5% Dextrose solution to produce a final concentration of 0.3 to 0.74 mg/mL.
   If a dose greater than 200 mg of TAXOTERE is required, use a larger volume of the infusion vehicle so that a concentration of 0.74 mg/mL TAXOTERE is not exceeded.
2. Thoroughly mix the infusion by manual rotation.
3. As with all parenteral products, TAXOTERE should be inspected visually for particulate matter or discoloration prior to administration whenever the solution and container permit. If the TAXOTERE for Injection initial diluted solution or final dilution for infusion is not clear or appears to have precipitation, these should be discarded.

The final TAXOTERE dilution for infusion should be administered intravenously as a 1-hour infusion under ambient room temperature and lighting conditions.

Contact of the TAXOTERE concentrate with plasticized PVC equipment or devices used to prepare solutions for infusion is not recommended. In order to minimize patient exposure to the plasticizer DEHP (di-2-ethylhexyl phthalate), which may be leached from PVC infusion bags or sets, the final TAXOTERE dilution for infusion should be stored in bottles (glass, polypropylene) or plastic bags (polypropylene, polyolefin) and administered through polyethylene-lined administration sets.

Stability: TAXOTERE infusion solution, if stored between 2 and 25°C (36 and 77°F) is stable for 4 hours. Fully prepared TAXOTERE infusion solution (in either 0.9% Sodium Chloride solution or 5% Dextrose solution) should be used within 4 hours (including the 1 hour i.v. administration).

HOW SUPPLIED

TAXOTERE for Injection Concentrate is supplied in a single-dose vial as a sterile, pyrogen-free, non-aqueous, viscous solution with an accompanying sterile, non-pyrogenic, diluent (13% ethanol in Water for Injection) vial. The following strengths are available:

TAXOTERE 80 MG (NDC 0075-8001-80)

TAXOTERE (docetaxel) 80 mg Concentrate for Infusion: 80 mg docetaxel in 2 mL polysorbate 80 and diluent for TAXOTERE 80 mg. 13% (w/w) ethanol in Water for Injection. Both items are in a blister pack in one carton.

TAXOTERE 20 MG (NDC 0075-8001-20)

TAXOTERE (docetaxel) 20 mg Concentrate for Infusion: 20 mg docetaxel in 0.5 mL polysorbate 80 and diluent for TAXOTERE 20 mg. 13% (w/w) ethanol in Water for Injection. Both items are in a blister pack in one carton.

Storage: Store between 2 and 25°C (36 and 77°F). Retain in the original package to protect from bright light. Freezing does not adversely affect the product.

Handling and Disposal: Procedures for proper handling and disposal of anticancer drugs should be considered. Several guidelines on this subject have been published[1–7]. There is no general agreement that all of the procedures recommended in the guidelines are necessary or appropriate.

REFERENCES

1. OSHA Work-Practice Guidelines for Controlling Occupational Exposure to Hazardous Drugs. *Am J Health-Syst Pharm.* 1996; 53: 1669–1685.
2. American Society of Hospital Pharmacists Technical Assistance Bulletin on Handling Cytotoxic and Hazardous Drugs. *Am J Hosp Pharm.* 1990; 47(95): 1033–1049.
3. AMA Council Report. Guidelines for Handling Parenteral Antineoplastics. *JAMA.* 1985; 253 (11): 1590–1592.
4. Recommendations for the Safe Handling of Parenteral Antineoplastic Drugs. NIH Publication No. 83-2621. For sale by the Superintendent of Documents, US Government Printing Office, Washington, DC 20402.
5. National Study Commission on Cytotoxic Exposure—Recommendations for Handling Cytotoxic Agents. Available from Louis P. Jeffry, Chairman, National Study Commission on Cytotoxic Exposure. Massachusetts College of Pharmacy and Allied Health Sciences, 179 Longwood Avenue, Boston, MA 02115.
6. Clinical Oncological Society of Australia. Guidelines and Recommendations for Safe Handling of Antineoplastic Agents. *Med J Austr.* 1983; 426–428.
7. Jones, RB, et al. Safe Handling of Chemotherapeutic Agents: A Report from the Mt. Sinai Medical Center. *CA-A Cancer Journal for Clinicians.* 1983; Sept/Oct: 258–263.

Prescribing Information as of November 2001
Manufactured by Aventis Pharma Rhone-Poulenc Rorer Exports Ltd.
Dagenham, Essex RM10 7XS
United Kingdom
Manufactured for
Aventis Pharmaceuticals Products Inc.
Bridgewater, NJ 08807 USA
www.aventispharma-us.com
Rev. 11/01

Patient Information Leaflet

Questions and Answers About Taxotere® for Injection Concentrate

(generic name = docetaxel)
(pronounced as TAX-O-TEER)

What is Taxotere?

Taxotere is a medication to treat breast cancer and non-small cell lung cancer. It has severe side effects in some patients. This leaflet is designed to help you understand how

Continued on next page

Taxotere—Cont.

to use Taxotere and avoid its side effects to the fullest extent possible. The more you understand your treatment, the better you will be able to participate in your care. If you have questions or concerns, be sure to ask your doctor or nurse. They are always your best source of information about your condition and treatment.

What is the most important information about Taxotere?

- Since this drug, like many other cancer drugs, affects your blood cells, your doctor will ask for routine blood tests. These will include regular checks of your white blood cell counts. About 5% of people with low blood counts have developed life-threatening infections. The earliest sign of infection may be fever, so if you experience a fever, tell your doctor right away.
- Occasionally, serious allergic reactions have occurred with this medicine. If you have any allergies, tell your doctor before receiving this medicine.
- A small number of people who take Taxotere have severe fluid retention, which can be life-threatening. To help avoid this problem, you must take another medication called dexamethasone (DECKS-A-METH-A-SONE) prior to each Taxotere treatment. You must follow the schedule and take the exact dose of dexamethasone prescribed (see schedule at end of brochure). If you forget to take a dose or do not take it on schedule you must tell the doctor or nurse prior to your Taxotere treatment.
- If you are using any other medicines, tell your doctor before receiving your infusions of Taxotere.

How does Taxotere work?

Taxotere works by attacking cancer cells in your body. Different cancer medications attack cancer cells in different ways.

Here's how Taxotere works: Every cell in your body contains a supporting structure (like a skeleton). If this "skeleton" is damaged, it cannot grow or reproduce. Taxotere makes the "skeleton" in cancer cells very stiff, so that the cells can no longer grow.

How will I receive Taxotere?

Taxotere is given by an infusion directly into your vein. Your treatment will take about 1 hour. Generally, people receive Taxotere every 3 weeks. The amount of Taxotere and the frequency of your infusions will be determined by your doctor.

As part of your treatment, to reduce side effects your doctor will prescribe another medicine called dexamethasone. Your doctor will tell you how and when to take this medicine. It is important that you take the dexamethasone on the schedule set by your doctor. If you forget to take your medication, or do not take it on schedule, make sure to tell your doctor or nurse **BEFORE** you receive your Taxotere treatment. **Included with this information leaflet is a chart to help you remember when to take your dexamethasone.**

What should be avoided while receiving Taxotere?

Taxotere can interact with other medicines. Use only medicines that are prescribed for you by your doctor and **be sure** to tell your doctor all the medicines that you use, including nonprescription drugs.

What are the possible side effects of Taxotere?

Low Blood Cell Count—Many cancer medications, including Taxotere, cause a temporary drop in the number of white blood cells. These cells help protect your body from infection. Your doctor will routinely check your blood count and tell you if it is too low. Although most people receiving Taxotere do not have an infection even if they have a low white blood cell count, the risk of infection is increased.

Fever is often one of the most common and earliest signs of infection. Your doctor will recommend that you take your temperature frequently, especially during the days after treatment with Taxotere. If you have a fever, tell your doctor or nurse immediately.

Allergic Reactions—This type of reaction, which occurs during the infusion of Taxotere, is infrequent. If you feel a warm sensation, a tightness in your chest, or itching during or shortly after your treatment, tell your doctor or nurse immediately.

Fluid Retention—This means that your body is holding extra water. If this fluid retention is in the chest or around the heart it can be life-threatening. If you notice swelling in the feet and legs or a slight weight gain, this may be the first warning sign. Fluid retention usually does not start immediately; but, if it occurs, it may start around your 5th treatment. Generally, fluid retention will go away within weeks or months after your treatments are completed.

Dexamethasone tablets may protect patients from significant fluid retention. It is important that you take this medicine on schedule. If you have not taken dexamethasone on schedule, you must tell your doctor or nurse before receiving your next Taxotere treatment.

Hair Loss—Loss of hair occurs in most patients taking Taxotere (including the hair on your head, underarm hair, pubic hair, eyebrows, and eyelashes). Hair loss will begin after the first few treatments and varies from patient to patient. Once you have completed all your treatments, hair generally grows back.

Your doctor or nurse can refer you to a store that carries wigs, hairpieces, and turbans for patients with cancer.

Treatment Emergent Adverse Events in Non-Small Cell Lung Cancer Patients Receiving TAXOTERE Regardless of Relationship to Treatment*

Adverse Event	TAXOTERE 75 mg/m² n=176 %	Best Supportive Care n=49 %	Vinorelbine/ Ifosfamide n=119 %
Neutropenia			
Any	84.1	14.3	83.2
Grade 3/4	65.3	12.2	57.1
Leukopenia			
Any	83.5	6.1	89.1
Grade 3/4	49.4	0	42.9
Thrombocytopenia			
Any	8.0	0	7.6
Grade 3/4	2.8	0	1.7
Anemia			
Any	91.0	55.1	90.8
Grade 3/4	9.1	12.2	14.3
Febrile Neutropenia**	6.3	NA†	0.8
Infection			
Any	33.5	28.6	30.3
Grade 3/4	10.2	6.1	9.2
Treatment Related Mortality	2.8	NA†	3.4
Hypersensitivity Reactions			
Any	5.7	0	0.8
Grade 3/4	2.8	0	0
Fluid Retention			
Any	33.5	ND††	22.7
Severe	2.8		3.4
Neurosensory			
Any	23.3	14.3	28.6
Grade 3/4	1.7	6.1	5.0
Neuromotor			
Any	15.9	8.2	10.1
Grade 3/4	4.5	6.1	3.4
Skin			
Any	19.9	6.1	16.8
Grade 3/4	0.6	2.0	0.8
Gastrointestinal			
Nausea			
Any	33.5	30.6	31.1
Grade 3/4	5.1	4.1	7.6
Vomiting			
Any	21.6	26.5	21.8
Grade 3/4	2.8	2.0	5.9
Diarrhea			
Any	22.7	6.1	11.8
Grade 3/4	2.8	0	4.2
Alopecia	56.3	34.7	49.6
Asthenia			
Any	52.8	57.1	53.8
Severe***	18.2	38.8	22.7
Stomatitis			
Any	26.1	6.1	7.6
Grade 3/4	1.7	0	0.8
Pulmonary			
Any	40.9	49.0	45.4
Grade 3/4	21.0	28.6	18.5
Nail Disorder			
Any	11.4	0	1.7
Severe***	1.1	0	0
Myalgia			
Any	6.3	0	2.5
Severe***	0	0	0
Arthralgia			
Any	3.4	2.0	1.7
Severe***	0	0	0.8
Taste Perversion			
Any	5.7	0	0
Severe***	0.6	0	0

***Normal Baseline LFTs: Transaminases ≤ 1.5 times ULN or alkaline phosphatase ≤ 2.5 times ULN or isolated elevations of transaminases or alkaline phosphatase up to 5 times ULN**

**** Febrile Neutropenia: ANC grade 4 with fever > 38°C with IV antibiotics and/or hospitalization**

***** COSTART term and grading system**

† Not Applicable; †† Not Done

Fatigue—A number of patients (about 10%) receiving Taxotere feel very tired following their treatments. If you feel tired or weak, allow yourself extra rest before your next treatment. If it is bothersome or lasts for longer than 1 week, inform your doctor or nurse.

Muscle Pain—This happens about 20% of the time, but is rarely severe. You may feel pain in your muscles or joints. Tell your doctor or nurse if this happens. They may suggest ways to make you more comfortable.

Rash—This side effect occurs commonly but is severe in about 5%. You may develop a rash that looks like a blotchy, hive-like reaction. This usually occurs on the hands and feet but may also appear on the arms, face, or body. Generally, it will appear between treatments and will go away before the next treatment. Inform your doctor or nurse if you experience a rash. They can help you avoid discomfort.

Odd Sensations—About half of patients getting Taxotere will feel numbness, tingling, or burning sensations in their hands and feet. If you do experience this, tell your doctor or nurse. Generally, these go away within a few weeks or months after your treatments are completed. About 14% of patients may also develop weakness in their hands and feet.

Nail Changes—Color changes to your fingernails or toenails may occur while taking Taxotere. In extreme, but rare, cases nails may fall off. After you have finished Taxotere treatments, your nails will generally grow back.

Other Possible Side Effects—Less severe side effects include nausea and vomiting. Severe diarrhea may occasionally occur. If you experience these or any other unusual effects, tell your doctor or nurse.

If you are interested in learning more about this drug, ask your doctor for a copy of the package insert.

Aventis Pharmaceuticals Products Inc.
Bridgewater, NJ 08807 USA
www.aventispharma-us.com

Rev. 11/01

Date ______________

Day 1

Start
Dexamethasone tablets
2 times per day
AM
PM

Date ______________

Day 2

Taxotere Treatment Day

Take
Dexamethasone tablets
2 times per day
AM
PM

Date ______________

Day 3

Take
Dexamethasone tablets
2 times per day
AM
PM

Berlex Laboratories

15049 SAN PABLO AVENUE, P.O. BOX 4099
RICHMOND, CA 94804-0099

Direct Inquiries to:
888-BERLEX-4

FLUDARA® ℞

[flū 'dər-ă]
(fludarabine phosphate)
FOR INJECTION
FOR INTRAVENOUS USE ONLY
Rx only

Prescribing information for this product, which appears on pages 995–997 of the 2002 PDR, has been completely revised as follows. Please write "See Supplement A" next to the product heading.

WARNING: FLUDARA FOR INJECTION should be administered under the supervision of a qualified physician experienced in the use of antineoplastic therapy. FLUDARA FOR INJECTION can severely suppress bone marrow function. When used at high doses in dose-ranging studies in patients with acute leukemia, FLUDARA FOR INJECTION was associated with severe neurologic effects, including blindness, coma, and death. This severe central nervous system toxicity occurred in 36% of patients treated with doses approximately four times greater (96 mg/m²/day for 5–7 days) than the recommended dose. Similar severe central nervous system toxicity has been rarely (≤0.2%) reported in patients treated at doses in the range of the dose recommended for chronic lymphocytic leukemia.

Instances of life-threatening and sometimes fatal autoimmune hemolytic anemia have been reported to occur after one or more cycles of treatment with FLUDARA FOR INJECTION. Patients undergoing treatment with FLUDARA FOR INJECTION should be evaluated and closely monitored for hemolysis.

In a clinical investigation using FLUDARA FOR INJECTION in combination with pentostatin (deoxycoformycin) for the treatment of refractory chronic lymphocytic leukemia (CLL), there was an unacceptably high incidence of fatal pulmonary toxicity. Therefore, the use of FLUDARA FOR INJECTION in combination with pentostatin is not recommended.

DESCRIPTION

FLUDARA FOR INJECTION contains fludarabine phosphate, a fluorinated nucleotide analog of the antiviral agent vidarabine, 9-β-D-arabinofuranosyladenine (ara-A) that is relatively resistant to deamination by adenosine deaminase. Each vial of sterile lyophilized solid cake contains 50 mg of the active ingredient fludarabine phosphate, 50 mg of mannitol, and sodium hydroxide to adjust pH to 7.7. The pH range for the final product is 7.2–8.2. Reconstitution with 2 mL of Sterile Water for Injection USP results in a solution containing 25 mg/mL of fludarabine phosphate intended for intravenous administration.

The chemical name for fludarabine phosphate is 9H-Purin-6-amine, 2-fluoro-9-(5-O-phosphono-β-D-arabinofuranosyl) (2-fluoro-ara-AMP).

The molecular formula of fludarabine phosphate is $C_{10}H_{13}FN_5O_7P$ (MW 365.2) and the structure is:

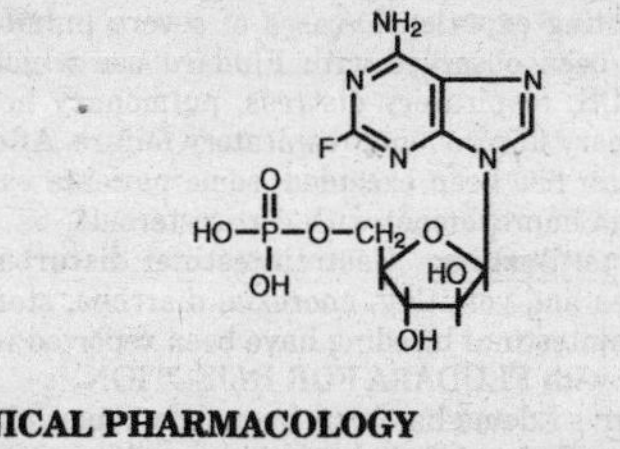

CLINICAL PHARMACOLOGY

Fludarabine phosphate is rapidly dephosphorylated to 2-fluoro-ara-A and then phosphorylated intracellularly by deoxycytidine kinase to the active triphosphate, 2-fluoro-ara-ATP. This metabolite appears to act by inhibiting DNA polymerase alpha, ribonucleotide reductase and DNA primase, thus inhibiting DNA synthesis. The mechanism of action of this antimetabolite is not completely characterized and may be multi-faceted.

Phase I studies in humans have demonstrated that fludarabine phosphate is rapidly converted to the active metabolite, 2-fluoro-ara-A, within minutes after intravenous infusion. Consequently, clinical pharmacology studies have focused on 2-fluoro-ara-A pharmacokinetics. After the five daily doses of 25 mg 2-fluoro-ara-AMP/m² to cancer patients infused over 30 minutes, 2-fluoro-ara-A concentrations show a moderate accumulation. During a 5-day treatment schedule, 2-fluoro-ara-A plasma trough levels increased by a factor of about 2. The terminal half-life of 2-fluoro-ara-A was estimated as approximately 20 hours. *In vitro*, plasma protein binding of fludarabine ranged between 19% and 29%.

A correlation was noted between the degree of absolute granulocyte count nadir and increased area under the concentration × time curve (AUC).

Special Populations

Patients with Renal Impairment

The total body clearance of the principal metabolite 2-fluoro-ara-A correlated with the creatinine clearance, indicating the importance of the renal excretion pathway for the elimination of the drug. Renal clearance represents approximately 40% of the total body clearance. Patients with moderate renal impairment (17–41 mL/min/m²) receiving 20% reduced Fludara dose had a similar exposure (AUC; 21 versus 20 nM•h/mL) compared to patients with normal renal function receiving the recommended dose. The mean total body clearance was 172 mL/min for normal and 124 mL/min for patients with moderately impaired renal function.

Clinical Studies

Two single-arm open-label studies of FLUDARA FOR INJECTION have been conducted in patients with CLL refractory to at least one prior standard alkylating-agent containing regimen. In a study conducted by M.D. Anderson Cancer Center (MDAH), 48 patients were treated with a dose of 22–40 mg/m² daily for 5 days every 28 days. Another study conducted by the Southwest Oncology Group (SWOG) involved 31 patients treated with a dose of 15–25 mg/m² daily for 5 days every 28 days. The overall objective response rates were 48% and 32% in the MDAH and SWOG studies, respectively. The complete response rate in both studies was 13%; the partial response rate was 35% in the MDAH study and 19% in the SWOG study. These response rates were obtained using standardized response criteria developed by the National Cancer Institute CLL Working Group[1] and were achieved in heavily pre-treated patients. The ability of FLUDARA FOR INJECTION to induce a significant rate of response in refractory patients suggests minimal cross-resistance with commonly used anti-CLL agents.

The median time to response in the MDAH and SWOG studies was 7 weeks (range of 1 to 68 weeks) and 21 weeks (range of 1 to 53 weeks) respectively. The median duration of disease control was 91 weeks (MDAH) and 65 weeks (SWOG). The median survival of all refractory CLL patients treated with FLUDARA FOR INJECTION was 43 weeks and 52 weeks in the MDAH and SWOG studies, respectively.

Rai stage improved to Stage II or better in 7 of 12 MDAH responders (58%) and in 5 of 7 SWOG responders (71%) who were Stage III or IV at baseline. In the combined studies, mean hemoglobin concentration improved from 9.0 g/dL at baseline to 11.8 g/dL at the time of response in a subgroup of anemic patients. Similarly, average platelet count improved from 63,500/mm³ to 103,300/mm³ at the time of response in a subgroup of patients who were thrombocytopenic at baseline.

INDICATIONS AND USAGE

FLUDARA FOR INJECTION is indicated for the treatment of patients with B-cell chronic lymphocytic leukemia (CLL) who have not responded to or whose disease has progressed during treatment with at least one standard alkylating-agent containing regimen. The safety and effectiveness of FLUDARA FOR INJECTION in previously untreated or non-refractory patients with CLL have not been established.

CONTRAINDICATIONS

FLUDARA FOR INJECTION is contraindicated in those patients who are hypersensitive to this drug or its components.

WARNINGS

(See boxed warning)

There are clear dose-dependent toxic effects seen with FLUDARA FOR INJECTION. Dose levels approximately 4 times greater (96 mg/m²/day for 5 to 7 days) than that recommended for CLL (25 mg/m²/day for 5 days) were associated with a syndrome characterized by delayed blindness, coma and death. Symptoms appeared from 21 to 60 days following the last dose. Thirteen of 36 patients (36%) who received FLUDARA FOR INJECTION at high doses (96 mg/m²/day for 5 to 7 days) developed this severe neurotoxicity. This syndrome has been reported rarely in patients treated with doses in the range of the recommended CLL dose of 25 mg/m²/day for 5 days every 28 days. The effect of chronic administration of FLUDARA FOR INJECTION on the central nervous system is unknown; however, patients have received the recommended dose for up to 15 courses of therapy.

Severe bone marrow suppression, notably anemia, thrombocytopenia and neutropenia, has been reported in patients treated with FLUDARA FOR INJECTION. In a Phase I study in solid tumor patients, the median time to nadir counts was 13 days (range, 3–25 days) for granulocytes and 16 days (range, 2–32) for platelets. Most patients had hematologic impairment at baseline either as a result of disease or as a result of prior myelosuppressive therapy. Cumulative myelosuppression may be seen. While chemotherapy-induced myelosuppression is often reversible, administration of FLUDARA FOR INJECTION requires careful hematologic monitoring.

Several instances of trilineage bone marrow hypoplasia or aplasia resulting in pancytopenia, sometimes resulting in death, have been reported. The duration of clinically significant cytopenia in the reported cases has ranged from approximately 2 months to approximately 1 year. These episodes have occurred both in previously treated or untreated patients.

Instances of life-threatening and sometimes fatal autoimmune hemolytic anemia have been reported to occur after one or more cycles of treatment with FLUDARA FOR INJECTION in patients with or without a previous history of autoimmune hemolytic anemia or a positive Coombs' test and who may or may not be in remission from their disease. Steroids may or may not be effective in controlling these hemolytic episodes. The majority of patients rechallenged with FLUDARA FOR INJECTION developed a recurrence in the hemolytic process. The mechanism(s) which predispose patients to the development of this complication has not been identified. Patients undergoing treatment with FLUDARA FOR INJECTION should be evaluated and closely monitored for hemolysis.

Transfusion-associated graft-versus-host disease has been observed rarely after transfusion of non-irradiated blood in FLUDARA FOR INJECTION treated patients. Consideration should, therefore, be given to the use of irradiated blood products in those patients requiring transfusions while undergoing treatment with FLUDARA FOR INJECTION.

In a clinical investigation using FLUDARA FOR INJECTION in combination with pentostatin (deoxycoformycin) for the treatment of refractory chronic lymphocytic leukemia (CLL), there was an unacceptably high incidence of fatal pulmonary toxicity. Therefore, the use of FLUDARA FOR INJECTION in combination with pentostatin is not recommended.

Of the 133 CLL patients in the two trials, there were 29 fatalities during study. Approximately 50% of the fatalities were due to infection and 25% due to progressive disease.

Pregnancy Category D: FLUDARA FOR INJECTION may cause fetal harm when administered to a pregnant woman. Fludarabine phosphate was teratogenic in rats and in rabbits. Fludarabine phosphate was administered intravenously at doses of 0, 1, 10 or 30 mg/kg/day to pregnant rats on days 6 to 15 of gestation. At 10 and 30 mg/kg/day in rats, there was an increased incidence of various skeletal malformations. Fludarabine phosphate was administered intravenously at doses of 0, 1, 5 or 8 mg/kg/day to pregnant rabbits on days 6 to 15 of gestation. Dose-related teratogenic effects manifested by external deformities and skeletal malformations were observed in the rabbits at 5 and 8 mg/kg/day. Drug-related deaths or toxic effects on maternal and fetal weights were not observed. There are no adequate and well-controlled studies in pregnant women.

If FLUDARA FOR INJECTION is used during pregnancy, or if the patient becomes pregnant while taking this drug, the patient should be apprised of the potential hazard to the fetus. Women of childbearing potential should be advised to avoid becoming pregnant.

Continued on next page

Fludara—Cont.

PRECAUTIONS

General: FLUDARA FOR INJECTION is a potent antineoplastic agent with potentially significant toxic side effects. Patients undergoing therapy should be closely observed for signs of hematologic and nonhematologic toxicity. Periodic assessment of peripheral blood counts is recommended to detect the development of anemia, neutropenia and thrombocytopenia.

Tumor lysis syndrome associated with FLUDARA FOR INJECTION treatment has been reported in CLL patients with large tumor burdens. Since FLUDARA FOR INJECTION can induce a response as early as the first week of treatment, precautions should be taken in those patients at risk of developing this complication.

There are inadequate data on dosing of patients with renal insufficiency. FLUDARA FOR INJECTION must be administered cautiously in patients with renal insufficiency. The total body clearance of 2-fluoro-ara-A has been shown to be directly correlated with creatinine clearance. Patients with moderate impairment of renal function (creatinine clearance 30–70 mL/min/1.73 m^2) should have their Fludara dose reduced by 20% and be monitored closely. Fludara is not recommended for patients with severely impaired renal function (creatinine clearance less than 30 mL/min/1.73 m^2).

Laboratory Tests: During treatment, the patient's hematologic profile (particularly neutrophils and platelets) should be monitored regularly to determine the degree of hematopoietic suppression.

Drug Interactions: The use of FLUDARA FOR INJECTION in combination with pentostatin is not recommended due to the risk of severe pulmonary toxicity (see WARNINGS section).

Carcinogenesis: No animal carcinogenicity studies with FLUDARA FOR INJECTION have been conducted.

Mutagenesis: Fludarabine phosphate was not mutagenic to bacteria (Ames test) or mammalian cells (HGRPT assay in Chinese hamster ovary cells) either in the presence or absence of metabolic activation. Fludarabine phosphate was clastogenic *in vitro* to Chinese hamster ovary cells (chromosome aberrations in the presence of metabolic activation) and induced sister chromatid exchanges both with and without metabolic activation. In addition, fludarabine phosphate was clastogenic *in vivo* (mouse micronucleus assay) but was not mutagenic to germ cells (dominant lethal test in male mice).

Impairment of Fertility: Studies in mice, rats and dogs have demonstrated dose-related adverse effects on the male reproductive system. Observations consisted of a decrease in mean testicular weights in mice and rats with a trend toward decreased testicular weights in dogs and degeneration and necrosis of spermatogenic epithelium of the testes in mice, rats and dogs. The possible adverse effects on fertility in humans have not been adequately evaluated.

Pregnancy: Pregnancy Category D: (See WARNINGS section).

Nursing Mothers: It is not known whether this drug is excreted in human milk. Because many drugs are excreted in human milk and because of the potential for serious adverse reactions in nursing infants from FLUDARA FOR INJECTION, a decision should be made to discontinue nursing or discontinue the drug, taking into account the importance of the drug for the mother.

Pediatric Use: The safety and effectiveness of FLUDARA FOR INJECTION in children have not been established.

ADVERSE REACTIONS

The most common adverse events include myelosuppression (neutropenia, thrombocytopenia and anemia), fever and chills, infection, and nausea and vomiting. Other commonly reported events include malaise, fatigue, anorexia, and weakness. Serious opportunistic infections have occurred in CLL patients treated with FLUDARA FOR INJECTION. The most frequently reported adverse events and those reactions which are more clearly related to the drug are arranged below according to body system.

Hematopoietic Systems: Hematologic events (neutropenia, thrombocytopenia, and/or anemia) were reported in the majority of CLL patients treated with FLUDARA FOR INJECTION. During FLUDARA FOR INJECTION treatment of 133 patients with CLL, the absolute neutrophil count decreased to less than 500/mm^3 in 59% of patients, hemoglobin decreased from pretreatment values by at least 2 grams percent in 60%, and platelet count decreased from pretreatment values by at least 50% in 55%. Myelosuppression may be severe, cumulative, and may affect multiple cell lines. Bone marrow fibrosis occurred in one CLL patient treated with FLUDARA FOR INJECTION.

Several instances of trilineage bone marrow hypoplasia or aplasia resulting in pancytopenia, sometimes resulting in death, have been reported in postmarketing surveillance. The duration of clinically significant cytopenia in the reported cases has ranged from approximately 2 months to approximately 1 year. These episodes have occurred both in previously treated or untreated patients.

Life-threatening and sometimes fatal autoimmune hemolytic anemia have been reported to occur in patients receiving FLUDARA FOR INJECTION (see WARNINGS section). The majority of patients rechallenged with FLUDARA FOR INJECTION developed a recurrence in the hemolytic process.

Metabolic: Tumor lysis syndrome has been reported in CLL patients treated with FLUDARA FOR INJECTION. This complication may include hyperuricemia, hyperphosphatemia, hypocalcemia, metabolic acidosis, hyperkalemia, hematuria, urate crystalluria, and renal failure. The onset of this syndrome may be heralded by flank pain and hematuria.

Nervous System: (See WARNINGS section) Objective weakness, agitation, confusion, visual disturbances, and coma have occurred in CLL patients treated with FLUDARA FOR INJECTION at the recommended dose. Peripheral neuropathy has been observed in patients treated with FLUDARA FOR INJECTION and one case of wrist-drop was reported.

Pulmonary System: Pneumonia, a frequent manifestation of infection in CLL patients, occurred in 16%, and 22% of those treated with FLUDARA FOR INJECTION in the MDAH and SWOG studies, respectively. Pulmonary hypersensitivity reactions to FLUDARA FOR INJECTION characterized by dyspnea, cough and interstitial pulmonary infiltrate have been observed.

In post-marketing experience, cases of severe pulmonary toxicity have been observed with Fludara use which resulted in ARDS, respiratory distress, pulmonary hemorrhage, pulmonary fibrosis, and respiratory failure. After an infectious origin has been excluded, some patients experienced symptom improvement with corticosteroids.

Gastrointestinal System: Gastrointestinal disturbances such as nausea and vomiting, anorexia, diarrhea, stomatitis, and gastrointestinal bleeding have been reported in patients treated with FLUDARA FOR INJECTION.

Cardiovascular: Edema has been frequently reported. One patient developed a pericardial effusion possibly related to treatment with FLUDARA FOR INJECTION. No other severe cardiovascular events were considered to be drug related.

Genitourinary System: Rare cases of hemorrhagic cystitis have been reported in patients treated with FLUDARA FOR INJECTION.

Skin: Skin toxicity, consisting primarily of skin rashes, has been reported in patients treated with FLUDARA FOR INJECTION.

Data in the following table are derived from the 133 patients with CLL who received FLUDARA FOR INJECTION in the MDAH and SWOG studies.

PERCENT OF CLL PATIENTS REPORTING NON-HEMATOLOGIC ADVERSE EVENTS

ADVERSE EVENTS	MDAH (N=101)	SWOG (N=32)
ANY ADVERSE EVENT	88%	91%
BODY AS A WHOLE	72	84
FEVER	60	69
CHILLS	11	19
FATIGUE	10	38
INFECTION	33	44
PAIN	20	22
MALAISE	8	6
DIAPHORESIS	1	13
ALOPECIA	0	3
ANAPHYLAXIS	1	0
HEMORRHAGE	1	0
HYPERGLYCEMIA	1	6
DEHYDRATION	1	0
NEUROLOGICAL	21	69
WEAKNESS	9	65
PARESTHESIA	4	12
HEADACHE	3	0
VISUAL DISTURBANCE	3	15
HEARING LOSS	2	6
SLEEP DISORDER	1	3
DEPRESSION	1	0
CEREBELLAR SYNDROME	1	0
IMPAIRED MENTATION	1	0
PULMONARY	35	69
COUGH	10	44
PNEUMONIA	16	22
DYSPNEA	9	22
SINUSITIS	5	0
PHARYNGITIS	0	9
UPPER RESPIRATORY INFECTION	2	16
ALLERGIC PNEUMONITIS	0	6
EPISTAXIS	1	0
HEMOPTYSIS	1	6
BRONCHITIS	1	0
HYPOXIA	1	0
GASTROINTESTINAL	46	63
NAUSEA/VOMITING	36	31
DIARRHEA	15	13
ANOREXIA	7	34
STOMATITIS	9	0
GI BLEEDING	3	13
ESOPHAGITIS	3	0
MUCOSITIS	2	0
LIVER FAILURE	1	0
ABNORMAL LIVER FUNCTION TEST	1	3
CHOLELITHIASIS	0	3
CONSTIPATION	1	3
DYSPHAGIA	1	0
CUTANEOUS	17	18
RASH	15	15
PRURITUS	1	3
SEBORRHEA	1	0
GENITOURINARY	12	22
DYSURIA	4	3
URINARY INFECTION	2	15
HEMATURIA	2	3
RENAL FAILURE	1	0
ABNORMAL RENAL FUNCTION TEST	1	0
PROTEINURIA	1	0
HESITANCY	0	3
CARDIOVASCULAR	12	38
EDEMA	8	19
ANGINA	0	6
CONGESTIVE HEART FAILURE	0	3
ARRHYTHMIA	0	3
SUPRAVENTRICULAR TACHYCARDIA	0	3
MYOCARDIAL INFARCTION	0	3
DEEP VENOUS THROMBOSIS	1	3
PHLEBITIS	1	3
TRANSIENT ISCHEMIC ATTACK	1	0
ANEURYSM	1	0
CEREBROVASCULAR ACCIDENT	0	3
MUSCULOSKELETAL	7	16
MYALGIA	4	16
OSTEOPOROSIS	2	0
ARTHRALGIA	1	0
TUMOR LYSIS SYNDROME	1	0

More than 3000 patients received FLUDARA FOR INJECTION in studies of other leukemias, lymphomas, and other solid tumors. The spectrum of adverse effects reported in these studies was consistent with the data presented above.

OVERDOSAGE

High doses of FLUDARA FOR INJECTION (see WARNINGS section) have been associated with an irreversible central nervous system toxicity characterized by delayed blindness, coma, and death. High doses are also associated with severe thrombocytopenia and neutropenia due to bone marrow suppression. There is no known specific antidote for FLUDARA FOR INJECTION overdosage. Treatment consists of drug discontinuation and supportive therapy.

DOSAGE AND ADMINISTRATION

Usual Dose:

The recommended dose of FLUDARA FOR INJECTION is 25 mg/m^2 administered intravenously over a period of approximately 30 minutes daily for five consecutive days. Each 5 day course of treatment should commence every 28 days. Dosage may be decreased or delayed based on evidence of hematologic or nonhematologic toxicity. Physicians should consider delaying or discontinuing the drug if neurotoxicity occurs.

A number of clinical settings may predispose to increased toxicity from FLUDARA FOR INJECTION. These include advanced age, renal insufficiency, and bone marrow impairment. Such patients should be monitored closely for excessive toxicity and the dose modified accordingly.

The optimal duration of treatment has not been clearly established. It is recommended that three additional cycles of FLUDARA FOR INJECTION be administered following the achievement of a maximal response and then the drug should be discontinued.

Renal Insufficiency

Patients with moderate impairment of renal function (creatinine clearance 30–70 mL/min/1.73 m^2) should have a 20% dose reduction of FLUDARA FOR INJECTION. FLUDARA FOR INJECTION should not be administered to patients with severely impaired renal function (creatinine clearance less than 30 mL/min/1.73 m^2).

Preparation of Solutions:

FLUDARA FOR INJECTION should be prepared for parenteral use by aseptically adding Sterile Water for Injection USP. When reconstituted with 2 mL of Sterile Water for Injection, USP, the solid cake should fully dissolve in 15 seconds or less; each mL of the resulting solution will contain 25 mg of fludarabine phosphate, 25 mg of mannitol, and sodium hydroxide to adjust the pH to 7.7. The pH range for the final product is 7.2–8.2. In clinical studies, the product has been diluted in 100 cc or 125 cc of 5% Dextrose Injection USP or 0.9% Sodium Chloride USP.

Reconstituted FLUDARA FOR INJECTION contains no antimicrobial preservative and thus should be used within 8 hours of reconstitution. Care must be taken to assure the sterility of prepared solutions. Parenteral drug products should be inspected visually for particulate matter and discoloration prior to administration.

Handling and Disposal:

Procedures for proper handling and disposal should be considered. Consideration should be given to handling and disposal according to guidelines issued for cytotoxic drugs. Several guidelines on this subject have been published.[2–9] There is no general agreement that all of the procedures recommended in the guidelines are necessary or appropriate.

Caution should be exercised in the handling and preparation of FLUDARA FOR INJECTION solution. The use of latex gloves and safety glasses is recommended to avoid exposure in case of breakage of the vial or other accidental spillage. If the solution contacts the skin or mucous membranes, wash thoroughly with soap and water; rinse eyes thoroughly with plain water. Avoid exposure by inhalation or by direct contact of the skin or mucous membranes.

HOW SUPPLIED

FLUDARA FOR INJECTION is supplied as a white, lyophilized solid cake. Each vial contains 50 mg of fludarabine phosphate, 50 mg of mannitol, and sodium hydroxide to adjust pH to 7.7. The pH range for the final product is 7.2–8.2. Store under refrigeration, between 2°–8°C (36°–46°F).

FLUDARA FOR INJECTION is supplied in a clear glass single dose vial (6 mL capacity) and packaged in a single dose vial carton in a shelf pack of five.

NDC 50419-511-06

Manufactured by: Ben Venue Laboratories, Bedford, OH 44146

Manufactured for: Berlex Laboratories, Richmond, CA 94804

U.S. Patent Number: 4,357,324

REFERENCES

1. Cheson B.D., Bennett J.M., Rai K.R. et al. Guidelines for clinical protocols for chronic lymphocytic leukemia: Recommendations of the National Cancer Institute-Sponsored Working Group. Amer J Hematol. 1988;29:152–163.
2. ONS Clinical Practice Committee. Cancer Chemotherapy Guidelines and Recommendations for Practice. Pittsburgh, Pa: Oncology Nursing Society. 1999:32–41.
3. Recommendations for the Safe Handling of Parenteral Antineoplastic Drugs.Washington, DC; Division of Safety, Clinical Center Pharmacy Department and Cancer Nursing Services, National Institute of Health; 1992. US Department of Health and Human Services, Public Health Service Publication NIH 92–2621.
4. AMA Council on Scientific Affairs. Guidelines for Handling Parenteral Antineoplastics. JAMA. 1985;253: 1590–1591.
5. National Study Commission on Cytotoxic Exposure—Recommendations for Handling Cytotoxic Agents. 1987. Available from Louis P. Jeffrey, Sc.D., Chairman, National Study Commission on Cytotoxic Exposure, Massachusetts College of Pharmacy and Allied Health Sciences, 179 Longwood Avenue, Boston, MA 02115.
6. Clinical Oncological Society of Australia: Guidelines and Recommendations for Safe Handling of Antineoplastic Agents. Med J Australia. 1983;1:426–428.
7. Jones, R.B, Frank R, Mass T. Safe Handling of Chemotherapeutic Agents: A Report from the Mount Sinai Medical Center. CA Cancer J Clin. 1983; 33:258–263.
8. American Society of Hospital Pharmacists. ASHP Technical Assistance Bulletin on Handling Cytotoxic and Hazardous Drugs. Am J Hosp Pharm. 1990; 47:1033–1049.
9. Controlling Occupational Exposure to Hazardous Drugs (OSHA Work-Practice Guidelines). Am J Health-Syst Pharm. 1996;53:1669–1685.

6063506
Rev. 12/01

Bristol-Myers Squibb Company

P.O. BOX 4500
PRINCETON, NJ 08543-4500

For Medical Information Contact:
Generally:
Bristol-Myers Squibb Drug Information Department
P.O. Box 4500
Princeton, NJ 08543-4500
(800) 321–1335

Adverse Drug Experiences
and Product Defects Reporting call
between 8:30 AM–4:30 PM EST:
(609) 818-3737

Sales and Ordering:
Orders may be placed by:
1. Calling your purchase orders toll-free between 8:30 AM–5:00 PM EST:
(800) 631-5244
2. Mailing your purchase orders to:
Bristol-Myers Squibb U.S. Pharmaceuticals
Attn: Customer Service
P.O. Box 5250
Princeton, NJ 08543-5250
3. Faxing your purchase orders to:
(800) 523-2965
4. Transmitting computer-to-computer on the NWDA and UCS formats through Ordernet Services use: DEA# PE0048579

PRAVACHOL® ℞
[prā-vă-chol]
(pravastatin sodium) Tablets
Rx only

Prescribing information for this product, which appears on pages 1099–1103 of the 2002 PDR, has been revised as follows. Please write "See Supplement A" next to the product heading.

The following dosing information has been added to the **HOW SUPPLIED** *section:*

80 mg tablets: Yellow, oval-shaped, biconvex with BMS embossed on one side and 80 engraved on the opposite side. They are supplied in bottles of 90 (NDC 0003-5195-10) and bottles of 500 (NDC 0003-5195-12). Bottles contain a desiccant canister.

Unimatic® unit-dose packs containing 100 tablets are also available for the **20 mg** (NDC 0003-5178-06) potency.

Centocor, Inc.

200 GREAT VALLEY PARKWAY
MALVERN, PA 19355
USA

Direct General Inquiries to:
Ph: (610) 651-6000
(888) 874-3083
Fax: (610) 651-6100

Medical Emergency Contact:
Ph: 1-800-457-6399

For Medical Information/Adverse Experience Reporting Contact:
Medical Information
Ph: (800) 457-6399

REMICADE® ℞
infliximab recombinant
for IV injection

Prescribing information for this product, which appears on pages 1178–1182 of the 2002 PDR, has been completely revised as follows. Please write "See Supplement A" next to the product heading.

> **WARNING**
>
> **RISK OF INFECTIONS**
>
> **Tuberculosis (frequently disseminated or extrapulmonary at clinical presentation), invasive fungal infections, and other opportunistic infections, have been observed in patients receiving REMICADE. Some of these infections have been fatal (see *WARNINGS*).**
>
> **Patients should be evaluated for latent tuberculosis infection with a tuberculin skin test.[1] Treatment of latent tuberculosis infection should be initiated prior to therapy with REMICADE.**

DESCRIPTION

REMICADE is a chimeric IgG1κ monoclonal antibody with an approximate molecular weight of 149,100 dåltons. It is composed of human constant and murine variable regions. Infliximab binds specifically to human tumor necrosis factor alpha (TNFα) with an association constant of 10^{10} M^{-1}. Infliximab is produced by a recombinant cell line cultured by continuous perfusion and is purified by a series of steps that includes measures to inactivate and remove viruses.

REMICADE is supplied as a sterile, white, lyophilized powder for intravenous infusion. Following reconstitution with 10 mL of Sterile Water for Injection, USP, the resulting pH is approximately 7.2. Each single-use vial contains 100 mg infliximab, 500 mg sucrose, 0.5 mg polysorbate 80, 2.2 mg monobasic sodium phosphate, monohydrate, and 6.1 mg dibasic sodium phosphate, dihydrate. No preservatives are present.

CLINICAL PHARMACOLOGY

General

Infliximab neutralizes the biological activity of TNFα by binding with high affinity to the soluble and transmembrane forms of TNFα and inhibits binding of TNFα with its receptors.[2-5] Infliximab does not neutralize TNFβ (lymphotoxin α), a related cytokine that utilizes the same receptors as TNFα. Biological activities attributed to TNFα include: induction of pro-inflammatory cytokines such as interleukins (IL) 1 and 6, enhancement of leukocyte migration by increasing endothelial layer permeability and expression of adhesion molecules by endothelial cells and leukocytes, activation of neutrophil and eosinophil functional activity, induction of acute phase reactants and other liver proteins, as well as tissue degrading enzymes produced by synoviocytes and/or chondrocytes. Cells expressing transmembrane TNFα bound by infliximab can be lysed *in vitro* by complement or effector cells.[3] Infliximab inhibits the functional activity of TNFα in a wide variety of *in vitro* bioassays utilizing human fibroblasts, endothelial cells, neutrophils,[4] B and T lymphocytes and epithelial cells. Anti-TNFα antibodies reduce disease activity in the cotton-top tamarin colitis model, and decrease synovitis and joint erosions in a murine model of collagen-induced arthritis. Infliximab prevents disease in transgenic mice that develop polyarthritis as a result of constitutive expression of human TNFα, and, when administered after disease onset, allows eroded joints to heal.

Pharmacodynamics

Elevated concentrations of TNFα have been found in the joints of rheumatoid arthritis patients[6] and the stools of Crohn's disease patients[7] and correlate with elevated disease activity. In rheumatoid arthritis, treatment with REMICADE reduced infiltration of inflammatory cells into inflamed areas of the joint as well as expression of molecules mediating cellular adhesion [E-selectin, intercellular adhesion molecule-1 (ICAM-1) and vascular cell adhesion molecule-1 (VCAM-1)], chemoattraction [IL-8 and monocyte chemotactic protein (MCP-1)] and tissue degradation [matrix metalloproteinase (MMP) 1 and 3].[5] In Crohn's disease, treatment with REMICADE reduced infiltration of inflammatory cells and TNFα production in inflamed areas of the intestine, and reduced the proportion of mononuclear cells from the lamina propria able to express TNFα and interferon.[5] After treatment with REMICADE, patients with rheumatoid arthritis or Crohn's disease exhibited decreased levels of serum IL-6 and C-reactive protein (CRP) compared to baseline. Peripheral blood lymphocytes from REMICADE-treated patients showed no significant decrease in number or in proliferative responses to *in vitro* mitogenic stimulation when compared to cells from untreated patients.

Pharmacokinetics

Single intravenous (IV) infusions of 3 mg/kg to 20 mg/kg showed a linear relationship between the dose administered and the maximum serum concentration. The volume of distribution at steady state was independent of dose and indicated that infliximab was distributed primarily within the vascular compartment. Median pharmacokinetic results for doses of 3 mg/kg to 10 mg/kg in rheumatoid arthritis and 5 mg/kg in Crohn's disease indicate that the terminal half-life of infliximab is 8.0 to 9.5 days.

Following an initial dose of REMICADE, repeated infusions at 2 and 6 weeks resulted in predictable concentration-time profiles following each treatment. No systemic accumulation of infliximab occurred upon continued repeated treatment with 3 mg/kg or 10 mg/kg at 4- or 8-week intervals. No major differences in clearance or volume of distribution were observed in patient subgroups defined by age or weight. It is not known if there are differences in clearance or volume of distribution between gender subgroups or in patients with marked impairment of hepatic or renal function.

CLINICAL STUDIES

Rheumatoid Arthritis

The safety and efficacy of REMICADE when given in conjunction with methotrexate (MTX) were assessed in a multicenter, randomized, double-blind, placebo-controlled study of 428 patients with active rheumatoid arthritis despite treatment with MTX (the Anti-TNF Trial in Rheumatoid Arthritis with Concomitant Therapy or ATTRACT). Patients enrolled had a median age of 54 years, median disease duration of 8.4 years, median swollen and tender joint count of 20 and 31 respectively, and were on a median dose of 15 mg/wk of MTX. Patients received either placebo + MTX or one of 4 doses/schedules of REMICADE + MTX: 3 mg/kg or 10 mg/kg of REMICADE by IV infusion at weeks 0, 2 and 6 followed by additional infusions every 4 or 8 weeks in combination with MTX. Concurrent use of stable doses of folic acid, oral corticosteroids (≤10 mg/day) and/or nonsteroidal anti-inflammatory drugs was also permitted.

Data on use of REMICADE without concurrent MTX are limited (see *ADVERSE REACTIONS, Immunogenicity*).[8,9]

Clinical response

All doses/schedules of REMICADE + MTX resulted in improvement in signs and symptoms as measured by the American College of Rheumatology response criteria (ACR 20)[10] with a higher percentage of patients achieving an ACR 20, 50 and 70 compared to placebo + MTX (Table 1). This improvement was observed at week 2 and maintained through week 102. Greater effects on each component of the ACR 20 were observed in all patients treated with REMICADE + MTX compared to placebo + MTX (Table 2). Approximately 10% of patients treated with REMICADE achieved a major clinical response, defined as maintenance of an ACR 70 response over a 6-month period compared to 0% of placebo-treated patients (p≤0.018).

[See table 1 at top of next page]
[See table 2 at top of next page]

Radiographic response

Structural damage in both hands and feet was assessed radiographically at week 54 by the change from baseline in the van der Heijde-modified Sharp score, a composite score of structural damage that measures the number and size of joint erosions and the degree of joint space narrowing in hands/wrists and feet.[12] Approximately 80% of patients had paired x-ray data at 54 weeks and approximately 70% at 102 weeks. The inhibition of progression of structural damage was observed at 54 weeks (Table 3) and maintained through 102 weeks.

[See table 3 at top of next page]

Physical function response

Physical function and disability were assessed using the Health Assessment Questionnaire (HAQ)[11] and the general health-related quality of life questionnaire SF-36.[13] All doses/schedules of REMICADE + MTX showed significantly greater improvement from baseline in HAQ and SF-36 physical component summary score averaged over time through week 54 compared to placebo + MTX, and no worsening in the SF-36 mental component summary score.

The median (interquartile range) improvement from baseline to week 54 in HAQ was 0.1 (-0.1, 0.5) for the placebo + MTX group and 0.4 (0.1, 0.9) for REMICADE + MTX (p<0.001). Both HAQ and SF-36 effects were maintained through week 102. Approximately 80% of patients in all doses/schedules of REMICADE + MTX remained in the trial through 102 weeks.

Active Crohn's Disease

The safety and efficacy of REMICADE were assessed in a randomized, double-blind, placebo-controlled dose ranging study of 108 patients with moderate to severe active Crohn's disease[14] [Crohn's Disease Activity Index (CDAI) ≥220 and

Continued on next page

Remicade—Cont.

≤400]. All patients had experienced an inadequate response to prior conventional therapies, including corticosteroids (60% of patients), 5-aminosalicylates (5-ASA) (60%) and/or 6-mercaptopurine/azathioprine (6-MP/AZA) (37%). Concurrent use of stable dose regimens of corticosteroids, 5-ASA, 6-MP and/or AZA was permitted and 92% of patients continued to receive at least one of these medications.

The study was divided into three phases. In the first phase, patients were randomized to receive a single IV dose of placebo, 5, 10 or 20 mg/kg of REMICADE. The primary endpoint was the proportion of patients who experienced a clinical response, defined as a decrease in CDAI by ≥70 points from baseline at the 4-week evaluation and without an increase in Crohn's disease medications or surgery for Crohn's disease. Patients who responded at week 4 were followed to week 12. Secondary endpoints included the proportion of patients who were in clinical remission at week 4 (CDAI <150), and clinical response over time.

At week four, 4 of 25 (16%) of the placebo patients achieved a clinical response vs. 22 of 27 (82%) of the patients receiving 5 mg/kg REMICADE ($p < 0.001$, two-sided, Fisher's Exact test). One of 25 (4%) placebo patients and 13 of 27 (48%) patients receiving 5 mg/kg REMICADE achieved a CDAI <150 at week 4. The maximum response to any dose of REMICADE was observed within 2 to 4 weeks. The proportion of patients responding gradually diminished over the 12 weeks of the evaluation period. There was no evidence of a dose response; doses higher than 5 mg/kg did not result in a greater proportion of responders. Results are shown in Figure 1.

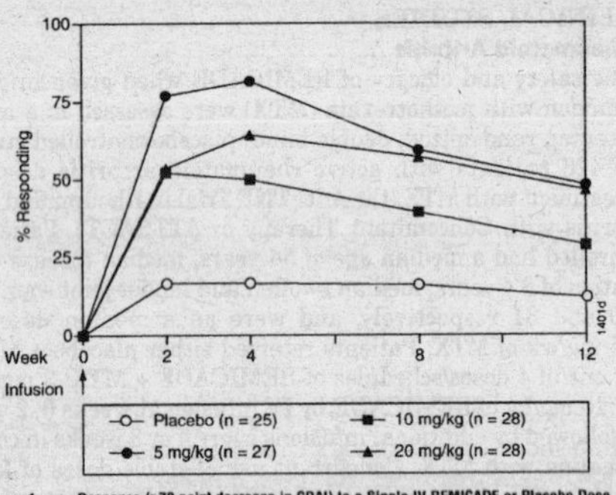

Figure 1 Response (≥70 point decrease in CDAI) to a Single IV REMICADE or Placebo Dose

During the 12-week period following infusion, patients treated with REMICADE compared to placebo demonstrated improvement in outcomes measured by the Inflammatory Bowel Disease Questionnaire.

In the second phase, 29 patients who did not respond to the single dose of 5, 10 or 20 mg/kg of REMICADE entered the open label phase and received a single 10 mg/kg dose of REMICADE 4 weeks after the initial dose. Ten of 29 (34%) patients experienced a response 4 weeks after receiving the second dose.

Patients who remained in clinical response at week 8 during the first or second phase were eligible for the retreatment phase. Seventy-three patients were re-randomized at week 12 to receive 4 infusions of placebo or 10 mg/kg REMICADE at 8-week intervals (weeks 12, 20, 28, 36) and were followed to week 48. In the limited data set available, no significant differences were observed between the REMICADE and placebo re-treated groups.

Fistulizing Crohn's Disease

The safety and efficacy of REMICADE were assessed in a randomized, double-blind, placebo-controlled study of 94 patients with fistulizing Crohn's disease with fistula(s) that were of at least 3 months duration.[15] Concurrent use of stable doses of corticosteroids, 5-ASA, antibiotics, MTX, 6-MP and/or AZA was permitted, and 83% of patients continued to receive at least one of these medications. Fifty-two (55%) had multiple cutaneously draining fistulas, 90% of patients had fistula(s) in the perianal area and 10% had abdominal fistula(s).

Patients received 3 doses of placebo, 5 or 10 mg/kg REMICADE at weeks 0, 2 and 6 and were followed up to 26 weeks. The primary endpoint was the proportion of patients who experienced a clinical response, defined as ≥50% reduction from baseline in the number of fistula(s) draining upon gentle compression, on at least two consecutive visits, without an increase in medication or surgery for Crohn's disease.

Eight of 31 (26%) patients in the placebo arm achieved a clinical response vs. 21 of the 31 (68%) patients in the 5 mg/kg REMICADE arm ($p = 0.002$, two-sided, Fisher's Exact test). Eighteen of 32 (56%) patients in the 10 mg/kg arm achieved a clinical response.

The median time to onset of response in the REMICADE-treated group was 2 weeks. The median duration of response was 12 weeks; after 22 weeks there was no difference between either dose of REMICADE and placebo in the proportion of patients in response (Figure 2). New fistula(s) developed in approximately 15% of both REMICADE- and placebo-treated patients.

[See figure at top of next column]

Seven of 60 (12%) evaluable REMICADE-treated patients, compared to 1 of 31 (3.5%) placebo-treated patients, developed an abscess in the area of fistulas between 8 and 16

Table 1

PERCENTAGE OF PATIENTS WHO ACHIEVED AN ACR RESPONSE AT WEEKS 30 AND 54

		REMICADE + MTX			
		3 mg/kg[a]		10 mg/kg[a]	
Response	Placebo + MTX (n=88)	q 8 wks (n=86)	q 4 wks (n=86)	q 8 wks (n=87)	q 4 wks (n=81)
ACR 20					
Week 30	20%	50%	50%	52%	58%
Week 54	17%	42%	48%	59%	59%
ACR 50					
Week 30	5%	27%	29%	31%	26%
Week 54	9%	21%	34%	40%	38%
ACR 70					
Week 30	0%	8%	11%	18%	11%
Week 54	2%	11%	18%	26%	19%

[a] $p < 0.05$ for each outcome compared to placebo

Table 2

COMPONENTS OF ACR 20 AT BASELINE AND 54 WEEKS

	Placebo + MTX (n=88)		REMICADE + MTX[a] (n=340)	
Parameter (medians)	Baseline	Week 54	Baseline	Week 54
No. of Tender Joints	24	16	32	8
No. of Swollen Joints	19	13	20	7
Pain[b]	6.7	6.1	6.8	3.3
Physician's Global Assessment[b]	6.5	5.2	6.2	2.1
Patient's Global Assessment[b]	6.2	6.2	6.3	3.2
Disability Index (HAQ)[c]	1.8	1.5	1.8	1.3
CRP (mg/dL)	3.0	2.3	2.4	0.6

[a] All doses/schedules of REMICADE + MTX
[b] Visual Analog Scale (0=best, 10=worst)
[c] Health Assessment Questionnaire, measurement of 8 categories: dressing and grooming, arising, eating, walking, hygiene, reach, grip, and activities (0=best, 3=worst)[11]

Table 3

RADIOGRAPHIC CHANGE FROM BASELINE TO WEEK 54

Median (10, 90 percentiles)	Placebo + MTX (n=64)	REMICADE + MTX 3 mg/kg q 8 wks (n=71)	3 mg/kg q 4 wks (n=71)	10 mg/kg q 8 wks (n=77)	10 mg/kg q 4 wks (n=66)	p-value[a]
Total Score						
Baseline	55 (14, 188)	57 (15, 187)	45 (8, 162)	56 (6, 143)	43 (7, 178)	
Change from baseline	4.0 (-1.0, 19.0)	0.5 (-3.0, 5.5)	0.1 (-5.2, 9.0)	0.5 (-4.8, 5.0)	-0.5 (-5.7, 4.0)	p<0.001
Erosion Score						
Baseline	25 (8, 110)	29 (9, 100)	22 (3, 91)	22 (3, 80)	26 (4, 104)	
Change from baseline	2.0 (-1.0, 9.7)	0.0 (-3.0 4.3)	-0.3 (-3.1, 2.5)	0.5 (-3.0, 2.5)	-0.5 (-2.7, 2.5)	p<0.001
JSN Score						
Baseline	26 (3, 88)	29 (4, 80)	20 (3, 83)	24 (1, 79)	25 (3, 77)	
Change from baseline	1.5 (-0.8, 8.0)	0.0 (-2.5, 4.5)	0.0 (-3.4, 5.0)	0.0 (-3.0, 2.5)	0.0 (-3.0, 3.5)	p<0.001

[a] For comparisons of each dose against placebo

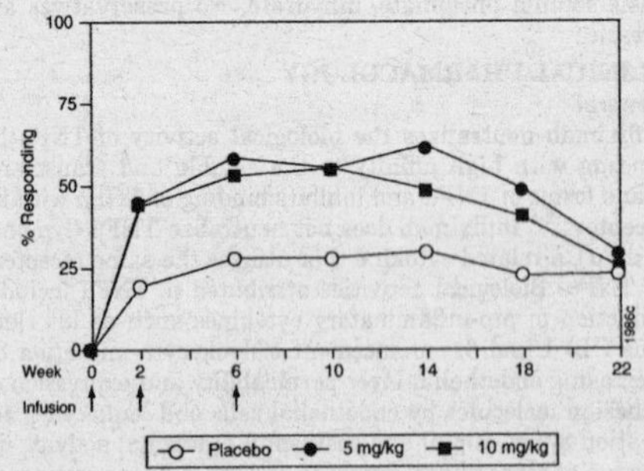

Figure 2 Response (fistula(s) closure) with Three Doses of REMICADE or Placebo

weeks after the last infusion of REMICADE. Six of the REMICADE patients who developed an abscess had experienced a clinical response (see *ADVERSE REACTIONS, Infections*).

Dose regimens other than dosing at weeks 0, 2 and 6 have not been studied. Studies have not been done to assess the effects of REMICADE on healing of the internal fistular canal, on closure of non-cutaneously draining fistulas (e.g., entero-entero), or on cutaneously draining fistulas in locations other than perianal and periabdominal.

INDICATIONS AND USAGE

Rheumatoid Arthritis

REMICADE, in combination with methotrexate, is indicated for reducing signs and symptoms, inhibiting the progression of structural damage and improving physical function in patients with moderately to severely active rheumatoid arthritis who have had an inadequate response to methotrexate.

Crohn's Disease

REMICADE is indicated for the reduction in signs and symptoms of Crohn's disease in patients with moderately to severely active Crohn's disease who have had an inadequate response to conventional therapy.

The safety and efficacy of therapy continued beyond a single dose have not been established (see *DOSAGE AND ADMINISTRATION*).

REMICADE is indicated for the reduction in the number of draining enterocutaneous fistulas in patients with fistulizing Crohn's disease.

The safety and efficacy of therapy continued beyond three doses have not been established (see *DOSAGE AND ADMINISTRATION*).

CONTRAINDICATIONS

REMICADE is contraindicated in patients with moderate or severe (NYHA Class III/IV) congestive heart failure (see *WARNINGS, Congestive Heart Failure*).

REMICADE should not be administered to patients with known hypersensitivity to any murine proteins or other component of the product.

WARNINGS

RISK OF INFECTIONS

(See boxed *WARNING*)

SERIOUS INFECTIONS, INCLUDING SEPSIS HAVE BEEN REPORTED IN PATIENTS RECEIVING TNF-BLOCKING AGENTS. SOME OF THESE INFECTIONS HAVE BEEN FATAL. MANY OF THE SERIOUS INFECTIONS IN PATIENTS TREATED WITH REMICADE HAVE OCCURRED IN PATIENTS ON CONCOMITANT IMMUNOSUPPRESSIVE THERAPY THAT, IN ADDITION TO THEIR CROHN'S DISEASE OR RHEUMATOID ARTHRITIS, COULD PREDISPOSE THEM TO INFECTIONS.

REMICADE SHOULD NOT BE GIVEN TO PATIENTS WITH A CLINICALLY IMPORTANT, ACTIVE INFECTION. CAUTION SHOULD BE EXERCISED WHEN CONSIDERING THE USE OF REMICADE IN PATIENTS WITH A CHRONIC INFECTION OR A HISTORY OF RECURRENT INFECTION. PATIENTS

SHOULD BE MONITORED FOR SIGNS AND SYMPTOMS OF INFECTION WHILE ON OR AFTER TREATMENT WITH REMICADE. NEW INFECTIONS SHOULD BE CLOSELY MONITORED. IF A PATIENT DEVELOPS A SERIOUS INFECTION, REMICADE THERAPY SHOULD BE DISCONTINUED (see *ADVERSE REACTIONS, Infections*).

CASES OF HISTOPLASMOSIS, LISTERIOSIS, PNEUMOCYSTOSIS AND TUBERCULOSIS, HAVE BEEN OBSERVED IN PATIENTS RECEIVING REMICADE. FOR PATIENTS WHO HAVE RESIDED IN REGIONS WHERE HISTOPLASMOSIS IS ENDEMIC, THE BENEFITS AND RISKS OF REMICADE TREATMENT SHOULD BE CAREFULLY CONSIDERED BEFORE INITIATION OF REMICADE THERAPY.

Congestive Heart Failure

Doses greater than 5 mg/kg should not be administered to patients with congestive heart failure (CHF). REMICADE should be used with caution in patients with mild heart failure (NYHA Class I/II). Patients should be closely monitored, and REMICADE must not be continued in patients who develop new or worsening symptoms of heart failure (see *CONTRAINDICATIONS* and *ADVERSE REACTIONS, Congestive Heart Failure*).

Hypersensitivity

REMICADE has been associated with hypersensitivity reactions that vary in their time of onset. Most hypersensitivity reactions, which include urticaria, dyspnea, and/or hypotension, have occurred during or within 2 hours of infliximab infusion. However, in some cases, serum sickness-like reactions have been observed in Crohn's disease patients 3 to 12 days after REMICADE therapy was reinstituted following an extended period without REMICADE treatment. Symptoms associated with these reactions include fever, rash, headache, sore throat, myalgias, polyarthralgias, hand and facial edema and/or dysphagia. These reactions were associated with marked increase in antibodies to infliximab, loss of detectable serum concentrations of REMICADE, and possible loss of drug efficacy. REMICADE should be discontinued for severe reactions. Medications for the treatment of hypersensitivity reactions (e.g., acetaminophen, antihistamines, corticosteroids and/or epinephrine) should be available for immediate use in the event of a reaction (see *ADVERSE REACTIONS, Infusion-related Reactions*).

Neurologic Events

Infliximab and other agents that inhibit TNF have been associated in rare cases with optic neuritis, seizure and new onset or exacerbation of clinical symptoms and/or radiographic evidence of central nervous system demyelinating disorders, including multiple sclerosis. Prescribers should exercise caution in considering the use of REMICADE in patients with pre-existing or recent onset of central nervous system demyelinating or seizure disorders.

PRECAUTIONS

Autoimmunity

Treatment with REMICADE may result in the formation of autoantibodies and, rarely, in the development of a lupus-like syndrome. If a patient develops symptoms suggestive of a lupus-like syndrome following treatment with REMICADE, treatment should be discontinued (see *ADVERSE REACTIONS, Autoantibodies/Lupus-like Syndrome*).

Malignancy

Patients with long duration of Crohn's disease or rheumatoid arthritis and chronic exposure to immunosuppressant therapies are more prone to develop lymphomas (see *ADVERSE REACTIONS, Malignancies/Lymphoproliferative Disease*). The impact of treatment with REMICADE on these phenomena is unknown.

Vaccinations

No data are available on the response to vaccination or on the secondary transmission of infection by live vaccines in patients receiving anti-TNF therapy. It is recommended that live vaccines not be given concurrently.

Drug Interactions

Specific drug interaction studies, including interactions with MTX, have not been conducted. The majority of patients in rheumatoid arthritis or Crohn's disease clinical studies received one or more concomitant medications. In rheumatoid arthritis, concomitant medications besides MTX were nonsteroidal anti-inflammatory agents, folic acid, corticosteroids and/or narcotics. Concomitant Crohn's disease medications were antibiotics, antivirals, corticosteroids, 6-MP/AZA and aminosalicylates. Patients with Crohn's disease who received immunosuppressants tended to experience fewer infusion reactions compared to patients on no immunosuppressants (see *ADVERSE REACTIONS, Immunogenicity* and *Infusion-related Reactions*).

Carcinogenesis, Mutagenesis and Impairment of Fertility

A repeat dose toxicity study was conducted with mice given cV1q anti-mouse TNFα to evaluate tumorigenicity. cV1q is an analogous antibody that inhibits the function of TNFα in mice. Animals were assigned to 1 of 3 dose groups: control, 10 mg/kg or 40 mg/kg cV1q given weekly for 6 months. The weekly doses of 10 mg/kg and 40 mg/kg are 2 and 8 times, respectively, the human dose of 5 mg/kg for Crohn's disease. Results indicated that cV1q did not cause tumorigenicity in mice. No clastogenic or mutagenic effects of infliximab were observed in the *in vivo* mouse micronucleus test or the *Salmonella-Escherichia coli* (Ames) assay, respectively. Chromosomal aberrations were not observed in an assay performed using human lymphocytes. The significance of these findings for human risk is unknown. It is not known whether infliximab can impair fertility in humans. No impairment of fertility was observed in a fertility and general reproduction toxicity study with the analogous mouse antibody used in the 6-month chronic toxicity study.

Pregnancy Category B

Since infliximab does not cross-react with TNFα in species other than humans and chimpanzees, animal reproduction studies have not been conducted with REMICADE. No evidence of maternal toxicity, embryotoxicity or teratogenicity was observed in a developmental toxicity study conducted in mice using an analogous antibody that selectively inhibits the functional activity of mouse TNFα. Doses of 10 to 15 mg/kg in pharmacodynamic animal models with the anti-TNF analogous antibody produced maximal pharmacologic effectiveness. Doses up to 40 mg/kg were shown to produce no adverse effects in animal reproduction studies. It is not known whether REMICADE can cause fetal harm when administered to a pregnant woman or can affect reproduction capacity. REMICADE should be given to a pregnant woman only if clearly needed.

Nursing Mothers

It is not known whether infliximab is excreted in human milk or absorbed systemically after ingestion. Because many drugs and immunoglobulins are excreted in human milk, and because of the potential for adverse reactions in nursing infants from REMICADE, a decision should be made whether to discontinue nursing or to discontinue the drug, taking into account the importance of the drug to the mother.

Pediatric Use

Safety and effectiveness of REMICADE in patients with juvenile rheumatoid arthritis and in pediatric patients with Crohn's disease have not been established.

Geriatric Use

In the ATTRACT study, no overall differences were observed in effectiveness or safety in 72 patients aged 65 or older compared to younger patients. In Crohn's disease studies, there were insufficient numbers of patients aged 65 and over to determine whether they respond differently from patients aged 18 to 65. Because there is a higher incidence of infections in the elderly population in general, caution should be used in treating the elderly (see *ADVERSE REACTIONS, Infections*).

ADVERSE REACTIONS

A total of 771 patients were treated with REMICADE in clinical studies. Approximately 8% of patients discontinued REMICADE because of adverse experiences. The most common reason for discontinuation of treatment was infusion-related reactions (dyspnea, urticaria, hypotension, flushing and headache). Adverse events have been reported in a higher proportion of patients receiving the 10 mg/kg dose than the 3 mg/kg dose.

Infusion-related Reactions

Acute infusion reactions

An infusion reaction was defined as any adverse event occurring during the infusion or within 1 to 2 hours after the infusion. Twenty percent of REMICADE-treated patients in all clinical studies experienced an infusion reaction compared to 9% of placebo-treated patients. Among the 6443 REMICADE infusions, 3% were accompanied by nonspecific symptoms such as fever or chills, 1% were accompanied by cardiopulmonary reactions (primarily chest pain, hypotension, hypertension or dyspnea), <1% were accompanied by pruritus, urticaria, or the combined symptoms of pruritus/urticaria and cardiopulmonary reactions. Serious infusion reactions occurred in <1% of patients and included anaphylaxis, convulsions, erythematous rash and hypotension. Two percent of patients discontinued REMICADE because of infusion reactions, and all patients recovered with treatment and/or discontinuation of infusion. REMICADE infusions beyond the initial infusion in rheumatoid arthritis patients were not associated with a higher incidence of reactions.

Patients who became positive for antibodies to infliximab were more likely (approximately 3-fold) to have an infusion reaction than were those who were negative. Use of concomitant immunosuppressant agents appeared to reduce the frequency of antibodies to infliximab and infusion reactions (see *ADVERSE REACTIONS, Immunogenicity* and *PRECAUTIONS, Drug Interactions*).

In post-marketing experience, cases of anaphylactic-like reactions, including laryngeal/pharyngeal edema and severe bronchospasm, and seizure have been associated with REMICADE administration.

Reactions following readministration

In a clinical study of 40 patients with Crohn's disease retreated with infliximab following a 2 to 4 year period without infliximab treatment, 10 patients experienced adverse events manifesting 3 to 12 days following infusion of which 6 were considered serious. Signs and symptoms included myalgia and/or arthralgia with fever and/or rash, with some patients also experiencing pruritus, facial, hand or lip edema, dysphagia, urticaria, sore throat, and headache. Patients experiencing these adverse events had not experienced infusion-related adverse events associated with their initial infliximab therapy. Of the 40 patients enrolled, these adverse events occurred in 9 of 23 (39%) who had received liquid formulation which is no longer in use and 1 of 17 (6%) who received lyophilized formulation. The clinical data are not adequate to determine if occurrence of these reactions is due to differences in formulation. Patients' signs and symptoms improved substantially or resolved with treatment in all cases. There are insufficient data on the incidence of these events after drug-free intervals of less than 2 years. However, these events have been observed infrequently in clinical studies and post-marketing surveillance at intervals of less than 1 year.

Infections

In REMICADE clinical studies, treated infections were reported in 39% of REMICADE-treated patients (average of 56 weeks of follow-up) and in 26% of placebo-treated patients (average of 41 weeks of follow-up). When longer observation of patients on REMICADE was accounted for, the event rate was similar for both groups. The infections most frequently reported were respiratory tract infections (including sinusitis, pharyngitis, and bronchitis) and urinary tract infections. No increased risk of serious infections or sepsis were observed with REMICADE compared to placebo in the ATTRACT study. Among REMICADE-treated patients, these serious infections included pneumonia, cellulitis, skin ulceration, sepsis, and bacterial infection. In the ATTRACT study, one patient died with miliary tuberculosis and one died with disseminated coccidioidomycosis. Other cases of tuberculosis, including disseminated tuberculosis, also have been reported post-marketing. Most of the cases of tuberculosis occurred within the first two months after initiation of therapy with infliximab and may reflect recrudescence of latent disease (see *WARNINGS, RISK OF INFECTIONS*). Twelve percent of patients with fistulizing Crohn's disease developed a new abscess 8 to 16 weeks after the last infusion of REMICADE (see *CLINICAL STUDIES, Fistulizing Crohn's Disease*).

In post-marketing experience, infections have been observed with various pathogens including viral, bacterial, fungal, and protozoal organisms. Infections have been noted in all organ systems and have been reported in patients receiving REMICADE alone or in combination with immunosuppressive agents.

Autoantibodies/Lupus-like Syndrome

In the ATTRACT study through week 102, 62% of REMICADE-treated patients developed antinuclear antibodies (ANA) between screening and last evaluation, compared to 27% of placebo-treated patients. Anti-dsDNA antibodies developed in approximately 15% of REMICADE-treated patients, compared to none of the placebo-treated patients. No association was seen between REMICADE dose/schedule and development of ANA or anti-dsDNA.

Of Crohn's disease patients treated with REMICADE who were evaluated for ANA, 34% developed ANA between screening and last evaluation. Anti-dsDNA antibodies developed in approximately 9% of Crohn's disease patients treated with REMICADE. The development of anti-dsDNA antibodies was not related to either the dose or duration of REMICADE treatment. However, baseline therapy with an immunosuppressant in Crohn's disease patients was associated with reduced development of anti-dsDNA antibodies (3% compared to 21% in patients not receiving any immunosuppressant). Crohn's disease patients were approximately 2 times more likely to develop anti-dsDNA antibodies if they were ANA-positive at study entry.

In clinical studies, 4 patients developed clinical symptoms consistent with a lupus-like syndrome, 3 with rheumatoid arthritis and 1 with Crohn's disease. All 4 patients improved following discontinuation of therapy and appropriate medical treatment. No patients had central nervous system or renal involvement. No cases of lupus-like reactions have been observed in up to three years of long-term follow-up (see *PRECAUTIONS, Autoimmunity*).

Malignancies/Lymphoproliferative Disease

In completed clinical studies of REMICADE for up to 102 weeks, 12 of 771 patients developed 13 new or recurrent malignancies. These were non-Hodgkin's B-cell lymphoma, breast cancer, melanoma, squamous, rectal adenocarcinoma and basal cell carcinoma. There are insufficient data to determine whether REMICADE contributed to the development of these malignancies. The observed rates and incidences were similar to those expected for the populations studied[16,17] (see *PRECAUTIONS, Malignancy*).

Immunogenicity

Treatment with REMICADE can be associated with the development of antibodies to infliximab. Approximately 10% of patients were antibody positive. Patients who were antibody-positive were more likely to experience an infusion reaction (see *ADVERSE REACTIONS, Infusion-related Reactions*). Antibody development was lower among rheumatoid arthritis and Crohn's disease patients receiving immunosuppressant therapies such as 6-MP, AZA or MTX. With repeated dosing of REMICADE, serum concentrations of infliximab were higher in rheumatoid arthritis patients who received concomitant MTX. Because immunogenicity analyses are product-specific, comparison of antibody rates to those from other products is not appropriate.

Congestive Heart Failure

In a phase II study evaluating REMICADE in NYHA Class III/IV CHF patients (left ventricular ejection fraction ≤35%), higher incidences of mortality and hospitalization due to worsening heart failure were seen in REMICADE-treated patients, especially those treated with 10 mg/kg. One hundred and fifty patients were treated with 3 infusions of REMICADE 5 mg/kg, 10 mg/kg, or placebo over 6 weeks. At 28 weeks, 4 of 101 patients treated with REMICADE (1 at 5 mg/kg and 3 at 10 mg/kg) died compared with no deaths among the 49 placebo-treated patients. In follow-up, at 38 weeks, 9 patients treated with REMICADE (2 at 5 mg/kg and 7 at 10 mg/kg) died compared with one death among the placebo-treated patients. At 28 weeks, 14

Continued on next page

Remicade—Cont.

of 101 patients treated with REMICADE (3 at 5 mg/kg and 11 at 10 mg/kg) were hospitalized for worsening CHF compared with 5 of the 49 placebo-treated patients (see *CONTRAINDICATIONS* and *WARNINGS*, *Congestive Heart Failure*).

Other Adverse Reactions

Adverse events occurring at a frequency of at least 5% in all patients treated with REMICADE are shown in Table 4. [See table below]

In clinical studies, serious adverse events (all occurred at frequencies <2%) by body system in all patients treated with REMICADE were as follows:

Autoimmunity: lupus erythematosus syndrome, rheumatoid nodules, worsening rheumatoid arthritis

Body as a whole: abdominal hernia, asthenia, chest pain, diaphragmatic hernia, drug overdose, edema, fall, pain

Blood: pancytopenia, splenic infarction, splenomegaly

Cardiovascular: circulatory failure, hypertension, hypotension, syncope

Central & Peripheral Nervous: cerebral hypoxia, convulsions, dizziness, encephalopathy, headache, hemiparesis, spinal stenosis, upper motor neuron lesion

Ear and Hearing: ceruminosis

Eye and Vision: endophthalmitis

Gastrointestinal: abdominal pain, appendicitis, Crohn's disease, diarrhea, diverticulitis, enteritis, gastric ulcer, gastrointestinal hemorrhage, intestinal obstruction, intestinal perforation, intestinal stenosis, nausea, pancreatitis, peritonitis, proctalgia, vomiting

Heart Rate and Rhythm: arrhythmia, atrioventricular block, bradycardia, cardiac arrest, palpitation, tachycardia, ventricular fibrillation

Liver and Biliary: biliary pain, cholecystitis, cholelithiasis, hepatitis cholestatic

Metabolic and Nutritional: dehydration, diabetes mellitus, hyperglycemia, hypoglycemia, pancreatic insufficiency, weight decrease

Musculoskeletal: arthralgia, arthritis, back pain, bone fracture, bursitis, hemarthrosis, intervertebral disk herniation, joint cyst, joint degeneration, joint dislocation, loosening of total hip prosthesis, myalgia, osteoarthritis, osteomyelitis, osteoporosis, spondylolisthesis, symphyseolysis, synovitis, tendon disorder, tendon injury

Myo-, Endo-, Pericardial and Coronary Valve: cardiac failure, mitral insufficiency, myocardial ischemia

Neoplasms: basal cell, breast, lymphoma, melanoma, rectal adenocarcinoma, squamous skin

Platelet, Bleeding and Clotting: thrombocytopenia

Psychiatric: abnormal thinking, anxiety, confusion, delirium, depression, somnolence, suicide attempt

Red Blood Cell: anemia

Reproductive: endometriosis, vaginal hemorrhage

Resistance Mechanism: abscess, bacterial infection, cellulitis, empyema, fever, fungal infection, herpes zoster, infection, inflammation, sepsis, tuberculosis, viremia

Respiratory: adult respiratory distress syndrome, bronchitis, coughing, dyspnea, pleural effusion, pleurisy, pneumonia, pneumothorax, pulmonary edema, pulmonary infiltration, respiratory insufficiency, respiratory tract fistula, sinusitis, upper respiratory tract infection

Skin and Appendages: furunculosis, increased sweating, injection site inflammation, rash, ulceration

Urinary: azotemia, dysuria, hydronephrosis, increased creatinine, kidney infarction, pyelonephritis, renal calculus, renal failure, ureteral obstruction, urinary tract infection

Vascular (Extracardiac): abdominal aortic perforation, arterial stenosis, brain hemorrhage, brain infarction, intermittent claudication, peripheral ischemia, pulmonary embolism, thrombophlebitis

White Cell and Reticuloendothelial: leukopenia, lymphadenopathy, lymphangitis

A greater proportion of patients enrolled into the ATTRACT study who received REMICADE + MTX experienced transient mild (<2 times the upper limit of normal) or moderate (≥2 but <3 times the upper limit of normal) elevations in AST or ALT (49% and 47%, respectively) compared to patients treated with placebo + MTX (27% and 35%, respectively). Six (1.8%) patients treated with REMICADE + MTX experienced more prolonged elevations in their ALT.

Additional adverse events reported from worldwide post-marketing experience with REMICADE include demyelinating disorders (such as multiple sclerosis and optic neuritis), Guillain-Barré syndrome, interstitial pneumonitis/fibrosis, and neuropathies (see *ADVERSE REACTIONS, Infections* and *Infusion-related Reactions*).

OVERDOSAGE

Single doses up to 20 mg/kg have been administered without any direct toxic effect. In case of overdosage, it is recommended that the patient be monitored for any signs or symptoms of adverse reactions or effects and appropriate symptomatic treatment instituted immediately.

DOSAGE AND ADMINISTRATION

Rheumatoid Arthritis

The recommended dose of REMICADE is 3 mg/kg given as an intravenous infusion followed with additional similar doses at 2 and 6 weeks after the first infusion then every 8 weeks thereafter. REMICADE should be given in combination with methotrexate. For patients who have an incomplete response, consideration may be given to adjusting the dose up to 10 mg/kg or treating as often as every 4 weeks.

Crohn's Disease

The recommended dose of REMICADE is 5 mg/kg given as a single intravenous infusion for treatment of moderately to severely active Crohn's disease. In patients with fistulizing disease, an initial 5 mg/kg dose should be followed with additional 5 mg/kg doses at 2 and 6 weeks after the first infusion.

There are insufficient safety and efficacy data for the use of REMICADE in Crohn's disease beyond the recommended duration (see *WARNINGS, Hypersensitivity; ADVERSE REACTIONS, Infusion-related Reactions;* and *INDICATIONS AND USAGE*).

Preparation and administration instructions:

Use aseptic technique.

REMICADE vials do not contain antibacterial preservatives. Therefore, the vials after reconstitution should be used immediately, not re-entered or stored. The diluent to be used for reconstitution is 10 mL of Sterile Water for Injection, USP. The total dose of the reconstituted product must be further diluted to 250 mL with 0.9% Sodium Chloride Injection, USP. The infusion concentration should range between 0.4 mg/mL and 4 mg/mL. The REMICADE infusion should begin within 3 hours of preparation.

1. Calculate the dose and the number of REMICADE vials needed. Each REMICADE vial contains 100 mg of infliximab. Calculate the total volume of reconstituted REMICADE solution required.
2. Reconstitute each REMICADE vial with 10 mL of Sterile Water for Injection, USP, using a syringe equipped with a 21-gauge or smaller needle. Remove the flip-top from the vial and wipe the top with an alcohol swab. Insert the syringe needle into the vial through the center of the rubber stopper and direct the stream of Sterile Water for Injection, USP, to the glass wall of the vial. Do not use the vial if the vacuum is not present. Gently swirl the solution by rotating the vial to dissolve the lyophilized powder. Avoid prolonged or vigorous agitation. DO NOT SHAKE. Foaming of the solution on reconstitution is not unusual. Allow the reconstituted solution to stand for 5 minutes. The solution should be colorless to light yellow and opalescent, and the solution may develop a few translucent particles as infliximab is a protein. Do not use if opaque particles, discoloration, or other foreign particles are present.
3. Dilute the total volume of the reconstituted REMICADE solution dose to 250 mL with 0.9% Sodium Chloride Injection, USP, by withdrawing a volume of 0.9% Sodium Chloride Injection, USP, equal to the volume of reconstituted REMICADE from the 0.9% Sodium Chloride Injection, USP, 250 mL bottle or bag. Slowly add the total volume of reconstituted REMICADE solution to the 250 mL infusion bottle or bag. Gently mix.
4. The infusion solution must be administered over a period of not less than 2 hours and must use an infusion set with an in-line, sterile, non-pyrogenic, low-protein-binding filter (pore size of 1.2-µm or less). Any unused portion of the infusion solution should not be stored for reuse.
5. No physical biochemical compatibility studies have been conducted to evaluate the co-administration of REMICADE with other agents. REMICADE should not be infused concomitantly in the same intravenous line with other agents.
6. Parenteral drug products should be inspected visually for particulate matter and discoloration prior to administration, whenever solution and container permit. If visibly opaque particles, discoloration or other foreign particulates are observed, the solution should not be used.

Storage

Store the lyophilized product under refrigeration at 2°C to 8°C (36°F to 46°F). Do not freeze. Do not use beyond the expiration date. This product contains no preservative.

HOW SUPPLIED

REMICADE lyophilized concentrate for IV injection is supplied in individually-boxed single-use vials in the following strength:

NDC 57894-030-01 — 100 mg infliximab in a 20-mL vial

REFERENCES

1. American Thoracic Society, Centers for Disease Control and Prevention. Targeted tuberculin testing and treatment of latent tuberculosis infection. *Am J Respir Crit Care Med* 2000;161:S221-S247.
2. Knight DM, Trinh H, Le J, et al. Construction and initial characterization of a mouse-human chimeric anti-TNF antibody. *Molec Immunol* 1993;30:1443-1453.
3. Scallon BJ, Moore MA, Trinh H, et al. Chimeric anti-TNFα monoclonal antibody cA2 binds recombinant transmembrane TNFα and activates immune effector functions. *Cytokine* 1995;7:251-259.
4. Siegel SA, Shealy DJ, Nakada MT, et al. The mouse/human chimeric monoclonal antibody cA2 neutralizes TNF *in vitro* and protects transgenic mice from cachexia and TNF lethality *in vivo*. *Cytokine* 1995;7:15-25.
5. Data on file.
6. Chu CQ, Field M, Feldmann M, et al. Localization of tumor necrosis factor α in synovial tissues and at the cartilage-pannus junction in patients with rheumatoid arthritis. *Arthritis and Rheum* 1991;34:1125-1132.
7. Braegger CP, Nicholls S, Murch SH, et al. Tumour necrosis factor alpha in stool as a marker of intestinal inflammation. *Lancet* 1992;339:89-91.
8. Maini RN, Breedveld FC, Kalden JR, et al. Therapeutic efficacy of multiple intravenous infusions of anti-tumor necrosis factor α monoclonal antibody combined with low-dose weekly methotrexate in rheumatoid arthritis. *Arthritis Rheum* 1998;41(9):1552-1563.
9. Elliott MJ, Maini RN, Feldmann M, et al. Randomised double-blind comparison of chimeric monoclonal antibody to tumour necrosis factor alpha (cA2) vs. placebo in rheumatoid arthritis. *Lancet* 1994;344(8930):1105-1110.
10. Felson DT, Anderson JJ, Boers M, et al. American College of Rheumatology preliminary definition of improvement in rheumatoid arthritis. *Arthritis Rheum* 1995;38(6):727-735.
11. Fries JF, Spitz PW, Young DY. The dimensions of health outcomes: the health assessment questionnaire, disability and pain scales. *J Rheumatol* 1982;9(5):789-793.
12. Van der Heijde DM, van Leeuwen MA, van Riel PL, et al. Biannual radiographic assessments of hands and feet in a three-year prospective followup of patients with early rheumatoid arthritis. *Arthritis Rheum* 1992;35(1):26-34.
13. Ware JE Jr, Sherbourne CD. The MOS 36-item short-form health survey (SF-36). I. Conceptual framework and item selection. *Med Care* 1992;30(6):473-483.
14. **Targan SR, Hanauer SR, van Deventer SJH, et al. A short-term study of chimeric monoclonal antibody cA2**

Table 4

ADVERSE EVENTS IN RHEUMATOID ARTHRITIS AND CROHN'S DISEASE STUDIES AT A RATE OF AT LEAST 5%

	RHEUMATOID ARTHRITIS		CROHN'S DISEASE	
	Placebo (n=133)	REMICADE (n=555)	Placebo (n=56)	REMICADE (n=199)
Avg. weeks of follow-up	52	68	15	27
Respiratory				
Upper respiratory infection	23%	33%	9%	16%
Coughing	7%	16%	0%	5%
Sinusitis	6%	16%	2%	5%
Pharyngitis	9%	14%	5%	9%
Rhinitis	8%	11%	4%	6%
Bronchitis	9%	11%	2%	7%
Dyspnea	3%	6%	0%	3%
Gastrointestinal				
Nausea	20%	21%	4%	17%
Diarrhea	14%	16%	2%	3%
Abdominal Pain	9%	15%	4%	12%
Vomiting	11%	11%	0%	9%
Dyspepsia	6%	9%	0%	5%
Ulcerative stomatitis	2%	7%	4%	2%
Other				
Headache	16%	26%	21%	23%
Rash	6%	15%	5%	6%
Urinary tract infection	8%	13%	4%	3%
Dizziness	11%	12%	9%	8%
Pain	12%	12%	5%	9%
Arthralgia	5%	11%	2%	5%
Fever	8%	11%	7%	10%
Back pain	4%	10%	4%	5%
Fatigue	5%	10%	5%	11%
Hypertension	5%	8%	2%	1%
Pruritus	2%	8%	2%	5%
Worsening of rheumatoid arthritis	7%	8%	0%	0%
Peripheral edema	6%	7%	2%	1%
Chest pain	5%	6%	5%	6%
Depression	3%	6%	0%	2%
Moniliasis	2%	6%	0%	5%
Urticaria	1%	6%	0%	3%

to tumor necrosis factor α for Crohn's disease. *N Engl J Med* 1997;337(15):1029-1035.
15. Present DH, Rutgeerts P, Targan S, et al. Infliximab for the treatment of fistulas in patients with Crohn's disease. *N Engl J Med* 1999;340:1398-1405.
16. Greenstein AJ, Mullin GE, Strauchen JA, et al. Lymphoma in inflammatory bowel disease. *Cancer* 1992;69:1119-1121.
17. Jones M, Symmons D, Finn J, et al. Does exposure to immunosuppressive therapy increase the 10 year malignancy and mortality risks in rheumatoid arthritis? A matched cohort study. *Br J Rheum* 1996;35:738-745.

Malvern, PA 19355, USA Revised March 2002
1-800-457-6399 IN02075

Cephalon, Inc.

145 BRANDYWINE PARKWAY
WEST CHESTER, PA 19380

For Medical Information/ADVERSE EXPERIENCE REPORTING CONTACT:
(800) 896-5855
Fax 610-738-6669

ACTIQ® Ⓒ℞

[*act' ĭc*]
(oral transmucosal fentanyl citrate)

Prescribing information for this product, which appears on pages 1184–1188 of the 2002 PDR, has been completely revised as follows. Please write "See Supplement A" next to the product heading.

PHYSICIANS AND OTHER HEALTHCARE PROVIDERS MUST BECOME FAMILIAR WITH THE IMPORTANT WARNINGS IN THIS LABEL.
***Actiq* is indicated only for the management of breakthrough cancer pain in patients with malignancies who are already receiving and who are tolerant to opioid therapy for their underlying persistent cancer pain.**
Patients considered opioid tolerant are those who are taking at least 60 mg morphine/day, 50 mcg transdermal fentanyl/hour, or an equianalgesic dose of another opioid for a week or longer.
Because life-threatening hypoventilation could occur at any dose in patients not taking chronic opiates, *Actiq* is contraindicated in the management of acute or postoperative pain. This product must not be used in opioid non-tolerant patients.
Actiq is intended to be used only in the care of cancer patients and only by oncologists and pain specialists who are knowledgeable of and skilled in the use of Schedule II opioids to treat cancer pain.
Patients and their caregivers must be instructed that *Actiq* contains a medicine in an amount which can be fatal to a child. Patients and their caregivers must be instructed to keep all units out of the reach of children and to discard open units properly. (See Information for Patients and Their Caregivers for disposal instructions.)

WARNING: May be habit forming

DESCRIPTION

Actiq (oral transmucosal fentanyl citrate) is a solid formulation of fentanyl citrate, a potent opioid analgesic, intended for oral transmucosal administration. *Actiq* is formulated as a white to off-white solid drug matrix on a handle that is radiopaque and is fracture resistant (ABS plastic) under normal conditions when used as directed.
Actiq is designed to be dissolved slowly in the mouth in a manner to facilitate transmucosal absorption. The handle allows the *Actiq* unit to be removed from the mouth if signs of excessive opioid effects appear during administration.
Active Ingredient: Fentanyl citrate, USP is N-(1-Phenethyl-4-piperidyl) propionanilide citrate (1:1). Fentanyl is a highly lipophilic compound (octanol-water partition coefficient at pH 7.4 is 816:1) that is freely soluble in organic solvents and sparingly soluble in water (1:40). The molecular weight of the free base is 336.5 (the citrate salt is 528.6). The pKa of the tertiary nitrogens are 7.3 and 8.4. The compound has the following structural formula:

CH_3CH_2CON – N – CH_2CH_2 · $HO\text{-}C(CH_2COOH)_2\text{-}COOH$

Actiq is available in six strengths equivalent to 200, 400, 600, 800, 1200, or 1600 mcg fentanyl base that is identified by the text on the foil pouch, the shelf carton, and the dosage unit handle.
Inactive Ingredients: Sucrose, liquid glucose, artificial raspberry flavor, and white dispersion G.B. dye.

Table 1.
Pharmacokinetic Parameters in Adult Subjects Receiving 200, 400, 800, and 1600 mcg Units of *Actiq*

Pharmacokinetic Parameter	200 mcg	400 mcg	800 mcg	1600 mcg
T_{max}, minute median (range)	40 (20-120)	25 (20-240)	25 (20-120)	20 (20-480)
C_{max}, ng/mL mean (% CV)	0.39 (23)	0.75 (33)	1.55 (30)	2.51 (23)
AUC_{0-1440}, ng/mL minute mean (% CV)	102 (65)	243 (67)	573 (64)	1026 (67)
$t_{1/2}$, minute mean (% CV)	193 (48)	386 (115)	381 (55)	358 (45)

CLINICAL PHARMACOLOGY AND PHARMACOKINETICS

Pharmacology:
Fentanyl, a pure opioid agonist, acts primarily through interaction with opioid mu-receptors located in the brain, spinal cord and smooth muscle. The primary site of therapeutic action is the central nervous system (CNS). The most clinically useful pharmacologic effects of the interaction of fentanyl with mu-receptors are analgesia and sedation.
Other opioid effects may include somnolence, hypoventilation, bradycardia, postural hypotension, pruritus, dizziness, nausea, diaphoresis, flushing, euphoria and confusion or difficulty in concentrating at clinically relevant doses.

Clinical Pharmacology

Analgesia:
The analgesic effects of fentanyl are related to the blood level of the drug, if proper allowance is made for the delay into and out of the CNS (a process with a 3-to-5-minute half-life). In opioid non-tolerant individuals, fentanyl provides effects ranging from analgesia at blood levels of 1 to 2 ng/mL, all the way to surgical anesthesia and profound respiratory depression at levels of 10-20 ng/mL.
In general, the minimum effective concentration and the concentration at which toxicity occurs rise with increasing tolerance to any and all opioids. The rate of development of tolerance varies widely among individuals. As a result, the dose of *Actiq* should be individually titrated to achieve the desired effect (see **DOSAGE AND ADMINISTRATION**).

Gastrointestinal (GI) Tract and Other Smooth Muscle:
Opioids increase the tone and decrease contractions of the smooth muscle of the gastrointestinal (GI) tract. This results in prolongation in GI transit time and may be responsible for the constipating effect of opioids. Because opioids may increase biliary tract pressure, some patients with biliary colic may experience worsening of pain.
While opioids generally increase the tone of urinary tract smooth muscle, the overall effect tends to vary, in some cases producing urinary urgency, in others, difficulty in urination.

Respiratory System:
All opioid mu-receptor agonists, including fentanyl, produce dose dependent respiratory depression. The risk of respiratory depression is less in patients receiving chronic opioid therapy who develop tolerance to respiratory depression and other opioid effects. During the titration phase of the clinical trials, somnolence, which may be a precursor to respiratory depression, did increase in patients who were treated with higher doses of *Actiq*. In studies of opioid non-tolerant subjects, respiratory rate and oxygen saturation typically decrease as fentanyl blood concentration increases. Typically, peak respiratory depressive effects (decrease in respiratory rate) are seen 15 to 30 minutes from the start of oral transmucosal fentanyl citrate (OTFC®) administration and may persist for several hours.
Serious or fatal respiratory depression can occur, even at recommended doses, in vulnerable individuals. As with other potent opioids, fentanyl has been associated with cases of serious and fatal respiratory depression in opioid non-tolerant individuals.
Fentanyl depresses the cough reflex as a result of its CNS activity. Although not observed with *Actiq* in clinical trials, fentanyl given rapidly by intravenous injection in large doses may interfere with respiration by causing rigidity in the muscles of respiration. Therefore, physicians and other healthcare providers should be aware of this potential complication. **(See BOX WARNING, CONTRAINDICATIONS, WARNINGS, PRECAUTIONS, ADVERSE REACTIONS, and OVERDOSAGE for additional information on hypoventilation.)**

Pharmacokinetics

Absorption:
The absorption pharmacokinetics of fentanyl from the oral transmucosal dosage form is a combination of an initial rapid absorption from the buccal mucosa and a more prolonged absorption of swallowed fentanyl from the GI tract. Both the blood fentanyl profile and the bioavailability of fentanyl will vary depending on the fraction of the dose that is absorbed through the oral mucosa and the fraction swallowed.
Absolute bioavailability, as determined by area under the concentration-time curve, of 15 mcg/kg in 12 adult males was 50% compared to intravenous fentanyl.
Normally, approximately 25% of the total dose of *Actiq* is rapidly absorbed from the buccal mucosa and becomes systemically available. The remaining 75% of the total dose is swallowed with the saliva and then is slowly absorbed from the GI tract. About 1/3 of this amount (25% of the total dose) escapes hepatic and intestinal first-pass elimination and becomes systemically available. Thus, the generally observed 50% bioavailability of *Actiq* is divided equally between rapid transmucosal and slower GI absorption. Therefore, a unit dose of *Actiq*, if chewed and swallowed, might result in lower peak concentrations and lower bioavailability than when consumed as directed.
Dose proportionality among four of the available strengths of *Actiq* (200, 400, 800, and 1600 mcg) has been demonstrated in a balanced crossover design in adult subjects. Mean serum fentanyl levels following these four doses of *Actiq* are shown in Figure 1. The curves for each dose level are similar in shape with increasing dose levels producing increasing serum fentanyl levels. C_{max} and $AUC_{0 \to \infty}$ increased in a dose-dependent manner that is approximately proportional to the *Actiq* administered.

Figure 1.
Mean Serum Fentanyl Concentration (ng/mL) in Adult Subjects Comparing 4 Doses of *Actiq*

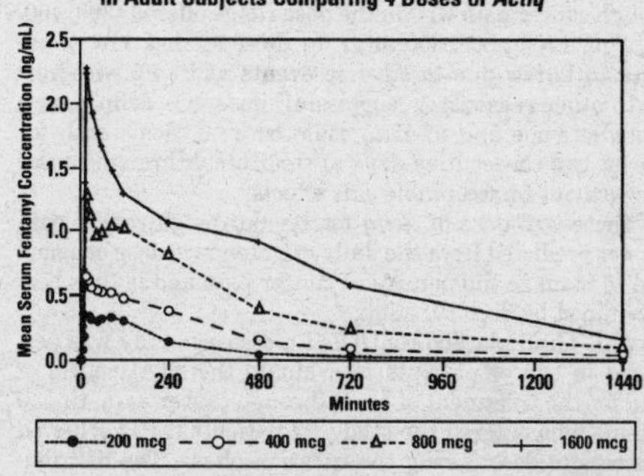

The pharmacokinetic parameters of the four strengths of *Actiq* tested in the dose-proportionality study are shown in Table 1. The mean C_{max} ranged from 0.39 - 2.51 ng/mL. The median time of maximum plasma concentration (T_{max}) across these four doses of *Actiq* varied from 20 - 40 minutes (range of 20-480 minutes) after a standardized consumption time of 15 minutes.
[See table 1 above]

Distribution:
Fentanyl is highly lipophilic. Animal data showed that following absorption, fentanyl is rapidly distributed to the brain, heart, lungs, kidneys and spleen followed by a slower redistribution to muscles and fat. The plasma protein binding of fentanyl is 80-85%. The main binding protein is alpha-1-acid glycoprotein, but both albumin and lipoproteins contribute to some extent. The free fraction of fentanyl increases with acidosis. The mean volume of distribution at steady state (V_{ss}) was 4 L/kg.

Metabolism:
Fentanyl is metabolized in the liver and in the intestinal mucosa to norfentanyl by cytochrome P450 3A4 isoform. Norfentanyl was not found to be pharmacologically active in animal studies (see **PRECAUTIONS: Drug Interactions** for additional information).

Elimination:
Fentanyl is primarily (more than 90%) eliminated by biotransformation to N-dealkylated and hydroxylated inactive metabolites. Less than 7% of the dose is excreted unchanged in the urine, and only about 1% is excreted unchanged in the feces. The metabolites are mainly excreted in the urine, while fecal excretion is less important. The total plasma clearance of fentanyl was 0.5 L/hr/kg (range 0.3 - 0.7 L/hr/kg). The terminal elimination half-life after *OTFC* administration is about 7 hours.

Special Populations:

Elderly Patients:
Elderly patients have been shown to be twice as sensitive to the effects of fentanyl when administered intravenously, compared with the younger population. While a formal study evaluating the safety profile of *Actiq* in the elderly population has not been performed, in the 257 opioid tolerant cancer patients studied with *Actiq*, approximately 20% were over age 65 years. No difference was noted in the safety profile in this group compared to those aged less than 65 years, though they did titrate to lower doses than younger patients (see **PRECAUTIONS**).

Patients with Renal or Hepatic Impairment:
Actiq should be administered with caution to patients with liver or kidney dysfunction because of the importance of these organs in the metabolism and excretion of drugs and effects on plasma-binding proteins (see **PRECAUTIONS**). Although fentanyl kinetics are known to be altered in both hepatic and renal disease due to alterations in metabolic clearance and plasma proteins, individualized doses of *Actiq* have been used successfully for breakthrough cancer pain in patients with hepatic and renal disorders. The duration of effect for the initial dose of fentanyl is determined by redis-

Continued on next page

Actiq—Cont.

tribution of the drug, such that diminished metabolic clearance may only become significant with repeated dosing or with excessively large single doses. For these reasons, while doses titrated to clinical effect are recommended for all patients, special care should be taken in patients with severe hepatic or renal disease.

Gender

Both male and female opioid-tolerant cancer patients were studied for the treatment of breakthrough cancer pain. No clinically relevant gender differences were noted either in dosage requirement or in observed adverse events.

CLINICAL TRIALS

Breakthrough Cancer Pain:

Actiq was investigated in clinical trials involving 257 opioid tolerant adult cancer patients experiencing breakthrough cancer pain. Breakthrough cancer pain was defined as a transient flare of moderate-to-severe pain occurring in cancer patients experiencing persistent cancer pain otherwise controlled with maintenance doses of opioid medications including at least 60 mg morphine/day, 50 mcg transdermal fentanyl/hour, or an equianalgesic dose of another opioid for a week or longer.

In two dose titration studies 95 of 127 patients (75%) who were on stable doses of either long-acting oral opioids or transdermal fentanyl for their persistent cancer pain titrated to a successful dose of *Actiq* to treat their breakthrough cancer pain within the dose range offered (200, 400, 600, 800, 1200 and 1600 mcg). In these studies 11% of patients withdrew due to adverse events and 14% withdrew due to other reasons. A "successful" dose was defined as a dose where one unit of *Actiq* could be used consistently for at least two consecutive days to treat breakthrough cancer pain without unacceptable side effects.

The successful dose of *Actiq* for breakthrough cancer pain was not predicted from the daily maintenance dose of opioid used to manage the persistent cancer pain and is thus best determined by dose titration.

A double-blind placebo controlled crossover study was performed in cancer patients to evaluate the effectiveness of *Actiq* for the treatment of breakthrough cancer pain. Of 130 patients who entered the study, 92 patients (71%) achieved a successful dose during the titration phase. The distribution of successful doses is shown in Table 2.

Table 2.
Successful Dose of *Actiq* Following Initial Titration

Actiq Dose	Total No (%) (N=92)
200 mcg	13 (14)
400 mcg	19 (21)
600 mcg	14 (15)
800 mcg	18 (20)
1200 mcg	13 (14)
1600 mcg	15 (16)
Mean±SD	789±468 mcg

On average, patients over 65 years of age titrated to a mean dose that was about 200 mcg less than the mean dose to which younger adult patients were titrated.

Actiq produced statistically significantly more pain relief compared with placebo at 15, 30, 45 and 60 minutes following administration (see Figure 2).

Figure 2
Pain Relief (PR) Scores (Mean±SD) During the Double-Blind Phase-All Patients with Evaluable Episodes on Both *Actiq* and Placebo (N=86)

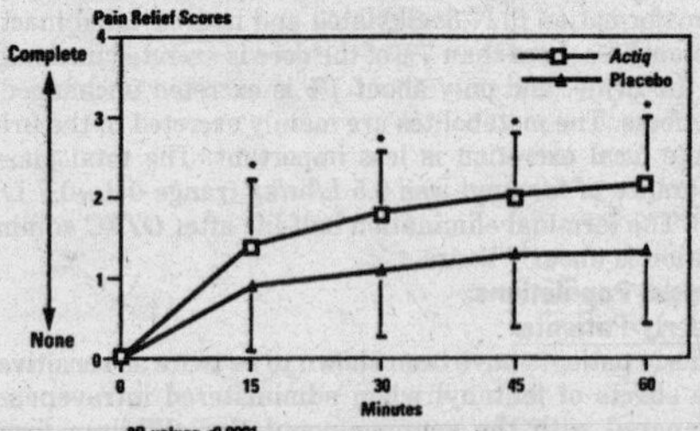

In this same study patients also rated the performance of medication to treat their breakthrough cancer pain using a different scale ranging from "poor" to "excellent." On average, placebo was rated "fair" and *Actiq* was rated "good."

INDICATIONS AND USAGE

(See BOX WARNING and CONTRAINDICATIONS)

Actiq is indicated only for the management of breakthrough cancer pain in patients with malignancies who are **already receiving and who are tolerant to opioid therapy for their underlying persistent cancer pain.** Patients considered opioid tolerant are those who are taking at least 60 mg morphine/day, 50 mcg transdermal fentanyl/hour, or an equianalgesic dose of another opioid for a week or longer.

Because life-threatening hypoventilation could occur at any dose in patients not taking chronic opiates, *Actiq* is contraindicated in the management of acute or postoperative pain. This product **must not** be used in opioid non-tolerant patients.

Actiq is intended to be used only in the care of cancer patients and only by oncologists and pain specialists who are knowledgeable of and skilled in the use of Schedule II opioids to treat cancer pain.

Actiq should be individually titrated to a dose that provides adequate analgesia and minimizes side effects. If signs of excessive opioid effects appear before the unit is consumed, the dosage unit should be removed from the patient's mouth immediately, disposed of properly, and subsequent doses should be decreased (see **DOSAGE AND ADMINISTRATION**).

Patients and their caregivers must be instructed that *Actiq* contains a medicine in an amount that can be fatal to a child. Patients and their caregivers must be instructed to keep all units out of the reach of children and to discard opened units properly in a secured container.

CONTRAINDICATIONS

Because life-threatening hypoventilation could occur at any dose in patients not taking chronic opiates, *Actiq* is contraindicated in the management of acute or postoperative pain. The risk of respiratory depression begins to increase with fentanyl plasma levels of 2.0 ng/mL in opioid nontolerant individuals (see **Pharmacokinetics**). This product **must not** be used in opioid non-tolerant patients.

Patients considered opioid tolerant are those who are taking at least 60 mg morphine/day, 50 mcg transdermal fentanyl/hour, or an equianalgesic dose of another opioid for a week or longer.

Actiq is contraindicated in patients with known intolerance or hypersensitivity to any of its components or the drug fentanyl.

WARNINGS

See BOX WARNING

The concomitant use of other CNS depressants, including other opioids, sedatives or hypnotics, general anesthetics, phenothiazines, tranquilizers, skeletal muscle relaxants, sedating antihistamines, potent inhibitors of cytochrome P450 3A4 isoform (e.g., erythromycin, ketoconazole, and certain protease inhibitors), and alcoholic beverages may produce increased depressant effects. Hypoventilation, hypotension, and profound sedation may occur.

Actiq is not recommended for use in patients who have received MAO inhibitors within 14 days, because severe and unpredictable potentiation by MAO inhibitors has been reported with opioid analgesics.

Pediatric Use: The appropriate dosing and safety of *Actiq* in opioid tolerant children with breakthrough cancer pain have not been established below the age of 16 years.

Patients and their caregivers must be instructed that *Actiq* contains a medicine in an amount which can be fatal to a child. Patients and their caregivers must be instructed to keep both used and unused dosage units out of the reach of children. While all units should be disposed of immediately after use, partially consumed units represent a special risk to children. In the event that a unit is not completely consumed it must be properly disposed as soon as possible. (See **SAFETY AND HANDLING, PRECAUTIONS,** and **PATIENT LEAFLET** for specific patient instructions.)

Physicians and dispensing pharmacists must specifically question patients or caregivers about the presence of children in the home on a full time or visiting basis and counsel them regarding the dangers to children from inadvertent exposure.

PRECAUTIONS

General

The initial dose of *Actiq* to treat episodes of breakthrough cancer pain should be 200 mcg. Each patient should be individually titrated to provide adequate analgesia while minimizing side effects.

Opioid analgesics impair the mental and/or physical ability required for the performance of potentially dangerous tasks (e.g., driving a car or operating machinery). Patients taking *Actiq* should be warned of these dangers and should be counseled accordingly.

The use of concomitant CNS active drugs requires special patient care and observation. (See **WARNINGS**.)

Hypoventilation (Respiratory Depression)

As with all opioids, there is a risk of clinically significant hypoventilation in patients using *Actiq*. Accordingly, all patients should be followed for symptoms of respiratory depression. Hypoventilation may occur more readily when opioids are given in conjunction with other agents that depress respiration.

Chronic Pulmonary Disease

Because potent opioids can cause hypoventilation, *Actiq* should be titrated with caution in patients with chronic obstructive pulmonary disease or pre-existing medical conditions predisposing them to hypoventilation. In such patients, even normal therapeutic doses of *Actiq* may further decrease respiratory drive to the point of respiratory failure.

Head Injuries and Increased Intracranial Pressure

Actiq should only be administered with extreme caution in patients who may be particularly susceptible to the intracranial effects of CO_2 retention such as those with evidence of increased intracranial pressure or impaired consciousness. Opioids may obscure the clinical course of a patient with a head injury and should be used only if clinically warranted.

Cardiac Disease

Intravenous fentanyl may produce bradycardia. Therefore, *Actiq* should be used with caution in patients with bradyarrhythmias.

Hepatic or Renal Disease

Actiq should be administered with caution to patients with liver or kidney dysfunction because of the importance of these organs in the metabolism and excretion of drugs and effects on plasma binding proteins (see **PHARMACOKINETICS**).

Information for Patients and Their Caregivers

Patients and their caregivers must be instructed that *Actiq* contains medicine in an amount that could be fatal to a child. Patients and their caregivers must be instructed to keep both used and unused dosage units out of the reach of children. Partially consumed units represent a special risk to children. In the event that a unit is not completely consumed it must be properly disposed as soon as possible. (See **SAFETY AND HANDLING, WARNINGS,** and **PATIENT LEAFLET** for specific patient instructions.)

Frequent consumption of sugar-containing products may increase the risk of dental caries (each *Actiq* unit contains approximately 2 grams of sugar [sucrose, liquid glucose]). The occurrence of dry mouth associated with the use of opioid medications (such as fentanyl) may add to this risk. Therefore, patients using *Actiq* should consult their dentist to ensure appropriate oral hygiene.

Diabetic patients should be advised that *Actiq* contains approximately 2 grams of sugar per unit.

Patients and their caregivers should be provided with an *Actiq* Welcome Kit, which contains educational materials and safe storage containers to help patients store *Actiq* and other medicines out of the reach of children. Patients and their caregivers should also have an opportunity to watch the patient safety video, which provides proper product use, storage, handling and disposal directions. Patients should also have an opportunity to discuss the video with their health care providers. Health care professionals should call 1-800-896-5855 to obtain a supply of welcome kits or videos for patient viewing.

Disposal of Used *Actiq* Units

Patients must be instructed to dispose of completely used and partially used *Actiq* units.

1) After consumption of the unit is complete and the matrix is totally dissolved, throw away the handle in a trash container that is out of the reach of children.
2) If any of the drug matrix remains on the handle, place the handle under hot running tap water until all of the drug matrix is dissolved, and then dispose of the handle in a place that is out of the reach of children.
3) Handles in the child-resistant container should be disposed of (as described in steps 1 and 2) at least once a day.

If the patient does not entirely consume the unit and the remaining drug cannot be immediately dissolved under hot running water, the patient or caregiver must temporarily store the *Actiq* unit in the specially provided child-resistant container out of the reach of children until proper disposal is possible.

Disposal of Unopened *Actiq* Units When No Longer Needed

Patients and members of their household must be advised to dispose of any unopened units remaining from a prescription as soon as they are no longer needed.

To dispose of the unused *Actiq* units:

1) Remove the *Actiq* unit from its pouch using scissors, and hold the *Actiq* by its handle over the toilet bowl.
2) Using wire-cutting pliers cut off the drug matrix end so that it falls into the toilet.
3) Dispose of the handle in a place that is out of the reach of children.
4) Repeat steps 1, 2, and 3 for each *Actiq* unit. Flush the toilet twice after 5 units have been cut and deposited into the toilet.

Do not flush the entire *Actiq* units, *Actiq* handles, foil pouches, or cartons down the toilet. The handle should be disposed of where children cannot reach it (see **SAFETY AND HANDLING**).

Detailed instructions for the proper storage, administration, disposal, and important instructions for managing an overdose of *Actiq* are provided in the *Actiq* Patient Leaflet. Patients should be encouraged to read this information in its entirety and be given an opportunity to have their questions answered.

In the event that a caregiver requires additional assistance in disposing of excess unusable units that remain in the home after a patient has expired, they should be instructed to call the toll-free number (1-800-896-5855) or seek assistance from their local DEA office.

Laboratory Tests

The effects of *Actiq* on laboratory tests have not been evaluated.

Drug Interactions

See **WARNINGS.**

Fentanyl is metabolized in the liver and intestinal mucosa to norfentanyl by the cytochrome P450 3A4 isoform. Drugs that inhibit P450 3A4 activity may increase the bioavailability of swallowed fentanyl (by decreasing intestinal and hepatic first pass metabolism) and may decrease the systemic clearance of fentanyl. The expected clinical results would be increased or prolonged opioid effects. Drugs that induce cytochrome P450 3A4 activity may have the opposite effects. However, no *in vitro* or *in vivo* studies have been performed to assess the impact of those potential interactions on the administration of *Actiq*. Thus patients who begin or end therapy with potent inhibitors of CYP450 3A4 such as macrolide antibiotics (e.g., erythromycin), azole antifungal agents (e.g., ketoconazole and itraconazole), and protease inhibitors (e.g., ritanovir) while receiving *Actiq* should be monitored for a change in opioid effects and, if warranted, the dose of *Actiq* should be adjusted.

Carcinogenesis, Mutagenesis, and Impairment of Fertility
Because animal carcinogenicity studies have not been conducted with fentanyl citrate, the potential carcinogenic effect of *Actiq* is unknown.

Standard mutagenicity testing of fentanyl citrate has been conducted. There was no evidence of mutagenicity in the Ames *Salmonella* or *Escherichia* mutagenicity assay, the *in-vitro* mouse lymphoma mutagenesis assay, and the *in-vivo* micronucleus cytogenetic assay in the mouse.

Reproduction studies in rats revealed a significant decrease in the pregnancy rate of all experimental groups. This decrease was most pronounced in the high dose group (1.25 mg/kg subcutaneously) in which one of twenty animals became pregnant.

Pregnancy - Category C
Fentanyl has been shown to impair fertility and to have an embryocidal effect with an increase in resorptions in rats when given for a period of 12 to 21 days in doses of 30 mcg/kg IV or 160 mcg/kg subcutaneously.

No evidence of teratogenic effects has been observed after administration of fentanyl citrate to rats. There are no adequate and well-controlled studies in pregnant women. *Actiq* should be used during pregnancy only if the potential benefit justifies the potential risk to the fetus.

Labor and Delivery
Actiq is not indicated for use in labor and delivery.

Nursing Mothers
Fentanyl is excreted in human milk; therefore *Actiq* should not be used in nursing women because of the possibility of sedation and/or respiratory depression in their infants.

Pediatric Use
See **WARNINGS.**

Geriatric Use
Of the 257 patients in clinical studies of *Actiq* in breakthrough cancer pain, 61 (24%) were 65 and over, while 15 (6%) were 75 and over.

Those patients over the age of 65 titrated to a mean dose that was about 200 mcg less than the mean dose titrated to by younger patients. Previous studies with intravenous fentanyl showed that elderly patients are twice as sensitive to the effects of fentanyl as the younger population.

No difference was noted in the safety profile of the group over 65 as compared to younger patients in *Actiq* clinical trials. However, greater sensitivity in older individuals cannot be ruled out. Therefore, caution should be exercised in individually titrating *Actiq* in elderly patients to provide adequate efficacy while minimizing risk.

ADVERSE REACTIONS

Pre-Marketing Clinical Trial Experience

The safety of *Actiq* has been evaluated in 257 opioid tolerant chronic cancer pain patients. The duration of *Actiq* use varied during the open-label study. Some patients were followed for over 21 months. The average duration of therapy in the open-label study was 129 days.

The adverse events seen with *Actiq* are typical opioid side effects. Frequently, these adverse events will cease or decrease in intensity with continued use of *Actiq*, as the patient is titrated to the proper dose. Opioid side effects should be expected and managed accordingly.

The most serious adverse effects associated with all opioids are respiratory depression (potentially leading to apnea or respiratory arrest), circulatory depression, hypotension, and shock. All patients should be followed for symptoms of respiratory depression.

Because the clinical trials of *Actiq* were designed to evaluate safety and efficacy in treating breakthrough cancer pain, all patients were also taking concomitant opioids, such as sustained-release morphine or transdermal fentanyl, for their persistent cancer pain. The adverse event data presented here reflect the actual percentage of patients experiencing each adverse effect among patients who received *Actiq* for breakthrough cancer pain along with a concomitant opioid for persistent cancer pain. There has been no attempt to correct for concomitant use of other opioids, duration of *Actiq* therapy, or cancer-related symptoms. Adverse events are included regardless of causality or severity.

Three short-term clinical trials with similar titration schemes were conducted in 257 patients with malignancy and breakthrough cancer pain. Data are available for 254 of these patients. The goal of titration in these trials was to find the dose of *Actiq* that provided adequate analgesia with acceptable side effects (successful dose). Patients were titrated from a low dose to a successful dose in a manner similar to current titration dosing guidelines. Table 3 lists by dose groups, adverse events with an overall frequency of 1% or greater that occurred during titration and are commonly associated with opioid administration or are of particular clinical interest. The ability to assign a dose-response relationship to these adverse events is limited by the titration schemes used in these studies. Adverse events are listed in descending order of frequency within each body system.

[See table 3 above]

Table 3.
Percent of Patients with Specific Adverse Events Commonly Associated with Opioid Administration or of Particular Clinical Interest Which Occurred During Titration (Events in 1% or More of Patients)

Dose Group	200-600 mcg	800-1400 mcg	1600 mcg	>1600 mcg	Any
Number of Patients	**230**	**138**	**54**	**41**	**254**
Body As A Whole					
Asthenia	6	4	0	7	9
Headache	3	4	6	5	6
Accidental Injury	1	1	4	0	2
Digestive					
Nausea	14	15	11	22	23
Vomiting	7	6	6	15	12
Constipation	1	4	2	0	4
Nervous					
Dizziness	10	16	6	15	17
Somnolence	9	9	11	20	17
Confusion	1	6	2	0	4
Anxiety	3	0	2	0	3
Abnormal Gait	0	1	4	0	2
Dry Mouth	1	1	2	0	2
Nervousness	1	1	0	0	2
Vasodilatation	2	0	2	0	2
Hallucinations	0	1	2	2	1
Insomnia	0	1	2	0	1
Thinking Abnormal	0	1	2	0	1
Vertigo	1	0	0	0	1
Respiratory					
Dyspnea	2	3	6	5	4
Skin					
Pruritus	1	0	0	5	2
Rash	1	1	0	2	2
Sweating	1	1	2	2	2
Special Senses					
Abnormal Vision	1	0	2	0	2

The following adverse events not reflected in Table 3 occurred during titration with an overall frequency of 1% or greater and are listed in descending order of frequency within each body system.

Body as a Whole: Pain, fever, abdominal pain, chills, back pain, chest pain, infection
Cardiovascular: Migraine
Digestive: Diarrhea, dyspepsia, flatulence
Metabolic and Nutritional: Peripheral edema, dehydration
Nervous: Hypesthesia
Respiratory: Pharyngitis, cough increased

The following events occurred during titration with an overall frequency of less than 1% and are listed in descending order of frequency within each body system.

Body as a Whole: Flu syndrome, abscess, bone pain
Cardiovascular: Deep thrombophlebitis, hypertension, hypotension
Digestive: Anorexia, eructation, esophageal stenosis, fecal impaction, gum hemorrhage, mouth ulceration, oral moniliasis
Hemic and Lymphatic: Anemia, leukopenia
Metabolic and Nutritional: Edema, hypercalcemia, weight loss
Musculoskeletal: Myalgia, pathological fracture, myasthenia
Nervous: Abnormal dreams, urinary retention, agitation, amnesia, emotional lability, euphoria, incoordination, libido decreased, neuropathy, paresthesia, speech disorder
Respiratory: Hemoptysis, pleural effusion, rhinitis, asthma, hiccup, pneumonia, respiratory insufficiency, sputum increased
Skin and Appendages: Alopecia, exfoliative dermatitis
Special Senses: Taste perversion
Urogenital: Vaginal hemorrhage, dysuria, hematuria, urinary incontinence, urinary tract infection

A long-term extension study was conducted in 156 patients with malignancy and breakthrough cancer pain who were treated for an average of 129 days. Data are available for 152 of these patients. Table 4 lists by dose groups, adverse events with an overall frequency of 1% or greater that occurred during the long-term extension study and are commonly associated with opioid administration or are of particular clinical interest. Adverse events are listed in descending order of frequency within each body system.

[See table 4 at top of next page]

The following events not reflected in Table 4 occurred with an overall frequency of 1% or greater in the long-term extension study and are listed in descending order of frequency within each body system.

Body as a Whole: Pain, fever, back pain, abdominal pain, chest pain, flu syndrome, chills, infection, abdomen enlarged, bone pain, ascites, sepsis, neck pain, viral infection, fungal infection, cachexia, cellulitis, malaise, pelvic pain
Cardiovascular: Deep thrombophlebitis, migraine, palpitation, vascular disorder
Digestive: Diarrhea, anorexia, dyspepsia, dysphagia, oral moniliasis, mouth ulceration, rectal disorder, stomatitis, flatulence, gastrointestinal hemorrhage, gingivitis, jaundice, periodontal abscess, eructation, glossitis, rectal hemorrhage
Hemic and Lymphatic: Anemia, leukopenia, thrombocytopenia, ecchymosis, lymphadenopathy, lymphedema, pancytopenia
Metabolic and Nutritional: Peripheral edema, edema, dehydration, weight loss, hyperglycemia, hypokalemia, hypercalcemia, hypomagnesemia
Musculoskeletal: Myalgia, pathological fracture, joint disorder, leg cramps, arthralgia, bone disorder
Nervous: Hypesthesia, paresthesia, hypokinesia, neuropathy, speech disorder
Respiratory: Cough increased, pharyngitis, pneumonia, rhinitis, sinusitis, bronchitis, epistaxis, asthma, hemoptysis, sputum increased
Skin and Appendages: Skin ulcer, alopecia
Special Senses: Tinnitus, conjunctivitis, ear disorder, taste perversion
Urogenital: Urinary tract infection, urinary incontinence, breast pain, dysuria, hematuria, scrotal edema, hydronephrosis, kidney failure, urinary urgency, urination impaired, breast neoplasm, vaginal hemorrhage, vaginitis

The following events occurred with a frequency of less than 1% in the long-term extension study and are listed in descending order of frequency within each body system.

Body as a Whole: Allergic reaction, cyst, face edema, flank pain, granuloma, bacterial infection, injection site pain, mucous membrane disorder, neck rigidity

Continued on next page

Actiq—Cont.

Cardiovascular: Angina pectoris, hemorrhage, hypotension, peripheral vascular disorder, postural hypotension, tachycardia
Digestive: Cheilitis, esophagitis, fecal incontinence, gastroenteritis, gastrointestinal disorder, gum hemorrhage, hemorrhage of colon, hepatorenal syndrome, liver tenderness, tooth caries, tooth disorder
Hemic and Lymphatic: Bleeding time increased
Metabolic and Nutritional: Acidosis, generalized edema, hypocalcemia, hypoglycemia, hyponatremia, hypoproteinemia, thirst
Musculoskeletal: Arthritis, muscle atrophy, myopathy, synovitis, tendon disorder
Nervous: Acute brain syndrome, agitation, cerebral ischemia, facial paralysis, foot drop, hallucinations, hemiplegia, miosis, subdural hematoma
Respiratory: Hiccup, hyperventilation, lung disorder, pneumothorax, respiratory failure, voice alteration
Skin and Appendages: Herpes zoster, maculopapular rash, skin discoloration, urticaria, vesiculobullous rash
Special Senses: Ear pain, eye hemorrhage, lacrimation disorder, partial permanent deafness, partial transitory deafness
Urogenital: Kidney pain, nocturia, oliguria, polyuria, pyelonephritis

DRUG ABUSE AND DEPENDENCE

Fentanyl is a mu-opioid agonist and a Schedule II controlled substance that can produce drug dependence of the morphine type. *Actiq* may be subject to misuse, abuse and addiction.

The administration of *Actiq* should be guided by the response of the patient. Physical dependence, per se, is not ordinarily a concern when one is treating a patient with chronic cancer pain, and fear of tolerance and physical dependence should not deter using doses that adequately relieve the pain.

Opioid analgesics may cause physical dependence. Physical dependence results in withdrawal symptoms in patients who abruptly discontinue the drug. Withdrawal also may be precipitated through the administration of drugs with opioid antagonist activity, e.g., naloxone, nalmefene, or mixed agonist/antagonist analgesics (pentazocine, butorphanol, buprenorphine, nalbuphine).

Physical dependence usually does not occur to a clinically significant degree until after several weeks of continued opioid usage. Tolerance, in which increasingly larger doses are required in order to produce the same degree of analgesia, is initially manifested by a shortened duration of analgesic effect, and subsequently, by decreases in the intensity of analgesia.

The handling of *Actiq* should be managed to minimize the risk of diversion, including restriction of access and accounting procedures as appropriate to the clinical setting and as required by law (see **SAFETY AND HANDLING**).

OVERDOSAGE

Clinical Presentation

The manifestations of *Actiq* overdosage are expected to be similar in nature to intravenous fentanyl and other opioids, and are an extension of its pharmacological actions with the most serious significant effect being hypoventilation (see **CLINICAL PHARMACOLOGY**).

General

Immediate management of opioid overdose includes removal of the *Actiq* unit, if still in the mouth, ensuring a patent airway, physical and verbal stimulation of the patient, and assessment of level of consciousness, ventilatory and circulatory status.

Treatment of Overdosage (Accidental Ingestion) in the Opioid NON-Tolerant Person

Ventilatory support should be provided, intravenous access obtained, and naloxone or other opioid antagonists should be employed as clinically indicated. The duration of respiratory depression following overdose may be longer than the effects of the opioid antagonist's action (e.g., the half-life of naloxone ranges from 30 to 81 minutes) and repeated administration may be necessary. Consult the package insert of the individual opioid antagonist for details about such use.

Treatment of Overdose in Opioid-Tolerant Patients

Ventilatory support should be provided and intravenous access obtained as clinically indicated. Judicious use of naloxone or another opioid antagonist may be warranted in some instances, but it is associated with the risk of precipitating an acute withdrawal syndrome.

General Considerations for Overdose

Management of severe *Actiq* overdose includes: securing a patent airway, assisting or controlling ventilation, establishing intravenous access, and GI decontamination by lavage and/or activated charcoal, once the patient's airway is secure. In the presence of hypoventilation or apnea, ventilation should be assisted or controlled and oxygen administered as indicated.

Patients with overdose should be carefully observed and appropriately managed until their clinical condition is well controlled.

Although muscle rigidity interfering with respiration has not been seen following the use of *Actiq*, this is possible with fentanyl and other opioids. If it occurs, it should be managed by the use of assisted or controlled ventilation, by an opioid antagonist, and as a final alternative, by a neuromuscular blocking agent.

Table 4.
Percent of Patients with Adverse Events Commonly Associated with Opioid Administration or of Particular Clinical Interest Which Occurred During Long-Term Treatment (Events in 1% or More of Patients)

Dose Group	200-600 mcg	800-1400 mcg	1600 mcg	>1600 mcg	Any
Number of Patients	**98**	**83**	**53**	**27**	**152**
Body As A Whole					
Asthenia	25	30	17	15	38
Headache	12	17	13	4	20
Accidental Injury	4	6	4	7	9
Hypertonia	2	2	2	0	3
Digestive					
Nausea	31	36	25	26	45
Vomiting	21	28	15	7	31
Constipation	14	11	13	4	20
Intestinal Obstruction	0	2	4	0	3
Cardiovascular					
Hypertension	1	1	0	0	1
Nervous					
Dizziness	12	10	9	0	16
Anxiety	9	8	8	7	15
Somnolence	8	13	8	7	15
Confusion	2	5	13	7	10
Depression	9	4	2	7	9
Insomnia	5	1	8	4	7
Abnormal Gait	5	1	0	0	4
Dry Mouth	3	1	2	4	4
Nervousness	2	2	0	4	3
Stupor	4	1	0	0	3
Vasodilatation	1	1	4	0	3
Thinking Abnormal	2	1	0	0	2
Abnormal Dreams	1	1	0	0	1
Convulsion	0	1	2	0	1
Myoclonus	0	0	4	0	1
Tremor	0	1	2	0	1
Vertigo	0	0	4	0	1
Respiratory					
Dyspnea	15	16	8	7	22
Skin					
Rash	3	5	8	4	8
Sweating	3	2	2	0	4
Pruritus	2	0	2	0	2
Special Senses					
Abnormal Vision	2	2	0	0	3
Urogenital					
Urinary Retention	1	2	0	0	2

DOSAGE AND ADMINISTRATION

***Actiq* is contraindicated in non-opioid tolerant individuals.** *Actiq* should be individually titrated to a dose that provides adequate analgesia and minimizes side effects (see **Dose Titration**).

As with all opioids, the safety of patients using such products is dependent on health care professionals prescribing them in strict conformity with their approved labeling with respect to patient selection, dosing, and proper conditions for use.

Physicians and dispensing pharmacists must specifically question patients and caregivers about the presence of children in the home on a full time or visiting basis and counsel accordingly regarding the dangers to children of inadvertent exposure to *Actiq*.

Administration of *Actiq*

The foil package should be opened with scissors immediately prior to product use. The patient should place the *Actiq* unit in his or her mouth between the cheek and lower gum, occasionally moving the drug matrix from one side to the other using the handle. The *Actiq* unit should be sucked, not chewed. A unit dose of *Actiq*, if chewed and swallowed, might result in lower peak concentrations and lower bioavailability than when consumed as directed.

The *Actiq* unit should be consumed over a 15-minute period. Longer or shorter consumption times may produce less efficacy than reported in *Actiq* clinical trials. If signs of excessive opioid effects appear before the unit is consumed, the drug matrix should be removed from the patient's mouth immediately and future doses should be decreased.

Patients and caregivers must be instructed that *Actiq* contains medicine in an amount that could be fatal to a child. While all units should be disposed of immediately after use, partially used units represent a special risk and must be disposed of as soon as they are consumed and/or no longer needed. Patients and caregivers should be advised to dispose of any units remaining from a prescription as soon as they are no longer needed (see **Disposal Instructions**).

Dose Titration

Starting Dose: *The initial dose of Actiq to treat episodes of breakthrough cancer pain should be 200 mcg.* Patients should be prescribed an initial titration supply of six 200 mcg *Actiq* units, thus limiting the number of units in the home during titration. Patients should use up all units before increasing to a higher dose.

From this initial dose, patients should be closely followed and the dosage level changed until the patient reaches a dose that provides adequate analgesia using a single *Actiq* dosage unit per breakthrough cancer pain episode.

Patients should record their use of *Actiq* over several episodes of breakthrough cancer pain and review their experience with their physicians to determine if a dosage adjustment is warranted.

Redosing Within a Single Episode: Until the appropriate dose is reached, patients may find it necessary to use an additional *Actiq* unit during a single episode. Redosing may start 15 minutes after the previous unit has been completed (30 minutes after the start of the previous unit). While patients are in the titration phase and consuming units which individually may be subtherapeutic, no more than two units should be taken for each individual breakthrough cancer pain episode.

Increasing the Dose: If treatment of several consecutive breakthrough cancer pain episodes requires more than one *Actiq* per episode, an increase in dose to the next higher available strength should be considered. At each new dose of *Actiq* during titration, it is recommended that six units of the titration dose be prescribed. Each new dose of *Actiq* used in the titration period should be evaluated over several episodes of breakthrough cancer pain (generally 1-2 days) to determine whether it provides adequate efficacy with acceptable side effects. The incidence of side effects is likely to be greater during this initial titration period compared to later, after the effective dose is determined.

Daily Limit: Once a successful dose has been found (i.e., an average episode is treated with a single unit), patients should limit consumption to four or fewer units per day. If consumption increases above four units/day, the dose of the long-acting opioid used for persistent cancer pain should be re-evaluated.

***Actiq* Titration Process**
See BOX WARNING

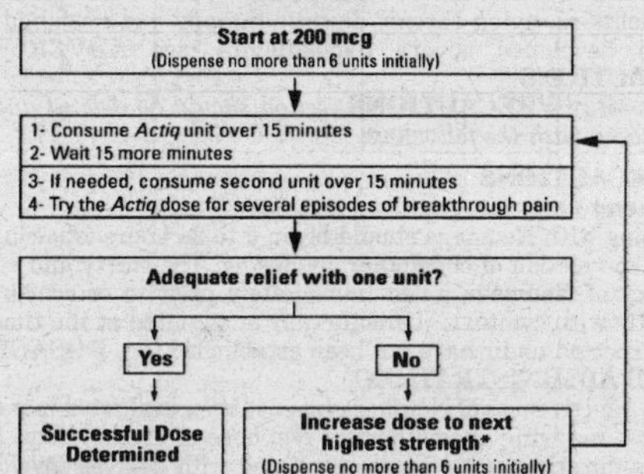
Start at 200 mcg
(Dispense no more than 6 units initially)
1- Consume Actiq unit over 15 minutes
2- Wait 15 more minutes
3- If needed, consume second unit over 15 minutes
4- Try the Actiq dose for several episodes of breakthrough pain
Adequate relief with one unit?
Yes
No
Successful Dose Determined
Increase dose to next highest strength*
(Dispense no more than 6 units initially)

*Available dosage strengths include: 200, 400, 600, 800, 1200, and 1600 mcg.

Dosage Adjustment

Experience in a long-term study of *Actiq* used in the treatment of breakthrough cancer pain suggests that dosage adjustment of both *Actiq* and the maintenance (around-the-clock) opioid analgesic may be required in some patients to continue to provide adequate relief of breakthrough cancer pain.

Generally, the *Actiq* dose should be increased when patients require more than one dosage unit per breakthrough cancer pain episode for several consecutive episodes. When titrating to an appropriate dose, small quantities (six units) should be prescribed at each titration step. Physicians should consider increasing the around-the-clock opioid dose used for persistent cancer pain in patients experiencing more than four breakthrough cancer pain episodes daily.

Discontinuation of *Actiq*

For patients requiring discontinuation of opioids, a gradual downward titration is recommended because it is not known at what dose level the opioid may be discontinued without producing the signs and symptoms of abrupt withdrawal.

SAFETY AND HANDLING

Actiq is supplied in individually sealed child-resistant foil pouches. The amount of fentanyl contained in *Actiq* can be fatal to a child. Patients and their caregivers must be instructed to keep *Actiq* out of the reach of children (see **BOX WARNING, WARNINGS, PRECAUTIONS,** and **PATIENT LEAFLET**).

Store at 25°C (77°F) with excursions permitted between 15° and 30°C (59° to 86°F) until ready to use. (See USP Controlled Room Temperature.)

Actiq should be protected from freezing and moisture. Do not store above 25°C. Do not use if the foil pouch has been opened.

DISPOSAL OF *ACTIQ*

Patients must be advised to dispose of any units remaining from a prescription as soon as they are no longer needed. While all units should be disposed of immediately after use, partially consumed units represent a special risk because they are no longer protected by the child resistant pouch, yet may contain enough medicine to be fatal to a child (see **Information for Patients**).

A temporary storage bottle is provided as part of the *Actiq* Welcome Kit (see **Information for Patients and Their Caregivers**). This container is to be used by patients or their caregivers in the event that a partially consumed unit cannot be disposed of promptly. Instructions for usage of this container are included in the patient leaflet.

Patients and members of their household must be advised to dispose of any units remaining from a prescription as soon as they are no longer needed. Instructions are included in **Information for Patients and Their Caregivers** and in the patient leaflet. If additional assistance is required, referral to the *Actiq* 800# (1-800-896-5855) should be made.

HOW SUPPLIED

Actiq is supplied in six dosage strengths. Each unit is individually wrapped in a child-resistant, protective foil pouch. These foil pouches are packed 24 per shelf carton for use when patients have been titrated to the appropriate dose.

Patients should be prescribed an initial titration supply of six 200 mcg *Actiq* units. At each new dose of *Actiq* during titration, it is recommended that only six units of the next higher dose be prescribed.

Each dosage unit has a white to off-white color. The dosage strength of each unit is marked on the handle, the foil pouch and the carton. See foil pouch and carton for product information.

Dosage Strength (fentanyl base)	Carton/Foil Pouch Color	NDC Number
200 mcg	Gray	NDC 63459-302-24
400 mcg	Blue	NDC 63459-304-24
600 mcg	Orange	NDC 63459-306-24
800 mcg	Purple	NDC 63459-308-24
1200 mcg	Green	NDC 63459-312-24
1600 mcg	Burgundy	NDC 63459-316-24

Note: Colors are a secondary aid in product identification. Please be sure to confirm the printed dosage before dispensing.

℞ only.

DEA order form required. A Schedule C-II narcotic.

Manufactured for:
Cephalon, Inc., West Chester, PA 19380
U. S. Patent No. 4,671,953
Printed in USA
ACT099-Rev. Mar 2002
ACTIQ® is a registered trademark of Anesta Corp., a wholly owned subsidiary of Cephalon, Inc.

ENDO PHARMACEUTICALS INC.

100 Painters Drive
Chadds Ford, PA 19317
Endo Laboratories
Endo Generic Products

Direct Inquiries to:
Customer Service:
(800) 462-3636
Fax: 877-329-3636

For Medical Information/Adverse Drug Experience Reporting Contact:
(800) 462-3636

PERCOCET® Ⓒ ℞
[perk' ō-sĕt]
(Oxycodone and Acetaminophen Tablets, USP)

DESCRIPTION

Each tablet, for oral administration, contains oxycodone hydrochloride and acetaminophen in the following strengths:

Oxycodone Hydrochloride	7.5 mg*
Acetaminophen, USP	325 mg

*7.5 mg oxycodone HCl is equivalent to 6.7228 mg of oxycodone.

Oxycodone Hydrochloride	10 mg*
Acetaminophen, USP	325 mg

*10 mg oxycodone HCl is equivalent to 8.9637 mg of oxycodone.

Both strengths of PERCOCET also contain the following inactive ingredients: Colloidal silicon dioxide, croscarmellose sodium, crospovidone, microcrystalline cellulose, povidone, pregelatinized starch, and stearic acid. In addition, the 7.5 mg/325 mg strength contains FD&C Yellow No. 6 Aluminum Lake and the 10 mg/325 mg strength contains D&C Yellow No. 10 Aluminum Lake.

Acetaminophen, 4′-hydroxyacetanilide, is a non-opiate, non-salicylate analgesic and antipyretic which occurs as a white, odorless, crystalline powder, possessing a slightly bitter taste. The molecular formula for acetaminophen is $C_8H_9NO_2$ and the molecular weight is 151.17. It may be represented by the following structural formula:

Oxycodone, 14-hydroxydihydrocodeinone, is a semisynthetic opioid analgesic which occurs as a white, odorless, crystalline powder having a saline, bitter taste. The molecular formula for oxycodone hydrochloride is $C_{18}H_{21}NO_4 \cdot HCl$ and the molecular weight 351.83. It is derived from the opium alkaloid thebaine, and may be represented by the following structural formula:

CLINICAL PHARMACOLOGY

The principal ingredient, oxycodone, is a semisynthetic opioid analgesic with multiple actions qualitatively similar to those of morphine; the most prominent involves the central nervous system and organs composed of smooth muscle. The principal actions of therapeutic value of the oxycodone in PERCOCET are analgesia and sedation.

Oxycodone is similar to codeine and methadone in that it retains at least one-half of its analgesic activity when administered orally.

Acetaminophen is a non-opiate, non-salicylate analgesic and antipyretic.

INDICATIONS AND USAGE

PERCOCET is indicated for the relief of moderate to moderately severe pain.

CONTRAINDICATIONS

PERCOCET should not be administered to patients who are hypersensitive to oxycodone, acetaminophen, or any other components of this product.

WARNINGS

Drug Dependence

Oxycodone can produce drug dependence of the morphine type and, therefore, has the potential for being abused. Psychic dependence, physical dependence and tolerance may develop upon repeated administration of PERCOCET (Oxycodone and Acetaminophen Tablets, USP), and it should be prescribed and administered with the same degree of caution appropriate to the use of other oral opioid-containing medications. Like other opioid-containing medications, PERCOCET is subject to the Federal Controlled Substances Act (Schedule II).

PRECAUTIONS

General

Head Injury and Increased Intracranial Pressure: The respiratory depressant effects of opioids and their capacity to elevate cerebrospinal fluid pressure may be markedly exaggerated in the presence of head injury, other intracranial lesions or a pre-existing increase in intracranial pressure. Furthermore, opioids produce adverse reactions which may obscure the clinical course of patients with head injuries.

Acute Abdominal Conditions: The administration of PERCOCET or other opioids may obscure the diagnosis or clinical course in patients with acute abdominal conditions.

Special Risk Patients: PERCOCET should be given with caution to certain patients such as the elderly or debilitated, and those with severe impairment of hepatic or renal function, hypothyroidism, Addison's disease, and prostatic hypertrophy or urethral stricture.

Information for Patients

Oxycodone may impair the mental and/or physical abilities required for the performance of potentially hazardous tasks such as driving a car or operating machinery. The patient using PERCOCET should be cautioned accordingly.

Drug Interactions

Patients receiving other opioid analgesics, general anesthetics, phenothiazines, other tranquilizers, sedative-hypnotics or other CNS depressants (including alcohol) concomitantly with PERCOCET may exhibit an additive CNS depression. When such combined therapy is contemplated, the dose of one or both agents should be reduced.

The concurrent use of anticholinergics with opioids may produce paralytic ileus.

Continued on next page

7.5 mg/325 mg Peach oval-shaped tablet debossed with "PERCOCET" on one side and "7.5/325" on the other.	Bottles of 100 Bottles of 500 Unit dose package of 100 tablets	NDC 63481-628-70 NDC 63481-628-85 NDC 63481-628-75
10 mg/325 mg Yellow capsule-shaped tablet debossed with "PERCOCET" on one side and "10/325" on the other.	Bottles of 100 Bottles of 500 Unit dose package of 100 tablets	NDC 63481-629-70 NDC 63481-629-85 NDC 63481-629-75

Percocet—Cont.

Usage in Pregnancy
Teratogenic Effects; Pregnancy Category C: Animal reproductive studies have not been conducted with PERCOCET. It is also not known whether PERCOCET can cause fetal harm when administered to a pregnant woman or can affect reproductive capacity. PERCOCET should not be given to a pregnant woman unless in the judgment of the physician, the potential benefits outweigh the possible hazards.
Nonteratogenic Effects: Use of opioids during pregnancy may produce physical dependence in the neonate.
Labor and Delivery: As with all opioids, administration of PERCOCET to the mother shortly before delivery may result in some degree of respiratory depression in the newborn and the mother, especially if higher doses are used.
Nursing Mothers
It is not known whether PERCOCET is excreted in human milk. Because many drugs are excreted in human milk, caution should be exercised when PERCOCET is administered to a nursing woman.
Pediatric Use
Safety and effectiveness in pediatric patients have not been established.

ADVERSE REACTIONS
The most frequently observed adverse reactions include lightheadedness, dizziness, sedation, nausea and vomiting. These effects seem to be more prominent in ambulatory than in nonambulatory patients, and some of these adverse reactions may be alleviated if the patient lies down.
Other adverse reactions include euphoria, dysphoria, constipation, skin rash and pruritus. At higher doses, oxycodone has most of the disadvantages of morphine including respiratory depression.

DRUG ABUSE AND DEPENDENCE
PERCOCET (Oxycodone and Acetaminophen Tablets, USP) is a Schedule II controlled substance.
Oxycodone can produce drug dependence and has the potential for being abused (See WARNINGS).

OVERDOSAGE
Acetaminophen
Signs and Symptoms: In acute acetaminophen overdosage, dose-dependent, potentially fatal hepatic necrosis is the most serious adverse effect. Renal tubular necrosis, hypoglycemic coma and thrombocytopenia may also occur.
In adults, hepatic toxicity has rarely been reported with acute overdoses of less than 10 grams and fatalities with less than 15 grams. Importantly, young children seem to be more resistant than adults to the hepatotoxic effect of an acetaminophen overdose. Despite this, the measures outlined below should be initiated in any adult or child suspected of having ingested an acetaminophen overdose.
Early symptoms following a potentially hepatotoxic overdose may include: nausea, vomiting, diaphoresis and general malaise. Clinical and laboratory evidence of hepatic toxicity may not be apparent until 48 to 72 hours post-ingestion.
Treatment: The stomach should be emptied promptly by lavage or by induction of emesis with syrup of ipecac. Patient's estimates of the quantity of a drug ingested are notoriously unreliable. Therefore, if an acetaminophen overdose is suspected, a serum acetaminophen assay should be obtained as early as possible, but no sooner than four hours following ingestion. Liver function studies should be obtained initially and repeated at 24-hour intervals.
The antidote, N-acetylcysteine, should be administered as early as possible, preferably within 16 hours of the overdose ingestion for optimal results, but in any case, within 24 hours. Following recovery, there are no residual, structural, or functional hepatic abnormalities.
Oxycodone
Signs and Symptoms: Serious overdosage with oxycodone is characterized by respiratory depression (a decrease in respiratory rate and/or tidal volume, Cheyne-Stokes respiration, cyanosis), extreme somnolence progressing to stupor or coma, skeletal muscle flaccidity, cold and clammy skin, and sometimes bradycardia and hypotension. In severe overdosage, apnea, circulatory collapse, cardiac arrest and death may occur.
Treatment: Primary attention should be given to the reestablishment of adequate respiratory exchange through provision of a patent airway and the institution of assisted or controlled ventilation. The opioid antagonist naloxone hydrochloride is a specific antidote against respiratory depression which may result from overdosage or unusual sensitivity to opioids, including oxycodone. Therefore, an appropriate dose of naloxone hydrochloride (usual initial adult dose 0.4 mg to 2 mg) should be administered preferably by the intravenous route, and simultaneously with efforts at respiratory resuscitation (see package insert). Since the duration of action of oxycodone may exceed that of the antagonist, the patient should be kept under continued surveillance and repeated doses of the antagonist should be administered as needed to maintain adequate respiration.
An antagonist should not be administered in the absence of clinically significant respiratory or cardiovascular depression. Oxygen, intravenous fluids, vasopressors and other supportive measures should be employed as indicated.
Gastric emptying may be useful in removing unabsorbed drug.

DOSAGE AND ADMINISTRATION
Dosage should be adjusted according to the severity of the pain and the response of the patient. It may occasionally be necessary to exceed the usual dosage recommended below in cases of more severe pain or in those patients who have become tolerant to the analgesic effect of opioids. PERCOCET (Oxycodone and Acetaminophen Tablets, USP) is given orally. The usual adult dosage is one tablet every 6 hours as needed for pain. The total daily dose of acetaminophen should not exceed 4 grams (maximal daily dose of PERCOCET 7.5 mg/325 mg and PERCOCET 10 mg/325 mg is 8 tablets and 6 tablets, respectively).

HOW SUPPLIED
PERCOCET (Oxycodone and Acetaminophen Tablets, USP) is supplied as follows:
[See table at bottom of previous page]
Store at controlled room temperature, 15° to 30°C (59° to 86°F) [see USP].
Dispense in a tight, light-resistant container as defined in the USP, with a child-resistant closure (as required).
DEA Order Form Required.
Manufactured for:
Endo Pharmaceuticals Inc.
Chadds Ford, Pennsylvania 19317
PERCOCET® is a Registered Trademark of Endo Pharmaceuticals Inc.

Printed in U.S.A. 6556-00/August, 2001
4091-42

Forest Pharmaceuticals, Inc.

(Subsidiary of Forest Laboratories, Inc.)
13600 SHORELINE DRIVE
ST. LOUIS, MO 63045

Direct Inquiries to:
Professional Affairs Department
13600 Shoreline Drive
St. Louis, MO 63045
(800) 678-1605

CELEXA™ ℞
(citalopram hydrobromide)

Prescribing information for this product, which appears on pages 1365–1369 of the 2002 PDR, has been revised as follows. Please write "See Supplement A" next to the product heading.
In the **CLINICAL PHARMACOLOGY: Pharmacokinetics: Drug-Drug Interactions** *section, the first and second paragraphs have been revised as follows:*
In vitro enzyme inhibition data did not reveal an inhibitory effect of citalopram on CYP3A4, -2C9, or –2E1, but did suggest that it is a weak inhibitor of CYP-1A2, -2D6, and –2C19. Citalopram would be expected to have little inhibitory effect on *in vivo* metabolism mediated by these cytochromes. However, *in vivo* data to address this question are limited.
Since CYP3A4 and 2C19 are the primary enzymes involved in the metabolism of citalopram, it is expected that potent inhibitors of 3A4, e.g., ketoconazole, itraconazole, and macrolide antibiotics, and potent inhibitors of CYP2C19, e.g., omeprazole, might decrease the clearance of citalopram. However, coadministration of citalopram and the potent 3A4 inhibitor ketoconazole did not significantly affect the pharmacokinetics of citalopram. Because citalopram is metabolized by multiple enzyme systems, inhibition of a single enzyme may not appreciably decrease citalopram clearance. Citalopram steady state levels were not significantly different in poor metabolizers and extensive 2D6 metabolizers after multiple dose administration of Celexa, suggesting that coadministration, with Celexa, of a drug that inhibits CYP2D6, is unlikely to have clinically significant effects on citalopram metabolism. See Drug Interactions under Precautions for more detailed information on available drug interaction data.
In the **PRECAUTIONS—Drug Interactions** *section, the following subsection has been added between the* Lithium *and* Sumatriptan *paragraphs:*
Theophylline—Combined administration of Celexa (40 mg/day for 21 days) and the CYP1A2 substrate theophylline (single dose of 300 mg) did not affect the pharmacokinetics of theophylline. The effect of theophylline on the pharmacokinetics of citalopram was not evaluated.
In the **PRECAUTIONS—Drug Interactions** *section, the following subsections have been added between the* Carbamazepine *and* CYP3A4 and 2C19 Inhibitors *paragraphs:*
Triazolam—Combined administration of Celexa (titrated to 40 mg/day for 28 days) and the CYP3A4 substrate triazolam (single dose of 0.25 mg) did not significantly affect the pharmacokinetics of either citalopram or triazolam.
Ketoconazole—Combined administration of Celexa (40 mg) and ketoconazole (200 mg) decreased the Cmax and AUC of ketoconazole by 21% and 10% respectively, and did not significantly affect the pharmacokinetics of citalopram.
In the **PRECAUTIONS—Drug Interactions** *section, the following subsection, between the* Ketoconazole *and* Metoprolol *paragraphs, has been revised as follows:*
CYP3A4 and 2C19 Inhibitors—*In vitro* studies indicated that CYP3A4 and 2C19 are the primary enzymes involved in the metabolism of citalopram. However, coadministration of citalopram (40 mg) and ketoconazole (200 mg), a potent inhibitor of CYP3A4, did not significantly affect the pharmacokinetics of citalopram. Because citalopram is metabolized by multiple enzyme systems, inhibition of a single enzyme may not appreciably decrease citalopram clearance.
In the **HOW SUPPLIED** *section, under* Oral Solution: (120 mL) NDC 0456-4130-04 *was deleted and* (240 mL) NDC 0456-4130-08 *was added.*
3/02

Genetics Institute

87 CAMBRIDGE PARK DRIVE
CAMBRIDGE, MA 02140

A Subsidiary of American Home Products
Direct Inquiries to:
1-888-638-6342

NEUMEGA® ℞
[*nū-mā-gă*]
(Oprelvekin)

Prescribing information for this product, which appears on pages 1434–1437 of the 2002 PDR, has been revised as follows. Please write "See Supplement A" next to the product heading.
The entire **WARNINGS** *section should be deleted and replaced with the following:*

WARNINGS
Neumega is known to cause fluid retention (See **CLINICAL PHARMACOLOGY: Pharmacodynamics**). Neumega should be used with caution in patients with clinically evident congestive heart failure, patients who may be susceptible to developing congestive heart failure, patients receiving aggressive hydration, patients with a history of heart failure who are well-compensated and receiving appropriate medical therapy, and patients with pleural or pericardial effusions (see **PRECAUTIONS: Fluid Retention** and **Cardiovascular Events**).
Close monitoring of fluid and electrolyte status should be performed in patients receiving chronic diuretic therapy. Sudden deaths have occurred in Oprelvekin-treated patients receiving chronic diuretic therapy and ifosfamide who developed severe hypokalemia (see **ADVERSE REACTIONS**).
The entire **PRECAUTIONS** *section should be deleted and replaced with the following:*

PRECAUTIONS
General
Dosing with Neumega should begin 6 to 24 hours following the completion of chemotherapy dosing. The safety and efficacy of Neumega given immediately prior to or concurrently with cytotoxic chemotherapy or initiated at the time of expected nadir have not been established (see **DOSAGE AND ADMINISTRATION**).
The effectiveness of Neumega has not been evaluated in patients receiving chemotherapy regimens of greater than 5 days duration or regimens associated with delayed myelosuppression (eg, nitrosoureas, mitomycin-C).
The parenteral administration of Neumega should be attended by appropriate precautions in case allergic reactions occur (see **CONTRAINDICATIONS**).
Administration of Neumega should be permanently discontinued in patients who experience clinically significant allergic reactions (see **CONTRAINDICATIONS** and **PRECAUTIONS, Antibody Formation/Allergic Reactions**).
Fluid Retention
Patients receiving Neumega have commonly experienced mild to moderate fluid retention which can result in peripheral edema or dyspnea on exertion. Fluid retention has also been associated with weight gain, pulmonary edema, capillary leak syndrome, and exacerbation of pre-existing pleural effusions.
Fluid retention is reversible within several days following discontinuation of Neumega. During dosing with Neumega, fluid balance should be monitored and appropriate medical management is advised. If a diuretic is used, fluid and electrolyte balance should be carefully monitored. Pre-existing fluid collections, including pericardial effusions or ascites, should be monitored. Drainage should be considered if medically indicated.
Neumega should be used with caution in patients who may develop fluid retention as a result of associated medical conditions or whose medical condition may be exacerbated by fluid retention.
Moderate decreases in hemoglobin concentration, hematocrit, and red blood cell count (~10% to 15%) without a decrease in red blood cell mass have been observed. These changes are predominantly due to an increase in plasma volume (dilutional anemia) that is primarily related to renal sodium and water retention. The decrease in hemoglobin concentration typically begins within 3 to 5 days of the initiation of Neumega, and is reversible over approximately a week following discontinuation of Neumega.
Cardiovascular Events
Neumega should be used with caution in patients with a history of atrial arrhythmia, and only after consideration of the potential risks in relation to anticipated benefit. In clinical trials, atrial arrhythmias (atrial fibrillation or atrial flutter) occurred in 15% (23/157) of patients treated with Neumega at doses of 50 μg/kg. Arrhythmias were usually brief in duration; conversion to sinus rhythm typically

occurred spontaneously or after rate-control drug therapy. Approximately one-half (11/24) of the patients who were rechallenged had recurrent atrial arrhythmias. Clinical sequelae, including stroke, have been reported in patients receiving Neumega who experienced atrial arrhythmias.
Neumega has not been shown to be directly arrhythmogenic in preclinical trials. In some patients, development of atrial arrhythmias may be due to increased plasma volume associated with fluid retention (see **PRECAUTIONS: Fluid Retention**). A retrospective analysis of data from clinical trials of Neumega suggests that advancing age and other conditions such as history of atrial fibrillation/flutter, cardiac disorder, alcohol use (moderate or more) and cardiac medication use may be associated with an increased risk of atrial arrhythmias. Ventricular arrhythmias have not been attributed to the use of Neumega.

Ophthalmologic Events
Transient, mild visual blurring has been reported by patients treated with Neumega. Papilledema has been reported in 2% (9/398) [95% CI, 1.04%-4.21%] of patients receiving Neumega in clinical trials, following repeated cycles of exposure. In clinical trials, the incidence of papilledema was higher 14% (5/36) [95% CI, 4.66%-29.58%] in children than in adults 1% (3/362) [95% CI, 0.17%-2.38%]. Nonhuman primates treated with Neumega at a dose of 1,000 μg/kg SC once daily for 4 to 13 weeks developed papilledema which was not associated with inflammation or any other histologic abnormality and was reversible after dosing was discontinued. Neumega should be used with caution in patients with preexisting papilledema, or with tumors involving the central nervous system since it is possible that papilledema could worsen or develop during treatment.

Nervous System Events
Stroke has been reported in patients who develop atrial fibrillation/flutter while receiving Neumega (see **PRECAUTIONS: Cardiovascular Events**).

Antibody Formation/Allergic Reactions
In clinical trials with Neumega, a small proportion (1%) of patients developed antibodies to Oprelvekin. The clinical relevance of the presence of these antibodies is unknown. No anaphylactoid or other severe allergic reactions were reported in clinical trials following single or repeated doses of Neumega. Rash and rare cases of hives have been reported (see **ADVERSE REACTIONS**), but a relationship between these reactions and the development of serum antibodies has not been established.
The data reflect the percentage of patients whose test results were considered positive for antibodies to Neumega in an ELISA assay, and are highly dependent on the sensitivity and specificity of the assay. Additionally the observed incidence of antibody positivity in an assay may be influenced by several factors including sample handling, concomitant medications, and underlying disease. For these reasons, comparisons of the incidence of antibodies to Neumega with incidence of antibodies to other products may be misleading.

Chronic Administration
Neumega has been administered safely using the recommended dosage schedule (see **DOSAGE AND ADMINISTRATION**) for up to 6 cycles following chemotherapy. The safety and efficacy of chronic administration of Neumega have not been established. Continuous dosage (2 to 13 weeks) in nonhuman primates produced joint capsule and tendon fibrosis and periosteal hyperostosis (see **PRECAUTIONS: Pediatric Use**). The relevance of these findings to humans is unclear.

Information for Patients
In situations when the physician determines that Neumega may be used outside of the hospital or office setting, persons who will be administering Neumega should be instructed as to the proper dose, and the method for reconstituting and administering Neumega (see **DOSAGE AND ADMINISTRATION**). If home use is prescribed, patients should be instructed in the importance or proper disposal and cautioned against the reuse of needles, syringes, drug product, and diluent. A puncture resistant container should be used by the patient for the disposal of used needles.
Patients should be informed of the most common adverse reactions associated with Neumega administration, including those symptoms related to fluid retention (see **ADVERSE REACTIONS** and **PRECAUTIONS**). Mild to moderate peripheral edema and shortness of breath on exertion can occur within the first week of treatment and may continue for the duration of administration of Neumega. Patients who have preexisting pleural or other effusions or a history of congestive heart failure should be advised to contact their physician for worsening of dyspnea. Most patients who receive Neumega develop anemia. Patients should be advised to contact their physician if symptoms attributable to atrial arrhythmia develop. Female patients of childbearing potential should be advised of the possible risks to the fetus of Neumega (see **PRECAUTIONS: Pregnancy Category C**).

Laboratory Monitoring
A complete blood count should be obtained prior to chemotherapy and at regular intervals during Neumega therapy (see **DOSAGE AND ADMINISTRATION**). Platelet counts should be monitored during the time of the expected nadir and until adequate recovery has occurred (post-nadir counts ≥50,000).

Drug Interactions
Most patients in trials evaluating Neumega were treated concomitantly with Filgrastim (granulocyte colony-stimulating factor [G-CSF]) with no adverse effect of Neumega on the activity of G-CSF. No information is available on the clinical use of Sargramostim (granulocyte-macrophage colony-stimulating factor [GM-CSF]) with Neumega. However, in a study in nonhuman primates in which Neumega and GM-CSF were coadministered, there were no adverse interactions between Neumega and GM-CSF and no apparent difference in the pharmacokinetic profile of Neumega.
Drug interactions between Neumega and other drugs have not been fully evaluated. Based on in vitro and nonclinical in vivo evaluations of Neumega, drug-drug interactions with known substrates of P450 enzymes would not be predicted.

Carcinogenesis, Mutagenesis, Impairment of Fertility
No trials have been performed to assess the carcinogenic potential of Neumega. In vitro, Neumega did not stimulate the growth of tumor colony-forming cells harvested from patients with a variety of human malignancies. Neumega has been shown to be non-genotoxic in in vitro trials. These data suggest that Neumega is not mutagenic. Although prolonged estrus cycles have been noted at 2 to 20 times the human dose, no effects on fertility have been observed in rats treated with Neumega at doses up to 1000 μg/kg/day.

Pregnancy Category C
Neumega has been shown to have embryocidal effects in pregnant rats and rabbits when given in doses of 0.2 to 20 times the human dose. There are no adequate and well-controlled trials of Neumega in pregnant women. Neumega should be used during pregnancy only if the potential benefit justifies the potential risk to the the fetus.
Neumega has been tested in trials of fertility, early embryonic development, and pre and postnatal development in rats and in trials of organogenesis (teratogenicity) in rats and rabbits. Parental toxicity has been observed when Neumega is given at doses of 2 to 20 times the human dose (≥100 μg/kg/day) in the rat and at 0.02 to 2.0 times the human dose (≥1 μg/kg/day) in the rabbit. Findings in pregnant rats consisted of transient hypoactivity and dyspnea after administration (maternal toxicity), as well as prolonged estrus cycle, increased early embryonic deaths and decreased numbers of live fetuses. In addition, low fetal body weights and a reduced number of ossified sacral and caudal vertebrae (ie, retarded fetal development) occurred in rats at 20 times the human dose. Findings in pregnant rabbits consisted of decreased fecal/urine eliminations (the only toxicity noted at 1 μg/kg/day in dams) as well as decreased food consumption, body weight loss, abortion, increased embryonic and fetal deaths, and decreased numbers of live fetuses. No teratogenic effects of Neumega were observed in rabbits at doses up to 0.6 times the human dose (30 μg/kg/day).
Adverse effects in the first generation offspring of rats given Neumega at maternally toxic doses ≥2 times the human dose (≥100 μg/kg/day) during both gestation and lactation included increased newborn mortality, decreased viability index on day 4 of lactation, and decreased body weights during lactation. In rats given 20 times the human dose (1000 μg/kg/day) during both gestation and lactation, maternal toxicity and growth retardation of the first generation offspring resulted in an increased rate of fetal death of the second generation offspring.

Nursing Mothers
It is not known if Neumega is excreted in human milk. Because many drugs are excreted in human milk and because of the potential for serious adverse reactions in nursing infants from Neumega, a decision should be made whether to discontinue nursing or to discontinue the drug, taking into account the importance of the drug to the mother.

Pediatric Use
There are no controlled clinical trials that have established a safe and effective dose of Neumega in chidren. Therefore, the administration of Neumega in chidren, particularly those <12 years of age, should be restricted to controlled clinical trial settings with closely monitored safety assessments. Preliminary data from a safety and pharmacokinetic trial identified papilledema in 4 of 16 children receiving doses of 100 μg/kg/day (25%; 95% CI, 7%-52%).
Limited data from the safety and pharmacokinetic trial are available for pediatric populations receiving doses of 50 μg/kg/day. Adequate pharmacokinetic data for doses of 50 μg/kg/day were obtained for seven individuals ≤12 years of age and four individuals >12 and <17 years of age. Children (≤12 years of age) given doses of 50 μg/kg/day did not achieve effective serum levels. For adolescents (13 to 16 years of age, N=2) and young adults (≥17 years of age, N=2) effective serum levels appeared to be achieved (see **CLINICAL PHARMACOLOGY: Pharmacokinetics** and **DOSAGE AND ADMINISTRATION**).
Adverse events in this pediatric open-label, non-comparative study were generally similar to those observed using Neumega at a dose of 50 μg/kg in the randomized chemotherapy trials in adults (see **ADVERSE REACTIONS**). However, the incidence of papilledema [14% (5/36)], tachycardia [46% (13/28)], and conjunctival injection [50% (14/28)] were higher in the pediatric subjects than in adults. There was no evidence of a dose-response relationship for any of the Neumega-associated adverse events among the pediatric patients.
No trials have been performed to assess the long-term effects of Neumega on growth and development. In growing rodents treated with 100, 300, or 1000 μg/kg/day for a minimum of 28 days, thickening of femoral and tibial growth plates was noted, which did not completely resolve after a 28-day non-treatment period. In a nonhuman primate toxicology study of Neumega, animals treated for 2 to 13 weeks at doses of 10 to 1000 μg/kg showed partially reversible joint capsule and tendon fibrosis and periosteal hyperostosis. The clinical significance of these findings is not known. An asymptomatic, laminated periosteal reaction in the diaphyses of the femur, tibia, and fibula has been observed in one patient during pediatric trials involving multiple courses of Neumega treatment. The relationship of these findings to treatment with Neumega is unclear.

Use in Patients with Renal Impairment
Neumega is eliminated primarily by the kidneys. The pharmacokinetics of Neumega have not been studied in patients with mild or moderate renal impairment (creatinine clearance ≥15 mL/min). Fluid retention associated with Neumega treatment has not been studied in patients with renal impairment, but fluid balance should be carefully monitored in these patients (see **PRECAUTIONS: Fluid Retention**).

The entire **ADVERSE REACTIONS** *section should be deleted and replaced with the following:*

ADVERSE REACTIONS

Three hundred eight subjects, with ages ranging from 8 months to 75 years, have been exposed to Neumega treatment. Subjects have received up to six (eight in pediatric patients) sequential courses of Neumega treatment, with each course lasting from 1 to 28 days. Apart from the sequelae of the underlying malignancy or cytotoxic chemotherapy, most adverse events were mild or moderate in severity and reversible after discontinuation of Neumega dosing.
In general, the incidence and type of adverse events were similar between Neumega 50 μg/kg and placebo groups. The following adverse events, occurring in ≥10% of patients, were observed at equal or greater frequency in placebo-treated patients: asthenia, pain, chills, abdominal pain, infection, anorexia, constipation, dyspepsia, ecchymosis, myalgia, bone pain, nervousness, and alopecia. Selected adverse events that occurred in Neumega-treated patients are listed in Table 3.

TABLE 3
SELECTED ADVERSE EVENTS

Body System Adverse Event	Placebo n=67 (%)	50 μg/kg n=69 (%)
Body as a Whole		
Edema*	10 (15)	41 (59)
Neutropenic fever	28 (42)	33 (48)
Headache	24 (36)	28 (41)
Fever	19 (28)	25 (36)
Cardiovascular System		
Tachycardia*	2 (3)	14 (20)
Vasodilatation	6 (9)	13 (19)
Palpitations*	2 (3)	10 (14)
Syncope	4 (6)	9 (13)
Atrial fibrillation/ flutter*	1 (1)	8 (12)
Digestive System		
Nausea/vomiting	47 (70)	53 (77)
Mucositis	25 (37)	30 (43)
Diarrhea	22 (33)	30 (43)
Oral moniliasis*	1 (1)	10 (14)
Nervous System		
Dizziness	19 (28)	26 (38)
Insomnia	18 (27)	23 (33)
Respiratory System		
Dyspnea*	15 (22)	33 (48)
Rhinitis	21 (31)	29 (42)
Cough increased	15 (22)	20 (29)
Pharyngitis	11 (16)	17 (25)
Pleural effusions*	0 (0)	7 (10)
Skin and Appendages		
Rash	11 (16)	17 (25)
Special Senses		
Conjunctival injection*	2 (3)	13 (19)

*Occurred in significantly more Neumega-treated patients than in placebo-treated patients.

The following adverse events also occurred more frequently in cancer patients receiving Neumega than in those receiving placebo: amblyopia, paresthesia, dehydration, skin discoloration, exfoliative dermatitis, and eye hemorrhage; a statistically significant association of Neumega to these events has not been established. Other than a higher incidence of severe asthenia in Neumega treated patients (10 [14%] in Neumega patients versus 2 [3%] in placebo patients), the incidence of severe or life-threatening adverse events was comparable in the Neumega and placebo treatment groups.
The incidence of fever, neutropenic fever, flu-like symptoms, thrombocytosis, thrombotic events, the average number of units of red blood cells transfused per patient, and the duration of neutropenia <500 cells/μL were similar in the Neumega 50 μg/kg and placebo groups.
Two patients with cancer treated with Neumega experienced sudden death which the investigator considered possibly or probably related to Neumega. Both deaths occurred in patients with severe hypokalemia (<3.0 mEq/L) who had received high doses of ifosfamide and were receiving daily doses of a diuretic. The relationship of these deaths to Neumega remains unclear.

Abnormal Laboratory Values
The most common laboratory abnormality reported in patients in clinical trials was a decrease in hemoglobin con-

Continued on next page

Neumega—Cont.

centration predominantly as a result of expansion of the plasma volume (see **PRECAUTIONS: Fluid Retention**). The increase in plasma volume is also associated with a decrease in the serum concentration of albumin and several other proteins (eg, transferrin and gamma globulins). A parallel decrease in calcium without clinical effects has been documented.

After daily SC injections, treatment with Neumega resulted in a two-fold increase in plasma fibrinogen. Other acute-phase proteins also increased. These protein levels returned to normal after dosing with Neumega was discontinued. Von Willebrand factor (vWF) concentrations increased with a normal multimer pattern in healthy subjects receiving Neumega.

The entire **DOSAGE AND ADMINISTRATION** *section should be deleted and replaced with the following:*

DOSAGE AND ADMINISTRATION

The recommended dose of Neumega in adults is 50 μg/kg given once daily. Neumega should be administered subcutaneously as a single injection in either the abdomen, thigh, or hip (or upper arm if not self-injecting). The safety and effectiveness of Neumega have not been established in children (see **PRECAUTIONS: Pediatric Use**).

Dosing should be initiated 6 to 24 hours after the completion of chemotherapy. Platelet counts should be monitored periodically to assess the optimal duration of therapy. Dosing should be continued until the post-nadir platelet count is ≥50,000 cells/μL. In controlled clinical trials, doses were administered in courses of 10 to 21 days. Dosing beyond 21 days per treatment course is not recommended.

Treatment with Neumega should be discontinued at least 2 days before starting the next planned cycle of chemotherapy.

Preparation of Neumega

1. Neumega is a sterile, white, preservative-free lyophilized powder for subcutaneous injection upon reconstitution. Neumega (5 mg vials) should be reconstituted aseptically with 1.0 mL of Sterile Water for Injection, USP (without preservative). The reconstituted Neumega solution is clear, colorless, isotonic, with a pH of 7.0, and contains 5 mg/mL of Neumega. The single-use vial should not be re-entered or reused. Any unused portion of either reconstituted Neumega solution or Sterile Water for Injection, USP should be discarded.
2. During reconstitution, the Sterile Water for Injection, USP should be directed at the side of the vial and the contents gently swirled. EXCESSIVE OR VIGOROUS AGITATION SHOULD BE AVOIDED.
3. Parenteral drug products should be inspected visually for particulate matter and discoloration prior to administration, whenever solution and container permit. If particulate matter is present or the solution is discolored, the vial should not be used.
4. Because neither Neumega powder for injection nor its accompanying diluent, Sterile Water for Injection, USP contains a preservative, Neumega should be used as soon as possible following reconstitution. Neumega may be used within 3 hours of reconstitution when stored either at 2°C to 8°C (36°F to 46°F) or at room temperature up to 25°C (77°F). DO NOT FREEZE OR SHAKE THE RECONSTITUTED SOLUTION.

4004G029 Rev. 8/01

GlaxoSmithKline

FIVE MOORE DRIVE
RESEARCH TRIANGLE PARK, NC 27709

For Medical Emergencies, Medical Information for Healthcare Professionals, and Consumer Inquiries, Contact:
1-888-825-5249
www.druginfo.gsk.com

AGENERASE® ℞

[a-jin' ə-rās]
(amprenavir)
Capsules

Prescribing information for this product, which appears on pages 1454–1459 of the 2002 PDR, has been completely revised as follows. Please write "See Supplement A" next to the product heading.

> Because of the potential risk of toxicity from the large amount of the excipient propylene glycol contained in **AGENERASE Oral Solution**, that formulation is contraindicated in infants and children below the age of 4 years and certain other patient populations and should be used with caution in others. Consult the complete prescribing information for **AGENERASE Oral Solution** for full information.

DESCRIPTION

AGENERASE (amprenavir) is an inhibitor of the human immunodeficiency virus (HIV) protease. The chemical name of amprenavir is (3*S*)-tetrahydro-3-furyl *N*-[(1*S*,2*R*)-3-(4-amino-*N*-isobutylbenzenesulfonamido)-1-benzyl-2-hydroxypropyl]carbamate. Amprenavir is a single stereoisomer with the (3*S*)(1*S*,2*R*) configuration. It has a molecular formula of $C_{25}H_{35}N_3O_6S$ and a molecular weight of 505.64. Amprenavir is a white to cream-colored solid with a solubility of approximately 0.04 mg/mL in water at 25°C.

AGENERASE Capsules are available for oral administration in strengths of 50 and 150 mg. Each 50-mg capsule contains the inactive ingredients d-alpha tocopheryl polyethylene glycol 1000 succinate (TPGS), polyethylene glycol 400 (PEG 400) 246.7 mg, and propylene glycol 19 mg. Each 150-mg capsule contains the inactive ingredients TPGS, PEG 400 740 mg, and propylene glycol 57 mg. The capsule shell contains the inactive ingredients d-sorbitol and sorbitans solution, gelatin, glycerin, and titanium dioxide. The soft gelatin capsules are printed with edible red ink. Each 150-mg AGENERASE Capsule contains 109 IU vitamin E in the form of TPGS. The total amount of vitamin E in the recommended daily adult dose of AGENERASE is 1744 IU.

MICROBIOLOGY

Mechanism of Action: Amprenavir is an inhibitor of HIV-1 protease. Amprenavir binds to the active site of HIV-1 protease and thereby prevents the processing of viral gag and gag-pol polyprotein precursors, resulting in the formation of immature non-infectious viral particles.

Antiviral Activity *in Vitro*: The *in vitro* antiviral activity of amprenavir was evaluated against HIV-1 IIIB in both acutely and chronically infected lymphoblastic cell lines (MT-4, CEM-CCRF, H9) and in peripheral blood lymphocytes. The 50% inhibitory concentration (IC_{50}) of amprenavir ranged from 0.012 to 0.08 μM in acutely infected cells and was 0.41 μM in chronically infected cells (1 μM = 0.50 mcg/mL). Amprenavir exhibited synergistic anti-HIV-1 activity in combination with abacavir, zidovudine, didanosine, or saquinavir, and additive anti-HIV-1 activity in combination with indinavir, nelfinavir, and ritonavir *in vitro*. These drug combinations have not been adequately studied in humans. The relationship between *in vitro* anti-HIV-1 activity of amprenavir and the inhibition of HIV-1 replication in humans has not been defined.

Resistance: HIV-1 isolates with a decreased susceptibility to amprenavir have been selected *in vitro* and obtained from patients treated with amprenavir. Genotypic analysis of isolates from amprenavir-treated patients showed mutations in the HIV-1 protease gene resulting in amino acid substitutions primarily at positions V32I, M46I/L, I47V, I50V, I54L/M, and I84V as well as mutations in the p7/p1 and p1/p6 gag cleavage sites. Phenotypic analysis of HIV-1 isolates from 21 nucleoside reverse transcriptase inhibitor-(NRTI-) experienced, protease inhibitor-naive patients treated with amprenavir in combination with NRTIs for 16 to 48 weeks identified isolates from 15 patients who exhibited a 4- to 17-fold decrease in susceptibility to amprenavir *in vitro* compared to wild-type virus. Clinical isolates that exhibited a decrease in amprenavir susceptibility harbored one or more amprenavir-associated mutations. The clinical relevance of the genotypic and phenotypic changes associated with amprenavir therapy is under evaluation.

Cross-Resistance: Varying degrees of HIV-1 cross-resistance among protease inhibitors have been observed. Five of 15 amprenavir-resistant isolates exhibited 4- to

Table 1: Average (%CV) Pharmacokinetic Parameters After 1200 mg b.i.d. of Amprenavir Capsules (n = 54)

C_{max} (mcg/mL)	T_{max} (hours)	AUC_{0-12} (mcg•h/mL)	C_{avg} (mcg/mL)	C_{min} (mcg/mL)	CL/F (mL/min/kg)
7.66 (54%)	1.0 (42%)	17.7 (47%)	1.48 (47%)	0.32 (77%)	19.5 (46%)

Table 2: Average (%CV) Pharmacokinetic Parameters in Children Ages 4 to 12 Years Receiving 20 mg/kg b.i.d. or 15 mg/kg t.i.d. of AGENERASE Oral Solution

Dose	n	C_{max} (mcg/mL)	T_{max} (hours)	AUC_{ss}* (mcg•h/mL)	C_{avg} (mcg/mL)	C_{min} (mcg/mL)	CL/F (mL/min/kg)
20 mg/kg b.i.d.	20	6.77 (51%)	1.1 (21%)	15.46 (59%)	1.29 (59%)	0.24 (98%)	29 (58%)
15 mg/kg t.i.d.	17	3.99 (37%)	1.4 (90%)	8.73 (36%)	1.09 (36%)	0.27 (95%)	32 (34%)

*AUC is 0 to 12 hours for b.i.d. and 0 to 8 hours for t.i.d., therefore the C_{avg} is a better comparison of the exposures.

Table 3: Drug Interactions: Pharmacokinetic Parameters for Amprenavir in the Presence of the Coadministered Drug

Co-administered Drug	Dose of Coadministered Drug	Dose of AGENERASE	n	% Change in **Amprenavir** Pharmacokinetic Parameters* (90% CI)		
				C_{max}	AUC	C_{min}
Abacavir	300 mg b.i.d. for 3 weeks	900 mg b.i.d. for 3 weeks	4	↑47 (↓15 to ↑154)	↑29 (↓18 to ↑103)	↑27 (↓46 to ↑197)
Clarithromycin	500 mg b.i.d. for 4 days	1200 mg b.i.d. for 4 days	12	↑15 (↑1 to ↑31)	↑18 (↑8 to ↑29)	↑39 (↑31 to ↑47)
Indinavir	800 mg t.i.d. for 2 weeks (fasted)	750 or 800 mg t.i.d. for 2 weeks (fasted)	9	↑18 (↓13 to ↑58)	↑33 (↑2 to ↑73)	↑25 (↓27 to ↑116)
Ketoconazole	400 mg single dose	1200 mg single dose	12	↓16 (↓25 to ↓6)	↑31 (↑20 to ↑42)	NA
Lamivudine	150 mg single dose	600 mg single dose	11	⇔ (↓17 to ↑9)	⇔ (↓15 to ↑14)	NA
Nelfinavir	750 mg t.i.d. for 2 weeks (fed)	750 or 800 mg t.i.d. for 2 weeks (fed)	6	↓14 (↓38 to ↑20)	⇔ (↓19 to ↑47)	↑189 (↑52 to ↑448)
Rifabutin	300 mg q.d. for 10 days	1200 mg b.i.d. for 10 days	5	⇔ (↓21 to ↑10)	↓15 (↓28 to 0)	↓15 (↓38 to ↑17)
Rifampin	300 mg q.d. for 4 days	1200 mg b.i.d. for 4 days	11	↓70 (↓76 to ↓62)	↓82 (↓84 to ↓78)	↓92 (↓95 to ↓89)
Ritonavir	100 mg b.i.d. for 2 to 4 weeks	600 mg b.i.d.	18	↓30† (↓44 to ↓14)	↑64† (↑37 to ↑97)	↑508† (↑394 to ↑649)
Ritonavir	200 mg q.d. for 2 to 4 weeks	1200 mg q.d.	12	⇔† (↓17 to ↑30)	↑62† (↑35 to ↑94)	↑319† (↑190 to ↑508)
Saquinavir	800 mg t.i.d. for 2 weeks (fed)	750 or 800 mg t.i.d. for 2 weeks (fed)	7	↓37 (↓54 to ↓14)	↓32 (↓49 to ↓9)	↓14 (↓52 to ↑54)
Zidovudine	300 mg single dose	600 mg single dose	12	⇔ (↓5 to ↑24)	↑13 (↓2 to ↑31)	NA

*Based on total-drug concentrations.
†Compared to amprenavir 1200 mg b.i.d. in the same patients.
↑ = Increase; ↓ = Decrease; ⇔ = No change (↑ or ↓ <10%); NA = C_{min} not calculated for single-dose study.

8-fold decrease in susceptibility to ritonavir. However, amprenavir-resistant isolates were susceptible to either indinavir or saquinavir.

CLINICAL PHARMACOLOGY

Pharmacokinetics in Adults: The pharmacokinetic properties of amprenavir have been studied in asymptomatic, HIV-infected adult patients after administration of single oral doses of 150 to 1200 mg and multiple oral doses of 300 to 1200 mg twice daily.

Absorption and Bioavailability: Amprenavir was rapidly absorbed after oral administration in HIV-1-infected patients with a time to peak concentration (T_{max}) typically between 1 and 2 hours after a single oral dose. The absolute oral bioavailability of amprenavir in humans has not been established. Increases in the area under the plasma concentration versus time curve (AUC) after single oral doses between 150 and 1200 mg were slightly greater than dose proportional. Increases in AUC were dose proportional after 3 weeks of dosing with doses from 300 to 1200 mg twice daily. The pharmacokinetic parameters after administration of amprenavir 1200 mg b.i.d. for 3 weeks to HIV-infected subjects are shown in Table 1.

[See table 1 at top of previous page]

The relative bioavailability of AGENERASE Capsules and Oral Solution was assessed in healthy adults. AGENERASE Oral Solution was 14% less bioavailable compared to the capsules.

Effects of Food on Oral Absorption: The relative bioavailability of AGENERASE Capsules was assessed in the fasting and fed states in healthy volunteers (standardized high-fat meal: 967 kcal, 67 grams fat, 33 grams protein, 58 grams carbohydrate). Administration of a single 1200-mg dose of amprenavir in the fed state compared to the fasted state was associated with changes in C_{max} (fed: 6.18 ± 2.92 mcg/mL, fasted: 9.72 ± 2.75 mcg/mL), T_{max} (fed: 1.51 ± 0.68, fasted: 1.05 ± 0.63), and $AUC_{0-\infty}$ (fed: 22.06 ± 11.6 mcg•h/mL, fasted: 28.05 ± 10.1 mcg•h/mL). AGENERASE may be taken with or without food, but should not be taken with a high-fat meal (see DOSAGE AND ADMINISTRATION).

Distribution: The apparent volume of distribution (V_z/F) is approximately 430 L in healthy adult subjects. *In vitro* binding is approximately 90% to plasma proteins. The high affinity binding protein for amprenavir is alpha$_1$-acid glycoprotein (AAG). The partitioning of amprenavir into erythrocytes is low, but increases as amprenavir concentrations increase, reflecting the higher amount of unbound drug at higher concentrations.

Metabolism: Amprenavir is metabolized in the liver by the cytochrome P450 3A4 (CYP3A4) enzyme system. The 2 major metabolites result from oxidation of the tetrahydrofuran and aniline moieties. Glucuronide conjugates of oxidized metabolites have been identified as minor metabolites in urine and feces.

Elimination: Excretion of unchanged amprenavir in urine and feces is minimal. Approximately 14% and 75% of an administered single dose of ^{14}C-amprenavir can be accounted for as radiocarbon in urine and feces, respectively. Two metabolites accounted for >90% of the radiocarbon in fecal samples. The plasma elimination half-life of amprenavir ranged from 7.1 to 10.6 hours.

Special Populations: ***Hepatic Insufficiency:*** AGENERASE has been studied in adult patients with impaired hepatic function using a single 600-mg oral dose. The $AUC_{0-\infty}$ was significantly greater in patients with moderate cirrhosis (25.76 ± 14.68 mcg•h/mL) compared with healthy volunteers (12.00 ± 4.38 mcg•h/mL). The $AUC_{0-\infty}$ and C_{max} were significantly greater in patients with severe cirrhosis ($AUC_{0-\infty}$: 38.66 ± 16.08 mcg•h/mL; C_{max}: 9.43 ± 2.61 mcg/mL) compared with healthy volunteers ($AUC_{0-\infty}$: 12.00 ± 4.38 mcg•h/mL; C_{max}: 4.90 ± 1.39 mcg/mL). Patients with impaired hepatic function require dosage adjustment (see DOSAGE AND ADMINISTRATION).

Renal Insufficiency: The impact of renal impairment on amprenavir elimination in adult patients has not been studied. The renal elimination of unchanged amprenavir represents <3% of the administered dose.

Pediatric Patients: The pharmacokinetics of amprenavir have been studied after either single or repeat doses of AGENERASE Capsules or Oral Solution in 84 pediatric patients. Twenty HIV-1-infected children ranging in age from 4 to 12 years received single doses from 5 mg/kg to 20 mg/kg using 25-mg or 150-mg capsules. The C_{max} of amprenavir increased less than proportionally with dose. The $AUC_{0-\infty}$ increased proportionally at doses between 5 and 20 mg/kg. Amprenavir is 14% less bioavailable from the liquid formulation than from the capsules; therefore **AGENERASE Capsules and AGENERASE Oral Solution are not interchangeable on a milligram-per-milligram basis. AGENERASE Oral Solution** is contraindicated in infants and children below the age of 4 years due to the potential risk of toxicity from the large amount of the excipient propylene glycol. Please see the complete prescribing information for **AGENERASE Oral Solution** for full information.

[See table 2 at top of previous page]

Geriatric Patients: The pharmacokinetics of amprenavir have not been studied in patients over 65 years of age.

Gender: The pharmacokinetics of amprenavir do not differ between males and females.

Race: The pharmacokinetics of amprenavir do not differ between Blacks and non-Blacks.

Drug Interactions: See also CONTRAINDICATIONS, WARNINGS, and PRECAUTIONS: Drug Interactions.

Amprenavir is metabolized in the liver by the cytochrome P450 enzyme system. Amprenavir inhibits CYP3A4. Caution should be used when coadministering medications that are substrates, inhibitors, or inducers of CYP3A4, or potentially toxic medications that are metabolized by CYP3A4. Amprenavir does not inhibit CYP2D6, CYP1A2, CYP2C9, CYP2C19, CYP2E1, or uridine glucuronosyltransferase (UDPGT).

Drug interaction studies were performed with amprenavir capsules and other drugs likely to be coadministered or drugs commonly used as probes for pharmacokinetic interactions. The effects of coadministration of amprenavir on the AUC, C_{max}, and C_{min} are summarized in Table 3 (effect of other drugs on amprenavir) and Table 4 (effect of amprenavir on other drugs). For information regarding clinical recommendations, see PRECAUTIONS.

[See table 3 at top of previous page]
[See table 4 above]

Table 4: Drug Interactions: Pharmacokinetic Parameters for Coadministered Drug in the Presence of Amprenavir

Co-administered Drug	Dose of Coadministered Drug	Dose of AGENERASE	n	% Change in Pharmacokinetic Parameters of Coadministered Drug (90% CI)		
				C_{max}	AUC	C_{min}
Clarithromycin	500 mg b.i.d. for 4 days	1200 mg b.i.d. for 4 days	12	↓10 (↓24 to ↑7)	⇔ (↓17 to ↑11)	⇔ (↓13 to ↑20)
Ketoconazole	400 mg single dose	1200 mg single dose	12	↑19 (↑8 to ↑33)	↑44 (↑31 to ↑59)	NA
Lamivudine	150 mg single dose	600 mg single dose	11	⇔ (↓17 to ↑3)	⇔ (↓11 to 0)	NA
Rifabutin	300 mg q.d. for 10 days	1200 mg b.i.d. for 10 days	5	↑119 (↑82 to ↑164)	↑193 (↑156 to ↑235)	↑271 (↑171 to ↑409)
Rifampin	300 mg q.d. for 4 days	1200 mg b.i.d. for 4 days	11	⇔ (↓13 to ↑12)	⇔ (↓10 to ↑13)	ND
Zidovudine	300 mg single dose	600 mg single dose	12	↑40 (↑14 to ↑71)	↑31 (↑19 to ↑45)	NA

↑ = Increase; ↓ = Decrease; ⇔ = No change (↑ or ↓ <10%); NA = C_{min} not calculated for single-dose study; ND = Interaction cannot be determined as C_{min} was below the lower limit of quantitation.

Table 5: Outcomes of Randomized Treatment Through Week 48 (PROAB3006)

Outcome	AGENERASE (n = 254)	Indinavir (n = 250)
HIV RNA <400 copies/mL*	30%	49%
HIV RNA ≥400 copies/mL[†,‡]	38%	26%
Discontinued due to adverse events*[,‡]	16%	12%
Discontinued due to other reasons[‡,§]	16%	13%

*Corresponds to rates at Week 48 in Figure 1.
[†]Virological failures at or before Week 48.
[‡]Considered to be treatment failure in the analysis.
[§]Includes discontinuations due to consent withdrawn, loss to follow-up, protocol violations, non-compliance, pregnancy, never treated, and other reasons.

Table 6: Drugs That are Contraindicated with AGENERASE

Drug Class	Drugs Within Class That Are CONTRAINDICATED with AGENERASE
Ergot derivatives	Dihydroergotamine, ergonovine, ergotamine, methylergonovine
GI motility agent	Cisapride
Neuroleptic	Pimozide
Sedatives/hypnotics	Midazolam, triazolam

Table 7: Drugs That Should Not Be Coadministered with AGENERASE

Drug Class/Drug Name	Clinical Comment
Antimycobacterials: Rifampin	May lead to loss of virologic response and possible resistance to AGENERASE or to the class of protease inhibitors.
Ergot derivatives: Dihydroergotamine, ergonovine, ergotamine, methylergonovine	**CONTRAINDICATED** due to potential for serious and/or life-threatening reactions such as acute ergot toxicity characterized by peripheral vasospasm and ischemia of the extremities and other tissues.
GI motility agents: Cisapride	**CONTRAINDICATED** due to potential for serious and/or life-threatening reactions such as cardiac arrhythmias.
Herbal Products: St. John's wort (hypericum perforatum)	May lead to loss of virologic response and possible resistance to AGENERASE or to the class of protease inhibitors.
HMG Co-Reductase Inhibitors: Lovastatin, simvastatin	Potential for serious reactions such as risk of myopathy including rhabdomyolysis.
Neuroleptic: Pimozide	**CONTRAINDICATED** due to potential for serious and/or life-threatening reactions such as cardiac arrhythmias.
Sedatives/hypnotics: Midazolam, triazolam	**CONTRAINDICATED** due to potential for serious and/or life-threatening reactions such as prolonged or increased sedation or respiratory depression.

Nucleoside Reverse Transcriptase Inhibitors (NRTIs): There was no effect of amprenavir on abacavir in subjects receiving both agents based on historical data.

HIV Protease Inhibitors: The effect of amprenavir on total drug concentrations of other HIV protease inhibitors in subjects receiving both agents was evaluated using comparisons to historical data. Indinavir steady-state C_{max}, AUC, and C_{min} were decreased by 22%, 38%, and 27%, respectively, by concomitant amprenavir. Similar decreases in C_{max} and AUC were seen after the first dose. Saquinavir steady-state C_{max}, AUC, and C_{min} were increased 21%, decreased 19%, and decreased 48%, respectively, by concomitant amprenavir. Nelfinavir steady-state C_{max}, AUC, and

Continued on next page

Agenerase Capsules—Cont.

C_{min} were increased by 12%, 15%, and 14%, respectively, by concomitant amprenavir.

For information regarding clinical recommendations, see PRECAUTIONS: Drug Interactions.

INDICATIONS AND USAGE

AGENERASE (amprenavir) is indicated in combination with other antiretroviral agents for the treatment of HIV-1 infection.

The following points should be considered when initiating therapy with AGENERASE:

In a study of NRTI-experienced, protease inhibitor-naive patients, AGENERASE was found to be significantly less effective than indinavir (see Description of Clinical Studies). Mild to moderate gastrointestinal adverse events led to discontinuation of AGENERASE primarily during the first 12 weeks of therapy (see ADVERSE REACTIONS).

There are no data on response to therapy with AGENERASE in protease inhibitor-experienced patients.

Description of Clinical Studies: ***Therapy-Naive Adults:*** PROAB3001, a randomized, double-blind, placebo-controlled, multicenter study, compared treatment with AGENERASE Capsules (1200 mg twice daily) plus lamivudine (150 mg twice daily) plus zidovudine (300 mg twice daily) versus lamivudine (150 mg twice daily) plus zidovudine (300 mg twice daily) in 232 patients. Through 24 weeks of therapy, 53% of patients assigned to AGENERASE/zidovudine/lamivudine achieved HIV RNA <400 copies/mL. Through week 48, the antiviral response was 41%. Through 24 weeks of therapy, 11% of patients assigned to zidovudine/lamivudine achieved HIV RNA <400 copies/mL. Antiviral response beyond week 24 is not interpretable because the majority of patients discontinued or changed their antiretroviral therapy.

NRTI-Experienced Adults: PROAB3006, a randomized, open-label multicenter study, compared treatment with AGENERASE Capsules (1200 mg twice daily) plus NRTIs versus indinavir (800 mg every 8 hours) plus NRTIs in 504 NRTI-experienced, protease inhibitor-naive patients, median age 37 years (range 20 to 71 years), 72% Caucasian, 80% male, with a median CD4 cell count of 404 cells/mm^3 (range 9 to 1706 cells/mm^3) and a median plasma HIV-1 RNA level of 3.93 $\log_{10}$ copies/mL (range 2.60 to 7.01 $\log_{10}$ copies/mL) at baseline. Through 48 weeks of therapy, the median CD4 cell count increase from baseline in the amprenavir group was significantly lower than in the indinavir group, 97 cells/mm^3 versus 144 cells/mm^3, respectively. There was also a significant difference in the proportions of patients with plasma HIV-1 RNA levels <400 copies/mL through 48 weeks (see Figure 1 and Table 5).

Figure 1: Virologic Response Through Week 48, PROAB3006*,†

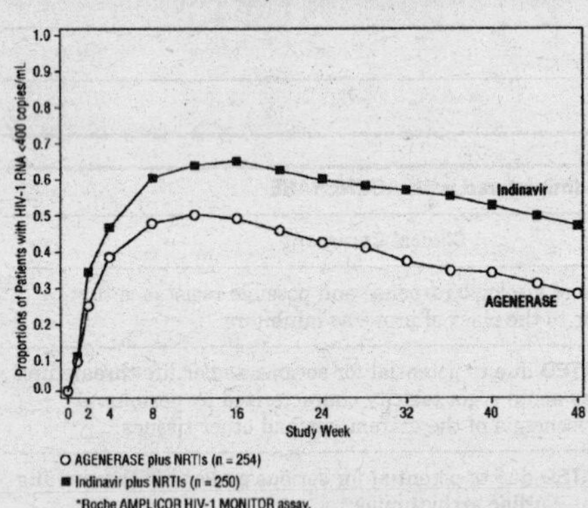

HIV-1 RNA status and reasons for discontinuation of randomized treatment at 48 weeks are summarized (Table 5).

[See table 5 at top of previous page]

CONTRAINDICATIONS

Coadministration of AGENERASE is contraindicated with drugs that are highly dependent on CYP3A4 for clearance and for which elevated plasma concentrations are associated with serious and/or life-threatening events. These drugs are listed in Table 6.

[See table 6 at top of previous page]

If AGENERASE is coadministered with ritonavir, the antiarrhythmic agents flecainide and propafenone are also contraindicated.

Because of the potential toxicity from the large amount of the excipient propylene glycol contained in **AGENERASE Oral Solution**, that formulation is contraindicated in certain patient populations and should be used with caution in others. Consult the complete prescribing information for **AGENERASE Oral Solution** for full information.

AGENERASE is contraindicated in patients with previously demonstrated clinically significant hypersensitivity to any of the components of this product.

WARNINGS

ALERT: Find out about medicines that should not be taken with AGENERASE.

Serious and/or life-threatening drug interactions could occur between amprenavir and amiodarone, lidocaine (systemic), tricyclic antidepressants, and quinidine. Concentration monitoring of these agents is recommended if these agents are used concomitantly with AGENERASE (see CONTRAINDICATIONS).

Rifampin should not be used in combination with amprenavir because it reduces plasma concentrations and AUC of amprenavir by about 90%.

Concomitant use of AGENERASE and St. John's wort (hypericum perforatum) or products containing St. John's wort is not recommended. Coadministration of protease inhibitors, including AGENERASE, with St. John's wort is expected to substantially decrease protease inhibitor concentrations and may result in suboptimal levels of amprenavir and lead to loss of virologic response and possible resistance to AGENERASE or to the class of protease inhibitors.

Concomitant use of AGENERASE with lovastatin or simvastatin is not recommended. Caution should be exercised if HIV protease inhibitors, including AGENERASE, are used concurrently with other HMG-CoA reductase inhibitors that are also metabolized by the CYP3A4 pathway (e.g., atorvastatin). The risk of myopathy, including rhabdomyolysis, may be increased when HIV protease inhibitors, including amprenavir, are used in combination with these drugs.

Particular caution should be used when prescribing sildenafil in patients receiving amprenavir. Coadministration of AGENERASE with sildenafil is expected to substantially increase sildenafil concentrations and may result in an increase in sildenafil-associated adverse events, including hypotension, visual changes, and priapism (see PRECAUTIONS: Drug Interactions and Information for Patients, and the complete prescribing information for sildenafil).

Because of the potential toxicity from the large amount of the excipient propylene glycol contained in **AGENERASE Oral Solution**, that formulation is contraindicated in certain patient populations and should be used with caution in others. Consult the complete prescribing information for **AGENERASE Oral Solution** for full information.

Severe and life-threatening skin reactions, including Stevens-Johnson syndrome, have occurred in patients treated with AGENERASE (see ADVERSE REACTIONS).

Acute hemolytic anemia has been reported in a patient treated with AGENERASE.

New onset diabetes mellitus, exacerbation of pre-existing diabetes mellitus, and hyperglycemia have been reported during post-marketing surveillance in HIV-infected patients receiving protease inhibitor therapy. Some patients required either initiation or dose adjustments of insulin or oral hypoglycemic agents for treatment of these events. In some cases, diabetic ketoacidosis has occurred. In those patients who discontinued protease inhibitor therapy, hyperglycemia persisted in some cases. Because these events have been reported voluntarily during clinical practice, estimates of frequency cannot be made and causal relationships between protease inhibitor therapy and these events have not been established.

PRECAUTIONS

General: AGENERASE Capsules and AGENERASE Oral Solution are not interchangeable on a milligram-per-milligram basis (see CLINICAL PHARMACOLOGY: Pediatric Patients).

Amprenavir is a sulfonamide. The potential for cross-sensitivity between drugs in the sulfonamide class and amprenavir is unknown. AGENERASE should be used with caution in patients with a known sulfonamide allergy.

AGENERASE is principally metabolized by the liver. AGENERASE, when used alone and in combination with low-dose ritonavir, has been associated with elevations of SGOT (AST) and SGPT (ALT) in some patients. Caution should be exercised when administering AGENERASE to patients with hepatic impairment (see DOSAGE AND ADMINISTRATION). Appropriate laboratory testing should be conducted prior to initiating therapy with AGENERASE and at periodic intervals during treatment.

Formulations of AGENERASE provide high daily doses of vitamin E (see Information for Patients, DESCRIPTION, and DOSAGE AND ADMINISTRATION). The effects of long-term, high-dose vitamin E administration in humans is not well characterized and has not been specifically studied in HIV-infected individuals. High vitamin E doses may exacerbate the blood coagulation defect of vitamin K deficiency caused by anticoagulant therapy or malabsorption.

Patients with Hemophilia: There have been reports of spontaneous bleeding in patients with hemophilia A and B treated with protease inhibitors. In some patients, additional factor VIII was required. In many of the reported cases, treatment with protease inhibitors was continued or restarted. A causal relationship between protease inhibitor therapy and these episodes has not been established.

Fat Redistribution: Redistribution/accumulation of body fat, including central obesity, dorsocervical fat enlargement

Table 8: Established and Other Potentially Significant Drug Interactions: Alteration in Dose or Regimen May be Recommended Based on Drug Interaction Studies or Predicted Interaction

Concomitant Drug Class: Drug Name	Effect on Concentration of Amprenavir or Concomitant Drug	Clinical Comment
	HIV-Antiviral Agents	
Non-nucleoside Reverse Transcriptase Inhibitors: Efavirenz, nevirapine	↓ Amprenavir	Appropriate doses of the combinations with respect to safety and efficacy have not been established.
Non-nucleoside Reverse Transcriptase Inhibitor: Delavirdine	↑ Amprenavir	Appropriate doses of the combination with respect to safety and efficacy have not been established.
Nucleoside Reverse Transcriptase Inhibitor: Didanosine (buffered formulation only)	↓ Amprenavir	Take AGENERASE at least 1 hour before or after the buffered formulation of didanosine.
HIV-Protease Inhibitors: Indinavir*, lopinavir/ritonavir, nelfinavir*	↑ Amprenavir Amprenavir's effect on other protease inhibitors is not well established.	Appropriate doses of the combinations with respect to safety and efficacy have not been established.
HIV-Protease Inhibitor: Ritonavir*	↑ Amprenavir	The dose of amprenavir should be reduced when used in combination with ritonavir (see Dosage and Administration). Also, see the full prescribing information for NORVIR® for additional drug interaction information.
HIV-Protease Inhibitor: Saquinavir*	↓ Amprenavir Amprenavir's effect on saquinavir is not well established.	Appropriate doses of the combination with respect to safety and efficacy have not been established.
	Other Agents	
Antacids	↓ Amprenavir	Take AGENERASE at least 1 hour before or after antacids.
Antiarrhythmics: Amiodarone, lidocaine (systemic), and quinidine	↑ Antiarrhythmics	Caution is warranted and therapeutic concentration monitoring is recommended for antiarrhythmics when coadministered with AGENERASE, if available.
Antiarrhythmic: Bepridil	↑ Bepridil	Use with caution. Increased bepridil exposure may be associated with life-threatening reactions such as cardiac arrhythmias.
Anticoagulant: Warfarin		Concentrations of warfarin may be affected. It is recommended that INR (international normalized ratio) be monitored.

(Table continued on next page)

(buffalo hump), peripheral wasting, facial wasting, breast enlargement, and "cushingoid appearance," have been observed in patients receiving antiretroviral therapy. The mechanism and long-term consequences of these events are currently unknown. A causal relationship has not been established.

Lipid Elevations: Treatment with AGENERASE alone or in combination with ritonavir has resulted in increases in the concentration of total cholesterol and triglycerides. Triglyceride and cholesterol testing should be performed prior to initiation of therapy with AGENERASE and at periodic intervals during treatment. Lipid disorders should be managed as clinically appropriate. See PRECAUTIONS Table 8: Established and Other Potentially Significant Drug Interactions for additional information on potential drug interactions with AGENERASE and HMG-CoA reductase inhibitors.

Resistance/Cross-Resistance: Because the potential for HIV cross-resistance among protease inhibitors has not been fully explored, it is unknown what effect amprenavir therapy will have on the activity of subsequently administered protease inhibitors. It is also unknown what effect previous treatment with other protease inhibitors will have on the activity of amprenavir (see MICROBIOLOGY).

Information for Patients: A statement to patients and healthcare providers is included on the product's bottle label: **ALERT: Find out about medicines that should NOT be taken with AGENERASE.** A Patient Package Insert (PPI) for AGENERASE Capsules is available for patient information. Patients treated with AGENERASE Capsules should be cautioned against switching to **AGENERASE Oral Solution** because of the increased risk of adverse events from the large amount of propylene glycol in **AGENERASE Oral Solution**. Please see the complete prescribing information for **AGENERASE Oral Solution** for full information.

Patients should be informed that AGENERASE is not a cure for HIV infection and that they may continue to develop opportunistic infections and other complications associated with HIV disease. The long-term effects of AGENERASE (amprenavir) are unknown at this time. Patients should be told that there are currently no data demonstrating that therapy with AGENERASE can reduce the risk of transmitting HIV to others through sexual contact.

Patients should remain under the care of a physician while using AGENERASE. Patients should be advised to take AGENERASE every day as prescribed. AGENERASE must always be used in combination with other antiretroviral drugs. Patients should not alter the dose or discontinue therapy without consulting their physician. If a dose is missed, patients should take the dose as soon as possible and then return to their normal schedule. However, if a dose is skipped, the patient should not double the next dose.

Patients should inform their doctor if they have a sulfa allergy. The potential for cross-sensitivity between drugs in the sulfonamide class and amprenavir is unknown.

AGENERASE may interact with many drugs; therefore, patients should be advised to report to their doctor the use of any other prescription or nonprescription medication or herbal products, particularly St. John's wort.

Patients taking antacids (or the buffered formulation of didanosine) should take AGENERASE at least 1 hour before or after antacid (or the buffered formulation of didanosine) use.

Patients receiving sildenafil should be advised that they may be at an increased risk of sildenafil-associated adverse events, including hypotension, visual changes, and priapism, and should promptly report any symptoms to their doctor.

Patients receiving hormonal contraceptives should be instructed that alternate contraceptive measures should be used during therapy with AGENERASE.

High-fat meals may decrease the absorption of AGENERASE and should be avoided. AGENERASE may be taken with meals of normal fat content.

Patients should be informed that redistribution or accumulation of body fat may occur in patients receiving antiretroviral therapy and that the cause and long-term health effects of these conditions are not known at this time.

Adult and pediatric patients should be advised not to take supplemental vitamin E since the vitamin E content of AGENERASE Capsules and Oral Solution exceeds the Reference Daily Intake (adults 30 IU, pediatrics approximately 10 IU).

Laboratory Tests: The combination of AGENERASE and low-dose ritonavir has been associated with elevations of cholesterol and triglycerides, SGOT (AST), and SGPT (ALT) in some patients. Appropriate laboratory testing should be considered prior to initiating combination therapy with AGENERASE and ritonavir and at periodic intervals or if any clinical signs or symptoms of hyperlipidemia or elevated liver function tests occur during therapy. For comprehensive information concerning laboratory test alterations associated with ritonavir, physicians should refer to the complete prescribing information for NORVIR® (ritonavir).

Drug Interactions: See also CONTRAINDICATIONS, WARNINGS, and CLINICAL PHARMACOLOGY: Drug Interactions.

AGENERASE is an inhibitor of cytochrome P450 3A4 metabolism and therefore should not be administered concurrently with medications with narrow therapeutic windows that are substrates of CYP3A4. There are other agents that may result in serious and/or life-threatening drug interactions (see CONTRAINDICATIONS and WARNINGS).

[See table 7 at top of page 157]
[See table 8 on previous page and above]

Table 8: Established and Other Potentially Significant Drug Interactions: Alteration in Dose or Regimen May be Recommended Based on Drug Interaction Studies or Predicted Interaction — *(cont.)*

Concomitant Drug Class: Drug Name	Effect on Concentration of Amprenavir or Concomitant Drug	Clinical Comment
	Other Agents — (continued)	
Anticonvulsants: Carbamazepine, phenobarbital, phenytoin	↓ Amprenavir	Use with caution. AGENERASE may be less effective due to decreased amprenavir plasma concentrations in patients taking these agents concomitantly.
Antifungals: Ketoconazole, itraconazole	↑ Ketoconazole ↑ Itraconazole	Increase monitoring for adverse events due to ketoconazole or itraconazole. Dose reduction of ketoconazole or itraconazole may be needed for patients receiving more than 400 mg ketoconazole or itraconazole per day.
Antimycobacterial: Rifabutin*	↑ Rifabutin and rifabutin metabolite	A dosage reduction of rifabutin to at least half the recommended dose is required when AGENERASE and rifabutin are coadministered.* A complete blood count should be performed weekly and as clinically indicated in order to monitor for neutropenia in patients receiving amprenavir and rifabutin.
Benzodiazepines: Alprazolam, clorazepate, diazepam, flurazepam	↑ Benzodiazepines	Clinical significance is unknown; however, a decrease in benzodiazepine dose may be needed.
Calcium Channel Blockers: Diltiazem, felodipine, nifedipine, nicardipine, nimodipine, verapamil, amlodipine, nisoldipine, isradipine	↑ Calcium channel blockers	Caution is warranted and clinical monitoring of patients is recommended.
Corticosteroid: Dexamethasone	↓ Amprenavir	Use with caution. AGENERASE may be less effective due to decreased amprenavir plasma concentrations in patients taking these agents concomitantly.
Erectile Dysfunction Agent: Sildenafil	↑ Sildenafil	Use with caution at reduced doses of 25 mg every 48 hours with increased monitoring for adverse events.
HMG-CoA Reductase Inhibitors: Atorvastatin	↑ Atorvastatin	Use lowest possible dose of atorvastatin with careful monitoring or consider other HMG-CoA reductase inhibitors such as pravastatin or fluvastatin in combination with AGENERASE.
Immunosuppressants: Cyclosporine, tacrolimus, rapamycin	↑ Immunosuppressants	Therapeutic concentration monitoring is recommended for immunosuppressant agents when coadministered with AGENERASE.
Oral Contraceptive: Ethinyl estradiol	Effect on ethinyl estradiol is not known.	Alternative or additional contraceptive measures should be used when estrogen-based oral contraceptives and AGENERASE are coadministered.
Tricyclic Antidepressants: Amitriptyline, imipramine	↑ Tricyclics	Therapeutic concentration monitoring is recommended for tricyclic antidepressants when coadministered with AGENERASE.

*See CLINICAL PHARMACOLOGY for magnitude of interaction, Tables 3 and 4.

Table 9: Selected Clinical Adverse Events of All Grades Reported in >5% of Adult Patients

	PROAB3001 Therapy-Naive Patients		PROAB3006 NRTI-Experienced Patients	
Adverse Event	AGENERASE/ Lamivudine/ Zidovudine (n = 113)	Lamivudine/ Zidovudine (n = 109)	AGENERASE/ NRTI (n = 245)	Indinavir/NRTI (n = 241)
Digestive				
Nausea	74%	50%	43%	35%
Vomiting	34%	17%	24%	20%
Diarrhea or loose stools	39%	35%	60%	41%
Taste disorders	10%	6%	2%	8%
Skin				
Rash	27%	6%	20%	15%
Nervous				
Paresthesia, oral/perioral	26%	6%	31%	2%
Paresthesia, peripheral	10%	4%	14%	10%
Psychiatric				
Depressive or mood disorders	16%	4%	9%	13%

Carcinogenesis and Mutagenesis: Long-term carcinogenicity studies of amprenavir in rodents are in progress. Amprenavir was not mutagenic or genotoxic in a battery of *in vitro* and *in vivo* assays including bacterial reverse mutation (Ames), mouse lymphoma, rat micronucleus, and chromosome aberrations in human lymphocytes.

Fertility: The effects of amprenavir on fertility and general reproductive performance were investigated in male rats (treated for 28 days before mating at doses producing up to twice the expected clinical exposure based on AUC comparisons) and female rats (treated for 15 days before mating through day 17 of gestation at doses producing up to 2 times the expected clinical exposure). Amprenavir did not impair mating or fertility of male or female rats and did not affect the development and maturation of sperm from treated rats. The reproductive performance of the F1 generation born to female rats given amprenavir was not different from control animals.

Pregnancy and Reproduction: Pregnancy Category C. Embryo/fetal development studies were conducted in rats (dosed from 15 days before pairing to day 17 of gestation) and rabbits (dosed from day 8 to day 20 of gestation). In pregnant rabbits, amprenavir administration was associated with abortions and an increased incidence of 3 minor skeletal variations resulting from deficient ossification of the femur, humerus trochlea, and humerus. Systemic exposure at the highest tested dose was approximately one twentieth of the exposure seen at the recommended human dose. In rat fetuses, thymic elongation and incomplete ossification of bones were attributed to amprenavir. Both findings were

Continued on next page

Agenerase Capsules—Cont.

seen at systemic exposures that were one half of that associated with the recommended human dose.
Pre- and post-natal developmental studies were performed in rats dosed from day 7 of gestation to day 22 of lactation. Reduced body weights (10% to 20%) were observed in the offspring. The systemic exposure associated with this finding was approximately twice the exposure in humans following administration of the recommended human dose. The subsequent development of these offspring, including fertility and reproductive performance, was not affected by the maternal administration of amprenavir.
There are no adequate and well-controlled studies in pregnant women. AGENERASE should be used during pregnancy only if the potential benefit justifies the potential risk to the fetus. **AGENERASE Oral Solution** is contraindicated during pregnancy due to the potential risk of toxicity to the fetus from the high propylene glycol content.
Antiretroviral Pregnancy Registry: To monitor maternal-fetal outcomes of pregnant women exposed to AGENERASE, an Antiretroviral Pregnancy Registry has been established. Physicians are encouraged to register patients by calling 1-800-258-4263.
Nursing Mothers: The Centers for Disease Control and Prevention recommend that HIV-infected mothers not breastfeed their infants to avoid risking postnatal transmission of HIV. Although it is not known if amprenavir is excreted in human milk, amprenavir is secreted into the milk of lactating rats. Because of both the potential for HIV transmission and the potential for serious adverse reactions in nursing infants, **mothers should be instructed not to breastfeed if they are receiving AGENERASE.**
Pediatric Use: Two hundred fifty-one patients aged 4 and above have received amprenavir as single or multiple doses in studies. An adverse event profile similar to that seen in adults was seen in pediatric patients.
AGENERASE Capsules have not been evaluated in pediatric patients below the age of 4 years (see CLINICAL PHARMACOLOGY and DOSAGE AND ADMINISTRATION).
AGENERASE Oral Solution is contraindicated in infants and children below the age of 4 years due to the potential risk of toxicity from the large amount of the excipient propylene glycol. Please see the complete prescribing information for **AGENERASE Oral Solution** for full information.
Geriatric Use: Clinical studies of AGENERASE did not include sufficient numbers of patients aged 65 and over to determine whether they respond differently from younger adults. In general, dose selection for an elderly patient should be cautious, reflecting the greater frequency of decreased hepatic, renal, or cardiac function, and of concomitant disease or other drug therapy.

ADVERSE REACTIONS

In clinical studies, adverse events leading to amprenavir discontinuation occurred primarily during the first 12 weeks of therapy, and were mostly due to gastrointestinal events (nausea, vomiting, diarrhea, and abdominal pain/discomfort), which were mild to moderate in severity.
Skin rash occurred in 22% of patients treated with amprenavir in studies PROAB3001 and PROAB3006. Rashes were usually maculopapular and of mild or moderate intensity, some with pruritus. Rashes had a median onset of 11 days after amprenavir initiation and a median duration of 10 days. Skin rashes led to amprenavir discontinuation in approximately 3% of patients. In some patients with mild or moderate rash, amprenavir dosing was often continued without interruption; if interrupted, reintroduction of amprenavir generally did not result in rash recurrence.
Severe or life-threatening rash (Grade 3 or 4), including cases of Stevens-Johnson syndrome, occurred in approximately 1% of recipients of AGENERASE (see WARNINGS). Amprenavir therapy should be discontinued for severe or life-threatening rashes and for moderate rashes accompanied by systemic symptoms.
[See table 9 at top of previous page]
Among amprenavir-treated patients in Phase 3 studies, 2 patients developed de novo diabetes mellitus, 1 patient developed a dorsocervical fat enlargement (buffalo hump), and 9 patients developed fat redistribution.
[See table 10 below]
In studies PROAB3001 and PROAB3006, no increased frequency of Grade 3 or 4 AST, ALT, amylase, or bilirubin elevations was seen compared to controls.
Pediatric Patients: An adverse event profile similar to that seen in adults was seen in pediatric patients.
Concomitant Therapy with Ritonavir:
[See table 11 below]
Treatment with AGENERASE in combination with ritonavir has resulted in increases in the concentration of total cholesterol and triglycerides (see PRECAUTIONS Lipid Elevations and Laboratory Tests).

OVERDOSAGE

There is no known antidote for AGENERASE. It is not known whether amprenavir can be removed by peritoneal dialysis or hemodialysis. If overdosage occurs, the patient should be monitored for evidence of toxicity and standard supportive treatment applied as necessary.

DOSAGE AND ADMINISTRATION

AGENERASE may be taken with or without food; however, a high-fat meal decreases the absorption of amprenavir and should be avoided (see CLINICAL PHARMACOLOGY: Effects of Food on Oral Absorption). **Adult and pediatric patients should be advised not to take supplemental vitamin E since the vitamin E content of AGENERASE Capsules exceeds the Reference Daily Intake (adults 30 IU, pediatrics approximately 10 IU) (see DESCRIPTION).**
Adults: The recommended oral dose of AGENERASE Capsules for adults is 1200 mg (eight 150-mg capsules) twice daily in combination with other antiretroviral agents.
Concomitant Therapy: If AGENERASE and ritonavir are used in combination, the recommended dosage regimens are: AGENERASE 1200 mg with ritonavir 200 mg once daily or AGENERASE 600 mg with ritonavir 100 mg twice daily.
Pediatric Patients: For adolescents (13 to 16 years), the recommended oral dose of AGENERASE Capsules is 1200 mg (eight 150-mg capsules) twice daily in combination with other antiretroviral agents. For patients between 4 and 12 years of age or for patients 13 to 16 years of age with weight of <50 kg, the recommended oral dose of AGENERASE Capsules is 20 mg/kg twice daily or 15 mg/kg 3 times daily (to a maximum daily dose of 2400 mg) in combination with other antiretroviral agents. Before using **AGENERASE Oral Solution**, the complete prescribing information should be consulted.
AGENERASE Capsules and AGENERASE Oral Solution are not interchangeable on a milligram-per-milligram basis (see CLINICAL PHARMACOLOGY).
Patients with Hepatic Impairment: AGENERASE Capsules should be used with caution in patients with moderate or severe hepatic impairment. Patients with a Child-Pugh score ranging from 5 to 8 should receive a reduced dose of AGENERASE Capsules of 450 mg twice daily, and patients with a Child-Pugh score ranging from 9 to 12 should receive a reduced dose of AGENERASE Capsules of 300 mg twice daily (see CLINICAL PHARMACOLOGY: Hepatic Insufficiency).

HOW SUPPLIED

AGENERASE Capsules, 50 mg, are oblong, opaque, off-white to cream-colored soft gelatin capsules printed with "GX CC1" on one side.
Bottles of 480 with child-resistant closures (NDC 0173-0679-00).
AGENERASE Capsules, 150 mg, are oblong, opaque, off-white to cream-colored soft gelatin capsules printed with "GX CC2" on one side.
Bottles of 240 with child-resistant closures (NDC 0173-0672-00).
Store at controlled room temperature of 25°C (77°F) (see USP).
Manufactured by R.P. Scherer, Beinheim, France
for GlaxoSmithKline, Research Triangle Park, NC 27709
Licensed from Vertex Pharmaceuticals Incorporated
Cambridge, MA 02139
AGENERASE is a registered trademark of the GlaxoSmithKline group of companies.

February 2002/RL-1061

Table 10: Selected Laboratory Abnormalities of All Grades Reported in ≥5% of Adult Patients

	PROAB3001 Therapy-Naive Patients		PROAB3006 NRTI-Experienced Patients	
Laboratory Abnormality (non-fasting specimens)	AGENERASE/ Lamivudine/ Zidovudine (n = 111)	Lamivudine/ Zidovudine (n = 108)	AGENERASE/ NRTI (n = 237)	Indinavir/NRTI (n = 239)
Hyperglycemia (>116 mg/dL)	45%	31%	53%	58%
Hypertriglyceridemia (>213 mg/dL)	41%	27%	56%	52%
Hypercholesterolemia (>283 mg/dL)	7%	3%	13%	15%

Table 11: Selected Clinical Adverse Events of all Grades Reported in ≥5% of Adult Patients in Ongoing, Open-Label Clinical Trials of AGENERASE in Combination with Ritonavir

	AGENERASE 1200 mg plus Ritonavir 200 mg q.d.* (n = 101)	AGENERASE 600 mg plus Ritonavir 100 mg b.i.d.† (n = 215)
Diarrhea/loose stools	25%	7%
Nausea	23%	7%
Vomiting	10%	4%
Abdominal symptoms	13%	3%
Headache	15%	3%
Paresthesias	8%	2%
Rash	9%	2%
Fatigue	5%	4%

*Data from 2 ongoing, open-label studies in treatment-naive patients also receiving abacavir/lamivudine.
†Data from 3 ongoing, open-label studies in treatment-naive and treatment-experienced patients receiving combination antiretroviral therapy.

AGENERASE® ℞

[ă-jin' ə-rās]
(amprenavir)
Oral Solution

Prescribing information for this product, which appears on pages 1459–1463 of the 2002 PDR, has been completely revised as follows. Please write "See Supplement A" next to the product heading.

> Because of the potential risk of toxicity from the large amount of the excipient propylene glycol, AGENERASE Oral Solution is contraindicated in infants and children below the age of 4 years, pregnant women, patients with hepatic or renal failure, and patients treated with disulfiram or metronidazole (see CONTRAINDICATIONS AND WARNINGS).
> AGENERASE Oral Solution should be used only when AGENERASE Capsules or other protease inhibitor formulations are not therapeutic options.

DESCRIPTION

AGENERASE (amprenavir) is an inhibitor of the human immunodeficiency virus (HIV) protease. The chemical name of amprenavir is (3*S*)-tetrahydro-3-furyl *N*-[(1*S*,2*R*)-3-(4-amino-*N*-isobutylbenzenesulfonamido)-1-benzyl-2-hydroxypropyl]carbamate. Amprenavir is a single stereoisomer with the (3*S*)(1*S*,2*R*) configuration. It has a molecular formula of $C_{25}H_{35}N_3O_6S$ and a molecular weight of 505.64. Amprenavir is a white to cream-colored solid with a solubility of approximately 0.04 mg/mL in water at 25°C.
AGENERASE Oral Solution is for oral administration. One milliliter (1 mL) of AGENERASE Oral Solution contains 15 mg of amprenavir in solution and the inactive ingredients acesulfame potassium, artificial grape bubblegum flavor, citric acid (anhydrous), d-alpha tocopheryl polyethylene glycol 1000 succinate (TPGS), menthol, natural peppermint flavor, polyethylene glycol 400 (PEG 400) (170 mg), propylene glycol (550 mg), saccharin sodium, sodium chloride, and sodium citrate (dihydrate). Solutions of sodium hydroxide and/or diluted hydrochloric acid may have been added to adjust pH. Each mL of AGENERASE Oral Solution contains 46 IU vitamin E in the form of TPGS. Propylene glycol is in the formulation to achieve adequate solubility of amprenavir. The recommended daily dose of AGENERASE Oral Solution of 22.5 mg/kg twice daily corresponds to a propylene glycol intake of 1650 mg/kg per day. Acceptable intake of propylene glycol for pharmaceuticals has not been established.

Table 1: Average (%CV) Pharmacokinetic Parameters After 1200 mg b.i.d. of Amprenavir Capsules (n = 54)

C_{max} (mcg/mL)	T_{max} (hours)	AUC_{0-12} (mcg•h/mL)	C_{avg} (mcg/mL)	C_{min} (mcg/mL)	CL/F (mL/min/kg)
7.66 (54%)	1.0 (42%)	17.7 (47%)	1.48 (47%)	0.32 (77%)	19.5 (46%)

Table 2: Average (%CV) Pharmacokinetic Parameters in Children Ages 4 to 12 Years Receiving 20 mg/kg b.i.d. or 15 mg/kg t.i.d. of AGENERASE Oral Solution

Dose	n	C_{max} (mcg/mL)	T_{max} (hours)	AUC_{ss}* (mcg•h/mL)	C_{avg} (mcg/mL)	C_{min} (mcg/mL)	CL/F (mL/min/kg)
20 mg/kg b.i.d.	20	6.77 (51%)	1.1 (21%)	15.46 (59%)	1.29 (59%)	0.24 (98%)	29 (58%)
15 mg/kg t.i.d.	17	3.99 (37%)	1.4 (90%)	8.73 (36%)	1.09 (36%)	0.27 (95%)	32 (34%)

*AUC is 0 to 12 hours for b.i.d. and 0 to 8 hours for t.i.d., therefore the C_{avg} is a better comparison of the exposures.

Table 3: Drug Interactions: Pharmacokinetic Parameters for Amprenavir in the Presence of the Coadministered Drug

Co-administered Drug	Dose of Coadministered Drug	Dose of AGENERASE	n	% Change in **Amprenavir** Pharmacokinetic Parameters* (90% CI)		
				C_{max}	AUC	C_{min}
Abacavir	300 mg b.i.d. for 3 weeks	900 mg b.i.d. for 3 weeks	4	↑47 (↓15 to ↑154)	↑29 (↓18 to ↑103)	↑27 (↓46 to ↑197)
Clarithromycin	500 mg b.i.d. for 4 days	1200 mg b.i.d. for 4 days	12	↑15 (↑1 to ↑31)	↑18 (↑8 to ↑29)	↑39 (↑31 to ↑47)
Indinavir	800 mg t.i.d. for 2 weeks (fasted)	750 or 800 mg t.i.d. for 2 weeks (fasted)	9	↑18 (↓13 to ↑58)	↑33 (↑2 to ↑73)	↑25 (↓27 to ↑116)
Ketoconazole	400 mg single dose	1200 mg single dose	12	↓16 (↓25 to ↓6)	↑31 (↑20 to ↑42)	NA
Lamivudine	150 mg single dose	600 mg single dose	11	⇔ (↓17 to ↑9)	⇔ (↓15 to ↑14)	NA
Nelfinavir	750 mg t.i.d. for 2 weeks (fed)	750 or 800 mg t.i.d. for 2 weeks (fed)	6	↓14 (↓38 to ↑20)	⇔ (↓19 to ↑47)	↑189 (↑52 to ↑448)
Rifabutin	300 mg q.d. for 10 days	1200 mg b.i.d. for 10 days	5	⇔ (↓21 to ↑10)	↓15 (↓28 to 0)	↓15 (↓38 to ↑17)
Rifampin	300 mg q.d. for 4 days	1200 mg b.i.d. for 4 days	11	↓70 (↓76 to ↓62)	↓82 (↓84 to ↓78)	↓92 (↓95 to ↓89)
Ritonavir	100 mg b.i.d. for 2 to 4 weeks	600 mg b.i.d.	18	↓30† (↓44 to ↓14)	↑64† (↑37 to ↑97)	↑508† (↑394 to ↑649)
Ritonavir	200 mg q.d. for 2 to 4 weeks	1200 mg q.d.	12	⇔† (↓17 to ↑30)	↑62† (↑35 to ↑94)	↑319† (↑190 to ↑508)
Saquinavir	800 mg t.i.d. for 2 weeks (fed)	750 or 800 mg t.i.d. for 2 weeks (fed)	7	↓37 (↓54 to ↓14)	↓32 (↓49 to ↓9)	↓14 (↓52 to ↑54)
Zidovudine	300 mg single dose	600 mg single dose	12	⇔ (↓5 to ↑24)	↑13 (↓2 to ↑31)	NA

*Based on total-drug concentrations.
†Compared to amprenavir capsules 1200 mg b.i.d. in the same patients.
↑ = Increase; ↓ = Decrease; ⇔ = No change (↑ or ↓ <10%); NA = C_{min} not calculated for single-dose study.

MICROBIOLOGY

Mechanism of Action: Amprenavir is an inhibitor of HIV-1 protease. Amprenavir binds to the active site of HIV-1 protease and thereby prevents the processing of viral gag and gag-pol polyprotein precursors, resulting in the formation of immature non-infectious viral particles.

Antiviral Activity *in Vitro*: The *in vitro* antiviral activity of amprenavir was evaluated against HIV-1 IIIB in both acutely and chronically infected lymphoblastic cell lines (MT-4, CEM-CCRF, H9) and in peripheral blood lymphocytes. The 50% inhibitory concentration (IC_{50}) of amprenavir ranged from 0.012 to 0.08 µM in acutely infected cells and was 0.41 µM in chronically infected cells (1 µM = 0.50 mcg/mL). Amprenavir exhibited synergistic anti-HIV-1 activity in combination with abacavir, zidovudine, didanosine, or saquinavir, and additive anti-HIV-1 activity in combination with indinavir, nelfinavir, and ritonavir *in vitro*. These drug combinations have not been adequately studied in humans. The relationship between *in vitro* anti-HIV-1 activity of amprenavir and the inhibition of HIV-1 replication in humans has not been defined.

Resistance: HIV-1 isolates with a decreased susceptibility to amprenavir have been selected *in vitro* and obtained from patients treated with amprenavir. Genotypic analysis of isolates from amprenavir-treated patients showed mutations in the HIV-1 protease gene resulting in amino acid substitutions primarily at positions V32I, M46I/L, I47V, I50V, I54L/M, and I84V as well as mutations in the p7/p1 and p1/p6 gag cleavage sites. Phenotypic analysis of HIV-1 isolates from 21 nucleoside reverse transcriptase inhibitor-(NRTI-) experienced, protease inhibitor-naive patients treated with amprenavir in combination with NRTIs for 16 to 48 weeks identified isolates from 15 patients who exhibited a 4- to 17-fold decrease in susceptibility to amprenavir *in vitro* compared to wild-type virus. Clinical isolates that exhibited a decrease in amprenavir susceptibility harbored one or more amprenavir-associated mutations. The clinical relevance of the genotypic and phenotypic changes associated with amprenavir therapy is under evaluation.

Cross-Resistance: Varying degrees of HIV-1 cross-resistance among protease inhibitors have been observed. Five of 15 amprenavir-resistant isolates exhibited 4- to 8-fold decrease in susceptibility to ritonavir. However, amprenavir-resistant isolates were susceptible to either indinavir or saquinavir.

CLINICAL PHARMACOLOGY

Pharmacokinetics in Adults: The pharmacokinetic properties of amprenavir have been studied in asymptomatic, HIV-infected adult patients after administration of single oral doses of 150 to 1200 mg and multiple oral doses of 300 to 1200 mg twice daily.

Absorption and Bioavailability: Amprenavir was rapidly absorbed after oral administration in HIV-1-infected patients with a time to peak concentration (T_{max}) typically between 1 and 2 hours after a single oral dose. The absolute oral bioavailability of amprenavir in humans has not been established.

Increases in the area under the plasma concentration versus time curve (AUC) after single oral doses between 150 and 1200 mg were slightly greater than dose proportional. Increases in AUC were dose proportional after 3 weeks of dosing with doses from 300 to 1200 mg twice daily. The pharmacokinetic parameters after administration of amprenavir 1200 mg b.i.d. for 3 weeks to HIV-infected subjects are shown in Table 1.

[See table above]

The relative bioavailability of AGENERASE Capsules and Oral Solution was assessed in healthy adults. AGENERASE Oral Solution was 14% less bioavailable compared to the capsules.

Effects of Food on Oral Absorption: The relative bioavailability of AGENERASE Capsules was assessed in the fasting and fed states in healthy volunteers (standardized high-fat meal: 967 kcal, 67 grams fat, 33 grams protein, 58 grams carbohydrate). Administration of a single 1200-mg dose of amprenavir in the fed state compared to the fasted state was associated with changes in C_{max} (fed: 6.18 ± 2.92 mcg/mL, fasted: 9.72 ± 2.75 mcg/mL), T_{max} (fed: 1.51 ± 0.68, fasted: 1.05 ± 0.63), and $AUC_{0-\infty}$ (fed: 22.06 ± 11.6 mcg•h/mL, fasted: 28.05 ± 10.1 mcg•h/mL). AGENERASE may be taken with or without food, but should not be taken with a high-fat meal (see DOSAGE AND ADMINISTRATION).

Distribution: The apparent volume of distribution (V_z/F) is approximately 430 L in healthy adult subjects. *In vitro* binding is approximately 90% to plasma proteins. The high affinity binding protein for amprenavir is $alpha_1$-acid glycoprotein (AAG). The partitioning of amprenavir into erythrocytes is low, but increases as amprenavir concentrations increase, reflecting the higher amount of unbound drug at higher concentrations.

Metabolism: Amprenavir is metabolized in the liver by the cytochrome P450 3A4 (CYP3A4) enzyme system. The 2 major metabolites result from oxidation of the tetrahydrofuran and aniline moieties. Glucuronide conjugates of oxidized metabolites have been identified as minor metabolites in urine and feces.

AGENERASE Oral Solution contains a large amount of propylene glycol, which is hepatically metabolized by the alcohol and aldehyde dehydrogenase enzyme pathway. Alcohol dehydrogenase (ADH) is present in the human fetal liver at 2 months of gestational age, but at only 3% of adult activity. Although the data are limited, it appears that by 12 to 30 months of postnatal age, ADH activity is equal to or greater than that observed in adults. Additionally, certain patient groups (females, Asians, Eskimos, Native Americans) may be at increased risk of propylene glycol-associated adverse events due to diminished ability to metabolize propylene glycol (see CLINICAL PHARMACOLOGY: Special Populations: Gender and Race).

Elimination: Excretion of unchanged amprenavir in urine and feces is minimal. Approximately 14% and 75% of an administered single dose of ^{14}C-amprenavir can be accounted for as radiocarbon in urine and feces, respectively. Two metabolites accounted for >90% of the radiocarbon in fecal samples. The plasma elimination half-life of amprenavir ranged from 7.1 to 10.6 hours.

Special Populations: *Hepatic Insufficiency:* AGENERASE Oral Solution is contraindicated in patients with hepatic failure.

Patients with hepatic impairment are at increased risk of propylene glycol-associated adverse events (see WARNINGS). AGENERASE Oral Solution should be used with caution in patients with hepatic impairment. AGENERASE Capsules have been studied in adult patients with impaired hepatic function using a single 600-mg oral dose. The $AUC_{0-\infty}$ was significantly greater in patients with moderate cirrhosis (25.76 ± 14.68 mcg•h/mL) compared with healthy volunteers (12.00 ± 4.38 mcg•h/mL). The $AUC_{0-\infty}$ and C_{max} were significantly greater in patients with severe cirrhosis ($AUC_{0-\infty}$: 38.66 ± 16.08 mcg•h/mL; C_{max}: 9.43 ± 2.61 mcg/mL) compared with healthy volunteers ($AUC_{0-\infty}$: 12.00 ± 4.38 mcg•h/mL; C_{max}: 4.90 ± 1.39 mcg/mL). Patients with impaired hepatic function require dosage adjustment (see DOSAGE AND ADMINISTRATION).

Renal Insufficiency: AGENERASE Oral Solution is contraindicated in patients with renal failure.

Patients with renal impairment are at increased risk of propylene glycol-associated adverse events. Additionally, because metabolites of the excipient propylene glycol in AGENERASE Oral Solution may alter acid-base balance, patients with renal impairment should be monitored for potential adverse events (see WARNINGS). AGENERASE Oral Solution should be used with caution in patients with renal impairment. The impact of renal impairment on amprenavir elimination has not been studied. The renal elimination of unchanged amprenavir represents <3% of the administered dose.

Pediatric Patients: AGENERASE Oral Solution is contraindicated in infants and children below 4 years of age (see CONTRAINDICATIONS and WARNINGS).

The pharmacokinetics of amprenavir have been studied after either single or repeat doses of AGENERASE Capsules or Oral Solution in 84 pediatric patients. Twenty HIV-1-infected children ranging in age from 4 to 12 years received single doses from 5 mg/kg to 20 mg/kg using 25-mg or 150-mg capsules. The C_{max} of amprenavir increased less than proportionally with dose. The $AUC_{0-\infty}$ increased proportionally at doses between 5 and 20 mg/kg. Amprenavir is

Continued on next page

Agenerase Oral Solution—Cont.

14% less bioavailable from the liquid formulation than from the capsules; therefore **AGENERASE Capsules and AGENERASE Oral Solution are not interchangeable on a milligram-per-milligram basis.**

[See table 2 at top of previous page]

Geriatric Patients: The pharmacokinetics of amprenavir have not been studied in patients over 65 years of age.

Gender: The pharmacokinetics of amprenavir do not differ between males and females. Females may have a lower amount of alcohol dehydrogenase compared with males and may be at increased risk of propylene glycol-associated adverse events; no data are available on propylene glycol metabolism in females.

Race: The pharmacokinetics of amprenavir do not differ between Blacks and non-Blacks. Certain ethnic populations (Asians, Eskimos, and Native Americans) may be at increased risk of propylene glycol-associated adverse events because of alcohol dehydrogenase polymorphisms; no data are available on propylene glycol metabolism in these groups.

Drug Interactions: See also CONTRAINDICATIONS, WARNINGS, and PRECAUTIONS: Drug Interactions.

Amprenavir is metabolized in the liver by the cytochrome P450 enzyme system. Amprenavir inhibits CYP3A4. Caution should be used when coadministering medications that are substrates, inhibitors, or inducers of CYP3A4, or potentially toxic medications that are metabolized by CYP3A4. Amprenavir does not inhibit CYP2D6, CYP1A2, CYP2C9, CYP2C19, CYP2E1, or uridine glucuronosyltransferase (UDPGT).

Drug interaction studies were performed with amprenavir capsules and other drugs likely to be coadministered or drugs commonly used as probes for pharmacokinetic interactions. The effects of coadministration of amprenavir on the AUC, C_{max}, and C_{min} are summarized in Table 3 (effect of other drugs on amprenavir) and Table 4 (effect of amprenavir on other drugs). For information regarding clinical recommendations, see PRECAUTIONS.

[See table 3 at top of previous page]

[See table 4 below]

Table 4: Drug Interactions: Pharmacokinetic Parameters for Coadministered Drug in the Presence of Amprenavir

Co-administered Drug	Dose of Co-administered Drug	Dose of AGENERASE	n	% Change in Pharmacokinetic Parameters of **Coadministered Drug** (90% CI) C_{max}	AUC	C_{min}
Clarithromycin	500 mg b.i.d. for 4 days	1200 mg b.i.d. for 4 days	12	↓10 (↓24 to ↑7)	⇔ (↓17 to ↑11)	⇔ (↓13 to ↑20)
Ketoconazole	400 mg single dose	1200 mg single dose	12	↑19 (↑8 to ↑33)	↑44 (↑31 to ↑59)	NA
Lamivudine	150 mg single dose	600 mg single dose	11	⇔ (↓17 to ↑3)	⇔ (↓11 to 0)	NA
Rifabutin	300 mg q.d. for 10 days	1200 mg b.i.d. for 10 days	5	↑119 (↑82 to ↑164)	↑193 (↑156 to ↑235)	↑271 (↑171 to ↑409)
Rifampin	300 mg q.d. for 4 days	1200 mg b.i.d. for 4 days	11	⇔ (↓13 to ↑12)	⇔ (↓10 to ↑13)	ND
Zidovudine	300 mg single dose	600 mg single dose	12	↑40 (↑14 to ↑71)	↑31 (↑19 to ↑45)	NA

↑ = Increase; ↓ = Decrease; ⇔ = No change (↑ or ↓ <10%); NA = C_{min} not calculated for single-dose study; ND = Interaction cannot be determined as C_{min} was below the lower limit of quantitation.

Table 5: Outcomes of Randomized Treatment Through Week 48 (PROAB3006)

Outcome	AGENERASE (n = 254)	Indinavir (n = 250)
HIV RNA <400 copies/mL*	30%	49%
HIV RNA ≥400 copies/mL[†,‡]	38%	26%
Discontinued due to adverse events[*,‡]	16%	12%
Discontinued due to other reasons[‡,§]	16%	13%

*Corresponds to rates at Week 48 in Figure 1.
†Virological failures at or before Week 48.
‡Considered to be treatment failure in the analysis.
§Includes discontinuations due to consent withdrawn, loss to follow-up, protocol violations, non-compliance, pregnancy, never treated, and other reasons.

Table 7: Drugs That Should Not Be Coadministered with AGENERASE Oral Solution

Drug Class/Drug Name	Clinical Comment
Alcohol-dependence treatment: Disulfiram	**CONTRAINDICATED** due to potential risk of toxicity from the large amount of the excipient, propylene glycol, in AGENERASE Oral Solution.
Antibiotic: Metronidazole	**CONTRAINDICATED** due to potential risk of toxicity from the large amount of the excipient, propylene glycol, in AGENERASE Oral Solution.
Antimycobacterials: Rifampin	May lead to loss of virologic response and possible resistance to AGENERASE or to the class of protease inhibitors.
Ergot derivatives: Dihydroergotamine, ergonovine, ergotamine, methylergonovine	**CONTRAINDICATED** due to potential for serious and/or life-threatening reactions such as acute ergot toxicity characterized by peripheral vasospasm and ischemia of the extremities and other tissues.
GI motility agents: Cisapride	**CONTRAINDICATED** due to potential for serious and/or life-threatening reactions such as cardiac arrhythmias.
Herbal Products: St. John's wort (hypericum perforatum)	May lead to loss of virologic response and possible resistance to AGENERASE or to the class of protease inhibitors.
HIV-Protease Inhibitor: Ritonavir oral solution	Concurrent use of AGENERASE Oral Solution and NORVIR (ritonavir) Oral Solution is not recommended because the large amount of propylene glycol in AGENERASE Oral Solution and ethanol in NOVIR Oral Solution may compete for the same metabolic pathway for elimination.
HMG Co-Reductase Inhibitors: Lovastatin, simvastatin	Potential for serious reactions such as risk of myopathy including rhabdomyolysis.
Neuroleptic: Pimozide	**CONTRAINDICATED** due to potential for serious and/or life-threatening reactions such as cardiac arrhythmias.
Sedative/hypnotics: Midazolam, triazolam	**CONTRAINDICATED** due to potential for serious and/or life-threatening reactions such as prolonged or increased sedation or respiratory depression.

Nucleoside Reverse Transcriptase Inhibitors (NRTIs): There was no effect of amprenavir on abacavir in subjects receiving both agents based on historical data.

HIV Protease Inhibitors: Concurrent use of AGENERASE Oral Solution and NORVIR® (ritonavir) Oral Solution is not recommended because the large amount of propylene glycol in AGENERASE Oral Solution and ethanol in NORVIR Oral Solution may compete for the same metabolic pathway for elimination. This combination has not been studied in pediatric patients.

The effect of amprenavir on total drug concentrations of other HIV protease inhibitors in subjects receiving both agents was evaluated using comparisons to historical data. Indinavir steady-state C_{max}, AUC, and C_{min} were decreased by 22%, 38%, and 27%, respectively, by concomitant amprenavir. Similar decreases in C_{max} and AUC were seen after the first dose. Saquinavir steady-state C_{max}, AUC, and C_{min} were increased 21%, decreased 19%, and decreased 48%, respectively, by concomitant amprenavir. Nelfinavir steady-state C_{max}, AUC, and C_{min} were increased by 12%, 15%, and 14%, respectively, by concomitant amprenavir.

For information regarding clinical recommendations, see PRECAUTIONS: Drug Interactions.

INDICATIONS AND USAGE

AGENERASE (amprenavir) is indicated in combination with other antiretroviral agents for the treatment of HIV-1 infection.

The following points should be considered when initiating therapy with AGENERASE:

In a study of NRTI-experienced, protease inhibitor-naive patients, AGENERASE was found to be significantly less effective than indinavir (see Description of Clinical Studies).

Mild to moderate gastrointestinal adverse events led to discontinuation of AGENERASE primarily during the first 12 weeks of therapy (see ADVERSE REACTIONS).

There are no data on response to therapy with AGENERASE in protease inhibitor-experienced patients.

AGENERASE Oral Solution should be used only when AGENERASE Capsules or other protease inhibitor formulations are not therapeutic options.

Description of Clinical Studies: ***Therapy-Naive Adults:*** PROAB3001, a randomized, double-blind, placebo-controlled, multicenter study, compared treatment with AGENERASE Capsules (1200 mg twice daily) plus lamivudine (150 mg twice daily) plus zidovudine (300 mg twice daily) versus lamivudine (150 mg twice daily) plus zidovudine (300 mg twice daily) in 232 patients. Through 24 weeks of therapy, 53% of patients assigned to AGENERASE/zidovudine/lamivudine achieved HIV RNA <400 copies/mL. Through week 48, the antiviral response was 41%. Through 24 weeks of therapy, 11% of patients assigned to zidovudine/lamivudine achieved HIV RNA <400 copies/mL. Antiviral response beyond week 24 is not interpretable because the majority of patients discontinued or changed their antiretroviral therapy.

NRTI-Experienced Adults: PROAB3006, a randomized, open-label multicenter study, compared treatment with AGENERASE Capsules (1200 mg twice daily) plus NRTIs versus indinavir (800 mg every 8 hours) plus NRTIs in 504 NRTI-experienced, protease inhibitor-naive patients, median age 37 years (range 20 to 71 years), 72% Caucasian, 80% male, with a median CD4 cell count of 404 cells/mm^3 (range 9 to 1706 cells/mm^3) and a median plasma HIV-1 RNA level of 3.93 log_{10} copies/mL (range 2.60 to 7.01 log_{10} copies/mL) at baseline. Through 48 weeks of therapy, the median CD4 cell count increase from baseline in the amprenavir group was significantly lower than in the indinavir group, 97 cells/mm^3 versus 144 cells/mm^3, respectively. There was also a significant difference in the proportions of patients with plasma HIV-1 RNA levels <400 copies/mL through 48 weeks (see Figure 1 and Table 5).

[See figure at top of next column]

HIV-1 RNA status and reasons for discontinuation of randomized treatment at 48 weeks are summarized (Table 5).

[See table 5 below]

CONTRAINDICATIONS

Because of the potential risk of toxicity from the large amount of the excipient propylene glycol, AGENERASE Oral Solution is contraindicated in infants and children below the age of 4 years, pregnant women, patients with hepatic or renal failure, and patients treated with disulfiram or metronidazole (see WARNINGS and PRECAUTIONS).

Coadministration of AGENERASE is contraindicated with drugs that are highly dependent on CYP3A4 for clearance and for which elevated plasma concentrations are associated with serious and/or life-threatening events. These drugs are listed in Table 6.

Figure 1: Virologic Response Through Week 48, PROAB3006*,†

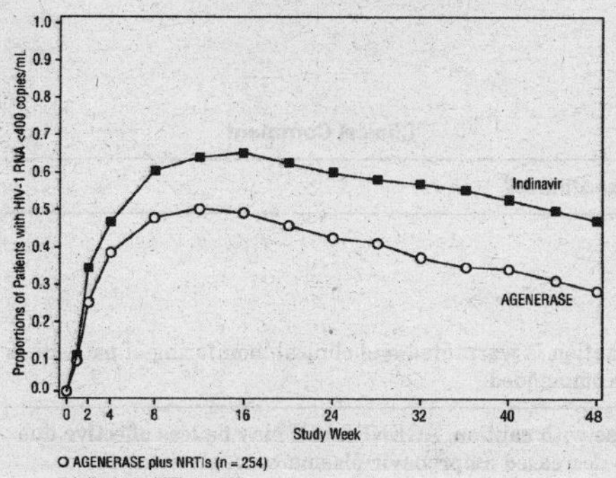

Table 6: Drugs That are Contraindicated with AGENERASE Oral Solution

Drug Class	Drugs Within Class That Are CONTRAINDICATED with AGENERASE
Alcohol-dependence treatment	Disulfiram
Antibiotic	Metronidazole
Ergot derivatives	Dihydroergotamine, ergonovine, ergotamine, methylergonovine
GI motility agent	Cisapride
Neuroleptic	Pimozide
Sedatives/hypnotics	Midazolam, triazolam

If AGENERASE Capsules are coadministered with ritonavir capsules, the antiarrhythmic agents flecainide and propafenone are also contraindicated.

AGENERASE is contraindicated in patients with previously demonstrated clinically significant hypersensitivity to any of the components of this product.

WARNINGS

ALERT: Find out about medicines that should not be taken with AGENERASE.

Because of the potential risk of toxicity from the large amount of the excipient propylene glycol, AGENERASE Oral Solution is contraindicated in infants and children below the age of 4 years, pregnant women, patients with hepatic or renal failure, and patients treated with disulfiram or metronidazole (see CLINICAL PHARMACOLOGY, CONTRAINDICATIONS, and PRECAUTIONS).

Because of the possible toxicity associated with the large amount of propylene glycol and the lack of information on chronic exposure to large amounts of propylene glycol, AGENERASE Oral Solution should be used only when AGENERASE Capsules or other protease inhibitor formulations are not therapeutic options. Certain ethnic populations (Asians, Eskimos, Native Americans) and women may be at increased risk of propylene glycol-associated adverse events due to diminished ability to metabolize propylene glycol; no data are available on propylene glycol metabolism in these groups (see CLINICAL PHARMACOLOGY: Special Populations: Gender and Race).

If patients require treatment with AGENERASE Oral Solution, they should be monitored closely for propylene glycol-associated adverse events, including seizures, stupor, tachycardia, hyperosmolality, lactic acidosis, renal toxicity, and hemolysis. Patients should be switched from AGENERASE Oral Solution to AGENERASE Capsules as soon as they are able to take the capsule formulation.

Concurrent use of AGENERASE Oral Solution and NORVIR (ritonavir) Oral Solution is not recommended because the large amount of propylene glycol in AGENERASE Oral Solution and ethanol in NORVIR Oral Solution may compete for the same metabolic pathway for elimination.

Use of alcoholic beverages is not recommended in patients treated with AGENERASE Oral Solution.

Serious and/or life-threatening drug interactions could occur between amprenavir and amiodarone, lidocaine (systemic), tricyclic antidepressants, and quinidine. Concentration monitoring of these agents is recommended if these agents are used concomitantly with AGENERASE (see CONTRAINDICATIONS).

Rifampin should not be used in combination with amprenavir because it reduces plasma concentrations and AUC of amprenavir by about 90%.

Concomitant use of AGENERASE and St. John's wort (hypericum perforatum) or products containing St. John's wort is not recommended. Coadministration of protease inhibitors, including AGENERASE, with St. John's wort is expected to substantially decrease protease inhibitor concentrations and may result in suboptimal levels of amprenavir and lead to loss of virologic response and possible resistance to AGENERASE or to the class of protease inhibitors.

Table 8: Established and Other Potentially Significant Drug Interactions: Alteration in Dose or Regimen May be Recommended Based on Drug Interaction Studies or Predicted Interaction

Concomitant Drug Class: Drug Name	Effect on Concentration of Amprenavir or Concomitant Drug	Clinical Comment
HIV-Antiviral Agents		
Non-nucleoside Reverse Transcriptase Inhibitors: Efavirenz, nevirapine	↓Amprenavir	Appropriate doses of the combinations with respect to safety and efficacy have not been established.
Non-nucleoside Reverse Transcriptase Inhibitor: Delavirdine	↑Amprenavir	Appropriate doses of the combination with respect to safety and efficacy have not been established.
Nucleoside Reverse Transcriptase Inhibitor: Didanosine (buffered formulation only)	↓Amprenavir	Take AGENERASE at least 1 hour before or after the buffered formulation of didanosine.
HIV-Protease Inhibitors: Indinavir*, lopinavir/ritonavir, nelfinavir*	↑Amprenavir Amprenavir's effect on other protease inhibitors is not well established.	Appropriate doses of the combinations with respect to safety and efficacy have not been established.
HIV-Protease Inhibitor: Ritonavir Capsules*	↑Amprenavir	The dose of amprenavir should be reduced when used in combination with ritonavir capsules (see Dosage and Administration). Also, see the full prescribing information for NORVIR for additional drug interaction information. Concurrent use of AGENERASE Oral Solution and NORVIR (ritonavir) Oral Solution is not recommended because the large amount of propylene glycol in AGENERASE Oral Solution and ethanol in NORVIR Oral Solution may compete for the same metabolic pathway for elimination.
HIV-Protease Inhibitor: Saquinavir*	↓Amprenavir Amprenavir's effect on saquinavir is not well established.	Appropriate doses of the combination with respect to safety and efficacy have not been established.
Other Agents		
Antacids	↓Amprenavir	Take AGENERASE at least 1 hour before or after antacids.
Antiarrhythmics: Amiodarone, lidocaine (systemic), and quinidine	↑Antiarrhythmics	Caution is warranted and therapeutic concentration monitoring is recommended for antiarrhythmics when coadministered with AGENERASE, if available.
Antiarrhythmic: Bepridil	↑Bepridil	Use with caution. Increased bepridil exposure may be associated with life-threatening reactions such as cardiac arrhythmias.
Anticoagulant: Warfarin		Concentrations of warfarin may be affected. It is recommended that INR (international normalized ratio) be monitored.
Anticonvulsants: Carbamazepine, phenobarbital, phenytoin	↓Amprenavir	Use with caution. AGENERASE may be less effective due to decreased amprenavir plasma concentrations in patients taking these agents concomitantly.
Antifungals: Ketoconazole, itraconazole	↑Ketoconazole ↑Itraconazole	Increase monitoring for adverse events due to ketoconazole or itraconazole. Dose reduction of ketoconazole or itraconazole may be needed for patients receiving more than 400 mg ketoconazole or itraconazole per day.
Antimycobacterial: Rifabutin*	↑Rifabutin and rifabutin metabolite	A dosage reduction of rifabutin to at least half the recommended dose is required when AGENERASE and rifabutin are coadministered.* A complete blood count should be performed weekly and as clinically indicated in order to monitor for neutropenia in patients receiving amprenavir and rifabutin.
Benzodiazepines: Alprazolam, clorazepate, diazepam, flurazepam	↑Benzodiazepines	Clinical significance is unknown; however, a decrease in benzodiazepine dose may be needed.

(Table continued on next page)

Concomitant use of AGENERASE with lovastatin or simvastatin is not recommended. Caution should be exercised if HIV protease inhibitors, including AGENERASE, are used concurrently with other HMG-CoA reductase inhibitors that are also metabolized by the CYP3A4 pathway (e.g., atorvastatin). The risk of myopathy, including rhabdomyolysis, may be increased when HIV protease inhibitors, including amprenavir, are used in combination with these drugs.

Particular caution should be used when prescribing sildenafil in patients receiving amprenavir. Coadministration of AGENERASE with sildenafil is expected to substantially increase sildenafil concentrations and may result in an increase in sildenafil-associated adverse events, including hypotension, visual changes, and priapism (see PRECAUTIONS: Drug Interactions and Information for Patients, and the complete prescribing information for sildenafil).

Severe and life-threatening skin reactions, including Stevens-Johnson syndrome, have occurred in patients treated with AGENERASE (see ADVERSE REACTIONS).

Acute hemolytic anemia has been reported in a patient treated with AGENERASE.

New onset diabetes mellitus, exacerbation of pre-existing diabetes mellitus, and hyperglycemia have been reported during post-marketing surveillance in HIV-infected patients receiving protease inhibitor therapy. Some patients required either initiation or dose adjustments of insulin or oral hypoglycemic agents for treatment of these events. In some cases, diabetic ketoacidosis has occurred. In those patients who discontinued protease inhibitor therapy, hyperglycemia persisted in some cases. Because these events have been reported voluntarily during clinical practice, es-

Continued on next page

Agenerase Oral Solution—Cont.

timates of frequency cannot be made and causal relationships between protease inhibitor therapy and these events have not been established.

PRECAUTIONS

General: AGENERASE Capsules and AGENERASE Oral Solution are not interchangeable on a milligram-per-milligram basis (see CLINICAL PHARMACOLOGY: Pediatric Patients and CONTRAINDICATIONS).

Amprenavir is a sulfonamide. The potential for cross-sensitivity between drugs in the sulfonamide class and amprenavir is unknown. AGENERASE should be used with caution in patients with a known sulfonamide allergy.

AGENERASE is principally metabolized by the liver. AGENERASE, when used alone and in combination with low-dose ritonavir, has been associated with elevations of SGOT (AST) and SGPT (ALT) in some patients. Caution should be exercised when administering AGENERASE to patients with hepatic impairment (see DOSAGE AND ADMINISTRATION). Appropriate laboratory testing should be conducted prior to initiating therapy with AGENERASE and at periodic intervals during treatment.

Formulations of AGENERASE provide high daily doses of vitamin E (see Information for Patients, DESCRIPTION, and DOSAGE AND ADMINISTRATION). The effects of long-term, high-dose vitamin E administration in humans is not well characterized and has not been specifically studied in HIV-infected individuals. High vitamin E doses may exacerbate the blood coagulation defect of vitamin K deficiency caused by anticoagulant therapy or malabsorption.

Patients with Hemophilia: There have been reports of spontaneous bleeding in patients with hemophilia A and B treated with protease inhibitors. In some patients, additional factor VIII was required. In many of the reported cases, treatment with protease inhibitors was continued or restarted. A causal relationship between protease inhibitor therapy and these episodes has not been established.

Fat Redistribution: Redistribution/accumulation of body fat, including central obesity, dorsocervical fat enlargement (buffalo hump), peripheral wasting, facial wasting, breast enlargement, and "cushingoid appearance," have been observed in patients receiving antiretroviral therapy. The mechanism and long-term consequences of these events are currently unknown. A causal relationship has not been established.

Lipid Elevations: Treatment with AGENERASE alone or in combination with ritonavir capsules has resulted in increases in the concentration of total cholesterol and triglycerides. Triglyceride and cholesterol testing should be performed prior to initiation of therapy with AGENERASE and at periodic intervals during treatment. Lipid disorders should be managed as clinically appropriate. See PRECAUTIONS Table 8: Established and Other Potentially Significant Drug Interactions for additional information on potential drug interactions with AGENERASE and HMG-CoA reductase inhibitors.

Resistance/Cross-Resistance: Because the potential for HIV cross-resistance among protease inhibitors has not been fully explored, it is unknown what effect amprenavir therapy will have on the activity of subsequently administered protease inhibitors. It is also unknown what effect previous treatment with other protease inhibitors will have on the activity of amprenavir (see MICROBIOLOGY).

Information for Patients: A statement to patients and health care providers is included on the product's bottle label: **ALERT: Find out about medicines that should NOT be taken with AGENERASE.** A Patient Package Insert (PPI) for AGENERASE Oral Solution is available for patient information.

AGENERASE Oral Solution is contraindicated in infants and children below the age of 4 years, pregnant women, patients with hepatic or renal failure, and patients treated with disulfiram or metronidazole. AGENERASE Oral Solution should be used only when AGENERASE Capsules or other protease inhibitor formulations are not therapeutic options.

Patients treated with AGENERASE Capsules should be cautioned against switching to AGENERASE Oral Solution because of the increased risk of adverse events from the large amount of propylene glycol in AGENERASE Oral Solution.

Women, Asians, Eskimos, or Native Americans, as well as patients who have hepatic or renal insufficiency, should be informed that they may be at increased risk of adverse events from the large amount of propylene glycol in AGENERASE Oral Solution.

Patients should be informed that AGENERASE is not a cure for HIV infection and that they may continue to develop opportunistic infections and other complications associated with HIV disease. The long-term effects of AGENERASE (amprenavir) are unknown at this time. Patients should be told that there are currently no data demonstrating that therapy with AGENERASE can reduce the risk of transmitting HIV to others through sexual contact. Patients should remain under the care of a physician while using AGENERASE. Patients should be advised to take AGENERASE every day as prescribed. AGENERASE must always be used in combination with other antiretroviral drugs. Patients should not alter the dose or discontinue therapy without consulting their physician. If a dose is missed, patients should take the dose as soon as possible and then return to their normal schedule. However, if a dose is skipped, the patient should not double the next dose.

Table 8: Established and Other Potentially Significant Drug Interactions: Alteration in Dose or Regimen May be Recommended Based on Drug Interaction Studies or Predicted Interaction — *(cont.)*

Concomitant Drug Class: Drug Name	Effect on Concentration of Amprenavir or Concomitant Drug	Clinical Comment
Other Agents — (continued)		
Calcium Channel Blockers: Diltiazem, felodipine, nifedipine, nicardipine, nimodipine, verapamil, amlodipine, nisoldipine, isradipine	↑ Calcium channel blockers	Caution is warranted and clinical monitoring of patients is recommended.
Corticosteroid: Dexamethasone	↓ Amprenavir	Use with caution. AGENERASE may be less effective due to decreased amprenavir plasma concentrations in patients taking these agents concomitantly.
Erectile Dysfunction Agent: Sildenafil	↑ Sildenafil	Use with caution at reduced doses of 25 mg every 48 hours with increased monitoring for adverse events.
HMG-CoA Reductase Inhibitors: Atorvastatin	↑ Atorvastatin	Use lowest possible dose of atorvastatin with careful monitoring or consider other HMG-CoA reductase inhibitors such as pravastatin or fluvastatin in combination with AGENERASE.
Immunosuppressants: Cyclosporine, tacrolimus, rapamycin	↑ Immunosuppressants	Therapeutic concentration monitoring is recommended for immunosuppressant agents when coadministered with AGENERASE.
Oral Contraceptive: Ethinyl estradiol	Effect on ethinyl estradiol is not known.	Alternative or additional contraceptive measures should be used when estrogen-based oral contraceptives and AGENERASE are coadministered.
Tricyclic Antidepressants: Amitriptyline, imipramine	↑ Tricyclics	Therapeutic concentration monitoring is recommended for tricyclic antidepressants when coadministered with AGENERASE.

*See CLINICAL PHARMACOLOGY for magnitude of interaction, Tables 3 and 4.

Table 9: Selected Clinical Adverse Events of All Grades Reported in >5% of Adult Patients

	PROAB3001 Therapy-Naive Patients		PROAB3006 NRTI-Experienced Patients	
Adverse Event	AGENERASE*/ Lamivudine/ Zidovudine (n = 113)	Lamivudine/ Zidovudine (n = 109)	AGENERASE*/ NRTI (n = 245)	Indinavir/NRTI (n = 241)
Digestive				
Nausea	74%	50%	43%	35%
Vomiting	34%	17%	24%	20%
Diarrhea or loose stools	39%	35%	60%	41%
Taste disorders	10%	6%	2%	8%
Skin				
Rash	27%	6%	20%	15%
Nervous				
Paresthesia, oral/perioral	26%	6%	31%	2%
Paresthesia, peripheral	10%	4%	14%	10%
Psychiatric				
Depressive or mood disorders	16%	4%	9%	13%

*AGENERASE Capsules.

Table 10: Selected Laboratory Abnormalities of All Grades Reported in ≥5% of Adult Patients

	PROAB3001 Therapy-Naive Patients		PROAB3006 NRTI-Experienced Patients	
Laboratory Abnormality (non-fasting specimens)	AGENERASE*/ Lamivudine/ Zidovudine (n = 111)	Lamivudine/ Zidovudine (n = 108)	AGENERASE*/ NRTI (n = 237)	Indinavir/NRTI (n = 239)
Hyperglycemia (>116 mg/dL)	45%	31%	53%	58%
Hypertriglyceridemia (>213 mg/dL)	41%	27%	56%	52%
Hypercholesterolemia (>283 mg/dL)	7%	3%	13%	15%

*AGENERASE Capsules.

Patients should inform their doctor if they have a sulfa allergy. The potential for cross-sensitivity between drugs in the sulfonamide class and amprenavir is unknown.

AGENERASE may interact with many drugs; therefore, patients should be advised to report to their doctor the use of any other prescription or nonprescription medication or herbal products, particularly St. John's wort.

Patients taking antacids (or the buffered formulation of didanosine) should take AGENERASE at least 1 hour before or after antacid (or the buffered formulation of didanosine) use.

Patients should be advised that drinking alcoholic beverages is not recommended while taking AGENERASE Oral Solution.

Patients receiving sildenafil should be advised that they may be at an increased risk of sildenafil-associated adverse events including hypotension, visual changes, and priapism, and should promptly report any symptoms to their doctor.

Patients receiving hormonal contraceptives should be instructed that alternate contraceptive measures should be used during therapy with AGENERASE.

High-fat meals may decrease the absorption of AGENERASE and should be avoided. AGENERASE may be taken with meals of normal fat content.

Patients should be informed that redistribution or accumulation of body fat may occur in patients receiving antiretroviral therapy and that the cause and long-term health effects of these conditions are not known at this time.

Adult and pediatric patients should be advised not to take supplemental vitamin E since the vitamin E content of AGENERASE exceeds the Reference Daily Intake (adults 30 IU, pediatrics approximately 10 IU).

Laboratory Tests: The combination of AGENERASE and low-dose ritonavir has been associated with elevations of cholesterol and triglycerides, SGOT (AST), and SGPT (ALT) in some patients. Appropriate laboratory testing should be considered prior to initiating combination therapy with AGENERASE and ritonavir capsules and at periodic intervals or if any clinical signs or symptoms of hyperlipidemia or elevated liver function tests occur during therapy. For comprehensive information concerning laboratory test alterations associated with ritonavir, physicians should refer to the complete prescribing information for NORVIR (ritonavir).

Drug Interactions: See also CONTRAINDICATIONS, WARNINGS, and CLINICAL PHARMACOLOGY: Drug Interactions.

AGENERASE is an inhibitor of cytochrome P450 3A4 metabolism and therefore should not be administered concurrently with medications with narrow therapeutic windows that are substrates of CYP3A4. There are other agents that may result in serious and/or life-threatening drug interactions (see CONTRAINDICATIONS and WARNINGS).

Use of alcoholic beverages is not recommended in patients treated with AGENERASE Oral Solution.

[See table 7 at bottom of page 162]

[See table 8 on pages 163 and 164]

Carcinogenesis and Mutagenesis: Long-term carcinogenicity studies of amprenavir in rodents are in progress. Amprenavir was not mutagenic or genotoxic in a battery of *in vitro* and *in vivo* assays including bacterial reverse mutation (Ames), mouse lymphoma, rat micronucleus, and chromosome aberrations in human lymphocytes.

Fertility: The effects of amprenavir on fertility and general reproductive performance were investigated in male rats (treated for 28 days before mating at doses producing up to twice the expected clinical exposure based on AUC comparisons) and female rats (treated for 15 days before mating through day 17 of gestation at doses producing up to 2 times the expected clinical exposure). Amprenavir did not impair mating or fertility of male or female rats and did not affect the development and maturation of sperm from treated rats. The reproductive performance of the F1 generation born to female rats given amprenavir was not different from control animals.

Pregnancy and Reproduction: AGENERASE Oral Solution is contraindicated during pregnancy due to the potential risk of toxicity to the fetus from the high propylene glycol content. Therefore, if AGENERASE is used in pregnant women, the AGENERASE Capsules formulation should be used (see complete prescribing information for AGENERASE Capsules).

Antiretroviral Pregnancy Registry: To monitor maternal-fetal outcomes of pregnant women exposed to AGENERASE, an Antiretroviral Pregnancy Registry has been established. Physicians are encouraged to register patients by calling 1-800-258-4263.

Nursing Mothers: The Centers for Disease Control and Prevention recommend that HIV-infected mothers not breastfeed their infants to avoid risking postnatal transmission of HIV. Although it is not known if amprenavir is excreted in human milk, amprenavir is secreted into the milk of lactating rats. Because of both the potential for HIV transmission and the potential for serious adverse reactions in nursing infants, **mothers should be instructed not to breastfeed if they are receiving AGENERASE.**

Pediatric Use: AGENERASE Oral Solution is contraindicated in infants and children below the age of 4 years due to the potential risk of toxicity from the excipient propylene glycol (see CONTRAINDICATIONS and WARNINGS). Alcohol dehydrogenase (ADH), which metabolizes propylene glycol, is present in the human fetal liver at 2 months of gestational age, but at only 3% of adult activity. Although the data are limited, it appears that by 12 to 30 months of postnatal age, ADH activity is equal to or greater than that observed in adults.

Two hundred fifty-one patients aged 4 and above have received amprenavir as single or multiple doses in studies. An adverse event profile similar to that seen in adults was seen in pediatric patients.

Concurrent use of AGENERASE Oral Solution and NORVIR (ritonavir) Oral Solution is not recommended because the large amount of propylene glycol in AGENERASE Oral Solution and ethanol in NORVIR Oral Solution may compete for the same metabolic pathway for elimination. This combination has not been studied in pediatric patients.

Geriatric Use: Clinical studies of AGENERASE did not include sufficient numbers of patients aged 65 and over to determine whether they respond differently from younger adults. In general, dose selection for an elderly patient should be cautious, reflecting the greater frequency of decreased hepatic, renal, or cardiac function, and of concomitant disease or other drug therapy.

ADVERSE REACTIONS

In clinical studies, adverse events leading to amprenavir discontinuation occurred primarily during the first 12 weeks of therapy, and were mostly due to gastrointestinal events (nausea, vomiting, diarrhea, and abdominal pain/discomfort), which were mild to moderate in severity.

Skin rash occurred in 22% of patients treated with amprenavir in studies PROAB3001 and PROAB3006. Rashes were usually maculopapular and of mild or moderate intensity, some with pruritus. Rashes had a median onset of 11 days after amprenavir initiation and a median duration of 10 days. Skin rashes led to amprenavir discontinuation in approximately 3% of patients. In some patients with mild or moderate rash, amprenavir dosing was often continued without interruption; if interrupted, reintroduction of amprenavir generally did not result in rash recurrence.

Severe or life-threatening rash (Grade 3 or 4), including cases of Stevens-Johnson syndrome, occurred in approximately 1% of recipients of AGENERASE (see WARNINGS). Amprenavir therapy should be discontinued for severe or life-threatening rashes and for moderate rashes accompanied by systemic symptoms.

[See table 9 at top of previous page]

Among amprenavir-treated patients in Phase 3 studies, 2 patients developed de novo diabetes mellitus, 1 patient developed a dorsocervical fat enlargement (buffalo hump), and 9 patients developed fat redistribution.

[See table 10 at top of previous page]

In studies PROAB3001 and PROAB3006, no increased frequency of Grade 3 or 4 AST, ALT, amylase, or bilirubin elevations was seen compared to controls.

Pediatric Patients: An adverse event profile similar to that seen in adults was seen in pediatric patients.

Concomitant Therapy with Ritonavir:

[See table 11 above]

Table 11: Selected Clinical Adverse Events of All Grades Reported in ≥5% of Adult Patients in Ongoing, Open-Label Clinical Trials of AGENERASE Capsules in Combination with Ritonavir Capsules

Adverse Event	AGENERASE 1200 mg plus Ritonavir 200 mg q.d.* (n = 101)	AGENERASE 600 mg plus Ritonavir 100 mg b.i.d.† (n = 215)
Diarrhea/loose stools	25%	7%
Nausea	23%	7%
Vomiting	10%	4%
Abdominal symptoms	13%	3%
Headache	15%	3%
Paresthesias	8%	2%
Rash	9%	2%
Fatigue	5%	4%

*Data from 2 ongoing, open-label studies in treatment-naive patients also receiving abacavir/lamivudine.

†Data from 3 ongoing, open-label studies in treatment-naive and treatment-experienced patients receiving combination antiretroviral therapy.

Treatment with AGENERASE in combination with ritonavir capsules has resulted in increases in the concentration of total cholesterol and triglycerides (see PRECAUTIONS Lipid Elevations and Laboratory Tests).

OVERDOSAGE

There is no known antidote for AGENERASE. It is not known whether amprenavir can be removed by peritoneal dialysis or hemodialysis. If overdosage occurs, the patient should be monitored for evidence of toxicity and standard supportive treatment applied as necessary.

AGENERASE Oral Solution contains large amounts of propylene glycol. In the event of overdosage, monitoring and management of acid-base abnormalities is recommended. Propylene glycol can be removed by hemodialysis.

DOSAGE AND ADMINISTRATION

AGENERASE may be taken with or without food; however, a high-fat meal decreases the absorption of amprenavir and should be avoided (see CLINICAL PHARMACOLOGY: Effects of Food on Oral Absorption). **Adult and pediatric patients should be advised not to take supplemental vitamin E since the vitamin E content of AGENERASE Oral Solution exceeds the Reference Daily Intake (adults 30 IU, pediatrics approximately 10 IU) (see DESCRIPTION).**

The recommended dose of AGENERASE Oral Solution based on body weight and age is shown in Table 12. **Consideration should be given to switching patients from AGENERASE Oral Solution to AGENERASE Capsules as soon as they are able to take the capsule formulation (see WARNINGS).**

[See table 12 above]

Table 12: Recommended Dosages of AGENERASE Oral Solution

Age/Weight Criteria	Dose	
	b.i.d.	t.i.d.
4–12 years or 13–16 years and <50 kg	22.5 mg/kg (1.5 mL/kg) (maximum dose 2800 mg per day)	17 mg/kg (1.1 mL/kg) (maximum dose 2800 mg per day)
13–16 years and ≥50 kg or >16 years	1400 mg	NA

Concomitant Therapy: Concurrent use of AGENERASE Oral Solution and NORVIR (ritonavir) Oral Solution is not recommended because the large amount of propylene glycol in AGENERASE Oral Solution and ethanol in NORVIR Oral Solution may compete for the same metabolic pathway for elimination.

Patients with Hepatic Impairment: AGENERASE Oral Solution is contraindicated in patients with hepatic failure (see CONTRAINDICATIONS).

Patients with hepatic impairment are at increased risk of propylene glycol-associated adverse events (see WARNINGS). AGENERASE Oral Solution should be used with caution in patients with hepatic impairment. Based on a study with AGENERASE Capsules, adult patients with a Child-Pugh score ranging from 5 to 8 should receive a reduced dose of AGENERASE Oral Solution of 513 mg (34 mL) twice daily, and adult patients with a Child-Pugh score ranging from 9 to 12 should receive a reduced dose of AGENERASE Oral Solution of 342 mg (23 mL) twice daily (see CLINICAL PHARMACOLOGY: Hepatic Insufficiency). AGENERASE Oral Solution has not been studied in children with hepatic impairment.

Renal Insufficiency: AGENERASE Oral Solution is contraindicated in patients with renal failure (see CONTRAINDICATIONS).

Patients with renal impairment are at increased risk of propylene glycol-associated adverse events. AGENERASE Oral Solution should be used with caution in patients with renal impairment (see WARNINGS).

AGENERASE Capsules and AGENERASE Oral Solution are not interchangeable on a milligram-per-milligram basis (see CLINICAL PHARMACOLOGY).

HOW SUPPLIED

AGENERASE Oral Solution, a clear, pale yellow to yellow, grape bubblegum-peppermint-flavored liquid, contains 15 mg of amprenavir in each 1 mL.

Bottles of 240 mL with child-resistant closures (NDC 0173-0687-00). This product does not require reconstitution.

Store at controlled room temperature of 25°C (77°F) (see USP).

GlaxoSmithKline, Research Triangle Park, NC 27709

Licensed from Vertex Pharmaceuticals Incorporated Cambridge, MA 02139

AGENERASE is a registered trademark of the GlaxoSmithKline group of companies.

February 2002/RL-1062

ALKERAN® ℞

[ăl' kur-ăn]

(melphalan hydrochloride)
for Injection

Prescribing information for this product, which appears on pages 1465–1466 of the 2002 PDR, has been revised as follows. Please write "See Supplement A" next to the product heading.

In **CLINICAL PHARMACOLOGY: Pharmacokinetics,** *"ng" was changed to "mcg" in the sentence* "Mean (±SD) peak melphalan plasma concentrations in myeloma patients given IV melphalan at doses of 10 or 20 mg/m^2 were 1.2 ± 0.4 and 2.8 ± 1.9 mcg/mL, respectively."

The **ADVERSE REACTIONS (see OVERDOSAGE): Gastrointestinal** *subsection was revised to:* Gastrointestinal disturbances such as nausea and vomiting, diarrhea, and oral ulceration occur infrequently. Hepatic disorders ranging from abnormal liver function tests to clinical manifestations such as hepatitis and jaundice have been reported. Hepatic veno-occlusive disease has been reported.

Continued on next page

Alkeran For Injection—Cont.

Reference no. 7 was revised to "Controlling Occupational Exposure to Hazardous Drugs. (OSHA Work-Practice Guidelines.) *Am J Health-Syst Pharm.* 1996;53:1669–1685."
November 2001/RL-1026

ALKERAN® ℞

[*ăl'-kur-ăn*]
(melphalan)
2-mg Scored Tablets

Prescribing information for this product, which appears on pages 1466–1467 of the 2002 PDR, has been completely revised as follows. Please write "See Supplement A" next to the product heading.

> **WARNING:** ALKERAN (melphalan) should be administered under the supervision of a qualified physician experienced in the use of cancer chemotherapeutic agents. Severe bone marrow suppression with resulting infection or bleeding may occur. Melphalan is leukemogenic in humans.
> Melphalan produces chromosomal aberrations in vitro and in vivo and, therefore, should be considered potentially mutagenic in humans.

DESCRIPTION

ALKERAN (melphalan), also known as L-phenylalanine mustard, phenylalanine mustard, L-PAM, or L-sarcolysin, is a phenylalanine derivative of nitrogen mustard. Melphalan is a bifunctional alkylating agent which is active against selective human neoplastic diseases. It is known chemically as 4-[bis(2-chloroethyl)amino]-*L*-phenylalanine. The molecular formula is $C_{13}H_{18}Cl_2N_2O_2$ and the molecular weight is 305.20.

Melphalan is the active L-isomer of the compound and was first synthesized in 1953 by Bergel and Stock; the D-isomer, known as medphalan, is less active against certain animal tumors, and the dose needed to produce effects on chromosomes is larger than that required with the L-isomer. The racemic (DL−) form is known as merphalan or sarcolysin. Melphalan is practically insoluble in water and has a pKa_1 of ~2.5.

ALKERAN (melphalan) is available in tablet form for oral administration. Each film-coated tablet contains 2 mg melphalan and the inactive ingredients colloidal silicon dioxide, crospovidone, hypromellose, macrogol/PEG 400, magnesium stearate, microcrystalline cellulose, and titanium dioxide.

CLINICAL PHARMACOLOGY

Melphalan is an alkylating agent of the bischloroethylamine type. As a result, its cytotoxicity appears to be related to the extent of its interstrand cross-linking with DNA, probably by binding at the N^7 position of guanine. Like other bifunctional alkylating agents, it is active against both resting and rapidly dividing tumor cells.

Pharmacokinetics: The pharmacokinetics of ALKERAN after oral administration has been extensively studied in adult patients. Plasma melphalan levels are highly variable after oral dosing, both with respect to the time of the first appearance of melphalan in plasma (range approximately 0 to 6 hours) and to the peak plasma concentration (C_{max}) (range 70 to 4000 ng/mL, depending upon the dose) achieved. These results may be due to incomplete intestinal absorption, a variable "first pass" hepatic metabolism, or to rapid hydrolysis. Five patients were studied after both oral and intravenous (IV) dosing with 0.6 mg/kg as a single bolus dose by each route. The areas under the plasma concentration-time curves (AUC) after oral administration averaged 61% ± 26% (± standard deviation [SD]; range 25% to 89%) of those following IV administration. In 18 patients given a single oral dose of 0.6 mg/kg of ALKERAN, the terminal elimination plasma half-life ($t_{1/2}$) of parent drug was 1.5 ± 0.83 hours. The 24-hour urinary excretion of parent drug in these patients was 10% ± 4.5%, suggesting that renal clearance is not a major route of elimination of parent drug. In a separate study in 18 patients given single oral doses of 0.2 to 0.25 mg/kg of ALKERAN, C_{max} and AUC, when dose adjusted to a dose of 14 mg, were (mean ± SD) 212 ± 74 ng/mL and 498 ± 137 ng•h/mL, respectively. Elimination phase $t_{½}$ in these patients was approximately 1 hour and the median t_{max} was 1 hour.

One study using universally labeled ^{14}C-melphalan, found substantially less radioactivity in the urine of patients given the drug by mouth (30% of administered dose in 9 days) than in the urine of those given it intravenously (35% to 65% in 7 days). Following either oral or IV administration, the pattern of label recovery was similar, with the majority being recovered in the first 24 hours. Following oral administration, peak radioactivity occurred in plasma at 2 hours and then disappeared with a half-life of approximately 160 hours. In one patient where parent drug (rather than just radiolabel) was determined, the melphalan half-disappearance time was 67 minutes.

The steady-state volume of distribution of melphalan is 0.5 L/kg. Penetration into cerebrospinal fluid (CSF) is low. The extent of melphalan binding to plasma proteins ranges from 60% to 90%. Serum albumin is the major binding protein, while α_1-acid glycoprotein appears to account for about 20% of the plasma protein binding. Approximately 30% of melphalan is (covalently) irreversibly bound to plasma proteins. Interactions with immunoglobulins have been found to be negligible.

Melphalan is eliminated from plasma primarily by chemical hydrolysis to monohydroxymelphalan and dihydroxymelphalan. Aside from these hydrolysis products, no other melphalan metabolites have been observed in humans. Although the contribution of renal elimination to melphalan clearance appears to be low, one pharmacokinetic study showed a significant positive correlation between the elimination rate constant for melphalan and renal function and a significant negative correlation between renal function and the area under the plasma melphalan concentration/time curve.

INDICATIONS AND USAGE

ALKERAN Tablets are indicated for the palliative treatment of multiple myeloma and for the palliation of non-resectable epithelial carcinoma of the ovary.

CONTRAINDICATIONS

ALKERAN should not be used in patients whose disease has demonstrated a prior resistance to this agent. Patients who have demonstrated hypersensitivity to melphalan should not be given the drug.

WARNINGS

ALKERAN should be administered in carefully adjusted dosage by or under the supervision of experienced physicians who are familiar with the drug's actions and the possible complications of its use.

As with other nitrogen mustard drugs, excessive dosage will produce marked bone marrow suppression. Bone marrow suppression is the most significant toxicity associated with ALKERAN in most patients. Therefore, the following tests should be performed at the start of therapy and prior to each subsequent course of ALKERAN: platelet count, hemoglobin, white blood cell count, and differential. Thrombocytopenia and/or leukopenia are indications to withhold further therapy until the blood counts have sufficiently recovered. Frequent blood counts are essential to determine optimal dosage and to avoid toxicity (see PRECAUTIONS: Laboratory Tests). Dose adjustment on the basis of blood counts at the nadir and day of treatment should be considered.

Hypersensitivity reactions, including anaphylaxis, have occurred rarely (see ADVERSE REACTIONS). These reactions have occurred after multiple courses of treatment and have recurred in patients who experienced a hypersensitivity reaction to IV ALKERAN. If a hypersensitivity reaction occurs, oral or IV ALKERAN should not be readministered.

Carcinogenesis: Secondary malignancies, including acute nonlymphocytic leukemia, myeloproliferative syndrome, and carcinoma have been reported in patients with cancer treated with alkylating agents (including melphalan). Some patients also received other chemotherapeutic agents or radiation therapy. Precise quantitation of the risk of acute leukemia, myeloproliferative syndrome, or carcinoma is not possible. Published reports of leukemia in patients who have received melphalan (and other alkylating agents) suggest that the risk of leukemogenesis increases with chronicity of treatment and with cumulative dose. In one study, the 10-year cumulative risk of developing acute leukemia or myeloproliferative syndrome after melphalan therapy was 19.5% for cumulative doses ranging from 730 mg to 9652 mg. In this same study, as well as in an additional study, the 10-year cumulative risk of developing acute leukemia or myeloproliferative syndrome after melphalan therapy was less than 2% for cumulative doses under 600 mg. This does not mean that there is a cumulative dose below which there is no risk of the induction of secondary malignancy. The potential benefits from melphalan therapy must be weighed on an individual basis against the possible risk of the induction of a second malignancy.

Adequate and well-controlled carcinogenicity studies have not been conducted in animals. However, i.p. administration of melphalan in rats (5.4 to 10.8 mg/m^2) and in mice (2.25 to 4.5 mg/m^2) 3 times per week for 6 months followed by 12 months post-dose observation produced peritoneal sarcoma and lung tumors, respectively.

Mutagenesis: ALKERAN has been shown to cause chromatid or chromosome damage in humans. Intramuscular administration of ALKERAN at 6 and 60 mg/m^2 produced structural aberrations of the chromatid and chromosomes in bone marrow cells of Wistar rats.

Impairment of Fertility: ALKERAN causes suppression of ovarian function in premenopausal women, resulting in amenorrhea in a significant number of patients. Reversible and irreversible testicular suppression have also been reported.

Pregnancy: Pregnancy Category D. ALKERAN may cause fetal harm when administered to a pregnant woman. Melphalan was embryolethal and teratogenic in rats following oral (6 to 18 mg/m^2 per day for 10 days) and intraperitoneal (18 mg/m^2) administration. Malformations resulting from melphalan included alterations of the brain (underdevelopment, deformation, meningocele, and encephalocele) and eye (anophthalmia and microphthalmos), reduction of the mandible and tail, as well as hepatocele (exomphaly).

There are no adequate and well-controlled studies in pregnant women. If this drug is used during pregnancy, or if the patient becomes pregnant while taking this drug, the patient should be apprised of the potential hazard to the fetus. Women of childbearing potential should be advised to avoid becoming pregnant.

PRECAUTIONS

General: In all instances where the use of ALKERAN is considered for chemotherapy, the physician must evaluate the need and usefulness of the drug against the risk of adverse events. ALKERAN should be used with extreme caution in patients whose bone marrow reserve may have been compromised by prior irradiation or chemotherapy, or whose marrow function is recovering from previous cytotoxic therapy. If the leukocyte count falls below 3000 cells/mcL, or the platelet count below 100,000 cells/mcL, ALKERAN should be discontinued until the peripheral blood cell counts have recovered.

A recommendation as to whether or not dosage reduction should be made routinely in patients with renal insufficiency cannot be made because:

a) There is considerable inherent patient-to-patient variability in the systemic availability of melphalan in patients with normal renal function.
b) Only a small amount of the administered dose appears as parent drug in the urine of patients with normal renal function.

Patients with azotemia should be closely observed, however, in order to make dosage reductions, if required, at the earliest possible time.

Information for Patients: Patients should be informed that the major toxicities of ALKERAN are related to bone marrow suppression, hypersensitivity reactions, gastrointestinal toxicity, and pulmonary toxicity. The major long-term toxicities are related to infertility and secondary malignancies. Patients should never be allowed to take the drug without close medical supervision and should be advised to consult their physician if they experience skin rash, vasculitis, bleeding, fever, persistent cough, nausea, vomiting, amenorrhea, weight loss, or unusual lumps/masses. Women of childbearing potential should be advised to avoid becoming pregnant.

Laboratory Tests: Periodic complete blood counts with differentials should be performed during the course of treatment with ALKERAN. At least one determination should be obtained prior to each treatment course. Patients should be observed closely for consequences of bone marrow suppression, which include severe infections, bleeding, and symptomatic anemia (see WARNINGS).

Drug Interactions: There are no known drug/drug interactions with oral ALKERAN.

Carcinogenesis, Mutagenesis, Impairment of Fertility: See WARNINGS section.

Pregnancy: *Teratogenic Effects:* Pregnancy Category D: See WARNINGS section.

Nursing Mothers: It is not known whether this drug is excreted in human milk. ALKERAN should not be given to nursing mothers.

Pediatric Use: The safety and effectiveness of ALKERAN in pediatric patients have not been established.

Geriatric Use: Clinical experience with ALKERAN has not identified differences in responses between the elderly and younger patients. In general, dose selection for an elderly patient should be cautious, reflecting the greater frequency of decreased hepatic, renal, or cardiac function, and of concomitant disease or other drug therapy.

ADVERSE REACTIONS

Hematologic: The most common side effect is bone marrow suppression. Although bone marrow suppression frequently occurs, it is usually reversible if melphalan is withdrawn early enough. However, irreversible bone marrow failure has been reported.

Gastrointestinal: Gastrointestinal disturbances such as nausea and vomiting, diarrhea, and oral ulceration occur infrequently. Hepatic disorders ranging from abnormal liver function tests to clinical manifestations such as hepatitis and jaundice have been reported.

Miscellaneous: Other reported adverse reactions include: pulmonary fibrosis and interstitial pneumonitis, skin hypersensitivity, vasculitis, alopecia, and hemolytic anemia. Allergic reactions, including rare anaphylaxis, have occurred after multiple courses of treatment.

OVERDOSAGE

Overdoses, including doses up to 50 mg/day for 16 days, have been reported. Immediate effects are likely to be vomiting, ulceration of the mouth, diarrhea, and hemorrhage of the gastrointestinal tract. The principal toxic effect is bone marrow suppression. Hematologic parameters should be closely followed for 3 to 6 weeks. An uncontrolled study suggests that administration of autologous bone marrow or hematopoietic growth factors (i.e., sargramostim, filgrastim) may shorten the period of pancytopenia. General supportive measures, together with appropriate blood transfusions and antibiotics, should be instituted as deemed necessary by the physician. This drug is not removed from plasma to any significant degree by hemodialysis.

DOSAGE AND ADMINISTRATION

Multiple Myeloma: The usual oral dose is 6 mg (3 tablets) daily. The entire daily dose may be given at one time. The dose is adjusted, as required, on the basis of blood counts done at approximately weekly intervals. After 2 to 3 weeks of treatment, the drug should be discontinued for up to 4 weeks, during which time the blood count should be followed carefully. When the white blood cell and platelet counts are rising, a maintenance dose of 2 mg daily may be instituted. Because of the patient-to-patient variation in melphalan plasma levels following oral administration of the drug, several investigators have recommended that the dosage of ALKERAN be cautiously escalated until some myelosuppression is observed in order to assure that potentially therapeutic levels of the drug have been reached.

Other dosage regimens have been used by various investigators. Osserman and Takatsuki have used an initial course of 10 mg/day for 7 to 10 days. They report that maximal suppression of the leukocyte and platelet counts occurs within 3 to 5 weeks and recovery within 4 to 8 weeks. Continuous maintenance therapy with 2 mg/day is instituted when the white blood cell count is greater than 4000 cells/

mcL and the platelet count is greater than 100,000 cells/mcL. Dosage is adjusted to between 1 and 3 mg/day depending upon the hematological response. It is desirable to try to maintain a significant degree of bone marrow depression so as to keep the leukocyte count in the range of 3000 to 3500 cells/mcL.

Hoogstraten et al have started treatment with 0.15 mg/kg per day for 7 days. This is followed by a rest period of at least 14 days, but it may be as long as 5 to 6 weeks. Maintenance therapy is started when the white blood cell and platelet counts are rising. The maintenance dose is 0.05 mg/kg per day or less and is adjusted according to the blood count.

Available evidence suggests that about one third to one half of the patients with multiple myeloma show a favorable response to oral administration of the drug.

One study by Alexanian et al has shown that the use of ALKERAN in combination with prednisone significantly improves the percentage of patients with multiple myeloma who achieve palliation. One regimen has been to administer courses of ALKERAN at 0.25 mg/kg per day for 4 consecutive days (or, 0.20 mg/kg per day for 5 consecutive days) for a total dose of 1 mg/kg per course. These 4- to 5-day courses are then repeated every 4 to 6 weeks if the granulocyte count and the platelet count have returned to normal levels. It is to be emphasized that response may be very gradual over many months; it is important that repeated courses or continuous therapy be given since improvement may continue slowly over many months, and the maximum benefit may be missed if treatment is abandoned too soon.

In patients with moderate to severe renal impairment, currently available pharmacokinetic data do not justify an absolute recommendation on dosage reduction to those patients, but it may be prudent to use a reduced dose initially.

Epithelial Ovarian Cancer: One commonly employed regimen for the treatment of ovarian carcinoma has been to administer ALKERAN at a dose of 0.2 mg/kg daily for 5 days as a single course. Courses are repeated every 4 to 5 weeks depending upon hematologic tolerance.

Administration Precautions: Procedures for proper handling and disposal of anticancer drugs should be considered. Several guidelines on this subject have been published.[1–7] There is no general agreement that all of the procedures recommended in the guidelines are necessary or appropriate.

HOW SUPPLIED

ALKERAN is supplied as white, film-coated, round, biconvex tablets containing 2 mg melphalan in amber glass bottles with child-resistant closures. One side is engraved with "GX EH3" and the other side is engraved with an "A." Bottle of 50 (NDC 0173-0045-35).

Store in a refrigerator, 2° to 8°C (36° to 46°F). Protect from light.

REFERENCES

1. Recommendations for the safe handling of parenteral antineoplastic drugs. Washington, DC: Division of Safety, National Institutes of Health; 1983. US Dept of Health and Human Services, Public Health Service publication NIH 83–2621.
2. AMA Council on Scientific Affairs. Guidelines for handling parenteral antineoplastics. *JAMA.* 1985;253:1590-1591.
3. National Study Commission on Cytotoxic Exposure. Recommendations for handling cytotoxic agents. 1987. Available from Louis P. Jeffrey, Chairman, National Study Commission on Cytotoxic Exposure. Massachusetts College of Pharmacy and Allied Health Sciences, 179 Longwood Avenue, Boston, MA 02115.
4. Clinical Oncological Society of Australia. Guidelines and recommendations for safe handling of antineoplastic agents. *Med J Australia.* 1983;1:426–428.
5. Jones RB, Frank R, Mass T. Safe handling of chemotherapeutic agents: a report from the Mount Sinai Medical Center. *CA-A Cancer J for Clin.* 1983;33:258–263.
6. American Society of Hospital Pharmacists. ASHP technical assistance bulletin on handling cytotoxic and hazardous drugs. *Am J Hosp Pharm.* 1990;47:1033–1049.
7. Controlling Occupational Exposure to Hazardous Drugs. (OSHA Work-Practice Guidelines.) *Am J Health-Syst Pharm.* 1996;53:1669–1685.

GlaxoSmithKline, Research Triangle Park, NC 27709
 November 2001/RL-1025

AMOXIL® ℞
[ə-mäx' ĭl]
brand of amoxicillin
capsules, tablets, chewable tablets, and powder for oral suspension

Prescribing information for these products, which appears on pages 1471–1474 of the 2002 PDR, has been revised as follows. Please write "See Supplement A" next to the product heading.

The first paragraph of the **DESCRIPTION: Chewable Tablets** *subsection was revised as follows to delete the 125- and 250-mg tablets:*

Chewable Tablets: Each cherry-banana-peppermint-flavored tablet contains 200 mg or 400 mg amoxicillin as the trihydrate.

The fourth paragraph of the **CLINICAL PHARMACOLOGY** *section was revised as follows:*

Vial Size	Amount of Diluent	Approximate Concentration	Approximate Available Volume
1 gram	2.5 mL	330 mg/mL	3.0 mL

Orally administered doses of amoxicillin suspension, 125 mg/5 mL and 250 mg/5 mL, result in average peak blood levels 1 to 2 hours after administration in the range of 1.5 µg/mL to 3.0 µg/mL and 3.5 µg/mL to 5.0 µg/mL, respectively.

"Acute generalized exanthematous pustulosis" *was added to the* **ADVERSE REACTIONS:** Hypersensitivity Reactions *subsection.*

The following subsection was added to **ADVERSE REACTIONS:**

Miscellaneous: Superficial tooth discoloration has been reported very rarely in children. Good oral hygiene may help to prevent tooth discoloration as it can usually be removed by brushing.

The **DOSAGE AND ADMINISTRATION: Directions For Mixing Oral Suspension** *subsection was revised to:*

Prepare suspension at time of dispensing as follows: Tap bottle until all powder flows freely. Add approximately $^{1}/_{3}$ of the total amount of water for reconstitution (see table below) and shake vigorously to wet powder. Add remainder of the water and again shake vigorously.

125 mg/5 mL

Bottle Size	Amount of Water Required for Reconstitution
80 mL	62 mL
150 mL	116 mL

Each teaspoonful (5 mL) will contain 125 mg amoxicillin.

200 mg/5 mL

Bottle Size	Amount of Water Required for Reconstitution
50 mL	39 mL
75 mL	57 mL
100 mL	76 mL

Each teaspoonful (5 mL) will contain 200 mg amoxicillin.

250 mg/5 mL

Bottle Size	Amount of Water Required for Reconstitution
100 mL	74 mL
150 mL	111 mL

Each teaspoonful (5 mL) will contain 250 mg amoxicillin.

400 mg/5 mL

Bottle Size	Amount of Water Required for Reconstitution
50 mL	36 mL
75 mL	54 mL
100 mL	71 mL

Each teaspoonful (5 mL) will contain 400 mg amoxicillin.

The **HOW SUPPLIED** *section was revised to delete the following packs:*

Amoxil (amoxicillin) Capsules.

250-mg Capsule

NDC 0029-6006-30 bottles of 100

500-mg Capsule

NDC 0029-6007-30 bottles of 100

Amoxil (amoxicillin) Chewable Tablets.

125-mg Tablet

NDC 0029-6004-39 bottles of 60

250-mg Tablet

NDC 0029-6005-13 bottles of 30
NDC 0029-6005-30 bottles of 100

Amoxil (amoxicillin) for Oral Suspension.

125 mg/5 mL

NDC 0029-6008-23 100-mL bottle

250 mg/5 mL

NDC 0029-6009-21 80-mL bottle

400 mg/5 mL

NDC 0029-6048-18 200-mg unit dose bottle
NDC 0029-6049-18 400-mg unit dose bottle

The storage information in the **HOW SUPPLIED** *section was revised to:*

Store at or below 20°C (68°F)
- 250-mg and 500-mg capsules
- 125-mg and 250-mg unreconstituted powder

Store at or below 25°C (77°F)
- 200-mg and 400-mg unreconstituted powder
- 200-mg and 400-mg chewable tablets
- 500-mg and 875-mg tablets

Dispense in a tight container.

GlaxoSmithKline, Research Triangle Park, NC 27709

March 2001/AM:L20

ANCEF® ℞
[an' sef]
brand of cefazolin for injection

Prescribing information for this product, which appears on pages 1474–1476 of the 2002 PDR, has been revised as follows. Please write "See Supplement A" next to the product heading.

The ANCEF® brand of cefazolin injection has been discontinued.

The **DESCRIPTION** *section was revised to:*

Ancef (cefazolin for injection) is a semi-synthetic cephalosporin for parenteral administration. It is the sodium salt of 3-{[(5-methyl-1,3,4-thiadiazol-2-yl)thio]-methyl}-8-oxo-7-[2-(1H-tetrazol-1-yl)acetamido]-5-thia-1-azabicyclo[4.2.0]oct-2-ene-2-carboxylic acid.

The sodium content is 48 mg per gram of cefazolin.

Ancef in lyophilized form is supplied in vials equivalent to 1 gram of cefazolin; in "Piggyback" Vials for intravenous admixture equivalent to 1 gram of cefazolin; and in Pharmacy Bulk Vials equivalent to 10 grams of cefazolin.

The **ADVERSE REACTIONS: Hepatic and Renal** *subsection was revised to the following 2 subsections:*

Hepatic: Transient rise in SGOT, SGPT and alkaline phosphatase levels has been observed. As with other cephalosporins, very rare reports of hepatitis have been received.

Renal: As with other cephalosporins, very rare reports of increased BUN and creatinine levels, as well as renal failure, have been received.

The **DOSAGE AND ADMINISTRATION:** RECONSTITUTION: **Single-Dose Vials** *table was revised as follows to delete the 500-mg vial size:*

[See table above]

The **DOSAGE AND ADMINISTRATION:** ADMINISTRATION *section was revised to delete the* **DIRECTIONS FOR USE OF ANCEF (CEFAZOLIN INJECTION) GALAXY® CONTAINER (PL 2040 PLASTIC)** *subsection.*

The **HOW SUPPLIED** *section was revised to:*

Ancef (cefazolin for injection)

Each vial contains cefazolin sodium equivalent to 1 gram of cefazolin.

NDC 0007-3130-16 (package of 25 vials)

Each vial contains cefazolin sodium equivalent to 1 gram of cefazolin.

NDC 0007-3137-05 (package of 10 "piggyback" vials)

Each vial contains cefazolin sodium equivalent to 10 grams of cefazolin.

NDC 0007-3135-05 (package of 10 pharmacy bulk vials)

As with other cephalosporins, *Ancef* tends to darken depending on storage conditions; within the stated recommendations, however, product potency is not adversely affected. Before reconstitution protect from light and store at Controlled Room Temperature 20° to 25°C (68° to 77°F).

GlaxoSmithKline, Research Triangle Park, NC 27709

January 2002/AF:L55

AUGMENTIN® ℞
[äg-ment' in]
amoxicillin/clavulanate potassium
Powder for Oral Suspension and Chewable Tablets

Prescribing information for these products, which appears on pages 1482–1485 of the 2002 PDR, has been revised as follows. Please write "See Supplement A" next to the product heading.

The following sentence was added to the end of the **PRECAUTIONS: Labor and Delivery** *subsection:*

In a single study in women with premature rupture of fetal membranes, it was reported that prophylactic treatment with *Augmentin* may be associated with an increased risk of necrotizing enterocolitis in neonates.

Added "acute generalized exanthematous pustulosis" *to the* **ADVERSE REACTIONS: Hypersensitivity Reactions** *subsection.*

Revised the first sentence of the **OVERDOSAGE** *section to:*

Following overdosage, patients have experienced primarily gastrointestinal symptoms including stomach and abdominal pain, vomiting, and diarrhea.

GlaxoSmithKline, Research Triangle Park, NC 27709
January 2002/AG:PL9

AUGMENTIN® ℞
[äg-mint' in]
amoxicillin/clavulanate potassium
Tablets

Prescribing information for this product, which appears on pages 1485–1487 of the 2002 PDR, has been revised as follows. Please write "See Supplement A" next to the product heading.

The following sentence was added to the end of the **PRECAUTIONS: Labor and Delivery** *subsection:*

In a single study in women with premature rupture of fetal membranes, it was reported that prophylactic treatment with *Augmentin* may be associated with an increased risk of necrotizing enterocolitis in neonates.

Added "acute generalized exanthemous pustulosis" *to the* **ADVERSE REACTIONS: Hypersensitivity Reactions** *subsection.*

Continued on next page

Augmentin Tablets—Cont.

Revised the first sentence of the **OVERDOSAGE** *section to:*
Following overdosage, patients have experienced primarily gastrointestinal symptoms including stomach and abdominal pain, vomiting, and diarrhea.
GlaxoSmithKline, Research Triangle Park, NC 27709
January 2002/AG:AL9

BACTROBAN OINTMENT® ℞

[*bac 'trō-ban*]
brand of
mupirocin ointment, 2%
For Dermatologic Use

Prescribing information for this product, which appears on pages 1496–1497 of the 2002 PDR, has been revised as follows. Please write "See Supplement A" next to the product heading.
Add the following sentence to the end of the first paragraph of the **ADVERSE REACTIONS** *section:*
Systemic reactions to *Bactroban Ointment* have occurred rarely.
GlaxoSmithKline, Research Triangle Park, NC 27709

April 2001/BC:L12C

BECONASE® ℞

[*be 'kō-nāz"*]
(beclomethasone dipropionate, USP)
Inhalation Aerosol

For Nasal Inhalation Only

Prescribing information for this product, which appears on pages 1497–1498 of the 2002 PDR, has been revised as follows. Please write "See Supplement A" next to the product heading.
The sentence "Beclomethasone 17,21-dipropionate is a diester of beclomethasone, a synthetic halogenated corticosteroid." *was added to the* **DESCRIPTION** *section.*
The **CLINICAL PHARMACOLOGY** *section was revised to:*
Mechanism of Action: Following topical administration, beclomethasone dipropionate produces anti-inflammatory and vasoconstrictor effects. The mechanisms responsible for the anti-inflammatory action of beclomethasone dipropionate are unknown. Corticosteroids have been shown to have a wide range of effects on multiple cell types (e.g., mast cells, eosinophils, neutrophils, macrophages, and lymphocytes) and mediators (e.g., histamine, eicosanoids, leukotrienes, and cytokines) involved in inflammation. The direct relationship of these findings to the effects of beclomethasone dipropionate on allergic rhinitis symptoms is not known.
Biopsies of nasal mucosa obtained during clinical studies showed no histopathologic changes when beclomethasone dipropionate was administered intranasally.
Beclomethasone dipropionate is a pro-drug with weak glucocorticoid receptor binding affinity. It is hydrolyzed via esterase enzymes to its active metabolite beclomethasone-17-monopropionate (B-17-MP), which has high topical anti-inflammatory activity.
Pharmacokinetics: ***Absorption:*** Beclomethasone dipropionate is sparingly soluble in water. When given by nasal inhalation in the form of an aqueous or aerosolized suspension, the drug is deposited primarily in the nasal passages. The majority of the drug is eventually swallowed. Following intranasal administration of aqueous beclomethasone dipropionate, the systemic absorption was assessed by measuring the plasma concentrations of its active metabolite B-17-MP, for which the absolute bioavailability following intranasal administration is 44% (43% of the administered dose came from the swallowed portion and only 1% of the total dose was bioavailable from the nose). The absorption of unchanged beclomethasone dipropionate following oral and intranasal dosing was undetectable (plasma concentrations <50 pg/mL).
Distribution: The tissue distribution at steady-state for beclomethasone dipropionate is moderate (20 L) but more extensive for B-17-MP (424 L). There is no evidence of tissue storage of beclomethasone dipropionate or its metabolites. Plasma protein binding is moderately high (87%).
Metabolism: Beclomethasone dipropionate is cleared very rapidly from the systemic circulation by metabolism mediated via esterase enzymes that are found in most tissues. The main product of metabolism is the active metabolite (B-17-MP). Minor inactive metabolites, beclomethasone-21-monopropionate (B-21-MP) and beclomethasone (BOH), are also formed, but these contribute little to systemic exposure.
Elimination: The elimination of beclomethasone dipropionate and B-17-MP after intravenous administration are characterized by high plasma clearance (150 and 120 L/hour) with corresponding terminal elimination half-lives of 0.5 and 2.7 hours. Following oral administration of tritiated beclomethasone dipropionate, approximately 60% of the dose was excreted in the feces within 96 hours, mainly as free and conjugated polar metabolites. Approximately 12% of the dose was excreted as free and conjugated polar metabolites in the urine. The renal clearance of beclomethasone dipropionate and its metabolites is negligible.
Pharmacodynamics: The effects of beclomethasone dipropionate on hypothalamic-pituitary-adrenal (HPA) function have been evaluated in adult volunteers by other routes of administration. Studies with beclomethasone dipropionate by the intranasal route may demonstrate that there is more or that there is less absorption by this route of administration. There was no suppression of early morning plasma cortisol concentrations when beclomethasone dipropionate was administered in a dose of 1000 mcg/day for 1 month as an oral aerosol or for 3 days by intramuscular injection. However, partial suppression of plasma cortisol concentrations was observed when beclomethasone dipropionate was administered in doses of 2000 mcg/day either by oral aerosol or intramuscular injection. Immediate suppression of plasma cortisol concentrations was observed after single doses of 4000 mcg of beclomethasone dipropionate. Suppression of HPA function (reduction of early morning plasma cortisol levels) has been reported in adult patients who received 1600-mcg daily doses of oral beclomethasone dipropionate for 1 month. In clinical studies using beclomethasone dipropionate intranasally, there was no evidence of adrenal insufficiency.
GlaxoSmithKline, Research Triangle Park, NC 27709
August 2001/RL-1008

BECONASE AQ® ℞

[*be' kō-nāz"*]
(beclomethasone dipropionate, monohydrate)
Nasal Spray, 0.042%*
***Calculated on the dried basis.** **SHAKE WELL**
For Intranasal Use Only **BEFORE USE.**

Prescribing information for this product, which appears on pages 1498–1499 of the 2002 PDR, has been revised as follows. Please write "See Supplement A" next to the product heading.
The sentence "Beclomethasone 17,21-dipropionate is a diester of beclomethasone, a synthetic halogenated corticosteroid." *was added to the* **DESCRIPTION** *section.*
The **CLINICAL PHARMACOLOGY** *section was revised to:*
Mechanism of Action: Following topical administration, beclomethasone dipropionate produces anti-inflammatory and vasoconstrictor effects. The mechanisms responsible for the anti-inflammatory action of beclomethasone dipropionate are unknown. Corticosteroids have been shown to have a wide range of effects on multiple cell types (e.g., mast cells, eosinophils, neutrophils, macrophages, and lymphocytes) and mediators (e.g., histamine, eicosanoids, leukotrienes, and cytokines) involved in inflammation. The direct relationship of these findings to the effects of beclomethasone dipropionate on allergic rhinitis symptoms is not known.
Biopsies of nasal mucosa obtained during clinical studies showed no histopathologic changes when beclomethasone dipropionate was administered intranasally.
Beclomethasone dipropionate is a pro-drug with weak glucocorticoid receptor binding affinity. It is hydrolyzed via esterase enzymes to its active metabolite beclomethasone-17-monopropionate (B-17-MP), which has high topical anti-inflammatory activity.
Pharmacokinetics: ***Absorption:*** Beclomethasone dipropionate is sparingly soluble in water. When given by nasal inhalation in the form of an aqueous or aerosolized suspension, the drug is deposited primarily in the nasal passages. The majority of the drug is eventually swallowed. Following intranasal administration of aqueous beclomethasone dipropionate, the systemic absorption was assessed by measuring the plasma concentrations of its active metabolite B-17-MP, for which the absolute bioavailability following intranasal administration is 44% (43% of the administered dose came from the swallowed portion and only 1% of the total dose was bioavailable from the nose). The absorption of unchanged beclomethasone dipropionate following oral and intranasal dosing was undetectable (plasma concentrations <50 pg/mL).
Distribution: The tissue distribution at steady-state for beclomethasone dipropionate is moderate (20 L) but more extensive for B-17-MP (424 L). There is no evidence of tissue storage of beclomethasone dipropionate or its metabolites. Plasma protein binding is moderately high (87%).
Metabolism: Beclomethasone dipropionate is cleared very rapidly from the systemic circulation by metabolism mediated via esterase enzymes that are found in most tissues. The main product of metabolism is the active metabolite (B-17-MP). Minor inactive metabolites, beclomethasone-21-monopropionate (B-21-MP) and beclomethasone (BOH), are also formed, but these contribute little to systemic exposure.
Elimination: The elimination of beclomethasone dipropionate and B-17-MP after intravenous administration are characterized by high plasma clearance (150 and 120 L/hour) with corresponding terminal elimination half-lives of 0.5 and 2.7 hours. Following oral administration of tritiated beclomethasone dipropionate, approximately 60% of the dose was excreted in the feces within 96 hours, mainly as free and conjugated polar metabolites. Approximately 12% of the dose was excreted as free and conjugated polar metabolites in the urine. The renal clearance of beclomethasone dipropionate and its metabolites is negligible.
Pharmacodynamics: The effects of beclomethasone dipropionate on hypothalamic-pituitary-adrenal (HPA) function have been evaluated in adult volunteers by other routes of administration. Studies with beclomethasone dipropionate by the intranasal route may demonstrate that there is more or that there is less absorption by this route of administration. There was no suppression of early morning plasma cortisol concentrations when beclomethasone dipropionate was administered in a dose of 1000 mcg/day for 1 month as an oral aerosol or for 3 days by intramuscular injection. However, partial suppression of plasma cortisol concentrations was observed when beclomethasone dipropionate was administered in doses of 2000 mcg/day either by oral aerosol or intramuscular injection. Immediate suppression of plasma cortisol concentrations was observed after single doses of 4000 mcg of beclomethasone dipropionate. Suppression of HPA function (reduction of early morning plasma cortisol levels) has been reported in adult patients who received 1600-mcg daily doses of oral beclomethasone dipropionate for 1 month. In clinical studies using beclomethasone dipropionate intranasally, there was no evidence of adrenal insufficiency. The effect of BECONASE AQ Nasal Spray on HPA function was not evaluated but would not be expected to differ from intranasal beclomethasone dipropionate aerosol.
In 1 study in children with asthma, the administration of inhaled beclomethasone at recommended daily doses for at least 1 year was associated with a reduction in nocturnal cortisol secretion. The clinical significance of this finding is not clear. It reinforces other evidence, however, that topical beclomethasone may be absorbed in amounts that can have systemic effects and that physicians should be alert for evidence of systemic effects, especially in chronically treated patients (see PRECAUTIONS).
The following subsection was added to **PRECAUTIONS:**
Geriatric Use: Clinical studies of BECONASE AQ Nasal Spray did not include sufficient numbers of subjects aged 65 and over to determine whether they respond differently from younger subjects. Other reported clinical experience has not identified differences in responses between the elderly and younger patients. In general, dose selection for an elderly patient should be cautious, starting at the low end of the dosing range, reflecting the greater frequency of decreased hepatic, renal, or cardiac function, and of concomitant disease or other drug therapy.
GlaxoSmithKline, Research Triangle Park, NC 27709
August 2001/RL-1009

CEFTIN® Tablets ℞

[*sef ' tin*]
(cefuroxime axetil tablets)

CEFTIN® for Oral Suspension

(cefuroxime axetil powder for oral suspension)

Marketing of these products, which appear on pages 1898–1902 of the 2002 PDR, has been transferred from LifeCycle Ventures, Inc. to GlaxoSmithKline.

DESCRIPTION
CEFTIN Tablets and CEFTIN for Oral Suspension contain cefuroxime as cefuroxime axetil. CEFTIN is a semisynthetic, broad-spectrum cephalosporin antibiotic for oral administration.
Chemically, cefuroxime axetil, the 1-(acetyloxy) ethyl ester of cefuroxime, is (*RS*)-1-hydroxyethyl (6*R*,7*R*)-7-[2-(2-furyl) glyoxylamido]-3-(hydroxymethyl)-8-oxo-5-thia-1-azabicyclo [4.2.0]oct-2-ene-2-carboxylate, 7^2-(*Z*)-(*O*-methyl-oxime), 1-acetate 3-carbamate. Its molecular formula is $C_{20}H_{22}N_4O_{10}S$, and it has a molecular weight of 510.48.
Cefuroxime axetil is in the amorphous form.
CEFTIN Tablets are film-coated and contain the equivalent of 125, 250, or 500 mg of cefuroxime as cefuroxime axetil. CEFTIN Tablets contain the inactive ingredients colloidal silicon dioxide, croscarmellose sodium, FD&C Blue No. 1 (250- and 500-mg tablets only), hydrogenated vegetable oil, hydroxypropyl methylcellulose, methylparaben, microcrystalline cellulose, propylene glycol, propylparaben, sodium benzoate (125-mg tablets only), sodium lauryl sulfate, and titanium dioxide.
CEFTIN for Oral Suspension, when reconstituted with water, provides the equivalent of 125 mg or 250 mg of cefuroxime (as cefuroxime axetil) per 5 mL of suspension. CEFTIN for Oral Suspension contains the inactive ingredients povidone K30, stearic acid, sucrose, and tutti-frutti flavoring.

CLINICAL PHARMACOLOGY
Absorption and Metabolism: After oral administration, cefuroxime axetil is absorbed from the gastrointestinal tract and rapidly hydrolyzed by nonspecific esterases in the intestinal mucosa and blood to cefuroxime. Cefuroxime is subsequently distributed throughout the extracellular fluids. The axetil moiety is metabolized to acetaldehyde and acetic acid.
Pharmacokinetics: Approximately 50% of serum cefuroxime is bound to protein. Serum pharmacokinetic parameters for CEFTIN Tablets and CEFTIN for Oral Suspension are shown in Tables 1 and 2.
[See table at top of next page]
[See table at top of next page]
Comparative Pharmacokinetic Properties: A 250 mg/5 mL-dose of CEFTIN Suspension is bioequivalent to 2 times 125 mg/5 mL-dose of CEFTIN Suspension when administered with food (see Table 3). **CEFTIN for Oral Suspension was not bioequivalent to CEFTIN Tablets when tested in healthy adults. The tablet and powder for oral suspension formulations are NOT substitutable on a milligram-per-milligram basis.** The area under the curve for the suspension averaged 91% of that for the tablet, and the peak plasma concentration for the suspension averaged 71% of the peak plasma concentration of the tablets. Therefore, the safety and effectiveness of both the tablet and oral suspension formulations had to be established in separate clinical trials.

[See table 3 above]

Food Effect on Pharmacokinetics: Absorption of the tablet is greater when taken after food (absolute bioavailability of CEFTIN Tablets increases from 37% to 52%). Despite this difference in absorption, the clinical and bacteriologic responses of patients were independent of food intake at the time of tablet administration in 2 studies where this was assessed.

All pharmacokinetic and clinical effectiveness and safety studies in pediatric patients using the suspension formulation were conducted in the fed state. No data are available on the absorption kinetics of the suspension formulation when administered to fasted pediatric patients.

Renal Excretion: Cefuroxime is excreted unchanged in the urine; in adults, approximately 50% of the administered dose is recovered in the urine within 12 hours. The pharmacokinetics of cefuroxime in the urine of pediatric patients have not been studied at this time. Until further data are available, the renal pharmacokinetic properties of cefuroxime axetil established in adults should not be extrapolated to pediatric patients.

Because cefuroxime is renally excreted, the serum half-life is prolonged in patients with reduced renal function. In a study of 20 elderly patients (mean age = 83.9 years) having a mean creatinine clearance of 34.9 mL/min, the mean serum elimination half-life was 3.5 hours. Despite the lower elimination of cefuroxime in geriatric patients, dosage adjustment based on age is not necessary (see PRECAUTIONS: Geriatric Use).

Microbiology: The in vivo bactericidal activity of cefuroxime axetil is due to cefuroxime's binding to essential target proteins and the resultant inhibition of cell-wall synthesis.

Cefuroxime has bactericidal activity against a wide range of common pathogens, including many beta-lactamase–producing strains. Cefuroxime is stable to many bacterial beta-lactamases, especially plasmid-mediated enzymes that are commonly found in enterobacteriaceae.

Cefuroxime has been demonstrated to be active against most strains of the following microorganisms both in vitro and in clinical infections as described in the INDICATIONS AND USAGE section (see INDICATIONS AND USAGE section).

Aerobic Gram-Positive Microorganisms:

Staphylococcus aureus (including beta-lactamase–producing strains)
Streptococcus pneumoniae
Streptococcus pyogenes

Aerobic Gram-Negative Microorganisms:

Escherichia coli
Haemophilus influenzae (including beta-lactamase–producing strains)
Haemophilus parainfluenzae
Klebsiella pneumoniae
Moraxella catarrhalis (including beta-lactamase–producing strains)
Neisseria gonorrhoeae (including beta-lactamase–producing strains)

Spirochetes:

Borrelia burgdorferi.

Cefuroxime has been shown to be active in vitro against most strains of the following microorganisms; however, the clinical significance of these findings is unknown.

Cefuroxime exhibits in vitro minimum inhibitory concentrations (MICs) of 4.0 mcg/mL or less (systemic susceptible breakpoint) against most (≥90%) strains of the following microorganisms; however, the safety and effectiveness of cefuroxime in treating clinical infections due to these microorganisms have not been established in adequate and well-controlled trials.

Aerobic Gram-Positive Microorganisms:

Staphylococcus epidermidis
Staphylococcus saprophyticus
Streptococcus agalactiae

NOTE: Certain strains of enterococci, e.g., *Enterococcus faecalis* (formerly *Streptococcus faecalis*), are resistant to cefuroxime. Methicillin-resistant staphylococci are resistant to cefuroxime.

Aerobic Gram-Negative Microorganisms:

Morganella morganii
Proteus inconstans
Proteus mirabilis
Providencia rettgeri

NOTE: *Pseudomonas* spp., *Campylobacter* spp., *Acinetobacter calcoaceticus*, and most strains of *Serratia* spp. and *Proteus vulgaris* are resistant to most first- and second-generation cephalosporins. Some strains of *Morganella morganii, Enterobacter cloacae,* and *Citrobacter* spp. have been shown by in vitro tests to be resistant to cefuroxime and other cephalosporins.

Anaerobic Microorganisms:

Peptococcus niger

NOTE: Most strains of *Clostridium difficile* and *Bacteroides fragilis* are resistant to cefuroxime.

Susceptibility Tests: ***Dilution Techniques:*** Quantitative methods that are used to determine MICs provide reproducible estimates of the susceptibility of bacteria to antimicrobial compounds. One such standardized procedure uses a standardized dilution method[1] (broth, agar, or microdilution) or equivalent with cefuroxime powder. The MIC values obtained should be interpreted according to the following criteria:

Table 1. Postprandial Pharmacokinetics of Cefuroxime Administered as CEFTIN Tablets to Adults*

Dose† (Cefuroxime Equivalent)	Peak Plasma Concentration (mcg/mL)	Time of Peak Plasma Concentration (hr)	Mean Elimination Half-Life (hr)	AUC (mcg-hr mL)
125 mg	2.1	2.2	1.2	6.7
250 mg	4.1	2.5	1.2	12.9
500 mg	7.0	3.0	1.2	27.4
1,000 mg	13.6	2.5	1.3	50.0

*Mean values of 12 healthy adult volunteers.
†Drug administered immediately after a meal.

Table 2. Postprandial Pharmacokinetics of Cefuroxime Administered as CEFTIN for Oral Suspension to Pediatric Patients*

Dose† (Cefuroxime Equivalent)	n	Peak Plasma Concentration (mcg/mL)	Time of Peak Plasma Concentration (hr)	Mean Elimination Half-Life (hr)	AUC (mcg-hr mL)
10 mg/kg	8	3.3	3.6	1.4	12.4
15 mg/kg	12	5.1	2.7	1.9	22.5
20 mg/kg	8	7.0	3.1	1.9	32.8

*Mean age = 23 months.
†Drug administered with milk or milk products.

Table 3. Pharmacokinetics of Cefuroxime Administered as 250 mg/5 mL or 2 × 125 mg/5 mL CEFTIN for Oral Suspension to Adults* With Food

Dose (Cefuroxime Equivalent)	Peak Plasma Concentration (mcg/mL)	Time of Peak Plasma Concentration (hr)	Mean Elimination Half-Life (hr)	AUC (mcg-hr mL)
250 mg/5 mL	2.23	3	1.40	8.92
2 × 125 mg/5 mL	2.37	3	1.44	9.75

*Mean values of 18 healthy adult volunteers.

Table 4. Adverse Reactions—CEFTIN Tablets Multiple-Dose Dosing Regimens—Clinical Trials

Incidence	Adverse reaction	%
Incidence ≥1%	Diarrhea/loose stools	3.7%
	Nausea/vomiting	3.0%
	Transient elevation in AST	2.0%
	Transient elevation in ALT	1.6%
	Eosinophilia	1.1%
	Transient elevation in LDH	1.0%
Incidence <1% but >0.1%	Abdominal pain	
	Abdominal cramps	
	Flatulence	
	Indigestion	
	Headache	
	Vaginitis	
	Vulvar itch	
	Rash	
	Hives	
	Itch	
	Dysuria	
	Chills	
	Chest Pain	
	Shortness of breath	
	Mouth ulcers	
	Swollen tongue	
	Sleepiness	
	Thirst	
	Anorexia	
	Positive Coombs test	

MIC (mcg/mL)	Interpretation
≤4	(S) Susceptible
8–16	(I) Intermediate
≥32	(R) Resistant

A report of "Susceptible" indicates that the pathogen, if in the blood, is likely to be inhibited by usually achievable concentrations of the antimicrobial compound in blood. A report of "Intermediate" indicates that inhibitory concentrations of the antibiotic may be achieved if high dosage is used or if the infection is confined to tissues or fluids in which high antibiotic concentrations are attained. This category also provides a buffer zone that prevents small, uncontrolled technical factors from causing major discrepancies in interpretation. A report of "Resistant" indicates that usually achievable concentrations of the antimicrobial compound in the blood are unlikely to be inhibitory and that other therapy should be selected.

Standardized susceptibility test procedures require the use of laboratory control microorganisms. Standard cefuroxime powder should give the following MIC values:

Microorganism	MIC (mcg/mL)
Escherichia coli ATCC 25922	2–8
Staphylococcus aureus ATCC 29213	0.5–2

Diffusion Techniques: Quantitative methods that require measurement of zone diameters provide estimates of the susceptibility of bacteria to antimicrobial compounds. One such standardized procedure[2] that has been recommended (for use with disks) to test the susceptibility of microorganisms to cefuroxime uses the 30-mcg cefuroxime disk. Interpretation involves correlation of the diameter obtained in the disk test with the MIC for cefuroxime.

Reports from the laboratory providing results of the standard single-disk susceptibility test with a 30-mcg cefuroxime disk should be interpreted according to the following criteria:

Zone Diameter (mm)	Interpretation
≥23	(S) Susceptible
15–22	(I) Intermediate
≤14	(R) Resistant

Interpretation should be as stated above for results using dilution techniques.

As with standard dilution techniques, diffusion methods require the use of laboratory control microorganisms. The 30-mcg cefuroxime disk provides the following zone diameters in these laboratory test quality control strains:

Microorganism	Zone Diameter (mm)
Escherichia coli ATCC 25922	20–26
Staphylococcus aureus ATCC 25923	27–35

INDICATIONS AND USAGE

NOTE: CEFTIN TABLETS AND CEFTIN FOR ORAL SUSPENSION ARE NOT BIOEQUIVALENT AND ARE NOT SUBSTITUTABLE ON A MILLIGRAM-PER-MILLIGRAM BASIS (SEE CLINICAL PHARMACOLOGY).

CEFTIN Tablets: CEFTIN Tablets are indicated for the treatment of patients with mild to moderate infections caused by susceptible strains of the designated microorganisms in the conditions listed below:

Continued on next page

Ceftin—Cont.

1. **Pharyngitis/Tonsillitis** caused by *Streptococcus pyogenes.* **NOTE:** The usual drug of choice in the treatment and prevention of streptococcal infections, including the prophylaxis of rheumatic fever, is penicillin given by the intramuscular route. CEFTIN Tablets are generally effective in the eradication of streptococci from the nasopharynx; however, substantial data establishing the efficacy of cefuroxime in the subsequent prevention of rheumatic fever are not available. Please also note that in all clinical trials, all isolates had to be sensitive to both penicillin and cefuroxime. There are no data from adequate and well-controlled trials to demonstrate the effectiveness of cefuroxime in the treatment of penicillin-resistant strains of *Streptococcus pyogenes.*
2. **Acute Bacterial Otitis Media** caused by *Streptococcus pneumoniae, Haemophilus influenzae* (including beta-lactamase–producing strains), *Moraxella catarrhalis* (including beta-lactamase–producing strains), or *Streptococcus pyogenes.*
3. **Acute Bacterial Maxillary Sinusitis** caused by *Streptococcus pneumoniae* or *Haemophilus influenzae* (non-beta-lactamase–producing strains only). (See CLINICAL STUDIES section.)
   NOTE: In view of the insufficient numbers of isolates of beta-lactamase–producing strains of *Haemophilus influenzae* and *Moraxella catarrhalis* that were obtained from clinical trials with CEFTIN Tablets for patients with acute bacterial maxillary sinusitis, it was not possible to adequately evaluate the effectiveness of CEFTIN Tablets for sinus infections known, suspected, or considered potentially to be caused by beta-lactamase–producing *Haemophilus influenzae* or *Moraxella catarrhalis.*
4. **Acute Bacterial Exacerbations of Chronic Bronchitis and Secondary Bacterial Infections of Acute Bronchitis** caused by *Streptococcus pneumoniae, Haemophilus influenzae* (beta-lactamase negative strains), or *Haemophilus parainfluenzae* (beta-lactamase negative strains). (See DOSAGE AND ADMINISTRATION section and CLINICAL STUDIES section.)
5. **Uncomplicated Skin and Skin-Structure Infections** caused by *Staphylococcus aureus* (including beta-lactamase–producing strains) or *Streptococcus pyogenes.*
6. **Uncomplicated Urinary Tract Infections** caused by *Escherichia coli* or *Klebsiella pneumoniae.*
7. **Uncomplicated Gonorrhea,** urethral and endocervical, caused by penicillinase-producing and non-penicillinase–producing strains of *Neisseria gonorrhoeae* and uncomplicated gonorrhea, rectal, in females, caused by non-penicillinase–producing strains of *Neisseria gonorrhoeae.*
8. **Early Lyme Disease (erythema migrans)** caused by *Borrelia burgdorferi.*

CEFTIN for Oral Suspension: CEFTIN for Oral Suspension is indicated for the treatment of pediatric patients 3 months to 12 years of age with mild to moderate infections caused by susceptible strains of the designated microorganisms in the conditions listed below. The safety and effectiveness of CEFTIN for Oral Suspension in the treatment of infections other than those specifically listed below have not been established either by adequate and well-controlled trials or by pharmacokinetic data with which to determine an effective and safe dosing regimen.

1. **Pharyngitis/Tonsillitis** caused by *Streptococcus pyogenes.* **NOTE:** The usual drug of choice in the treatment and prevention of streptococcal infections, including the prophylaxis of rheumatic fever, is penicillin given by the intramuscular route. CEFTIN for Oral Suspension is generally effective in the eradication of streptococci from the nasopharynx; however, substantial data establishing the efficacy of cefuroxime in the subsequent prevention of rheumatic fever are not available. Please also note that in all clinical trials, all isolates had to be sensitive to both penicillin and cefuroxime. There are no data from adequate and well-controlled trials to demonstrate the effectiveness of cefuroxime in the treatment of penicillin-resistant strains of *Streptococcus pyogenes.*
2. **Acute Bacterial Otitis Media** caused by *Streptococcus pneumoniae, Haemophilus influenzae* (including beta-lactamase–producing strains), *Moraxella catarrhalis* (including beta-lactamase–producing strains), or *Streptococcus pyogenes.*
3. **Impetigo** caused by *Staphylococcus aureus* (including beta-lactamase–producing strains) or *Streptococcus pyogenes.*

Culture and susceptibility testing should be performed when appropriate to determine susceptibility of the causative microorganism(s) to cefuroxime. Therapy may be started while awaiting the results of this testing. Antimicrobial therapy should be appropriately adjusted according to the results of such testing.

CONTRAINDICATIONS

CEFTIN products are contraindicated in patients with known allergy to the cephalosporin group of antibiotics.

WARNINGS

CEFTIN TABLETS AND CEFTIN FOR ORAL SUSPENSION ARE NOT BIOEQUIVALENT AND ARE THEREFORE NOT SUBSTITUTABLE ON A MILLIGRAM-PER-MILLIGRAM BASIS (SEE CLINICAL PHARMACOLOGY).

BEFORE THERAPY WITH CEFTIN PRODUCTS IS INSTITUTED, CAREFUL INQUIRY SHOULD BE MADE TO DETERMINE WHETHER THE PATIENT HAS HAD PREVIOUS HYPERSENSITIVITY REACTIONS TO CEFTIN PRODUCTS, OTHER CEPHALOSPORINS, PENICILLINS, OR OTHER DRUGS. IF THIS PRODUCT IS TO BE GIVEN TO PENICILLIN-SENSITIVE PATIENTS, CAUTION SHOULD BE EXERCISED BECAUSE CROSS-HYPERSENSITIVITY AMONG BETA-LACTAM ANTIBIOTICS HAS BEEN CLEARLY DOCUMENTED AND MAY OCCUR IN UP TO 10% OF PATIENTS WITH A HISTORY OF PENICILLIN ALLERGY. IF A CLINICALLY SIGNIFICANT ALLERGIC REACTION TO CEFTIN PRODUCTS OCCURS, DISCONTINUE THE DRUG AND INSTITUTE APPROPRIATE THERAPY. SERIOUS ACUTE HYPERSENSITIVITY REACTIONS MAY REQUIRE TREATMENT WITH EPINEPHRINE AND OTHER EMERGENCY MEASURES, INCLUDING OXYGEN, INTRAVENOUS FLUIDS, INTRAVENOUS ANTIHISTAMINES, CORTICOSTEROIDS, PRESSOR AMINES, AND AIRWAY MANAGEMENT, AS CLINICALLY INDICATED.

Pseudomembranous colitis has been reported with nearly all antibacterial agents, including cefuroxime, and may range from mild to life threatening. Therefore, it is important to consider this diagnosis in patients who present with diarrhea subsequent to the administration of antibacterial agents.

Treatment with antibacterial agents alters normal flora of the colon and may permit overgrowth of clostridia. Studies indicate that a toxin produced by *Clostridium difficile* is one primary cause of antibiotic-associated colitis.

After the diagnosis of pseudomembranous colitis has been established, appropriate therapeutic measures should be initiated. Mild cases of pseudomembranous colitis usually respond to drug discontinuation alone. In moderate to severe cases, consideration should be given to management with fluids and electrolytes, protein supplementation, and treatment with an antibacterial drug effective against *Clostridium difficile.*

Table 5. Adverse Reactions—CEFTIN Tablets 1-g Single-Dose Regimen for Uncomplicated Gonorrhea—Clinical Trials

Incidence ≥1%	Nausea/vomiting	6.8%
	Diarrhea	4.2%
Incidence <1% but >0.1%	Abdominal pain	
	Dyspepsia	
	Erythema	
	Rash	
	Pruritus	
	Vaginal candidiasis	
	Vaginal itch	
	Vaginal discharge	
	Headache	
	Dizziness	
	Somnolence	
	Muscle cramps	
	Muscle stiffness	
	Muscle spasm of neck	
	Tightness/pain in chest	
	Bleeding/pain in urethra	
	Kidney pain	
	Tachycardia	
	Lockjaw-type reaction	

Table 6. Adverse Reactions—CEFTIN for Oral Suspension Multiple-Dose Dosing Regimens—Clinical Trials

Incidence ≥1%	Diarrhea/loose stools	8.6%
	Dislike of taste	5.0%
	Diaper rash	3.4%
	Nausea/vomiting	2.6%
Incidence <1% but >0.1%	Abdominal pain	
	Flatulence	
	Gastrointestinal infection	
	Candidiasis	
	Vaginal irritation	
	Rash	
	Hyperactivity	
	Irritable behavior	
	Eosinophilia	
	Positive direct Coombs test	
	Elevated liver enzymes	
	Viral illness	
	Upper respiratory infection	
	Sinusitis	
	Cough	
	Urinary tract infection	
	Joint swelling	
	Arthralgia	
	Fever	
	Ptyalism	

PRECAUTIONS

General: As with other broad-spectrum antibiotics, prolonged administration of cefuroxime axetil may result in overgrowth of nonsusceptible microorganisms. If superinfection occurs during therapy, appropriate measures should be taken.

Cephalosporins, including cefuroxime axetil, should be given with caution to patients receiving concurrent treatment with potent diuretics because these diuretics are suspected of adversely affecting renal function.

Cefuroxime axetil, as with other broad-spectrum antibiotics, should be prescribed with caution in individuals with a history of colitis. The safety and effectiveness of cefuroxime axetil have not been established in patients with gastrointestinal malabsorption. Patients with gastrointestinal malabsorption were excluded from participating in clinical trials of cefuroxime axetil.

Information for Patients/Caregivers (Pediatric):

1. During clinical trials, the tablet was tolerated by pediatric patients old enough to swallow the cefuroxime axetil tablet whole. The crushed tablet has a strong, persistent, bitter taste and should not be administered to pediatric patients in this manner. Pediatric patients who cannot swallow the tablet whole should receive the oral suspension.
2. Discontinuation of therapy due to taste and/or problems of administering this drug occurred in 1.4% of pediatric patients given the oral suspension. Complaints about taste (which may impair compliance) occurred in 5% of pediatric patients.

Drug/Laboratory Test Interactions: A false-positive reaction for glucose in the urine may occur with copper reduction tests (Benedict's or Fehling's solution or with CLINITEST® tablets), but not with enzyme-based tests for glycosuria (e.g., CLINISTIX®). As a false-negative result may occur in the ferricyanide test, it is recommended that either the glucose oxidase or hexokinase method be used to determine blood/plasma glucose levels in patients receiving cefuroxime axetil. The presence of cefuroxime does not interfere with the assay of serum and urine creatinine by the alkaline picrate method.

Drug/Drug Interactions: Concomitant administration of probenecid with cefuroxime axetil tablets increases the area under the serum concentration versus time curve by 50%. The peak serum cefuroxime concentration after a 1.5-g single dose is greater when taken with 1 g of probenecid (mean = 14.8 mcg/mL) than without probenecid (mean = 12.2 mcg/mL).

Drugs that reduce gastric acidity may result in a lower bioavailability of CEFTIN compared with that of fasting state and tend to cancel the effect of postprandial absorption.

Carcinogenesis, Mutagenesis, Impairment of Fertility: Although lifetime studies in animals have not been performed to evaluate carcinogenic potential, no mutagenic potential was found for cefuroxime axetil in the micronucleus test and a battery of bacterial mutation tests. Reproduction studies in rats at doses up to 1,000 mg/kg/day (9 times the recommended maximum human dose based on mg/m^2) have revealed no evidence of impaired fertility.

Pregnancy: *Teratogenic Effects:* Pregnancy Category B. Reproduction studies have been performed in rats and mice at doses up to 3,200 mg/kg/day (23 times the recommended maximum human dose based on mg/m^2) and have revealed no evidence of harm to the fetus due to cefuroxime axetil. There are, however, no adequate and well-controlled studies in pregnant women. Because animal reproduction studies are not always predictive of human response, this drug should be used during pregnancy only if clearly needed.

Labor and Delivery: Cefuroxime axetil has not been studied for use during labor and delivery.

Nursing Mothers: Because cefuroxime is excreted in human milk, consideration should be given to discontinuing nursing temporarily during treatment with cefuroxime axetil.
Pediatric Use: The safety and effectiveness of CEFTIN have been established for pediatric patients aged 3 months to 12 years for acute bacterial maxillary sinusitis based upon its approval in adults. Use of CEFTIN in pediatric patients is supported by pharmacokinetic and safety data in adults and pediatric patients, and by clinical and microbiological data from adequate and well-controlled studies of the treatment of acute bacterial maxillary sinusitis in adults and of acute otitis media with effusion in pediatric patients. It is also supported by post-marketing adverse events surveillance (see CLINICAL PHARMACOLOGY, INDICATIONS AND USAGE, ADVERSE REACTIONS, DOSAGE AND ADMINISTRATION, and CLINICAL STUDIES).
Geriatric Use: In clinical trials when 12- to 64-year-old patients and geriatric patients (65 years of age or older) were treated with usual recommended dosages (i.e., 125 to 500 mg b.i.d., depending on type of infections), no overall differences in effectiveness were observed between the 2 age-groups. The geriatric patients reported somewhat fewer gastrointestinal events and less frequent vaginal candidiasis compared with patients aged 12 to 64 years old; however, no clinically significant differences were reported between the 2 age-groups. Therefore, no adjustment of the usual adult dose is necessary based on age alone.

ADVERSE REACTIONS

CEFTIN TABLETS IN CLINICAL TRIALS: Multiple-Dose Dosing Regimens: ***7 to 10 Days Dosing:*** Using multiple doses of cefuroxime axetil tablets, 912 patients were treated with the recommended dosages of cefuroxime axetil (125 to 500 mg twice a day). There were no deaths or permanent disabilities thought related to drug toxicity. Twenty (2.2%) patients discontinued medication due to adverse events thought by the investigators to be possibly, probably, or almost certainly related to drug toxicity. Seventeen (85%) of the 20 patients who discontinued therapy did so because of gastrointestinal disturbances, including diarrhea, nausea, vomiting, and abdominal pain. The percentage of cefuroxime axetil tablet-treated patients who discontinued study drug because of adverse events was very similar at daily doses of 1,000, 500, and 250 mg (2.3%, 2.1%, and 2.2%, respectively). However, the incidence of gastrointestinal adverse events increased with the higher recommended doses.
The following adverse events were thought by the investigators to be possibly, probably, or almost certainly related to cefuroxime axetil tablets in multiple-dose clinical trials (n = 912 cefuroxime axetil-treated patients).
[See table 4 at top of page 169]
5-Day Experience (see CLINICAL STUDIES section): In clinical trials using CEFTIN in a dose of 250 mg b.i.d. in the treatment of secondary bacterial infections of acute bronchitis, 399 patients were treated for 5 days and 402 patients were treated for 10 days. No difference in the occurrence of adverse events was found between the 2 regimens.
In Clinical Trials for Early Lyme Disease With 20 Days Dosing: Two multicenter trials assessed cefuroxime axetil tablets 500 mg twice a day for 20 days. The most common drug-related adverse experiences were diarrhea (10.6% of patients), Jarisch-Herxheimer reaction (5.6%), and vaginitis (5.4%). Other adverse experiences occurred with frequencies comparable to those reported with 7 to 10 days dosing.
Single-Dose Regimen for Uncomplicated Gonorrhea: In clinical trials using a single dose of cefuroxime axetil tablets, 1,061 patients were treated with the recommended dosage of cefuroxime axetil (1,000 mg) for the treatment of uncomplicated gonorrhea. There were no deaths or permanent disabilities thought related to drug toxicity in these studies.
The following adverse events were thought by the investigators to be possibly, probably, or almost certainly related to cefuroxime axetil in 1,000-mg single-dose clinical trials of cefuroxime axetil tablets in the treatment of uncomplicated gonorrhea conducted in the US.
[See table 5 at top of previous page]

CEFTIN FOR ORAL SUSPENSION IN CLINICAL TRIALS

In clinical trials using multiple doses of cefuroxime axetil powder for oral suspension, pediatric patients (96.7% of whom were younger than 12 years of age) were treated with the recommended dosages of cefuroxime axetil (20 to 30 mg/kg/day divided twice a day up to a maximum dose of 500 or 1,000 mg/day, respectively). There were no deaths or permanent disabilities in any of the patients in these studies. Eleven US patients (1.2%) discontinued medication due to adverse events thought by the investigators to be possibly, probably, or almost certainly related to drug toxicity. The discontinuations were primarily for gastrointestinal disturbances, usually diarrhea or vomiting. During clinical trials, discontinuation of therapy due to the taste and/or problems with administering this drug occurred in 13 (1.4%) pediatric patients enrolled at centers in the United States.
The following adverse events were thought by the investigators to be possibly, probably, or almost certainly related to cefuroxime axetil for oral suspension in multiple-dose clinical trials (n = 931 cefuroxime axetil-treated US patients).
[See table 6 at top of previous page]

OBSERVED DURING CLINICAL PRACTICE

In addition to adverse events reported from clinical trials, the following events have been identified during post-approval use of CEFTIN. Because they are reported voluntarily from a population of unknown size, estimates of frequency cannot be made. These events have been chosen for inclusion due to combination of their seriousness, frequency of reporting, or potential causal connection to CEFTIN.

Table 7. CEFTIN Tablets (May be administered without regard to meals.)

Population/Infection	Dosage	Duration (days)
Adolescents and Adults (13 years and older)		
Pharyngitis/tonsillitis	250 mg b.i.d.	10
Acute bacterial maxillary sinusitis	250 mg b.i.d.	10
Acute bacterial exacerbations of chronic bronchitis	250 or 500 mg b.i.d.	10*
Secondary bacterial infections of acute bronchitis	250 or 500 mg b.i.d.	5–10
Uncomplicated skin and skin-structure infections	250 or 500 mg b.i.d.	10
Uncomplicated urinary tract infections	125 or 250 mg b.i.d.	7–10
Uncomplicated gonorrhea	1,000 mg once	single dose
Early Lyme disease	500 mg b.i.d.	20
Pediatric Patients (who can swallow tablets whole)		
Pharyngitis/tonsillitis	125 mg b.i.d.	10
Acute otitis media	250 mg b.i.d.	10
Acute bacterial maxillary sinusitis	250 mg b.i.d.	10

*The safety and effectiveness of CEFTIN administered for less than 10 days in patients with acute exacerbations of chronic bronchitis have not been established.

Table 8. CEFTIN for Oral Suspension (Must be administered with food. Shake well each time before using.)

Population/Infection	Dosage	Daily Maximum Dose	Duration (days)
Pediatric Patients (3 months to 12 years)			
Pharyngitis/tonsillitis	20 mg/kg/day divided b.i.d.	500 mg	10
Acute otitis media	30 mg/kg/day divided b.i.d.	1,000 mg	10
Acute bacterial maxillary sinusitis	30 mg/kg/day divided b.i.d.	1,000 mg	10
Impetigo	30 mg/kg/day divided b.i.d.	1,000 mg	10

Table 9. Amount of Water Required for Reconstitution of Labeled Volumes of CEFTIN for Oral Suspension

CEFTIN for Oral Suspension	Labeled Volume After Reconstitution	Amount of Water Required for Reconstitution
125 mg/5 mL	100 mL	37 mL
250 mg/5 mL	50 mL 100 mL	19 mL 35 mL

Table 10. Clinical Effectiveness of CEFTIN Tablets Compared to Beta-Lactamase Inhibitor-Containing Control Drug in the Treatment of Acute Bacterial Maxillary Sinusitis

	US Patients*		South American Patients†	
	CEFTIN n = 49	Control n = 43	CEFTIN n = 87	Control n = 89
Clinical success (cure + improvement)	65%	53%	77%	74%
Clinical cure	53%	44%	72%	64%
Clinical improvement	12%	9%	5%	10%

*95% Confidence interval around the success difference [−0.08, +0.32].
†95% Confidence interval around the success difference [−0.10, +0.16].

Table 11. Clinical Effectiveness of CEFTIN Tablets Compared to Doxycycline in the Treatment of Early Lyme Disease

	Part I (1 Month Posttreatment)*		Part II (1 Year Posttreatment)†	
	CEFTIN n = 125	Doxycycline n = 108	CEFTIN n = 105‡	Doxycycline n = 83‡
Satisfactory clinical outcome§	91%	93%	84%	87%
Clinical cure/success	72%	73%	73%	73%
Clinical improvement	19%	19%	10%	13%

*95% confidence interval around the satisfactory difference for Part I (−0.08, +0.05).
†95% confidence interval around the satisfactory difference for Part II (−0.13, +0.07).
‡ n's include patients assessed as unsatisfactory clinical outcomes (failure + recurrence) in Part I (CEFTIN - 11 [5 failure, 6 recurrence]; doxycycline - 8 [6 failure, 2 recurrence]).
§ Satisfactory clinical outcome inclues cure + improvement (Part I) and success + improvement (Part II).

Blood and Lymphatic: Increased prothrombin time.
General: The following hypersensitivity reactions have been reported: anaphylaxis, angioedema, pruritus, rash, serum sickness-like reaction, urticaria.
Gastrointestinal: Pseudomembranous colitis (see WARNINGS).
Hematologic: Hemolytic anemia, leukopenia, pancytopenia, thrombocytopenia.
Hepatobiliary Tract and Pancreas: Hepatic impairment including hepatitis and cholestasis, jaundice.
Neurologic: Seizure.
Skin: Erythema multiforme, Stevens-Johnson syndrome, toxic epidermal necrolysis.
Urologic: Renal dysfunction.

CEPHALOSPORIN-CLASS ADVERSE REACTIONS

In addition to the adverse reactions listed above that have been observed in patients treated with cefuroxime axetil, the following adverse reactions and altered laboratory tests have been reported for cephalosporin-class antibiotics: renal dysfunction, toxic nephropathy, hepatic cholestasis, aplastic anemia, hemolytic anemia, hemorrhage, increased prothrombin time, increased BUN, increased creatinine, false-positive test for urinary glucose, increased alkaline phosphatase, neutropenia, thrombocytopenia, leukopenia, elevated bilirubin, pancytopenia, and agranulocytosis.
Several cephalosporins have been implicated in triggering seizures, particularly in patients with renal impairment when the dosage was not reduced (see DOSAGE AND ADMINISTRATION and OVERDOSAGE). If seizures associated with drug therapy occur, the drug should be discontinued. Anticonvulsant therapy can be given if clinically indicated.

OVERDOSAGE

Overdosage of cephalosporins can cause cerebral irritation leading to convulsions. Serum levels of cefuroxime can be reduced by hemodialysis and peritoneal dialysis.

Continued on next page

Ceftin—Cont.

DOSAGE AND ADMINISTRATION

NOTE: CEFTIN TABLETS AND CEFTIN FOR ORAL SUSPENSION ARE NOT BIOEQUIVALENT AND ARE NOT SUBSTITUTABLE ON A MILLIGRAM-PER-MILLIGRAM BASIS (SEE CLINICAL PHARMACOLOGY).

[See table 7 at top of previous page]

CEFTIN for Oral Suspension: CEFTIN for Oral Suspension may be administered to pediatric patients ranging in age from 3 months to 12 years, according to dosages in Table 8:

[See table 8 at top of previous page]

Patients With Renal Failure: The safety and efficacy of cefuroxime axetil in patients with renal failure have not been established. Since cefuroxime is renally eliminated, its half-life will be prolonged in patients with renal failure.

Directions for Mixing CEFTIN for Oral Suspension: Prepare a suspension at the time of dispensing as follows:

1. Shake the bottle to loosen the powder.
2. Remove the cap.
3. Add the total amount of water for reconstitution (see Table 9) and replace the cap.
4. Invert the bottle and vigorously rock the bottle from side to side so that water rises through the powder.
5. Once the sound of the powder against the bottle disappears, turn the bottle upright and vigorously shake it in a diagonal direction.

[See table 9 at top of previous page]

NOTE: SHAKE THE ORAL SUSPENSION WELL BEFORE EACH USE. Replace cap securely after each opening. The reconstituted suspension should be stored between 2° and 25°C (36° and 77°F) (either in the refrigerator or at room temperature). DISCARD AFTER 10 DAYS.

HOW SUPPLIED

CEFTIN Tablets: CEFTIN Tablets, 125 mg of cefuroxime (as cefuroxime axetil), are white, capsule-shaped, film-coated tablets engraved with "395" on one side and "Glaxo" on the other side as follows:

60 Tablets/Bottle NDC 0173-0395-01

CEFTIN Tablets, 250 mg of cefuroxime (as cefuroxime axetil), are light blue, capsule-shaped, film-coated tablets engraved with "387" on one side and "Glaxo" on the other side as follows:

20 Tablets/Bottle NDC 0173-0387-00
60 Tablets/Bottle NDC 0173-0387-42
Unit Dose Packs of 100 NDC 0173-0387-01

CEFTIN Tablets, 500 mg of cefuroxime (as cefuroxime axetil), are dark blue, capsule-shaped, film-coated tablets engraved with "394" on one side and "Glaxo" on the other side as follows:

20 Tablets/Bottle NDC 0173-0394-00
60 Tablets/Bottle NDC 0173-0394-42
Unit Dose Packs of 50 NDC 0173-0394-01

Store the tablets between 15° and 30°C (59° and 86°F). Replace cap securely after each opening. Protect unit dose packs from excessive moisture.

CEFTIN for Oral Suspension: CEFTIN for Oral Suspension is provided as dry, white to pale yellow, tutti-frutti–flavored powder. When reconstituted as directed, CEFTIN for Oral Suspension provides the equivalent of 125 mg or 250 mg of cefuroxime (as cefuroxime axetil) per 5 mL of suspension. It is supplied in amber glass bottles as follows:

125 mg/5 mL:
100-mL Suspension NDC 0173-0406-00
250 mg/5 mL:
50-mL Suspension NDC 0173-0554-00
100-mL Suspension NDC 0173-0555-00

Before reconstitution, store dry powder between 2° and 30°C (36° and 86°F).

After reconstitution, store suspension between 2° and 25°C (36° and 77°F), in a refrigerator or at room temperature. DISCARD AFTER 10 DAYS.

CLINICAL STUDIES

CEFTIN Tablets: ***Acute Bacterial Maxillary Sinusitis:*** One adequate and well-controlled study was performed in patients with acute bacterial maxillary sinusitis. In this study each patient had a maxillary sinus aspirate collected by sinus puncture before treatment was initiated for presumptive acute bacterial sinusitis. All patients had to have radiographic and clinical evidence of acute maxillary sinusitis. As shown in the following summary of the study, the general clinical effectiveness of CEFTIN Tablets was comparable to an oral antimicrobial agent that contained a specific beta-lactamase inhibitor in treating acute maxillary sinusitis. However, sufficient microbiology data were obtained to demonstrate the effectiveness of CEFTIN Tablets in treating acute bacterial maxillary sinusitis due only to *Streptococcus pneumoniae* or non-beta-lactamase–producing *Haemophilus influenzae*. An insufficient number of beta-lactamase-producing *Haemophilus influenzae* and *Moraxella catarrhalis* isolates were obtained in this trial to adequately evaluate the effectiveness of CEFTIN Tablets in the treatment of acute bacterial maxillary sinusitis due to these 2 organisms. This study enrolled 317 adult patients, 132 patients in the United States and 185 patients in South America. Patients were randomized in a 1:1 ratio to cefuroxime axetil 250 mg b.i.d. or an oral antimicrobial agent that contained a specific beta-lactamase inhibitor. An intent-to-treat analysis of the submitted clinical data yielded the following results:

[See table 10 at top of previous page]

In this trial and in a supporting maxillary puncture trial, 15 evaluable patients had non-beta-lactamase–producing *Haemophilus influenzae* as the identified pathogen. Ten (10) of these 15 patients (67%) had their pathogen (non-beta-lactamase–producing *Haemophilus influenzae*) eradicated. Eighteen (18) evaluable patients had *Streptococcus pneumoniae* as the identified pathogen. Fifteen (15) of these 18 patients (83%) had their pathogen (*Streptococcus pneumoniae*) eradicated.

Safety: The incidence of drug-related gastrointestinal adverse events was statistically significantly higher in the control arm (an oral antimicrobial agent that contained a specific beta-lactamase inhibitor) versus the cefuroxime axetil arm (12% versus 1%, respectively; $P<.001$), particularly drug-related diarrhea (8% versus 1%, respectively; $P = .001$).

Early Lyme Disease: Two adequate and well-controlled studies were performed in patients with early Lyme disease. In these studies all patients had to present with physician-documented erythema migrans, with or without systemic manifestations of infection. Patients were randomized in a 1:1 ratio to a 20-day course of treatment with cefuroxime axetil 500 mg b.i.d. or doxycycline 100 mg t.i.d. Patients were assessed at 1 month posttreatment for success in treating early Lyme disease (Part I) and at 1 year posttreatment for success in preventing the progression to the sequelae of late Lyme disease (Part II).

A total of 355 adult patients (181 treated with cefuroxime axetil and 174 treated with doxycycline) were enrolled in the 2 studies. In order to objectively validate the clinical diagnosis of early Lyme disease in these patients, 2 approaches were used: 1) blinded expert reading of photographs, when available, of the pretreatment erythema migrans skin lesion; and 2) serologic confirmation (using enzyme-linked immunosorbent assay [ELISA] and immunoblot assay ["Western" blot]) of the presence of antibodies specific to *Borrelia burgdorferi*, the etiologic agent of Lyme disease. By these procedures, it was possible to confirm the physician diagnosis of early Lyme disease in 281 (79%) of the 355 study patients. The efficacy data summarized below are specific to this "validated" patient subset, while the safety data summarized below reflect the entire patient population for the 2 studies.

Analysis of the submitted clinical data for evaluable patients in the "validated" patient subset yielded the following results:

[See table 11 at top of previous page]

CEFTIN and doxycycline were effective in prevention of the development of sequelae of late Lyme disease.

Safety: Drug-related adverse events affecting the skin were reported significantly more frequently by patients treated with doxycycline than by patients treated with cefuroxime axetil (12% versus 3%, respectively; $P = .002$), primarily reflecting the statistically significantly higher incidence of drug-related photosensitivity reactions in the doxycycline arm versus the cefuroxime axetil arm (9% versus 0%, respectively; $P<.001$). While the incidence of drug-related gastrointestinal adverse events was similar in the 2 treatment groups (cefuroxime axetil - 13%; doxycycline - 11%), the incidence of drug-related diarrhea was statistically significantly higher in the cefuroxime axetil arm versus the doxycycline arm (11% versus 3%, respectively; $P = .005$).

Secondary Bacterial Infections of Acute Bronchitis: Four randomized, controlled clinical studies were performed comparing 5 days versus 10 days of CEFTIN for the treatment of patients with secondary bacterial infections of acute bronchitis. These studies enrolled a total of 1253 patients (CAE-516 n = 360; CAE-517 n = 177; CAEA4001 n = 362; CAEA4002 n = 354). The protocols for CAE-516 and CAE-517 were identical and compared CEFTIN 250 mg b.i.d. for 5 days, CEFTIN 250 mg b.i.d. for 10 days, and AUGMENTIN® 500 mg t.i.d. for 10 days. These 2 studies were conducted simultaneously. CAEA4001 and CAEA4002 compared CEFTIN 250 mg b.i.d. for 5 days, CEFTIN 250 mg b.i.d. for 10 days, and CECLOR® 250 mg t.i.d. for 10 days. They were otherwise identical to CAE-516 and CAE-517 and were conducted over the following 2 years. Patients were required to have polymorphonuclear cells present on the Gram stain of their screening sputum specimen, but isolation of a bacterial pathogen from the sputum culture was not required for inclusion. The following table demonstrates the results of the clinical outcome analysis of the pooled studies CAE-516/CAE-517 and CAEA4001/CAEA4002, respectively:

[See table 12 below]

The response rates for patients who were both clinically and bacteriologically evaluable were consistent with those reported for the clinically evaluable patients.

Safety: In these clinical trials, 399 patients were treated with CEFTIN for 5 days and 402 patients with CEFTIN for 10 days. No difference in the occurrence of adverse events was observed between the 2 regimens.

Table 12. Clinical Effectiveness of CEFTIN Tablets 250 mg b.i.d. in Secondary Bacterial Infections of Acute Bronchitis: Comparison of 5 Versus 10 Days' Treatment Duration

	CAE-516 and CAE-517*		CAEA4001 and CAEA4002†	
	5 Day (n = 127)	10 Day (n = 139)	5 Day (n = 173)	10 Day (n = 192)
Clinical success (cure + improvement)	80%	87%	84%	82%
Clinical cure	61%	70%	73%	72%
Clinical improvement	19%	17%	11%	10%

*95% Confidence interval around the success difference [−0.164, +0.029].
†95% Confidence interval around the success difference [−0.061, +0.103].

REFERENCES

1. National Committee for Clinical Laboratory Standards. *Methods for Dilution Antimicrobial Susceptibility Tests for Bacteria that Grow Aerobically.* 3rd ed. Approved Standard NCCLS Document M7-A3, Vol. 13, No. 25. Villanova, Pa: NCCLS; 1993.
2. National Committee for Clinical Laboratory Standards. *Performance Standards for Antimicrobial Disk Susceptibility Tests.* 4th ed. Approved Standard NCCLS Document M2-A4, Vol. 10, No. 7. Villanova, Pa: NCCLS; 1990.

GlaxoSmithKline, Research Triangle Park, NC 27709

November 2001/RL-1033

COMBIVIR® Tablets ℞

[*kom 'bə-vir*]
(lamivudine/zidovudine tablets)

Prescribing information for this product, which appears on pages 1502–1505 of the 2002 PDR, has been revised as follows. Please write "See Supplement A" next to the product heading.

The following paragraph was added to the **CLINICAL PHARMACOLOGY: Special Populations** *subsection:*

Impaired Hepatic Function: COMBIVIR: A reduction in the daily dose of zidovudine may be necessary in patients with mild to moderate impaired hepatic function or liver cirrhosis. Because COMBIVIR is a fixed-dose combination that cannot be adjusted for this patient population, COMBIVIR is not recommended for patients with impaired hepatic function.

The first paragraph of the **WARNINGS** *section was revised to:*

COMBIVIR is a fixed-dose combination of lamivudine and zidovudine. Ordinarily, COMBIVIR should not be administered concomitantly with lamivudine, zidovudine, or TRIZIVIR®, a fixed-dose combination of abacavir, lamivudine, and zidovudine.

The following subsection was added to **WARNINGS:**

Posttreatment Exacerbations of Hepatitis: In clinical trials in non-HIV-infected patients treated with lamivudine for chronic hepatitis B (HBV), clinical and laboratory evidence of excerbations of hepatitis have occurred after discontinuation of lamivudine. These exacerbations have been detected primarily by serum ALT elevations in addition to re-emergence of HBV DNA. Although most events appear to have been self-limited, fatalities have been reported in some cases. Similar events have been reported from post-marketing experience after changes from lamivudine-containing HIV treatment regimens to non-lamivudine-containing regimens in patients infected with both HIV and HBV. The causal relationship to discontinuation of lamivudine treatment is unknown. Patients should be closely monitored with both clinical and laboratory followup for at least several months after stopping treatment. There is insufficient evidence to determine whether re-initiation of lamivudine alters the course of posttreatment exacerbations of hepatitis.

The **PRECAUTIONS** *section was revised to:*

Patients with HIV and Hepatitis B Virus Coinfection: Safety and efficacy of lamivudine have not been established for treatment of chronic hepatitis B in patients dually infected with HIV and HBV. In non-HIV-infected patients treated with lamivudine for chronic hepatitis B, emergence of lamivudine-resistant HBV has been detected and has been associated with diminished treatment response (see EPIVIR-HBV package insert for additional information). Emergence of hepatitis B virus variants associated with resistance to lamivudine has also been reported in HIV-infected patients who have received lamivudine-containing antiretroviral regimens in the presence of concurrent infection with hepatitis B virus.

Patients with Impaired Renal Function: Reduction of the dosages of lamivudine and zidovudine is recommended for patients with impaired renal function. Patients with creatinine clearance <50 mL/min should not receive COMBIVIR.

Information for Patients: COMBIVIR is not a cure for HIV infection and patients may continue to experience illnesses associated with HIV infection, including opportunistic infections. Patients should be advised that the use of COMBIVIR has not been shown to reduce the risk of transmission of HIV to others through sexual contact or blood contamination. Patients should be informed that the major toxicities of COMBIVIR are neutropenia and/or anemia. They should be told of the extreme importance of having their blood counts followed closely while on therapy, especially for patients with advanced HIV disease. Patients should be advised of the importance of taking COMBIVIR as it is prescribed.

Drug Interactions: ***Lamivudine:*** Trimethoprim (TMP) 160 mg/sulfamethoxazole (SMX) 800 mg once daily has been shown to increase lamivudine exposure (AUC). The effect of higher doses of TMP/SMX on lamivudine pharmacokinetics has not been investigated (see CLINICAL PHARMACOLOGY).

Lamivudine and zalcitabine may inhibit the intracellular phosphorylation of one another. Therefore, use of COMBIVIR in combination with zalcitabine is not recommended.

Zidovudine: Coadministration of ganciclovir, interferon-alpha, and other bone marrow suppressive or cytotoxic agents may increase the hematologic toxicity of zidovudine. Concomitant use of COMBIVIR with stavudine should be avoided since an antagonistic relationship with zidovudine has been demonstrated in vitro. In addition, concomitant use of zidovudine with doxorubicin or ribavirin should be avoided because an antagonistic relationship has been demonstrated in vitro.

See CLINICAL PHARMACOLOGY for additional drug interactions.

Carcinogenesis, Mutagenesis, and Impairment of Fertility:
Carcinogenicity:

Lamivudine: Long-term carcinogenicity studies with lamivudine in mice and rats showed no evidence of carcinogenic potential at exposures up to 10 times (mice) and 58 times (rats) those observed in humans at the recommended therapeutic dose for HIV infection.

Zidovudine: Zidovudine was administered orally at 3 dosage levels to separate groups of mice and rats (60 females and 60 males in each group). Initial single daily doses were 30, 60, and 120 mg/kg per day in mice and 80, 220, and 600 mg/kg per day in rats. The doses in mice were reduced to 20, 30, and 40 mg/kg per day after day 90 because of treatment-related anemia, whereas in rats only the high dose was reduced to 450 mg/kg per day on day 91 and then to 300 mg/kg per day on day 279.

In mice, 7 late-appearing (after 19 months) vaginal neoplasms (5 nonmetastasizing squamous cell carcinomas, 1 squamous cell papilloma, and 1 squamous polyp) occurred in animals given the highest dose. One late-appearing squamous cell papilloma occurred in the vagina of a middle-dose animal. No vaginal tumors were found at the lowest dose.

In rats, 2 late-appearing (after 20 months), nonmetastasizing vaginal squamous cell carcinomas occurred in animals given the highest dose. No vaginal tumors occurred at the low or middle dose in rats. No other drug-related tumors were observed in either sex of either species.

At doses that produced tumors in mice and rats, the estimated drug exposure (as measured by AUC) was approximately 3 times (mouse) and 24 times (rat) the estimated human exposure at the recommended therapeutic dose of 100 mg every 4 hours.

Two transplacental carcinogenicity studies were conducted in mice. One study administered zidovudine at doses of 20 mg/kg per day or 40 mg/kg per day from gestation day 10 through parturition and lactation with dosing continuing in offspring for 24 months postnatally. The doses of zidovudine employed in this study produced zidovudine exposures approximately 3 times the estimated human exposure at recommended doses. After 24 months, at the highest dose, an increase in incidence of vaginal tumors was noted with no increase in tumors in the liver or lung or any other organ in either gender. These findings are consistent with results of the standard oral carcinogenicity study in mice, as described earlier. A second study administered zidovudine at maximum tolerated doses of 12.5 mg/day or 25 mg/day (~1000 mg/kg nonpregnant body weight or ~450 mg/kg of term body weight) to pregnant mice from days 12 through 18 of gestation. There was an increase in the number of tumors in the lung, liver, and female reproductive tracts in the offspring of mice receiving the higher dose level of zidovudine.

It is not known how predictive the results of rodent carcinogenicity studies may be for humans.

Mutagenicity: Lamivudine: Lamivudine was negative in a microbial mutagenicity screen, in an in vitro cell transformation assay, in a rat micronucleus test, in a rat bone marrow cytogenetic assay, and in an assay for unscheduled DNA synthesis in rat liver. It was mutagenic in a L5178Y/TK$^{+/-}$ mouse lymphoma assay and clastogenic in a cytogenetic assay using cultured human lymphocytes.

Zidovudine: Zidovudine was mutagenic in a L5178Y/TK$^{+/-}$ mouse lymphoma assay, positive in an in vitro cell transformation assay, clastogenic in a cytogenetic assay using cultured human lymphocytes, and positive in mouse and rat micronucleus tests after repeated doses. It was negative in a cytogenetic study in rats given a single dose.

Impairment of Fertility: Lamivudine: In a study of reproductive performance, lamivudine, administered to male and female rats at doses up to 130 times the usual adult dose based on body surface area considerations, revealed no evidence of impaired fertility (judged by conception rates) and no effect on the survival, growth, and development to weaning of the offspring.

Zidovudine: Zidovudine, administered to male and female rats at doses up to 7 times the usual adult dose based on body surface area considerations, had no effect on fertility judged by conception rates.

Pregnancy: Pregnancy Category C.

COMBIVIR: There are no adequate and well-controlled studies of COMBIVIR in pregnant women. Reproduction studies with lamivudine and zidovudine have been performed in animals (see Lamivudine and Zidovudine sections below). COMBIVIR should be used during pregnancy only if the potential benefits outweigh the risks.

Lamivudine: Reproduction studies with orally administered lamivudine have been performed in rats and rabbits at doses up to 4000 mg/kg per day and 1000 mg/kg per day, respectively, producing plasma levels up to approximately 35 times that for the adult HIV dose. No evidence of teratogenicity due to lamivudine was observed. Evidence of early embryolethality was seen in the rabbit at exposure levels similar to those observed in humans, but there was no indication of this effect in the rat at exposure levels up to 35 times that in humans. Studies in pregnant rats and rabbits showed that lamivudine is transferred to the fetus through the placenta.

Zidovudine: Reproduction studies with orally administered zidovudine in the rat and in the rabbit at doses up to 500 mg/kg per day revealed no evidence of teratogenicity with zidovudine. Zidovudine treatment resulted in embryo/fetal toxicity as evidenced by an increase in the incidence of fetal resorptions in rats given 150 or 450 mg/kg per day and rabbits given 500 mg/kg per day. The doses used in the teratology studies resulted in peak zidovudine plasma concentrations (after one half of the daily dose) in rats 66 to 226 times, and in rabbits 12 to 87 times, mean steady-state peak human plasma concentrations (after one sixth of the daily dose) achieved with the recommended daily dose (100 mg every 4 hours). In an additional teratology study in rats, a dose of 3000 mg/kg per day (very near the oral median lethal dose in rats of 3683 mg/kg) caused marked maternal toxicity and an increase in the incidence of fetal malformations. This dose resulted in peak zidovudine plasma concentrations 350 times peak human plasma concentrations. No evidence of teratogenicity was seen in this experiment at doses of 600 mg/kg per day or less. Two rodent carcinogenicity studies were conducted (see Carcinogenesis, Mutagenesis, Impairment of Fertility).

Antiretroviral Pregnancy Registry: To monitor maternal-fetal outcomes of pregnant women exposed to COMBIVIR and other antiretroviral agents, an Antiretroviral Pregnancy Registry has been established. Physicians are encouraged to register patients by calling 1-800-258-4263.

Nursing Mothers: The Centers for Disease Control and Prevention recommend that HIV-infected mothers not breastfeed their infants to avoid risking postnatal transmission of HIV infection. No specific studies of lamivudine and zidovudine excretion in breast milk after dosing with COMBIVIR have been performed, although zidovudine is excreted in breast milk after dosing with RETROVIR (see CLINICAL PHARMACOLOGY: Pharmacokinetics: Nursing Mothers). Although it is not known if lamivudine is excreted in human milk, a study in which lactating rats were administered 45 mg/kg of lamivudine showed that lamivudine concentrations in milk were slightly greater than those in plasma.

Because of both the potential for HIV transmission and the potential for serious adverse reactions in nursing infants, **mothers should be instructed not to breastfeed if they are receiving COMBIVIR.**

Pediatric Use: COMBIVIR should not be administered to pediatric patients less than 12 years of age because it is a fixed-dose combination that cannot be adjusted for this patient population.

Geriatric Use: Clinical studies of COMBIVIR did not include sufficient numbers of subjects aged 65 and over to determine whether they respond differently from younger subjects. In general, dose selection for an elderly patient should be cautious, reflecting the greater frequency of decreased hepatic, renal, or cardiac function, and of concomitant disease or other drug therapy. COMBIVIR is not recommended for patients with impaired renal function (i.e., creatinine clearance ≤50 mL/min; see PRECAUTIONS: Patients with Impaired Renal Function and DOSAGE AND ADMINISTRATION).

The **ADVERSE REACTIONS: Observed During Clinical Practice** *subsection was revised to:*

In addition to adverse events reported from clinical trials, the following events have been identified during post-approval use of EPIVIR, RETROVIR, and/or COMBIVIR. Because they are reported voluntarily from a population of unknown size, estimates of frequency cannot be made. These events have been chosen for inclusion due to a combination of their seriousness, frequency of reporting, or potential causal connection to EPIVIR, RETROVIR, and/or COMBIVIR.

Cardiovascular: Cardiomyopathy.
Digestive: Stomatitis.
Endocrine and Metabolic: Hyperglycemia.
General: Vasculitis, weakness.
Hemic and Lymphatic: Anemia, lymphadenopathy, pure red cell aplasia, splenomegaly.
Hepatic and Pancreatic: Lactic acidosis and hepatic steatosis, pancreatitis, posttreatment exacerbation of hepatitis B (see WARNINGS).
Hypersensitivity: Sensitization reactions (including anaphylaxis), urticaria.
Musculoskeletal: Muscle weakness, CPK elevation, rhabdomyolysis.
Nervous: Paresthesia, peripheral neuropathy, seizures.
Respiratory: Abnormal breath sounds/wheezing.
Skin: Alopecia, erythema multiforme, Stevens-Johnson syndrome.

GlaxoSmithKline, Research Triangle Park, NC 27709
Manufactured under agreement from
Shire PLC, Basing Stoke, UK

August 2001/RL-979

COMPAZINE® ℞

[komp 'ə-zēn]

brand of prochlorperazine
antiemetic • antipsychotic • tranquilizer

Prescribing information for this product, which appears on pages 1505–1508 of the 2002 PDR, has been revised. Please write "See Supplement A" next to the product heading.

The second paragraph in the **INDICATIONS** *section was revised to:*

For management of the manifestations of psychotic disorders such as schizophrenia.

The **WARNINGS: Tardive Dyskinesia** *subsection was revised to:*

Tardive dyskinesia, a syndrome consisting of potentially irreversible, involuntary, dyskinetic movements, may develop in patients treated with antipsychotic drugs. Although the prevalence of the syndrome appears to be highest among the elderly, especially elderly women, it is impossible to rely upon prevalence estimates to predict, at the inception of antipsychotic treatment, which patients are likely to develop the syndrome. Whether antipsychotic drug products differ in their potential to cause tardive dyskinesia is unknown.

Both the risk of developing the syndrome and the likelihood that it will become irreversible are believed to increase as the duration of treatment and the total cumulative dose of antipsychotic drugs administered to the patient increase. However, the syndrome can develop, although much less commonly, after relatively brief treatment periods at low doses.

There is no known treatment for established cases of tardive dyskinesia, although the syndrome may remit, partially or completely, if antipsychotic treatment is withdrawn. Antipsychotic treatment itself, however, may suppress (or partially suppress) the signs and symptoms of the syndrome and thereby may possibly mask the underlying disease process.

The effect that symptomatic suppression has upon the long-term course of the syndrome is unknown. Given these considerations, antipsychotics should be prescribed in a manner that is most likely to minimize the occurrence of tardive dyskinesia. Chronic antipsychotic treatment should generally be reserved for patients who suffer from a chronic illness that, 1) is known to respond to antipsychotic drugs, and 2) for whom alternative, equally effective, but potentially less harmful treatments are *not* available or appropriate. In patients who do require chronic treatment, the smallest dose and the shortest duration of treatment producing a satisfactory clinical response should be sought. The need for continued treatment should be reassessed periodically.

If signs and symptoms of tardive dyskinesia appear in a patient on antipsychotics, drug discontinuation should be considered. However, some patients may require treatment despite the presence of the syndrome.

For further information about the description of tardive dyskinesia and its clinical detection, please refer to the sections on PRECAUTIONS and ADVERSE REACTIONS.

The fifth paragraph of the **WARNINGS: Neuroleptic Malignant Syndrome (NMS)** *subsection was revised to:*

An encephalopathic syndrome (characterized by weakness, lethargy, fever, tremulousness and confusion, extrapyramidal symptoms, leukocytosis, elevated serum enzymes, BUN and FBS) has occurred in a few patients treated with lithium plus an antipsychotic. In some instances, the syndrome was followed by irreversible brain damage. Because of a possible causal relationship between these events and the concomitant administration of lithium and antipsychotics, patients receiving such combined therapy should be monitored closely for early evidence of neurologic toxicity and treatment discontinued promptly if such signs appear. This encephalopathic syndrome may be similar to or the same as neuroleptic malignant syndrome (NMS).

The following paragraphs were revised in the **PRECAUTIONS** *section:*

Antipsychotic drugs elevate prolactin levels; the elevation persists during chronic administration. Tissue culture experiments indicate that approximately one third of human breast cancers are prolactin-dependent *in vitro*, a factor of potential importance if the prescribing of these drugs is contemplated in a patient with a previously detected breast cancer. Although disturbances such as galactorrhea, amenorrhea, gynecomastia and impotence have been reported, the clinical significance of elevated serum prolactin levels is unknown for most patients. An increase in mammary neoplasms has been found in rodents after chronic administration of antipsychotic drugs. Neither clinical nor epidemiologic studies conducted to date, however, have shown an association between chronic administration of these drugs and mammary tumorigenesis; the available evidence is considered too limited to be conclusive at this time.

Continued on next page

Compazine—Cont.

Chromosomal aberrations in spermatocytes and abnormal sperm have been demonstrated in rodents treated with certain antipsychotics.

Long-Term Therapy: Given the likelihood that some patients exposed chronically to antipsychotics will develop tardive dyskinesia, it is advised that all patients in whom chronic use is contemplated be given, if possible, full information about this risk. The decision to inform patients and/or their guardians must obviously take into account the clinical circumstances and the competency of the patient to understand the information provided.

To lessen the likelihood of adverse reactions related to cumulative drug effect, patients with a history of long-term therapy with Compazine (prochlorperazine) and/or other antipsychotics should be evaluated periodically to decide whether the maintenance dosage could be lowered or drug therapy discontinued.

The following sentence was revised in the **ADVERSE REACTIONS: Tardive Dyskinesia** *subsection:*

Although its prevalence appears to be highest among elderly patients, especially elderly women, it is impossible to rely upon prevalence estimates to predict at the inception of antipsychotic treatment which patients are likely to develop the syndrome.

The following subsection heading was revised in the **DOSAGE AND ADMINISTRATION—ADULTS: Oral Dosage** *section:*

Psychotic Disorders including Schizophrenia

The following sentence was revised in the **DOSAGE AND ADMINISTRATION—ADULTS: I.M. Dosage** *subsection:*

For immediate control of adult schizophrenic patients with severe symptomatology, inject an initial dose of 10 to 20 mg (2 to 4 mL) *deeply* into the upper outer quadrant of the buttock.

The following sentence was revised in the **DOSAGE AND ADMINISTRATION—CHILDREN: I.M. Dosage** *subsection:*

2. In Psychotic Children including Schizophrenia in Children:

GlaxoSmithKline, Research Triangle Park, NC 27709
January 2002/CZ:L94

COREG®

℞

[*kor' eg*]
brand of
carvedilol
Tablets

Prescribing information for this product, which appears on pages 1508–1511 of the 2002 PDR, has been completely revised as follows. Please write "See Supplement A" next to the product heading.

DESCRIPTION

Carvedilol is a nonselective β-adrenergic blocking agent with α_1-blocking activity. It is (±)-1-(Carbazol-4-yloxy)-3-[[2-(o-methoxyphenoxy)ethyl]amino]-2-propanol. It is a racemic mixture.

Tablets for Oral Administration:

Coreg (carvedilol) is a white, oval, film-coated tablet containing 3.125 mg, 6.25 mg, 12.5 mg or 25 mg of carvedilol. The 6.25 mg, 12.5 mg and 25 mg tablets are Tiltab® tablets. Inactive ingredients consist of colloidal silicon dioxide, crospovidone, hydroxypropyl methylcellulose, lactose, magnesium stearate, polyethylene glycol, polysorbate 80, povidone, sucrose and titanium dioxide.

Carvedilol is a white to off-white powder with a molecular weight of 406.5 and a molecular formula of $C_{24}H_{26}N_2O_4$. It is freely soluble in dimethylsulfoxide; soluble in methylene chloride and methanol; sparingly soluble in 95% ethanol and isopropanol; slightly soluble in ethyl ether; and practically insoluble in water, gastric fluid (simulated, TS, pH 1.1) and intestinal fluid (simulated, TS without pancreatin, pH 7.5).

CLINICAL PHARMACOLOGY

Coreg is a racemic mixture in which nonselective β-adrenoreceptor blocking activity is present in the S(-) enantiomer and α-adrenergic blocking activity is present in both R(+) and S(-) enantiomers at equal potency. *Coreg* has no intrinsic sympathomimetic activity.

Pharmacokinetics

Coreg is rapidly and extensively absorbed following oral administration, with absolute bioavailability of approximately 25% to 35% due to a significant degree of first-pass metabolism. Following oral administration, the apparent mean terminal elimination half-life of carvedilol generally ranges from 7 to 10 hours. Plasma concentrations achieved are proportional to the oral dose administered. When administered with food, the rate of absorption is slowed, as evidenced by a delay in the time to reach peak plasma levels, with no significant difference in extent of bioavailability. Taking *Coreg* with food should minimize the risk of orthostatic hypotension.

Carvedilol is extensively metabolized. Following oral administration of radiolabelled carvedilol to healthy volunteers, carvedilol accounted for only about 7% of the total radioactivity in plasma as measured by area under the curve (AUC). Less than 2% of the dose was excreted unchanged in the urine. Carvedilol is metabolized primarily by aromatic ring oxidation and glucuronidation. The oxidative metabolites are further metabolized by conjugation via glucuronidation and sulfation. The metabolites of carvedilol are excreted primarily via the bile into the feces. Demethylation and hydroxylation at the phenol ring produce three active metabolites with β-receptor blocking activity. Based on preclinical studies, the 4'-hydroxyphenyl metabolite is approximately 13 times more potent than carvedilol for β-blockade. Compared to carvedilol, the three active metabolites exhibit weak vasodilating activity. Plasma concentrations of the active metabolites are about one-tenth of those observed for carvedilol and have pharmacokinetics similar to the parent.

Carvedilol undergoes stereoselective first-pass metabolism with plasma levels of R(+)-carvedilol approximately 2 to 3 times higher than S(-)-carvedilol following oral administration in healthy subjects. The mean apparent terminal elimination half-lives for R(+)-carvedilol range from 5 to 9 hours compared with 7 to 11 hours for the S(-)-enantiomer.

The primary P450 enzymes responsible for the metabolism of both R(+) and S(-)-carvedilol in human liver microsomes were CYP2D6 and CYP2C9 and to a lesser extent CYP3A4, 2C19, 1A2, and 2E1. CYP2D6 is thought to be the major enzyme in the 4'- and 5'-hydroxylation of carvedilol, with a potential contribution from 3A4. CYP2C9 is thought to be of primary importance in the O-methylation pathway of S(-)-carvedilol.

Carvedilol is subject to the effects of genetic polymorphism with poor metabolizers of debrisoquin (a marker for cytochrome P450 2D6) exhibiting 2- to 3-fold higher plasma concentrations of R(+)-carvedilol compared to extensive metabolizers. In contrast, plasma levels of S(-)-carvedilol are increased only about 20% to 25% in poor metabolizers, indicating this enantiomer is metabolized to a lesser extent by cytochrome P450 2D6 than R(+)-carvedilol. The pharmacokinetics of carvedilol do not appear to be different in poor metabolizers of S-mephenytoin (patients deficient in cytochrome P450 2C19).

Carvedilol is more than 98% bound to plasma proteins, primarily with albumin. The plasma-protein binding is independent of concentration over the therapeutic range. Carvedilol is a basic, lipophilic compound with a steady-state volume of distribution of approximately 115 L, indicating substantial distribution into extravascular tissues. Plasma clearance ranges from 500 to 700 mL/min.

Congestive Heart Failure: Steady-state plasma concentrations of carvedilol and its enantiomers increased proportionally over the 6.25 to 50 mg dose range in patients with congestive heart failure. Compared to healthy subjects, congestive heart failure patients had increased mean AUC and C_{max} values for carvedilol and its enantiomers, with up to 50% to 100% higher values observed in 6 patients with NYHA class IV heart failure. The mean apparent terminal elimination half-life for carvedilol was similar to that observed in healthy subjects.

Pharmacokinetic Drug-Drug Interactions: Since carvedilol undergoes substantial oxidative metabolism, the metabolism and pharmacokinetics of carvedilol may be affected by induction or inhibition of cytochrome P450 enzymes.

Rifampin: In a pharmacokinetic study conducted in 8 healthy male subjects, rifampin (600 mg daily for 12 days) decreased the AUC and C_{max} of carvedilol by about 70%.

Cimetidine: In a pharmacokinetic study conducted in 10 healthy male subjects, cimetidine (1000 mg/day) increased the steady-state AUC of carvedilol by 30% with no change in C_{max}.

Glyburide: In 12 healthy subjects, combined administration of carvedilol (25 mg once daily) and a single dose of glyburide did not result in a clinically relevant pharmacokinetic interaction for either compound.

Hydrochlorothiazide: A single oral dose of carvedilol 25 mg did not alter the pharmacokinetics of a single oral dose of hydrochlorothiazide 25 mg in 12 patients with hypertension. Likewise, hydrochlorothiazide had no effect on the pharmacokinetics of carvedilol.

Digoxin: Following concomitant administration of carvedilol (25 mg once daily) and digoxin (0.25 mg once daily) for 14 days, steady-state AUC and trough concentrations of digoxin were increased by 14% and 16%, respectively, in 12 hypertensive patients.

Torsemide: In a study of 12 healthy subjects, combined oral administration of carvedilol 25 mg once daily and torsemide 5 mg once daily for 5 days did not result in any significant differences in their pharmacokinetics compared with administration of the drugs alone.

Warfarin: Carvedilol (12.5 mg twice daily) did not have an effect on the steady-state prothrombin time ratios and did not alter the pharmacokinetics of R(+)- and S(-)-warfarin following concomitant administration with warfarin in 9 healthy volunteers.

Table 1. Results of COPERNICUS

End point	Placebo N=1,133	Carvedilol N=1,156	Hazard ratio (95% CI)	% Reduction	Nominal *P* value
Mortality	190	130	0.65 (0.52 – 0.81)	35	0.00013
Mortality + all hospitalization	507	425	0.76 (0.67 – 0.87)	24	0.00004
Mortality + CV hospitalization	395	314	0.73 (0.63 – 0.84)	27	0.00002
Mortality + CHF hospitalization	357	271	0.69 (0.59 – 0.81)	31	0.000004

Special Populations

Elderly: Plasma levels of carvedilol average about 50% higher in the elderly compared to young subjects.

Hepatic Impairment: Compared to healthy subjects, patients with cirrhotic liver disease exhibit significantly higher concentrations of carvedilol (approximately 4- to 7-fold) following single-dose therapy (see WARNINGS, Hepatic Injury).

Renal Insufficiency: Although carvedilol is metabolized primarily by the liver, plasma concentrations of carvedilol have been reported to be increased in patients with renal impairment. Based on mean AUC data, approximately 40% to 50% higher plasma concentrations of carvedilol were observed in hypertensive patients with moderate to severe renal impairment compared to a control group of hypertensive patients with normal renal function. However, the ranges of AUC values were similar for both groups. Changes in mean peak plasma levels were less pronounced, approximately 12% to 26% higher in patients with impaired renal function. Consistent with its high degree of plasma protein-binding, carvedilol does not appear to be cleared significantly by hemodialysis.

Pharmacodynamics and Clinical Trials

Congestive Heart Failure

Pharmacodynamics

The basis for the beneficial effects of Coreg (carvedilol) in congestive heart failure is not established.

Two placebo-controlled studies compared the acute hemodynamic effects of *Coreg* to baseline measurements in 59 and 49 patients with NYHA class II-IV heart failure receiving diuretics, ACE inhibitors, and digitalis. There were significant reductions in systemic blood pressure, pulmonary artery pressure, pulmonary capillary wedge pressure, and heart rate. Initial effects on cardiac output, stroke volume index, and systemic vascular resistance were small and variable.

These studies measured hemodynamic effects again at 12 to 14 weeks. *Coreg* significantly reduced systemic blood pressure, pulmonary artery pressure, right atrial pressure, systemic vascular resistance, and heart rate, while stroke volume index was increased.

Among 839 patients with NYHA class II-III heart failure treated for 26 to 52 weeks in 4 U.S. placebo-controlled trials, average left ventricular ejection fraction (EF) measured by radionuclide ventriculography increased by 9 EF units (%) in *Coreg* patients and by 2 EF units in placebo patients at a target dose of 25-50 mg b.i.d. The effects of carvedilol on ejection fraction were related to dose. Doses of 6.25 mg b.i.d., 12.5 mg b.i.d. and 25 mg b.i.d. were associated with placebo-corrected increases in EF of 5 EF units, 6 EF units and 8 EF units, respectively; each of these effects were nominally statistically significant.

Hypertension

Pharmacodynamics

The mechanism by which β-blockade produces an antihypertensive effect has not been established.

β-adrenoreceptor blocking activity has been demonstrated in animal and human studies showing that carvedilol (1) reduces cardiac output in normal subjects; (2) reduces exercise- and/or isoproterenol-induced tachycardia and (3) reduces reflex orthostatic tachycardia. Significant β-adrenoreceptor blocking effect is usually seen within 1 hour of drug administration.

α_1-adrenoreceptor blocking activity has been demonstrated in human and animal studies, showing that carvedilol (1) attenuates the pressor effects of phenylephrine; (2) causes vasodilation and (3) reduces peripheral vascular resistance. These effects contribute to the reduction of blood pressure and usually are seen within 30 minutes of drug administration.

Due to the α_1-receptor blocking activity of carvedilol, blood pressure is lowered more in the standing than in the supine position, and symptoms of postural hypotension (1.8%), including rare instances of syncope, can occur. Following oral administration, when postural hypotension has occurred, it has been transient and is uncommon when *Coreg* (carvedilol) is administered with food at the recommended starting dose and titration increments are closely followed (see DOSAGE AND ADMINISTRATION).

In hypertensive patients with normal renal function, therapeutic doses of *Coreg* decreased renal vascular resistance with no change in glomerular filtration rate or renal plasma flow. Changes in excretion of sodium, potassium, uric acid and phosphorus in hypertensive patients with normal renal function were similar after *Coreg* and placebo.

Coreg has little effect on plasma catecholamines, plasma aldosterone or electrolyte levels, but it does significantly reduce plasma renin activity when given for at least 4 weeks. It also increases levels of atrial natriuretic peptide.

CLINICAL TRIALS

Congestive Heart Failure

A total of 3,946 patients with mild to severe heart failure were evaluated in placebo-controlled studies of carvedilol.

In the largest study (COPERNICUS), 2,289 patients with heart failure at rest or with minimal exertion and left ventricular ejection fraction <25% (mean 20%), despite digitalis (66%), diuretics (99%), and ACE inhibitors (89%) were randomized to placebo or carvedilol. Carvedilol was titrated from a starting dose of 3.125 mg twice daily to the maximum tolerated dose or up to 25 mg twice daily over a minimum of 6 weeks. Most subjects achieved the target dose of 25 mg. The study was conducted in Eastern and Western Europe, the United States, Israel, and Canada. Similar numbers of subjects per group (about 100) withdrew during the titration period.

The primary end point of the trial was all-cause mortality, but cause-specific mortality and the risk of death or hospitalization (total, cardiovascular [CV] or congestive heart failure [CHF]) were also examined. The developing trial data were followed by a data monitoring committee, and mortality analyses were adjusted for these multiple looks. The trial was stopped after a median follow-up of 10 months because of an observed 35% reduction in mortality (from 19.7% per patient year on placebo to 12.8% on carvedilol, hazard ratio 0.65, 95% CI 0.52 – 0.81, p=0.0014, adjusted) (see Figure 1). The results of COPERNICUS are shown in Table 1.

[See table 1 at top of previous page]

Figure 1. Survival analysis for COPERNICUS (intent-to-treat)

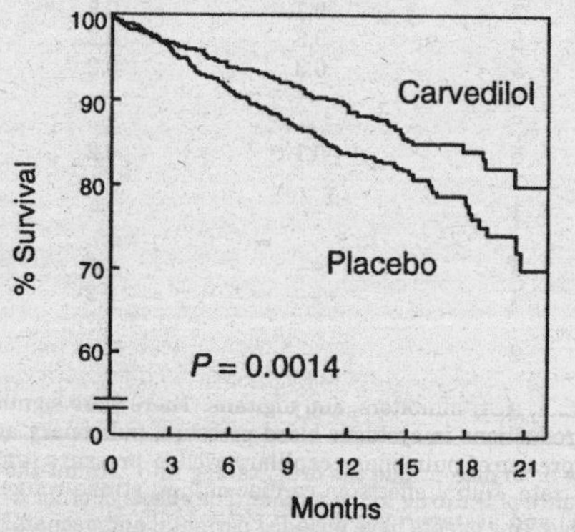

Effects were similar in patients with and without diabetes based on data from both COPERNICUS and the U.S. trials described below.

The effect on mortality was principally the result of a reduction in the rate of sudden death among patients without worsening heart failure.

Patients' global assessments showed significant improvement following treatment with carvedilol in COPERNICUS. The protocol also specified that hospitalizations would be assessed. Fewer patients on *Coreg* than on placebo were hospitalized for any reason (198 vs. 268, p=0.0001), for cardiovascular reasons (246 vs. 314, p=0.0003), or for worsening heart failure (372 vs. 432, p=0.0029).

Coreg (carvedilol) had a consistent and beneficial effect on all-cause mortality as well as the combined end points of all-cause mortality plus hospitalization (total, CV or for heart failure) in the overall study population and in all subgroups examined, including men and women, elderly and non-elderly, blacks and non-blacks.

Carvedilol was also studied in five other multicenter, placebo-controlled studies.

Four U.S. multicenter, double-blind, placebo-controlled studies enrolled 1,094 patients (696 randomized to carvedilol) with NYHA class II-III heart failure and ejection fraction <0.35. The vast majority were on digitalis, diuretics, and an ACE inhibitor at study entry. Patients were assigned to the studies based upon exercise ability. An Australia-New Zealand double-blind, placebo-controlled study enrolled 415 patients (half randomized to carvedilol) with less severe heart failure. All protocols excluded patients expected to undergo cardiac transplantation during the 7.5 to 15 months of double-blind follow-up. All randomized patients had tolerated a 2-week course on carvedilol 6.25 mg b.i.d.

In each study, there was a primary end point, either progression of heart failure (one U.S. study) or exercise tolerance (two U.S. studies meeting enrollment goals and the Australia-New Zealand study). There were many secondary end points specified in these studies, including NYHA classification, patient and physician global assessments, and cardiovascular hospitalization. Death was not a specified end point in any study, but it was analyzed in all studies. Other analyses not prospectively planned included the sum of deaths and total cardiovascular hospitalizations. In situations where the primary end points of a trial do not show a significant benefit of treatment, assignment of significance values to the other results is complex, and such values need to be interpreted cautiously.

The results of the U.S. and Australia-New Zealand trials were as follows:

Slowing Progression of Heart Failure: One U.S. multicenter study (366 subjects) had as its primary end point the sum of cardiovascular mortality, cardiovascular hospitalization, and sustained increase in heart failure medications. Heart failure progression was reduced, during an average follow-up of 7 months, by 48% (p=0.008).

In the Australia-New Zealand study, death and total hospitalizations were reduced by about 25% over 18 to 24 months. In the three largest U.S. studies, death and total hospitalizations were reduced by 19%, 39% and 49%, nominally statistically significant in the last two studies. The Australia-New Zealand results were statistically borderline.

Functional Measures: None of the multicenter studies had NYHA classification as a primary end point, but all such studies had it as a secondary end point. There was at least a trend toward improvement in NYHA class in all studies. Exercise tolerance was the primary end point in 3 studies; in none was a statistically significant effect found.

Subjective Measures: Quality of life, as measured with a standard questionnaire (a primary end point in one study), was unaffected by carvedilol. However, patients' and investigators' global assessments showed significant improvement in most studies.

Mortality: Overall, in these four U.S. trials, mortality was reduced, nominally significantly so in 2 studies.

Hypertension

Coreg (carvedilol) was studied in two placebo-controlled trials that utilized twice-daily dosing, at total daily doses of 12.5 to 50 mg. In these and other studies, the starting dose did not exceed 12.5 mg. At 50 mg per day, *Coreg* reduced sitting trough (12-hour) blood pressure by about 9/5.5 mm Hg; at 25 mg/day the effect was about 7.5/3.5 mm Hg. Comparisons of trough to peak blood pressure showed a trough to peak ratio for blood pressure response of about 65%. Heart rate fell by about 7.5 beats per minute at 50 mg/day. In general, as is true for other β-blockers, responses were smaller in black than non-black patients. There were no age- or gender-related differences in response.

The peak antihypertensive effect occurred 1 to 2 hours after a dose. The dose-related blood pressure response was accompanied by a dose-related increase in adverse effects (see ADVERSE REACTIONS).

INDICATIONS AND USAGE

Congestive Heart Failure

Coreg is indicated for the treatment of mild to severe heart failure of ischemic or cardiomyopathic origin, usually in addition to diuretics, ACE inhibitor, and digitalis, to increase survival and, also, to reduce the risk of hospitalization.

Coreg may be used in patients unable to tolerate an ACE inhibitor and may also be used in patients who are or are not receiving digitalis, hydralazine or nitrate therapy.

Hypertension

Coreg (carvedilol) is also indicated for the management of essential hypertension. It can be used alone or in combination with other antihypertensive agents, especially thiazide-type diuretics (see PRECAUTIONS, Drug Interactions).

CONTRAINDICATIONS

Coreg is contraindicated in patients with bronchial asthma (two cases of death from status asthmaticus have been reported in patients receiving single doses of *Coreg*) or related bronchospastic conditions, second- or third-degree AV block, sick sinus syndrome or severe bradycardia (unless a permanent pacemaker is in place), or in patients with cardiogenic shock or who have decompensated heart failure requiring the use of intravenous inotropic therapy. Such patients should first be weaned from intravenous therapy before initiating *Coreg*.

Use of *Coreg* in patients with clinically manifest hepatic impairment is not recommended.

Coreg is contraindicated in patients with hypersensitivity to the drug.

WARNINGS

Hepatic Injury: Mild hepatocellular injury, confirmed by rechallenge, has occurred rarely with *Coreg* therapy in the treatment of hypertension. In controlled studies of hypertensive patients, the incidence of liver function abnormalities reported as adverse experiences was 1.1% (13 of 1,142 patients) in patients receiving *Coreg* and 0.9% (4 of 462 patients) in those receiving placebo. One patient receiving carvedilol in a placebo-controlled trial withdrew for abnormal hepatic function.

In controlled studies of primarily mild-to-moderate congestive heart failure, the incidence of liver function abnormalities reported as adverse experiences was 5.0% (38 of 765 patients) in patients receiving *Coreg* and 4.6% (20 of 437 patients) in those receiving placebo. Three patients receiving *Coreg* (0.4%) and two patients receiving placebo (0.5%) in placebo-controlled trials withdrew for abnormal hepatic function. Similarly, in a long-term, placebo-controlled trial in severe heart failure, there was no difference in the incidence of liver function abnormalities reported as adverse experiences between patients receiving *Coreg* and those receiving placebo. No patients receiving *Coreg* and one patient receiving placebo (0.09%) withdrew for hepatitis. In addition, patients treated with *Coreg* had lower values for hepatic transaminases than patients treated with placebo, possibly because *Coreg*-induced improvements in cardiac function led to less hepatic congestion and/or improved hepatic blood flow.

Hepatic injury has been reversible and has occurred after short- and/or long-term therapy with minimal clinical symptomatology. No deaths due to liver function abnormalities have been reported in association with the use of *Coreg*.

At the first symptom/sign of liver dysfunction (e.g., pruritus, dark urine, persistent anorexia, jaundice, right upper quadrant tenderness or unexplained "flu-like" symptoms), laboratory testing should be performed. If the patient has laboratory evidence of liver injury or jaundice, carvedilol should be stopped and not restarted.

Peripheral Vascular Disease: β-blockers can precipitate or aggravate symptoms of arterial insufficiency in patients with peripheral vascular disease. Caution should be exercised in such individuals.

Anesthesia and Major Surgery: If *Coreg* treatment is to be continued perioperatively, particular care should be taken when anesthetic agents which depress myocardial function, such as ether, cyclopropane and trichloroethylene, are used. See OVERDOSAGE for information on treatment of bradycardia and hypertension.

Diabetes and Hypoglycemia: In general, β-blockers may mask some of the manifestations of hypoglycemia, particularly tachycardia. Nonselective β-blockers may potentiate insulin-induced hypoglycemia and delay recovery of serum glucose levels. Patients subject to spontaneous hypoglycemia, or diabetic patients receiving insulin or oral hypoglycemic agents, should be cautioned about these possibilities. In congestive heart failure patients, there is a risk of worsening hyperglycemia (see PRECAUTIONS).

Thyrotoxicosis: β-adrenergic blockade may mask clinical signs of hyperthyroidism, such as tachycardia. Abrupt withdrawal of β-blockade may be followed by an exacerbation of the symptoms of hyperthyroidism or may precipitate thyroid storm.

PRECAUTIONS

General

Since Coreg (carvedilol) has β-blocking activity, it should not be discontinued abruptly, particularly in patients with ischemic heart disease. Instead, it should be discontinued over 1 to 2 weeks, whenever possible.

In clinical trials, *Coreg* caused bradycardia in about 2% of hypertensive patients and 9% of congestive heart failure patients. If pulse rate drops below 55 beats/min., the dosage should be reduced.

In clinical trials of primarily mild-to-moderate heart failure, hypotension and postural hypotension occurred in 9.7% and syncope in 3.4% of patients receiving *Coreg* compared to 3.6% and 2.5% of placebo patients, respectively. The risk for these events was highest during the first 30 days of dosing, corresponding to the up-titration period and was a cause for discontinuation of therapy in 0.7% of *Coreg* patients, compared to 0.4% of placebo patients. In a long-term, placebo-controlled trial in severe heart failure (COPERNICUS), hypotension and postural hypotension occurred in 15.1% and syncope in 2.9% of heart failure patients receiving *Coreg* compared to 8.7% and 2.3% of placebo patients, respectively. These events were a cause for discontinuation of therapy in 1.1% of *Coreg* patients, compared to 0.8% of placebo patients.

Postural hypotension occurred in 1.8% and syncope in 0.1% of hypertensive patients, primarily following the initial dose or at the time of dose increase and was a cause for discontinuation of therapy in 1% of patients.

To decrease the likelihood of syncope or excessive hypotension, treatment should be initiated with 3.125 mg b.i.d. for congestive heart failure patients and 6.25 mg b.i.d. for hypertensive patients. Dosage should then be increased slowly, according to recommendations in the DOSAGE AND ADMINISTRATION section, and the drug should be taken with food. During initiation of therapy, the patient should be cautioned to avoid situations such as driving or hazardous tasks, where injury could result should syncope occur.

Rarely, use of carvedilol in patients with congestive heart failure has resulted in deterioration of renal function. Patients at risk appear to be those with low blood pressure (systolic BP<100 mm Hg), ischemic heart disease and diffuse vascular disease, and/or underlying renal insufficiency. Renal function has returned to baseline when carvedilol was stopped. In patients with these risk factors it is recommended that renal function be monitored during up-titration of carvedilol and the drug discontinued or dosage reduced if worsening of renal function occurs.

Worsening cardiac failure or fluid retention may occur during up-titration of carvedilol. If such symptoms occur, diuretics should be increased and the carvedilol dose should not be advanced until clinical stability resumes (see DOSAGE AND ADMINISTRATION). Occasionally it is necessary to lower the carvedilol dose or temporarily discontinue it. Such episodes do not preclude subsequent successful titration of, or a favorable response to, carvedilol. In a placebo-controlled trial of patients with severe heart failure, worsening heart failure during the first 3 months was reported to a similar degree with carvedilol and with placebo. When treatment was maintained beyond 3 months, worsening heart failure was reported less frequently in patients treated with carvedilol than with placebo. Worsening heart failure observed during long-term therapy is more likely to be related to the patients' underlying disease than to treatment with carvedilol.

In patients with pheochromocytoma, an α-blocking agent should be initiated prior to the use of any β-blocking agent. Although carvedilol has both α- and β-blocking pharmacologic activities, there has been no experience with its use in this condition. Therefore, caution should be taken in the administration of carvedilol to patients suspected of having pheochromocytoma.

Agents with non-selective β-blocking activity may provoke chest pain in patients with Prinzmetal's variant angina. There has been no clinical experience with carvedilol in

Continued on next page

Coreg—Cont.

these patients although the α-blocking activity may prevent such symptoms. However, caution should be taken in the administration of carvedilol to patients suspected of having Prinzmetal's variant angina.

In congestive heart failure patients with diabetes, carvedilol therapy may lead to worsening hyperglycemia, which responds to intensification of hypoglycemic therapy. It is recommended that blood glucose be monitored when carvedilol dosing is initiated, adjusted, or discontinued.

Risk of Anaphylactic Reaction

While taking β-blockers, patients with a history of severe anaphylactic reaction to a variety of allergens may be more reactive to repeated challenge, either accidental, diagnostic or therapeutic. Such patients may be unresponsive to the usual doses of epinephrine used to treat allergic reaction.

Nonallergic Bronchospasm (e.g., chronic bronchitis and emphysema)

Patients with bronchospastic disease should, in general, not receive β-blockers. *Coreg* may be used with caution, however, in patients who do not respond to, or cannot tolerate, other antihypertensive agents. It is prudent, if Coreg (carvedilol) is used, to use the smallest effective dose, so that inhibition of endogenous or exogenous β-agonists is minimized.

In clinical trials of patients with congestive heart failure, patients with bronchospastic disease were enrolled if they did not require oral or inhaled medication to treat their bronchospastic disease. In such patients, it is recommended that carvedilol be used with caution. The dosing recommendations should be followed closely and the dose should be lowered if any evidence of bronchospasm is observed during up-titration.

Information for Patients

Patients taking *Coreg* should be advised of the following:

- they should not interrupt or discontinue using *Coreg* without a physician's advice.
- congestive heart failure patients should consult their physician if they experience signs or symptoms of worsening heart failure such as weight gain or increasing shortness of breath.
- they may experience a drop in blood pressure when standing, resulting in dizziness and, rarely, fainting. Patients should sit or lie down when these symptoms of lowered blood pressure occur.
- if patients experience dizziness or fatigue, they should avoid driving or hazardous tasks.
- they should consult a physician if they experience dizziness or faintness, in case the dosage should be adjusted.
- they should take *Coreg* with food.
- diabetic patients should report any changes in blood sugar levels to their physician.
- contact lens wearers may experience decreased lacrimation.

Drug Interactions

(Also see CLINICAL PHARMACOLOGY, Pharmacokinetic Drug-Drug Interactions.)

Inhibitors of CYP2D6; poor metabolizers of debrisoquin: Interactions of carvedilol with strong inhibitors of CYP2D6 (such as quinidine, fluoxetine, paroxetine, and propafenone) have not been studied, but these drugs would be expected to increase blood levels of the R(+) enantiomer of carvedilol (see CLINICAL PHARMACOLOGY). Retrospective analysis of side effects in clinical trials showed that poor 2D6 metabolizers had a higher rate of dizziness during up-titration, presumably resulting from vasodilating effects of the higher concentrations of the α-blocking R(+) enantiomer.

Catecholamine-depleting agents: Patients taking both agents with β-blocking properties and a drug that can deplete catecholamines (e.g., reserpine and monoamine oxidase inhibitors) should be observed closely for signs of hypotension and/or severe bradycardia.

Clonidine: Concomitant administration of clonidine with agents with β-blocking properties may potentiate blood-pressure- and heart-rate-lowering effects. When concomitant treatment with agents with β-blocking properties and clonidine is to be terminated, the β-blocking agent should be discontinued first. Clonidine therapy can then be discontinued several days later by gradually decreasing the dosage.

Cyclosporin: Modest increases in mean trough cyclosporin concentrations were observed following initiation of carvedilol treatment in 21 renal transplant patients suffering from chronic vascular rejection. In about 30% of patients, the dose of cyclosporin had to be reduced in order to maintain cyclosporin concentrations within the therapeutic range, while in the remainder no adjustment was needed. On the average for the group, the dose of cyclosporin was reduced about 20% in these patients. Due to wide interindividual variability in the dose adjustment required, it is recommended that cyclosporin concentrations be monitored closely after initiation of carvedilol therapy and that the dose of cyclosporin be adjusted as appropriate.

Digoxin: Digoxin concentrations are increased by about 15% when digoxin and carvedilol are administered concomitantly. Both digoxin and *Coreg* slow AV conduction. Therefore, increased monitoring of digoxin is recommended when initiating, adjusting or discontinuing *Coreg*.

Inducers and inhibitors of hepatic metabolism: Rifampin reduced plasma concentrations of carvedilol by about 70%. Cimetidine increased AUC by about 30% but caused no change in C_{max}.

Calcium channel blockers: Isolated cases of conduction disturbance (rarely with hemodynamic compromise) have been observed when *Coreg* is co-administered with diltiazem. As with other agents with β-blocking properties, if Coreg (carvedilol) is to be administered orally with calcium channel blockers of the verapamil or diltiazem type, it is recommended that ECG and blood pressure be monitored.

Insulin or oral hypoglycemics: Agents with β-blocking properties may enhance the blood-sugar-reducing effect of insulin and oral hypoglycemics. Therefore, in patients taking insulin or oral hypoglycemics, regular monitoring of blood glucose is recommended.

Carcinogenesis, Mutagenesis, Impairment of Fertility

In 2-year studies conducted in rats given carvedilol at doses up to 75 mg/kg/day (12 times the maximum recommended human dose [MRHD] when compared on a mg/m² basis) or in mice given up to 200 mg/kg/day (16 times the MRHD on a mg/m² basis), carvedilol had no carcinogenic effect.

Carvedilol was negative when tested in a battery of genotoxicity assays, including the Ames and the CHO/HGPRT assays for mutagenicity and the *in vitro* hamster micronucleus and *in vivo* human lymphocyte cell tests for clastogenicity.

At doses ≥200 mg/kg/day (≥32 times the MRHD as mg/m²) carvedilol was toxic to adult rats (sedation, reduced weight gain) and was associated with a reduced number of successful matings, prolonged mating time, significantly fewer corpora lutea and implants per dam and complete resorption of 18% of the litters. The no-observed-effect dose level for overt toxicity and impairment of fertility was 60 mg/kg/day (10 times the MRHD as mg/m²).

Pregnancy: Teratogenic Effects. Pregnancy Category C.

Studies performed in pregnant rats and rabbits given carvedilol revealed increased post-implantation loss in rats at doses of 300 mg/kg/day (50 times the MRHD as mg/m²) and in rabbits at doses of 75 mg/kg/day (25 times the MRHD as mg/m²). In the rats, there was also a decrease in fetal body weight at the maternally toxic dose of 300 mg/kg/day (50 times the MRHD as mg/m²), which was accompanied by an elevation in the frequency of fetuses with delayed skeletal development (missing or stunted 13th rib). In rats the no-observed-effect level for developmental toxicity was 60 mg/kg/day (10 times the MRHD as mg/m²); in rabbits it was 15 mg/kg/day (5 times the MRHD as mg/m²). There are no adequate and well-controlled studies in pregnant women. *Coreg* should be used during pregnancy only if the potential benefit justifies the potential risk to the fetus.

Nursing Mothers

It is not known whether this drug is excreted in human milk. Studies in rats have shown that carvedilol and/or its metabolites (as well as other β-blockers) cross the placental barrier and are excreted in breast milk. There was increased mortality at one week post-partum in neonates from rats treated with 60 mg/kg/day (10 times the MRHD as mg/m²) and above during the last trimester through day 22 of lactation. Because many drugs are excreted in human milk and because of the potential for serious adverse reactions in nursing infants from β-blockers, especially bradycardia, a decision should be made whether to discontinue nursing or to discontinue the drug, taking into account the importance of the drug to the mother. The effects of other α- and β-blocking agents have included perinatal and neonatal distress.

Pediatric Use

Safety and efficacy in patients younger than 18 years of age have not been established.

Geriatric Use

Of the 765 patients with congestive heart failure randomized to *Coreg* in U.S. clinical trials, 31% (235) were 65 years of age or older. Of the 1,156 patients randomized to *Coreg* in a long-term, placebo-controlled trial in severe heart failure, 47% (547) were 65 years of age or older. Of 3,025 patients receiving *Coreg* in congestive heart failure trials worldwide, 42% were 65 years of age or older. There were no notable differences in efficacy or the incidence of adverse events between older and younger patients.

Of the 2,065 hypertensive patients in U.S. clinical trials of efficacy or safety who were treated with Coreg (carvedilol), 21% (436) were 65 years of age or older. Of 3,722 patients receiving *Coreg* in hypertension clinical trials conducted worldwide, 24% were 65 years of age or older. There were no notable differences in efficacy or the incidence of adverse events between older and younger patients. With the exception of dizziness (incidence 8.8% in the elderly vs. 6% in younger patients), there were no events for which the incidence in the elderly exceeded that in the younger population by greater than 2.0%.

Similar results were observed in a postmarketing surveillance study of 3,328 *Coreg* patients, of whom approximately 20% were 65 years of age or older.

ADVERSE REACTIONS

Congestive Heart Failure

Coreg has been evaluated for safety in congestive heart failure in more than 3,000 patients worldwide of whom more than 2,100 participated in placebo-controlled clinical trials. Approximately 60% of the total treated population received *Coreg* for at least 6 months and 30% received *Coreg* for at least 12 months. The adverse experience profile of *Coreg* in patients with congestive heart failure was consistent with the pharmacology of the drug and the health status of the patients. In U.S. clinical trials in mild-to-moderate heart failure that compared *Coreg* in daily doses up to 100 mg (n=765) to placebo (n=437), 5.4% of *Coreg* patients discontinued treatment for adverse experiences vs. 8.0% of placebo patients. In a multinational clinical trial in severe heart failure (COPERNICUS) that compared *Coreg* in daily doses up to 50 mg (n=1,156) with placebo (n=1,133), 9.4% of *Coreg* patients discontinued treatment for adverse experiences vs. 11.2% of placebo patients.

Table 2 shows adverse events reported in patients with mild-to-moderate heart failure enrolled in U.S. placebo-controlled clinical trials. Shown are adverse events that occurred more frequently in drug-treated patients than placebo-treated patients with an incidence of >2% regardless of causality. Median study medication exposure was 6.33 months for both carvedilol and placebo patients.

Table 2. Adverse Events (% Occurrence and % Withdrawals) Occurring More Frequently with *Coreg* Than with Placebo in Patients with Mild-to-Moderate Heart Failure Enrolled in U.S. Heart Failure Trials (Incidence >2%, Regardless of Causality)

	Adverse Reactions		Withdrawals	
	Coreg (n=765) % occurrence	Placebo (n=437) % occurrence	*Coreg* (n=765) % withdrawals	Placebo (n=437) % withdrawals
Autonomic Nervous System				
Sweating increased	3	2	—	—
Body as a Whole				
Fatigue	24	22	0.7	0.7
Pain	9	8	—	0.2
Digoxin level increased	5	4	—	0.2
Edema generalized	5	3	—	—
Edema dependent	4	2	—	—
Fever	3	2	—	—
Edema legs	2	—	0.1	0.2
Cardiovascular				
Bradycardia	9	1	0.8	—
Hypotension	9	3	0.4	0.2
AV block	3	1	—	—
Central Nervous System				
Dizziness	32	19	0.4	—
Headache	8	7	0.3	—
Gastrointestinal				
Diarrhea	12	6	0.3	—
Nausea	9	5	—	—
Vomiting	6	4	0.1	—
Metabolic				
Hyperglycemia	12	8	0.1	—
Weight increase	10	7	0.1	0.5
BUN increased	6	5	0.3	0.2
NPN increased	6	5	0.3	0.2
Hypercholesterolemia	4	3	—	—
Musculoskeletal				
Arthralgia	6	5	0.1	0.2
Resistance Mechanism				
Infection	2	1	—	—
Respiratory				
Sinusitis	5	4	—	—
Bronchitis	5	4	—	0.2
Urinary/Renal				
Hematuria	3	2	—	—
Vision				
Vision abnormal	5	2	0.1	—

[See table 2 at top of previous page]

Incidence >2%, Regardless of Causality; Withdrawal Rates due to Adverse Events

In addition to the events in Table 2, asthenia, chest pain, injury, cardiac failure, syncope, hypertension, abdominal pain, flatulence, anorexia, dyspepsia, palpitation, extrasystoles, gout, hyperkalemia, dehydration, back pain, myalgia, arthritis, angina pectoris, insomnia, depression, anemia, upper respiratory tract infection, viral infection, dyspnea, coughing, rales, pharyngitis, rhinitis, rash, urinary tract infection, and leg cramps were also reported, but rates were equal or greater in placebo-treated patients.

The following adverse events were reported with a frequency of >1% but ≤2% and more frequently with Coreg (carvedilol) in U.S. placebo-controlled trials in patients with mild-to-moderate heart failure:

Incidence >1% to ≤2%

Body as a Whole: Allergy, malaise, hypovolemia.
Cardiovascular: Fluid overload, postural hypotension, aggravated angina pectoris.
Central and Peripheral Nervous System: Hypesthesia, vertigo, paresthesia.
Gastrointestinal: Melena, periodontitis.
Liver and Biliary System: SGPT increased, SGOT increased.
Metabolic and Nutritional: Hyperuricemia, hypoglycemia, hyponatremia, increased alkaline phosphatase, glycosuria, hypervolemia.
Platelet, Bleeding and Clotting: Prothrombin decreased, purpura, thrombocytopenia.
Psychiatric: Somnolence.
Reproductive, male: Impotence.
Urinary System: Renal insufficiency, albuminuria.

Table 3 shows adverse events reported in patients with severe heart failure enrolled in the COPERNICUS trial. Shown are adverse events that occurred more frequently in drug-treated patients than placebo-treated patients with an incidence >2%, regardless of causality. Median study medication exposure was 10.4 months for both carvedilol and placebo patients.

[See table 3 above]

In addition to the events in Table 3, atrial fibrillation, heart failure, peripheral vascular disorder, unstable angina pectoris and ventricular tachycardia, abdominal pain, pain in the extremity, anemia, gout, hypokalemia, dyspnea, bronchitis, lung edema, pneumonia, abnormal kidney function and urinary tract infection were also reported but rates were equal or greater in placebo patients.

The following adverse events were reported with a frequency of >1% but ≤2% and more frequently with *Coreg* in the COPERNICUS trial:

Incidence >1% to ≤2%

Cardiovascular: Palpitation, postural hypotension.
Metabolic and Nutritional: Diabetes mellitus, GGT increased, weight loss.
Musculoskeletal: Muscle cramps.
Nervous System: Paresthesia.
Respiratory: Sinusitis.
Urogenital: Kidney failure.

Rates of adverse events were generally similar across demographic subsets (men and women, elderly and non-elderly, blacks and non-blacks).

POSTMARKETING EXPERIENCE

The following adverse reaction has been reported in postmarketing experience: reports of aplastic anemia have been rare and received only when carvedilol was administered concomitantly with other medications associated with the event.

Hypertension

Coreg (carvedilol) has been evaluated for safety in hypertension in more than 2,193 patients in U.S. clinical trials and in 2,976 patients in international clinical trials. Approximately 36% of the total treated population received *Coreg* for at least 6 months. In general, *Coreg* was well tolerated at doses up to 50 mg daily. Most adverse events reported during *Coreg* therapy were of mild to moderate severity. In U.S. controlled clinical trials directly comparing *Coreg* monotherapy in doses up to 50 mg (n=1,142) to placebo (n=462), 4.9% of *Coreg* patients discontinued for adverse events vs. 5.2% of placebo patients. Although there was no overall difference in discontinuation rates, discontinuations were more common in the carvedilol group for postural hypotension (1% vs. 0). The overall incidence of adverse events in U.S. placebo-controlled trials was found to increase with increasing dose of *Coreg*. For individual adverse events this could only be distinguished for dizziness, which increased in frequency from 2% to 5% as total daily dose increased from 6.25 mg to 50 mg.

Table 4 shows adverse events in U.S. placebo-controlled clinical trials for hypertension that occurred with an incidence of greater than 1% regardless of causality, and that were more frequent in drug-treated patients than placebo-treated patients.

[See table 4 above]

In addition to the events in Table 4, abdominal pain, back pain, chest pain, dependent edema, dyspepsia, dyspnea, fatigue, headache, injury, nausea, pain, rhinitis, sinusitis, somnolence and upper respiratory tract infection were also reported, but rates were equal or greater in placebo-treated patients.

The following adverse events not described above were reported as possibly or probably related to *Coreg* in worldwide open or controlled trials with Coreg (carvedilol) in patients with hypertension or congestive heart failure.

Table 3. Adverse Events (% Occurrence and % Withdrawals) Occurring More Frequently with *Coreg* Than with Placebo in the COPERNICUS trial (Incidence >2%, Regardless of Causality)

	Adverse Reactions		Withdrawals	
	Coreg **(n=1,156)** % occurrence	**Placebo (n=1,133)** % occurrence	***Coreg*** **(n=1,156)** % withdrawals	**Placebo (n=1,133)** % withdrawals
Body as a Whole				
Asthenia	11	9	0.4	0.7
Infection	3	2	—	—
Back pain	3	1	—	—
Cardiovascular				
Hypotension	14	8	0.6	0.4
Bradycardia	10	3	0.6	—
Syncope	8	5	0.4	0.4
Angina pectoris	6	4	0.1	0.1
Hypertension	3	2	—	0.1
Gastrointestinal				
Diarrhea	5	3	0.3	—
Nausea	4	3	—	0.1
Metabolic and Nutritional				
Weight gain	12	11	0.1	0.1
Peripheral edema	7	6	0.2	0.1
Generalized edema	6	5	0.2	0.2
Hyperglycemia	5	3	0.0	0.1
Hyperkalemia	3	2	0.2	0.1
Creatinine increased	3	1	—	0.1
Nervous System				
Dizziness	24	17	1.3	0.6
Headache	5	3	—	0.1
Respiratory				
Upper respiratory infection	14	13	0.1	—
Cough increased	5	4	0.1	0.2
Rales	4	2	0.1	—
Special senses				
Blurred vision	3	2	0.2	0.1

Table 4. Adverse Events in U.S. Placebo-Controlled Hypertension Trials Incidence ≥1%, Regardless of Causality; Withdrawal Rates due to Adverse Events

	Adverse Reactions		Withdrawals	
	Coreg **(n=1,142)** % occurrence	**Placebo (n=462)** % occurrence	***Coreg*** **(n=1,142)** % withdrawals	**Placebo (n=462)** % withdrawals
Cardiovascular				
Bradycardia	2	—	0.4	—
Postural hypotension	2	—	1.0	—
Peripheral edema	1	—	0.2	—
Central Nervous System				
Dizziness	6	5	0.4	1.3
Insomnia	2	1	—	0.2
Gastrointestinal				
Diarrhea	2	1	0.1	—
Hematologic				
Thrombocytopenia	1	—	—	—
Metabolic				
Hypertriglyceridemia	1	—	—	—
Resistance Mechanism				
Viral infection	2	1	—	—
Respiratory				
Pharyngitis	2	1	—	—
Urinary/Renal				
Urinary tract infection	2	1	—	—

Incidence >0.1% to ≤1%

Cardiovascular: Peripheral ischemia, tachycardia.
Central and Peripheral Nervous System: Hypokinesia.
Gastrointestinal: Bilirubinemia, increased hepatic enzymes (0.2% of hypertension patients and 0.4% of congestive heart failure patients were discontinued from therapy because of increases in hepatic enzymes; see WARNINGS, Hepatic Injury).
Psychiatric: Nervousness, sleep disorder, aggravated depression, impaired concentration, abnormal thinking, paroniria, emotional lability.
Respiratory System: Asthma (see CONTRAINDICATIONS).
Reproductive: Male: decreased libido.
Skin and Appendages: Pruritus, rash erythematous, rash maculopapular, rash psoriaform, photosensitivity reaction.
Special Senses: Tinnitus.
Urinary System: Micturition frequency increased.
Autonomic Nervous System: Dry mouth, sweating increased.
Metabolic and Nutritional: Hypokalemia, hypertriglyceridemia.
Hematologic: Anemia, leukopenia.

Rates of adverse events were generally similar across demographic subsets (men and women, elderly and non-elderly, blacks and non-blacks).

The following events were reported in ≤0.1% of patients and are potentially important: complete AV block, bundle branch block, myocardial ischemia, cerebrovascular disorder, convulsions, migraine, neuralgia, paresis, anaphylactoid reaction, alopecia, exfoliative dermatitis, amnesia, GI hemorrhage, bronchospasm, pulmonary edema, decreased hearing, respiratory alkalosis, increased BUN, decreased HDL, pancytopenia and atypical lymphocytes.

Other adverse events occurred sporadically in single patients and cannot be distinguished from concurrent disease states or medications.

Coreg (carvedilol) therapy has not been associated with clinically significant changes in routine laboratory tests in hypertensive patients. No clinically relevant changes were noted in serum potassium, fasting serum glucose, total triglycerides, total cholesterol, HDL cholesterol, uric acid, blood urea nitrogen or creatinine.

OVERDOSAGE

The acute oral LD_{50} doses in male and female mice and male and female rats are over 8000 mg/kg. Overdosage may cause severe hypotension, bradycardia, cardiac insufficiency, cardiogenic shock and cardiac arrest. Respiratory problems, bronchospasms, vomiting, lapses of consciousness and generalized seizures may also occur.

The patient should be placed in a supine position and, where necessary, kept under observation and treated under intensive-care conditions. Gastric lavage or pharmacologically induced emesis may be used shortly after ingestion. The following agents may be administered: for excessive bradycardia: atropine, 2 mg IV.

to support cardiovascular function: glucagon, 5 to 10 mg IV rapidly over 30 seconds, followed by a continuous infusion of 5 mg/hour; sympathomimetics (dobutamine, isoprenaline, adrenaline) at doses according to body weight and effect.

If peripheral vasodilation dominates, it may be necessary to administer adrenaline or noradrenaline with continuous monitoring of circulatory conditions. For therapy-resistant bradycardia, pacemaker therapy should be performed. For bronchospasm, β-sympathomimetics (as aerosol or IV) or aminophylline IV should be given. In the event of seizures, slow IV injection of diazepam or clonazepam is recommended.

NOTE: In the event of severe intoxication where there are symptoms of shock, treatment with antidotes must be con-

Continued on next page

Coreg—Cont.

tinued for a sufficiently long period of time consistent with the 7- to 10-hour half-life of carvedilol.
Cases of overdosage with *Coreg* alone or in combination with other drugs have been reported. Quantities ingested in some cases exceeded 1000 milligrams. Symptoms experienced included low blood pressure and heart rate. Standard supportive treatment was provided and individuals recovered.

DOSAGE AND ADMINISTRATION

Congestive Heart Failure
DOSAGE MUST BE INDIVIDUALIZED AND CLOSELY MONITORED BY A PHYSICIAN DURING UP-TITRATION. Prior to initiation of *Coreg*, it is recommended that fluid retention be minimized. The recommended starting dose of *Coreg* is 3.125 mg, twice daily for two weeks. Patients who tolerate a dose of 3.125 mg twice daily may have their dose increased to 6.25, 12.5 and 25 mg twice daily over successive intervals of at least two weeks. Patients should be maintained on lower doses if higher doses are not tolerated. A maximum dose of 50 mg b.i.d. has been administered to patients with mild-to-moderate heart failure weighing over 85 kg (187 lbs).
Patients should be advised that initiation of treatment and (to a lesser extent) dosage increases may be associated with transient symptoms of dizziness or lightheadedness (and rarely syncope) within the first hour after dosing. Thus during these periods they should avoid situations such as driving or hazardous tasks, where symptoms could result in injury. In addition, Coreg (carvedilol) should be taken with food to slow the rate of absorption. Vasodilatory symptoms often do not require treatment, but it may be useful to separate the time of dosing of *Coreg* from that of the ACE inhibitor or to reduce temporarily the dose of the ACE inhibitor. The dose of *Coreg* should not be increased until symptoms of worsening heart failure or vasodilation have been stabilized.
Fluid retention (with or without transient worsening heart failure symptoms) should be treated by an increase in the dose of diuretics.
The dose of *Coreg* should be reduced if patients experience bradycardia (heart rate <55 beats/min).
Episodes of dizziness or fluid retention during initiation of Coreg can generally be managed without discontinuation of treatment and do not preclude subsequent successful titration of, or a favorable response to, carvedilol.

Hypertension
DOSAGE MUST BE INDIVIDUALIZED. The recommended starting dose of *Coreg* is 6.25 mg twice daily. If this dose is tolerated, using standing systolic pressure measured about 1 hour after dosing as a guide, the dose should be maintained for 7 to 14 days, and then increased to 12.5 mg twice daily if needed, based on trough blood pressure, again using standing systolic pressure one hour after dosing as a guide for tolerance. This dose should also be maintained for 7 to 14 days and can then be adjusted upward to 25 mg twice daily if tolerated and needed. The full antihypertensive effect of *Coreg* is seen within 7 to 14 days. Total daily dose should not exceed 50 mg. *Coreg* should be taken with food to slow the rate of absorption and reduce the incidence of orthostatic effects.
Addition of a diuretic to *Coreg*, or *Coreg* to a diuretic can be expected to produce additive effects and exaggerate the orthostatic component of *Coreg* action.
Coreg (carvedilol) should not be given to patients with severe hepatic impairment (see CONTRAINDICATIONS).

HOW SUPPLIED

Tablets: White, oval, film-coated tablets: 3.125 mg–engraved with 39 and SB, in bottles of 100; 6.25 mg–engraved with 4140 and SB, in bottles of 100; 12.5 mg–engraved with 4141 and SB, in bottles of 100; 25 mg–engraved with 4142 and SB, in bottles of 100. The 6.25 mg, 12.5 mg and 25 mg tablets are Tiltab® tablets.
Store below 30°C (86°F). Protect from moisture. Dispense in a tight, light-resistant container.
3.125 mg 100's: NDC 0007-4139-20
6.25 mg 100's: NDC 0007-4140-20
12.5 mg 100's: NDC 0007-4141-20
25 mg 100's: NDC 0007-4142-20
Coreg is a registered trademark.
GlaxoSmithKline, Research Triangle Park, NC 27709

November 2001/CO:L6B

ENGERIX-B® ℞

[en 'jur-ix bee]
Hepatitis B Vaccine (Recombinant)

Prescribing information for this product, which appears on pages 1517–1520 of the 2002 PDR, has been revised as follows. Please write "See Supplement A" next to the product heading.

The **STORAGE** *section was revised to:*
Store refrigerated between 2° and 8°C (36° and 46°F). *Do not freeze;* discard if product has been frozen. Do not dilute to administer.
The **HOW SUPPLIED** *section was revised to:*
Engerix-B [Hepatitis B Vaccine (Recombinant)] is supplied as a slightly turbid white suspension in vials and prefilled Tip-Lok® syringes.
Adult Dose
20 mcg/mL in Single-Dose Vials in packages of 1 and 25 vials.
NDC 58160-857-01 (package of 1)
NDC 58160-857-16 (package of 25)
20 mcg/mL in Single-Dose Prefilled Disposable Tip-Lok® Syringes (packaged without needles).
NDC 58160-857-46 (package of 5)
NDC 58160-857-50 (package of 25)
Pediatric/Adolescent Doses
10 mcg/0.5 mL in Single-Dose Vials in packages of 1 and 10 vials.
NDC 58160-856-01 (package of 1)
NDC 58160-856-11 (package of 10)
10 mcg/0.5 mL in Single-Dose Prefilled Disposable Tip-Lok® Syringes (packaged without needles)
NDC 58160-856-46 (package of 5)
NDC 58160-856-50 (package of 25)
10 mcg/0.5 mL in Single-Dose Prefilled Disposable Tip-Lok® Syringes with 1-inch 25-gauge SafetyGlide™ needles.
NDC 58160-856-56 (package of 25)
10 mcg/0.5 mL in Single-Dose Prefilled Disposable Tip-Lok® Syringes with 1-inch 23-gauge SafetyGlide™ needles.
NDC 58160-856-58 (package of 25)
10 mcg/0.5 mL in Single-Dose Prefilled Disposable Tip-Lok® Syringes with 5/8-inch 25-gauge SafetyGlide™ needles.
NDC 58160-856-57 (package of 25)
The following sentence was added to the end of the product information:
SafetyGlide is a trademark of Becton, Dickinson and Company.
U.S. License No. 1090
Manufactured by GlaxoSmithKline Biologicals
Rixensart, Belgium
Distributed by GlaxoSmithKline
GlaxoSmithKline, Research Triangle Park, NC 27709

November 2001/EB:L33

EPIVIR® Tablets ℞

[ep'ə-vir]
(lamivudine tablets)

EPIVIR® Oral Solution ℞

(lamivudine oral solution)

Prescribing information for these products, which appears on pages 1520–1524 of the 2002 PDR, has been revised as follows. Please write "See Supplement A" next to the product heading.

The second paragraph of the **MICROBIOLOGY: Drug Resistance** *subsection was revised to:*
Susceptibility of clinical isolates to lamivudine and zidovudine was monitored in controlled clinical trials. In patients receiving lamivudine monotherapy or combination therapy with lamivudine plus zidovudine, HIV-1 isolates from most patients became phenotypically and genotypically resistant to lamivudine within 12 weeks. In some patients harboring zidovudine-resistant virus at baseline, phenotypic sensitivity to zidovudine was restored by 12 weeks of treatment with lamivudine and zidovudine. Combination therapy with lamivudine plus zidovudine delayed the emergence of mutations conferring resistance to zidovudine.
The following was added as the third paragraph of the **CLINICAL PHARMACOLOGY: Drug Interactions** *subsection:*
Lamivudine and zalcitabine may inhibit the intracellular phosphorylation of one another. Therefore, use of lamivudine in combination with zalcitabine is not recommended.
The last sentence of the **WARNINGS: Important Differences Among Lamivudine-Containing Products** *subsection was revised to:*
COMBIVIR (a fixed-dose combination tablet of lamivudine and zidovudine) should not be administered concomitantly with EPIVIR, EPIVIR-HBV, RETROVIR, or TRIZIVIR®.
The following sentence was added to the end of the **PRECAUTIONS: Patients with HIV and Hepatitis B Virus Coinfection** *subsection:*
Posttreatment exacerbations of hepatitis have also been reported (see WARNINGS).
The **PRECAUTIONS: Drug Interactions** *subsection was revised to:*
TMP 160 mg/SMX 800 mg once daily has been shown to increase lamivudine exposure (AUC) by 44% (see CLINICAL PHARMACOLOGY). No change in dose of either drug is recommended. There is no information regarding the effect on lamivudine pharmacokinetics of higher doses of TMP/SMX such as those used to treat *Pneumocystis carinii* pneumonia. No data are available regarding the potential for interaction with other drugs that have renal clearance mechanisms similar to that of lamivudine.
Lamivudine and zalcitabine may inhibit the intracellular phosphorylation of one another. Therefore, use of lamivudine in combination with zalcitabine is not recommended.
The **ADVERSE REACTIONS: Observed During Clinical Practice:** ***Hemic and Lymphatic*** *subsection was revised to:*
Anemia, lymphadenopathy, pure red cell aplasia, splenomegaly.
In **HOW SUPPLIED,** *the storage statement for EPIVIR Tablets was revised to:*
Store at 25°C (77°F), excursions permitted to 15° to 30°C (59° to 86°F) [see USP Controlled Room Temperature].
The storage statement for EPIVIR Oral Solution was revised to:
Store in tightly closed bottles at 25°C (77°F) [see USP Controlled Room Temperature].
GlaxoSmithKline, Research Triangle Park, NC 27709
Manufactured under agreement from
Shire PLC, Basing Stoke, UK

August 2001/RL-981

EPIVIR-HBV® ℞

[ep'ə-vir]
(lamivudine)
Tablets

EPIVIR-HBV® ℞

(lamivudine)
Oral Solution

Prescribing information for these products, which appears on pages 1524–1527 of the 2002 PDR, has been completely revised as follows. Please write "See Supplement A" next to the product heading.

WARNING: LACTIC ACIDOSIS AND SEVERE HEPATOMEGALY WITH STEATOSIS, INCLUDING FATAL CASES, HAVE BEEN REPORTED WITH THE USE OF NUCLEOSIDE ANALOGUES ALONE OR IN COMBINATION, INCLUDING LAMIVUDINE AND OTHER ANTIRETROVIRALS (SEE WARNINGS). HUMAN IMMUNODEFICIENCY VIRUS (HIV) COUNSELING AND TESTING SHOULD BE OFFERED TO ALL PATIENTS BEFORE BEGINNING EPIVIR-HBV AND PERIODICALLY DURING TREATMENT (SEE WARNINGS), BECAUSE EPIVIR-HBV TABLETS AND ORAL SOLUTION CONTAIN A LOWER DOSE OF THE SAME ACTIVE INGREDIENT (LAMIVUDINE) AS EPIVIR® TABLETS AND ORAL SOLUTION USED TO TREAT HIV INFECTION. IF TREATMENT WITH EPIVIR-HBV IS PRESCRIBED FOR CHRONIC HEPATITIS B FOR A PATIENT WITH UNRECOGNIZED OR UNTREATED HIV INFECTION, RAPID EMERGENCE OF HIV RESISTANCE IS LIKELY BECAUSE OF SUBTHERAPEUTIC DOSE AND INAPPROPRIATE MONOTHERAPY.

DESCRIPTION

EPIVIR-HBV is a brand name for lamivudine, a synthetic nucleoside analogue with activity against HBV and HIV. Lamivudine was initially developed for the treatment of HIV infection as EPIVIR®. Please see the complete prescribing information for EPIVIR Tablets and Oral Solution for additional information. The chemical name of lamivudine is (2R,cis)-4-amino-1-(2-hydroxymethyl-1,3-oxathiolan-5-yl)-(1H)-pyrimidin-2-one. Lamivudine is the (-)enantiomer of a dideoxy analogue of cytidine. Lamivudine has also been referred to as (-)2′,3′-dideoxy, 3′-thiacytidine. It has a molecular formula of $C_8H_{11}N_3O_3S$ and a molecular weight of 229.3.
Lamivudine is a white to off-white crystalline solid with a solubility of approximately 70 mg/mL in water at 20°C.
EPIVIR-HBV Tablets are for oral administration. Each tablet contains 100 mg of lamivudine and the inactive ingredients hypromellose, macrogol 400, magnesium stearate, microcrystalline cellulose, polysorbate 80, red iron oxide, sodium starch glycolate, titanium dioxide, and yellow iron oxide.
EPIVIR-HBV Oral Solution is for oral administration. One milliliter (1 mL) of EPIVIR-HBV Oral Solution contains 5 mg of lamivudine (5 mg/mL) in an aqueous solution and the inactive ingredients artificial strawberry and banana flavors, citric acid (anhydrous), methylparaben, propylene glycol, propylparaben, sodium citrate (dihydrate), and sucrose.

MICROBIOLOGY

Mechanism of Action: Lamivudine is a synthetic nucleoside analogue. Lamivudine is phosphorylated intracellularly to lamivudine triphosphate, L-TP. Incorporation of the monophosphate form into viral DNA by hepatitis B virus (HBV) polymerase results in DNA chain termination. L-TP also inhibits the RNA- and DNA-dependent DNA polymerase activities of HIV-1 reverse transcriptase (RT). L-TP is a weak inhibitor of mammalian alpha-, beta-, and gamma-DNA polymerases.
Antiviral Activity *In Vitro*: *In vitro* activity of lamivudine against HBV was assessed in HBV DNA-transfected 2.2.15 cells, HB611 cells, and infected human primary hepatocytes. IC_{50} values (the concentration of drug needed to reduce the level of extracellular HBV DNA by 50%) varied from 0.01 μM (2.3 ng/mL) to 5.6 μM (1.3 mcg/mL) depending upon the duration of exposure of cells to lamivudine, the cell model system, and the protocol used. See the EPIVIR package insert for information regarding activity of lamivudine against HIV.
Drug Resistance: ***HBV:*** Genotypic analysis of viral isolates obtained from patients who show renewed evidence of replication of HBV while receiving lamivudine suggests that a reduction in sensitivity of HBV to lamivudine is associated with mutations resulting in a methionine to valine or isoleucine substitution in the YMDD motif of the catalytic domain of HBV polymerase (position 552) and a leucine to methionine substitution at position 528. It is not known whether other HBV mutations may be associated with reduced lamivudine susceptibility *in vitro*.

In 4 controlled clinical trials in adults, YMDD-mutant HBV were detected in 81 of 335 patients receiving lamivudine 100 mg once daily for 52 weeks. The prevalence of YMDD mutations was less than 10% in each of these trials for patients studied at 24 weeks and increased to an average of 24% (range in 4 studies: 16% to 32%) at 52 weeks. In limited data from a long-term follow-up trial in patients who continued 100 mg/day lamivudine after one of these studies, YMDD mutations further increased from 16% at 1 year to 42% at 2 years. In small numbers of patients receiving lamivudine for longer periods, further increases in the appearance of YMDD mutations were observed.

In a controlled trial in pediatric patients, YMDD-mutant HBV were detected in 31 of 166 (19%) patients receiving lamivudine for 52 weeks. For a subgroup who remained on lamivudine therapy in a follow-up study, YMDD mutations increased from 24% at 12 months to 45% (53 of 118) at 18 months of lamivudine treatment.

Mutant viruses were associated with evidence of diminished treatment response at 52 weeks relative to lamivudine-treated patients without evidence of YMDD mutations in both adult and pediatric studies (see PRECAUTIONS). The long-term clinical significance of YMDD-mutant HBV is not known.

HIV: In studies of HIV-1-infected patients who received lamivudine monotherapy or combination therapy with lamivudine plus zidovudine for at least 12 weeks, HIV-1 isolates with reduced *in vitro* susceptibility to lamivudine were detected in most patients (see WARNINGS).

CLINICAL PHARMACOLOGY

Pharmacokinetics in Adults: The pharmacokinetic properties of lamivudine have been studied as single and multiple oral doses ranging from 5 to 600 mg per day administered to HBV-infected patients.

The pharmacokinetic properties of lamivudine have also been studied in asymptomatic, HIV-infected adult patients after administration of single intravenous (IV) doses ranging from 0.25 to 8 mg/kg, as well as single and multiple (twice-daily regimen) oral doses ranging from 0.25 to 10 mg/kg.

Absorption and Bioavailability: Lamivudine was rapidly absorbed after oral administration in HBV-infected patients and in healthy subjects. Following single oral doses of 100 mg, the peak serum lamivudine concentration (C_{max}) in HBV-infected patients (steady state) and healthy subjects (single dose) was 1.28 ± 0.56 mcg/mL and 1.05 ± 0.32 mcg/mL (mean ± SD), respectively, which occurred between 0.5 and 2 hours after administration. The area under the plasma concentration versus time curve ($AUC_{[0-24\ h]}$) following 100 mg lamivudine oral single and repeated daily doses to steady state was 4.3 ± 1.4 (mean ± SD) and 4.7 ± 1.7 mcg•h/mL, respectively. The relative bioavailability of the tablet and solution were then demonstrated in healthy subjects. Although the solution demonstrated a slightly higher peak serum concentration (C_{max}), there was no significant difference in systemic exposure (AUC_∞) between the solution and the tablet. Therefore, the solution and the tablet may be used interchangeably.

After oral administration of lamivudine once daily to HBV-infected adults, the AUC and peak serum levels (C_{max}) increased in proportion to dose over the range from 5 mg to 600 mg once daily.

The 100-mg tablet was administered orally to 24 healthy subjects on 2 occasions, once in the fasted state and once with food (standard meal: 967 kcal; 67 grams fat, 33 grams protein, 58 grams carbohydrate). There was no significant difference in systemic exposure (AUC_∞) in the fed and fasted states; therefore, EPIVIR-HBV Tablets and Oral Solution may be administered with or without food.

Lamivudine was rapidly absorbed after oral administration in HIV-infected patients. Absolute bioavailability in 12 adult patients was 86% ± 16% (mean ± SD) for the 150-mg tablet and 87% ± 13% for the 10-mg/mL oral solution.

Distribution: The apparent volume of distribution after IV administration of lamivudine to 20 asymptomatic HIV-infected patients was 1.3 ± 0.4 L/kg, suggesting that lamivudine distributes into extravascular spaces. Volume of distribution was independent of dose and did not correlate with body weight.

Binding of lamivudine to human plasma proteins is low (<36%) and independent of dose. *In vitro* studies showed that, over the concentration range of 0.1 to 100 mcg/mL, the amount of lamivudine associated with erythrocytes ranged from 53% to 57% and was independent of concentration.

Metabolism: Metabolism of lamivudine is a minor route of elimination. In man, the only known metabolite of lamivudine is the trans-sulfoxide metabolite. In 9 healthy subjects receiving 300 mg of lamivudine as single oral doses, a total of 4.2% (range 1.5% to 7.5%) of the dose was excreted as the trans-sulfoxide metabolite in the urine, the majority of which was excreted in the first 12 hours.

Serum concentrations of the trans-sulfoxide metabolite have not been determined.

Elimination: The majority of lamivudine is eliminated unchanged in urine. In 9 healthy subjects given a single 300-mg oral dose of lamivudine, renal clearance was 199.7 ± 56.9 mL/min (mean ± SD). In 20 HIV-infected patients given a single IV dose, renal clearance was 280.4 ± 75.2 mL/min (mean ± SD), representing 71% ± 16% (mean ± SD) of total clearance of lamivudine.

In most single-dose studies in HIV- or HBV-infected patients or healthy subjects with serum sampling for 24 hours after dosing, the observed mean elimination half-life ($t_{1/2}$) ranged from 5 to 7 hours. In HIV-infected patients, total clearance was 398.5 ± 69.1 mL/min (mean ± SD). Oral clearance and elimination half-life were independent of dose and body weight over an oral dosing range from 0.25 to 10 mg/kg.

Table 1: Pharmacokinetic Parameters (Mean ± SD) Dose-Normalized to a Single 100-mg Oral Dose of Lamivudine in Patients With Varying Degrees of Renal Function

Parameter	Creatinine Clearance Criterion (Number of Subjects)		
	≥80 mL/min (n = 9)	20-59 mL/min (n = 8)	<20 mL/min (n = 6)
Creatinine clearance (mL/min)	97 (range 82-117)	39 (range 25-49)	15 (range 13-19)
C_{max} (mcg/mL)	1.31 ± 0.35	1.85 ± 0.40	1.55 ± 0.31
AUC_∞ (mcg•h/mL)	5.28 ± 1.01	14.67 ± 3.74	27.33 ± 6.56
Cl/F (mL/min)	326.4 ± 63.8	120.1 ± 29.5	64.5 ± 18.3

Special Populations: ***Adults With Impaired Renal Function:*** The pharmacokinetic properties of lamivudine have been determined in healthy subjects and in subjects with impaired renal function, with and without hemodialysis (Table 1):

[See table 1 above]

Exposure (AUC_∞), C_{max}, and half-life increased with diminishing renal function (as expressed by creatinine clearance). Apparent total oral clearance (Cl/F) of lamivudine decreased as creatinine clearance decreased. T_{max} was not significantly affected by renal function. Based on these observations, it is recommended that the dosage of lamivudine be modified in patients with renal impairment (see DOSAGE AND ADMINISTRATION).

Hemodialysis increases lamivudine clearance from a mean of 64 to 88 mL/min; however, the length of time of hemodialysis (4 hours) was insufficient to significantly alter mean lamivudine exposure after a single-dose administration. Therefore, it is recommended, following correction of dose for creatinine clearance, that no additional dose modification is made after routine hemodialysis.

It is not known whether lamivudine can be removed by peritoneal dialysis or continuous (24-hour) hemodialysis.

The effect of renal impairment on lamivudine pharmacokinetics in pediatric patients with chronic hepatitis B is not known.

Adults With Impaired Hepatic Function: The pharmacokinetic properties of lamivudine have been determined in adults with impaired hepatic function (Table 2). Patients were stratified by severity of hepatic functional impairment.

[See table 2 at top of next page]

Pharmacokinetic parameters were not altered by diminishing hepatic function. Therefore, no dose adjustment for lamivudine is required for patients with impaired hepatic function. Safety and efficacy of EPIVIR-HBV have not been established in the presence of decompensated liver disease (see PRECAUTIONS).

Post-Hepatic Transplant: Fourteen HBV-infected patients received liver transplant following lamivudine therapy and completed pharmacokinetic assessments at enrollment, 2 weeks after 100-mg once-daily dosing (pre-transplant), and 3 months following transplant; there were no significant differences in pharmacokinetic parameters. The overall exposure of lamivudine is primarily affected by renal dysfunction; consequently, transplant patients with reduced renal function had generally higher exposure than patients with normal renal function. Safety and efficacy of EPIVIR-HBV have not been established in this population (see PRECAUTIONS).

Pediatric Patients: Lamivudine pharmacokinetics were evaluated in a 28-day dose-ranging study in 53 pediatric patients with chronic hepatitis B. Patients aged 2 to 12 years were randomized to receive lamivudine 0.35 mg/kg twice daily, 3 mg/kg once daily, 1.5 mg/kg twice daily, or 4 mg/kg twice daily. Patients aged 13 to 17 years received lamivudine 100 mg once daily. Lamivudine was rapidly absorbed (T_{max} 0.5 to 1 hour). In general, both C_{max} and exposure (AUC) showed dose proportionality in the dosing range studied. Weight-corrected oral clearance was highest at age 2 and declined from 2 to 12 years, where values were then similar to those seen in adults. A dose of 3 mg/kg given once daily produced a steady-state lamivudine AUC (mean 5953 ng•h/mL ± 1562 SD) similar to that associated with a dose of 100 mg/day in adults.

Gender: There are no significant gender differences in lamivudine pharmacokinetics.

Race: There are no significant racial differences in lamivudine pharmacokinetics.

Drug Interactions: Multiple doses of lamivudine and a single dose of interferon were coadministered to 19 healthy male subjects in a pharmacokinetics study. Results indicated a small (10%) reduction in lamivudine AUC, but no change in interferon pharmacokinetic parameters when the 2 drugs were given in combination. All other pharmacokinetic parameters (C_{max}, T_{max}, and $t_{1/2}$) were unchanged. There was no significant pharmacokinetic interaction between lamivudine and interferon alfa in this study.

Lamivudine and zidovudine were coadministered to 12 asymptomatic HIV-positive adult patients in a single-center, open-label, randomized, crossover study. No significant differences were observed in AUC_∞ or total clearance for lamivudine or zidovudine when the 2 drugs were administered together. Coadministration of lamivudine with zidovudine resulted in an increase of 39% ± 62% (mean ± SD) in C_{max} of zidovudine.

Lamivudine and trimethoprim/sulfamethoxazole (TMP/SMX) were coadministered to 14 HIV-positive patients in a single-center, open-label, randomized, crossover study. Each patient received treatment with a single 300-mg dose of lamivudine and TMP 160 mg/SMX 800 mg once a day for 5 days with concomitant administration of lamivudine 300 mg with the fifth dose in a crossover design. Coadministration of TMP/SMX with lamivudine resulted in an increase of 44% ± 23% (mean ± SD) in lamivudine AUC_∞, a decrease of 29% ± 13% in lamivudine oral clearance, and a decrease of 30% ± 36% in lamivudine renal clearance. The pharmacokinetic properties of TMP and SMX were not altered by coadministration with lamivudine (see PRECAUTIONS: Drug Interactions).

Lamivudine and zalcitabine may inhibit the intracellular phosphorylation of one another. Therefore, use of lamivudine in combination with zalcitabine is not recommended.

INDICATIONS AND USAGE

EPIVIR-HBV is indicated for the treatment of chronic hepatitis B associated with evidence of hepatitis B viral replication and active liver inflammation. This indication is based on 1-year histologic and serologic responses in adult patients with compensated chronic hepatitis B, and more limited information from a study in pediatric patients ages 2 to 17 years (see Description of Clinical Studies below).

Description of Clinical Studies: ***Adults:*** The safety and efficacy of EPIVIR-HBV were evaluated in 4 controlled studies in 967 patients with compensated chronic hepatitis B. All patients were 16 years of age or older and had chronic hepatitis B virus infection (serum HBsAg positive for at least 6 months) accompanied by evidence of HBV replication (serum HBeAg positive and positive for serum HBV DNA, as measured by a research solution-hybridization assay) and persistently elevated ALT levels and/or chronic inflammation on liver biopsy compatible with a diagnosis of chronic viral hepatitis. Three of these studies provided comparisons of EPIVIR-HBV 100 mg once daily versus placebo, and results of these comparisons are summarized below.

- Study 1 was a randomized, double-blind study of EPIVIR-HBV 100 mg once daily versus placebo for 52 weeks, followed by a 16-week no-treatment period, in treatment-naive US patients.
- Study 2 was a randomized, double-blind, 3-arm study that compared EPIVIR-HBV 25 mg once daily versus EPIVIR-HBV 100 mg once daily versus placebo for 52 weeks in Asian patients.
- Study 3 was a randomized, partially-blind, 3-arm study conducted primarily in North America and Europe in patients who had ongoing evidence of active chronic hepatitis B despite previous treatment with interferon alfa. The study compared EPIVIR-HBV 100 mg once daily for 52 weeks, followed by either EPIVIR-HBV 100 mg or matching placebo once daily for 16 weeks (Arm 1), versus placebo once daily for 68 weeks (Arm 2). (A third arm using a combination of interferon and lamivudine is not presented here because there was not sufficient information to evaluate this regimen.)

Principal endpoint comparisons for the histologic and serologic outcomes in lamivudine (100 mg daily) and placebo recipients in placebo-controlled studies are shown in the following tables.

[See table 3 at top of next page]
[See table 4 at top of next page]

Normalization of serum ALT levels was more frequent with lamivudine treatment compared with placebo in Studies 1-3.

The majority of lamivudine-treated patients showed a decrease of HBV DNA to below the assay limit early in the course of therapy. However, reappearance of assay-detectable HBV DNA during lamivudine treatment was observed in approximately one third of patients after this initial response.

Pediatrics: The safety and efficacy of EPIVIR-HBV were evaluated in a double-blind clinical trial in 286 patients ranging from 2 to 17 years of age, who were randomized (2:1) to receive 52 weeks of lamivudine (3 mg/kg once daily to a maximum of 100 mg once daily) or placebo. All patients

Continued on next page

Epivir-HBV—Cont.

had compensated chronic hepatitis B accompanied by evidence of hepatitis B virus replication (positive serum HBeAg and positive for serum HBV DNA by a research branched-chain DNA assay) and persistently elevated serum ALT levels. The combination of loss of HBeAg and reduction of HBV DNA to below the assay limit of the research assay, evaluated at Week 52, was observed in 23% of lamivudine subjects and 13% of placebo subjects. Normalization of serum ALT was achieved and maintained to Week 52 more frequently in patients treated with EPIVIR-HBV compared with placebo (55% versus 13%). As in the adult controlled trials, most lamivudine-treated subjects had decreases in HBV DNA below the assay limit early in treatment, but about one third of subjects with this initial response had reappearance of assay-detectable HBV DNA during treatment. Adolescents (ages 13 to 17 years) showed less evidence of treatment effect than younger children.

Table 2: Pharmacokinetic Parameters (Mean ± SD) Dose-Normalized to a Single 100-mg Dose of Lamivudine in 3 Groups of Subjects With Normal or Impaired Hepatic Function

Parameter	Normal (n = 8)	Impairment* Moderate (n = 8)	Impairment* Severe (n = 8)
C_{max} (mcg/mL)	0.92 ± 0.31	1.06 ± 0.58	1.08 ± 0.27
AUC_{∞} (mcg•h/mL)	3.96 ± 0.58	3.97 ± 1.36	4.30 ± 0.63
T_{max} (h)	1.3 ± 0.8	1.4 ± 0.8	1.4 ± 1.2
Cl/F (mL/min)	424.7 ± 61.9	456.9 ± 129.8	395.2 ± 51.8
Clr (mL/min)	279.2 ± 79.2	323.5 ± 100.9	216.1 ± 58.0

*Hepatic impairment assessed by aminopyrine breath test.

Table 3: Histologic Response at Week 52 Among Adult Patients Receiving EPIVIR-HBV 100 mg Once Daily or Placebo

Assessment	Study 1 EPIVIR-HBV (n = 62)	Study 1 Placebo (n = 63)	Study 2 EPIVIR-HBV (n = 131)	Study 2 Placebo (n = 68)	Study 3 EPIVIR-HBV (n = 110)	Study 3 Placebo (n = 54)
Improvement*	55%	25%	56%	26%	56%	26%
No Improvement	27%	59%	36%	62%	25%	54%
Missing Data	18%	16%	8%	12%	19%	20%

*Improvement was defined as a ≥2-point decrease in the Knodell Histologic Activity Index (HAI)[1] at Week 52 compared with pretreatment HAI. Patients with missing data at baseline were excluded.

Table 4: HBeAg Seroconversion* at Week 52 Among Adult Patients Receiving EPIVIR-HBV 100 mg Once Daily or Placebo

Seroconversion	Study 1 EPIVIR-HBV (n = 63)	Study 1 Placebo (n = 69)	Study 2 EPIVIR-HBV (n = 140)	Study 2 Placebo (n = 70)	Study 3 EPIVIR-HBV (n = 108)	Study 3 Placebo (n = 53)
Responder	17%	6%	16%	4%	15%	13%
Nonresponder	67%	78%	80%	91%	69%	68%
Missing Data	16%	16%	4%	4%	17%	19%

*Three-component seroconversion was defined as Week 52 values showing loss of HBeAg, gain of HBeAb, and reduction of HBV DNA to below the solution hybridization assay limit. Subjects with negative baseline HBeAg or HBV DNA assay were excluded from the analysis.

CONTRAINDICATIONS

EPIVIR-HBV Tablets and EPIVIR-HBV Oral Solution are contraindicated in patients with previously demonstrated clinically significant hypersensitivity to any of the components of the products.

WARNINGS

Lactic Acidosis/Severe Hepatomegaly with Steatosis: Lactic acidosis and severe hepatomegaly with steatosis, including fatal cases, have been reported with the use of nucleoside analogues alone or in combination, including lamivudine and other antiretrovirals. A majority of these cases have been in women. Obesity and prolonged nucleoside exposure may be risk factors. Most of these reports have described patients receiving nucleoside analogues for treatment of HIV infection, but there have been reports of lactic acidosis in patients receiving lamivudine for hepatitis B. Particular caution should be exercised when administering EPIVIR or EPIVIR-HBV to any patient with known risk factors for liver disease; however, cases have also been reported in patients with no known risk factors. Treatment with EPIVIR or EPIVIR-HBV should be suspended in any patient who develops clinical or laboratory findings suggestive of lactic acidosis or pronounced hepatotoxicity (which may include hepatomegaly and steatosis even in the absence of marked transaminase elevations).

Important Differences Between Lamivudine-Containing Products, HIV Testing, and Risk of Emergence of Resistant HIV: EPIVIR-HBV Tablets and Oral Solution contain a lower dose of the same active ingredient (lamivudine) as EPIVIR Tablets and Oral Solution, COMBIVIR® (lamivudine/zidovudine) Tablets, and TRIZIVIR® (abacavir, lamivudine, and zidovudine) Tablets used to treat HIV infection. The formulation and dosage of lamivudine in EPIVIR-HBV are not appropriate for patients dually infected with HBV and HIV. If a decision is made to administer lamivudine to such patients, the higher dosage indicated for HIV therapy should be used as part of an appropriate combination regimen, and the prescribing information for EPIVIR, COMBIVIR, or TRIZIVIR as well as for EPIVIR-HBV should be consulted. HIV counseling and testing should be offered to all patients before beginning EPIVIR-HBV and periodically during treatment because of the risk of rapid emergence of resistant HIV and limitation of treatment options if EPIVIR-HBV is prescribed to treat chronic hepatitis B in a patient who has unrecognized or untreated HIV infection or acquires HIV infection during treatment.

Posttreatment Exacerbations of Hepatitis: Clinical and laboratory evidence of exacerbations of hepatitis have occurred after discontinuation of EPIVIR-HBV (these have been primarily detected by serum ALT elevations, in addition to the re-emergence of HBV DNA commonly observed after stopping treatment; see Table 7 for more information regarding frequency of posttreatment ALT elevations). Although most events appear to have been self-limited, fatalities have been reported in some cases. The causal relationship to discontinuation of lamivudine treatment is unknown. Patients should be closely monitored with both clinical and laboratory follow-up for at least several months after stopping treatment. There is insufficient evidence to determine whether re-initiation of therapy alters the course of posttreatment exacerbations of hepatitis.

Pancreatitis: Pancreatitis has been reported in patients receiving lamivudine, particularly in HIV-infected pediatric patients with prior nucleoside exposure.

PRECAUTIONS

General: Patients should be assessed before beginning treatment with EPIVIR-HBV by a physician experienced in the management of chronic hepatitis B.

Emergence of Resistance-Associated HBV Mutations: In controlled clinical trials, YMDD-mutant HBV were detected in patients with on-lamivudine re-appearance of HBV DNA after an initial decline below the solution hybridization assay limit (see MICROBIOLOGY: Drug Resistance). These mutations can be detected by a research assay and have been associated with reduced susceptibility to lamivudine *in vitro*. Lamivudine-treated patients (adult and pediatric) with YMDD-mutant HBV at 52 weeks showed diminished treatment responses in comparison to lamivudine-treated patients without evidence of YMDD mutations, including lower rates of HBeAg seroconversion and HBeAg loss (no greater than placebo recipients), more frequent return of positive HBV DNA by solution hybridization or branched-chain DNA assay, and more frequent ALT elevations. In the controlled trials, when patients developed YMDD-mutant HBV, they had a rise in HBV DNA and ALT from their own previous on-treatment levels. Progression of hepatitis B, including death, has been reported in some patients with YMDD-mutant HBV, including patients from the liver transplant setting and from other clinical trials. The long-term clinical significance of YMDD-mutant HBV is not known. Increased clinical and laboratory monitoring may aid in treatment decisions if emergence of viral mutants is suspected.

Limitations of Populations Studied: Safety and efficacy of EPIVIR-HBV have not been established in patients with decompensated liver disease or organ transplants; pediatric patients <2 years of age; patients dually infected with HBV and HCV, hepatitis delta, or HIV; or other populations not included in the principal phase III controlled studies. There are no studies in pregnant women and no data regarding effect on vertical transmission, and appropriate infant immunizations should be used to prevent neonatal acquisition of HBV.

Assessing Patients During Treatment: Patients should be monitored regularly during treatment by a physician experienced in the management of chronic hepatitis B. The safety and effectiveness of treatment with EPIVIR-HBV beyond 1 year have not been established. During treatment, combinations of such events such as return of persistently elevated ALT, increasing levels of HBV DNA over time after an initial decline below assay limit, progression of clinical signs or symptoms of hepatic disease, and/or worsening of hepatic necroinflammatory findings may be considered as potentially reflecting loss of therapeutic response. Such observations should be taken into consideration when determining the advisability of continuing therapy with EPIVIR-HBV.

The optimal duration of treatment, the durability of HBeAg seroconversions occurring during treatment, and the relationship between treatment response and long-term outcomes such as hepatocellular carcinoma or decompensated cirrhosis are not known.

Patients with Impaired Renal Function: Reduction of the dosage of EPIVIR-HBV is recommended for patients with impaired renal function (see CLINICAL PHARMACOLOGY and DOSAGE AND ADMINISTRATION).

Information for Patients: A Patient Package Insert (PPI) for EPIVIR-HBV is available for patient information.

Patients should remain under the care of a physician while taking EPIVIR-HBV. They should discuss any new symptoms or concurrent medications with their physician.

Patients should be advised that EPIVIR-HBV is not a cure for hepatitis B, that the long-term treatment benefits of EPIVIR-HBV are unknown at this time, and, in particular, that the relationship of initial treatment response to outcomes such as hepatocellular carcinoma and decompensated cirrhosis is unknown. Patients should be informed that deterioration of liver disease has occurred in some cases if treatment was discontinued, and that they should discuss any change in regimen with their physician. Patients should be informed that emergence of resistant hepatitis B virus and worsening of disease can occur during treatment, and they should promptly report any new symptoms to their physician.

Patients should be counseled on the importance of testing for HIV to avoid inappropriate therapy and development of resistant HIV, and HIV counseling and testing should be offered before starting EPIVIR-HBV and periodically during therapy. Patients should be advised that EPIVIR-HBV Tablets and EPIVIR-HBV Oral Solution contain a lower dose of the same active ingredient (lamivudine) as EPIVIR Tablets, EPIVIR Oral Solution, COMBIVIR Tablets, and TRIZIVIR Tablets. EPIVIR-HBV should not be taken concurrently with EPIVIR, COMBIVIR, or TRIZIVIR (see WARNINGS). Patients infected with both HBV and HIV who are planning to change their HIV treatment regimen to a regimen that does not include EPIVIR, COMBIVIR, or TRIZIVIR should discuss continued therapy for hepatitis B with their physician.

Patients should be advised that treatment with EPIVIR-HBV has not been shown to reduce the risk of transmission of HBV to others through sexual contact or blood contamination (see Pregnancy section).

Drug Interactions: TMP 160 mg/SMX 800 mg once daily has been shown to increase lamivudine exposure (AUC) by 44% (see CLINICAL PHARMACOLOGY). No change in dose of either drug is recommended. There is no information regarding the effect on lamivudine pharmacokinetics of higher doses of TMP/SMX such as those used to treat *Pneumocystis carinii* pneumonia. No data are available regarding the potential for interaction with other drugs that have renal clearance mechanisms similar to that of lamivudine. Lamivudine and zalcitabine may inhibit the intracellular phosphorylation of one another. Therefore, use of lamivudine in combination with zalcitabine is not recommended.

Carcinogenesis, Mutagenesis, and Impairment of Fertility: Lamivudine long-term carcinogenicity studies in mice and rats showed no evidence of carcinogenic potential at exposures up to 34 times (mice) and 200 times (rats) those observed in humans at the recommended therapeutic dose for chronic hepatitis B. Lamivudine was not active in a microbial mutagenicity screen or an *in vitro* cell transformation assay, but showed weak *in vitro* mutagenic activity in a cytogenetic assay using cultured human lymphocytes and in the mouse lymphoma assay. However, lamivudine showed no evidence of *in vivo* genotoxic activity in the rat at oral doses of up to 2000 mg/kg producing plasma levels of 60 to 70 times those in humans at the recommended dose for chronic hepatitis B. In a study of reproductive performance, lamivudine administered to rats at doses up to 4000 mg/kg per day, producing plasma levels 80 to 120 times those in humans, revealed no evidence of impaired fertility and no effect on the survival, growth, and development to weaning of the offspring.

Pregnancy: Pregnancy Category C. Reproduction studies have been performed in rats and rabbits at orally administered doses up to 4000 mg/kg per day and 1000 mg/kg per day, respectively, producing plasma levels up to approximately 60 times that for the adult HBV dose. No evidence of teratogenicity due to lamivudine was observed. Evidence of early embryolethality was seen in the rabbit at exposure levels similar to those observed in humans, but there was no indication of this effect in the rat at exposures up to 60 times that in humans. Studies in pregnant rats and rabbits showed that lamivudine is transferred to the fetus through the placenta. There are no adequate and well-controlled studies in pregnant women. Because animal reproductive toxicity studies are not always predictive of human response, lamivudine should be used during pregnancy only if the potential benefits outweigh the risks.

Lamivudine has not been shown to affect the transmission of HBV from mother to infant, and appropriate infant immunizations should be used to prevent neonatal acquisition of HBV.

Pregnancy Registry: To monitor maternal-fetal outcomes of pregnant women exposed to lamivudine, a Pregnancy Registry has been established. Physicians are encouraged to register patients by calling 1-800-258-4263.

Nursing Mothers: A study in lactating rats showed that lamivudine concentrations in milk were similar to those in plasma. Although it is not known if lamivudine is excreted in human milk, there is the potential for adverse effects from lamivudine in nursing infants. Mothers should be instructed not to breastfeed if they are receiving lamivudine.

Pediatric Use: ***HBV:*** Safety and efficacy of lamivudine for treatment of chronic hepatitis B in children have been studied in pediatric patients from 2 to 17 years of age in a controlled clinical trial (see CLINICAL PHARMACOLOGY, INDICATIONS AND USAGE, and DOSAGE AND ADMINISTRATION).

Safety and efficacy in pediatric patients <2 years of age have not been established.

HIV: See the complete prescribing information for EPIVIR Tablets and Oral Solution for additional information on pharmacokinetics of lamivudine in HIV-infected children.

Geriatric Use: Clinical studies of EPIVIR-HBV did not include sufficient numbers of subjects aged 65 and over to determine whether they respond differently from younger subjects. In general, dose selection for an elderly patient should be cautious, reflecting the greater frequency of decreased hepatic, renal, or cardiac function, and of concomitant disease or other drug therapy. In particular, because lamivudine is substantially excreted by the kidney and elderly patients are more likely to have decreased renal function, renal function should be monitored and dosage adjustments should be made accordingly (see PRECAUTIONS: Patients with Impaired Renal Function and DOSAGE AND ADMINISTRATION).

ADVERSE REACTIONS

Several serious adverse events reported with lamivudine (lactic acidosis and severe hepatomegaly with steatosis, posttreatment exacerbations of hepatitis B, pancreatitis, and emergence of viral mutants associated with reduced drug susceptibility and diminished treatment response) are also described in WARNINGS and PRECAUTIONS.

Clinical Trials In Chronic Hepatitis B: ***Adults:*** Selected clinical adverse events observed with a ≥5% frequency during therapy with EPIVIR-HBV compared with placebo are listed in Table 5. Frequencies of specified laboratory abnormalities during therapy with EPIVIR-HBV compared with placebo are listed in Table 6.

[See table 5 above]

[See table 6 above]

Table 5: Selected Clinical Adverse Events (≥5% Frequency) in 3 Placebo-Controlled Clinical Trials in Adults During Treatment* (Studies 1-3)

Adverse Event	EPIVIR-HBV (n = 332)	Placebo (n = 200)
Non-site specific		
Malaise and fatigue	24%	28%
Fever or chills	7%	9%
Ear, nose, and throat		
Ear, nose, and throat infections	25%	21%
Sore throat	13%	8%
Gastrointestinal		
Nausea and vomiting	15%	17%
Abdominal discomfort and pain	16%	17%
Diarrhea	14%	12%
Musculoskeletal		
Myalgia	14%	17%
Arthralgia	7%	5%
Neurological		
Headache	21%	21%
Skin		
Skin rashes	5%	5%

*Includes patients treated for 52 to 68 weeks.

Table 6: Frequencies of Specified Laboratory Abnormalities in 3 Placebo-Controlled Trials in Adults During Treatment* (Studies 1-3)

Test (Abnormal Level)	Patients with Abnormality/Patients with Observations	
	EPIVIR-HBV	Placebo
ALT >3 × baseline†	37/331 (11%)	26/199 (13%)
Albumin <2.5 g/dL	0/331 (0%)	2/199 (1%)
Amylase >3 × baseline	2/259 (<1%)	4/167 (2%)
Serum Lipase ≥2.5 × ULN‡	19/189 (10%)	9/127 (7%)
CPK ≥7 × baseline	31/329 (9%)	9/198 (5%)
Neutrophils <750/mm^3	0/331 (0%)	1/199 (<1%)
Platelets <50,000/mm^3	10/272 (4%)	5/168 (3%)

*Includes patients treated for 52 to 68 weeks.
†See Table 7 for posttreatment ALT values.
‡Includes observations during and after treatment in the 2 placebo-controlled trials that collected this information.
ULN = Upper limit of normal.

In patients followed for up to 16 weeks after discontinuation of treatment, posttreatment ALT elevations were observed more frequently in patients who had received EPIVIR-HBV than in patients who had received placebo. A comparison of ALT elevations between weeks 52 and 68 in patients who discontinued EPIVIR-HBV at week 52 and patients in the same studies who received placebo throughout the treatment course is shown in Table 7.

[See table 7 above]

Table 7: Posttreatment ALT Elevations in 2 Placebo-Controlled Studies in Adults With No-Active-Treatment Follow-up (Studies 1 and 3)

Abnormal Value	Patients with ALT Elevation/ Patients with Observations*	
	EPIVIR-HBV	Placebo
ALT ≥2 × baseline value	37/137 (27%)	22/116 (19%)
ALT ≥3 × baseline value†	29/137 (21%)	9/116 (8%)
ALT ≥2 × baseline value and absolute ALT >500 IU/L	21/137 (15%)	8/116 (7%)
ALT ≥2 × baseline value; and bilirubin >2 × ULN and ≥2 × baseline value	1/137 (0.7%)	1/116 (0.9%)

*Each patient may be represented in one or more category.
†Comparable to a Grade 3 toxicity in accordance with modified WHO criteria.
ULN = Upper limit of normal.

Lamivudine in Patients with HIV: In HIV-infected patients, safety information reflects a higher dose of lamivudine (150 mg b.i.d.) than the dose used to treat chronic hepatitis B in HIV-negative patients. In clinical trials using lamivudine as part of a combination regimen for treatment of HIV infection, several clinical adverse events occurred more often in lamivudine-containing treatment arms than in comparator arms. These included nasal signs and symptoms (20% vs. 11%), dizziness (10% vs. 4%), and depressive disorders (9% vs. 4%). Pancreatitis was observed in 3 of the 656 adult patients (<0.5%) who received EPIVIR in controlled clinical trials. Laboratory abnormalities reported more often in lamivudine-containing arms included neutropenia and elevations of liver function tests (also more frequent in lamivudine-containing arms for a retrospective analysis of HIV/HBV dually infected patients in one study), and amylase elevations. Please see the complete prescribing information for EPIVIR Tablets and Oral Solution for more information.

Pediatric Patients with Hepatitis B: Most commonly observed adverse events in the pediatric trials were similar to those in adult trials; in addition, respiratory symptoms (cough, bronchitis, and viral respiratory infections) were reported in both lamivudine and placebo recipients. Posttreatment transaminase elevations were observed in some patients followed after cessation of lamivudine.

Pediatric Patients with HIV Infection: In early open-label studies of lamivudine in children with HIV, peripheral neuropathy and neutropenia were reported, and pancreatitis was observed in 14% to 15% of patients.

Observed During Clinical Practice: The following events have been identified during post-approval use of lamivudine in clinical practice. Because they are reported voluntarily from a population of unknown size, estimates of frequency cannot be made. These events have been chosen for inclusion due to either their seriousness, frequency of reporting, potential causal connection to lamivudine, or a combination of these factors. Post-marketing experience with lamivudine at this time is largely limited to use in HIV-infected patients.

Digestive: Stomatitis.
Endocrine and Metabolic: Hyperglycemia.
General: Weakness.
Hemic and Lymphatic: Anemia, pure red cell aplasia, lymphadenopathy, splenomegaly.
Hepatic and Pancreatic: Lactic acidosis and steatosis, pancreatitis, posttreatment exacerbation of hepatitis (see WARNINGS and PRECAUTIONS).
Hypersensitivity: Anaphylaxis, urticaria.
Musculoskeletal: Rhabdomyolysis.
Nervous: Paresthesia, peripheral neuropathy.
Respiratory: Abnormal breath sounds/wheezing.
Skin: Alopecia, pruritus, rash.

OVERDOSAGE

There is no known antidote for EPIVIR-HBV. One case of an adult ingesting 6 g of EPIVIR was reported; there were no clinical signs or symptoms noted and hematologic tests remained normal. It is not known whether lamivudine can be removed by peritoneal dialysis or hemodialysis.

DOSAGE AND ADMINISTRATION

Adults: The recommended oral dose of EPIVIR-HBV for treatment of chronic hepatitis B in adults is 100 mg once daily (see paragraph below and WARNINGS). Safety and effectiveness of treatment beyond 1 year have not been established and the optimum duration of treatment is not known (see PRECAUTIONS).

The formulation and dosage of lamivudine in EPIVIR-HBV are not appropriate for patients dually infected with HBV and HIV. If lamivudine is administered to such patients, the higher dosage indicated for HIV therapy should be used as part of an appropriate combination regimen, and the prescribing information for EPIVIR as well as EPIVIR-HBV should be consulted.

Continued on next page

Epivir-HBV—Cont.

Pediatric Patients: The recommended oral dose of EPIVIR-HBV for pediatric patients 2 to 17 years of age with chronic hepatitis B is 3 mg/kg once daily up to a maximum daily dose of 100 mg. Safety and effectiveness of treatment beyond 1 year have not been established and the optimum duration of treatment is not known (see PRECAUTIONS).
EPIVIR-HBV is available in a 5-mg/mL oral solution when a liquid formulation is needed. (Please see information above regarding distinctions between different lamivudine-containing products.)
Dose Adjustment: It is recommended that doses of EPIVIR-HBV be adjusted in accordance with renal function (Table 8) (see CLINICAL PHARMACOLOGY: Special Populations).

Table 8: Adjustment of Adult Dosage of EPIVIR-HBV in Accordance With Creatinine Clearance

Creatinine Clearance (mL/min)	Recommended Dosage of EPIVIR-HBV
≥50	100 mg once daily
30-49	100 mg first dose, then 50 mg once daily
15-29	100 mg first dose, then 25 mg once daily
5-14	35 mg first dose, then 15 mg once daily
<5	35 mg first dose, then 10 mg once daily

Although there are insufficient data to recommend a specific dose adjustment of EPIVIR-HBV in pediatric patients with renal impairment, a dose reduction should be considered.
No additional dosing of EPIVIR-HBV is required after routine (4-hour) hemodialysis. Insufficient data are available to recommend a dosage of EPIVIR-HBV in patients undergoing peritoneal dialysis (see CLINICAL PHARMACOLOGY: Special Populations).

HOW SUPPLIED

EPIVIR-HBV Tablets, 100 mg, are butterscotch-colored, film-coated, biconvex, capsule-shaped tablets imprinted with "GX CG5" on one side.
Bottles of 60 tablets (NDC 0173-0662-00) with child-resistant closures.
Store at 25°C (77°F), excursions permitted to 15° to 30°C (59° to 86°F) [see USP Controlled Room Temperature].
EPIVIR-HBV Oral Solution, a clear, colorless to pale yellow, strawberry-banana-flavored liquid, contains 5 mg of lamivudine in each 1 mL in plastic bottles of 240 mL.
Bottles of 240 mL (NDC 0173-0663-00) with child-resistant closures. This product does not require reconstitution.
Store at controlled room temperature of 20° to 25°C (68° to 77°F) (see USP) in tightly closed bottles.

REFERENCES

1. Knodell RG, Ishak KG, Black WC, et al. Formulation and application of a numerical scoring system for assessing histological activity in asymptomatic chronic active hepatitis. *Hepatology*. 1982;1:431-435.

GlaxoSmithKline, Research Triangle Park, NC 27709
Manufactured under agreement from
Shire Pharmaceuticals Group plc, Basingstoke, UK

August 2001/RL-986

FLOVENT® 44 mcg ℞
[flō' vĕnt]
(fluticasone propionate, 44 mcg)
Inhalation Aerosol

FLOVENT® 110 mcg ℞
(fluticasone propionate, 110 mcg)
Inhalation Aerosol

FLOVENT® 220 mcg ℞
(fluticasone propionate, 220 mcg)
Inhalation Aerosol

For Oral Inhalation Only

Prescribing information for these products, which appears on pages 1535–1537 of the 2002 PDR, has been revised as follows. Please write "See Supplement A" next to the product heading.
The **ADVERSE REACTIONS: Observed During Clinical Practice** *subsection was revised to:*
In addition to adverse experiences reported from clinical trials, the following experiences have been identified during postapproval use of fluticasone propionate. Because they are reported voluntarily from a population of unknown size, estimates of frequency cannot be made. These experiences have been chosen for inclusion due to either their seriousness, frequency of reporting, causal connection to fluticasone propionate or a combination of these factors.
Ear, Nose, and Throat: Aphonia, facial and oropharyngeal edema, hoarseness, laryngitis, and throat soreness and irritation.
Endocrine and Metabolic: Cushingoid features, growth velocity reduction in children/adolescents, hyperglycemia, osteoporosis, and weight gain.
Eye: Cataracts.
Psychiatry: Agitation, aggression, depression, and restlessness.
Respiratory: Asthma exacerbation, bronchospasm, chest tightness, cough, dyspnea, immediate bronchospasm, paradoxical bronchospasm, pneumonia, and wheeze.
Skin: Contusions, ecchymoses, and pruritus.
Eosinophilic Conditions: In rare cases, patients on inhaled fluticasone propionate may present with systemic eosinophilic conditions, with some patients presenting with clinical features of vasculitis consistent with Churg-Strauss syndrome, a condition that is often treated with systemic corticosteroid therapy. These events usually, but not always, have been associated with the reduction and/or withdrawal of oral corticosteroid therapy following the introduction of fluticasone propionate. Cases of serious eosinophilic conditions have also been reported with other inhaled corticosteroids in this clinical setting. Physicians should be alert to eosinophilia, vasculitic rash, worsening pulmonary symptoms, cardiac complications, and/or neuropathy presenting in their patients. A causal relationship between fluticasone propionate and these underlying conditions has not been established (see PRECAUTIONS: Eosinophilic Conditions).
GlaxoSmithKline, Research Triangle Park, NC 27709

September 2001/RL-978

FLOVENT® ROTADISK® 50 mcg ℞
[flō' vĕnt]
(fluticasone propionate inhalation powder, 50 mcg)

FLOVENT® ROTADISK® 100 mcg ℞
(fluticasone propionate inhalation powder, 100 mcg)

FLOVENT® ROTADISK® 250 mcg ℞
(fluticasone propionate inhalation powder, 250 mcg)

For Oral Inhalation Only
For Use With the DISKHALER® Inhalation Device

Prescribing information for these products, which appears on pages 1537–1541 of the 2002 PDR, has been revised as follows. Please write "See Supplement A" next to the product heading.
The **ADVERSE REACTIONS: Observed During Clinical Practice** *subsection was revised to:*
In addition to adverse experiences reported from clinical trials, the following experiences have been identified during postapproval use of fluticasone propionate in clinical practice. Because they are reported voluntarily from a population of unknown size, estimates of frequency cannot be made. These events have been chosen for inclusion due to either their seriousness, frequency of reporting, or causal connection to fluticasone propionate or a combination of these factors.
Ear, Nose, and Throat: Aphonia, facial and oropharyngeal edema, hoarseness, and throat soreness and irritation.
Endocrine and Metabolic: Cushingoid features, growth velocity reduction in children/adolescents, hyperglycemia, osteoporosis, and weight gain.
Eye: Cataracts.
Psychiatry: Agitation, aggression, depression, and restlessness.
Respiratory: Asthma exacerbation, bronchospasm, chest tightness, cough, immediate bronchospasm, paradoxical bronchospasm, pneumonia, and wheeze.
Skin: Contusions, ecchymoses, and pruritus.
Eosinophilic Conditions: In rare cases, patients on inhaled fluticasone propionate may present with systemic eosinophilic conditions, with some patients presenting with clinical features of vasculitis consistent with Churg-Strauss syndrome, a condition that is often treated with systemic corticosteroid therapy. These events usually, but not always, have been associated with the reduction and/or withdrawal of oral corticosteroid therapy following the introduction of fluticasone propionate. Cases of serious eosinophilic conditions have also been reported with other inhaled corticosteroids in this clinical setting. Physicians should be alert to eosinophilia, vasculitic rash, worsening pulmonary symptoms, cardiac complications, and/or neuropathy presenting in their patients. A causal relationship between fluticasone propionate and these underlying conditions has not been established (see PRECAUTIONS: Eosinophilic Conditions).
GlaxoSmithKline, Research Triangle Park, NC 27709

September 2001/RL-971

HYCAMTIN® ℞
[hī-kam' tin]
brand of topotecan hydrochloride
for Injection
(for intravenous use)

Prescribing information for this product, which appears on pages 1546–1549 of the 2002 PDR, has been revised as follows. Please write "See Supplement A" next to the product heading.
The following subsection was added to **PRECAUTIONS:**
Information for Patients: As with other chemotherapeutic agents, *Hycamtin* may cause asthenia or fatigue; if these symptoms occur, caution should be observed when driving or operating machinery.
The first paragraph of the **DOSAGE AND ADMINISTRATION** *section was revised to:*
Prior to administration of the first course of *Hycamtin,* patients must have a baseline neutrophil count of >1500 cells/mm^3 and a platelet count of >100,000 cells/mm^3. The recommended dose of Hycamtin (topotecan hydrochloride) is 1.5 mg/m^2 by intravenous infusion over 30 minutes daily for 5 consecutive days, starting on day 1 of a 21-day course. In the absence of tumor progression, a minimum of four courses is recommended because tumor response may be delayed. The median time to response in three ovarian clinical trials was 9 to 12 weeks and median time to response in four small cell lung cancer trials was 5 to 7 weeks. In the event of severe neutropenia during any course, the dose should be reduced by 0.25 mg/m^2 for subsequent courses. Doses should be similarly reduced if the platelet count falls below 25,000 cells/mm^3. Alternatively, in the event of severe neutropenia, G-CSF may be administered following the subsequent course (before resorting to dose reduction) starting from day 6 of the course (24 hours after completion of topotecan administration).
GlaxoSmithKline, Research Triangle Park, NC 27709

November 2001/HY:L12

INFANRIX® ℞
[in' fan-rix]
Diphtheria and Tetanus Toxoids and Acellular Pertussis Vaccine Adsorbed

Prescribing information for this product, which appears on pages 1562–1567 of the 2002 PDR, has been revised as follows. Please write "See Supplement A" next to the product heading.
The fifth paragraph of the **DESCRIPTION** *section was revised as follows to delete thimerosal as a component of the early stages of manufacturing:*
Each 0.5 mL dose also contains 2.5 mg 2-phenoxyethanol as a preservative, 4.5 mg sodium chloride, water for injection and not more than 0.02% (w/v) residual formaldehyde.
The **STORAGE** *section was revised to:*
Store *Infanrix* refrigerated between 2° and 8°C (36° and 46°F). **Do not freeze.** Discard if the vaccine has been frozen. Do not use after expiration date shown on the label.
The **HOW SUPPLIED** *section was revised to:*
Infanrix (Diptheria and Tetanus Toxoids and Acellular Pertussis Vaccine Adsorbed) is supplied as a turbid white suspension in vials and prefilled syringes containing a 0.5 mL single dose.
Single-Dose Vials
NDC 58160-840-11 (package of 10)
Single-Dose Prefilled Disposable Tip-Lok® Syringes (packaged without needles)
NDC 58160-840-50 (package of 25)
Manufactured by GlaxoSmithKline Biologicals
Rixensart, Belgium, U.S. License 1090, and
Chiron Behring GmbH & Co
Marburg, Germany, U.S. License 0097
Distributed by GlaxoSmithKline
Research Triangle Park, NC 27709
Infanrix is a registered trademark of GlaxoSmithKline.
December 2001/IN:L6

LEUKERAN® ℞
[lū 'kūh-răn]
(chlorambucil)
Tablets

Prescribing information for this product, which appears on pages 1591–1592 of the 2002 PDR, has been completely revised as follows. Please write "See Supplement A" next to the product heading.

> **WARNING**
> LEUKERAN (chlorambucil) can severely suppress bone marrow function. Chlorambucil is a carcinogen in humans. Chlorambucil is probably mutagenic and teratogenic in humans. Chlorambucil produces human infertility (see WARNINGS and PRECAUTIONS).

DESCRIPTION

LEUKERAN (chlorambucil) was first synthesized by Everett et al. It is a bifunctional alkylating agent of the nitrogen mustard type that has been found active against selected human neoplastic diseases. Chlorambucil is known chemically as 4-[bis(2-chlorethyl)amino]benzenebutanoic acid.
Chlorambucil hydrolyzes in water and has a pKa of 5.8.
LEUKERAN (chlorambucil) is available in tablet form for oral administration. Each film-coated tablet contains 2 mg chlorambucil and the inactive ingredients colloidal silicon dioxide, hypromellose, lactose (anhydrous), macrogol/PEG 400, microcrystalline cellulose, red iron oxide, stearic acid, titanium dioxide, and yellow iron oxide.

CLINICAL PHARMACOLOGY

Chlorambucil is rapidly and completely absorbed from the gastrointestinal tract. After single oral doses of 0.6 to 1.2 mg/kg, peak plasma chlorambucil levels (C_{max}) are reached within 1 hour and the terminal elimination half-life ($t_{1/2}$) of the parent drug is estimated at 1.5 hours. Chlorambucil undergoes rapid metabolism to phenylacetic acid mustard, the major metabolite, and the combined chlorambucil and phenylacetic acid mustard urinary excretion is extremely low—less than 1% in 24 hours. In a study of 12 patients given single oral doses of 0.2 mg/kg of LEUKERAN, the mean dose (12 mg) adjusted (±SD) plasma chlorambucil C_{max} was 492 ± 160 ng/mL, the AUC was 883 ± 329 ng•h/mL, $t_{1/2}$ was 1.3 ± 0.5 hours, and the t_{max} was 0.83 ± 0.53 hours. For the major metabolite, phenylacetic acid mustard, the mean dose (12 mg) adjusted (±SD) plasma C_{max} was 306 ± 73 ng/mL, the AUC was 1204 ± 285 ng•h/mL, the $t_{1/2}$ was 1.8 ± 0.4 hours, and the t_{max} was 1.9 ± 0.7 hours.

Chlorambucil and its metabolites are extensively bound to plasma and tissue proteins. In vitro, chlorambucil is 99% bound to plasma proteins, specifically albumin. Cerebrospinal fluid levels of chlorambucil have not been determined. Evidence of human teratogenicity suggests that the drug crosses the placenta.

Chlorambucil is extensively metabolized in the liver primarily to phenylacetic acid mustard, which has antineoplastic activity. Chlorambucil and its major metabolite spontaneously degrade in vivo forming monohydroxy and dihydroxy derivatives. After a single dose of radiolabeled chlorambucil (^{14}C), approximately 15% to 60% of the radioactivity appears in the urine after 24 hours. Again, less than 1% of the urinary radioactivity is in the form of chlorambucil or phenylacetic acid mustard. In summary, the pharmacokinetic data suggest that oral chlorambucil undergoes rapid gastrointestinal absorption and plasma clearance and that it is almost completely metabolized, having extremely low urinary excretion.

INDICATIONS AND USAGE

LEUKERAN (chlorambucil) is indicated in the treatment of chronic lymphatic (lymphocytic) leukemia, malignant lymphomas including lymphosarcoma, giant follicular lymphoma, and Hodgkin's disease. It is not curative in any of these disorders but may produce clinically useful palliation.

CONTRAINDICATIONS

Chlorambucil should not be used in patients whose disease has demonstrated a prior resistance to the agent. Patients who have demonstrated hypersensitivity to chlorambucil should not be given the drug. There may be cross-hypersensitivity (skin rash) between chlorambucil and other alkylating agents.

WARNINGS

Because of its carcinogenic properties, chlorambucil should not be given to patients with conditions other than chronic lymphatic leukemia or malignant lymphomas. Convulsions, infertility, leukemia, and secondary malignancies have been observed when chlorambucil was employed in the therapy of malignant and non-malignant diseases.

There are many reports of acute leukemia arising in patients with both malignant and non-malignant diseases following chlorambucil treatment. In many instances, these patients also received other chemotherapeutic agents or some form of radiation therapy. The quantitation of the risk of chlorambucil-induction of leukemia or carcinoma in humans is not possible. Evaluation of published reports of leukemia developing in patients who have received chlorambucil (and other alkylating agents) suggests that the risk of leukemogenesis increases with both chronicity of treatment and large cumulative doses. However, it has proved impossible to define a cumulative dose below which there is no risk of the induction of secondary malignancy. The potential benefits from chlorambucil therapy must be weighed on an individual basis against the possible risk of the induction of a secondary malignancy.

Chlorambucil has been shown to cause chromatid or chromosome damage in humans. Both reversible and permanent sterility have been observed in both sexes receiving chlorambucil.

A high incidence of sterility has been documented when chlorambucil is administered to prepubertal and pubertal males. Prolonged or permanent azoospermia has also been observed in adult males. While most reports of gonadal dysfunction secondary to chlorambucil have related to males, the induction of amenorrhea in females with alkylating agents is well documented and chlorambucil is capable of producing amenorrhea. Autopsy studies of the ovaries from women with malignant lymphoma treated with combination chemotherapy including chlorambucil have shown varying degrees of fibrosis, vasculitis, and depletion of primordial follicles.

Rare instances of skin rash progressing to erythema multiforme, toxic epidermal necrolysis, or Stevens-Johnson syndrome have been reported. Chlorambucil should be discontinued promptly in patients who develop skin reactions.

Pregnancy: Pregnancy Category D. Chlorambucil can cause fetal harm when administered to a pregnant woman. Unilateral renal agenesis has been observed in 2 offspring whose mothers received chlorambucil during the first trimester. Urogenital malformations, including absence of a kidney, were found in fetuses of rats given chlorambucil. There are no adequate and well-controlled studies in pregnant women. If this drug is used during pregnancy, or if the patient becomes pregnant while taking this drug, the patient should be apprised of the potential hazard to the fetus. Women of childbearing potential should be advised to avoid becoming pregnant.

PRECAUTIONS

General: Many patients develop a slowly progressive lymphopenia during treatment. The lymphocyte count usually rapidly returns to normal levels upon completion of drug therapy. Most patients have some neutropenia after the third week of treatment and this may continue for up to 10 days after the last dose. Subsequently, the neutrophil count usually rapidly returns to normal. Severe neutropenia appears to be related to dosage and usually occurs only in patients who have received a total dosage of 6.5 mg/kg or more in one course of therapy with continuous dosing. About one quarter of all patients receiving the continuous-dose schedule, and one third of those receiving this dosage in 8 weeks or less may be expected to develop severe neutropenia.

While it is not necessary to discontinue chlorambucil at the first evidence of a fall in neutrophil count, it must be remembered that the fall may continue for 10 days after the last dose, and that as the total dose approaches 6.5 mg/kg, there is a risk of causing irreversible bone marrow damage. The dose of chlorambucil should be decreased if leukocyte or platelet counts fall below normal values and should be discontinued for more severe depression.

Chlorambucil should **not** be given at full dosages before 4 weeks after a full course of radiation therapy or chemotherapy because of the vulnerability of the bone marrow to damage under these conditions. If the pretherapy leukocyte or platelet counts are depressed from bone marrow disease process prior to institution of therapy, the treatment should be instituted at a reduced dosage.

Persistently low neutrophil and platelet counts or peripheral lymphocytosis suggest bone marrow infiltration. If confirmed by bone marrow examination, the daily dosage of chlorambucil should not exceed 0.1 mg/kg. Chlorambucil appears to be relatively free from gastrointestinal side effects or other evidence of toxicity apart from the bone marrow depressant action. In humans, single oral doses of 20 mg or more may produce nausea and vomiting.

Children with nephrotic syndrome and patients receiving high pulse doses of chlorambucil may have an increased risk of seizures. As with any potentially epileptogenic drug, caution should be exercised when administering chlorambucil to patients with a history of seizure disorder or head trauma, or who are receiving other potentially epileptogenic drugs.

Information for Patients: Patients should be informed that the major toxicities of chlorambucil are related to hypersensitivity, drug fever, myelosuppression, hepatotoxicity, infertility, seizures, gastrointestinal toxicity, and secondary malignancies. Patients should never be allowed to take the drug without medical supervision and should consult their physician if they experience skin rash, bleeding, fever, jaundice, persistent cough, seizures, nausea, vomiting, amenorrhea, or unusual lumps/masses. Women of childbearing potential should be advised to avoid becoming pregnant.

Laboratory Tests: Patients must be followed carefully to avoid life-endangering damage to the bone marrow during treatment. Weekly examination of the blood should be made to determine hemoglobin levels, total and differential leukocyte counts, and quantitative platelet counts. Also, during the first 3 to 6 weeks of therapy, it is recommended that white blood cell counts be made 3 or 4 days after each of the weekly complete blood counts. Galton et al have suggested that in following patients it is helpful to plot the blood counts on a chart at the same time that body weight, temperature, spleen size, etc., are recorded. It is considered dangerous to allow a patient to go more than 2 weeks without hematological and clinical examination during treatment.

Drug Interactions: There are no known drug/drug interactions with chlorambucil.

Carcinogenesis, Mutagenesis, Impairment of Fertility: See WARNINGS section for information on carcinogenesis, mutagenesis, and impairment of fertility.

Pregnancy: ***Teratogenic Effects:*** Pregnancy Category D: See WARNINGS section.

Nursing Mothers: It is not known whether this drug is excreted in human milk. Because many drugs are excreted in human milk and because of the potential for serious adverse reactions in nursing infants from chlorambucil, a decision should be made whether to discontinue nursing or to discontinue the drug, taking into account the importance of the drug to the mother.

Pediatric Use: The safety and effectiveness in pediatric patients have not been established.

ADVERSE REACTIONS

Hematologic: The most common side effect is bone marrow suppression. Although bone marrow suppression frequently occurs, it is usually reversible if the chlorambucil is withdrawn early enough. However, irreversible bone marrow failure has been reported.

Gastrointestinal: Gastrointestinal disturbances such as nausea and vomiting, diarrhea, and oral ulceration occur infrequently.

CNS: Tremors, muscular twitching, myoclonia, confusion, agitation, ataxia, flaccid paresis, and hallucinations have been reported as rare adverse experiences to chlorambucil which resolve upon discontinuation of drug. Rare, focal and/or generalized seizures have been reported to occur in both children and adults at both therapeutic daily doses and pulse-dosing regimens, and in acute overdose (see PRECAUTIONS: General).

Dermatologic: Allergic reactions such as urticaria and angioneurotic edema have been reported following initial or subsequent dosing. Skin hypersensitivity (including rare reports of skin rash progressing to erythema multiforme, toxic epidermal necrolysis, and Stevens-Johnson syndrome) has been reported (see WARNINGS).

Miscellaneous: Other reported adverse reactions include: pulmonary fibrosis, hepatotoxicity and jaundice, drug fever, peripheral neuropathy, interstitial pneumonia, sterile cystitis, infertility, leukemia, and secondary malignancies (see WARNINGS).

OVERDOSAGE

Reversible pancytopenia was the main finding of inadvertent overdoses of chlorambucil. Neurological toxicity ranging from agitated behavior and ataxia to multiple grand mal seizures has also occurred. As there is no known antidote, the blood picture should be closely monitored and general supportive measures should be instituted, together with appropriate blood transfusions, if necessary. Chlorambucil is not dialyzable.

Oral LD_{50} single doses in mice are 123 mg/kg. In rats, a single intraperitoneal dose of 12.5 mg/kg of chlorambucil produces typical nitrogen-mustard effects; these include atrophy of the intestinal mucous membrane and lymphoid tissues, severe lymphopenia becoming maximal in 4 days, anemia, and thrombocytopenia. After this dose, the animals begin to recover within 3 days and appear normal in about a week, although the bone marrow may not become completely normal for about 3 weeks. An intraperitoneal dose of 18.5 mg/kg kills about 50% of the rats with development of convulsions. As much as 50 mg/kg has been given orally to rats as a single dose, with recovery. Such a dose causes bradycardia, excessive salivation, hematuria, convulsions, and respiratory dysfunction.

DOSAGE AND ADMINISTRATION

The usual oral dosage is 0.1 to 0.2 mg/kg body weight daily for 3 to 6 weeks as required. This usually amounts to 4 to 10 mg per day for the average patient. The entire daily dose may be given at one time. These dosages are for initiation of therapy or for short courses of treatment. The dosage must be carefully adjusted according to the response of the patient and must be reduced as soon as there is an abrupt fall in the white blood cell count. Patients with Hodgkin's disease usually require 0.2 mg/kg daily, whereas patients with other lymphomas or chronic lymphocytic leukemia usually require only 0.1 mg/kg daily. When lymphocytic infiltration of the bone marrow is present, or when the bone marrow is hypoplastic, the daily dose should not exceed 0.1 mg/kg (about 6 mg for the average patient).

Alternate schedules for the treatment of chronic lymphocytic leukemia employing intermittent, biweekly, or once-monthly pulse doses of chlorambucil have been reported. Intermittent schedules of chlorambucil begin with an initial single dose of 0.4 mg/kg. Doses are generally increased by 0.1 mg/kg until control of lymphocytosis or toxicity is observed. Subsequent doses are modified to produce mild hematologic toxicity. It is felt that the response rate of chronic lymphocytic leukemia to the biweekly or once-monthly schedule of chlorambucil administration is similar or better to that previously reported with daily administration and that hematologic toxicity was less than or equal to that encountered in studies using daily chlorambucil.

Radiation and cytotoxic drugs render the bone marrow more vulnerable to damage, and chlorambucil should be used with particular caution within 4 weeks of a full course of radiation therapy or chemotherapy. However, small doses of palliative radiation over isolated foci remote from the bone marrow will not usually depress the neutrophil and platelet count. In these cases chlorambucil may be given in the customary dosage.

It is presently felt that short courses of treatment are safer than continuous maintenance therapy, although both methods have been effective. It must be recognized that continuous therapy may give the appearance of "maintenance" in patients who are actually in remission and have no immediate need for further drug. If maintenance dosage is used, it should not exceed 0.1 mg/kg daily and may well be as low as 0.03 mg/kg daily. A typical maintenance dose is 2 mg to 4 mg daily, or less, depending on the status of the blood counts. It may, therefore, be desirable to withdraw the drug after maximal control has been achieved, since intermittent therapy reinstituted at time of relapse may be as effective as continuous treatment.

Procedures for proper handling and disposal of anticancer drugs should be considered. Several guidelines on this subject have been published.[1–7]

There is no general agreement that all of the procedures recommended in the guidelines are necessary or appropriate.

HOW SUPPLIED

Leukeran is supplied as brown, film-coated, round, biconvex tablets containing 2 mg chlorambucil in amber glass bottles with child-resistant closures. One side is engraved with "GX EG3" and the other side is engraved with an "L."

Bottle of 50 (NDC 0173-0635-35).

Store in a refrigerator, 2° to 8°C (36° to 46°F).

REFERENCES

1. Recommendations for the safe handling of parenteral antineoplastic drugs. Washington, DC: Division of Safety; National Institutes of Health; 1983. US Dept of Health and Human Services, Public Health Service publication NIH 83-2621.
2. AMA Council on Scientific Affairs. Guidelines for handling parenteral antineoplastics. *JAMA.* 1985;253:1590-1591.
3. National Study Commission on Cytotoxic Exposure. Recommendations for handling cytotoxic agents. 1987. Available from Louis P. Jeffrey, Chairman, National Study Commission on Cytotoxic Exposure. Massachusetts College of Pharmacy and Allied Health Sciences, 179 Longwood Avenue, Boston, MA 02115.

Continued on next page

Leukeran—Cont.

4. Clinical Oncological Society of Australia. Guidelines and recommendations for safe handling of antineoplastic agents. *Med J Australia*. 1983;1:426-428.
5. Jones RB, Frank R, Mass T. Safe handling of chemotherapeutic agents: a report from the Mount Sinai Medical Center. *CA-A Cancer J for Clin*. 1983;33:258-263.
6. American Society of Hospital Pharmacists. ASHP technical assistance bulletin on handling cytotoxic and hazardous drugs. *Am J Hosp Pharm*. 1990;47:1033-1049.
7. Controlling Occupational Exposure to Hazardous Drugs. (OSHA Work-Practice Guidelines.) *Am J Health-Syst Pharm*. 1996;53:1669-1685.

GlaxoSmithKline, Research Triangle Park, NC 27709

August 2001/RL-974

MALARONE™ ℞

[*mal' ə-rōn*]

(atovaquone and proguanil hydrochloride)

Tablets

MALARONE™ ℞

(atovaquone and proguanil hydrochloride)

Pediatric Tablets

Prescribing information for these products, which appears on pages 1596–1598 of the 2002 PDR, has been revised as follows. Please write "See Supplement A" next to the product heading.

The following pack was added to the **HOW SUPPLIED** *section:*

Unit Dose Pack of 24 (NDC 0173-0675-02).

GlaxoSmithKline, Research Triangle Park, NC 27709

September 2001/RL-998

NAVELBINE® ℞

[*na 'vəl-bēn*]

(vinorelbine tartrate)

Injection

Prescribing information for this product, which appears on pages 1604–1607 of the 2002 PDR, has been completely revised as follows. Please write "See Supplement A" next to the product heading.

WARNING: NAVELBINE (vinorelbine tartrate) Injection should be administered under the supervision of a physician experienced in the use of cancer chemotherapeutic agents. This product is for intravenous (IV) use only. Intrathecal administration of other vinca alkaloids has resulted in death. Syringes containing this product should be labeled "WARNING—FOR IV USE ONLY. FATAL if given intrathecally."

Severe granulocytopenia resulting in increased susceptibility to infection may occur. Granulocyte counts should be ≥1000 cells/mm^3 prior to the administration of NAVELBINE. The dosage should be adjusted according to complete blood counts with differentials obtained on the day of treatment. Caution—It is extremely important that the intravenous needle or catheter be properly positioned before NAVELBINE is injected. Administration of NAVELBINE may result in extravasation causing local tissue necrosis and/or thrombophlebitis (see DOSAGE AND ADMINISTRATION: Administration Precautions).

DESCRIPTION

NAVELBINE (vinorelbine tartrate) Injection is for intravenous administration. Each vial contains vinorelbine tartrate equivalent to 10 mg (1-mL vial) or 50 mg (5-mL vial) vinorelbine in Water for Injection. No preservatives or other additives are present. The aqueous solution is sterile and nonpyrogenic.

Vinorelbine tartrate is a semi-synthetic vinca alkaloid with antitumor activity. The chemical name is 3′,4′-didehydro-4′-deoxy-C′-norvincaleukoblastine [*R*-(*R**,*R**)-2,3-dihydroxybutanedioate (1:2)(salt)].

Vinorelbine tartrate is a white to yellow or light brown amorphous powder with the molecular formula $C_{45}H_{54}N_4O_8 \bullet 2C_4H_6O_6$ and molecular weight of 1079.12. The aqueous solubility is >1000 mg/mL in distilled water. The pH of NAVELBINE Injection is approximately 3.5.

CLINICAL PHARMACOLOGY

Vinorelbine is a vinca alkaloid that interferes with microtubule assembly. The vinca alkaloids are structurally similar compounds comprised of 2 multiringed units, vindoline and catharanthine. Unlike other vinca alkaloids, the catharanthine unit is the site of structural modification for vinorelbine. The antitumor activity of vinorelbine is thought to be due primarily to inhibition of mitosis at metaphase through its interaction with tubulin. Like other vinca alkaloids, vinorelbine may also interfere with: 1) amino acid, cyclic AMP, and glutathione metabolism, 2) calmodulin-dependent Ca^{++}-transport ATPase activity, 3) cellular respiration, and 4) nucleic acid and lipid biosynthesis. In intact tectal plates from mouse embryos, vinorelbine, vincristine, and vinblastine inhibited mitotic microtubule formation at the same concentration (2 μM), inducing a blockade of cells at metaphase. Vincristine produced depolymerization of axonal microtubules at 5 μM, but vinblastine and vinorelbine did not have this effect until concentrations of 30 μM and 40 μM, respectively. These data suggest relative selectivity of vinorelbine for mitotic microtubules.

Pharmacokinetics: The pharmacokinetics of vinorelbine were studied in 49 patients who received doses of 30 mg/m^2 in 4 clinical trials. Doses were administered by 15- to 20-minute constant-rate infusions. Following intravenous administration, vinorelbine concentration in plasma decays in a triphasic manner. The initial rapid decline primarily represents distribution of drug to peripheral compartments followed by metabolism and excretion of the drug during subsequent phases. The prolonged terminal phase is due to relatively slow efflux of vinorelbine from peripheral compartments. The terminal phase half-life averages 27.7 to 43.6 hours and the mean plasma clearance ranges from 0.97 to 1.26 L/h per kg. Steady-state volume of distribution (V_{ss}) values range from 25.4 to 40.1 L/kg.

Vinorelbine demonstrated high binding to human platelets and lymphocytes. The free fraction was approximately 0.11 in pooled human plasma over a concentration range of 234 to 1169 ng/mL. The binding to plasma constituents in cancer patients ranged from 79.6% to 91.2%. Vinorelbine binding was not altered in the presence of cisplatin, 5-fluorouracil, or doxorubicin.

Vinorelbine undergoes substantial hepatic elimination in humans, with large amounts recovered in feces after intravenous administration to humans. Two metabolites of vinorelbine have been identified in human blood, plasma, and urine; vinorelbine N-oxide and deacetylvinorelbine. Deacetylvinorelbine has been demonstrated to be the primary metabolite of vinorelbine in humans, and has been shown to possess antitumor activity similar to vinorelbine. Therapeutic doses of NAVELBINE (30 mg/m^2) yield very small, if any, quantifiable levels of either metabolite in blood or urine. The metabolism of vinca alkaloids has been shown to be mediated by hepatic cytochrome P450 isoenzymes in the CYP3A subfamily. This metabolic pathway may be impaired in patients with hepatic dysfunction or who are taking concomitant potent inhibitors of these isoenzymes (see PRECAUTIONS). The effects of renal or hepatic dysfunction on the disposition of vinorelbine have not been assessed, but based on experience with other anticancer vinca alkaloids, dose adjustments are recommended for patients with impaired hepatic function (see DOSAGE AND ADMINISTRATION).

The disposition of radiolabeled vinorelbine given intravenously was studied in a limited number of patients. Approximately 18% and 46% of the administered dose was recovered in the urine and in the feces, respectively. Incomplete recovery in humans is consistent with results in animals where recovery is incomplete, even after prolonged sampling times. A separate study of the urinary excretion of vinorelbine using specific chromatographic analytical methodology showed that 10.9% ± 0.7% of a 30-mg/m^2 intravenous dose was excreted unchanged in the urine.

The influence of age on the pharmacokinetics of vinorelbine was examined using data from 44 cancer patients (average age, 56.7 ± 7.8 years; range, 41 to 74 years; with 12 patients ≥60 years and 6 patients ≥65 years) in 3 studies. CL (the mean plasma clearance), $t_{1/2}$ (the terminal phase half-life), and V_Z (the volume of distribution during terminal phase) were independent of age. A separate pharmacokinetic study was conducted in 10 elderly patients with metastatic breast cancer (age range, 66 to 81 years; 3 patients >75 years; normal liver function tests) receiving vinorelbine 30 mg/m^2 intravenously. CL, V_{ss}, and $t_{1/2}$ were similar to those reported for younger adult patients in previous studies. No relationship between age, systemic exposure ($AUC_{0-\infty}$), and hematological toxicity was observed.

The pharmacokinetics of vinorelbine are not influenced by the concurrent administration of cisplatin with NAVELBINE (see PRECAUTIONS: Drug Interactions).

Clinical Trials: Data from 1 randomized clinical study (211 evaluable patients) with single-agent NAVELBINE and 2 randomized clinical trials (1044 patients) using NAVELBINE combined with cisplatin support the use of NAVELBINE in patients with advanced nonsmall cell lung cancer (NSCLC).

Single-Agent NAVELBINE: Single-agent NAVELBINE was studied in a North American, randomized clinical trial in which patients with Stage IV NSCLC, no prior chemotherapy, and Karnofsky Performance Status ≥70 were treated with NAVELBINE (30 mg/m^2) weekly or 5-fluorouracil (5-FU) (425 mg/m^2 IV bolus) plus leucovorin (LV) (20 mg/m^2 IV bolus) daily for 5 days every 4 weeks. A total of 211 patients were randomized at a 2:1 ratio to NAVELBINE (143) or 5-FU/LV (68). NAVELBINE showed improved survival time compared to 5-FU/LV. In an intent-to-treat analysis, the median survival time was 30 weeks versus 22 weeks for patients receiving NAVELBINE versus 5-FU/LV, respectively (*P* = 0.06). The 1-year survival rates were 24% (±4% SE) for NAVELBINE and 16% (±5% SE) for the 5-FU/LV group, using the Kaplan-Meier product-limit estimates. The median survival time with 5-FU/LV was similar to or slightly better than that usually observed in untreated patients with advanced NSCLC, suggesting that the difference was not related to some unknown detrimental effect of 5-FU/LV therapy. The response rates (all partial responses) for NAVELBINE and 5-FU/LV were 12% and 3%, respectively.

NAVELBINE in Combination with Cisplatin: NAVELBINE plus Cisplatin versus Single-Agent Cisplatin: A Phase III open-label, randomized study was conducted which compared NAVELBINE (25 mg/m^2 per week) plus cisplatin (100 mg/m^2 every 4 weeks) to single-agent cisplatin (100 mg/m^2 every 4 weeks) in patients with Stage IV or Stage IIIb NSCLC patients with malignant pleural effusion or multiple lesions in more than one lobe who were not previously treated with chemotherapy. Patients included in the study had a performance status of 0 or 1, and 34% had received prior surgery and/or radiotherapy. Characteristics of the 432 randomized patients are provided in Table 1. Two hundred and twelve patients received NAVELBINE plus cisplatin and 210 received single-agent cisplatin. The primary objective of this trial was to compare survival between the 2 treatment groups. Survival (Figure 1) for patients receiving NAVELBINE plus cisplatin was significantly better compared to the patients who received single-agent cisplatin. The results of this trial are summarized in Table 1.

NAVELBINE plus Cisplatin versus Vindesine plus Cisplatin versus Single-Agent NAVELBINE: In a large European clinical trial, 612 patients with Stage III or IV NSCLC, no prior chemotherapy, and WHO Performance Status of 0, 1, or 2 were randomized to treatment with single-agent

Table 1: Randomized Clinical Trials of NAVELBINE in Combination with Cisplatin in NSCLC

	NAVELBINE/Cisplatin vs. Single-Agent Cisplatin		NAVELBINE/Cisplatin vs. Vindesine/Cisplatin vs. Single-Agent NAVELBINE		
	NAVELBINE/ Cisplatin	Cisplatin	NAVELBINE/ Cisplatin	Vindesine/ Cisplatin	NAVELBINE
Demographics					
Number of patients	214	218	206	200	206
Number of males	146	141	182	179	188
Number of females	68	77	24	21	18
Median age (years)	63	64	59	59	60
Range (years)	33-84	37-81	32-75	31-75	30-74
Stage of disease					
Stage IIIA	NA	NA	11%	11%	10%
Stage IIIB	8%	8%	28%	25%	32%
Stage IV	92%	92%	50%	55%	47%
Local recurrence	NA	NA	2%	3%	3%
Metastatic after surgery	NA	NA	9%	8%	9%
Histology					
Adenocarcinoma	54%	52%	32%	40%	28%
Squamous	19%	22%	56%	50%	56%
Large cell	14%	14%	13%	11%	16%
Unspecified	13%	13%	NA	NA	NA
Results					
Median survival (months)	7.8	6.2	9.2*†	7.4	7.2
P value	*P* = 0.01		**P* = 0.09 vs. vindesine/cisplatin; † = 0.05 vs. single-agent NAVELBINE		
12-Month survival rate	38%	22%	35%	27%	30%
Overall response	19%	8%	28%‡§	19%	14%
P value	*P* < 0.001		‡*P* = 0.03 vs. vindesine/cisplatin; §*P*<0.001 vs. single-agent NAVELBINE		

NAVELBINE (30 mg/m^2 per week), NAVELBINE (30 mg/m^2 per week) plus cisplatin (120 mg/m^2 days 1 and 29, then every 6 weeks), and vindesine (3 mg/m^2 per week for 7 weeks, then every other week) plus cisplatin (120 mg/m^2 days 1 and 29, then every 6 weeks). Patient characteristics are provided in Table 1. Survival was longer in patients treated with NAVELBINE plus cisplatin compared to those treated with vindesine plus cisplatin (Figure 2). Study results are summarized in Table 1.

Dose-Ranging Study: A dose-ranging study of NAVELBINE (20, 25, or 30 mg/m^2 per week) plus cisplatin (120 mg/m^2 days 1 and 29, then every 6 weeks) in 32 patients with NSCLC demonstrated a median survival of 10.2 months. There were no responses at the lowest dose level; the response rate was 33% in the 21 patients treated at the 2 highest dose levels.

[See table at top of previous page]

Figure 1: Overall Survival NAVELBINE/Cisplatin versus Single-Agent Cisplatin

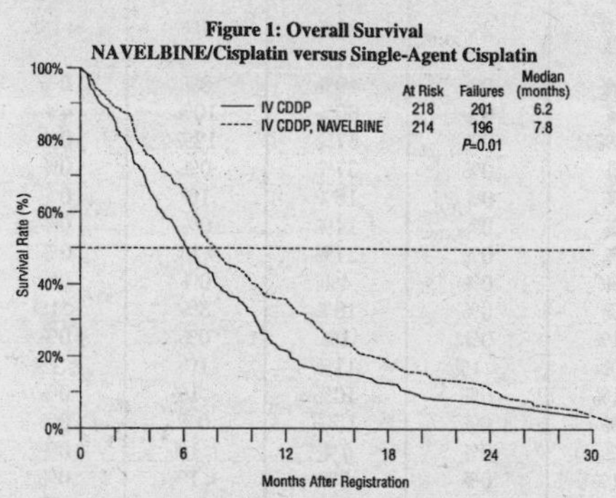

Figure 2: Overall Survival NAVELBINE/Cisplatin versus Vindesine/Cisplatin versus Single-Agent NAVELBINE

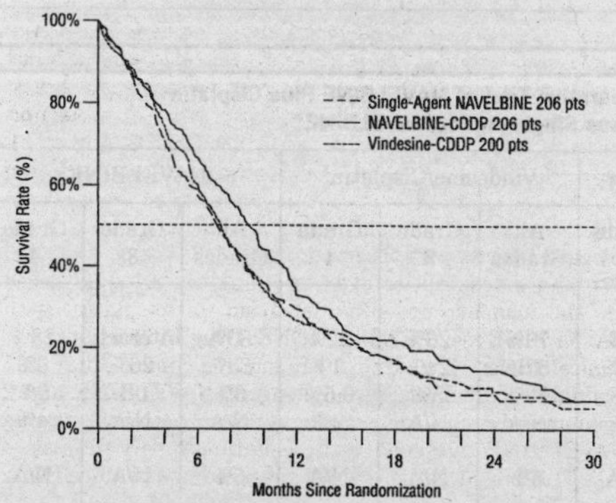

Table 2: Summary of Adverse Events in 365 Patients Receiving Single-Agent NAVELBINE*†

Adverse Event		All Patients (n = 365)	NSCLC (n = 143)
Bone Marrow			
Granulocytopenia	<2000 cells/mm^3	90%	80%
	<500 cells/mm^3	36%	29%
Leukopenia	<4000 cells/mm^3	92%	81%
	<1000 cells/mm^3	15%	12%
Thrombocytopenia	<100,000 cells/mm^3	5%	4%
	<50,000 cells/mm^3	1%	1%
Anemia	<11 g/dL	83%	77%
	<8 g/dL	9%	1%
Hospitalizations due to granulocytopenic complications		9%	8%

Adverse Event	All Grades		Grade 3		Grade 4	
	All Patients	NSCLC	All Patients	NSCLC	All Patients	NSCLC
Clinical Chemistry Elevations						
Total Bilirubin (n = 351)	13%	9%	4%	3%	3%	2%
SGOT (n = 346)	67%	54%	5%	2%	1%	1%
General						
Asthenia	36%	27%	7%	5%	0%	0%
Injection Site Reactions	28%	38%	2%	5%	0%	0%
Injection Site Pain	16%	13%	2%	1%	0%	0%
Phlebitis	7%	10%	<1%	1%	0%	0%
Digestive						
Nausea	44%	34%	2%	1%	0%	0%
Vomiting	20%	15%	2%	1%	0%	0%
Constipation	35%	29%	3%	2%	0%	0%
Diarrhea	17%	13%	1%	1%	0%	0%
Peripheral Neuropathy‡	25%	20%	1%	1%	<1%	0%
Dyspnea	7%	3%	2%	2%	1%	0%
Alopecia	12%	12%	≤1%	1%	0%	0%

* None of the reported toxicities were influenced by age. Grade based on modified criteria from the National Cancer Institute.

† Patients with NSCLC had not received prior chemotherapy. The majority of the remaining patients had received prior chemotherapy.

‡ Incidence of paresthesia plus hypesthesia.

INDICATIONS AND USAGE

NAVELBINE is indicated as a single agent or in combination with cisplatin for the first-line treatment of ambulatory patients with unresectable, advanced nonsmall cell lung cancer (NSCLC). In patients with Stage IV NSCLC, NAVELBINE is indicated as a single agent or in combination with cisplatin. In Stage III NSCLC, NAVELBINE is indicated in combination with cisplatin.

CONTRAINDICATIONS

Administration of NAVELBINE is contraindicated in patients with pretreatment granulocyte counts <1000 cells/mm^3 (see WARNINGS).

WARNINGS

NAVELBINE should be administered in carefully adjusted doses by or under the supervision of a physician experienced in the use of cancer chemotherapeutic agents.

Patients treated with NAVELBINE should be frequently monitored for myelosuppression both during and after therapy. Granulocytopenia is dose-limiting. Granulocyte nadirs occur between 7 and 10 days after dosing with granulocyte count recovery usually within the following 7 to 14 days. Complete blood counts with differentials should be performed and results reviewed prior to administering each dose of NAVELBINE. NAVELBINE should not be administered to patients with granulocyte counts <1000 cells/mm^3. Patients developing severe granulocytopenia should be monitored carefully for evidence of infection and/or fever. See DOSAGE AND ADMINISTRATION for recommended dose adjustments for granulocytopenia.

Acute shortness of breath and severe bronchospasm have been reported infrequently, following the administration of NAVELBINE and other vinca alkaloids, most commonly when the vinca alkaloid was used in combination with mitomycin. These adverse events may require treatment with supplemental oxygen, bronchodilators, and/or corticosteroids, particularly when there is pre-existing pulmonary dysfunction.

Reported cases of interstitial pulmonary changes and acute respiratory distress syndrome (ARDS), most of which were fatal, occurred in patients treated with single-agent NAVELBINE. The mean time to onset of these symptoms after vinorelbine administration was 1 week (range 3 to 8 days). Patients with alterations in their baseline pulmonary symptoms or with new onset of dyspnea, cough, hypoxia, or other symptoms should be evaluated promptly.

NAVELBINE has been reported to cause severe constipation (e.g., Grade 3–4), paralytic ileus, intestinal obstruction, necrosis, and/or perforation. Some events have been fatal.

Pregnancy: Pregnancy Category D. NAVELBINE may cause fetal harm if administered to a pregnant woman. A single dose of vinorelbine has been shown to be embryo- and/or fetotoxic in mice and rabbits at doses of 9 mg/m^2 and 5.5 mg/m^2, respectively (one third and one sixth the human dose). At nonmaternotoxic doses, fetal weight was reduced and ossification was delayed. There are no studies in pregnant women. If NAVELBINE is used during pregnancy, or if the patient becomes pregnant while receiving this drug, the patient should be apprised of the potential hazard to the fetus. Women of childbearing potential should be advised to avoid becoming pregnant during therapy with NAVELBINE.

PRECAUTIONS

General: Most drug-related adverse events of NAVELBINE are reversible. If severe adverse events occur, NAVELBINE should be reduced in dosage or discontinued and appropriate corrective measures taken. Reinstitution of therapy with NAVELBINE should be carried out with caution and alertness as to possible recurrence of toxicity.

NAVELBINE should be used with extreme caution in patients whose bone marrow reserve may have been compromised by prior irradiation or chemotherapy, or whose marrow function is recovering from the effects of previous chemotherapy (see DOSAGE AND ADMINISTRATION).

Administration of NAVELBINE to patients with prior radiation therapy may result in radiation recall reactions (see ADVERSE REACTIONS and Drug Interactions).

Patients with a prior history or pre-existing neuropathy, regardless of etiology, should be monitored for new or worsening signs and symptoms of neuropathy while receiving NAVELBINE.

Care must be taken to avoid contamination of the eye with concentrations of NAVELBINE used clinically. Severe irritation of the eye has been reported with accidental exposure to another vinca alkaloid. If exposure occurs, the eye should immediately be thoroughly flushed with water.

Information for Patients: Patients should be informed that the major acute toxicities of NAVELBINE are related to bone marrow toxicity, specifically granulocytopenia with increased susceptibility to infection. They should be advised to report fever or chills immediately. Women of childbearing potential should be advised to avoid becoming pregnant during treatment. Patients should be advised to contact their physician if they experience increased shortness of breath, cough, or other new pulmonary symptoms, or if they experience symptoms of abdominal pain or constipation.

Laboratory Tests: Since dose-limiting clinical toxicity is the result of depression of the white blood cell count, it is imperative that complete blood counts with differentials be obtained and reviewed on the day of treatment prior to each dose of NAVELBINE (see ADVERSE REACTIONS: Hematologic).

Hepatic: There is no evidence that the toxicity of NAVELBINE is enhanced in patients with elevated liver enzymes. No data are available for patients with severe baseline cholestasis, but the liver plays an important role in the metabolism of NAVELBINE. Because clinical experience in patients with severe liver disease is limited, caution should be exercised when administering NAVELBINE to patients with severe hepatic injury or impairment (see DOSAGE AND ADMINISTRATION).

Drug Interactions: Acute pulmonary reactions have been reported with NAVELBINE and other anticancer vinca alkaloids used in conjunction with mitomycin. Although the pharmacokinetics of vinorelbine are not influenced by the concurrent administration of cisplatin, the incidence of granulocytopenia with NAVELBINE used in combination with cisplatin is significantly higher than with single-agent NAVELBINE. Patients who receive NAVELBINE and paclitaxel, either concomitantly or sequentially, should be monitored for signs and symptoms of neuropathy. Administration of NAVELBINE to patients with prior or concomitant radiation therapy may result in radiosensitizing effects.

Caution should be exercised in patients concurrently taking drugs known to inhibit drug metabolism by hepatic cytochrome P450 isoenzymes in the CYP3A subfamily, or in patients with hepatic dysfunction. Concurrent administration of vinorelbine tartrate with an inhibitor of this metabolic pathway may cause an earlier onset and/or an increased severity of side effects.

Carcinogenesis, Mutagenesis, Impairment of Fertility: The carcinogenic potential of NAVELBINE has not been studied. Vinorelbine has been shown to affect chromosome number and possibly structure in vivo (polyploidy in bone marrow cells from Chinese hamsters and a positive micronucleus test in mice). It was not mutagenic in the Ames test and gave inconclusive results in the mouse lymphoma TK Locus assay. The significance of these or other short-term test results for human risk is unknown. Vinorelbine did not affect fertility to a statistically significant extent when administered to rats on either a once-weekly (9 mg/m^2, approximately one third the human dose) or alternate-day schedule (4.2 mg/m^2, approximately one seventh the human dose) prior to and during mating. However, biweekly administration for 13 or 26 weeks in the rat at 2.1 and 7.2 mg/m^2 (approximately one fifteenth and one fourth the human dose) resulted in decreased spermatogenesis and prostate/seminal vesicle secretion.

Pregnancy: Pregnancy Category D. See WARNINGS section.

Nursing Mothers: It is not known whether the drug is excreted in human milk. Because many drugs are excreted in human milk and because of the potential for serious adverse reactions in nursing infants from NAVELBINE, it is recommended that nursing be discontinued in women who are receiving therapy with NAVELBINE.

Pediatric Use: Safety and effectiveness in pediatric patients have not been established.

Geriatric Use: Of the total number of patients in North American clinical studies of IV NAVELBINE, approximately one third were 65 years of age or greater. No overall differences in effectiveness or safety were observed between

Continued on next page

Navelbine—Cont.

Table 3: Selected Adverse Events From a Comparative Trial of NAVELBINE plus Cisplatin versus Single-Agent Cisplatin*

	NAVELBINE 25 mg/m² plus Cisplatin 100 mg/m² (n = 212)			Cisplatin 100 mg/m² (n = 210)		
Adverse Event	All Grades	Grade 3	Grade 4	All Grades	Grade 3	Grade 4
Bone Marrow						
Granulocytopenia	89%	22%	60%	26%	4%	1%
Anemia	88%	21%	3%	72%	7%	<1%
Leukopenia	88%	39%	19%	31%	<1%	0%
Thrombocytopenia	29%	4%	1%	21%	1%	<1%
Febrile neutropenia	N/A	N/A	11%	N/A	N/A	0%
Hepatic						
Elevated transaminase	1%	0%	0%	<1%	<1%	0%
Renal						
Elevated creatinine	37%	2%	2%	28%	4%	<1%
Non-Laboratory						
Malaise/fatigue/lethargy	67%	12%	0%	49%	8%	0%
Vomiting	60%	7%	6%	60%	10%	4%
Nausea	58%	14%	0%	57%	12%	0%
Anorexia	46%	0%	0%	37%	0%	0%
Constipation	35%	3%	0%	16%	1%	0%
Alopecia	34%	0%	0%	14%	0%	0%
Weight loss	34%	1%	0%	21%	<1%	0%
Fever without infection	20%	2%	0%	4%	0%	0%
Hearing	18%	4%	0%	18%	3%	<1%
Local (injection site reactions)	17%	<1%	0%	1%	0%	0%
Diarrhea	17%	2%	<1%	11%	1%	<1%
Paresthesias	17%	<1%	0%	10%	<1%	0%
Taste alterations	17%	0%	0%	15%	0%	0%
Peripheral numbness	11%	2%	0%	7%	<1%	0%
Myalgia/arthralgia	12%	<1%	0%	3%	<1%	0%
Phlebitis/thrombosis/embolism	10%	3%	0%	<1%	0%	<1%
Weakness	12%	2%	<1%	7%	2%	0%
Dizziness/vertigo	9%	<1%	0%	3%	<1%	0%
Infection	11%	5%	<1%	<1%	<1%	0%
Respiratory infection	10%	4%	<1%	3%	3%	0%

*Graded according to the standard SWOG criteria.

Table 4: Selected Adverse Events From a Comparative Trial of NAVELBINE Plus Cisplatin versus Vindesine Plus Cisplatin versus Single-Agent NAVELBINE*

	NAVELBINE/Cisplatin†			Vindesine/Cisplatin‡			NAVELBINE§		
Adverse Event	All Grades	Grade 3	Grade 4	All Grades	Grade 3	Grade 4	All Grades	Grade 3	Grade 4
Bone Marrow									
Neutropenia	95%	20%	58%	79%	26%	22%	85%	25%	28%
Leukopenia	94%	40%	17%	82%	24%	3%	83%	26%	6%
Thrombocytopenia	15%	3%	1%	10%	3%	0.5%	3%	0%	0%
Febrile neutropenia	N/A	N/A	4%	N/A	N/A	2%	N/A	N/A	4%
Hepatic									
Elevated bilirubin‖	6%	N/A	N/A	5%	N/A	N/A	5%	N/A	N/A
Renal									
Elevated creatinine‖	46%	N/A	N/A	37%	N/A	N/A	13%	N/A	N/A
Non-Laboratory									
Nausea/vomiting	74%	27%	3%	72%	24%	1%	31%	1%	1%
Alopecia	51%	7%	0.5%	56%	14%	0%	30%	2%	0%
Ototoxicity	10%	1%	1%	14%	1%	0%	1%	0%	0%
Local reactions	17%	2%	0.5%	7%	0%	0%	22%	2%	0%
Diarrhea	25%	1.5%	0%	24%	1%	0%	12%	0%	0.5%
Neurotoxicity¶	44%	7%	0%	58%	16%	1%	44%	8%	0.5%

*Grade based on criteria from the World Health Organization (WHO).
†n = 194 to 207; all patients receiving NAVELBINE/cisplatin with laboratory and non-laboratory data.
‡n = 173 to 192; all patients receiving vindesine/cisplatin with laboratory and non-laboratory data.
§n = 165 to 201; all patients receiving NAVELBINE with laboratory and non-laboratory data.
‖ Categorical toxicity grade not specified.
¶Neurotoxicity includes peripheral neuropathy and constipation.

these patients and younger adult patients. Other reported clinical experience has not identified differences in responses between the elderly and younger adult patients, but greater sensitivity of some older individuals cannot be ruled out.
The pharmacokinetics of vinorelbine in elderly and younger adult patients are similar (see CLINICAL PHARMACOLOGY).

ADVERSE REACTIONS

The pattern of adverse reactions is similar whether NAVELBINE is used as a single agent or in combination. Adverse reactions from studies with single-agent and combination use of NAVELBINE are summarized in Tables 2–4.
Single-Agent NAVELBINE: Data in the following table are based on the experience of 365 patients (143 patients with NSCLC; 222 patients with advanced breast cancer) treated with IV NAVELBINE as a single agent in 3 clinical studies. The dosing schedule in each study was 30 mg/m² NAVELBINE on a weekly basis.
[See table 2 at top of previous page]
Hematologic: Granulocytopenia is the major dose-limiting toxicity with NAVELBINE. Dose adjustments are required for hematologic toxicity and hepatic insufficiency (see DOSAGE AND ADMINISTRATION). Granulocytopenia was generally reversible and not cumulative over time. Granulocyte nadirs occurred 7 to 10 days after the dose, with granulocyte recovery usually within the following 7 to 14 days. Granulocytopenia resulted in hospitalizations for fever and/or sepsis in 8% of patients. Septic deaths occurred in approximately 1% of patients. Prophylactic hematologic growth factors have not been routinely used with NAVELBINE. If medically necessary, growth factors may be administered at recommended doses no earlier than 24 hours after the administration of cytotoxic chemotherapy. Growth factors should not be administered in the period 24 hours before the administration of chemotherapy.
Whole blood and/or packed red blood cells were administered to 18% of patients who received NAVELBINE.
Neurologic: Loss of deep tendon reflexes occurred in less than 5% of patients. The development of severe peripheral neuropathy was infrequent (1%) and generally reversible.
Skin: Like other anticancer vinca alkaloids, NAVELBINE is a moderate vesicant. Injection site reactions, including erythema, pain at injection site, and vein discoloration, occurred in approximately one third of patients; 5% were severe. Chemical phlebitis along the vein proximal to the site of injection was reported in 10% of patients.
Gastrointestinal: Prophylactic administration of antiemetics was not routine in patients treated with single-agent NAVELBINE. Due to the low incidence of severe nausea and vomiting with single-agent NAVELBINE, the use of serotonin antagonists is generally not required.
Hepatic: Transient elevations of liver enzymes were reported without clinical symptoms.
Cardiovascular: Chest pain was reported in 5% of patients. Most reports of chest pain were in patients who had either a history of cardiovascular disease or tumor within the chest. There have been rare reports of myocardial infarction.
Pulmonary: Shortness of breath was reported in 3% of patients; it was severe in 2% (see WARNINGS). Interstitial pulmonary changes were documented.
Other: Fatigue occurred in 27% of patients. It was usually mild or moderate but tended to increase with cumulative dosing.
Other toxicities that have been reported in less than 5% of patients include jaw pain, myalgia, arthralgia, and rash. Hemorrhagic cystitis and the syndrome of inappropriate ADH secretion were each reported in <1% of patients.
Combination Use: Adverse events for combination use are summarized in Tables 3 and 4.
NAVELBINE in Combination with Cisplatin:
NAVELBINE plus Cisplatin versus Single-Agent Cisplatin (Table 3): Myelosuppression was the predominant toxicity in patients receiving combination therapy, Grade 3 and 4 granulocytopenia of 82% compared to 5% in the single-agent cisplatin arm. Fever and/or sepsis related to granulocytopenia occurred in 11% of patients on NAVELBINE and cisplatin compared to 0% on the cisplatin arm.
Four patients on the combination died of granulocytopenia-related sepsis. During this study, the use of granulocyte colony-stimulating factor ([G-CSF] filgrastim) was permitted, but not mandated, after the first course of treatment for patients who experienced Grade 3 or 4 granulocytopenia (≤1000 cells/mm³) or in those who developed neutropenic fever between cycles of chemotherapy. Beginning 24 hours after completion of chemotherapy, G-CSF was started at a dose of 5 mcg/kg per day and continued until the total granulocyte count was >1000 cells/mm³ on 2 successive determinations. G-CSF was not administered on the day of treatment.
Grade 3 and 4 anemia occurred more frequently in the combination arm compared to control, 24% vs. 8%, respectively. Thrombocytopenia occurred in 6% of patients treated with NAVELBINE plus cisplatin compared to 2% of patients treated with cisplatin.
The incidence of severe non-hematologic toxicity was similar among the patients in both treatment groups. Patients receiving NAVELBINE plus cisplatin compared to single-agent cisplatin experienced more Grade 3 and/or 4 peripheral numbness (2% vs. <1%), phlebitis/thrombosis/embolism (3% vs. <1%), and infection (6% vs. <1%). Grade 3–4 constipation and/or ileus occurred in 3% of patients treated with combination therapy and in 1% of patients treated with cisplatin.
Seven deaths were reported on the combination arm; 2 were related to cardiac ischemia, 1 massive cerebrovascular accident, 1 multisystem failure due to an overdose of NAVELBINE, and 3 from febrile neutropenia. One death, secondary to respiratory infection unrelated to granulocytopenia, occurred with single-agent cisplatin.
NAVELBINE plus Cisplatin versus Vindesine plus Cisplatin versus Single-Agent NAVELBINE (Table 4): Myelosuppression, specifically Grade 3 and 4 granulocytopenia, was significantly greater with the combination of NAVELBINE plus cisplatin (79%) than with either single-agent NAVELBINE (53%) or vindesine plus cisplatin (48%), $P<0.0001$. Hospitalization due to documented sepsis occurred in 4.4% of patients treated with NAVELBINE plus cisplatin; 2% of patients treated with vindesine and cisplatin, and 4% of patients treated with single-agent NAVELBINE. Grade 3 and 4 thrombocytopenia was infrequent in patients receiving combination chemotherapy and no events were reported with single-agent NAVELBINE.
The incidence of Grade 3 and/or 4 nausea and vomiting, alopecia, and renal toxicity were reported more frequently in the cisplatin-containing combinations compared to single-agent NAVELBINE. Severe local reactions occurred in 2% of patients treated with combinations containing NAVELBINE; none were observed in the vindesine plus cisplatin arm. Grade 3 and 4 neurotoxicity was significantly more frequent in patients receiving vindesine plus cisplatin (17%) compared to NAVELBINE plus cisplatin (7%) and single-agent NAVELBINE (9%) ($P < 0.005$). Cisplatin did not appear to increase the incidence of neurotoxicity observed with single-agent NAVELBINE.
[See table 3 above]
[See table 4 above]
Observed During Clinical Practice: In addition to the adverse events reported from clinical trials, the following events have been identified during post-approval use of NAVELBINE. Because they are reported voluntarily from a population of unknown size, estimates of frequency cannot be made. These events have been chosen for inclusion due to a combination of their seriousness, frequency of reporting, or potential causal connection to NAVELBINE.
Body as a Whole: Systemic allergic reactions reported as anaphylaxis, pruritus, urticaria, and angioedema; flushing; and radiation recall events such as dermatitis and esophagitis (see PRECAUTIONS) have been reported.
Hematologic: Thromboembolic events, including pulmonary embolus and deep venous thrombosis, have been reported primarily in seriously ill and debilitated patients with known predisposing risk factors for these events.
Neurologic: Peripheral neurotoxicities such as, but not limited to, muscle weakness and disturbance of gait, have been observed in patients with and without prior symptoms. There may be increased potential for neurotoxicity in patients with pre-existing neuropathy, regardless of etiology, who receive NAVELBINE. Vestibular and auditory deficits have been observed with NAVELBINE, usually when used in combination with cisplatin.
Skin: Injection site reactions, including localized rash and urticaria, blister formation, and skin sloughing have been

observed in clinical practice. Some of these reactions may be delayed in appearance.

Gastrointestinal: Dysphagia, mucositis, and pancreatitis have been reported.

Cardiovascular: Hypertension, hypotension, vasodilation, tachycardia, and pulmonary edema have been reported.

Pulmonary: Pneumonia has been reported.

Musculoskeletal: Headache has been reported, with and without other musculoskeletal aches and pains.

Other: Pain in tumor-containing tissue, back pain, and abdominal pain have been reported. Electrolyte abnormalities, including hyponatremia with or without the syndrome of inappropriate ADH secretion, have been reported in seriously ill and debilitated patients.

Combination Use: Patients with prior exposure to paclitaxel and who have demonstrated neuropathy should be monitored closely for new or worsening neuropathy. Patients who have experienced neuropathy with previous drug regimens should be monitored for symptoms of neuropathy while receiving NAVELBINE. NAVELBINE may result in radiosensitizing effects with prior or concomitant radiation therapy (see PRECAUTIONS).

OVERDOSAGE

There is no known antidote for overdoses of NAVELBINE. Overdoses involving quantities up to 10 times the recommended dose (30 mg/m^2) have been reported. The toxicities described were consistent with those listed in the ADVERSE REACTIONS section including paralytic ileus, stomatitis, and esophagitis. Bone marrow aplasia, sepsis, and paresis have also been reported. Fatalities have occurred following overdose of NAVELBINE. If overdosage occurs, general supportive measures together with appropriate blood transfusions, growth factors, and antibiotics should be instituted as deemed necessary by the physician.

DOSAGE AND ADMINISTRATION

Single-Agent NAVELBINE: The usual initial dose of single-agent NAVELBINE is 30 mg/m^2 administered weekly. The recommended method of administration is an intravenous injection over 6 to 10 minutes. In controlled trials, single-agent NAVELBINE was given weekly until progression or dose-limiting toxicity.

NAVELBINE in Combination with Cisplatin: NAVELBINE may be administered weekly at a dose of 25 mg/m^2 in combination with cisplatin given every 4 weeks at a dose of 100 mg/m^2.

Blood counts should be checked weekly to determine whether dose reductions of NAVELBINE and/or cisplatin are necessary. In the SWOG study, most patients required a 50% dose reduction of NAVELBINE at day 15 of each cycle and a 50% dose reduction of cisplatin by cycle 3.

NAVELBINE may also be administered weekly at a dose of 30 mg/m^2 in combination with cisplatin, given on days 1 and 29, then every 6 weeks at a dose of 120 mg/m^2.

Dose Modifications for NAVELBINE: The dosage should be adjusted according to hematologic toxicity or hepatic insufficiency, whichever results in the lower dose for the corresponding starting dose of NAVELBINE (see Table 5).

Dose Modifications for Hematologic Toxicity: Granulocyte counts should be ≥1000 cells/mm^3 prior to the administration of NAVELBINE. Adjustments in the dosage of NAVELBINE should be based on granulocyte counts obtained on the day of treatment according to Table 5.

Table 5: Dose Adjustments Based on Granulocyte Counts

Granulocytes on Day of Treatment (cells/mm^3)	Percentage of Starting Dose of NAVELBINE
≥1500	100%
1000 to 1499	50%
<1000	Do not administer. Repeat granulocyte count in 1 week. If 3 consecutive weekly doses are held because granulocyte count is <1000 cells/mm^3, discontinue NAVELBINE.

Note: For patients who, during treatment with NAVELBINE experienced fever and/or sepsis while granulocytopenic or had 2 consecutive weekly doses held due to granulocytopenia, subsequent doses of NAVELBINE should be:

≥1500	75%
1000 to 1499	37.5%
<1000	See above

Dose Modifications for Hepatic Insufficiency: NAVELBINE should be administered with caution to patients with hepatic insufficiency. In patients who develop hyperbilirubinemia during treatment with NAVELBINE, the dose should be adjusted for total bilirubin according to Table 6.

Table 6: Dose Modification Based on Total Bilirubin

Total Bilirubin (mg/dL)	Percentage of Starting Dose of NAVELBINE
≤2.0	100%
2.1 to 3.0	50%
>3.0	25%

Dose Modifications for Concurrent Hematologic Toxicity and Hepatic Insufficiency: In patients with both hematologic toxicity and hepatic insufficiency, the lower of the doses based on the corresponding starting dose of NAVELBINE determined from Table 5 and Table 6 should be administered.

Dose Modifications for Renal Insufficiency: No dose adjustments for NAVELBINE are required for renal insufficiency. Appropriate dose reductions for cisplatin should be made when NAVELBINE is used in combination.

Dose Modifications for Neurotoxicity: If Grade ≥2 neurotoxicity develops, NAVELBINE should be discontinued.

Administration Precautions: Caution—NAVELBINE must be administered intravenously. It is extremely important that the intravenous needle or catheter be properly positioned before any NAVELBINE is injected. Leakage into surrounding tissue during intravenous administration of NAVELBINE may cause considerable irritation, local tissue necrosis, and/or thrombophlebitis. If extravasation occurs, the injection should be discontinued immediately, and any remaining portion of the dose should then be introduced into another vein. Since there are no established guidelines for the treatment of extravasation injuries with NAVELBINE, institutional guidelines may be used. The *ONS Chemotherapy Guidelines* provide additional recommendations for the prevention of extravasation injuries.[1]

As with other toxic compounds, caution should be exercised in handling and preparing the solution of NAVELBINE. Skin reactions may occur with accidental exposure. The use of gloves is recommended. If the solution of NAVELBINE contacts the skin or mucosa, immediately wash the skin or mucosa thoroughly with soap and water. Severe irritation of the eye has been reported with accidental contamination of the eye with another vinca alkaloid. If this happens with NAVELBINE, the eye should be flushed with water immediately and thoroughly.

Procedures for proper handling and disposal of anticancer drugs should be used. Several guidelines on this subject have been published.[2–8] There is no general agreement that all of the procedures recommended in the guidelines are necessary or appropriate.

NAVELBINE Injection is a clear, colorless to pale yellow solution. Parenteral drug products should be visually inspected for particulate matter and discoloration prior to administration whenever solution and container permit. If particulate matter is seen, NAVELBINE should not be administered.

Preparation for Administration: NAVELBINE Injection must be diluted in either a syringe or IV bag using one of the recommended solutions. The diluted NAVELBINE should be administered over 6 to 10 minutes into the side port of a free-flowing IV **closest to the IV bag** followed by flushing with at least 75 to 125 mL of one of the solutions. Diluted NAVELBINE may be used for up to 24 hours under normal room light when stored in polypropylene syringes or polyvinyl chloride bags at 5° to 30°C (41° to 86°F).

Syringe: The calculated dose of NAVELBINE should be diluted to a concentration between 1.5 and 3.0 mg/mL. The following solutions may be used for dilution:

5% Dextrose Injection, USP

0.9% Sodium Chloride Injection, USP

IV Bag: The calculated dose of NAVELBINE should be diluted to a concentration between 0.5 and 2 mg/mL. The following solutions may be used for dilution:

5% Dextrose Injection, USP

0.9% Sodium Chloride Injection, USP

0.45% Sodium Chloride Injection, USP

5% Dextrose and 0.45% Sodium Chloride Injection, USP

Ringer's Injection, USP

Lactated Ringer's Injection, USP

Stability: Unopened vials of NAVELBINE are stable until the date indicated on the package when stored under refrigeration at 2° to 8°C (36° to 46°F) and protected from light in the carton. Unopened vials of NAVELBINE are stable at temperatures up to 25°C (77°F) for up to 72 hours. This product should not be frozen.

HOW SUPPLIED

NAVELBINE Injection is a clear, colorless to pale yellow solution in Water for Injection, containing 10 mg vinorelbine per mL. NAVELBINE Injection is available in single-use, clear glass vials with elastomeric stoppers and royal blue caps, individually packaged in a carton in the following vial sizes:

10 mg/1 mL Single-Use Vial, Carton of 1 (NDC 0173-0656-01).

50 mg/5 mL Single-Use Vial, Carton of 1 (NDC 0173-0656-44).

Store the vials under refrigeration at 2° to 8°C (36° to 46°F) in the carton. Protect from light. DO NOT FREEZE.

REFERENCES

1. ONS Clinical Practice Committee. Cancer Chemotherapy Guidelines and Recommendations for Practice. Pittsburgh, Pa: Oncology Nursing Society; 1999:32–41.
2. Recommendations for the safe handling of parenteral antineoplastic drugs. Washington, DC: Division of Safety, National Institutes of Health; 1983. US Dept of Health and Human Services, Public Health Service publication NIH 83–2621.
3. AMA Council on Scientific Affairs. Guidelines for handling parenteral antineoplastics. *JAMA*. 1985;253: 1590–1591.
4. National Study Commission on Cytotoxic Exposure. Recommendations for handling cytotoxic agents. 1987. Available from Louis P. Jeffrey, Chairman, National Study Commission on Cytotoxic Exposure. Massachusetts College of Pharmacy and Allied Health Sciences, 179 Longwood Avenue, Boston, MA 02115.
5. Clinical Oncological Society of Australia. Guidelines and recommendations for safe handling of antineoplastic agents. *Med J Australia*. 1983;1:426–428.
6. Jones RB, Frank R, Mass T. Safe handling of chemotherapeutic agents: a report from the Mount Sinai Medical Center. *CA-A Cancer J for Clin*. 1983;33:258–263.
7. American Society of Hospital Pharmacists. ASHP technical assistance bulletin on handling cytotoxic and hazardous drugs. *Am J Hosp Pharm*. 1990;47:1033–1049.
8. Controlling Occupational Exposure to Hazardous Drugs. (OSHA Work-Practice Guidelines.) *Am J Health-Syst Pharm*. 1996;53:1669–1685.

Manufactured by Pierre Fabre Médicament Production
64320 Idron, FRANCE
for GlaxoSmithKline, Research Triangle Park, NC 27709
Under license of Pierre Fabre Médicament -
Centre National de la Recherche Scientifique-France

October 2001/RL-1010

PARNATE® ℞

[*par' nāt*]
brand of tranylcypromine sulfate
tablets 10 mg

Prescribing information for this product, which appears on pages 1607–1609 of the 2002 PDR, has been revised as follows. Please write "See Supplement A" next to the product heading.

The following subsections of **CONTRAINDICATIONS** *were revised:*

3. In combination with MAO inhibitors or with dibenzazepine-related entities

Parnate (tranylcypromine sulfate) should not be administered together or in rapid succession with other MAO inhibitors or with dibenzazepine-related entities. Hypertensive crises or severe convulsive seizures may occur in patients receiving such combinations.

In patients being transferred to *Parnate* from another MAO inhibitor or from a dibenzazepine-related entity, allow a medication-free interval of at least a week, then initiate *Parnate* using half the normal starting dosage for at least the first week of therapy. Similarly, at least a week should elapse between the discontinuance of *Parnate* and the administration of another MAO inhibitor or a dibenzazepine-related entity, or the readministration of *Parnate*.

The following list includes some other MAO inhibitors, dibenzazepine-related entities and tricyclic antidepressants, and the companies which market them.

Other MAO Inhibitors

Generic Name	Source
Furazolidone	
Isocarboxazid	Marplan® (Oxford Pharm Services)
Pargyline HCl	
Pargyline HCl and methyclothiazide	
Phenelzine sulfate	Nardil® (Parke-Davis)
Procarbazine HCl	Matulane® (Sigma Tau)

Dibenzazepine-Related and Other Tricyclics

Generic Name	Source
Amitriptyline HCl	Elavil® (Zeneca)
Perphenazine and amitriptyline HCl	Etrafon® (Schering) Triavil® (Lotus Biochemical)
Clomipramine hydrochloride	Anafranil® (Geneva)
Desipramine HCl	Norpramin® (Aventis)
Imipramine HCl	Janimine™ (Geneva) Tofranil® (Novartis) (Geneva)
Nortriptyline HCl	Pamelor® (Mallinckrodt)
Protriptyline HCl	Vivactil® (Merck & Co., Inc.)
Doxepin HCL	Sinequan® (Pfizer)
Carbamazepine	Tegretol® (Novartis)
Cyclobenzaprine HCl	Flexeril® (Merck & Co., Inc.)
Amoxapine	(Geneva)
Maprotiline HCl	(Mylan)
Trimipramine maleate	Surmontil® (Wyeth-Ayerst Pharmaceuticals)

4. In combination with bupropion

The concurrent administration of a MAO inhibitor and buproprion hydrochloride (Wellbutrin®, Wellbutrin SR®, Zyban®, GlaxoSmithKline) is contraindicated. At least 14

Continued on next page

Parnate—Cont.

days should elapse between discontinuation of a MAO inhibitor and initiation of treatment with bupropion hydrochloride.

5. In combination with dexfenfluramine hydrochloride

Because dexfenfluramine hydrochloride is a serotonin releaser and reuptake inhibitor, it should not be used concomitantly with Parnate (tranylcypromine sulfate).

6. In combination with selective serotonin reuptake inhibitors (SSRIs)

As a general rule, *Parnate* should not be administered in combination with any SSRI. There have been reports of serious, sometimes fatal, reactions (including hyperthermia, rigidity, myoclonus, autonomic instability with possible rapid fluctuations of vital signs, and mental status changes that include extreme agitation progressing to delirium and coma) in patients receiving fluoxetine (Prozac®, Eli Lilly and Company) in combination with a monoamine oxidase inhibitor (MAOI), and in patients who have recently discontinued fluoxetine and are then started on a MAOI. Some cases presented with features resembling neuroleptic malignant syndrome. Therefore, fluoxetine and other SSRIs should not be used in combination with a MAOI, or within 14 days of discontinuing therapy with a MAOI. Since fluoxetine and its major metabolite have very long elimination half-lives, at least 5 weeks should be allowed after stopping fluoxetine before starting a MAOI.

At least 2 weeks should be allowed after stopping sertraline (Zoloft®, Pfizer) or paroxetine (Paxil®, GlaxoSmithKline) before starting a MAOI.

8. In combination with sympathomimetics

Parnate (tranylcypromine sulfate) should not be administered in combination with sympathomimetics, including amphetamines, and over-the-counter drugs such as cold, hay fever or weight-reducing preparations that contain vasoconstrictors.

During *Parnate* therapy, it appears that certain patients are particularly vulnerable to the effects of sympathomimetics when the activity of certain enzymes is inhibited. Use of sympathomimetics and compounds such as guanethidine, methyldopa, reserpine, dopamine, levodopa and tryptophan with *Parnate* may precipitate hypertension, headache and related symptoms. The combination of MAOIs and tryptophan has been reported to cause behavioral and neurologic syndromes including disorientation, confusion, amnesia, delirium, agitation, hypomanic signs, ataxia, myoclonus, hyperreflexia, shivering, ocular oscillations and Babinski's signs.

The following paragraph in **ADVERSE REACTIONS** *was revised to add alopecia:*

Rare instances of hepatitis, skin rash and alopecia have been reported.

GlaxoSmithKline, Research Triangle Park, NC 27709

August 2001/PT:L65

PAXIL® ℞

[*pax'il*]

brand of paroxetine hydrochloride tablets and oral suspension

Prescribing information for these products, which appears on pages 1609–1615 of the 2002 PDR, has been completely revised as follows. Please write "See Supplement A" next to the product heading.

DESCRIPTION

Paxil (paroxetine hydrochloride) is an orally administered psychotropic drug. It is the hydrochloride salt of a phenylpiperidine compound identified chemically as (-)-*trans*-4*R*-(4'-fluorophenyl)-3*S*-[(3',4'-methylenedioxyphenoxy) methyl] piperidine hydrochloride hemihydrate and has the empirical formula of $C_{19}H_{20}FNO_3HCl \cdot 1/2H_2O$. The molecular weight is 374.8 (329.4 as free base).

Paroxetine hydrochloride is an odorless, off-white powder, having a melting point range of 120° to 138°C and a solubility of 5.4 mg/mL in water.

Tablets

Each film-coated tablet contains paroxetine hydrochloride equivalent to paroxetine as follows: 10 mg–yellow (scored); 20 mg–pink (scored); 30 mg–blue, 40 mg–green. Inactive ingredients consist of dibasic calcium phosphate dihydrate, hydroxypropyl methylcellulose, magnesium stearate, polyethylene glycols, polysorbate 80, sodium starch glycolate, titanium dioxide and one or more of the following: D&C Red No. 30, D&C Yellow No. 10, FD&C Blue No. 2, FD&C Yellow No. 6.

Suspension for Oral Administration

Each 5 mL of orange-colored, orange-flavored liquid contains paroxetine hydrochloride equivalent to paroxetine, 10 mg. Inactive ingredients consist of polacrilin potassium, microcrystalline cellulose, propylene glycol, glycerin, sorbitol, methyl paraben, propyl paraben, sodium citrate dihydrate, citric acid anhydrate, sodium saccharin, flavorings, FD&C Yellow No. 6 and simethicone emulsion, USP.

CLINICAL PHARMACOLOGY

Pharmacodynamics

The efficacy of paroxetine in the treatment of major depressive disorder, social anxiety disorder, obsessive compulsive disorder (OCD), panic disorder (PD), generalized anxiety disorder (GAD) and posttraumatic stress disorder (PTSD) is presumed to be linked to potentiation of serotonergic activity in the central nervous system resulting from inhibition of neuronal reuptake of serotonin (5-hydroxy-tryptamine, 5-HT). Studies at clinically relevant doses in humans have demonstrated that paroxetine blocks the uptake of serotonin into human platelets. *In vitro* studies in animals also suggest that paroxetine is a potent and highly selective inhibitor of neuronal serotonin reuptake and has only very weak effects on norepinephrine and dopamine neuronal reuptake. *In vitro* radioligand binding studies indicate that paroxetine has little affinity for muscarinic, alpha$_1$-, alpha$_2$-, beta-adrenergic-, dopamine (D_2)-, 5-HT$_1$-, 5-HT$_2$- and histamine (H_1)-receptors; antagonism of muscarinic, histaminergic and alpha$_1$-adrenergic receptors has been associated with various anticholinergic, sedative and cardiovascular effects for other psychotropic drugs.

Because the relative potencies of paroxetine's major metabolites are at most 1/50 of the parent compound, they are essentially inactive.

Pharmacokinetics

Paroxetine is equally bioavailable from the oral suspension and tablet.

Paroxetine hydrochloride is completely absorbed after oral dosing of a solution of the hydrochloride salt. In a study in which normal male subjects (n=15) received 30 mg tablets daily for 30 days, steady-state paroxetine concentrations were achieved by approximately 10 days for most subjects, although it may take substantially longer in an occasional patient. At steady state, mean values of C_{max}, T_{max}, C_{min} and $T_{1/2}$ were 61.7 ng/mL (CV 45%), 5.2 hr. (CV 10%), 30.7 ng/mL (CV 67%) and 21.0 hr. (CV 32%), respectively. The steady-state C_{max} and C_{min} values were about 6 and 14 times what would be predicted from single-dose studies. Steady-state drug exposure based on AUC_{0-24} was about 8 times greater than would have been predicted from single-dose data in these subjects. The excess accumulation is a consequence of the fact that one of the enzymes that metabolizes paroxetine is readily saturable.

In steady-state dose proportionality studies involving elderly and nonelderly patients, at doses of 20 to 40 mg daily for the elderly and 20 to 50 mg daily for the nonelderly, some nonlinearity was observed in both populations, again reflecting a saturable metabolic pathway. In comparison to C_{min} values after 20 mg daily, values after 40 mg daily were only about 2 to 3 times greater than doubled.

The effects of food on the bioavailability of paroxetine were studied in subjects administered a single dose with and without food. AUC was only slightly increased (6%) when drug was administered with food but the C_{max} was 29% greater, while the time to reach peak plasma concentration decreased from 6.4 hours post-dosing to 4.9 hours.

Paroxetine is extensively metabolized after oral administration. The principal metabolites are polar and conjugated products of oxidation and methylation, which are readily cleared. Conjugates with glucuronic acid and sulfate predominate, and major metabolites have been isolated and identified. Data indicate that the metabolites have no more than 1/50 the potency of the parent compound at inhibiting serotonin uptake. The metabolism of paroxetine is accomplished in part by cytochrome $P_{450}IID_6$. Saturation of this enzyme at clinical doses appears to account for the nonlinearity of paroxetine kinetics with increasing dose and increasing duration of treatment. The role of this enzyme in paroxetine metabolism also suggests potential drug-drug interactions (see PRECAUTIONS).

Approximately 64% of a 30 mg oral solution dose of paroxetine was excreted in the urine with 2% as the parent compound and 62% as metabolites over a 10-day post-dosing period. About 36% was excreted in the feces (probably via the bile), mostly as metabolites and less than 1% as the parent compound over the 10-day post-dosing period.

Distribution: Paroxetine distributes throughout the body, including the CNS, with only 1% remaining in the plasma.

Protein Binding: Approximately 95% and 93% of paroxetine is bound to plasma protein at 100 ng/mL and 400 ng/mL, respectively. Under clinical conditions, paroxetine concentrations would normally be less than 400 ng/mL. Paroxetine does not alter the *in vitro* protein binding of phenytoin or warfarin.

Renal and Liver Disease: Increased plasma concentrations of paroxetine occur in subjects with renal and hepatic impairment. The mean plasma concentrations in patients with creatinine clearance below 30 mL/min. was approximately 4 times greater than seen in normal volunteers. Patients with creatinine clearance of 30 to 60 mL/min. and patients with hepatic functional impairment had about a 2-fold increase in plasma concentrations (AUC, C_{max}).

The initial dosage should therefore be reduced in patients with severe renal or hepatic impairment, and upward titration, if necessary, should be at increased intervals (see DOSAGE AND ADMINISTRATION).

Elderly Patients: In a multiple-dose study in the elderly at daily paroxetine doses of 20, 30 and 40 mg, C_{min} concentrations were about 70% to 80% greater than the respective C_{min} concentrations in nonelderly subjects. Therefore the initial dosage in the elderly should be reduced (see DOSAGE AND ADMINISTRATION).

Clinical Trials

Major Depressive Disorder

The efficacy of Paxil (paroxetine hydrochloride) as a treatment for major depressive disorder has been established in 6 placebo-controlled studies of patients with major depressive disorder (ages 18 to 73). In these studies *Paxil* was shown to be significantly more effective than placebo in treating major depressive disorder by at least 2 of the following measures: Hamilton Depression Rating Scale (HDRS), the Hamilton depressed mood item, and the Clinical Global Impression (CGI)-Severity of Illness. Paxil (paroxetine hydrochloride) was significantly better than placebo in improvement of the HDRS sub-factor scores, including the depressed mood item, sleep disturbance factor and anxiety factor.

A study of outpatients with major depressive disorder who had responded to *Paxil* (HDRS total score <8) during an initial 8-week open-treatment phase and were then randomized to continuation on *Paxil* or placebo for 1 year demonstrated a significantly lower relapse rate for patients taking *Paxil* (15%) compared to those on placebo (39%). Effectiveness was similar for male and female patients.

Obsessive Compulsive Disorder

The effectiveness of *Paxil* in the treatment of obsessive compulsive disorder (OCD) was demonstrated in two 12-week multicenter placebo-controlled studies of adult outpatients (Studies 1 and 2). Patients in all studies had moderate to severe OCD (DSM-IIIR) with mean baseline ratings on the Yale Brown Obsessive Compulsive Scale (YBOCS) total score ranging from 23 to 26. Study 1, a dose-range finding study where patients were treated with fixed doses of 20, 40 or 60 mg of paroxetine/day demonstrated that daily doses of paroxetine 40 and 60 mg are effective in the treatment of OCD. Patients receiving doses of 40 and 60 mg paroxetine experienced a mean reduction of approximately 6 and 7 points, respectively, on the YBOCS total score which was significantly greater than the approximate 4 point reduction at 20 mg and a 3 point reduction in the placebo-treated patients. Study 2 was a flexible-dose study comparing paroxetine (20 to 60 mg daily) with clomipramine (25 to 250 mg daily). In this study, patients receiving paroxetine experienced a mean reduction of approximately 7 points on the YBOCS total score which was significantly greater than the mean reduction of approximately 4 points in placebo-treated patients.

The following table provides the outcome classification by treatment group on Global Improvement items of the Clinical Global Impression (CGI) scale for Study 1.

Outcome Classification (%) on CGI-Global Improvement Item for Completers in Study 1				
Outcome Classification	Placebo (n=74)	*Paxil* 20 mg (n=75)	*Paxil* 40 mg (n=66)	*Paxil* 60 mg (n=66)
Worse	14%	7%	7%	3%
No Change	44%	35%	22%	19%
Minimally Improved	24%	33%	29%	34%
Much Improved	11%	18%	22%	24%
Very Much Improved	7%	7%	20%	20%

Subgroup analyses did not indicate that there were any differences in treatment outcomes as a function of age or gender.

The long-term maintenance effects of *Paxil* in OCD were demonstrated in a long-term extension to Study 1. Patients who were responders on paroxetine during the 3-month double-blind phase and a 6-month extension on open-label paroxetine (20 to 60 mg/day) were randomized to either paroxetine or placebo in a 6-month double-blind relapse prevention phase. Patients randomized to paroxetine were significantly less likely to relapse than comparably treated patients who were randomized to placebo.

Panic Disorder

The effectiveness of *Paxil* in the treatment of panic disorder was demonstrated in three 10- to 12-week multicenter, placebo-controlled studies of adult outpatients (Studies 1-3). Patients in all studies had panic disorder (DSM-IIIR), with or without agoraphobia. In these studies, *Paxil* was shown to be significantly more effective than placebo in treating panic disorder by at least 2 out of 3 measures of panic attack frequency and on the Clinical Global Impression Severity of Illness score.

Study 1 was a 10-week dose-range finding study; patients were treated with fixed paroxetine doses of 10, 20, or 40 mg/day or placebo. A significant difference from placebo was observed only for the 40 mg/day group. At endpoint, 76% of patients receiving paroxetine 40 mg/day were free of panic attacks, compared to 44% of placebo-treated patients.

Study 2 was a 12-week flexible-dose study comparing paroxetine (10 to 60 mg daily) and placebo. At endpoint, 51% of paroxetine patients were free of panic attacks compared to 32% of placebo-treated patients.

Study 3 was a 12-week flexible-dose study comparing paroxetine (10 to 60 mg daily) to placebo in patients concurrently receiving standardized cognitive behavioral therapy. At endpoint, 33% of the paroxetine-treated patients showed a reduction to 0 or 1 panic attacks compared to 14% of placebo patients.

In both Studies 2 and 3, the mean paroxetine dose for completers at endpoint was approximately 40 mg/day of paroxetine.

Long-term maintenance effects of *Paxil* in panic disorder were demonstrated in an extension to Study 1. Patients who were responders during the 10-week double-blind phase and during a 3-month double-blind extension phase were randomized to either paroxetine (10, 20, or 40 mg/day) or placebo in a 3-month double-blind relapse prevention phase.

Patients randomized to paroxetine were significantly less likely to relapse than comparably treated patients who were randomized to placebo.
Subgroup analyses did not indicate that there were any differences in treatment outcomes as a function of age or gender.

Social Anxiety Disorder

The effectiveness of *Paxil* in the treatment of social anxiety disorder was demonstrated in three 12-week, multicenter, placebo-controlled studies (Studies 1-3) of adult outpatients with social anxiety disorder (DSM-IV). In these studies, the effectiveness of *Paxil* compared to placebo was evaluated on the basis of (1) the proportion of responders, as defined by a Clinical Global Impression (CGI) Improvement score of 1 (very much improved) or 2 (much improved), and (2) change from baseline in the Liebowitz Social Anxiety Scale (LSAS).
Studies 1 and 2 were flexible-dose studies comparing paroxetine (20 to 50 mg daily) and placebo. Paroxetine demonstrated statistically significant superiority over placebo on both the CGI Improvement responder criterion and the Liebowitz Social Anxiety Scale (LSAS). In Study 1, for patients who completed to week 12, 69% of paroxetine-treated patients compared to 29% of placebo-treated patients were CGI Improvement responders. In Study 2, CGI Improvement responders were 77% and 42% for the paroxetine- and placebo-treated patients, respectively.
Study 3 was a 12-week study comparing fixed paroxetine doses of 20, 40 or 60 mg/day with placebo. Paroxetine 20 mg was demonstrated to be significantly superior to placebo on both the LSAS Total Score and the CGI Improvement responder criterion; there were trends for superiority over placebo for the 40 and 60 mg/day dose groups. There was no indication in this study of any additional benefit for doses higher than 20 mg/day.
Subgroup analyses generally did not indicate differences in treatment outcomes as a function of age, race, or gender.

Generalized Anxiety Disorder

The effectiveness of *Paxil* in the treatment of Generalized Anxiety Disorder (GAD) was demonstrated in two 8-week, multicenter, placebo-controlled studies (Studies 1 and 2) of adult outpatients with Generalized Anxiety Disorder (DSM-IV).
Study 1 was an 8-week study comparing fixed paroxetine doses of 20 mg or 40 mg/day with placebo. *Paxil* 20 mg or 40 mg were both demonstrated to be significantly superior to placebo on the Hamilton Rating Scale for Anxiety (HAM-A) total score. There was not sufficient evidence in this study to suggest a greater benefit for the 40 mg/day dose compared to the 20 mg/day dose. Study 2 was a flexible-dose study comparing paroxetine (20 mg to 50 mg daily) and placebo. *Paxil* demonstrated statistically significant superiority over placebo on the Hamilton Rating Scale for Anxiety (HAM-A) total score. A third study, also flexible dose comparing paroxetine (20 mg to 50 mg daily), did not demonstrate statistically significant superiority of *Paxil* over placebo on the Hamilton Rating Scale for Anxiety (HAM-A) total score, the primary outcome.
Subgroup analyses did not indicate differences in treatment outcomes as a function of race or gender. There were insufficient elderly patients to conduct subgroup analyses on the basis of age.

Posttraumatic Stress Disorder

The effectiveness of *Paxil* in the treatment of Posttraumatic Stress Disorder (PTSD) was demonstrated in two 12-week, multicenter, placebo-controlled studies (Studies 1 and 2) of adult outpatients who met DSM-IV criteria for PTSD. The mean duration of PTSD symptoms for the 2 studies combined was 13 years (ranging from .1 years to 57 years). The percentage of patients with secondary major depressive disorder or non-PTSD anxiety disorders in the combined two studies was 41% (356 out of 858 patients) and 40% (345 out of 858 patients), respectively. Study outcome was assessed by i) the Clinician-Administered PTSD Scale Part 2 (CAPS-2) score and ii) the Clinical Global Impression-Global Improvement Scale (CGI-I). The CAPS-2 is a multi-item instrument that measures three aspects of PTSD with the following symptom clusters: reexperiencing/intrusion, avoidance/numbing and hyperarousal. The two primary outcomes for each trial were i) change from baseline to endpoint on the CAPS-2 total score (17 items), and ii) proportion of responders on the CGI-I, where responders were defined as patients having a score of 1 (very much improved) or 2 (much improved).
Study 1 was a 12-week study comparing fixed paroxetine doses of 20 or 40 mg/day to placebo. *Paxil* 20 mg and 40 mg were demonstrated to be significantly superior to placebo on change from baseline for the CAPS-2 total score and on proportion of responders on the CGI-I. There was not sufficient evidence in this study to suggest a greater benefit for the 40 mg/day dose compared to the 20 mg/day dose.
Study 2 was a 12-week flexible-dose study comparing paroxetine (20 to 50 mg daily) to placebo. *Paxil* was demonstrated to be significantly superior to placebo on change from baseline for the CAPS-2 total score and on proportion of responders on the CGI-I.
A third study, also a flexible-dose study comparing paroxetine (20 mg to 50 mg daily) to placebo, demonstrated *Paxil* to be significantly superior to placebo on change from baseline for CAPS-2 total score, but not on proportion of responders on the CGI-I.
The majority of patients in these trials were women (68% women: 377 out of 551 subjects in Study 1 and 66% women: 202 out of 303 subjects in Study 2). Subgroup analyses did not indicate differences in treatment outcomes as a function of gender. There were an insufficient number of patients who were 65 years and older or were non-Caucasian to conduct subgroup analyses on the basis of age or race, respectively.

INDICATIONS AND USAGE

Major Depressive Disorder

Paxil (paroxetine hydrochloride) is indicated for the treatment of major depressive disorder.
The efficacy of *Paxil* in the treatment of a major depressive episode was established in 6-week controlled trials of outpatients whose diagnoses corresponded most closely to the DSM-III category of major depressive disorder (see CLINICAL PHARMACOLOGY). A major depressive episode implies a prominent and relatively persistent depressed or dysphoric mood that usually interferes with daily functioning (nearly every day for at least 2 weeks); it should include at least 4 of the following 8 symptoms: change in appetite, change in sleep, psychomotor agitation or retardation, loss of interest in usual activities or decrease in sexual drive, increased fatigue, feelings of guilt or worthlessness, slowed thinking or impaired concentration, and a suicide attempt or suicidal ideation.
The effects of *Paxil* in hospitalized depressed patients have not been adequately studied.
The efficacy of *Paxil* in maintaining a response in major depressive disorder for up to 1 year was demonstrated in a placebo-controlled trial (see CLINICAL PHARMACOLOGY). Nevertheless, the physician who elects to use *Paxil* for extended periods should periodically re-evaluate the long-term usefulness of the drug for the individual patient.

Obsessive Compulsive Disorder

Paxil is indicated for the treatment of obsessions and compulsions in patients with obsessive compulsive disorder (OCD) as defined in the DSM-IV. The obsessions or compulsions cause marked distress, are time-consuming, or significantly interfere with social or occupational functioning.
The efficacy of *Paxil* was established in two 12-week trials with obsessive compulsive outpatients whose diagnoses corresponded most closely to the DSM-IIIR category of obsessive compulsive disorder (see CLINICAL PHARMACOLOGY—Clinical Trials).
Obsessive compulsive disorder is characterized by recurrent and persistent ideas, thoughts, impulses or images (obsessions) that are ego-dystonic and/or repetitive, purposeful and intentional behaviors (compulsions) that are recognized by the person as excessive or unreasonable.
Long-term maintenance of efficacy was demonstrated in a 6-month relapse prevention trial. In this trial, patients assigned to paroxetine showed a lower relapse rate compared to patients on placebo (see CLINICAL PHARMACOLOGY). Nevertheless, the physician who elects to use *Paxil* for extended periods should periodically re-evaluate the long-term usefulness of the drug for the individual patient (see DOSAGE AND ADMINISTRATION).

Panic Disorder

Paxil is indicated for the treatment of panic disorder, with or without agoraphobia, as defined in DSM-IV. Panic disorder is characterized by the occurrence of unexpected panic attacks and associated concern about having additional attacks, worry about the implications or consequences of the attacks, and/or a significant change in behavior related to the attacks.
The efficacy of Paxil (paroxetine hydrochloride) was established in three 10- to 12-week trials in panic disorder patients whose diagnoses corresponded to the DSM-IIIR category of panic disorder (see CLINICAL PHARMACOLOGY—Clinical Trials).
Panic disorder (DSM-IV) is characterized by recurrent unexpected panic attacks, i.e., a discrete period of intense fear or discomfort in which four (or more) of the following symptoms develop abruptly and reach a peak within 10 minutes: (1) palpitations, pounding heart, or accelerated heart rate; (2) sweating; (3) trembling or shaking; (4) sensations of shortness of breath or smothering; (5) feeling of choking; (6) chest pain or discomfort; (7) nausea or abdominal distress; (8) feeling dizzy, unsteady, lightheaded, or faint; (9) derealization (feelings of unreality) or depersonalization (being detached from oneself); (10) fear of losing control; (11) fear of dying; (12) paresthesias (numbness or tingling sensations); (13) chills or hot flushes.
Long-term maintenance of efficacy was demonstrated in a 3-month relapse prevention trial. In this trial, patients with panic disorder assigned to paroxetine demonstrated a lower relapse rate compared to patients on placebo (see CLINICAL PHARMACOLOGY). Nevertheless, the physician who prescribes *Paxil* for extended periods should periodically re-evaluate the long-term usefulness of the drug for the individual patient.

Social Anxiety Disorder

Paxil is indicated for the treatment of social anxiety disorder, also known as social phobia, as defined in DSM-IV (300.23). Social anxiety disorder is characterized by a marked and persistent fear of one or more social or performance situations in which the person is exposed to unfamiliar people or to possible scrutiny by others. Exposure to the feared situation almost invariably provokes anxiety, which may approach the intensity of a panic attack. The feared situations are avoided or endured with intense anxiety or distress. The avoidance, anxious anticipation, or distress in the feared situation(s) interferes significantly with the person's normal routine, occupational or academic functioning, or social activities or relationships, or there is marked distress about having the phobias. Lesser degrees of performance anxiety or shyness generally do not require psychopharmacological treatment.
The efficacy of *Paxil* (paroxetine hydrochloride) was established in three 12-week trials in adult patients with social anxiety disorder (DSM-IV). *Paxil* has not been studied in children or adolescents with social phobia (see CLINICAL PHARMACOLOGY—Clinical Trials).
The effectiveness of *Paxil* in long-term treatment of social anxiety disorder, i.e., for more than 12 weeks, has not been systematically evaluated in adequate and well-controlled trials. Therefore, the physician who elects to prescribe *Paxil* for extended periods should periodically re-evaluate the long-term usefulness of the drug for the individual patient (see DOSAGE AND ADMINISTRATION).

Generalized Anxiety Disorder

Paxil is indicated for the treatment of Generalized Anxiety Disorder (GAD), as defined in DSM-IV. Anxiety or tension associated with the stress of everyday life usually does not require treatment with an anxiolytic.
The efficacy of *Paxil* in the treatment of GAD was established in two 8-week placebo-controlled trials in adults with GAD. Paxil has not been studied in children or adolescents with Generalized Anxiety Disorder (see CLINICAL PHARMACOLOGY—Clinical Trials).
Generalized Anxiety Disorder (DSM-IV) is characterized by excessive anxiety and worry (apprehensive expectation) that is persistent for at least 6 months and which the person finds difficult to control. It must be associated with at least 3 of the following 6 symptoms: restlessness or feeling keyed up or on edge, being easily fatigued, difficulty concentrating or mind going blank, irritability, muscle tension, sleep disturbance.
The effectiveness of *Paxil* in the long-term treatment of GAD, that is, for more than 8 weeks, has not been systematically evaluated in controlled trials. The physician who elects to use *Paxil* for extended periods should periodically re-evaluate the long-term usefulness of the drug for the individual patient (see DOSAGE AND ADMINISTRATION).

Posttraumatic Stress Disorder

Paxil is indicated for the treatment of Posttraumatic Stress Disorder (PTSD).
The efficacy of Paxil in the treatment of PTSD was established in two 12-week placebo-controlled trials in adults with PTSD (DSM-IV) (see CLINICAL PHARMACOLOGY—Clinical Trials).
PTSD, as defined by DSM-IV, requires exposure to a traumatic event that involved actual or threatened death or serious injury, or threat to the physical integrity of self or others, and a response which involves intense fear, helplessness, or horror. Symptoms that occur as a result of exposure to the traumatic event include reexperiencing of the event in the form of intrusive thoughts, flashbacks or dreams, and intense psychological distress and physiological reactivity on exposure to cues to the event; avoidance of situations reminiscent of the traumatic event, inability to recall details of the event, and/or numbing of general responsiveness manifested as diminished interest in significant activities, estrangement from others, restricted range of affect, or sense of foreshortened future; and symptoms of autonomic arousal including hypervigilance, exaggerated startle response, sleep disturbance, impaired concentration, and irritability or outbursts of anger. A PTSD diagnosis requires that the symptoms are present for at least a month and that they cause clinically significant distress or impairment in social, occupational, or other important areas of functioning.
The efficacy of *Paxil* in longer-term treatment of PTSD, i.e., for more than 12 weeks, has not been systematically evaluated in placebo-controlled trials. Therefore, the physician who elects to prescribe *Paxil* for extended periods should periodically re-evaluate the long-term usefulness of the drug for the individual patient (see DOSAGE AND ADMINISTRATION).

CONTRAINDICATIONS

Concomitant use in patients taking either monoamine oxidase inhibitors (MAOIs) or thioridazine is contraindicated (see WARNINGS and PRECAUTIONS).
Paxil is contraindicated in patients with a hypersensitivity to paroxetine or any of the inactive ingredients in *Paxil*.

WARNINGS

Potential for Interaction with Monoamine Oxidase Inhibitors

In patients receiving another serotonin reuptake inhibitor drug in combination with a monoamine oxidase inhibitor (MAOI), there have been reports of serious, sometimes fatal, reactions including hyperthermia, rigidity, myoclonus, autonomic instability with possible rapid fluctuations of vital signs, and mental status changes that include extreme agitation progressing to delirium and coma. These reactions have also been reported in patients who have recently discontinued that drug and have been started on an MAOI. Some cases presented with features resembling neuroleptic malignant syndrome. While there are no human data showing such an interaction with *Paxil*, limited animal data on the effects of combined use of paroxetine and MAOIs suggest that these drugs may act synergistically to elevate blood pressure and evoke behavioral excitation. Therefore, it is recommended that Paxil (paroxetine hydrochloride) not be used in combination with an MAOI, or within 14 days of discontinuing treatment with an MAOI. At least 2 weeks should be allowed after stopping *Paxil* before starting an MAOI.

Potential Interaction with Thioridazine

Thioridazine administration alone produces prolongation of the QTc interval, which is associated with serious ven-

Continued on next page

Paxil—Cont.

tricular arrhythmias, such as torsade de pointes-type arrhythmias, and sudden death. This effect appears to be dose related.

An *in vivo* study suggests that drugs which inhibit $P_{450}IID_6$, such as paroxetine, will elevate plasma levels of thioridazine. Therefore, it is recommended that paroxetine not be used in combination with thioridazine (see CONTRAINDICATIONS and PRECAUTIONS).

PRECAUTIONS

General

Activation of Mania/Hypomania: During premarketing testing, hypomania or mania occurred in approximately 1.0% of *Paxil*-treated unipolar patients compared to 1.1% of active-control and 0.3% of placebo-treated unipolar patients. In a subset of patients classified as bipolar, the rate of manic episodes was 2.2% for *Paxil* and 11.6% for the combined active-control groups. As with all drugs effective in the treatment of major depressive disorder, *Paxil* should be used cautiously in patients with a history of mania.

Seizures: During premarketing testing, seizures occurred in 0.1% of *Paxil*-treated patients, a rate similar to that associated with other drugs effective in the treatment of major depressive disorder. *Paxil* should be used cautiously in patients with a history of seizures. It should be discontinued in any patient who develops seizures.

Suicide: The possibility of a suicide attempt is inherent in major depressive disorder and may persist until significant remission occurs. Close supervision of high-risk patients should accompany initial drug therapy. Prescriptions for *Paxil* should be written for the smallest quantity of tablets consistent with good patient management, in order to reduce the risk of overdose.

Because of well-established comorbidity between major depressive disorder and other psychiatric disorders, the same precautions observed when treating patients with major depressive disorder should be observed when treating patients with other psychiatric disorders.

***Discontinuation of Treatment with* Paxil:** Recent clinical trials supporting the various approved indications of *Paxil* employed a taper phase regimen, rather than an abrupt discontinuation of treatment. The taper phase regimen used in GAD and PTSD clinical trials involved an incremental decrease in the daily dose by 10 mg/day at weekly intervals. When a daily dose of 20 mg/day was reached, patients were continued on this dose for 1 week before treatment was stopped.

With this regimen in those studies, the following adverse events were reported at an incidence of 2% or greater for *Paxil* and were at least twice that reported for placebo: abnormal dreams (2.3% vs 0.5%), paresthesia (2.0% vs 0.4%), and dizziness (7.1% vs 1.5%). In the majority of patients, these events were mild to moderate and were self-limiting and did not require medical intervention. During *Paxil* marketing, there have been spontaneous reports of similar adverse events, which may have no causal relationship to the drug, upon the discontinuation of *Paxil* (particularly when abrupt), including the following: dizziness, sensory disturbances (e.g., paresthesias such as electric shock sensations), agitation, anxiety, nausea, and sweating. These events are generally self-limiting. Similar events have been reported for other selective serotonin reuptake inhibitors.

Patients should be monitored for these symptoms when discontinuing treatment, regardless of the indication for which *Paxil* is being prescribed. A gradual reduction in the dose rather than abrupt cessation is recommended whenever possible. If intolerable symptoms occur following a decrease in the dose or upon discontinuation of treatment, then resuming the previously prescribed dose may be considered. Subsequently, the physician may continue decreasing the dose but at a more gradual rate (see DOSAGE AND ADMINISTRATION).

Hyponatremia: Several cases of hyponatremia have been reported. The hyponatremia appeared to be reversible when *Paxil* was discontinued. The majority of these occurrences have been in elderly individuals, some in patients taking diuretics or who were otherwise volume depleted.

Abnormal Bleeding: There have been several reports of abnormal bleeding (mostly ecchymosis and purpura) associated with paroxetine treatment, including a report of impaired platelet aggregation. While a causal relationship to paroxetine is unclear, impaired platelet aggregation may result from platelet serotonin depletion and contribute to such occurrences.

Use in Patients with Concomitant Illness: Clinical experience with *Paxil* in patients with certain concomitant systemic illness is limited. Caution is advisable in using *Paxil* in patients with diseases or conditions that could affect metabolism or hemodynamic responses.

As with other SSRIs, mydriasis has been infrequently reported in premarketing studies with *Paxil*. A few cases of acute angle closure glaucoma associated with paroxetine therapy have been reported in the literature. As mydriasis can cause acute angle closure in patients with narrow angle glaucoma, caution should be used when *Paxil* is prescribed for patients with narrow angle glaucoma.

Paxil has not been evaluated or used to any appreciable extent in patients with a recent history of myocardial infarction or unstable heart disease. Patients with these diagnoses were excluded from clinical studies during the product's premarket testing. Evaluation of electrocardiograms of 682 patients who received *Paxil* in double-blind, placebo-controlled trials, however, did not indicate that *Paxil* is associated with the development of significant ECG abnormalities. Similarly, Paxil (paroxetine hydrochloride) does not cause any clinically important changes in heart rate or blood pressure.

Increased plasma concentrations of paroxetine occur in patients with severe renal impairment (creatinine clearance <30 mL/min.) or severe hepatic impairment. A lower starting dose should be used in such patients (see DOSAGE AND ADMINISTRATION).

Information for Patients

Physicians are advised to discuss the following issues with patients for whom they prescribe *Paxil*:

Interference with Cognitive and Motor Performance: Any psychoactive drug may impair judgment, thinking or motor skills. Although in controlled studies *Paxil* has not been shown to impair psychomotor performance, patients should be cautioned about operating hazardous machinery, including automobiles, until they are reasonably certain that *Paxil* therapy does not affect their ability to engage in such activities.

Completing Course of Therapy: While patients may notice improvement with *Paxil* therapy in 1 to 4 weeks, they should be advised to continue therapy as directed.

Concomitant Medication: Patients should be advised to inform their physician if they are taking, or plan to take, any prescription or over-the-counter drugs, since there is a potential for interactions.

Alcohol: Although *Paxil* has not been shown to increase the impairment of mental and motor skills caused by alcohol, patients should be advised to avoid alcohol while taking *Paxil*.

Pregnancy: Patients should be advised to notify their physician if they become pregnant or intend to become pregnant during therapy.

Nursing: Patients should be advised to notify their physician if they are breast-feeding an infant (see PRECAUTIONS—Nursing Mothers).

Laboratory Tests

There are no specific laboratory tests recommended.

Drug Interactions

Tryptophan: As with other serotonin reuptake inhibitors, an interaction between paroxetine and tryptophan may occur when they are co-administered. Adverse experiences, consisting primarily of headache, nausea, sweating and dizziness, have been reported when tryptophan was administered to patients taking Paxil (paroxetine hydrochloride). Consequently, concomitant use of *Paxil* with tryptophan is not recommended.

Monoamine Oxidase Inhibitors: See CONTRAINDICATIONS and WARNINGS.

Thioridazine: See CONTRAINDICATIONS and WARNINGS.

Warfarin: Preliminary data suggest that there may be a pharmacodynamic interaction (that causes an increased bleeding diathesis in the face of unaltered prothrombin time) between paroxetine and warfarin. Since there is little clinical experience, the concomitant administration of *Paxil* and warfarin should be undertaken with caution.

Sumatriptan: There have been rare postmarketing reports describing patients with weakness, hyperreflexia, and incoordination following the use of a selective serotonin reuptake inhibitor (SSRI) and sumatriptan. If concomitant treatment with sumatriptan and an SSRI (e.g., fluoxetine, fluvoxamine, paroxetine, sertraline) is clinically warranted, appropriate observation of the patient is advised.

Drugs Affecting Hepatic Metabolism: The metabolism and pharmacokinetics of paroxetine may be affected by the induction or inhibition of drug-metabolizing enzymes.

Cimetidine–Cimetidine inhibits many cytochrome P_{450} (oxidative) enzymes. In a study where *Paxil* (30 mg q.d.) was dosed orally for 4 weeks, steady-state plasma concentrations of paroxetine were increased by approximately 50% during co-administration with oral cimetidine (300 mg t.i.d.) for the final week. Therefore, when these drugs are administered concurrently, dosage adjustment of Paxil (paroxetine hydrochloride) after the 20 mg starting dose should be guided by clinical effect. The effect of paroxetine on cimetidine's pharmacokinetics was not studied.

Phenobarbital–Phenobarbital induces many cytochrome P_{450} (oxidative) enzymes. When a single oral 30 mg dose of *Paxil* was administered at phenobarbital steady state (100 mg q.d. for 14 days), paroxetine AUC and $T_{1/2}$ were reduced (by an average of 25% and 38%, respectively) compared to paroxetine administered alone. The effect of paroxetine on phenobarbital pharmacokinetics was not studied. Since *Paxil* exhibits nonlinear pharmacokinetics, the results of this study may not address the case where the two drugs are both being chronically dosed. No initial *Paxil* dosage adjustment is considered necessary when co-administered with phenobarbital; any subsequent adjustment should be guided by clinical effect.

Phenytoin–When a single oral 30 mg dose of *Paxil* was administered at phenytoin steady state (300 mg q.d. for 14 days), paroxetine AUC and $T_{1/2}$ were reduced (by an average of 50% and 35%, respectively) compared to *Paxil* administered alone. In a separate study, when a single oral 300 mg dose of phenytoin was administered at paroxetine steady state (30 mg q.d. for 14 days), phenytoin AUC was slightly reduced (12% on average) compared to phenytoin administered alone. Since both drugs exhibit nonlinear pharmacokinetics, the above studies may not address the case where the two drugs are both being chronically dosed. No initial dosage adjustments are considered necessary when these drugs are co-administered; any subsequent adjustments should be guided by clinical effect (see ADVERSE REACTIONS–Postmarketing Reports).

Drugs Metabolized by Cytochrome P_{450} IID_6: Many drugs, including most drugs effective in the treatment of major depressive disorder (paroxetine, other SSRIs and many tricyclics), are metabolized by the cytochrome P_{450} isozyme $P_{450}IID_6$. Like other agents that are metabolized by $P_{450}IID_6$, paroxetine may significantly inhibit the activity of this isozyme. In most patients (>90%), this $P_{450}IID_6$ isozyme is saturated early during *Paxil* dosing. In one study, daily dosing of *Paxil* (20 mg q.d.) under steady-state conditions increased single dose desipramine (100 mg) C_{max}, AUC and $T_{1/2}$ by an average of approximately two-, five- and three-fold, respectively. Concomitant use of *Paxil* with other drugs metabolized by cytochrome $P_{450}IID_6$ has not been formally studied but may require lower doses than usually prescribed for either *Paxil* or the other drug.

Therefore, co-administration of *Paxil* with other drugs that are metabolized by this isozyme, including certain drugs effective in the treatment of major depressive disorder (e.g., nortriptyline, amitriptyline, imipramine, desipramine and fluoxetine), phenothiazines and Type 1C antiarrhythmics (e.g., propafenone, flecainide and encainide), or that inhibit this enzyme (e.g., quinidine), should be approached with caution.

However, due to the risk of serious ventricular arrhythmias and sudden death potentially associated with elevated plasma levels of thioridazine, paroxetine and thioridazine should not be co-administered (see CONTRAINDICATIONS and WARNINGS).

At steady state, when the $P_{450}IID_6$ pathway is essentially saturated, paroxetine clearance is governed by alternative P_{450} isozymes which, unlike $P_{450}IID_6$, show no evidence of saturation (see PRECAUTIONS–Tricyclic Antidepressants).

Drugs Metabolized by Cytochrome P_{450} $IIIA_4$: An *in vivo* interaction study involving the co-administration under steady-state conditions of paroxetine and terfenadine, a substrate for cytochrome $P_{450}IIIA_4$, revealed no effect of paroxetine on terfenadine pharmacokinetics. In addition, *in vitro* studies have shown ketoconazole, a potent inhibitor of $P_{450}IIIA_4$ activity, to be at least 100 times more potent than paroxetine as an inhibitor of the metabolism of several substrates for this enzyme, including terfenadine, astemizole, cisapride, triazolam, and cyclosporin. Based on the assumption that the relationship between paroxetine's *in vitro* K_i and its lack of effect on terfenadine's *in vivo* clearance predicts its effect on other $IIIA_4$ substrates, paroxetine's extent of inhibition of $IIIA_4$ activity is not likely to be of clinical significance.

Tricyclic Antidepressants (TCAs): Caution is indicated in the co-administration of tricyclic antidepressants (TCAs) with *Paxil*, because paroxetine may inhibit TCA metabolism. Plasma TCA concentrations may need to be monitored, and the dose of TCA may need to be reduced, if a TCA is co-administered with *Paxil* (see PRECAUTIONS–*Drugs Metabolized by Cytochrome $P_{450}IID_6$*).

Drugs Highly Bound to Plasma Protein: Because paroxetine is highly bound to plasma protein, administration of *Paxil* to a patient taking another drug that is highly protein bound may cause increased free concentrations of the other drug, potentially resulting in adverse events. Conversely, adverse effects could result from displacement of paroxetine by other highly bound drugs.

Alcohol: Although *Paxil* does not increase the impairment of mental and motor skills caused by alcohol, patients should be advised to avoid alcohol while taking Paxil (paroxetine hydrochloride).

Lithium: A multiple-dose study has shown that there is no pharmacokinetic interaction between *Paxil* and lithium carbonate. However, since there is little clinical experience, the concurrent administration of paroxetine and lithium should be undertaken with caution.

Digoxin: The steady-state pharmacokinetics of paroxetine was not altered when administered with digoxin at steady state. Mean digoxin AUC at steady state decreased by 15% in the presence of paroxetine. Since there is little clinical experience, the concurrent administration of paroxetine and digoxin should be undertaken with caution.

Diazepam: Under steady-state conditions, diazepam does not appear to affect paroxetine kinetics. The effects of paroxetine on diazepam were not evaluated.

Procyclidine: Daily oral dosing of *Paxil* (30 mg q.d.) increased steady-state AUC_{0-24}, C_{max} and C_{min} values of procyclidine (5 mg oral q.d.) by 35%, 37% and 67%, respectively, compared to procyclidine alone at steady state. If anticholinergic effects are seen, the dose of procyclidine should be reduced.

Beta-Blockers: In a study where propranolol (80 mg b.i.d.) was dosed orally for 18 days, the established steady-state plasma concentrations of propranolol were unaltered during co-administration with *Paxil* (30 mg q.d.) for the final 10 days. The effects of propranolol on paroxetine have not been evaluated (see ADVERSE REACTIONS–Postmarketing Reports).

Theophylline: Reports of elevated theophylline levels associated with *Paxil* treatment have been reported. While this interaction has not been formally studied, it is recommended that theophylline levels be monitored when these drugs are concurrently administered.

Electroconvulsive Therapy (ECT): There are no clinical studies of the combined use of ECT and *Paxil*.

Carcinogenesis, Mutagenesis, Impairment of Fertility

Carcinogenesis: Two-year carcinogenicity studies were conducted in rodents given paroxetine in the diet at 1, 5, and 25 mg/kg/day (mice) and 1, 5, and 20 mg/kg/day (rats). These doses are up to 2.4 (mouse) and 3.9 (rat) times the maximum recommended human dose (MRHD) for major depressive disorder, social anxiety disorder GAD and PTSD on a mg/m^2 basis. Because the MRHD for major depressive disorder is slightly less than that for OCD (50 mg vs. 60 mg), the doses used in these carcinogenicity studies were only 2.0 (mouse) and 3.2 (rat) times the MRHD for OCD. There was a significantly greater number of male rats in the high-dose group with reticulum cell sarcomas (1/100, 0/50, 0/50 and 4/50 for control, low-, middle- and high-dose groups, respectively) and a significantly increased linear trend across dose groups for the occurrence of lymphoreticular tumors in male rats. Female rats were not affected. Although there was a dose-related increase in the number of tumors in mice, there was no drug-related increase in the number of mice with tumors. The relevance of these findings to humans is unknown.

Mutagenesis: Paroxetine produced no genotoxic effects in a battery of 5 *in vitro* and 2 *in vivo* assays that included the following: bacterial mutation assay, mouse lymphoma mutation assay, unscheduled DNA synthesis assay, and tests for cytogenetic aberrations *in vivo* in mouse bone marrow and *in vitro* in human lymphocytes and in a dominant lethal test in rats.

Impairment of Fertility: A reduced pregnancy rate was found in reproduction studies in rats at a dose of paroxetine of 15 mg/kg/day which is 2.9 times the MRHD for major depressive disorder, social anxiety disorder, GAD and PTSD or 2.4 times the MRHD for OCD on a mg/m^2 basis. Irreversible lesions occurred in the reproductive tract of male rats after dosing in toxicity studies for 2 to 52 weeks. These lesions consisted of vacuolation of epididymal tubular epithelium at 50 mg/kg/day and atrophic changes in the seminiferous tubules of the testes with arrested spermatogenesis at 25 mg/kg/day (9.8 and 4.9 times the MRHD for major depressive disorder, social anxiety disorder and GAD; 8.2 and 4.1 times the MRHD for OCD and PD on a mg/m^2 basis).

Pregnancy

Teratogenic Effects–Pregnancy Category C

Reproduction studies were performed at doses up to 50 mg/kg/day in rats and 6 mg/kg/day in rabbits administered during organogenesis. These doses are equivalent to 9.7 (rat) and 2.2 (rabbit) times the maximum recommended human dose (MRHD) for major depressive disorder, social anxiety disorder, GAD, and PTSD (50 mg) and 8.1 (rat) and 1.9 (rabbit) times the MRHD for OCD, on a mg/m^2 basis. These studies have revealed no evidence of teratogenic effects. However, in rats, there was an increase in pup deaths during the first 4 days of lactation when dosing occurred during the last trimester of gestation and continued throughout lactation. This effect occurred at a dose of 1 mg/kg/day or 0.19 times (mg/m^2) the MRHD for depression, social anxiety disorder, GAD, and PTSD and at 0.16 times (mg/m^2) the MRHD for OCD. The no-effect dose for rat pup mortality was not determined. The cause of these deaths is not known. There are no adequate and well-controlled studies in pregnant women. Because animal reproduction studies are not always predictive of human response, this drug should be used during pregnancy only if the potential benefit justifies the potential risk to the fetus.

Labor and Delivery

The effect of paroxetine on labor and delivery in humans is unknown.

Nursing Mothers

Like many other drugs, paroxetine is secreted in human milk, and caution should be exercised when Paxil (paroxetine hydrochloride) is administered to a nursing woman.

Pediatric Use

Safety and effectiveness in the pediatric population have not been established.

Geriatric Use

In worldwide premarketing *Paxil* clinical trials, 17% of *Paxil*-treated patients (approximately 700) were 65 years of age or older. Pharmacokinetic studies revealed a decreased clearance in the elderly, and a lower starting dose is recommended; there were, however, no overall differences in the adverse event profile between elderly and younger patients, and effectiveness was similar in younger and older patients (see CLINICAL PHARMACOLOGY and DOSAGE AND ADMINISTRATION).

ADVERSE REACTIONS

Associated with Discontinuation of Treatment

Twenty percent (1,199/6,145) of *Paxil* patients in worldwide clinical trials in major depressive disorder and 16.1% (84/522), 11.8% (64/542), 9.4% (44/469), 10.7% (79/735) and 11.7% (79/676) of *Paxil* patients in worldwide trials in social anxiety disorder, OCD, panic disorder, GAD and PTSD, respectively, discontinued treatment due to an adverse event. The most common events (≥1%) associated with discontinuation and considered to be drug related (i.e., those events associated with dropout at a rate approximately twice or greater for *Paxil* compared to placebo) included the following:

[See first table above]

	Major Depressive Disorder		OCD		Panic Disorder		Social Anxiety Disorder		Generalized Anxiety Disorder		PTSD	
	Paxil	Placebo	*Paxil*	Placebo	*Paxil*	Placebo	*Paxil*	Placebo	*Paxil*	Placebo	*Paxil*	Placebo
CNS												
Somnolence	2.3%	0.7%	—		1.9%	0.3%	3.4%	0.3%	2.0%	0.2%	2.8%	0.6%
Insomnia	—	—	1.7%	0%	1.3%	0.3%	3.1%	0%			—	—
Agitation	1.1%	0.5%	—								—	—
Tremor	1.1%	0.3%	—				1.7%	0%			1.0%	0.2%
Anxiety	—	—	—				1.1%	0%			—	—
Dizziness	—	—	1.5%	0%			1.9%	0%	1.0%	0.2%	—	—
Gastrointestinal												
Constipation	—		1.1%	0%							—	—
Nausea	3.2%	1.1%	1.9%	0%	3.2%	1.2%	4.0%	0.3%	2.0%	0.2%	2.2%	0.6%
Diarrhea	1.0%	0.3%	—									
Dry mouth	1.0%	0.3%	—								—	—
Vomiting	1.0%	0.3%	—				1.0%	0%			—	—
Flatulence							1.0%	0.3%			—	—
Other												
Asthenia	1.6%	0.4%	1.9%	0.4%			2.5%	0.6%	1.8%	0.2%	1.6%	0.2%
Abnormal ejaculation[1]	1.6%	0%	2.1%	0%			4.9%	0.6%	2.5%	0.5%	—	—
Sweating	1.0%	0.3%	—				1.1%	0%	1.1%	0.2%	—	—
Impotence[1]	—		1.5%	0%							—	—
Libido Decreased							1.0%	0%			—	—

Where numbers are not provided the incidence of the adverse events in Paxil (paroxetine hydrochloride) patients was not >1% or was not greater than or equal to two times the incidence of placebo.

1. Incidence corrected for gender.

Table 1. Treatment-Emergent Adverse Experience Incidence in Placebo-Controlled Clinical Trials for Major Depressive Disorder[1]

Body System	Preferred Term	*Paxil* (n=421)	Placebo (n=421)
Body as a Whole	Headache	18%	17%
	Asthenia	15%	6%
Cardiovascular	Palpitation	3%	1%
	Vasodilation	3%	1%
Dermatologic	Sweating	11%	2%
	Rash	2%	1%
Gastrointestinal	Nausea	26%	9%
	Dry Mouth	18%	12%
	Constipation	14%	9%
	Diarrhea	12%	8%
	Decreased Appetite	6%	2%
	Flatulence	4%	2%
	Oropharynx Disorder[2]	2%	0%
	Dyspepsia	2%	1%
Musculoskeletal	Myopathy	2%	1%
	Myalgia	2%	1%
	Myasthenia	1%	0%
Nervous System	Somnolence	23%	9%
	Dizziness	13%	6%
	Insomnia	13%	6%
	Tremor	8%	2%
	Nervousness	5%	3%
	Anxiety	5%	3%
	Paresthesia	4%	2%
	Libido Decreased	3%	0%
	Drugged Feeling	2%	1%
	Confusion	1%	0%
Respiration	Yawn	4%	0%
Special Senses	Blurred Vision	4%	1%
	Taste Perversion	2%	0%
Urogenital System	Ejaculatory Disturbance[3,4]	13%	0%
	Other Male Genital Disorders[3,5]	10%	0%
	Urinary Frequency	3%	1%
	Urination Disorder[6]	3%	0%
	Female Genital Disorders[3,7]	2%	0%

1. Events reported by at least 1% of patients treated with Paxil (paroxetine hydrochloride) are included, except the following events which had an incidence on placebo ≥ *Paxil:* abdominal pain, agitation, back pain, chest pain, CNS stimulation, fever, increased appetite, myoclonus, pharyngitis, postural hypotension, respiratory disorder (includes mostly "cold symptoms" or "URI"), trauma and vomiting.
2. Includes mostly "lump in throat" and "tightness in throat."
3. Percentage corrected for gender.
4. Mostly "ejaculatory delay."
5. Includes "anorgasmia," "erectile difficulties," "delayed ejaculation/orgasm," and "sexual dysfunction," and "impotence."
6. Includes mostly "difficulty with micturition" and "urinary hesitancy."
7. Includes mostly "anorgasmia" and "difficulty reaching climax/orgasm."

Commonly Observed Adverse Events

Major Depressive Disorder

The most commonly observed adverse events associated with the use of paroxetine (incidence of 5% or greater and incidence for *Paxil* at least twice that for placebo, derived from Table 1 above) were: asthenia, sweating, nausea, decreased appetite, somnolence, dizziness, insomnia, tremor, nervousness, ejaculatory disturbance and other male genital disorders.

Obsessive Compulsive Disorder

The most commonly observed adverse events associated with the use of paroxetine (incidence of 5% or greater and incidence for *Paxil* at least twice that of placebo, derived from Table 2 below) were: nausea, dry mouth, decreased appetite, constipation, dizziness, somnolence, tremor, sweating, impotence and abnormal ejaculation.

Panic Disorder

The most commonly observed adverse events associated with the use of paroxetine (incidence of 5% or greater and incidence for *Paxil* at least twice that for placebo, derived from Table 2 below) were: asthenia, sweating, decreased appetite, libido decreased, tremor, abnormal ejaculation, female genital disorders and impotence.

Social Anxiety Disorder

The most commonly observed adverse events associated with the use of paroxetine (incidence of 5% or greater and incidence for *Paxil* at least twice that for placebo, derived from Table 2 below) were: sweating, nausea, dry mouth, constipation, decreased appetite, somnolence, tremor, libido decreased, yawn, abnormal ejaculation, female genital disorders and impotence.

Generalized Anxiety Disorder

The most commonly observed adverse events associated with the use of paroxetine (incidence of 5% or greater and incidence for *Paxil* at least twice that for placebo, derived from Table 3 below) were: asthenia, infection, constipation, decreased appetite, dry mouth, nausea, libido decreased, somnolence, tremor, sweating, and abnormal ejaculation.

Posttraumatic Stress Disorder

The most commonly observed adverse events associated with the use of paroxetine (incidence of 5% or greater and incidence for *Paxil* at least twice that for placebo, derived from Table 3 below) were: asthenia, sweating, nausea, dry mouth, diarrhea, decreased appetite, somnolence, libido decreased, abnormal ejaculation, female genital disorders, and impotence.

Continued on next page

Paxil—Cont.

Incidence in Controlled Clinical Trials

The prescriber should be aware that the figures in the tables following cannot be used to predict the incidence of side effects in the course of usual medical practice where patient characteristics and other factors differ from those which prevailed in the clinical trials. Similarly, the cited frequencies cannot be compared with figures obtained from other clinical investigations involving different treatments, uses and investigators. The cited figures, however, do provide the prescribing physician with some basis for estimating the relative contribution of drug and nondrug factors to the side effect incidence rate in the populations studied.

Major Depressive Disorder

Table 1 enumerates adverse events that occurred at an incidence of 1% or more among paroxetine-treated patients who participated in short-term (6-week) placebo-controlled trials in which patients were dosed in a range of 20 to 50 mg/day. Reported adverse events were classified using a standard COSTART-based Dictionary terminology.

[See table 1 at top of previous page]

Obsessive Compulsive Disorder, Panic Disorder and Social Anxiety Disorder

Table 2 enumerates adverse events that occurred at a frequency of 2% or more among OCD patients on *Paxil* who participated in placebo-controlled trials of 12-weeks duration in which patients were dosed in a range of 20 to 60 mg/day or among patients with panic disorder on *Paxil* who participated in placebo-controlled trials of 10- to 12-weeks duration in which patients were dosed in a range of 10 to 60 mg/day or among patients with social anxiety disorder on Paxil (paroxetine hydrochloride) who participated in placebo-controlled trials of 12-weeks duration in which patients were dosed in a range of 20 to 50 mg/day.

[See table above]

Generalized Anxiety Disorder and Posttraumatic Stress Disorder

Table 3 enumerates adverse events that occurred at a frequency of 2% or more among GAD patients on *Paxil* who participated in placebo-controlled trials of 8 weeks duration in which patients were dosed in a range of 10 mg/day to 50 mg/day or among PTSD patients on *Paxil* who participated in placebo-controlled trials of 12-weeks duration in which patients were dosed in a range of 20 mg/day to 50 mg/day.

[See table 3 at bottom of next page]

Dose Dependency of Adverse Events: A comparison of adverse event rates in a fixed-dose study comparing *Paxil* 10, 20, 30 and 40 mg/day with placebo in the treatment of major depressive disorder revealed a clear dose dependency for some of the more common adverse events associated with *Paxil* use, as shown in the following table:

[See table at bottom of next page]

In a fixed-dose study comparing placebo and *Paxil* 20, 40 and 60 mg in the treatment of OCD, there was no clear relationship between adverse events and the dose of Paxil (paroxetine hydrochloride) to which patients were assigned. No new adverse events were observed in the *Paxil* 60 mg dose group compared to any of the other treatment groups.

In a fixed-dose study comparing placebo and *Paxil* 10, 20 and 40 mg in the treatment of panic disorder, there was no clear relationship between adverse events and the dose of *Paxil* to which patients were assigned, except for asthenia, dry mouth, anxiety, libido decreased, tremor and abnormal ejaculation. In flexible dose studies, no new adverse events were observed in patients receiving *Paxil* 60 mg compared to any of the other treatment groups.

In a fixed-dose study comparing placebo and *Paxil* 20, 40 and 60 mg in the treatment of social anxiety disorder, for most of the adverse events, there was no clear relationship between adverse events and the dose of Paxil (paroxetine hydrochloride) to which patients were assigned.

In a fixed-dose study comparing placebo and *Paxil* 20 and 40 mg in the treatment of generalized anxiety disorder, for most of the adverse events, there was no clear relationship between adverse events and the dose of Paxil (paroxetine hydrochloride) to which patients were assigned, except for the following adverse events: asthenia, constipation, and abnormal ejaculation.

In a fixed-dose study comparing placebo and *Paxil* 20 and 40 mg in the treatment of posttraumatic stress disorder, for most of the adverse events, there was no clear relationship between adverse events and the dose of *Paxil* to which patients were assigned, except for impotence and abnormal ejaculation.

Adaptation to Certain Adverse Events: Over a 4- to 6-week period, there was evidence of adaptation to some adverse events with continued therapy (e.g., nausea and dizziness), but less to other effects (e.g., dry mouth, somnolence and asthenia).

Male and Female Sexual Dysfunction with SSRIs: Although changes in sexual desire, sexual performance and sexual satisfaction often occur as manifestations of a psychiatric disorder, they may also be a consequence of pharmacologic treatment. In particular, some evidence suggests that selective serotonin reuptake inhibitors (SSRIs) can cause such untoward sexual experiences.

Reliable estimates of the incidence and severity of untoward experiences involving sexual desire, performance and satisfaction are difficult to obtain, however, in part because patients and physicians may be reluctant to discuss them.

Table 2. Treatment-Emergent Adverse Experience Incidence in Placebo-Controlled Clinical Trials for Obsessive Compulsive Disorder, Panic Disorder and Social Anxiety Disorder[1]

Body System	Preferred Term	Obsessive Compulsive Disorder *Paxil* (n=542)	Obsessive Compulsive Disorder Placebo (n=265)	Panic Disorder *Paxil* (n=469)	Panic Disorder Placebo (n=324)	Social Anxiety Disorder *Paxil* (n=425)	Social Anxiety Disorder Placebo (n=339)
Body as a Whole	Asthenia	22%	14%	14%	5%	22%	14%
	Abdominal Pain	—	—	4%	3%	—	—
	Chest Pain	3%	2%	—	—	—	—
	Back Pain	—	—	3%	2%	—	—
	Chills	2%	1%	2%	1%	—	—
	Trauma	—	—	—	—	3%	1%
Cardiovascular	Vasodilation	4%	1%	—	—	—	—
	Palpitation	2%	0%	—	—	—	—
Dermatologic	Sweating	9%	3%	14%	6%	9%	2%
	Rash	3%	2%	—	—	—	—
Gastrointestinal	Nausea	23%	10%	23%	17%	25%	7%
	Dry Mouth	18%	9%	18%	11%	9%	3%
	Constipation	16%	6%	8%	5%	5%	2%
	Diarrhea	10%	10%	12%	7%	9%	6%
	Decreased Appetite	9%	3%	7%	3%	8%	2%
	Dyspepsia	—	—	—	—	4%	2%
	Flatulence	—	—	—	—	4%	2%
	Increased Appetite	4%	3%	2%	1%	—	—
	Vomiting	—	—	—	—	2%	1%
Musculoskeletal	Myalgia	—	—	—	—	4%	3%
Nervous System	Insomnia	24%	13%	18%	10%	21%	16%
	Somnolence	24%	7%	19%	11%	22%	5%
	Dizziness	12%	6%	14%	10%	11%	7%
	Tremor	11%	1%	9%	1%	9%	1%
	Nervousness	9%	8%	—	—	8%	7%
	Libido Decreased	7%	4%	9%	1%	12%	1%
	Agitation	—	—	5%	4%	3%	1%
	Anxiety	—	—	5%	4%	5%	4%
	Abnormal Dreams	4%	1%	—	—	—	—
	Concentration Impaired	3%	2%	—	—	4%	1%
	Depersonalization	3%	0%	—	—	—	—
	Myoclonus	3%	0%	3%	2%	2%	1%
	Amnesia	2%	1%	—	—	—	—
Respiratory System	Rhinitis	—	—	3%	0%	—	—
	Pharyngitis	—	—	—	—	4%	2%
	Yawn	—	—	—	—	5%	1%
Special Senses	Abnormal Vision	4%	2%	—	—	4%	1%
	Taste Perversion	2%	0%	—	—	—	—
Urogenital System	Abnormal Ejaculation[2]	23%	1%	21%	1%	28%	1%
	Dysmenorrhea	—	—	—	—	5%	4%
	Female Genital Disorder[2]	3%	0%	9%	1%	9%	1%
	Impotence[2]	8%	1%	5%	0%	5%	1%
	Urinary Frequency	3%	1%	2%	0%	—	—
	Urination Impaired	3%	0%	—	—	—	—
	Urinary Tract Infection	2%	1%	2%	1%	—	—

1. Events reported by at least 2% of OCD, panic disorder, and social anxiety disorder *Paxil*-treated patients are included, except the following events which had an incidence on placebo ≥*Paxil*: [OCD]: abdominal pain, agitation, anxiety, back pain, cough increased, depression, headache, hyperkinesia, infection, paresthesia, pharyngitis, respiratory disorder, rhinitis and sinusitis. [panic disorder]: abnormal dreams, abnormal vision, chest pain, cough increased, depersonalization, depression, dysmenorrhea, dyspepsia, flu syndrome, headache, infection, myalgia, nervousness, palpitation, paresthesia, pharyngitis, rash, respiratory disorder, sinusitis, taste perversion, trauma, urination impaired and vasodilation. [social anxiety disorder]: abdominal pain, depression, headache, infection, respiratory disorder and sinusitis.
2. Percentage corrected for gender.

Accordingly, estimates of the incidence of untoward sexual experience and performance cited in product labeling, are likely to underestimate their actual incidence.

In placebo-controlled clinical trials involving more than 3,200 patients, the ranges for the reported incidence of sexual side effects in males and females with major depressive disorder, OCD, panic disorder, social anxiety disorder, GAD and PTSD are displayed in Table 5 below.

[See table at bottom of next page]

There are no adequate and well-controlled studies examining sexual dysfunction with paroxetine treatment.

Paroxetine treatment has been associated with several cases of priapism. In those cases with a known outcome, patients recovered without sequelae.

While it is difficult to know the precise risk of sexual dysfunction associated with the use of SSRIs, physicians should routinely inquire about such possible side effects.

Weight and Vital Sign Changes: Significant weight loss may be an undesirable result of treatment with *Paxil* for some patients but, on average, patients in controlled trials had minimal (about 1 pound) weight loss vs. smaller changes on placebo and active control. No significant changes in vital signs (systolic and diastolic blood pressure, pulse and temperature) were observed in patients treated with *Paxil* in controlled clinical trials.

ECG Changes: In an analysis of ECGs obtained in 682 patients treated with *Paxil* and 415 patients treated with placebo in controlled clinical trials, no clinically significant changes were seen in the ECGs of either group.

Liver Function Tests: In placebo-controlled clinical trials, patients treated with *Paxil* exhibited abnormal values on liver function tests at no greater rate than that seen in placebo-treated patients. In particular, the *Paxil*-vs.-placebo comparisons for alkaline phosphatase, SGOT, SGPT and bilirubin revealed no differences in the percentage of patients with marked abnormalities.

Other Events Observed During the Premarketing Evaluation of Paxil (paroxetine hydrochloride)

During its premarketing assessment in major depressive disorder, multiple doses of *Paxil* were administered to 6,145 patients in phase 2 and 3 studies. The conditions and duration of exposure to *Paxil* varied greatly and included (in overlapping categories) open and double-blind studies, uncontrolled and controlled studies, inpatient and outpatient studies, and fixed-dose and titration studies. During premarketing clinical trials in OCD, panic disorder, social anxiety disorder, generalized anxiety disorder and posttraumatic stress disorder, 542, 469, 522, 735 and 676 patients, respectively, received multiple doses of *Paxil*. Untoward events associated with this exposure were recorded by clinical investigators using terminology of their own choosing. Consequently, it is not possible to provide a meaningful estimate of the proportion of individuals experiencing adverse events without first grouping similar types of untoward events into a smaller number of standardized event categories.

In the tabulations that follow, reported adverse events were classified using a standard COSTART-based Dictionary terminology. The frequencies presented, therefore, represent the proportion of the 9,089 patients exposed to multiple doses of Paxil (paroxetine hydrochloride) who experienced an event of the type cited on at least one occasion while receiving *Paxil*. All reported events are included except those already listed in Tables 1–3, those reported in terms so general as to be uninformative and those events where a drug cause was remote. It is important to emphasize that although the events reported occurred during treatment with paroxetine, they were not necessarily caused by it.

Events are further categorized by body system and listed in order of decreasing frequency according to the following definitions: frequent adverse events are those occurring on one or more occasions in at least 1/100 patients (only those not already listed in the tabulated results from placebo-controlled trials appear in this listing); infrequent adverse events are those occurring in 1/100 to 1/1000 patients; rare events are those occurring in fewer than 1/1000 patients. Events of major clinical importance are also described in the PRECAUTIONS section.

Body as a Whole: *infrequent:* allergic reaction, chills, face edema, malaise, neck pain; *rare:* adrenergic syndrome, cellulitis, moniliasis, neck rigidity, pelvic pain, peritonitis, sepsis, ulcer.

Cardiovascular System: *frequent:* hypertension, tachycardia; *infrequent:* bradycardia, hematoma, hypotension, migraine, syncope; *rare:* angina pectoris, arrhythmia nodal, atrial fibrillation, bundle branch block, cerebral ischemia, cerebrovascular accident, congestive heart failure, heart block, low cardiac output, myocardial infarct, myocardial ischemia, pallor, phlebitis, pulmonary embolus, supraventricular extrasystoles, thrombophlebitis, thrombosis, varicose vein, vascular headache, ventricular extrasystoles.

Digestive System: *infrequent:* bruxism, colitis, dysphagia, eructation, gastritis, gastroenteritis, gingivitis, glossitis, increased salivation, liver function tests abnormal, rectal hemorrhage, ulcerative stomatitis; *rare:* aphthous stomatitis, bloody diarrhea, bulimia, cardiospasm, cholelithiasis, duodenitis, enteritis, esophagitis, fecal impactions, fecal incontinence, gum hemorrhage, hematemesis, hepatitis, ileitis, ileus, intestinal obstruction, jaundice, melena, mouth ulceration, peptic ulcer, salivary gland enlargement, sialadenitis, stomach ulcer, stomatitis, tongue discoloration, tongue edema, tooth caries.

Endocrine System: *rare:* diabetes mellitus, goiter, hyperthyroidism, hypothyroidism, thyroiditis.

Hemic and Lymphatic Systems: *infrequent:* anemia, leukopenia, lymphadenopathy, purpura; *rare:* abnormal erythrocytes, basophilia, bleeding time increased, eosinophilia, hypochromic anemia, iron deficiency anemia, leukocytosis, lymphedema, abnormal lymphocytes, lymphocytosis, microcytic anemia, monocytosis, normocytic anemia, thrombocythemia, thrombocytopenia.

Metabolic and Nutritional: *frequent:* weight gain; *infrequent:* edema, peripheral edema, SGOT increased, SGPT increased, thirst, weight loss; *rare:* alkaline phosphatase increased, bilirubinemia, BUN increased, creatinine phosphokinase increased, dehydration, gamma globulins increased, gout, hypercalcemia, hypercholesteremia, hyperglycemia, hyperkalemia, hyperphosphatemia, hypocalcemia, hypoglycemia, hypokalemia, hyponatremia, ketosis, lactic dehydrogenase increased, non-protein nitrogen (NPN) increased.

Musculoskeletal System: *frequent:* arthralgia; *infrequent:* arthritis, arthrosis; *rare:* bursitis, myositis, osteoporosis, generalized spasm, tenosynovitis, tetany.

Nervous System: *frequent:* emotional lability, vertigo; *infrequent:* abnormal thinking, alcohol abuse, ataxia, dystonia, dyskinesia, euphoria, hallucinations, hostility, hypertonia, hypesthesia, hypokinesia, incoordination, lack of emotion, libido increased, manic reaction, neurosis, paralysis, paranoid reaction; *rare:* abnormal gait, akinesia, antisocial reaction, aphasia, choreoathetosis, circumoral paresthesias, convulsion, delirium, delusions, diplopia, drug dependence, dysarthria, extrapyramidal syndrome, fasciculations, grand mal convulsion, hyperalgesia, hysteria, manic-depressive reaction, meningitis, myelitis, neuralgia, neuropathy, nystagmus, peripheral neuritis, psychotic depression, psychosis, reflexes decreased, reflexes increased, stupor, torticollis, trismus, withdrawal syndrome.

Respiratory System: *infrequent:* asthma, bronchitis, dyspnea, epistaxis, hyperventilation, pneumonia, respiratory flu; *rare:* emphysema, hemoptysis, hiccups, lung fibrosis, pulmonary edema, sputum increased, stridor, voice alteration.

Skin and Appendages: *frequent:* pruritus; *infrequent:* acne, alopecia, contact dermatitis, dry skin, ecchymosis, eczema, herpes simplex, photosensitivity, urticaria; *rare:* angioedema, erythema nodosum, erythema multiforme, exfoliative dermatitis, fungal dermatitis, furunculosis; herpes zoster, hirsutism, maculopapular rash, seborrhea, skin discoloration, skin hypertrophy, skin ulcer, sweating decreased, vesiculobullous rash.

Special Senses: *frequent:* tinnitus; *infrequent:* abnormality of accommodation, conjunctivitis, ear pain, eye pain, keratoconjunctivitis, mydriasis, otitis media; *rare:* amblyopia, anisocoria, blepharitis, cataract, conjunctival edema, corneal ulcer, deafness, exophthalmos, eye hemorrhage, glaucoma, hyperacusis, night blindness, otitis externa, parosmia, photophobia, ptosis, retinal hemorrhage, taste loss, visual field defect.

Urogenital System: *infrequent:* amenorrhea, breast pain, cystitis, dysuria, hematuria, menorrhagia, nocturia, polyuria, pyuria, urinary incontinence, urinary retention, urinary urgency, vaginitis; *rare:* abortion, breast atrophy, breast enlargement, endometrial disorder, epididymitis, female lactation, fibrocystic breast, kidney calculus, kidney pain, leukorrhea, mastitis, metrorrhagia, nephritis, oliguria, salpingitis, urethritis, urinary casts, uterine spasm, urolith, vaginal hemorrhage, vaginal moniliasis.

Postmarketing Reports

Voluntary reports of adverse events in patients taking Paxil (paroxetine hydrochloride) that have been received since market introduction and not listed above that may have no causal relationship with the drug include acute pancreatitis, elevated liver function tests (the most severe cases were deaths due to liver necrosis, and grossly elevated transaminases associated with severe liver dysfunction), Guillain-Barré syndrome, toxic epidermal necrolysis, priapism, syndrome of inappropriate ADH secretion, symptoms suggestive of prolactinemia and galactorrhea, neuroleptic malignant syndrome-like events; extrapyramidal symptoms which have included akathisia, bradykinesia, cogwheel rigidity, dystonia, hypertonia, oculogyric crisis which has been associated with concomitant use of pimozide, tremor and trismus; serotonin syndrome, associated in some cases with concomitant use of serotonergic drugs and with drugs which may have impaired *Paxil* metabolism (symptoms have included agitation, confusion, diaphoresis, hallucinations, hyperreflexia, myoclonus, shivering, tachycardia and tremor), status epilepticus, acute renal failure, pulmonary hypertension, allergic alveolitis, anaphylaxis, eclampsia, laryngismus, optic neuritis, porphyria, ventricular fibrillation, ventricular tachycardia (including torsade de pointes), thrombocytopenia, hemolytic anemia, and events related to impaired hematopoiesis (including aplastic anemia, pancytopenia, bone marrow aplasia, and agranulocytosis). There has been a case report of an elevated phenytoin level after 4 weeks of *Paxil* and phenytoin co-administration. There has been a case report of severe hypotension when *Paxil* was added to chronic metoprolol treatment.

DRUG ABUSE AND DEPENDENCE

Controlled Substance Class: Paxil (paroxetine hydrochloride) is not a controlled substance.

Physical and Psychologic Dependence: *Paxil* has not been systematically studied in animals or humans for its potential for abuse, tolerance or physical dependence. While the clinical trials did not reveal any tendency for any drug-seeking behavior, these observations were not systematic and it is not possible to predict on the basis of this limited

Continued on next page

Table 3. Treatment-Emergent Adverse Experience Incidence in Placebo-Controlled Clinical Trials for Generalized Anxiety Disorder and Posttraumatic Stress Disorder[1]

		Generalized Anxiety Disorder		Posttraumatic Stress Disorder	
Body System	**Preferred Term**	***Paxil* (n=735)**	**Placebo (n=529)**	***Paxil* (n=676)**	**Placebo (n=504)**
Body as a Whole	Asthenia	14%	6%	12%	4%
	Headache	17%	14%	—	—
	Infection	6%	3%	5%	4%
	Abdominal Pain			4%	3%
	Trauma			6%	5%
Cardiovascular	Vasodilation	3%	1%	2%	1%
Dermatologic	Sweating	6%	2%	5%	1%
Gastrointestinal	Nausea	20%	5%	19%	8%
	Dry Mouth	11%	5%	10%	5%
	Constipation	10%	2%	5%	3%
	Diarrhea	9%	7%	11%	5%
	Decreased Appetite	5%	1%	6%	3%
	Vomiting	3%	2%	3%	2%
	Dyspepsia	—	—	5%	3%
Nervous System	Insomnia	11%	8%	12%	11%
	Somnolence	15%	5%	16%	5%
	Dizziness	6%	1%	6%	5%
	Tremor	5%	1%	4%	1%
	Nervousness	4%	3%	—	—
	Libido Decreased	9%	2%	5%	2%
	Abnormal Dreams			3%	2%
Respiratory System	Respiratory Disorder	7%	3%	—	—
	Sinusitis	4%	3%	—	—
	Yawn	4%	—	2%	<1%
Special Senses	Abnormal Vision	2%	1%	3%	1%
Urogenital System	Abnormal Ejaculation[2]	25%	2%	13%	2%
	Female Genital Disorder[2]	4%	3%	5%	1%
	Impotence[2]	4%	3%	9%	1%

1. Events reported by at least 2% of GAD and PTSD *Paxil*-treated patients are included, except the following events which had an incidence on placebo ≥*Paxil: [GAD]*: abdominal pain, back pain, trauma, dyspepsia, myalgia, and pharyngitis. [PTSD]: back pain, headache, anxiety, depression, nervousness, respiratory disorder, pharyngitis and sinusitis.
2. Percentage corrected for gender.

Table 4. Treatment-Emergent Adverse Experience Incidence in Dose-Comparison Trial in the Treatment of Major Depressive Disorder*

	Placebo	*Paxil*			
Body System/ Preferred Term	**n=51**	**10 mg n=102**	**20 mg n=104**	**30 mg n=101**	**40 mg n=102**
Body as a Whole					
Asthenia	0.0%	2.9%	10.6%	13.9%	12.7%
Dermatology					
Sweating	2.0%	1.0%	6.7%	8.9%	11.8%
Gastrointestinal					
Constipation	5.9%	4.9%	7.7%	9.9%	12.7%
Decreased Appetite	2.0%	2.0%	5.8%	4.0%	4.9%
Diarrhea	7.8%	9.8%	19.2%	7.9%	14.7%
Dry Mouth	2.0%	10.8%	18.3%	15.8%	20.6%
Nausea	13.7%	14.7%	26.9%	34.7%	36.3%
Nervous System					
Anxiety	0.0%	2.0%	5.8%	5.9%	5.9%
Dizziness	3.9%	6.9%	6.7%	8.9%	12.7%
Nervousness	0.0%	5.9%	5.8%	4.0%	2.9%
Paresthesia	0.0%	2.9%	1.0%	5.0%	5.9%
Somnolence	7.8%	12.7%	18.3%	20.8%	21.6%
Tremor	0.0%	0.0%	7.7%	7.9%	14.7%
Special Senses					
Blurred Vision	2.0%	2.9%	2.9%	2.0%	7.8%
Urogenital System					
Abnormal Ejaculation	0.0%	5.8%	6.5%	10.6%	13.0%
Impotence	0.0%	1.9%	4.3%	6.4%	1.9%
Male Genital Disorders	0.0%	3.8%	8.7%	6.4%	3.7%

* Rule for including adverse events in table: incidence at least 5% for one of paroxetine groups and ≥ twice the placebo incidence for at least one paroxetine group.

Table 5. Incidence of Sexual Adverse Events in Controlled Clinical Trials

	Paxil	Placebo
n (males)	**1446**	**1042**
Decreased Libido	6-15%	0-5%
Ejaculatory Disturbance	13-28%	0-2%
Impotence	2-8%	0-3%
n (females)	**1822**	**1340**
Decreased Libido	0-9%	0-2%
Orgasmic Disturbance	2-9%	0-1%

Paxil—Cont.

experience the extent to which a CNS-active drug will be misused, diverted and/or abused once marketed. Consequently, patients should be evaluated carefully for history of drug abuse, and such patients should be observed closely for signs of *Paxil* misuse or abuse (e.g., development of tolerance, incrementations of dose, drug-seeking behavior).

OVERDOSAGE

Human Experience: Since the introduction of *Paxil* in the U.S., 342 spontaneous cases of deliberate or accidental overdosage during paroxetine treatment have been reported worldwide (circa 1999). These include overdoses with paroxetine alone and in combination with other substances. Of these, 48 cases were fatal and, of the fatalities, 17 appeared to involve paroxetine alone. Eight fatal cases which documented the amount of paroxetine ingested were generally confounded by the ingestion of other drugs or alcohol or the presence of significant comorbid conditions. Of 145 nonfatal cases with known outcome, most recovered without sequelae. The largest known ingestion involved 2,000 mg of paroxetine (33 times the maximum recommended daily dose) in a patient who recovered.

Commonly reported adverse events associated with paroxetine overdosage include somnolence, coma, nausea, tremor, tachycardia, confusion, vomiting, and dizziness. Other notable signs and symptoms observed with overdoses involving paroxetine (alone or with other substances) include mydriasis, convulsions (including status epilepticus), ventricular dysrhythmias (including torsade de pointes), hypertension, aggressive reactions, syncope, hypotension, stupor, bradycardia, dystonia, rhabdomyolysis, symptoms of hepatic dysfunction (including hepatic failure, hepatic necrosis, jaundice, hepatitis, and hepatic steatosis), serotonin syndrome, manic reactions, myoclonus, acute renal failure, and urinary retention.

Overdosage Management: Treatment should consist of those general measures employed in the management of overdosage with any drugs effective in the treatment of major depressive disorder.

Ensure an adequate airway, oxygenation, and ventilation. Monitor cardiac rhythm and vital signs. General supportive and symptomatic measures are also recommended. Induction of emesis is not recommended. Gastric lavage with a large-bore orogastric tube with appropriate airway protection, if needed, may be indicated if performed soon after ingestion, or in symptomatic patients.

Activated charcoal should be administered. Due to the large volume of distribution of this drug, forced diuresis, dialysis, hemoperfusion and exchange transfusion are unlikely to be of benefit. No specific antidotes for paroxetine are known.

A specific caution involves patients who are taking or have recently taken paroxetine who might ingest excessive quantities of a tricyclic antidepressant. In such a case, accumulation of the parent tricyclic and/or an active metabolite may increase the possibility of clinically significant sequelae and extend the time needed for close medical observation (see Drugs Metabolized by Cytochrome $P_{450}IID_6$ under PRECAUTIONS).

In managing overdosage, consider the possibility of multiple drug involvement. The physician should consider contacting a poison control center for additional information on the treatment of any overdose. Telephone numbers for certified poison control centers are listed in the *Physicians' Desk Reference* (PDR).

DOSAGE AND ADMINISTRATION

Major Depressive Disorder

Usual Initial Dosage: Paxil (paroxetine hydrochloride) should be administered as a single daily dose with or without food, usually in the morning. The recommended initial dose is 20 mg/day. Patients were dosed in a range of 20 to 50 mg/day in the clinical trials demonstrating the effectiveness of *Paxil* in the treatment of major depressive disorder. As with all drugs effective in the treatment of major depressive disorder, the full effect may be delayed. Some patients not responding to a 20 mg dose may benefit from dose increases, in 10 mg/day increments, up to a maximum of 50 mg/day. Dose changes should occur at intervals of at least 1 week.

Maintenance Therapy: There is no body of evidence available to answer the question of how long the patient treated with *Paxil* should remain on it. It is generally agreed that acute episodes of major depressive disorder require several months or longer of sustained pharmacologic therapy. Whether the dose needed to induce remission is identical to the dose needed to maintain and/or sustain euthymia is unknown.

Systematic evaluation of the efficacy of Paxil (paroxetine hydrochloride) has shown that efficacy is maintained for periods of up to 1 year with doses that averaged about 30 mg.

Obsessive Compulsive Disorder

Usual Initial Dosage: Paxil (paroxetine hydrochloride) should be administered as a single daily dose with or without food, usually in the morning. The recommended dose of *Paxil* in the treatment of OCD is 40 mg daily. Patients should be started on 20 mg/day and the dose can be increased in 10 mg/day increments. Dose changes should occur at intervals of at least 1 week. Patients were dosed in a range of 20 to 60 mg/day in the clinical trials demonstrating the effectiveness of *Paxil* in the treatment of OCD. The maximum dosage should not exceed 60 mg/day.

Maintenance Therapy: Long-term maintenance of efficacy was demonstrated in a 6-month relapse prevention trial. In this trial, patients with OCD assigned to paroxetine demonstrated a lower relapse rate compared to patients on placebo (see CLINICAL PHARMACOLOGY). OCD is a chronic condition, and it is reasonable to consider continuation for a responding patient. Dosage adjustments should be made to maintain the patient on the lowest effective dosage, and patients should be periodically reassessed to determine the need for continued treatment.

Panic Disorder

Usual Initial Dosage: *Paxil* should be administered as a single daily dose with or without food, usually in the morning. The target dose of *Paxil* in the treatment of panic disorder is 40 mg/day. Patients should be started on 10 mg/day. Dose changes should occur in 10 mg/day increments and at intervals of at least 1 week. Patients were dosed in a range of 10 to 60 mg/day in the clinical trials demonstrating the effectiveness of *Paxil*. The maximum dosage should not exceed 60 mg/day.

Maintenance Therapy: Long-term maintenance of efficacy was demonstrated in a 3-month relapse prevention trial. In this trial, patients with panic disorder assigned to paroxetine demonstrated a lower relapse rate compared to patients on placebo (see CLINICAL PHARMACOLOGY). Panic disorder is a chronic condition, and it is reasonable to consider continuation for a responding patient. Dosage adjustments should be made to maintain the patient on the lowest effective dosage, and patients should be periodically reassessed to determine the need for continued treatment.

Social Anxiety Disorder

Usual Initial Dosage: *Paxil* should be administered as a single daily dose with or without food, usually in the morning. The recommended and initial dosage is 20 mg/day. In clinical trials the effectiveness of *Paxil* was demonstrated in patients dosed in a range of 20 to 60 mg/day. While the safety of *Paxil* has been evaluated in patients with social anxiety disorder at doses up to 60 mg/day, available information does not suggest any additional benefit for doses above 20 mg/day. (See CLINICAL PHARMACOLOGY).

Maintenance Therapy: There is no body of evidence available to answer the question of how long the patient treated with *Paxil* should remain on it. Although the efficacy of *Paxil* beyond 12 weeks of dosing has not been demonstrated in controlled clinical trials, social anxiety disorder is recognized as a chronic condition, and it is reasonable to consider continuation of treatment for a responding patient. Dosage adjustments should be made to maintain the patient on the lowest effective dosage, and patients should be periodically reassessed to determine the need for continued treatment.

Generalized Anxiety Disorder

Usual Initial Dosage: *Paxil* should be administered as a single daily dose with or without food, usually in the morning. In clinical trials the effectiveness of *Paxil* was demonstrated in patients dosed in a range of 20 to 50 mg/day. The recommended starting dosage and the established effective dosage is 20 mg/day. There is not sufficient evidence to suggest a greater benefit to doses higher than 20 mg/day. Dose changes should occur in 10 mg/day increments and at intervals of at least 1 week.

Maintenance Therapy: There is no body of evidence available to answer the question of how long the patient treated with *Paxil* should remain on it. Although the efficacy of *Paxil* beyond 8 weeks of dosing has not been demonstrated in controlled clinical trials, generalized anxiety disorder is recognized as a chronic condition, and it is reasonable to consider continuation of treatment for a responding patient. Dosage adjustments should be made to maintain the patient on the lowest effective dosage, and patients should be periodically reassessed to determine the need for continued treatment.

Posttraumatic Stress Disorder

Usual Initial Dosage: Paxil should be administered as a single daily dose with or without food., usually in the morning. The recommended starting dosage and the established effective dosage is 20 mg/day. In one clinical trial, the effectiveness of *Paxil* was demonstrated in patients dosed in a range of 20 to 50 mg/day. However, in a fixed dose study, there was not sufficient evidence to suggest a greater benefit for a dose of 40 mg/day compared to 20 mg/day. Dose changes, if indicated, should occur in 10 mg/day increments and at intervals of at least 1 week.

Maintenance Therapy: There is no body of evidence available to answer the question of how long the patient treated with *Paxil* should remain on it. Although the efficacy of *Paxil* beyond 12 weeks of dosing has not been demonstrated in controlled clinical trials, PTSD is recognized as a chronic condition, and it is reasonable to consider continuation of treatment for a responding patient. Dosage adjustments should be made to maintain the patient on the lowest effective dosage, and patients should be periodically reassessed to determine the need for continued treatment.

Dosage for Elderly or Debilitated, and Patients with Severe Renal or Hepatic Impairment: The recommended initial dose is 10 mg/day for elderly patients, debilitated patients, and/or patients with severe renal or hepatic impairment. Increases may be made if indicated. Dosage should not exceed 40 mg/day.

Switching Patients to or from a Monoamine Oxidase Inhibitor: At least 14 days should elapse between discontinuation of a MAOI and initiation of *Paxil* therapy. Similarly, at least 14 days should be allowed after stopping Paxil (paroxetine hydrochloride) before starting a MAOI.

Discontinuation of Treatment with Paxil: Symptoms associated with discontinuation of *Paxil* have been reported (see PRECAUTIONS). Patients should be monitored for these symptoms when discontinuing treatment, regardless of the indication for which *Paxil* is being prescribed. A gradual reduction in the dose rather than abrupt cessation is recommended whenever possible. If intolerable symptoms occur following a decrease in the dose or upon discontinuation of treatment, then resuming the previously prescribed dose may be considered. Subsequently, the physician may continue decreasing the dose but at a more gradual rate.

NOTE: SHAKE SUSPENSION WELL BEFORE USING.

HOW SUPPLIED

Tablets: Film-coated, modified-oval as follows:
10 mg yellow, scored tablets engraved on the front with PAXIL and on the back with 10.
NDC 0029-3210-13 Bottles of 30
20 mg pink, scored tablets engraved on the front with PAXIL and on the back with 20.
NDC 0029-3211-13 Bottles of 30
NDC 0029-3211-20 Bottles of 100
NDC 0029-3211-21 SUP 100's (intended for institutional use only)
30 mg blue tablets engraved on the front with PAXIL and on the back with 30.
NDC 0029-3212-13 Bottles of 30
40 mg green tablets engraved on the front with PAXIL and on the back with 40.
NDC 0029-3213-13 Bottles of 30
Store tablets between 15° and 30°C (59° and 86°F).
Oral Suspension: Orange-colored, orange-flavored, 10 mg/5 mL, in 250 mL white bottles.
NDC 0029-3215-48
Store suspension at or below 25°C (77°F).
GlaxoSmithKline, Research Triangle Park, NC 27709

January 2002/PX: L22

PURINETHOL® ℞
[*pur 'ĭn-thawl*]
(mercaptopurine)
50-mg Scored Tablets

Prescribing information for this product, which appears on pages 1615–1617 of the 2002 PDR, has been revised as follows. Please write "See Supplement A" next to the product heading.

The following paragraph was added to the end of the **CONTRAINDICATIONS** *section:*

PURINETHOL should not be used in patients who have a hypersensitivity to mercaptopurine or any component of the formulation.

The third paragraph of the **WARNINGS** *section was revised to:*

There are individuals with an inherited deficiency of the enzyme thiopurine methyltransferase (TPMT) who may be unusually sensitive to the myelosuppressive effects of mercaptopurine and prone to developing rapid bone marrow suppression following the initiation of treatment.[6,7] Substantial dosage reductions may be required to avoid the development of life-threatening bone marrow suppression in these patients. This toxicity may be more profound in patients treated with concomitant allopurinol (see PRECAUTIONS: Drug Interactions). This problem could be exacerbated by coadministration with drugs that inhibit TPMT, such as olsalazine, mesalazine, or sulphasalazine.

The **PRECAUTIONS: Drug Interactions** *subsection was revised to:*

When allopurinol and mercaptopurine are administered concomitantly, it is imperative that the dose of mercaptopurine be reduced to one third to one quarter of the usual dose. Failure to observe this dosage reduction will result in a delayed catabolism of mercaptopurine and the strong likelihood of inducing severe toxicity.

There is usually complete cross-resistance between mercaptopurine and thioguanine.

The dosage of mercaptopurine may need to be reduced when this agent is combined with other drugs whose primary or secondary toxicity is myelosuppression. Enhanced marrow suppression has been noted in some patients also receiving trimethoprim-sulfamethoxazole.[17,18]

Inhibition of the anticoagulant effect of warfarin, when given with mercaptopurine, has been reported. As there is in vitro evidence that aminosalicylate derivatives (e.g., olsalazine, mesalazine, or sulphasalazine) inhibit the TPMT enzyme, they should be administered with caution to patients receiving concurrent mercaptopurine therapy (see WARNINGS).

The first sentence of the **ADVERSE REACTIONS: Renal** *subsection was revised to:*

Hyperuricemia and/or hyperuricosuria may occur in patients receiving PURINETHOL as a consequence of rapid cell lysis accompanying the antineoplastic effect.

The following sentence was added to the **OVERDOSAGE** *section:*

Hematologic toxicity is likely to be more profound with chronic overdosage than with a single ingestion of PURINETHOL.

The following subsections were added to the **DOSAGE AND ADMINISTRATION** *section:*

Dosage in Renal Impairment: Consideration should be given to reducing the dosage in patients with impaired renal function.

Dosage in Hepatic Impairment: Consideration should be given to reducing the dosage in patients with impaired hepatic function.

The following **REFERENCE,** *which refers to proper handling and disposal of anticancer drugs in the DOSAGE AND ADMINISTRATION: Maintenance Therapy subsection, was revised to:*

32. Controlling Occupational Exposure to Hazardous Drugs. (OSHA Work-Practice Guidelines.) *Am J Health-Syst Pharm.* 1996;53:1669–1685.

Manufactured by Catalytica Pharmaceuticals, Inc.
Greenville, NC 27834
for GlaxoSmithKline, Research Triangle Park, NC 27709

September 2001/RL-995

RETROVIR® ℞
[re 'trō-vir]
(zidovudine)
Tablets

RETROVIR® ℞
(zidovudine)
Capsules

RETROVIR® ℞
(zidovudine)
Syrup

Prescribing information for these products, which appears on pages 1625–1629 of the 2002 PDR, has been revised as follows. Please write "See Supplement A" next to the product heading.

The following subsection was added to **PRECAUTIONS:**

Geriatric Use: Clinical studies of RETROVIR did not include sufficient numbers of subjects aged 65 and over to determine whether they respond differently from younger subjects. Other reported clinical experience has not identified differences in responses between the elderly and younger patients. In general, dose selection for an elderly patient should be cautious, reflecting the greater frequency of decreased hepatic, renal, or cardiac function, and of concomitant disease or other drug therapy.

The following subsections of **ADVERSE REACTIONS: Observed During Clinical Practice** *were added or revised:*

Endocrine: Gynecomastia.

Gastrointestinal: Constipation, dysphagia, flatulence, oral mucosa pigmentation, mouth ulcer.

Hemic and Lymphatic: Aplastic anemia, hemolytic anemia, leukopenia, lymphadenopathy, pancytopenia with marrow hypoplasia, pure red cell aplasia.

GlaxoSmithKline, Research Triangle Park, NC 27709

December 2001/RL-1040

RETROVIR® ℞
[re'trō-vir]
(zidovudine)
IV infusion

FOR INTRAVENOUS INFUSION ONLY

Prescribing information for this product, which appears on pages 1629–1633 of the 2002 PDR, has been completely revised as follows. Please write "See Supplement A" next to the product heading.

> **WARNING**
> **RETROVIR (ZIDOVUDINE) HAS BEEN ASSOCIATED WITH HEMATOLOGIC TOXICITY, INCLUDING NEUTROPENIA AND SEVERE ANEMIA, PARTICULARLY IN PATIENTS WITH ADVANCED HIV DISEASE (SEE WARNINGS). PROLONGED USE OF RETROVIR HAS BEEN ASSOCIATED WITH SYMPTOMATIC MYOPATHY. LACTIC ACIDOSIS AND SEVERE HEPATOMEGALY WITH STEATOSIS, INCLUDING FATAL CASES, HAVE BEEN REPORTED WITH THE USE OF NUCLEOSIDE ANALOGUES ALONE OR IN COMBINATION, INCLUDING RETROVIR AND OTHER ANTIRETROVIRALS (SEE WARNINGS).**

DESCRIPTION

RETROVIR is the brand name for zidovudine (formerly called azidothymidine [AZT]), a pyrimidine nucleoside analogue active against human immunodeficiency virus (HIV). RETROVIR IV Infusion is a sterile solution for intravenous infusion only. Each mL contains 10 mg zidovudine in Water for Injection. Hydrochloric acid and/or sodium hydroxide may have been added to adjust the pH to approximately 5.5. RETROVIR IV Infusion contains no preservatives.

The chemical name of zidovudine is 3′-azido-3′-deoxythymidine.

Zidovudine is a white to beige, odorless, crystalline solid with a molecular weight of 267.24 and a solubility of 20.1 mg/mL in water at 25°C. The molecular formula is $C_{10}H_{13}N_5O_4$.

MICROBIOLOGY

Mechanism of Action: Zidovudine is a synthetic nucleoside analogue of the naturally occurring nucleoside, thymidine, in which the 3′-hydroxy (−OH) group is replaced by an azido ($-N_3$) group. Within cells, zidovudine is converted to the active metabolite, zidovudine 5′-triphosphate (AztTP), by the sequential action of the cellular enzymes. Zidovudine 5′-triphosphate inhibits the activity of the HIV reverse transcriptase both by competing for utilization with the natural substrate, deoxythymidine 5′-triphosphate (dTTP), and by its incorporation into viral DNA. The lack of a 3′-OH group in the incorporated nucleoside analogue prevents the formation of the 5′ to 3′ phosphodiester linkage essential for DNA chain elongation and, therefore, the viral DNA growth is terminated. The active metabolite AztTP is also a weak inhibitor of the cellular DNA polymerase-alpha and mitochondrial polymerase-gamma and has been reported to be incorporated into the DNA of cells in culture.

In Vitro HIV Susceptibility: The in vitro anti-HIV activity of zidovudine was assessed by infecting cell lines of lymphoblastic and monocytic origin and peripheral blood lymphocytes with laboratory and clinical isolates of HIV. The IC_{50} and IC_{90} values (50% and 90% inhibitory concentrations) were 0.003 to 0.013 and 0.03 to 0.13 mcg/mL, respectively (1 nM = 0.27 ng/mL). The IC_{50} and IC_{90} values of HIV isolates recovered from 18 untreated AIDS/ARC patients were in the range of 0.003 to 0.013 mcg/mL and 0.03 to 0.3 mcg/mL, respectively. Zidovudine showed antiviral activity in all acutely infected cell lines; however, activity was substantially less in chronically infected cell lines. In drug combination studies with zalcitabine, didanosine, lamivudine, saquinavir, indinavir, ritonavir, nevirapine, delavirdine, or interferon-alpha, zidovudine showed additive to synergistic activity in cell culture. The relationship between the in vitro susceptibility of HIV to reverse transcriptase inhibitors and the inhibition of HIV replication in humans has not been established.

Drug Resistance: HIV isolates with reduced sensitivity to zidovudine have been selected in vitro and were also recovered from patients treated with RETROVIR. Genetic analysis of the isolates showed mutations that result in 5 amino acid substitutions (Met41→Leu, A67→Asn, Lys70→Arg, Thr215→Tyr or Phe, and Lys219→Gln) in the viral reverse transcriptase. In general, higher levels of resistance were associated with greater number of mutations, with 215 mutation being the most significant.

Cross-Resistance: The potential for cross-resistance between HIV reverse transcriptase inhibitors and protease inhibitors is low because of the different enzyme targets involved. Combination therapy with zidovudine plus zalcitabine or didanosine does not appear to prevent the emergence of zidovudine-resistant isolates. Combination therapy with RETROVIR plus EPIVIR® delayed the emergence of mutations conferring resistance to zidovudine. In some patients harboring zidovudine-resistant virus, combination therapy with RETROVIR plus EPIVIR restored phenotypic sensitivity to zidovudine by 12 weeks of treatment. HIV isolates with multidrug resistance to zidovudine, didanosine, zalcitabine, stavudine, and lamivudine were recovered from a small number of patients treated for ≥1 year with the combination of zidovudine and didanosine or zalcitabine. The pattern of resistant mutations in the combination therapy was different (Ala62→Val, Val75→Ile, Phe77→116Tyr, and Gln→151Met) from monotherapy, with mutation 151 being most significant for multidrug resistance. Site-directed mutagenesis studies showed that these mutations could also result in resistance to zalcitabine, lamivudine, and stavudine.

CLINICAL PHARMACOLOGY

Pharmacokinetics: ***Adults:*** The pharmacokinetics of zidovudine have been evaluated in 22 adult HIV-infected patients in a Phase 1 dose-escalation study. Following intravenous (IV) dosing, dose-independent kinetics was observed over the range of 1 to 5 mg/kg. The major metabolite of zidovudine is 3′-azido-3′-deoxy-5′-*O*-β-*D*-glucopyranuronosylthymidine (GZDV). GZDV area under the curve (AUC) is about 3-fold greater than the zidovudine AUC. Urinary recovery of zidovudine and GZDV accounts for 18% and 60%, respectively, following IV dosing. A second metabolite, 3′-amino-3′-deoxythymidine (AMT), has been identified in the plasma following single-dose IV administration of zidovudine. The AMT AUC was one fifth of the zidovudine AUC.

The mean steady-state peak and trough concentrations of zidovudine at 2.5 mg/kg every 4 hours were 1.06 and 0.12 mcg/mL, respectively.

The zidovudine cerebrospinal fluid (CSF)/plasma concentration ratio was determined in 39 patients receiving chronic therapy with RETROVIR. The median ratio measured in 50 paired samples drawn 1 to 8 hours after the last dose of RETROVIR was 0.6.

Table 1. Zidovudine Pharmacokinetic Parameters Following Intravenous Administration in HIV-Infected Patients

Parameter	Mean ± SD (except where noted)
Apparent volume of distribution (L/kg)	1.6 ± 0.6 (n = 11)
Plasma protein binding (%)	<38
CSF:plasma ratio*	0.6 [0.04 to 2.62] (n = 39)
Systemic clearance (L/hr/kg)	1.6 (0.8 to 2.7) (n = 18)
Renal clearance (L/hr/kg)	0.34 ± 0.05 (n = 16)
Elimination half-life (hr)†	1.1 (0.5 to 2.9) (n = 19)

*Median [range].
†Approximate range.

Adults with Impaired Renal Function: Zidovudine clearance was decreased resulting in increased zidovudine and GZDV half-life and AUC in patients with impaired renal function (n = 14) following a single 200-mg oral dose (Table 2). Plasma concentrations of AMT were not determined. A dose adjustment should not be necessary for patients with creatinine clearance (CrCl) ≥15 mL/min.

[See table 2 at top of next page]

The pharmacokinetics and tolerance of oral zidovudine were evaluated in a multiple-dose study in patients undergoing hemodialysis (n = 5) or peritoneal dialysis (n = 6) receiving escalating doses up to 200 mg 5 times daily for 8 weeks. Daily doses of 500 mg or less were well tolerated despite significantly elevated GZDV plasma concentrations. Apparent zidovudine oral clearance was approximately 50% of that reported in patients with normal renal function. Hemodialysis and peritoneal dialysis appeared to have a negligible effect on the removal of zidovudine, whereas GZDV elimination was enhanced. A dosage adjustment is recommended for patients undergoing hemodialysis or peritoneal dialysis (see DOSAGE AND ADMINISTRATION: Dose Adjustment).

Adults with Impaired Hepatic Function: Data describing the effect of hepatic impairment on the pharmacokinetics of zidovudine are limited. However, because zidovudine is eliminated primarily by hepatic metabolism, it is expected that zidovudine clearance would be decreased and plasma concentrations would be increased following administration of the recommended adult doses to patients with hepatic impairment (see DOSAGE AND ADMINISTRATION: Dose Adjustment).

Pediatrics: Zidovudine pharmacokinetics have been evaluated in HIV-infected pediatric patients (Table 3).

Patients from 3 Months to 12 Years of Age: Overall, zidovudine pharmacokinetics in pediatric patients >3 months of age are similar to those in adult patients. Proportional increases in plasma zidovudine concentrations were observed following administration of oral solution from 90 to 240 mg/m^2 every 6 hours. Oral bioavailability, terminal half-life, and oral clearance were comparable to adult values. As in adult patients, the major route of elimination was by metabolism to GZDV. After intravenous dosing, about 29% of the dose was excreted in the urine unchanged and about 45% of the dose was excreted as GZDV (see DOSAGE AND ADMINISTRATION: Pediatrics).

Patients Younger Than 3 Months of Age: Zidovudine pharmacokinetics have been evaluated in pediatric patients from birth to 3 months of life. Zidovudine elimination was determined immediately following birth in 8 neonates who were exposed to zidovudine in utero. The half-life was 13.0 ± 5.8 hours. In neonates ≤14 days old, bioavailability was greater, total body clearance was slower, and half-life was longer than in pediatric patients >14 days old. For dose recommendations for neonates, see DOSAGE AND ADMINISTRATION: Neonatal Dosing.

[See table 3 at top of next page]

Pregnancy: Zidovudine pharmacokinetics have been studied in a Phase 1 study of 8 women during the last trimester of pregnancy. As pregnancy progressed, there was no evidence of drug accumulation. Zidovudine pharmacokinetics were similar to that of nonpregnant adults. Consistent with passive transmission of the drug across the placenta, zidovudine concentrations in neonatal plasma at birth were essentially equal to those in maternal plasma at delivery. Although data are limited, methadone maintenance therapy in 5 pregnant women did not appear to alter zidovudine pharmacokinetics. However, in another patient population, a potential for interaction has been identified (see PRECAUTIONS).

Nursing Mothers: **The Centers for Disease Control and Prevention recommend that HIV-infected mothers not breast-feed their infants to avoid risking postnatal transmission of HIV.** After administration of a single dose of 200 mg zidovudine to 13 HIV-infected women, the mean concentration of zidovudine was similar in human milk and serum (see PRECAUTIONS: Nursing Mothers).

Geriatric Patients: Zidovudine pharmacokinetics have not been studied in patients over 65 years of age.

Gender: A pharmacokinetic study in healthy male (n = 12) and female (n = 12) subjects showed no differences in zidovudine exposure (AUC) when a single dose of zidovudine was administered as the 300-mg RETROVIR Tablet.

Drug Interactions: See Table 4 and PRECAUTIONS: Drug Interactions.

Zidovudine Plus Lamivudine: No clinically significant alterations in lamivudine or zidovudine pharmacokinetics were observed in 12 asymptomatic HIV-infected adult patients given a single oral dose of zidovudine (200 mg) in combination with multiple oral doses of lamivudine (300 mg every 12 hours).

[See table 4 at top of next page]

Continued on next page

Retrovir Infusion—Cont.

INDICATIONS AND USAGE

RETROVIR IV Infusion in combination with other antiretroviral agents is indicated for the treatment of HIV infection.

Maternal-Fetal HIV Transmission: RETROVIR is also indicated for the prevention of maternal-fetal HIV transmission as part of a regimen that includes oral RETROVIR beginning between 14 and 34 weeks of gestation, intravenous RETROVIR during labor, and administration of RETROVIR Syrup to the neonate after birth. The efficacy of this regimen for preventing HIV transmission in women who have received RETROVIR for a prolonged period before pregnancy has not been evaluated. The safety of RETROVIR for the mother or fetus during the first trimester of pregnancy has not been assessed (see Description of Clinical Studies).

Description of Clinical Studies: Therapy with RETROVIR has been shown to prolong survival and decrease the incidence of opportunistic infections in patients with advanced HIV disease at the initiation of therapy and to delay disease progression in asymptomatic HIV-infected patients. RETROVIR in combination with other antiretroviral agents has been shown to be superior to monotherapy in one or more of the following endpoints: delaying death, delaying development of AIDS, increasing CD4 cell counts, and decreasing plasma HIV-1 RNA. The complete prescribing information for each drug should be consulted before combination therapy that includes RETROVIR is initiated.

Pregnant Women and Their Neonates: The utility of RETROVIR for the prevention of maternal-fetal HIV transmission was demonstrated in a randomized, double-blind, placebo-controlled trial (ACTG 076) conducted in HIV-infected pregnant women with CD4 cell counts of 200 to 1,818 cells/mm^3 (median in the treated group: 560 cells/mm^3) who had little or no previous exposure to RETROVIR. Oral RETROVIR was initiated between 14 and 34 weeks of gestation (median 11 weeks of therapy) followed by intravenous administration of RETROVIR during labor and delivery. Following birth, neonates received oral RETROVIR Syrup for 6 weeks. The study showed a statistically significant difference in the incidence of HIV infection in the neonates (based on viral culture from peripheral blood) between the group receiving RETROVIR and the group receiving placebo. Of 363 neonates evaluated in the study, the estimated risk of HIV infection was 7.8% in the group receiving RETROVIR and 24.9% in the placebo group, a relative reduction in transmission risk of 68.7%. RETROVIR was well tolerated by mothers and infants. There was no difference in pregnancy-related adverse events between the treatment groups.

CONTRAINDICATIONS

RETROVIR IV Infusion is contraindicated for patients who have potentially life-threatening allergic reactions to any of the components of the formulation.

WARNINGS

COMBIVIR® and TRIZIVIR® are combination product tablets that contain zidovudine as one of their components. RETROVIR should not be administered concomitantly with COMBIVIR or TRIZIVIR.

The incidence of adverse reactions appears to increase with disease progression; patients should be monitored carefully, especially as disease progression occurs.

Bone Marrow Suppression: RETROVIR should be used with caution in patients who have bone marrow compromise evidenced by granulocyte count <1,000 cells/mm^3 or hemoglobin <9.5 g/dL. In patients with advanced symptomatic HIV disease, anemia and neutropenia were the most significant adverse events observed. There have been reports of pancytopenia associated with the use of RETROVIR, which was reversible in most instances, after discontinuance of the drug. However, significant anemia, in many cases requiring dose adjustment, discontinuation of RETROVIR, and/or blood transfusions, has occurred during treatment with RETROVIR alone or in combination with other antiretrovirals.

Frequent blood counts are strongly recommended in patients with advanced HIV disease who are treated with RETROVIR. For HIV-infected individuals and patients with asymptomatic or early HIV disease, periodic blood counts are recommended. If anemia or neutropenia develops, dosage adjustments may be necessary (see DOSAGE AND ADMINISTRATION).

Myopathy: Myopathy and myositis with pathological changes, similar to that produced by HIV disease, have been associated with prolonged use of RETROVIR.

Lactic Acidosis/Severe Hepatomegaly with Steatosis: Lactic acidosis and severe hepatomegaly with steatosis, including fatal cases, have been reported with the use of nucleoside analogues alone or in combination, including zidovudine and other antiretrovirals. A majority of these cases have been in women. Obesity and prolonged exposure to antiretroviral nucleoside analogues may be risk factors. Particular caution should be exercised when administering RETROVIR to any patient with known risk factors for liver disease; however, cases have also been reported in patients with no known risk factors. Treatment with RETROVIR should be suspended in any patient who develops clinical or laboratory findings suggestive of lactic acidosis or pronounced hepatotoxicity (which may include hepatomegaly and steatosis even in the absence of marked transaminase elevations).

PRECAUTIONS

General: Zidovudine is eliminated from the body primarily by renal excretion following metabolism in the liver (glucuronidation). In patients with severely impaired renal function (CrCl<15 mL/min), dosage reduction is recommended. Although the data are limited, zidovudine concentrations appear to be increased in patients with severely impaired hepatic function, which may increase the risk of hematologic toxicity (see CLINICAL PHARMACOLOGY: Pharmacokinetics and DOSAGE AND ADMINISTRATION).

Information for Patients: RETROVIR is not a cure for HIV infection, and patients may continue to acquire illnesses associated with HIV infection, including opportunistic infections. Therefore, patients should be advised to seek medical care for any significant change in their health status.

The safety and efficacy of RETROVIR in treating women, intravenous drug users, and racial minorities is not significantly different than that observed in white males.

Patients should be informed that the major toxicities of RETROVIR are neutropenia and/or anemia. The frequency and severity of these toxicities are greater in patients with more advanced disease and in those who initiate therapy later in the course of their infection. They should be told that if toxicity develops, they may require transfusions or drug discontinuation. They should be told of the extreme importance of having their blood counts followed closely while on therapy, especially for patients with advanced symptomatic HIV disease. They should be cautioned about the use of other medications, including ganciclovir and interferon-alpha, which may exacerbate the toxicity of RETROVIR (see PRECAUTIONS: Drug Interactions). Patients should be informed that other adverse effects of RETROVIR include nausea and vomiting. Patients should also be encouraged to contact their physician if they experience muscle weakness, shortness of breath, symptoms of hepatitis or pancreatitis, or any other unexpected adverse events while being treated with RETROVIR.

Pregnant women considering the use of RETROVIR during pregnancy for prevention of HIV transmission to their infants should be advised that transmission may still occur in some cases despite therapy. The long-term consequences of in utero and neonatal exposure to RETROVIR are unknown, including the possible risk of cancer.

HIV-infected pregnant women should be advised not to breastfeed to avoid postnatal transmission of HIV to a child who may not yet be infected.

Patients should be advised that therapy with RETROVIR has not been shown to reduce the risk of transmission of HIV to others through sexual contact or blood contamination.

Drug Interactions: See CLINICAL PHARMACOLOGY section (Table 4) for information on zidovudine concentrations when coadministered with other drugs. For patients experiencing pronounced anemia or other severe zidovudine-associated events while receiving chronic administration of zidovudine and some of the drugs (e.g., fluconazole, valproic acid) listed in Table 4, zidovudine dose reduction may be considered.

Antiretroviral Agents: Concomitant use of zidovudine with stavudine should be avoided since an antagonistic relationship has been demonstrated in vitro.

Some nucleoside analogues affecting DNA replication, such as ribavirin, antagonize the in vitro antiviral activity of RETROVIR against HIV; concomitant use of such drugs should be avoided.

Doxorubicin: Concomitant use of zidovudine with doxorubicin should be avoided since an antagonistic relationship has been demonstrated in vitro (see CLINICAL PHARMACOLOGY for additional drug interactions).

Phenytoin: Phenytoin plasma levels have been reported to be low in some patients receiving RETROVIR, while in 1 case a high level was documented. However, in a pharmacokinetic interaction study in which 12 HIV-positive volunteers received a single 300-mg phenytoin dose alone and during steady-state zidovudine conditions (200 mg every 4

Table 2. Zidovudine Pharmacokinetic Parameters in Patients With Severe Renal Impairment*

Parameter	Control Subjects (Normal Renal Function) (n = 6)	Patients With Renal Impairment (n = 14)
CrCl (mL/min)	120 ± 8	18 ± 2
Zidovudine AUC (ng•hr/mL)	1,400 ± 200	3,100 ± 300
Zidovudine half-life (hr)	1.0 ± 0.2	1.4 ± 0.1

*Data are expressed as mean ± standard deviation.

Table 3. Zidovudine Pharmacokinetic Parameters in Pediatric Patients*

Parameter	Birth to 14 Days of Age	14 Days to 3 Months of Age	3 Months to 12 Years of Age
Oral bioavailability (%)	89 ± 19 (n = 15)	61 ± 19 (n = 17)	65 ± 24 (n = 18)
CSF:plasma ratio	no data	no data	0.26 ± 0.17† (n = 28)
CL (L/hr/kg)	0.65 ± 0.29 (n = 18)	1.14 ± 0.24 (n = 16)	1.85 ± 0.47 (n =20)
Elimination half-life (hr)	3.1 ± 1.2 (n = 21)	1.9 ± 0.7 (n = 18)	1.5 ± 0.7 (n = 21)

*Data presented as mean ± standard deviation except where noted.
†CSF ratio determined at steady-state on constant intravenous infusion.

Table 4. Effect of Coadministered Drugs on Zidovudine AUC*
Note: ROUTINE DOSE MODIFICATION OF ZIDOVUDINE IS NOT WARRANTED WITH COADMINISTRATION OF THE FOLLOWING DRUGS.

Coadministered Drug and Dose	Zidovudine Oral Dose	n	Zidovudine Concentrations: AUC	Zidovudine Concentrations: Variability	Concentration of Coadministered Drug
Atovaquone 750 mg q 12 hr with food	200 mg q 8 hr	14	↑ AUC 31%	Range 23% to 78%†	↔
Fluconazole 400 mg daily	200 mg q 8 hr	12	↑ AUC 74%	95% CI: 54% to 98%	Not Reported
Methadone 30 to 90 mg daily	200 mg q 4 hr	9	↑ AUC 43%	Range 16% to 64%†	↔
Nelfinavir 750 mg q 8 hr × 7 to 10 days	single 200 mg	11	↓ AUC 35%	Range 28% to 41%	↔
Probenecid 500 mg q 6 hr × 2 days	2 mg/kg q 8 hr × 3 days	3	↑ AUC 106%	Range 100% to 170%†	Not Assessed
Ritonavir 300 mg q 6 hr × 4 days	200 mg q 8 hr × 4 days	9	↓ AUC 25%	95% CI: 15% to 34%	↔
Valproic acid 250 mg or 500 mg q 8 hr × 4 days	100 mg q 8 hr × 4 days	6	↑ AUC 80%	Range 64% to 130%†	Not Assessed

↑ = Increase; ↓ = Decrease; ↔ = no significant change; AUC = area under the concentration versus time curve; CI = confidence interval.
*This table is not all inclusive.
†Estimated range of percent difference.

hours), no change in phenytoin kinetics was observed. Although not designed to optimally assess the effect of phenytoin on zidovudine kinetics, a 30% decrease in oral zidovudine clearance was observed with phenytoin.

Overlapping Toxicities: Coadministration of ganciclovir, interferon-alpha, and other bone marrow suppressive or cytotoxic agents may increase the hematologic toxicity of zidovudine.

Carcinogenesis, Mutagenesis, Impairment of Fertility: Zidovudine was administered orally at 3 dosage levels to separate groups of mice and rats (60 females and 60 males in each group). Initial single daily doses were 30, 60, and 120 mg/kg/day in mice and 80, 220, and 600 mg/kg/day in rats. The doses in mice were reduced to 20, 30, and 40 mg/kg/day after day 90 because of treatment-related anemia, whereas in rats only the high dose was reduced to 450 mg/kg/day on day 91, and then to 300 mg/kg/day on day 279.

In mice, 7 late-appearing (after 19 months) vaginal neoplasms (5 nonmetastasizing squamous cell carcinomas, 1 squamous cell papilloma, and 1 squamous polyp) occurred in animals given the highest dose. One late-appearing squamous cell papilloma occurred in the vagina of a middle-dose animal. No vaginal tumors were found at the lowest dose.

In rats, 2 late-appearing (after 20 months), nonmetastasizing vaginal squamous cell carcinomas occurred in animals given the highest dose. No vaginal tumors occurred at the low or middle dose in rats. No other drug-related tumors were observed in either sex of either species.

At doses that produced tumors in mice and rats, the estimated drug exposure (as measured by AUC) was approximately 3 times (mouse) and 24 times (rat) the estimated human exposure at the recommended therapeutic dose of 100 mg every 4 hours.

Two transplacental carcinogenicity studies were conducted in mice. One study administered zidovudine at doses of 20 mg/kg/day or 40 mg/kg/day from gestation day 10 through parturition and lactation with dosing continuing in offspring for 24 months postnatally. The doses of zidovudine employed in this study produced zidovudine exposures approximately 3 times the estimated human exposure at recommended doses. After 24 months, an increase in incidence of vaginal tumors was noted with no increase in tumors in the liver or lung or any other organ in either gender. These findings are consistent with results of the standard oral carcinogenicity study in mice, as described earlier. A second study administered zidovudine at maximum tolerated doses of 12.5 mg/day or 25 mg/day (~1,000 mg/kg nonpregnant body weight or ~450 mg/kg of term body weight) to pregnant mice from days 12 through 18 of gestation. There was an increase in the number of tumors in the lung, liver, and female reproductive tracts in the offspring of mice receiving the higher dose level of zidovudine. It is not known how predictive the results of rodent carcinogenicity studies may be for humans.

Zidovudine was mutagenic in a 5178Y/TK$^{+/-}$ mouse lymphoma assay, positive in an in vitro cell transformation assay, clastogenic in a cytogenetic assay using cultured human lymphocytes, and positive in mouse and rat micronucleus tests after repeated doses. It was negative in a cytogenetic study in rats given a single dose.

Zidovudine, administered to male and female rats at doses up to 7 times the usual adult dose based on body surface area considerations, had no effect on fertility judged by conception rates.

Pregnancy: Pregnancy Category C. Oral teratology studies in the rat and in the rabbit at doses up to 500 mg/kg/day revealed no evidence of teratogenicity with zidovudine. Zidovudine treatment resulted in embryo/fetal toxicity as evidenced by an increase in the incidence of fetal resorptions in rats given 150 or 450 mg/kg/day and rabbits given 500 mg/kg/day. The doses used in the teratology studies resulted in peak zidovudine plasma concentrations (after one half of the daily dose) in rats 66 to 226 times, and in rabbits 12 to 87 times, mean steady-state peak human plasma concentrations (after one sixth of the daily dose) achieved with the recommended daily dose (100 mg every 4 hours). In an in vitro experiment with fertilized mouse oocytes, zidovudine exposure resulted in a dose-dependent reduction in blastocyst formation. In an additional teratology study in rats, a dose of 3,000 mg/kg/day (very near the oral median lethal dose in rats of 3,683 mg/kg) caused marked maternal toxicity and an increase in the incidence of fetal malformations. This dose resulted in peak zidovudine plasma concentrations 350 times peak human plasma concentrations. (Estimated area-under-the-curve [AUC] in rats at this dose level was 300 times the daily AUC in humans given 600 mg per day.) No evidence of teratogenicity was seen in this experiment at doses of 600 mg/kg/day or less.

Two rodent transplacental carcinogenicity studies were conducted (see Carcinogenesis, Mutagenesis, Impairment of Fertility).

A randomized, double-blind, placebo-controlled trial was conducted in HIV-infected pregnant women to determine the utility of RETROVIR for the prevention of maternal-fetal HIV transmission (see INDICATIONS AND USAGE: Description of Clinical Studies). Congenital abnormalities occurred with similar frequency between neonates born to mothers who received RETROVIR and neonates born to mothers who received placebo. Abnormalities were either problems in embryogenesis (prior to 14 weeks) or were recognized on ultrasound before or immediately after initiation of study drug.

Antiretroviral Pregnancy Registry: To monitor maternal-fetal outcomes of pregnant women exposed to RETROVIR, an Antiretroviral Pregnancy Registry has been established. Physicians are encouraged to register patients by calling 1-800-258-4263.

Nursing Mothers: The Centers for Disease Control and Prevention recommend that HIV-infected mothers not breastfeed their infants to avoid risking postnatal transmission of HIV.

Zidovudine is excreted in human milk (see CLINICAL PHARMACOLOGY: Pharmacokinetics: Nursing Mothers). Because of both the potential for HIV transmission and the potential for serious adverse reactions in nursing infants, **mothers should be instructed not to breastfeed if they are receiving RETROVIR** (see Pediatric Use and INDICATIONS AND USAGE: Maternal-Fetal HIV Transmission).

Pediatric Use: RETROVIR has been studied in HIV-infected pediatric patients over 3 months of age who had HIV-related symptoms or who were asymptomatic with abnormal laboratory values indicating significant HIV-related immunosuppression. RETROVIR has also been studied in neonates perinatally exposed to HIV (see ADVERSE REACTIONS, DOSAGE AND ADMINISTRATION, INDICATIONS AND USAGE: Description of Clinical Studies, and CLINICAL PHARMACOLOGY: Pharmacokinetics).

Geriatric Use: Clinical studies of RETROVIR did not include sufficient numbers of subjects aged 65 and over to determine whether they respond differently from younger subjects. Other reported clinical experience has not identified differences in responses between the elderly and younger patients. In general, dose selection for an elderly patient should be cautious, reflecting the greater frequency of decreased hepatic, renal, or cardiac function, and of concomitant disease or other drug therapy.

ADVERSE REACTIONS

The adverse events reported during intravenous administration of RETROVIR IV Infusion are similar to those reported with oral administration; neutropenia and anemia were reported most frequently. Long-term intravenous administration beyond 2 to 4 weeks has not been studied in adults and may enhance hematologic adverse events. Local reaction, pain, and slight irritation during intravenous administration occur infrequently.

Adults: The frequency and severity of adverse events associated with the use of RETROVIR are greater in patients with more advanced infection at the time of initiation of therapy.

Table 5 summarizes events reported at a statistically significantly greater incidence for patients receiving RETROVIR orally in a monotherapy study:

Table 5. Percentage (%) of Patients with Adverse Events* in Asymptomatic HIV Infection (ACTG 019)

Adverse Event	RETROVIR 500 mg/day (n = 453)	Placebo (n = 428)
Body as a Whole		
Asthenia	8.6%	5.8%
Headache	62.5%	52.6%
Malaise	53.2%	44.9%
Gastrointestinal		
Anorexia	20.1%	10.5%
Constipation	6.4†%	3.5%
Nausea	51.4%	29.9%
Vomiting	17.2%	9.8%

*Reported in ≥5% of study population.
†Not statistically significant versus placebo.

In addition to the adverse events listed in Table 5, other adverse events observed in clinical studies were abdominal cramps, abdominal pain, arthralgia, chills, dyspepsia, fatigue, hyperbilirubinemia, insomnia, musculoskeletal pain, myalgia, and neuropathy.

Selected laboratory abnormalities observed during a clinical study of monotherapy with oral RETROVIR are shown in Table 6.

Table 6. Frequencies of Selected (Grade 3/4) Laboratory Abnormalities in Patients with Asymptomatic HIV Infection (ACTG 019)

Adverse Event	RETROVIR 500 mg/day (n = 453)	Placebo (n = 428)
Anemia (Hgb<8 g/dL)	1.1%	0.2%
Granulocytopenia (<750 cells/mm^3)	1.8%	1.6%
Thrombocytopenia (platelets <50,000/mm^3)	0%	0.5%
ALT (>5 × ULN)	3.1%	2.6%
AST (>5 × ULN)	0.9%	1.6%
Alkaline phosphatase (>5 × ULN)	0%	0%

ULN = Upper limit of normal.

Pediatrics: ***Study ACTG300:*** Selected clinical adverse events and physical findings with a ≥5% frequency during therapy with EPIVIR 4 mg/kg twice daily plus RETROVIR 160 mg/m^2 orally 3 times daily compared with didanosine in therapy-naive (≤56 days of antiretroviral therapy) pediatric patients are listed in Table 7.

Table 7. Selected Clinical Adverse Events and Physical Findings (≥5% Frequency) in Pediatric Patients in Study ACTG300

Adverse Event	EPIVIR plus RETROVIR (n = 236)	Didanosine (n = 235)
Body as a Whole		
Fever	25%	32%
Digestive		
Hepatomegaly	11%	11%
Nausea & vomiting	8%	7%
Diarrhea	8%	6%
Stomatitis	6%	12%
Splenomegaly	5%	8%
Respiratory		
Cough	15%	18%
Abnormal breath sounds/wheezing	7%	9%
Ear, Nose and Throat		
Signs or symptoms of ears*	7%	6%
Nasal discharge or congestion	8%	11%
Other		
Skin rashes	12%	14%
Lymphadenopathy	9%	11%

*Includes pain, discharge, erythema, or swelling of an ear.

Selected laboratory abnormalities experienced by therapy-naive (≤56 days of antiretroviral therapy) pediatric patients are listed in Table 8.

Table 8. Frequencies of Selected (Grade 3/4) Laboratory Abnormalities in Pediatric Patients in Study ACTG300

Test (Abnormal Level)	EPIVIR plus RETROVIR	Didanosine
Neutropenia (ANC<400 cells/mm^3)	8%	3%
Anemia (Hgb<7.0 g/dL)	4%	2%
Thrombocytopenia (platelets<50,000/mm^3)	1%	3%
ALT (>10 × ULN)	1%	3%
AST (>10 × ULN)	2%	4%
Lipase (>2.5 ×ULN)	3%	3%
Total amylase (>2.5 × ULN)	3%	3%

ULN = Upper limit of normal.
ANC = Absolute neutrophil count.

Additional adverse events reported in open-label studies in pediatric patients receiving RETROVIR 180 mg/m^2 every 6 hours were congestive heart failure, decreased reflexes, ECG abnormality, edema, hematuria, left ventricular dilation, macrocytosis, nervousness/irritability, and weight loss. The clinical adverse events reported among adult recipients of RETROVIR may also occur in pediatric patients.

Use for the Prevention of Maternal-Fetal Transmission of HIV: In a randomized, double-blind, placebo-controlled trial in HIV-infected women and their neonates conducted to determine the utility of RETROVIR for the prevention of maternal-fetal HIV transmission, RETROVIR Syrup at 2 mg/kg was administered every 6 hours for 6 weeks to neonates beginning within 12 hours following birth. The most commonly reported adverse experiences were anemia (hemoglobin <9.0 g/dL) and neutropenia (<1,000 cells/mm^3). Anemia occurred in 22% of the neonates who received RETROVIR and in 12% of the neonates who received placebo. The mean difference in hemoglobin values was less than 1.0 g/dL for neonates receiving RETROVIR compared to neonates receiving placebo. No neonates with anemia required transfusion and all hemoglobin values spontaneously returned to normal within 6 weeks after completion of therapy with RETROVIR. Neutropenia was reported with similar frequency in the group that received RETROVIR (21%) and in the group that received placebo (27%). The long-term consequences of in utero and infant exposure to RETROVIR are unknown.

Observed During Clinical Practice: In addition to adverse events reported from clinical trials, the following events have been identified during use of RETROVIR in clinical practice. Because they are reported voluntarily from a population of unknown size, estimates of frequency cannot be made. These events have been chosen for inclusion due to either their seriousness, frequency of reporting, potential causal connection to RETROVIR, or a combination of these factors.

Body as a Whole: Back pain, chest pain, flu-like syndrome, generalized pain.

Cardiovascular: Cardiomyopathy, syncope.

Endocrine: Gynecomastia.

Eye: Macular edema.

Gastrointestinal: Constipation, dysphagia, flatulence, oral mucosal pigmentation, mouth ulcer.

General: Sensitization reactions including anaphylaxis and angioedema, vasculitis.

Hemic and Lymphatic: Aplastic anemia, hemolytic anemia, leukopenia, lymphadenopathy, pancytopenia with marrow hypoplasia, pure red cell aplasia.

Continued on next page

Retrovir Infusion—Cont.

Hepatobiliary Tract and Pancreas: Hepatitis, hepatomegaly with steatosis, jaundice, lactic acidosis, pancreatitis.
Musculoskeletal: Increased CPK, increased LDH, muscle spasm, myopathy and myositis with pathological changes (similar to that produced by HIV disease), rhabdomyolysis, tremor.
Nervous: Anxiety, confusion, depression, dizziness, loss of mental acuity, mania, paresthesia, seizures, somnolence, vertigo.
Respiratory: Cough, dyspnea, rhinitis, sinusitis.
Skin: Changes in skin and nail pigmentation, pruritus, rash, Stevens-Johnson syndrome, toxic epidermal necrolysis, sweat, urticaria.
Special Senses: Amblyopia, hearing loss, photophobia, taste perversion.
Urogenital: Urinary frequency, urinary hesitancy.

OVERDOSAGE

Acute overdoses of zidovudine have been reported in pediatric patients and adults. These involved exposures up to 50 grams. No specific symptoms or signs have been identified following acute overdosage with zidovudine apart from those listed as adverse events such as fatigue, headache, vomiting, and occasional reports of hematological disturbances. All patients recovered without permanent sequelae. Hemodialysis and peritoneal dialysis appear to have a negligible effect on the removal of zidovudine, while elimination of its primary metabolite, GZDV, is enhanced.

DOSAGE AND ADMINISTRATION

Adults: The recommended intravenous dose is 1 mg/kg infused over 1 hour. This dose should be administered 5 to 6 times daily (5 to 6 mg/kg daily). The effectiveness of this dose compared to higher dosing regimens in improving the neurologic dysfunction associated with HIV disease is unknown. A small randomized study found a greater effect of higher doses of RETROVIR on improvement of neurological symptoms in patients with pre-existing neurological disease.
Patients should receive RETROVIR IV Infusion only until oral therapy can be administered. The intravenous dosing regimen equivalent to the oral administration of 100 mg every 4 hours is approximately 1 mg/kg intravenously every 4 hours.
Maternal-Fetal HIV Transmission: The recommended dosing regimen for administration to pregnant women (>14 weeks of pregnancy) and their neonates is:
Maternal Dosing: 100 mg orally 5 times per day until the start of labor. During labor and delivery, intravenous RETROVIR should be administered at 2 mg/kg (total body weight) over 1 hour followed by a continuous intravenous infusion of 1 mg/kg/hour (total body weight) until clamping of the umbilical cord.
Neonatal Dosing: 2 mg/kg orally every 6 hours starting within 12 hours after birth and continuing through 6 weeks of age. Neonates unable to receive oral dosing may be administered RETROVIR intravenously at 1.5 mg/kg, infused over 30 minutes, every 6 hours. (See PRECAUTIONS if hepatic disease or renal insufficiency is present.)
Monitoring of Patients: Hematologic toxicities appear to be related to pretreatment bone marrow reserve and to dose and duration of therapy. In patients with poor bone marrow reserve, particularly in patients with advanced symptomatic HIV disease, frequent monitoring of hematologic indices is recommended to detect serious anemia or neutropenia (see WARNINGS). In patients who experience hematologic toxicity, reduction in hemoglobin may occur as early as 2 to 4 weeks, and neutropenia usually occurs after 6 to 8 weeks.
Dose Adjustment: ***Anemia:*** Significant anemia (hemoglobin of <7.5 g/dL or reduction of >25% of baseline) and/or significant neutropenia (granulocyte count of <750 cells/mm^3 or reduction of >50% from baseline) may require a dose interruption until evidence of marrow recovery is observed (see WARNINGS). In patients who develop significant anemia, dose interruption does not necessarily eliminate the need for transfusion. If marrow recovery occurs following dose interruption, resumption in dose may be appropriate using adjunctive measures such as epoetin alfa at recommended doses, depending on hematologic indices such as serum erythropoetin level and patient tolerance.
For patients experiencing pronounced anemia while receiving chronic coadministration of zidovudine and some of the drugs (e.g., fluconazole, valproic acid) listed in Table 4, zidovudine dose reduction may be considered.
End-Stage Renal Disease: In patients maintained on hemodialysis or peritoneal dialysis (CrCl <15 mL/min), recommended dosing is 1 mg/kg every 6 to 8 hours (see CLINICAL PHARMACOLOGY: Pharmacokinetics).
Hepatic Impairment: There are insufficient data to recommend dose adjustment of RETROVIR in patients with mild to moderate impaired hepatic function or liver cirrhosis. Since RETROVIR is primarily eliminated by hepatic metabolism, a reduction in the daily dose may be necessary in these patients. Frequent monitoring of hematologic toxicities is advised (see CLINICAL PHARMACOLOGY: Pharmacokinetics and PRECAUTIONS: General).
Method of Preparation: RETROVIR IV Infusion must be diluted prior to administration. The calculated dose should be removed from the 20-mL vial and added to 5% Dextrose Injection solution to achieve a concentration no greater than 4 mg/mL. Admixture in biologic or colloidal fluids (e.g., blood products, protein solutions, etc.) is not recommended.
After dilution, the solution is physically and chemically stable for 24 hours at room temperature and 48 hours if refrigerated at 2° to 8°C (36° to 46°F). Care should be taken during admixture to prevent inadvertent contamination. As an additional precaution, the diluted solution should be administered within 8 hours if stored at 25°C (77°F) or 24 hours if refrigerated at 2° to 8°C to minimize potential administration of a microbially contaminated solution.
Parenteral drug products should be inspected visually for particulate matter and discoloration prior to administration whenever solution and container permit. Should either be observed, the solution should be discarded and fresh solution prepared.
Administration: RETROVIR IV Infusion is administered intravenously at a constant rate over 1 hour. Rapid infusion or bolus injection should be avoided. RETROVIR IV Infusion should not be given intramuscularly.

HOW SUPPLIED

RETROVIR IV Infusion, 10 mg zidovudine in each mL.
20-mL Single-Use Vial, Tray of 10 (NDC 0173-0107-93).
Store vials at 15° to 25°C (59° to 77°F) and protect from light.
Manufactured by Catalytica Pharmaceuticals, Inc.
Greenville, NC 27834
for GlaxoSmithKline, Research Triangle Park, NC 27709

December 2001/RL-1041

SEREVENT® DISKUS® ℞

[sĕr' ə-vent dĭsk' us]
(salmeterol xinafoate inhalation powder)

FOR ORAL INHALATION ONLY

Prescribing information for this product, which appears on pages 1637–1640 of the 2002 PDR, has been completely revised as follows. Please write "See Supplement A" next to the product heading.

DESCRIPTION

SEREVENT DISKUS (salmeterol xinafoate inhalation powder) contains salmeterol xinafoate as the racemic form of the 1-hydroxy-2-naphthoic acid salt of salmeterol. The active component of the formulation is salmeterol base, a highly selective beta$_2$-adrenergic bronchodilator. The chemical name of salmeterol xinafoate is 4-hydroxy-α^1-[[[6-(4-phenylbutoxy)hexyl]amino]methyl]-1,3-benzenedimethanol, 1-hydroxy-2-naphthalenecarboxylate.
Salmeterol xinafoate is a white to off-white powder with a molecular weight of 603.8, and the empirical formula is $C_{25}H_{37}NO_4 \bullet C_{11}H_8O_3$. It is freely soluble in methanol; slightly soluble in ethanol, chloroform, and isopropanol; and sparingly soluble in water.
SEREVENT DISKUS is a specially designed plastic inhalation delivery system containing a double-foil blister strip of a powder formulation of salmeterol xinafoate intended for oral inhalation only. The DISKUS®, which is the delivery component, is an integral part of the drug product. Each blister on the double-foil strip within the unit contains 50 mcg of salmeterol administered as the salmeterol xinafoate salt in 12.5 mg of formulation containing lactose. After a blister containing medication is opened by activating the DISKUS, the medication is dispersed into the airstream created by the patient inhaling through the mouthpiece.
Under standardized in vitro test conditions, SEREVENT DISKUS delivers 47 mcg when tested at a flow rate of 60 L/min for 2 seconds. In adult patients with obstructive lung disease and severely compromised lung function (mean forced expiratory volume in 1 second [FEV$_1$] 20% to 30% of predicted), mean peak inspiratory flow (PIF) through a DISKUS was 82.4 L/min (range, 46.1 to 115.3 L/min).
The actual amount of drug delivered to the lung will depend on patient factors, such as inspiratory flow profile.

CLINICAL PHARMACOLOGY

Mechanism of Action: Salmeterol is a selective, long-acting beta-adrenergic agonist. In vitro studies and in vivo pharmacologic studies demonstrate that salmeterol is selective for beta$_2$-adrenoceptors compared with isoproterenol, which has approximately equal agonist activity on beta$_1$- and beta$_2$-adrenoceptors. In vitro studies show salmeterol to be at least 50 times more selective for beta$_2$-adrenoceptors than albuterol. Although beta$_2$-adrenoceptors are the predominant adrenergic receptors in bronchial smooth muscle and beta$_1$-adrenoceptors are the predominant receptors in the heart, there are also beta$_2$-adrenoceptors in the human heart comprising 10% to 50% of the total beta-adrenoceptors. The precise function of these receptors has not been established, but they raise the possibility that even highly selective beta$_2$-agonists may have cardiac effects.
The pharmacologic effects of beta$_2$-adrenoceptor agonist drugs, including salmeterol, are at least in part attributable to stimulation of intracellular adenyl cyclase, the enzyme that catalyzes the conversion of adenosine triphosphate (ATP) to cyclic-3′,5′-adenosine monophosphate (cyclic AMP). Increased cyclic AMP levels cause relaxation of bronchial smooth muscle and inhibition of release of mediators of immediate hypersensitivity from cells, especially from mast cells.
In vitro tests show that salmeterol is a potent and long-lasting inhibitor of the release of mast cell mediators, such as histamine, leukotrienes, and prostaglandin D$_2$, from human lung. Salmeterol inhibits histamine-induced plasma protein extravasation and inhibits platelet-activating factor-induced eosinophil accumulation in the lungs of guinea pigs when administered by the inhaled route. In humans, single doses of salmeterol administered via inhalation aerosol attenuate allergen-induced bronchial hyper-responsiveness.
Pharmacokinetics: Salmeterol xinafoate, an ionic salt, dissociates in solution so that the salmeterol and 1-hydroxy-2-naphthoic acid (xinafoate) moieties are absorbed, distributed, metabolized, and excreted independently. Salmeterol acts locally in the lung; therefore, plasma levels do not predict therapeutic effect.
Absorption: Because of the small therapeutic dose, systemic levels of salmeterol are low or undetectable after inhalation of recommended doses (50 mcg of salmeterol inhalation powder twice daily). Following chronic administration of an inhaled dose of 50 mcg of salmeterol inhalation powder twice daily, salmeterol was detected in plasma within 5 to 45 minutes in 7 patients with asthma; plasma concentrations were very low, with mean peak concentrations of 167 pg/mL at 20 minutes and no accumulation with repeated doses.
Distribution: The percentage of salmeterol bound to human plasma proteins averages 96% in vitro over the concentration range of 8 to 7,722 ng of salmeterol base per milliliter, much higher concentrations than those achieved following therapeutic doses of salmeterol.
Metabolism: Salmeterol base is extensively metabolized by hydroxylation, with subsequent elimination predominantly in the feces. No significant amount of unchanged salmeterol base has been detected in either urine or feces.
Elimination: In 2 healthy subjects who received 1 mg of radiolabeled salmeterol (as salmeterol xinafoate) orally, approximately 25% and 60% of the radiolabeled salmeterol was eliminated in urine and feces, respectively, over a period of 7 days. The terminal elimination half-life was about 5.5 hours (1 volunteer only).
The xinafoate moiety has no apparent pharmacologic activity. The xinafoate moiety is highly protein bound (>99%) and has a long elimination half-life of 11 days.
Special Populations: The pharmacokinetics of salmeterol base has not been studied in elderly patients nor in patients with hepatic or renal impairment. Since salmeterol is predominantly cleared by hepatic metabolism, liver function impairment may lead to accumulation of salmeterol in plasma. Therefore, patients with hepatic disease should be closely monitored.
Pharmacodynamics: Inhaled salmeterol, like other beta-adrenergic agonist drugs, can in some patients produce dose-related cardiovascular effects and effects on blood glucose and/or serum potassium (see PRECAUTIONS). The cardiovascular effects (heart rate, blood pressure) associated with salmeterol inhalation aerosol occur with similar frequency, and are of similar type and severity, as those noted following albuterol administration.
The effects of rising doses of salmeterol and standard inhaled doses of albuterol were studied in volunteers and in patients with asthma. Salmeterol doses up to 84 mcg administered as inhalation aerosol resulted in heart rate increases of 3 to 16 beats/min, about the same as albuterol dosed at 180 mcg by inhalation aerosol (4 to 10 beats/min). Adolescent and adult patients receiving 50-mcg doses of salmeterol inhalation powder (n = 60) underwent continuous electrocardiographic monitoring during two 12-hour periods after the first dose and after 1 month of therapy, and no clinically significant dysrhythmias were noted. Also, pediatric patients receiving 50-mcg doses of salmeterol inhalation powder (n = 67) underwent continuous electrocardiographic monitoring during two 12-hour periods after the first dose and after 3 months of therapy, and no clinically significant dysrhythmias were noted.
In 24-week clinical studies in patients with chronic obstructive pulmonary disease (COPD), the incidence of clinically significant abnormalities on the predose electrocardiograms (ECGs) at Weeks 12 and 24 in patients who received salmeterol 50 mcg was not different compared with placebo. No effect of treatment with salmeterol 50 mcg was observed on pulse rate and systolic and diastolic blood pressure in a subset of patients with COPD who underwent 12-hour serial vital sign measurements after the first dose (n = 91) and after 12 weeks of therapy (n = 74). Median changes from baseline in pulse rate and systolic and diastolic blood pressure were similar for patients receiving either salmeterol or placebo (see ADVERSE REACTIONS).
Studies in laboratory animals (minipigs, rodents, and dogs) have demonstrated the occurrence of cardiac arrhythmias and sudden death (with histologic evidence of myocardial necrosis) when beta-agonists and methylxanthines are administered concurrently. The clinical significance of these findings is unknown.

CLINICAL TRIALS

Asthma: During the initial treatment day in several multiple-dose clinical trials with salmeterol inhalation powder in patients with asthma, the median time to onset of clinically significant bronchodilatation (≥15% improvement in FEV$_1$) ranged from 30 to 48 minutes after a 50-mcg dose.
One hour after a single dose of 50 mcg of salmeterol inhalation powder, the majority of patients had ≥15% improvement in FEV$_1$. Maximum improvement in FEV$_1$ generally occurred within 180 minutes, and clinically significant improvement continued for 12 hours in most patients.
In 2 randomized, double-blind studies, salmeterol inhalation powder was compared with albuterol inhalation aerosol and placebo in adolescent and adult patients with mild-to-moderate asthma (protocol defined as 50% to 80% predicted

FEV_1, actual mean of 67.7% at baseline), including patients who did and who did not receive concurrent inhaled corticosteroids. The efficacy of salmeterol inhalation powder was demonstrated over the 12-week period with no change in effectiveness over this time period (see Figure 1). There were no gender- or age-related differences in safety or efficacy. No development of tachyphylaxis to the bronchodilator effect has been noted in these studies. FEV_1 measurements (mean change from baseline) from these two 12-week studies are shown below for both the first and last treatment days.

Figure 1. Serial 12-Hour FEV_1 From 2 12-Week Clinical Trials in Patients with Asthma

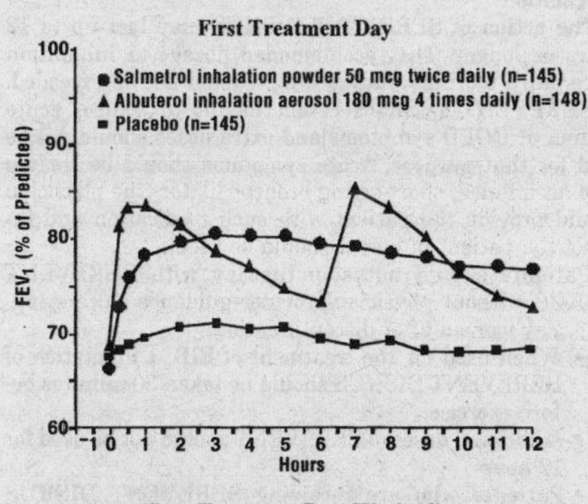

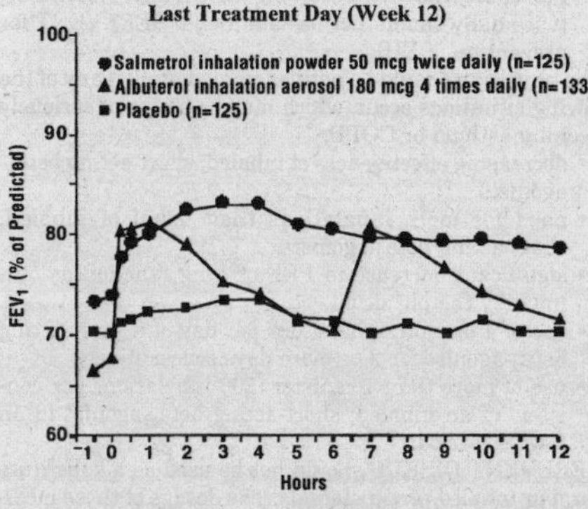

During daily treatment with salmeterol inhalation powder for 12 weeks in adolescent and adult patients with mild-to-moderate asthma, the following treatment effects were seen:

[See table 1 above]

Safe usage with maintenance of efficacy for periods up to 1 year has been documented.

Salmeterol inhalation powder and salmeterol inhalation aerosol were compared to placebo in 2 additional randomized, double-blind clinical trials in adolescent and adult patients with mild-to-moderate asthma. Salmeterol inhalation powder 50 mcg administered via the DISKUS and salmeterol inhalation aerosol 42 mcg, both administered twice daily, produced significant improvements in pulmonary function compared with placebo over the 12-week period. While no statistically significant differences were observed between the active treatments for any of the efficacy assessments or safety evaluations performed, there were some efficacy measures on which the metered-dose inhaler appeared to provide better results. Similar findings were noted in 2 randomized, single-dose, crossover comparisons of salmeterol inhalation powder and salmeterol inhalation aerosol for the prevention of exercise-induced bronchospasm. Therefore, while salmeterol inhalation powder was comparable to salmeterol inhalation aerosol in clinical trials in mild-to-moderate patients with asthma, it should not be assumed that the SEREVENT® (salmeterol xinafoate) Inhalation Aerosol and SEREVENT DISKUS drug products will produce clinically equivalent outcomes in all patients.

In a randomized, double-blind, controlled study (n = 449), 50 mcg of salmeterol inhalation powder, via the DISKUS, was administered twice daily to pediatric patients with asthma who did and who did not receive concurrent inhaled corticosteroids. The efficacy of salmeterol inhalation powder was demonstrated over the 12-week treatment period with respect to periodic serial peak expiratory flow (PEF) (36% to 39% postdose increase from baseline) and FEV_1 (32% to 33% postdose increase from baseline). Salmeterol was effective in demographic subgroup analyses (gender and age) and was effective when coadministered with other inhaled asthma medications such as short-acting bronchodilators and inhaled corticosteroids. A second randomized, double-blind, placebo-controlled study (n = 207) with 50 mcg of salmeterol inhalation powder via an alternate device supported the findings of the trial with the DISKUS.

Effects in Patients With Asthma on Concomitant Inhaled Corticosteroids: In 4 clinical trials in adult and adolescent patients with asthma (n = 1922), the effect of adding salmeterol to inhaled corticosteroid therapy was evaluated. The studies utilized the inhalation aerosol formulation of salmeterol xinafoate for a treatment period of 6 months. They compared the addition of salmeterol therapy to an increase (at least doubling) of the inhaled corticosteroid dose. Two randomized, double-blind, controlled, parallel-group clinical trials (n = 997) enrolled patients (ages 18 to 82 years) with persistent asthma who were previously maintained but not adequately controlled on inhaled corticosteroid therapy. During the 2-week run-in period all patients were switched to beclomethasone dipropionate 168 mcg twice daily. Patients still not adequately controlled were randomized to either the addition of salmeterol inhalation aerosol 42 mcg twice daily or an increase of beclomethasone dipropionate to 336 mcg twice daily. As compared to the doubled dose of beclomethasone dipropionate, the addition of salmeterol resulted in statistically significantly greater improvements in pulmonary function and asthma symptoms, and statistically significantly greater reduction in supplemental albuterol use. The percent of patients who experienced asthma exacerbations overall was not different between groups (i.e., 16.2% in the salmeterol group versus 17.9% in the higher dose beclomethasone dipropionate group).

Two randomized, double-blind, parallel-group clinical trials (n = 925) enrolled patients (ages 12 to 78 years) with persistent asthma who were previously maintained but not adequately controlled on prior therapy. During the 2- to 4-week run-in period, all patients were switched to fluticasone propionate 88 mcg twice daily. Patients still not adequately controlled were randomized to either the addition of salmeterol inhalation aerosol 42 mcg twice daily or an increase of fluticasone propionate to 220 mcg twice daily. As compared to the increased (2.5 times) dose of fluticasone propionate, the addition of salmeterol resulted in statistically significantly greater improvements in pulmonary function and asthma symptoms, and statistically significantly greater reductions in supplemental albuterol use. Fewer patients receiving salmeterol experienced asthma exacerbations than those receiving the higher dose of fluticasone propionate (8.8% versus 13.8%)

In 2 randomized, single-dose, crossover studies in adolescents and adults with exercise-induced bronchospasm (EIB) (n = 53), 50 mcg of salmeterol inhalation powder prevented EIB when dosed 30 minutes prior to exercise. For many patients, this protective effect against EIB was still apparent up to 8.5 hours following a single dose.

[See table 2 above]

In 2 randomized studies in children 4 to 11 years old with asthma and EIB (n = 50), a single 50-mcg dose of salmeterol inhalation powder prevented EIB when dosed 30 minutes prior to exercise, with protection lasting up to 11.5 hours in repeat testing following this single dose in many patients.

Chronic Obstructive Pulmonary Disease (COPD): In 2 clinical trials evaluating twice-daily treatment with salmeterol inhalation powder 50 mcg (n = 336) compared to placebo (n = 366) in patients with chronic bronchitis with airflow limitation, with or without emphysema, improvements in pulmonary function endpoints were greater with salmeterol 50 mcg than with placebo. Treatment with salmeterol did not result in significant improvements in secondary endpoints assessing COPD symptoms in either clinical trial. Both trials were randomized, double-blind, parallel-group studies of 24 weeks' duration and were identical in design, patient entrance criteria, and overall conduct.

Table 1. Daily Efficacy Measurements in 2 12-Week Clinical Trials (Combined Data)

Parameter	Time	Placebo	Salmeterol Inhalation Powder	Albuterol Inhalation Aerosol
No. of randomized subjects		152	149	148
Mean AM peak expiratory flow rate (L/min)	baseline 12 weeks	394 396	395 427*	394 394
Mean % days with no asthma symptoms	baseline 12 weeks	14 20	13 33	12 21
Mean % nights with no awakenings	baseline 12 weeks	70 73	63 85*	68 71
Rescue medications (mean no. of inhalations per day)	baseline 12 weeks	4.2 3.3	4.3 1.6†	4.3 2.2
Asthma exacerbations		14%	15%	16%

* Statistically superior to placebo and albuterol ($p<0.001$).
† Statistically superior to placebo ($p<0.001$).

Table 2. Results of 2 Exercise-Induced Bronchospasm Studies in Adolescents and Adults

		Placebo (n = 52)		Salmeterol Inhalation Powder (n = 52)	
		n	% Total	n	% Total
0.5-Hour postdose exercise challenge	% Fall in FEV_1				
	<10%	15	29	31	60
	≥10%,<20%	3	6	11	21
	≥20%	34	65	10	19
Mean maximal % fall in FEV_1 (SE)		−25% (1.8)		−11% (1.9)	
8.5-Hour postdose exercise challenge	% Fall in FEV_1				
	<10%	12	23	26	50
	≥10%,<20%	7	13	12	23
	≥20%	33	63	14	27
Mean maximal % fall in FEV_1 (SE)		−27% (1.5)		−16% (2.0)	

Figure 2 displays the integrated 2-hour postdose FEV_1 results from the 2 clinical trials. The percent change in FEV_1 refers to the change from baseline, defined as the predose value on Treatment Day 1. To account for patient withdrawals during the study, Endpoint (last evaluable FEV_1) data are provided. Patients receiving salmeterol 50 mcg had significantly greater improvements in 2-hour postdose FEV_1 at Endpoint (216 mL, 20%) compared to placebo (43 mL, 5%). Improvement was apparent on the first day of treatment and maintained throughout the 24 weeks of treatment.

Figure 2. Mean Percent Change From Baseline in Postdose FEV_1 Integrated Data from 2 Trials of Patients With Chronic Bronchitis and Airflow Limitation

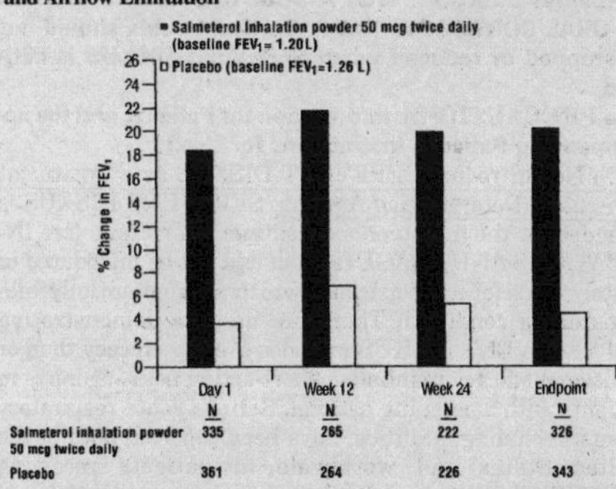

Onset of Action and Duration of Effect: The onset of action and duration of effect of salmeterol were evaluated in a subset of patients (n = 87) from 1 of the 2 clinical trials discussed above. Following the first 50-mcg dose, significant improvement in pulmonary function (mean FEV_1 increase of 12% or more and at least 200 mL) occurred at 2 hours. The mean time to peak bronchodilator effect was 4.75 hours. As seen in Figure 3, evidence of bronchodilatation was seen throughout the 12-hour period. Figure 3 also demonstrates that the bronchodilating effect after 12 weeks of treatment was similar to that observed after the first dose. The mean time to peak bronchodilator effect after 12 weeks of treatment was 3.27 hours.

[See figure at top of next column]

INDICATIONS AND USAGE

Asthma: SEREVENT DISKUS is indicated for long-term, twice-daily (morning and evening) administration in the maintenance treatment of asthma and in the prevention of bronchospasm in patients 4 years of age and older with reversible obstructive airway disease, including patients with symptoms of nocturnal asthma, who require regular treatment with inhaled, short-acting beta$_2$-agonists. It is not indicated for patients whose asthma can be managed by occasional use of inhaled, short-acting beta$_2$-agonists.

Continued on next page

Serevent Diskus—Cont.

Figure 3. Serial 12-Hour FEV_1 on the First Day and at Week 12 of Treatment

Day 1 ● Salmeterol inhalation powder 50 mcg twice daily (n=87)
Day 1 ■ Placebo (n=95)
Week 12 ○ Salmeterol inhalation powder 50 mcg twice daily (n=73)
Week 12 □ Placebo (n=65)

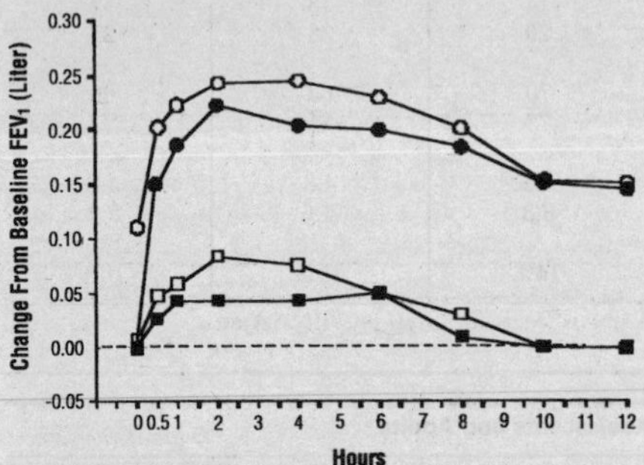

SEREVENT DISKUS is also indicated for prevention of exercise-induced bronchospasm in patients 4 years of age and older.

SEREVENT DISKUS may be used alone or in combination with inhaled or systemic corticosteroid therapy.

Chronic Obstructive Pulmonary Disease (COPD): SEREVENT DISKUS is indicated for the long-term, twice-daily (morning and evening) administration in the maintenance treatment of bronchospasm associated with COPD (including emphysema and chronic bronchitis).

CONTRAINDICATIONS

SEREVENT DISKUS is contraindicated in patients with a history of hypersensitivity to salmeterol or any other component of the drug product.

WARNINGS

IMPORTANT INFORMATION: SEREVENT DISKUS SHOULD NOT BE INITIATED IN PATIENTS WITH SIGNIFICANTLY WORSENING OR ACUTELY DETERIORATING ASTHMA, WHICH MAY BE A LIFE-THREATENING CONDITION. Serious acute respiratory events, including fatalities, have been reported both in the United States and worldwide when SEREVENT has been initiated in this situation. Although it is not possible from these reports to determine whether SEREVENT contributed to these adverse events or simply failed to relieve the deteriorating asthma, the use of SEREVENT DISKUS in this setting is inappropriate.

SEREVENT DISKUS SHOULD NOT BE USED TO TREAT ACUTE SYMPTOMS. It is crucial to inform patients of this and prescribe an inhaled, short-acting $beta_2$-agonist for this purpose as well as warn them that increasing inhaled $beta_2$-agonist use is a signal of deteriorating asthma.

SEREVENT DISKUS IS NOT A SUBSTITUTE FOR INHALED OR ORAL CORTICOSTEROIDS. Corticosteroids should not be stopped or reduced when SEREVENT DISKUS is initiated.

(See PRECAUTIONS: Information for Patients and the accompanying Patient's Instructions for Use.)

1. Do Not Introduce SEREVENT DISKUS as a Treatment for Acutely Deteriorating Asthma: SEREVENT DISKUS is intended for the maintenance treatment of asthma (see INDICATIONS AND USAGE) and should not be introduced in acutely deteriorating asthma, which is a potentially life-threatening condition. There are no data demonstrating that SEREVENT DISKUS provides greater efficacy than or additional efficacy to inhaled, short-acting $beta_2$-agonists in patients with worsening asthma. Serious acute respiratory events, including fatalities, have been reported both in the United States and worldwide in patients receiving SEREVENT. In most cases, these have occurred in patients with severe asthma (e.g., patients with a history of corticosteroid dependence, low pulmonary function, intubation, mechanical ventilation, frequent hospitalizations, or previous life-threatening acute asthma exacerbations) and/or in some patients in whom asthma has been acutely deteriorating (e.g., unresponsive to usual medications; increasing need for inhaled, short-acting $beta_2$-agonists; increasing need for systemic corticosteroids; significant increase in symptoms; recent emergency room visits; sudden or progressive deterioration in pulmonary function). However, they have occurred in a few patients with less severe asthma as well. It was not possible from these reports to determine whether SEREVENT contributed to these events or simply failed to relieve the deteriorating asthma.

2. Do Not Use SEREVENT DISKUS to Treat Acute Symptoms: An inhaled, short-acting $beta_2$-agonist, not SEREVENT DISKUS, should be used to relieve acute asthma or COPD symptoms. When prescribing SEREVENT DISKUS, the physician must also provide the patient with an inhaled, short-acting $beta_2$-agonist (e.g., albuterol) for treatment of symptoms that occur acutely, despite regular twice-daily (morning and evening) use of SEREVENT DISKUS.

When beginning treatment with SEREVENT DISKUS, patients who have been taking inhaled, short-acting $beta_2$-agonists on a regular basis (e.g., 4 times a day) should be instructed to discontinue the regular use of these drugs and use them only for symptomatic relief of acute asthma or COPD symptoms (see PRECAUTIONS: Information for Patients).

3. Watch for Increasing Use of Inhaled, Short-Acting $Beta_2$-Agonists, Which Is a Marker of Deteriorating Asthma or COPD: The patient's condition may deteriorate acutely over a period of hours or chronically over several days or longer. If the patient's inhaled, short-acting $beta_2$-agonist becomes less effective or the patient needs more inhalations than usual, or the patient develops a significant decrease in PEF or lung function, these may be markers of destabilization of their disease. In this setting, the patient requires immediate reevaluation with reassessment of the treatment regimen, giving special consideration to the possible need for corticosteroids. If the patient uses 4 or more inhalations per day of an inhaled, short-acting $beta_2$-agonist for 2 or more consecutive days, or if more than 1 canister (200 inhalations per canister) of inhaled, short-acting $beta_2$-agonist is used in an 8-week period in conjunction with SEREVENT DISKUS, then the patient should consult the physician for reevaluation. **Increasing the daily dosage of SEREVENT DISKUS in this situation is not appropriate. SEREVENT DISKUS should not be used more frequently than twice daily (morning and evening) at the recommended dose of 1 inhalation.**

4. Do Not Use SEREVENT DISKUS as a Substitute for Oral or Inhaled Corticosteroids: The use of beta-adrenergic agonist bronchodilators alone may not be adequate to control asthma in many patients. Early consideration should be given to adding anti-inflammatory agents, e.g., corticosteroids. There are no data demonstrating that SEREVENT DISKUS has a clinical anti-inflammatory effect and could be expected to take the place of corticosteroids. Patients who already require oral or inhaled corticosteroids for treatment of asthma should be continued on a suitable dose to maintain clinical stability even if they feel better as a result of initiating SEREVENT DISKUS. Any change in corticosteroid dosage should be made ONLY after clinical evaluation (see PRECAUTIONS: Information for Patients).

5. Do Not Exceed Recommended Dosage: As with other inhaled $beta_2$-adrenergic drugs, SEREVENT DISKUS should not be used more often or at higher doses than recommended. Fatalities have been reported in association with excessive use of inhaled sympathomimetic drugs. Large doses of inhaled or oral salmeterol (12 to 20 times the recommended dose) have been associated with clinically significant prolongation of the QTc interval, which has the potential for producing ventricular arrhythmias.

6. Paradoxical Bronchospasm: As with other inhaled asthma and COPD medications, SEREVENT DISKUS can produce paradoxical bronchospasm, which may be life threatening. If paradoxical bronchospasm occurs following dosing with SEREVENT DISKUS, it should be treated with a short-acting, inhaled bronchodilator; SEREVENT DISKUS should be discontinued immediately; and alternative therapy should be instituted.

7. Immediate Hypersensitivity Reactions: Immediate hypersensitivity reactions may occur after administration of SEREVENT DISKUS, as demonstrated by cases of urticaria, angioedema, rash, and bronchospasm.

8. Upper Airway Symptoms: Symptoms of laryngeal spasm, irritation, or swelling, such as stridor and choking, have been reported in patients receiving SEREVENT DISKUS.

9. Cardiovascular Disorders: SEREVENT DISKUS, like all sympathomimetic amines, should be used with caution in patients with cardiovascular disorders, especially coronary insufficiency, cardiac arrhythmias, and hypertension. SEREVENT DISKUS, like all other beta-adrenergic agonists, can produce a clinically significant cardiovascular effect in some patients as measured by pulse rate, blood pressure, and/or symptoms. Although such effects are uncommon after administration of SEREVENT DISKUS at recommended doses, if they occur, the drug may need to be discontinued. In addition, beta-agonists have been reported to produce electrocardiogram (ECG) changes, such as flattening of the T wave, prolongation of the QTc interval, and ST segment depression. The clinical significance of these findings is unknown.

PRECAUTIONS

General: 1. Cardiovascular and Other Effects: No effect on the cardiovascular system is usually seen after the administration of inhaled salmeterol at recommended doses, but the cardiovascular and central nervous system effects seen with all sympathomimetic drugs (e.g., increased blood pressure, heart rate, excitement) can occur after use of salmeterol and may require discontinuation of the drug. Salmeterol, like all sympathomimetic amines, should be used with caution in patients with cardiovascular disorders, especially coronary insufficiency, cardiac arrhythmias, and hypertension; in patients with convulsive disorders or thyrotoxicosis; and in patients who are unusually responsive to sympathomimetic amines.

As has been described with other beta-adrenergic agonist bronchodilators, clinically significant changes in systolic and/or diastolic blood pressure, pulse rate, and electrocardiograms have been seen infrequently in individual patients in controlled clinical studies with salmeterol.

2. Metabolic Effects: Doses of the related $beta_2$-adrenoceptor agonist albuterol, when administered intravenously, have been reported to aggravate preexisting diabetes mellitus and ketoacidosis. Beta-adrenergic agonist medications may produce significant hypokalemia in some patients, possibly through intracellular shunting, which has the potential to produce adverse cardiovascular effects. The decrease in serum potassium is usually transient, not requiring supplementation.

Clinically significant changes in blood glucose and/or serum potassium were seen rarely during clinical studies with long-term administration of salmeterol at recommended doses.

Information for Patients: Patients being treated with SEREVENT DISKUS should receive the following information and instructions. This information is intended to aid them in the safe and effective use of this medication. It is not a disclosure of all possible adverse or intended effects. It is important that patients understand how to use the DISKUS appropriately and how to use SEREVENT DISKUS in relation to other asthma or COPD medications they are taking. Patients should be given the following information:

1. The action of SEREVENT DISKUS may last up to 12 hours or longer. The recommended dosage (1 inhalation twice daily, morning and evening) should not be exceeded.
2. SEREVENT DISKUS is not meant to relieve acute asthma or COPD symptoms and extra doses should not be used for that purpose. Acute symptoms should be treated with an inhaled, short-acting bronchodilator (the physician should provide the patient with such medication and instruct the patient in how it should be used).
3. Patients should not stop therapy with SEREVENT DISKUS without physician/provider guidance since symptoms may worsen after discontinuation.
4. • When used for the treatment of EIB, 1 inhalation of SEREVENT DISKUS should be taken 30 minutes before exercise.
   • Additional doses of SEREVENT should not be used for 12 hours.
   • Patients who are receiving SEREVENT DISKUS twice daily should not use additional SEREVENT for prevention of EIB.
5. The physician should be notified immediately if any of the following situations occur, which may be a sign of seriously worsening asthma or COPD:
   • decreasing effectiveness of inhaled, short-acting $beta_2$-agonists,
   • need for more inhalations than usual of inhaled, short-acting $beta_2$-agonists,
   • significant decrease in PEF or lung function as outlined by the physician,
   • use of 4 or more inhalations per day of a short-acting $beta_2$-agonist for 2 or more days consecutively,
   • use of more than 1 canister (200 inhalations per canister) of an inhaled, short-acting $beta_2$-agonist in an 8-week period.
6. SEREVENT DISKUS should not be used as a substitute for oral or inhaled corticosteroids. The dosage of these medications should not be changed and they should not be stopped without consulting the physician, even if the patient feels better after initiating treatment with SEREVENT DISKUS.
7. Patients should be cautioned regarding adverse effects associated with $beta_2$-agonists, such as palpitations, chest pain, rapid heart rate, tremor, or nervousness.
8. When patients are prescribed SEREVENT DISKUS, other medications for asthma and COPD should be used only as directed by the physician.
9. SEREVENT DISKUS should not be used with a spacer device.
10. If you are pregnant or nursing, contact your physician about the use of SEREVENT DISKUS.
11. Effective and safe use of SEREVENT DISKUS includes an understanding of the way that it should be used:
   • Never exhale into the DISKUS.
   • Never attempt to take the DISKUS apart.
   • Always activate and use the DISKUS in a level, horizontal position.
   • Never wash the mouthpiece or any part of the DISKUS. KEEP IT DRY.
   • Always keep the DISKUS in a dry place.
   • Discard **6 weeks** after removal from the moisture-protective foil overwrap pouch or after all blisters have been used (when the dose indicator reads "0"), whichever comes first.
12. For the proper use of SEREVENT DISKUS and to attain maximum benefit, the patient should read and follow carefully the Patient's Instructions for Use accompanying the product.

Drug Interactions: ***Short-Acting Beta-Agonists:*** In the two 12-week, repetitive-dose adolescent and adult clinical trials in patients with asthma (n = 149), the mean daily need for additional $beta_2$-agonist in patients using salmeterol inhalation powder was approximately 1½ inhalations/day. Twenty-six percent (26%) of the patients in these trials used between 8 and 24 inhalations of short-acting beta-agonist per day on 1 or more occasions. Nine percent (9%) of the patients in these trials averaged over 4 inhalations/day over the course of the 12-week trials. No increase in frequency of cardiovascular events was observed among the 3 patients who averaged 8 to 11 inhalations per day; however, the safety of concomitant use of more than 8 inhalations per day of short-acting $beta_2$-agonist with salmeterol inhalation powder has not been established. In 29 patients who experienced worsening of asthma while receiving salmeterol inhalation powder during these trials, albuterol therapy administered via either nebulizer or inhalation aerosol (1 dose in most cases) led to improvement in FEV_1 and no increase in occurrence of cardiovascular adverse events.

In 2 clinical trials in patients with COPD, the mean daily need for additional $beta_2$-agonist for patients using salmeterol inhalation powder was approximately 4 inhalations/day. Twenty-four percent (24%) of the patients using salmeterol inhalation powder in these trials averaged 6 or more inhalations of albuterol per day over the course of the 24-week trials. No increase in frequency of cardiovascular events was observed among patients who averaged 6 or more inhalations per day.

Monoamine Oxidase Inhibitors and Tricyclic Antidepressants: Salmeterol should be administered with extreme caution to patients being treated with monoamine oxidase inhibitors or tricyclic antidepressants, or within 2 weeks of discontinuation of such agents, because the action of salmeterol on the vascular system may be potentiated by these agents.

Corticosteroids and Cromoglycate: In clinical trials, inhaled corticosteroids and/or inhaled cromolyn sodium did not alter the safety profile of salmeterol when administered concurrently.

Methylxanthines: The concurrent use of intravenously or orally administered methylxanthines (e.g., aminophylline, theophylline) by patients receiving salmeterol has not been completely evaluated. In 1 clinical asthma trial, 87 patients receiving SEREVENT Inhalation Aerosol 42 mcg twice daily concurrently with a theophylline product had adverse event rates similar to those in 71 patients receiving SEREVENT Inhalation Aerosol without theophylline. Resting heart rates were slightly higher in the patients on theophylline but were little affected by therapy with SEREVENT Inhalation Aerosol.

In 2 clinical trials in patients with COPD, 39 subjects receiving salmeterol inhalation powder concurrently with a theophylline product had adverse event rates similar to those in 302 patients receiving salmeterol inhalation powder without theophylline. Based on the available data, the concomitant administration of methylxanthines with salmeterol inhalation powder did not alter the observed adverse event profile.

Beta-Adrenergic Receptor Blocking Agents: Beta-blockers not only block the pulmonary effect of beta-agonists, such as SEREVENT DISKUS, but may also produce severe bronchospasm in patients with asthma or COPD. Therefore, patients with asthma or COPD should not normally be treated with beta-blockers. However, under certain circumstances, e.g., as prophylaxis after myocardial infarction, there may be no acceptable alternatives to the use of beta-adrenergic blocking agents in patients with asthma or COPD. In this setting, cardioselective beta-blockers could be considered, although they should be administered with caution.

Diuretics: The ECG changes and/or hypokalemia that may result from the administration of nonpotassium-sparing diuretics (such as loop or thiazide diuretics) can be acutely worsened by beta-agonists, especially when the recommended dose of the beta-agonist is exceeded. Although the clinical significance of these effects is not known, caution is advised in the coadministration of beta-agonists with nonpotassium-sparing diuretics.

Carcinogenesis, Mutagenesis, Impairment of Fertility: In an 18-month carcinogenicity study in CD-mice, salmeterol xinafoate at oral doses of 1.4 mg/kg and above (approximately 20 times the maximum recommended daily inhalation dose in adults and children based on comparison of the area under the plasma concentration versus time curves [AUCs]) caused a dose-related increase in the incidence of smooth muscle hyperplasia, cystic glandular hyperplasia, leiomyomas of the uterus, and cysts in the ovaries. The incidence of leiomyosarcomas was not statistically significant. No tumors were seen at 0.2 mg/kg (approximately 3 times the maximum recommended daily inhalation doses in adults and children based on comparison of the AUCs).

In a 24-month oral and inhalation carcinogenicity study in Sprague Dawley rats, salmeterol caused a dose-related increase in the incidence of mesovarian leiomyomas and ovarian cysts at doses of 0.68 mg/kg and above (approximately 55 times the maximum recommended daily inhalation dose in adults and approximately 25 times the maximum recommended daily inhalation dose in children on a mg/m^2 basis). No tumors were seen at 0.21 mg/kg (approximately 15 times the maximum recommended daily inhalation dose in adults and approximately 8 times the maximum recommended daily inhalation dose in children on a mg/m^2 basis). These findings in rodents are similar to those reported previously for other beta-adrenergic agonist drugs. The relevance of these findings to human use is unknown.

Salmeterol produced no detectable or reproducible increases in microbial and mammalian gene mutation in vitro. No clastogenic activity occurred in vitro in human lymphocytes or in vivo in a rat micronucleus test. No effects on fertility were identified in male and female rats treated with salmeterol at oral doses up to 2 mg/kg (approximately 160 times the maximum recommended daily inhalation dose in adults on a mg/m^2 basis).

Pregnancy: ***Teratogenic Effects:*** Pregnancy Category C. No teratogenic effects occurred in rats at oral doses up to 2 mg/kg (approximately 160 times the maximum recommended daily inhalation dose in adults on a mg/m^2 basis). In pregnant Dutch rabbits administered oral doses of 1 mg/kg and above (approximately 50 times the maximum recommended daily inhalation dose in adults based on comparison of the AUCs), salmeterol exhibited fetal toxic effects characteristically resulting from beta-adrenoceptor stimulation. These included precocious eyelid openings, cleft palate, sternebral fusion, limb and paw flexures, and delayed ossification of the frontal cranial bones. No significant effects occurred at an oral dose of 0.6 mg/kg (approximately 20 times the maximum recommended daily inhalation dose in adults based on comparison of the AUCs).

Table 3. Adverse Experience Incidence in Two 12-Week Adolescent and Adult Clinical Trials in Patients With Asthma

Adverse Experience Type	Percent of Patients: Placebo (N = 152)	Salmeterol Inhalation Powder 50 mcg Twice Daily (N = 149)	Albuterol Inhalation Aerosol 180 mcg 4 Times Daily (N = 150)
Ear, nose, and throat			
Nasal/sinus congestion, pallor	6	9	8
Rhinitis	4	5	4
Neurological			
Headache	9	13	12
Respiratory			
Asthma	1	3	<1
Tracheitis/bronchitis	4	7	3
Influenza	2	5	5

Table 4. Adverse Experience Incidence in Two 12-Week Pediatric Clinical Trials in Patients With Asthma

Adverse Experience Type	Percent of Patients: Placebo (N = 215)	Salmeterol Inhalation Powder 50 mcg Twice Daily (N = 211)	Albuterol Inhalation Powder 200 mcg 4 Times Daily (N = 115)
Ear, nose, and throat			
Ear signs and symptoms	3	4	9
Pharyngitis	3	6	3
Neurological			
Headache	14	17	20
Respiratory			
Asthma	2	4	<1
Skin			
Skin rashes	3	4	2
Urticaria	0	3	2

New Zealand White rabbits were less sensitive since only delayed ossification of the frontal bones was seen at an oral dose of 10 mg/kg (approximately 1,600 times the maximum recommended daily inhalation dose in adults on a mg/m^2 basis). Extensive use of other beta-agonists has provided no evidence that these class effects in animals are relevant to their use in humans. There are no adequate and well-controlled studies with SEREVENT DISKUS in pregnant women. SEREVENT DISKUS should be used during pregnancy only if the potential benefit justifies the potential risk to the fetus.

Salmeterol xinafoate crossed the placenta following oral administration of 10 mg/kg to mice and rats (approximately 410 and 810 times, respectively, the maximum recommended daily inhalation dose in adults on a mg/m^2 basis).

Use in Labor and Delivery: There are no well-controlled human studies that have investigated effects of salmeterol on preterm labor or labor at term. Because of the potential for beta-agonist interference with uterine contractility, use of SEREVENT DISKUS during labor should be restricted to those patients in whom the benefits clearly outweigh the risks.

Nursing Mothers: Plasma levels of salmeterol after inhaled therapeutic doses are very low. In rats, salmeterol xinafoate is excreted in the milk. However, since there are no data from controlled trials on the use of salmeterol by nursing mothers, a decision should be made whether to discontinue nursing or to discontinue SEREVENT DISKUS, taking into account the importance of SEREVENT DISKUS to the mother. Caution should be exercised when SEREVENT DISKUS is administered to a nursing woman.

Pediatric Use: The safety and efficacy of salmeterol inhalation powder has been evaluated in over 2,500 patients aged 4 to 11 years with asthma, 346 of whom were administered salmeterol inhalation powder for 1 year. Based on available data, no adjustment of salmeterol dosage in pediatric patients is warranted for either asthma or EIB (see DOSAGE AND ADMINISTRATION).

In 2 randomized, double-blind, controlled clinical trials of 12 weeks' duration, salmeterol 50-mcg powder was administered to 211 pediatric asthma patients who did and who did not receive concurrent inhaled corticosteroids. The efficacy of salmeterol inhalation powder was demonstrated over the 12-week treatment period with respect to PEF and FEV_1. Salmeterol inhalation powder was effective in demographic subgroups (gender and age) of the population. Salmeterol was effective when coadministered with other inhaled asthma medications, such as short-acting bronchodilators and inhaled corticosteroids. Salmeterol inhalation powder was well tolerated in the pediatric population, and there were no safety issues identified specific to the administration of salmeterol inhalation powder to pediatric patients.

In 2 randomized studies in children 4 to 11 years old with asthma and EIB, a single 50-mcg dose of salmeterol inhalation powder prevented EIB when dosed 30 minutes prior to exercise, with protection lasting up to 11.5 hours in repeat testing following this single dose in many patients.

Geriatric Use: Of the total number of adolescent and adult patients with asthma who received salmeterol inhalation powder in chronic dosing clinical trials, 209 were 65 years of age and older. Of the total number of patients with COPD who received salmeterol inhalation powder in chronic dosing clinical trials, 167 were 65 years of age or older and 45 were 75 years of age or older. No apparent differences in the safety of SEREVENT inhalation powder were observed when geriatric patients were compared with younger patients in clinical trials. As with other beta$_2$-agonists, however, special caution should be observed when using SEREVENT DISKUS in geriatric patients who have concomitant cardiovascular disease that could be adversely affected by this class of drug. Data from the trials in patients with COPD suggested a greater effect on FEV_1 of salmeterol inhalation powder in the <65 years age-group, as compared with the ≥65 years age-group. However, based on available data, no adjustment of salmeterol dosage in geriatric patients is warranted.

ADVERSE REACTIONS

Adverse reactions to salmeterol are similar in nature to reactions to other selective beta$_2$-adrenoceptor agonists, i.e., tachycardia; palpitations; immediate hypersensitivity reactions, including urticaria, angioedema, rash, bronchospasm (see WARNINGS); headache; tremor; nervousness; and paradoxical bronchospasm (see WARNINGS).

Asthma: Two multicenter, 12-week, controlled studies have evaluated twice-daily doses of salmeterol inhalation powder in patients 12 years of age and older with asthma. Table 3 reports the incidence of adverse experiences in these 2 studies.

[See table 3 above]

Table 3 includes all experiences (whether considered drug-related or nondrug-related by the investigator) that occurred at a rate of 3% or greater in the group receiving salmeterol inhalation powder and were more common than in the placebo group.

Pharyngitis, sinusitis, upper respiratory tract infection, and cough occurred at ≥3% but were more common in the placebo group. However, throat irritation has been described at rates exceeding that of placebo in other controlled clinical trials.

Other adverse experiences that occurred in the group receiving salmeterol inhalation powder in these studies with an incidence of 1% to 3% and that occurred at a greater incidence than with placebo were:

Ear, Nose, and Throat: Sinus headache.

Gastrointestinal: Nausea.

Mouth and Teeth: Oral mucosal abnormality.

Musculoskeletal: Pain in joint.

Neurological: Sleep disturbance, paresthesia.

Skin: Contact dermatitis, eczema.

Miscellaneous: Localized aches and pains, pyrexia of unknown origin.

Two multicenter, 12-week, controlled studies have evaluated twice-daily doses of salmeterol inhalation powder in patients aged 4 to 11 years with asthma. Table 4 includes all experiences (whether considered drug-related or nondrug-related by the investigator) that occurred at a rate of 3% or greater in the group receiving salmeterol inhalation powder and were more common than in the placebo group.

[See table 4 above]

Continued on next page

Serevent Diskus—Cont.

The following experiences were reported at an incidence of 1% to 2% (3 to 4 patients) in the salmeterol group and with a higher incidence than in the albuterol and placebo groups: gastrointestinal signs and symptoms, lower respiratory signs and symptoms, photodermatitis, and arthralgia and articular rheumatism.

In clinical trials evaluating concurrent therapy of salmeterol with inhaled corticosteroids, adverse experiences were consistent with those previously reported for salmeterol, or might otherwise be expected with the use of inhaled corticosteroids.

Chronic Obstructive Pulmonary Disease (COPD): Two multicenter, 24-week, controlled studies have evaluated twice-daily doses of salmeterol inhalation powder administered via the DISKUS in patients with COPD. For presentation (Table 5), the placebo data from a third trial, identical in design, patient entrance criteria, and overall conduct but comparing fluticasone propionate with placebo, were integrated with the placebo data from these 2 studies (total N = 341 for salmeterol and 576 for placebo).

[See table 5 below]

Other experiences occurring in the group treated with salmeterol inhalation powder that occurred at a frequency of 1% to <3% and were more common than in the placebo group were as follows:

Endocrine and Metabolic: Hyperglycemia.

Eye: Keratitis and conjunctivitis.

Gastrointestinal: Candidiasis mouth/throat, dyspeptic symptoms, hyposalivation, dental discomfort and pain, gastrointestinal infections.

Lower Respiratory: Lower respiratory signs and symptoms.

Musculoskeletal: Arthralgia and articular rheumatism; muscle pain; bone and skeletal pain; musculoskeletal inflammation; muscle stiffness, tightness, and rigidity.

Neurology: Migraines.

Non-Site Specific: Pain, edema and swelling.

Psychiatry: Anxiety.

Skin: Skin rashes.

Observed During Clinical Practice: In addition to adverse experiences reported from clinical trials, the following experiences have been identified during postapproval use of salmeterol. Because they are reported voluntarily from a population of unknown size, estimates of frequency cannot be made. These experiences have been chosen for inclusion due either their seriousness, frequency of reporting, or causal connection to salmeterol or a combination of these factors.

In extensive US and worldwide postmarketing experience with salmeterol, serious exacerbations of asthma, including some that have been fatal, have been reported. In most cases, these have occurred in patients with severe asthma and/or in some patients in whom asthma has been acutely deteriorating (see WARNINGS no. 1), but they have also occurred in a few patients with less severe asthma. It was not possible from these reports to determine whether salmeterol contributed to these events or simply failed to relieve the deteriorating asthma.

Respiratory: Reports of upper airway symptoms of laryngeal spasm, irritation, or swelling such as stridor or choking; oropharyngeal irritation.

Cardiovascular: Arrhythmias (including atrial fibrillation, supraventricular tachycardia, extrasystoles), and anaphylaxis.

OVERDOSAGE

The expected signs and symptoms with overdosage of SEREVENT DISKUS are those of excessive beta-adrenergic stimulation and/or occurrence or exaggeration of any of the signs and symptoms listed under ADVERSE REACTIONS, e.g., seizures, angina, hypertension or hypotension, tachycardia with rates up to 200 beats/min, arrhythmias, nervousness, headache, tremor, muscle cramps, dry mouth, palpitation, nausea, dizziness, fatigue, malaise, and insomnia.

Overdosage with SEREVENT DISKUS may be expected to result in exaggeration of the pharmacologic adverse effects associated with beta-adrenoceptor agonists, including tachycardia and/or arrhythmia, tremor, headache, and muscle cramps. Overdosage with SEREVENT DISKUS can lead to clinically significant prolongation of the QTc interval, which can produce ventricular arrhythmias. Other signs of overdosage may include hypokalemia and hyperglycemia.

As with all sympathomimetic medications, cardiac arrest and even death may be associated with abuse of SEREVENT DISKUS.

Treatment consists of discontinuation of SEREVENT DISKUS together with appropriate symptomatic therapy. The judicious use of a cardioselective beta-receptor blocker may be considered, bearing in mind that such medication can produce bronchospasm. There is insufficient evidence to determine if dialysis is beneficial for overdosage of SEREVENT DISKUS. Cardiac monitoring is recommended in cases of overdosage.

No deaths were seen in rats at an inhalation dose of 2.9 mg/kg (approximately 240 times the maximum recommended daily inhalation dose in adults and approximately 110 times the maximum recommended daily inhalation dose in children on a mg/m^2 basis) and in dogs at an inhalation dose of 0.7 mg/kg (approximately 190 times the maximum recommended daily inhalation dose in adults and approximately 90 times the maximum recommended daily inhalation dose in children on a mg/m^2 basis). By the oral route, no deaths occurred in mice at 150 mg/kg (approximately 6,100 times the maximum recommended daily inhalation dose in adults and approximately 2,900 times the maximum recommended daily inhalation dose in children on a mg/m^2 basis) and in rats at 1,000 mg/kg (approximately 81,000 times the maximum recommended daily inhalation dose in adults and approximately 38,000 times the maximum recommended daily inhalation dose in children on a mg/m^2 basis).

DOSAGE AND ADMINISTRATION

SEREVENT DISKUS should be administered by the orally inhaled route only (see Patient's Instructions for Use). The patient must not exhale into the DISKUS and the DISKUS should only be activated and used in a level, horizontal position.

Asthma: For maintenance of bronchodilatation and prevention of symptoms of asthma, including the symptoms of nocturnal asthma, the usual dosage for adults and children 4 years of age and older is 1 inhalation (50 mcg) twice daily (morning and evening, approximately 12 hours apart). If a previously effective dosage regimen fails to provide the usual response, medical advice should be sought immediately as this is often a sign of destabilization of asthma. Under these circumstances, the therapeutic regimen should be reevaluated and additional therapeutic options, such as inhaled or systemic corticosteroids, should be considered. If symptoms arise in the period between doses, an inhaled, short-acting beta$_2$-agonist should be taken for immediate relief.

Chronic Obstructive Pulmonary Disease (COPD): For maintenance treatment of bronchospasm associated with COPD (including chronic bronchitis and emphysema), the usual dosage for adults is 1 inhalation (50 mcg) twice daily (morning and evening, approximately 12 hours apart).

For both asthma and COPD, adverse effects are more likely to occur with higher doses of salmeterol, and more frequent administration or administration of a larger number of inhalations is not recommended.

To gain full therapeutic benefit, SEREVENT DISKUS should be administered twice daily (morning and evening) in the treatment of reversible airway obstruction.

Geriatric Use: Based on available data for SEREVENT DISKUS, no dosage adjustment is recommended.

Prevention of Exercise-Induced Bronchospasm (EIB): One inhalation of SEREVENT DISKUS at least 30 minutes before exercise has been shown to protect patients against EIB. When used intermittently as needed for prevention of EIB, this protection may last up to 9 hours in adolescents and adults and up to 12 hours in patients 4 to 11 years of age. Additional doses of SEREVENT should not be used for 12 hours after the administration of this drug. Patients who are receiving SEREVENT DISKUS twice daily should not use additional SEREVENT for prevention of EIB. If regular, twice-daily dosing is not effective in preventing EIB, other appropriate therapy for EIB should be considered.

HOW SUPPLIED

SEREVENT DISKUS is supplied as a disposable, teal green-colored unit containing 60 blisters. The drug product is packaged within a teal green-colored, plastic-coated, moisture-protective foil pouch (NDC 0173-0521-00).

SEREVENT DISKUS is also supplied in an institutional pack of 1 teal green-colored, disposable unit containing 28 blisters. The drug product is packaged within a teal green-colored, plastic-coated, moisture-protective foil pouch (NDC 0173-0520-00).

Store at controlled room temperature (see USP), 20° to 25°C (68° to 77°F) in a dry place away from direct heat or sunlight. Keep out of reach of children. SEREVENT DISKUS should be discarded 6 weeks after removal from the moisture-protective foil overwrap pouch or after all blisters have been used (when the dose indicator reads "0"), whichever comes first. The DISKUS is not reusable. Do not attempt to take the DISKUS apart.

GlaxoSmithKline, Research Triangle Park, NC 27709

March 2002/RL-1068

Table 5. Adverse Experiences With ≥3% Incidence in US Controlled Clinical Trials With Salmeterol Inhalation Powder in Patients With Chronic Obstructive Pulmonary Disease*

Adverse Experience Type	Percent of Patients: Placebo (N = 576)	Percent of Patients: Salmeterol Inhalation Powder 50 mcg Twice Daily (N = 341)
Cardiovascular		
Hypertension	2	4
Ear, nose, and throat		
Throat irritation	6	7
Nasal congestion/blockage	3	4
Sinusitis	2	4
Ear signs and symptoms	1	3
Gastrointestinal		
Nausea and vomiting	3	3
Lower respiratory		
Cough	4	5
Rhinitis	2	4
Viral respiratory infection	4	5
Musculoskeletal		
Musculoskeletal pain	10	12
Muscle cramps and spasms	1	3
Neurological		
Headache	11	14
Dizziness	2	4
Average duration of exposure (days)	128.9	138.5

*Table 5 includes all events (whether considered drug-related or nondrug-related by the investigator) that occurred at a rate of 3% or greater in the group treated with salmeterol inhalation powder and were more common in the group treated with salmeterol inhalation powder than in the placebo group.

STELAZINE® ℞

[stel' ə-zēn]

brand of trifluoperazine hydrochloride

Antianxiety/Antipsychotic

Prescribing information for this product, which appears on pages 1640–1642 of the 2002 PDR, has been revised as follows. Please write "See Supplement A" next to the product heading.

The last paragraph of the **DESCRIPTION** *section was revised to:*

N.B.: The Concentrate is for use in severe neuropsychiatric conditions including schizophrenia when oral medication is preferred and other oral forms are considered impractical.

The first paragraph of the **INDICATIONS** *section was revised to:*

For the management of the manifestations of psychotic disorders such as schizophrenia.

The **WARNINGS: Tardive Dyskinesia** *subsection was revised to:*

Tardive dyskinesia, a syndrome consisting of potentially irreversible, involuntary, dyskinetic movements, may develop in patients treated with antipsychotic drugs. Although the prevalence of the syndrome appears to be highest among the elderly, especially elderly women, it is impossible to rely upon prevalence estimates to predict, at the inception of antipsychotic treatment, which patients are likely to develop the syndrome. Whether antipsychotic drug products differ in their potential to cause tardive dyskinesia is unknown.

Both the risk of developing the syndrome and the likelihood that it will become irreversible are believed to increase as the duration of treatment and the total cumulative dose of antipsychotic drugs administered to the patient increase. However, the syndrome can develop, although much less commonly, after relatively brief treatment periods at low doses.

There is no known treatment for established cases of tardive dyskinesia, although the syndrome may remit, partially or completely, if antipsychotic treatment is withdrawn. Antipsychotic treatment itself, however, may suppress (or partially suppress) the signs and symptoms of the syndrome and thereby may possibly mask the underlying disease process. The effect that symptomatic suppression has upon the long-term course of the syndrome is unknown.

Given these considerations, antipsychotics should be prescribed in a manner that is most likely to minimize the occurrence of tardive dyskinesia. Chronic antipsychotic treatment should generally be reserved for patients who suffer from a chronic illness that 1) is known to respond to antipsychotic drugs, and, 2) for whom alternative, equally effective, but potentially less harmful treatments are *not* available or appropriate. In patients who do require chronic treatment, the smallest dose and the shortest duration of treatment producing a satisfactory clinical response should be sought. The need for continued treatment should be reassessed periodically.

If signs and symptoms of tardive dyskinesia appear in a patient on antipsychotics, drug discontinuation should be considered. However, some patients may require treatment despite the presence of the syndrome.

For further information about the description of tardive dyskinesia and its clinical detection, please refer to the sections on PRECAUTIONS and ADVERSE REACTIONS.

The **WARNINGS: Neuroleptic Malignant Syndrome (NMS)** *subsection was revised to:*

A potentially fatal symptom complex sometimes referred to as Neuroleptic Malignant Syndrome (NMS) has been reported in association with antipsychotic drugs. Clinical manifestations of NMS are hyperpyrexia, muscle rigidity, altered mental status and evidence of autonomic instability (irregular pulse or blood pressure, tachycardia, diaphoresis, and cardiac dysrhythmias).

The diagnostic evaluation of patients with this syndrome is complicated. In arriving at a diagnosis, it is important to identify cases where the clinical presentation includes both serious medical illness (e.g., pneumonia, systemic infection, etc.) and untreated or inadequately treated extrapyramidal signs and symptoms (EPS). Other important considerations in the differential diagnosis include central anticholinergic toxicity, heat stroke, drug fever and primary central nervous system (CNS) pathology.

The management of NMS should include 1) immediate discontinuation of antipsychotic drugs and other drugs not essential to concurrent therapy, 2) intensive symptomatic treatment and medical monitoring, and 3) treatment of any concomitant serious medical problems for which specific treatments are available. There is no general agreement about specific pharmacological treatment regimens for uncomplicated NMS.

If a patient requires antipsychotic drug treatment after recovery from NMS, the potential reintroduction of drug therapy should be carefully considered. The patient should be carefully monitored, since recurrences of NMS have been reported.

An encephalopathic syndrome (characterized by weakness, lethargy, fever, tremulousness and confusion, extrapyramidal symptoms, leukocytosis, elevated serum enzymes, BUN and FBS) has occurred in a few patients treated with lithium plus an antipsychotic. In some instances, the syndrome was followed by irreversible brain damage. Because of a possible causal relationship between these events and the concomitant administration of lithium and antipsychotics, patients receiving such combined therapy should be monitored closely for early evidence of neurologic toxicity and treatment discontinued promptly if such signs appear. This encephalopathic syndrome may be similar to or the same as neuroleptic malignant syndrome (NMS).

Patients who have demonstrated a hypersensitivity reaction (e.g., blood dyscrasias, jaundice) with a phenothiazine should not be re-exposed to any phenothiazine, including Stelazine (trifluoperazine HCl), unless in the judgment of the physician the potential benefits of treatment outweigh the possible hazard.

Stelazine Concentrate contains sodium bisulfite, a sulfite that may cause allergic-type reactions including anaphylactic symptoms and life-threatening or less severe asthmatic episodes in certain susceptible people. The overall prevalence of sulfite sensitivity in the general population is unknown and probably low. Sulfite sensitivity is seen more frequently in asthmatic than in non-asthmatic people.

Stelazine (trifluoperazine HCl) may impair mental and/or physical abilities, especially during the first few days of therapy. Therefore, caution patients about activities requiring alertness (e.g., operating vehicles or machinery).

If agents such as sedatives, narcotics, anesthetics, tranquilizers or alcohol are used either simultaneously or successively with the drug, the possibility of an undesirable additive depressant effect should be considered.

The following paragraphs in the **PRECAUTIONS: General** *subsection were revised to:*

Given the likelihood that some patients exposed chronically to antipsychotics will develop tardive dyskinesia, it is advised that all patients in whom chronic use is contemplated be given, if possible, full information about this risk.

Antipsychotic drugs elevate prolactin levels; the elevation persists during chronic administration. Tissue culture experiments indicate that approximately 1/3 of human breast cancers are prolactin-dependent in vitro, a factor of potential importance if the prescribing of these drugs is contemplated in a patient with a previously detected breast cancer. Although disturbances such as galactorrhea, amenorrhea, gynecomastia and impotence have been reported, the clinical significance of elevated serum prolactin levels is unknown for most patients. An increase in mammary neoplasms has been found in rodents after chronic administration of antipsychotic drugs. Neither clinical nor epidemiologic studies conducted to date, however, have shown an association between chronic administration of these drugs and mammary tumorigenesis; the available evidence is considered too limited to be conclusive at this time. Chromosomal aberrations in spermatocytes and abnormal sperm have been demonstrated in rodents treated with certain antipsychotics.

The **PRECAUTIONS: Long-Term Therapy** *subsection was revised to:*

To lessen the likelihood of adverse reactions related to cumulative drug effect, patients with a history of long-term therapy with Stelazine (trifluoperazine HCl) and/or other antipsychotics should be evaluated periodically to decide whether the maintenance dosage could be lowered or drug therapy discontinued.

The **ADVERSE REACTIONS: Tardive Dyskinesia** *subsection was revised to:*

As with all antipsychotic agents, tardive dyskinesia may appear in some patients on long-term therapy or may appear after drug therapy has been discontinued. The syndrome can also develop, although much less frequently, after relatively brief treatment periods at low doses. This syndrome appears in all age groups. Although its prevalence appears to be highest among elderly patients, especially elderly women, it is impossible to rely upon prevalence estimates to predict at the inception of antipsychotic treatment which patients are likely to develop the syndrome. The symptoms are persistent and in some patients appear to be irreversible. The syndrome is characterized by rhythmical involuntary movements of the tongue, face, mouth or jaw (e.g., protrusion of tongue, puffing of cheeks, puckering of mouth, chewing movements). Sometimes these may be accompanied by involuntary movements of extremities. In rare instances, these involuntary movements of the extremities are the only manifestations of tardive dyskinesia. A variant of tardive dyskinesia, tardive dystonia, has also been described.

The fourth paragraph in the **ADVERSE REACTIONS: Adverse Reactions Reported with Stelazine (trifluoperazine HCl) or Other Phenothiazine Derivatives** *subsection was revised to:*

EKG changes—particularly nonspecific, usually reversible Q and T wave distortions—have been observed in some patients receiving phenothiazine antipsychotics. Although phenothiazines cause neither psychic nor physical dependence, sudden discontinuance in long-term psychiatric patients may cause temporary symptoms, e.g., nausea and vomiting, dizziness, tremulousness.

The following subhead in **DOSAGE AND ADMINISTRATION—ADULTS** *was revised to:*

Psychotic Disorders including Schizophrenia

The following subhead in **DOSAGE AND ADMINISTRATION** *was revised to:*

PSYCHOTIC CHILDREN INCLUDING SCHIZOPHRENIA IN CHILDREN.

GlaxoSmithKline, Research Triangle Park, NC 27709

January 2002/SZ:L73

TABLOID® brand Thioguanine ℞
[tab 'loid]
40-mg Scored Tablets

Prescribing information for this product, which appears on pages 1642–1644 of the 2002 PDR, has been revised as follows. Please write "See Supplement A" next to the product heading.

The following was added as the third paragraph in the **WARNINGS** *section:*

There are individuals with an inherited deficiency of the enzyme thiopurine methyltransferase (TPMT) who may be unusually sensitive to the myelosuppressive effects of mercaptopurine and prone to developing rapid bone marrow suppression following the initiation of treatment. This problem could be exacerbated by coadministration with drugs that inhibit TPMT, such as olsalazine, mesalazine, or sulphasalazine.

The following was added as the third paragraph in the **PRECAUTIONS: Drug Interactions** *subsection:*

As there is in vitro evidence that aminosalicylate derivatives (e.g., olsalazine, mesalazine, or sulphasalazine) inhibit the TPMT enzyme, they should be administered with caution to patients receiving concurrent thioguanine therapy (see WARNINGS).

The following **REFERENCE,** *which refers to proper handling and disposal of anticancer drugs in the DOSAGE AND ADMINISTRATION section, was revised to:*

23. Controlling Occupational Exposure to Hazardous Drugs. (OSHA Work-Practice Guidelines.) *Am J Health-Syst Pharm.* 1996;53:1669–1685.

Manufactured by Catalytica Pharmaceuticals, Inc.
Greenville, NC 27834
for GlaxoSmithKline, Research Triangle Park, NC 27709

May 2001/RL-911

TAZICEF® ℞
[taz 'i-sef]
(ceftazidime for injection)

For Intravenous or Intramuscular Use

Prescribing information for this product, which appears on pages 1647–1650 of the 2002 PDR, has been completely revised as follows. Please write "See Supplement A" next to the product heading.

DESCRIPTION

Ceftazidime is a semisynthetic, broad-spectrum, beta-lactam antibiotic for parenteral administration. It is the pentahydrate of pyridinium, 1-[[7-[[(2-amino-4-thiazolyl)[(1-carboxy-1-methylethoxy)imino]acetyl]amino]-2-carboxy-8-oxo-5-thia-1-azabicyclo[4.2.0]oct-2-en-3-yl]methyl]-, hydroxide, inner salt, [6R-[6α,7β(Z)]].

The empirical formula is $C_{22}H_{32}N_6O_{12}S_2$, representing a molecular weight of 636.6.

TAZICEF is a sterile, dry powdered mixture of ceftazidime pentahydrate and sodium carbonate. The sodium carbonate at a concentration of 118 mg/g of ceftazidime activity has been admixed to facilitate dissolution. The total sodium content of the mixture is approximately 54 mg (2.3 mEq)/g of ceftazidime activity.

TAZICEF in sterile crystalline form is supplied in vials equivalent to 1 g, 2 g, or 6 g of anhydrous ceftazidime and in ADD-Vantage® vials equivalent to 1 or 2 g of anhydrous ceftazidime. Solutions of TAZICEF range in color from light yellow to amber, depending on the diluent and volume used. The pH of freshly constituted solutions usually ranges from 5 to 8.

TAZICEF is available as a frozen, iso-osmotic, sterile, nonpyrogenic solution with 1 or 2 g of ceftazidime as ceftazidime sodium premixed with approximately 2.2 or 1.6 g, respectively, of dextrose hydrous, USP. Dextrose has been added to adjust the osmolality. Sodium hydroxide is used to adjust pH and neutralize ceftazidime pentahydrate free acid to the sodium salt. The pH may have been adjusted with hydrochloric acid. Solutions of premixed TAZICEF range in color from light yellow to amber. The solution is intended for intravenous (IV) use after thawing to room temperature. The osmolality of the solution is approximately 300 mOsmol/kg, and the pH of thawed solutions ranges from 5 to 7.5.

The plastic container for the frozen solution is fabricated from a specially designed multilayer plastic, PL 2040. Solutions are in contact with the polyethylene layer of this container and can leach out certain chemical components of the plastic in very small amounts within the expiration period. The suitability of the plastic has been confirmed in tests in animals according to USP biological tests for plastic containers as well as by tissue culture toxicity studies.

CLINICAL PHARMACOLOGY

After IV administration of 500-mg and 1-g doses of ceftazidime over 5 minutes to normal adult male volunteers, mean peak serum concentrations of 45 and 90 mcg/mL, respectively, were achieved. After IV infusion of 500-mg, 1-g, and 2-g doses of ceftazidime over 20 to 30 minutes to normal adult male volunteers, mean peak serum concentrations of 42, 69, and 170 mcg/mL, respectively, were achieved. The average serum concentrations following IV infusion of 500-mg, 1-g, and 2-g doses to these volunteers over an 8-hour interval are given in Table 1.

[See table 1 at top of next page]

The absorption and elimination of ceftazidime were directly proportional to the size of the dose. The half-life following IV administration was approximately 1.9 hours. Less than 10% of ceftazidime was protein bound. The degree of protein binding was independent of concentration. There was no evidence of accumulation of ceftazidime in the serum in individuals with normal renal function following multiple IV doses of 1 and 2 g every 8 hours for 10 days.

Following intramuscular (IM) administration of 500-mg and 1-g doses of ceftazidime to normal adult volunteers, the mean peak serum concentrations were 17 and 39 mcg/mL, respectively, at approximately 1 hour. Serum concentrations remained above 4 mcg/mL for 6 and 8 hours after the IM administration of 500-mg and 1-g doses, respectively. The half-life of ceftazidime in these volunteers was approximately 2 hours.

The presence of hepatic dysfunction had no effect on the pharmacokinetics of ceftazidime in individuals administered 2 g intravenously every 8 hours for 5 days. Therefore, a dosage adjustment from the normal recommended dosage is not required for patients with hepatic dysfunction, provided renal function is not impaired.

Approximately 80% to 90% of an IM or IV dose of ceftazidime is excreted unchanged by the kidneys over a 24-hour period. After the IV administration of single 500-mg or 1-g doses, approximately 50% of the dose appeared in the urine in the first 2 hours. An additional 20% was excreted between 2 and 4 hours after dosing, and approximately another 12% of the dose appeared in the urine between 4 and 8 hours later. The elimination of ceftazidime by the kidneys resulted in high therapeutic concentrations in the urine.

The mean renal clearance of ceftazidime was approximately 100 mL/min. The calculated plasma clearance of approximately 115 mL/min indicated nearly complete elimination of ceftazidime by the renal route. Administration of probenecid before dosing had no effect on the elimination kinetics of ceftazidime. This suggested that ceftazidime is eliminated by glomerular filtration and is not actively secreted by renal tubular mechanisms.

Since ceftazidime is eliminated almost solely by the kidneys, its serum half-life is significantly prolonged in patients with impaired renal function. Consequently, dosage adjustments in such patients as described in the DOSAGE AND ADMINISTRATION section are suggested.

Therapeutic concentrations of ceftazidime are achieved in the following body tissues and fluids.

[See table 2 at top of next page]

Microbiology: Ceftazidime is bactericidal in action, exerting its effect by inhibition of enzymes responsible for cell-wall synthesis. A wide range of gram-negative organisms is susceptible to ceftazidime in vitro, including strains resis-

Continued on next page

Tazicef—Cont.

tant to gentamicin and other aminoglycosides. In addition, ceftazidime has been shown to be active against gram-positive organisms. It is highly stable to most clinically important beta-lactamases, plasmid or chromosomal, which are produced by both gram-negative and gram-positive organisms and, consequently, is active against many strains resistant to ampicillin and other cephalosporins.

Ceftazidime has been shown to be active against the following organisms both in vitro and in clinical infections (see INDICATIONS AND USAGE).

Aerobes, Gram-negative: *Citrobacter* spp., including *Citrobacter freundii* and *Citrobacter diversus*; *Enterobacter* spp., including *Enterobacter cloacae* and *Enterobacter aerogenes*; *Escherichia coli*; *Haemophilus influenzae*, including ampicillin-resistant strains; *Klebsiella* spp. (including *Klebsiella pneumoniae*); *Neisseria meningitidis*; *Proteus mirabilis*; *Proteus vulgaris*; *Pseudomonas* spp. (including *Pseudomonas aeruginosa*); and *Serratia* spp.

Aerobes, Gram-positive: *Staphylococcus aureus*, including penicillinase- and non-penicillinase-producing strains; *Streptococcus agalactiae* (group B streptococci); *Streptococcus pneumoniae*; and *Streptococcus pyogenes* (group A beta-hemolytic streptococci).

Anaerobes: *Bacteroides* spp. (NOTE: many strains of *Bacteroides fragilis* are resistant.)

Ceftazidime has been shown to be active in vitro against most strains of the following organisms; however, the clinical significance of these data is unknown: *Acinetobacter* spp., *Clostridium* spp. (not including *Clostridium difficile*), *Haemophilus parainfluenzae, Morganella morganii* (formerly *Proteus morganii*), *Neisseria gonorrhoeae, Peptococcus* spp., *Peptostreptococcus* spp., *Providencia* spp. (including *Providencia rettgeri*, formerly *Proteus rettgeri*), *Salmonella* spp., *Shigella* spp., *Staphylococcus epidermidis*, and *Yersinia enterocolitica*.

Ceftazidime and the aminoglycosides have been shown to be synergistic in vitro against *Pseudomonas aeruginosa* and the enterobacteriaceae. Ceftazidime and carbenicillin have also been shown to be synergistic in vitro against *Pseudomonas aeruginosa*.

Ceftazidime is not active in vitro against methicillin-resistant staphylococci, *Streptococcus faecalis* and many other enterococci, *Listeria monocytogenes, Campylobacter* spp., or *Clostridium difficile*.

Susceptibility Tests: ***Diffusion Techniques:*** Quantitative methods that require measurement of zone diameters give an estimate of antibiotic susceptibility. One such procedure[1–3] has been recommended for use with disks to test susceptibility to ceftazidime.

Reports from the laboratory giving results of the standard single-disk susceptibility test with a 30-mcg ceftazidime disk should be interpreted according to the following criteria:

Susceptible organisms produce zones of 18 mm or greater, indicating that the test organism is likely to respond to therapy.

Organisms that produce zones of 15 to 17 mm are expected to be susceptible if high dosage is used or if the infection is confined to tissues and fluids (e.g., urine) in which high antibiotic levels are attained.

Resistant organisms produce zones of 14 mm or less, indicating that other therapy should be selected.

Organisms should be tested with the ceftazidime disk since ceftazidime has been shown by in vitro tests to be active against certain strains found resistant when other beta-lactam disks are used.

Standardized procedures require the use of laboratory control organisms. The 30-mcg ceftazidime disk should give zone diameters between 25 and 32 mm for *Escherichia coli* ATCC 25922. For *Pseudomonas aeruginosa* ATCC 27853, the zone diameters should be between 22 and 29 mm. For *Staphylococcus aureus* ATCC 25923, the zone diameters should be between 16 and 20 mm.

Dilution Techniques: In other susceptibility testing procedures, e.g., ICS agar dilution or the equivalent, a bacterial isolate may be considered susceptible if the minimum inhibitory concentration (MIC) value for ceftazidime is not more than 16 mcg/mL. Organisms are considered resistant to ceftazidime if the MIC is ≥64 mcg/mL. Organisms having an MIC value of <64 mcg/mL but >16 mcg/mL are expected to be susceptible if high dosage is used or if the infection is confined to tissues and fluids (e.g., urine) in which high antibiotic levels are attained.

As with standard diffusion methods, dilution procedures require the use of laboratory control organisms. Standard ceftazidime powder should give MIC values in the range of 4 to 16 mcg/mL for *Staphylococcus aureus* ATCC 25923. For *Escherichia coli* ATCC 25922, the MIC range should be between 0.125 and 0.5 mcg/mL. For *Pseudomonas aeruginosa* ATCC 27853, the MIC range should be between 0.5 and 2 mcg/mL.

INDICATIONS AND USAGE

TAZICEF is indicated for the treatment of patients with infections caused by susceptible strains of the designated organisms in the following diseases:

1. **Lower Respiratory Tract Infections,** including pneumonia, caused by *Pseudomonas aeruginosa* and other *Pseudomonas* spp.; *Haemophilus influenzae*, including ampicillin-resistant strains; *Klebsiella* spp.; *Enterobacter* spp.; *Proteus mirabilis*; *Escherichia coli*; *Serratia* spp.; *Citrobacter* spp.; *Streptococcus pneumoniae*; and *Staphylococcus aureus* (methicillin-susceptible strains).

Table 1. Average Serum Concentrations of Ceftazidime

Ceftazidime IV Dose	Serum Concentrations (mcg/mL)				
	0.5 hr	1 hr	2 hr	4 hr	8 hr
500 mg	42	25	12	6	2
1 g	60	39	23	11	3
2 g	129	75	42	13	5

Table 2. Ceftazidime Concentrations in Body Tissues and Fluids

Tissue or Fluid	Dose/Route	No. of Patients	Time of Sample Postdose	Average Tissue or Fluid Level (mcg/mL or mcg/g)
Urine	500 mg IM	6	0–2 hr	2,100.0
	2 g IV	6	0–2 hr	12,000.0
Bile	2 g IV	3	90 min	36.4
Synovial fluid	2 g IV	13	2 hr	25.6
Peritoneal fluid	2 g IV	8	2 hr	48.6
Sputum	1 g IV	8	1 hr	9.0
Cerebrospinal fluid	2 g q8h IV	5	120 min	9.8
(inflamed meninges)	2 g q8h IV	6	180 min	9.4
Aqueous humor	2 g IV	13	1–3 hr	11.0
Blister fluid	1 g IV	7	2–3 hr	19.7
Lymphatic fluid	1 g IV	7	2–3 hr	23.4
Bone	2 g IV	8	0.67 hr	31.1
Heart muscle	2 g IV	35	30–280 min	12.7
Skin	2 g IV	22	30–180 min	6.6
Skeletal muscle	2 g IV	35	30–280 min	9.4
Myometrium	2 g IV	31	1–2 hr	18.7

2. **Skin and Skin-Structure Infections** caused by *Pseudomonas aeruginosa*; *Klebsiella* spp.; *Escherichia coli*; *Proteus* spp., including *Proteus mirabilis* and indole-positive *Proteus*; *Enterobacter* spp.; *Serratia* spp.; *Staphylococcus aureus* (methicillin-susceptible strains); and *Streptococcus pyogenes* (group A beta-hemolytic streptococci).
3. **Urinary Tract Infections,** both complicated and uncomplicated, caused by *Pseudomonas aeruginosa*; *Enterobacter* spp.; *Proteus* spp., including *Proteus mirabilis* and indole-positive *Proteus*; *Klebsiella* spp.; and *Escherichia coli*.
4. **Bacterial Septicemia** caused by *Pseudomonas aeruginosa*, *Klebsiella* spp., *Haemophilus influenzae*, *Escherichia coli*, *Serratia* spp., *Streptococcus pneumoniae*, and *Staphylococcus aureus* (methicillin-susceptible strains).
5. **Bone and Joint Infections** caused by *Pseudomonas aeruginosa*, *Klebsiella* spp., *Enterobacter* spp., and *Staphylococcus aureus* (methicillin-susceptible strains).
6. **Gynecologic Infections,** including endometritis, pelvic cellulitis, and other infections of the female genital tract caused by *Escherichia coli*.
7. **Intra-abdominal Infections,** including peritonitis caused by *Escherichia coli*, *Klebsiella* spp., and *Staphylococcus aureus* (methicillin-susceptible strains) and polymicrobial infections caused by aerobic and anaerobic organisms and *Bacteroides* spp. (many strains of *Bacteroides fragilis* are resistant).
8. **Central Nervous System Infections,** including meningitis, caused by *Haemophilus influenzae* and *Neisseria meningitidis*. Ceftazidime has also been used successfully in a limited number of cases of meningitis due to *Pseudomonas aeruginosa* and *Streptococcus pneumoniae*.

Specimens for bacterial cultures should be obtained before therapy in order to isolate and identify causative organisms and to determine their susceptibility to ceftazidime. Therapy may be instituted before results of susceptibility studies are known; however, once these results become available, the antibiotic treatment should be adjusted accordingly.

TAZICEF may be used alone in cases of confirmed or suspected sepsis. Ceftazidime has been used successfully in clinical trials as empiric therapy in cases where various concomitant therapies with other antibiotics have been used.

TAZICEF may also be used concomitantly with other antibiotics, such as aminoglycosides, vancomycin, and clindamycin; in severe and life-threatening infections; and in the immunocompromised patient. When such concomitant treatment is appropriate, prescribing information in the labeling for the other antibiotics should be followed. The dose depends on the severity of the infection and the patient's condition.

CONTRAINDICATIONS

TAZICEF is contraindicated in patients who have shown hypersensitivity to ceftazidime or the cephalosporin group of antibiotics.

WARNINGS

BEFORE THERAPY WITH TAZICEF IS INSTITUTED, CAREFUL INQUIRY SHOULD BE MADE TO DETERMINE WHETHER THE PATIENT HAS HAD PREVIOUS HYPERSENSITIVITY REACTIONS TO CEFTAZIDIME, CEPHALOSPORINS, PENICILLINS, OR OTHER DRUGS. IF THIS PRODUCT IS TO BE GIVEN TO PENICILLIN-SENSITIVE PATIENTS, CAUTION SHOULD BE EXERCISED BECAUSE CROSS-HYPERSENSITIVITY AMONG BETA-LACTAM ANTIBIOTICS HAS BEEN CLEARLY DOCUMENTED AND MAY OCCUR IN UP TO 10% OF PATIENTS WITH A HISTORY OF PENICILLIN ALLERGY. IF AN ALLERGIC REACTION TO TAZICEF OCCURS, DISCONTINUE THE DRUG. SERIOUS ACUTE HYPERSENSITIVITY REACTIONS MAY REQUIRE TREATMENT WITH EPINEPHRINE AND OTHER EMERGENCY MEASURES, INCLUDING OXYGEN, IV FLUIDS, IV ANTIHISTAMINES, CORTICOSTEROIDS, PRESSOR AMINES, AND AIRWAY MANAGEMENT, AS CLINICALLY INDICATED.

Pseudomembranous colitis has been reported with nearly all antibacterial agents, including ceftazidime, and may range in severity from mild to life threatening. Therefore, it is important to consider this diagnosis in patients who present with diarrhea subsequent to the administration of antibacterial agents.

Treatment with antibacterial agents alters the normal flora of the colon and may permit overgrowth of clostridia. Studies indicate that a toxin produced by *Clostridium difficile* is one primary cause of "antibiotic-associated colitis."

After the diagnosis of pseudomembranous colitis has been established, appropriate therapeutic measures should be initiated. Mild cases of pseudomembranous colitis usually respond to drug discontinuation alone. In moderate to severe cases, consideration should be given to management with fluids and electrolytes, protein supplementation, and treatment with an antibacterial drug clinically effective against *Clostridium difficile* colitis.

Elevated levels of ceftazidime in patients with renal insufficiency can lead to seizures, encephalopathy, coma, asterixis, neuromuscular excitability, and myoclonia (see PRECAUTIONS).

PRECAUTIONS

General: High and prolonged serum ceftazidime concentrations can occur from usual dosages in patients with transient or persistent reduction of urinary output because of renal insufficiency. The total daily dosage should be reduced when ceftazidime is administered to patients with renal insufficiency (see DOSAGE AND ADMINISTRATION). Elevated levels of ceftazidime in these patients can lead to seizures, encephalopathy, coma, asterixis, neuromuscular excitability, and myoclonia. Continued dosage should be determined by degree of renal impairment, severity of infection, and susceptibility of the causative organisms.

As with other antibiotics, prolonged use of TAZICEF may result in overgrowth of nonsusceptible organisms. Repeated evaluation of the patient's condition is essential. If superinfection occurs during therapy, appropriate measures should be taken.

Inducible type I beta-lactamase resistance has been noted with some organisms (e.g., *Enterobacter* spp., *Pseudomonas* spp., and *Serratia* spp.). As with other extended-spectrum beta-lactam antibiotics, resistance can develop during therapy, leading to clinical failure in some cases. When treating infections caused by these organisms, periodic susceptibility testing should be performed when clinically appropriate. If patients fail to respond to monotherapy, an aminoglycoside or similar agent should be considered.

Cephalosporins may be associated with a fall in prothrombin activity. Those at risk include patients with renal and hepatic impairment, or poor nutritional state, as well as patients receiving a protracted course of antimicrobial therapy. Prothrombin time should be monitored in patients at risk and exogenous vitamin K administered as indicated.

TAZICEF should be prescribed with caution in individuals with a history of gastrointestinal disease, particularly colitis.

Distal necrosis can occur after inadvertent intra-arterial administration of ceftazidime.

Drug Interactions: Nephrotoxicity has been reported following concomitant administration of cephalosporins with aminoglycoside antibiotics or potent diuretics such as furosemide. Renal function should be carefully monitored, especially if higher dosages of the aminoglycosides are to be administered or if therapy is prolonged, because of the potential nephrotoxicity and ototoxicity of aminoglycosidic antibiotics. Nephrotoxicity and ototoxicity were not noted when ceftazidime was given alone in clinical trials.

Chloramphenicol has been shown to be antagonistic to beta-lactam antibiotics, including ceftazidime, based on in vitro studies and time kill curves with enteric gram-negative bacilli. Due to the possibility of antagonism in vivo, particularly when bactericidal activity is desired, this drug combination should be avoided.

Drug/Laboratory Test Interactions: The administration of ceftazidime may result in a false-positive reaction for glucose in the urine when using CLINITEST® tablets, Benedict's solution, or Fehling's solution. It is recommended that glucose tests based on enzymatic glucose oxidase reactions (such as CLINISTIX®) be used.

Carcinogenesis, Mutagenesis, Impairment of Fertility: Long-term studies in animals have not been performed to evaluate carcinogenic potential. However, a mouse Micronucleus test and an Ames test were both negative for mutagenic effects.

Pregnancy: ***Teratogenic Effects:*** Pregnancy Category B. Reproduction studies have been performed in mice and rats at doses up to 40 times the human dose and have revealed no evidence of impaired fertility or harm to the fetus due to TAZICEF. There are, however, no adequate and well-controlled studies in pregnant women. Because animal reproduction studies are not always predictive of human response, this drug should be used during pregnancy only if clearly needed.

Nursing Mothers: Ceftazidime is excreted in human milk in low concentrations. Caution should be exercised when TAZICEF is administered to a nursing woman.

Pediatric Use: (see DOSAGE AND ADMINISTRATION).

Geriatric Use: Of the 2,221 subjects who received ceftazidime in 11 clinical studies, 824 (37%) were 65 and over while 391 (18%) were 75 and over. No overall differences in safety or effectiveness were observed between these subjects and younger subjects, and other reported clinical experience has not identified differences in responses between the elderly and younger patients, but greater susceptibility of some older individuals to drug effects cannot be ruled out. This drug is known to be substantially excreted by the kidney, and the risk of toxic reactions to this drug may be greater in patients with impaired renal function. Because elderly patients are more likely to have decreased renal function, care should be taken in dose selection, and it may be useful to monitor renal function (see DOSAGE AND ADMINISTRATION).

ADVERSE REACTIONS

Ceftazidime is generally well tolerated. The incidence of adverse reactions associated with the administration of ceftazidime was low in clinical trials. The most common were local reactions following IV injection and allergic and gastrointestinal reactions. Other adverse reactions were encountered infrequently. No disulfiramlike reactions were reported.

The following adverse effects from clinical trials were considered to be either related to ceftazidime therapy or were of uncertain etiology:

Local Effects, reported in fewer than 2% of patients, were phlebitis and inflammation at the site of injection (1 in 69 patients).

Hypersensitivity Reactions, reported in 2% of patients, were pruritus, rash, and fever. Immediate reactions, generally manifested by rash and/or pruritus, occurred in 1 in 285 patients. Toxic epidermal necrolysis, Stevens-Johnson syndrome, and erythema multiforme have also been reported with cephalosporin antibiotics, including ceftazidime. Angioedema and anaphylaxis (bronchospasm and/or hypotension) have been reported very rarely.

Gastrointestinal Symptoms, reported in fewer than 2% of patients, were diarrhea (1 in 78), nausea (1 in 156), vomiting (1 in 500), and abdominal pain (1 in 416). The onset of pseudomembranous colitis symptoms may occur during or after treatment (see WARNINGS).

Central Nervous System Reactions (fewer than 1%) included headache, dizziness, and paresthesia. Seizures have been reported with several cephalosporins, including ceftazidime. In addition, encephalopathy, coma, asterixis, neuromuscular excitability, and myoclonia have been reported in renally impaired patients treated with unadjusted dosing regimens of ceftazidime (see PRECAUTIONS: General).

Less Frequent Adverse Events (fewer than 1%) were candidiasis (including oral thrush) and vaginitis.

Hematologic: Rare cases of hemolytic anemia have been reported.

Laboratory Test Changes noted during clinical trials with TAZICEF were transient and included: eosinophilia (1 in 13), positive Coombs' test without hemolysis (1 in 23), thrombocytosis (1 in 45), and slight elevations in one or more of the hepatic enzymes, aspartate aminotransferase (AST, SGOT) (1 in 16), alanine aminotransferase (ALT, SGPT) (1 in 15), LDH (1 in 18), GGT (1 in 19), and alkaline phosphatase (1 in 23). As with some other cephalosporins, transient elevations of blood urea, blood urea nitrogen, and/or serum creatinine were observed occasionally. Transient leukopenia, neutropenia, agranulocytosis, thrombocytopenia, and lymphocytosis were seen very rarely.

POSTMARKETING EXPERIENCE WITH TAZICEF PRODUCTS

In addition to the adverse events reported during clinical trials, the following events have been observed during clinical practice in patients treated with TAZICEF and were reported spontaneously. For some of these events, data are insufficient to allow an estimate of incidence or to establish causation.

Table 3. Recommended Dosage Schedule

	Dose	Frequency
Adults		
Usual recommended dosage	**1 gram IV or IM**	**q8–12hr**
Uncomplicated urinary tract infections	250 mg IV or IM	q12hr
Bone and joint infections	2 grams IV	q12hr
Complicated urinary tract infections	500 mg IV or IM	q8–12hr
Uncomplicated pneumonia; mild skin and skin-structure infections	500 mg–1 gram IV or IM	q8hr
Serious gynecologic and intra-abdominal infections	2 grams IV	q8hr
Meningitis	2 grams IV	q8hr
Very severe life-threatening infections, especially in immunocompromised patients	2 grams IV	q8hr
Lung infections caused by *Pseudomonas* spp. in patients with cystic fibrosis with normal renal function*	30–50 mg/kg IV to a maximum of 6 grams per day	q8hr
Neonates (0–4 weeks)	30 mg/kg IV	q12hr
Infants and children (1 month–12 years)	30–50 mg/kg IV to a maximum of 6 grams per day†	q8hr

*Although clinical improvement has been shown, bacteriologic cures cannot be expected in patients with chronic respiratory disease and cystic fibrosis.

†The higher dose should be reserved for immunocompromised pediatric patients or pediatric patients with cystic fibrosis or meningitis.

General: Anaphylaxis; allergic reactions, which, in rare instances, were severe (e.g., cardiopulmonary arrest); urticaria; pain at injection site.

Hepatobiliary Tract: Hyperbilirubinemia, jaundice.

Renal and Genitourinary: Renal impairment.

Cephalosporin-Class Adverse Reactions: In addition to the adverse reactions listed above that have been observed in patients treated with ceftazidime, the following adverse reactions and altered laboratory tests have been reported for cephalosporin-class antibiotics:

Adverse Reactions: Colitis, toxic nephropathy, hepatic dysfunction including cholestasis, aplastic anemia, hemorrhage.

Altered Laboratory Tests: Prolonged prothrombin time, false-positive test for urinary glucose, pancytopenia.

OVERDOSAGE

Ceftazidime overdosage has occurred in patients with renal failure. Reactions have included seizure activity, encephalopathy, asterixis, neuromuscular excitability, and coma. Patients who receive an acute overdosage should be carefully observed and given supportive treatment. In the presence of renal insufficiency, hemodialysis or peritoneal dialysis may aid in the removal of ceftazidime from the body.

DOSAGE AND ADMINISTRATION

Dosage: The usual adult dosage is 1 gram administered intravenously or intramuscularly every 8 to 12 hours. The dosage and route should be determined by the susceptibility of the causative organisms, the severity of infection, and the condition and renal function of the patient.

The guidelines for dosage of TAZICEF are listed in Table 3. The following dosage schedule is recommended.

[See table 3 above]

Impaired Hepatic Function: No adjustment in dosage is required for patients with hepatic dysfunction.

Impaired Renal Function: Ceftazidime is excreted by the kidneys, almost exclusively by glomerular filtration. Therefore, in patients with impaired renal function (glomerular filtration rate [GFR] <50 mL/min), it is recommended that the dosage of ceftazidime be reduced to compensate for its slower excretion. In patients with suspected renal insufficiency, an initial loading dose of 1 gram of TAZICEF may be given. An estimate of GFR should be made to determine the appropriate maintenance dosage. The recommended dosage is presented in Table 4.

Table 4. Recommended Maintenance Dosages of TAZICEF in Renal Insufficiency

NOTE: IF THE DOSE RECOMMENDED IN TABLE 3 ABOVE IS LOWER THAN THAT RECOMMENDED FOR PATIENTS WITH RENAL INSUFFICIENCY AS OUTLINED IN TABLE 4, THE LOWER DOSE SHOULD BE USED.

Creatinine Clearance (mL/min)	Recommened Dose of TAZICEF	Frequency of Dosing
50–31	1 gram	q12hr
30–16	1 gram	q24hr
15–6	500 mg	q24hr
<5	500 mg	q48hr

When only serum creatinine is available, the following formula (Cockcroft's equation)[4] may be used to estimate creatinine clearance. The serum creatinine should represent a steady state of renal function:

[See table at bottom of next page]

In patients with severe infections who would normally receive 6 grams of TAZICEF daily were it not for renal insufficiency, the unit dose given in the table above may be increased by 50% or the dosing frequency may be increased appropriately. Further dosing should be determined by therapeutic monitoring, severity of the infection, and susceptibility of the causative organism.

In pediatric patients as for adults, the creatinine clearance should be adjusted for body surface area or lean body mass, and the dosing frequency should be reduced in cases of renal insufficiency.

In patients undergoing hemodialysis, a loading dose of 1 gram is recommended, followed by 1 gram after each hemodialysis period.

TAZICEF can also be used in patients undergoing intraperitoneal dialysis and continuous ambulatory peritoneal dialysis. In such patients, a loading dose of 1 gram of TAZICEF may be given, followed by 500 mg every 24 hours. In addition to IV use, TAZICEF can be incorporated in the dialysis fluid at a concentration of 250 mg for 2 L of dialysis fluid.

Note: Generally TAZICEF should be continued for 2 days after the signs and symptoms of infection have disappeared, but in complicated infections longer therapy may be required.

Administration: TAZICEF may be given intravenously or by deep IM injection into a large muscle mass such as the upper outer quadrant of the gluteus maximus or lateral part of the thigh. Intra-arterial administration should be avoided (see PRECAUTIONS).

Intramuscular Administration: For IM administration, TAZICEF should be constituted with one of the following diluents: Sterile Water for Injection, Bacteriostatic Water for Injection, or 0.5% or 1% Lidocaine Hydrochloride Injection. Refer to Table 5.

Intravenous Administration: The IV route is preferable for patients with bacterial septicemia, bacterial meningitis, peritonitis, or other severe or life-threatening infections, or for patients who may be poor risks because of lowered resistance resulting from such debilitating conditions as malnutrition, trauma, surgery, diabetes, heart failure, or malignancy, particularly if shock is present or pending.

For direct intermittent IV administration, constitute TAZICEF as directed in Table 5 with Sterile Water for Injection. Slowly inject directly into the vein over a period of 3 to 5 minutes or give through the tubing of an administration set while the patient is also receiving one of the compatible IV fluids (see COMPATIBILITY AND STABILITY).

For IV infusion, constitute the 1—gram infusion pack with 100 mL of Sterile Water for Injection or one of the compatible IV fluids listed under the COMPATIBILITY AND STABILITY section. Alternatively, constitute the 1-gram or 2-gram vial and add an appropriate quantity of the resulting solution to an IV container with one of the compatible IV fluids.

Intermittent IV infusion with a Y-type administration set can be accomplished with compatible solutions. However, during infusion of a solution containing ceftazidime, it is desirable to discontinue the other solution.

ADD-Vantage vials are to be constituted only with 50 or 100 mL of 5% Dextrose Injection, 0.9% Sodium Chloride Injection, or 0.45% Sodium Chloride Injection in Abbott ADD-Vantage flexible diluent containers (see Instructions for Constitution). ADD-Vantage vials that have been joined to Abbott ADD-Vantage diluent containers and activated to dissolve the drug are stable for 24 hours at room temperature or for 7 days under refrigeration. Joined vials that have not been activated may be used within a 14-day period; this period corresponds to that for use of Abbott ADD-Vantage containers following removal of the outer packaging (overwrap).

Freezing solutions of TAZICEF in the ADD-Vantage system is not recommended.

[See table 5 at bottom of next page]

All vials of TAZICEF as supplied are under reduced pressure. When TAZICEF is dissolved, carbon dioxide is released and a positive pressure develops. For ease of use please follow the recommended techniques of constitution described on the detachable Instructions for Constitution section of this insert.

Solutions of TAZICEF, like those of most beta-lactam antibiotics, should not be added to solutions of aminoglycoside antibiotics because of potential interaction.

However, if concurrent therapy with TAZICEF and an aminoglycoside is indicated, each of these antibiotics can be administered separately to the same patient.

Continued on next page

Tazicef—Cont.

COMPATIBILITY AND STABILITY

Intramuscular: TAZICEF, when constituted as directed with Sterile Water for Injection, Bacteriostatic Water for Injection, or 0.5% or 1% Lidocaine Hydrochloride Injection, maintains satisfactory potency for 24 hours at room temperature or for 7 days under refrigeration. Solutions in Sterile Water for Injection that are frozen immediately after constitution in the original container are stable for 3 months when stored at −20°C. Once thawed, solutions should not be refrozen. Thawed solutions may be stored for up to 8 hours at room temperature or for 4 days in a refrigerator.

Intravenous: TAZICEF, when constituted as directed with Sterile Water for Injection, maintains satisfactory potency for 24 hours at room temperature or for 7 days under refrigeration. Solutions in Sterile Water for Injection in the infusion vial or in 0.9% Sodium Chloride Injection in VIAFLEX® small-volume containers that are frozen immediately after constitution are stable for 6 months when stored at −20°C. Do not force thaw by immersion in water baths or by microwave irradiation. Once thawed, solutions should not be refrozen. Thawed solutions may be stored for up to 24 hours at room temperature or for 7 days in a refrigerator. More concentrated solutions in Sterile Water for Injection in the original container that are frozen immediately after constitution are stable for 3 months when stored at −20°C. Once thawed, solutions should not be refrozen. Thawed solutions may be stored for up to 8 hours at room temperature or for 4 days in a refrigerator.

TAZICEF is compatible with the more commonly used IV infusion fluids. Solutions at concentrations between 1 and 40 mg/mL in 0.9% Sodium Chloride Injection; 1/6 M Sodium Lactate Injection; 5% Dextrose Injection; 5% Dextrose and 0.225% Sodium Chloride Injection; 5% Dextrose and 0.45% Sodium Chloride Injection; 5% Dextrose and 0.9% Sodium Chloride Injection; 10% Dextrose Injection; Ringer's Injection, USP; Lactated Ringer's Injection, USP; 10% Invert Sugar in Water for Injection; and NORMOSOL®-M in 5% Dextrose Injection may be stored for up to 24 hours at room temperature or for 7 days if refrigerated.

The 1- and 2-g TAZICEF ADD-Vantage vials, when diluted in 50 or 100 mL of 5% Dextrose Injection, 0.9% Sodium Chloride Injection, or 0.45% Sodium Chloride Injection, may be stored for up to 24 hours at room temperature or for 7 days under refrigeration.

TAZICEF is less stable in Sodium Bicarbonate Injection than in other IV fluids. It is not recommended as a diluent. Solutions of TAZICEF in 5% Dextrose Injection and 0.9% Sodium Chloride Injection are stable for at least 6 hours at room temperature in plastic tubing, drip chambers, and volume control devices of common IV infusion sets.

Ceftazidime at a concentration of 4 mg/mL has been found compatible for 24 hours at room temperature or for 7 days under refrigeration in 0.9% Sodium Chloride Injection or 5% Dextrose Injection when admixed with: cefuroxime sodium (ZINACEF®) 3 mg/mL; heparin 10 or 50 U/mL; or potassium chloride 10 or 40 mEq/L.

Vancomycin solution exhibits a physical incompatibility when mixed with a number of drugs, including ceftazidime. The likelihood of precipitation with ceftazidime is dependent on the concentrations of vancomycin and ceftazidime present. It is therefore recommended, when both drugs are to be administered by intermittent IV infusion, that they be given separately, flushing the IV lines (with one of the compatible IV fluids) between the administration of these two agents.

Note: Parenteral drug products should be inspected visually for particulate matter before administration whenever solution and container permit.

As with other cephalosporins, TAZICEF powder as well as solutions tend to darken, depending on storage conditions; within the stated recommendations, however, product potency is not adversely affected.

HOW SUPPLIED

TAZICEF in the dry state should be stored between 15° and 30°C (59° and 86°F) and protected from light. TAZICEF is a dry, white to off-white powder supplied in vials and infusion packs as follows:

NDC 0074-5082-16 1-g* Vial (Tray of 25)
NDC 0074-5084-11 2-g* Vial (Tray of 10)
NDC 0074-5083-11 1-g* Infusion Pack (Tray of 10)
NDC 0074-5086-11 6-g* Pharmacy Bulk Package (Tray of 10)
NDC 0074-5092-16 1-g ADD-Vantage® Vial (Tray of 25)
NDC 0074-5093-11 2-g ADD-Vantage® Vial (Tray of 10)
(The above ADD-Vantage vials are to be used only with Abbott ADD-Vantage diluent containers.)
*Equivalent to anhydrous ceftazidime.

REFERENCES

1. Bauer AW, Kirby WMM, Sherris JC, Turck M. Antibiotic susceptibility testing by a standardized single disk method. *Am J Clin Pathol.* 1966;45:493–496.
2. National Committee for Clinical Laboratory Standards. *Approved Standard: Performance Standards for Antimicrobial Disc Susceptibility Tests.* (M2-A3). December 1984.
3. Certification procedure for antibiotic sensitivity discs (21 CFR 460.1). *Federal Register.* May 30, 1974;39:19182–19184.
4. Cockcroft DW, Gault MH. Prediction of creatinine clearance from serum creatinine. *Nephron.* 1976;16:31–41.

Manufactured by GlaxoSmithKline, Research Triangle Park, NC 27709
for ABBOTT LABORATORIES, North Chicago, IL 60064
ZINACEF is a registered trademark of the GlaxoSmithKline group of companies.
ADD-Vantage is a registered trademark of Abbott Laboratories.
CLINITEST and CLINISTIX are registered trademarks of Ames Division, Miles Laboratories, Inc.
VIAFLEX is a registered trademark of Baxter International Inc.
April 2002/RL-1091

THORAZINE® ℞

[*thor 'ə-zēn*]
brand of chlorpromazine
antipsychotic • tranquilizer • antiemetic

Prescribing information for this product, which appears on pages 1656–1658 of the 2002 PDR, has been revised as follows. Please write "See Supplement A" next to the product heading.

The first paragraph of the **INDICATIONS** *section was revised to:*

For the treatment of schizophrenia.

The **WARNINGS: Tardive Dyskinesia** *subsection was revised to:*

Tardive dyskinesia, a syndrome consisting of potentially irreversible, involuntary, dyskinetic movements, may develop in patients treated with antipsychotic drugs. Although the prevalence of the syndrome appears to be highest among the elderly, especially elderly women, it is impossible to rely upon prevalence estimates to predict, at the inception of antipsychotic treatment, which patients are likely to develop the syndrome. Whether antipsychotic drug products differ in their potential to cause tardive dyskinesia is unknown.

Both the risk of developing the syndrome and the likelihood that it will become irreversible are believed to increase as the duration of treatment and the total cumulative dose of antipsychotic drugs administered to the patient increase. However, the syndrome can develop, although much less commonly, after relatively brief treatment periods at low doses.

There is no known treatment for established cases of tardive dyskinesia, although the syndrome may remit, partially or completely, if antipsychotic treatment is withdrawn. Antipsychotic treatment itself, however, may suppress (or partially suppress) the signs and symptoms of the syndrome and thereby may possibly mask the underlying disease process. The effect that symptomatic suppression has upon the long-term course of the syndrome is unknown.

Given these considerations, antipsychotics should be prescribed in a manner that is most likely to minimize the occurrence of tardive dyskinesia. Chronic antipsychotic treatment should generally be reserved for patients who suffer from a chronic illness that, 1) is known to respond to antipsychotic drugs, and, 2) for whom alternative, equally effective, but potentially less harmful treatments are *not* available or appropriate. In patients who do require chronic treatment, the smallest dose and the shortest duration of treatment producing a satisfactory clinical response should be sought. The need for continued treatment should be reassessed periodically.

If signs and symptoms of tardive dyskinesia appear in a patient on antipsychotics, drug discontinuation should be considered. However, some patients may require treatment despite the presence of the syndrome.

For further information about the description of tardive dyskinesia and its clinical detection, please refer to the sections on PRECAUTIONS and ADVERSE REACTIONS.

The **WARNINGS: Neuroleptic Malignant Syndrome (NMS)** *subsection was revised to:*

A potentially fatal symptom complex sometimes referred to as Neuroleptic Malignant Syndrome (NMS) has been reported in association with antipsychotic drugs. Clinical manifestations of NMS are hyperpyrexia, muscle rigidity, altered mental status and evidence of autonomic instability (irregular pulse or blood pressure, tachycardia, diaphoresis and cardiac dysrhythmias.)

The diagnostic evaluation of patients with this syndrome is complicated. In arriving at a diagnosis, it is important to identify cases where the clinical presentation includes both serious medical illness (e.g., pneumonia, systemic infection, etc.) and untreated or inadequately treated extrapyramidal signs and symptoms (EPS). Other important considerations in the differential diagnosis include central anticholinergic toxicity, heat stroke, drug fever and primary central nervous system (CNS) pathology.

The management of NMS should include 1) immediate discontinuation of antipsychotic drugs and other drugs not essential to concurrent therapy, 2) intensive symptomatic treatment and medical monitoring, and 3) treatment of any concomitant serious medical problems for which specific treatments are available. There is no general agreement about specific pharmacological treatment regimens for uncomplicated NMS.

If a patient requires antipsychotic drug treatment after recovery from NMS, the potential reintroduction of drug therapy should be carefully considered. The patient should be carefully monitored, since recurrences of NMS have been reported.

An encephalopathic syndrome (characterized by weakness, lethargy, fever, tremulousness and confusion, extrapyramidal symptoms, leukocytosis, elevated serum enzymes, BUN and FBS) has occurred in a few patients treated with lithium plus an antipsychotic. In some instances, the syndrome was followed by irreversible brain damage. Because of a possible causal relationship between these events and the concomitant administration of lithium and antipsychotics, patients receiving such combined therapy should be monitored closely for early evidence of neurologic toxicity and treatment discontinued promptly if such signs appear. This encephalopathic syndrome may be similar to or the same as neuroleptic malignant syndrome (NMS).

Thorazine (chlorpromazine) ampuls and multi-dose vials contain sodium bisulfite and sodium sulfite, sulfites that may cause allergic-type reactions including anaphylactic symptoms and life-threatening or less severe asthmatic episodes in certain susceptible people. The overall prevalence of sulfite sensitivity in the general population is unknown and probably low. Sulfite sensitivity is seen more frequently in asthmatic than in nonasthmatic people.

Patients with bone marrow depression or who have previously demonstrated a hypersensitivity reaction (e.g., blood dyscrasias, jaundice) with a phenothiazine should not receive any phenothiazine, including *Thorazine*, unless in the judgment of the physician the potential benefits of treatment outweigh the possible hazard.

Thorazine may impair mental and/or physical abilities, especially during the first few days of therapy. Therefore, caution patients about activities requiring alertness (e.g., operating vehicles or machinery).

The use of alcohol with this drug should be avoided due to possible additive effects and hypotension.

Thorazine may counteract the antihypertensive effect of guanethidine and related compounds.

The following paragraphs in the **PRECAUTIONS: General** *subsection were revised to:*

Given the likelihood that some patients exposed chronically to antipsychotics will develop tardive dyskinesia, it is advised that all patients in whom chronic use is contemplated be given, if possible, full information about this risk. The decision to inform patients and/or their guardians must obviously take into account the clinical circumstances and the competency of the patient to understand the information provided.

Antipsychotic drugs elevate prolactin levels; the elevation persists during chronic administration. Tissue culture experiments indicate that approximately 1/3 of human breast cancers are prolactin-dependent *in vitro*, a factor of potential importance if the prescribing of these drugs is contemplated in a patient with a previously detected breast cancer. Although disturbances such as galactorrhea, amenorrhea, gynecomastia and impotence have been reported, the clinical significance of elevated serum prolactin levels is unknown for most patients. An increase in mammary neoplasms has been found in rodents after chronic administration of antipsychotic drugs. Neither clinical nor epidemiologic studies conducted to date, however, have shown an association between chronic administration of these drugs and mammary tumorigenesis; the available evidence is considered too limited to be conclusive at this time.

$$\text{Males: Creatinine clearance (mL/min)} = \frac{\text{Weight (kg)} \times (140 - \text{age})}{72 \times \text{serum creatinine (mg/dL)}}$$

Females: 0.85 × male value

Table 5. Preparation of Solutions of TAZICEF

Size	Amount of Diluent to be Added (mL)	Approximate Available Volume (mL)	Approximate Ceftazidime Concentration (mg/mL)
Intramuscular			
1-gram vial	3.0	3.6	280
Intravenous			
1-gram vial	10.0	10.6	100
2-gram vial	10.0	11.5	170
Infusion pack			
1-gram vial	100*	100	10
Pharmacy bulk package 6-gram vial	26	30	200

***Note:** Addition should be in two stages (see Instructions for Constitution).

Chromosomal aberrations in spermatocytes and abnormal sperm have been demonstrated in rodents treated with certain antipsychotics.
The **PRECAUTIONS: Long-Term Therapy** *subsection was revised to:*
To lessen the likelihood of adverse reactions related to cumulative drug effect, patients with a history of long-term therapy with *Thorazine* and/or other antipsychotics should be evaluated periodically to decide whether the maintenance dosage could be lowered or drug therapy discontinued.
The following paragraph in the **ADVERSE REACTIONS: Cardiovascular** *subsection was revised to:*
EKG Changes—particularly nonspecific, usually reversible Q and T wave distortions–have been observed in some patients receiving phenothiazine antipsychotics, including Thorazine (chlorpromazine).
The following sentence in the **ADVERSE REACTIONS: CNS Reactions: Pseudo-parkinsonism** *subsection was revised to:*
(Note: Levodopa has not been found effective in antipsychotic -induced pseudo-parkinsonism.)
The following sentence in the **ADVERSE REACTIONS: CNS Reactions: *Tardive Dyskinesia*** *subsection was revised to:*
Although its prevalence appears to be highest among elderly patients, especially elderly women, it is impossible to rely upon prevalence estimates to predict at the inception of antipsychotic treatment which patients are likely to develop the syndrome.
The following subhead in **DOSAGE AND ADMINISTRATION—ADULTS: Psychotic Disorders** *was revised to:*
HOSPITALIZED PATIENTS: ACUTE SCHIZOPHRENIC OR MANIC STATES
The following sentence in the **DOSAGE AND ADMINISTRATION—PEDIATRIC PATIENTS (6 months to 12 years of age): HOSPITALIZED PATIENTS** *subsection was revised to:*
In severe behavior disorders, higher dosages (50 to 100 mg daily, and in older children, 200 mg daily or more) may be necessary.
GlaxoSmithKline, Research Triangle Park, NC 27709

January 2002/TZ:L85

TIMENTIN® ℞

[*tī-mĕn' tĭn*]
brand of sterile ticarcillin disodium
and clavulanate potassium
for Intravenous Administration

Prescribing information for this product, which appears on pages 1658–1661 of the 2002 PDR, has been revised as follows. Please write "See Supplement A" next to the product heading.
The following sentence in the fifth paragraph of the **CLINICAL PHARMACOLOGY** *section was revised to:*
Neither component of *Timentin* is highly protein bound; ticarcillin has been found to be approximately 45% bound to human serum protein and clavulanic acid approximately 25% bound.
GlaxoSmithKline, Research Triangle Park, NC 27709

April 2001/TI:L10IV

TIMENTIN® ℞

[*tī-mĕn' tĭn*]
brand of sterile ticarcillin disodium
and clavulanate potassium
for Intravenous Administration
ADD-Vantage® ANTIBIOTIC VIAL

Prescribing information for this product, which appears on pages 1661–1664 of the 2002 PDR, has been revised as follows. Please write "See Supplement A" next to the product heading.
The following sentence in the fifth paragraph of the **CLINICAL PHARMACOLOGY** *section was revised to:*
Neither component of *Timentin* is highly protein bound; ticarcillin has been found to be approximately 45% bound to human serum protein and clavulanic acid approximately 25% bound.
GlaxoSmithKline, Research Triangle Park, NC 27709

April 2001/TI:L9AV

TIMENTIN® ℞

[*tī-mĕn' tĭn*]
brand of ticarcillin disodium
and clavulanate potassium
Injection

Galaxy® (PL 2040) Plastic Container
(Product Package)

Prescribing information for this product, which appears on pages 1664–1666 of the 2002 PDR, has been revised as follows. Please write "See Supplement A" next to the product heading.
The following sentence in the sixth paragraph of the **CLINICAL PHARMACOLOGY** *section was revised to:*
Neither component of *Timentin* is highly protein bound; ticarcillin has been found to be approximately 45% bound to human serum protein and clavulanic acid approximately 25% bound.
GlaxoSmithKline, Research Triangle Park, NC 27709

April 2001/TI:L12G

TIMENTIN® ℞

[*tī-mĕn' tĭn*]
brand of sterile ticarcillin disodium
and clavulanate potassium
for Intravenous Administration

PHARMACY BULK PACKAGE
NOT FOR DIRECT INFUSION

Prescribing information for this product, which appears on pages 1666–1669 of the 2002 PDR, has been revised as follows. Please write "See Supplement A" next to the product heading.
The sixth paragraph of the **CLINICAL PHARMACOLOGY** *section was revised to:*
Neither component of *Timentin* is highly protein bound; ticarcillin has been found to be approximately 45% bound to human serum protein and clavulanic acid approximately 25% bound.
GlaxoSmithKline, Research Triangle Park, NC 27709

April 2001/TI:L10PB

TRIZIVIR® ℞

[*trī zə-vir*]
(abacavir sulfate, lamivudine, and zidovudine)
Tablets

Prescribing information for this product, which appears on pages 1669–1674 of the 2002 PDR, has been revised as follows. Please write "See Supplement A" next to the product heading.
The following subsection was added to **CLINICAL PHARMACOLOGY: Special Populations: *Impaired Hepatic Function:***
TRIZIVIR: A reduction in the daily dose of zidovudine may be necessary in patients with mild to moderate impaired hepatic function or liver cirrhosis. Because TRIZIVIR is a fixed-dose combination that cannot be adjusted for this patient population, TRIZIVIR is not recommended for patients with impaired hepatic function.
The following subsection was added to **WARNINGS:**
Posttreatment Exacerbations of Hepatitis: In clinical trials in non-HIV-infected patients treated with lamivudine for chronic hepatitis B (HBV), clinical and laboratory evidence of exacerbations of hepatitis have occurred after discontinuation of lamivudine. These exacerbations have been detected primarily by serum ALT elevations in addition to re-emergence of HBV DNA. Although most events appear to have been self-limited, fatalities have been reported in some cases. Similar events have been reported from post-marketing experience after changes from lamivudine-containing HIV treatment regimens to non-lamivudine-containing regimens in patients infected with both HIV and HBV. The causal relationship to discontinuation of lamivudine treatment is unknown. Patients should be closely monitored with both clinical and laboratory followup for at least several months after stopping treatment. There is insufficient evidence to determine whether re-initiation of lamivudine alters the course of posttreatment exacerbations of hepatitis.
The **PRECAUTIONS: Patients with HIV and Hepatitis B Virus Coinfection: Lamivudine** *subsection was revised to:*
Safety and efficacy of lamivudine have not been established for treatment of chronic hepatitis B in patients dually infected with HIV and HBV. In non-HIV-infected patients treated with lamivudine for chronic hepatitis B, emergence of lamivudine-resistant HBV has been detected and has been associated with diminished treatment response (see EPIVIR-HBV package insert for additional information). Emergence of hepatitis B virus variants associated with resistance to lamivudine has also been reported in HIV-infected patients who have received lamivudine-containing antiretroviral regimens in the presence of concurrent infection with hepatitis B virus.
The **PRECAUTIONS: Drug Interactions: *Lamivudine*** *subsection was revised to:*
Trimethoprim (TMP) 160 mg/sulfamethoxazole (SMX) 800 mg once daily has been shown to increase lamivudine exposure (AUC). The effect of higher doses of TMP/SMX on lamivudine pharmacokinetics has not been investigated (see CLINICAL PHARMACOLOGY).
Lamivudine and zalcitabine may inhibit the intracellular phosphorylation of one another. Therefore, use of TRIZIVIR in combination with zalcitabine is not recommended.
The **PRECAUTIONS: Carcinogenesis, Mutagenesis, and Impairment of Fertility: *Carcinogenicity: Abacavir*** *subsection was revised to:*
Abacavir was administered orally at 3 dosage levels to separate groups of mice (60 females and 60 males per group) and rats (56 females and 56 males in each group) in carcinogenicity studies. Single doses were 55, 110, and 330 mg/kg per day in mice and 30, 120, and 600 mg/kg per day in rats. Results showed an increase in the incidence of malignant and non-malignant tumors. Malignant tumors occurred in the preputial gland of males and the clitoral gland of females of both species, and in the liver of female rats. In addition, non-malignant tumors also occurred in the liver and thyroid gland of female rats.
The **PRECAUTIONS: Carcinogenesis, Mutagenesis, and Impairment of Fertility: *Carcinogenicity: Lamivudine*** *subsection was revised to:*
Long-term carcinogenicity studies with lamivudine in mice and rats showed no evidence of carcinogenic potential at exposures up to 10 times (mice) and 58 times (rats) those observed in humans at the recommended therapeutic dose for HIV infection.
The **PRECAUTIONS: Pregnancy: *Lamivudine*** *subsection was revised to:*
Studies in pregnant rats and rabbits showed that lamivudine is transferred to the fetus through the placenta. Reproduction studies with orally administered lamivudine have been performed in rats and rabbits at doses up to 4000 mg/kg per day and 1000 mg/kg per day, respectively, producing plasma levels up to approximately 35 times that for the adult HIV dose. No evidence of teratogenicity due to lamivudine was observed. Evidence of early embryolethality was seen in the rabbit at exposure levels similar to those observed in humans, but there was no indication of this effect in the rat at exposure levels up to 35 times that in humans.
The first paragraph of the **PRECAUTIONS: Nursing Mothers: Abacavir, Lamivudine, and Zidovudine** *subsection was revised to:*
Zidovudine is excreted in breast milk; abacavir and lamivudine are secreted into the milk of lactating rats.
The **ADVERSE REACTIONS: Observed During Clinical Practice** *subsection was revised to:*
The following events have been identified during post-approval use of abacavir, lamivudine, and/or zidovudine. Because they are reported voluntarily from a population of unknown size, estimates of frequency cannot be made. These events have been chosen for inclusion due to a combination of their seriousness, frequency of reporting, or potential causal connection to lamivudine and/or zidovudine.
Abacavir: Suspected Stevens-Johnson syndrome (SJS) has been reported in patients receiving abacavir in combination with medications known to be associated with SJS. Because of the overlap of clinical signs and symptoms between hypersensitivity to abacavir and SJS, and the possibility of multiple drug sensitivities in some patients, abacavir should be discontinued and not restarted in such cases.
Lamivudine and Zidovudine:
Cardiovascular: Cardiomyopathy.
Digestive: Stomatitis.
Endocrine and Metabolic: Gynecomastia, hyperglycemia.
Gastrointestinal: Oral mucosal pigmentation.
General: Vasculitis, weakness.
Hemic and Lymphatic: Aplastic anemia, anemia, lymphadenopathy, pure red cell aplasia, splenomegaly.
Hepatic and Pancreatic: Lactic acidosis and hepatic steatosis, pancreatitis, posttreatment exacerbation of hepatitis B (see WARNINGS).
Hypersensitivity: Sensitization reactions (including anaphylaxis), urticaria.
Musculoskeletal: Muscle weakness, CPK elevation, rhabdomyolysis.
Nervous: Paresthesia, peripheral neuropathy, seizures.
Respiratory: Abnormal breath sounds/wheezing.
Skin: Alopecia, erythema multiforme, Stevens-Johnson syndrome.
The following section was added to the end of the labeling after the **HOW SUPPLIED** *section:*
ANIMAL TOXICOLOGY
Myocardial degeneration was found in mice and rats following administration of abacavir for 2 years. The systemic exposures were equivalent to 7 to 24 times the expected systemic exposure in humans. The clinical relevance of this finding has not been determined.
GlaxoSmithKline, Research Triangle Park, NC 27709
Lamivudine is manufactured under agreement from
Shire Pharmaceuticals Group plc, Basingstoke, UK

January 2002/RL-1054

TWINRIX® ℞

[*twin'rix*]
Hepatitis A Inactivated
& Hepatitis B (Recombinant) Vaccine

Prescribing information for this product, which appears on pages 1674–1676 of the 2002 PDR, has been revised as follows. Please write "See Supplement A" next to the product heading.
The third paragraph of the **DESCRIPTION** *section was revised to:*
Twinrix [Hepatitis A Inactivated & Hepatitis B (Recombinant) Vaccine] is supplied as a sterile suspension for intramuscular administration. The vaccine is ready for use without reconstitution; it must be shaken before administration since a fine white deposit with a clear colorless supernatant may form on storage. After shaking, the vaccine is a slightly turbid white suspension.

Continued on next page

Twinrix—Cont.

The following sentence was revised in the **DOSAGE AND ADMINISTRATION: Preparation for Administration** *subsection:*
With thorough agitation, *Twinrix* is a slightly turbid white suspension.
The following sentence was revised in the **HOW SUPPLIED** *section:*
Twinrix [Hepatitis A Inactivated & Hepatitis B (Recombinant) Vaccine] is supplied as a slightly turbid white suspension in vials and prefilled Tip-Lok® syringes containing a 1.0 mL single dose.
U.S. License No. 1090
Manufactured by GlaxoSmithKline Biologicals
Rixensart, Belgium
Distributed by GlaxoSmithKline
Research Triangle Park, NC 27709
Twinrix and *Tip-Lok* are registered trademarks of GlaxoSmithKline.

September 2001/TW:L2

VALTREX® ℞

[*val' trĕx*]
(valacyclovir hydrochloride)
Caplets

Prescribing information for this product, which appears on pages 1676–1679 of the 2002 PDR, has been completely revised as follows. Please write "See Supplement A" next to the product heading.

DESCRIPTION

VALTREX (valacyclovir hydrochloride) is the hydrochloride salt of *L*-valyl ester of the antiviral drug acyclovir (ZOVIRAX® Brand, GlaxoSmithKline).
VALTREX Caplets are for oral administration. Each caplet contains valacyclovir hydrochloride equivalent to 500 mg or 1 gram valacyclovir and the inactive ingredients carnauba wax, colloidal silicon dioxide, crospovidone, FD&C Blue No. 2 Lake, hydroxypropyl methylcellulose, magnesium stearate, microcrystalline cellulose, polyethylene glycol, polysorbate 80, povidone, and titanium dioxide. The blue, film-coated caplets are printed with edible white ink.
The chemical name of valacyclovir hydrochloride is *L*-valine, 2-[(2-amino-1,6-dihydro-6-oxo-9*H*-purin-9-yl)methoxy] ethyl ester, monohydrochloride.
Valacyclovir hydrochloride is a white to off-white powder with the molecular formula $C_{13}H_{20}N_6O_4 \bullet HCl$ and a molecular weight of 360.80. The maximum solubility in water at 25°C is 174 mg/mL. The pk_a's for valacyclovir hydrochloride are 1.90, 7.47, and 9.43.

MICROBIOLOGY

Mechanism of Antiviral Action: Valacyclovir hydrochloride is rapidly converted to acyclovir which has demonstrated antiviral activity against herpes simplex virus types 1 (HSV-1) and 2 (HSV-2) and varicella-zoster virus (VZV) both in vitro and in vivo.
The inhibitory activity of acyclovir is highly selective due to its affinity for the enzyme thymidine kinase (TK) encoded by HSV and VZV. This viral enzyme converts acyclovir into acyclovir monophosphate, a nucleotide analogue. The monophosphate is further converted into diphosphate by cellular guanylate kinase and into triphosphate by a number of cellular enzymes. In vitro, acyclovir triphosphate stops replication of herpes viral DNA. This is accomplished in 3 ways: 1) competitive inhibition of viral DNA polymerase, 2) incorporation and termination of the growing viral DNA chain, and 3) inactivation of the viral DNA polymerase. The greater antiviral activity of acyclovir against HSV compared to VZV is due to its more efficient phosphorylation by the viral TK.
Antiviral Activities: The quantitative relationship between the in vitro susceptibility of herpesviruses to antivirals and the clinical response to therapy has not been established in humans, and virus sensitivity testing has not been standardized. Sensitivity testing results, expressed as the concentration of drug required to inhibit by 50% the growth of virus in cell culture (IC_{50}), vary greatly depending upon a number of factors. Using plaque-reduction assays, the IC_{50} against herpes simplex virus isolates ranges from 0.02 to 13.5 mcg/mL for HSV-1 and from 0.01 to 9.9 mcg/mL for HSV-2. The IC_{50} for acyclovir against most laboratory strains and clinical isolates of VZV ranges from 0.12 to 10.8 mcg/mL. Acyclovir also demonstrates activity against the Oka vaccine strain of VZV with a mean IC_{50} of 1.35 mcg/mL.
Drug Resistance: Resistance of HSV and VZV to acyclovir can result from qualitative and quantitative changes in the viral TK and/or DNA polymerase. Clinical isolates of VZV with reduced susceptibility to acyclovir have been recovered from patients with AIDS. In these cases, TK-deficient mutants of VZV have been recovered.
Resistance of HSV and VZV to acyclovir occurs by the same mechanisms. While most of the acyclovir-resistant mutants isolated thus far from immunocompromised patients have been found to be TK-deficient mutants, other mutants involving the viral TK gene (TK partial and TK altered) and DNA polymerase have also been isolated. TK-negative mutants may cause severe disease in immunocompromised patients. The possibility of viral resistance to valacyclovir (and therefore, to acyclovir) should be considered in patients who show poor clinical response during therapy.

CLINICAL PHARMACOLOGY

After oral administration, valacyclovir hydrochloride is rapidly absorbed from the gastrointestinal tract and nearly completely converted to acyclovir and *L*-valine by first-pass intestinal and/or hepatic metabolism.
Pharmacokinetics: The pharmacokinetics of valacyclovir and acyclovir after oral administration of VALTREX have been investigated in 14 volunteer studies involving 283 adults.
Absorption and Bioavailability: The absolute bioavailability of acyclovir after administration of VALTREX is 54.5% ± 9.1% as determined following a 1-gram oral dose of VALTREX and a 350-mg intravenous acyclovir dose to 12 healthy volunteers. Acyclovir bioavailability from the administration of VALTREX is not altered by administration with food (30 minutes after an 873 Kcal breakfast, which included 51 grams of fat).
There was a lack of dose proportionality in acyclovir maximum concentration (C_{max}) and area under the acyclovir concentration-time curve (AUC) after single-dose administration of 100 mg, 250 mg, 500 mg, 750 mg, and 1 gram of VALTREX to 8 healthy volunteers. The mean C_{max} (± SD) was 0.83 (± 0.14), 2.15 (± 0.50), 3.28 (± 0.83), 4.17 (± 1.14), and 5.65 (± 2.37) mcg/mL, respectively; and the mean AUC (± SD) was 2.28 (± 0.40), 5.76 (± 0.60), 11.59 (± 1.79), 14.11 (± 3.54), and 19.52 (± 6.04) h•mcg/mL, respectively.
There was also a lack of dose proportionality in acyclovir C_{max} and AUC after the multiple-dose administration of 250 mg, 500 mg, and 1 gram of VALTREX administered 4 times daily for 11 days in parallel groups of 8 healthy volunteers. The mean C_{max} (± SD) was 2.11 (± 0.33), 3.69 (± 0.87), and 4.96 (± 0.64) mcg/mL, respectively, and the mean AUC (± SD) was 5.66 (± 1.09), 9.88 (± 2.01), and 15.70 (± 2.27) h•mcg/mL, respectively.
There is no accumulation of acyclovir after the administration of valacyclovir at the recommended dosage regimens in healthy volunteers with normal renal function.
Distribution: The binding of valacyclovir to human plasma proteins ranged from 13.5% to 17.9%.
Metabolism: After oral administration, valacyclovir hydrochloride is rapidly absorbed from the gastrointestinal tract. Valacyclovir is converted to acyclovir and *L*-valine by first-pass intestinal and/or hepatic metabolism. Acyclovir is converted to a small extent to inactive metabolites by aldehyde oxidase and by alcohol and aldehyde dehydrogenase. Neither valacyclovir nor acyclovir is metabolized by cytochrome P450 enzymes. Plasma concentrations of unconverted valacyclovir are low and transient, generally becoming non-quantifiable by 3 hours after administration. Peak plasma valacyclovir concentrations are generally less than 0.5 mcg/mL at all doses. After single-dose administration of 1 gram of VALTREX, average plasma valacyclovir concentrations observed were 0.5, 0.4, and 0.8 mcg/mL in patients with hepatic dysfunction, renal insufficiency, and in healthy volunteers who received concomitant cimetidine and probenecid, respectively.
Elimination: The pharmacokinetic disposition of acyclovir delivered by valacyclovir is consistent with previous experience from intravenous and oral acyclovir. Following the oral administration of a single 1-gram dose of radiolabeled valacyclovir to 4 healthy subjects, 45.60% and 47.12% of administered radioactivity was recovered in urine and feces over 96 hours, respectively. Acyclovir accounted for 88.60% of the radioactivity excreted in the urine. Renal clearance of acyclovir following the administration of a single 1-gram dose of VALTREX to 12 healthy volunteers was approximately 255 ± 86 mL/min which represents 41.9% of total acyclovir apparent plasma clearance.
The plasma elimination half-life of acyclovir typically averaged 2.5 to 3.3 hours in all studies of VALTREX in volunteers with normal renal function.
End-Stage Renal Disease (ESRD): Following administration of VALTREX to volunteers with ESRD, the average acyclovir half-life is approximately 14 hours. During hemodialysis, the acyclovir half-life is approximately 4 hours. Approximately one third of acyclovir in the body is removed by dialysis during a 4-hour hemodialysis session. Apparent plasma clearance of acyclovir in dialysis patients was 86.3 ± 21.3 mL/min/1.73 m^2, compared to 679.16 ± 162.76 mL/min/1.73 m^2 in healthy volunteers.
Reduction in dosage is recommended in patients with renal impairment (see DOSAGE AND ADMINISTRATION).
Geriatrics: After single-dose administration of 1 gram of VALTREX in healthy geriatric volunteers, the half-life of acyclovir was 3.11 ± 0.51 hours, compared to 2.91 ± 0.63 hours in healthy volunteers. The pharmacokinetics of acyclovir following single- and multiple-dose oral administration of VALTREX in geriatric volunteers varied with renal function. Dose reduction may be required in geriatric patients, depending on the underlying renal status of the patient (see PRECAUTIONS and DOSAGE AND ADMINISTRATION).
Pediatrics: Valacyclovir pharmacokinetics have not been evaluated in pediatric patients.
Liver Disease: Administration of VALTREX to patients with moderate (biopsy-proven cirrhosis) or severe (with and without ascites and biopsy-proven cirrhosis) liver disease indicated that the rate but not the extent of conversion of valacyclovir to acyclovir is reduced, and the acyclovir half-life is not affected. Dosage modification is not recommended for patients with cirrhosis.
HIV Disease: In 9 patients with advanced HIV disease (CD4 cell counts <150 cells/mm^3) who received VALTREX at a dosage of 1 gram 4 times daily for 30 days, the pharmacokinetics of valacyclovir and acyclovir were not different from that observed in healthy volunteers (see WARNINGS).
Drug Interactions: The pharmacokinetics of digoxin was not affected by coadministration of VALTREX 1 gram 3 times daily, and the pharmacokinetics of acyclovir after a single dose of VALTREX (1 gram) was unchanged by coadministration of digoxin (2 doses of 0.75 mg), single doses of antacids (Al^{3+} or Mg^{++}), or multiple doses of thiazide diuretics. Acyclovir C_{max} and AUC following a single dose of VALTREX (1 gram) increased by 8% and 32%, respectively, after a single dose of cimetidine (800 mg), or by 22% and 49%, respectively, after probenecid (1 gram), or by 30% and 78%, respectively, after a combination of cimetidine and probenecid, primarily due to a reduction in renal clearance of acyclovir. These effects are not considered to be of clinical significance in subjects with normal renal function. Therefore, no dosage adjustment is recommended when VALTREX is coadministered with digoxin, antacids, thiazide diuretics, cimetidine, or probenecid in subjects with normal renal function.
Clinical Trials: ***Herpes Zoster Infections:*** Two randomized double-blind clinical trials in immunocompetent adults with localized herpes zoster were conducted. VALTREX was compared to placebo in patients less than 50 years of age, and to ZOVIRAX in patients greater than 50 years of age. All patients were treated within 72 hours of appearance of zoster rash. In patients less than 50 years of age, the median time to cessation of new lesion formation was 2 days for those treated with VALTREX compared to 3 days for those treated with placebo. In patients greater than 50 years of age, the median time to cessation of new lesions was 3 days in patients treated with either VALTREX or ZOVIRAX. In patients less than 50 years of age, no difference was found with respect to the duration of pain after healing (post-herpetic neuralgia) between the recipients of VALTREX and placebo. In patients greater than 50 years of age, among the 83% who reported pain after healing (post-herpetic neuralgia), the median duration of pain after healing [95% confidence interval] in days was: 40 [31, 51], 43 [36, 55], and 59 [41, 77] for 7-day VALTREX, 14-day VALTREX, and 7-day ZOVIRAX, respectively.
Genital Herpes Infections: Initial Episode: Six hundred and forty-three immunocompetent adults with first episode genital herpes who presented within 72 hours of symptom onset were randomized in a double-blind trial to receive 10 days of VALTREX 1 gram b.i.d. (n = 323) or ZOVIRAX 200 mg 5 times a day (n = 320). For both treatment groups: the median time to lesion healing was 9 days, the median time to cessation of pain was 5 days, the median time to cessation of viral shedding was 3 days.
Recurrent Episodes: Three double-blind trials (2 of them placebo-controlled) in immunocompetent adults with recurrent genital herpes were conducted. Patients self-initiated therapy within 24 hours of the first sign or symptom of a recurrent genital herpes episode.
In 1 study, patients were randomized to receive 5 days of treatment with either VALTREX 500 mg b.i.d. (n = 360) or placebo (n = 259). The median time to lesion healing was 4 days in the group receiving VALTREX 500 mg versus 6 days in the placebo group, and the median time to cessation of viral shedding in patients with at least 1 positive culture (42% of the overall study population) was 2 days in the group receiving VALTREX 500 mg versus 4 days in the placebo group. The median time to cessation of pain was 3 days in the group receiving VALTREX 500 mg versus 4 days in the placebo group. Results supporting efficacy were replicated in a second trial.
In a third study, patients were randomized to receive VALTREX 500 mg b.i.d. for 5 days (n = 398) or VALTREX 500 mg b.i.d. for 3 days (and matching placebo b.i.d. for 2 additional days) (n = 402). The median time to lesion healing was about 4½ days in both treatment groups. The median time to cessation of pain was about 3 days in both treatment groups.
Suppressive Therapy: One thousand four hundred seventy-nine (1479) immunocompetent adults with a history of 6 or more recurrences per year were randomized into

Table 1: Proportions of Patients Recurrence Free at 6 and 12 Months

	6 Months			12 Months		
Treatment Arm	VALTREX 1 gram q.d. (n = 269)	ZOVIRAX 400 mg b.i.d. (n = 267)	Placebo (n = 134)	VALTREX 1 gram q.d. (n = 269)	ZOVIRAX 400 mg b.i.d. (n = 267)	Placebo (n = 134)
Recurrence free (%)	55	54	7	34	34	4
Recurrences (%)	35	36	83	46	46	85
Unknowns (%)	10	10	10	19	19	10

a double-blind, placebo-controlled study. Outcomes for the overall study population are shown in Table 1.
[See table 1 at top of previous page]
Subjects with 9 or fewer recurrences per year showed comparable results with VALTREX 500 mg once daily.

INDICATIONS AND USAGE

Herpes Zoster: VALTREX is indicated for the treatment of herpes zoster (shingles).

Genital Herpes: VALTREX is indicated for the treatment or suppression of genital herpes.

CONTRAINDICATIONS

VALTREX is contraindicated in patients with a known hypersensitivity or intolerance to valacyclovir, acyclovir, or any component of the formulation.

WARNINGS

Thrombotic thrombocytopenic purpura/hemolytic uremic syndrome (TTP/HUS), in some cases resulting in death, has occurred in patients with advanced HIV disease and also in allogeneic bone marrow transplant and renal transplant recipients participating in clinical trials of VALTREX at doses of 8 grams per day.

PRECAUTIONS

Dosage reduction is recommended when administering VALTREX to patients with renal impairment (see DOSAGE AND ADMINISTRATION). Acute renal failure and central nervous system symptoms have been reported in patients with underlying renal disease who have received inappropriately high doses of VALTREX for their level of renal function. Similar caution should be exercised when administering VALTREX to geriatric patients (see Geriatric Use) and patients receiving potentially nephrotoxic agents.

Precipitation of acyclovir in renal tubules may occur when the solubility (2.5 mg/mL) is exceeded in the intratubular fluid. In the event of acute renal failure and anuria, the patient may benefit from hemodialysis until renal function is restored (see DOSAGE AND ADMINISTRATION).

The efficacy of VALTREX has not been established for the treatment of disseminated herpes zoster or in immunocompromised patients.

Information for Patients: ***Herpes Zoster:*** There are no data on treatment initiated more than 72 hours after onset of the zoster rash. Patients should be advised to initiate treatment as soon as possible after a diagnosis of herpes zoster.

Genital Herpes: Patients should be informed that VALTREX is not a cure for genital herpes. There are no data evaluating whether VALTREX will prevent transmission of infection to others. Because genital herpes is a sexually transmitted disease, patients should avoid contact with lesions or intercourse when lesions and/or symptoms are present to avoid infecting partners. Genital herpes can also be transmitted in the absence of symptoms through asymptomatic viral shedding. If medical management of a genital herpes recurrence is indicated, patients should be advised to initiate therapy at the first sign or symptom of an episode.

There are no data on the effectiveness of treatment initiated more than 72 hours after the onset of signs and symptoms of a first episode of genital herpes or more than 24 hours of the onset of signs and symptoms of a recurrent episode.

There are no data on the safety or effectiveness of chronic suppressive therapy of more than 1 year's duration.

Drug Interactions: See CLINICAL PHARMACOLOGY: Pharmacokinetics.

Carcinogenesis, Mutagenesis, Impairment of Fertility: The data presented below include references to the steady-state acyclovir AUC observed in humans treated with 1 gram VALTREX given orally 3 times a day to treat herpes zoster. Plasma drug concentrations in animal studies are expressed as multiples of human exposure to acyclovir (see CLINICAL PHARMACOLOGY: Pharmacokinetics).

Valacyclovir was noncarcinogenic in lifetime carcinogenicity bioassays at single daily doses (gavage) of up to 120 mg/kg per day for mice and 100 mg/kg per day for rats. There was no significant difference in the incidence of tumors between treated and control animals, nor did valacyclovir shorten the latency of tumors. Plasma concentrations of acyclovir were equivalent to human levels in the mouse bioassay and 1.4 to 2.3 times human levels in the rat bioassay.

Valacyclovir was tested in 5 genetic toxicity assays. An Ames assay was negative in the absence or presence of metabolic activation. Also negative were an in vitro cytogenetic study with human lymphocytes and a rat cytogenetic study at a single oral dose of 3000 mg/kg (8 to 9 times human plasma levels).

In the mouse lymphoma assay, valacyclovir was not mutagenic in the absence of metabolic activation. In the presence of metabolic activation (76% to 88% conversion to acyclovir), valacyclovir was mutagenic.

Valacyclovir was not mutagenic in a mouse micronucleus assay at 250 mg/kg but positive at 500 mg/kg (acyclovir concentrations 26 to 51 times human plasma levels).

Valacyclovir did not impair fertility or reproduction in rats at 200 mg/kg per day (6 times human plasma levels).

Pregnancy: ***Teratogenic Effects:*** Pregnancy Category B. Valacyclovir was not teratogenic in rats or rabbits given 400 mg/kg (which results in exposures of 10 and 7 times human plasma levels, respectively) during the period of major organogenesis.

There are no adequate and well-controlled studies of VALTREX or ZOVIRAX in pregnant women. A prospective epidemiologic registry of acyclovir use during pregnancy was established in 1984 and completed in April 1999. There were 749 pregnancies followed in women exposed to systemic acyclovir during the first trimester of pregnancy resulting in 756 outcomes. The occurrence rate of birth defects approximates that found in the general population. However, the small size of the registry is insufficient to evaluate the risk for less common defects or to permit reliable or definitive conclusions regarding the safety of acyclovir in pregnant women and their developing fetuses. VALTREX should be used during pregnancy only if the potential benefit justifies the potential risk to the fetus.

Nursing Mothers: There is no experience with VALTREX. However, acyclovir concentrations have been documented in breast milk in 2 women following oral administration of ZOVIRAX and ranged from 0.6 to 4.1 times corresponding plasma levels. These concentrations would potentially expose the nursing infant to a dose of acyclovir as high as 0.3 mg/kg per day. VALTREX should be administered to a nursing mother with caution and only when indicated.

Pediatric Use: Safety and effectiveness of VALTREX in pre-pubertal pediatric patients have not been established.

Geriatric Use: Of the total number of subjects in clinical studies of VALTREX, 852 were 65 and over, and 346 were 75 and over. In a clinical study of herpes zoster, the duration of pain after healing (post-herpetic neuralgia) was longer in patients 65 and older compared with younger adults. Elderly patients are more likely to have reduced renal function and require dose reduction. Elderly patients are also more likely to have renal or CNS adverse events. With respect to CNS adverse events observed during clinical practice, agitation, hallucinations, confusion, delirium, and encephalopathy were reported more frequently in elderly patients (see CLINICAL PHARMACOLOGY, ADVERSE REACTIONS: Observed During Clinical Practice, and DOSAGE AND ADMINISTRATION).

ADVERSE REACTIONS

Frequently reported adverse events in clinical trials of VALTREX are listed in Tables 2 and 3.

Table 2: Incidence (%) of Adverse Events in Herpes Zoster Study Populations

Adverse Event	VALTREX 1 gram t.i.d. (n = 967)	Placebo (n = 195)
Nausea	15%	8%
Headache	14%	12%
Vomiting	6%	3%
Dizziness	3%	2%
Abdominal Pain	3%	2%

Table 3: Incidence (%) of Adverse Events in Genital Herpes Study Populations

	Genital Herpes Treatment			Genital Herpes Suppression		
Adverse Event	VALTREX 1 gram b.i.d. (n = 1194)	VALTREX 500 mg b.i.d. (n = 1159)	Placebo (n = 439)	VALTREX 1 gram q.d. (n = 269)	VALTREX 500 mg q.d. (n = 266)	Placebo (n = 134)
Nausea	6%	5%	8%	11%	11%	8%
Headache	16%	15%	14%	35%	38%	34%
Vomiting	1%	<1%	<1%	3%	3%	2%
Dizziness	3%	2%	3%	4%	2%	1%
Abdominal Pain	2%	1%	3%	11%	9%	6%
Dysmenorrhea	<1%	<1%	1%	8%	5%	4%
Arthralgia	<1%	<1%	<1%	6%	5%	4%
Depression	1%	0%	<1%	7%	5%	5%

[See table 3 above]
Laboratory abnormalities reported in clinical trials of VALTREX are listed in Table 4.
[See table 4 above]

Table 4: Incidence (%) of Laboratory Abnormalities in Herpes Zoster and Genital Herpes Study Populations

	Herpes Zoster		Genital Herpes Treatment			Genital Herpes Suppression		
Laboratory Abnormality	VALTREX 1 gram t.i.d.	Placebo	VALTREX 1 gram b.i.d.	VALTREX 500 mg b.i.d.	Placebo	VALTREX 1 gram q.d.	VALTREX 500 mg q.d.	Placebo
Anemia	0.8%	0%	0.3%	0.2%	0%	0%	0.8%	0.8%
Leukopenia	1.3%	0.6%	0.7%	0.6%	0.2%	0.7%	0.8%	1.5%
Thrombocytopenia	1.0%	1.2%	0.3%	0.1%	0.7%	0.4%	1.1%	1.5%
AST (SGOT)	1.0%	0%	1.0%	*	0.5%	4.1%	3.8%	3.0%
Serum Creatinine	0.2%	0%	0.7%	0%	0%	0%	0%	0%

*Data were not collected prospectively.

Observed During Clinical Practice: The following events have been identified during post-approval use of VALTREX in clinical practice. Because they are reported voluntarily from a population of unknown size, estimates of frequency cannot be made. These events have been chosen for inclusion due to either their seriousness, frequency of reporting, causal connection to VALTREX, or a combination of these factors.

General: Facial edema, hypertension, tachycardia.

Allergic: Acute hypersensitivity reactions including anaphylaxis, angioedema, dyspnea, pruritus, rash, and urticaria.

CNS Symptoms: Aggressive behavior; agitation; coma; confusion; decreased consciousness; encephalopathy; mania; and psychosis, including auditory and visual hallucinations (see PRECAUTIONS).

Eye: Visual abnormalities.

Gastrointestinal: Diarrhea.

Hepatobiliary Tract and Pancreas: Liver enzyme abnormalities, hepatitis.

Renal: Elevated creatinine, renal failure.

Hematologic: Thrombocytopenia, aplastic anemia.

Skin: Erythema multiforme, rashes including photosensitivity.

Renal Impairment: Renal failure and CNS symptoms have been reported in patients with renal impairment who received VALTREX or acyclovir at greater than the recommended dose. **Dose reduction is recommended in this patient population (see DOSAGE AND ADMINISTRATION).**

OVERDOSAGE

Caution should be exercised to prevent inadvertent overdose (see PRECAUTIONS). Precipitation of acyclovir in renal tubules may occur when the solubility (2.5 mg/mL) is exceeded in the intratubular fluid. In the event of acute renal failure and anuria, the patient may benefit from hemodialysis until renal function is restored (see DOSAGE AND ADMINISTRATION).

Table 5: Dosages for Patients with Renal Impairment

		Creatinine Clearance (mL/min)		
Indications	Normal Dosage Regimen (Creatinine Clearance ≥50)	30-49	10-29	<10
Herpes zoster	1 gram every 8 hours	1 gram every 12 hours	1 gram every 24 hours	500 mg every 24 hours
Genital herpes				
Initial treatment	1 gram every 12 hours	no reduction	1 gram every 24 hours	500 mg every 24 hours
Recurrent episodes	500 gram every 12 hours	no reduction	500 mg every 24 hours	500 mg every 24 hours
Suppressive therapy	1 gram every 24 hours	no reduction	500 mg every 24 hours	500 mg every 24 hours
Suppressive therapy	500 mg every 24 hours	no reduction	500 mg every 48 hours	500 mg every 48 hours

Continued on next page

Valtrex—Cont.

DOSAGE AND ADMINISTRATION

VALTREX Caplets may be given without regard to meals.

Herpes Zoster: The recommended dosage of VALTREX for the treatment of herpes zoster is 1 gram orally 3 times daily for 7 days. Therapy should be initiated at the earliest sign or symptom of herpes zoster and is most effective when started within 48 hours of the onset of zoster rash. No data are available on efficacy of treatment started greater than 72 hours after rash onset.

Genital Herpes: ***Initial Episodes:*** The recommended dosage of VALTREX for treatment of initial genital herpes is 1 gram twice daily for 10 days.

There are no data on the effectiveness of treatment with VALTREX when initiated more than 72 hours after the onset of signs and symptoms. Therapy was most effective when administered within 48 hours of the onset of signs and symptoms.

Recurrent Episodes: The recommended dosage of VALTREX for the treatment of recurrent genital herpes is 500 mg twice daily for 3 days.

If medical management of a genital herpes recurrence is indicated, patients should be advised to initiate therapy at the first sign or symptom of an episode. There are no data on the effectiveness of treatment with VALTREX when initiated more than 24 hours after the onset of signs or symptoms.

Suppressive Therapy: The recommended dosage of VALTREX for chronic suppressive therapy of recurrent genital herpes is 1 gram once daily. In patients with a history of 9 or fewer recurrences per year, an alternative dose is 500 mg once daily. The safety and efficacy of therapy with VALTREX beyond 1 year have not been established.

Patients with Acute or Chronic Renal Impairment: In patients with reduced renal function, reduction in dosage is recommended (see Table 5).

[See table at top of previous page]

Hemodialysis: During hemodialysis, the half-life of acyclovir after administration of VALTREX is approximately 4 hours. About one third of acyclovir in the body is removed by dialysis during a 4-hour hemodialysis session. Patients requiring hemodialysis should receive the recommended dose of VALTREX after hemodialysis.

Peritoneal Dialysis: There is no information specific to administration of VALTREX in patients receiving peritoneal dialysis. The effect of chronic ambulatory peritoneal dialysis (CAPD) and continuous arteriovenous hemofiltration/dialysis (CAVHD) on acyclovir pharmacokinetics has been studied. The removal of acyclovir after CAPD and CAVHD is less pronounced than with hemodialysis, and the pharmacokinetic parameters closely resemble those observed in patients with ESRD not receiving hemodialysis. Therefore, supplemental doses of VALTREX should not be required following CAPD or CAVHD.

HOW SUPPLIED

VALTREX Caplets (blue, film-coated, capsule-shaped tablets) containing valacyclovir hydrochloride equivalent to 500 mg valacyclovir and printed with "VALTREX 500 mg"—Bottle of 42 (NDC 0173-0933-03) and unit dose pack of 100 (NDC 0173-0933-56).

VALTREX Caplets (blue, film-coated, capsule-shaped tablets) containing valacyclovir hydrochloride equivalent to 1 gram valacyclovir and printed with "VALTREX 1 gram"—Bottle of 21 (NDC 0173-0565-02).

Store at 15° to 25°C (59° to 77°F).

GlaxoSmithKline, Research Triangle Park, NC 27709

August 2001/RL-953

VENTOLIN® ℞
[vent 'ō-lin]
(albuterol, USP)
Inhalation Aerosol

Bronchodilator Aerosol
For Oral Inhalation Only

Prescribing information for this product, which appears on pages 1679–1680 of the 2002 PDR, has been revised as follows. Please write "See Supplement A" next to the product heading.

The following subsection was added to the **PRECAUTIONS** *section:*

Geriatric Use: Clinical studies of VENTOLIN Inhalation Aerosol did not include sufficient numbers of subjects aged 65 and over to determine whether they respond differently from younger subjects. Other reported clinical experience has not identified differences in responses between the elderly and younger patients. In general, dose selection for an elderly patient should be cautious, starting at the low end of the dosing range, reflecting the greater frequency of decreased hepatic, renal, or cardiac function, and of concomitant disease or other drug therapy.

GlaxoSmithKline, Research Triangle Park, NC 27709
August 2001/RL-963

WELLBUTRIN® ℞
[wel 'byü-trin]
(bupropion hydrochloride)
Tablets

Prescribing information for this product, which appears on pages 1680–1684 of the 2002 PDR, has been revised as follows. Please write "See Supplement A" next to the product heading.

The fourth paragraph of the **WARNINGS: Seizures** *subsection was revised to:*

The risk of seizure appears to be strongly associated with dose. Sudden and large increments in dose may contribute to increased risk. While many seizures occurred early in the course of treatment, some seizures did occur after several weeks at fixed dose. WELLBUTRIN should be discontinued and not restarted in patients who experience a seizure while on treatment.

The following paragraph was added to the **PRECAUTIONS: Information for Patients** *subsection:*

Patients should be told that WELLBUTRIN should be discontinued and not restarted if they experience a seizure while on treatment.

Manufactured by Catalytica Pharmaceuticals, Inc.
Greenville, NC 27834
for GlaxoSmithKline, Research Triangle Park, NC 27709

August 2001/RL-932

WELLBUTRIN SR® ℞
[wel' byü-trin]
(bupropion hydrochloride)
Sustained-Release Tablets

Prescribing information for this product, which appears on pages 1684–1688 of the 2002 PDR, has been revised as follows. Please write "See Supplement A" next to the product heading.

The first paragraph of the **WARNINGS: Seizures** *subsection was revised to:*

Bupropion is associated with a dose-related risk of seizures. The risk of seizures is also related to patient factors, clinical situations, and concomitant medications, which must be considered in selection of patients for therapy with WELLBUTRIN SR. WELLBUTRIN SR should be discontinued and not restarted in patients who experience a seizure while on treatment.

The following paragraph was added to the **PRECAUTIONS: Information for Patients** *subsection:*

Patients should be told that WELLBUTRIN SR should be discontinued and not restarted if they experience a seizure while on treatment.

Distributed by GlaxoSmithKline
Research Triangle Park, NC 27709
Manufactured by GlaxoSmithKline
Research Triangle Park, NC 27709
or Catalytica Pharmaceuticals, Inc.
Greenville, NC 27834

August 2001/RL-933

ZANTAC® ℞
[zan 'tak]
(ranitidine hydrochloride)
Injection

ZANTAC® ℞
(ranitidine hydrochloride)
Injection Premixed

Prescribing information for these products, which appears on pages 1688–1690 of the 2002 PDR, has been revised as follows. Please write "See Supplement A" next to the product heading.

The **ADVERSE REACTIONS: Integumentary** *subsection was revised to:*

Rash, including rare cases of erythema multiforme. Rare cases of alopecia and vasculitis.

ZANTAC® Injection:
GlaxoSmithKline, Research Triangle Park, NC 27709
ZANTAC® Injection Premixed:
Manufactured for GlaxoSmithKline
Research Triangle Park, NC 27709
by Abbott Laboratories, North Chicago, IL 60064
ZANTAC is a registered trademark of Warner-Lambert Company, used under license.

January 2002/RL-1049

ZANTAC® 150 ℞
[zan 'tak]
(ranitidine hydrochloride)
Tablets, USP

ZANTAC® 300 ℞
(ranitidine hydrochloride)
Tablets, USP

ZANTAC® 150 ℞
(ranitidine hydrochloride effervescent)
EFFERdose® Tablets

ZANTAC® 150 ℞
(ranitidine hydrochloride effervescent)
EFFERdose® Granules

ZANTAC® ℞
(ranitidine hydrochloride)
Syrup, USP

Prescribing information for these products, which appears on pages 1690–1692 of the 2002 PDR, has been revised as follows. Please write "See Supplement A" next to the product heading.

The following subsection was added to **CLINICAL PHARMACOLOGY: Pharmacokinetics*:*** ***Geriatrics:*** The plasma half-life is prolonged and total clearance is reduced in the elderly population due to a decrease in renal function. The elimination half-life is 3 to 4 hours. Peak levels average 526 ng/mL following a 150-mg twice daily dose and occur in about 3 hours (see PRECAUTIONS: Geriatric Use and DOSAGE AND ADMINISTRATION: Dosage Adjustment for Patients with Impaired Renal Function).

The **PRECAUTIONS: Use in Elderly Patients** *subsection was revised to:*

Geriatric Use: Of the total number of subjects enrolled in US and foreign controlled clinical trials of oral formulations of ZANTAC, for which there were subgroup analyses, 4197 were 65 and over, while 899 were 75 and over. No overall differences in safety or effectiveness were observed between these subjects and younger subjects, and other reported clinical experience has not identified differences in responses between the elderly and younger patients, but greater sensitivity of some older individuals cannot be ruled out.

This drug is known to be substantially excreted by the kidney and the risk of toxic reactions to this drug may be greater in patients with impaired renal function. Because elderly patients are more likely to have decreased renal function, caution should be exercised in dose selection, and it may be useful to monitor renal function (see CLINICAL PHARMACOLOGY: Pharmacokinetics: Geriatric Use and DOSAGE AND ADMINISTRATION: Dosage Adjustment for Patients with Impaired Renal Function).

The **ADVERSE REACTIONS: Integumentary** *subsection was revised to:*

Rash, including rare cases of erythema multiforme. Rare cases of alopecia and vasculitis.

The following was added as the second paragraph of the **DOSAGE AND ADMINISTRATION: Dosage Adjustment for Patients With Impaired Renal Function** *subsection:*

Elderly patients are more likely to have decreased renal function, therefore caution should be exercised in dose selection, and it may be useful to monitor renal function (see CLINICAL PHARMACOLOGY: Pharmacokinetics: Geriatric Use and PRECAUTIONS: Geriatric Use).

In **HOW SUPPLIED,** *the description of ZANTAC Syrup was revised to:*

ZANTAC Syrup, a clear, peppermint-flavored liquid, contains 16.8 mg of ranitidine HCl equivalent to 15 mg of ranitidine per 1 mL (75 mg/5mL) in bottles of 16 fluid ounces (one pint) (NDC 0173-0383-54).

ZANTAC® 150 Tablets/ZANTAC® 300 Tablets/ZANTAC® 150 EFFERdose® Tablets/ZANTAC® 150 EFFERdose® Granules:
GlaxoSmithKline, Research Triangle Park, NC 27709
ZANTAC® Syrup: Manufactured for GlaxoSmithKline
Research Triangle Park, NC 27709
by Roxane Laboratories, Inc., Columbus, OH 43216
ZANTAC and EFFERdose are registered trademarks of Warner-Lambert Company, used under license.

January 2002/RL-1048

ZIAGEN® ℞
[zi' ə-jin]
(abacavir sulfate)
Tablets

ZIAGEN® ℞
(abacavir sulfate)
Oral Solution

Prescribing information for these products, which appears on pages 1692–1696 of the 2002 PDR, has been revised as follows. Please write "See Supplement A" next to the product heading.

The following subsection was added to **ADVERSE REACTIONS:**

Observed During Clinical Practice: In addition to adverse events reported from clinical trials, the following events have been identified during use of abacavir in clinical practice. Because they are reported voluntarily from a population of unknown size, estimates of frequency cannot be made. These events have been chosen for inclusion due to either their seriousness, frequency of reporting, potential causal connection to abacavir, or a combination of these factors.

Suspected Stevens-Johnson syndrome (SJS) has been reported in patients receiving abacavir in combination with medications known to be associated with SJS. Because of

the overlap of clinical signs and symptoms between hypersensitivity to abacavir and SJS, and the possibility of multiple drug sensitivities in some patients, abacavir should be discontinued and not restarted in such cases.
GlaxoSmithKline, Research Triangle Park, NC 27709

December 2001/RL-1053

ZINACEF® ℞
[*zin 'a-sef*]
(cefuroxime for injection)

ZINACEF® ℞
(cefuroxime injection)

Prescribing information for these products, which appears on pages 1696–1698 of the 2002 PDR, has been revised as follows. Please write "See Supplement A" next to the product heading.
The subhead **General** *was added to the beginning of the* **PRECAUTIONS** *section, and the following was added as the last paragraph:*
Cephalosporins may be associated with a fall in prothrombin activity. Those at risk include patients with renal or hepatic impairment, or poor nutritional state, as well as patients receiving a protracted course of antimicrobial therapy, and patients previously stabilized on anticoagulant therapy.
Prothrombin time should be monitored in patients at risk and exogenous Vitamin K administered as indicated.
The **PRECAUTIONS: Carcinogenesis, Mutagenesis, Impairment of Fertility** *subsection was revised to:*
Although lifetime studies in animals have not been performed to evaluate carcinogenic potential, no mutagenic activity was found for cefuroxime in the mouse lymphoma assay and a battery of bacterial mutation tests. Positive results were obtained in an *in vitro* chromosome aberration assay, however, negative results were found in an *in vivo* micronucleus test at doses up to 10 g/kg. Reproduction studies in mice at doses up to 3200 mg/kg per day (3.1 times the recommended maximum human dose based on mg/m^2) have revealed no impairment of fertility.
Reproductive studies revealed no impairment of fertility in animals.
The **PRECAUTIONS: Pregnancy: Teratogenic Effects** *subsection was revised to:*
Pregnancy Category B. Reproduction studies have been performed in mice at doses up to 6400 mg/kg per day (6.3 times the recommended maximum human dose based on mg/m^2) and rabbits at doses up to 400 mg/kg per day (2.1 times the recommended maximum human dose based on mg/m^2) and have revealed no evidence of impaired fertility or harm to the fetus due to cefuroxime. There are, however, no adequate and well-controlled studies in pregnant women. Because animal reproduction studies are not always predictive of human response, this drug should be used during pregnancy only if clearly needed.
The following subsection was added to **ADVERSE REACTIONS:**
Postmarketing Experience with ZINACEF Products: In addition to the adverse events reported during clinical trials, the following events have been observed during clinical practice in patients treated with ZINACEF and were reported spontaneously. Data are generally insufficient to allow an estimate of incidence or to establish causation.
The following sentence was revised in the **ADVERSE REACTIONS: Cephalosporin-class Adverse Reactions** *subsection:*
Several cephalosporins, including ZINACEF, have been implicated in triggering seizures, particularly in patients with renal impairment when the dosage was not reduced (see DOSAGE AND ADMINISTRATION).
ZINACEF® (cefuroxime for injection):
GlaxoSmithKline, Research Triangle Park, NC 27709
ZINACEF® (cefuroxime injection):
Manufactured for GlaxoSmithKline, Research Triangle Park, NC 27709
by Baxter Healthcare Corporation, Deerfield, IL 60015
July 2001/RL-964

ZOFRAN® ℞
[*zō' fran*]
(ondansetron hydrochloride)
Tablets

ZOFRAN ODT® ℞
(ondansetron)
Orally Disintegrating Tablets

ZOFRAN® ℞
(ondansetron hydrochloride)
Oral Solution

Prescribing information for these products, which appears on pages 1703–1706 of the 2002 PDR, has been completely revised as follows. Please write "See Supplement A" next to the product heading.

DESCRIPTION
The active ingredient in ZOFRAN Tablets and ZOFRAN Oral Solution is ondansetron hydrochloride (HCl) as the dihydrate, the racemic form of ondansetron and a selective blocking agent of the serotonin 5-HT$_3$ receptor type. Chemically it is (±) 1, 2, 3, 9-tetrahydro-9-methyl-3-[(2-methyl-1H-imidazol-1-yl)methyl]-4H-carbazol-4-one, monohydrochloride, dihydrate.
The empirical formula is $C_{18}H_{19}N_3O \bullet HCl \bullet 2H_2O$, representing a molecular weight of 365.9. Ondansetron HCl dihydrate is a white to off-white powder that is soluble in water and normal saline.
The active ingredient in ZOFRAN ODT Orally Disintegrating Tablets is ondansetron base, the racemic form of ondansetron, and a selective blocking agent of the serotonin 5-HT$_3$ receptor type. Chemically it is (±) 1, 2, 3, 9-tetrahydro-9-methyl-3-[(2-methyl-1H-imidazol-1-yl) methyl]-4H-carbazol-4-one.
The empirical formula is $C_{18}H_{19}N_3O$ representing a molecular weight of 293.4.
Each 4-mg ZOFRAN Tablet for oral administration contains ondansetron HCl dihydrate equivalent to 4 mg of ondansetron. Each 8-mg ZOFRAN Tablet for oral administration contains ondansetron HCl dihydrate equivalent to 8 mg of ondansetron. Each 24-mg ZOFRAN Tablet for oral administration contains ondansetron HCl dihydrate equivalent to 24 mg of ondansetron. Each tablet also contains the inactive ingredients lactose, microcrystalline cellulose, pregelatinized starch, hydroxypropyl methylcellulose, magnesium stearate, titanium dioxide, triacetin, iron oxide yellow (8-mg tablet only), and iron oxide red (24-mg tablet only).
Each 4-mg ZOFRAN ODT Orally Disintegrating Tablet for oral administration contains 4 mg ondansetron base. Each 8-mg ZOFRAN ODT Orally Disintegrating Tablet for oral administration contains 8 mg ondansetron base. Each ZOFRAN ODT Tablet also contains the inactive ingredients aspartame, gelatin, mannitol, methylparaben sodium, propylparaben sodium, and strawberry flavor. ZOFRAN ODT Tablets are a freeze-dried, orally administered formulation of ondansetron which rapidly disintegrates on the tongue and does not require water to aid dissolution or swallowing.
Each 5 mL of ZOFRAN Oral Solution contains 5 mg of ondansetron HCl dihydrate equivalent to 4 mg of ondansetron. ZOFRAN Oral Solution contains the inactive ingredients citric acid anhydrous, purified water, sodium benzoate, sodium citrate, sorbitol, and strawberry flavor.

CLINICAL PHARMACOLOGY
Pharmacodynamics: Ondansetron is a selective 5-HT$_3$ receptor antagonist. While its mechanism of action has not been fully characterized, ondansetron is not a dopamine-receptor antagonist. Serotonin receptors of the 5-HT$_3$ type are present both peripherally on vagal nerve terminals and centrally in the chemoreceptor trigger zone of the area postrema. It is not certain whether ondansetron's antiemetic action is mediated centrally, peripherally, or in both sites. However, cytotoxic chemotherapy appears to be associated with release of serotonin from the enterochromaffin cells of the small intestine. In humans, urinary 5-HIAA (5-hydroxyindoleacetic acid) excretion increases after cisplatin administration in parallel with the onset of emesis. The released serotonin may stimulate the vagal afferents through the 5-HT$_3$ receptors and initiate the vomiting reflex.
In animals, the emetic response to cisplatin can be prevented by pretreatment with an inhibitor of serotonin synthesis, bilateral abdominal vagotomy and greater splanchnic nerve section, or pretreatment with a serotonin 5-HT$_3$ receptor antagonist.
In normal volunteers, single intravenous doses of 0.15 mg/kg of ondansetron had no effect on esophageal motility, gastric motility, lower esophageal sphincter pressure, or small intestinal transit time. Multiday administration of ondansetron has been shown to slow colonic transit in normal volunteers. Ondansetron has no effect on plasma prolactin concentrations.
Ondansetron does not alter the respiratory depressant effects produced by alfentanil or the degree of neuromuscular blockade produced by atracurium. Interactions with general or local anesthetics have not been studied.
Pharmacokinetics: Ondansetron is extensively metabolized in humans, with approximately 5% of a radiolabeled dose recovered from the urine as the parent compound. The primary metabolic pathway is hydroxylation on the indole ring followed by subsequent glucuronide or sulfate conjugation. Although some nonconjugated metabolites have pharmacologic activity, these are not found in plasma at concentrations likely to significantly contribute to the biological activity of ondansetron.
In vitro metabolism studies have shown that ondansetron is a substrate for human hepatic cytochrome P-450 enzymes, including CYP1A2, CYP2D6, and CYP3A4. In terms of overall ondansetron turnover, CYP3A4 played the predominant role. Because of the multiplicity of metabolic enzymes capable of metabolizing ondansetron, it is likely that inhibition or loss of one enzyme (e.g., CYP2D6 genetic deficiency) will be compensated by others and may result in little change in overall rates of ondansetron elimination. Ondansetron elimination may be affected by cytochrome P-450 inducers. In a pharmacokinetic study of 16 epileptic patients maintained chronically on carbamazepine or phenytoin, reduction in AUC, C_{max} and $T_{½}$ of ondansetron was observed. This resulted in a significant increase in clearance. However, on the basis of available data, no dosage adjustment is recommended (see PRECAUTIONS: Drug Interactions).
Ondansetron is well absorbed from the gastrointestinal tract and undergoes some first-pass metabolism. Mean bioavailability in healthy subjects, following administration of a single 8-mg tablet, is approximately 56%.
Ondansetron systemic exposure does not increase proportionately to dose. AUC from a 16-mg tablet was 24% greater than predicted from an 8-mg tablet dose. This may reflect some reduction of first-pass metabolism at higher oral doses. Bioavailability is also slightly enhanced by the presence of food but unaffected by antacids.
Gender differences were shown in the disposition of ondansetron given as a single dose. The extent and rate of ondansetron's absorption is greater in women than men. Slower clearance in women, a smaller apparent volume of distribution (adjusted for weight), and higher absolute bioavailability resulted in higher plasma ondansetron levels. These higher plasma levels may in part be explained by differences in body weight between men and women. It is not known whether these gender-related differences were clinically important. More detailed pharmacokinetic information is contained in Tables 1 and 2 taken from two studies.
[See table 1 above]

Table 1: Pharmacokinetics in Normal Volunteers: Single 8-mg ZOFRAN Tablet Dose

Age-group (years)	Mean Weight (kg)	n	Peak Plasma Concentration (ng/mL)	Time of Peak Plasma Concentration (h)	Mean Elimination Half-life (h)	Systemic Plasma Clearance L/h/kg	Absolute Bioavailability
18–40 M	69.0	6	26.2	2.0	3.1	0.403	0.483
F	62.7	5	42.7	1.7	3.5	0.354	0.663
61–74 M	77.5	6	24.1	2.1	4.1	0.384	0.585
F	60.2	6	52.4	1.9	4.9	0.255	0.643
≥75 M	78.0	5	37.0	2.2	4.5	0.277	0.619
F	67.6	6	46.1	2.1	6.2	0.249	0.747

[See table 2 above]

Table 2: Pharmacokinetics in Normal Volunteers: Single 24-mg ZOFRAN Tablet Dose

Age-group (years)	Mean Weight (kg)	n	Peak Plasma Concentration (ng/mL)	Time of Peak Plasma Concentration (h)	Mean Elimination Half-life (h)
18–43 M	84.1	8	125.8	1.9	4.7
F	71.8	8	194.4	1.6	5.8

A reduction in clearance and increase in elimination half-life are seen in patients over 75 years of age. In clinical trials with cancer patients, safety and efficacy was similar in patients over 65 years of age and those under 65 years of age; there was an insufficient number of patients over 75 years of age to permit conclusions in that age-group. No dosage adjustment is recommended in the elderly.
In patients with mild-to-moderate hepatic impairment, clearance is reduced twofold and mean half-life is increased to 11.6 hours compared to 5.7 hours in normals. In patients with severe hepatic impairment (Child-Pugh[1] score of 10 or greater), clearance is reduced twofold to threefold and apparent volume of distribution is increased with a resultant increase in half-life to 20 hours. In patients with severe hepatic impairment, a total daily dose of 8 mg should not be exceeded.
Due to the very small contribution (5%) of renal clearance to the overall clearance, renal impairment was not expected to significantly influence the total clearance of ondansetron. However, ondansetron oral mean plasma clearance was reduced by about 50% in patients with severe renal impairment (creatinine clearance <30 mL/min). This reduction in clearance is variable and was not consistent with an increase in half-life. No reduction in dose or dosing frequency in these patients is warranted.
Plasma protein binding of ondansetron as measured in vitro was 70% to 76% over the concentration range of 10 to 500 ng/mL. Circulating drug also distributes into erythrocytes.
Four- and 8-mg doses of either ZOFRAN Oral Solution or ZOFRAN ODT Orally Disintegrating Tablets are bioequivalent to corresponding doses of ZOFRAN Tablets and may be used interchangeably. One 24-mg ZOFRAN Tablet is bioequivalent to and interchangeable with three 8-mg ZOFRAN Tablets.

Continued on next page

Zofran—Cont.

CLINICAL TRIALS

Chemotherapy-Induced Nausea and Vomiting: ***Highly Emetogenic Chemotherapy:*** In two randomized, double-blind, monotherapy trials, a single 24-mg ZOFRAN Tablet was superior to a relevant historical placebo control in the prevention of nausea and vomiting associated with highly emetogenic cancer chemotherapy, including cisplatin ≥50 mg/m^2. Steroid administration was excluded from these clinical trials. More than 90% of patients receiving a cisplatin dose ≥50 mg/m^2 in the historical placebo comparator experienced vomiting in the absence of antiemetic therapy.

The first trial compared oral doses of ondansetron 24 mg once a day, 8 mg twice a day, and 32 mg once a day in 357 adult cancer patients receiving chemotherapy regimens containing cisplatin ≥50 mg/m^2. A total of 66% of patients in the ondansetron 24 mg once a day group, 55% in the ondansetron 8 mg twice a day group, and 55% in the ondansetron 32 mg once a day group completed the 24-hour study period with zero emetic episodes and no rescue antiemetic medications, the primary endpoint of efficacy. Each of the three treatment groups was shown to be statistically significantly superior to a historical placebo control.

In the same trial, 56% of patients receiving oral ondansetron 24 mg once a day experienced no nausea during the 24-hour study period, compared with 36% of patients in the oral ondansetron 8 mg twice a day group (p = 0.001) and 50% in the oral ondansetron 32 mg once a day group.

In a second trial, efficacy of the oral ondansetron 24 mg once a day regimen in the prevention of nausea and vomiting associated with highly emetogenic cancer chemotherapy, including cisplatin ≥50 mg/m^2, was confirmed.

Moderately Emetogenic Chemotherapy: In one double-blind US study in 67 patients, ZOFRAN Tablets 8 mg administered twice a day were significantly more effective than placebo in preventing vomiting induced by cyclophosphamide-based chemotherapy containing doxorubicin. Treatment response is based on the total number of emetic episodes over the 3-day study period. The results of this study are summarized in Table 3:

[See table 3 above]

Table 3: Emetic Episodes: Treatment Response

	Ondansetron 8-mg b.i.d. ZOFRAN Tablets*	Placebo	*P* Value
Number of patients	33	34	
Treatment response			
0 Emetic episodes	20 (61%)	2 (6%)	<0.001
1–2 Emetic episodes	6 (18%)	8 (24%)	
More than 2 emetic episodes/withdrawn	7 (21%)	24 (71%)	<0.001
Median number of emetic episodes	0.0	Undefined†	
Median time to first emetic episode (h)	Undefined‡	6.5	

*The first dose was administered 30 minutes before the start of emetogenic chemotherapy, with a subsequent dose 8 hours after the first dose. An 8-mg ZOFRAN Tablet was administered twice a day for 2 days after completion of chemotherapy.

† Median undefined since at least 50% of the patients were withdrawn or had more than two emetic episodes.

‡ Median undefined since at least 50% of patients did not have any emetic episodes.

In one double-blind US study in 336 patients, ZOFRAN Tablets 8 mg administered twice a day were as effective as ZOFRAN Tablets 8 mg administered three times a day in preventing nausea and vomiting induced by cyclophosphamide-based chemotherapy containing either methotrexate or doxorubicin. Treatment response is based on the total number of emetic episodes over the 3-day study period. The results of this study are summarized in Table 4:

[See table 4 above]

Table 4: Emetic Episodes: Treatment Response

	Ondansetron	
	8-mg b.i.d. ZOFRAN Tablets*	8-mg t.i.d. ZOFRAN Tablets†
Number of patients	165	171
Treatment response		
0 Emetic episodes	101 (61%)	99 (58%)
1–2 Emetic episodes	16 (10%)	17 (10%)
More than 2 emetic episodes/withdrawn	48 (29%)	55 (32%)
Median number of emetic episodes	0.0	0.0
Median time to first emetic episode (h)	Undefined‡	Undefined‡
Median nausea scores (0–100)§	6	6

*The first dose was administered 30 minutes before the start of emetogenic chemotherapy, with a subsequent dose 8 hours after the first dose. An 8-mg ZOFRAN Tablet was administered twice a day for 2 days after completion of chemotherapy.

† The first dose was administered 30 minutes before the start of emetogenic chemotherapy, with subsequent doses 4 and 8 hours after the first dose. An 8-mg ZOFRAN Tablet was administered three times a day for 2 days after completion of chemotherapy.

‡ Median undefined since at least 50% of patients did not have any emetic episodes.

§ Visual analog scale assessment: 0 = no nausea, 100 = nausea as bad as it can be.

Re-treatment: In uncontrolled trials, 148 patients receiving cyclophosphamide-based chemotherapy were re-treated with ZOFRAN Tablets 8 mg t.i.d. of oral ondansetron during subsequent chemotherapy for a total of 396 re-treatment courses. No emetic episodes occurred in 314 (79%) of the re-treatment courses, and only one to two emetic episodes occurred in 43 (11%) of the re-treatment courses.

Pediatric Studies: Three open-label, uncontrolled, foreign trials have been performed with 182 pediatric patients 4 to 18 years old with cancer who were given a variety of cisplatin or noncisplatin regimens. In these foreign trials, the initial dose of ZOFRAN® (ondansetron HCl) Injection ranged from 0.04 to 0.87 mg/kg for a total dose of 2.16 to 12 mg. This was followed by the administration of ZOFRAN Tablets ranging from 4 to 24 mg daily for 3 days. In these studies, 58% of the 170 evaluable patients had a complete response (no emetic episodes) on day 1. Two studies showed the response rates for patients less than 12 years of age who received ZOFRAN Tablets 4 mg three times a day to be similar to those in patients 12 to 18 years of age who received ZOFRAN Tablets 8 mg three times daily. Thus, prevention of emesis in these pediatric patients was essentially the same as for patients older than 18 years of age. Overall, ZOFRAN Tablets were well tolerated in these pediatric patients.

Radiation-Induced Nausea and Vomiting: ***Total Body Irradiation:*** In a randomized, double-blind study in 20 patients, ZOFRAN Tablets (8 mg given 1.5 hours before each fraction of radiotherapy for 4 days) were significantly more effective than placebo in preventing vomiting induced by total body irradiation. Total body irradiation consisted of 11 fractions (120 cGy per fraction) over 4 days for a total of 1320 cGy. Patients received three fractions for 3 days, then two fractions on day 4.

Single High-Dose Fraction Radiotherapy: Ondansetron was significantly more effective than metoclopramide with respect to complete control of emesis (0 emetic episodes) in a double-blind trial in 105 patients receiving single high-dose radiotherapy (800 to 1000 cGy) over an anterior or posterior field size of ≥80 cm^2 to the abdomen. Patients received the first dose of ZOFRAN Tablets (8 mg) or metoclopramide (10 mg) 1 to 2 hours before radiotherapy. If radiotherapy was given in the morning, two additional doses of study treatment were given (one tablet late afternoon and one tablet before bedtime). If radiotherapy was given in the afternoon, patients took only one further tablet that day before bedtime. Patients continued the oral medication on a t.i.d. basis for 3 days.

Daily Fractionated Radiotherapy: Ondansetron was significantly more effective than prochlorperazine with respect to complete control of emesis (0 emetic episodes) in a double-blind trial in 135 patients receiving a 1- to 4-week course of fractionated radiotherapy (180 cGy doses) over a field size of ≥100 cm^2 to the abdomen. Patients received the first dose of ZOFRAN Tablets (8 mg) or prochlorperazine (10 mg) 1 to 2 hours before the patient received the first daily radiotherapy fraction, with two subsequent doses on a t.i.d. basis. Patients continued the oral medication on a t.i.d. basis on each day of radiotherapy.

Postoperative Nausea and Vomiting: Surgical patients who received ondansetron 1 hour before the induction of general balanced anesthesia (barbiturate: thiopental, methohexital, or thiamylal; opioid: alfentanil, sufentanil, morphine, or fentanyl; nitrous oxide; neuromuscular blockade: succinylcholine/curare or gallamine and/or vecuronium, pancuronium, or atracurium; and supplemental isoflurane or enflurane) were evaluated in two double-blind studies (one US study, one foreign) involving 865 patients. ZOFRAN Tablets (16 mg) were significantly more effective than placebo in preventing postoperative nausea and vomiting.

The study populations in all trials thus far consisted of women undergoing inpatient surgical procedures. No studies have been performed in males. No controlled clinical study comparing ZOFRAN Tablets to ZOFRAN Injection has been performed.

INDICATIONS AND USAGE

1. Prevention of nausea and vomiting associated with highly emetogenic cancer chemotherapy, including cisplatin ≥50 mg/m^2.
2. Prevention of nausea and vomiting associated with initial and repeat courses of moderately emetogenic cancer chemotherapy.
3. Prevention of nausea and vomiting associated with radiotherapy in patients receiving either total body irradiation, single high-dose fraction to the abdomen, or daily fractions to the abdomen.
4. Prevention of postoperative nausea and/or vomiting. As with other antiemetics, routine prophylaxis is not recommended for patients in whom there is little expectation that nausea and/or vomiting will occur postoperatively. In patients where nausea and/or vomiting must be avoided postoperatively, ZOFRAN Tablets, ZOFRAN ODT Orally Disintegrating Tablets, and ZOFRAN Oral Solution are recommended even where the incidence of postoperative nausea and/or vomiting is low.

CONTRAINDICATIONS

ZOFRAN Tablets, ZOFRAN ODT Orally Disintegrating Tablets, and ZOFRAN Oral Solution are contraindicated for patients known to have hypersensitivity to the drug.

WARNINGS

Hypersensitivity reactions have been reported in patients who have exhibited hypersensitivity to other selective 5-HT_3 receptor antagonists.

PRECAUTIONS

Ondansetron is not a drug that stimulates gastric or intestinal peristalsis. It should not be used instead of nasogastric suction. The use of ondansetron in patients following abdominal surgery or in patients with chemotherapy-induced nausea and vomiting may mask a progressive ileus and/or gastric distension.

Information for Patients: ***Phenylketonurics:*** Phenylketonuric patients should be informed that ZOFRAN ODT Orally Disintegrating Tablets contain phenylalanine (a component of aspartame). Each 4-mg and 8-mg orally disintegrating tablet contains <0.03 mg phenylalanine.

Patients should be instructed not to remove ZOFRAN ODT Tablets from the blister until just prior to dosing. The tablet should not be pushed through the foil. With dry hands, the blister backing should be peeled completely off the blister. The tablet should be gently removed and immediately placed on the tongue to dissolve and be swallowed with the saliva. Peelable illustrated stickers are affixed to the product carton that can be provided with the prescription to ensure proper use and handling of the product.

Drug Interactions: Ondansetron does not itself appear to induce or inhibit the cytochrome P-450 drug-metabolizing enzyme system of the liver. Because ondansetron is metabolized by hepatic cytochrome P-450 drug-metabolizing enzymes, inducers or inhibitors of these enzymes may change the clearance and, hence, the half-life of ondansetron. On the basis of available data, no dosage adjustment is recommended for patients on these drugs. Tumor response to chemotherapy in the P 388 mouse leukemia model is not affected by ondansetron. In humans, carmustine, etoposide, and cisplatin do not affect the pharmacokinetics of ondansetron.

In a crossover study in 76 pediatric patients, I.V. ondansetron did not increase blood levels of high-dose methotrexate.

Use in Surgical Patients: The coadministration of ondansetron had no effect on the pharmacokinetics and pharmacodynamics of temazepam.

Carcinogenesis, Mutagenesis, Impairment of Fertility: Carcinogenic effects were not seen in 2-year studies in rats and mice with oral ondansetron doses up to 10 and 30 mg/kg per day, respectively. Ondansetron was not mutagenic in standard tests for mutagenicity. Oral administration of ondansetron up to 15 mg/kg per day did not affect fertility or general reproductive performance of male and female rats.

Pregnancy: ***Teratogenic Effects:*** Pregnancy Category B. Reproduction studies have been performed in pregnant rats and rabbits at daily oral doses up to 15 and 30 mg/kg per day, respectively, and have revealed no evidence of impaired fertility or harm to the fetus due to ondansetron. There are, however, no adequate and well-controlled studies in pregnant women. Because animal reproduction studies are not always predictive of human response, this drug should be used during pregnancy only if clearly needed.

Nursing Mothers: Ondansetron is excreted in the breast milk of rats. It is not known whether ondansetron is excreted in human milk. Because many drugs are excreted in human milk, caution should be exercised when ondansetron is administered to a nursing woman.

Pediatric Use: Little information is available about dosage in pediatric patients 4 years of age or younger (see CLINICAL PHARMACOLOGY and DOSAGE AND ADMINISTRATION sections for use in pediatric patients 4 to 18 years of age).

Geriatric Use: Of the total number of subjects enrolled in cancer chemotherapy-induced and postoperative nausea and vomiting in US- and foreign-controlled clinical trials, for which there were subgroup analyses, 938 were 65 years of age and over. No overall differences in safety or effectiveness were observed between these subjects and younger subjects, and other reported clinical experience has not identified differences in responses between the elderly and younger patients, but greater sensitivity of some older individuals cannot be ruled out. Dosage adjustment is not needed in patients over the age of 65 (see CLINICAL PHARMACOLOGY).

ADVERSE REACTIONS

The following have been reported as adverse events in clinical trials of patients treated with ondansetron, the active ingredient of ZOFRAN. A causal relationship to therapy with ZOFRAN has been unclear in many cases.

Chemotherapy-Induced Nausea and Vomiting: The adverse events in Table 5 have been reported in ≥5% of adult patients receiving a single 24-mg ZOFRAN Tablet in two trials. These patients were receiving concurrent highly emetogenic cisplatin-based chemotherapy regimens (cisplatin dose ≥50 mg/m^2).

[See table 5 above]

The adverse events in Table 6 have been reported in ≥5% of adults receiving either 8 mg of ZOFRAN Tablets two or three times a day for 3 days or placebo in four trials. These patients were receiving concurrent moderately emetogenic chemotherapy, primarily cyclophosphamide-based regimens.

[See table 6 above]

Central Nervous System: There have been rare reports consistent with, but not diagnostic of, extrapyramidal reactions in patients receiving ondansetron.

Hepatic: In 723 patients receiving cyclophosphamide-based chemotherapy in US clinical trials, AST and/or ALT values have been reported to exceed twice the upper limit of normal in approximately 1% to 2% of patients receiving ZOFRAN Tablets. The increases were transient and did not appear to be related to dose or duration of therapy. On repeat exposure, similar transient elevations in transaminase values occurred in some courses, but symptomatic hepatic disease did not occur. The role of cancer chemotherapy in these biochemical changes cannot be clearly determined.

There have been reports of liver failure and death in patients with cancer receiving concurrent medications including potentially hepatotoxic cytotoxic chemotherapy and antibiotics. The etiology of the liver failure is unclear.

Integumentary: Rash has occurred in approximately 1% of patients receiving ondansetron.

Other: Rare cases of anaphylaxis, bronchospasm, tachycardia, angina (chest pain), hypokalemia, electrocardiographic alterations, vascular occlusive events, and grand mal seizures have been reported. Except for bronchospasm and anaphylaxis, the relationship to ZOFRAN was unclear.

Radiation-Induced Nausea and Vomiting: The adverse events reported in patients receiving ZOFRAN Tablets and concurrent radiotherapy were similar to those reported in patients receiving ZOFRAN Tablets and concurrent chemotherapy. The most frequently reported adverse events were headache, constipation, and diarrhea.

Postoperative Nausea and Vomiting: The adverse events in Table 7 have been reported in ≥5% of patients receiving ZOFRAN Tablets at a dosage of 16 mg orally in clinical trials. With the exception of headache, rates of these events were not significantly different in the ondansetron and placebo groups. These patients were receiving multiple concomitant perioperative and postoperative medications.

[See table above]

Preliminary observations in a small number of subjects suggest a higher incidence of headache when ZOFRAN ODT Orally Disintegrating Tablets are taken with water, when compared to without water.

Observed During Clinical Practice: In addition to adverse events reported from clinical trials, the following events have been identified during post-approval use of oral formulations of ZOFRAN. Because they are reported voluntarily from a population of unknown size, estimates of frequency cannot be made. The events have been chosen for inclusion due to a combination of their seriousness, frequency of reporting, or potential causal connection to ZOFRAN.

General: Flushing. Rare cases of hypersensitivity reactions, sometimes severe (e.g., anaphylaxis/anaphylactoid reactions, angioedema, bronchospasm, shortness of breath, hypotension, laryngeal edema, stridor) have also been reported. Laryngospasm, shock, and cardiopulmonary arrest have occurred during allergic reactions in patients receiving injectable ondansetron.

Hepatobiliary: Liver enzyme abnormalities

Lower Respiratory: Hiccups

Neurology: Oculogyric crisis, appearing alone, as well as with other dystonic reactions

Skin: Urticaria

DRUG ABUSE AND DEPENDENCE

Animal studies have shown that ondansetron is not discriminated as a benzodiazepine nor does it substitute for benzodiazepines in direct addiction studies.

Table 5: Principal Adverse Events in US Trials: Single Day Therapy With 24-mg ZOFRAN Tablets (Highly Emetogenic Chemotherapy)

Event	Ondansetron 24 mg q.d. n = 300	Ondansetron 8 mg b.i.d. n = 124	Ondansetron 32 mg q.d. n = 117
Headache	33 (11%)	16 (13%)	17 (15%)
Diarrhea	13 (4%)	9 (7%)	3 (3%)

Table 6: Principal Adverse Events in US Trials: 3 Days of Therapy With 8 mg ZOFRAN Tablets (Moderately Emetogenic Chemotherapy)

Event	Ondansetron 8 mg b.i.d. n = 242	Ondansetron 8 mg t.i.d. n = 415	Placebo n = 262
Headache	58 (24%)	113 (27%)	34 (13%)
Malaise/fatigue	32 (13%)	37 (9%)	6 (2%)
Constipation	22 (9%)	26 (6%)	1 (<1%)
Diarrhea	15 (6%)	16 (4%)	10 (4%)
Dizziness	13 (5%)	18 (4%)	12 (5%)

Table 7: Frequency of Adverse Events From Controlled Studies With ZOFRAN Tablets (Postoperative Nausea and Vomiting)

Adverse Event	Ondansetron 16 mg (n = 550)	Placebo (n = 531)
Wound problem	152 (28%)	162 (31%)
Drowsiness/sedation	112 (20%)	122 (23%)
Headache	49 (9%)	27 (5%)
Hypoxia	49 (9%)	35 (7%)
Pyrexia	45 (8%)	34 (6%)
Dizziness	36 (7%)	34 (6%)
Gynecological disorder	36 (7%)	33 (6%)
Anxiety/agitation	33 (6%)	29 (5%)
Bradycardia	32 (6%)	30 (6%)
Shiver(s)	28 (5%)	30 (6%)
Urinary retention	28 (5%)	18 (3%)
Hypotension	27 (5%)	32 (6%)
Pruritus	27 (5%)	20 (4%)

OVERDOSAGE

There is no specific antidote for ondansetron overdose. Patients should be managed with appropriate supportive therapy. Individual intravenous doses as large as 150 mg and total daily intravenous doses as large as 252 mg have been inadvertently administered without significant adverse events. These doses are more than 10 times the recommended daily dose.

In addition to the adverse events listed above, the following events have been described in the setting of ondansetron overdose: "Sudden blindness" (amaurosis) of 2 to 3 minutes' duration plus severe constipation occurred in one patient that was administered 72 mg of ondansetron intravenously as a single dose. Hypotension (and faintness) occurred in a patient that took 48 mg of ZOFRAN Tablets. Following infusion of 32 mg over only a 4-minute period, a vasovagal episode with transient second-degree heart block was observed. In all instances, the events resolved completely.

DOSAGE AND ADMINISTRATION

Instructions for Use/Handling ZOFRAN ODT Orally Disintegrating Tablets: Do not attempt to push ZOFRAN ODT Tablets through the foil backing. With dry hands, PEEL BACK the foil backing of one blister and GENTLY remove the tablet. IMMEDIATELY place the ZOFRAN ODT Tablet on top of the tongue where it will dissolve in seconds, then swallow with saliva. Administration with liquid is not necessary.

Prevention of Nausea and Vomiting Associated With Highly Emetogenic Cancer Chemotherapy: The recommended adult oral dosage of ZOFRAN is a single 24-mg tablet administered 30 minutes before the start of single-day highly emetogenic chemotherapy, including cisplatin ≥50 mg/m^2. Multiday, single-dose administration of ZOFRAN 24-mg Tablets has not been studied.

Pediatric Use: There is no experience with the use of 24-mg ZOFRAN Tablets in pediatric patients.

Geriatric Use: The dosage recommendation is the same as for the general population.

Prevention of Nausea and Vomiting Associated With Moderately Emetogenic Cancer Chemotherapy: The recommended adult oral dosage is one 8-mg ZOFRAN Tablet or one 8-mg ZOFRAN ODT Tablet or 10 mL (2 teaspoonfuls equivalent to 8 mg of ondansetron) of ZOFRAN Oral Solution given twice a day. The first dose should be administered 30 minutes before the start of emetogenic chemotherapy, with a subsequent dose 8 hours after the first dose. One 8-mg ZOFRAN Tablet or one 8-mg ZOFRAN ODT Tablet or 10 mL (2 teaspoonfuls equivalent to 8 mg of ondansetron) of ZOFRAN Oral Solution should be administered twice a day (every 12 hours) for 1 to 2 days after completion of chemotherapy.

Pediatric Use: For pediatric patients 12 years of age and older, the dosage is the same as for adults. For pediatric patients 4 through 11 years of age, the dosage is one 4-mg ZOFRAN Tablet or one 4-mg ZOFRAN ODT Tablet or 5 mL (1 teaspoonful equivalent to 4 mg of ondansetron) of ZOFRAN Oral Solution given three times a day. The first dose should be administered 30 minutes before the start of emetogenic chemotherapy, with subsequent doses 4 and 8 hours after the first dose. One 4-mg ZOFRAN Tablet or one 4-mg ZOFRAN ODT Tablet or 5 mL (1 teaspoonful equivalent to 4 mg of ondansetron) of ZOFRAN Oral Solution should be administered three times a day (every 8 hours) for 1 to 2 days after completion of chemotherapy.

Geriatric Use: The dosage is the same as for the general population.

Prevention of Nausea and Vomiting Associated With Radiotherapy, Either Total Body Irradiation, or Single High-Dose Fraction or Daily Fractions to the Abdomen: The recommended oral dosage is one 8-mg ZOFRAN Tablet or one 8-mg ZOFRAN ODT Tablet or 10 mL (2 teaspoonfuls equivalent to 8 mg of ondansetron) of ZOFRAN Oral Solution given three times a day.

For total body irradiation, one 8-mg ZOFRAN Tablet or one 8-mg ZOFRAN ODT Tablet or 10 mL (2 teaspoonfuls equivalent to 8 mg of ondansetron) of ZOFRAN Oral Solution should be administered 1 to 2 hours before each fraction of radiotherapy administered each day.

For single high-dose fraction radiotherapy to the abdomen, one 8-mg ZOFRAN Tablet or one 8-mg ZOFRAN ODT Tablet or 10 mL (2 teaspoonfuls equivalent to 8 mg of ondansetron) of ZOFRAN Oral Solution should be administered 1 to 2 hours before radiotherapy, with subsequent doses every 8 hours after the first dose for 1 to 2 days after completion of radiotherapy.

For daily fractionated radiotherapy to the abdomen, one 8-mg ZOFRAN Tablet or one 8-mg ZOFRAN ODT Tablet or 10 mL (2 teaspoonfuls equivalent to 8 mg of ondansetron) of ZOFRAN Oral Solution should be administered 1 to 2 hours before radiotherapy, with subsequent doses every 8 hours after the first dose for each day radiotherapy is given.

Pediatric Use: There is no experience with the use of ZOFRAN Tablets, ZOFRAN ODT Tablets, or ZOFRAN Oral Solution in the prevention of radiation-induced nausea and vomiting in pediatric patients.

Geriatric Use: The dosage recommendation is the same as for the general population.

Postoperative Nausea and Vomiting: The recommended dosage is 16 mg given as two 8-mg ZOFRAN Tablets or two 8-mg ZOFRAN ODT Tablets or 20 mL (4 teaspoonfuls equivalent to 16 mg of ondansetron) of ZOFRAN Oral Solution 1 hour before induction of anesthesia.

Pediatric Use: There is no experience with the use of ZOFRAN Tablets, ZOFRAN ODT Tablets, or ZOFRAN Oral Solution in the prevention of postoperative nausea and vomiting in pediatric patients.

Geriatric Use: The dosage is the same as for the general population.

Dosage Adjustment for Patients With Impaired Renal Function: The dosage recommendation is the same as for the general population. There is no experience beyond first-day administration of ondansetron.

Dosage Adjustment for Patients With Impaired Hepatic Function: In patients with severe hepatic impairment (Child-Pugh[1] score of 10 or greater), clearance is reduced and apparent volume of distribution is increased with a resultant increase in plasma half-life. In such patients, a total daily dose of 8 mg should not be exceeded.

HOW SUPPLIED

ZOFRAN Tablets, 4 mg (ondansetron HCl dihydrate equivalent to 4 mg of ondansetron), are white, oval, film-coated

Continued on next page

Zofran—Cont.

tablets engraved with "Zofran" on one side and "4" on the other in daily unit dose packs of 3 tablets (NDC 0173-0446-04), bottles of 30 tablets (NDC 0173-0446-00), and unit dose packs of 100 tablets (NDC 0173-0446-02).
ZOFRAN Tablets, 8 mg (ondansetron HCl dihydrate equivalent to 8 mg of ondansetron), are yellow, oval, film-coated tablets engraved with "Zofran" on one side and "8" on the other in daily unit dose packs of 3 tablets (NDC 0173-0447-04), bottles of 30 tablets (NDC 0173-0447-00), and unit dose packs of 100 tablets (NDC 0173-0447-02).
Bottles: Store between 2° and 30°C (36° and 86°F). Protect from light. Dispense in tight, light-resistant container as defined in the USP.
Unit Dose Packs: Store between 2° and 30°C (36° and 86°F). Protect from light. Store blisters in cartons.
ZOFRAN Tablets, 24 mg (ondansetron HCl dihydrate equivalent to 24 mg of ondansetron), are pink, oval, film-coated tablets engraved with "GX CF7" on one side and "24" on the other in daily unit dose packs of 1 tablet (NDC 0173-0680-00).
Store between 2° and 30°C (36° and 86°F).
ZOFRAN ODT Orally Disintegrating Tablets, 4 mg (as 4 mg ondansetron base) are white, round and plano-convex tablets debossed with a "Z4" on one side in unit dose packs of 30 tablets (NDC 0173-0569-00).
ZOFRAN ODT Orally Disintegrating Tablets, 8 mg (as 8 mg ondansetron base) are white, round and plano-convex tablets debossed with a "Z8" on one side in unit dose packs of 10 tablets (NDC 0173-0570-04) and 30 tablets (NDC 0173-0570-00).
Store between 2° and 30°C (36° and 86°F).
ZOFRAN Oral Solution, a clear, colorless to light yellow liquid with a characteristic strawberry odor, contains 5 mg of ondansetron HCl dihydrate equivalent to 4 mg of ondansetron per 5 mL in amber glass bottles of 50 mL with child-resistant closures (NDC 0173-0489-00).
Store upright between 15° and 30°C (59° and 86°F). Protect from light. Store bottles upright in cartons.

REFERENCE

1. Pugh RNH, Murray-Lyon IM, Dawson JL, Pietroni MC, Williams R. Transection of the oesophagus for bleeding oesophageal varices. *Brit J Surg.* 1973;60:646–649.

ZOFRAN Tablets and Oral Solution:
GlaxoSmithKline, Research Triangle Park, NC 27709
ZOFRAN ODT Orally Disintegrating Tablets:
Manufactured for GlaxoSmithKline
Research Triangle Park, NC 27709
by Scherer DDS, Blagrove, Swindon, Wiltshire, UK
SN5 8RU

May 2001/RL-931

ZOVIRAX® ℞
[*zō-vī'rax*]
(acyclovir)
Capsules
ZOVIRAX® ℞
(acyclovir)
Tablets
ZOVIRAX® ℞
(acyclovir)
Suspension

Prescribing information for these products, which appears on pages 1706–1707 of the 2002 PDR, has been revised as follows. Please write "See Supplement A" next to the product heading.
The **VIROLOGY: Mechanism of Antiviral Action** *subsection was revised to:*
Acyclovir is a synthetic purine nucleoside analogue with in vitro and in vivo inhibitory activity against herpes simplex virus types 1 (HSV-1), 2 (HSV-2), and varicella-zoster virus (VZV).
The first sentence of the **VIROLOGY: Drug Resistance** *subsection was revised to:*
Resistance of HSV and VZV to acyclovir can result from qualitative and quantitative changes in the viral TK and/or DNA polymerase.
The following was added to the **CLINICAL PHARMACOLOGY: Special Populations** *subsection:*
Geriatrics: Acyclovir plasma concentrations are higher in geriatric patients compared to younger adults, in part due to age-related changes in renal function. Dosage reduction may be required in geriatric patients with underlying renal impairment (see PRECAUTIONS: Geriatric Use).
The **PRECAUTIONS: Carcinogenesis, Mutagenesis, Impairment of Fertility** *subsection was revised to:*
The data presented below include references to peak steady-state plasma acyclovir concentrations observed in humans treated with 800 mg given orally 5 times a day (dosing appropriate for treatment of herpes zoster) or 200 mg given orally 5 times a day (dosing appropriate for treatment of genital herpes). Plasma drug concentrations in animal studies are expressed as multiples of human exposure to acyclovir at the higher and lower dosing schedules (see CLINICAL PHARMACOLOGY: Pharmacokinetics).
Acyclovir was tested in lifetime bioassays in rats and mice at single daily doses of up to 450 mg/kg administered by gavage. There was no statistically significant difference in the incidence of tumors between treated and control animals, nor did acyclovir shorten the latency of tumors. Maximum plasma concentrations were 3 to 6 times human levels in the mouse bioassay and 1 to 2 times human levels in the rat bioassay.
Acyclovir was tested in 16 in vitro and in vivo genetic toxicity assays. Acyclovir was positive in 5 of the assays.
Acyclovir did not impair fertility or reproduction in mice (450 mg/kg per day, PO) or in rats (25 mg/kg per day, SC). In the mouse study, plasma levels were 9 to 18 times human levels, while in the rat study, they were 8 to 15 times human levels. At higher doses (50 mg/kg per day, SC) in rats and rabbits (11 to 22 and 16 to 31 times human levels, respectively) implantation efficacy, but not litter size, was decreased. In a rat peri- and post-natal study at 50 mg/kg per day, SC, there was a statistically significant decrease in group mean numbers of corpora lutea, total implantation sites, and live fetuses. No testicular abnormalities were seen in dogs given 50 mg/kg per day, IV for 1 month (21 to 41 times human levels) or in dogs given 60 mg/kg per day orally for 1 year (6 to 12 times human levels). Testicular atrophy and aspermatogenesis were observed in rats and dogs at higher dose levels.
The first sentence of the **PRECAUTIONS: Pregnancy: Teratogenic Effects** *subsection was revised to:*
Acyclovir administered during organogenesis was not teratogenic in the mouse (450 mg/kg per day, PO), rabbit (50 mg/kg per day, SC and IV), or rat (50 mg/kg per day, SC).
The **PRECAUTIONS: Pediatric Use** *subsection was revised to:*
Safety and effectiveness of oral formulations of acyclovir in pediatric patients less than 2 years of age have not been established.
The **PRECAUTIONS: Geriatric Use** *subsection was revised to:*
Of 376 subjects who received ZOVIRAX in a clinical study of herpes zoster treatment in immunocompetent subjects greater than or equal to 50 years of age, 244 were 65 and over while 111 were 75 and over. No overall differences in effectiveness for time to cessation of new lesion formation or time to healing were reported between geriatric subjects and younger adult subjects. The duration of pain after healing was longer in patients 65 and over. Nausea, vomiting, and dizziness were reported more frequently in elderly subjects. Elderly patients are more likely to have reduced renal function and require dose reduction. Elderly patients are also more likely to have renal or CNS adverse events. With respect to CNS adverse events observed during clinical practice, somnolence, hallucinations, confusion, and coma were reported more frequently in elderly patients (see CLINICAL PHARMACOLOGY, ADVERSE REACTIONS: Observed During Clinical Practice, and DOSAGE AND ADMINISTRATION).
The **ADVERSE REACTIONS: Observed During Clinical Practice: Hemic and Lymphatic:** *subsection was revised to:*
Hematologic and Lymphatic: Anemia, leukocytoclastic vasculitis, leukopenia, lymphadenopathy, thrombocytopenia.
The following sentence was revised in the **OVERDOSAGE** *section:*
Adverse events that have been reported in association with overdosage include agitation, coma, seizures, and lethargy.
GlaxoSmithKline, Research Triangle Park, NC 27709

November 2001/RL-1032

ZOVIRAX® ℞
[*zō-vī' răx*]
(acyclovir sodium)
for Injection
FOR INTRAVENOUS INFUSION ONLY

Prescribing information for this product, which appears on pages 1708–1710 of the 2002 PDR, has been revised as follows. Please write "See Supplement A" next to the product heading.
The first paragraph of the **VIROLOGY: Mechanism of Antiviral Action** *subsection was revised to:*
Acyclovir is a synthetic purine nucleoside analogue with in vitro and in vivo inhibitory activity against herpes simplex virus types 1 (HSV-1), 2 (HSV-2), and varicella-zoster virus (VZV).
The first sentence of the **VIROLOGY: Drug Resistance** *subsection was revised to:*
Resistance of HSV and VZV to acyclovir can result from qualitative and quantitative changes in the viral TK and/or DNA polymerase.
The following was added to the **CLINICAL PHARMACOLOGY: Special Populations** *subsection:*
Geriatrics: Acyclovir plasma concentrations are higher in geriatric patients compared to younger adults, in part due to age-related changes in renal function. Dosage reduction may be required in geriatric patients with underlying renal impairment (see PRECAUTIONS: Geriatric Use).
The **PRECAUTIONS: Carcinogenesis, Mutagenesis, Impairment of Fertility** *subsection was revised to:*
The data presented below include references to peak steady-state plasma acyclovir concentrations observed in humans treated with 30 mg/kg per day (10 mg/kg every 8 hours, dosing appropriate for treatment of herpes zoster or herpes encephalitis), or 15 mg/kg per day (5 mg/kg every 8 hours, dosing appropriate for treatment of primary genital herpes or herpes simplex infections in immunocompromised patients). Plasma drug concentrations in animal studies are expressed as multiples of human exposure to acyclovir at the higher and lower dosing schedules (see CLINICAL PHARMACOLOGY: Pharmacokinetics).
Acyclovir was tested in lifetime bioassays in rats and mice at single daily doses of up to 450 mg/kg administered by gavage. There was no statistically significant difference in the incidence of tumors between treated and control animals, nor did acyclovir shorten the latency of tumors. At 450 mg/kg per day, plasma concentrations in both the mouse and rat bioassay were lower than concentrations in humans.
Acyclovir was tested in 16 in vitro and in vivo genetic toxicity assays. Acyclovir was positive in 5 of the assays.
Acyclovir did not impair fertility or reproduction in mice (450 mg/kg per day, PO) or in rats (25 mg/kg per day, SC). In the mouse study, plasma levels were the same as human levels, while in the rat study, they were 1 to 2 times human levels. At higher doses (50 mg/kg per day, SC) in rats and rabbits (1 to 2 and 1 to 3 times human levels, respectively) implantation efficacy, but not litter size, was decreased. In a rat peri- and post-natal study at 50 mg/kg per day, SC, there was a statistically significant decrease in group mean numbers of corpora lutea, total implantation sites, and live fetuses.
No testicular abnormalities were seen in dogs given 50 mg/kg per day, IV for 1 month (1 to 3 times human levels) or in dogs given 60 mg/kg per day orally for 1 year (the same as human levels). Testicular atrophy and aspermatogenesis were observed in rats and dogs at higher dose levels.
The **PRECAUTIONS: Pregnancy: Teratogenic Effects** *subsection was revised to:*
Pregnancy Category B. Acyclovir administered during organogenesis was not teratogenic in the mouse (450 mg/kg per day, PO), rabbit (50 mg/kg per day, SC and IV), or rat (50 mg/kg per day, SC). These exposures resulted in plasma levels the same as, 4 and 9, and 1 and 2 times, respectively, human levels. There are no adequate and well-controlled studies in pregnant women. A prospective epidemiologic registry of acyclovir use during pregnancy was established in 1984 and completed in April 1999. There were 749 pregnancies followed in women exposed to systemic acyclovir during the first trimester of pregnancy resulting in 756 outcomes. The occurrence rate of birth defects approximates that found in the general population. However, the small size of the registry is insufficient to evaluate the risk for less common defects or to permit reliable or definitive conclusions regarding the safety of acyclovir in pregnant women and their developing fetuses. Acyclovir should be used during pregnancy only if the potential benefit justifies the potential risk to the fetus.
The **PRECAUTIONS: Geriatric Use** *subsection was revised to:*
Clinical studies of ZOVIRAX for Injection did not include sufficient numbers of patients aged 65 and over to determine whether they respond differently from younger patients. Other reported clinical experience has identified differences in the severity of CNS adverse events between elderly and younger patients (see ADVERSE REACTIONS: Observed During Clinical Practice). In general, dose selection for an elderly patient should be cautious, reflecting the greater frequency of decreased renal function, and of concomitant disease or other drug therapy. This drug is known to be substantially excreted by the kidney, and the risk of toxic reactions to this drug may be greater in patients with impaired renal function. Because elderly patients are more likely to have decreased renal function, care should be taken in dose selection, and it may be useful to monitor renal function.
The **ADVERSE REACTIONS: Observed During Clinical Practice** *subsection was revised to:*
In addition to adverse events reported from clinical trials, the following events have been identified during post-approval use of ZOVIRAX for Injection in clinical practice. Because they are reported voluntarily from a population of unknown size, estimates of frequency cannot be made. These events have been chosen for inclusion due to either their seriousness, frequency of reporting, potential causal connection to ZOVIRAX, or a combination of these factors.
General: Anaphylaxis, angioedema, fever, headache, pain, peripheral edema.
Digestive: Diarrhea, gastrointestinal distress, nausea.
Cardiovascular: Hypotension.
Hematologic and Lymphatic: Disseminated intravascular coagulation, hemolysis, leukocytoclastic vasculitis, leukopenia, lymphadenopathy.
Hepatobiliary Tract and Pancreas: Elevated liver function tests, hepatitis, hyperbilirubinemia, jaundice.
Musculoskeletal: Myalgia.
Nervous: Aggressive behavior, agitation, ataxia, coma, confusion, delirium, dizziness, encephalopathy, hallucinations, obtundation, paresthesia, psychosis, seizure, somnolence, tremor. These symptoms may be marked, particularly in older adults (see PRECAUTIONS).
Skin: Alopecia, erythema multiforme, photosensitive rash, pruritus, rash, Stevens-Johnson syndrome, toxic epidermal necrolysis, urticaria. Severe local inflammatory reactions, including tissue necrosis, have occurred following infusion of ZOVIRAX into extravascular tissues.
Special Senses: Visual abnormalities.
Urogenital: Renal failure, elevated blood urea nitrogen, elevated creatinine (see WARNINGS).
The following sentence was revised in the **OVERDOSAGE** *section:*
Adverse events that have been reported in association with overdosage include agitation, coma, seizures, and lethargy.

Manufactured by Catalytica Pharmaceuticals, Inc.
Greenville, NC 27834
for GlaxoSmithKline, Research Triangle Park, NC 27709

January 2002/RL-1060

ZYBAN® ℞
[zī' ban]
(bupropion hydrochloride)
Sustained-Release Tablets

Prescribing information for this product, which appears on pages 1710–1715 of the 2002 PDR, has been revised as follows. Please write "See Supplement A" next to the product heading.

The following sentence was added to the end of the first paragraph of the **WARNINGS** *section:*

ZYBAN should be discontinued and not restarted in patients who experience a seizure while on treatment.

The following sentence was added to the first paragraph of the **DOSAGE AND ADMINISTRATION: ZYBAN:** ***Usual Dosage for Adults*** *subsection:*

ZYBAN should be swallowed whole and not crushed, divided, or chewed.

The following subsections were revised in the **PATIENT INFORMATION** *section:*

IMPORTANT WARNING:

There is a chance that approximately 1 out of every 1000 people taking bupropion hydrochloride, the active ingredient in ZYBAN, will have a seizure. The chance of this happening increases if you:

- have a seizure disorder (for example, epilepsy);
- have or have had an eating disorder (for example, bulimia or anorexia nervosa);
- take more than the recommended amount of ZYBAN; or
- take other medicines with the same active ingredient that is in ZYBAN, such as WELLBUTRIN® (bupropion hydrochloride) Tablets and WELLBUTRIN SR® (bupropion hydrochloride) Sustained-Release Tablets. (Both of these medicines are used to treat depression.)

You can reduce the chance of experiencing a seizure by following your doctor's directions on how to take ZYBAN. If you experience a seizure while taking ZYBAN, stop taking the tablets immediately, contact your doctor, and do not restart ZYBAN. In addition, tell your doctor if you have or have had other medical conditions. You should also discuss with your doctor whether ZYBAN is right for you.

2. Who should not take ZYBAN?

You should not take ZYBAN if you:

- have or have had a seizure disorder (for example, epilepsy);
- are already taking WELLBUTRIN, WELLBUTRIN SR, or any other medicines that contain bupropion hydrochloride;
- have or have had an eating disorder (for example, bulimia or anorexia nervosa);
- are currently taking or have recently taken a monoamine oxidase inhibitor (MAOI);
- are allergic to bupropion.

5. Are there any concerns for patients with liver or kidney problems?

If you have liver or kidney problems, tell your doctor before taking ZYBAN. Depending on the severity of your condition, your doctor may need to adjust your dosage.

10. Can ZYBAN be used at the same time as nicotine patches?

Yes, ZYBAN and nicotine patches can be used at the same time but should only be used together under the supervision of your doctor. Using ZYBAN and nicotine patches together may raise your blood pressure, sometimes severely. Tell your doctor if you are planning to use nicotine replacement therapy because your doctor will probably want to check your blood pressure regularly to make sure that it stays within acceptable levels.

DO NOT SMOKE AT ANY TIME if you are using a nicotine patch or any other nicotine product along with ZYBAN. It is possible to get too much nicotine and have serious side effects.

11. What are possible side effects of ZYBAN?

Like all medicines, ZYBAN may cause side effects. Do not rely on this summary alone for information about side effects. Your doctor can discuss with you a more complete list of side effects that may be relevant to you.

- Hypertension (high blood pressure), in some cases severe, has been reported in patients taking ZYBAN alone and in combination with nicotine replacement therapy (for example, a nicotine patch, see Question #10).
- The most common side effects include dry mouth and difficulty sleeping. These side effects are generally mild and often disappear after a few weeks. If you have difficulty sleeping, avoid taking your medicine too close to bedtime.
- The most common side effects that caused people to stop taking ZYBAN during clinical studies were shakiness and skin rash.
- Stop taking ZYBAN and contact your doctor or health care professional if you have signs of an allergic reaction such as a rash, hives, or difficulty in breathing. It is not possible to predict whether a mild rash will develop into a more serious reaction. Therefore, if you experience a skin rash, hives, fever, swollen lymph glands, painful sores in the mouth or around the eyes, or swelling of lips or tongue, tell a doctor immediately, since these symptoms may be the first signs of a serious reaction. Discuss any other troublesome side effects with your doctor.
- Use caution before driving a car or operating complex, hazardous machinery until you know if ZYBAN affects your ability to perform these tasks.

Manufactured by Catalytica Pharmaceuticals, Inc.
Greenville, NC 27834
for GlaxoSmithKline, Research Triangle Park, NC 27709

August 2001/RL-934

Janssen Pharmaceutica Products, L.P.

1125 TRENTON-HARBOURTON ROAD
P.O. BOX 200
TITUSVILLE, NJ 08560-0200

For Medical Information Monday through Friday 9 am-5 pm EST Contact:
(800) JANSSEN
FAX: (609) 730-2461
After Hours and Weekends:
(800) JANSSEN

REMINYL® ℞
[rĕm ĭ-nil]
(GALANTAMINE HBr)
TABLETS AND ORAL SOLUTION

Prescribing information for this product, which appears on pages 1792–1796 of the 2002 PDR, has been completely revised as follows. Please write "See Supplement A" next to the product heading.

DESCRIPTION

REMINYL® (galantamine hydrobromide) is a reversible, competitive acetylcholinesterase inhibitor. It is known chemically as (4a*S*,6*R*,8a*S*)-4a,5,9,10,11,12-hexahydro-3-methoxy-11-methyl-6*H*-benzofuro[3a,3,2-*ef*][2]benzazepin-6-ol hydrobromide. It has an empirical formula of $C_{17}H_{21}NO_3$ •HBr and a molecular weight of 368.27. Galantamine hydrobromide is a white to almost white powder and is sparingly soluble in water. The structural formula for galantamine hydrobromide is:

REMINYL® for oral use is available in circular biconvex film-coated tablets of 4 mg (off-white), 8 mg (pink), and 12 mg (orange-brown). Each 4, 8, and 12 mg (base equivalent) tablet contains 5.126, 10.253, and 15.379 mg of galantamine hydrobromide, respectively. Inactive ingredients include colloidal silicon dioxide, crospovidone, hydroxypropyl methylcellulose, lactose monohydrate, magnesium stearate, microcrystalline cellulose, propylene glycol, talc, and titanium dioxide. The 4 mg tablets contain yellow ferric oxide. The 8 mg tablets contain red ferric oxide. The 12 mg tablets contain red ferric oxide and FD&C yellow #6 aluminum lake.

REMINYL® is also available as a 4 mg/mL oral solution. The inactive ingredients for this solution are methyl parahydroxybenzoate, propyl parahydroxybenzoate, sodium saccharin, sodium hydroxide and purified water.

CLINICAL PHARMACOLOGY

Mechanism of Action

Although the etiology of cognitive impairment in Alzheimer's disease (AD) is not fully understood, it has been reported that acetylcholine-producing neurons degenerate in the brains of patients with Alzheimer's disease. The degree of this cholinergic loss has been correlated with degree of cognitive impairment and density of amyloid plaques (a neuropathological hallmark of Alzheimer's disease).

Galantamine, a tertiary alkaloid, is a competitive and reversible inhibitor of acetylcholinesterase. While the precise mechanism of galantamine's action is unknown, it is postulated to exert its therapeutic effect by enhancing cholinergic function. This is accomplished by increasing the concentration of acetylcholine through reversible inhibition of its hydrolysis by cholinesterase. If this mechanism is correct, galantamine's effect may lessen as the disease process advances and fewer cholinergic neurons remain functionally intact. There is no evidence that galantamine alters the course of the underlying dementing process.

Pharmacokinetics

Galantamine is well absorbed with absolute oral bioavailability of about 90%. It has a terminal elimination half-life of about 7 hours and pharmacokinetics are linear over the range of 8-32 mg/day.

The maximum inhibition of anticholinesterase activity of about 40% was achieved about one hour after a single oral dose of 8 mg galantamine in healthy male subjects.

Absorption and Distribution

Galantamine is rapidly and completely absorbed with time to peak concentration about 1 hour. Bioavailability of the tablet was the same as the bioavailability of an oral solution. Food did not affect the AUC of galantamine but C_{max} decreased by 25% and T_{max} was delayed by 1.5 hours. The mean volume of distribution of galantamine is 175 L.

The plasma protein binding of galantamine is 18% at therapeutically relevant concentrations. In whole blood, galantamine is mainly distributed to blood cells (52.7%). The blood to plasma concentration ratio of galantamine is 1.2.

Metabolism and Elimination

Galantamine is metabolized by hepatic cytochrome P450 enzymes, glucuronidated, and excreted unchanged in the urine. *In vitro* studies indicate that cytochrome CYP2D6 and CYP3A4 were the major cytochrome P450 isoenzymes involved in the metabolism of galantamine, and inhibitors of both pathways increase oral bioavailability of galantamine modestly (See **PRECAUTIONS, Drug-Drug Interactions**). O-demethylation, mediated by CYP2D6 was greater in extensive metabolizers of CYP2D6 than in poor metabolizers. In plasma from both poor and extensive metabolizers, however, unchanged galantamine and its glucuronide accounted for most of the sample radioactivity.

In studies of oral ^{3}H-galantamine, unchanged galantamine and its glucuronide, accounted for most plasma radioactivity in poor and extensive CYP2D6 metabolizers. Up to 8 hours post-dose, unchanged galantamine accounted for 39-77% of the total radioactivity in the plasma, and galantamine glucuronide for 14-24%. By 7 days, 93-99% of the radioactivity had been recovered, with about 95% in urine and about 5% in the feces. Total urinary recovery of unchanged galantamine accounted for, on average, 32% of the dose and that of galantamine glucuronide for another 12% on average.

After i.v. or oral administration, about 20% of the dose was excreted as unchanged galantamine in the urine in 24 hours, representing a renal clearance of about 65 mL/min, about 20-25% of the total plasma clearance of about 300 mL/min.

Special Populations

CYP2D6 poor metabolizers

Approximately 7% of the normal population has a genetic variation that leads to reduced levels of activity of CYP2D6 isozyme. Such individuals have been referred to as poor metabolizers. After a single oral dose of 4 mg or 8 mg galantamine, CYP2D6 poor metabolizers demonstrated a similar C_{max} and about 35% AUC_{∞} increase of unchanged galantamine compared to extensive metabolizers.

A total of 356 patients with Alzheimer's disease enrolled in two phase 3 studies were genotyped with respect to CYP2D6 (n=210 hetero-extensive metabolizers, 126 homo-extensive metabolizers, and 20 poor metabolizers). Population pharmacokinetic analysis indicated that there was a 25% decrease in median clearance in poor metabolizers compared to extensive metabolizers. Dosage adjustment is not necessary in patients identified as poor metabolizers as the dose of drug is individually titrated to tolerability.

Hepatic Impairment: Following a single 4 mg dose of galantamine, the pharmacokinetics of galantamine in subjects with mild hepatic impairment (n=8; Child-Pugh score of 5-6) were similar to those in healthy subjects. In patients with moderate hepatic impairment (n=8; Child-Pugh score of 7-9), galantamine clearance was decreased by about 25% compared to normal volunteers. Exposure would be expected to increase further with increasing degree of hepatic impairment (See **PRECAUTIONS** and **DOSAGE AND ADMINISTRATION**).

Renal Impairment: Following a single 8 mg dose of galantamine, AUC increased by 37% and 67% in moderate and severely renal-impaired patients compared to normal volunteers. (See **PRECAUTIONS** and **DOSAGE AND ADMINISTRATION**).

Elderly: Data from clinical trials in patients with Alzheimer's disease indicate that galantamine concentrations are 30-40% higher than in healthy young subjects.

Gender and Race: No specific pharmacokinetic study was conducted to investigate the effect of gender and race on the disposition of REMINYL® (galantamine hydrobromide), but a population pharmacokinetic analysis indicates (n= 539 males and 550 females) that galantamine clearance is about 20% lower in females than in males (explained by lower body weight in females) and race (n= 1029 White, 24 Black, 13 Asian and 23 other) did not affect the clearance of REMINYL®.

Drug-Drug Interactions

Multiple metabolic pathways and renal excretion are involved in the elimination of galantamine so no single pathway appears predominant. Based on *in vitro* studies, CYP2D6 and CYP3A4 were the major enzymes involved in the metabolism of galantamine. CYP2D6 was involved in the formation of O-desmethyl-galantamine, whereas CYP3A4 mediated the formation of galantamine-N-oxide. Galantamine is also glucuronidated and excreted unchanged in urine.

(A) Effect of other drugs on the metabolism of REMINYL®: Drugs that are potent inhibitors for CYP2D6 or CYP3A4 may increase the AUC of galantamine. Multiple dose pharmacokinetic studies demonstrated that the AUC of galantamine increased 30% and 40%, respectively, during coadministration of ketoconazole and paroxetine. As coadministered with erythromycin, another CYP3A4 inhibitor, the galantamine AUC increased only 10%. Population PK analysis with a database of 852 patients with Alzheimer's

Continued on next page

Reminyl—Cont.

disease showed that the clearance of galantamine was decreased about 25-33% by concurrent administration of amitriptyline (n = 17), fluoxetine (n = 48), fluvoxamine (n = 14), and quinidine (n = 7), known inhibitors of CYP2D6.

Concurrent administration of H_2-antagonists demonstrated that ranitidine did not affect the pharmacokinetics of galantamine, and cimetidine increased the galantamine AUC by approximately 16%.

(B) Effect of REMINYL® on the metabolism of other drugs: *In vitro* studies show that galantamine did not inhibit the metabolic pathways catalyzed by CYP1A2, CYP2A6, CYP3A4, CYP4A, CYP2C, CYP2D6 and CYP2E1. This indicated that the inhibitory potential of galantamine towards the major forms of cytochrome P450 is very low. Multiple doses of galantamine (24 mg/day) had no effect on the pharmacokinetics of digoxin and warfarin (R- and S-forms). Galantamine had no effect on the increased prothrombin time induced by warfarin.

CLINICAL TRIALS

The effectiveness of REMINYL® (galantamine hydrobromide) as a treatment for Alzheimer's disease is demonstrated by the results of 4 randomized, double-blind, placebo-controlled clinical investigations in patients with probable Alzheimer's disease [diagnosed by NINCDS-ADRDA criteria, with Mini-Mental State Examination scores that were $\geq$10 and $\leq$24]. Doses studied were 8-32 mg/day given as twice daily doses. In 3 of the 4 studies patients were started on a low dose of 8 mg, then titrated weekly by 8 mg/day to 24 or 32 mg as assigned. In the fourth study (USA 4-week Dose-Escalation Fixed-Dose Study) dose escalation of 8 mg/day occurred over 4 week intervals. The mean age of patients participating in the 4 REMINYL® trials was 75 years with a range of 41 to 100. Approximately 62% of patients were women and 38% were men. The racial distribution was White 94%, Black 3% and other races 3%. Two other studies examined a three times daily dosing regimen; these also showed or suggested benefit but did not suggest an advantage over twice daily dosing.

Study Outcome Measures: In each study, the primary effectiveness of REMINYL® was evaluated using a dual outcome assessment strategy as measured by the Alzheimer's Disease Assessment Scale (ADAS-cog) and the Clinician's Interview Based Impression of Change (CIBIC-plus).

The ability of REMINYL® to improve cognitive performance was assessed with the cognitive sub-scale of the Alzheimer's Disease Assessment Scale (ADAS-cog), a multi-item instrument that has been extensively validated in longitudinal cohorts of Alzheimer's disease patients. The ADAS-cog examines selected aspects of cognitive performance including elements of memory, orientation, attention, reasoning, language and praxis. The ADAS-cog scoring range is from 0 to 70, with higher scores indicating greater cognitive impairment. Elderly normal adults may score as low as 0 or 1, but it is not unusual for non-demented adults to score slightly higher.

The patients recruited as participants in each study had mean scores on ADAS-cog of approximately 27 units, with a range from 5 to 69. Experience gained in longitudinal studies of ambulatory patients with mild to moderate Alzheimer's disease suggests that they gain 6 to 12 units a year on the ADAS-cog. Lesser degrees of change, however, are seen in patients with very mild or very advanced disease because the ADAS-cog is not uniformly sensitive to change over the course of the disease. The annualized rate of decline in the placebo patients participating in REMINYL® trials was approximately 4.5 units per year.

The ability of REMINYL® to produce an overall clinical effect was assessed using a Clinician's Interview Based Impression of Change that required the use of caregiver information, the CIBIC-plus. The CIBIC-plus is not a single instrument and is not a standardized instrument like the ADAS-cog. Clinical trials for investigational drugs have used a variety of CIBIC formats, each different in terms of depth and structure. As such, results from a CIBIC-plus reflect clinical experience from the trial or trials in which it was used and can not be compared directly with the results of CIBIC-plus evaluations from other clinical trials. The CIBIC-plus used in the trials was a semi-structured instrument based on a comprehensive evaluation at baseline and subsequent time-points of 4 major areas of patient function: general, cognitive, behavioral and activities of daily living. It represents the assessment of a skilled clinician based on his/her observation at an interview with the patient, in combination with information supplied by a caregiver familiar with the behavior of the patient over the interval rated. The CIBIC-plus is scored as a seven point categorical rating, ranging from a score of 1, indicating "markedly improved", to a score of 4, indicating "no change" to a score of 7, indicating "marked worsening". The CIBIC-plus has not been systematically compared directly to assessments not using information from caregivers (CIBIC) or other global methods.

U.S.Twenty-One-Week Fixed-Dose Study

In a study of 21 weeks duration, 978 patients were randomized to doses of 8, 16, or 24 mg of REMINYL® per day, or to placebo, each given in 2 divided doses. Treatment was initiated at 8 mg/day for all patients randomized to REMINYL®, and increased by 8 mg/day every 4 weeks. Therefore, the maximum titration phase was 8 weeks and the minimum maintenance phase was 13 weeks (in patients randomized to 24 mg/day of REMINYL®).

Effects on the ADAS-cog: Figure 1 illustrates the time course for the change from baseline in ADAS-cog scores for all four dose groups over the 21 weeks of the study. At 21 weeks of treatment, the mean differences in the ADAS-cog change scores for the REMINYL®-treated patients compared to the patients on placebo were 1.7, 3.3, and 3.6 units for the 8, 16 and 24 mg/day treatments, respectively. The 16 mg/day and 24 mg/day treatments were statistically significantly superior to placebo and to the 8 mg/day treatment. There was no statistically significant difference between the 16 mg/day and 24 mg/day dose groups.

Figure 1: Time-course of the Change from Baseline in ADAS-cog Score for Patients Completing 21 Weeks (5 Months) of Treatment

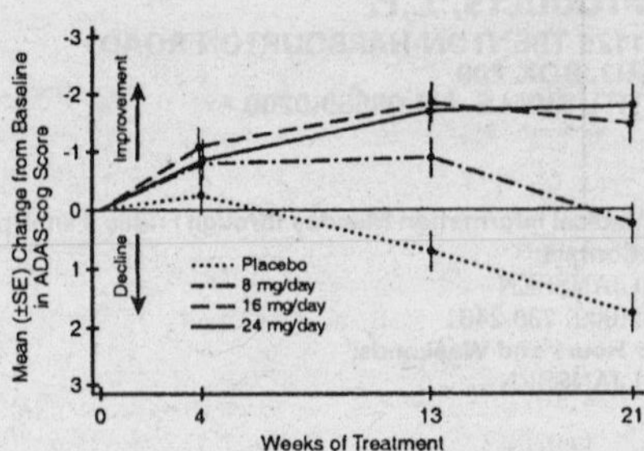

Figure 2 illustrates the cumulative percentages of patients from each of the four treatment groups who had attained at least the measure of improvement in ADAS-cog score shown on the X axis. Three change scores (10-point, 7-point and 4-point reductions) and no change in score from baseline have been identified for illustrative purposes, and the percent of patients in each group achieving that result is shown in the inset table.

The curves demonstrate that both patients assigned to galantamine and placebo have a wide range of responses, but that the REMINYL® groups are more likely to show the greater improvements.

Figure 2: Cumulative Percentage of Patients Completing 21 Weeks of Double-blind Treatment with Specified Changes from Baseline in ADAS-cog Scores.
The Percentages of Randomized Patients who Completed the Study were: Placebo 84%, 8 mg/day 77%, 16 mg/day 78% and 24 mg/day 78%.

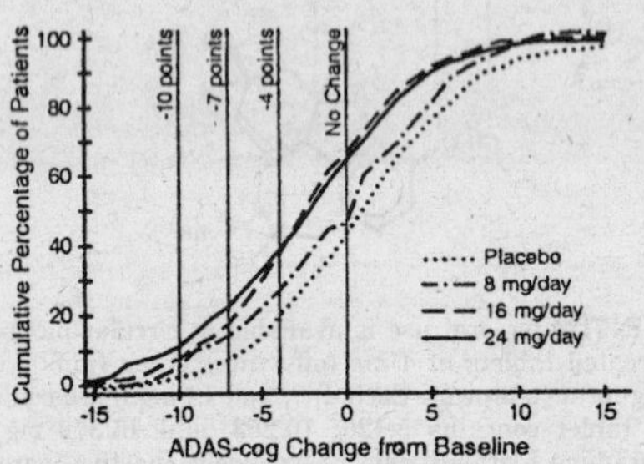

	Change in ADAS-cog			
Treatment	-10	-7	-4	0
Placebo	3.6%	7.6%	19.6%	41.8%
8 mg/day	5.9%	13.9%	25.7%	46.5%
16 mg/day	7.2%	15.9%	35.6%	65.4%
24 mg/day	10.4%	22.3%	37.0%	64.9%

Effects on the CIBIC-plus: Figure 3 is a histogram of the percentage distribution of CIBIC-plus scores attained by patients assigned to each of the four treatment groups who completed 21 weeks of treatment. The REMINYL®-placebo differences for these groups of patients in mean rating were 0.15, 0.41 and 0.44 units for the 8, 16 and 24 mg/day treatments, respectively. The 16 mg/day and 24 mg/day treatments were statistically significantly superior to placebo. The differences vs. the 8 mg/day treatment for the 16 and 24 mg/day treatments were 0.26 and 0.29, respectively. There were no statistically significant differences between the 16 mg/day and 24 mg/day dose groups.

Figure 3: Distribution of CIBIC-plus Ratings at Week 21

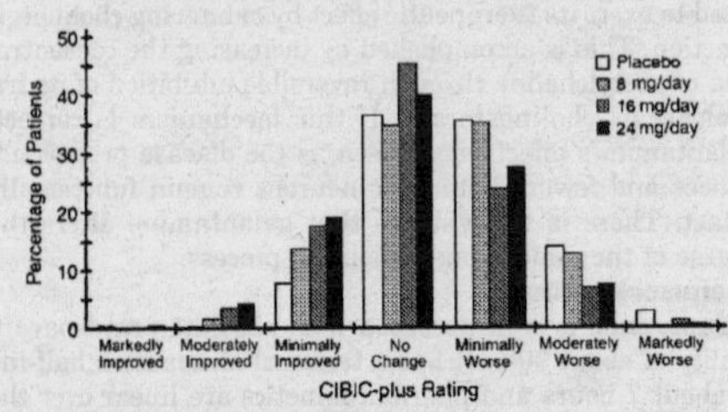

U.S.Twenty-Six-Week Fixed-Dose Study

In a study of 26 weeks duration, 636 patients were randomized to either a dose of 24 mg or 32 mg of REMINYL® per day, or to placebo, each given in two divided doses. The 26-week study was divided into a 3-week dose titration phase and a 23-week maintenance phase.

Effects on the ADAS-cog: Figure 4 illustrates the time course for the change from baseline in ADAS-cog scores for all three dose groups over the 26 weeks of the study. At 26 weeks of treatment, the mean differences in the ADAS-cog change scores for the REMINYL®-treated patients compared to the patients on placebo were 3.9 and 3.8 units for the 24 mg/day and 32 mg/day treatments, respectively. Both treatments were statistically significantly superior to placebo, but were not significantly different from each other.

Figure 4: Time-course of the Change from Baseline in ADAS-cog Score for Patients Completing 26 Weeks of Treatment

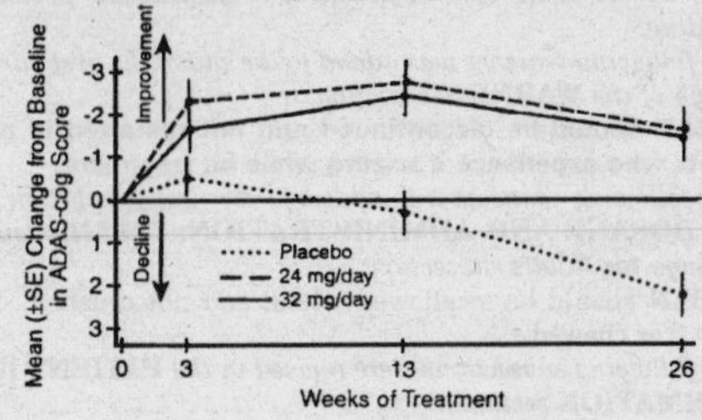

Figure 5 illustrates the cumulative percentages of patients from each of the three treatment groups who had attained at least the measure of improvement in ADAS-cog score shown on the X axis. Three change scores (10-point, 7-point and 4-point reductions) and no change in score from baseline have been identified for illustrative purposes, and the percent of patients in each group achieving that result is shown in the inset table.

The curves demonstrate that both patients assigned to REMINYL® and placebo have a wide range of responses, but that the REMINYL® groups are more likely to show the greater improvements. A curve for an effective treatment would be shifted to the left of the curve for placebo, while an ineffective or deleterious treatment would be superimposed upon, or shifted to the right of the curve for placebo, respectively.

Figure 5: Cumulative Percentage of Patients Completing 26 Weeks of Double-blind Treatment with Specified Changes from Baseline in ADAS-cog Scores.
The Percentages of Randomized Patients who Completed the Study were: Placebo 81%, 24 mg/day 68%, and 32 mg/day 58%.

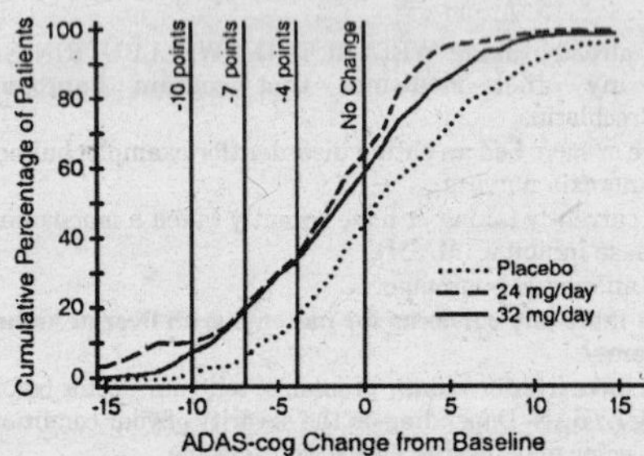

	Change in ADAS-cog			
Treatment	-10	-7	-4	0
Placebo	2.1%	5.7%	16.6%	43.9%
24 mg/day	7.6%	18.3%	33.6%	64.1%
32 mg/day	11.1%	19.7%	33.3%	58.1%

Effects on the CIBIC-plus: Figure 6 is a histogram of the percentage distribution of CIBIC-plus scores attained by patients assigned to each of the three treatment groups who completed 26 weeks of treatment. The mean REMINYL®-placebo differences for these groups of patients in the mean rating were 0.28 and 0.29 units for 24 and 32 mg/day of REMINYL®, respectively. The mean ratings for both groups were statistically significantly superior to placebo, but were not significantly different from each other.

Figure 6: Distribution of CIBIC-plus Ratings at Week 26

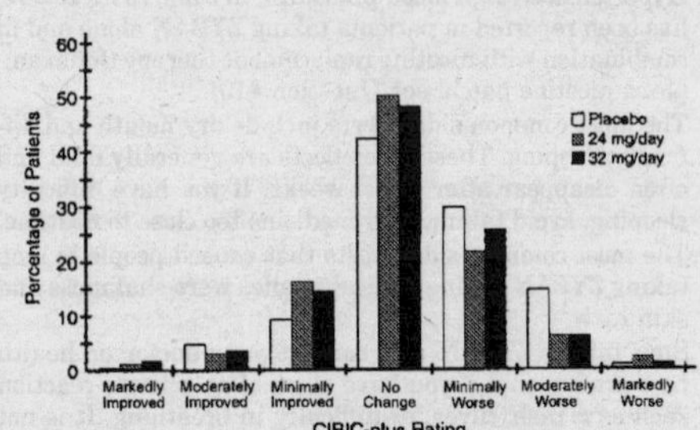

International Twenty-Six-Week Fixed-Dose Study

In a study of 26 weeks duration identical in design to the USA 26-Week Fixed-Dose Study, 653 patients were randomized to either a dose of 24 mg or 32 mg of REMINYL® per day, or to placebo, each given in two divided doses. The 26-week study was divided into a 3-week dose titration phase and a 23-week maintenance phase.

Effects on the ADAS-cog: Figure 7 illustrates the time course for the change from baseline in ADAS-cog scores for all three dose groups over the 26 weeks of the study. At 26 weeks of treatment, the mean differences in the ADAS-cog change scores for the REMINYL®-treated patients compared to the patients on placebo were 3.1 and 4.1 units for the 24 mg/day and 32 mg/day treatments, respectively. Both treatments were statistically significantly superior to placebo, but were not significantly different from each other.

Figure 7: Time-course of the Change from Baseline in ADAS-cog Score for Patients Completing 26 Weeks of Treatment

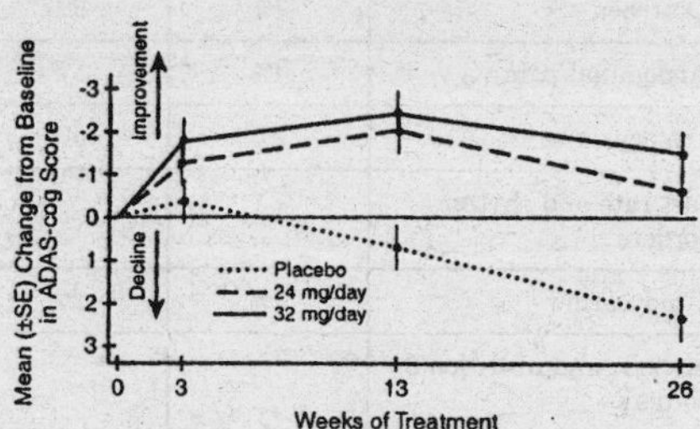

Figure 8 illustrates the cumulative percentages of patients from each of the three treatment groups who had attained at least the measure of improvement in ADAS-cog score shown on the X axis. Three change scores (10-point, 7-point and 4-point reductions) and no change in score from baseline have been identified for illustrative purposes, and the percent of patients in each group achieving that result is shown in the inset table.

The curves demonstrate that both patients assigned to REMINYL® and placebo have a wide range of responses, but that the REMINYL® groups are more likely to show the greater improvements.

Figure 8: Cumulative Percentage of Patients Completing 26 Weeks of Double-blind Treatment with Specified Changes from Baseline in ADAS-cog Scores. The Percentages of Randomized Patients who Completed the Study were: Placebo 87%, 24 mg/day 80%, and 32 mg/day 75%.

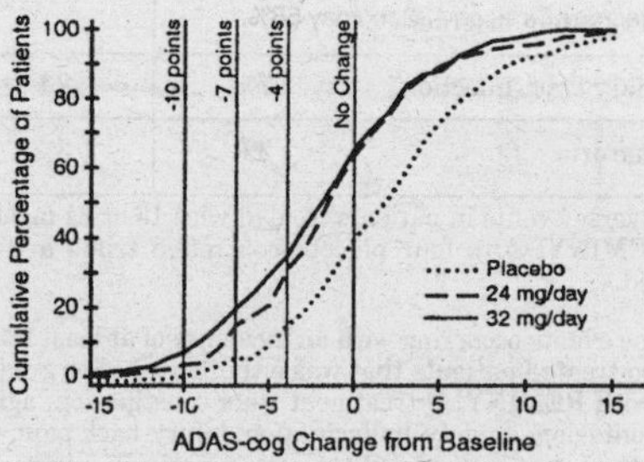

Treatment	Change in ADAS-cog -10	-7	-4	0
Placebo	1.2%	5.8%	15.2%	39.8%
24 mg/day	4.5%	15.4%	30.8%	65.4%
32 mg/day	7.9%	19.7%	34.9%	63.8%

Effects on the CIBIC-plus: Figure 9 is a histogram of the percentage distribution of CIBIC-plus scores attained by patients assigned to each of the three treatment groups who completed 26 weeks of treatment. The mean REMINYL®-placebo differences for these groups of patients in the mean rating of change from baseline were 0.34 and 0.47 for 24 and 32 mg/day of REMINYL®, respectively. The mean ratings for the REMINYL® groups were statistically significantly superior to placebo, but were not significantly different from each other.

Figure 9: Distribution of CIBIC-plus Rating at Week 26

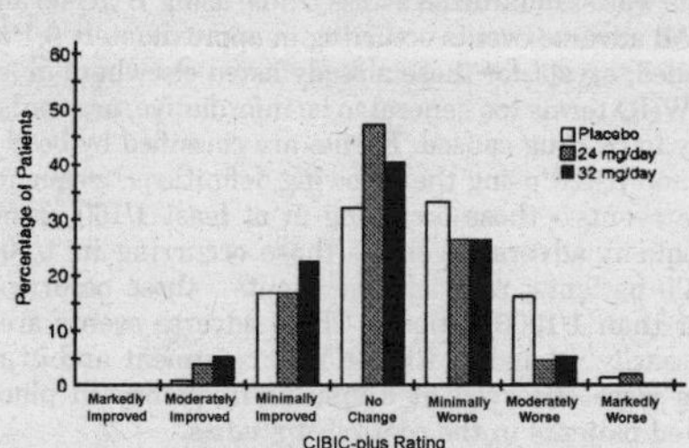

International Thirteen-Week Flexible-Dose Study

In a study of 13 weeks duration, 386 patients were randomized to either a flexible dose of 24-32 mg/day of REMINYL® or to placebo, each given in two divided doses. The 13-week study was divided into a 3-week dose titration phase and a 10-week maintenance phase. The patients in the active treatment arm of the study were maintained at either 24 mg/day or 32 mg/day at the discretion of the investigator.

Effects on the ADAS-cog: Figure 10 illustrates the time course for the change from baseline in ADAS-cog scores for both dose groups over the 13 weeks of the study. At 13 weeks of treatment, the mean difference in the ADAS-cog change scores for the treated patients compared to the patients on placebo was 1.9. REMINYL® at a dose of 24-32 mg/day was statistically significantly superior to placebo.

Figure 10: Time-course of the Change from Baseline in ADAS-cog Score for Patients Completing 13 Weeks of Treatment

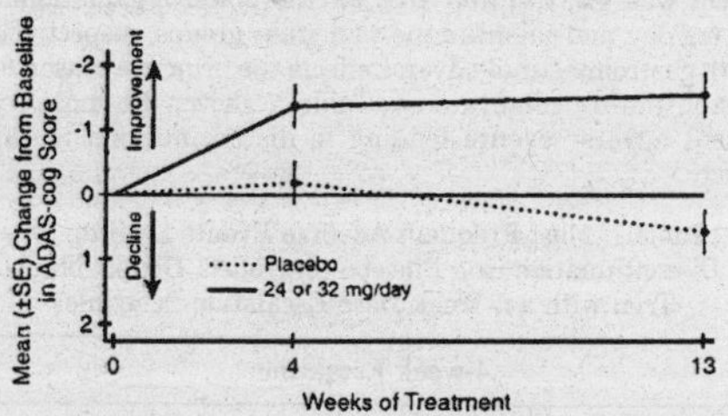

Figure 11 illustrates the cumulative percentages of patients from each of the two treatment groups who had attained at least the measure of improvement in ADAS-cog score shown on the X axis. Three change scores (10-point, 7-point and 4-point reductions) and no change in score from baseline have been identified for illustrative purposes, and the percent of patients in each group achieving that result is shown in the inset table.

The curves demonstrate that both patients assigned to REMINYL® and placebo have a wide range of responses, but that the REMINYL® group is more likely to show the greater improvement.

Figure 11: Cumulative Percentage of Patients Completing 13 Weeks of Double-blind Treatment with Specified Changes from Baseline in ADAS-cog Scores. The Percentages of Randomized Patients who Completed the Study were: Placebo 90%, 24-32 mg/day 67%.

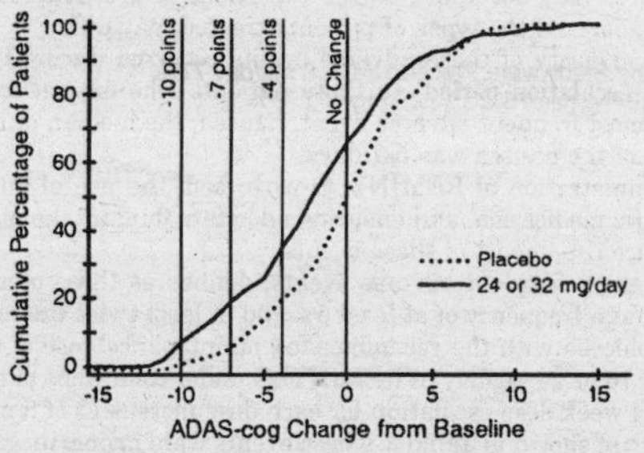

Treatment	Change in ADAS-cog -10	-7	-4	0
Placebo	1.9%	5.6%	19.4%	50.0%
24 or 32 mg/day	7.1%	18.8%	32.9%	65.3%

Effects on the CIBIC-plus: Figure 12 is a histogram of the percentage distribution of CIBIC-plus scores attained by patients assigned to each of the two treatment groups who completed 13 weeks of treatment. The mean REMINYL®-placebo differences for the group of patients in the mean rating of change from baseline was 0.37 units. The mean rating for the 24-32 mg/day group was statistically significantly superior to placebo.

Figure 12: Distribution of CIBIC-plus Ratings at Week 13

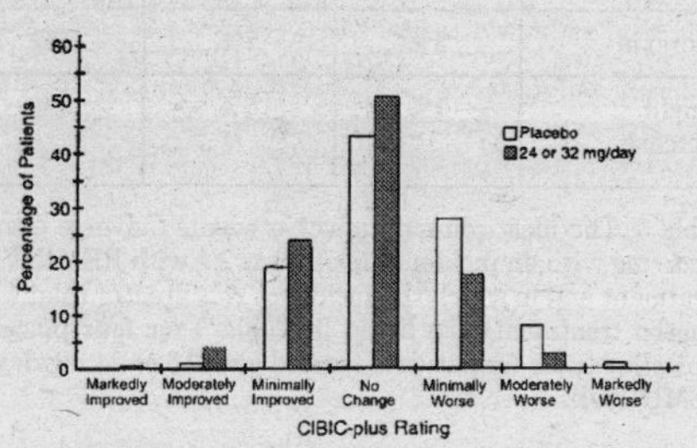

Age, gender and race: Patient's age, gender, or race did not predict clinical outcome of treatment.

INDICATIONS AND USAGE

REMINYL® (galantamine hydrobromide) is indicated for the treatment of mild to moderate dementia of the Alzheimer's type.

CONTRAINDICATIONS

REMINYL® (galantamine hydrobromide) is contraindicated in patients with known hypersensitivity to galantamine hydrobromide or to any excipients used in the formulation.

WARNINGS

Anesthesia

Galantamine, as a cholinesterase inhibitor, is likely to exaggerate the neuromuscular blockade effects of succinylcholine-type and similar neuromuscular blocking agents during anesthesia.

Cardiovascular Conditions

Because of their pharmacological action, cholinesterase inhibitors have vagotonic effects on the sinoatrial and atrioventricular nodes, leading to bradycardia and AV block. These actions may be particularly important to patients with supraventricular cardiac conduction disorders or to patients taking other drugs concomitantly that significantly slow heart rate. Postmarketing surveillance of marketed anticholinesterase inhibitors has shown, however, that bradycardia and all types of heart block have been reported in patients both with and without known underlying cardiac conduction abnormalities. Therefore all patients should be considered at risk for adverse effects on cardiac conduction.

In randomized controlled trials, bradycardia was reported more frequently in galantamine-treated patients than in placebo-treated patients, but rarely led to treatment discontinuation. The overall frequency of this event was 2-3% for galantamine doses up to 24 mg/day compared with <1% for placebo. No increased incidence of heart block was observed at the recommended doses.

Patients treated with galantamine up to 24 mg/day using the recommended dosing schedule showed a dose-related increase in risk of syncope (placebo 0.7% [2/286]; 4 mg BID 0.4% [3/692]; 8 mg BID 1.3% [7/552]; 12 mg BID 2.2% [6/273]).

Gastrointestinal Conditions

Through their primary action, cholinomimetics may be expected to increase gastric acid secretion due to increased cholinergic activity. Therefore, patients should be monitored closely for symptoms of active or occult gastrointestinal bleeding, especially those with an increased risk for developing ulcers, e.g., those with a history of ulcer disease or patients using concurrent nonsteroidal anti-inflammatory drugs (NSAIDS). Clinical studies of REMINYL® (galantamine hydrobromide) have shown no increase, relative to placebo, in the incidence of either peptic ulcer disease or gastrointestinal bleeding.

REMINYL®, as a predictable consequence of its pharmacological properties, has been shown to produce nausea, vomiting, diarrhea, anorexia, and weight loss. (See **ADVERSE REACTIONS**)

Genitourinary

Although this was not observed in clinical trials with REMINYL®, cholinomimetics may cause bladder outflow obstruction.

Neurological Conditions

Seizures: Cholinesterase inhibitors are believed to have some potential to cause generalized convulsions. However, seizure activity may also be a manifestation of Alzheimer's disease. In clinical trials, there was no increase in the incidence of convulsions with REMINYL® compared to placebo.

Pulmonary Conditions

Because of its cholinomimetic action, galantamine should be prescribed with care to patients with a history of severe asthma or obstructive pulmonary disease.

PRECAUTIONS

Information for Patients and Caregivers: Caregivers should be instructed in the recommended administration (twice per day, preferably with morning and evening meal) and dose escalation (dose increases should follow minimum of four weeks at prior dose).

Patients and caregivers should be advised that the most frequent adverse events associated with use of the drug can be minimized by following the recommended dosage and administration.

Patients and caregivers should be informed that if therapy has been interrupted for several days or longer, the patient should be restarted at the lowest dose and the dose escalated to the current dose.

Caregivers should be instructed in the correct procedure for administering REMINYL® (galantamine hydrobromide) Oral Solution. In addition, they should be informed of the existence of an Instruction Sheet (included with the product) describing how the solution is to be administered. They should be urged to read this sheet prior to administering REMINYL® Oral Solution. Caregivers should direct questions about the administration of the solution to either their physician or pharmacist.

Special Populations

Hepatic Impairment

In patients with moderately impaired hepatic function, dose titration should proceed cautiously (See **CLINICAL PHARMACOLOGY** and **DOSAGE AND ADMINISTRATION**). The use of REMINYL® (galantamine hydrobromide) in patients with severe hepatic impairment is not recommended.

Renal Impairment

In patients with moderately impaired renal function, dose titration should proceed cautiously (See **CLINICAL PHARMACOLOGY** and **DOSAGE AND ADMINISTRATION**). In patients with severely impaired renal function (CL_{cr} < 9 mL/min) the use of REMINYL® is not recommended.

Continued on next page

Reminyl—Cont.

Drug-Drug Interactions
Use with Anticholinergics
REMINYL® has the potential to interfere with the activity of anticholinergic medications.
Use with Cholinomimetics and Other Cholinesterase Inhibitors
A synergistic effect is expected when cholinesterase inhibitors are given concurrently with succinylcholine, other cholinesterase inhibitors, similar neuromuscular blocking agents or cholinergic agonists such as bethanechol.
A) Effect of Other Drugs on Galantamine
In vitro
CYP3A4 and CYP2D6 are the major enzymes involved in the metabolism of galantamine. CYP3A4 mediates the formation of galantamine-N-oxide; CYP2D6 leads to the formation of O-desmethyl-galantamine. Because galantamine is also glucuronidated and excreted unchanged, no single pathway appears predominant.
In vivo
Cimetidine and Ranitidine: Galantamine was administered as a single dose of 4 mg on day 2 of a 3-day treatment with either cimetidine (800 mg daily) or ranitidine (300 mg daily). Cimetidine increased the bioavailability of galantamine by approximately 16%. Ranitidine had no effect on the PK of galantamine.
Ketoconazole: Ketoconazole, a strong inhibitor of CYP3A4 and an inhibitor of CYP2D6, at a dose of 200 mg BID for 4 days, increased the AUC of galantamine by 30%.
Erythromycin: Erythromycin, a moderate inhibitor of CYP3A4, at a dose of 500 mg QID for 4 days, affected the AUC of galantamine minimally (10% increase).
Paroxetine: Paroxetine, a strong inhibitor of CYP2D6, at 20 mg/day for 16 days, increased the oral bioavailability of galantamine by about 40%.
B) Effect of Galantamine on Other Drugs
In vitro
Galantamine did not inhibit the metabolic pathways catalyzed by CYP1A2, CYP2A6, CYP3A4, CYP4A, CYP2C, CYP2D6 or CYP2E1. This indicates that the inhibitory potential of galantamine towards the major forms of cytochrome P450 is very low.
In vivo
Warfarin: Galantamine at 24 mg/day had no effect on the pharmacokinetics of R-and-S-warfarin (25 mg single dose) or on the prothrombin time. The protein binding of warfarin was unaffected by galantamine.
Digoxin: Galantamine at 24 mg/day had no effect on the steady-state pharmacokinetics of digoxin (0.375 mg once daily) when they were coadministered. In this study, however, one healthy subject was hospitalized for 2nd and 3rd degree heart block and bradycardia.
Carcinogenesis, Mutagenesis and Impairment of Fertility
In a 24-month oral carcinogenicity study in rats, a slight increase in endometrial adenocarcinomas was observed at 10 mg/kg/day (4 times the Maximum Recommended Human Dose [MRHD] on a mg/m^2 basis or 6 times on an exposure [AUC] basis and 30 mg/kg/day (12 times MRHD on a mg/m^2 basis or 19 times on an AUC basis). No increase in neoplastic changes was observed in females at 2.5 mg/kg/day (equivalent to the MRHD on a mg/m^2 basis or 2 times on an AUC basis) or in males up to the highest dose tested of 30 mg/kg/day (12 times the MRHD on a mg/m^2 and AUC basis).
Galantamine was not carcinogenic in a 6-month oral carcinogenicity study in transgenic (P 53-deficient) mice up to 20 mg/kg/day, or in a 24-month oral carcinogenicity study in male and female mice up to 10 mg/kg/day (2 times the MRHD on a mg/m^2 basis and equivalent on an AUC basis).
Galantamine produced no evidence of genotoxic potential when evaluated in the *in vitro* Ames *S. typhimurium* or *E. coli* reverse mutation assay, *in vitro* mouse lymphoma assay, *in vivo* micronucleus test in mice, or *in vitro* chromosome aberration assay in Chinese hamster ovary cells.
No impairment of fertility was seen in rats given up to 16 mg/kg/day (7 times the MRHD on a mg/m^2 basis) for 14 days prior to mating in females and for 60 days prior to mating in males.
Pregnancy
Pregnancy Category B: In a study in which rats were dosed from day 14 (females) or day 60 (males) prior to mating through the period of organogenesis, a slightly increased incidence of skeletal variations was observed at doses of 8 mg/kg/day (3 times the Maximum Recommended Human Dose [MRHD] on a mg/m^2 basis) and 16 mg/kg/day. In a study in which pregnant rats were dosed from the beginning of organogenesis through day 21 post-partum, pup weights were decreased at 8 and 16 mg/kg/day, but no adverse effects on other postnatal developmental parameters were seen. The doses causing the above effects in rats produced slight maternal toxicity. No major malformations were caused in rats given up to 16 mg/kg/day. No drug related teratogenic effects were observed in rabbits given up to 40 mg/kg/day (32 times the MRHD on a mg/m^2 basis) during the period of organogenesis.
There are no adequate and well-controlled studies of REMINYL® in pregnant women. REMINYL® should be used during pregnancy only if the potential benefit justifies the potential risk to the fetus.
Nursing Mothers
It is not known whether galantamine is excreted in human breast milk. REMINYL® has no indication for use in nursing mothers.
Pediatric Use
There are no adequate and well-controlled trials documenting the safety and efficacy of galantamine in any illness occurring in children. Therefore, use of REMINYL® in children is not recommended.

ADVERSE REACTIONS

Adverse Events Leading to Discontinuation: In two large scale, placebo-controlled trials of 6 months duration, in which patients were titrated weekly from 8 to 16 to 24, and to 32 mg/day, the risk of discontinuation because of an adverse event in the galantamine group exceeded that in the placebo group by about threefold. In contrast, in a 5-month trial with escalation of the dose by 8 mg/day every 4 weeks, the overall risk of discontinuation because of an adverse event was 7%, 7%, and 10% for the placebo, galantamine 16 mg/day, and galantamine 24 mg/day groups, respectively, with gastrointestinal adverse effects the principle reason for discontinuing galantamine. Table 1 shows the most frequent adverse events leading to discontinuation in this study.

Table 1: Most Frequent Adverse Events Leading to Discontinuation in a Placebo-controlled, Double-blind Trial with a 4-Week Dose Escalation Schedule

	4-week Escalation		
	Placebo	16 mg/day	24 mg/day
Adverse Event	N=286	N=279	N=273
Nausea	<1%	2%	4%
Vomiting	0%	1%	3%
Anorexia	<1%	1%	<1%
Dizziness	<1%	2%	1%
Syncope	0%	0%	1%

Adverse Events Reported in Controlled Trials: The reported adverse events in REMINYL® (galantamine hydrobromide) trials reflect experience gained under closely monitored conditions in a highly selected patient population. In actual practice or in other clinical trials, these frequency estimates may not apply, as the conditions of use, reporting behavior and the types of patients treated may differ.
The majority of these adverse events occurred during the dose-escalation period. In those patients who experienced the most frequent adverse event, nausea, the median duration of the nausea was 5-7 days.
Administration of REMINYL® with food, the use of antiemetic medication, and ensuring adequate fluid intake may reduce the impact of these events.
The most frequent adverse events, defined as those occurring at a frequency of at least 5% and at least twice the rate on placebo with the recommended maintenance dose of either 16 or 24 mg/day of REMINYL® under conditions of every 4 week dose-escalation for each dose increment of 8 mg/day, are shown in Table 2. These events were primarily gastrointestinal and tended to be less frequent with the 16 mg/day recommended initial maintenance dose.

Table 2: The Most Frequent Adverse Events in the Placebo-controlled Trial with Dose Escalation Every 4 Weeks Occurring in at Least 5% of Patients Receiving REMINYL® and at Least Twice the Rate on Placebo.

	Placebo	REMINYL® 16 mg/day	REMINYL® 24 mg/day
Adverse Event	N=286	N=279	N=273
Nausea	5%	13%	17%
Vomiting	1%	6%	10%
Diarrhea	6%	12%	6%
Anorexia	3%	7%	9%
Weight decrease	1%	5%	5%

Table 3: The most common adverse events (adverse events occurring with an incidence of at least 2% with REMINYL® treatment and in which the incidence was greater than with placebo treatment) are listed in Table 3 for four placebo-controlled trials for patients treated with 16 or 24 mg/day of REMINYL®.

Table 3: Adverse Events Reported in at Least 2% of Patients with Alzheimer's Disease Administered REMINYL® and at a Frequency Greater than with Placebo

Body System Adverse Event	Placebo (N=801)	REMINYL®[a] (N=1040)
Body as a whole – general disorders		
Fatigue	3%	5%
Syncope	1%	2%
Central & peripheral nervous system disorders		
Dizziness	6%	9%
Headache	5%	8%
Tremor	2%	3%
Gastrointestinal system disorders		
Nausea	9%	24%
Vomiting	4%	13%
Diarrhea	7%	9%
Abdominal pain	4%	5%
Dyspepsia	2%	5%
Heart rate and rhythm disorders		
Bradycardia	1%	2%
Metabolic and nutritional disorders		
Weight decrease	2%	7%
Psychiatric disorders		
Anorexia	3%	9%
Depression	5%	7%
Insomnia	4%	5%
Somnolence	3%	4%
Red blood cell disorders		
Anemia	2%	3%
Respiratory system disorders		
Rhinitis	3%	4%
Urinary system disorders		
Urinary tract infection	7%	8%
Hematuria	2%	3%

a: Adverse events in patients treated with 16 or 24 mg/day of REMINYL® in four placebo-controlled trials are included.

Adverse events occurring with an incidence of at least 2% in placebo-treated patients that was either equal to or greater than with REMINYL® treatment were constipation, agitation, confusion, anxiety, hallucination, injury, back pain, peripheral edema, asthenia, chest pain, urinary incontinence, upper respiratory tract infection, bronchitis, coughing, hypertension, fall, and purpura.
There were no important differences in adverse event rate related to dose or sex. There were too few non-Caucasian patients to assess the effects of race on adverse event rates.
No clinically relevant abnormalities in laboratory values were observed.
Other Adverse Events Observed During Clinical Trials
REMINYL® was administered to 3055 patients with Alzheimer's disease. A total of 2357 patients received galantamine in placebo-controlled trials and 761 patients with Alzheimer's disease received galantamine 24 mg/day, the maximum recommended maintenance dose. About 1000 patients received galantamine for at least one year and approximately 200 patients received galantamine for two years.
To establish the rate of adverse events, data from all patients receiving any dose of galantamine in 8 placebo-controlled trials and 6 open-label extension trials were pooled. The methodology to gather and codify these adverse events was standardized across trials, using WHO terminology. All adverse events occurring in approximately 0.1% are included, except for those already listed elsewhere in labeling, WHO terms too general to be informative, or events unlikely to be drug caused. Events are classified by body system and listed using the following definitions: frequent adverse events - those occurring in at least 1/100 patients; infrequent adverse events - those occurring in 1/100 to 1/1000 patients; rare adverse events - those occurring in fewer than 1/1000 patients. These adverse events are not necessarily related to REMINYL® treatment and in most cases were observed at a similar frequency in placebo-treated patients in the controlled studies.
Body As a Whole – General Disorders: *Frequent:* chest pain
Cardiovascular System Disorders: *Infrequent:* postural hypotension, hypotension, dependent edema, cardiac failure
Central & Peripheral Nervous System Disorders: *Infrequent:* vertigo, hypertonia, convulsions, involuntary muscle

contractions, paresthesia, ataxia, hypokinesia, hyperkinesia, apraxia, aphasia

Gastrointestinal System Disorders: *Frequent:* flatulence; *Infrequent:* gastritis, melena, dysphagia, rectal hemorrhage, dry mouth, saliva increased, diverticulitis, gastroenteritis, hiccup; *rare:* esophageal perforation

Heart Rate & Rhythm Disorders: *Infrequent:* AV block, palpitation, atrial fibrillation, QT prolonged, bundle branch block, supraventricular tachycardia, T-wave inversion, ventricular tachycardia

Metabolic & Nutritional Disorders: *Infrequent:* hyperglycemia, alkaline phosphatase increased

Platelet, Bleeding & Clotting Disorders: *Infrequent:* purpura, epistaxis, thrombocytopenia

Psychiatric Disorders: *Infrequent:* apathy, paroniria, paranoid reaction, libido increased, delirium

Urinary System Disorders: *Frequent:* incontinence; *Infrequent:* hematuria, micturition frequency, cystitis, urinary retention, nocturia, renal calculi

OVERDOSAGE

Because strategies for the management of overdose are continually evolving, it is advisable to contact a poison control center to determine the latest recommendations for the management of an overdose of any drug.

As in any case of overdose, general supportive measures should be utilized. Signs and symptoms of significant overdosing of galantamine are predicted to be similar to those of overdosing of other cholinomimetics. These effects generally involve the central nervous system, the parasympathetic nervous system, and the neuromuscular junction. In addition to muscle weakness or fasciculations, some or all of the following signs of cholinergic crisis may develop: severe nausea, vomiting, gastrointestinal cramping, salivation, lacrimation, urination, defecation, sweating, bradycardia, hypotension, respiratory depression, collapse and convulsions. Increasing muscle weakness is a possibility and may result in death if respiratory muscles are involved.

Tertiary anticholinergics such as atropine may be used as an antidote for REMINYL® (galantamine hydrobromide) overdosage. Intravenous atropine sulfate titrated to effect is recommended at an initial dose of 0.5 to 1.0 mg i.v. with subsequent doses based upon clinical response. Atypical responses in blood pressure and heart rate have been reported with other cholinomimetics when coadministered with quaternary anticholinergics. It is not known whether REMINYL® and/or its metabolites can be removed by dialysis (hemodialysis, peritoneal dialysis, or hemofiltration). Dose-related signs of toxicity in animals included hypoactivity, tremors, clonic convulsions, salivation, lacrimation, chromodacryorrhea, mucoid feces, and dyspnea.

In a postmarketing report, one patient who had been taking 4 mg of galantamine daily for a week inadvertantly ingested eight 4 mg tablets (32 mg total) on a single day. Subsequently, she developed bradycardia, QT prolongation, ventricular tachycardia and torsades de pointes accompanied by a brief loss of consciousness for which she required hospital treatment.

DOSAGE AND ADMINISTRATION

The dosage of REMINYL® (galantamine hydrobromide) shown to be effective in controlled clinical trials is 16-32 mg/day given as twice daily dosing. As the dose of 32 mg/day is less well tolerated than lower doses and does not provide increased effectiveness, the recommended dose range is 16-24 mg/day given in a BID regimen. The dose of 24 mg/day did not provide a statistically significant greater clinical benefit than 16 mg/day. It is possible, however, that a daily dose of 24 mg of REMINYL® might provide additional benefit for some patients.

The recommended starting dose of REMINYL® is 4 mg twice a day (8 mg/day). After a minimum of 4 weeks of treatment, if this dose is well tolerated, the dose should be increased to 8 mg twice a day (16 mg/day). A further increase to 12 mg twice a day (24 mg/day) should be attempted only after a minimum of 4 weeks at the previous dose.

REMINYL® should be administered twice a day, preferably with morning and evening meals.

Patients and caregivers should be informed that if therapy has been interrupted for several days or longer, the patient should be restarted at the lowest dose and the dose escalated to the current dose.

Caregivers should be instructed in the correct procedure for administering REMINYL® Oral Solution. In addition, they should be informed of the existence of an Instruction Sheet (included with the product) describing how the solution is to be administered. They should be urged to read this sheet prior to administering REMINYL® Oral Solution. Caregivers should direct questions about the administration of the solution to either their physician or pharmacist.

The abrupt withdrawal of REMINYL® in those patients who had been receiving doses in the effective range was not associated with an increased frequency of adverse events in comparison with those continuing to receive the same doses of that drug. The beneficial effects of REMINYL® are lost, however, when the drug is discontinued.

Doses in Special Populations

Galantamine plasma concentrations may be increased in patients with moderate to severe hepatic impairment. In patients with moderately impaired hepatic function (Child-Pugh score of 7-9), the dose should generally not exceed 16 mg/day. The use of REMINYL® in patients with severe hepatic impairment (Child-Pugh score of 10-15) is not recommended.

For patients with moderate renal impairment the dose should generally not exceed 16 mg/day. In patients with severe renal impairment (creatinine clearance < 9 mL/min), the use of REMINYL® is not recommended.

HOW SUPPLIED

REMINYL® (galantamine hydrobromide) tablets are imprinted "JANSSEN" on one side, and "G" and the strength "4", "8", or "12" on the other.

4 mg off-white tablet: bottles of 60 NDC 50458-390-60
8 mg pink tablet: bottles of 60 NDC 50458-391-60
12 mg orange-brown tablet: bottles of 60 NDC 50458-392-60

REMINYL® (galantamine hydrobromide) 4 mg/mL oral solution (NDC 50458-399-10) is a clear colorless solution supplied in 100 mL bottles with a calibrated (in milligrams and milliliters) pipette. The minimum calibrated volume is 0.5 mL, while the maximum calibrated volume is 4 mL.

Storage and Handling

REMINYL® tablets should be stored at 25°C (77°F); excursions permitted to 15-30°C (59-86°F) [see USP Controlled Room Temperature].

REMINYL® Oral Solution should be stored at 25°C (77°F); excursions permitted to 15-30°C (59-86°F) [see USP Controlled Room Temperature]. DO NOT FREEZE.

Keep out of reach of children.

7517304
October 2001
US Patent No. 4,663,318

REMINYL® tablets are manufactured by:
Janssen-Cilag SpA
Latina, Italy
REMINYL® oral solution is manufactured by:
Janssen Pharmaceutica N.V.
Beerse, Belgium
REMINYL® tablets and oral solution are distributed by:
Janssen Pharmaceutica Products, L.P.
Titusville, NJ 08560
Janssen Pharmaceutica Products, L.P.

RISPERDAL® ℞

[ris 'pər dăl]
(risperidone)
Tablets/Oral Solution

Prescribing information for this product, which appears on pages 1796–1800 of the 2002 PDR, has been completely revised as follows. Please write "See Supplement A" next to the product heading.

DESCRIPTION

RISPERDAL® (risperidone) is a psychotropic agent belonging to a new chemical class, the benzisoxazole derivatives. The chemical designation is 3-[2-[4-(6-fluoro-1,2-benzisoxazol-3-yl)-1-piperidinyl]ethyl]-6,7,8,9-tetrahydro-2-methyl-4*H*-pyrido[1,2-a]pyrimidin-4-one. Its molecular formula is $C_{23}H_{27}FN_4O_2$ and its molecular weight is 410.49. The structural formula is:

Risperidone is a white to slightly beige powder. It is practically insoluble in water, freely soluble in methylene chloride, and soluble in methanol and 0.1 N HCl.

RISPERDAL® tablets are available in 0.25 mg (dark yellow), 0.5 mg (red-brown), 1 mg (white), 2 mg (orange), 3 mg (yellow), and 4 mg (green) strengths. Inactive ingredients are colloidal silicon dioxide, hydroxypropyl methylcellulose, lactose, magnesium stearate, microcrystalline cellulose, propylene glycol, sodium lauryl sulfate, and starch (corn). Tablets of 0.25, 0.5, 2, 3, and 4 mg also contain talc and titanium dioxide. The 0.25 mg tablets contain yellow iron oxide; the 0.5 mg tablets contain red iron oxide, the 2 mg tablets contain FD&C Yellow No. 6 Aluminum Lake; the 3 mg and 4 mg tablets contain D&C Yellow No. 10; the 4 mg tablets contain FD&C Blue No. 2 Aluminum Lake.

RISPERDAL® is also available as a 1 mg/mL oral solution. The inactive ingredients for this solution are tartaric acid, benzoic acid, sodium hydroxide and purified water.

CLINICAL PHARMACOLOGY

Pharmacodynamics

The mechanism of action of RISPERDAL® (risperidone), as with other drugs used to treat schizophrenia, is unknown. However, it has been proposed that this drug's therapeutic activity in schizophrenia is mediated through a combination of dopamine type 2 (D_2) and serotonin type 2 ($5HT_2$) antagonism. Antagonism at receptors other than D_2 and $5HT_2$ may explain some of the other effects of RISPERDAL®.

RISPERDAL® is a selective monoaminergic antagonist with high affinity (Ki of 0.12 to 7.3 nM) for the serotonin type 2 ($5HT_2$), dopamine type 2 (D_2), α_1 and α_2 adrenergic, and H_1 histaminergic receptors. RISPERDAL® antagonizes other receptors, but with lower potency. RISPERDAL® has low to moderate affinity (Ki of 47 to 253 nM) for the serotonin $5HT_{1C}$, $5HT_{1D}$, and $5HT_{1A}$ receptors, weak affinity (Ki of 620 to 800 nM) for the dopamine D_1 and haloperidol-sensitive sigma site, and no affinity (when tested at concentrations $>10^{-5}$ M) for cholinergic muscarinic or β_1 and β_2 adrenergic receptors.

Pharmacokinetics

Risperidone is well absorbed, as illustrated by a mass balance study involving a single 1 mg oral dose of ^{14}C-risperidone as a solution in three healthy male volunteers. Total recovery of radioactivity at one week was 85%, including 70% in the urine and 15% in the feces.

Risperidone is extensively metabolized in the liver by cytochrome $P_{450}IID_6$ to a major active metabolite, 9-hydroxyrisperidone, which is the predominant circulating specie, and appears approximately equi-effective with risperidone with respect to receptor binding activity and some effects in animals. (A second minor pathway is *N*-dealkylation). Consequently, the clinical effect of the drug likely results from the combined concentrations of risperidone plus 9-hydroxyrisperidone. Plasma concentrations of risperidone, 9-hydroxyrisperidone, and risperidone plus 9-hydroxyrisperidone are dose proportional over the dosing range of 1 to 16 mg daily (0.5 to 8 mg BID). The relative oral bioavailability of risperidone from a tablet was 94% (CV=10%) when compared to a solution. Food does not affect either the rate or extent of absorption of risperidone. Thus, risperidone can be given with or without meals. The absolute oral bioavailability of risperidone was 70% (CV=25%).

The enzyme catalyzing hydroxylation of risperidone to 9-hydroxyrisperidone is cytochrome $P_{450}IID_6$, also called debrisoquin hydroxylase, the enzyme responsible for metabolism of many neuroleptics, antidepressants, antiarrhythmics, and other drugs. Cytochrome $P_{450}IID_6$ is subject to genetic polymorphism (about 6-8% of Caucasians, and a very low percent of Asians have little or no activity and are "poor metabolizers") and to inhibition by a variety of substrates and some non-substrates, notably quinidine. Extensive metabolizers convert risperidone rapidly into 9-hydroxyrisperidone, while poor metabolizers convert it much more slowly. Extensive metabolizers, therefore, have lower risperidone and higher 9-hydroxyrisperidone concentrations than poor metabolizers. Following oral administration of solution or tablet, mean peak plasma concentrations occurred at about 1 hour. Peak 9-hydroxyrisperidone occurred at about 3 hours in extensive metabolizers, and 17 hours in poor metabolizers. The apparent half-life of risperidone was three hours (CV=30%) in extensive metabolizers and 20 hours (CV=40%) in poor metabolizers. The apparent half-life of 9-hydroxyrisperidone was about 21 hours (CV=20%) in extensive metabolizers and 30 hours (CV=25%) in poor metabolizers. Steady-state concentrations of risperidone are reached in 1 day in extensive metabolizers and would be expected to reach steady state in about 5 days in poor metabolizers. Steady-state concentrations of 9-hydroxyrisperidone are reached in 5–6 days (measured in extensive metabolizers).

Because risperidone and 9-hydroxyrisperidone are approximately equi-effective, the sum of their concentrations is pertinent. The pharmacokinetics of the sum of risperidone and 9-hydroxyrisperidone, after single and multiple doses, were similar in extensive and poor metabolizers, with an overall mean elimination half-life of about 20 hours. In analyses comparing adverse reaction rates in extensive and poor metabolizers in controlled and open studies, no important differences were seen.

Risperidone could be subject to two kinds of drug-drug interactions. First, inhibitors of cytochrome $P_{450}IID_6$ could interfere with conversion of risperidone to 9-hydroxyrisperidone. This in fact occurs with quinidine, giving essentially all recipients a risperidone pharmacokinetic profile typical of poor metabolizers. The favorable and adverse effects of risperidone in patients receiving quinidine have not been evaluated, but observations in a modest number (n=70) of poor metabolizers given risperidone do not suggest important differences between poor and extensive metabolizers. It would also be possible for risperidone to interfere with metabolism of other drugs metabolized by cytochrome $P_{450}IID_6$. Relatively weak binding of risperidone to the enzyme suggests this is unlikely (See PRECAUTIONS and DRUG INTERACTIONS).

The plasma protein binding of risperidone was about 90% over the in vitro concentration range of 0.5 to 200 ng/mL and increased with increasing concentrations of α_1-acid glycoprotein. The plasma binding of 9-hydroxyrisperidone was 77%. Neither the parent nor the metabolite displaced each other from the plasma binding sites. High therapeutic concentrations of sulfamethazine (100 µg/mL), warfarin (10 µg/mL) and carbamazepine (10 µg/mL) caused only a slight increase in the free fraction of risperidone at 10 ng/mL and 9-hydroxyrisperidone at 50 ng/mL, changes of unknown clinical significance.

Special Populations

Renal Impairment: In patients with moderate to severe renal disease, clearance of the sum of risperidone and its active metabolite decreased by 60% compared to young healthy subjects. RISPERDAL® doses should be reduced in patients with renal disease (See PRECAUTIONS and DOSAGE AND ADMINISTRATION).

Hepatic Impairment: While the pharmacokinetics of risperidone in subjects with liver disease were comparable to those in young healthy subjects, the mean free fraction of risperidone in plasma was increased by about 35% because of the diminished concentration of both albumin and α_1-acid glycoprotein. RISPERDAL® doses should be reduced in pa-

Continued on next page

Risperdal—Cont.

tients with liver disease (See PRECAUTIONS and DOSAGE AND ADMINISTRATION).

Elderly: In healthy elderly subjects renal clearance of both risperidone and 9-hydroxyrisperidone was decreased, and elimination half-lives were prolonged compared to young healthy subjects. Dosing should be modified accordingly in the elderly patients (See DOSAGE AND ADMINISTRATION).

Race and Gender Effects: No specific pharmacokinetic study was conducted to investigate race and gender effects, but a population pharmacokinetic analysis did not identify important differences in the disposition of risperidone due to gender (whether corrected for body weight or not) or race.

Clinical Trials

The efficacy of RISPERDAL® in the treatment of schizophrenia was established in four short-term (4 to 8-week) controlled trials of psychotic inpatients who met DSM-III-R criteria for schizophrenia.

Several instruments were used for assessing psychiatric signs and symptoms in these studies, among them the Brief Psychiatric Rating Scale (BPRS), a multi-item inventory of general psychopathology traditionally used to evaluate the effects of drug treatment in schizophrenia. The BPRS psychosis cluster (conceptual disorganization, hallucinatory behavior, suspiciousness, and unusual thought content) is considered a particularly useful subset for assessing actively psychotic schizophrenic patients. A second traditional assessment, the Clinical Global Impression (CGI), reflects the impression of a skilled observer, fully familiar with the manifestations of schizophrenia, about the overall clinical state of the patient. In addition, two more recently developed, but less well evaluated scales, were employed; these included the Positive and Negative Syndrome Scale (PANSS) and the Scale for Assessing Negative Symptoms (SANS).

The results of the trials follow:

(1) In a 6-week, placebo-controlled trial (n=160) involving titration of RISPERDAL® in doses up to 10 mg/day (BID schedule), RISPERDAL® was generally superior to placebo on the BPRS total score, on the BPRS psychosis cluster, and marginally superior to placebo on the SANS.

(2) In an 8-week, placebo-controlled trial (n=513) involving 4 fixed doses of RISPERDAL® (2, 6, 10, and 16 mg/day, on a BID schedule), all 4 RISPERDAL® groups were generally superior to placebo on the BPRS total score, BPRS psychosis cluster, and CGI severity score; the 3 highest RISPERDAL® dose groups were generally superior to placebo on the PANSS negative subscale. The most consistently positive responses on all measures were seen for the 6 mg dose group, and there was no suggestion of increased benefit from larger doses.

(3) In an 8-week, dose comparison trial (n=1356) involving 5 fixed doses of RISPERDAL® (1, 4, 8, 12, and 16 mg/day, on a BID schedule), the four highest RISPERDAL® dose groups were generally superior to the 1 mg RISPERDAL® dose group on BPRS total score, BPRS psychosis cluster, and CGI severity score. None of the dose groups were superior to the 1 mg group on the PANSS negative subscale. The most consistently positive responses were seen for the 4 mg dose group.

(4) In a 4-week, placebo-controlled dose comparison trial (n=246) involving 2 fixed doses of RISPERDAL® (4 and 8 mg/day on a QD schedule), both RISPERDAL® dose groups were generally superior to placebo on several PANSS measures, including a response measure (> 20% reduction in PANSS total score), PANSS total score, and the BPRS psychosis cluster (derived from PANSS). The results were generally stronger for the 8 mg than for the 4 mg dose group.

Long-Term Efficacy

In a longer-term trial, 365 adult outpatients predominantly meeting DSM-IV criteria for schizophrenia and who had been clinically stable for at least 4 weeks on an antipsychotic medication were randomized to RISPERDAL® (2–8 mg/day) or to an active comparator, for 1 to 2 years of observation for relapse. Patients receiving RISPERDAL® experienced a significantly longer time to relapse over this time period compared to those receiving the active comparator.

INDICATIONS AND USAGE

RISPERDAL® (risperidone) is indicated for the treatment of schizophrenia.

The efficacy of RISPERDAL® in schizophrenia was established in short-term (6 to 8-weeks) controlled trials of schizophrenic inpatients (See CLINICAL PHARMACOLOGY).

The efficacy of RISPERDAL® in delaying relapse was demonstrated in schizophrenic patients who had been clinically stable for at least 4 weeks before initiation of treatment with RISPERDAL® or an active comparator and who were then observed for relapse during a period of 1 to 2 years (See Clinical Trials, under CLINICAL PHARMACOLOGY). Nevertheless, the physician who elects to use RISPERDAL® for extended periods should periodically re-evaluate the long-term usefulness of the drug for the individual patient (See DOSAGE AND ADMINISTRATION).

CONTRAINDICATIONS

RISPERDAL® (risperidone) is contraindicated in patients with a known hypersensitivity to the product.

WARNINGS

Neuroleptic Malignant Syndrome (NMS)

A potentially fatal symptom complex sometimes referred to as Neuroleptic Malignant Syndrome (NMS) has been reported in association with antipsychotic drugs. Clinical manifestations of NMS are hyperpyrexia, muscle rigidity, altered mental status and evidence of autonomic instability (irregular pulse or blood pressure, tachycardia, diaphoresis and cardiac dysrhythmia). Additional signs may include elevated creatine phosphokinase, myoglobinuria (rhabdomyolysis), and acute renal failure.

The diagnostic evaluation of patients with this syndrome is complicated. In arriving at a diagnosis, it is important to identify cases where the clinical presentation includes both serious medical illness (e.g., pneumonia, systemic infection, etc.) and untreated or inadequately treated extrapyramidal signs and symptoms (EPS). Other important considerations in the differential diagnosis include central anticholinergic toxicity, heat stroke, drug fever, and primary central nervous system pathology.

The management of NMS should include: 1) immediate discontinuation of antipsychotic drugs and other drugs not essential to concurrent therapy; 2) intensive symptomatic treatment and medical monitoring; and 3) treatment of any concomitant serious medical problems for which specific treatments are available. There is no general agreement about specific pharmacological treatment regimens for uncomplicated NMS.

If a patient requires antipsychotic drug treatment after recovery from NMS, the potential reintroduction of drug therapy should be carefully considered. The patient should be carefully monitored, since recurrences of NMS have been reported.

Tardive Dyskinesia

A syndrome of potentially irreversible, involuntary, dyskinetic movements may develop in patients treated with antipsychotic drugs. Although the prevalence of the syndrome appears to be highest among the elderly, especially elderly women, it is impossible to rely upon prevalence estimates to predict, at the inception of antipsychotic treatment, which patients are likely to develop the syndrome. Whether antipsychotic drug products differ in their potential to cause tardive dyskinesia is unknown.

The risk of developing tardive dyskinesia and the likelihood that it will become irreversible are believed to increase as the duration of treatment and the total cumulative dose of antipsychotic drugs administered to the patient increase. However, the syndrome can develop, although much less commonly, after relatively brief treatment periods at low doses.

There is no known treatment for established cases of tardive dyskinesia, although the syndrome may remit, partially or completely, if antipsychotic treatment is withdrawn. Antipsychotic treatment, itself, however, may suppress (or partially suppress) the signs and symptoms of the syndrome and thereby may possibly mask the underlying process. The effect that symptomatic suppression has upon the long-term course of the syndrome is unknown.

Given these considerations, RISPERDAL® (risperidone) should be prescribed in a manner that is most likely to minimize the occurrence of tardive dyskinesia. Chronic antipsychotic treatment should generally be reserved for patients who suffer from a chronic illness that (1) is known to respond to antipsychotic drugs, and (2) for whom alternative, equally effective, but potentially less harmful treatments are not available or appropriate. In patients who do require chronic treatment, the smallest dose and the shortest duration of treatment producing a satisfactory clinical response should be sought. The need for continued treatment should be reassessed periodically.

If signs and symptoms of tardive dyskinesia appear in a patient on RISPERDAL®, drug discontinuation should be considered. However, some patients may require treatment with RISPERDAL® despite the presence of the syndrome.

Potential for Proarrhythmic Effects: Risperidone and/or 9-hydroxyrisperidone appears to lengthen the QT interval in some patients, although there is no average increase in treated patients, even at 12–16 mg/day, well above the recommended dose. Other drugs that prolong the QT interval have been associated with the occurrence of torsades de pointes, a life-threatening arrhythmia. Bradycardia, electrolyte imbalance, concomitant use with other drugs that prolong QT, or the presence of congenital prolongation in QT can increase the risk for occurrence of this arrhythmia.

PRECAUTIONS

General

Orthostatic Hypotension: RISPERDAL® (risperidone) may induce orthostatic hypotension associated with dizziness, tachycardia, and in some patients, syncope, especially during the initial dose-titration period, probably reflecting its alpha-adrenergic antagonistic properties. Syncope was reported in 0.2% (6/2607) of RISPERDAL® treated patients in phase 2–3 studies. The risk of orthostatic hypotension and syncope may be minimized by limiting the initial dose to 2 mg total (either QD or 1 mg BID) in normal adults and 0.5 mg BID in the elderly and patients with renal or hepatic impairment (See DOSAGE AND ADMINISTRATION). Monitoring of orthostatic vital signs should be considered in patients for whom this is of concern. A dose reduction should be considered if hypotension occurs. RISPERDAL® should be used with particular caution in patients with known cardiovascular disease (history of myocardial infarction or ischemia, heart failure, or conduction abnormalities), cerebrovascular disease, and conditions which would predispose patients to hypotension e.g., dehydration and hypovolemia. Clinically significant hypotension has been observed with concomitant use of RISPERDAL® and antihypertensive medication.

Seizures: During premarketing testing, seizures occurred in 0.3% (9/2607) of RISPERDAL® treated patients, two in association with hyponatremia. RISPERDAL® should be used cautiously in patients with a history of seizures.

Dysphagia: Esophageal dysmotility and aspiration have been associated with antipsychotic drug use. Aspiration pneumonia is a common cause of morbidity and mortality in patients with advanced Alzheimer's dementia. RISPERDAL® and other antipsychotic drugs should be used cautiously in patients at risk for aspiration pneumonia.

Hyperprolactinemia: As with other drugs that antagonize dopamine D_2 receptors, risperidone elevates prolactin levels and the elevation persists during chronic administration. Tissue culture experiments indicate that approximately one-third of human breast cancers are prolactin dependent in vitro, a factor of potential importance if the prescription of these drugs is contemplated in a patient with previously detected breast cancer. Although disturbances such as galactorrhea, amenorrhea, gynecomastia, and impotence have been reported with prolactin-elevating compounds, the clinical significance of elevated serum prolactin levels is unknown for most patients. As is common with compounds which increase prolactin release, an increase in pituitary gland, mammary gland, and pancreatic islet cell hyperplasia and/or neoplasia was observed in the risperidone carcinogenicity studies conducted in mice and rats (See CARCINOGENESIS). However, neither clinical studies nor epidemiologic studies conducted to date have shown an association between chronic administration of this class of drugs and tumorigenesis in humans; the available evidence is considered too limited to be conclusive at this time.

Potential for Cognitive and Motor Impairment: Somnolence was a commonly reported adverse event associated with RISPERDAL® treatment, especially when ascertained by direct questioning of patients. This adverse event is dose related, and in a study utilizing a checklist to detect adverse events, 41% of the high dose patients (RISPERDAL® 16 mg/day) reported somnolence compared to 16% of placebo patients. Direct questioning is more sensitive for detecting adverse events than spontaneous reporting, by which 8% of RISPERDAL® 16 mg/day patients and 1% of placebo patients reported somnolence as an adverse event. Since RISPERDAL® has the potential to impair judgment, thinking, or motor skills, patients should be cautioned about operating hazardous machinery, including automobiles, until they are reasonably certain that RISPERDAL® therapy does not affect them adversely.

Priapism: Rare cases of priapism have been reported. While the relationship of the events to RISPERDAL® use has not been established, other drugs with alpha-adrenergic blocking effects have been reported to induce priapism, and it is possible that RISPERDAL® may share this capacity. Severe priapism may require surgical intervention.

Thrombotic Thrombocytopenic Purpura (TTP): A single case of TTP was reported in a 28 year-old female patient receiving RISPERDAL® in a large, open premarketing experience (approximately 1300 patients). She experienced jaundice, fever, and bruising, but eventually recovered after receiving plasmapheresis. The relationship to RISPERDAL® therapy is unknown.

Antiemetic effect: Risperidone has an antiemetic effect in animals; this effect may also occur in humans, and may mask signs and symptoms of overdosage with certain drugs or of conditions such as intestinal obstruction, Reye's syndrome, and brain tumor.

Body Temperature Regulation: Disruption of body temperature regulation has been attributed to antipsychotic agents. Both hyperthermia and hypothermia have been reported in association with RISPERDAL® use. Caution is advised when prescribing for patients who will be exposed to temperature extremes.

Suicide: The possibility of a suicide attempt is inherent in schizophrenia, and close supervision of high risk patients should accompany drug therapy. Prescriptions for RISPERDAL® should be written for the smallest quantity of tablets consistent with good patient management, in order to reduce the risk of overdose.

Use in Patients with Concomitant Illness: Clinical experience with RISPERDAL® in patients with certain concomitant systemic illnesses is limited. Caution is advisable in using RISPERDAL® in patients with diseases or conditions that could affect metabolism or hemodynamic responses.

RISPERDAL® has not been evaluated or used to any appreciable extent in patients with a recent history of myocardial infarction or unstable heart disease. Patients with these diagnoses were excluded from clinical studies during the product's premarket testing. The electrocardiograms of approximately 380 patients who received RISPERDAL® and 120 patients who received placebo in two double-blind, placebo-controlled trials were evaluated and the data revealed one finding of potential concern, i.e., 8 patients taking RISPERDAL® whose baseline QTc interval was less than 450 msec were observed to have QTc intervals greater than 450 msec during treatment; no such prolongations were seen in the smaller placebo group. There were 3 such episodes in the approximately 125 patients who received haloperidol. Because of the risks of orthostatic hypotension and QT prolongation, caution should be observed in cardiac patients (See WARNINGS and PRECAUTIONS).

Increased plasma concentrations of risperidone and 9-hydroxyrisperidone occur in patients with severe renal impairment (creatinine clearance <30 mL/min/1.73 m^2), and an increase in the free fraction of the risperidone is seen in patients with severe hepatic impairment. A lower starting dose should be used in such patients (See DOSAGE AND ADMINISTRATION).

Information for Patients

Physicians are advised to discuss the following issues with patients for whom they prescribe RISPERDAL®:

Orthostatic Hypotension: Patients should be advised of the risk of orthostatic hypotension, especially during the period of initial dose titration.

Interference With Cognitive and Motor Performance: Since RISPERDAL® has the potential to impair judgment, thinking, or motor skills, patients should be cautioned about operating hazardous machinery, including automobiles, until they are reasonably certain that RISPERDAL® therapy does not affect them adversely.

Pregnancy: Patients should be advised to notify their physician if they become pregnant or intend to become pregnant during therapy.

Nursing: Patients should be advised not to breast feed an infant if they are taking RISPERDAL®.

Concomitant Medication: Patients should be advised to inform their physicians if they are taking, or plan to take, any prescription or over-the-counter drugs, since there is a potential for interactions.

Alcohol: Patients should be advised to avoid alcohol while taking RISPERDAL®.

Laboratory Tests

No specific laboratory tests are recommended.

Drug Interactions

The interactions of RISPERDAL® and other drugs have not been systematically evaluated. Given the primary CNS effects of risperidone, caution should be used when RISPERDAL® is taken in combination with other centrally acting drugs and alcohol.

Because of its potential for inducing hypotension, RISPERDAL® may enhance the hypotensive effects of other therapeutic agents with this potential.

RISPERDAL® may antagonize the effects of levodopa and dopamine agonists.

Chronic administration of carbamazepine with risperidone may increase the clearance of risperidone.

Chronic administration of clozapine with risperidone may decrease the clearance of risperidone.

Fluoxetine may increase the plasma concentration of the anti-psychotic fraction (risperidone plus 9-hydroxyrisperidone) by raising the concentration of risperidone, although not the active metabolite, 9-hydroxyrisperidone.

Drugs that Inhibit Cytochrome $P_{450}IID_6$ and Other P_{450} Isozymes: Risperidone is metabolized to 9-hydroxyrisperidone by cytochrome $P_{450}IID_6$, an enzyme that is polymorphic in the population and that can be inhibited by a variety of psychotropic and other drugs (See CLINICAL PHARMACOLOGY). Drug interactions that reduce the metabolism of risperidone to 9-hydroxyrisperidone would increase the plasma concentrations of risperidone and lower the concentrations of 9-hydroxyrisperidone. Analysis of clinical studies involving a modest number of poor metabolizers (n=70) does not suggest that poor and extensive metabolizers have different rates of adverse effects. No comparison of effectiveness in the two groups has been made.

In vitro studies showed that drugs metabolized by other P_{450} isozymes, including 1A1, 1A2, IIC9, MP, and IIIA4, are only weak inhibitors of risperidone metabolism.

Drugs Metabolized by Cytochrome $P_{450}IID_6$: In vitro studies indicate that risperidone is a relatively weak inhibitor of cytochrome $P_{450}IID_6$. Therefore, RISPERDAL® is not expected to substantially inhibit the clearance of drugs that are metabolized by this enzymatic pathway. However, clinical data to confirm this expectation are not available.

Carcinogenesis, Mutagenesis, Impairment of Fertility

Carcinogenesis: Carcinogenicity studies were conducted in Swiss albino mice and Wistar rats. Risperidone was administered in the diet at doses of 0.63, 2.5, and 10 mg/kg for 18 months to mice and for 25 months to rats. These doses are equivalent to 2.4, 9.4 and 37.5 times the maximum human dose (16 mg/day) on a mg/kg basis or 0.2, 0.75 and 3 times the maximum human dose (mice) or 0.4, 1.5, and 6 times the maximum human dose (rats) on a mg/m^2 basis. A maximum tolerated dose was not achieved in male mice. There were statistically significant increases in pituitary gland adenomas, endocrine pancreas adenomas and mammary gland adenocarcinomas. The following table summarizes the multiples of the human dose on a mg/m^2 (mg/kg) basis at which these tumors occurred.

[See table above]

TUMOR TYPE	SPECIES	SEX	MULTIPLE OF MAXIMUM HUMAN DOSE in mg/m^2 (mg/kg)	
			LOWEST EFFECT LEVEL	HIGHEST NO EFFECT LEVEL
Pituitary adenomas	mouse	female	0.75 (*9.4*)	0.2 (*2.4*)
Endocrine pancreas adenomas	rat	male	1.5 (*9.4*)	0.4 (*2.4*)
Mammary gland adenocarcinomas	mouse	female	0.2 (*2.4*)	none
	rat	female	0.4 (*2.4*)	none
	rat	male	6 (*37.5*)	1.5 (*9.4*)
Mammary gland neoplasms, Total	rat	male	1.5 (*9.4*)	0.4 (*2.4*)

Antipsychotic drugs have been shown to chronically elevate prolactin levels in rodents. Serum prolactin levels were not measured during the risperidone carcinogenicity studies; however, measurements during subchronic toxicity studies showed that risperidone elevated serum prolactin levels 5 to 6 fold in mice and rats at the same doses used in the carcinogenicity studies. An increase in mammary, pituitary, and endocrine pancreas neoplasms has been found in rodents after chronic administration of other antipsychotic drugs and is considered to be prolactin mediated. The relevance for human risk of the findings of prolactin-mediated endocrine tumors in rodents is unknown (See Hyperprolactinemia under PRECAUTIONS, GENERAL).

Mutagenesis: No evidence of mutagenic potential for risperidone was found in the Ames reverse mutation test, mouse lymphoma assay, in vitro rat hepatocyte DNA-repair assay, in vivo micronucleus test in mice, the sex-linked recessive lethal test in Drosophila, or the chromosomal aberration test in human lymphocytes or Chinese hamster cells.

Impairment of Fertility: Risperidone (0.16 to 5 mg/kg) was shown to impair mating, but not fertility, in Wistar rats in three reproductive studies (two Segment I and a multigenerational study) at doses 0.1 to 3 times the maximum recommended human dose on a mg/m^2 basis. The effect appeared to be in females since impaired mating behavior was not noted in the Segment I study in which males only were treated. In a subchronic study in Beagle dogs in which risperidone was administered at doses of 0.31 to 5 mg/kg, sperm motility and concentration were decreased at doses 0.6 to 10 times the human dose on a mg/m^2 basis. Dose-related decreases were also noted in serum testosterone at the same doses. Serum testosterone and sperm parameters partially recovered but remained decreased after treatment was discontinued. No no-effect doses were noted in either rat or dog.

Pregnancy

Pregnancy Category C: The teratogenic potential of risperidone was studied in three Segment II studies in Sprague-Dawley and Wistar rats and in one Segment II study in New Zealand rabbits. The incidence of malformations was not increased compared to control in offspring of rats or rabbits given 0.4 to 6 times the human dose on a mg/m^2 basis. In three reproductive studies in rats (two Segment III and a multigenerational study), there was an increase in pup deaths during the first 4 days of lactation at doses 0.1 to 3 times the human dose on a mg/m^2 basis. It is not known whether these deaths were due to a direct effect on the fetuses or pups or to effects on the dams. There was no no-effect dose for increased rat pup mortality. In one Segment III study, there was an increase in stillborn rat pups at a dose 1.5 times higher than the human dose on a mg/m^2 basis.

Placental transfer of risperidone occurs in rat pups. There are no adequate and well-controlled studies in pregnant women. However, there was one report of a case of agenesis of the corpus callosum in an infant exposed to risperidone in utero. The causal relationship to RISPERDAL® therapy is unknown.

RISPERDAL® should be used during pregnancy only if the potential benefit justifies the potential risk to the fetus.

Labor and Delivery

The effect of RISPERDAL® on labor and delivery in humans is unknown.

Nursing Mothers

In animal studies, risperidone and 9-hydroxyrisperidone were excreted in breast milk. It has been demonstrated that risperidone and 9-hydroxyrisperidone are also excreted in human breast milk. Therefore, women receiving RISPERDAL® should not breast feed.

Pediatric Use

Safety and effectiveness in children have not been established.

Geriatric Use

Clinical studies of RISPERDAL® did not include sufficient numbers of patients aged 65 and over to determine whether they respond differently from younger patients. Other reported clinical experience has not identified differences in responses between elderly and younger patients. In general, a lower starting dose is recommended for an elderly patient, reflecting a decreased pharmacokinetic clearance in the elderly, as well as a greater frequency of decreased hepatic, renal, or cardiac function, and of concomitant disease or other drug therapy (See CLINICAL PHARMACOLOGY and DOSAGE AND ADMINISTRATION). While elderly patients exhibit a greater tendency to orthostatic hypotension, its risk in the elderly may be minimized by limiting the initial dose to 0.5 mg BID followed by careful titration (See PRECAUTIONS). Monitoring of orthostatic vital signs should be considered in patients for whom this is of concern.

This drug is known to be substantially excreted by the kidney, and the risk of toxic reactions to this drug may be greater in patients with impaired renal function. Because elderly patients are more likely to have decreased renal function, care should be taken in dose selection, and it may be useful to monitor renal function (See DOSAGE AND ADMINISTRATION).

ADVERSE REACTIONS

Associated with Discontinuation of Treatment

Approximately 9% (244/2607) of RISPERDAL® (risperidone)-treated patients in phase 2–3 studies discontinued treatment due to an adverse event, compared with about 7% on placebo and 10% on active control drugs. The more common events (≥ 0.3%) associated with discontinuation and considered to be possibly or probably drug-related included:

Adverse Event	RISPERDAL®	Placebo
Extrapyramidal symptoms	2.1%	0%
Dizziness	0.7%	0%
Hyperkinesia	0.6%	0%
Somnolence	0.5%	0%
Nausea	0.3%	0%

Suicide attempt was associated with discontinuation in 1.2% of RISPERDAL®-treated patients compared to 0.6% of placebo patients, but, given the almost 40-fold greater exposure time in RISPERDAL® compared to placebo patients, it is unlikely that suicide attempt is a RISPERDAL® related adverse event (See PRECAUTIONS). Discontinuation for extrapyramidal symptoms was 0% in placebo patients but 3.8% in active-control patients in the phase 2–3 trials.

Incidence in Controlled Trials

Commonly Observed Adverse Events in Controlled Clinical Trials: In two 6 to 8-week placebo-controlled trials, spontaneously-reported, treatment-emergent adverse events with an incidence of 5% or greater in at least one of the RISPERDAL® groups and at least twice that of placebo were: anxiety, somnolence, extrapyramidal symptoms, dizziness, constipation, nausea, dyspepsia, rhinitis, rash, and tachycardia.

Adverse events were also elicited in one of these two trials (i.e., in the fixed-dose trial comparing RISPERDAL® at doses of 2, 6, 10, and 16 mg/day with placebo) utilizing a checklist for detecting adverse events, a method that is more sensitive than spontaneous reporting. By this method, the following additional common and drug-related adverse events were present at at least 5% and twice the rate of placebo: increased dream activity, increased duration of sleep, accommodation disturbances, reduced salivation, micturition disturbances, diarrhea, weight gain, menorrhagia, diminished sexual desire, erectile dysfunction, ejaculatory dysfunction, and orgastic dysfunction.

Adverse Events Occurring at an Incidence of 1% or More Among RISPERDAL®-Treated Patients: The table that follows enumerates adverse events that occurred at an incidence of 1% or more, and were at least as frequent among RISPERDAL®-treated patients treated at doses of ≤ 10 mg/day than among placebo-treated patients in the pooled results of two 6 to 8-week controlled trials. Patients received RISPERDAL® doses of 2, 6, 10, or 16 mg/day in the dose comparison trial, or up to a maximum dose of 10 mg/day in the titration study. This table shows the percentage of patients in each dose group (≤ 10 mg/day or 16 mg/day) who spontaneously reported at least one episode of an event at some time during their treatment. Patients given doses of 2, 6, or 10 mg did not differ materially in these rates. Reported adverse events were classified using the World Health Organization preferred terms.

The prescriber should be aware that these figures cannot be used to predict the incidence of side effects in the course of usual medical practice where patient characteristics and other factors differ from those which prevailed in this clinical trial. Similarly, the cited frequencies cannot be compared with figures obtained from other clinical investigations involving different treatments, uses and investigators. The cited figures, however, do provide the prescribing physician with some basis for estimating the relative contribution of drug and nondrug factors to the side effect incidence rate in the population studied.

Table 1: **Treatment-Emergent Adverse Experience Incidence in 6 to 8-Week Controlled Clinical Trials[1]**

Body System/ Preferred Term	RISPERDAL® ≤10 mg/day (N=324)	RISPERDAL® 16 mg/day (N=77)	Placebo (N=142)
Psychiatric Disorders			
Insomnia	26%	23%	19%
Agitation	22%	26%	20%
Anxiety	12%	20%	9%
Somnolence	3%	8%	1%
Aggressive reaction	1%	3%	1%
Nervous System			
Extrapyramidal symptoms[2]	17%	34%	16%
Headache	14%	12%	12%
Dizziness	4%	7%	1%

Continued on next page

Risperdal—Cont.

Gastrointestinal System			
Constipation	7%	13%	3%
Nausea	6%	4%	3%
Dyspepsia	5%	10%	4%
Vomiting	5%	7%	4%
Abdominal pain	4%	1%	0%
Saliva increased	2%	0%	1%
Toothache	2%	0%	0%
Respiratory System			
Rhinitis	10%	8%	4%
Coughing	3%	3%	1%
Sinusitis	2%	1%	1%
Pharyngitis	2%	3%	0%
Dyspnea	1%	0%	0%
Body as a Whole			
Back pain	2%	0%	1%
Chest pain	2%	3%	1%
Fever	2%	3%	0%
Dermatological			
Rash	2%	5%	1%
Dry skin	2%	4%	0%
Seborrhea	1%	0%	0%
Infections			
Upper respiratory	3%	3%	1%
Visual			
Abnormal vision	2%	1%	1%
Musculo-Skeletal			
Arthralgia	2%	3%	0%
Cardiovascular			
Tachycardia	3%	5%	0%

[1] Events reported by at least 1% of patients treated with RISPERDAL® ≤ 10 mg/day are included, and are rounded to the nearest %. Comparative rates for RISPERDAL® 16 mg/day and placebo are provided as well. Events for which the RISPERDAL® incidence (in both dose groups) was equal to or less than placebo are not listed in the table, but included the following: nervousness, injury, and fungal infection.

[2] Includes tremor, dystonia, hypokinesia, hypertonia, hyperkinesia, oculogyric crisis, ataxia, abnormal gait, involuntary muscle contractions, hyporeflexia, akathisia and extrapyramidal disorders. Although the incidence of 'extrapyramidal symptoms' does not appear to differ for the '≤ 10 mg/day' group and placebo, the data for individual dose groups in fixed dose trials do suggest a dose/response relationship (See DOSE DEPENDENCY OF ADVERSE EVENTS).

Dose Dependency of Adverse Events:

Extrapyramidal symptoms: Data from two fixed dose trials provided evidence of dose-relatedness for extrapyramidal symptoms associated with risperidone treatment.

Two methods were used to measure extrapyramidal symptoms (EPS) in an 8-week trial comparing four fixed doses of risperidone (2, 6, 10, and 16 mg/day), including (1) a parkinsonism score (mean change from baseline) from the Extrapyramidal Symptom Rating Scale and (2) incidence of spontaneous complaints of EPS:

Dose Groups	Placebo	Ris 2	Ris 6	Ris 10	Ris 16
Parkinsonism	1.2	0.9	1.8	2.4	2.6
EPS Incidence	13%	13%	16%	20%	31%

Similar methods were used to measure extrapyramidal symptoms (EPS) in an 8-week trial comparing five fixed doses of risperidone (1, 4, 8, 12, and 16 mg/day):

Dose Groups	Ris 1	Ris 4	Ris 8	Ris 12	Ris 16
Parkinsonism	0.6	1.7	2.4	2.9	4.1
EPS Incidence	7%	12%	18%	18%	21%

Other Adverse Events: Adverse event data elicited by a checklist for side effects from a large study comparing 5 fixed doses of RISPERDAL® (1, 4, 8, 12, and 16 mg/day) were explored for dose-relatedness of adverse events. A Cochran-Armitage Test for trend in these data revealed a positive trend ($p<0.05$) for the following adverse events: sleepiness, increased duration of sleep, accommodation disturbances, orthostatic dizziness, palpitations, weight gain, erectile dysfunction, ejaculatory dysfunction, orgastic dysfunction, asthenia/lassitude/increased fatiguability, and increased pigmentation.

Vital Sign Changes: RISPERDAL® is associated with orthostatic hypotension and tachycardia (See PRECAUTIONS).

Weight Changes: The proportions of RISPERDAL® and placebo-treated patients meeting a weight gain criterion of ≥ 7% of body weight were compared in a pool of 6 to 8-week placebo-controlled trials, revealing a statistically significantly greater incidence of weight gain for RISPERDAL® (18%) compared to placebo (9%).

Laboratory Changes: A between group comparison for 6 to 8-week placebo-controlled trials revealed no statistically significant RISPERDAL®/placebo differences in the proportions of patients experiencing potentially important changes in routine serum chemistry, hematology, or urinalysis parameters. Similarly, there were no RISPERDAL®/placebo differences in the incidence of discontinuations for changes in serum chemistry, hematology, or urinalysis. However, RISPERDAL® administration was associated with increases in serum prolactin (See PRECAUTIONS).

ECG Changes: The electrocardiograms of approximately 380 patients who received RISPERDAL® and 120 patients who received placebo in two double-blind, placebo-controlled trials were evaluated and revealed one finding of potential concern; i.e., 8 patients taking RISPERDAL® whose baseline QTc interval was less than 450 msec were observed to have QTc intervals greater than 450 msec during treatment (See WARNINGS). Changes of this type were not seen among about 120 placebo patients, but were seen in patients receiving haloperidol (3/126).

Other Events Observed During the Pre-Marketing Evaluation of RISPERDAL®

During its premarketing assessment, multiple doses of RISPERDAL® (risperidone) were administered to 2607 patients in phase 2 and 3 studies. The conditions and duration of exposure to RISPERDAL® varied greatly, and included (in overlapping categories) open and double-blind studies, uncontrolled and controlled studies, inpatient and outpatient studies, fixed-dose and titration studies, and short-term or longer-term exposure. In most studies, untoward events associated with this exposure were obtained by spontaneous report and recorded by clinical investigators using terminology of their own choosing. Consequently, it is not possible to provide a meaningful estimate of the proportion of individuals experiencing adverse events without first grouping similar types of untoward events into a smaller number of standardized event categories. In two large studies, adverse events were also elicited utilizing the UKU (direct questioning) side effect rating scale, and these events were not further categorized using standard terminology (Note: These events are marked with an asterisk in the listings that follow).

In the listings that follow, spontaneously reported adverse events were classified using World Health Organization (WHO) preferred terms. The frequencies presented, therefore, represent the proportion of the 2607 patients exposed to multiple doses of RISPERDAL® who experienced an event of the type cited on at least one occasion while receiving RISPERDAL®. All reported events are included except those already listed in Table 1, those events for which a drug cause was remote, and those event terms which were so general as to be uninformative. It is important to emphasize that, although the events reported occurred during treatment with RISPERDAL®, they were not necessarily caused by it.

Events are further categorized by body system and listed in order of decreasing frequency according to the following definitions: frequent adverse events are those occurring in at least 1/100 patients (only those not already listed in the tabulated results from placebo-controlled trials appear in this listing); infrequent adverse events are those occurring in 1/100 to 1/1000 patients; rare events are those occurring in fewer than 1/1000 patients.

Psychiatric Disorders: *Frequent:* increased dream activity*, diminished sexual desire*, nervousness. *Infrequent:* impaired concentration, depression, apathy, catatonic reaction, euphoria, increased libido, amnesia. *Rare:* emotional lability, nightmares, delirium, withdrawal syndrome, yawning.

Central and Peripheral Nervous System Disorders: *Frequent:* increased sleep duration*. *Infrequent:* dysarthria, vertigo, stupor, paraesthesia, confusion. *Rare:* aphasia, cholinergic syndrome, hypoesthesia, tongue paralysis, leg cramps, torticollis, hypotonia, coma, migraine, hyperreflexia, choreoathetosis.

Gastro-intestinal Disorders: *Frequent:* anorexia, reduced salivation*. *Infrequent:* flatulence, diarrhea, increased appetite, stomatitis, melena, dysphagia, hemorrhoids, gastritis. *Rare:* fecal incontinence, eructation, gastroesophageal reflux, gastroenteritis, esophagitis, tongue discoloration, cholelithiasis, tongue edema, diverticulitis, gingivitis, discolored feces, GI hemorrhage, hematemesis.

Body as a Whole/General Disorders: *Frequent:* fatigue. *Infrequent:* edema, rigors, malaise, influenza-like symptoms. *Rare:* pallor, enlarged abdomen, allergic reaction, ascites, sarcoidosis, flushing.

Respiratory System Disorders: *Infrequent:* hyperventilation, bronchospasm, pneumonia, stridor. *Rare:* asthma, increased sputum, aspiration.

Skin and Appendage Disorders: *Frequent:* increased pigmentation*, photosensitivity*. *Infrequent:* increased sweating, acne, decreased sweating, alopecia, hyperkeratosis, pruritus, skin exfoliation. *Rare:* bullous eruption, skin ulceration, aggravated psoriasis, furunculosis, verruca, dermatitis lichenoid, hypertrichosis, genital pruritus, urticaria.

Cardiovascular Disorders: *Infrequent:* palpitation, hypertension, hypotension, AV block, myocardial infarction. *Rare:* ventricular tachycardia, angina pectoris, premature atrial contractions, T wave inversions, ventricular extrasystoles, ST depression, myocarditis.

Vision Disorders: *Infrequent:* abnormal accommodation, xerophthalmia. *Rare:* diplopia, eye pain, blepharitis, photopsia, photophobia, abnormal lacrimation.

Metabolic and Nutritional Disorders: *Infrequent:* hyponatremia, weight increase, creatine phosphokinase increase, thirst, weight decrease, diabetes mellitus. *Rare:* decreased serum iron, cachexia, dehydration, hypokalemia, hypoproteinemia, hyperphosphatemia, hypertriglyceridemia, hyperuricemia, hypoglycemia.

Urinary System Disorders: *Frequent:* polyuria/polydipsia*. *Infrequent:* urinary incontinence, hematuria, dysuria. *Rare:* urinary retention, cystitis, renal insufficiency.

Musculo-skeletal System Disorders: *Infrequent:* myalgia. *Rare:* arthrosis, synostosis, bursitis, arthritis, skeletal pain.

Reproductive Disorders, Female: *Frequent:* menorrhagia*, orgastic dysfunction*, dry vagina*. *Infrequent:* nonpuerperal lactation, amenorrhea, female breast pain, leukorrhea, mastitis, dysmenorrhea, female perineal pain, intermenstrual bleeding, vaginal hemorrhage.

Liver and Biliary System Disorders: *Infrequent:* increased SGOT, increased SGPT. *Rare:* hepatic failure, cholestatic hepatitis, cholecystitis, cholelithiasis, hepatitis, hepatocellular damage.

Platelet, Bleeding and Clotting Disorders: *Infrequent:* epistaxis, purpura. *Rare:* hemorrhage, superficial phlebitis, thrombophlebitis, thrombocytopenia.

Hearing and Vestibular Disorders: *Rare:* tinnitus, hyperacusis, decreased hearing.

Red Blood Cell Disorders: *Infrequent:* anemia, hypochromic anemia. *Rare:* normocytic anemia.

Reproductive Disorders, Male: *Frequent:* erectile dysfunction*. *Infrequent:* ejaculation failure.

White Cell and Resistance Disorders: *Rare:* leukocytosis, lymphadenopathy, leucopenia, Pelger-Huet anomaly.

Endocrine Disorders: *Rare:* gynecomastia, male breast pain, antidiuretic hormone disorder.

Special Senses: *Rare:* bitter taste.

* Incidence based on elicited reports.

Postintroduction Reports: Adverse events reported since market introduction which were temporally (but not necessarily causally) related to RISPERDAL® therapy, include the following: anaphylactic reaction, angioedema, apnea, atrial fibrillation, cerebrovascular disorder, including cerebrovascular accident, diabetes mellitus aggravated, including diabetic ketoacidosis, intestinal obstruction, jaundice, mania, pancreatitis, Parkinson's disease aggravated, pulmonary embolism. There have been rare reports of sudden death and/or cardiopulmonary arrest in patients receiving RISPERDAL®. A causal relationship with RISPERDAL® has not been established. It is important to note that sudden and unexpected death may occur in psychotic patients whether they remain untreated or whether they are treated with other antipsychotic drugs.

DRUG ABUSE AND DEPENDENCE

Controlled Substance Class: RISPERDAL® (risperidone) is not a controlled substance.

Physical and Psychologic Dependence: RISPERDAL® has not been systematically studied in animals or humans for its potential for abuse, tolerance or physical dependence. While the clinical trials did not reveal any tendency for any drug-seeking behavior, these observations were not systematic and it is not possible to predict on the basis of this limited experience the extent to which a CNS-active drug will be misused, diverted and/or abused once marketed. Consequently, patients should be evaluated carefully for a history of drug abuse, and such patients should be observed closely for signs of RISPERDAL® misuse or abuse (e.g., development of tolerance, increases in dose, drug-seeking behavior).

OVERDOSAGE

Human Experience: Premarketing experience included eight reports of acute RISPERDAL® (risperidone) overdosage with estimated doses ranging from 20 to 300 mg and no fatalities. In general, reported signs and symptoms were those resulting from an exaggeration of the drug's known pharmacological effects, i.e., drowsiness and sedation, tachycardia and hypotension, and extrapyramidal symptoms. One case, involving an estimated overdose of 240 mg, was associated with hyponatremia, hypokalemia, prolonged QT, and widened QRS. Another case, involving an estimated overdose of 36 mg, was associated with a seizure. Postmarketing experience includes reports of acute RISPERDAL® overdosage, with estimated doses of up to 360 mg. In general, the most frequently reported signs and symptoms are those resulting from an exaggeration of the drug's known pharmacological effects, i.e., drowsiness, sedation, tachycardia and hypotension. Other adverse events reported since market introduction which were temporally, (but not necessarily causally) related to RISPERDAL® overdose, include prolonged QT interval, convulsions, cardiopulmonary arrest, and rare fatality associated with multiple drug overdose.

Management of Overdosage: In case of acute overdosage, establish and maintain an airway and ensure adequate oxygenation and ventilation. Gastric lavage (after intubation, if patient is unconscious) and administration of activated charcoal together with a laxative should be considered. The possibility of obtundation, seizures or dystonic reaction of the head and neck following overdose may create a risk of aspiration with induced emesis. Cardiovascular monitoring should commence immediately and should include continuous electrocardiographic monitoring to detect possible arrhythmias. If antiarrhythmic therapy is administered, disopyramide, procainamide and quinidine carry a theoretical hazard of QT-prolonging effects that might be additive to those of risperidone. Similarly, it is reasonable to expect that the alpha-blocking properties of bretylium might be additive to those of risperidone, resulting in problematic hypotension.

There is no specific antidote to RISPERDAL®. Therefore appropriate supportive measures should be instituted. The possibility of multiple drug involvement should be considered. Hypotension and circulatory collapse should be treated with appropriate measures such as intravenous fluids and/or sympathomimetic agents (epinephrine and dopamine should not be used, since beta stimulation may worsen hypotension in the setting of risperidone-induced alpha blockade). In cases of severe extrapyramidal symptoms, anticholinergic medication should be administered. Close medical supervision and monitoring should continue until the patient recovers.

DOSAGE AND ADMINISTRATION

Usual Initial Dose: RISPERDAL® (risperidone) can be administered on either a BID or a QD schedule. In early short-term clinical trials, RISPERDAL® was generally administered at 1 mg BID initially, with increases in increments of 1 mg BID on the second and third day, as tolerated, to a target dose of 3 mg BID by the third day. Subsequent short-term controlled trials have indicated that total daily risperidone doses of up to 8 mg on a QD regimen are also safe and effective. In a long-term controlled trial in stable patients, RISPERDAL® was administered on a QD schedule at 1 mg QD initially, with increases to 2 mg QD on the second day and to a target dose of 4 mg QD on the third day. However, regardless of which regimen is employed, in some patients a slower titration may be medically appropriate. Further dosage adjustments, if indicated, should generally occur at intervals of not less than 1 week, since steady state for the active metabolite would not be achieved for approximately 1 week in the typical patient. When dosage adjustments are necessary, small dose increments/decrements of 1–2 mg are recommended.

Efficacy in schizophrenia was demonstrated in a dose range of 4 to 16 mg/day in short-term clinical trials supporting effectiveness of RISPERDAL®, however, maximal effect was generally seen in a range of 4 to 8 mg/day. Doses above 6 mg/day for BID dosing were not demonstrated to be more efficacious than lower doses, were associated with more extrapyramidal symptoms and other adverse effects, and are not generally recommended. In a single study supporting QD dosing, the efficacy results were generally stronger for 8 mg than for 4 mg. The safety of doses above 16 mg/day has not been evaluated in clinical trials.

Maintenance Therapy: While there is no body of evidence available to answer the question of how long the schizophrenic patient treated with RISPERDAL® should remain on it, the effectiveness of RISPERDAL® 2 mg/day to 8 mg/day at delaying relapse was demonstrated in a controlled trial in patients who had been clinically stable for at least 4 weeks and were then followed for a period of 1 to 2 years. In this trial, RISPERDAL® was administered on a QD schedule, at 1 mg QD initially, with increases to 2 mg QD on the second day and to a target dose of 4 mg QD on the third day (See Clinical Trials, under CLINICAL PHARMACOLOGY). Nevertheless, patients should be periodically reassessed to determine the need for maintenance treatment with appropriate dose.

Pediatric Use: Safety and effectiveness in pediatric patients have not been established.

Dosage in Special Populations: The recommended initial dose is 0.5 mg BID in patients who are elderly or debilitated, patients with severe renal or hepatic impairment, and patients either predisposed to hypotension or for whom hypotension would pose a risk. Dosage increases in these patients should be in increments of no more than 0.5 mg BID. Increases to dosages above 1.5 mg BID should generally occur at intervals of at least 1 week. In some patients, slower titration may be medically appropriate.

Elderly or debilitated patients, and patients with renal impairment, may have less ability to eliminate RISPERDAL® than normal adults. Patients with impaired hepatic function may have increases in the free fraction of the risperidone, possibly resulting in an enhanced effect (See CLINICAL PHARMACOLOGY). Patients with a predisposition to hypotensive reactions or for whom such reactions would pose a particular risk likewise need to be titrated cautiously and carefully monitored (See PRECAUTIONS). If a once-a-day dosing regimen in the elderly or debilitated patient is being considered, it is recommended that the patient be titrated on a twice-a-day regimen for 2–3 days at the target dose. Subsequent switches to a once-a-day dosing regimen can be done thereafter.

Reinitiation of Treatment in Patients Previously Discontinued: Although there are no data to specifically address reinitiation of treatment, it is recommended that when restarting patients who have had an interval off RISPERDAL®, the initial titration schedule should be followed.

Switching from Other Antipsychotics: There are no systematically collected data to specifically address switching schizophrenic patients from other antipsychotics to RISPERDAL®, or concerning concomitant administration with other antipsychotics. While immediate discontinuation of the previous antipsychotic treatment may be acceptable for some schizophrenic patients, more gradual discontinuation may be most appropriate for others. In all cases, the period of overlapping antipsychotic administration should be minimized. When switching schizophrenic patients from depot antipsychotics, if medically appropriate, initiate RISPERDAL® therapy in place of the next scheduled injection. The need for continuing existing EPS medication should be reevaluated periodically.

HOW SUPPLIED

RISPERDAL® (risperidone) tablets are imprinted "JANSSEN", and either "Ris" and the strength "0.25", "0.5", or "R" and the strength "1", "2", "3", or "4".

0.25 mg dark yellow tablet: bottles of 60 NDC 50458-301-04, bottles of 500 NDC 50458-301-50.

0.5 mg red-brown tablet: bottles of 60 NDC 50458-302-06, bottles of 500 NDC 50458-302-50.

1 mg white tablet: bottles of 60 NDC 50458-300-06, blister pack of 100 NDC 50458-300-01, bottles of 500 NDC 50458-300-50.

2 mg orange tablet: bottles of 60 NDC 50458-320-06, blister pack of 100 NDC 50458-320-01, bottles of 500 NDC 50458-320-50.

3 mg yellow tablet: bottles of 60 NDC 50458-330-06, blister pack of 100 NDC 50458-330-01, bottles of 500 NDC 50458-330-50.

4 mg green tablet: bottles of 60 NDC 50458-350-06, blister pack of 100 NDC 50458-350-01.

RISPERDAL® (risperidone) 1 mg/mL oral solution (NDC 50458-305-03) is supplied in 30 mL bottles with a calibrated (in milligrams and milliliters) pipette. The minimum calibrated volume is 0.25 mL, while the maximum calibrated volume is 3 mL.

Tests indicate that RISPERDAL® (risperidone) oral solution is compatible in the following beverages: water, coffee, orange juice, and low-fat milk; it is NOT compatible with either cola or tea, however.

Storage and Handling

RISPERDAL® tablets should be stored at controlled room temperature 15°–25°C (59°–77°F). Protect from light and moisture.

Keep out of reach of children.

RISPERDAL® 1 mg/mL oral solution should be stored at controlled room temperature 15°–25°C (59°–77°F). Protect from light and freezing.

Keep out of reach of children.

7503220

US Patent 4,804,663

February 2002

RISPERDAL® tablets are manufactured by:
JOLLC, Gurabo, Puerto Rico or
Janssen-Cilag, SpA, Latina, Italy

RISPERDAL® oral solution is manufactured by:
Janssen Pharmaceutica N.V.
Beerse, Belgium

RISPERDAL® tablets and oral solution are distributed by:
Janssen Pharmaceutica Products, L.P.
Titusville, NJ 08560

SPORANOX ℞

[*spɔr 'ah-näks"*]
(itraconazole)
Capsules

Prescribing information for this product, which appears on pages 1800–1804 of the 2002 PDR, has been completely revised as follows. Please write "See Supplement A" next to the product heading.

Congestive Heart Failure

SPORANOX® (itraconazole) Capsules should not be administered for the treatment of onychomycosis in patients with evidence of ventricular dysfunction such as congestive heart failure (CHF) or a history of CHF. If signs or symptoms of congestive heart failure occur during administration of SPORANOX® Capsules, discontinue administration. When itraconazole was administered intravenously to dogs and healthy human volunteers, negative inotropic effects were seen. (See CLINICAL PHARMACOLOGY: Special Populations, CONTRAINDICATIONS, WARNINGS, PRECAUTIONS: Drug Interactions and ADVERSE REACTIONS: Post-marketing Experience for more information.)

Drug Interactions: Coadministration of cisapride, pimozide, quinidine, or dofetilide with SPORANOX® (itraconazole) Capsules, Injection or Oral Solution is contraindicated. SPORANOX®, a potent cytochrome P450 3A4 isoenzyme system (CYP3A4) inhibitor, may increase plasma concentrations of drugs metabolized by this pathway. Serious cardiovascular events, including QT prolongation, torsades de pointes, ventricular tachycardia, cardiac arrest, and/or sudden death have occurred in patients using cisapride, pimozide, or quinidine, concomitantly with SPORANOX® and/or other CYP3A4 inhibitors. See CONTRAINDICATIONS, WARNINGS, and PRECAUTIONS: Drug Interactions for more information.

DESCRIPTION

SPORANOX® is the brand name for itraconazole, a synthetic triazole antifungal agent. Itraconazole is a 1:1:1:1 racemic mixture of four diastereomers (two enantiomeric pairs), each possessing three chiral centers. It may be represented by the following structural formula and nomenclature:

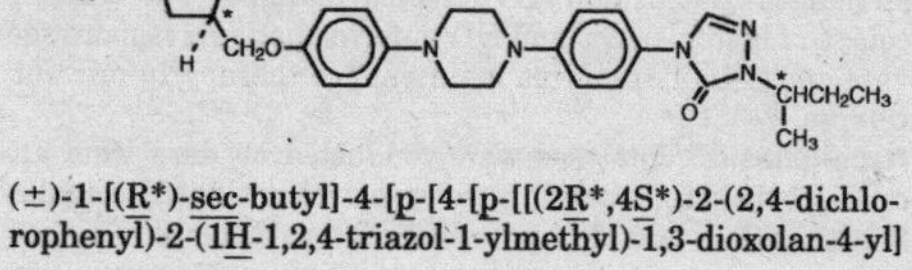

(±)-1-[(R*)-sec-butyl]-4-[p-[4-[p-[[(2R*,4S*)-2-(2,4-dichlorophenyl)-2-(1H-1,2,4-triazol-1-ylmethyl)-1,3-dioxolan-4-yl]methoxy]phenyl]-1-piperazinyl]phenyl]-Δ^2 1,2,4-triazolin-5-one mixture with (±)-1-[(R*)-sec-butyl]-4-[p-[4-[p-[[(2S*,4R*)-2-(2,4-dichlorophenyl)-2-(1H-1,2,4-triazol-1-ylmethyl)-1,3-dioxolan-4-yl]methoxy]phenyl]-1-piperazinyl]phenyl]-Δ^2-1,2,4-triazolin-5-one

or

(±)-1-[(RS)-sec-butyl]-4-[p-[4-[p-[[(2R,4S)-2-(2,4-dichlorophenyl)-2-(1H-1,2,4-triazol-1-ylmethyl)-1,3-dioxolan-4-yl]methoxy]phenyl]-1-piperazinyl]phenyl]-Δ^2-1,2,4-triazolin-5-one

Itraconazole has a molecular formula of $C_{35}H_{38}C_{12}N_8O_4$ and a molecular weight of 705.64. It is a white to slightly yellowish powder. It is insoluble in water, very slightly soluble in alcohols, and freely soluble in dichloromethane. It has a pKa of 3.70 (based on extrapolation of values obtained from methanolic solutions) and a log (n-octanol/water) partition coefficient of 5.66 at pH 8.1.

SPORANOX® Capsules contain 100 mg of itraconazole coated on sugar spheres. Inactive ingredients are gelatin, hydroxypropyl methylcellulose, polyethylene glycol (PEG) 20,000, starch, sucrose, titanium dioxide, FD&C Blue No. 1, FD&C Blue No. 2, D&C Red No. 22 and D&C Red No. 28.

CLINICAL PHARMACOLOGY

Pharmacokinetics and Metabolism: NOTE: The plasma concentrations reported below were measured by high-performance liquid chromatography (HPLC) specific for itraconazole. When itraconazole in plasma is measured by a bioassay, values reported are approximately 3.3 times higher than those obtained by HPLC due to the presence of the bioactive metabolite, hydroxyitraconazole. (See MICROBIOLOGY.)

The pharmacokinetics of itraconazole after intravenous administration and its absolute oral bioavailability from an oral solution were studied in a randomized crossover study in 6 healthy male volunteers. The observed absolute oral bioavailability of itraconazole was 55%.

The oral bioavailability of itraconazole is maximal when SPORANOX® (itraconazole) Capsules are taken with a full meal. The pharmacokinetics of itraconazole were studied in 6 healthy male volunteers who received, in a crossover design, single 100-mg doses of itraconazole as a polyethylene glycol capsule, with or without a full meal. The same 6 volunteers also received 50 mg or 200 mg with a full meal in a crossover design. In this study, only itraconazole plasma concentrations were measured. The respective pharmacokinetic parameters for itraconazole are presented in the table below:

[See table at top of next page]

Doubling the SPORANOX® dose results in approximately a three-fold increase in the itraconazole plasma concentrations.

Values given in the table below represent data from a crossover pharmacokinetics study in which 27 healthy male volunteers each took a single 200-mg dose of SPORANOX® Capsules with or without a full meal:

[See table at top of next page]

Absorption of itraconazole under fasted conditions in individuals with relative or absolute achlorhydria, such as patients with AIDS or volunteers taking gastric acid secretion suppressors (e.g., H_2 receptor antagonists), was increased when SPORANOX® Capsules were administered with a cola beverage. Eighteen men with AIDS received single 200-mg doses of SPORANOX® Capsules under fasted conditions with 8 ounces of water or 8 ounces of a cola beverage in a crossover design. The absorption of itraconazole was increased when SPORANOX® Capsules were coadministered with a cola beverage, with AUC_{0-24} and C_{max} increasing 75% ± 121% and 95% ± 128%, respectively.

Thirty healthy men received single 200-mg doses of SPORANOX® Capsules under fasted conditions either 1) with water; 2) with water, after ranitidine 150 mg b.i.d. for 3 days; or 3) with cola, after ranitidine 150 mg b.i.d. for 3 days. When SPORANOX® Capsules were administered after ranitidine pretreatment, itraconazole was absorbed to a lesser extent than when SPORANOX® Capsules were administered alone, with decreases in AUC_{0-24} and C_{max} of 39% ± 37% and 42% ± 39%, respectively. When SPORANOX® Capsules were administered with cola after ranitidine pretreatment, itraconazole absorption was comparable to that observed when SPORANOX® Capsules were administered alone. (See PRECAUTIONS: Drug Interactions.)

Steady-state concentrations were reached within 15 days following oral doses of 50 mg to 400 mg daily. Values given in the table below are data at steady-state from a pharmacokinetics study in which 27 healthy male volunteers took 200-mg SPORANOX® Capsules b.i.d.(with a full meal) for 15 days:

	Itraconazole	Hydroxyitraconazole
C_{max} (ng/mL)	2282 ± 514*	3488 ± 742
C_{min} (ng/mL)	1855 ± 535	3349 ± 761
T_{max} (hours)	4.6 ± 1.8	3.4 ± 3.4
AUC_{0-12h} (ng•h/mL)	22569 ± 5375	38572 ± 8450
$t_{½}$ (hours)	64 ± 32	56 ± 24

* mean ± standard deviation

Continued on next page

Sporanox—Cont.

The plasma protein binding of itraconazole is 99.8% and that of hydroxyitraconazole is 99.5%. Following intravenous administration, the volume of distribution of itraconazole averaged 796 ± 185 liters.

Itraconazole is metabolized predominately by the cytochrome P450 3A4 isoenzyme system (CYP3A4), resulting in the formation of several metabolites, including hydroxyitraconazole, the major metabolite. Results of a pharmacokinetics study suggest that itraconazole may undergo saturable metabolism with multiple dosing. Fecal excretion of the parent drug varies between 3–18% of the dose. Renal excretion of the parent drug is less than 0.03% of the dose. About 40% of the dose is excreted as inactive metabolites in the urine. No single excreted metabolite represents more than 5% of a dose. Itraconazole total plasma clearance averaged 381 ± 95 mL/minute following intravenous administration. (See CONTRAINDICATIONS and PRECAUTIONS: Drug Interactions for more information.)

Special Populations:

Renal Insufficiency: A pharmacokinetic study using a single 200-mg dose of itraconazole (four 50-mg capsules) was conducted in three groups of patients with renal impairment (uremia: n=7; hemodialysis: n=7; and continuous ambulatory peritoneal dialysis: n=5). In uremic subjects with a mean creatinine clearance of 13 mL/min. × 1.73 m^2, the bioavailability was slightly reduced compared with normal population parameters. This study did not demonstrate any significant effect of hemodialysis or continuous ambulatory peritoneal dialysis on the pharmacokinetics of itraconazole (T_{max}, C_{max}, and AUC_{0-8}). Plasma concentration-versus-time profiles showed wide intersubject variation in all three groups.

Hepatic Insufficiency: A pharmacokinetic study using a single 100-mg dose of itraconazole (one 100-mg capsule) was conducted in 6 healthy and 12 cirrhotic subjects. No statistically significant differences in AUC were seen between these two groups. A statistically significant reduction in mean C_{max} (47%) and a twofold increase in the elimination half-life (37 ± 17 hours) of itraconazole were noted in cirrhotic subjects compared with healthy subjects. Patients with impaired hepatic function should be carefully monitored when taking itraconazole. The prolonged elimination half-life of itraconazole observed in cirrhotic patients should be considered when deciding to initiate therapy with other medications metabolized by CYP3A4. (See BOX WARNING, CONTRAINDICATIONS, and PRECAUTIONS: Drug Interactions.)

Decreased Cardiac Contractility: When itraconazole was administered intravenously to anesthetized dogs, a dose-related negative inotropic effect was documented. In a healthy volunteer study of SPORANOX® Injection (intravenous infusion), transient, asymptomatic decreases in left ventricular ejection fraction were observed using gated SPECT imaging; these resolved before the next infusion, 12 hours later. If signs or symptoms of congestive heart failure appear during administration of SPORANOX® Capsules, SPORANOX should be discontinued. (See CONTRAINDICATIONS, WARNINGS, PRECAUTIONS: Drug Interactions and ADVERSE REACTIONS: Post-marketing Experience for more information.)

MICROBIOLOGY

Mechanism of Action: In vitro studies have demonstrated that itraconazole inhibits the cytochrome P450-dependent synthesis of ergosterol, which is a vital component of fungal cell membranes.

Activity In Vitro and In Vivo: Itraconazole exhibits in vitro activity against *Blastomyces dermatitidis, Histoplasma capsulatum, Histoplasma duboisii, Aspergillus flavus, Aspergillus fumigatus, Candida albicans*, and *Cryptococcus neoformans*. Itraconazole also exhibits varying in vitro activity against *Sporothrix schenckii, Trichophyton species, Candida krusei*, and other *Candida* species. The bioactive metabolite, hydroxyitraconazole, has not been evaluated against *Histoplasma capsulatum* and *Blastomyces dermatitidis*. Correlation between minimum inhibitory concentration (MIC) results in vitro and clinical outcome has yet to be established for azole antifungal agents.

Itraconazole administered orally was active in a variety of animal models of fungal infection using standard laboratory strains of fungi. Fungistatic activity has been demonstrated against disseminated fungal infections caused by *Blastomyces dermatitidis, Histoplasma duboisii, Aspergillus fumigatus, Coccidioides immitis, Cryptococcus neoformans, Paracoccidioides brasiliensis, Sporothrix schenckii, Trichophyton rubrum*, and *Trichophyton mentagrophytes*.

Itraconazole administered at 2.5 mg/kg and 5 mg/kg via the oral and parenteral routes increased survival rates and sterilized organ systems in normal and immunosuppressed guinea pigs with disseminated *Aspergillus fumigatus* infections. Oral itraconazole administered daily at 40 mg/kg and 80 mg/kg increased survival rates in normal rabbits with disseminated disease and in immunosuppressed rats with pulmonary *Aspergillus fumigatus* infection, respectively. Itraconazole has demonstrated antifungal activity in a variety of animal models infected with *Candida albicans* and other *Candida* species.

Resistance: Isolates from several fungal species with decreased susceptibility to itraconazole have been isolated in vitro and from patients receiving prolonged therapy.

Several in vitro studies have reported that some fungal clinical isolates, including *Candida* species, with reduced susceptibility to one azole antifungal agent may also be less

	50 mg (fed)	100 mg (fed)	100 mg (fasted)	200 mg (fed)
C_{max} (ng/mL)	45 ± 16*	132 ± 67	38 ± 20	289 ± 100
T_{max} (hours)	3.2 ± 1.3	4.0 ± 1.1	3.3 ± 1.0	4.7 ± 1.4
$AUC_{0-\infty}$ (ng•h/mL)	567 ± 264	1899 ± 838	722 ± 289	5211 ± 2116

* mean ± standard deviation

	Itraconazole		Hydroxyitraconazole	
	Fed	Fasted	Fed	Fasted
C_{max} (ng/mL)	239 ± 85*	140 ± 65	397 ± 103	286 ± 101
T_{max} (hours)	4.5 ± 1.1	3.9 ± 1.0	5.1 ± 1.6	4.5 ± 1.1
$AUC_{0-\infty}$ (ng•h/mL)	3423 ± 1154	2094 ± 905	7978 ± 2648	5191 ± 2489
$t_{1/2}$ (hours)	21 ± 5	21 ± 7	12 ± 3	12 ± 3

* mean ± standard deviation

susceptible to other azole derivatives. The finding of cross-resistance is dependent on a number of factors, including the species evaluated, its clinical history, the particular azole compounds compared, and the type of susceptibility test that is performed. The relevance of these in vitro susceptibility data to clinical outcome remains to be elucidated.

Studies (both in vitro and in vivo) suggest that the activity of amphotericin B may be suppressed by prior azole antifungal therapy. As with other azoles, itraconazole inhibits the ^{14}C-demethylation step in the synthesis of ergosterol, a cell wall component of fungi. Ergosterol is the active site for amphotericin B. In one study the antifungal activity of amphotericin B against *Aspergillus fumigatus* infections in mice was inhibited by ketoconazole therapy. The clinical significance of test results obtained in this study is unknown.

INDICATIONS AND USAGE

SPORANOX® (itraconazole) Capsules are indicated for the treatment of the following fungal infections in immunocompromised and non-immunocompromised patients:

1. Blastomycosis, pulmonary and extrapulmonary
2. Histoplasmosis, including chronic cavitary pulmonary disease and disseminated, non-meningeal histoplasmosis, and
3. Aspergillosis, pulmonary and extrapulmonary, in patients who are intolerant of or who are refractory to amphotericin B therapy.

Specimens for fungal cultures and other relevant laboratory studies (wet mount, histopathology, serology) should be obtained before therapy to isolate and identify causative organisms. Therapy may be instituted before the results of the cultures and other laboratory studies are known; however, once these results become available, antiinfective therapy should be adjusted accordingly.

SPORANOX® Capsules are also indicated for the treatment of the following fungal infections in non-immunocompromised patients:

1. Onychomycosis of the toenail, with or without fingernail involvement, due to dermatophytes (tinea unguium), and
2. Onychomycosis of the fingernail due to dermatophytes (tinea unguium).

Prior to initiating treatment, appropriate nail specimens for laboratory testing (KOH preparation, fungal culture, or nail biopsy) should be obtained to confirm the diagnosis of onychomycosis.

(See CLINICAL PHARMACOLOGY: Special Populations, CONTRAINDICATIONS, WARNINGS, and ADVERSE REACTIONS: Post-marketing Experience for more information.)

Description of Clinical Studies:

Blastomycosis: Analyses were conducted on data from two open-label, non-concurrently controlled studies (N=73 combined) in patients with normal or abnormal immune status. The median dose was 200 mg/day. A response for most signs and symptoms was observed within the first 2 weeks, and all signs and symptoms cleared between 3 and 6 months. Results of these two studies demonstrated substantial evidence of the effectiveness of itraconazole for the treatment of blastomycosis compared with the natural history of untreated cases.

Histoplasmosis: Analyses were conducted on data from two open-label, non-concurrently controlled studies (N=34 combined) in patients with normal or abnormal immune status (not including HIV-infected patients). The median dose was 200 mg/day. A response for most signs and symptoms was observed within the first 2 weeks, and all signs and symptoms cleared between 3 and 12 months. Results of these two studies demonstrated substantial evidence of the effectiveness of itraconazole for the treatment of histoplasmosis, compared with the natural history of untreated cases.

Histoplasmosis in HIV-infected patients: Data from a small number of HIV-infected patients suggested that the response rate of histoplasmosis in HIV-infected patients is similar to that of non-HIV-infected patients. The clinical course of histoplasmosis in HIV-infected patients is more severe and usually requires maintenance therapy to prevent relapse.

Aspergillosis: Analyses were conducted on data from an open-label, "single-patient-use" protocol designed to make itraconazole available in the U.S. for patients who either failed or were intolerant of amphotericin B therapy (N=190). The findings were corroborated by two smaller open-label studies (N=31 combined) in the same patient population. Most adult patients were treated with a daily dose of 200 to 400 mg, with a median duration of 3 months. Results of these studies demonstrated substantial evidence of effectiveness of itraconazole as a second-line therapy for the treatment of aspergillosis compared with the natural history of the disease in patients who either failed or were intolerant of amphotericin B therapy.

Onychomycosis of the toenail: Analyses were conducted on data from three double-blind, placebo-controlled studies (N=214 total; 110 given SPORANOX® Capsules) in which patients with onychomycosis of the toenails received 200 mg of SPORANOX® Capsules once daily for 12 consecutive weeks. Results of these studies demonstrated mycologic cure, defined as simultaneous occurrence of negative KOH plus negative culture, in 54% of patients. Thirty-five percent (35%) of patients were considered an overall success (mycologic cure plus clear or minimal nail involvement with significantly decreased signs) and 14% of patients demonstrated mycologic cure plus clinical cure (clearance of all signs, with or without residual nail deformity). The mean time to overall success was approximately 10 months. Twenty-one percent (21%) of the overall success group had a relapse (worsening of the global score or conversion of KOH or culture from negative to positive).

Onychomycosis of the fingernail: Analyses were conducted on data from a double-blind, placebo-controlled study (N=73 total; 37 given SPORANOX® Capsules) in which patients with onychomycosis of the fingernails received a 1-week course (pulse) of 200 mg of SPORANOX® Capsules b.i.d., followed by a 3-week period without SPORANOX®, which was followed by a second 1-week pulse of 200 mg of SPORANOX® Capsules b.i.d. Results demonstrated mycologic cure in 61% of patients. Fifty-six percent (56%) of patients were considered an overall success and 47% of patients demonstrated mycologic cure plus clinical cure. The mean time to overall success was approximately 5 months. None of the patients who achieved overall success relapsed.

CONTRAINDICATIONS

Congestive Heart Failure: SPORANOX® (itraconazole) Capsules should not be administered for the treatment of onychomycosis in patients with evidence of ventricular dysfunction such as congestive heart failure (CHF) or a history of CHF. (See CLINICAL PHARMACOLOGY: Special Populations, WARNINGS, PRECAUTIONS: Drug Interactions—Calcium Channel Blockers, and ADVERSE REACTIONS: Post-marketing Experience.)

Drug Interactions: Concomitant administration of SPORANOX® (itraconazole) Capsules, Injection, or Oral Solution and certain drugs metabolized by the cytochrome P450 3A4 isoenzyme system (CYP3A4) may result in increased plasma concentrations of those drugs, leading to potentially serious and/or life-threatening adverse events. Cisapride, oral midazolam, pimozide, quinidine, dofetilide, and triazolam are contraindicated with SPORANOX®. HMG CoA-reductase inhibitors metabolized by CYP3A4, such as lovastatin and simvastatin, are also contraindicated with SPORANOX®. (See BOX WARNING, and PRECAUTIONS: Drug Interactions.)

SPORANOX® should not be administered for the treatment of onychomycosis to pregnant patients or to women contemplating pregnancy.

SPORANOX® is contraindicated for patients who have shown hypersensitivity to itraconazole or its excipients. There is no information regarding cross-hypersensitivity between itraconazole and other azole antifungal agents. Caution should be used when prescribing SPORANOX® to patients with hypersensitivity to other azoles.

WARNINGS

SPORANOX® (itraconazole) Capsules and SPORANOX® Oral Solution should not be used interchangeably. This is because drug exposure is greater with the Oral Solution than with the Capsules when the same dose of drug is given. In addition, the topical effects of mucosal exposure may be different between the two formulations. Only the Oral Solution has been demonstrated effective for oral and/or esophageal candidiasis.

Hepatic Effects: SPORANOX® has been associated with rare cases of serious hepatotoxicity, including liver failure and death. Some of these cases had neither pre-existing liver disease nor a serious underlying medical condition. If clinical signs or symptoms develop that are consistent with liver disease, treatment should be discontinued and liver function testing performed. The risks and benefits of SPORANOX® use should be reassessed. (See PRECAUTIONS: Information for Patients and ADVERSE REACTIONS.)

Cardiac Dysrhythmias: Life-threatening cardiac dysrhythmias and/or sudden death have occurred in patients using cisapride, pimozide, or quinidine concomitantly with SPORANOX® and/or other CYP3A4 inhibitors. Concomitant administration of these drugs with SPORANOX® is contraindicated. (See BOX WARNING, CONTRAINDICATIONS, and PRECAUTIONS: Drug Interactions.)

Cardiac Disease: SPORANOX® Capsules should not be administered for the treatment of onychomycosis in patients with evidence of ventricular dysfunction such as congestive heart failure (CHF) or a history of CHF. SPORANOX® Capsules should not be used for other indications in patients with evidence of ventricular dysfunction unless the benefit clearly outweighs the risk.

For patients with risk factors for congestive heart failure, physicians should carefully review the risks and benefits of SPORANOX® therapy. These risk factors include cardiac disease such as ischemic and valvular disease; significant pulmonary disease such as chronic obstructive pulmonary disease; and renal failure and other edematous disorders. Such patients should be informed of the signs and symptoms of CHF, should be treated with caution, and should be monitored for signs and symptoms of CHF during treatment. If signs or symptoms of CHF appear during administration of SPORANOX® Capsules, discontinue administration.

When itraconazole was administered intravenously to anesthetized dogs, a dose-related negative inotropic effect was documented. In a healthy volunteer study of SPORANOX® Injection (intravenous infusion), transient, asymptomatic decreases in left ventricular ejection fraction were observed using gated SPECT imaging; these resolved before the next infusion, 12 hours later.

Cases of CHF, peripheral edema, and pulmonary edema have been reported in the post-marketing period among patients being treated for onychomycosis and/or systemic fungal infections. (See CLINICAL PHARMACOLOGY: Special Populations, CONTRAINDICATIONS, PRECAUTIONS: Drug Interactions, and ADVERSE REACTIONS: Post-marketing Experience for more information.)

PRECAUTIONS

General: Rare cases of serious hepatotoxicity have been observed with Sporanox® treatment, including some cases within the first week. In patients with raised liver enzymes or active liver disease, or who have experienced liver toxicity with other drugs, treatment should not be started unless the expected benefit exceeds the risk. Liver function monitoring should be done in patients with pre-existing hepatic function abnormalities or those who have experienced liver toxicity with other medications and should be considered in all patients receiving SPORANOX®. Treatment should be stopped immediately and liver function testing should be conducted in patients who develop signs and symptoms suggestive of liver dysfunction.

If neuropathy occurs that may be attributable to SPORANOX® capsules, the treatment should be discontinued.

SPORANOX® (itraconazole) Capsules should be administered after a full meal. (See CLINICAL PHARMACOLOGY: Pharmacokinetics and Metabolism.)

Under fasted conditions, itraconazole absorption was decreased in the presence of decreased gastric acidity. The absorption of itraconazole may be decreased with the concomitant administration of antacids or gastric acid secretion suppressors. Studies conducted under fasted conditions demonstrated that administration with 8 ounces of a cola beverage resulted in increased absorption of itraconazole in AIDS patients with relative or absolute achlorhydria. This increase relative to the effects of a full meal is unknown. (See CLINICAL PHARMACOLOGY: Pharmacokinetics and Metabolism.)

Information for Patients:

- The topical effects of mucosal exposure may be different between the SPORANOX® Capsules and Oral Solution. Only the Oral Solution has been demonstrated effective for oral and/or esophageal candidiasis. SPORANOX® Capsules should not be used interchangeably with SPORANOX® Oral Solution.
- Instruct patients to take SPORANOX® Capsules with a full meal.
- Instruct patients about the signs and symptoms of congestive heart failure, and if these signs or symptoms occur during SPORANOX® administration, they should discontinue SPORANOX® and contact their healthcare provider immediately.
- Instruct patients to stop SPORANOX® treatment immediately and contact their healthcare provider if any signs and symptoms suggestive of liver dysfunction develop. Such signs and symptoms may include unusual fatigue, anorexia, nausea and/or vomiting, jaundice, dark urine, or pale stools.
- Instruct patients to contact their physician before taking any concomitant medications with itraconazole to ensure there are no potential drug interactions.

Drug Interactions: Itraconazole and its major metabolite, hydroxyitraconazole, are inhibitors of CYP3A4. Therefore, the following drug interactions may occur (See Table 1 below and the following drug class subheadings that follow):

1. SPORANOX® may decrease the elimination of drugs metabolized by CYP3A4, resulting in increased plasma concentrations of these drugs when they are administered with SPORANOX®. These elevated plasma concentrations may increase or prolong both therapeutic and adverse effects of these drugs. Whenever possible, plasma concentrations of these drugs should be monitored, and dosage adjustments made after concomitant SPORANOX® therapy is initiated. When appropriate, clinical monitoring for signs or symptoms of increased or prolonged pharmacologic effects is advised. Upon discontinuation, depending on the dose and duration of treatment, itraconazole plasma concentrations decline gradually (especially in patients with hepatic cirrhosis or in those receiving CYP3A4 inhibitors). This is particularly important when initiating therapy with drugs whose metabolism is affected by itraconazole.
2. Inducers of CYP3A4 may decrease the plasma concentrations of itraconazole. SPORANOX® may not be effective in patients concomitantly taking SPORANOX® and one of these drugs. Therefore, administration of these drugs with SPORANOX® is not recommended.
3. Other inhibitors of CYP3A4 may increase the plasma concentrations of itraconazole. Patients who must take SPORANOX® concomitantly with one of these drugs should be monitored closely for signs or symptoms of increased or prolonged pharmacologic effects of SPORANOX®.

Table 1. Selected Drugs that are predicted to alter the plasma concentration of itraconazole or have their plasma concentration altered by SPORANOX®[1]

Drug plasma concentration increased by itraconazole	
Antiarrhythmics	digoxin, dofetilide,[2] quinidine[2]
Anticonvulsants	carbamazepine
Antimycobacterials	rifabutin
Antineoplastics	busulfan, docetaxel, vinca alkaloids
Antipsychotics	pimozide[2]
Benzodiazepines	alprazolam, diazepam, midazolam,[2,3] triazolam[2]
Calcium Channel Blockers	dihydropyridines, verapamil
Gastrointestinal Motility Agents	cisapride[2]
HMG CoA-Reductase Inhibitors	atorvastatin, cerivastatin, lovastatin,[2] simvastatin[2]
Immunosuppressants	cyclosporine, tacrolimus, sirolimus
Oral Hypoglycemics	oral hypoglycemics
Protease Inhibitors	indinavir, ritonavir, saquinavir
Other	alfentanil, buspirone, methylprednisolone, trimetrexate, warfarin

Decrease plasma concentration of itraconazole	
Anticonvulsants	carbamazepine, phenobarbital, phenytoin
Antimycobacterials	isoniazid, rifabutin, rifampin
Gastric Acid Suppressors/ Neutralizers	antacids, H_2-receptor antagonists, proton pump inhibitors
Non-nucleoside Reverse Transcriptase Inhibitors	nevirapine

Increase plasma concentration of itraconazole	
Macrolide Antibiotics	clarithromycin, erythromycin
Protease Inhibitors	indinavir, ritonavir

[1]This list is not all-inclusive.
[2] Contraindicated with SPORANOX® based on clinical and/or pharmacokinetics studies. (See WARNINGS and below.)
[3] For information on parenterally administered midazolam, see the Benzodiazepine paragraph below.

Antiarrhythmics: The class IA antiarrhythmic quinidine and class III antiarrhythmic dofetilide are known to prolong the QT interval. Coadministration of quinidine or dofetilide with SPORANOX® may increase plasma concentrations of quinidine or dofetilide which could result in serious cardiovascular events. Therefore, concomitant administration of SPORANOX® and quinidine or dofetilide is contraindicated. (See BOX WARNING, CONTRAINDICATIONS, and WARNINGS.)

Concomitant administration of digoxin and SPORANOX® has led to increased plasma concentrations of digoxin.

Anticonvulsants: Reduced plasma concentrations of itraconazole were reported when SPORANOX® was administered concomitantly with phenytoin. Carbamazepine, phenobarbital, and phenytoin are all inducers of CYP3A4. Although interactions with carbamazepine and phenobarbital have not been studied, concomitant administration of SPORANOX® and these drugs would be expected to result in decreased plasma concentrations of itraconazole. In addition, in vivo studies have demonstrated an increase in plasma carbamazepine concentrations in subjects concomitantly receiving ketoconazole. Although there are no data regarding the effect of itraconazole on carbamazepine metabolism, because of the similarities between ketoconazole and itraconazole, concomitant administration of SPORANOX® and carbamazepine may inhibit the metabolism of carbamazepine.

Antimycobacterials: Drug interaction studies have demonstrated that plasma concentrations of azole antifungal agents and their metabolites, including itraconazole and hydroxyitraconazole, were significantly decreased when these agents were given concomitantly with rifabutin or rifampin. In vivo data suggest that rifabutin is metabolized in part by CYP3A4. SPORANOX® may inhibit the metabolism of rifabutin. Although no formal study data are available for isoniazid, similar effects should be anticipated. Therefore, the efficacy of SPORANOX® could be substantially reduced if given concomitantly with one of these agents. Coadministration is not recommended.

Antineoplastics: SPORANOX® may inhibit the metabolism of busulfan, docetaxel, and vinca alkaloids.

Antipsychotics: Pimozide is known to prolong the QT interval and is partially metabolized by CYP3A4. Coadministration of pimozide with SPORANOX® could result in serious cardiovascular events. Therefore, concomitant administration of SPORANOX® and pimozide is contraindicated. (See BOX WARNING, CONTRAINDICATIONS, and WARNINGS.)

Benzodiazepines: Concomitant administration of SPORANOX® and alprazolam, diazepam, oral midazolam, or triazolam could lead to increased plasma concentrations of these benzodiazepines. Increased plasma concentrations could potentiate and prolong hypnotic and sedative effects. Concomitant administration of SPORANOX® and oral midazolam or triazolam is contraindicated. (See CONTRAINDICATIONS and WARNINGS.) If midazolam is administered parenterally, special precaution and patient monitoring is required since the sedative effect may be prolonged.

Calcium Channel Blockers: Edema has been reported in patients concomitantly receiving SPORANOX® and dihydropyridine calcium channel blockers. Appropriate dosage adjustment may be necessary.

Calcium channel blockers can have a negative inotropic effect which may be additive to those of itraconazole; itraconazole can inhibit the metabolism of calcium channel blockers such as dihydropyridines (e.g., nifedipine and felodipine) and verapamil. Therefore, caution should be used when co-administering itraconazole and calcium channel blockers. (See CLINICAL PHARMACOLOGY: Special Populations, CONTRAINDICATIONS, WARNINGS, and ADVERSE REACTIONS: Post-marketing Experience for more information).

Gastric Acid Suppressors/Neutralizers: Reduced plasma concentrations of itraconazole were reported when SPORANOX® Capsules were administered concomitantly with H_2-receptor antagonists. Studies have shown that absorption of itraconazole is impaired when gastric acid production is decreased. Therefore, SPORANOX® should be administered with a cola beverage if the patient has achlorhydria or is taking H_2-receptor antagonists or other gastric acid suppressors. Antacids should be administered at least 1 hour before or 2 hours after administration of SPORANOX® Capsules. In a clinical study, when SPORANOX® Capsules were administered with omeprazole (a proton pump inhibitor), the bioavailability of itraconazole was significantly reduced.

Gastrointestinal Motility Agents: Coadministration of SPORANOX® with cisapride can elevate plasma cisapride concentrations which could result in serious cardiovascular events. Therefore, concomitant administration of SPORANOX® with cisapride is contraindicated. (See BOX WARNING, CONTRAINDICATIONS, and WARNINGS.)

HMG CoA-Reductase Inhibitors: Human pharmacokinetic data suggest that SPORANOX® inhibits the metabolism of atorvastatin, cerivastatin, lovastatin, and simvastatin, which may increase the risk of skeletal muscle toxicity, including rhabdomyolysis. Concomitant administration of SPORANOX® with HMG CoA-reductase inhibitors, such as lovastatin and simvastatin, is contraindicated. (See CONTRAINDICATIONS and WARNINGS.)

Immunosuppressants: Concomitant administration of SPORANOX® and cyclosporine or tacrolimus has led to increased plasma concentrations of these immunosuppressants. Concomitant administration of SPORANOX® and sirolimus could increase plasma concentrations of sirolimus.

Continued on next page

Sporanox—Cont.

Macrolide Antibiotics: Erythromycin and clarithromycin are known inhibitors of CYP3A4 (See Table 1) and may increase plasma concentrations of itraconazole. In a small pharmacokinetic study involving HIV infected patients, clarithromycin was shown to increase plasma concentrations of itraconazole. Similarly, following administration of 1 gram of erythromycin ethyl succinate and 200 mg itraconazole as single doses, the mean C_{max} and $AUC_{0-\infty}$ of itraconazole increased by 44% (90% CI: 119–175%) and 36% (90% CI: 108–171%), respectively.

Non-nucleoside Reverse Transcriptase Inhibitors: Nevirapine is an inducer of CYP3A4. In vivo studies have shown that nevirapine induces the metabolism of ketoconazole, significantly reducing the bioavailability of ketoconazole. Studies involving nevirapine and itraconazole have not been conducted. However, because of the similarities between ketoconazole and itraconazole, concomitant administration of SPORANOX® and nevirapine is not recommended.

In a clinical study, when 8 HIV-infected subjects were treated concomitantly with SPORANOX® Capsules 100 mg twice daily and the nucleoside reverse transcriptase inhibitor zidovudine 8 ± 0.4 mg/kg/day, the pharmacokinetics of zidovudine were not affected. Other nucleoside reverse transcriptase inhibitors have not been studied.

Oral Hypoglycemic Agents: Severe hypoglycemia has been reported in patients concomitantly receiving azole antifungal agents and oral hypoglycemic agents. Blood glucose concentrations should be carefully monitored when SPORANOX® and oral hypoglycemic agents are coadministered.

Polyenes: Prior treatment with itraconazole, like other azoles, may reduce or inhibit the activity of polyenes such as amphotericin B. However, the clinical significance of this drug effect has not been clearly defined.

Protease Inhibitors: Concomitant administration of SPORANOX® and protease inhibitors metabolized by CYP3A4, such as indinavir, ritonavir, and saquinavir, may increase plasma concentrations of these protease inhibitors. In addition, concomitant administration of SPORANOX® and indinavir and ritonavir (but not saquinavir) may increase plasma concentrations of itraconazole. Caution is advised when SPORANOX® and protease inhibitors must be given concomitantly.

Other:

- In vitro data suggest that alfentanil is metabolized by CYP3A4. Administration with SPORANOX® may increase plasma concentrations of alfentanil.
- Human pharmacokinetic data suggest that concomitant administration of SPORANOX® and buspirone results in significant increases in plasma concentrations of buspirone.
- SPORANOX® may inhibit the metabolism of methylprednisolone.
- In vitro data suggest that trimetrexate is extensively metabolized by CYP3A4. In vitro animal models have demonstrated that ketoconazole potently inhibits the metabolism of trimetrexate. Although there are no data regarding the effect of itraconazole on trimetrexate metabolism, because of the similarities between ketoconazole and itraconazole, concomitant administration of SPORANOX® and trimetrexate may inhibit the metabolism of trimetrexate.
- SPORANOX® enhances the anticoagulant effect of coumarin-like drugs, such as warfarin.

Carcinogenesis, Mutagenesis, and Impairment of Fertility: Itraconazole showed no evidence of carcinogenicity potential in mice treated orally for 23 months at dosage levels up to 80 mg/kg/day (approximately 10× the maximum recommended human dose [MRHD]). Male rats treated with 25 mg/kg/day (3.1× MRHD) had a slightly increased incidence of soft tissue sarcoma. These sarcomas may have been a consequence of hypercholesterolemia, which is a response of rats, but not dogs or humans, to chronic itraconazole administration. Female rats treated with 50 mg/kg/day (6.25× MRHD) had an increased incidence of squamous cell carcinoma of the lung (2/50) as compared to the untreated group. Although the occurrence of squamous cell carcinoma in the lung is extremely uncommon in untreated rats, the increase in this study was not statistically significant.

Itraconazole produced no mutagenic effects when assayed in DNA repair test (unscheduled DNA synthesis) in primary rat hepatocytes, in Ames tests with *Salmonella typhimurium* (6 strains) and *Escherichia coli*, in the mouse lymphoma gene mutation tests, in a sex-linked recessive lethal mutation (*Drosophila melanogaster*) test, in chromosome aberration tests in human lymphocytes, in a cell transformation test with C3H/10T½ C18 mouse embryo fibroblasts cells, in a dominant lethal mutation test in male and female mice, and in micronucleus tests in mice and rats.

Itraconazole did not affect the fertility of male or female rats treated orally with dosage levels of up to 40 mg/kg/day (5× MRHD), even though parental toxicity was present at this dosage level. More severe signs of parental toxicity, including death, were present in the next higher dosage level, 160 mg/kg/day (20× MRHD).

Pregnancy: Teratogenic effects. Pregnancy Category C: Itraconazole was found to cause a dose-related increase in maternal toxicity, embryotoxicity, and teratogenicity in rats at dosage levels of approximately 40–160 mg/kg/day (5–20× MRHD), and in mice at dosage levels of approximately 80 mg/kg/day (10× MRHD). In rats, the teratogenicity consisted of major skeletal defects; in mice, it consisted of encephaloceles and/or macroglossia.

There are no studies in pregnant women. SPORANOX® should be used for the treatment of systemic fungal infections in pregnancy only if the benefit outweighs the potential risk. SPORANOX® should not be administered for the treatment of onychomycosis to pregnant patients or to women contemplating pregnancy. SPORANOX® should not be administered to women of childbearing potential for the treatment of onychomycosis unless they are using effective measures to prevent pregnancy and they begin therapy on the second or third day following the onset of menses. Effective contraception should be continued throughout SPORANOX® therapy and for 2 months following the end of treatment.

Nursing Mothers: Itraconazole is excreted in human milk; therefore, the expected benefits of SPORANOX® therapy for the mother should be weighed against the potential risk from exposure of itraconazole to the infant. The U.S. Public Health Service Centers for Disease Control and Prevention advises HIV-infected women not to breast-feed to avoid potential transmission of HIV to uninfected infants.

Pediatric Use: The efficacy and safety of SPORANOX® have not been established in pediatric patients. No pharmacokinetic data on SPORANOX® Capsules are available in children. A small number of patients ages 3 to 16 years have been treated with 100 mg/day of itraconazole capsules for systemic fungal infections, and no serious unexpected adverse events have been reported. SPORANOX® Oral Solution (5 mg/kg/day) has been administered to pediatric patients (N=26; ages 6 months to 12 years) for 2 weeks and no serious unexpected adverse events were reported.

The long-term effects of itraconazole on bone growth in children are unknown. In three toxicology studies using rats, itraconazole induced bone defects at dosage levels as low as 20 mg/kg/day (2.5× MRHD). The induced defects included reduced bone plate activity, thinning of the zona compacta of the large bones, and increased bone fragility. At a dosage level of 80 mg/kg/day (10× MRHD) over 1 year or 160 mg/kg/day (20× MRHD) for 6 months, itraconazole induced small tooth pulp with hypocellular appearance in some rats. No such bone toxicity has been reported in adult patients.

HIV-Infected Patients: Because hypochlorhydria has been reported in HIV-infected individuals, the absorption of itraconazole in these patients may be decreased.

ADVERSE REACTIONS

SPORANOX® has been associated with rare cases of serious hepatotoxicity, including liver failure and death. Some of these cases had neither pre-existing liver disease nor a serious underlying medical condition. If clinical signs or symptoms develop that are consistent with liver disease, treatment should be discontinued and liver function testing performed. The risks and benefits of SPORANOX® use should be reassessed. (See WARNINGS: Hepatic Effects and PRECAUTIONS: Information for Patients.)

Adverse Events in the Treatment of Systemic Fungal Infections

Adverse event data were derived from 602 patients treated for systemic fungal disease in U.S. clinical trials who were immunocompromised or receiving multiple concomitant medications. Treatment was discontinued in 10.5% of patients due to adverse events. The median duration before discontinuation of therapy was 81 days (range: 2 to 776 days). The table lists adverse events reported by at least 1% of patients.

Clinical Trials of Systemic Fungal Infections: Adverse Events Occurring with an Incidence of Greater than or Equal to 1%

Body System/Adverse Event	Incidence (%) (N=602)
Gastrointestinal	
Nausea	11
Vomiting	5
Diarrhea	3
Abdominal Pain	2
Anorexia	1
Body as a Whole	
Edema	4
Fatigue	3
Fever	3
Malaise	1
Skin and Appendages	
Rash*	9
Pruritus	3
Central/Peripheral Nervous System	
Headache	4
Dizziness	2
Psychiatric	
Libido Decreased	1
Somnolence	1
Cardiovascular	
Hypertension	3
Metabolic/Nutritional	
Hypokalemia	2
Urinary System	
Albuminuria	1
Liver and Biliary System	
Hepatic Function Abnormal	3
Reproductive System, Male	
Impotence	1

*Rash tends to occur more frequently in immunocompromised patients receiving immunosuppressive medications.

Adverse events infrequently reported in all studies included constipation, gastritis, depression, insomnia, tinnitus, menstrual disorder, adrenal insufficiency, gynecomastia, and male breast pain.

Adverse Events Reported in Toenail Onychomycosis Clinical Trials

Patients in these trials were on a continuous dosing regimen of 200 mg once daily for 12 consecutive weeks.

The following adverse events led to temporary or permanent discontinuation of therapy.

Clinical Trials of Onychomycosis of the Toenail: Adverse Events Leading to Temporary or Permanent Discontinuation of Therapy

Adverse Event	Incidence (%) Itraconazole (N=112)
Elevated Liver Enzymes (greater than twice the upper limit of normal)	4
Gastrointestinal Disorders	4
Rash	3
Hypertension	2
Orthostatic Hypotension	1
Headache	1
Malaise	1
Myalgia	1
Vasculitis	1
Vertigo	1

The following adverse events occurred with an incidence of greater than or equal to 1% (N=112): headache: 10%; rhinitis: 9%; upper respiratory tract infection: 8%; sinusitis, injury: 7%; diarrhea, dyspepsia, flatulence, abdominal pain, dizziness, rash: 4%; cystitis, urinary tract infection, liver function abnormality, myalgia, nausea: 3%; appetite increased, constipation, gastritis, gastroenteritis, pharyngitis, asthenia, fever, pain, tremor, herpes zoster, abnormal dreaming: 2%.

Adverse Events Reported in Fingernail Onychomycosis Clinical Trials

Patients in these trials were on a pulse regimen consisting of two 1-week treatment periods of 200 mg twice daily, separated by a 3-week period without drug.

The following adverse events led to temporary or permanent discontinuation of therapy.

Clinical Trials of Onychomycosis of the Fingernail: Adverse Events Leading to Temporary or Permanent Discontinuation of Therapy

Adverse Event	Incidence (%) Itraconazole (N=37)
Rash/Pruritus	3
Hypertriglyceridemia	3

The following adverse events occurred with an incidence of greater than or equal to 1% (N=37): headache: 8%; pruritus, nausea, rhinitis: 5%; rash, bursitis, anxiety, depression, constipation, abdominal pain, dyspepsia, ulcerative stomatitis, gingivitis, hypertriglyceridemia, sinusitis, fatigue, malaise, pain, injury: 3%.

Post-marketing Experience

Worldwide post-marketing experiences with the use of SPORANOX® include adverse events of gastrointestinal origin, such as dyspepsia, nausea, vomiting, diarrhea, abdominal pain and constipation. Other reported adverse events include peripheral edema, congestive heart failure and pulmonary edema, headache, dizziness, peripheral neuropathy, menstrual disorders, reversible increases in hepatic enzymes, hepatitis, liver failure, hypokalemia, hypertriglyceridemia, alopecia, allergic reactions (such as pruritus, rash, urticaria, angioedema, anaphylaxis), Stevens-Johnson syndrome, and neutropenia. (See CLINICAL PHARMACOLOGY: Special Populations, CONTRAINDICATIONS, WARNINGS, and PRECAUTIONS: Drug Interactions for more information).

OVERDOSAGE

Itraconazole is not removed by dialysis. In the event of accidental overdosage, supportive measures, including gastric lavage with sodium bicarbonate, should be employed.

Limited data exist on the outcomes of patients ingesting high doses of itraconazole. In patients taking either 1000 mg of SPORANOX® (itraconazole) Oral Solution or up to 3000 mg of SPORANOX® (itraconazole) Capsules, the adverse event profile was similar to that observed at recommended doses.

DOSAGE AND ADMINISTRATION

SPORANOX® (itraconazole) Capsules should be taken with a full meal to ensure maximal absorption.

SPORANOX® Capsules is a different preparation than SPORANOX® Oral Solution and should not be used interchangeably.

Treatment of Blastomycosis and Histoplasmosis: The recommended dose is 200 mg once daily (2 capsules). If there is no obvious improvement, or there is evidence of progressive fungal disease, the dose should be increased in 100-mg increments to a maximum of 400 mg daily. Doses above 200 mg/day should be given in two divided doses.

Treatment of Aspergillosis: A daily dose of 200 to 400 mg is recommended.

Treatment in Life-Threatening Situations: In life-threatening situations, a loading dose should be used whether given as oral capsules or intravenously.

- IV Injection: the recommended intravenous dose is 200 mg b.i.d. for four consecutive doses, followed by 200 mg once daily thereafter. Each intravenous dose should be infused over 1 hour. The safety and efficacy of SPORANOX® Injection administered for greater than 14 days is not known. See complete prescribing information for SPORANOX® (itraconazole) Injection.
- Capsules: although clinical studies did not provide for a loading dose, it is recommended, based on pharmacokinetic data, that a loading dose of 200 mg (2 capsules) three times daily (600 mg/day) be given for the first 3 days of treatment.

Treatment should be continued for a minimum of three months and until clinical parameters and laboratory tests indicate that the active fungal infection has subsided. An inadequate period of treatment may lead to recurrence of active infection.

SPORANOX® Capsules and SPORANOX® Oral Solution should not be used interchangeably. Only the oral solution has been demonstrated effective for oral and/or esophageal candidiasis.

Treatment of Onychomycosis: Toenails with or without fingernail involvement: The recommended dose is 200 mg (2 capsules) once daily for 12 consecutive weeks.

Treatment of Onychomycosis: Fingernails only: The recommended dosing regimen is 2 treatment pulses, each consisting of 200 mg (2 capsules) b.i.d. (400 mg/day) for 1 week. The pulses are separated by a 3-week period without SPORANOX®.

HOW SUPPLIED

SPORANOX® (itraconazole) Capsules are available containing 100 mg of itraconazole, with a blue opaque cap and pink transparent body, imprinted with "JANSSEN" and "SPORANOX 100." The capsules are supplied in unit-dose blister packs of 3 × 10 capsules (NDC 50458-290-01), bottles of 30 capsules (NDC 50458-290-04) and in the PulsePak® containing 7 blister packs × 4 capsules each (NDC 50458-290-28).

Store at controlled room temperature 15°–25°C (59°–77°F). Protect from light and moisture.

Keep out of reach of children.

 7501618

U.S. Patent Nos. 4,267,179; 5,633,015

Revised February 2002

Distributed by:
JANSSEN PHARMACEUTICA PRODUCTS, L.P.
Titusville, New Jersey 08560, USA
Capsule contents manufactured by:
JANSSEN PHARMACEUTICA N.V.
Beerse, Belgium

To keep your **PDR** up to date throughout the year, note these revisions on the corresponding pages of the annual volume. Simply write **"See Supplement A"** next to the product heading.

Key Pharmaceuticals, Inc.

GALLOPING HILL ROAD
KENILWORTH, NJ 07033

For Medical Information Contact:
Generally:
Drug Information Services
(800) 526-4099
(9:00 AM to 5:00 PM EST)

After Hours and Weekends:
(908) 298-4000

K-DUR® ℞

[kā'-dūr]

(Potassium Chloride) USP
Extended Release Tablets

Prescribing information for this product, which appears on pages 1832–1833 of the 2002 PDR, has been completely revised as follows. Please write "See Supplement A" next to the product heading.

DESCRIPTION

The K-DUR® 20 product is an immediately dispersing extended release oral dosage form of potassium chloride containing 1500 mg of microencapsulated potassium chloride, USP equivalent to 20 mEq of potassium in a tablet.

The K-DUR® 10 product is an immediately dispersing extended release oral dosage form of potassium chloride containing 750 mg of microencapsulated potassium chloride, USP equivalent to 10 mEq of potassium in a tablet.

These formulations are intended to slow the release of potassium so that the likelihood of a high localized concentration of potassium chloride within the gastrointestinal tract is reduced.

K-DUR is an electrolyte replenisher. The chemical name of the active ingredient is potassium chloride, and the structural formula is KCl. Potassium chloride, USP occurs as a white, granular powder or as colorless crystals. It is odorless and has a saline taste. Its solutions are neutral to litmus. It is freely soluble in water and insoluble in alcohol.

K-DUR is a tablet formulation (not enteric coated or wax matrix) containing individually microencapsulated potassium chloride crystals which disperse upon tablet disintegration. In simulated gastric fluid at 37°C and in the absence of outside agitation, K-DUR begins disintegrating into microencapsulated crystals within seconds and completely disintegrates within 1 minute. The microencapsulated crystals are formulated to provide an extended release of potassium chloride.

Inactive Ingredients: Crospovidone, Ethylcellulose, Hydroxypropyl Cellulose, Magnesium Stearate, and Microcrystalline Cellulose.

CLINICAL PHARMACOLOGY

The potassium ion is the principal intracellular cation of most body tissues. Potassium ions participate in a number of essential physiological processes including the maintenance of intracellular tonicity; the transmission of nerve impulses; the contraction of cardiac, skeletal, and smooth muscle; and the maintenance of normal renal function.

The intracellular concentration of potassium is approximately 150 to 160 mEq per liter. The normal adult plasma concentration is 3.5 to 5 mEq per liter. An active ion transport system maintains this gradient across the plasma membrane.

Potassium is a normal dietary constituent and under steady-state conditions the amount of potassium absorbed from the gastrointestinal tract is equal to the amount excreted in the urine. The usual dietary intake of potassium is 50 to 100 mEq per day.

Potassium depletion will occur whenever the rate of potassium loss through renal excretion and/or loss from the gastrointestinal tract exceeds the rate of potassium intake. Such depletion usually develops as a consequence of therapy with diuretics, primary or secondary hyperaldosteronism, diabetic ketoacidosis, or inadequate replacement of potassium in patients on prolonged parenteral nutrition.]Depletion can develop rapidly with severe diarrhea, especially if associated with vomiting. Potassium depletion due to these causes is usually accompanied by a concomitant loss of chloride and is manifested by hypokalemia and metabolic alkalosis. Potassium depletion may produce weakness, fatigue, disturbances or cardiac rhythm (primarily ectopic beats), prominent U-waves in the electrocardiogram, and in advanced cases, flaccid paralysis and/or impaired ability to concentrate urine.

If potassium depletion associated with metabolic alkalosis cannot be managed by correcting the fundamental cause of the deficiency, eg, where the patient requires long-term diuretic therapy, supplemental potassium in the form of high-potassium food or potassium chloride may be able to restore normal potassium levels.

In rare circumstances (eg, patients with renal tubular acidosis) potassium depletion may be associated with metabolic acidosis and hyperchloremia. In such patients potassium replacement should be accomplished with potassium salts other than the chloride, such as potassium bicarbonate, potassium citrate, potassium acetate, or potassium gluconate.

INDICATIONS AND USAGE

BECAUSE OF REPORTS OF INTESTINAL AND GASTRIC ULCERATION AND BLEEDING WITH CONTROLLED RELEASE POTASSIUM CHLORIDE PREPARATIONS, THESE DRUGS SHOULD BE RESERVED FOR THOSE PATIENTS WHO CANNOT TOLERATE OR REFUSE TO TAKE LIQUID OR EFFERVESCENT POTASSIUM PREPARATIONS OR FOR PATIENTS IN WHOM THERE IS A PROBLEM OF COMPLIANCE WITH THESE PREPARATIONS.

1. For the treatment of patients with hypokalemia with or without metabolic alkalosis, in digitalis intoxication, and in patients with hypokalemic familial periodic paralysis. If hypokalemia is the result of diuretic therapy, consideration should be given to the use of a lower dose of diuretic, which may be sufficient without leading to hypokalemia.
2. For the prevention of hypokalemia in patients who would be at particular risk if hypokalemia were to develop, eg, digitalized patients or patients with significant cardiac arrhythmias.

The use of potassium salts in patients receiving diuretics for uncomplicated essential hypertension is often unnecessary when such patients have a normal dietary pattern and when low doses of the diuretic are used. Serum potassium should be checked periodically, however, and if hypokalemia occurs, dietary supplementation with potassium-containing foods may be adequate to control milder cases. In more severe cases, and if dose adjustment of the diuretic is ineffective or unwarranted, supplementation with potassium salts may be indicated.

CONTRAINDICATIONS

Potassium supplements are contraindicated in patients with hyperkalemia since a further increase in serum potassium concentration in such patients can produce cardiac arrest. Hyperkalemia may complicate any of the following conditions: chronic renal failure, systemic acidosis, such as diabetic acidosis, acute dehydration, extensive tissue breakdown as in severe burns, adrenal insufficiency, or the administration of a potassium-sparing diuretic (eg, spironolactone, triamterene, amiloride) (see **OVERDOSAGE**).

Controlled release formulations of potassium chloride have produced esophageal ulceration in certain cardiac patients with esophageal compression due to enlarged left atrium. Potassium supplementation, when indicated in such patients, should be given as a liquid preparation or as an aqueous (water) suspension of K-DUR (see **PRECAUTIONS: Information for Patients**, and **DOSAGE AND ADMINISTRATION** sections).

All solid oral dosage forms of potassium chloride are contraindicated in any patient in whom there is structural, pathological (eg, diabetic gastroparesis), or pharmacologic (use of anticholinergic agents or other agents with anticholinergic properties at sufficient doses to exert anticholinergic effects) cause for arrest or delay in tablet passage through the gastrointestinal tract.

WARNINGS

Hyperkalemia (see **OVERDOSAGE**): In patients with impaired mechanisms for excreting potassium, the administration of potassium salts can produce hyperkalemia and cardiac arrest. This occurs most commonly in patients given potassium by the intravenous route but may also occur in patients given potassium orally. Potentially fatal hyperkalemia can develop rapidly and be asymptomatic. The use of potassium salts in patients with chronic renal disease, or any other condition which impairs potassium excretion, requires particularly careful monitoring of the serum potassium concentration and appropriate dosage adjustment.

Interaction with Potassium-Sparing Diuretics: Hypokalemia should not be treated by the concomitant administration of potassium salts and a potassium-sparing diuretic (eg, spironolactone, triamterene, or amiloride) since the simultaneous administration of these agents can produce severe hyperkalemia.

Interaction with Angiotensin-Converting Enzyme Inhibitors: Angiotensin-converting enzyme (ACE) inhibitors (eg, captopril, enalapril) will produce some potassium retention by inhibiting aldosterone production. Potassium supplements should be given to patients receiving ACE inhibitors only with close monitoring.

Gastrointestinal Lesions: Solid oral dosage forms of potassium chloride can produce ulcerative and/or stenotic lesions of the gastrointestinal tract. Based on spontaneous adverse reaction reports, enteric-coated preparations of potassium chloride are associated with an increased frequency of small bowel lesions (40–50 per 100,000 patient years) compared to sustained release wax matrix formulations (less than one per 100,000 patient years). Because of the lack of extensive marketing experience with microencapsulated products, a comparison between such products and wax matrix or enteric-coated products is not available. K-DUR is a tablet formulated to provide a controlled rate of release of microencapsulated potassium chloride and thus to minimize the possibility of a high local concentration of potassium near the gastrointestinal wall.

Prospective trials have been conducted in normal human volunteers in which the upper gastrointestinal tract was evaluated by endoscopic inspection before and after 1 week of solid oral potassium chloride therapy. The ability of this model to predict events occurring in usual clinical practice is unknown. Trials which approximated usual clinical practice did not reveal any clear differences between the wax matrix and microencapsulated dosage forms. In contrast,

Continued on next page

K-Dur—Cont.

there was a higher incidence of gastric and duodenal lesions in subjects receiving a high dose of a wax matrix controlled-release formulation under conditions which did not resemble usual or recommended clinical practice (ie, 96 mEq per day in divided doses of potassium chloride administered to fasted patients, in the presence of an anticholinergic drug to delay gastric emptying). The upper gastrointestinal lesions observed by endoscopy were asymptomatic and were not accompanied by evidence of bleeding (Hemoccult testing). The relevance of these findings to the usual conditions (ie, nonfasting, no anticholinergic agent, smaller doses) under which controlled release potassium chloride products are used is uncertain; epidemiologic studies have not identified an elevated risk, compared to microencapsulated products, for upper gastrointestinal lesions in patients receiving wax matrix formulations. K-DUR should be discontinued immediately and the possibility of ulceration, obstruction, or perforation considered if severe vomiting, abdominal pain, distention, or gastrointestinal bleeding occurs.

Metabolic Acidosis: Hypokalemia in patients with metabolic acidosis should be treated with an alkalinizing potassium salt such as potassium bicarbonate, potassium citrate, potassium acetate, or potassium gluconate.

PRECAUTIONS

General: The diagnosis of potassium depletion is ordinarily made by demonstrating hypokalemia in a patient with a clinical history suggesting some cause for potassium depletion. In interpreting the serum potassium level, the physician should bear in mind that acute alkalosis per se can produce hypokalemia in the absence of a deficit in total body potassium while acute acidosis per se can increase the serum potassium concentration into the normal range even in the presence of a reduced total body potassium. The treatment of potassium depletion, particularly in the presence of cardiac disease, renal disease, or acidosis requires careful attention to acid-base balance and appropriate monitoring of serum electrolytes, the electrocardiogram, and the clinical status of the patient.

Information for Patients: Physicians should consider reminding the patient of the following:

To take each dose with meals and with a full glass of water or other liquid.

To take each dose without crushing, chewing, or sucking the tablets. If those patients are having difficulty swallowing whole tablets, they may try one of the following alternate methods of administration:

a. Break the tablet in half, and take each half separately with a glass of water.

b. Prepare an aqueous (water) suspension as follows:

1. Place the whole tablet(s) in approximately ½ glass of water (4 fluid ounces).
2. Allow approximately 2 minutes for the tablet(s) to disintegrate.
3. Stir for about half a minute after the tablet(s) has disintegrated.
4. Swirl the suspension and consume the entire contents of the glass immediately by drinking or by the use of a straw.
5. Add another 1 fluid ounce of water, swirl, and consume immediately.
6. Then, add an additional 1 fluid ounce of water, swirl, and consume immediately.

Aqueous suspension of K-DUR tablets that is not taken immediately should be discarded. The use of other liquids for suspending K-DUR tablets is not recommended.

To take this medicine following the frequency and amount prescribed by the physician. This is especially important if the patient is also taking diuretics and/or digitalis preparations.

To check with the physician at once if tarry stools or other evidence of gastrointestinal bleeding is noticed.

Laboratory Tests: When blood is drawn for analysis of plasma potassium it is important to recognize that artifactual elevations can occur after improper venipuncture technique or as a result of *in vitro* hemolysis of the sample.

Drug Interactions: Potassium-sparing diuretics, angiotensin-converting enzyme inhibitors (see **WARNINGS**).

Carcinogenesis, Mutagenesis, Impairment of Fertility: Carcinogenicity, mutagenicity, and fertility studies in animals have not been performed. Potassium is a normal dietary constituent.

Pregnancy Category C: Animal reproduction studies have not been conducted with K-DUR. It is unlikely that potassium supplementation that does not lead to hyperkalemia would have an adverse effect on the fetus or would affect reproductive capacity.

Nursing Mothers: The normal potassium ion content of human milk is about 13 mEq per liter. Since oral potassium becomes part of the body potassium pool, so long as body potassium is not excessive, the contribution of potassium chloride supplementation should have little or no effect on the level in human milk.

Pediatric Use: Safety and effectiveness in pediatric patients have not been established.

ADVERSE REACTIONS

One of the most severe adverse effects is hyperkalemia (see **CONTRAINDICATIONS, WARNINGS**, and **OVERDOSAGE**). There have also been reports of upper and lower gastrointestinal conditions including obstruction, bleeding, ulceration, and perforation (see **CONTRAINDICATIONS** and **WARNINGS**).

The most common adverse reactions to oral potassium salts are nausea, vomiting, flatulence, abdominal pain/discomfort, and diarrhea. These symptoms are due to irritation of the gastrointestinal tract and are best managed by diluting the preparation further, taking the dose with meals or reducing the amount taken at one time.

OVERDOSAGE

The administration of oral potassium salts to persons with normal excretory mechanisms for potassium rarely causes serious hyperkalemia. However, if excretory mechanisms are impaired or if potassium is administered too rapidly intravenously, potentially fatal hyperkalemia can result (see **CONTRAINDICATIONS** and **WARNINGS**). It is important to recognize that hyperkalemia is usually asymptomatic and may be manifested only by an increased serum potassium concentration (6.5–8.0 mEq/L) and characteristic electrocardiographic changes (peaking of T-waves, loss of P-waves, depression of S-T segment and prolongation of the QT-interval). Late manifestations include muscle paralysis and cardiovascular collapse from cardiac arrest (9–12 mEq/L).

Treatment measures for hyperkalemia include the following:

1. Elimination of foods and medications containing potassium and of any agents with potassium-sparing properties.
2. Intravenous administration of 300 to 500 mL/hr of 10% dextrose solution containing 10–20 units of crystalline insulin per 1,000 mL.
3. Correction of acidosis, if present, with intravenous sodium bicarbonate.
4. Use of exchange resins, hemodialysis, or peritoneal dialysis.

In treating hyperkalemia, it should be recalled that in patients who have been stabilized on digitalis, too rapid a lowering of the serum potassium concentration can produce digitalis toxicity.

DOSAGE AND ADMINISTRATION

The usual dietary intake of potassium by the average adult is 50 to 100 mEq per day. Potassium depletion sufficient to cause hypokalemia usually requires the loss of 200 or more mEq of potassium from the total body store.

Dosage must be adjusted to the individual needs of each patient. The dose for the prevention of hypokalemia is typically in the range of 20 mEq per day. Doses of 40–100 mEq per day or more are used for the treatment of potassium depletion. Dosage should be divided if more than 20 mEq per day is given such that no more than 20 mEq is given in a single dose.

Each K-DUR 20 tablet provides 20 mEq of potassium chloride.

Each K-DUR 10 tablet provides 10 mEq of potassium chloride.

K-DUR tablets should be taken with meals and with a glass of water or other liquid. This product should not be taken on an empty stomach because of its potential for gastric irritation (see **WARNINGS**).

Patients having difficulty swallowing whole tablets may try one of the following alternate methods of administration:

a. Break the tablet in half, and take each half separately with a glass of water.

b. Prepare an aqueous (water) suspension as follows:

1. Place the whole tablet(s) in approximately ½ glass of water (4 fluid ounces).
2. Allow approximately 2 minutes for the tablet(s) to disintegrate.
3. Stir for about half a minute after the tablet(s) has disintegrated.
4. Swirl the suspension and consume the entire contents of the glass immediately by drinking or by the use of a straw.
5. Add another 1 fluid ounce of water, swirl, and consume immediately.
6. Then, add an additional 1 fluid ounce of water, swirl, and consume immediately.

Aqueous suspension of K-DUR tablets that is not taken immediately should be discarded. The use of other liquids for suspending K-DUR tablets is not recommended.

HOW SUPPLIED

K-DUR 20 mEq Extended Release Tablets are available in bottles of 100 (NDC 0085-0787-01); bottles of 500 (NDC 0085-0787-06); bottles of 1000 (NDC 0085-0787-10); and boxes of 100 for unit dose dispensing (NDC 0085-0787-81). K-DUR 20 mEq tablets are white to off-white mottled capsule-shaped tablets, imprinted "K-DUR 20" and scored on the other side for flexibility of dosing.

K-DUR 10 mEq Extended Release Tablets are available in bottles of 100 (NDC 0085-0263-01) and boxes of 100 for unit dose dispensing (NDC 0085-0263- 81). K-DUR 10 mEq tablets are white to off-white mottled capsule-shaped tablets, imprinted K-DUR 10 on one side and plain on the other side.

Storage Conditions: Keep tightly closed. Store at controlled room temperature 15°–30°C (59°–86°F).

Rx only.

Key Pharmaceuticals, Inc.,
Kenilworth, NJ 07033 USA.

Rev. 9/01 B-14274782
24206718T

NITRO-DUR® ℞

[*nītrō-dur*]
(nitroglycerin)
Transdermal Infusion System

Prescribing information for this product, which appears on pages 1834–1835 of the 2002 PDR, has been completely revised as follows. Please write "See Supplement A" next to the product heading.

DESCRIPTION

Nitroglycerin is 1,2,3-propanetriol trinitrate, an organic nitrate whose structural formula is:

$$H_2CONO_2$$
$$HCONO_2$$
$$H_2CONO_2$$

and whose molecular weight is 227.09. The organic nitrates are vasodilators, active on both arteries and veins.

The NITRO-DUR (nitroglycerin) Transdermal Infusion System is a flat unit designed to provide continuous controlled release of nitroglycerin through intact skin. The rate of release of nitroglycerin is linearly dependent upon the area of the applied system; each cm^2 of applied system delivers approximately 0.02 mg of nitroglycerin per hour. Thus, the 5-, 10-, 15-, 20-, 30-, and 40-cm^2 systems deliver approximately 0.1, 0.2, 0.3, 0.4, 0.6, and 0.8 mg of nitroglycerin per hour, respectively.

The remainder of the nitroglycerin in each system serves as a reservoir and is not delivered in normal use. After 12 hours, for example, each system has delivered approximately 6% of its original content of nitroglycerin.

The NITRO-DUR transdermal system contains nitroglycerin in acrylic-based polymer adhesives with a resinous cross-linking agent to provide a continuous source of active ingredient. Each unit is sealed in a paper polyethylene-foil pouch.

Cross section of the system.

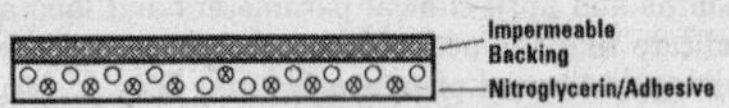

CLINICAL PHARMACOLOGY

The principal pharmacological action of nitroglycerin is relaxation of vascular smooth muscle and consequent dilatation of peripheral arteries and veins, especially the latter. Dilatation of the veins promotes peripheral pooling of blood and decreases venous return to the heart, thereby reducing left ventricular end-diastolic pressure and pulmonary capillary wedge pressure (preload). Arteriolar relaxation reduces systemic vascular resistance, systolic arterial pressure, and mean arterial pressure (afterload). Dilatation of the coronary arteries also occurs. The relative importance of preload reduction, afterload reduction, and coronary dilatation remains undefined.

Dosing regimens for most chronically used drugs are designed to provide plasma concentrations that are continuously greater than a minimally effective concentration. This strategy is inappropriate for organic nitrates. Several well-controlled clinical trials have used exercise testing to assess the antianginal efficacy of continuously delivered nitrates. In the large majority of these trials, active agents were indistinguishable from placebo after 24 hours (or less) of continuous therapy. Attempts to overcome nitrate tolerance by dose escalation, even to doses far in excess of those used acutely, have consistently failed. Only after nitrates have been absent from the body for several hours has their antianginal efficacy been restored.

Pharmacokinetics:

The volume of distribution of nitroglycerin is about 3 L/kg, and nitroglycerin is cleared from this volume at extremely rapid rates, with a resulting serum half-life of about 3 minutes. The observed clearance rates (close to 1 L/kg/min) greatly exceed hepatic blood flow; known sites of extrahepatic metabolism include red blood cells and vascular walls. The first products in the metabolism of nitroglycerin are inorganic nitrate and the 1,2- and 1,3-dinitroglycerols. The dinitrates are less effective vasodilators than nitroglycerin, but they are longer-lived in the serum, and their net contribution to the overall effect of chronic nitroglycerin regimens is not known. The dinitrates are further metabolized to (nonvasoactive) mononitrates and, ultimately, to glycerol and carbon dioxide.

To avoid development of tolerance to nitroglycerin, drug-free intervals of 10 to 12 hours are known to be sufficient; shorter intervals have not been well studied. In one well-controlled clinical trial, subjects receiving nitroglycerin appeared to exhibit a rebound or withdrawal effect, so that their exercise tolerance at the end of the daily drug-free interval was *less* than that exhibited by the parallel group receiving placebo.

In healthy volunteers, steady-state plasma concentrations of nitroglycerin are reached by about 2 hours after application of a patch and are maintained for the duration of wearing the system (observations have been limited to 24 hours). Upon removal of the patch, the plasma concentration declines with a half-life of about an hour.

Clinical Trials:

Regimens in which nitroglycerin patches were worn for 12 hours daily have been studied in well-controlled trials up to 4 weeks in duration. Starting about 2 hours after applica-

tion and continuing until 10 to 12 hours after application, patches that deliver at least 0.4 mg of nitroglycerin per hour have consistently demonstrated greater antianginal activity than placebo. Lower-dose patches have not been as well studied, but in one large, well-controlled trial in which higher-dose patches were also studied, patches delivering 0.2 mg/hr had significantly *less* antianginal activity than placebo.
It is reasonable to believe that the rate of nitroglycerin absorption from patches may vary with the site of application, but this relationship has not been adequately studied.

INDICATIONS AND USAGE

Transdermal nitroglycerin is indicated for the prevention of angina pectoris due to coronary artery disease. The onset of action of transdermal nitroglycerin is not sufficiently rapid for this product to be useful in aborting an acute attack.

CONTRAINDICATIONS

Allergic reactions to organic nitrates are extremely rare, but they do occur. Nitroglycerin is contraindicated in patients who are allergic to it. Allergy to the adhesives used in nitroglycerin patches has also been reported, and it similarly constitutes a contraindication to the use of this product.

WARNINGS

Amplification of the vasodilatory effects of the NITRO-DUR patch by sildenafil can result in severe hypotension. The time course and dose dependence of this interaction have not been studied. Appropriate supportive care has not been studied, but it seems reasonable to treat this as a nitrate overdose, with elevation of the extremities and with central volume expansion.
The benefits of transdermal nitroglycerin in patients with acute myocardial infarction or congestive heart failure have not been established. If one elects to use nitroglycerin in these conditions, careful clinical or hemodynamic monitoring must be used to avoid the hazards of hypotension and tachycardia.
A cardioverter/defibrillator should not be discharged through a paddle electrode that overlies a NITRO-DUR patch. The arcing that may be seen in this situation is harmless in itself, but it may be associated with local current concentration that can cause damage to the paddles and burns to the patient.

PRECAUTIONS

General:
Severe hypotension, particularly with upright posture, may occur with even small doses of nitroglycerin. This drug should therefore be used with caution in patients who may be volume depleted or who, for whatever reason, are already hypotensive. Hypotension induced by nitroglycerin may be accompanied by paradoxical bradycardia and increased angina pectoris.
Nitrate therapy may aggravate the angina caused by hypertrophic cardiomyopathy.
As tolerance to other forms of nitroglycerin develops, the effects of sublingual nitroglycerin on exercise tolerance, although still observable, is somewhat blunted.
In industrial workers who have had long-term exposure to unknown (presumably high) doses of organic nitrates, tolerance clearly occurs. Chest pain, acute myocardial infarction, and even sudden death have occurred during temporary withdrawal of nitrates from these workers, demonstrating the existence of true physical dependence.
Several clinical trials in patients with angina pectoris have evaluated nitroglycerin regimens which incorporated a 10- to 12-hour, nitrate-free interval. In some of these trials, an increase in the frequency of anginal attacks during the nitrate-free interval was observed in a small number of patients. In one trial, patients had decreased exercise tolerance at the end of the nitrate-free interval. Hemodynamic rebound has been observed only rarely; on the other hand, few studies were so designed that rebound, if it had occurred, would have been detected. The importance of these observations to the routine, clinical use of transdermal nitroglycerin is unknown.
Information for Patients:
Daily headaches sometimes accompany treatment with nitroglycerin. In patients who get these headaches, the headaches may be a marker of the activity of the drug. Patients should resist the temptation to avoid headaches by altering the schedule of their treatment with nitroglycerin, since loss of headache may be associated with simultaneous loss of antianginal efficacy.
Treatment with nitroglycerin may be associated with lightheadedness on standing, especially just after rising from a recumbent or seated position. This effect may be more frequent in patients who have also consumed alcohol.
After normal use, there is enough residual nitroglycerin in discarded patches that they are a potential hazard to children and pets.
A patient leaflet is supplied with the systems.
Drug Interactions:
The vasodilating effects of nitroglycerin may be additive with those of other vasodilators. Alcohol, in particular, has been found to exhibit additive effects of this variety.
Carcinogenesis, Mutagenesis, Impairment of Fertility:
Animal carcinogenesis studies with topically applied nitroglycerin have not been performed.
Rats receiving up to 434 mg/kg/day of dietary nitroglycerin for 2 years developed dose-related fibrotic and neoplastic changes in liver, including carcinomas, and interstitial cell tumors in testes. At high dose, the incidences of hepatocellular carcinomas in both sexes were 52% vs 0% in controls, and incidences of testicular tumors were 52% vs 8% in controls. Lifetime dietary administration of up to 1058 mg/kg/day of nitroglycerin was not tumorigenic in mice.
Nitroglycerin was weakly mutagenic in Ames tests performed in two different laboratories. Nevertheless, there was no evidence of mutagenicity in an *in vivo* dominant lethal assay with male rats treated with doses up to about 363 mg/kg/day, po, or in *in vitro* cytogenetic tests in rat and dog tissues.
In a three-generation reproduction study, rats received dietary nitroglycerin at doses up to about 434 mg/kg/day for 6 months prior to mating of the F_0 generation with treatment continuing through successive F_1 and F_2 generations. The high dose was associated with decreased feed intake and body weight gain in both sexes at all matings. No specific effect on the fertility of the F_0 generation was seen. Infertility noted in subsequent generations, however, was attributed to increased interstitial cell tissue and aspermatogenesis in the high-dose males. In this three-generation study there was no clear evidence of teratogenicity.
Pregnancy: Pregnancy Category C:
Animal teratology studies have not been conducted with nitroglycerin transdermal systems. Teratology studies in rats and rabbits, however, were conducted with topically applied nitroglycerin ointment at doses up to 80 mg/kg/day and 240 mg/kg/day, respectively. No toxic effects on dams or fetuses were seen at any dose tested. There are no adequate and well-controlled studies in pregnant women. Nitroglycerin should be given to a pregnant woman only if clearly needed.
Nursing Mothers:
It is not known whether nitroglycerin is excreted in human milk. Because many drugs are excreted in human milk, caution should be exercised when nitroglycerin is administered to a nursing woman.
Pediatric Use:
Safety and effectiveness in pediatric patients have not been established.

ADVERSE REACTIONS

Adverse reactions to nitroglycerin are generally dose related, and almost all of these reactions are the result of nitroglycerin's activity as a vasodilator. Headache, which may be severe, is the most commonly reported side effect. Headache may be recurrent with each daily dose, especially at higher doses. Transient episodes of lightheadedness, occasionally related to blood pressure changes, may also occur. Hypotension occurs infrequently, but in some patients it may be severe enough to warrant discontinuation of therapy. Syncope, crescendo angina, and rebound hypertension have been reported but are uncommon.
Allergic reactions to nitroglycerin are also uncommon, and the great majority of those reported have been cases of contact dermatitis or fixed drug eruptions in patients receiving nitroglycerin in ointments or patches. There have been a few reports of genuine anaphylactoid reactions, and these reactions can probably occur in patients receiving nitroglycerin by any route.
Extremely rarely, ordinary doses of organic nitrates have caused methemoglobinemia in normal-seeming patients. Methemoglobinemia is so infrequent at these doses that further discussion of its diagnosis and treatment is deferred (see **OVERDOSAGE**).
Application-site irritation may occur but is rarely severe.
In two placebo-controlled trials of intermittent therapy with nitroglycerin patches at 0.2 to 0.8 mg/hr, the most frequent adverse reactions among 307 subjects were as follows:

	Placebo	Patch
Headache	18%	63%
Lightheadedness	4%	6%
Hypotension, and/or Syncope	0%	4%
Increased Angina	2%	2%

OVERDOSAGE

Hemodynamic Effects:
The ill effects of nitroglycerin overdose are generally the results of nitroglycerin's capacity to induce vasodilatation, venous pooling, reduced cardiac output, and hypotension. These hemodynamic changes may have protean manifestations, including increased intracranial pressure, with any or all of persistent throbbing headache, confusion, and moderate fever; vertigo; palpitations; visual disturbances; nausea and vomiting (possibly with colic and even bloody diarrhea); syncope (especially in the upright posture); air hunger and dyspnea, later followed by reduced ventilatory effort; diaphoresis, with the skin either flushed or cold and clammy; heart block and bradycardia; paralysis; coma; seizures; and death.
Laboratory determinations of serum levels of nitroglycerin and its metabolites are not widely available, and such determinations have, in any event, no established role in the management of nitroglycerin overdose.
No data are available to suggest physiological maneuvers (eg, maneuvers to change the pH of the urine) that might accelerate elimination of nitroglycerin and its active metabolites. Similarly, it is not known which – if any – of these substances can usefully be removed from the body by hemodialysis.
No specific antagonist to the vasodilator effects of nitroglycerin is known, and no intervention has been subject to controlled study as a therapy of nitroglycerin overdose. Because the hypotension associated with nitroglycerin overdose is the result of venodilatation and arterial hypovolemia, prudent therapy in this situation should be directed toward increase in central fluid volume. Passive elevation of the patient's legs may be sufficient, but intravenous infusion of normal saline or similar fluid may also be necessary.
The use of epinephrine or other arterial vasoconstrictors in this setting is likely to do more harm than good.
In patients with renal disease or congestive heart failure, therapy resulting in central volume expansion is not without hazard. Treatment of nitroglycerin overdose in these patients may be subtle and difficult, and invasive monitoring may be required.
Methemoglobinemia:
Nitrate ions liberated during metabolism of nitroglycerin can oxidize hemoglobin into methemoglobin. Even in patients totally without cytochrome b_5 reductase activity, however, and even assuming that the nitrate moieties of nitroglycerin are quantitatively applied to oxidation of hemoglobin, about 1 mg/kg of nitroglycerin should be required before any of these patients manifests clinically significant (≥10%) methemoglobinemia. In patients with normal reductase function, significant production of methemoglobin should require even larger doses of nitroglycerin. In one study in which 36 patients received 2 to 4 weeks of continuous nitroglycerin therapy at 3.1 to 4.4 mg/hr, the average methemoglobin level measured was 0.2%; this was comparable to that observed in parallel patients who received placebo.
Notwithstanding these observations, there are case reports of significant methemoglobinemia in association with moderate overdoses of organic nitrates. None of the affected patients had been thought to be unusually susceptible.
Methemoglobin levels are available from most clinical laboratories. The diagnosis should be suspected in patients who exhibit signs of impaired oxygen delivery despite adequate cardiac output and adequate arterial PO_2. Classically, methemoglobinemic blood is described as chocolate brown, without color change on exposure to air.
When methemoglobinemia is diagnosed, the treatment of choice is methylene blue, 1-2 mg/kg intravenously.

DOSAGE AND ADMINISTRATION

The suggested starting dose is between 0.2 mg/hr* and 0.4 mg/hr*. Doses between 0.4 mg/hr* and 0.8 mg/hr* have shown continued effectiveness for 10 to 12 hours daily for at least 1 month (the longest period studied) of intermittent administration. Although the minimum nitrate-free interval has not been defined, data show that a nitrate-free interval of 10 to 12 hours is sufficient (see **CLINICAL PHARMACOLOGY**). Thus, an appropriate dosing schedule for nitroglycerin patches would include a daily patch-on period of 12 to 14 hours and a daily patch-off period of 10 to 12 hours.

*Release rates were formerly described in terms of drug delivered per 24 hours. In these terms, the supplied NITRO-DUR systems would be rated at 2.5 mg/24 hours (0.1 mg/hour), 5 mg/24 hours (0.2 mg/hour), 7.5 mg/24 hours (0.3 mg/hour), 10 mg/24 hours (0.4 mg/hour), and 15 mg/24 hours (0.6 mg/hour).

Although some well-controlled clinical trials using exercise tolerance testing have shown maintenance of effectiveness when patches are worn continuously, the large majority of such controlled trials have shown the development of tolerance (ie, complete loss of effect) within the first 24 hours after therapy was initiated. Dose adjustment, even to levels much higher than generally used, did not restore efficacy.

HOW SUPPLIED

NITRO-DUR

System Rated Release *In Vivo**	Total Nitro-glycerin Content	System Size	Package Size
0.1 mg/hr	20 mg	5 cm^2	Unit Dose 30 (NDC 0085-3305-30) Institutional Package 30 (NDC 0085-3305-35)
0.2 mg/hr	40 mg	10 cm^2	Unit Dose 30 (NDC 0085-3310-30) Institutional Package 30 (NDC 0085-3310-35)
0.3 mg/hr	60 mg	15 cm^2	Unit Dose 30 (NDC 0085-3315-30) Institutional Package 30 (NDC 0085-3315-35)
0.4 mg/hr	80 mg	20 cm^2	Unit Dose 30 (NDC 0085-3320-30) Institutional Package 30 (NDC 0085-3320-35)
0.6 mg/hr	120 mg	30 cm^2	Unit Dose 30 (NDC 0085-3330-30) Institutional Package 30 (NDC 0085-3330-35)
0.8 mg/hr	160 mg	40 cm^2	Unit Dose 30 (NDC 0085-0819-30) Institutional Package 30 (NDC 0085-0819-35)

*Release rates were formerly described in terms of drug delivered per 24 hours. In these terms, the supplied

Continued on next page

Nitro-Dur—Cont.

NITRO-DUR systems would be rated at 2.5 mg/24 hours (0.1 mg/hour), 5 mg/24 hours (0.2 mg/hour), 7.5 mg/24 hours (0.3 mg/hour), 10 mg/24 hours (0.4 mg/hour), and 15 mg/24 hours (0.6 mg/hour).

Store between 15° and 30°C (59° and 86°F). Do not refrigerate.

Rx only

Key Pharmaceuticals, Inc.
Kenilworth, NJ 07033 USA
Rev. 11/01 B-18143666
U.S. Patent No. 5,186,938

Merck & Co., Inc.
WEST POINT, PA 19486

For Medical Information Contact:
Generally:
Product and service information:
Call the Merck National Service Center, 8:00 AM to 7:00 PM (ET), Monday through Friday:
(800) NSC-MERCK
(800) 672-6372
FAX: (800) MERCK-68
FAX: (800) 637-2568
Adverse Drug Experiences:
Call the Merck National Service Center, 8:00 AM to 7:00 PM (ET), Monday through Friday:
(800) NSC-MERCK
(800) 672-6372
In Emergencies:
24-hour emergency information for healthcare professionals:
(800) NSC-MERCK
(800) 672-6372
Sales and Ordering:
For product orders and direct account inquiries only, call the Order Management Center,
8:00 AM to 7:00 PM (ET), Monday through Friday:
(800) MERCK RX
(800) 637-2579

AGGRASTAT® ℞
(tirofiban hydrochloride injection premixed)
AGGRASTAT® ℞
(tirofiban hydrochloride injection)

Prescribing information for this product, which appears on pages 2031–2035 of the 2002 PDR, has been revised as follows. Please write "See Supplement A" alongside product heading.
In the **DESCRIPTION** *section, in the fifth paragraph, at the end of the first sentence, delete* "or 500 mL" *and delete the last sentence.*
In the **PRECAUTIONS** *section, under the Bleeding Precautions subsection, in the Minimize Vascular and Other Trauma paragraph, after* "Other arterial and venous punctures," *add* "epidural procedures,".
In the **ADVERSE REACTIONS** *section, under Post-Marketing Experience, under Bleeding, after* "hemopericardium" *delete* "and", *after* "hemorrhage" *add* ", and spinal-epidural hematoma.", *and replace* "Fatal bleedings have been reported rarely;" *with* "Fatal bleeding events have been reported;".
In the **DOSAGE AND ADMINISTRATION** *section, under Directions for Use, in the paragraph beginning* "AGGRASTAT Injection Premixed...", *in the first sentence delete* "or 500 mL".
In the **HOW SUPPLIED** *section, replace* No. 3739 *with the following:*
No. 3739—AGGRASTAT Injection Premixed 12.5 mg tirofiban per 250 mL (50 mcg per mL) is a clear, non-preserved, sterile solution premixed in a vehicle made isoosmotic with sodium chloride, and is supplied as follows:
NDC 0006-3739-96, 250 mL single-dose IntraVia® containers (PL 2408 Plastic).
Revisions based on 9123310, issued January 2001.

AquaMEPHYTON® Injection ℞
(Phytonadione)
Aqueous Colloidal Solution of Vitamin K_1

Prescribing information for this product, which appears on pages 2042–2043 of the 2002 PDR, has been revised as follows. Please write "See Supplement A" alongside product heading.
In the boxed **WARNING** *title, add* **"AND INTRAMUSCULAR"** *after* **"INTRAVENOUS"**.
Also in the boxed **WARNING**, *after the first sentence, add* "Severe reactions, including fatalities, have also been reported following INTRAMUSCULAR administration.", *and replace the last sentence with* "Therefore the INTRAVENOUS and INTRAMUSCULAR routes should be restricted to those situations where the subcutaneous route is not feasible and the serious risk involved is considered justified."
In the **ADVERSE REACTIONS** *section, in the first paragraph, in the first sentence, after* "intravenous" *add* "and intramuscular", *and in the second sentence, delete* "at beginning of circular".
In the **DOSAGE AND ADMINISTRATION** *section, in the first paragraph, in the first sentence, after* "subcutaneous", *delete* "or intramuscular", *and after* "route", *add* "(see Box Warning.)".
In the **HOW SUPPLIED** *section, after the first paragraph, replace the copy with the following:*
No. 7780—10 mg of vitamin K_1 per mL
NDC 0006-7780-38 boxes of 5 × 1 mL ampuls
NDC 0006-7780-66 five boxes of 5 × 1 mL ampuls.
No. 7784—1 mg of vitamin K_1 per 0.5 mL
NDC 0006-7784-33 five boxes of 5 × 0.5 mL ampuls.
Also in the **HOW SUPPLIED** *section, under Storage, replace the sentence with* "Store in original carton. Protect from light."
Revisions based on 9073024, issued May 2001.

ATTENUVAX® ℞
(Measles Virus Vaccine Live)

Prescribing information for this product, which appears on pages 2044–2046 of the 2002 PDR, has been revised as follows. Please write "See Supplement A" alongside product heading.
In the **PRECAUTIONS** *section, at the end, add the following subsection:*
Geriatric Use
Clinical studies of ATTENUVAX did not include sufficient numbers of seronegative subjects aged 65 and over to determine whether they respond differently from younger subjects. Other reported clinical experience has not identified differences in responses between the elderly and younger subjects.
In the **ADVERSE REACTIONS** *section, under Immune System, at the end, add* "in individuals with or without an allergic history.".
Revisions based on 9243204, issued August 2001.

BLOCADREN® Tablets ℞
(timolol maleate)

Prescribing information for this product, which appears on pages 2046–2048 of the 2002 PDR, has been revised as follows. Please write "See Supplement A" alongside product heading.
In the **ADVERSE REACTIONS** *section, in the sixth paragraph, which begins* "The following additional adverse effects...", *after* "Body as a Whole:", *add* "anaphylaxis,".
In the **HOW SUPPLIED** *section, under* No. 3344, *delete* "(6505-01-132-0651, 10 mg 100's)" *and under* No. 3371, *delete* "(6505-01-132-0652, 20 mg 100's)".
Revisions based on 7901232, issued April 2001.

COGENTIN® Tablets ℞
(benztropine mesylate)
COGENTIN® Injection ℞
(benztropine mesylate)

Prescribing information for this product, which appears on pages 2055–2056 of the 2002 PDR, has been revised as follows. Please write "See Supplement A" alongside product heading.
In the **DESCRIPTION** *section, in the fourth paragraph, replace* "three" *with* "two" *and delete* ", 1 mg,".
Also in the **DESCRIPTION** *section, in the first sentence in the fifth paragraph, delete* ", 1".
In the **HOW SUPPLIED** *section, delete* No. 3334, *and under* No. 3172, *delete* "(6505-01-230-8726, 2 mg 100's)", *and under* No. 3275, *delete* "(6505-00-785-0307, tray of 6 × 2 mL ampuls).".
Revisions based on 7924124, issued June 2001.

COSOPT® Sterile Ophthalmic Solution ℞
(dorzolamide hydrochloride–timolol maleate ophthalmic solution)

Prescribing information for this product, which appears on pages 2065–2067 of the 2002 PDR, has been revised as follows. Please write "See Supplement A" alongside product heading.
In the **ADVERSE REACTIONS** *section, under Dorzolamide—Skin/Mucous Membranes, after* "dermatitis,", *add* "epistaxis,".
Also in the **ADVERSE REACTIONS** *section, under Timolol—Hypersensitivity, after* "including", *add* "anaphylaxis,".
Replace the **INSTRUCTIONS FOR USE** *section.*
INSTRUCTIONS FOR USE
Please follow these instructions carefully when using COSOPT*. Use COSOPT as prescribed by your doctor.

1. If you use other topically applied ophthalmic medications, they should be administered at least 10 minutes before or after COSOPT.
2. Wash hands before each use.
3. Before using the medication for the first time, be sure the Safety Strip on the front of the bottle is unbroken. A gap between the bottle and the cap is normal for an unopened bottle.

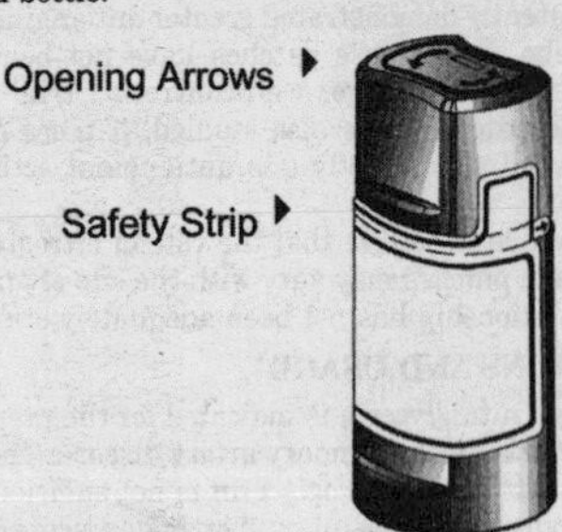

4. Tear off the Safety Strip to break the seal. [See first figure at top of next page]
5. To open the bottle, unscrew the cap by turning as indicated by the arrows.

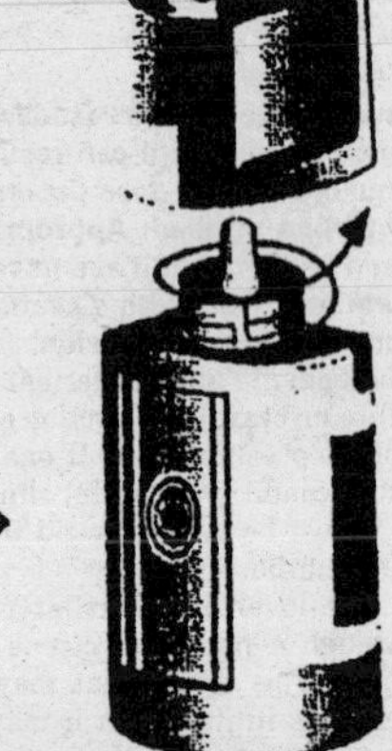

6. Tilt your head back and pull your lower eyelid down slightly to form a pocket between your eyelid and your eye.

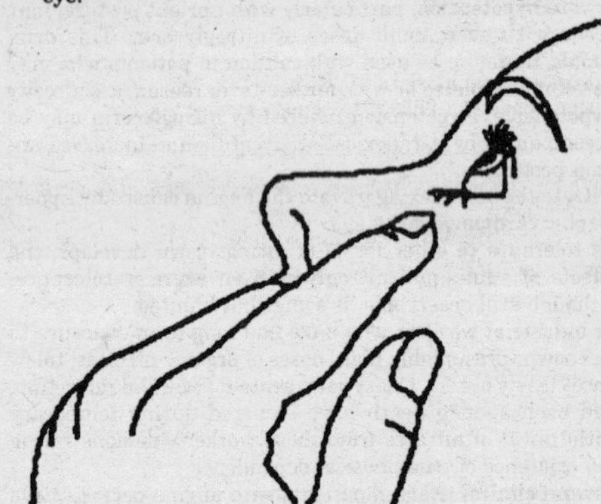

7. Invert the bottle, and press lightly with the thumb or index finger over the "Finger Push Area" (as shown) until a single drop is dispensed into the eye as directed by your doctor.

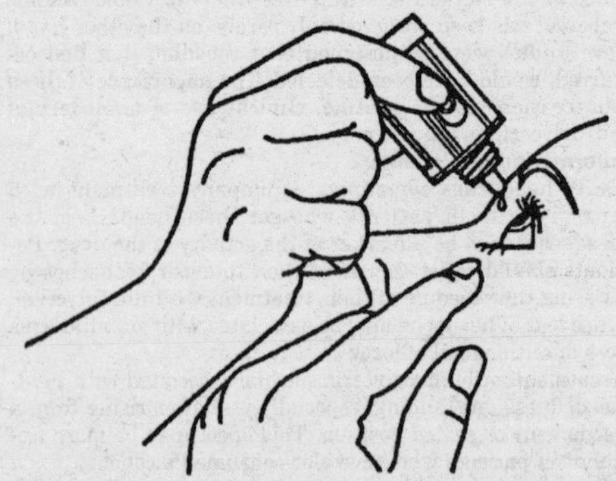

[See second figure at top of next column]

DO NOT TOUCH YOUR EYE OR EYELID WITH THE DROPPER TIP.
Ophthalmic medications, if handled improperly, can become contaminated by common bacteria known to cause eye infections. Serious damage to the eye and subsequent loss of vision may result from using contaminated ophthalmic medications. If you think your medication may be contaminated, or if you develop an eye infection, contact your doctor immediately concerning continued use of this bottle.

8. Repeat steps 6 & 7 with the other eye if instructed to do so by your doctor.
9. Replace the cap by turning until it is firmly touching the bottle. Do not overtighten the cap.

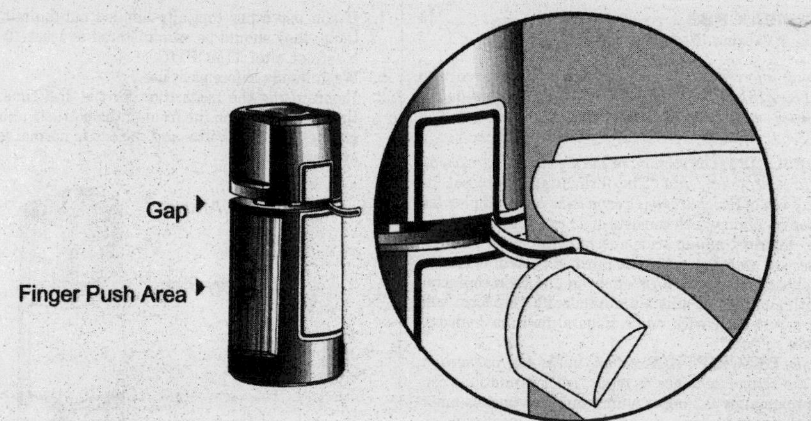

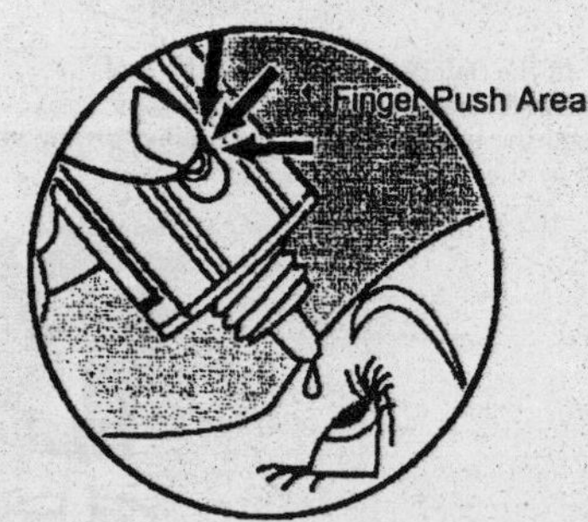

10. The dispenser tip is designed to provide a pre-measured drop; therefore, do NOT enlarge the hole of the dispenser tip.
11. After you have used all doses, there will be some COSOPT left in the bottle. You should not be concerned since an extra amount of COSOPT has been added and you will get the full amount of COSOPT that your doctor prescribed. Do not attempt to remove the excess medicine from the bottle.

WARNING: Keep out of reach of children.
If you have any questions about the use of COSOPT, please consult your doctor.

*Registered trademark of MERCK & CO., Inc.
Revisions based on 9359301, issued October 2001.

COZAAR® ℞
(losartan potassium tablets)

Prescribing information for this product, which appears on pages 2067–2070 of the 2002 PDR, has been revised as follows. Please write "See Supplement A" alongside product heading.
In the **PRECAUTIONS** *section, under Drug Interactions, at the end, add the following paragraph:*
As with other antihypertensive agents, the antihypertensive effect of losartan may be blunted by the non-steroidal anti-inflammatory drug indomethacin.
In the **ADVERSE REACTIONS** *section, under Post-Marketing Experience, under Hypersensitivity, after the first sentence, add* "Vasculitis, including Henoch-Schönlein purpura, has been reported."
In the **DOSAGE AND ADMINISTRATION** *section, at the beginning, add* "Dosing must be individualized." *Also, in the second paragraph, at the end, add* "The effect of losartan is substantially present within one week but in some studies the maximal effect occurred in 3–6 weeks (see CLINICAL PHARMACOLOGY, *Pharmacodynamics and Clinical Effects*)."
Revisions based on 7882919, issued November 2001.

CRIXIVAN® Capsules ℞
(indinavir sulfate)

Prescribing information for this product, which appears on pages 2070–2075 of the 2002 PDR has been revised as follows. Please write "See Supplement A" alongside product heading.
In the **CLINICAL PHARMACOLOGY** *section, under Drugs Requiring Dose Modification, after the Efavirenz subsection, add the following subsection:*
Sildenafil: The results of one published study in HIV-infected men (n=6) indicated that coadministration of indinavir (800 mg every 8 hours chronically) with a single 25 mg-dose of sildenafil resulted in an 11% increase in average AUC_{0-8hr} of indinavir and a 48% increase in average indinavir peak concentration (C_{max}) compared to 800 mg every 8 hours alone. Average sildenafil AUC was increased by 340% following coadministration of sildenafil and indinavir compared to historical data following administration of sildenafil alone (see PRECAUTIONS, *Drug Interactions*).
In the **WARNINGS** *section, under Drug Interactions, after the first paragraph, add the following paragraph:*
Particular caution should be used when prescribing sildenafil in patients receiving indinavir. Coadministration of CRIXIVAN with sildenafil is expected to substantially increase sildenafil plasma concentrations and may result in an increase in sildenafil-associated adverse events, including hypotension, visual changes, and priapism (see PRECAUTIONS, *Drug Interactions* and *Information for Patients*, and the manufacturer's complete prescribing information for sildenafil).
In the **PRECAUTIONS** *section, under Information for Patients, after the fifth paragraph, add the following paragraph:*
Patients receiving sildenafil should be advised that they may be at an increased risk of sildenafil-associated adverse events including hypotension, visual changes, and priapism, and should promptly report any symptoms to their doctors.
Also in the **PRECAUTIONS** *section, under Drug Interactions, after the Efavirenz subsection, add the following subsection:*
Erectile Dysfunction Agents
Particular caution should be used when prescribing sildenafil for patients receiving indinavir. The results of one published study in six HIV-infected subjects indicated that coadministration of indinavir (800 mg every 8 hours chronically) and sildenafil (25 mg as a single dose) resulted in increased indinavir and sildenafil concentrations. In two of the six subjects, prolonged clinical effects of sildenafil were noted for 72 hours after a single dose of sildenafil in combination with indinavir. Based on the results of this study, the dose of sildenafil should not exceed 25 mg in a 48-hour period. Patients receiving sildenafil should be advised that they are at an increased risk of sildenafil-associated adverse events including hypotension, visual changes, and priapism, and should promptly report any symptoms to their health care providers (see CLINICAL PHARMACOLOGY, *Drug Interactions* and WARNINGS).
Also in the **PRECAUTIONS** *section, at the end, add the following subsection:*
Geriatric Use
Clinical studies of CRIXIVAN did not include sufficient numbers of subjects aged 65 and over to determine whether they respond differently from younger subjects. In general, dose selection for an elderly patient should be cautious, reflecting the greater frequency of decreased hepatic, renal or cardiac function and of concomitant disease or other drug therapy.
Revisions based on 7979821, issued March 2001.
In the Patient Information, under **MEDICINES YOU SHOULD NOT TAKE WITH CRIXIVAN,** *at the end, add the following paragraph:*
Before you take VIAGRA® (sildenafil) with CRIXIVAN, talk to your doctor about possible drug interactions and side effects. If you take VIAGRA and CRIXIVAN together, you may be at increased risk of side effects of VIAGRA-associated adverse events such as low blood pressure, visual changes, and penile erection lasting more than 4 hours. If an erection lasts longer than 4 hours, you should seek immediate medical assistance to avoid permanent damage to your penis. Your doctor can explain these symptoms to you.
Revisions based on 9024515, issued March 2001.

DECADRON® Tablets ℞
(dexamethasone)

Prescribing information for this product, which appears on pages 2079–2081 of the 2002 PDR, has been revised as follows. Please write "See Supplement A" alongside product heading.
In the **PRECAUTIONS** *section, after the fifth paragraph, add the following paragraph:*
Co-administration of thalidomide with DECADRON tablets should be employed cautiously, as toxic epidermal necrolysis has been reported with concomitant use.
Revisions based on 7921149, issued February 2001.

DECADRON® Phosphate Injection ℞
(dexamethasone sodium phosphate)

Prescribing information for this product, which appears on pages 2081–2083 of the 2002 PDR, has been revised as follows. Please write "See Supplement A" alongside product heading.
In the **PRECAUTIONS** *section, after the sixth paragraph, add the following paragraph:*
Co-administration of thalidomide with DECADRON Phosphate injection should be employed cautiously, as toxic epidermal necrolysis has been reported with concomitant use.
In the **HOW SUPPLIED** *section, under* No. 7628X, *delete* "(6505-00-963-5355, 5 mL vial)", *and under* No. 7646, *delete* "(6505-01-153-3524, 5 mL vial)."
Revisions based on 9051533, issued February 2001.

HYZAAR® 50-12.5 ℞
(losartan potassium-hydrochlorothiazide tablets)
HYZAAR® 100-25 ℞
(losartan potassium-hydrochlorothiazide tablets)

Prescribing information for this product, which appears on pages 2109–2112 of the 2002 PDR has been revised as follows. Please write "See Supplement A" alongside product heading.
In the **PRECAUTIONS** *section, under Drug Interactions, Losartan Potassium, at the end, add the following paragraph:*
As with other antihypertensive agents, the antihypertensive effect of losartan may be blunted by the non-steroidal anti-inflammatory drug indomethacin.
In the **ADVERSE REACTIONS** *section, under Post-Marketing Experience, under Hypersensitivity, after the first sentence, add* "Vasculitis, including Henoch-Schönlein purpura, has been reported with losartan."
In the **DOSAGE AND ADMINISTRATION** *section, at the beginning, add* "Dosing must be individualized." *Also, under* **Dose Titration by Clinical Effect,** *in the first sentence, after"* (see above)", *add* "or hydrochlorothiazide alone,".
Revisions based on 7892818, issued November 2001.

INDOCIN® I.V. ℞
(indomethacin sodium trihydrate)

Prescribing information for this product, which appears on pages 2115–2117 of the 2002 PDR, has been revised as follows. Please write "See Supplement A" alongside product heading.
In the **DOSAGE AND ADMINISTRATION** *section, under Directions for Use, replace the last paragraph with the following:*
INDOCIN I.V. is not buffered. Further dilution with intravenous infusion solutions is not recommended.
In the **HOW SUPPLIED** *section, delete* "(6505-01-209-1192, 3 single dose vials)."
Revisions based on 9408717, issued May 2001.

M-M-R®II ℞
(Measles, Mumps, and Rubella Virus Vaccine Live)

Prescribing information for this product, which appears on pages 2118–2120 of the 2002 PDR, has been revised as follows. Please write "See Supplement A" alongside product heading.
In the **PRECAUTIONS** *section, at the end, add the following subsection:*
Geriatric Use
Clinical studies of M-M-R II did not include sufficient numbers of seronegative subjects aged 65 and over to determine whether they respond differently from younger subjects. Other reported clinical experience has not identified differences in responses between the elderly and younger subjects.
Revisions based on 9265206, issued August 2001.

MERUVAX®$_{II}$ ℞
(Rubella Virus Vaccine Live)
Wistar RA 27/3 Strain

Prescribing information for this product, which appears on pages 2130–2132 of the 2002 PDR, has been revised. Please write "See Supplement A" alongside product heading.
In the **PRECAUTIONS** *section, at the end, add the following subsection:*
Geriatric Use
Clinical studies of MERUVAX II did not include sufficient numbers of seronegative subjects aged 65 and over to determine whether they respond differently from younger subjects. Other reported clinical experience has not identified differences in responses between the elderly and younger subjects.
In the **ADVERSE REACTIONS** *section, under Immune System, at the end, add* "in individuals with or without an allergic history."
Revisions based on 9243403, issued August 2001.

Continued on next page

Information on the Merck & Co., Inc., products listed on these pages is from the prescribing information in use April 1, 2002.

Meruvax II—Cont.

MUMPSVAX® ℞
(Mumps Virus Vaccine Live)
Jeryl Lynn Strain

Prescribing information for this product, which appears on pages 2141–2142 of the 2002 PDR, has been revised. Please write "See Supplement A" alongside product heading.
In the **PRECAUTIONS** *section, at the end, add the following subsection:*
Geriatric Use
Clinical studies of MUMPSVAX did not include sufficient numbers of seronegative subjects aged 65 and over to determine whether they respond differently from younger subjects. Other reported clinical experience has not identified differences in responses between the elderly and younger subjects.
In the **ADVERSE REACTIONS** *section, under Immune System, at the end, add* "in individuals with or without an allergic history."
In the **DOSAGE AND ADMINISTRATION** *section, delete the entire 10 Dose Vial and 50 Dose Vial subsections.*
Revisions based on 9243503, issued August 2001.

PNEUMOVAX® 23 ℞
(pneumococcal vaccine polyvalent)

Prescribing information for this product, which appears on pages 2156–2158 of the 2002 PDR, has been revised as follows. Please write "See Supplement A" alongside product heading.
In the **PRECAUTIONS** *section, at the end, add the following subsection:*
Geriatric Use
Persons 65 years of age or older were enrolled in several clinical studies of PNEUMOVAX 23 that were conducted pre- and post-licensure. In the largest of these studies, the safety of PNEUMOVAX 23 in adults 65 years of age and older was compared to the safety of PNEUMOVAX 23 in adults 50 to 64 years of age. Of 1007 subjects enrolled in this study, 433 subjects were 65 to 74 years of age, and 195 subjects were 75 years of age or older. No overall difference in safety was observed between these subjects and younger subjects. However, since elderly individuals may not tolerate medical interventions as well as younger individuals, a higher frequency and/or a greater severity of reactions in some older individuals cannot be ruled out.
In the **HOW SUPPLIED** *section, delete the second paragraph.*
Revisions based on 7999818, issued February 2001.

PRINIVIL® Tablets ℞
(lisinopril)

Prescribing information for this product, which appears on pages 2164–2168 of the 2002 PDR, has been revised as follows. Please write "See Supplement A" alongside product heading.
In the **PRECAUTIONS** *section, in the Drug Interactions subsection, under Non-steroidal Anti-inflammatory Agents, in the second paragraph, delete the first sentence, and at the end of the second sentence, add* ", including lisinopril."
In the **HOW SUPPLIED** *section:*
Under No. 3658, delete "**NDC** 0006-0015-72 carton of 25 UNIBLISTER™ cards of 31 tablets each."
Under No. 3577, after the third **NDC** *entry, add* "**NDC** 0006-0019-54 unit of use bottles of 90" *and delete* "**NDC** 0006-0019-86 bottles of 5,000".
Under No. 3578, after the fourth **NDC** *entry, add* "**NDC** 0006-0106-54 unit of use bottles of 90" *and delete* "**NDC** 0006-0106-86 bottles of 5,000".
Under No. 3579, after the fourth **NDC** *entry, add* "**NDC** 0006-0207-54 unit of use bottles of 90" *and delete* "**NDC** 0006-0207-86 bottles of 5,000".
Revisions based on 7825247, issued January 2002.

PRINZIDE® Tablets ℞
(lisinopril-hydrochlorothiazide)

Prescribing information for this product, which appears on pages 2168–2172 of the 2002 PDR, has been revised as follows. Please write "See Supplement A" alongside product heading.
In the **PRECAUTIONS** *section, under Drug Interactions, in the Lisinopril subsection, under Non-steroidal Anti-inflammatory Agents, in the second paragraph, delete the first sentence, and at the end of the second sentence, add* ", including lisinopril."
In the **DOSAGE AND ADMINISTRATION** *section, under Dose Titration Guided by Clinical Effect, at the end, add* "Dosage higher than lisinopril 80 mg and hydrochlorothiazide 50 mg should not be used."
Revisions based on 7836333, issued February 2001.

RECOMBIVAX HB® ℞
Hepatitis B Vaccine (Recombinant)

Prescribing information for this product, which appears on pages 2178–2181 of the 2002 PDR, has been revised as follows. Please write "See Supplement A" alongside product heading.
In the **DESCRIPTION** *section, in the second paragraph, after the first sentence, add* "The fermentation process involves growth of *Saccharomyces cerevisiae* on a complex fermentation medium which consists of an extract of yeast, soy peptone, dextrose, amino acids and mineral salts." *Also, after the second sentence, add* "The purified protein is treated in phosphate buffer with formaldehyde and then coprecipitated with alum (potassium aluminum sulfate) to form bulk vaccine adjuvanted with amorphous aluminum hydroxyphosphate sulfate."
Also in the **DESCRIPTION** *section, in the last paragraph, change the second sentence to read:* "All formulations contain approximately 0.5 mg of aluminum (provided as amorphous aluminum hydroxyphosphate sulfate, previously referred to as aluminum hydroxide) per mL of vaccine." *Also, in the third sentence, change the parenthetic statement to read* "(provided as amorphous aluminum hydroxyphosphate sulfate)".
In the **PRECAUTIONS** *section, move the Carcinogenesis, Mutagenesis, Impairment of Fertility subsection to appear after the Drug Interactions subsection.*
Also in the **PRECAUTIONS** *section, at the end, add the following subsection:*
Geriatric Use
Clinical studies of RECOMBIVAX HB did not include sufficient numbers of subjects aged 65 and over to determine whether they respond differently from younger subjects. Other reports from the clinical literature indicate that hepatitis B vaccines are less immunogenic in adults aged 65 years or older than in younger individuals. No overall differences in safety were observed between these subjects and younger subjects.
In the **HOW SUPPLIED** *section, under* PEDIATRIC/ADOLESCENT FORMULATION (PRESERVATIVE-FREE), *at the end of the first and second paragraphs, after* "labels and cartons" *add* "and an orange banner on the vial labels and cartons stating "Preservative Free",".
Also in the **HOW SUPPLIED** *section, under* PEDIATRIC/ADOLESCENT FORMULATION (PRESERVATIVE-FREE), *at the end, add:*
No. 4982—RECOMBIVAX HB for use in infants, children, and adolescents is supplied as 5 mcg/0.5 mL of HBsAg in a 0.5 mL pre-filled single-dose glass syringe with a 1 inch, 23 gauge needle, in a box of 5 pre-filled single-dose syringes with 1 inch, 23 gauge needles, color coded with a yellow plunger rod and stripe on the syringe labels and cartons and an orange banner on the syringe labels and cartons stating "Preservative Free", **NDC** 0006-4982-00.
No. 4983—RECOMBIVAX HB for use in infants, children, and adolescents is supplied as 5 mcg/0.5 mL of HBsAg in a 0.5 mL pre-filled single-dose glass syringe with a 5/8 inch, 25 gauge needle, in a box of 5 pre-filled single-dose syringes with 5/8 inch, 25 gauge needles, color coded with a yellow plunger rod and stripe on the syringe labels and cartons and an orange banner on the syringe labels and cartons stating "Preservative Free", **NDC** 0006-4983-00.
No. 4994—RECOMBIVAX HB for use in infants, children, and adolescents is supplied as 5 mcg/0.5 mL of HBsAg in a 0.5 mL pre-filled single-dose Luer-Lok™ syringe in a box of 10 pre-filled single-dose syringes, color coded with a yellow plunger rod and stripe on the syringe labels and cartons and an orange banner on the syringe labels and cartons stating "Preservative Free", **NDC** 0006-4994-41.
Revisions based on 7994321, issued May 2001.

SINGULAIR® Tablets and Chewable Tablets ℞
(montelukast sodium)

Prescribing information for this product, which appears on pages 2181–2185 of the 2002 PDR, has been revised as follows. Please write "See Supplement A" alongside product heading.
In the **ADVERSE REACTIONS** *section, under Post-Marketing Experience, in the first paragraph, after* "dream abnormalities", *add* "and hallucinations,"
Revision based on 9088810, issued August 2001.
In the Patient Information, *under* **What are the possible side effects of SINGULAIR?**, *in the paragraph beginning* "Less common side effects...", *after* "• bad/vivid dreams", *add* "• hallucinations".
Revision based on 9094210, issued August 2001.

TIMOPTIC® Sterile Ophthalmic Solution ℞
0.25% and 0.5%
(timolol maleate ophthalmic solution)

Prescribing information for this product, which appears on pages 2190–2192 of the 2002 PDR, has been revised as follows. Please write "See Supplement A" alongside product heading.
Replace the **INSTRUCTIONS FOR USE** *section.*
INSTRUCTIONS FOR USE
Please follow these instructions carefully when using TIMOPTIC*. Use TIMOPTIC as prescribed by your doctor.

1. If you use other topically applied ophthalmic medications, they should be administered at least 10 minutes before or after TIMOPTIC.
2. Wash hands before each use.
3. Before using the medication for the first time, be sure the Safety Strip on the front of the bottle is unbroken. A gap between the bottle and the cap is normal for an unopened bottle.

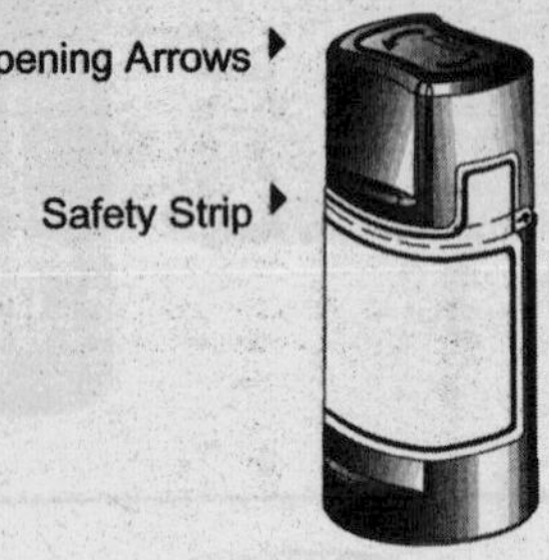

4. Tear off the Safety Strip to break the seal.
[See first figure at top of next page]
5. To open the bottle, unscrew the cap by turning as indicated by the arrows.

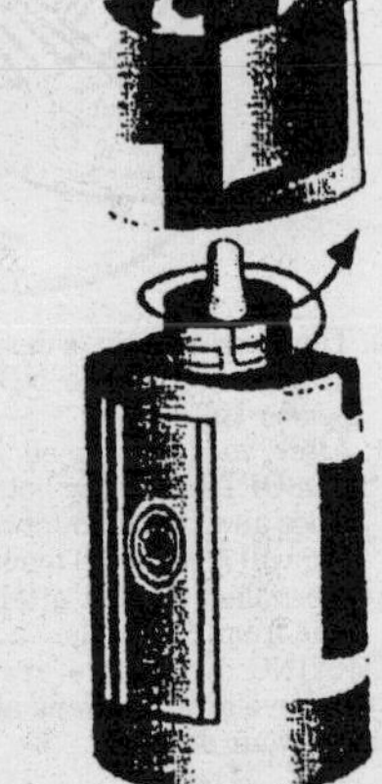

6. Tilt your head back and pull your lower eyelid down slightly to form a pocket between your eyelid and your eye.

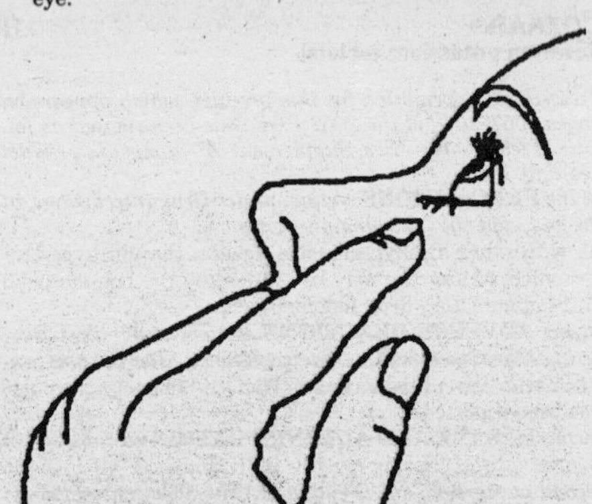

7. Invert the bottle, and press lightly with the thumb or index finger over the "Finger Push Area" (as shown) until a single drop is dispensed into the eye as directed by your doctor.

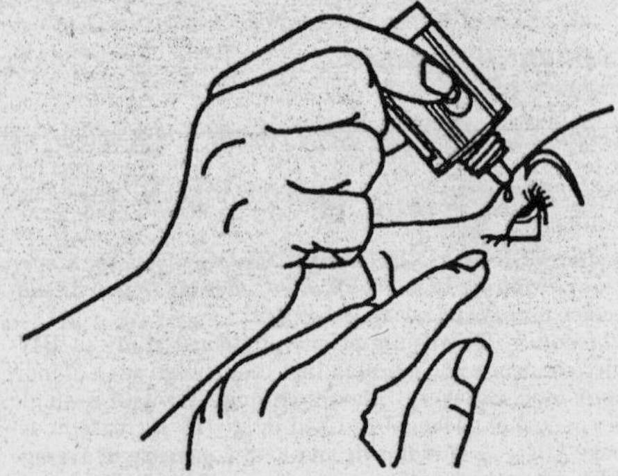

[See second figure at top of next page]
DO NOT TOUCH YOUR EYE OR EYELID WITH THE DROPPER TIP.
Ophthalmic medications, if handled improperly, can become contaminated by common bacteria known to cause eye infections. Serious damage to the eye and subsequent loss of vision may result from using contaminated ophthalmic medications. If you think your medication

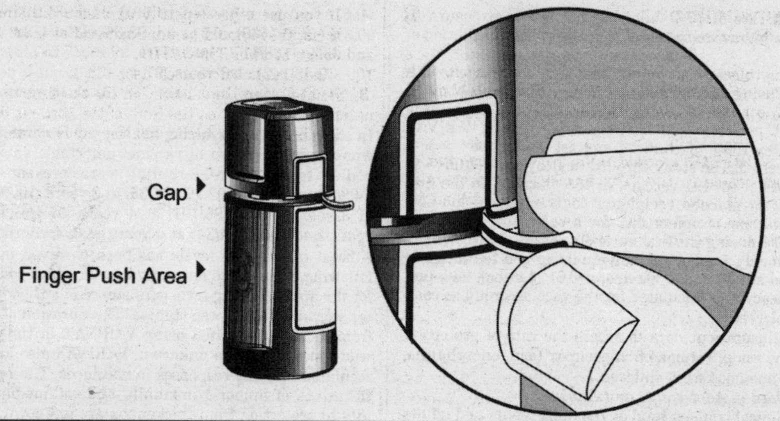

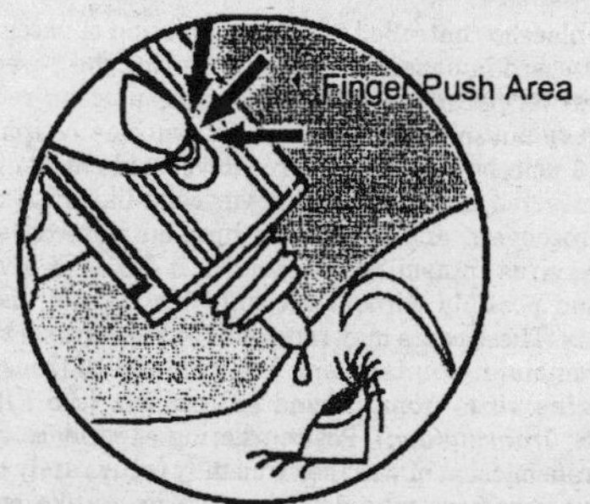

may be contaminated, or if you develop an eye infection, contact your doctor immediately concerning continued use of this bottle.

8. Repeat steps 6 & 7 with the other eye if instructed to do so by your doctor.
9. Replace the cap by turning until it is firmly touching the bottle. Do not overtighten the cap.
10. The dispenser tip is designed to provide a pre-measured drop; therefore, do NOT enlarge the hole of the dispenser tip.
11. After you have used all doses, there will be some TIMOPTIC left in the bottle. You should not be concerned since an extra amount of TIMOPTIC has been added and you will get the full amount of TIMOPTIC that your doctor prescribed. Do not attempt to remove excess medicine from the bottle.

WARNING: Keep out of reach of children.
If you have any questions about the use of TIMOPTIC, please consult your doctor.

*Registered trademark of MERCK & CO., Inc.
Revisions based on 9391001, issued October 2001.

TRUSOPT® Sterile Ophthalmic Solution 2% ℞
(dorzolamide hydrochloride ophthalmic solution)

Prescribing Information for this product, which appears on pages 2196–2198 of the 2002 PDR, has been revised as follows. Please write "See Supplement A" alongside product heading.

In the **ADVERSE REACTIONS** *section, under Clinical practice:, in the last sentence, after* "contact dermatitis," *add* "epistaxis,".

Replace the **INSTRUCTIONS FOR USE** *section.*
INSTRUCTIONS FOR USE
Please follow these instructions carefully when using TRUSOPT*. Use TRUSOPT as prescribed by your doctor.

1. If you use other topically applied ophthalmic medications, they should be administered at least 10 minutes before or after TRUSOPT.
2. Wash hands before each use.
3. Before using the medication for the first time, be sure the Safety Strip on the front of the bottle is unbroken. A gap between the bottle and the cap is normal for an unopened bottle.

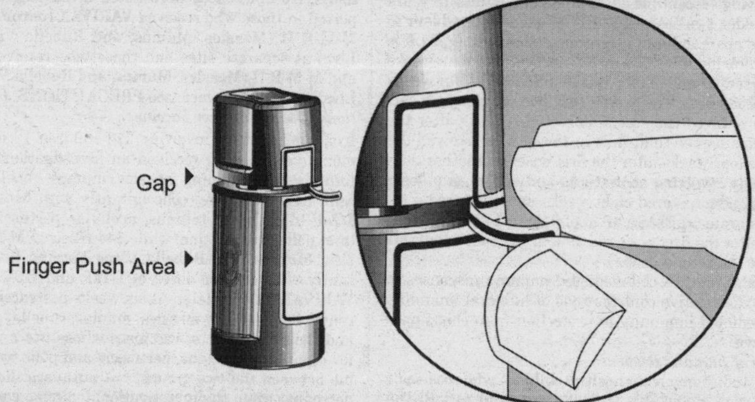

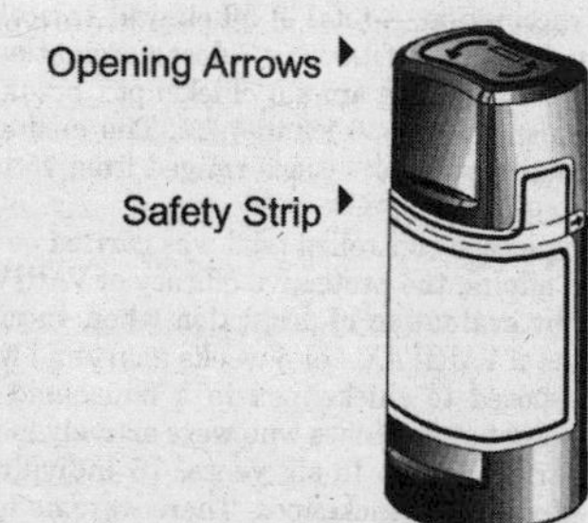

4. Tear off the Safety Strip to break the seal.
[See figure below]
5. To open the bottle, unscrew the cap by turning as indicated by the arrows.

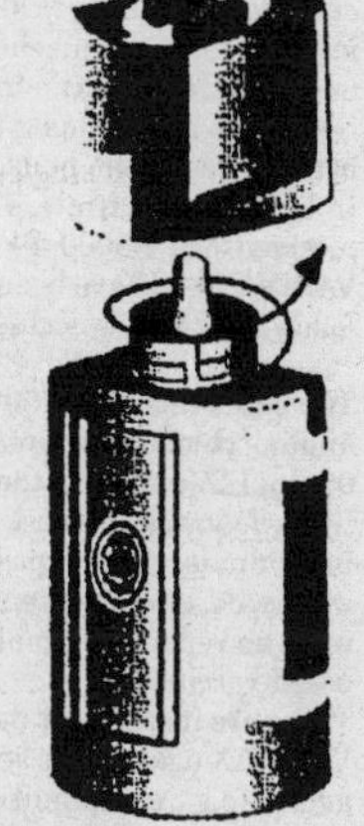

6. Tilt your head back and pull your lower eyelid down slightly to form a pocket between your eyelid and your eye.
[See first figure at top of next column]
7. Invert the bottle, and press lightly with the thumb or index finger over the "Finger Push Area" (as shown) until a single drop is dispensed into the eye as directed by your doctor.
[See second figure at top of next column]
[See third figure at top of next column]

DO NOT TOUCH YOUR EYE OR EYELID WITH THE DROPPER TIP.
Ophthalmic medications, if handled improperly, can become contaminated by common bacteria known to cause eye infections. Serious damage to the eye and subsequent loss of vision may result from using contaminated ophthalmic medications. If you think your medication may be contaminated, or if you develop an eye infection, contact your doctor immediately concerning continued use of this bottle.

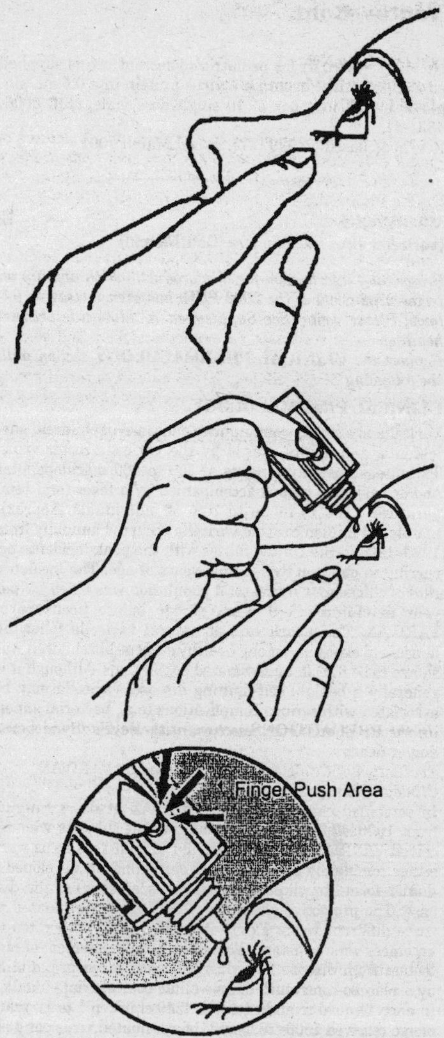

8. Repeat steps 6 & 7 with the other eye if instructed to do so by your doctor.
9. Replace the cap by turning until it is firmly touching the bottle. Do not overtighten the cap.
10. The dispenser tip is designed to provide a pre-measured drop; therefore, do NOT enlarge the hole of the dispenser tip.
11. After you have used all doses, there will be some TRUSOPT left in the bottle. You should not be concerned since an extra amount of TRUSOPT has been added and you will get the full amount of TRUSOPT that your doctor prescribed. Do not attempt to remove excess medicine from the bottle.

WARNING: Keep out of reach of children.
If you have any questions about the use of TRUSOPT, please consult your doctor.

*Registered trademark of MERCK & CO., Inc.
Revisions based on 9368203, issued October 2001.

VAQTA® ℞
(Hepatitis A Vaccine, Inactivated)

Prescribing information for this product, which appears on pages 2199–2202 of the 2002 PDR, has been revised as follows. Please write "See Supplement A" alongside product heading.

In the **ADVERSE REACTIONS** *section, at the end, add the following:*
Marketed Experience
The following additional adverse reactions have been reported with use of the marketed vaccine.
NERVOUS SYSTEM
Very rarely, Guillain-Barré syndrome.
In the **HOW SUPPLIED** *section, under* PEDIATRIC/ADOLESCENT FORMULATION, *Vials, at the end, add the following:*

Continued on next page

Information on the Merck & Co., Inc., products listed on these pages is from the prescribing information in use April 1, 2002.

Vaqta—Cont.

No. 4831 – VAQTA for pediatric/adolescent use is supplied as 25U/0.5 mL of hepatitis A virus protein in a 0.5 mL single-dose vial, in a box of 10 single-dose vials, **NDC** 0006-4831-41.
Revisions based on 9392702, issued March 2001.

VARIVAX® ℞
[varicella virus vaccine live (Oka/Merck)]

Prescribing information for this product, which appears on pages 2202–2204 of the 2002 PDR, has been revised as follows. Please write "See Supplement A" alongside product heading.
Replace the **CLINICAL PHARMACOLOGY** *section with the following.*

CLINICAL PHARMACOLOGY

Varicella is a highly communicable disease in children, adolescents, and adults caused by the varicella-zoster virus. The disease usually consists of 300 to 500 maculopapular and/or vesicular lesions accompanied by a fever (oral temperature ≥100°F) in up to 70% of individuals. Approximately 3.5 million cases of varicella occurred annually from 1980–1994 in the United States with the peak incidence occurring in children five to nine years of age. The incidence rate of chickenpox in the total population was 8.3–9.1% per year in children 1–9 years of age before licensure of VARIVAX. The attack rate of natural varicella following household exposure among healthy susceptible children was shown to be 87% in unvaccinated populations. Although it is generally a benign, self-limiting disease, varicella may be associated with serious complications (e.g., bacterial superinfection, pneumonia, encephalitis, Reye's Syndrome), and/or death.

Evaluation of Clinical Efficacy Afforded by VARIVAX

Clinical Data in Children

In combined clinical trials of VARIVAX at doses ranging from 1000–17,000 PFU, the majority of subjects who received VARIVAX and were exposed to wild-type virus were either completely protected from chickenpox or developed a milder form (for clinical description see below) of the disease. The protective efficacy of VARIVAX was evaluated in three different ways: 1) by comparing chickenpox rates in vaccinees versus historical controls, 2) by assessment of protection from disease following household exposure, and 3) by a placebo-controlled, double-blind clinical trial.

In early clinical trials, a total of 4240 children 1 to 12 years of age received 1000–1625 PFU of attenuated virus per dose of VARIVAX and have been followed for up to nine years post single-dose vaccination. In this group there was considerable variation in chickenpox rates among studies and study sites, and much of the reported data was acquired by passive follow-up. It was observed that 0.3%–3.8% of vaccinees per year reported chickenpox (called breakthrough cases). This represents an approximate 83% (95% confidence interval [CI], 82%, 84%) decrease from the age-adjusted expected incidence rates in susceptible subjects over this same period. In those who developed breakthrough chickenpox postvaccination, the majority experienced mild disease (median of the maximum number of lesions <50). In one study, a total of 47% (27/58) of breakthrough cases had <50 lesions compared with 8% (7/92) in unvaccinated individuals, and 7% (4/58) of breakthrough cases had >300 lesions compared with 50% (46/92) in unvaccinated individuals.

Among a subset of vaccinees who were actively followed in these early trials for up to nine years postvaccination, 179 individuals had household exposure to chickenpox. There were no reports of breakthrough chickenpox in 84% (150/179) of exposed children, while 16% (29/179) reported a mild form of chickenpox (38% [11/29] of the cases with a maximum total number of <50 lesions; no individuals with >300 lesions). This represents an 81% reduction in the expected number of varicella cases utilizing the historical attack rate of 87% following household exposure to chickenpox in unvaccinated individuals in the calculation of efficacy.

In later clinical trials with the current vaccine, a total of 1164 children 1 to 12 years of age received 2900–9000 PFU of attenuated virus per dose of VARIVAX and have been actively followed for up to six years post single-dose vaccination. It was observed that 0.2%–2.4% of vaccinees per year reported breakthrough chickenpox for up to six years post single-dose vaccination. This represents an approximate 93% (95% CI, 92%, 95%) decrease from the age-adjusted expected incidence rates in susceptible subjects over the same period. In those who developed breakthrough chickenpox postvaccination, the majority experienced mild disease with the median of the maximum total number of lesions <50. The severity of reported breakthrough chickenpox, as measured by number of lesions and maximum temperature, appeared not to increase with time since vaccination.

Among a subset of vaccinees who were actively followed in these later trials for up to five years postvaccination, 64 individuals were exposed to an unvaccinated individual with wild-type chickenpox in a household setting. There were no reports of breakthrough chickenpox in 91% (58/64) of exposed children, while 9% (6/64) reported a mild form of chickenpox (maximum total number of lesions <50, ranging from 6 to 40 lesions). This represents an 89% reduction in the expected number of varicella cases utilizing the historical attack rate of 87% following household exposure to chickenpox in unvaccinated individuals in the calculation of efficacy.

Although no placebo-controlled trial was carried out with VARIVAX using the current vaccine, a placebo-controlled trial was conducted using a formulation containing 17,000 PFU per dose. In this trial, a single dose of VARIVAX protected 96–100% of children against chickenpox over a two-year period. The study enrolled healthy individuals 1 to 14 years of age (n=491 vaccine, n=465 placebo). In the first year, 8.5% of placebo recipients contracted chickenpox, while no vaccine recipient did, for a calculated protection rate of 100% during the first varicella season. In the second year, when only a subset of individuals agreed to remain in the blinded study (n=163 vaccine, n=161 placebo), 96% protective efficacy was calculated for the vaccine group as compared to placebo.

There are insufficient data to assess the rate of protection against the complications of chickenpox (e.g., encephalitis, hepatitis, pneumonia) in children.

Clinical Data in Adolescents and Adults

In early clinical trials, a total of 796 adolescents and adults received 905–1230 PFU of attenuated virus per dose of VARIVAX and have been followed for up to six years following 2-dose vaccination. A total of 50 clinical varicella cases were reported >42 days following 2-dose vaccination. Based on passive follow-up, the annual chickenpox breakthrough event rate ranged from <0.1% to 1.9%. The median of the maximum total number of lesions ranged from 15 to 42 per year.

Although no placebo-controlled trial was carried out in adolescents and adults, the protective efficacy of VARIVAX was determined by evaluation of protection when vaccinees received 2 doses of VARIVAX 4 or 8 weeks apart and were subsequently exposed to chickenpox in a household setting. Among the subset of vaccinees who were actively followed in these early trials for up to six years, 76 individuals had household exposure to chickenpox. There were no reports of breakthrough chickenpox in 83% (63/76) of exposed vaccinees, while 17% (13/76) reported a mild form of chickenpox. Among 13 vaccinated individuals who developed breakthrough chickenpox after a household exposure, 62% (8/13) of the cases reported maximum total number of lesions <50, while no individual reported >75 lesions. The attack rate of unvaccinated adults exposed to a single contact in a household has not been previously studied. Utilizing the previously reported historical attack rate of 87% for natural varicella following household exposure to chickenpox among unvaccinated children in the calculation of efficacy, this represents an approximate 80% reduction in the expected number of cases in the household setting.

In later clinical trials, a total of 220 adolescents and adults received 3315–9000 PFU of attenuated virus per dose of VARIVAX and have been actively followed for up to six years following 2-dose vaccination. A total of 3 clinical varicella cases were reported >42 days following 2-dose vaccination. Two cases reported <50 lesions and none reported >75. The annual chickenpox breakthrough event rate ranged from 0% to 1.2%. Among the subset of vaccinees who were actively followed in these later trials for up to five years, 16 individuals were exposed to an unvaccinated individual with wild-type chickenpox in a household setting. There were no reports of breakthrough chickenpox among the exposed vaccinees.

There are insufficient data to assess the rate of protection of VARIVAX against the serious complications of chickenpox in adults (e.g., encephalitis, hepatitis, pneumonitis) and during pregnancy (congenital varicella syndrome).

Immunogenicity of VARIVAX

Clinical trials with several formulations of the vaccine containing attenuated virus ranging from 1000 to 17,000 PFU per dose have demonstrated that VARIVAX induces detectable immune responses in a high proportion of individuals and is generally well tolerated in healthy individuals ranging from 12 months to 55 years of age.

Seroconversion as defined by the acquisition of any detectable varicella antibodies (gpELISA >0.3, a highly sensitive assay which is not commercially available) was observed in 97% of vaccinees at approximately 4–6 weeks postvaccination in 6889 susceptible children 12 months to 12 years of age. Rates of breakthrough disease were significantly lower among children with varicella antibody titers ≥5 compared to children with titers <5. Titers ≥5 were induced in approximately 76% of children vaccinated with a single dose of vaccine at 1000–17,000 PFU per dose. In a multicenter study involving susceptible adolescents and adults 13 years of age and older, two doses of VARIVAX administered four to eight weeks apart induced a seroconversion rate (gpELISA >0.3) of approximately 75% in 539 individuals four weeks after the first dose and of 99% in 479 individuals four weeks after the second dose. The average antibody response in vaccinees who received the second dose eight weeks after the first dose was higher than that in those, who received the second dose four weeks after the first dose. In another multicenter study involving adolescents and adults, two doses of VARIVAX administered eight weeks apart induced a seroconversion rate (gpELISA >0.3) of 94% in 142 individuals six weeks after the first dose and 99% in 122 individuals six weeks after the second dose.

VARIVAX also induces cell-mediated immune responses in vaccinees. The relative contributions of humoral immunity and cell-mediated immunity to protection from chickenpox are unknown.

Persistence of Immune Response

In clinical studies involving healthy children who received 1 dose of vaccine, detectable varicella antibodies (gpELISA >0.6 units) were present in 99.0% (3886/3926) at 1 year, 99.3% (1555/1566) at 2 years, 98.6% (1106/1122) at 3 years, and 99.4 (1168/1175) at 4 years, 99.2% (737/743) at 5 years, 100% (142/142) at 6 years, 97.4% (38/39) at 7 years, 100% (34/34) at 8 years, and 100% (16/16) at 10 years postvaccination.

In clinical studies involving healthy adolescents and adults who received 2 doses of vaccine, detectable varicella antibodies (gpELISA >0.6 units) were present in 97.9% (568/580) at 1 year, 97.1% (34/35) at 2 years, 100% (144/144) at 3 years, 97.0% (98/101) at 4 years, 97.4% (76/78) at 5 years, and 100% (34/34) at 6 years postvaccination.

A boost in antibody levels has been observed in vaccinees following exposure to natural varicella which could account for the apparent long-term persistence of antibody levels after vaccination in these studies. The duration of protection from varicella obtained using VARIVAX in the absence of wild-type boosting in unknown. VARIVAX also induces cell-mediated immune responses in vaccinees. The relative contributions of humoral immunity and cell-mediated immunity to protection from chickenpox are unknown.

Transmission

In the placebo-controlled trial, transmission of vaccine virus was assessed in household settings (during the 8-week post-vaccination period) in 416 susceptible placebo recipients who were household contacts of 445 vaccine recipients. Of the 416 placebo recipients, three developed chickenpox and seroconverted, nine reported a varicella-like rash and did not seroconvert, and six had no rash but seroconverted. If vaccine virus transmission occurred, it did so at a very low rate and possibly without recognizable clinical disease in contacts. These cases may represent either natural varicella from community contacts or a low incidence of transmission of vaccine virus from vaccinated contacts (see PRECAUTIONS, *Transmission*). Postmarketing experience suggests that transmission of vaccine virus may occur rarely between healthy vaccinees who develop a varicella-like rash and healthy susceptible contacts. Transmission of vaccine virus from vaccinees without a varicella-like rash has been reported but has not been confirmed.

Herpes Zoster

Overall, 9454 healthy children (12 months to 12 years of age) and 1648 adolescents and adults (13 years of age and older) have been vaccinated with Oka/Merck live attenuated varicella vaccine in clinical trials. Eight cases of herpes zoster have been reported in children during 42,556 person years of follow-up in clinical trials, resulting in a calculated incidence of at least 18.8 cases per 100,000 person years. The completeness of this reporting has not been determined. One case of herpes zoster has been reported in the adolescent and adult age group during 5410 person years of follow-up in clinical trials resulting in a calculated incidence of 18.5 cases per 100,000 person years.

All nine cases were mild and without sequelae. Two cultures (one child and one adult) obtained from vesicles were positive for wild-type varicella zoster virus as confirmed by restriction endonuclease analysis. The long-term effect of VARIVAX on the incidence of herpes zoster, particularly in those vaccinees exposed to natural varicella, is unknown at present.

In children, the reported rate of zoster in vaccine recipients appears not to exceed that previously determined in a population-based study of healthy children who had experienced natural varicella. The incidence of zoster in adults who have had natural varicella infection is higher than that in children.

Reye's Syndrome

Reye's Syndrome has occurred in children and adolescents following natural varicella infection, the majority of whom had received salicylates. In clinical studies in healthy children and adolescents in the United States, physicians advised varicella vaccine recipients not to use salicylates for six weeks after vaccination. There were no reports of Reye's Syndrome in varicella vaccine recipients during these studies.

Studies with Other Vaccines

In combined clinical studies involving 1080 children 12 to 36 months of age, 653 received VARIVAX and M-M-R* II (Measles, Mumps, and Rubella Virus Vaccine Live) concomitantly at separate sites and 427 received the vaccines six weeks apart. Seroconversion rates and antibody levels were comparable between the two groups at approximately six weeks post-vaccination to each of the virus vaccine components. No differences were noted in adverse reactions reported in those who received VARIVAX concomitantly with M-M-R II (Measles, Mumps, and Rubella Virus Vaccine Live) at separate sites and those who received VARIVAX and M-M-R II (Measles, Mumps, and Rubella Virus Vaccine Live) at different times (see PRECAUTIONS, *Drug Interactions, Use with Other Vaccines*).

In a clinical study involving 318 children 12 months to 42 months of age, 160 received an investigational vaccine (a formulation combining measles, mumps, rubella, and varicella in one syringe) concomitantly with booster doses of DTaP (diphtheria, tetanus, acellular pertussis) and OPV (oral poliovirus vaccine) while 144 received M-M-R II (Measles, Mumps, and Rubella Virus Vaccine Live) concomitantly with booster doses of DTaP and OPV followed by VARIVAX 6 weeks later. At six weeks postvaccination, seroconversion rates for measles, mumps, rubella, and varicella and the percentage of vaccinees whose titers were boosted for diphtheria, tetanus, pertussis, and polio were comparable between the two groups, but anti-varicella levels were decreased when the investigational vaccine containing var-

icella was administered concomitantly with DTaP. No clinically significant differences were noted in adverse reactions between the two groups.
In another clinical study involving 307 children 12 to 18 months of age, 150 received an investigational vaccine (a formulation combining measles, mumps, rubella, and varicella in one syringe) concomitantly with a booster dose of PedvaxHIB* [Haemophilus b Conjugate Vaccine (Meningococcal Protein Conjugate)] while 130 received M-M-R II (Measles, Mumps, and Rubella Virus Vaccine Live) concomitantly with a booster dose of PedvaxHIB followed by VARIVAX 6 weeks later. At six weeks postvaccination, seroconversion rates for measles, mumps, rubella, and varicella, and geometric mean titers for PedvaxHIB were comparable between the two groups, but anti-varicella levels were decreased when the investigational vaccine containing varicella was administered concomitantly with PedvaxHIB. No clinically significant differences in adverse reactions were seen between the two groups.
In a clinical study involving 609 children 12 to 23 months of age, 305 received VARIVAX, M-M-R II (Measles, Mumps, and Rubella Virus Vaccine Live), and TETRAMUNE** (*Haemophilus influenzae* type b, diphtheria, tetanus, and pertussis vaccines) concomitantly at separate sites, and 304 received M-M-R II and TETRAMUNE concomitantly at separate sites, followed by VARIVAX 6 weeks later. At six weeks postvaccination, seroconversion rates for measles, mumps, rubella and varicella were similar between the two groups. Postvaccination GMTs for all antigens were similar in both treatment groups except for varicella, which was lower when VARIVAX was administered concomitantly with M-M-R II and TETRAMUNE, but within the range of GMTs seen in previous clinical experience when VARIVAX was administered alone. At 1 year postvaccination, GMTs for measles, mumps, rubella, varicella and *Haemophilus influenzae* type b were similar between the two groups. All three vaccines were well tolerated regardless of whether they were administered concomitantly at separate sites or 6 weeks apart. There were no clinically important differences in reaction rates when the three vaccines were administered concomitantly versus 6 weeks apart.
In a clinical study involving 822 children 12 to 15 months of age, 410 received COMVAX* [Haemophilus b Conjugate (Meningococcal Protein Conjugate) and Hepatitis B (Recombinant) vaccine], M-M-R II, and VARIVAX concomitantly at separate sites, and 412 received COMVAX followed by M-M-R II and VARIVAX given concomitantly at separate sites, 6 weeks later. At six weeks postvaccination, the immune responses for the subjects who received the concomitant injections of COMVAX, M-M-R II, and VARIVAX were similar to those of the subjects who received COMVAX followed 6 weeks later by M-M-R II and VARIVAX with respect to all antigens administered. All three vaccines were generally well tolerated regardless of whether they were administered concomitantly at separate sites or 6 weeks apart. There were no clinically important differences in reaction rates when the three vaccines were administered concomitantly versus 6 weeks apart.
VARIVAX is recommended for subcutaneous administration. However, during clinical trials, some children received VARIVAX intramuscularly resulting in seroconversion rates similar to those in children who received the vaccine by the subcutaneous route. Persistence of antibody and efficacy in those receiving intramuscular injections have not been defined.

*Registered trademark of MERCK & CO., Inc.
**Registered trademark of Lederle Laboratories

In the **WARNINGS** *section, replace the last sentence with the following:*
More information is available by contacting the VARIVAX coordinating center, Omnicare Clinical Research, Inc., 630 Allendale Road, King of Prussia, PA 19406, (484) 679-2856.
In the **PRECAUTIONS** *section, under Drug Interactions, Use with Other Vaccines, replace the first paragraph with the following:*
Results from clinical studies indicate that VARIVAX can be administered concomitantly with M-M-R II, COMVAX, or TETRAMUNE (see CLINICAL PHARMACOLOGY, *Studies with Other Vaccines*).
In the **ADVERSE REACTIONS** *section, under Body As A Whole, after* "Anaphylaxis," *add* "in individuals with or without an allergic history.", *and replace the Nervous/Psychiatric subsection with the following:*
Encephalitis; cerebrovascular accident; transverse myelitis; Guillain-Barré syndrome; Bell's palsy; ataxia; non-febrile seizures; dizziness; paresthesia.
Revisions based on 7999910, issued November 2000.

VASOTEC® I.V. Injection ℞
(enalaprilat)

Prescribing information for this product, which appears on pages 2207–2210 of the 2002 PDR, has been revised as follows. Please write "See Supplement A" alongside product heading.
Replace the **HOW SUPPLIED** *section with the following:*
HOW SUPPLIED
No. 3824—VASOTEC I.V., 1.25 mg per mL, is a clear, colorless solution and is supplied in vials containing 1 mL and 2 mL.
NDC 0006-3824-01, 1 mL vials
NDC 0006-3824-04, 2 mL vials.
Storage
Store at 25°C (77°F); excursions permitted to 15–30°C (59–86°F) [see USP Controlled Room Temperature].
Revision based on 7875731, issued August 2001.

VIOXX® ℞
(rofecoxib tablets and oral suspension)

Prescribing information for this product, which appears on pages 2213–2217 of the 2002 PDR, has been revised as follows. Please write "See Supplement A" alongside product heading.
In the **WARNINGS** *section, under Anaphylactoid Reactions, in the second sentence, replace* "anaphylactoid" *with* "anaphylactic/anaphylactoid".
In the **PRECAUTIONS** *section, under Hepatic Effects, in the first paragraph, at the end of the third sentence, add* ", including VIOXX."
In the **ADVERSE REACTIONS** *section, in the Gastrointestinal subsection, after* "gastrointestinal bleeding,", *add* "hepatic failure,". *In the Immune System subsection, replace* "anaphylactoid" *with* "anaphylactic/anaphylactoid" *and after* "angioedema," *add* "bronchospasm,". *In the Skin and Skin Appendages subsection, at the end, add* "and toxic epidermal necrolysis."
Revisions based on 9183809, issued July 2001.
In the Patient Information, under **What are the possible side effects of VIOXX?**, *in the paragraph beginning* "Serious allergic reactions . . .", *in the first sentence, after* "or swallowing", *add* "and wheezing". *In the paragraph beginning* "Severe liver problems," *in the first sentence, replace* "including hepatitis and jaundice," *with* "including hepatitis, jaundice and liver failure,". *In the paragraph beginning* "In addition, the following side effects . . .", *after* "confusion," *add* "depression,"; *after* "low blood cell counts," *add* "palpitations, pancreatitis,"; *and after* "(aseptic meningitis)", *add* ", vertigo."
Revisions based on 9183904, issued July 2001.

ZOCOR® Tablets ℞
(simvastatin)

Prescribing information for this product, which appears on pages 2219–2223 of the 2002 PDR, has been revised as follows. Please write "See Supplement A" alongside product heading.
In the **HOW SUPPLIED** *section, under* No. 3588, *at the end, add* "**NDC** 0006-0726-82 bottles of 1000."; *under* No. 3591, *at the end, add* "**NDC** 0006-0749-82 bottles of 1000."; *under* No. 6577, *at the end, add* "**NDC** 0006-0543-82 bottles of 1000."
Revisions based on 7825441, issued June 2001.

Novartis Pharmaceuticals Corporation

NOVARTIS PHARMACEUTICALS CORPORATION
One Health Plaza
East Hanover, NJ 07936
(for branded products)
For Information Contact *(branded products)*:
Customer Response Department
(888) NOW-NOVARTIS [888-669-6682]
Global Internet Address:
http: //www.novartis.com

CLOZARIL® ℞
[*klō' ză-ril*]
(clozapine) Tablets
Rx only

Prescribing information for this product, which appears on pages 2319–2323 of the 2002 PDR, has been completely revised as follows. Please write "See Supplement A" next to the product heading.

Prescribing Information
Before prescribing CLOZARIL® (clozapine), the physician should be thoroughly familiar with the details of this prescribing information.

WARNING

1. AGRANULOCYTOSIS
BECAUSE OF A SIGNIFICANT RISK OF AGRANULOCYTOSIS, A POTENTIALLY LIFE-THREATENING ADVERSE EVENT, CLOZAPINE SHOULD BE RESERVED FOR USE IN THE TREATMENT OF SEVERELY ILL SCHIZOPHRENIC PATIENTS WHO FAIL TO SHOW AN ACCEPTABLE RESPONSE TO ADEQUATE COURSES OF STANDARD ANTIPSYCHOTIC DRUG TREATMENT.
PATIENTS BEING TREATED WITH CLOZAPINE MUST HAVE A BASELINE WHITE BLOOD CELL (WBC) AND DIFFERENTIAL COUNT BEFORE INITIATION OF TREATMENT AS WELL AS REGULAR WBC COUNTS DURING TREATMENT AND FOR 4 WEEKS AFTER DISCONTINUATION OF TREATMENT.
CLOZAPINE IS AVAILABLE ONLY THROUGH A DISTRIBUTION SYSTEM THAT ENSURES MONITORING OF WBC COUNTS ACCORDING TO THE SCHEDULE DESCRIBED BELOW PRIOR TO DELIVERY OF THE NEXT SUPPLY OF MEDICATION. (SEE WARNINGS)
2. SEIZURES
SEIZURES HAVE BEEN ASSOCIATED WITH THE USE OF CLOZAPINE. DOSE APPEARS TO BE AN IMPORTANT PREDICTOR OF SEIZURE, WITH A GREATER LIKELIHOOD AT HIGHER CLOZAPINE DOSES. CAUTION SHOULD BE USED WHEN ADMINISTERING CLOZAPINE TO PATIENTS HAVING A HISTORY OF SEIZURES OR OTHER PREDISPOSING FACTORS. PATIENTS SHOULD BE ADVISED NOT TO ENGAGE IN ANY ACTIVITY WHERE SUDDEN LOSS OF CONSCIOUSNESS COULD CAUSE SERIOUS RISK TO THEMSELVES OR OTHERS. (SEE WARNINGS)
3. MYOCARDITIS
ANALYSES OF POSTMARKETING SAFETY DATABASES SUGGEST THAT CLOZAPINE IS ASSOCIATED WITH AN INCREASED RISK OF FATAL MYOCARDITIS, ESPECIALLY DURING, BUT NOT LIMITED TO, THE FIRST MONTH OF THERAPY. IN PATIENTS IN WHOM MYOCARDITIS IS SUSPECTED, CLOZAPINE TREATMENT SHOULD BE PROMPTLY DISCONTINUED. (SEE WARNINGS)
4. OTHER ADVERSE CARDIOVASCULAR AND RESPIRATORY EFFECTS
ORTHOSTATIC HYPOTENSION, WITH OR WITHOUT SYNCOPE, CAN OCCUR WITH CLOZAPINE TREATMENT. RARELY, COLLAPSE CAN BE PROFOUND AND BE ACCOMPANIED BY RESPIRATORY AND/OR CARDIAC ARREST. ORTHOSTATIC HYPOTENSION IS MORE LIKELY TO OCCUR DURING INITIAL TITRATION IN ASSOCIATION WITH RAPID DOSE ESCALATION. IN PATIENTS WHO HAVE HAD EVEN A BRIEF INTERVAL OFF CLOZAPINE, i.e., 2 OR MORE DAYS SINCE THE LAST DOSE, TREATMENT SHOULD BE STARTED WITH 12.5 mg ONCE OR TWICE DAILY. (SEE WARNINGS and DOSAGE AND ADMINISTRATION)
SINCE COLLAPSE, RESPIRATORY ARREST AND CARDIAC ARREST DURING INITIAL TREATMENT HAS OCCURRED IN PATIENTS WHO WERE BEING ADMINISTERED BENZODIAZEPINES OR OTHER PSYCHOTROPIC DRUGS, CAUTION IS ADVISED WHEN CLOZAPINE IS INITIATED IN PATIENTS TAKING A BENZODIAZEPINE OR ANY OTHER PSYCHOTROPIC DRUG. (SEE WARNINGS)

DESCRIPTION
CLOZARIL® (clozapine), an atypical antipsychotic drug, is a tricyclic dibenzodiazepine derivative, 8-chloro-11-(4-methyl-1-piperazinyl)-5*H*-dibenzo [*b,e*] [1,4] diazepine. The structural formula is:

$C_{18}H_{19}ClN_4$ Mol. wt. 326.83

CLOZARIL® (clozapine) is available in pale yellow tablets of 25 mg and 100 mg for oral administration.
25 mg and 100 mg Tablets
Active Ingredient: clozapine is a yellow, crystalline powder, very slightly soluble in water.
Inactive Ingredients: colloidal silicon dioxide, lactose, magnesium stearate, povidone, starch (corn), and talc.

CLINICAL PHARMACOLOGY
Pharmacodynamics
CLOZARIL® (clozapine) is classified as an 'atypical' antipsychotic drug because its profile of binding to dopamine receptors and its effects on various dopamine mediated behaviors differ from those exhibited by more typical antipsychotic drug products. In particular, although CLOZARIL® (clozapine) does interfere with the binding of dopamine at D_1, D_2, D_3 and D_5 receptors, and has a high affinity for the D_4 receptor, it does not induce catalepsy nor inhibit apomorphine-induced stereotypy. This evidence, consistent with the view that CLOZARIL® (clozapine) is preferentially more active at limbic than at striatal dopamine receptors, may explain the relative freedom of CLOZARIL® (clozapine) from extrapyramidal side effects.
CLOZARIL® (clozapine) also acts as an antagonist at adrenergic, cholinergic, histaminergic and serotonergic receptors.
Absorption, Distribution, Metabolism and Excretion
In man, CLOZARIL® (clozapine) tablets (25 mg and 100 mg) are equally bioavailable relative to a clozapine solution. Following a dosage of 100 mg b.i.d., the average steady state peak plasma concentration was 319 ng/mL (range: 102–771 ng/mL), occurring at the average of 2.5 hours (range: 1–6 hours) after dosing. The average minimum concentration at steady state was 122 ng/mL (range: 41–343 ng/mL), after 100 mg b.i.d. dosing. Food does not appear to affect the systemic bioavailability of CLOZARIL® (clozapine). Thus, CLOZARIL® (clozapine) may be administered with or without food.

Continued on next page

Clozaril—Cont.

Clozapine is approximately 97% bound to serum proteins. The interaction between CLOZARIL® (clozapine) and other highly protein-bound drugs has not been fully evaluated but may be important. (See PRECAUTIONS)

Clozapine is almost completely metabolized prior to excretion and only trace amounts of unchanged drug are detected in the urine and feces. Approximately 50% of the administered dose is excreted in the urine and 30% in the feces. The demethylated, hydroxylated and N-oxide derivatives are components in both urine and feces. Pharmacological testing has shown the desmethyl metabolite to have only limited activity, while the hydroxylated and N-oxide derivatives were inactive.

The mean elimination half-life of clozapine after a single 75 mg dose was 8 hours (range: 4–12 hours), compared to a mean elimination half-life, after achieving steady state with 100 mg b.i.d. dosing, of 12 hours (range: 4–66 hours). A comparison of single-dose and multiple-dose administration of clozapine showed that the elimination half-life increased significantly after multiple dosing relative to that after single-dose administration, suggesting the possibility of concentration dependent pharmacokinetics. However, at steady state, linearly dose-proportional changes with respect to AUC (area under the curve), peak and minimum clozapine plasma concentrations were observed after administration of 37.5 mg, 75 mg, and 150 mg b.i.d.

Human Pharmacology

In contrast to more typical antipsychotic drugs, CLOZARIL® (clozapine) therapy produces little or no prolactin elevation.

As is true of more typical antipsychotic drugs, clinical EEG studies have shown that CLOZARIL® (clozapine) increases delta and theta activity and slows dominant alpha frequencies. Enhanced synchronization occurs, and sharp wave activity and spike and wave complexes may also develop. Patients, on rare occasions, may report an intensification of dream activity during CLOZARIL® (clozapine) therapy. REM sleep was found to be increased to 85% of the total sleep time. In these patients, the onset of REM sleep occurred almost immediately after falling asleep.

INDICATIONS AND USAGE

CLOZARIL® (clozapine) is indicated for the management of severely ill schizophrenic patients who fail to respond adequately to standard drug treatment for schizophrenia. Because of the significant risk of agranulocytosis and seizure associated with its use, CLOZARIL® (clozapine) should be used only in patients who have failed to respond adequately to treatment with appropriate courses of standard drug treatments for schizophrenia, either because of insufficient effectiveness or the inability to achieve an effective dose due to intolerable adverse effects from those drugs. (See WARNINGS)

The effectiveness of CLOZARIL® (clozapine) in a treatment resistant schizophrenic population was demonstrated in a 6-week study comparing CLOZARIL® (clozapine) and chlorpromazine. Patients meeting DSM-III criteria for schizophrenia and having a mean BPRS total score of 61 were demonstrated to be treatment resistant by history and by open, prospective treatment with haloperidol before entering into the double-blind phase of the study. The superiority of CLOZARIL® (clozapine) to chlorpromazine was documented in statistical analyses employing both categorical and continuous measures of treatment effect.

Because of the significant risk of agranulocytosis and seizure, events which both present a continuing risk over time, the extended treatment of patients failing to show an acceptable level of clinical response should ordinarily be avoided. In addition, the need for continuing treatment in patients exhibiting beneficial clinical responses should be periodically re-evaluated.

CONTRAINDICATIONS

CLOZARIL® (clozapine) is contraindicated in patients with a previous hypersensitivity to clozapine or any other component of this drug, in patients with myeloproliferative disorders, uncontrolled epilepsy, or a history of CLOZARIL® (clozapine) induced agranulocytosis or severe granulocytopenia. As with more typical antipsychotic drugs, CLOZARIL® (clozapine) is contraindicated in severe central nervous system depression or comatose states from any cause.

CLOZARIL® (clozapine) should not be used simultaneously with other agents having a well-known potential to cause agranulocytosis or otherwise suppress bone marrow function. The mechanism of CLOZARIL® (clozapine) induced agranulocytosis is unknown; nonetheless, it is possible that causative factors may interact synergistically to increase the risk and/or severity of bone marrow suppression.

WARNINGS

General

BECAUSE OF THE SIGNIFICANT RISK OF AGRANULOCYTOSIS, A POTENTIALLY LIFE-THREATENING ADVERSE EVENT (SEE FOLLOWING), CLOZARIL® (clozapine) SHOULD BE RESERVED FOR USE IN THE TREATMENT OF SEVERELY ILL SCHIZOPHRENIC PATIENTS WHO FAIL TO SHOW AN ACCEPTABLE RESPONSE TO ADEQUATE COURSES OF STANDARD DRUG TREATMENT FOR SCHIZOPHRENIA, EITHER BECAUSE OF INSUFFICIENT EFFECTIVENESS OR THE INABILITY TO ACHIEVE AN EFFECTIVE DOSE DUE TO INTOLERABLE ADVERSE EFFECTS FROM THOSE DRUGS. CONSEQUENTLY, BEFORE INITIATING TREATMENT WITH CLOZARIL® (clozapine), IT IS STRONGLY RECOMMENDED THAT A PATIENT BE GIVEN AT LEAST 2 TRIALS, EACH WITH A DIFFERENT STANDARD DRUG PRODUCT FOR SCHIZOPHRENIA, AT AN ADEQUATE DOSE, AND FOR AN ADEQUATE DURATION.

PATIENTS WHO ARE BEING TREATED WITH CLOZARIL® (clozapine) MUST HAVE A BASELINE WHITE BLOOD CELL (WBC) AND DIFFERENTIAL COUNT BEFORE INITIATION OF TREATMENT, AND A WBC COUNT EVERY WEEK FOR THE FIRST SIX MONTHS. THEREAFTER, IF ACCEPTABLE WBC COUNTS (WBC greater than or equal to 3,000/mm^3, ANC ≥1500/mm^3) HAVE BEEN MAINTAINED DURING THE FIRST 6 MONTHS OF CONTINUOUS THERAPY, WBC COUNTS CAN BE MONITORED EVERY OTHER WEEK. WBC COUNTS MUST BE MONITORED WEEKLY FOR AT LEAST 4 WEEKS AFTER THE DISCONTINUATION OF CLOZARIL® (clozapine).

CLOZARIL® (clozapine) IS AVAILABLE ONLY THROUGH A DISTRIBUTION SYSTEM THAT ENSURES MONITORING OF WBC COUNTS ACCORDING TO THE SCHEDULE DESCRIBED BELOW PRIOR TO DELIVERY OF THE NEXT SUPPLY OF MEDICATION.

Agranulocytosis

Agranulocytosis, defined as an absolute neutrophil count (ANC) of less than 500/mm^3, has been estimated to occur in association with CLOZARIL® (clozapine) use at a cumulative incidence at 1 year of approximately 1.3%, based on the occurrence of 15 US cases out of 1743 patients exposed to CLOZARIL® (clozapine) during its clinical testing prior to domestic marketing. All of these cases occurred at a time when the need for close monitoring of WBC counts was already recognized. This reaction could prove fatal if not detected early and therapy interrupted. Of the 149 cases of agranulocytosis reported worldwide in association with CLOZARIL® (clozapine) use as of December 31, 1989, 32% were fatal. However, few of these deaths occurred since 1977, at which time the knowledge of CLOZARIL® (clozapine) induced agranulocytosis became more widespread, and close monitoring of WBC counts more widely practiced. Nevertheless, it is unknown at present what the case fatality rate will be for CLOZARIL® (clozapine) induced agranulocytosis, despite strict adherence to the required frequency of monitoring. In the U.S., under a weekly WBC monitoring system with CLOZARIL® (clozapine), there have been 585 cases of agranulocytosis as of August 21, 1997; 19 were fatal. During this period 150,409 patients received CLOZARIL® (clozapine). A hematologic risk analysis was conducted based upon the available information in the Clozaril® National Registry (CNR) for U.S. patients. Based upon a cut-off date of April 30, 1995, the incidence rates of agranulocytosis based upon a weekly monitoring schedule, rose steeply during the first two months of therapy, peaking in the third month. Among CLOZARIL® (clozapine) patients who continued the drug beyond the third month, the weekly incidence of agranulocytosis fell to a substantial degree, so that by the sixth month the weekly incidence of agranulocytosis was reduced to 3 per 1000 person-years. After six months, the weekly incidence of agranulocytosis declines still further, however, never reaches zero. It should be noted that any type of reduction in the frequency of monitoring WBC counts may result in an increase incidence of agranulocytosis.

Because of the substantial risk for developing agranulocytosis in association with CLOZARIL® (clozapine) use, which may persist over an extended period of time, patients must have a blood sample drawn for a WBC count before initiation of treatment with CLOZARIL® (clozapine), and must have subsequent WBC counts done at least weekly for the first 6 months of continuous treatment. If WBC counts remain acceptable (WBC greater than or equal to 3000/mm^3, ANC ≥1500/mm^3) during this period, WBC counts may be monitored every other week thereafter. After the discontinuation of CLOZARIL® (clozapine), weekly WBC counts should be continued for an additional 4 weeks.

If a patient is on CLOZARIL® (clozapine) therapy for less than 6 months with no abnormal blood events and there is a break on therapy which is less than or equal to 1 month, then patients can continue where they left off with weekly WBC testing for 6 months. When this 6-month period has been completed, the frequency of WBC count monitoring can be reduced to every other week. If a patient is on CLOZARIL® (clozapine) therapy for less than 6 months with no abnormal blood events and there is a break on therapy which is greater than 1 month, then patients should be tested weekly for an additional 6-month period before biweekly testing is initiated. If a patient is on CLOZARIL® (clozapine) therapy for less than 6 months and experiences an abnormal blood event as described below but remains a rechallengeable patient [patients cannot be reinitiated on CLOZARIL® (clozapine) therapy if WBC counts fall below 2000/mm^3 or the ANC falls below 1000/mm^3 during CLOZARIL® (clozapine) therapy], the patient must restart the 6-month period of weekly WBC monitoring at day 0.

If a patient is on CLOZARIL® (clozapine) therapy for 6 months or longer with no abnormal blood events and there is a break on therapy which is 1 year or less, then the patient can continue WBC count monitoring every other week if CLOZARIL® (clozapine) therapy is reinitiated. If a patient is on CLOZARIL® (clozapine) therapy for 6 months or longer with no abnormal blood events and there is a break on therapy which is greater than 1 year, then, if CLOZARIL® (clozapine) therapy is reinitiated, the patient must have WBC counts monitored weekly for an additional 6 months. If a patient is on CLOZARIL® (clozapine) therapy for 6 months or longer and subsequently has an abnormal blood event, but remains a rechallengeable patient, then the patient must restart weekly WBC count monitoring until an additional 6 months of CLOZARIL® (clozapine) therapy has been received. The distribution of CLOZARIL® (clozapine) is contingent upon performance of the required blood tests.

Treatment should not be initiated if the WBC count is less than 3500/mm^3, or if the patient has a history of a myeloproliferative disorder, or previous CLOZARIL® (clozapine) induced agranulocytosis or granulocytopenia. Patients should be advised to report immediately the appearance of lethargy, weakness, fever, sore throat or any other signs of infection. If, after the initiation of treatment, the total WBC count has dropped below 3500/mm^3 or it has dropped by a substantial amount from baseline, even if the count is above 3500/mm^3, or if immature forms are present, a repeat WBC count and a differential count should be done. A substantial drop is defined as a single drop of 3,000 or more in the WBC count or a cumulative drop of 3,000 or more within 3 weeks. If subsequent WBC counts and the differential count reveal a total WBC count between 3000 and 3500/mm^3 and an ANC above 1500/mm^3, twice weekly WBC counts and differential counts should be performed. If the total WBC count falls below 3000/mm^3 or the ANC below 1500/mm^3, CLOZARIL® (clozapine) therapy should be interrupted, WBC count and differential should be performed daily, and patients should be carefully monitored for flu-like symptoms or other symptoms suggestive of infection. CLOZARIL® (clozapine) therapy may be resumed if no symptoms of infection develop, and if the total WBC count returns to levels above 3000/mm^3 and the ANC returns to levels above 1500/mm^3. However, in this event, twice-weekly WBC counts and differential counts should continue until total WBC counts return to levels above 3500/mm^3.

If the total WBC count falls below 2000/mm^3 or the ANC falls below 1000/mm^3, bone marrow aspiration should be considered to ascertain granulopoietic status. Protective isolation with close observation may be indicated if granulopoiesis is determined to be deficient. Should evidence of infection develop, the patient should have appropriate cultures performed and an appropriate antibiotic regimen instituted.

Patients whose total WBC counts fall below 2000/mm^3, or ANCs below 1000/mm^3 during CLOZARIL® (clozapine) therapy should have daily WBC count and differential. These patients should not be rechallenged with CLOZARIL® (clozapine). Patients discontinued from CLOZARIL® (clozapine) therapy due to significant WBC suppression have been found to develop agranulocytosis upon rechallenge, often with a shorter latency on reexposure. To reduce the chances of rechallenge occurring in patients who have experienced significant bone marrow suppression during CLOZARIL® (clozapine) therapy, a single, national master file will be maintained confidentially.

Except for evidence of significant bone marrow suppression during initial CLOZARIL® (clozapine) therapy, there are no established risk factors, based on world-wide experience, for the development of agranulocytosis in association with CLOZARIL® (clozapine) use. However, a disproportionate number of the U.S. cases of agranulocytosis occurred in patients of Jewish background compared to the overall proportion of such patients exposed during domestic development of CLOZARIL® (clozapine). Most of the U.S. cases occurred within 4–10 weeks of exposure, but neither dose nor duration is a reliable predictor of this problem. No patient characteristics have been clearly linked to the development of agranulocytosis in association with CLOZARIL® (clozapine) use, but agranulocytosis associated with other antipsychotic drugs has been reported to occur with a greater frequency in women, the elderly and in patients who are cachectic or have serious underlying medical illness; such patients may also be at particular risk with CLOZARIL® (clozapine).

To reduce the risk of agranulocytosis developing undetected, CLOZARIL® (clozapine) is available only through a distribution system that ensures monitoring of WBC counts according to the schedule described above prior to delivery of the next supply of medication.

Interrupted Therapy (WBC <3000/mm^3 ANC <1500/mm^3) for Bi-Weekly Monitoring

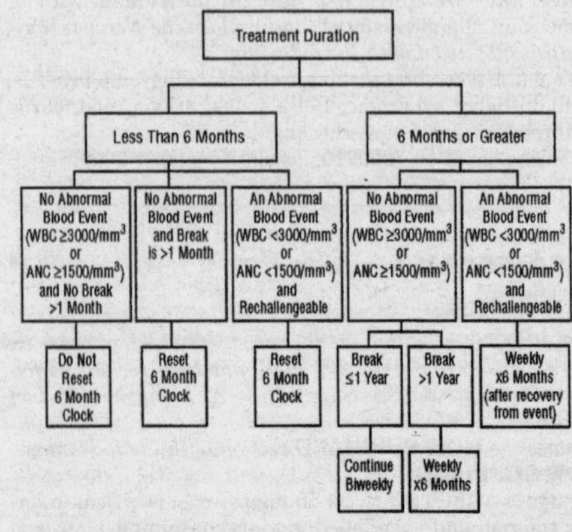

Eosinophilia

In clinical trials, 1% of patients developed eosinophilia, which, in rare cases, can be substantial. If a differential count reveals a total eosinophil count above 4,000/mm^3, CLOZARIL® (clozapine) therapy should be interrupted until the eosinophil count falls below 3,000/mm^3.

Seizures

Seizure has been estimated to occur in association with CLOZARIL® (clozapine) use at a cumulative incidence at one year of approximately 5%, based on the occurrence of one or more seizures in 61 of 1743 patients exposed to CLOZARIL® (clozapine) during its clinical testing prior to domestic marketing (i.e., a crude rate of 3.5%). Dose appears to be an important predictor of seizure, with a greater likelihood of seizure at the higher CLOZARIL® (clozapine) doses used.

Caution should be used in administering CLOZARIL® (clozapine) to patients having a history of seizures or other predisposing factors. Because of the substantial risk of seizure associated with CLOZARIL® (clozapine) use, patients should be advised not to engage in any activity where sudden loss of consciousness could cause serious risk to themselves or others, e.g., the operation of complex machinery, driving an automobile, swimming, climbing, etc.

Myocarditis

Post-marketing surveillance data from four countries that employ hematological monitoring of clozapine-treated patients revealed: 30 reports of myocarditis with 17 fatalities in 205,493 U.S. patients (August 2001); 7 reports of myocarditis with 1 fatality in 15,600 Canadian patients (April 2001); 30 reports of myocarditis with 8 fatalities in 24,108 U.K. patients (August 2001); 15 reports of myocarditis with 5 fatalities in 8,000 Australian patients (March 1999). These reports represent an incidence of 5.0, 16.3, 43.2, and 96.6 cases/100,000 patient years, respectively. The number of fatalities represent an incidence of 2.8, 2.3, 11.5, and 32.2 cases/100,000 patient years, respectively.

The overall incidence rate of myocarditis in patients with schizophrenia treated with antipsychotic agents is unknown. However, for the established market economies (WHO), the incidence of myocarditis is 0.3 cases/100,000 patient years and the fatality rate is 0.2 cases/100,000 patient years. Therefore, the rate of myocarditis in clozapine-treated patients appears to be 17–322 times greater than the general population and is associated with an increased risk of fatal myocarditis that is 14–161 times greater than the general population.

The total reports of myocarditis for these four countries was 82 of which 51 (62%) occurred within the first month of clozapine treatment, 25 (31%) occurred after the first month of therapy and 6 (7%) were unknown. The median duration of treatment was 3 weeks. Of 5 patients rechallenged with clozapine, 3 had a recurrence of myocarditis. Of the 82 reports, 31 (38%) were fatal and 25 patients who died had evidence of myocarditis at autopsy. These data also suggest that the incidence of fatal myocarditis may be highest during the first month of therapy.

Therefore, the possibility of myocarditis should be considered in patients receiving CLOZARIL® (clozapine) who present with unexplained fatigue, dyspnea, tachypnea, fever, chest pain, palpitations, other signs or symptoms of heart failure, or electrocardiographic findings such as ST-T wave abnormalities or arrhythmias. It is not known whether eosinophilia is a reliable predictor of myocarditis. Tachycardia, which has been associated with CLOZARIL® (clozapine) treatment, has also been noted as a presenting sign in patients with myocarditis. Therefore, tachycardia during the first month of therapy warrants close monitoring for other signs of myocarditis.

Prompt discontinuation of CLOZARIL® (clozapine) treatment is warranted upon suspicion of myocarditis. Patients with clozapine-related myocarditis should not be rechallenged with CLOZARIL® (clozapine).

Other Adverse Cardiovascular and Respiratory Effects

Orthostatic hypotension with or without syncope can occur with CLOZARIL® (clozapine) treatment and may represent a continuing risk in some patients. Rarely (approximately 1 case per 3,000 patients), collapse can be profound and be accompanied by respiratory and/or cardiac arrest. Orthostatic hypotension is more likely to occur during initial titration in association with rapid dose escalation and may even occur on first dose. In one report, initial doses as low as 12.5 mg were associated with collapse and respiratory arrest. When restarting patients who have had even a brief interval off CLOZARIL® (clozapine), i.e., 2 days or more since the last dose, it is recommended that treatment be reinitiated with one-half of a 25 mg tablet (12.5 mg) once or twice daily. (See DOSAGE AND ADMINISTRATION)

Some of the cases of collapse/respiratory arrest/cardiac arrest during initial treatment occurred in patients who were being administered benzodiazepines; similar events have been reported in patients taking other psychotropic drugs or even CLOZARIL® (clozapine) by itself. Although it has not been established that there is an interaction between CLOZARIL® (clozapine) and benzodiazepines or other psychotropics, caution is advised when clozapine is initiated in patients taking a benzodiazepine or any other psychotropic drug.

Tachycardia, which may be sustained, has also been observed in approximately 25% of patients taking CLOZARIL® (clozapine), with patients having an average increase in pulse rate of 10–15 bpm. The sustained tachycardia is not simply a reflex response to hypotension, and is present in all positions monitored. Either tachycardia or hypotension may pose a serious risk for an individual with compromised cardiovascular function.

A minority of CLOZARIL® (clozapine) treated patients experience ECG repolarization changes similar to those seen with other antipsychotic drugs, including S-T segment depression and flattening or inversion of T waves, which all normalize after discontinuation of CLOZARIL® (clozapine). The clinical significance of these changes is unclear. However, in clinical trials with CLOZARIL® (clozapine), several patients experienced significant cardiac events, including ischemic changes, myocardial infarction, arrhythmias and sudden death. In addition there have been postmarketing reports of congestive heart failure. Causality assessment was difficult in many of these cases because of serious preexisting cardiac disease and plausible alternative causes. Rare instances of sudden death have been reported in psychiatric patients, with or without associated antipsychotic drug treatment, and the relationship of these events to antipsychotic drug use is unknown.

CLOZARIL® (clozapine) should be used with caution in patients with known cardiovascular and/or pulmonary disease, and the recommendation for gradual titration of dose should be carefully observed.

Neuroleptic Malignant Syndrome (NMS)

A potentially fatal symptom complex sometimes referred to as Neuroleptic Malignant Syndrome (NMS) has been reported in association with antipsychotic drugs. Clinical manifestations of NMS are hyperpyrexia, muscle rigidity, altered mental status and evidence of autonomic instability (irregular pulse or blood pressure, tachycardia, diaphoresis, and cardiac dysrhythmias).

The diagnostic evaluation of patients with this syndrome is complicated. In arriving at a diagnosis, it is important to identify cases where the clinical presentation includes both serious medical illness (e.g., pneumonia, systemic infection, etc.) and untreated or inadequately treated extrapyramidal signs and symptoms (EPS). Other important considerations in the differential diagnosis include central anticholinergic toxicity, heat stroke, drug fever and primary central nervous system (CNS) pathology.

The management of NMS should include 1) immediate discontinuation of antipsychotic drugs and other drugs not essential to concurrent therapy, 2) intensive symptomatic treatment and medical monitoring, and 3) treatment of any concomitant serious medical problems for which specific treatments are available. There is no general agreement about specific pharmacological treatment regimens for uncomplicated NMS.

If a patient requires antipsychotic drug treatment after recovery from NMS, the potential reintroduction of drug therapy should be carefully considered. The patient should be carefully monitored, since recurrences of NMS have been reported.

There have been several reported cases of NMS in patients receiving CLOZARIL® (clozapine) alone or in combination with lithium or other CNS-active agents.

Tardive Dyskinesia

A syndrome consisting of potentially irreversible, involuntary, dyskinetic movements may develop in patients treated with antipsychotic drugs. Although the prevalence of the syndrome appears to be highest among the elderly, especially elderly women, it is impossible to rely upon prevalence estimates to predict, at the inception of treatment, which patients are likely to develop the syndrome.

There are several reasons for predicting that CLOZARIL® (clozapine) may be different from other antipsychotic drugs in its potential for inducing tardive dyskinesia, including the preclinical finding that it has a relatively weak dopamine-blocking effect and the clinical finding of a virtual absence of certain acute extrapyramidal symptoms, e.g., dystonia. A few cases of tardive dyskinesia have been reported in patients on CLOZARIL® (clozapine) who had been previously treated with other antipsychotic agents, so that a causal relationship cannot be established. There have been no reports of tardive dyskinesia directly attributable to CLOZARIL® (clozapine) alone. Nevertheless, it cannot be concluded, without more extended experience, that CLOZARIL® (clozapine) is incapable of inducing this syndrome.

Both the risk of developing the syndrome and the likelihood that it will become irreversible are believed to increase as the duration of treatment and the total cumulative dose of antipsychotic drugs administered to the patient increase. However, the syndrome can develop, although much less commonly, after relatively brief treatment periods at low doses. There is no known treatment for established cases of tardive dyskinesia, although the syndrome may remit, partially or completely, if antipsychotic drug treatment is withdrawn. Antipsychotic drug treatment, itself, however, may suppress (or partially suppress) the signs and symptoms of the syndrome and thereby may possibly mask the underlying process. The effect that symptom suppression has upon the long-term course of the syndrome is unknown.

Given these considerations, CLOZARIL® (clozapine) should be prescribed in a manner that is most likely to minimize the occurrence of tardive dyskinesia. As with any antipsychotic drug, chronic CLOZARIL® (clozapine) use should be reserved for patients who appear to be obtaining substantial benefit from the drug. In such patients, the smallest dose and the shortest duration of treatment should be sought. The need for continued treatment should be reassessed periodically.

If signs and symptoms of tardive dyskinesia appear in a patient on CLOZARIL® (clozapine), drug discontinuation should be considered. However, some patients may require treatment with CLOZARIL® (clozapine) despite the presence of the syndrome.

PRECAUTIONS

General

Because of the significant risk of agranulocytosis and seizure, both of which present a continuing risk over time, the extended treatment of patients failing to show an acceptable level of clinical response should ordinarily be avoided. In addition, the need for continuing treatment in patients exhibiting beneficial clinical responses should be periodically re-evaluated. Although it is not known whether the risk would be increased, it is prudent either to avoid CLOZARIL® (clozapine) or use it cautiously in patients with a previous history of agranulocytosis induced by other drugs.

Fever

During CLOZARIL® (clozapine) therapy, patients may experience transient temperature elevations above 100.4°F (38°C), with the peak incidence within the first 3 weeks of treatment. While this fever is generally benign and self limiting, it may necessitate discontinuing patients from treatment. On occasion, there may be an associated increase or decrease in WBC count. Patients with fever should be carefully evaluated to rule out the possibility of an underlying infectious process or the development of agranulocytosis. In the presence of high fever, the possibility of Neuroleptic Malignant Syndrome (NMS) must be considered. There have been several reports of NMS in patients receiving CLOZARIL® (clozapine), usually in combination with lithium or other CNS-active drugs. [See Neuroleptic Malignant Syndrome (NMS), under WARNINGS]

Pulmonary Embolism

The possibility of pulmonary embolism should be considered in patients receiving CLOZARIL® (clozapine) who present with deep vein thrombosis, acute dyspnea, chest pain or with other respiratory signs and symptoms. As of December 31, 1993 there were 18 cases of fatal pulmonary embolism in association with CLOZARIL® (clozapine) therapy in users 10–54 years of age. Based upon the extent of use observed in the Clozaril National Registry, the mortality rate associated with pulmonary embolus was 1 death per 3450 person-years of use. This rate was about 27.5 times higher than that in the general population of a similar age and gender (95% Confidence Interval; 17.1,42.2). Deep vein thrombosis has also been observed in association with CLOZARIL® (clozapine) therapy. Whether pulmonary embolus can be attributed to CLOZARIL® (clozapine) or some characteristic(s) of its users is not clear, but the occurrence of deep vein thrombosis or respiratory symptomatology should suggest its presence.

Hyperglycemia

Severe hyperglycemia, sometimes leading to ketoacidosis, has been reported during CLOZARIL® (clozapine) treatment in patients with no prior history of hyperglycemia. While a causal relationship to CLOZARIL® (clozapine) use has not been definitively established, glucose levels normalized in most patients after discontinuation of CLOZARIL® (clozapine), and a rechallenge in one patient produced a recurrence of hyperglycemia. The effect of CLOZARIL® (clozapine) on glucose metabolism in patients with diabetes mellitus has not been studied. The possibility of impaired glucose tolerance should be considered in patients receiving CLOZARIL® (clozapine) who develop symptoms of hyperglycemia, such as polydipsia, polyuria, polyphagia, and weakness. In patients with significant treatment-emergent hyperglycemia, the discontinuation of CLOZARIL® (clozapine) should be considered.

Hepatitis

Caution is advised in patients using CLOZARIL® (clozapine) who have concurrent hepatic disease. Hepatitis has been reported in both patients with normal and preexisting liver function abnormalities. In patients who develop nausea, vomiting, and/or anorexia during CLOZARIL® (clozapine) treatment, liver function tests should be performed immediately. If the elevation of these values is clinically relevant or if symptoms of jaundice occur, treatment with CLOZARIL® (clozapine) should be discontinued.

Anticholinergic Toxicity

Eye

CLOZARIL® (clozapine) has potent anticholinergic effects and care should be exercised in using this drug in the presence of narrow angle glaucoma.

Gastrointestinal

CLOZARIL® (clozapine) use has been associated with varying degrees of impairment of intestinal peristalsis, ranging from constipation to intestinal obstruction, fecal impaction and paralytic ileus (see ADVERSE REACTIONS). On rare occasions, these cases have been fatal. Constipation should be initially treated by ensuring adequate hydration, and use of ancillary therapy such as bulk laxatives. Consultation with a gastroenterologist is advisable in more serious cases.

Prostate

CLOZARIL® (clozapine) has potent anticholinergic effects and care should be exercised in using this drug in the presence of prostatic enlargement.

Interference with Cognitive and Motor Performance

Because of initial sedation, CLOZARIL® (clozapine) may impair mental and/or physical abilities, especially during the first few days of therapy. The recommendations for gradual dose escalation should be carefully adhered to, and patients cautioned about activities requiring alertness.

Use in Patients with Concomitant Illness

Clinical experience with CLOZARIL® (clozapine) in patients with concomitant systemic diseases is limited. Nevertheless, caution is advisable in using CLOZARIL® (clozapine) in patients with renal or cardiac disease.

Continued on next page

Clozaril—Cont.

Use in Patients Undergoing General Anesthesia
Caution is advised in patients being administered general anesthesia because of the CNS effects of CLOZARIL® (clozapine). Check with the anesthesiologist regarding continuation of CLOZARIL® (clozapine) therapy in a patient scheduled for surgery.

Information for Patients
Physicians are advised to discuss the following issues with patients for whom they prescribe CLOZARIL® (clozapine):

— Patients who are to receive CLOZARIL® (clozapine) should be warned about the significant risk of developing agranulocytosis. They should be informed that weekly blood tests are required for the first 6 months, if acceptable WBC counts (WBC greater than or equal to $3000/mm^3$, ANC $\geq 1500/mm^3$) have been maintained during the first 6 months of continuous therapy, then WBC counts can be monitored every other week in order to monitor for the occurrence of agranulocytosis, and that CLOZARIL® (clozapine) tablets will be made available only through a special program designed to ensure the required blood monitoring. Patients should be advised to report immediately the appearance of lethargy, weakness, fever, sore throat, malaise, mucous membrane ulceration or other possible signs of infection. Particular attention should be paid to any flu-like complaints or other symptoms that might suggest infection.

— Patients should be informed of the significant risk of seizure during CLOZARIL® (clozapine) treatment, and they should be advised to avoid driving and any other potentially hazardous activity while taking CLOZARIL® (clozapine).

— Patients should be advised of the risk of orthostatic hypotension, especially during the period of initial dose titration.

— Patients should be informed that if they stop taking CLOZARIL® (clozapine) for more than 2 days, they should not restart their medication at the same dosage, but should contact their physician for dosing instructions.

— Patients should notify their physician if they are taking, or plan to take, any prescription or over-the-counter drugs or alcohol.

— Patients should notify their physician if they become pregnant or intend to become pregnant during therapy.

— Patients should not breast feed an infant if they are taking CLOZARIL® (clozapine).

Drug Interactions
The risks of using CLOZARIL® (clozapine) in combination with other drugs have not been systematically evaluated.

Pharmacodynamic-related Interactions
The mechanism of CLOZARIL® (clozapine) induced agranulocytosis is unknown; nonetheless, the possibility that causative factors may interact synergistically to increase the risk and/or severity of bone marrow suppression warrants consideration. Therefore, CLOZARIL® (clozapine) should not be used with other agents having a well-known potential to suppress bone marrow function.

Given the primary CNS effects of CLOZARIL® (clozapine), caution is advised in using it concomitantly with other CNS-active drugs or alcohol.

Orthostatic hypotension in patients taking clozapine can, in rare cases (approximately 1 case per 3,000 patients), be accompanied by profound collapse and respiratory and/or cardiac arrest. Some of the cases of collapse/respiratory arrest/cardiac arrest during initial treatment occurred in patients who were being administered benzodiazepines; similar events have been reported in patients taking other psychotropic drugs or even CLOZARIL® (clozapine) by itself. Although it has not been established that there is an interaction between CLOZARIL® (clozapine) and benzodiazepines or other psychotropics, caution is advised when clozapine is initiated in patients taking a benzodiazepine or any other psychotropic drug.

CLOZARIL® (clozapine) may potentiate the hypotensive effects of antihypertensive drugs and the anticholinergic effects of atropine-type drugs. The administration of epinephrine should be avoided in the treatment of drug induced hypotension because of a possible reverse epinephrine effect.

Pharmacokinetic-related Interactions
Clozapine is a substrate for many CYP 450 isozymes, in particular 1A2, 2D6, and 3A4. The risk of metabolic interactions caused by an effect on an individual isoform is therefore minimized. Nevertheless, caution should be used in patients receiving concomitant treatment with other drugs which are either inhibitors or inducers of these enzymes.

Concomitant administration of drugs known to induce cytochrome P450 enzymes may decrease the plasma levels of clozapine. Phenytoin, nicotine, and rifampin may decrease CLOZARIL® (clozapine) plasma levels, resulting in a decrease in effectiveness of a previously effective CLOZARIL® (clozapine) dose.

Concomitant administration of drugs known to inhibit the activity of cytochrome P450 isozymes may increase the plasma levels of clozapine. Cimetidine, caffeine, and erythromycin may increase plasma levels of CLOZARIL® (clozapine), potentially resulting in adverse effects. Although concomitant use of CLOZARIL® (clozapine) and carbamazepine is not recommended, it should be noted that discontinuation of concomitant carbamazepine administration may result in an increase in CLOZARIL® (clozapine) plasma levels.

In a study of schizophrenic patients who received clozapine under steady state conditions, fluvoxamine or paroxetine was added in 16 and 14 patients, respectively. After 14 days of co-administration, mean trough concentrations of clozapine and its metabolites, *N*-desmethylclozapine and clozapine *N*-oxide, were elevated with fluvoxamine by about three-fold compared to baseline concentrations. Paroxetine produced only minor changes in the levels of clozapine and its metabolites. However, other published reports describe modest elevations (less than two-fold) of clozapine and metabolite concentrations when clozapine was taken with paroxetine, fluoxetine, and sertraline. Therefore, such combined treatment should be approached with caution and patients should be monitored closely when CLOZARIL® (clozapine) is combined with these drugs, particularly with fluvoxamine. A reduced CLOZARIL® (clozapine) dose should be considered.

A subset (3%–10%) of the population has reduced activity of certain drug metabolizing enzymes such as the cytochrome P450 isozyme P450 2D6. Such individuals are referred to as "poor metabolizers" of drugs such as debrisoquin, dextromethorphan, the tricyclic antidepressants, and clozapine. These individuals may develop higher than expected plasma concentrations of clozapine when given usual doses. In addition, certain drugs that are metabolized by this isozyme, including many antidepressants (clozapine, selective serotonin reuptake inhibitors, and others), may inhibit the activity of this isozyme, and thus may make normal metabolizers resemble poor metabolizers with regard to concomitant therapy with other drugs metabolized by this enzyme system, leading to drug interaction.

Concomitant use of clozapine with other drugs metabolized by cytochrome P450 2D6 may require lower doses than usually prescribed for either clozapine or the other drug. Therefore, co-administration of clozapine with other drugs that are metabolized by this isozyme, including antidepressants, phenothiazines, carbamazepine, and Type 1C antiarrhythmics (e.g., propafenone, flecainide and encainide), or that inhibit this enzyme (e.g., quinidine), should be approached with caution.

Carcinogenesis, Mutagenesis, Impairment of Fertility
No carcinogenic potential was demonstrated in long-term studies in mice and rats at doses approximately 7 times the typical human dose on a mg/kg basis. Fertility in male and female rats was not adversely affected by clozapine. Clozapine did not produce genotoxic or mutagenic effects when assayed in appropriate bacterial and mammalian tests.

Pregnancy Category B
Reproduction studies have been performed in rats and rabbits at doses of approximately 2–4 times the human dose and have revealed no evidence of impaired fertility or harm to the fetus due to clozapine. There are, however, no adequate and well-controlled studies in pregnant women. Because animal reproduction studies are not always predictive of human response, and in view of the desirability of keeping the administration of all drugs to a minimum during pregnancy, this drug should be used only if clearly needed.

Nursing Mothers
Animal studies suggest that clozapine may be excreted in breast milk and have an effect on the nursing infant. Therefore, women receiving CLOZARIL® (clozapine) should not breast feed.

Pediatric Use
Safety and effectiveness in pediatric patients have not been established.

Geriatric Use
Clinical studies of clozapine did not include sufficient numbers of subjects age 65 and over to determine whether they respond differently from younger subjects.

Orthostatic hypotension can occur with CLOZARIL® (clozapine) treatment and tachycardia, which may be sustained, has been observed in about 25% of patients taking CLOZARIL® (clozapine) (see WARNINGS, Other Adverse Cardiovascular and Respiratory Effects). Elderly patients, particularly those with compromised cardiovascular functioning, may be more susceptible to these effects.

Also, elderly patients may be particularly susceptible to the anticholinergic effects of CLOZARIL® (clozapine), such as urinary retention and constipation. (See PRECAUTIONS, Anticholinergic Toxicity)

Dose selection for an elderly patient should be cautious, reflecting the greater frequency of decreased hepatic, renal, or cardiac function, and of concomitant disease or other drug therapy. Other reported clinical experience does suggest that the prevalence of tardive dyskinesia appears to be highest among the elderly, especially elderly women. (See WARNINGS, Tardive Dyskinesia)

ADVERSE REACTIONS

Associated with Discontinuation of Treatment
Sixteen percent of 1080 patients who received CLOZARIL® (clozapine) in premarketing clinical trials discontinued treatment due to an adverse event, including both those that could be reasonably attributed to CLOZARIL® (clozapine) treatment and those that might more appropriately be considered intercurrent illness. The more common events considered to be causes of discontinuation included: CNS, primarily drowsiness/sedation, seizures, dizziness/syncope; cardiovascular, primarily tachycardia, hypotension and ECG changes; gastrointestinal, primarily nausea/vomiting; hematologic, primarily leukopenia/granulocytopenia/agranulocytosis; and fever. None of the events enumerated accounts for more than 1.7% of all discontinuations attributed to adverse clinical events.

Commonly Observed
Adverse events observed in association with the use of CLOZARIL® (clozapine) in clinical trials at an incidence of greater than 5% were: central nervous system complaints, including drowsiness/sedation, dizziness/vertigo, headache and tremor; autonomic nervous system complaints, including salivation, sweating, dry mouth and visual disturbances; cardiovascular findings, including tachycardia, hypotension and syncope; and gastrointestinal complaints, including constipation and nausea; and fever. Complaints of drowsiness/sedation tend to subside with continued therapy or dose reduction. Salivation may be profuse, especially during sleep, but may be diminished with dose reduction.

Incidence in Clinical Trials
The following table enumerates adverse events that occurred at a frequency of 1% or greater among CLOZARIL® (clozapine) patients who participated in clinical trials. These rates are not adjusted for duration of exposure.

Treatment-Emergent Adverse Experience Incidence Among Patients Taking CLOZARIL® (clozapine) in Clinical Trials (N = 842) (Percentage of Patients Reporting)

Body System Adverse Event[a]	Percent
Central Nervous System	
Drowsiness/Sedation	39
Dizziness/Vertigo	19
Headache	7
Tremor	6
Syncope	6
Disturbed sleep/Nightmares	4
Restlessness	4
Hypokinesia/Akinesia	4
Agitation	4
Seizures (convulsions)	3[b]
Rigidity	3
Akathisia	3
Confusion	3
Fatigue	2
Insomnia	2
Hyperkinesia	1
Weakness	1
Lethargy	1
Ataxia	1
Slurred speech	1
Depression	1
Epileptiform movements/Myoclonic jerks	1
Anxiety	1
Cardiovascular	
Tachycardia	25[b]
Hypotension	9
Hypertension	4
Chest pain/Angina	1
ECG change/Cardiac abnormality	1
Gastrointestinal	
Constipation	14
Nausea	5
Abdominal discomfort/Heartburn	4
Nausea/Vomiting	3
Vomiting	3
Diarrhea	2
Liver test abnormality	1
Anorexia	1
Urogenital	
Urinary abnormalities	2
Incontinence	1
Abnormal ejaculation	1
Urinary urgency/frequency	1
Urinary retention	1
Autonomic Nervous System	
Salivation	31
Sweating	6
Dry mouth	6
Visual disturbances	5
Integumentary (Skin)	
Rash	2
Musculoskeletal	
Muscle weakness	1
Pain (back, neck, legs)	1
Muscle spasm	1
Muscle pain, ache	1
Respiratory	
Throat discomfort	1
Dyspnea, shortness of breath	1
Nasal congestion	1
Hemic/Lymphatic	
Leukopenia/Decreased WBC/Neutropenia	3
Agranulocytosis	1[b]
Eosinophilia	1

Miscellaneous

Fever	5
Weight gain	4
Tongue numb/sore	1

[a] Events reported by at least 1% of CLOZARIL® (clozapine) patients are included.

[b] Rate based on population of approximately 1700 exposed during premarket clinical evaluation of CLOZARIL® (clozapine).

Other Events Observed During the Premarketing Evaluation of CLOZARIL® (clozapine)

This section reports additional, less frequent adverse events which occurred among the patients taking CLOZARIL® (clozapine) in clinical trials. Various adverse events were reported as part of the total experience in these clinical studies; a causal relationship to CLOZARIL® (clozapine) treatment cannot be determined in the absence of appropriate controls in some of the studies. The table above enumerates adverse events that occurred at a frequency of at least 1% of patients treated with CLOZARIL® (clozapine). The list below includes all additional adverse experiences reported as being temporally associated with the use of the drug which occurred at a frequency less than 1%, enumerated by organ system.

Central Nervous System: loss of speech, amentia, tics, poor coordination, delusions/hallucinations, involuntary movement, stuttering, dysarthria, amnesia/memory loss, histrionic movements, libido increase or decrease, paranoia, shakiness, Parkinsonism, and irritability.

Cardiovascular System: edema, palpitations, phlebitis/thrombophlebitis, cyanosis, premature ventricular contraction, bradycardia, and nose bleed.

Gastrointestinal System: abdominal distention, gastroenteritis, rectal bleeding, nervous stomach, abnormal stools, hematemesis, gastric ulcer, bitter taste, and eructation.

Urogenital System: dysmenorrhea, impotence, breast pain/discomfort, and vaginal itch/infection.

Autonomic Nervous System: numbness, polydypsia, hot flashes, dry throat, and mydriasis.

Integumentary (Skin): pruritus, pallor, eczema, erythema, bruise, dermatitis, petechiae, and urticaria.

Musculoskeletal System: twitching and joint pain.

Respiratory System: coughing, pneumonia/pneumonia-like symptoms, rhinorrhea, hyperventilation, wheezing, bronchitis, laryngitis, and sneezing.

Hemic and Lymphatic System: anemia and leukocytosis.

Miscellaneous: chills/chills with fever, malaise, appetite increase, ear disorder, hypothermia, eyelid disorder, bloodshot eyes, and nystagmus.

Postmarketing Clinical Experience

Postmarketing experience has shown an adverse experience profile similar to that presented above. Voluntary reports of adverse events temporally associated with CLOZARIL® (clozapine) not mentioned above that have been received since market introduction and that may have no causal relationship with the drug include the following:

Central Nervous System: delirium; EEG abnormal; exacerbation of psychosis; myoclonus; overdose; paresthesia; possible mild cataplexy; and status epilepticus.

Cardiovascular System: atrial or ventricular fibrillation and periorbital edema.

Gastrointestinal System: acute pancreatitis; dysphagia; fecal impaction; intestinal obstruction/paralytic ileus; and salivary gland swelling.

Hepatobiliary System: cholestasis; hepatitis; jaundice.

Hepatic System: cholestasis.

Urogenital System: acute interstitial nephritis and priapism.

Integumentary (Skin): hypersensitivity reactions: photosensitivity, vasculitis, erythema multiforme, and Stevens-Johnson Syndrome.

Musculoskeletal System: myasthenic syndrome and rhabdomyolysis.

Respiratory System: aspiration and pleural effusion.

Hemic and Lymphatic System: deep vein thrombosis; elevated hemoglobin/hematocrit; ESR increased; pulmonary embolism; sepsis; thrombocytosis; and thrombocytopenia.

Vision Disorders: narrow angle glaucoma

Miscellaneous: CPK elevation; hyperglycemia; hyperuricemia; hyponatremia; and weight loss.

DRUG ABUSE AND DEPENDENCE

Physical and psychological dependence have not been reported or observed in patients taking CLOZARIL® (clozapine).

OVERDOSAGE

Human Experience

The most commonly reported signs and symptoms associated with CLOZARIL® (clozapine) overdose are: altered states of consciousness, including drowsiness, delirium and coma; tachycardia; hypotension; respiratory depression or failure; hypersalivation. Aspiration pneumonia and cardiac arrhythmias have also been reported. Seizures have occurred in a minority of reported cases. Fatal overdoses have been reported with CLOZARIL® (clozapine), generally at doses above 2500 mg. There have also been reports of patients recovering from overdoses well in excess of 4 g.

Management of Overdose

Establish and maintain an airway; ensure adequate oxygenation and ventilation. Activated charcoal, which may be used with sorbitol, may be as or more effective than emesis or lavage, and should be considered in treating overdosage. Cardiac and vital signs monitoring is recommended along with general symptomatic and supportive measures. Additional surveillance should be continued for several days because of the risk of delayed effects. Avoid epinephrine and derivatives when treating hypotension, and quinidine and procainamide when treating cardiac arrhythmia.

There are no specific antidotes for CLOZARIL® (clozapine). Forced diuresis, dialysis, hemoperfusion and exchange transfusion are unlikely to be of benefit.

In managing overdosage, the physician should consider the possibility of multiple drug involvement.

Up-to-date information about the treatment of overdose can often be obtained from a certified Regional Poison Control Center. Telephone numbers of certified Poison Control Centers are listed in the Physicians' Desk Reference®.*

DOSAGE AND ADMINISTRATION

Upon initiation of CLOZARIL® (clozapine) therapy, up to a 1 week supply of additional CLOZARIL® (clozapine) tablets may be provided to the patient to be held for emergencies (e.g., weather, holidays).

Initial Treatment

It is recommended that treatment with CLOZARIL® (clozapine) begin with one-half of a 25 mg tablet (12.5 mg) once or twice daily and then be continued with daily dosage increments of 25–50 mg/day, if well-tolerated, to achieve a target dose of 300–450 mg/day by the end of 2 weeks. Subsequent dosage increments should be made no more than once or twice-weekly, in increments not to exceed 100 mg. Cautious titration and a divided dosage schedule are necessary to minimize the risks of hypotension, seizure, and sedation.

In the multicenter study that provides primary support for the effectiveness of CLOZARIL® (clozapine) in patients resistant to standard drug treatment for schizophrenia, patients were titrated during the first 2 weeks up to a maximum dose of 500 mg/day, on a t.i.d. basis, and were then dosed in a total daily dose range of 100–900 mg/day, on a t.i.d. basis thereafter, with clinical response and adverse effects as guides to correct dosing.

Therapeutic Dose Adjustment

Daily dosing should continue on a divided basis as an effective and tolerable dose level is sought. While many patients may respond adequately at doses between 300–600 mg/day, it may be necessary to raise the dose to the 600–900 mg/day range to obtain an acceptable response. [Note: In the multicenter study providing the primary support for the superiority of CLOZARIL® (clozapine) in treatment resistant patients, the mean and median CLOZARIL® (clozapine) doses were both approximately 600 mg/day.]

Because of the possibility of increased adverse reactions at higher doses, particularly seizures, patients should ordinarily be given adequate time to respond to a given dose level before escalation to a higher dose is contemplated. CLOZARIL® (clozapine) can cause EEG changes, including the occurrence of spike and wave complexes. It lowers the seizures threshold in a dose-dependent manner and may induce myoclonic jerks or generalized seizures. These symptoms may be likely to occur with rapid dose increase and in patients with pre-existing epilepsy. In this case, the dose should be reduced and, if necessary, anticonvulsant treatment initiated.

Dosing should not exceed 900 mg/day.

Because of the significant risk of agranulocytosis and seizure, events which both present a continuing risk over time, the extended treatment of patients failing to show an acceptable level of clinical response should ordinarily be avoided.

Maintenance Treatment

While the maintenance effectiveness of CLOZARIL® (clozapine) in schizophrenia is still under study, the effectiveness of maintenance treatment is well established for many other drugs used to treat schizophrenia. It is recommended that responding patients be continued on CLOZARIL® (clozapine), but at the lowest level needed to maintain remission. Because of the significant risk associated with the use of CLOZARIL® (clozapine), patients should be periodically reassessed to determine the need for maintenance treatment.

Discontinuation of Treatment

In the event of planned termination of CLOZARIL® (clozapine) therapy, gradual reduction in dose is recommended over a 1–2 week period. However, should a patient's medical condition require abrupt discontinuation (e.g., leukopenia), the patient should be carefully observed for the recurrence of psychotic symptoms and symptoms related to cholinergic rebound such as headache, nausea, vomiting, and diarrhea.

Reinitiation of Treatment in Patients Previously Discontinued

When restarting patients who have had even a brief interval off CLOZARIL® (clozapine), i.e., 2 days or more since the last dose, it is recommended that treatment be reinitiated with one-half of a 25 mg tablet (12.5 mg) once or twice daily (see WARNINGS). If that dose is well tolerated, it may be feasible to titrate patients back to a therapeutic dose more quickly than is recommended for initial treatment. However, any patient who has previously experienced respiratory or cardiac arrest with initial dosing, but was then able to be successfully titrated to a therapeutic dose, should be re-titrated with extreme caution after even 24 hours of discontinuation.

Certain additional precautions seem prudent when reinitiating treatment. The mechanisms underlying CLOZARIL® (clozapine) induced adverse reactions are unknown. It is conceivable, however, that re-exposure of a patient might enhance the risk of an untoward event's occurrence and increase its severity. Such phenomena, for example, occur when immune mediated mechanisms are responsible. Consequently, during the reinitiation of treatment, additional caution is advised. Patients discontinued for WBC counts below 2000/mm^3 or an ANC below 1000/mm^3 must *not* be restarted on CLOZARIL® (clozapine). (See WARNINGS)

HOW SUPPLIED

CLOZARIL® (clozapine) is available as 25 mg and 100 mg round, pale-yellow, uncoated tablets with a facilitated score on one side.

CLOZARIL® (clozapine) Tablets

25 mg

Engraved with "CLOZARIL" once on the periphery of one side.

Engraved with a facilitated score and "25" once on the other side.

Bottle of 100 .... NDC 0078-0126-05
Bottle of 500 .... NDC 0078-0126-08
Unit dose packages of 100: 2 × 5 strips,
10 blisters per strip .... NDC 0078-0126-06

100 mg

Engraved with "CLOZARIL" once on the periphery of one side.

Engraved with a facilitated score and "100" once on the other side.

Bottle of 100 .... NDC 0078-0127-05
Bottle of 500 .... NDC 0078-0127-08
Unit dose packages of 100: 2 × 5 strips,
10 blisters per strip .... NDC 0078-0127-06

Store and Dispense

Storage temperature should not exceed 86°F (30°C). Drug dispensing should not ordinarily exceed a weekly supply. If a patient is eligible for WBC testing every other week, then a two-week supply of CLOZARIL® (clozapine) can be dispensed. Dispensing should be contingent upon the results of a WBC count.

*Trademark of Medical Economics Company, Inc.

NOVARTIS
Novartis Pharmaceuticals Corporation
East Hanover, New Jersey 07936

T2002-02
REV: FEBRUARY 2002 Printed in U.S.A. 89004506

GLEEVEC™ ℞

[glē' vek]

(imatinib mesylate)

Capsules

Rx only

Prescribing information for this product, which appears on pages 2357–2360 of the 2002 PDR, has been completely revised as follows. Please write "See Supplement A" next to the product heading.

Prescribing Information

DESCRIPTION

Gleevec™ capsules contain imatinib mesylate equivalent to 100 mg of imatinib free base. Imatinib mesylate is designated chemically as 4-[(4-Methyl-1-piperazinyl)methyl]-N-[4-methyl-3-[[4-(3-pyridinyl)-2-pyrimidinyl]amino]-phenyl] benzamide methanesulfonate and its structural formula is

Imatinib mesylate is a white to off-white to brownish or yellowish tinged crystalline powder. Its molecular formula is $C_{29}H_{31}N_7O \bullet CH_4SO_3$ and its relative molecular mass is 589.7. Imatinib mesylate is very soluble in water and soluble in aqueous buffers ≤ pH 5.5 but is very slightly soluble to insoluble in neutral/alkaline aqueous buffers. In non-aqueous solvents, the drug substance is freely soluble to very slightly soluble in dimethyl sulfoxide, methanol and ethanol, but is insoluble in n-octanol, acetone and acetonitrile.

Inactive ingredients: colloidal silicon dioxide (NF), crospovidone (NF), magnesium stearate (NF) and microcrystalline cellulose (NF). Capsule shell: gelatin, iron oxide, red (E172); iron oxide, yellow (E172); titanium dioxide (E171).

CLINICAL PHARMACOLOGY

Mechanism of Action

Imatinib mesylate is a protein-tyrosine kinase inhibitor that inhibits the Bcr-Abl tyrosine kinase, the constitutive abnormal tyrosine kinase created by the Philadelphia chromosome abnormality in chronic myeloid leukemia (CML). It inhibits proliferation and induces apoptosis in Bcr-Abl positive cell lines as well as fresh leukemic cells from Philadel-

Continued on next page

Gleevec—Cont.

phia chromosome positive chronic myeloid leukemia. In colony formation assays using *ex vivo* peripheral blood and bone marrow samples, imatinib shows inhibition of Bcr-Abl positive colonies from CML patients.
In vivo, it inhibits tumor growth of Bcr-Abl transfected murine myeloid cells as well as Bcr-Abl positive leukemia lines derived from CML patients in blast crisis.
Imatinib is also an inhibitor of the receptor tyrosine kinases for platelet-derived growth factor (PDGF) and stem cell factor (SCF), c-kit, and inhibits PDGF- and SCF-mediated cellular events. *In vitro*, imatinib inhibits proliferation and induces apoptosis in gastrointestinal stromal tumor (GIST) cells, which express an activating c-kit mutation.

Pharmacokinetics

The pharmacokinetics of Gleevec™ (imatinib mesylate) have been evaluated in studies in healthy subjects and in population pharmacokinetic studies in over 500 patients. Imatinib is well absorbed after oral administration with C_{max} achieved within 2-4 hours post-dose. Mean absolute bioavailability for the capsule formulation is 98%. Following oral administration in healthy volunteers, the elimination half-lives of imatinib and its major active metabolite, the N-desmethyl derivative, were approximately 18 and 40 hours, respectively. Mean imatinib AUC increased proportionally with increasing dose in the range 25 mg -1000 mg. There was no significant change in the pharmacokinetics of imatinib on repeated dosing, and accumulation is 1.5-2.5 fold at steady state when Gleevec is dosed once daily. At clinically relevant concentrations of imatinib, binding to plasma proteins in *in vitro* experiments is approximately 95%, mostly to albumin and α_1-acid glycoprotein.
The pharmacokinetics of imatinib were similar in CML and GIST patients.

Metabolism and Elimination

CYP3A4 is the major enzyme responsible for metabolism of imatinib. Other cytochrome P450 enzymes, such as CYP1A2, CYP2D6, CYP2C9, and CYP2C19, play a minor role in its metabolism. The main circulating active metabolite in humans is the N-demethylated piperazine derivative, formed predominantly by CYP3A4. It shows *in vitro* potency similar to the parent imatinib. The plasma AUC for this metabolite is about 15% of the AUC for imatinib.
Elimination is predominately in the feces, mostly as metabolites. Based on the recovery of compound(s) after an oral ^{14}C-labelled dose of imatinib, approximately 81% of the dose was eliminated within 7 days, in feces (68% of dose) and urine (13% of dose). Unchanged imatinib accounted for 25% of the dose (5% urine, 20% feces), the remainder being metabolites.
Typically, clearance of imatinib in a 50-year-old patient weighing 50 kg is expected to be 8 L/h, while for a 50-year-old patient weighing 100 kg the clearance will increase to 14 L/h. However, the inter-patient variability of 40% in clearance does not warrant initial dose adjustment based on body weight and/or age but indicates the need for close monitoring for treatment related toxicity.

Special Populations

Pediatric: There are no pharmacokinetic data in pediatric patients.
Hepatic Insufficiency: No clinical studies were conducted with Gleevec in patients with impaired hepatic function.
Renal Insufficiency: No clinical studies were conducted with Gleevec in patients with decreased renal function (studies excluded patients with serum creatinine concentration more than 2 times the upper limit of the normal range). Imatinib and its metabolites are not significantly excreted via the kidney.

Drug-Drug Interactions

CYP3A4 Inhibitors: There was a significant increase in exposure to imatinib (mean C_{max} and AUC increased by 26% and 40%, respectively) in healthy subjects when Gleevec was co-administered with a single dose of ketoconazole (a CYP3A4 inhibitor). (See PRECAUTIONS.)
CYP3A4 Substrates: Imatinib increased the mean C_{max} and AUC of simvastatin (CYP3A4 substrate) by 2- and 3.5-fold, respectively, indicating an inhibition of CYP3A4 by imatinib. (See PRECAUTIONS.)
CYP3A4 Inducers: No formal study of CYP3A4 inducers has been conducted, but a patient on chronic therapy with phenytoin (a CYP3A4 inducer) given 350 mg daily dose of Gleevec had an AUC_{0-24} about one-fifth of the typical AUC_{0-24} of 20 μg•h/mL. This probably reflects the induction of CYP3A4 by phenytoin. (See PRECAUTIONS.)
In Vitro Studies of CYP Enzyme Inhibition: Human liver microsome studies demonstrated that imatinib is a potent competitive inhibitor of CYP2C9, CYP2D6, and CYP3A4/5 with K_i values of 27, 7.5, and 8 μM, respectively. Imatinib is likely to increase the blood level of drugs that are substrates of CYP2C9, CYP2D6 and CYP3A4/5. (See PRECAUTIONS.)

CLINICAL STUDIES

Chronic Myeloid Leukemia

Three international, open-label, single-arm studies were conducted in patients with Philadelphia chromosome positive (Ph+) chronic myeloid leukemia (CML): 1) in the chronic phase after failure of interferon-alfa (IFN) therapy, 2) in accelerated phase disease, or 3) in myeloid blast crisis. About 45% of patients were women and 6% were Black. In clinical studies 38%-40% of patients were ≥60 years of age and 10%-12% of patients were ≥70 years of age.

Chronic Phase, Prior Interferon-Treatment

532 patients were treated at a starting dose of 400 mg; dose escalation to 600 mg was allowed. The patients were distributed in three main categories according to their response to prior interferon: failure to achieve (within 6 months), or loss of a complete hematologic response (29%), failure to achieve (within 1 year) or loss of a major cytogenetic response (35%), or intolerance to interferon (36%). Patients had received a median of 14 months of prior IFN therapy at doses ≥25 $\times10^6$ IU/week and were all in late chronic phase, with a median time from diagnosis of 32 months. Effectiveness was evaluated on the basis of the rate of hematologic response and by bone marrow exams to assess the rate of major cytogenetic response (up to 35% Ph+ metaphases) or complete cytogenetic response (0% Ph+ metaphases). Efficacy results are reported in Table 1. Results were similar in the three subgroups described above.

Table 1 Response in CML Patients in Clinical Studies

	Chronic Phase IFN Failure (n=532) 400 mg	Accelerated Phase (n=235) 600 mg n=158 400 mg n=77	Myeloid Blast Crisis (n=260) 600 mg n=223 400 mg n=37
		% of patients [$CI_{95\%}$]	
Hematologic Response[1]	**93% [91.0-95.4]**	**69% [63.0-75.2]**	**31% [25.2-36.8]**
Complete hematologic response (CHR)	93%	37%	7%
No evidence of leukemia (NEL)	Not applicable	12%	5%
Return to chronic phase (RTC)	Not applicable	20%	19%
Major Cytogenetic Response[2] (unconfirmed[3])	**53% [48.7-57.3]** (61%)	**19% [14.3-24.8]** (25%)	**7% [4.2-10.7]** (15%)
Complete[4](unconfirmed[3])	32% (41%)	13% (17%)	1.5% (7%)

[1]**Hematologic response criteria (all responses to be confirmed after ≥4 weeks):**
CHR: Chronic phase study [WBC <10 $\times10^9$/L, platelet <450 $\times10^9$/L, myelocytes+metamyelocytes <5% in blood, no blasts and promyelocytes in blood, basophils <20%, no extramedullary involvement] and in the accelerated and blast crisis studies [ANC ≥1.5 $\times10^9$/L, platelets ≥100 $\times10^9$/L, no blood blasts, BM blasts <5% and no extramedullary disease]
NEL: same criteria as for CHR but ANC ≥1 $\times10^9$/L and platelets ≥20 $\times10^9$/L (accelerated and blast crisis studies)
RTC: <15% blasts BM and PB, <30% blasts+promyelocytes in BM and PB, <20% basophils in PB, no extramedullary disease other than spleen and liver (accelerated and blast crisis studies).
BM=bone marrow, PB=peripheral blood
[2]**Major Cytogenetic Response:** A major response combines both complete and partial responses: complete (0% Ph+ metaphases), partial (1%-35% Ph+ metaphases).
[3]Unconfirmed cytogenetic response is based on a single bone marrow cytogenetic evaluation, therefore unconfirmed complete or partial cytogenetic responses might have had a lesser cytogenetic response on a subsequent bone marrow evaluation.
[4]Complete cytogenetic response confirmed by a second bone marrow cytogenetic evaluation performed at least one month after the initial bone marrow study.

Accelerated Phase

235 patients with accelerated phase disease were enrolled. These patients met one or more of the following criteria ≥15% - <30% blasts in PB or BM; ≥30% blasts + promyelocytes in PB or BM; ≥20% basophils in PB; <100 $\times$ 10^9/L platelets. The first 77 patients were started at 400 mg, with the remaining 158 patients starting at 600 mg.
Effectiveness was evaluated primarily on the basis of the rate of hematologic response, reported as either complete hematologic response, no evidence of leukemia (i.e., clearance of blasts from the marrow and the blood, but without a full peripheral blood recovery as for complete responses), or return to chronic phase CML. Cytogenetic responses were also evaluated. Efficacy results are reported in Table 1. Response rates in accelerated phase CML were higher for the 600 mg dose group than for the 400 mg group: hematologic response (73% vs. 62%), confirmed and unconfirmed major cytogenetic response (28% vs. 18%).

Myeloid Blast Crisis

260 patients with myeloid blast crisis were enrolled. These patients had ≥30% blasts in PB or BM and/or extramedullary involvement other than spleen or liver; 95 (37%) had received prior chemotherapy for treatment of either accelerated phase or blast crisis ("pretreated patients") whereas 165 (63%) had not ("untreated patients"). The first 37 patients were started at 400 mg; the remaining 223 patients were started at 600 mg.
Effectiveness was evaluated primarily on the basis of rate of hematologic response, reported as either complete hematologic response, no evidence of leukemia, or return to chronic phase CML using the same criteria as for the study in accelerated phase. Cytogenetic responses were also assessed. Efficacy results are reported in Table 1. The hematologic response rate was higher in untreated patients than in treated patients (36% vs. 22% respectively) and in the group receiving an initial dose of 600 mg rather than 400 mg (33% vs. 16%). The confirmed and unconfirmed major cytogenetic response rate was also higher for the 600 mg dose group than for the 400 mg group (17% vs. 8%).
[See table above]
The median time to hematologic response was 1 month. Response duration cannot be precisely defined because follow-up on most patients is relatively short. In blast crisis, the estimated median duration of hematologic response is about 10 months. In accelerated phase, median duration of hematologic response is greater than 12 months but cannot yet be estimated. Follow-up is insufficient to estimate duration of cytogenetic response in all studies.
Efficacy results were similar in men and women and in patients younger and older than age 65. Responses were seen in Black patients, but there were too few Black patients to allow a quantitative comparison.

Gastrointestinal Stromal Tumors

One open-label, multinational study was conducted in patients with unresectable or metastatic malignant gastrointestinal stromal tumors (GIST). In this study 147 patients were enrolled and randomized to receive either 400 mg or 600 mg orally q.d. for up to 24 months. The study was not powered to show a statistically significant difference in response rates between the two dose groups. Patients ranged in age from 18 to 83 years old and had a pathologic diagnosis of Kit-positive unresectable and/or metastatic malignant GIST. Immunohistochemistry was routinely performed with Kit antibody (A-4052, rabbit polyclonal antiserum, 1:100; DAKO Corporation, Carpinteria, CA) according to analysis by an avidin-biotin-peroxidase complex method after antigen retrieval.
The primary outcome of the study was objective response rate. Tumors were required to be measurable at entry in at least one site of disease, and response characterization was based on Southwestern Oncology Group (SWOG) criteria. Results are shown in Table 2.

Table 2 Tumor Response in GIST

Total Patients N	Confirmed Partial Response N (%)	95% Confidence Interval
400 mg daily 73	24 (33%)	22%, 45%
600 mg daily 74	32 (43%)	32%, 55%
Total 147	56 (38%)	30%, 46%

A statistically significant difference in response rates between the two dose groups was not demonstrated. At the time of interim analysis, when the median follow-up was less than 7 months, 55 of 56 patients with a confirmed partial response (PR) had a maintained PR. The data were too immature to determine a meaningful response duration. No responses were observed in 12 patients with progressive disease on 400 mg daily whose doses were increased to 600 mg daily.

INDICATIONS AND USAGE

Gleevec™ (imatinib mesylate) is indicated for the treatment of patients with Philadelphia chromosome positive chronic myeloid leukemia (CML) in blast crisis, accelerated phase, or in chronic phase after failure of interferon-alpha therapy. Gleevec is also indicated for the treatment of patients with Kit (CD117) positive unresectable and/or metastatic malignant gastrointestinal stromal tumors (GIST). (See CLINICAL STUDIES: Gastrointestinal Stromal Tumors.)
The effectiveness of Gleevec is based on overall hematologic and cytogenetic response rates in CML and objective response rate in GIST (see CLINICAL STUDIES). There are no controlled trials demonstrating a clinical benefit, such as improvement in disease-related symptoms or increased survival.

CONTRAINDICATIONS

Use of Gleevec™ (imatinib mesylate) is contraindicated in patients with hypersensitivity to imatinib or to any other component of Gleevec.

WARNINGS

Pregnancy

Women of childbearing potential should be advised to avoid becoming pregnant.
Imatinib mesylate was teratogenic in rats when administered during organogenesis at doses ≥100 mg/kg, approximately equal to the maximum clinical dose of 800 mg/day, based on body surface area. Teratogenic effects included exencephaly or encephalocele, absent/reduced frontal and absent parietal bones. Female rats administered this dose also experienced significant post-implantation loss in the form of early fetal resorption. At doses higher than 100 mg/kg, total fetal loss was noted in all animals. These effects were not seen at doses ≤30 mg/kg (one-third the maximum human dose of 800 mg).

There are no adequate and well-controlled studies in pregnant women. If Gleevec™ (imatinib mesylate) is used during pregnancy, or if the patient becomes pregnant while taking (receiving) Gleevec, the patient should be apprised of the potential hazard to the fetus.

PRECAUTIONS

General

Fluid Retention and Edema: Gleevec™ (imatinib mesylate) is often associated with edema and occasionally serious fluid retention (see ADVERSE REACTIONS). Patients should be weighed and monitored regularly for signs and symptoms of fluid retention. An unexpected rapid weight gain should be carefully investigated and appropriate treatment provided. The probability of edema was increased with higher imatinib dose and age >65 years in the CML studies. Severe fluid retention (e.g., pleural effusion, pericardial effusion, pulmonary edema, and ascites) was reported in 2%-8% of patients taking Gleevec for CML. In addition, severe superficial edema was reported in 2%-5% of the patients with CML.

Severe superficial edema and severe fluid retention (pleural effusion, pulmonary edema and ascites) were reported in 1%-6% of patients taking Gleevec for GIST.

GI Irritation: Gleevec is sometimes associated with GI irritation. Gleevec should be taken with food and a large glass of water to minimize this problem.

Hemorrhage: In the GIST clinical trial seven patients (5%), four in the 600-mg dose group and three in the 400-mg dose group, had a total of eight events of CTC grade 3/4-gastrointestinal (GI) bleeds (3 patients), intra-tumoral bleeds (3 patients) or both (1 patient). Gastrointestinal tumor sites may have been the source of GI bleeds.

Hematologic Toxicity: Treatment with Gleevec is associated with neutropenia or thrombocytopenia. Complete blood counts should be performed weekly for the first month, biweekly for the second month, and periodically thereafter as clinically indicated (for example every 2-3 months). In CML, the occurrence of these cytopenias is dependent on the stage of disease and is more frequent in patients with accelerated phase CML or blast crisis than in patients with chronic phase CML. (See DOSAGE AND ADMINISTRATION.)

Hepatotoxicity: Hepatotoxicity, occasionally severe, may occur with Gleevec (see ADVERSE REACTIONS). Liver function (transaminases, bilirubin, and alkaline phosphatase) should be monitored before initiation of treatment and monthly or as clinically indicated. Laboratory abnormalities should be managed with interruption and/or dose reduction of the treatment with Gleevec. (See DOSAGE AND ADMINISTRATION.) Patients with hepatic impairment should be closely monitored because exposure to Gleevec may be increased. As there are no clinical studies of Gleevec in patients with impaired liver function, no specific advice concerning initial dosing adjustment can be given.

Toxicities From Long-Term Use: Because follow-up of most patients treated with imatinib is relatively short, there are no long-term safety data on Gleevec treatment. It is important to consider potential toxicities suggested by animal studies, specifically, *liver and kidney toxicity and immunosuppression*. Severe liver toxicity was observed in dogs treated for 2 weeks, with elevated liver enzymes, hepatocellular necrosis, bile duct necrosis, and bile duct hyperplasia. Renal toxicity was observed in monkeys treated for 2 weeks, with focal mineralization and dilation of the renal tubules and tubular nephrosis. Increased BUN and creatinine were observed in several of these animals. An increased rate of opportunistic infections was observed with chronic imatinib treatment. In a 39-week monkey study, treatment with imatinib resulted in worsening of normally suppressed malarial infections in these animals. Lymphopenia was observed in animals (as in humans).

Drug Interactions

Drugs that may alter imatinib plasma concentrations

Drugs that may **increase** imatinib plasma concentrations:
Caution is recommended when administering Gleevec with inhibitors of the CYP3A4 family (e.g., ketoconazole, itraconazole, erythromycin, clarithromycin). Substances that inhibit the cytochrome P450 isoenzyme (CYP3A4) activity may decrease metabolism and increase imatinib concentrations. There is a significant increase in exposure to imatinib when Gleevec is co-administered with ketoconazole (CYP3A4 inhibitor).

Drugs that may **decrease** imatinib plasma concentrations:
Substances that are inducers of CYP3A4 activity may increase metabolism and decrease imatinib plasma concentrations. Co-medications that induce CYP3A4 (e.g., dexamethasone, phenytoin, carbamazepine, rifampicin, phenobarbital or St. John's Wort) may reduce exposure to Gleevec. No formal study of CYP3A4 inducers has been conducted, but a patient on chronic therapy with phenytoin (a CYP3A4 inducer) given 350 mg daily dose of Gleevec had an $AUC_{0\text{-}24}$ about one-fifth of the typical $AUC_{0\text{-}24}$ of 20 μg•h/mL. This probably reflects the induction of CYP3A4 by phenytoin. (See PRECAUTIONS.)

Drugs that may have their plasma concentration altered by Gleevec

Imatinib increases the mean C_{max} and AUC of simvastatin (CYP3A4 substrate) 2- and 3.5- fold, respectively, suggesting an inhibition of the CYP3A4 by imatinib. Particular caution is recommended when administering Gleevec with CYP3A4 substrates that have a narrow therapeutic window (e.g., cyclosporine or pimozide). Gleevec will increase plasma concentration of other CYP3A4 metabolized drugs

Table 3 Adverse Experiences Reported in CML Clinical Trials (≥10% of all patients in any trial)[1]

	Myeloid Blast Crisis (n=260) %		Accelerated Phase (n=235) %		Chronic Phase, IFN Failure (n=532) %	
Preferred Term	**All Grades**	**Grade 3/4**	**All Grades**	**Grades 3/4**	**All Grades**	**Grade 3/4**
Nausea	70	4	71	5	60	2
Fluid retention	71	12	73	6	66	3
- Superficial edema	67	5	71	4	64	2
- Other fluid retention events[2]	22	8	10	3	7	2
Muscle cramps	27	0.8	42	0.4	55	1
Diarrhea	42	4	55	4	43	2
Vomiting	54	4	56	3	32	1
Hemorrhage	52	19	44	9	22	2
- CNS hemorrhage	7	5	2	0.9	1	1
- Gastrointestinal hemorrhage	8	3	5	3	2	0.4
Musculoskeletal pain	43	9	46	9	35	2
Skin rash	35	5	44	4	42	3
Headache	27	5	30	2	34	0.2
Fatigue	29	3	41	4	40	1
Arthralgia	25	4	31	6	36	1
Dyspepsia	11	0	21	0	24	0
Myalgia	8	0	22	2	25	0.2
Weight increase	5	0.8	14	3	30	5
Pyrexia	41	7	39	8	17	1
Abdominal pain	31	6	33	3	29	0.6
Cough	14	0.8	26	0.9	17	0
Dyspnea	14	4	20	7	9	0.6
Anorexia	14	2	17	2	6	0
Constipation	15	2	15	0.9	6	0.2
Nasopharingitis	8	0	16	0	18	0.2
Night sweats	12	0.8	14	1	10	0.2
Pruritus	8	1	13	0.9	12	0.8
Epistaxis	13	3	13	0	5	0.2
Hypokalemia	13	4	8	2	5	0.2
Petechiae	10	2	5	0.9	1	0
Pneumonia	12	6	8	6	3	0.8
Weakness	12	3	9	3	7	0.2
Upper respiratory tract infection	3	0	9	0.4	15	0
Dizziness	11	0.4	12	0	13	0.2
Insomnia	10	0	13	0	13	0.2
Sore throat	8	0	11	0	11	0
Ecchymosis	11	0.4	6	0.9	2	0
Rigors	10	0	11	0.4	8	0
Asthenia	5	2	11	2	6	0
Influenza	0.8	0.4	6	0	10	0.2

[1] All adverse events occurring in ≥10% of patients are listed regardless of suspected relationship to treatment.
[2] Other fluid retention events include pleural effusion, ascites, pulmonary edema, pericardial effusion, anasarca, edema aggravated, and fluid retention not otherwise specified.

Table 4 Lab Abnormalities in CML Clinical Trials

	Myeloid Blast Crisis (n=260) 600 mg n=223 400 mg n=37 %		Accelerated Phase (n=235) 600 mg n=158 400 mg n=77 %		Chronic Phase, IFN Failure (n=532) 400 mg %	
CTC Grade	**Grade 3**	**Grade 4**	**Grade 3**	**Grade 4**	**Grade 3**	**Grade 4**
Hematology Parameters						
• Neutropenia	16	48	23	36	27	8
• Thrombocytopenia	29	33	31	13	19	<1
• Anemia	41	11	34	6	6	1
Biochemistry Parameters						
• Elevated creatinine	1.5	0	1.3	0	0.2	0
• Elevated bilirubin	3.8	0	2.1	0	0.8	0
• Elevated alkaline phosphatase	4.6	0	5.1	0.4	0.2	0
• Elevated SGOT (AST)	1.9	0	3.0	0	2.3	0
• Elevated SGPT (ALT)	2.3	0.4	3.8	0	1.9	0

CTC grades: neutropenia (grade 3 ≥0.5 - 1.0 × 10^9/L), grade 4 <0.5 × 10^9L), thrombocytopenia (grade 3 ≥10 - 50 × 10^9/L, grade 4 <10 × 10^9/L), anemia (hemoglobin ≥65 - 80 g/L, grade 4 <65 g/L), elevated creatinine (grade 3 >3-6 × upper limit normal range (ULN), grade 4 >6 × ULN), elevated bilirubin (grade 3 >3-10 × ULN, grade 4 >10 × ULN), elevated alkaline phosphatase (grade 3 >5-20 × ULN, grade 4 >20 × ULN), elevated SGOT or SGPT (grade 3 >5-20 × ULN, grade 4 >20 × ULN)

(e.g., triazolo-benzodiazepines, dihydropyridine calcium channel blockers, certain HMG-CoA reductase inhibitors, etc.)

Because *warfarin* is metabolized by CYP2C9 and CYP3A4, patients who require anticoagulation should receive low-molecular weight or standard heparin.

In vitro, Gleevec inhibits the cytochrome P450 isoenzyme CYP2D6 activity at similar concentrations that affect CYP3A4 activity. Systemic exposure to substrates of CYP2D6 is expected to be increased when co-administered with Gleevec. No specific studies have been performed and caution is recommended.

Carcinogenesis, Mutagenesis, Impairment of Fertility

Carcinogenicity studies have not been performed with imatinib mesylate.

Positive genotoxic effects were obtained for imatinib in an *in vitro* mammalian cell assay (Chinese hamster ovary) for clastogenicity (chromosome aberrations) in the presence of metabolic activation. Two intermediates of the manufacturing process, which are also present in the final product, are positive for mutagenesis in the Ames assay. One of these intermediates was also positive in the mouse lymphoma assay. Imatinib was not genotoxic when tested in an *in vitro* bacterial cell assay (Ames test), an *in vitro* mammalian cell assay (mouse lymphoma) and an *in vivo* rat micronucleus assay.

In a study of fertility, in male rats dosed for 70 days prior to mating, testicular and epididymal weights and percent motile sperm were decreased at 60 mg/kg, approximately equal to the maximum clinical dose of 800 mg/day, based on body surface area. This was not seen at doses ≤20 mg/kg (one-fourth the maximum human dose of 800 mg). When female rats were dosed 14 days prior to mating and through to gestational day 6, there was no effect on mating or on number

Continued on next page

Gleevec—Cont.

of pregnant females. At a dose of 60 mg/kg (approximately equal to the human dose of 800 mg), female rats had significant post-implantation fetal loss and a reduced number of live fetuses. This was not seen at doses ≤20 mg/kg (one-fourth the maximum human dose of 800 mg).

Pregnancy

Pregnancy Category D. (See WARNINGS.)

Nursing Mothers

It is not known whether imatinib mesylate or its metabolites are excreted in human milk. However, in lactating female rats administered 100 mg/kg, a dose approximately equal to the maximum clinical dose of 800 mg/day based on body surface area, imatinib and/or its metabolites were extensively excreted in milk. It is estimated that approximately 1.5% of a maternal dose is excreted into milk, which is equivalent to a dose to the infant of 30% the maternal dose per unit body weight. Because many drugs are excreted in human milk and because of the potential for serious adverse reactions in nursing infants, women should be advised against breastfeeding while taking Gleevec.

Pediatric Use

The safety and effectiveness of Gleevec in pediatric patients have not been established.

Geriatric Use

In the CML clinical studies, approximately 40% of patients were older than 60 years and 10% were older than 70 years. No difference was observed in the safety profile in patients older than 65 years as compared to younger patients, with the exception of a higher frequency of edema. (See PRECAUTIONS.) The efficacy of Gleevec was similar in older and younger patients.

In the GIST study, 29% of patients were older than 60 years and 10% of patients were older than 70 years. No obvious differences in the safety or efficacy profile were noted in patients older than 65 years as compared to younger patients, but the small number of patients does not allow a formal analysis.

ADVERSE REACTIONS

Chronic Myeloid Leukemia

The majority of Gleevec-treated patients experienced adverse events at some time. Most events were of mild to moderate grade, but drug was discontinued for adverse events in 2% of patients in chronic phase, 3% in accelerated phase and 5% in blast crisis.

The most frequently reported drug-related adverse events were nausea, vomiting, diarrhea, edema, and muscle cramps (Table 3). Edema was most frequently periorbital or in lower limbs and was managed with diuretics, other supportive measures, or by reducing the dose of Gleevec™ (imatinib mesylate). (See DOSAGE AND ADMINISTRATION.) The frequency of severe superficial edema was 2%-5%.

A variety of adverse events represent local or general fluid retention including pleural effusion, ascites, pulmonary edema and rapid weight gain with or without superficial edema. These events appear to be dose related, were more common in the blast crisis and accelerated phase studies (where the dose was 600 mg/day), and are more common in the elderly. These events were usually managed by interrupting Gleevec treatment and with diuretics or other appropriate supportive care measures. However, a few of these events may be serious or life threatening, and one patient with blast crisis died with pleural effusion, congestive heart failure, and renal failure.

Adverse events, regardless of relationship to study drug, that were reported in at least 10% of the patients treated in the Gleevec studies are shown in Table 3.

[See table 3 at top of previous page]

Hematologic Toxicity

Cytopenias, and particularly neutropenia and thrombocytopenia, were a consistent finding in all studies, with a higher frequency at doses ≥750 mg (Phase I study). The occurrence of cytopenias in CML patients was also dependent on the stage of the disease, with a frequency of grade 3 or 4 neutropenia and thrombocytopenia between 2- and 3-fold higher in blast crisis and accelerated phase compared to chronic phase (see Table 4). The median duration of the neutropenic and thrombocytopenic episodes ranged usually from 2 to 3 weeks, and from 3 to 4 weeks, respectively. These events can usually be managed with either a reduction of the dose or an interruption of treatment with Gleevec, but in rare cases require permanent discontinuation of treatment.

Hepatotoxicity

Severe elevation of transaminases or bilirubin occurred in 1%-4% (see Table 4) and were usually managed with dose reduction or interruption (the median duration of these episodes was approximately one week). Treatment was discontinued permanently because of liver laboratory abnormalities in less than 0.5% of patients. However, one patient, who was taking acetaminophen regularly for fever, died of acute liver failure.

Adverse Effects in Subpopulations

With the exception of edema, where it was more frequent, there was no evidence of an increase in the incidence or severity of adverse events in older patients (≥65 years old). With the exception of a slight increase in the frequency of grade 1/2 periorbital edema, headache and fatigue in women, there was no evidence of a difference in the incidence or severity of adverse events between the sexes. No differences were seen related to race but the subsets were too small for proper evaluation.

[See table 4 at top of previous page]

Gastrointestinal Stromal Tumors

The majority of Gleevec-treated patients experienced adverse events at some time. The most frequently reported adverse events were edema, nausea, diarrhea, abdominal pain, muscle cramps, fatigue and rash. Most events were of mild to moderate severity. Drug was discontinued for adverse events in 6 patients (8%) in both dose levels studied. Superficial edema, most frequently periorbital or lower extremity edema, was managed with diuretics, other supportive measures, or by reducing the dose of Gleevec™ (imatinib mesylate). (See DOSAGE AND ADMINISTRATION.) Severe (CTC grade 3/4) superficial edema was observed in 3 patients (2%), including face edema in one patient. Grade 3/4 pleural effusion or ascites was observed in 3 patients (2%).

Adverse events, regardless of relationship to study drug, that were reported in at least 10% of the patients treated with Gleevec are shown in Table 5. No major differences were seen in the severity of adverse events between the 400 mg or 600 mg treatment groups, although overall incidence of diarrhea, muscle cramps, headache, dermatitis and edema was somewhat higher in the 600 mg treatment group.

[See table 5 above]

Table 5 Adverse Experiences Reported in GIST Trial (≥10% of all patients at either dose)[1)]

Initial dose (mg/day)	All CTC Grades		CTC Grade 3/4	
	400 mg (n=73)	600 mg (n=74)	400 mg (n=73)	600 mg (n=74)
Preferred Term	%	%	%	%
Fluid retention	71	76	6	3
- Superficial edema	71	76	4	0
- Pleural effusion or ascites	6	4	1	3
Diarrhea	56	60	1	4
Nausea	53	56	3	3
Fatigue	33	38	1	0
Muscle cramps	30	41	0	0
Abdominal pain	37	37	7	3
Skin Rash	26	38	3	3
Headache	25	35	0	0
Vomiting	22	23	1	3
Musculoskeletal pain	19	11	3	0
Flatulence	16	23	0	0
Any hemorrhage	18	19	5	8
- Tumor hemorrhage	1	4	1	4
- Cerebral hemorrhage	1	0	1	0
- GI tract hemorrhage	6	4	4	1
Nasopharyngitis	12	14	0	0
Pyrexia	12	5	0	0
Insomnia	11	11	0	0
Back pain	11	10	1	0
Lacrimation increased	6	11	0	0
Upper respiratory tract infection	6	11	0	0
Taste disturbance	1	14	0	0

[1)] All adverse events occurring in ≥10% of patients are listed regardless of suspected relationship to treatment.

Table 6 Laboratory Abnormalities in GIST Trial

Parameter	400 mg (n=73) %		600 mg (n=74) %	
CTC Grade	Grade 3	Grade 4	Grade 3	Grade 4
Hematology parameters				
• Anemia	3	0	4	1
• Thrombocytopenia	0	0	1	0
• Neutropenia	3	3	5	4
Biochemistry parameters				
• Elevated creatinine	0	1	3	0
• Reduced albumin	3	0	4	0
• Elevated bilirubin	1	0	1	3
• Elevated alkaline phosphatase	0	0	1	0
• Elevated SGOT (AST)	3	0	1	1
• Elevated SGPT (ALT)	3	0	4	0

CTC grades: neutropenia (grade 3 ≥0.5 - 1.0 × 10^9/L, grade 4 <0.5 × 10^9/L), thrombocytopenia (grade 3 ≥10 - 50 × 10^9/L, grade 4 <10 × 10^9/L), anemia (grade 3 ≥65 - 80 g/L, grade 4 <65 g/L), elevated creatinine (grade 3 >3 - 6 × upper limit normal range (ULN), grade 4 >6 × ULN), elevated bilirubin (grade 3 >3 - 10 × ULN, grade 4 >10 × ULN), elevated alkaline phosphatase, SGOT or SGPT (grade 3 >5 - 20 × ULN, grade 4 >20 × ULN), albumin (grade 3 <20 g/L)

Table 7 Dose Adjustments for Neutropenia and Thrombocytopenia

Chronic Phase CML or GIST (starting dose 400 mg)	ANC <1.0 ×10^9/L and/or Platelets <50 ×10^9/L	1. Stop Gleevec until ANC ≥1.5 ×10^9/L and platelets ≥75 ×10^9/L 2. Resume treatment with Gleevec at dose of 400 mg 3. If recurrence of ANC <1.0 ×10^9/L and/or platelets <50 ×10^9/L, repeat step 1 and resume Gleevec at reduced dose of 300 mg
Accelerated Phase CML and Blast Crisis or GIST (starting dose 600 mg)	[1]ANC <0.5 ×10^9/L and/or Platelets <10×10^9/L	1. Check if cytopenia is related to leukemia (marrow aspirate or biopsy) 2. If cytopenia is unrelated to leukemia, reduce dose of Gleevec to 400 mg 3. If cytopenia persist 2 weeks, reduce further to 300 mg 4. If cytopenia persist 4 weeks and is still unrelated to leukemia, stop Gleevec until ANC ≥1 ×10^9/L and platelets ≥20 ×10^9/L and then resume treatment at 300 mg

[1]occurring after at least 1 month of treatment

Clinically relevant or severe abnormalities of routine hematologic or biochemistry laboratory values are presented in Table 6.

[See table 6 above]

OVERDOSAGE

Experience with doses greater than 800 mg is limited. In the event of overdosage, the patient should be observed and appropriate supportive treatment given. An oral dose of 1200 mg/m²/day, approximately 2.5 times the human dose of 800 mg, based on body surface area, was not lethal to rats following 14 days of administration. A dose of 3600 mg/m²/day, approximately 7.5 times the human dose of 800 mg, was lethal to rats after 7-10 administrations, due to general deterioration of the animals with secondary degenerative histological changes in many tissues.

DOSAGE AND ADMINISTRATION

Therapy should be initiated by a physician experienced in the treatment of patients with chronic myeloid leukemia or gastrointestinal stromal tumors.

The prescribed dose should be administered orally, with a meal and a large glass of water. Doses of 400 mg or 600 mg

should be administered once daily, whereas a dose of 800 mg should be administered as 400 mg twice a day.
Treatment may be continued as long as there is no evidence of progressive disease or unacceptable toxicity.
The recommended dosage of Gleevec™ (imatinib mesylate) is 400 mg/day for patients in chronic phase CML and 600 mg/day for patients in accelerated phase or blast crisis.
The recommended dosage of Gleevec is 400 mg/day or 600 mg/day for patients with unresectable and/or metastatic, malignant GIST.
In CML, dose increase from 400 mg to 600 mg in patients with chronic phase disease, or from 600 mg to 800 mg (given as 400 mg twice daily) in patients in accelerated phase or blast crisis may be considered in the absence of severe adverse drug reaction and severe non-leukemia related neutropenia or thrombocytopenia in the following circumstances: disease progression (at any time); failure to achieve a satisfactory hematologic response after at least 3 months of treatment; loss of a previously achieved hematologic response.

Dose Adjustment for Hepatotoxicity and Other Non-Hematologic Adverse Reactions

If a severe non-hematologic adverse reaction develops (such as severe hepatotoxicity or severe fluid retention), Gleevec should be withheld until the event has resolved. Thereafter, treatment can be resumed as appropriate depending on the initial severity of the event.
If elevations in bilirubin >3 × institutional upper limit of normal (IULN) or in liver transaminases >5 × IULN occur, Gleevec should be withheld until bilirubin levels have returned to a <1.5 × IULN and transaminase levels to <2.5 × IULN. Treatment with Gleevec may then be continued at a reduced daily dose (i.e., 400 mg to 300 mg or 600 mg to 400 mg).

Hematologic Adverse Reactions

Dose reduction or treatment interruptions for severe neutropenia and thrombocytopenia are recommended as indicated in Table 7.
[See table 7 at top of previous page]

Pediatric

The safety and efficacy of Gleevec in patients under the age of 18 years have not been established.

HOW SUPPLIED

Each hard gelatin capsule contains 100 mg of imatinib free base.

100 mg Capsules

Orange to grayish orange opaque capsule with "NVR SI" printed in red ink.
Bottles of 120 capsules .... NDC 0078-0373-66

Storage

Store at 25°C (77°F); excursions permitted to 15°C-30°C (59°F-86°F). [See USP Controlled Room Temperature]
Dispense in a tight container, USP.

T2002-09
REV: JANUARY 2002 Printed in U.S.A. 89012403
NOVARTIS
Manufactured by:
Novartis Pharma AG
Basle, Switzerland
Distributed by:
Novartis Pharmaceuticals Corporation
East Hanover, New Jersey 07936

ZOMETA® ℞

[*zō' mĕ-tăh*]
(zoledronic acid for injection)
For Intravenous Infusion
Rx only
Prescribing Information

Prescribing information for this product, which appears on pages 3621–3623 of the 2002 PDR, has been completely revised as follows. Please write "See Supplement A" next to the product heading.

DESCRIPTION

Zometa® contains zoledronic acid, a bisphosphonic acid which is an inhibitor of osteoclastic bone resorption. Zoledronic acid is designated chemically as (1-Hydroxy-2-imidazol-1-yl-phosphonoethyl) phosphonic acid monohydrate and its structural formula is

Zoledronic acid is a white crystalline powder. Its molecular formula is $C_5H_{10}N_2O_7P_2 \bullet H_2O$ and its molar mass is 290.1g/Mol. Zoledronic acid is highly soluble in 0.1N sodium hydroxide solution, sparingly soluble in water and 0.1N hydrochloric acid, and practically insoluble in organic solvents. The pH of a 0.7% solution of zoledronic acid in water is approximately 2.0.
Zometa® (zoledronic acid for injection) is available in vials as a sterile powder for reconstitution for intravenous infusion. Each vial contains 4.264 mg of zoledronic acid monohydrate, corresponding to 4 mg zoledronic acid on an anhydrous basis.
Inactive Ingredients: mannitol, USP, as bulking agent, and sodium citrate, USP, as buffering agent.

CLINICAL PHARMACOLOGY

General

The principal pharmacologic action of zoledronic acid is inhibition of bone resorption. Although the antiresorptive mechanism is not completely understood, several factors are thought to contribute to this action. *In vitro*, zoledronic acid inhibits osteoclastic activity and induces osteoclast apoptosis. Zoledronic acid also blocks the osteoclastic resorption of mineralized bone and cartilage through its binding to bone. Zoledronic acid inhibits the increased osteoclastic activity and skeletal calcium release induced by various stimulatory factors released by tumors.

Pharmacokinetics

Distribution

Single or multiple (q 28 days) 5-minute or 15-minute infusions of 2, 4, 8 or 16 mg Zometa® (zoledronic acid for injection) were given to 64 patients with cancer and bone metastases. The post-infusion decline of zoledronic acid concentrations in plasma was consistent with a triphasic process showing a rapid decrease from peak concentrations at end-of-infusion to <1% of C_{max} 24 hours post infusion with population half-lives of $t_{1/2\alpha}$ 0.24 hours and $t_{1/2\beta}$ 1.87 hours for the early disposition phases of the drug. The terminal elimination phase of zoledronic acid was prolonged, with very low concentrations in plasma between days 2 and 28 post infusion, and a terminal elimination half-life $t_{1/2\gamma}$ of 146 hours. The area under the plasma concentration versus time curve (AUC_{0-24h}) of zoledronic acid was dose proportional from 2 to 16 mg. The accumulation of zoledronic acid measured over three cycles was low, with mean AUC_{0-24h} ratios for cycles 2 and 3 versus 1 of 1.13 ± 0.30 and 1.16 ± 0.36, respectively.
In vitro and *ex vivo* studies showed low affinity of zoledronic acid for the cellular components of human blood. Binding to human plasma proteins was approximately 22% and was independent of the concentration of zoledronic acid.

Metabolism

Zoledronic acid does not inhibit human P450 enzymes *in vitro*. Zoledronic acid does not undergo biotransformation *in vivo*. In animal studies, <3% of the administered intravenous dose was found in the feces, with the balance either recovered in the urine or taken up by bone, indicating that the drug is eliminated intact via the kidney. Following an intravenous dose of 20 nCi ^{14}C-zoledronic acid in a patient with cancer and bone metastases, only a single radioactive species with chromatographic properties identical to those of parent drug was recovered in urine, which suggests that zoledronic acid is not metabolized.

Excretion

In 64 patients with cancer and bone metastases on average (± s.d.) 39 ± 16% of the administered zoledronic acid dose was recovered in the urine within 24 hours, with only trace amounts of drug found in urine post day 2. The cumulative percent of drug excreted in the urine over 0–24 hours was independent of dose. The balance of drug not recovered in urine over 0–24 hours, representing drug presumably bound to bone, is slowly released back into the systemic circulation, giving rise to the observed prolonged low plasma concentrations. The 0–24 hour renal clearance of zoledronic acid was 3.7 ± 2.0 L/h.
Zoledronic acid clearance was independent of dose but dependent upon the patient's creatinine clearance. In a study in patients with cancer and bone metastases, increasing the infusion time of a 4 mg dose of zoledronic acid from 5 minutes (n=5) to 15 minutes (n=7) resulted in a 34% decrease in the zoledronic acid concentration at the end of the infusion ([mean ± SD] 403 ± 118 ng/mL vs 264 ± 86 ng/mL) and a 10% increase in the total AUC (378 ± 116 ng × h/mL vs 420 ± 218 ng × h/mL). The difference between the AUC means was not statistically significant.

Special Populations

Pharmacokinetic data in patients with hypercalcemia are not available.
Pediatrics: Pharmacokinetic data in pediatric patients are not available.
Geriatrics: The pharmacokinetics of zoledronic acid were not affected by age in patients with cancer and bone metastases who ranged in age from 38 years to 84 years.
Race: The pharmacokinetics of zoledronic acid were not affected by race in patients with cancer and bone metastases.
Hepatic Insufficiency: No clinical studies were conducted to evaluate the effect of hepatic impairment on the pharmacokinetics of zoledronic acid.
Renal Insufficiency: The pharmacokinetic studies conducted in 64 cancer patients represented typical clinical populations with normal to moderately impaired renal function. Compared to patients with normal renal function (N=37), patients with mild renal impairment (N=15) showed an average increase in plasma AUC of 15%, whereas patients with moderate renal impairment (N=11) showed an average increase in plasma AUC of 43%. Limited pharmacokinetic data are available for Zometa in patients with severe renal impairment (creatinine clearance <30 mL/min). Based on population PK/PD modeling, the risk of renal deterioration appears to increase with AUC, which is doubled at a creatinine clearance of 10 mL/min.
Creatinine clearance is calculated by the Cockcroft-Gault formula (Creatinine clearance [CL_{cr}, mL/min]=[140-age]*weight [kg]/X*[plasma creatinine concentration, where X=72 for males, and X=85 for females]). Zometa systemic clearance in individual patients can be calculated from the population clearance of Zometa, CL (L/h)=6.5(CL_{cr}/90)$^{0.4}$. These formulae can be used to predict the Zometa AUC in patients. CL = Dose/AUC. The average AUC in patients with normal renal function was 0.42 mg*h/L (%CV 33) following a 4-mg dose of Zometa. However, efficacy and safety of adjusted dosing based on these formulae have not been prospectively assessed. (See WARNINGS.)

Pharmacodynamics

Clinical studies in patients with hypercalcemia of malignancy (HCM) showed that single-dose infusions of Zometa are associated with decreases in serum calcium and phosphorus and increases in urinary calcium and phosphorus excretion.

Hypercalcemia of Malignancy

Osteoclastic hyperactivity resulting in excessive bone resorption is the underlying pathophysiologic derangement in hypercalcemia of malignancy (HCM, tumor-induced hypercalcemia) and metastatic bone disease. Excessive release of calcium into the blood as bone is resorbed results in polyuria and gastrointestinal disturbances, with progressive dehydration and decreasing glomerular filtration rate. This, in turn, results in increased renal resorption of calcium, setting up a cycle of worsening systemic hypercalcemia. Reducing excessive bone resorption and maintaining adequate fluid administration are, therefore, essential to the management of hypercalcemia of malignancy.
Patients who have hypercalcemia of malignancy can generally be divided into two groups according to the pathophysiologic mechanism involved: humoral hypercalcemia and hypercalcemia due to tumor invasion of bone. In humoral hypercalcemia, osteoclasts are activated and bone resorption is stimulated by factors such as parathyroid-hormone-related protein, which are elaborated by the tumor and circulate systemically. Humoral hypercalcemia usually occurs in squamous-cell malignancies of the lung or head and neck or in genitourinary tumors such as renal-cell carcinoma or ovarian cancer. Skeletal metastases may be absent or minimal in these patients.
Extensive invasion of bone by tumor cells can also result in hypercalcemia due to local tumor products that stimulate bone resorption by osteoclasts. Tumors commonly associated with locally mediated hypercalcemia include breast cancer and multiple myeloma.
Total serum calcium levels in patients who have hypercalcemia of malignancy may not reflect the severity of hypercalcemia, since concomitant hypoalbuminemia is commonly present. Ideally, ionized calcium levels should be used to diagnose and follow hypercalcemic conditions; however, these are not commonly or rapidly available in many clinical situations. Therefore, adjustment of the total serum calcium value for differences in albumin levels (corrected serum calcium, CSC) is often used in place of measurement of ionized calcium; several nomograms are in use for this type of calculation (see DOSAGE AND ADMINISTRATION).

Clinical Trials in Hypercalcemia of Malignancy

Two identical multicenter, randomized, double-blind, double-dummy studies of Zometa 4 mg given as a 5-minute intravenous infusion or pamidronate 90 mg given as a 2-hour intravenous infusion were conducted in 185 patients with hypercalcemia of malignancy (HCM). **NOTE: Administration of Zometa 4 mg given as a 5-minute intravenous infusion has been shown to result in an increased risk of renal toxicity, as measured by increases in serum creatinine, which can progress to renal failure. The incidence of renal toxicity and renal failure has been shown to be reduced when Zometa 4 mg is given as a 15-minute intravenous infusion. Zometa should be administered by intravenous infusion over no less than 15 minutes. (See WARNINGS and DOSAGE AND ADMINISTRATION.)** The treatment groups in the clinical studies were generally well balanced with regards to age, sex, race, and tumor types. The mean age of the study population was 59 years; 81% were Caucasian, 15% were Black, and 4% were of other races. Sixty percent of the patients were male. The most common tumor types were lung, breast, head and neck, and renal.
In these studies, HCM was defined as a corrected serum calcium (CSC) concentration of ≥12.0 mg/dL (3.00 mmol/L). The primary efficacy variable was the proportion of patients having a complete response, defined as the lowering of the CSC to ≤10.8 mg/dL (2.70 mmol/L) within 10 days after drug infusion.
To assess the effects of Zometa versus those of pamidronate, the two multicenter HCM studies were combined in a preplanned analysis. The results of the primary analysis revealed that the proportion of patients that had normalization of corrected serum calcium by Day 10 were 88% and 70% for Zometa 4 mg and pamidronate 90 mg, respectively (P=0.002). (See Figure 1.) **In these studies, no additional benefit was seen for Zometa 8 mg over Zometa 4 mg; however, the risk of renal toxicity of Zometa 8 mg was significantly greater than that seen with Zometa 4 mg.**

Figure 1
Proportion of Complete Responders by Day 10 in Pooled HCM Studies

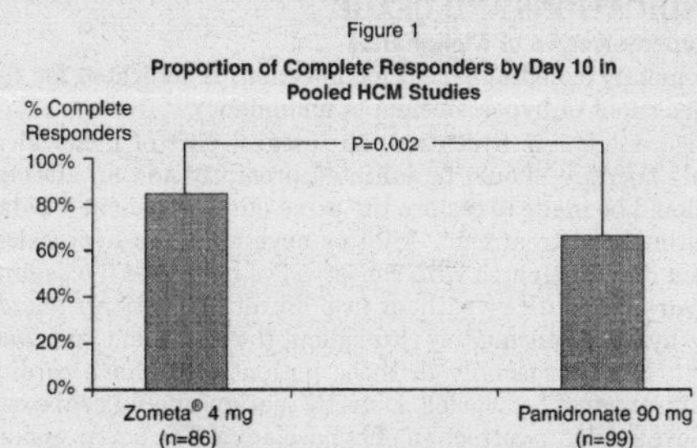

Secondary efficacy variables from the pooled HCM studies included the proportion of patients who had normalization of corrected serum calcium (CSC) by Day 4; the proportion

Continued on next page

Zometa—Cont.

of patients who had normalization of CSC by Day 7; time to relapse of HCM; and duration of complete response. Time to relapse of HCM was defined as the duration (in days) of normalization of serum calcium from study drug infusion until the last CSC value <11.6 mg/dL (<2.90 mmol/L). Patients who did not have a complete response were assigned a time to relapse of 0 days. Duration of complete response was defined as the duration (in days) from the occurrence of a complete response until the last CSC ≤10.8 mg/dL (2.70 mmol/L). The results of these secondary analyses for Zometa 4 mg and pamidronate 90 mg are shown in Table 1.

[See table 1 above]

Clinical Trials in Multiple Myeloma and Bone Metastases of Solid Tumors

Table 2 describes three randomized Zometa trials in patients with multiple myeloma and bone metastases of solid tumors. These include a pamidronate-controlled study in breast cancer and multiple myeloma, a placebo-controlled study in prostate cancer and a placebo-controlled study in other solid tumors. The prostate cancer study required documentation of previous bone metastases and 3 consecutive rising PSAs while on hormonal therapy. The other placebo-controlled solid tumor study included patients with bone metastases from malignancies other than breast cancer and prostate cancer, listed in Table 3.

[See table 2 above]

Table 3: Solid Tumor Patients by Cancer Type and Treatment Arm

Cancer type	Zometa® 4 mg N	Placebo N
NSCLC	124	121
Renal	26	19
Small cell lung	19	22
Colorectal	19	16
Unknown	17	14
Bladder	11	16
GI (other)	10	12
Head and neck	6	4
Genitourinary	6	6
Malignant melanoma	5	4
Hepatobiliary	3	4
Thyroid	2	4
Other	3	2
Sarcoma	2	3
Neuroendocrine/ carcinoid	2	3
Mesothelioma	1	0

The planned duration of therapy was 12 months for multiple myeloma and breast cancer, 15 months for prostate cancer, and 9 months for the other solid tumors.

The studies were amended twice because of renal toxicity. The Zometa infusion duration was increased from 5 minutes to 15 minutes. After all patients had been accrued, but while dosing and follow-up continued, patients in the 8-mg Zometa treatment arm were switched to 4 mg. Patients who were randomized to the Zometa 8-mg group are not included in these analyses.

Each study evaluated skeletal-related events (SREs), defined as any of the following: pathologic fracture, radiation therapy to bone, surgery to bone, or spinal cord compression. Change in antineoplastic therapy due to increased pain was a SRE in the prostate cancer study only. Planned analyses included the proportion of patients with a SRE during the study (the primary endpoint) and time to first SRE. Results for the two Zometa placebo-controlled studies are given in Table 4.

[See table 4 above]

In the breast cancer and myeloma trial, efficacy was determined by a non-inferiority analysis comparing Zometa to pamidronate 90 mg for the proportion of patients with a SRE. This analysis required an estimation of pamidronate efficacy. Historical data from 1128 patients in three pamidronate placebo-controlled trials demonstrated that pamidronate decreased the proportion of patients with a SRE by 13.1% (95% CI = 7.3%,18.9%). Results of the comparison of treatment with Zometa compared to pamidronate are given in Table 5.

[See table 5 above]

INDICATIONS AND USAGE

Hypercalcemia of Malignancy

Zometa® (zoledronic acid for injection) is indicated for the treatment of hypercalcemia of malignancy.

Vigorous saline hydration, an integral part of hypercalcemia therapy, should be initiated promptly and an attempt should be made to restore the urine output to about 2 L/day throughout treatment. Mild or asymptomatic hypercalcemia may be treated with conservative measures (i.e., saline hydration, with or without loop diuretics). Patients should be hydrated adequately throughout the treatment, but overhydration, especially in those patients who have cardiac failure, must be avoided. Diuretic therapy should not be employed prior to correction of hypovolemia. The safety and efficacy of Zometa in the treatment of hypercalcemia associated with hyperparathyroidism or with other non-tumor-related conditions has not been established.

Multiple Myeloma and Bone Metastases of Solid Tumors

Zometa is indicated for the treatment of patients with multiple myeloma and patients with documented bone metastases from solid tumors, in conjunction with standard antineoplastic therapy. Prostate cancer should have progressed after treatment with at least one hormonal therapy.

Table 1: Secondary Efficacy Variables in Pooled HCM Studies

	Zometa® 4 mg		Pamidronate 90 mg	
Complete response	N	Response rate	N	Response rate
By Day 4	86	45.3%	99	33.3%
By Day 7	86	82.6%*	99	63.6%
Duration of response	N	Median duration (days)	N	Median duration (days)
Time to replapse	86	30*	99	17
Duration of complete response	76	32	69	18

* P less than 0.05 vs. pamidronate 90 mg

Table 2: Overview of Phase III Studies

Study No.	No. of Patients	Treatment Duration	Zometa® Dose	Control	Patient Population
010	1648	12 months	4 and 8* mg Q3–4 weeks	Pamidronate 90 mg Q3–4 weeks	Multiple myeloma or metastatic breast cancer
039	643	15 months	4 and 8* mg Q3 weeks	Placebo	Metastatic prostate cancer
011	773	9 months	4 and 8* mg Q3 weeks	Placebo	Metastatic solid tumor other than breast or prostate cancer

* Patients who were randomized to the 8-mg Zometa group are not included in any of the analyses in this package insert.

Table 4: Zometa® Compared to Placebo in Patients with Bone Metastases from Prostate Cancer or Other Solid Tumors

		Analysis of Proportion of Patients with a SRE*			Analysis of Time to First SRE*			
Study	Study Arm	Proportion	Difference & 95% CI	P value	Median (days)	HR	95% CI of HR	P value
Prostate Cancer	Zometa 4 mg	33%	−11 (−20, −2)	0.021	NR	0.67	(0.49, 0.91)	0.011
	Placebo	44%	—	—	321	—	—	—
Solid Tumors	Zometa 4 mg	38%	−7 (−15, 2)	0.13	230	0.73	(0.55, 0.96)	0.023
	Placebo	44%	—	—	163	—	—	—

*SRE = Skeletal Related Event
NR = Not reached by 420 days
HR = Hazard Ratio

Table 5: Zometa® Compared to Pamidronate in Patients with Multiple Myeloma or Bone Metastases from Breast Cancer

		Analysis of Proportion of Patients with a SRE*			Analysis of Time to First SRE*			
Study	Study Arm	Proportion	Difference & 95% CI	P value	Median (days)	HR	95% CI of HR	P value
Multiple Myeloma and Breast Cancer	Zometa 4 mg	44%	−2 (−7.9, −3.7)	0.46	373	0.92	(0.77, 1.09)	0.322
	Pamidronate 90 mg	46%	—	—	363	—	—	—

*SRE = Skeletal Related Event
HR = Hazard Ratio

Table 6: Grade 3–4 Laboratory Abnormalities for Serum Creatinine, Serum Calcium, Serum Phosphorus, and Serum Magnesium in Two Clinical Trials in Patients with HCM

	Grade 3				Grade 4			
Laboratory Parameter	**Zometa® 4 mg** n/N	(%)	**Pamidronate 90 mg** n/N	(%)	**Zometa® 4 mg** n/N	(%)	**Pamidronate 90 mg** n/N	(%)
Serum Creatinine[1]	2/86	(2.3%)	3/100	(3.0%)	0/86	—	1/100	(1.0%)
Hypocalcemia[2]	1/86	(1.2%)	2/100	(2.0%)	0/86	—	0/100	—
Hypophosphatemia[3]	36/70	(51.4%)	27/81	(33.3%)	1/70	(1.4%)	4/81	(4.9%)
Hypomagnesemia[4]	0/71	—	0/84	—	0/71	—	1/84	(1.2%)

[1] Grade 3 (>3× Upper Limit of Normal); Grade 4 (>6× Upper Limit of Normal)
[2] Grade 3 (<7 mg/dL); Grade 4 (<6 mg/dL)
[3] Grade 3 (<2 mg/dL); Grade 4 (<1 mg/dL)
[4] Grade 3 (<0.8 mEq/L); Grade 4 (<0.5 mEq/L)

CONTRAINDICATIONS

Zometa® (zoledronic acid for injection) is contraindicated in patients with clinically significant hypersensitivity to zoledronic acid or other bisphosphonates, or any of the excipients in the formulation of Zometa.

WARNINGS

DUE TO THE RISK OF CLINICALLY SIGNIFICANT DETERIORATION IN RENAL FUNCTION, WHICH MAY PROGRESS TO RENAL FAILURE, SINGLE DOSES OF ZOMETA SHOULD NOT EXCEED 4 MG AND THE DURATION OF INFUSION SHOULD BE NO LESS THAN 15 MINUTES.

BECAUSE SAFETY AND PHARMACOKINETIC DATA ARE LIMITED IN PATIENTS WITH SEVERE RENAL IMPAIRMENT:

- **ZOMETA TREATMENT IS NOT RECOMMENDED IN PATIENTS WITH BONE METASTASES WITH SEVERE RENAL IMPAIRMENT.** In the clinical studies, patients with serum creatinine >3.0 mg/dL were excluded.
- **ZOMETA TREATMENT IN PATIENTS WITH HYPERCALCEMIA OF MALIGNANCY SHOULD BE CONSIDERED ONLY AFTER EVALUATING THE RISKS AND BENEFITS OF TREATMENT.** In the clinical studies, patients with serum creatinine >400 μmol/L or >4.5 mg/dL were excluded.

Bisphosphonates, including Zometa® (zoledronic acid for injection), have been associated with renal toxicity manifested as deterioration of renal function and potential renal failure. In clinical trials, the risk for renal function deterioration (defined as an increase in serum creatinine) was significantly increased in patients who received Zometa over 5 minutes compared to patients who received the same dose over 15 minutes. In addition, the risk for renal function deterioration and renal failure was significantly increased in patients who received Zometa 8 mg, even when given over 15 minutes. While this risk is reduced with the Zometa 4-mg dose administered over 15 minutes, deterioration in renal function can still occur. Risk factors for this deterioration include elevated baseline creatinine and multiple cycles of treatment with the bisphosphonate.

Patients who receive Zometa should have serum creatinine assessed prior to each treatment. Patients treated with

Zometa for bone metastases should have the dose withheld if renal function has deteriorated. (See DOSAGE AND ADMINISTRATION.) Patients with hypercalcemia of malignancy with evidence of deterioration in renal function should be appropriately evaluated as to whether the potential benefit of continued treatment with Zometa outweighs the possible risk.

PREGNANCY: ZOMETA SHOULD NOT BE USED DURING PREGNANCY.

Zometa may cause fetal harm when administered to a pregnant woman. In reproductive studies in the pregnant rat, subcutaneous doses equivalent to 2.4 or 4.8 times the human systemic exposure (an i.v. dose of 4 mg based on an AUC comparison) resulted in pre- and post-implantation losses, decreases in viable fetuses and fetal skeletal, visceral and external malformations. (See PRECAUTIONS, Pregnancy Category D.)

There are no studies in pregnant women using Zometa. If the patient becomes pregnant while taking this drug, the patient should be apprised of the potential harm to the fetus. Women of childbearing potential should be advised to avoid becoming pregnant.

PRECAUTIONS

General

Standard hypercalcemia-related metabolic parameters, such as serum levels of calcium, phosphate, and magnesium, as well as serum creatinine, should be carefully monitored following initiation of therapy with Zometa® (zoledronic acid for injection). If hypocalcemia, hypophosphatemia, or hypomagnesemia occur, short-term supplemental therapy may be necessary.

Patients with hypercalcemia of malignancy must be adequately rehydrated prior to administration of Zometa. Loop diuretics should not be used until the patient is adequately rehydrated and should be used with caution in combination with Zometa in order to avoid hypocalcemia. Zometa should be used with caution with other nephrotoxic drugs.

Renal Insufficiency: Limited clinical data are available regarding use of Zometa in patients with renal impairment. Zometa is excreted intact primarily via the kidney, and the risk of adverse reactions, in particular renal adverse reactions, may be greater in patients with impaired renal function. Serum creatinine should be monitored in all patients treated with Zometa prior to each dose.

Studies of Zometa in the treatment of hypercalcemia of malignancy excluded patients with serum creatinine ≥400 µmol/L or ≥4.5 mg/dL. Bone metastasis trials excluded patients with serum creatinine >265 µmol/L or >3.0 mg/dL. No clinical or pharmacokinetics data are available to guide dose selection or to provide guidance on how to safely use Zometa in patients with severe renal impairment. For hypercalcemia of malignancy, Zometa should be used in patients with severe renal impairment only if the expected clinical benefits outweigh the risk of renal failure and after considering other available treatment options. (See WARNINGS.) Dose adjustments of Zometa are not necessary in treating patients for hypercalcemia presenting with mild-to-moderate renal impairment prior to initiation of therapy (serum creatinine <400 µmol/L or <4.5 mg/dL). For bone metastases, the use of Zometa in patients with severe renal impairment is not recommended. In studies of patients with bone metastases, patients with a serum creatinine >3.0 mg/dL were excluded.

Patients receiving Zometa for hypercalcemia of malignancy with evidence of deterioration in renal function should be appropriately evaluated and consideration should be given as to whether the potential benefit of continued treatment with Zometa outweighs the possible risk. In patients receiving Zometa for bone metastases, who show evidence of deterioration in renal function, Zometa treatment should be withheld until renal function returns to baseline. (See WARNINGS and DOSAGE AND ADMINISTRATION.)

Hepatic Insufficiency: Only limited clinical data are available for use of Zometa to treat hypercalcemia of malignancy in patients with hepatic insufficiency, and these data are not adequate to provide guidance on dosage selection or how to safely use Zometa in these patients.

Patients with Asthma: While not observed in clinical trials with Zometa, administration of other bisphosphonates has been associated with bronchoconstriction in aspirin-sensitive asthmatic patients. Zometa should be used with caution in patients with aspirin-sensitive asthma.

Laboratory Tests

Serum creatinine should be monitored prior to each dose of Zometa. Serum calcium, electrolytes, phosphate, magnesium, and hematocrit/hemoglobin should also be monitored regularly. (See WARNINGS, PRECAUTIONS, DOSAGE AND ADMINISTRATION, and ADVERSE REACTIONS.)

Drug Interactions

In vitro studies indicate that zoledronic acid is approximately 56% bound to plasma proteins. *In vitro* studies also indicate that zoledronic acid does not inhibit microsomal CYP450 enzymes. *In vivo* studies showed that zoledronic acid is not metabolized, and is excreted into the urine as the intact drug. However, no *in vivo* drug interaction studies have been performed.

Caution is advised when bisphosphonates are administered with aminoglycosides, since these agents may have an additive effect to lower serum calcium level for prolonged periods. This has not been reported in Zometa clinical trials. Caution should also be exercised when Zometa is used in combination with loop diuretics due to an increased risk of hypocalcemia. Caution is indicated when Zometa is used with other potentially nephrotoxic drugs.

In multiple myeloma patients, the risk of renal dysfunction may be increased when Zometa is used in combination with thalidomide.

Carcinogenesis, Mutagenesis, Impairment of Fertility

Carcinogenesis: Standard lifetime carcinogenicity bioassays were conducted in mice and rats. Mice were given oral doses of zoledronic acid of 0.1, 0.5, or 2.0 mg/kg/day. There was an increased incidence of Harderian gland adenomas in males and females in all treatment groups (at doses ≥0.002 times a human intravenous dose of 4 mg, based on a comparison of relative body surface areas). Rats were given oral doses of zoledronic acid of 0.1, 0.5, or 2.0 mg/kg/day. No increased incidence of tumors was observed (at doses ≤0.2 times the human intravenous dose of 4 mg, based on a comparison of relative body surface areas).

Mutagenesis: Zoledronic acid was not genotoxic in the Ames bacterial mutagenicity assay, in the Chinese hamster ovary cell assay, or in the Chinese hamster gene mutation assay, with or without metabolic activation. Zoledronic acid was not genotoxic in the *in vivo* rat micronucleus assay.

Impairment of Fertility: Female rats were given subcutaneous doses of zoledronic acid of 0.01, 0.03, or 0.1 mg/kg/day beginning 15 days before mating and continuing through gestation. Effects observed in the high-dose group (with systemic exposure of 1.2 times the human systemic exposure following an intravenous dose of 4 mg, based on AUC comparison) included inhibition of ovulation and a decrease in the number of pregnant rats. Effects observed in both the mid-dose group (with systemic exposure of 0.2 times the human systemic exposure following an intravenous dose of 4 mg, based on an AUC comparison) and high-dose group included an increase in pre-implantation losses and a decrease in the number of implantations and live fetuses.

Pregnancy Category D *See WARNINGS.*

In female rats given subcutaneous doses of zoledronic acid of 0.01, 0.03, or 0.1 mg/kg/day beginning 15 days before mating and continuing through gestation, the number of stillbirths was increased and survival of neonates was decreased in the mid- and high-dose groups (≥0.2 times the human systemic exposure following an intravenous dose of 4 mg, based on an AUC comparison). Adverse maternal effects were observed in all dose groups (with a systemic exposure of ≥0.07 times the human systemic exposure following an intravenous dose of 4 mg, based on an AUC comparison) and included dystocia and periparturient mortality in pregnant rats allowed to deliver. Maternal mortality may have been related to drug-induced inhibition of skeletal calcium mobilization, resulting in periparturient hypocalcemia. This appears to be a bisphosphonate class effect.

In pregnant rats given a subcutaneous dose of zoledronic acid of 0.1, 0.2, or 0.4 mg/kg/day during gestation, adverse fetal effects were observed in the mid- and high-dose groups (with systemic exposures of 2.4 and 4.8 times, respectively, the human systemic exposure following an intravenous dose of 4 mg, based on an AUC comparison). These adverse effects included increases in pre- and post-implantation losses, decreases in viable fetuses, and fetal skeletal, visceral, and external malformations. Fetal skeletal effects observed in the high-dose group included unossified or incompletely ossified bones, thickened, curved or shortened bones, wavy ribs, and shortened jaw. Other adverse fetal effects observed in the high-dose group included reduced lens, rudimentary cerebellum, reduction or absence of liver lobes, reduction of lung lobes, vessel dilation, cleft palate, and edema. Skeletal variations were also observed in the low-dose group (with systemic exposure of 1.2 times the human systemic exposure following an intravenous dose of 4 mg, based on an AUC comparison). Signs of maternal toxicity were observed in the high-dose group and included reduced body weights and food consumption, indicating that maximal exposure levels were achieved in this study.

In pregnant rabbits given subcutaneous doses of zoledronic acid of 0.01, 0.03, or 0.1 mg/kg/day during gestation (≤0.5 times the human intravenous dose of 4 mg, based on a comparison of relative body surface areas), no adverse fetal effects were observed. Maternal mortality and abortion occurred in all treatment groups (at doses ≥0.05 times the human intravenous dose of 4 mg, based on a comparison of relative body surface areas). Adverse maternal effects were associated with, and may have been caused by, drug-induced hypocalcemia.

Nursing Mothers

It is not known whether Zometa is excreted in human milk. Because many drugs are excreted in human milk, and because Zometa binds to bone long-term, Zometa should not be administered to a nursing woman.

Pediatric Use

The safety and effectiveness of Zometa in pediatric patients have not been established. Because of long-term retention in bone, Zometa should only be used in children if the potential benefit outweighs the potential risk.

Geriatric Use

Clinical studies of Zometa in hypercalcemia of malignancy included 34 patients who were 65 years of age or older. No significant differences in response rate or adverse reactions were seen in geriatric patients receiving Zometa as compared to younger patients. Controlled clinical studies of Zometa in the treatment of multiple myeloma and bone metastases of solid tumors in patients over age 65 revealed similar efficacy and safety in older and younger patients. Because decreased renal function occurs more commonly in the elderly, special care should be taken to monitor renal function.

ADVERSE REACTIONS

Hypercalcemia of Malignancy

Adverse reactions to Zometa® (zoledronic acid for injection) are usually mild and transient and similar to those reported for other bisphosphonates. Intravenous administration has been most commonly associated with fever. Occasionally, patients experience a flu-like syndrome consisting of fever, chills, bone pain and/or arthralgias, and myalgias. Gastrointestinal reactions such as nausea and vomiting have been reported following intravenous infusion of Zometa. Local reactions at the infusion site, such as redness or swelling, were observed infrequently. In most cases, no specific treatment is required and the symptoms subside after 24–48 hours.

Rare cases of rash, pruritus, and chest pain have been reported following treatment with Zometa.

As with other bisphosphonates, cases of conjunctivitis and hypomagnesemia have been reported following treatment with Zometa.

Grade 3 and Grade 4 laboratory abnormalities for serum creatinine, serum calcium, serum phosphorus, and serum magnesium observed in two clinical trials of Zometa in patients with HCM are shown in Table 6.

[See table at top of previous page]

Table 7 provides adverse events that were reported by 10% or more of the 189 patients treated with Zometa 4 mg or pamidronate 90 mg from the two controlled multi-center HCM trials. Adverse events are listed regardless of presumed causality to study drug.

Table 7: Percentage of Patients with Adverse Events ≥10% Reported in Hypercalcemia of Malignancy Clinical Trials By Body System

	Zometa® 4 mg n (%)	Pamidronate 90 mg n (%)
Patients Studied		
Total no. of patients studied	86 (100)	103 (100)
Total no. of patients with any AE	81 (94.2)	95 (92.2)
Body as a Whole		
Fever	38 (44.2)	34 (33.0)
Progression of Cancer	14 (16.3)	21 (20.4)
Digestive		
Nausea	25 (29.1)	28 (27.2)
Constipation	23 (26.7)	13 (12.6)
Diarrhea	15 (17.4)	17 (16.5)
Abdominal Pain	14 (16.3)	13 (12.6)
Vomiting	12 (14.0)	17 (16.5)
Anorexia	8 (9.3)	14 (13.6)
Cardiovascular		
Hypotension	9 (10.5)	2 (1.9)
Hemic and Lymphatic System		
Anemia	19 (22.1)	18 (17.5)
Infections		
Moniliasis	10 (11.6)	4 (3.9)
Laboratory Abnormalities		
Hypophosphatemia	11 (12.8)	2 (1.9)
Hypokalemia	10 (11.6)	16 (15.5)
Hypomagnesemia	9 (10.5)	5 (4.9)
Musculoskeletal		
Skeletal Pain	10 (11.6)	10 (9.7)
Nervous		
Insomnia	13 (15.1)	10 (9.7)
Anxiety	12 (14.0)	8 (7.8)
Confusion	11 (12.8)	13 (12.6)
Agitation	11 (12.8)	8 (7.8)
Respiratory		
Dyspnea	19 (22.1)	20 (19.4)
Coughing	10 (11.6)	12 (11.7)
Urogenital		
Urinary Tract Infection	12 (14.0)	15 (14.6)

The following adverse events from the two controlled multicenter HCM trials (n=189) were reported by a greater percentage of patients treated with Zometa 4 mg than with pamidronate 90 mg and occurred with a frequency of greater than or equal to 5% but less than 10%. Adverse events are listed regardless of presumed causality to study drug.

Body as a Whole: asthenia, chest pain, leg edema, mucositis, metastases

Digestive System: dysphagia

Hemic and Lymphatic System: granulocytopenia, thrombocytopenia, pancytopenia

Infection: non-specific infection

Laboratory Abnormalities: hypocalcemia

Metabolic and Nutritional: dehydration

Musculoskeletal: arthralgias

Nervous System: headache, somnolence

Respiratory System: pleural effusion

NOTE: In the HCM clinical trials, pamidronate 90 mg was given as a 2-hour intravenous infusion. The relative safety of pamidronate 90 mg given as a 2-hour intravenous infusion compared to the same dose given as a 24-hour intravenous infusion has not been adequately studied in controlled clinical trials.

Multiple Myeloma and Bone Metastases of Solid Tumors

Table 8 provides adverse events that were reported by 10% or more of the 2185 patients treated with Zometa 4 mg, pa-

Continued on next page

Zometa—Cont.

midronate 90 mg or placebo from the four controlled multicenter Bone Metastases trials. Adverse events are listed regardless of presumed causality to study drug.
[See table 8 above]
Grade 3 and Grade 4 laboratory abnormalities for serum creatinine, serum calcium, serum phosphorus, and serum magnesium observed in four clinical trials of Zometa in patients with Bone Metastases are shown in Tables 9 and 10.
[See table 9 above]
[See table 10 above]
Among the less frequently occurring adverse events (<15% of patients), rigors, hypokalemia, influenza-like illness, and hypocalcemia showed a trend for more events with bisphosphonate administration (Zometa 4 mg and pamidronate groups) compared to the placebo group.
Less common adverse events reported more often with Zometa 4 mg than pamidronate included decreased weight, which was reported in 13.0% of patients in the Zometa 4 mg compared with 7.1% in the pamidronate group. The incidence of decreased weight, however, was similar for the placebo group (12.5%) and Zometa. Decreased appetite was reported in slightly more patients in the Zometa 4 mg (10.8%) compared with the pamidronate (7.3%) and placebo (8.6%) groups, but the clinical significance of these small differences is not clear.

Renal Toxicity
In the bone metastases trials renal deterioration was defined as an increase of 0.5 mg/dL for patients with normal baseline creatinine (<1.4 mg/dL) or an increase of 1.0 mg/dL for patients with an abnormal baseline creatinine (≥1.4 mg/dL). The following are data on the incidence of renal deterioration in patients receiving Zometa 4 mg over 15 minutes in these trials. (See Table 11.)
[See table at top of next page]
The risk of deterioration in renal function appeared to be related to time on study, whether patients were receiving Zometa (4 mg over 15 minutes), placebo, or pamidronate.

OVERDOSAGE

There is no experience of acute overdose with Zometa® (zoledronic acid for injection). Two patients received Zometa 32 mg over 5 minutes in clinical trials. Neither patient experienced any clinical or laboratory toxicity. Overdosage may cause clinically significant hypocalcemia, hypophosphatemia, and hypomagnesemia. Clinically relevant reductions in serum levels of calcium, phosphorus, and magnesium should be corrected by intravenous administration of calcium gluconate, potassium or sodium phosphate, and magnesium sulfate, respectively.
In controlled clinical trials, administration of Zometa 4 mg as an intravenous infusion over 5 minutes has been shown to increase the risk of renal toxicity compared to the same dose administered as a 15-minute intravenous infusion. In controlled clinical trials, Zometa 8 mg has been shown to be associated with an increased risk of renal toxicity compared to Zometa 4 mg, even when given as a 15-minute intravenous infusion, and was not associated with added benefit in patients with hypercalcemia of malignancy. **Single doses of Zometa should not exceed 4 mg and the duration of the intravenous infusion should be no less than 15 minutes. (See WARNINGS.)**

DOSAGE AND ADMINISTRATION

Hypercalcemia of Malignancy
Consideration should be given to the severity of, as well as the symptoms of, tumor-induced hypercalcemia when considering use of Zometa® (zoledronic acid for injection). Vigorous saline hydration alone may be sufficient to treat mild, asymptomatic hypercalcemia.
The maximum recommended dose of Zometa in hypercalcemia of malignancy (albumin-corrected serum calcium* ≥12 mg/dL [3.0 mmol/L]) is 4 mg. The 4-mg dose must be given as a single-dose intravenous infusion over **no less than 15 minutes.**
Patients should be adequately rehydrated prior to administration of Zometa. (See WARNINGS and PRECAUTIONS.)
Retreatment with Zometa 4 mg, may be considered if serum calcium does not return to normal or remain normal after initial treatment. It is recommended that a minimum of 7 days elapse before retreatment, to allow for full response to the initial dose. Renal function must be carefully monitored in all patients receiving Zometa and possible deterioration in renal function must be assessed prior to retreatment with Zometa. (See WARNINGS and PRECAUTIONS.)

*Albumin-corrected serum calcium (Cca, mg/dL) = Ca + 0.8 (mid-range albumin-measured albumin in mg/dL).

Multiple Myeloma and Metastatic Bone Lesions From Solid Tumors
The recommended dose of Zometa in patients with multiple myeloma and metastatic bone lesions from solid tumors is 4 mg infused over 15 minutes every three or four weeks. Duration of treatment in the clinical studies was 15 months for prostate cancer, 12 months for breast cancer and multiple myeloma, and 9 months for other solid tumors. Patients should also be administered an oral calcium supplement of 500 mg and a multiple vitamin containing 400 IU of Vitamin D daily.
Serum creatinine should be measured before each Zometa dose and treatment should be withheld for renal deterioration. In the clinical studies, renal deterioration was defined as follows:

- For patients with normal baseline creatinine, increase of 0.5 mg/dL
- For patients with abnormal baseline creatinine, increase of 1.0 mg/dL

In the clinical studies, Zometa treatment was resumed only when the creatinine returned to within 10% of the baseline value.

Table 8: Percentage of Patients with Adverse Events ≥10% Reported in Four Bone Metastases Clinical Trials By Body System

	Zometa® 4 mg n (%)	Pamidronate 90 mg n (%)	Placebo n (%)
Patients Studied			
Total no. of patients	1099 (100)	631 (100)	455 (100)
Total no. of patients with any AE	1081 (98)	622 (99)	444 (98)
Blood and Lymphatic			
Anemia	320 (29)	170 (27)	119 (26)
Neutropenia	121 (11)	87 (14)	34 (8)
Gastrointestinal			
Nausea	470 (43)	282 (45)	160 (35)
Vomiting	328 (30)	189 (30)	114 (25)
Constipation	307 (28)	148 (24)	161 (35)
Diarrhea	238 (22)	157 (25)	76 (17)
Abdominal Pain	128 (12)	70 (11)	43 (10)
General Disorders and Administration Site			
Fatigue	394 (36)	235 (37)	125 (28)
Pyrexia	326 (30)	175 (28)	83 (18)
Weakness	232 (21)	103 (16)	105 (23)
Edema Lower Limb	203 (19)	115 (18)	76 (17)
Rigors	107 (10)	64 (10)	21 (5)
Infections			
Urinary Tract Infection	115 (11)	53 (8)	39 (9)
Upper Respiratory Tract Infection	88 (8)	83 (13)	26 (6)
Metabolism			
Anorexia	220 (20)	76 (12)	98 (22)
Weight Decreased	143 (13)	45 (7)	57 (13)
Dehydration	135 (12)	57 (9)	54 (12)
Appetite Decreased	119 (11)	46 (7)	39 (9)
Musculoskeletal			
Bone Pain	579 (53)	345 (55)	272 (60)
Myalgia	232 (21)	148 (24)	68 (15)
Arthralgia	195 (18)	109 (17)	60 (13)
Back Pain	113 (10)	79 (13)	29 (6)
Neoplasms			
Malignant Neoplasm Aggravated	166 (15)	71 (11)	72 (16)
Nervous			
Headache	193 (18)	152 (24)	47 (10)
Dizziness (excluding vertigo)	158 (14)	79 (13)	52 (11)
Insomnia	154 (14)	106 (17)	67 (15)
Parethesia	129 (12)	85 (14)	28 (6)
Hypoesthesia	109 (10)	63 (10)	38 (8)
Psychiatric			
Depression	136 (12)	89 (14)	41 (9)
Anxiety	101 (9)	76 (12)	34 (8)
Respiratory			
Dyspnea	264 (24)	147 (23)	93 (20)
Cough	212 (19)	132 (21)	57 (13)
Skin			
Alopecia	119 (11)	83 (13)	30 (7)
Dermatitis	108 (10)	68 (11)	35 (8)

Table 9: Grade 3 Laboratory Abnormalities for Serum Creatinine, Serum Calcium, Serum Phosphorus, and Serum Magnesium in Four Clinical Trials in Patients with Bone Metastases

Laboratory Parameter	Grade 3 Zometa® 4 mg n/N	(%)	Pamidronate 90 mg n/N	(%)	Placebo n/N	(%)
Serum Creatinine[1]*	7/529	(1.3%)	4/268	(1.5%)	2/241	(0.8%)
Hypocalcemia[2]	7/1041	(0.7%)	4/610	(0.7%)	0/415	—
Hypophosphatemia[3]	96/1041	(9.2%)	40/611	(6.6%)	13/415	(3.1%)
Hypermagnesemia[4]	19/1039	(1.8%)	3/609	(0.5%)	8/415	(1.9%)
Hypomagnesemia[5]	0/1039	—	0/609	—	1/415	(0.2%)

[1] Grade 3 (>3× Upper Limit of Normal); Grade 4 (>6× Upper Limit of Normal)
* Serum creatinine data for all patients randomized after the 15-minute infusion amendment
[2] Grade 3 (<7 mg/dL); Grade 4 (<6 mg/dL)
[3] Grade 3 (<2 mg/dL); Grade 4 (<1 mg/dL)
[4] Grade 3 (>3 mEq/L); Grade 4 (>8 mEq/L)
[5] Grade 3 (<0.9 mEq/L); Grade 4 (<0.7 mEq/L)

Table 10: Grade 4 Laboratory Abnormalities for Serum Creatinine, Serum Calcium, Serum Phosphorus, and Serum Magnesium in Four Clinical Trials in Patients with Bone Metastases

Laboratory Parameter	Grade 4 Zometa® 4 mg n/N	(%)	Pamidronate 90 mg n/N	(%)	Placebo n/N	(%)
Serum Creatinine[1]*	2/529	(0.4%)	1/268	(0.4%)	0/241	—
Hypocalcemia[2]	6/1041	(0.6%)	2/610	(0.3%)	1/415	(0.2%)
Hypophosphatemia[3]	6/1041	(0.6%)	0/611	—	1/415	(0.2%)
Hypermagnesemia[4]	0/1039	—	0/609	—	2/415	(0.5%)
Hypomagnesemia[5]	2/1039	(0.2%)	2/609	(0.3%)	0/415	—

[1] Grade 3 (>3× Upper Limit of Normal); Grade 4 (>6× Upper Limit of Normal)
* Serum creatinine data for all patients randomized after the 15-minute infusion amendment
[2] Grade 3 (<7 mg/dL); Grade 4 (<6 mg/dL)
[3] Grade 3 (<2 mg/dL); Grade 4 (<1 mg/dL)
[4] Grade 3 (>3 mEq/L); Grade 4 (>8 mEq/L)
[5] Grade 3 (<0.9 mEq/L); Grade 4 (<0.7 mEq/L)

Preparation of Solution
Zometa is reconstituted by adding 5 mL of Sterile Water for Injection, USP, to each vial. The resulting solution allows for withdrawal of 4 mg of zoledronic acid. The drug must be completely dissolved before the solution is withdrawn.

Table 11: Percentage of Patients with Renal Function Deterioration Who Were Randomized Following the 15-Minute Infusion Amendment

Patient Population/Baseline Creatinine

Multiple Myeloma and Breast Cancer	**Zometa® 4 mg**		**Pamidronate 90 mg**	
	n/N	(%)	n/N	(%)
Normal	23/246	(9.3%)	20/246	(8.1%)
Abnormal	1/26	(3.8%)	2/22	(9.1%)
Total	24/272	(8.8%)	22/268	(8.2%)
Solid Tumors	**Zometa® 4 mg**		**Placebo**	
	n/N	(%)	n/N	(%)
Normal	17/154	(11%)	10/143	(7%)
Abnormal	1/11	(9.1%)	1/20	(5%)
Total	18/165	(10.9%)	11/163	(6.7%)
Prostate Cancer	**Zometa® 4 mg**		**Placebo**	
	n/N	(%)	n/N	(%)
Normal	10/82	(12.2%)	7/68	(10.3%)
Abnormal	4/10	(40%)	2/10	(20%)
Total	14/92	(15.2%)	9/78	(11.5%)

The maximum recommended 4 mg-dose must be further diluted in 100 mL of sterile 0.9% Sodium Chloride, USP, or 5% Dextrose Injection, USP. The dose must be given as a single intravenous infusion over no less than 15 minutes.

If not used immediately after reconstitution, for microbiological integrity, the solution should be refrigerated at 36°F–46°F (2°C–8°C). The total time between reconstitution, dilution, storage in the refrigerator, and end of administration must not exceed 24 hours.

Zometa must not be mixed with calcium-containing infusion solutions, such as Lactated Ringer's solution, and should be administered as a single intravenous solution in a line separate from all other drugs.

Method of Administration: **DUE TO THE RISK OF CLINICALLY SIGNIFICANT DETERIORATION IN RENAL FUNCTION, WHICH MAY PROGRESS TO RENAL FAILURE, SINGLE DOSES OF ZOMETA SHOULD NOT EXCEED 4 MG AND THE DURATION OF INFUSION SHOULD BE NO LESS THAN 15 MINUTES. (SEE WARNINGS.)**

There must be strict adherence to the intravenous administration recommendations for Zometa in order to decrease the risk of deterioration in renal function.

Note: **Parenteral drug products should be inspected visually for particulate matter and discoloration prior to administration, whenever solution and container permit.**

HOW SUPPLIED

Each vial contains 4.264 mg zoledronic acid monohydrate, corresponding to 4 mg zoledronic acid on an anhydrous basis, 220 mg of mannitol, USP and 24 mg of sodium citrate, USP.

Carton of 1 vial .... NDC 0078-0350-84

Store at 25°C (77°F); excursions permitted to 15°C–30°C (59°F–86°F).

T2002-21

REV: FEBRUARY 2002 Printed in U.S.A. 89008003

NOVARTIS
Manufactured by
Novartis Pharma AG
Basle, Switzerland for
Novartis Pharmaceuticals Corporation
East Hanover, NJ 07936

Ortho-McNeil Pharmaceutical

RARITAN, NJ 08869-0602

www.ortho-mcneil.com
For Medical Information Contact:
(800) 682-6532
In Emergencies:
(908) 218-7325
For Patient Education Materials Contact:
877-323-2200
For Customer Service (Sales and Ordering):
800-631-5273

TOPAMAX® ℞
[tō '-p-ă-măx]
(topiramate)
Tablets

TOPAMAX® ℞
(topiramate capsules)
Sprinkle Capsules
Prescribing Information

Prescribing information for this product, which appears on pages 2590–2595 of the 2002 PDR, has been completely revised as follows. Please write "See Supplement A" next to the product heading.

DESCRIPTION

Topiramate is a sulfamate-substituted monosaccharide that is intended for use as an antiepileptic drug. TOPAMAX® (topiramate) Tablets are available as 25 mg, 100 mg, and 200 mg round tablets for oral administration. TOPAMAX® (topiramate capsules) Sprinkle Capsules are available as 15 mg and 25 mg sprinkle capsules for oral administration as whole capsules or opened and sprinkled onto soft food.

Topiramate is a white crystalline powder with a bitter taste. Topiramate is most soluble in alkaline solutions containing sodium hydroxide or sodium phosphate and having a pH of 9 to 10. It is freely soluble in acetone, chloroform, dimethylsulfoxide, and ethanol. The solubility in water is 9.8 mg/mL. Its saturated solution has a pH of 6.3. Topiramate has the molecular formula $C_{12}H_{21}NO_8S$ and a molecular weight of 339.37. Topiramate is designated chemically as 2,3:4,5-Di-*O*-isopropylidene-β-D-fructopyranose sulfamate and has the following structural formula:

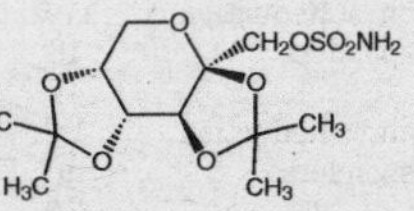

TOPAMAX® (topiramate) Tablets contain the following inactive ingredients: lactose monohydrate, pregelatinized starch, microcrystalline cellulose, sodium starch glycolate, magnesium stearate, purified water, carnauba wax, hydroxypropyl methylcellulose, titanium dioxide, polyethylene glycol, synthetic iron oxide (100 and 200 mg tablets) and polysorbate 80.

TOPAMAX® (topiramate capsules) Sprinkle Capsules contain topiramate coated beads in a hard gelatin capsule. The inactive ingredients are: sugar spheres (sucrose and starch), povidone, cellulose acetate, gelatin, silicone dioxide, sodium lauryl sulfate, titanium dioxide, and black pharmaceutical ink.

CLINICAL PHARMACOLOGY

Mechanism of Action:

The precise mechanism by which topiramate exerts its antiseizure effect is unknown; however, electrophysiological and biochemical studies of the effects of topiramate on cultured neurons have revealed three properties that may contribute to topiramate's antiepileptic efficacy. First, action potentials elicited repetitively by a sustained depolarization of the neurons are blocked by topiramate in a time-dependent manner, suggestive of a state-dependent sodium channel blocking action. Second, topiramate increases the frequency at which γ-aminobutyrate (GABA) activates $GABA_A$ receptors, and enhances the ability of GABA to induce a flux of chloride ions into neurons, suggesting that topiramate potentiates the activity of this inhibitory neurotransmitter. This effect was not blocked by flumazenil, a benzodiazepine antagonist, nor did topiramate increase the duration of the channel open time, differentiating topiramate from barbiturates that modulate $GABA_A$ receptors. Third, topiramate antagonizes the ability of kainate to activate the kainate/AMPA (α-amino-3-hydroxy-5-methylisoxazole-4-propionic acid; non-NMDA) subtype of excitatory amino acid (glutamate) receptor, but has no apparent effect on the activity of N-methyl-D-aspartate (NMDA) at the NMDA receptor subtype. These effects of topiramate are concentration-dependent within the range of 1 µM to 200 µM.

Topiramate also inhibits some isoenzymes of carbonic anhydrase (CA-II and CA-IV). This pharmacologic effect is generally weaker than that of acetazolamide, a known carbonic anhydrase inhibitor, and is not thought to be a major contributing factor to topiramates antiepileptic activity.

Pharmacodynamics:

Topiramate has anticonvulsant activity in rat and mouse maximal electroshock seizure (MES) tests. Topiramate is only weakly effective in blocking clonic seizures induced by the $GABA_A$ receptor antagonist, pentylenetetrazole. Topiramate is also effective in rodent models of epilepsy, which include tonic and absence-like seizures in the spontaneous epileptic rat (SER) and tonic and clonic seizures induced in rats by kindling of the amygdala or by global ischemia.

Pharmacokinetics:

The sprinkle formulation is bioequivalent to the immediate release tablet formulation and, therefore, may be substituted as a therapeutic equivalent.

Absorption of topiramate is rapid, with peak plasma concentrations occurring at approximately 2 hours following a 400 mg oral dose. The relative bioavailability of topiramate from the tablet formulation is about 80% compared to a solution. The bioavailability of topiramate is not affected by food.

The pharmacokinetics of topiramate are linear with dose proportional increases in plasma concentration over the dose range studied (200 to 800 mg/day). The mean plasma elimination half-life is 21 hours after single or multiple doses. Steady state is thus reached in about 4 days in patients with normal renal function. Topiramate is 13–17% bound to human plasma proteins over the concentration range of 1–250 µg/mL.

Metabolism and Excretion:

Topiramate is not extensively metabolized and is primarily eliminated unchanged in the urine (approximately 70% of an administered dose). Six metabolites have been identified in humans, none of which constitutes more than 5% of an administered dose. The metabolites are formed via hydroxylation, hydrolysis, and glucuronidation. There is evidence of renal tubular reabsorption of topiramate. In rats, given probenecid to inhibit tubular reabsorption, along with topiramate, a significant increase in renal clearance of topiramate was observed. This interaction has not been evaluated in humans. Overall, oral plasma clearance (CL/F) is approximately 20 to 30 mL/min in humans following oral administration.

Pharmacokinetic Interactions (see also Drug Interactions):

Antiepileptic Drugs

Potential interactions between topiramate and standard AEDs were assessed in controlled clinical pharmacokinetic studies in patients with epilepsy. The effect of these interactions on mean plasma AUCs are summarized under **PRECAUTIONS (Table 3).**

Special Populations:

Renal Impairment:

The clearance of topiramate was reduced by 42% in moderately renally impaired (creatinine clearance 30–69 mL/min/1.73m^2) and by 54% in severely renally impaired subjects (creatinine clearance <30 mL/min/1.73m^2) compared to normal renal function subjects (creatinine clearance >70 mL/min/1.73m^2). Since topiramate is presumed to undergo significant tubular reabsorption, it is uncertain whether this experience can be generalized to all situations of renal impairment. It is conceivable that some forms of renal disease could differentially affect glomerular filtration rate and tubular reabsorption resulting in a clearance of topiramate not predicted by creatinine clearance. In general, however, use of one-half the usual dose is recommended in patients with moderate or severe renal impairment.

Hemodialysis:

Topiramate is cleared by hemodialysis. Using a high efficiency, counterflow, single pass-dialysate hemodialysis procedure, topiramate dialysis clearance was 120 mL/min with blood flow through the dialyzer at 400 mL/min. This high clearance (compared to 20–30 mL/min total oral clearance in healthy adults) will remove a clinically significant amount of topiramate from the patient over the hemodialysis treatment period. Therefore, a supplemental dose may be required (see **DOSAGE AND ADMINISTRATION**).

Hepatic Impairment:

In hepatically impaired subjects, the clearance of topiramate may be decreased; the mechanism underlying the decrease is not well understood.

Age, Gender, and Race:

Clearance of topiramate in adults was not affected by age (18–67 years), gender, or race.

Pediatric Pharmacokinetics:

Pharmacokinetics of topiramate were evaluated in patients ages 4 to 17 years receiving one or two other antiepileptic drugs. Pharmacokinetic profiles were obtained after one week at doses of 1, 3, and 9 mg/kg/day. Clearance was independent of dose.

Pediatric patients have a 50% higher clearance and consequently shorter elimination half-life than adults. Consequently, the plasma concentration for the same mg/kg dose may be lower in pediatric patients compared to adults. As in adults, hepatic enzyme-inducing antiepileptic drugs decrease the steady state plasma concentrations of topiramate.

CLINICAL STUDIES

The results of controlled clinical trials established the efficacy of TOPAMAX® (topiramate) as adjunctive therapy in adults and pediatric patients ages 2–16 years with partial onset seizures or primary generalized tonic-clonic seizures, and in patients 2 years of age and older with seizures associated with Lennox-Gastaut syndrome.

The studies described in the following sections were conducted using TOPAMAX® (topiramate) Tablets.

Controlled Trials in Patients With Partial Onset Seizures

Adults With Partial Onset Seizures

The effectiveness of topiramate as an adjunctive treatment for adults with partial onset seizures was established in five multicenter, randomized, double-blind, placebo-controlled trials, two comparing several dosages of topiramate and placebo and three comparing a single dosage with placebo, in patients with a history of partial onset seizures, with or without secondarily generalized seizures.

Patients in these studies were permitted a maximum of two antiepileptic drugs (AEDs) in addition to TOPAMAX® Tablets or placebo. In each study, patients were stabilized on optimum dosages of their concomitant AEDs during an 8–12 week baseline phase. Patients who experienced at least 12 (or 8, for 8-week baseline studies) partial onset sei-

Continued on next page

Topamax—Cont.

zures, with or without secondary generalization, during the baseline phase were randomly assigned to placebo or a specified dose of TOPAMAX® Tablets in addition to their other AEDs.

Following randomization, patients began the double-blind phase of treatment. Patients received active drug beginning at 100 mg per day; the dose was then increased by 100 mg or 200 mg/day increments weekly or every other week until the assigned dose was reached, unless intolerance prevented increases. After titration, patients entered an 8- or 12-week stabilization period. The numbers of patients randomized to each dose, and the actual mean, and median doses in the stabilization period are shown in Table 1.

Pediatric Patients Ages 2–16 Years With Partial Onset Seizures

The effectiveness of topiramate as an adjunctive treatment for pediatric patients ages 2–16 years with partial onset seizures was established in a multicenter, randomized, double-blind, placebo-controlled trial, comparing topiramate and placebo in patients with a history of partial onset seizures, with or without secondarily generalized seizures.

Patients in this study were permitted a maximum of two antiepileptic drugs (AEDs) in addition to TOPAMAX® Tablets or placebo. In this study, patients were stabilized on optimum dosages of their concomitant AEDs during an 8-week baseline phase. Patients who experienced at least six partial onset seizures, with or without secondarily generalized seizures, during the baseline phase were randomly assigned to placebo or TOPAMAX® Tablets in addition to their other AEDs.

Following randomization, patients began the double-blind phase of treatment. Patients received active drug beginning at 25 or 50 mg per day; the dose was then increased by 25 mg to 150 mg/day increments every other week until the assigned dosage of 125, 175, 225, or 400 mg/day based on patients' weight to approximate a dosage of 6 mg/kg per day was reached, unless intolerance prevented increases. After titration, patients entered an 8-week stabilization period.

Controlled Trials in Patients With Primary Generalized Tonic-Clonic Seizures

The effectiveness of topiramate as an adjunctive treatment for primary generalized tonic-clonic seizures in patients 2 years old and older was established in a multicenter, randomized, double-blind, placebo-controlled trial, comparing a single dosage of topiramate and placebo.

Patients in this study were permitted a maximum of two antiepileptic drugs (AEDs) in addition to TOPAMAX® or placebo. Patients were stabilized on optimum dosages of their concomitant AEDs during an 8-week baseline phase. Patients who experienced at least three primary generalized tonic-clonic seizures during the baseline phase were randomly assigned to placebo or TOPAMAX® in addition to their other AEDs.

Following randomization, patients began the double-blind phase of treatment. Patients received active drug beginning at 50 mg per day for four weeks; the dose was then increased by 50 mg to 150 mg/day increments every other week until the assigned dose of 175, 225, or 400 mg/day based on patients' body weight to approximate a dosage of 6 mg/kg per day was reached, unless intolerance prevented increases. After titration, patients entered a 12-week stabilization period.

Controlled Trial in Patients With Lennox-Gastaut Syndrome

The effectiveness of topiramate as an adjunctive treatment for seizures associated with Lennox-Gastaut syndrome was established in a multicenter, randomized, double-blind, placebo-controlled trial comparing a single dosage of topiramate with placebo in patients 2 years of age and older.

Patients in this study were permitted a maximum of two antiepileptic drugs (AEDs) in addition to TOPAMAX® or placebo. Patients who were experiencing at least 60 seizures per month before study entry were stabilized on optimum dosages of their concomitant AEDs during a four week baseline phase. Following baseline, patients were randomly assigned to placebo or TOPAMAX® in addition to their other AEDs. Active drug was titrated beginning at 1 mg/kg per day for a week; the dose was then increased to 3 mg/kg per day for one week then to 6 mg/kg per day. After titration, patients entered an 8-week stabilization period. The primary measures of effectiveness were the percent reduction in drop attacks and a parental global rating of seizure severity.

[See table 1 above]

In all add-on trials, the reduction in seizure rate from baseline during the entire double-blind phase was measured. The median percent reductions in seizure rates and the responder rates (fraction of patients with at least a 50% reduction) by treatment group for each study are shown below in Table 2. As described above, a global improvement in seizure severity was also assessed in the Lennox-Gastaut trial.

[See table 2 above]

Subset analyses of the antiepileptic efficacy of TOPAMAX® Tablets in these studies showed no differences as a function of gender, race, age, baseline seizure rate, or concomitant AED.

Table 1: Topiramate Dose Summary During the Stabilization Periods of Each of Five Double-Blind, Placebo-Controlled, Add-On Trials in Adults with Partial Onset Seizures[b]

			Target Topiramate Dosage (mg/day)				
Protocol	Stabilization Dose	Placebo[a]	200	400	600	800	1,000
YD	N	42	42	40	41	—	—
	Mean Dose	5.9	200	390	556	—	—
	Median Dose	6.0	200	400	600	—	—
YE	N	44	—	—	40	45	40
	Mean Dose	9.7	—	—	544	739	796
	Median Dose	10.0	—	—	600	800	1,000
Y1	N	23	—	19	—	—	—
	Mean Dose	3.8	—	395	—	—	—
	Median Dose	4.0	—	400	—	—	—
Y2	N	30	—	—	28	—	—
	Mean Dose	5.7	—	—	522	—	—
	Median Dose	6.0	—	—	600	—	—
Y3	N	28	—	—	—	25	—
	Mean Dose	7.9	—	—	—	568	—
	Median Dose	8.0	—	—	—	600	—

[a] Placebo dosages are given as the number of tablets. Placebo target dosages were as follows: Protocol Y1, 4 tablets/day; Protocols YD and Y2, 6 tablets/day; Protocol Y3, 8 tablets/day; Protocol YE, 10 tablets/day.

[b] Dose-response studies were not conducted for other indications or pediatric partial onset seizures.

Table 2: Efficacy Results in Double-Blind, Placebo-Controlled, Add-On Trials

			Target Topiramate Dosage (mg/day)					
Protocol	Efficacy Results	Placebo	200	400	600	800	1,000	≈6 mg/kg/day*
Partial Onset Seizures Studies in Adults								
YD	N	45	45	45	46	—	—	—
	Median % Reduction	11.6	27.2[a]	47.5[b]	44.7[c]	—	—	—
	% Responders	18	24	44[d]	46[d]	—	—	—
YE	N	47	—	—	48	48	47	—
	Median % Reduction	1.7	—	—	40.8[c]	41.0[c]	36.0[c]	—
	% Responders	9	—	—	40[c]	41[c]	36[d]	—
Y1	N	24	—	23	—	—	—	—
	Median % Reduction	1.1	—	40.7[e]	—	—	—	—
	% Responders	8	—	35[d]	—	—	—	—
Y2	N	30	—	—	30	—	—	—
	Median % Reduction	−12.2	—	—	46.4[f]	—	—	—
	% Responders	10	—	—	47[c]	—	—	—
Y3	N	28	—	—	—	28	—	—
	Median % Reduction	−20.6	—	—	—	24.3[c]	—	—
	% Responders	0	—	—	—	43[c]	—	—
Studies in Pediatric Patients								
YP	N	45	—	—	—	—	—	41
	Median % Reduction	10.5	—	—	—	—	—	33.1[d]
	% Responders	20	—	—	—	—	—	39
Primary Generalized Tonic-Clonic[h]								
YTC	N	40	—	—	—	—	—	39
	Median % Reduction	9.0	—	—	—	—	—	56.7[d]
	% Responders	20	—	—	—	—	—	56[c]
Lennox-Gastaut Syndrome[i]								
YL	N	49	—	—	—	—	—	46
	Median % Reduction	−5.1	—	—	—	—	—	14.8[d]
	% Responders	14	—	—	—	—	—	28[g]
	Improvement in Seizure Severity[j]	28	—	—	—	—	—	52[d]

Comparisons with placebo: [a]p=0.080; [b]p≤0.010; [c]p≤0.001; [d]p≤0.050; [e]p=0.065; [f]p≤0.005; [g]p=0.071; [h]Median % reduction and % responders are reported for PGTC Seizures; [i]Median % reduction and % responders for drop attacks, i.e., toxic or atonic seizures; [j]Percent of subjects who were minimally, much, or very much improved from baseline

*For Protocols YP and YTC, protocol-specified target dosages (<9.3 mg/kg/day) were assigned based on subject's weight to approximate a dosage of 6 mg/kg per day; these dosages corresponded to mg/day dosages of 125, 175, 225, and 400 mg/day.

INDICATIONS AND USAGE

TOPAMAX® (topiramate) Tablets and TOPAMAX® (topiramate capsules) Sprinkle Capsules are indicated as adjunctive therapy for adults and pediatric patients ages 2–16 years with partial onset seizures, or primary generalized tonic-clonic seizures, and in patients 2 years of age and older with seizures associated with Lennox-Gastaut syndrome.

CONTRAINDICATIONS

TOPAMAX® is contraindicated in patients with a history of hypersensitivity to any component of this product.

WARNINGS

Acute Myopia and Secondary Angle Closure Glaucoma

A syndrome consisting of acute myopia associated with secondary angle closure glaucoma has been reported in patients receiving TOPAMAX®. Symptoms include acute onset of decreased visual acuity and/or ocular pain. Opthalmologic findings can include myopia, anterior chamber shallowing, ocular hyperemia (redness) and increased intraocular pressure. Mydriasis may or may not be present. This syndrome may be associated with supraciliary effusion resulting in anterior displacement of the lens and iris, with secondary angle closure glaucoma. Symptoms typically occur within 1 month of initiating TOPAMAX® therapy. In contrast to primary narrow angle glaucoma, which is rare under 40 years of age, secondary angle closure glaucoma associated with topiramate has been reported in pediatric patients as well as adults. The primary treatment to reverse symptoms is discontinuation of TOPAMAX® as rapidly as possible, according to the judgement of the treating physician. Other measures, in conjunction with discontinuation of TOPAMAX®, may be helpful.

Elevated intraocular pressure of any etiology, if left untreated, can lead to serious sequelae including permanent vision loss.

Withdrawal of AEDs

Antiepileptic drugs, including TOPAMAX®, should be withdrawn gradually to minimize the potential of increased seizure frequency.

Cognitive/Neuropsychiatric Adverse Events

Adults

Adverse events most often associated with the use of TOPAMAX® were central nervous system related. In adults, the most significant of these can be classified into two general categories: 1) psychomotor slowing, difficulty with concentration, and speech or language problems, in particular, word-finding difficulties and 2) somnolence or fatigue. Additional nonspecific CNS effects occasionally observed with topiramate as add-on therapy include dizziness or imbalance, confusion, memory problems, and exacerbation of mood disturbances (e.g., irritability and depression). Reports of psychomotor slowing, speech and language problems, and difficulty with concentration and attention were common in adults. Although in some cases these events were mild to moderate, they at times led to withdrawal from treatment. The incidence of psychomotor slowing is only marginally dose-related, but both language problems and difficulty with concentration or attention clearly increased in frequency with increasing dosage in the five double-blind trials [see **ADVERSE REACTIONS, Table 5**].

Somnolence and fatigue were the most frequently reported adverse events during clinical trials with TOPAMAX®. These events were generally mild to moderate and occurred early in therapy. While the incidence of somnolence does not appear to be dose-related, that of fatigue increases at dosages above 400 mg/day.

Pediatric Patients

In double-blind clinical studies, the incidences of cognitive/neuropsychiatric adverse events in pediatric patients were generally lower than previously observed in adults. These events included psychomotor slowing, difficulty with concentration/attention, speech disorders/related speech problems and language problems. The most frequently reported neuropsychiatric events in this population were somnolence and fatigue. No patients discontinued treatment due to adverse events in double-blind trials.

Sudden Unexplained Death in Epilepsy (SUDEP)

During the course of premarketing development of TOPAMAX® (topiramate) Tablets, 10 sudden and unexplained deaths were recorded among a cohort of treated patients (2,796 subject years of exposure). This represents an incidence of 0.0035 deaths per patient year. Although this rate exceeds that expected in a healthy population matched for age and sex, it is within the range of estimates for the incidence of sudden unexplained deaths in patients with epilepsy not receiving TOPAMAX® (ranging from 0.0005 for the general population of patients with epilepsy, to 0.003 for a clinical trial population similar to that in the TOPAMAX® program, to 0.005 for patients with refractory epilepsy).

PRECAUTIONS

General:

Kidney Stones

A total of 32/2,086 (1.5%) of adults exposed to topiramate during its development reported the occurrence of kidney stones, an incidence about 2–4 times that expected in a similar, untreated population. As in the general population, the incidence of stone formation among topiramate treated patients was higher in men. Kidney stones have also been reported in pediatric patients.

An explanation for the association of TOPAMAX® and kidney stones may lie in the fact that topiramate is a weak carbonic anhydrase inhibitor. Carbonic anhydrase inhibitors, e.g., acetazolamide or dichlorphenamide, promote stone formation by reducing urinary citrate excretion and by increasing urinary pH. The concomitant use of TOPAMAX® with other carbonic anhydrase inhibitors or potentially in patients on a ketogenic diet may create a physiological environment that increases the risk of kidney stone formation, and should therefore be avoided.

Increased fluid intake increases the urinary output, lowering the concentration of substances involved in stone formation. Hydration is recommended to reduce new stone formation.

Paresthesia

Paresthesia, an effect associated with the use of other carbonic anhydrase inhibitors, appears to be a common effect of TOPAMAX®.

Adjustment of Dose in Renal Failure

The major route of elimination of unchanged topiramate and its metabolites is via the kidney. Dosage adjustment may be required (see **DOSAGE AND ADMINISTRATION**).

Decreased Hepatic Function

In hepatically impaired patients, topiramate should be administered with caution as the clearance of topiramate may be decreased.

Information for Patients

Patients taking TOPAMAX® should be told to seek immediate medical attention if they experience blurred vision or periorbital pain.

Patients, particularly those with predisposing factors, should be instructed to maintain an adequate fluid intake in order to minimize the risk of renal stone formation [see **PRECAUTIONS: General**, for support regarding hydration as a preventative measure].

Patients should be warned about the potential for somnolence, dizziness, confusion, and difficulty concentrating and advised not to drive or operate machinery until they have gained sufficient experience on topiramate to gauge whether it adversely affects their mental and/or motor performance.

Additional food intake may be considered if the patient is losing weight while on this medication.

Please refer to the end of the product labeling for important information on how to take TOPAMAX® (topiramate capsules) Sprinkle Capsules.

Drug Interactions:

Antiepileptic Drugs

Potential interactions between topiramate and standard AEDs were assessed in controlled clinical pharmacokinetic studies in patients with epilepsy. The effects of these interactions on mean plasma AUCs are summarized in the following table:

In Table 3, the second column (AED concentration) describes what happens to the concentration of the AED listed in the first column when topiramate is added.

The third column (topiramate concentration) describes how the coadministration of a drug listed in the first column modifies the concentration of topiramate in experimental settings when TOPAMAX® was given alone.

[See table 3 above]

Other Drug Interactions

Digoxin: In a single-dose study, serum digoxin AUC was decreased by 12% with concomitant TOPAMAX® administration. The clinical relevance of this observation has not been established.

CNS Depressants: Concomitant administration of TOPAMAX® and alcohol or other CNS depressant drugs has not been evaluated in clinical studies. Because of the potential of topiramate to cause CNS depression, as well as other cognitive and/or neuropsychiatric adverse events, topiramate should be used with extreme caution if used in combination with alcohol and other CNS depressants.

Table 3: Summary of AED Interactions with TOPAMAX®

AED Co-administered	AED Concentration	Topiramate Concentration
Phenytoin	NC or 25% increase[a]	48% decrease
Carbamazepine (CBZ)	NC	40% decrease
CBZ epoxide[b]	NC	NE
Valproic acid	11% decrease	14% decrease
Phenobarbital	NC	NE
Primidone	NC	NE

a = Plasma concentration increased 25% in some patients, generally those on a b.i.d. dosing regimen of phenytoin.
b = is not administered but is an active metabolite of carbamazepine.
NC = Less than 10% change in plasma concentration.
AED = Antiepileptic drug.
NE = Not Evaluated.

Table 4: Incidence of Treatment-Emergent Adverse Events in Placebo-Controlled, Add-On Trials in Adults[a,b] Where Rate Was > 1% in Either Topiramate Group and Greater Than the Rate in Placebo-Treated Patients

		TOPAMAX® Dosage (mg/day)	
Body System/ Adverse Event[c]	Placebo (N=291)	200–400 (N=183)	600–1,000 (N=414)
Body as a Whole—General Disorders			
Fatigue	13	15	30
Asthenia	1	6	3
Back Pain	4	5	3
Chest Pain	3	4	2
Influenza-Like Symptoms	2	3	4
Leg Pain	2	2	4
Hot Flushes	1	2	1
Allergy	1	2	3
Edema	1	2	1
Body Odor	0	1	0
Rigors	0	1	<1
Central & Peripheral Nervous System Disorders			
Dizziness	15	25	32
Ataxia	7	16	14
Speech Disorders/Related Speech Problems	2	13	11
Paresthesia	4	11	19
Nystagmus	7	10	11
Tremor	6	9	9
Language Problems	1	6	10
Coordination Abnormal	2	4	4
Hypoaesthesia	1	2	1
Gait Abnormal	1	3	2
Muscle Contractions Involuntary	1	2	2
Stupor	0	2	1
Vertigo	1	1	2
Gastro-Intestinal System Disorders			
Nausea	8	10	12
Dyspepsia	6	7	6
Abdominal Pain	4	6	7
Constipation	2	4	3
Gastroenteritis	1	2	1
Dry Mouth	1	2	4
Gingivitis	<1	1	1
GI Disorder	<1	1	0
Hearing and Vestibular Disorders			
Hearing Decreased	1	2	1
Metabolic and Nutritional Disorders			
Weight Decrease	3	9	13
Muscle-Skeletal System Disorders			
Myalgia	1	2	2
Skeletal Pain	0	1	0
Platelet, Bleeding & Clotting Disorders			
Epistaxis	1	2	1
Psychiatric Disorders			
Somnolence	12	29	28
Nervousness	6	16	19
Psychomotor Slowing	2	13	21
Difficulty with Memory	3	12	14
Anorexia	4	10	12
Confusion	5	11	14
Depression	5	5	13
Difficulty with Concentration/Attention	2	6	14
Mood Problems	2	4	9
Agitation	2	3	3
Aggressive Reaction	2	3	3
Emotional Lability	1	3	3
Cognitive Problems	1	3	3
Libido Decreased	1	2	<1
Apathy	1	1	3
Depersonalization	1	1	2

(Table continued on next page)

Oral Contraceptives: In a pharmacokinetic interaction study with oral contraceptives using a combination product containing norethindrone and ethinyl estradiol, TOPAMAX® did not significantly affect the clearance of norethindrone. The mean oral clearance of ethinyl estradiol at 800 mg/day dose was increased by 47% (range: 13–107%). The mean total exposure to the estrogenic component decreased by 18%, 21%, and 30% at daily doses of 200, 400, and 800 mg/day, respectively. Therefore, efficacy of oral contraceptives may be compromised by topiramate. Patients taking oral contraceptives should be asked to report any change in their bleeding patterns. The effect of oral contraceptives on the pharmacokinetics of topiramate is not known.

Metformin: A drug-drug interaction study conducted in healthy volunteers evaluated the steady-state pharmacokinetics of metformin and topiramate in plasma when metformin was given alone and when metformin and topiramate were given simultaneously. The results of this study indicated that metformin mean C_{max} and mean AUC_{0-12h} increased by 18% and 25%, respectively, while mean CL/F decreased 20% when metformin was co-administered with topiramate. Topiramate did not affect metformin t_{max}. The clinical significance of the effect of topiramate on metformin pharmacokinetics is unclear. Oral plasma clearance of topiramate appears to be reduced when

Continued on next page

Topamax—Cont.

administered with metformin. The extent of change in the clearance is unknown. The clinical significance of the effect of metformin on topiramate pharmacokinetics is unclear. When TOPAMAX® is added or withdrawn in patients on metformin therapy, careful attention should be given to the routine monitoring for adequate control of their diabetic disease state.

Others: Concomitant use of TOPAMAX®, a weak carbonic anhydrase inhibitor, with other carbonic anhydrase inhibitors, e.g., acetazolamide or dichlorphenamide, may create a physiological environment that increases the risk of renal stone formation, and should therefore be avoided.

Laboratory Tests: There are no known interactions of topiramate with commonly used laboratory tests.

Carcinogenesis, Mutagenesis, Impairment of Fertility:
An increase in urinary bladder tumors was observed in mice given topiramate (20, 75, and 300 mg/kg) in the diet for 21 months. The elevated bladder tumor incidence, which was statistically significant in males and females receiving 300 mg/kg, was primarily due to the increased occurrence of a smooth muscle tumor considered histomorphologically unique to mice. Plasma exposures in mice receiving 300 mg/kg were approximately 0.5 to 1 times steady state exposures measured in patients receiving topiramate monotherapy at the recommended human dose (RHD) of 400 mg, and 1.5 to 2 times steady state topiramate exposures in patients receiving 400 mg of topiramate plus phenytoin. The relevance of this finding to human carcinogenic risk is uncertain. No evidence of carcinogenicity was seen in rats following oral administration of topiramate for 2 years at doses up to 120 mg/kg (approximately 3 times the RHD on a mg/m^2 basis).

Topiramate did not demonstrate genotoxic potential when tested in a battery of *in vitro* and *in vivo* assays. Topiramate was not mutagenic in the Ames test or the *in vitro* mouse lymphoma assay; it did not increase unscheduled DNA synthesis in rat hepatocytes *in vitro*; and it did not increase chromosomal aberrations in human lymphocytes *in vitro* or in rat bone marrow *in vivo*.

No adverse effects on male or female fertility were observed in rats at doses up to 100 mg/kg (2.5 times the RHD on a mg/m^2 basis).

Pregnancy: Pregnancy Category C.
Topiramate has demonstrated selective developmental toxicity, including teratogenicity, in several animal studies. When oral doses of 20, 100, or 500 mg/kg were administered to pregnant mice during the period of organogenesis, the incidence of fetal malformations (primarily craniofacial defects) was increased at all doses. The low dose is approximately 0.2 times the recommended human dose (RHD=400 mg/day) on a mg/m^2 basis. Fetal body weights and skeletal ossification were reduced at 500 mg/kg in conjunction with decreased maternal body weight gain.

In rat studies (oral doses of 20, 100, and 500 mg/kg or 0.2, 2.5, 30 and 400 mg/kg), the frequency of limb malformations (ectrodactyly, micromelia, and amelia) was increased among the offspring of dams treated with 400 mg/kg (10 times the RHD on a mg/m^2 basis) or greater during the organogenesis period of pregnancy. Embryotoxicity (reduced fetal body weights, increased incidence of structural variations) was observed at doses as low as 20 mg/kg (0.5 times the RHD on a mg/m^2 basis). Clinical signs of maternal toxicity were seen at 400 mg/kg and above, and maternal body weight gain was reduced during treatment with 100 mg/kg or greater.

In rabbit studies (20, 60, and 180 mg/kg or 10, 35, and 120 mg/kg orally during organogenesis), embryo/fetal mortality was increased at 35 mg/kg (2 times the RHD on a mg/m^2 basis) or greater, and teratogenic effects (primarily rib and vertebral malformations) were observed at 120 mg/kg (6 times the RHD on a mg/m^2 basis). Evidence of maternal toxicity (decreased body weight gain, clinical signs, and/or mortality) was seen at 35 mg/kg and above.

When female rats were treated during the latter part of gestation and throughout lactation (0.2, 4, 20, and 100 mg/kg or 2, 20, and 200 mg/kg), offspring exhibited decreased viability and delayed physical development at 200 mg/kg (5 times the RHD on a mg/m^2 basis) and reductions in pre- and/or postweaning body weight gain at 2 mg/kg (0.05 times the RHD on a mg/m^2 basis) and above. Maternal toxicity (decreased body weight gain, clinical signs) was evident at 100 mg/kg or greater.

In a rat embryo/fetal development study with a postnatal component (0.2, 2.5, 30 or 400 mg/kg during organogenesis; noted above), pups exhibited delayed physical development at 400 mg/kg (10 times the RHD on a mg/m^2 basis) and persistent reductions in body weight gain at 30 mg/kg (1 times the RHD on a mg/m^2 basis) and higher.

There are no studies using TOPAMAX® in pregnant women. TOPAMAX® should be used during pregnancy only if the potential benefit outweighs the potential risk to the fetus.

In post-marketing experience, cases of hypospadias have been reported in male infants exposed in utero to topiramate, with or without other anticonvulsants; however, a causal relationship with topiramate has not been established.

Labor and Delivery:
In studies of rats where dams were allowed to deliver pups naturally, no drug-related effects on gestation length or parturition were observed at dosage levels up to 200 mg/kg/day. The effect of TOPAMAX® on labor and delivery in humans is unknown.

Table 4: Incidence of Treatment-Emergent Adverse Events in Placebo-Controlled, Add-On Trials in Adults[a,b] Where Rate Was > 1% in Either Topiramate Group and Greater Than the Rate in Placebo-Treated Patients — *(cont.)*

Body System/ Adverse Event[c]	Placebo (N=291)	TOPAMAX® Dosage (mg/day) 200–400 (N=183)	600–1,000 (N=414)
Reproductive Disorders, Female			
Breast Pain	2	4	0
Amenorrhea	1	2	2
Menorrhagia	0	2	1
Menstrual Disorder	1	2	1
Reproductive Disorders, Male			
Prostatic Disorder	<1	2	0
Resistance Mechanism Disorders			
Infection	1	2	1
Infection Viral	1	2	<1
Moniliasis	<1	1	0
Respiratory System Disorders			
Pharyngitis	2	6	3
Rhinitis	6	7	6
Sinusitis	4	5	6
Dyspnea	1	1	2
Skin and Appendages Disorders			
Skin Disorder	<1	2	1
Sweating Increased	<1	1	<1
Rash Erythematous	<1	1	<1
Special Sense Other, Disorders			
Taste Perversion	0	2	4
Urinary System Disorders			
Hematuria	1	2	<1
Urinary Tract Infection	1	2	3
Micturition Frequency	1	1	2
Urinary Incontinence	<1	2	1
Urine Abnormal	0	1	<1
Vision Disorders			
Vision Abnormal	2	13	10
Diplopia	5	10	10
White Cell and RES Disorders			
Leukopenia	1	2	1

[a] Patients in these add-on trials were receiving 1 to 2 concomitant antiepileptic drugs in addition to TOPAMAX® or placebo.
[b] Values represent the percentage of patients reporting a given adverse event. Patients may have reported more than one adverse event during the study and can be included in more than one adverse event category.
[c] Adverse events reported by at least 1% of patients in the TOPAMAX® 200–400 mg/day group and more common than in the placebo group are listed in this table.

Table 5: Incidence (%) of Dose-Related Adverse Events From Placebo-Controlled, Add-On Trials in Adults with Partial Onset Seizures[a]

Adverse Event	Placebo (N = 216)	TOPAMAX® Dosage (mg/day) 200 (N = 45)	400 (N = 68)	600–1,000 (N = 414)
Fatigue	13	11	12	30
Nervousness	7	13	18	19
Difficulty with Concentration/Attention	1	7	9	14
Confusion	4	9	10	14
Depression	6	9	7	13
Anorexia	4	4	6	12
Language problems	<1	2	9	10
Anxiety	6	2	3	10
Mood problems	2	0	6	9
Weight decrease	3	4	9	13

[a] Dose-response studies were not conducted for other indications or for pediatric indications.

Nursing Mothers:
Topiramate is excreted in the milk of lactating rats. It is not known if topiramate is excreted in human milk. Since many drugs are excreted in human milk, and because the potential for serious adverse reactions in nursing infants to TOPAMAX® is unknown, the potential benefit to the mother should be weighed against the potential risk to the infant when considering recommendations regarding nursing.

Pediatric Use:
Safety and effectiveness in patients below the age of 2 years have not been established.

Geriatric Use:
In clinical trials, 2% of patients were over 60. No age related difference in effectiveness or adverse effects were seen. There were no pharmacokinetic differences related to age alone, although the possibility of age-associated renal functional abnormalities should be considered.

Race and Gender Effects:
Evaluation of effectiveness and safety in clinical trials has shown no race or gender related effects.

ADVERSE REACTIONS

The data described in the following section were obtained using TOPAMAX® (topiramate) Tablets.

The most commonly observed adverse events associated with the use of topiramate at dosages of 200 to 400 mg/day in controlled trials in adults with partial onset seizures, primary generalized tonic-clonic seizures, or Lennox-Gastaut syndrome, that were seen at greater frequency in topiramate-treated patients and did not appear to be dose-related were: somnolence, dizziness, ataxia, speech disorders and related speech problems, psychomotor slowing, abnormal vision, difficulty with memory, paresthesia and diplopia [see Table 4]. The most common dose-related adverse events at dosages of 200 to 1,000 mg/day were: fatigue, nervousness, difficulty with concentration or attention, confusion, depression, anorexia, language problems, anxiety, mood problems, and weight decrease [see Table 5].

Adverse events associated with the use of topiramate at dosages of 5 to 9 mg/kg/day in controlled trials in pediatric patients with partial onset seizures, primary generalized tonic-clonic seizures, or Lennox-Gastaut syndrome, that were seen at greater frequency in topiramate-treated patients were: fatigue, somnolence, anorexia, nervousness, difficulty with concentration/attention, difficulty with memory, aggressive reaction, and weight decrease [see Table 6].

In controlled clinical trials in adults, 11% of patients receiving topiramate 200 to 400 mg/day as adjunctive therapy discontinued due to adverse events. This rate appeared to increase at dosages above 400 mg/day. Adverse events associated with discontinuing therapy included somnolence, dizziness, anxiety, difficulty with concentration or attention, fatigue, and paresthesia and increased at dosages above 400 mg/day. None of the pediatric patients who received topiramate adjunctive therapy at 5 to 9 mg/kg/day in controlled clinical trials discontinued due to adverse events.

Approximately 28% of the 1,757 adults with epilepsy who received topiramate at dosages of 200 to 1,600 mg/day in clinical studies discontinued treatment because of adverse events; an individual patient could have reported more than one adverse event. These adverse events were: psychomotor slowing (4.0%), difficulty with memory (3.2%), fatigue (3.2%), confusion (3.1%), somnolence (3.2%), difficulty with concentration/attention (2.9%), anorexia (2.7%), depression (2.6%), dizziness (2.5%), weight decrease (2.5%), nervousness (2.3%), ataxia (2.1%), and paresthesia (2.0%). Approximately 11% of the 310 pediatric patients who received topiramate at dosages up to 30 mg/kg/day discontinued due to adverse events. Adverse events associated with discontinuing therapy included aggravated convulsions (2.3%), difficulty with concentration/attention (1.6%), language problems (1.3%), personality disorder (1.3%), and somnolence (1.3%).

Incidence in Controlled Clinical Trials—Add-On Therapy
Table 4 lists treatment-emergent adverse events that occurred in at least 1% of adults treated with 200 to 400 mg/day topiramate in controlled trials that were numerically more common at this dose than in the patients treated with placebo. In general, most patients who experienced adverse events during the first eight weeks of these trials no longer experienced them by their last visit. Table 6 lists treatment-emergent adverse events that occurred in at least 1% of pediatric patients treated with 5 to 9 mg/kg topiramate in controlled trials that were numerically more common than in patients treated with placebo.
The prescriber should be aware that these data were obtained when TOPAMAX® was added to concurrent antiepileptic drug therapy and cannot be used to predict the frequency of adverse events in the course of usual medical practice where patient characteristics and other factors may differ from those prevailing during clinical studies. Similarly, the cited frequencies cannot be directly compared with data obtained from other clinical investigations involving different treatments, uses, or investigators. Inspection of these frequencies, however, does provide the prescribing physician with a basis to estimate the relative contribution of drug and non-drug factors to the adverse event incidences in the population studied.
[See table 4 on pages 249 and 250]
[See table 5 at top of previous page]
[See table above]

Other Adverse Events Observed
Other events that occurred in more than 1% of adults treated with 200 to 400 mg of topiramate in placebo-controlled trials but with equal or greater frequency in the placebo group were: headache, injury, anxiety, rash, pain, convulsions aggravated, coughing, fever, diarrhea, vomiting, muscle weakness, insomnia, personality disorder, dysmenorrhea, upper respiratory tract infection, and eye pain.

Other Adverse Events Observed During All Clinical Trials
Topiramate, initiated as adjunctive therapy, has been administered to 1,757 adults and 310 pediatric patients with epilepsy during all clinical studies. During these studies, all adverse events were recorded by the clinical investigators using terminology of their own choosing. To provide a meaningful estimate of the proportion of individuals having adverse events, similar types of events were grouped into a smaller number of standardized categories using modified WHOART dictionary terminology. The frequencies presented represent the proportion of patients who experienced an event of the type cited on at least one occasion while receiving topiramate. Reported events are included except those already listed in the previous table or text, those too general to be informative, and those not reasonably associated with the use of the drug.
Events are classified within body system categories and enumerated in order of decreasing frequency using the following definitions: *frequent* occurring in at least 1/100 patients; *infrequent* occurring in 1/100 to 1/1000 patients; *rare* occurring in fewer than 1/1000 patients.

Autonomic Nervous System Disorders: *Infrequent:* vasodilation.

Body as a Whole: *Frequent:* fever. *Infrequent:* syncope, abdomen enlarged. *Rare:* alcohol intolerance.

Cardiovascular Disorders, General: *Infrequent:* hypotension, postural hypotension.

Central & Peripheral Nervous System Disorders: *Frequent:* hypertonia. *Infrequent:* neuropathy, apraxia, hyperaesthesia, dyskinesia, dysphonia, scotoma, ptosis, dystonia, visual field defect, encephalopathy, upper motor neuron lesion, EEG abnormal. *Rare:* cerebellar syndrome, tongue paralysis.

Gastrointestinal System Disorders: *Frequent:* diarrhea, vomiting, hemorrhoids. *Infrequent:* stomatitis, melena, gastritis, tongue edema, esophagitis.

Hearing and Vestibular Disorders: *Frequent:* tinnitus.

Heart Rate and Rhythm Disorders: *Infrequent:* AV block, bradycardia.

Liver and Biliary System Disorders: *Infrequent:* SGPT increased, SGOT increased, gamma-GT increased.

Metabolic and Nutritional Disorders: *Frequent:* dehydration. *Infrequent:* hypokalemia, alkaline phosphatase increased, hypocalcemia, hyperlipemia, acidosis, hyperglycemia, hyperchloremia, xerophthalmia. *Rare:* diabetes mellitus, hypernatremia, hyponatremia, hypocholesterolemia, hypophosphatemia, creatinine increased.

Musculoskeletal System Disorders: *Frequent:* arthralgia, muscle weakness. *Infrequent:* arthrosis.

Myo-, Endo-, Pericardial & Valve Disorders: *Infrequent:* angina pectoris.

Neoplasms: *Infrequent:* thrombocythemia. *Rare:* polycythemia.

Platelet, Bleeding, and Clotting Disorders: *Infrequent:* gingival bleeding, pulmonary embolism.

Psychiatric Disorders: *Frequent:* impotence, hallucination, euphoria, psychosis. *Infrequent:* paranoid reaction, delusion, paranoia, delirium, abnormal dreaming, neurosis, libido increased, manic reaction, suicide attempt.

Red Blood Cell Disorders: *Frequent:* anemia. *Rare:* marrow depression, pancytopenia.

Reproductive Disorders, Male: *Infrequent:* ejaculation disorder, breast discharge.

Skin and Appendages Disorders: *Frequent:* acne, urticaria. *Infrequent:* photosensitivity reaction, sweating decreased, abnormal hair texture. *Rare:* chloasma.

Special Senses Other, Disorders: *Infrequent:* taste loss, parosmia.

Table 6: Incidence (%) of Treatment-Emergent Adverse Events in Placebo-Controlled, Add-On Trials in Pediatric Patients Ages 2–16 Years[a,b] (Events that Occurred in at Least 1% of Topiramate-Treated Patients and Occurred More Frequently in Topiramate-Treated Than Placebo-Treated Patients)

Body System/ Adverse Event	Placebo (N=101)	Topiramate (N=98)
Body as a Whole—General Disorders		
Fatigue	5	16
Injury	13	14
Allergic Reaction	1	2
Back Pain	0	1
Pallor	0	1
Cardiovascular Disorders, General		
Hypertension	0	1
Central & Peripheral Nervous System Disorders		
Gait Abnormal	5	8
Ataxia	2	6
Hyperkinesia	4	5
Dizziness	2	4
Speech Disorders/Related Speech Problems	2	4
Hyporeflexia	0	2
Convulsions Grand Mal	0	1
Fecal Incontinence	0	1
Paresthesia	0	1
Gastro-Intestinal System Disorders		
Nausea	5	6
Saliva Increased	4	6
Constipation	4	5
Gastroenteritis	2	3
Dysphagia	0	1
Flatulence	0	1
Gastroesophageal Reflux	0	1
Glossitis	0	1
Gum Hyperplasia	0	1
Heart Rate and Rhythm Disorders		
Bradycardia	0	1
Metabolic and Nutritional Disorders		
Weight Decrease	1	9
Thirst	1	2
Hypoglycemia	0	1
Weight Increase	0	1
Platelet, Bleeding, & Clotting Disorders		
Purpura	4	8
Epistaxis	1	4
Hematoma	0	1
Prothrombin Increased	0	1
Thrombocytopenia	0	1
Psychiatric Disorders		
Somnolence	16	26
Anorexia	15	24
Nervousness	7	14
Personality Disorder (Behavior Problems)	9	11
Difficulty with Concentration/Attention	2	10
Aggressive Reaction	4	9
Insomnia	7	8
Difficulty with Memory NOS	0	5
Confusion	3	4
Psychomotor Slowing	2	3
Appetite Increased	0	1
Neurosis	0	1
Reproductive Disorders, Female		
Leukorrhoea	0	2
Resistance Mechanism Disorders		
Infection Viral	3	7
Respiratory System Disorders		
Pneumonia	1	5
Respiratory Disorder	0	1
Skin and Appendages Disorders		
Skin Disorder	2	3
Alopecia	1	2
Dermatitis	0	2
Hypertrichosis	1	2
Rash Erythematous	0	2
Eczema	0	1
Seborrhoea	0	1
Skin Discoloration	0	1
Urinary System Disorders		
Urinary Incontinence	2	4
Nocturia	0	1
Vision Disorders		
Eye Abnormality	1	2
Vision Abnormal	1	2
Diplopia	0	1
Lacrimation Abnormal	0	1
Myopia	0	1
White Cell and RES Disorders		
Leukopenia	0	2

[a] Patients in these add-on trials were receiving 1 to 2 concomitant antiepileptic drugs in addition to TOPAMAX® or placebo.
[b] Values represent the percentage of patients reporting a given adverse event. Patients may have reported more than one adverse event during the study and can be included in more than one adverse event category.

Urinary System Disorders: *Frequent:* dysuria, renal calculus. *Infrequent:* urinary retention, face edema, renal pain, albuminuria, polyuria, oliguria.

Vascular (Extracardiac) Disorders: *Infrequent:* flushing, deep vein thrombosis, phlebitis. *Rare:* vasospasm.

Vision Disorders: *Frequent:* conjunctivitis. *Infrequent:* abnormal accommodation, photophobia, strabismus, mydriasis. *Rare:* iritis.

White Cell and Reticuloendothelial System Disorders: *Infrequent:* lymphadenopathy, eosinophilia, lymphopenia, granulocytopenia, lymphocytosis.

Postmarketing and Other Experience
In addition to the adverse experiences reported during clinical testing of TOPAMAX®, the following adverse experiences have been reported in patients receiving marketed TOPAMAX® from worldwide use since approval. These adverse experiences have not been listed above and data are insufficient to support an estimate of their incidence or to establish causation. The listing is alphabetized: hepatic failure, hepatitis, pancreatitis, and renal tubular acidosis.

Continued on next page

Topamax—Cont.

DRUG ABUSE AND DEPENDENCE

The abuse and dependence potential of TOPAMAX® has not been evaluated in human studies.

OVERDOSAGE

In acute TOPAMAX® overdose, if the ingestion is recent, the stomach should be emptied immediately by lavage or by induction of emesis. Activated charcoal has not been shown to adsorb topiramate *in vitro*. Therefore, its use in overdosage is not recommended. Treatment should be appropriately supportive. Hemodialysis is an effective means of removing topiramate from the body. However, in the few cases of acute overdosage reported, hemodialysis has not been necessary.

DOSAGE AND ADMINISTRATION

TOPAMAX® has been shown to be effective in adults and pediatric patients ages 2–16 years with partial onset seizures or primary generalized tonic-clonic seizures, and in patients 2 years of age and older with seizures associated with Lennox-Gastaut syndrome. In the controlled add-on trials, no correlation has been demonstrated between trough plasma concentrations of topiramate and clinical efficacy. No evidence of tolerance has been demonstrated in humans. Doses above 400 mg/day (600, 800, or 1000 mg/day) have not been shown to improve responses in dose-response studies in adults with partial onset seizures.

It is not necessary to monitor topiramate plasma concentrations to optimize TOPAMAX® therapy. On occasion, the addition of TOPAMAX® to phenytoin may require an adjustment of the dose of phenytoin to achieve optimal clinical outcome. Addition or withdrawal of phenytoin and/or carbamazepine during adjunctive therapy with TOPAMAX® may require adjustment of the dose of TOPAMAX®. Because of the bitter taste, tablets should not be broken.

TOPAMAX® can be taken without regard to meals.

Adults (17 Years of Age and Over)

The recommended total daily dose of TOPAMAX® as adjunctive therapy is 400 mg/day in two divided doses. In studies of adults with partial onset seizures, a daily dose of 200 mg/day has inconsistent effects and is less effective than 400 mg/day. It is recommended that therapy be initiated at 25–50 mg/day followed by titration to an effective dose in increments of 25–50 mg/week. Titrating in increments of 25 mg/week may delay the time to reach an effective dose. Daily doses above 1,600 mg have not been studied.

In the study of primary generalized tonic-clonic seizures the initial titration rate was slower than in previous studies; the assigned dose was reached at the end of 8 weeks (see **CLINICAL STUDIES, Controlled Trials in Patients With Primary Generalized Tonic-Clonic Seizures**).

Pediatric Patients (Ages 2–16 Years)—Partial Seizures, Primary Generalized Tonic-Clonic Seizures, or Lennox-Gastaut Syndrome

The recommended total daily dose of TOPAMAX® (topiramate) as adjunctive therapy for patients with partial seizures, primary generalized tonic-clonic seizures, or seizures associated with Lennox-Gastaut Syndrome is approximately 5 to 9 mg/kg/day in two divided doses. Titration should begin at 25 mg (or less, based on a range of 1 to 3 mg/kg/day) nightly for the first week. The dosage should then be increased at 1- or 2-week intervals by increments of 1 to 3 mg/kg/day (administered in two divided doses), to achieve optimal clinical response. Dose titration should be guided by clinical outcome.

In the study of primary generalized tonic-clonic seizures the initial titration rate was slower than in previous studies; the assigned dose of 6 mg/kg/day was reached at the end of 8 weeks (see **CLINICAL STUDIES, Controlled Trials in Patients With Primary Generalized Tonic-Clonic Seizures**).

Administration of TOPAMAX® Sprinkle Capsules

TOPAMAX® (topiramate capsules) Sprinkle Capsules may be swallowed whole or may be administered by carefully opening the capsule and sprinkling the entire contents on a small amount (teaspoon) of soft food. This drug/food mixture should be swallowed immediately and not chewed. It should not be stored for future use.

Patients with Renal Impairment:

In renally impaired subjects (creatinine clearance less than 70 mL/min/1.73m²), one half of the usual adult dose is recommended. Such patients will require a longer time to reach steady-state at each dose.

Patients Undergoing Hemodialysis:

Topiramate is cleared by hemodialysis at a rate that is 4 to 6 times greater than a normal individual. Accordingly, a prolonged period of dialysis may cause topiramate concentration to fall below that required to maintain an anti-seizure effect. To avoid rapid drops in topiramate plasma concentration during hemodialysis, a supplemental dose of topiramate may be required. The actual adjustment should take into account 1) the duration of dialysis period, 2) the clearance rate of the dialysis system being used, and 3) the effective renal clearance of topiramate in the patient being dialyzed.

Patients with Hepatic Disease:

In hepatically impaired patients topiramate plasma concentrations may be increased. The mechanism is not well understood.

HOW SUPPLIED

TOPAMAX® (topiramate) Tablets is available as debossed, coated, round tablets in the following strengths and colors:
25 mg white (coded "TOP" on one side; "25" on the other)
100 mg yellow (coded "TOPAMAX" on one side; "100" on the other)
200 mg salmon (coded "TOPAMAX" on one side; "200" on the other)

They are supplied as follows:
25 mg tablets—bottles of 60 count with desiccant (NDC 0045-0639-65)
100 mg tablets bottles of 60 count with desiccant (NDC 0045-0641-65)
200 mg tablets bottles of 60 count with desiccant (NDC 0045-0642-65)

TOPAMAX® (topiramate capsules) Sprinkle Capsules contain small, white to off white spheres. The gelatin capsules are white and clear.

They are marked as follows:
15 mg capsule with "TOP" and "15 mg" on the side
25 mg capsule with "TOP" and "25 mg" on the side

The capsules are supplied as follows:
15 mg capsules—bottles of 60 (NDC 0045-0647-65)
25 mg capsules—bottles of 60 (NDC 0045-0645-65)

TOPAMAX® (topiramate) Tablets should be stored in tightly-closed containers at controlled room temperature, (59 to 86°F, 15 to 30°C). Protect from moisture.

TOPAMAX® (topiramate capsules) Sprinkle Capsules should be stored in tightly-closed containers at or below 25°C (77°F). Protect from moisture.

TOPAMAX® (topiramate) and TOPAMAX® (topiramate capsules) are trademarks of Ortho-McNeil Pharmaceutical.

HOW TO TAKE

TOPAMAX® (topiramate capsules) SPRINKLE CAPSULES

A Guide for Patients and Their Caregivers

Your doctor has given you a prescription for TOPAMAX® (topiramate capsules) Sprinkle Capsules. Here are your instructions for taking this medication. Please read these instructions prior to use.

To Take With Food

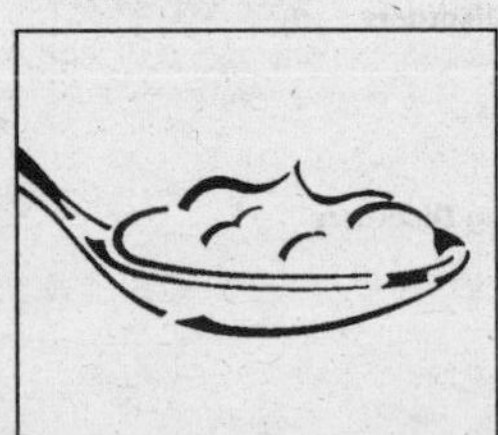

You may sprinkle the contents of TOPAMAX® Sprinkle Capsules on a small amount (teaspoon) of soft food, such as applesauce, custard, ice cream, oatmeal, pudding, or yogurt.

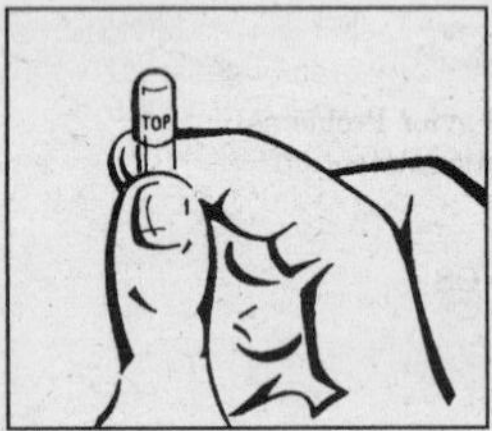

Hold the capsule upright so that you can read the word "TOP".

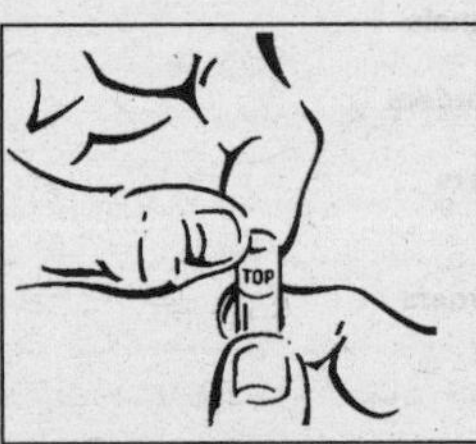

Carefully twist off the clear portion of the capsule. You may find it best to do this over the small portion of the food onto which you will be pouring the sprinkles.

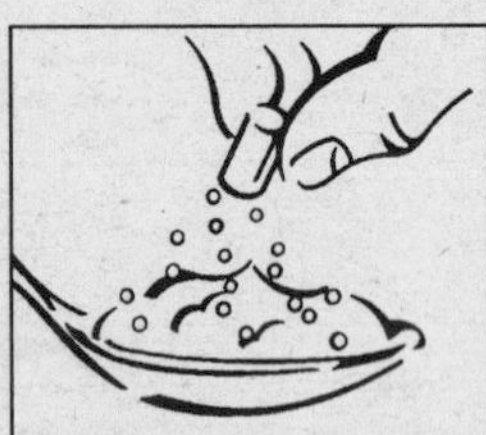

Sprinkle all of the capsule's contents onto a spoonful of soft food, taking care to see that the entire prescribed dosage is sprinkled onto the food.

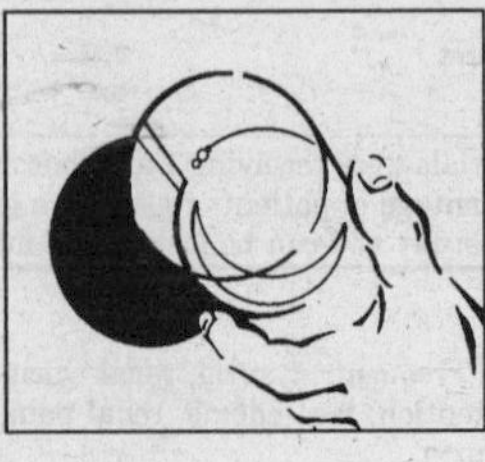

Be sure the patient swallows the entire spoonful of the sprinkle/food mixture immediately. Chewing should be avoided. It may be helpful to have the patient drink fluids immediately in order to make sure all of the mixture is swallowed.

IMPORTANT: Never store any sprinkle/food mixture for use at a later time.

To Take Without Food

TOPAMAX® Sprinkle Capsules may also be swallowed as whole capsules.

For more information about TOPAMAX® Sprinkle Capsules, ask your doctor or pharmacist.

Ortho-McNeil
OMP DIVISION
ORTHO-McNEIL PHARMACEUTICAL, INC.
Raritan, NJ 08869
© OMP 1999 Revised December 2001 7517103

Parke-Davis

A Warner-Lambert Division
A Pfizer Company
201 TABOR ROAD
MORRIS PLAINS, NEW JERSEY 07950

For Medical Information Contact:
During working hours:
Customer Service
Product/Medical Information
(800) 223-0432
FAX: (973) 385-2248
After Hours and Weekend Emergencies:
(973) 385-6089

Distribution:
1855 Shelby Oaks Drive North
Memphis, TN 38134
(901) 387-5200
Customer Service:
(800) 533-4535

EXPORT INQUIRIES:
Pfizer International Inc.
(212) 573-2323

ACCURETIC™ ℞

[*àk' kū rə tik*]
(quinapril HCl/hydrochlorothiazide) Tablets

Prescribing information for this product, which appears on pages 2614–2617 of the 2002 PDR, has been completely revised as follows. Please write "See Supplement A" next to the product heading.

USE IN PREGNANCY
When used in pregnancy during the second and third trimesters, ACE inhibitors can cause injury and even death to the developing fetus. When pregnancy is detected, ACCURETIC should be discontinued as soon as possible. See **WARNINGS: Fetal/Neonatal Morbidity and Mortality.**

DESCRIPTION

ACCURETIC is a fixed-combination tablet that combines an angiotensin-converting enzyme (ACE) inhibitor, quinapril hydrochloride, and a thiazide diuretic, hydrochlorothiazide. Quinapril hydrochloride is chemically described as [3S-[2[R*(R*)], 3R*]]-2-[2-[[1-(ethoxycarbonyl)-3-phenylpropyl] amino]-1-oxopropyl]-1,2,3,4-tetrahydro-3-isoquinolinecarboxylic acid, monohydrochloride. Its empirical formula is $C_{25}H_{30}N_2O_5$ HCl and its structural formula is:

• HCl M.W. = 474.98

Quinapril hydrochloride is a white to off-white amorphous powder that is freely soluble in aqueous solvents.

Hydrochlorothiazide is chemically described as: 6-Chloro-3,4-dihydro-2H-1,2,4-benzothiadiazine-7-sulfonamide 1,1-dioxide. Its empirical formula is $C_7H_8ClN_3O_4S_2$ and its structural formula is:

M.W. = 297.72

Hydrochlorothiazide is a white to off-white, crystalline powder which is slightly soluble in water but freely soluble in sodium hydroxide solution.

ACCURETIC is available for oral use as fixed combination tablets in three strengths of quinapril with hydrochlorothiazide: 10 mg with 12.5 mg (ACCURETIC 10/12.5), 20 mg with 12.5 mg (ACCURETIC 20/12.5), and 20 mg with 25 mg (ACCURETIC 20/25).

Inactive ingredients: candelilla wax, crospovidone, hydroxypropyl cellulose, hydroxypropylmethyl cellulose, iron oxide red, iron oxide yellow, lactose, magnesium carbonate, magnesium stearate, polyethylene glycol, povidone, and titanium dioxide.

CLINICAL PHARMACOLOGY

Mechanism of Action: The principal metabolite of quinapril, quinaprilat, is an inhibitor of ACE activity in human subjects and animals. ACE is peptidyl dipeptidase that catalyzes the conversion of angiotensin I to the vasoconstrictor, angiotensin II. The effect of quinapril in hypertension appears to result primarily from the inhibition of circulating and tissue ACE activity, thereby reducing angiotensin II formation. Quinapril inhibits the elevation in blood pressure caused by intravenously administered angiotensin I, but has no effect on the pressor response to angiotensin II, norepinephrine, or epinephrine. Angiotensin II also stimulates the secretion of aldosterone from the adrenal cortex, thereby facilitating renal sodium and fluid reabsorption. Reduced aldosterone secretion by quinapril may result in a small increase in serum potassium. In controlled hypertension trials, treatment with quinapril alone resulted in mean increases in potassium of 0.07 mmol/L (see **PRECAUTIONS**). Removal of angiotensin II negative feedback on renin secretion leads to increased plasma renin activity (PRA).

While the principal mechanism of antihypertensive effect is thought to be through the renin-angiotensin-aldosterone system, quinapril exerts antihypertensive actions even in patients with low renin hypertension. Quinapril was an effective antihypertensive in all races studied, although it was somewhat less effective in blacks (usually a predominantly low renin group) than in non-blacks. ACE is identical to kininase II, an enzyme that degrades bradykinin, a potent peptide vasodilator; whether increased levels of bradykinin play a role in the therapeutic effect of quinapril remains to be elucidated.

Hydrochlorothiazide is a thiazide diuretic. Thiazides affect the renal tubular mechanisms of electrolyte reabsorption, directly increasing excretion of sodium and chloride in approximately equivalent amounts. Indirectly, the diuretic action of hydrochlorothiazide reduces plasma volume, with consequent increases in plasma renin activity, increases in aldosterone secretion, increases in urinary potassium loss, and decreases in serum potassium. The renin-aldolsterone link is mediated by angiotensin, so coadministration of an ACE inhibitor tends to reverse the potassium loss associated with these diuretics.

The mechanism of the antihypertensive effect of thiazides is unknown.

Pharmacokinetics and Metabolism: The rate and extent of absorption of quinapril and hydrochlorothiazide from ACCURETIC tablets are not different, respectively, from the rate and extent of absorption of quinapril and hydrochlorothiazide from immediate-release monotherapy formulations, either administered concurrently or separately. Following oral administration of Accupril (quinapril monotherapy) tablets, peak plasma quinapril concentrations are observed within 1 hour. Based on recovery of quinapril and its metabolites in urine, the extent of absorption is at least 60%. The absorption of hydrochlorothiazide is somewhat slower (1 to 2.5 hours) and more complete (50% to 80%).

The rate of quinapril absorption was reduced by 14% when ACCURETIC tablets were administered with a high-fat meal as compared to fasting, while the extent of absorption was not affected. The rate of hydrochlorothiazide absorption was reduced by 12% when ACCURETIC tablets were administered with a high-fat meal, while the extent of absorption was not significantly affected. Therefore, ACCURETIC may be administered without regard to food.

Following absorption, quinapril is deesterified to its major active metabolite, quinaprilat (about 38% of oral dose), and to other minor inactive metabolites. Following multiple oral dosing of quinapril, there is an effective accumulation half-life of quinaprilat of approximately 3 hours, and peak plasma quinaprilat concentrations are observed approximately 2 hours postdose. Approximately 97% of either quinapril or quinaprilat circulating in plasma is bound to proteins. Hydrochlorothiazide is not metabolized. Its apparent volume of distribution is 3.6 to 7.8 L/kg, consistent with measured plasma protein binding of 67.9%. The drug also accumulates in red blood cells, so that whole blood levels are 1.6 to 1.8 times those measured in plasma.

Some placental passage occurred when quinapril was administered to pregnant rats. Studies in rats indicate that quinapril and its metabolites do not cross the blood-brain barrier. Hydrochlorothiazide crosses the placenta freely but not the blood-brain barrier.

Quinaprilat is eliminated primarily by renal excretion, up to 96% of an IV dose, and has an elimination half-life in plasma of approximately 2 hours and a prolonged terminal phase with a half-life of 25 hours. Hydrochlorothiazide is excreted unchanged by the kidney. When plasma levels have been followed for at least 24 hours, the plasma half-life has been observed to vary between 4 to 15 hours. At least 61% of the oral dose is eliminated unchanged within 24 hours.

In patients with renal insufficiency, the elimination half-life of quinaprilat increases as creatinine clearance decreases. There is a linear correlation between plasma quinaprilat clearance and creatinine clearance. In patients with end-stage renal disease, chronic hemodialysis or continuous ambulatory peritoneal dialysis have little effect on the elimination of quinapril and quinaprilat. Elimination of quinaprilat is reduced in elderly patients (≥65 years) and in those with heart failure; this reduction is attributable to decrease in renal function (see **DOSAGE AND ADMINISTRATION**). Quinaprilat concentrations are reduced in patients with alcoholic cirrhosis due to impaired deesterification of quinapril. In a study of patients with impaired renal function (mean creatinine clearance of 19 mL/min), the half-life of hydrochlorothiazide elimination was lengthened to 21 hours.

The pharmacokinetics of quinapril and quinaprilat are linear over a single-dose range of 5- to 80-mg doses and 40- to 160-mg in multiple daily doses.

Pharmacodynamics and Clinical Effects: Single doses of 20 mg of quinapril provide over 80% inhibition of plasma ACE for 24 hours. Inhibition of the pressor response to angiotensin I is shorter-lived, with a 20-mg dose giving 75% inhibition for about 4 hours, 50% inhibition for about 8 hours, and 20% inhibition at 24 hours. With chronic dosing, however, there is substantial inhibition of angiotensin II levels at 24 hours by doses of 20 to 80 mg.

Administration of 10 to 80 mg of quinapril to patients with mild to severe hypertension results in a reduction of sitting and standing blood pressure to about the same extent with minimal effect on heart rate. Symptomatic postural hypotension is infrequent, although it can occur in patients who are salt- and/or volume-depleted (see **WARNINGS**).

Antihypertensive activity commences within 1 hour with peak effects usually achieved by 2 to 4 hours after dosing. During chronic therapy, most of the blood pressure lowering effect of a given dose is obtained in 1 to 2 weeks. In multiple-dose studies, 10 to 80 mg per day in single or divided doses lowered systolic and diastolic blood pressure throughout the dosing interval, with a trough effect of about 5 to 11/3 to 7 mm Hg. The trough effect represents about 50% of the peak effect.

While the dose-response relationship is relatively flat, doses of 40 to 80 mg were somewhat more effective at trough than 10 to 20 mg, and twice-daily dosing tended to give a somewhat lower trough blood pressure than once-daily dosing with the same total dose. The antihypertensive effect of quinapril continues during long-term therapy, with no evidence of loss of effectiveness.

Hemodynamic assessments in patients with hypertension indicate that blood pressure reduction produced by quinapril is accompanied by a reduction in total peripheral resistance and renal vascular resistance with little or no change in heart rate, cardiac index, renal blood flow, glomerular filtration rate, or filtration fraction.

Therapeutic effects of quinapril appear to be the same for elderly (≥65 years of age) and younger adult patients given the same daily dosages, with no increase in adverse events in elderly patients. In patients with hypertension, quinapril 10 to 40 mg was similar in effectiveness to captopril, enalapril, propranolol, and thiazide diuretics.

After oral administration of hydrochlorothiazide, diuresis begins within 2 hours, peaks in about 4 hours, and lasts about 6 to 12 hours. Use of quinapril with a thiazide diuretic gives blood pressure lowering effect greater than that seen with either agent alone. In clinical trials of quinapril/hydrochlorothiazide using quinapril doses of 2.5 to 40 mg and hydrochlorothiazide doses of 6.25 to 25 mg, the antihypertensive effects were sustained for at least 24 hours, and increased with increasing dose of either component. Although quinapril monotherapy is somewhat less effective in blacks than in non-blacks, the efficacy of combination therapy appears to be independent of race. By blocking the renin-angiotensin-aldosterone axis, administration of quinapril tends to reduce the potassium loss associated with the diuretic. In clinical trials of ACCURETIC, the average change in serum potassium was near zero when 2.5 to 40 mg of quinapril was combined with hydrochlorothiazide 6.25 mg, and the average subject who received 10 to 20/12.5 to 25 mg experienced a milder reduction in serum potassium than that experienced by the average subject receiving the same dose of hydrochlorothiazide monotherapy.

INDICATIONS AND USAGE

ACCURETIC is indicated for the treatment of hypertension. This fixed combination is not indicated for the initial therapy of hypertension (see **DOSAGE AND ADMINISTRATION**).

In using ACCURETIC, consideration should be given to the fact that another angiotensin-converting enzyme inhibitor, captopril, has caused agranulocytosis, particularly in patients with renal impairment or collagen-vascular disease. Available data are insufficient to show that quinapril does not have a similar risk (see **WARNINGS: Neutropenia/Agranulocytosis**).

Angioedema in Black Patients: Black patients receiving ACE inhibitor monotherapy have been reported to have a higher incidence of angioedema compared to non-blacks. It should also be noted that in controlled clinical trials, ACE inhibitors have an effect on blood pressure that is less in black patients than in non-blacks.

CONTRAINDICATIONS

ACCURETIC is contraindicated in patients who are hypersensitive to quinapril or hydrochlorothiazide and in patients with a history of angioedema related to previous treatment with an ACE inhibitor.

Because of the hydrochlorothiazide components, this product is contraindicated in patients with anuria or hypersensitivity to other sulfonamide-derived drugs.

WARNINGS

Anaphylactoid and Possibly Related Reactions: Presumably because angiotensin converting inhibitors affect the metabolism of eicosanoids and polypeptides, including endogenous bradykinin, patients receiving ACE inhibitors (including quinapril) may be subject to a variety of adverse reactions, some of them serious.

Angioedema: Angioedema of the face, extremities, lips, tongue, glottis, and larynx has been reported in patients treated with ACE inhibitors and has been seen in 0.1% of patients receiving quinapril. In two similarly sized US postmarketing quinapril trials that, combined, enrolled over 3,000 black patients and over 19,000 non-blacks, angioedema was reported in 0.30% and 0.55% of blacks (in Study 1 and 2, respectively) and 0.39% and 0.17% of non-blacks. Angioedema associated with laryngeal edema can be fatal. If laryngeal stridor or angioedema of the face, tongue, or glottis occurs, treatment with ACCURETIC should be discontinued immediately, the patient treated in accordance with accepted medical care, and carefully observed until the swelling disappears. In instances where swelling is confined to the face and lips, the condition generally resolves without treatment; antihistamines may be useful in relieving symptoms. **Where there is involvement of the tongue, glottis, or larynx likely to cause airway obstruction, emergency therapy including, but not limited to, subcutaneous epinephrine solution 1:1000 (0.3 to 0.5 mL) should be promptly administered** (see **PRECAUTIONS** and **ADVERSE REACTIONS**).

Patients With a History of Angioedema: Patients with a history of angioedema unrelated to ACE inhibitor therapy may be at increased risk of angioedema while receiving an ACE inhibitor (see also **CONTRAINDICATIONS**).

Anaphylactoid Reactions During Desensitization: Two patients undergoing desensitizing treatment with Hymenoptera venom while receiving ACE inhibitors sustained life-threatening anaphylactoid reactions. In the same patients, these reactions were avoided when ACE inhibitors were temporarily withheld, but they reappeared upon inadvertent challenge.

Anaphylactoid Reactions During Membrane Exposure: Anaphylactoid reactions have been reported in patients dialyzed with high-flux membranes and treated concomitantly with an ACE inhibitor. Anaphylactoid reactions have also been reported in patients undergoing low-density lipoprotein apheresis with dextran sulfate absorption.

Hepatic Failure: Rarely, ACE inhibitors have been associated with a syndrome that starts with cholestatic jaundice and progresses to fulminant hepatic necrosis and (sometimes) death. The mechanism of this syndrome is not understood. Patients receiving ACE inhibitors who develop jaundice or marked elevations of hepatic enzymes should discontinue the ACE inhibitor and receive appropriate medical follow-up.

Hypotension: ACCURETIC can cause symptomatic hypotension, probably not more frequently than either monotherapy. It was reported in 1.2% of 1,571 patients receiving ACCURETIC during clinical trials. Like other ACE inhibitors, quinapril has been only rarely associated with hypotension in uncomplicated hypertensive patients.

Symptomatic hypotension sometimes associated with oliguria and/or progressive azotemia, and rarely acute renal failure and/or death, include patients with the following conditions or characteristics: heart failure, hyponatremia, high dose diuretic therapy, recent intensive diuresis or increase in diuretic dose, renal dialysis or severe volume and/or salt depletion of any etiology. Volume and/or salt depletion should be corrected before initiating therapy with ACCURETIC.

ACCURETIC should be used cautiously in patients receiving concomitant therapy with other antihypertensives. The thiazide component of ACCURETIC may potentiate the action of other antihypertensive drugs, especially ganglionic or peripheral adrenergic-blocking drugs. The antihypertensive effects of the thiazide component may also be enhanced in the postsympathectomy patients.

In patients at risk of excessive hypotension, therapy with ACCURETIC should be started under close medical supervision. Such patients should be followed closely for the first 2 weeks of treatment and whenever the dosage of quinapril or diuretic is increased. Similar considerations may apply to patients with ischemic heart or cerebrovascular disease in whom an excessive fall in blood pressure could result in myocardial infarction or cerebrovascular accident.

If excessive hypotension occurs, the patient should be placed in a supine position and, if necessary, treated with intravenous infusion of normal saline. ACCURETIC treatment usually can be continued following restoration of blood pressure and volume. If symptomatic hypotension develops, a dose reduction or discontinuation of ACCURETIC may be necessary.

Impaired Renal Function: ACCURETIC should be used with caution in patients with severe renal disease. Thiazides may precipitate azotemia in such patients, and the effects of repeated dosing may be cumulative.

When the renin-angiotensin-aldosterone system is inhibited by quinapril, changes in renal function may be anticipated in susceptible individuals. In patients with severe congestive heart failure, whose renal function may depend on the activity of the renin-angiotensin-aldosterone system, treatment with angiotensin-converting enzyme inhibitors (including quinapril) may be associated with oliguria and/or progressive azotemia and (rarely) with acute renal failure and/or death.

In clinical studies in hypertensive patients with unilateral renal artery stenosis, treatment with ACE inhibitors was associated with increases in blood urea nitrogen and serum creatinine; these increases were reversible upon discontinuation of ACE inhibitor, concomitant diuretic, or both. When such patients are treated with ACCURETIC, renal function should be monitored during the first few weeks of therapy.

Some quinapril-treated hypertensive patients with no apparent preexisting renal vascular diseases have developed increases in blood urea nitrogen and serum creatinine, usually minor and transient, especially when quinapril has been given concomitantly with a diuretic. This is more likely to occur in patients with pre-existing renal impairment. Dosage reduction of ACCURETIC may be required. **Evalua-**

Continued on next page

Accuretic—Cont.

tion of the hypertensive patients should also include assessment of the renal function (see **DOSAGE AND ADMINISTRATION**).

Neutropenia/Agranulocytosis: Another ACE inhibitor, captopril, has been shown to cause agranulocytosis and bone marrow depression rarely in patients with uncomplicated hypertension, but more frequently in patients with renal impairment, especially if they also have a collagen vascular disease, such as systemic lupus erythematosus or scleroderma. Agranulocytosis did occur during quinapril treatment in one patient with a history of neutropenia during previous captopril therapy. Available data from clinical trials of quinapril are insufficient to show that, in patients without prior reactions to other ACE inhibitors, quinapril does not cause agranulocytosis at similar rates. As with other ACE inhibitors, periodic monitoring of white blood cell counts in patients with collagen vascular disease and/or renal disease should be considered.

Fetal/Neonatal Morbidity and Mortality: ACE inhibitors can cause fetal and neonatal morbidity and death when administered to pregnant women. Several dozen cases have been reported in the world literature. When pregnancy is detected, ACCURETIC should be discontinued as soon as possible.

The use of ACE inhibitors during the second and third trimesters of pregnancy has been associated with fetal and neonatal injury, including hypotension, neonatal skull hypoplasia, anuria, reversible or irreversible renal failure, and death. Oligohydramnios has also been reported, presumably resulting from decreased fetal renal function; oligohydramnios in this setting has been associated with fetal limb contractures, craniofacial deformation, and hypoplastic lung development. Prematurity, intrauterine growth retardation, and patent ductus arteriosus have also been reported, although it is not clear whether these occurrences were due to the ACE inhibitor exposure.

These adverse effects do not appear to have resulted from intrauterine ACE inhibitor exposure that has been limited to the first trimester. Mothers whose embryos and fetuses are exposed to ACE inhibitors only during the first trimester should be so informed. Nonetheless, when patients become pregnant, physicians should make every effort to discontinue the use of quinapril as soon as possible.

Rarely (probably less often than once in every thousand pregnancies), no alternative ACE inhibitors will be found. In these rare cases, the mothers should be apprised of the potential hazards to their fetuses, and serial ultrasound examinations should be performed to assess the intraamniotic environment.

If oligohydramnios is observed, quinapril should be discontinued unless it is considered life-saving for the mother. Contraction stress testing (CST), a nonstress test (NST), or biophysical profiling (BPP) may be appropriate, depending upon the week of pregnancy. Patients and physicians should be aware, however, that oligohydramnios may not appear until after the fetus has sustained irreversible injury.

Infants with histories of *in utero* exposure to ACE inhibitors should be closely observed for hypotension, oliguria, and hyperkalemia. If oliguria occurs, attention should be directed toward support of blood pressure and renal perfusion. Exchange transfusion or peritoneal dialysis may be required as a means of reversing hypotension and/or substituting for disordered renal function. Removal of quinapril, which crosses the placenta, from the neonatal circulation is not significantly accelerated by these means.

Intrauterine exposure to thiazide diuretics is associated with fetal or neonatal jaundice, thrombocytopenia, and possibly other adverse reactions that occurred in adults.

No teratogenic effects of quinapril were seen in studies of pregnant rats and rabbits. On a mg/kg basis, the doses used were up to 180 times (in rats) and one time (in rabbits) the maximum recommended human dose. No teratogenic effects of ACCURETIC were seen in studies of pregnant rats and rabbits. On a mg/kg (quinapril/hydrochlorothiazide) basis, the doses used were up to 188/94 times (in rats) and 0.6/0.3 times (in rabbits) the maximum recommended human dose.

Impaired Hepatic Function: ACCURETIC should be used with caution in patients with impaired hepatic function or progressive liver disease, since minor alterations of fluid and electrolyte balance may precipitate hepatic coma. Also, since the metabolism of quinapril to quinaprilat is normally dependent upon hepatic esterases, patients with impaired liver function could develop markedly elevated plasma levels of quinapril. No normal pharmacokinetic studies have been carried out in hypertensive patients with impaired liver function.

Systemic Lupus Erythematosus: Thiazide diuretics have been reported to cause exacerbation or activation of systemic lupus erythematosus.

PRECAUTIONS

General

Derangements of Serum Electrolytes: In clinical trials, hyperkalemia (serum potassium ≥5.8 mmol/L) occurred in approximately 2% of patients receiving quinapril. In most cases, elevated serum potassium levels were isolated values which resolved despite continued therapy. Less than 0.1% of patients discontinued therapy due to hyperkalemia. Risk factors for the development of hyperkalemia include renal insufficiency, diabetes mellitus, and the concomitant use of potassium-sparing diuretics, potassium supplements, and/or potassium-containing salt substitutes.

Treatment with thiazide diuretics has been associated with hypokalemia, hyponatremia, and hypochloremic alkalosis. These disturbances have sometimes been manifest as one or more of dryness of mouth, thirst, weakness, lethargy, drowsiness, restlessness, muscle pains or cramps, muscular fatigue, hypotension, oliguria, tachycardia, nausea, and vomiting. Hypokalemia can also sensitize or exaggerate the response of the heart to the toxic effects of digitalis. The risk of hypokalemia is greatest in patients with cirrhosis of the liver, in patients experiencing a brisk diuresis, in patients who are receiving inadequate oral intake of electrolytes, and in patients receiving concomitant therapy with corticosteroids or ACTH.

The opposite effects of quinapril and hydrochlorothiazide on serum potassium will approximately balance each other in many patients, so that no net effect upon serum potassium will be seen. In other patients, one or the other effect may be dominant. Initial and periodic determinations of serum electrolytes to detect possible electrolyte imbalance should be performed at appropriate intervals.

Chloride deficits secondary to thiazide therapy are generally mild and require specific treatment only under extraordinary circumstances (eg, in liver disease or renal disease). Dilutional hyponatremia may occur in edematous patients in hot weather; appropriate therapy is water restriction rather than administration of salt, except in rare instances when the hyponatremia is life threatening. In actual salt depletion, appropriate replacement is the therapy of choice.

Calcium excretion is decreased by thiazides. In a few patients on prolonged thiazide therapy, pathological changes in the parathyroid gland have been observed, with hypercalcemia and hypophosphatemia. More serious complications of hyperparathyroidism (renal lithiasis, bone resorption, and peptic ulceration) have not been seen.

Thiazides increase the urinary excretion of magnesium, and hypomagnesemia may result.

Other Metabolic Disturbances: Thiazide diuretics tend to reduce glucose tolerance and to raise serum levels of cholesterol, triglycerides, and uric acid. These effects are usually minor, but frank gout or overt diabetes may be precipitated in susceptible patients.

Cough: Presumably due to the inhibition of the degradation of endogenous bradykinin, persistent nonproductive cough has been reported with all ACE inhibitors, resolving after discontinuation of therapy. ACE inhibitor-induced cough should be considered in the differential diagnosis of cough.

Surgery/Anesthesia: In patients undergoing surgery or during anesthesia with agents that produce hypotension, quinapril will block the angiotensin II formation that could otherwise occur secondary to compensatory renin release. Hypotension that occurs as a result of this mechanism can be corrected by volume expansion.

Information for Patients

Angioedema: Angioedema, including laryngeal edema, can occur with treatment with ACE inhibitors, especially following the first dose. Patients receiving ACCURETIC should be told to report immediately any signs or symptoms suggesting angioedema (swelling of face, eyes, lips, or tongue, or difficulty in breathing) and to take no more drug until after consulting with the prescribing physician.

Pregnancy: Female patients of childbearing age should be told about the consequences of second- and third-trimester exposure to ACE inhibitors, and they should also be told that these consequences do not appear to have resulted from intrauterine ACE-inhibitor exposure that has been limited to the first trimester. These patients should be asked to report pregnancies to their physicians as soon as possible.

Symptomatic Hypotension: A patient receiving ACCURETIC should be cautioned that lightheadedness can occur, especially during the first days of therapy, and that it should be reported to the prescribing physician. The patient should be told that if syncope occurs, ACCURETIC should be discontinued until the physician has been consulted.

All patients should be cautioned that inadequate fluid intake, excessive perspiration, diarrhea, or vomiting can lead to an excessive fall in blood pressure because of reduction in fluid volume, with the same consequences of lightheadedness and possible syncope.

Patients planning to undergo major surgery and/ or general or spinal anesthesia should be told to inform their physicians that they are taking an ACE inhibitor.

Hyperkalemia: A patient receiving ACCURETIC should be told not to use potassium supplements or salt substitutes containing potassium without consulting the prescribing physician.

Neutropenia: Patients should be told to promptly report any indication of infection (eg, sore throat, fever) which could be a sign of neutropenia.

NOTE: As with many other drugs, certain advice to patients being treated with quinapril is warranted. This information is intended to aid in the safe and effective use of this medication. It is not a disclosure of all possible adverse or intended effects.

Laboratory Tests

The hydrochlorothiazide component of ACCURETIC may decrease serum PBI levels without signs of thyroid disturbance.

Therapy with ACCURETIC should be interrupted for a few days before carrying out tests of parathyroid function.

Drug Interactions

Potassium Supplements and Potassium-Sparing Diuretics: As noted above ("Derangements of Serum Electrolytes"), the net effect of ACCURETIC may be to elevate a patient's serum potassium, to reduce it, or to leave it unchanged. Potassium-sparing diuretics (spironolactone, amiloride, triamterene, and others) or potassium supplements can increase the risk of hyperkalemia. If concomitant use of such agents is indicated, they should be given with caution, and the patients serum potassium should be monitored frequently.

Lithium: Increased serum lithium levels and symptoms of lithium toxicity have been reported in patients receiving ACE inhibitors during therapy with lithium. Because renal clearance of lithium is reduced by thiazides, the risk of lithium toxicity is presumably raised further when, as in therapy with ACCURETIC, a thiazide diuretic is coadministered with the ACE inhibitor. ACCURETIC and lithium should be coadministered with caution, and frequent monitoring of serum lithium levels is recommended.

Tetracycline and Other Drugs That Interact with Magnesium: Simultaneous administration of tetracycline with quinapril reduced the absorption of tetracycline by approximately 28% to 37%, possibly due to the high magnesium content in quinapril tablets. This interaction should be considered if coprescribing quinapril and tetracycline or other drugs that interact with magnesium.

Other Agents:

Drug interaction studies of quinapril and other agents showed:

- Multiple dose therapy with propranolol or cimetidine has no effect on the pharmacokinetics of single doses of quinapril.
- The anticoagulant effect of a single dose of warfarin (measured by prothrombin time) was not significantly changed by quinapril coadministration twice daily.
- Quinapril treatment did not affect the pharmacokinetics of digoxin.
- No pharmacokinetic interaction was observed when single doses of quinapril and hydrochlorothiazide were administered concomitantly.

When administered concurrently, the following drugs may interact with thiazide diuretics.

- Alcohol, Barbiturates, or Narcotics—potentiation of orthostatic hypotension may occur.
- Antidiabetic Drugs (oral hypoglycemic agents and insulin)—dosage adjustments of the antidiabetic drug may be required.
- Cholestyramine and Colestipol Resin—absorption of hydrochlorothiazide is impaired in the presence of anionic exchange resins. Single doses of either cholestyramine or colestipol resins bind the hydrochlorothiazide and reduce its absorption from the gastrointestinal tract by up to 85% and 43%, respectively.
- Corticosteroids, ACTH—intensified electrolyte depletion, particularly hypokalemia.
- Pressor Amines (eg, norepinephrine)—possible decreased response to pressor amines, but not sufficient to preclude their therapeutic use.
- Skeletal Muscle Relaxants, Nondepolarizing (eg, tubocurarine)—possible increased responsiveness to the muscle relaxant.
- Nonsteroidal Antiinflammatory Drugs—the diuretic, natriuretic, and antihypertensive effects of thiazide diuretics may be reduced by concurrent administration of nonsteroidal antiinflammatory agents.

Carcinogenesis, Mutagenesis, Impairment of Fertility

Carcinogenicity, mutagenicity, and fertility studies have not been conducted in animals with ACCURETIC.

Quinapril hydrochloride was not carcinogenic in mice or rats when given in doses up to 75 or 100 mg/kg/day (50 or 60 times the maximum human daily dose, respectively, on a mg/kg basis and 3.8 or 10 times the maximum human daily dose on a mg/m^2 basis) for 104 weeks. Female rats given the highest dose level had an increased incidence of mesenteric lymph node hemangiomas and skin/subcutaneous lipomas. Neither quinapril nor quinaprilat were mutagenic in the Ames bacterial assay with or without metabolic activation. Quinapril was also negative in the following genetic toxicology studies: *in vitro* mammalian cell point mutation, sister chromatid exchange in cultured mammalian cells, micronucleus test with mice, *in vitro* chromosome aberration with V79 cultured lung cells, and in an *in vivo* cytogenetic study with rat bone marrow. There were no adverse effects on fertility or reproduction in rats at doses up to 100 mg/kg/day (60 and 10 times the maximum daily human dose when based on mg/kg and mg/m^2, respectively).

Under the auspices of the National Toxicology Program, rats and mice received hydrochlorothiazide in their feed for 2 years, at doses up to 600 mg/kg/day in mice and up to 100 mg/kg/day in rats. These studies uncovered no evidence of a carcinogenic potential of hydrochlorothiazide in rats or female mice, but there was "equivocal" evidence of hepatocarcinogenicity in male mice. Hydrochlorothiazide was not genotoxic in *in vitro* assays using strains TA 98, TA 100, TA 1535, TA 1537, and TA 1538 of *Salmonella typhimurium* (the Ames test); in the Chinese hamster ovary (CHO) test for chromosomal aberrations; or *in vivo* assays using mouse germinal cell chromosomes, Chinese hamster bone marrow chromosomes, and the *Drosophila* sex-linked recessive lethal trait gene. Positive test results were obtained in the *in vitro* CHO sister chromatid exchange (clastogenicity) test and in the mouse lymphoma cell (mutagenicity) assays, using concentrations of hydrochlorothiazide of 43 to 1300 µg/mL. Positive test results were also obtained in the *Aspergillus nidulans* nondisjunction assay, using an unspecified concentration of hydrochlorothiazide.

Hydrochlorothiazide had no adverse effects on the fertility of mice and rats of either sex in studies wherein these species were exposed, via their diets, to doses of up to 100 and 4 mg/kg/day, respectively, prior to mating and throughout gestation.

Pregnancy

Pregnancy Categories C (first trimester) and D (second and third trimesters): See WARNINGS: Fetal/Neonatal Morbidity and Mortality.

Nursing Mothers

Because quinapril and hydrochlorothiazide are secreted in human milk, caution should be exercised when ACCURETIC is administered to a nursing woman.

Because of the potential for serious adverse reactions in nursing infants from hydrochlorothiazide and the unknown effects of quinapril in infants, a decision should be made whether to discontinue nursing or to discontinue ACCURETIC, taking into account the importance of the drug to the mother.

Geriatric Use

Clinical studies of quinapril HCl/hydrochlorothiazide did not include sufficient numbers of subjects aged 65 and over to determine whether they respond differently from younger subjects. Other reported clinical experience has not identified differences in responses between the elderly and younger patients. In general, dose selection for an elderly patient should be cautious, usually starting at the low end of the dosing range, reflecting the greater frequency of decreased hepatic, renal, or cardiac function, and of concomitant disease or other drug therapy.

Pediatric Use

Safety and effectiveness of ACCURETIC in children have not been established.

ADVERSE REACTIONS

ACCURETIC has been evaluated for safety in 1571 patients in controlled and uncontrolled studies. Of these, 498 were given quinapril plus hydrochlorothiazide for at least 1 year, with 153 patients extending combination therapy for over 2 years. In clinical trials with ACCURETIC, no adverse experience specific to the combination has been observed. Adverse experiences that have occurred have been limited to those that have been previously reported with quinapril or hydrochlorothiazide.

Adverse experiences were usually mild and transient, and there was no relationship between side effects and age, sex, race, or duration of therapy. Discontinuation of therapy because of adverse effects was required in 2.1% in patients in controlled studies. The most common reasons for discontinuation of therapy with ACCURETIC were cough (1.0%; see **PRECAUTIONS**) and headache (0.7%).

Adverse experiences probably or possibly related to therapy or of unknown relationship to therapy occurring in 1% or more of the 943 patients treated with quinapril plus hydrochlorothiazide in controlled trials are shown below.

[See first table above]

	Percent of Patients in Controlled Trials	
	Quinapril/HCTZ N = 943	Placebo N = 100
Headache	6.7	30.0
Dizziness	4.8	4.0
Coughing	3.2	2.0
Fatigue	2.9	3.0
Myalgia	2.4	5.0
Viral Infection	1.9	4.0
Rhinitis	2.0	3.0
Nausea and/or Vomiting	1.8	6.0
Abdominal Pain	1.7	4.0
Back Pain	1.5	2.0
Diarrhea	1.4	1.0
Upper Respiratory Infection	1.3	4.0
Insomnia	1.2	2.0
Somnolence	1.2	0.0
Bronchitis	1.2	1.0
Dyspepsia	1.2	2.0
Asthenia	1.1	1.0
Pharyngitis	1.1	2.0
Vasodilatation	1.0	1.0
Vertigo	1.0	2.0
Chest Pain	1.0	2.0

Clinical adverse experiences probably, possibly, or definitely related or of uncertain relationship to therapy occurring in ≥0.5% to <1.0% (except as noted) of the patients treated with quinapril/HCTZ in controlled and uncontrolled trials (N=1571) and less frequent, clinically significant events seen in clinical trials or postmarketing experience (the rarer events are in italics) include (listed by body system):

[See second table above]

BODY AS A WHOLE:	Asthenia, Malaise
CARDIOVASCULAR:	Palpitation, Tachycardia, *Heart Failure, Hyperkalemia, Myocardial Infarction, Cerebrovascular Accident, Hypertensive Crisis, Angina Pectoris, Orthostatic Hypotension, Cardiac Rhythm Disturbance*
GASTROINTESTINAL:	Mouth or Throat Dry, *Gastrointestinal Hemorrhage, Pancreatitis, Abnormal Liver Function Tests*
NERVOUS/PSYCHIATRIC:	Nervousness, Vertigo, *Paresthesia*
RESPIRATORY:	Sinusitis, Dyspnea
INTEGUMENTARY:	Pruritus, Sweating Increased, *Erythema Multiforme, Exfoliative Dermatitis, Photosensitivity Reaction, Alopecia, Pemphigus*
UROGENITAL SYSTEM:	*Acute Renal Failure, Impotence*
OTHER:	*Agranulocytosis, Thrombocytopenia, Arthralgia*
Angioedema:	Angioedema has been reported in 0.1% of patients receiving quinapril (0.1%) (see **WARNINGS**).
Fetal/Neonatal Morbidity and Mortality:	See **WARNINGS**: Fetal/Neonatal Morbidity and Mortality

Postmarketing Experience

The following serious nonfatal adverse events, regardless of their relationship to quinapril and HCTZ combination tablets, have been reported during extensive postmarketing experience:

BODY AS A WHOLE: Shock, accidental injury, neoplasm, cellulitis, ascites, generalized edema, and hernia.

CARDIOVASCULAR SYSTEM: Bradycardia, cor pulmonale, vasculitis, and deep thrombosis.

DIGESTIVE SYSTEM: Gastrointestinal carcinoma, cholestatic jaundice, hepatitis, esophagitis, vomiting, and diarrhea.

HEMIC SYSTEM: Anemia.

METABOLIC AND NUTRITIONAL DISORDERS: Weight loss.

MUSCULOSKELETAL SYSTEM: Myopathy, myositis, and arthritis.

NERVOUS SYSTEM: Paralysis, hemiplegia, speech disorder, abnormal gait, meningism, and amnesia.

RESPIRATORY SYSTEM: Pneumonia, asthma, respiratory infiltration, and lung disorder.

SKIN AND APPENDAGES: Urticaria, macropapular rash, and petechiases.

SPECIAL SENSES: Abnormal vision.

UROGENITAL SYSTEM: Kidney function abnormal, albuminuria, pyuria, hematuria, and nephrosis.

Quinapril monotherapy has been evaluated for safety in 4960 patients. In clinical trials adverse events which occurred with quinapril were also seen with ACCURETIC. In addition, the following were reported for quinapril at an incidence >0.5%: depression, back pain, constipation, syncope, and amblyopia.

Hydrochlorothiazide has been extensively prescribed for many years, but there has not been enough systematic collection of data to support an estimate of the frequency of the observed adverse reactions. Within organ-system groups, the reported reactions are listed here in decreasing order of severity, without regard to frequency.

[See third table above]

BODY AS A WHOLE:	Weakness.
CARDIOVASCULAR:	Orthostatic hypotension (may be potentiated by alcohol, barbiturates, or narcotics).
DIGESTIVE:	Pancreatitis, jaundice (intrahepatic cholestatic), sialadenitis, vomiting, diarrhea, cramping, nausea, gastric irritation, constipation, and anorexia.
NEUROLOGIC:	Vertigo, lightheadedness, transient blurred vision, headache, paresthesia, xanthopsia, weakness, and restlessness.
MUSCULOSKELETAL:	Muscle spasm.
HEMATOLOGIC:	Aplastic anemia, agranulocytosis, leukopenia, thrombocytopenia, and hemolytic anemia.
RENAL:	Renal failure, renal dysfunction, interstitial nephritis (see **WARNINGS**).
METABOLIC:	Hyperglycemia, glycosuria, and hyperuricemia.
HYPERSENSITIVITY:	Necrotizing angiitis, Stevens-Johnson syndrome, respiratory distress (including pneumonitis and pulmonary edema), purpura, urticaria, rash, and photosensitivity.

Clinical Laboratory Test Findings

Serum Electrolytes: See **PRECAUTIONS.**

Creatinine, Blood Urea Nitrogen: Increases (>1.25 times the upper limit of normal) in serum creatinine and blood urea nitrogen were observed in 3% and 4%, respectively, of patients treated with ACCURETIC. Most increases were minor and reversible, which can occur in patients with essential hypertension but most frequently in patients with renal artery stenosis (see **PRECAUTIONS**).

PBI and Tests of Parathyroid Function: See **PRECAUTIONS**.

Hematology: See **WARNINGS**.

Other (causal relationships unknown): Other clinically important changes in standard laboratory tests were rarely associated with ACCURETIC administration. Elevations in uric acid, glucose, magnesium, cholesterol, triglyceride, and calcium (see **PRECAUTIONS**) have been reported.

OVERDOSAGE

No specific information is available on the treatment of overdosage with ACCURETIC or quinapril monotherapy; treatment should be symptomatic and supportive. Therapy with ACCURETIC should be discontinued, and the patient should be observed. Dehydration, electrolyte imbalance, and hypotension should be treated by established procedures.

The oral median lethal dose of quinapril/hydrochlorothiazide in combination ranges from 1063/664 to 4640/2896 mg/kg in mice and rats. Doses of 1440 to 4280 mg/kg of quinapril cause significant lethality in mice and rats. In single-dose studies of hydrochlorothiazide, most rats survived doses up to 2.75 g/kg.

Data from human overdoses of ACE inhibitors are scanty; the most likely manifestation of human quinapril overdosage is hypotension. In human hydrochlorothiazide overdose, the most common signs and symptoms observed have been those of dehydration and electrolyte depletion (hypokalemia, hypochloremia, hyponatremia). If digitalis has also been administered, hypokalemia may accentuate cardiac arrhythmias.

Laboratory determinations of serum levels of quinapril and its metabolites are not widely available, and such determinations have, in any event, no established role in the management of quinapril overdose.

No data are available to suggest physiological maneuvers (eg, maneuvers to change the pH of the urine) that might accelerate elimination of quinapril and its metabolites. Hemodialysis and peritoneal dialysis have little effect on the elimination of quinapril and quinaprilat.

Angiotensin II could presumably serve as a specific antagonist-antidote in the setting of quinapril overdose, but angiotensin II is essentially unavailable outside of scattered research facilities. Because the hypotensive effect of quinapril is achieved through vasodilation and effective hypovolemia, it is reasonable to treat quinapril overdose by infusion of normal saline solution.

DOSAGE AND ADMINISTRATION

As individual monotherapy, quinapril is an effective treatment of hypertension in once-daily doses of 10 to 80 mg and hydrochlorothiazide is effective in doses of 12.5 to 50 mg. In clinical trials of quinapril/hydrochlorothiazide combination therapy using quinapril doses of 2.5 to 40 mg and hydrochlorothiazide doses of 6.25 to 25 mg, the antihypertensive effects increased with increasing dose of either component.

The side effects (see **WARNINGS**) of quinapril are generally rare and apparently independent of dose; those of hydrochlorothiazide are a mixture of dose-dependent phenomena (primarily hypokalemia) and dose-independent phenomena (eg, pancreatitis), the former much more common than the latter. Therapy with any combination of quinapril and hydrochlorothiazide will be associated with both sets of dose-independent side effects, but regimens that combine low doses of hydrochlorothiazide with quinapril produce minimal effects on serum potassium. In clinical trials of ACCURETIC, the average change in serum potassium was near zero in subjects who received HCTZ 6.25 mg in the combination, and the average subject who received 10 to 40/12.5 to 25 mg experienced a milder reduction in serum potassium than that experienced by the average subject receiving the same dose of hydrochlorothiazide monotherapy.

To minimize dose-independent side effects, it is usually appropriate to begin combination therapy only after a patient has failed to achieve the desired effect with monotherapy.

Therapy Guided by Clinical Effect

Patients whose blood pressures are not adequately controlled with quinapril monotherapy may instead be given

Continued on next page

Accuretic—Cont.

ACCURETIC 10/12.5 or 20/12.5. Further increases of either or both components could depend on clinical response. The hydrochlorothiazide dose should generally not be increased until 2 to 3 weeks have elapsed. Patients whose blood pressures are adequately controlled with 25 mg of daily hydrochlorothiazide, but who experience significant potassium loss with this regimen, may achieve blood pressure control with less electrolyte disturbance if they are switched to ACCURETIC 10/12.5 or 20/12.5.

Replacement Therapy

For convenience, patients who are adequately treated with 20 mg of quinapril and 25 mg of hydrochlorothiazide and experience no significant electrolyte disturbances may instead wish to receive ACCURETIC 20/25.

Use in Renal Impairment

Regimens of therapy with ACCURETIC need not take account of renal function as long as the patient's creatinine clearance is >30 mL/min/1.73 m^2 (serum creatinine roughly ≤3 mg/dL or 265 μmol/L). In patients with more severe renal impairment, loop diuretics are preferred to thiazides. Therefore, ACCURETIC is not recommended for use in these patients.

HOW SUPPLIED

ACCURETIC is available in tablets of three different strengths:

10/12.5 tablets: pink, scored elliptical, biconvex, film-coated tablets. Each tablet contains 10 mg of quinapril and 12.5 mg of hydrochlorothiazide.
N0071-0222-06: 30 tablets (3 blisters — 10 tablets each)
N0071-0222-23: 90 tablet bottles

20/12.5 tablets: pink, scored triangular, film-coated tablets. Each tablet contains 20 mg of quinapril and 12.5 mg of hydrochlorothiazide.
N0071-0220-06: 30 tablets (3 blisters — 10 tablets each)
N0071-0220-23: 90 tablet bottles

20/25 tablets: pink, scored round, biconvex, film-coated tablets. Each tablet contains 20 mg of quinapril and 25 mg of hydrochlorothiazide.
N0071-0223-06: 30 tablets (3 blisters — 10 tablets each)
N0071-0223-23: 90 tablet bottles

Dispense in well-closed containers as defined in the USP.

Store at Controlled Room Temperature 20–25°C (68–77°F) [see USP].

Rx only

69-5822-00-0

Manufactured by:
Parke Davis Pharmaceuticals, Ltd
Vega Baja, PR 00694
MADE IN GERMANY
Distributed by:
PARKE-DAVIS
Div of Pfizer Inc
NY, NY 10017

Revised September 2001

NEURONTIN® ℞
(gabapentin) capsules

NEURONTIN® ℞
(gabapentin) tablets

NEURONTIN® ℞
(gabapentin) oral solution

Prescribing information for this product, which appears on pages 2655–2658 of the 2002 PDR, has been completely revised as follows. Please write "See Supplement A" next to the product heading.

DESCRIPTION

Neurontin® (gabapentin) capsules, Neurontin® (gabapentin) tablets, and Neurontin® (gabapentin) oral solution are supplied as imprinted hard shell capsules containing 100 mg, 300 mg, and 400 mg of gabapentin, elliptical film-coated tablets containing 600 mg and 800 mg of gabapentin or an oral solution containing 250 mg/5 mL of gabapentin.

The inactive ingredients for the capsules are lactose, cornstarch, and talc. The 100 mg capsule shell contains gelatin and titanium dioxide. The 300 mg capsule shell contains gelatin, titanium dioxide, and yellow iron oxide. The 400 mg capsule shell contains gelatin, red iron oxide, titanium dioxide, and yellow iron oxide. The imprinting ink contains FD&C Blue No. 2 and titanium dioxide.

The inactive ingredients for the tablets are poloxamer 407, copolyvidonum, cornstarch, magnesium stearate, hydroxypropyl cellulose, talc, candelilla wax and purified water. The imprinting ink for the 600 mg tablets contains synthetic black iron oxide, pharmaceutical shellac, pharmaceutical glaze, propylene glycol, ammonium hydroxide, isopropyl alcohol and n-butyl alcohol. The imprinting ink for the 800 mg tablets contains synthetic yellow iron oxide, synthetic red iron oxide, hydroxypropyl methylcellulose, propylene glycol, methanol, isopropyl alcohol and deionized water.

The inactive ingredients for the oral solution are glycerin, xylitol, purified water and artificial cool strawberry anise flavor.

Gabapentin is described as 1-(aminomethyl)cyclohexaneacetic acid with an empirical formula of $C_9H_{17}NO_2$ and a molecular weight of 171.24. The molecular structure of gabapentin is:

CH_2NH_2

CH_2CO_2H

Gabapentin is a white to off-white crystalline solid. It is freely soluble in water and both basic and acidic aqueous solutions.

CLINICAL PHARMACOLOGY

Mechanism of Action

The mechanism by which gabapentin exerts its anticonvulsant action is unknown, but in animal test systems designed to detect anticonvulsant activity, gabapentin prevents seizures as do other marketed anticonvulsants. Gabapentin exhibits antiseizure activity in mice and rats in both the maximal electroshock and pentylenetetrazole seizure models and other preclinical models (e.g., strains with genetic epilepsy, etc.). The relevance of these models to human epilepsy is not known.

Gabapentin is structurally related to the neurotransmitter GABA (gamma-aminobutyric acid) but it does not interact with GABA receptors, it is not converted metabolically into GABA or a GABA agonist, and it is not an inhibitor of GABA uptake or degradation. Gabapentin was tested in radioligand binding assays at concentrations up to 100 μM and did not exhibit affinity for a number of other common receptor sites, including benzodiazepine, glutamate, N-methyl-D-aspartate (NMDA), quisqualate, kainate, strychnine-insensitive or strychnine-sensitive glycine, alpha 1, alpha 2, or beta adrenergic, adenosine A1 or A2, cholinergic muscarinic or nicotinic, dopamine D1 or D2, histamine H1, serotonin S1 or S2, opiate mu, delta or kappa, voltage-sensitive calcium channel sites labeled with nitrendipine or diltiazem, or at voltage-sensitive sodium channel sites with batrachotoxinin A 20-alpha-benzoate.

Several test systems ordinarily used to assess activity at the NMDA receptor have been examined. Results are contradictory. Accordingly, no general statement about the effects, if any, of gabapentin at the NMDA receptor can be made.

In vitro studies with radiolabeled gabapentin have revealed a gabapentin binding site in areas of rat brain including neocortex and hippocampus. A high-affinity binding protein in animal brain tissue has been identified as an auxiliary subunit of voltage-activated calcium channels. However, functional correlates of gabapentin binding, if any, remain to be elucidated.

Pharmacokinetics and Drug Metabolism

All pharmacological actions following gabapentin administration are due to the activity of the parent compound; gabapentin is not appreciably metabolized in humans.

Oral Bioavailability: Gabapentin bioavailability is not dose proportional; i.e., as dose is increased, bioavailability decreases. A 400 mg dose, for example, is about 25% less bioavailable than a 100 mg dose. Over the recommended dose range of 300 to 600 mg T.I.D., however, the differences in bioavailability are not large, and bioavailability is about 60 percent. Food has only a slight effect on the rate and extent of absorption of gabapentin (14% increase in AUC and C_{max}).

Distribution: Gabapentin circulates largely unbound (<3%) to plasma protein. The apparent volume of distribution of gabapentin after 150 mg intravenous administration is 58±6 L (Mean±SD). In patients with epilepsy, steady-state predose (C_{min}) concentrations of gabapentin in cerebrospinal fluid were approximately 20% of the corresponding plasma concentrations.

Elimination: Gabapentin is eliminated from the systemic circulation by renal excretion as unchanged drug. Gabapentin is not appreciably metabolized in humans.

Gabapentin elimination half-life is 5 to 7 hours and is unaltered by dose or following multiple dosing. Gabapentin elimination rate constant, plasma clearance, and renal clearance are directly proportional to creatinine clearance (see Special Populations: Patients With Renal Insufficiency, below). In elderly patients, and in patients with impaired renal function, gabapentin plasma clearance is reduced. Gabapentin can be removed from plasma by hemodialysis. Dosage adjustment in patients with compromised renal function or undergoing hemodialysis is recommended (see DOSAGE AND ADMINISTRATION, Table 3).

Special Populations: *Adult Patients With Renal Insufficiency:* Subjects (N=60) with renal insufficiency (mean creatinine clearance ranging from 13–114 mL/min) were administered single 400 mg oral doses of gabapentin. The mean gabapentin half-life ranged from about 6.5 hours (patients with creatinine clearance >60 mL/min) to 52 hours (creatinine clearance <30 mL/min) and gabapentin renal clearance from about 90 mL/min (>60 mL/min group) to about 10 mL/min (<30 mL/min). Mean plasma clearance (CL/F) decreased from approximately 190 mL/min to 20 mL/min.

Dosage adjustment in adult patients with compromised renal function is necessary (see DOSAGE AND ADMINISTRATION). Pediatric patients with renal insufficiency have not been studied.

Hemodialysis: In a study in anuric subjects (N=11), the apparent elimination half-life of gabapentin on nondialysis days was about 132 hours; dialysis three times a week (4 hours duration) lowered the apparent half-life of gabapentin by about 60%, from 132 hours to 51 hours. Hemodialysis thus has a significant effect on gabapentin elimination in anuric subjects.

Dosage adjustment in patients undergoing hemodialysis is necessary (see DOSAGE AND ADMINISTRATION).

Hepatic Disease: Because gabapentin is not metabolized, no study was performed in patients with hepatic impairment.

Age: The effect of age was studied in subjects 20–80 years of age. Apparent oral clearance (CL/F) of gabapentin decreased as age increased, from about 225 mL/min in those under 30 years of age to about 125 mL/min in those over 70 years of age. Renal clearance (CLr) and CLr adjusted for body surface area also declined with age; however, the decline in the renal clearance of gabapentin with age can largely be explained by the decline in renal function. Reduction of gabapentin dose may be required in patients who have age related compromised renal function. (See PRECAUTIONS, Geriatric Use, and DOSAGE AND ADMINISTRATION.)

Pediatric: Gabapentin pharmacokinetics were determined in 48 pediatric subjects between the ages of 1 month and 12 years following a dose of approximately 10 mg/kg. Peak plasma concentrations were similar across the entire age group and occurred 2 to 3 hours postdose. In general, pediatric subjects between 1 month and <5 years of age achieved approximately 30% lower exposure (AUC) than that observed in those 5 years of age and older. Accordingly, oral clearance normalized per body weight was higher in the younger children. Apparent oral clearance of gabapentin was directly proportional to creatinine clearance. Gabapentin elimination half-life averaged 4.7 hours and was similar across the age groups studied.

A population pharmacokinetic analysis was performed in 253 pediatric subjects between 1 month and 13 years of age. Patients received 10 to 65 mg/kg/day given T.I.D. Apparent oral clearance (CL/F) was directly proportional to creatinine clearance and this relationship was similar following a single dose and at steady state. Higher oral clearance values were observed in children <5 years of age compared to those observed in children 5 years of age and older, when normalized per body weight. The clearance was highly variable in infants <1 year of age. The normalized CL/F values observed in pediatric patients 5 years of age and older were consistent with values observed in adults after a single dose. The oral volume of distribution normalized per body weight was constant across the age range.

These pharmacokinetic data indicate that the effective daily dose in pediatric patients ages 3 and 4 years should be 40 mg/kg/day to achieve average plasma concentrations similar to those achieved in patients 5 years of age and older receiving gabapentin at 30 mg/kg/day. (See DOSAGE AND ADMINISTRATION).

Gender: Although no formal study has been conducted to compare the pharmacokinetics of gabapentin in men and women, it appears that the pharmacokinetic parameters for males and females are similar and there are no significant gender differences.

Race: Pharmacokinetic differences due to race have not been studied. Because gabapentin is primarily renally excreted and there are no important racial differences in creatinine clearance, pharmacokinetic differences due to race are not expected.

Clinical Studies

The effectiveness of Neurontin® as adjunctive therapy (added to other antiepileptic drugs) was established in multicenter placebo-controlled, double-blind, parallel-group clinical trials in adult and pediatric patients (3 years and older) with refractory partial seizures.

Evidence of effectiveness was obtained in three trials conducted in 705 patients (age 12 years and above) and one trial conducted in 247 pediatric patients (3 to 12 years of age). The patients enrolled had a history of at least 4 partial seizures per month in spite of receiving one or more antiepileptic drugs at therapeutic levels and were observed on their established antiepileptic drug regimen during a 12-week baseline period (6 weeks in the study of pediatric patients). In patients continuing to have at least 2 (or 4 in some studies) seizures per month, Neurontin® or placebo was then added on to the existing therapy during a 12-week treatment period. Effectiveness was assessed primarily on the basis of the percent of patients with a 50% or greater reduction in seizure frequency from baseline to treatment (the "responder rate") and a derived measure called response ratio, a measure of change defined as (T − B)/(T + B), where B is the patient's baseline seizure frequency and T is the patient's seizure frequency during treatment. Response ratio is distributed within the range −1 to +1. A zero value indicates no change while complete elimination of seizures would give a value of −1; increased seizure rates would give positive values. A response ratio of −0.33 corresponds to a 50% reduction in seizure frequency. The results given below are for all partial seizures in the intent-to-treat (all patients who received any doses of treatment) population in each study, unless otherwise indicated.

One study compared Neurontin® 1200 mg/day T.I.D. with placebo. Responder rate was 23% (14/61) in the Neurontin® group and 9% (6/66) in the placebo group; the difference between groups was statistically significant. Response ratio was also better in the Neurontin® group (−0.199) than in the placebo group (−0.044), a difference that also achieved statistical significance.

A second study compared primarily 1200 mg/day T.I.D. Neurontin® (N=101) with placebo (N=98). Additional smaller Neurontin® dosage groups (600 mg/day, N=53; 1800 mg/day, N=54) were also studied for information regarding dose response. Responder rate was higher in the Neurontin® 1200 mg/day group (16%) than in the placebo group (8%), but the difference was not statistically significant. The responder rate at 600 mg (17%) was also not significantly higher than in the placebo, but the responder rate in the 1800 mg group (26%) was statistically significantly superior to the placebo rate. Response ratio was better in the Neurontin® 1200 mg/day group (−0.103) than in the placebo group (−0.022); but this difference was also not statistically significant (p = 0.224). A better response was seen in the Neurontin® 600 mg/day group (−0.105) and 1800 mg/day group (−0.222) than in the 1200 mg/day group, with the 1800 mg/day group achieving statistical significance compared to the placebo group.

A third study compared Neurontin® 900 mg/day T.I.D. (N=111) and placebo (N=109). An additional Neurontin® 1200 mg/day dosage group (N=52) provided dose-response data. A statistically significant difference in responder rate was seen in the Neurontin® 900 mg/day group (22%) compared to that in the placebo group (10%). Response ratio was also statistically significantly superior in the Neurontin® 900 mg/day group (−0.119) compared to that in the placebo group (−0.027), as was response ratio in 1200 mg/day Neurontin® (−0.184) compared to placebo.

Analyses were also performed in each study to examine the effect of Neurontin® on preventing secondarily generalized tonic-clonic seizures. Patients who experienced a secondarily generalized tonic-clonic seizure in either the baseline or in the treatment period in all three placebo-controlled studies were included in these analyses. There were several response ratio comparisons that showed a statistically significant advantage for Neurontin® compared to placebo and favorable trends for almost all comparisons.

Analysis of responder rate using combined data from all three studies and all doses (N=162, Neurontin®; N=89, placebo) also showed a significant advantage for Neurontin® over placebo in reducing the frequency of secondarily generalized tonic-clonic seizures.

In two of the three controlled studies, more than one dose of Neurontin® was used. Within each study the results did not show a consistently increased response to dose. However, looking across studies, a trend toward increasing efficacy with increasing dose is evident (see Figure 1).

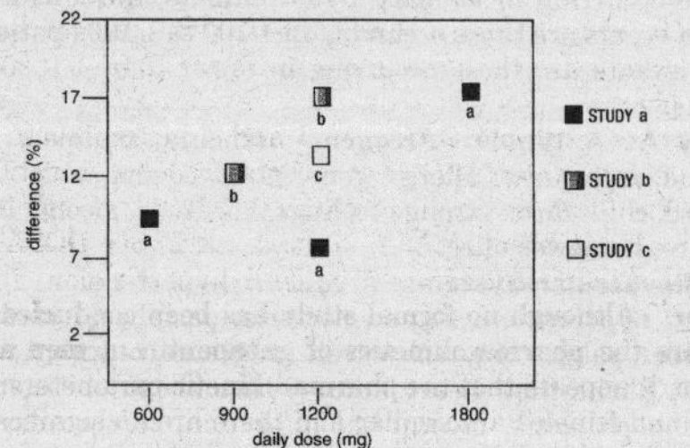

FIGURE 1. Responder Rate in Patients Receiving Neurontin® Expressed as a Difference from Placebo by Dose and Study

In the figure, treatment effect magnitude, measured on the Y axis in terms of the difference in the proportion of gabapentin and placebo assigned patients attaining a 50% or greater reduction in seizure frequency from baseline, is plotted against the daily dose of gabapentin administered (X axis).

Although no formal analysis by gender has been performed, estimates of response (Response Ratio) derived from clinical trials (398 men, 307 women) indicate no important gender differences exist. There was no consistent pattern indicating that age had any effect on the response to Neurontin®. There were insufficient numbers of patients of races other than Caucasian to permit a comparison of efficacy among racial groups.

A fourth study in pediatric patients age 3 to 12 years compared 25–35 mg/kg/day Neurontin (N=118) with placebo (N=127). For all partial seizures in the intent-to-treat population, the response ratio was statistically significantly better for the Neurontin group (−0.146) than for the placebo group (−0.079). For the same population, the responder rate for Neurontin (21%) was not significantly different from placebo (18%).

A study in pediatric patients age 1 month to 3 years compared 40 mg/kg/day Neurontin (N=38) with placebo (N=38) in patients who were receiving at least one marketed antiepileptic drug and had at least one partial seizure during the screening period (within 2 weeks prior to baseline). Patients had up to 48 hours of baseline and up to 72 hours of double-blind video EEG monitoring to record and count the occurrence of seizures. There were no statistically significant differences between treatments in either the response ratio or responder rate.

INDICATIONS AND USAGE

Neurontin® (gabapentin) is indicated as adjunctive therapy in the treatment of partial seizures with and without secondary generalization in patients over 12 years of age with epilepsy. Neurontin is also indicated as adjunctive therapy in the treatment of partial seizures in pediatric patients age 3–12 years.

CONTRAINDICATIONS

Neurontin® is contraindicated in patients who have demonstrated hypersensitivity to the drug or its ingredients.

WARNINGS

Neuropsychiatric Adverse Events—Pediatric Patients 3–12 years of age

Gabapentin use in pediatric patients with epilepsy 3–12 years of age is associated with the occurrence of central nervous system related adverse events. The most significant of these can be classified into the following categories: 1) emotional lability (primarily behavioral problems), 2) hostility, including aggressive behaviors, 3) thought disorder, including concentration problems and change in school performance, and 4) hyperkinesia (primarily restlessness and hyperactivity). Among the gabapentin-treated patients, most of the events were mild to moderate in intensity.

In controlled trials in pediatric patients 3–12 years of age the incidence of these adverse events was: emotional lability 6% (gabapentin-treated patients) vs 1.3% (placebo-treated patients); hostility 5.2% vs 1.3%; hyperkinesia 4.7% vs 2.9%; and thought disorder 1.7% vs 0%. One of these events, a report of hostility, was considered serious. Discontinuation of gabapentin treatment occurred in 1.3% of patients reporting emotional lability and hyperkinesia and 0.9% of gabapentin-treated patients reporting hostility and thought disorder. One placebo-treated patient (0.4%) withdrew due to emotional lability.

Withdrawal Precipitated Seizure, Status Epilepticus

Antiepileptic drugs should not be abruptly discontinued because of the possibility of increasing seizure frequency.

In the placebo-controlled studies in patients >12 years of age, the incidence of status epilepticus in patients receiving Neurontin® was 0.6% (3 of 543) versus 0.5% in patients receiving placebo (2 of 378). Among the 2074 patients >12 years of age treated with Neurontin® across all studies (controlled and uncontrolled) 31 (1.5%) had status epilepticus. Of these, 14 patients had no prior history of status epilepticus either before treatment or while on other medications. Because adequate historical data are not available, it is impossible to say whether or not treatment with Neurontin® is associated with a higher or lower rate of status epilepticus than would be expected to occur in a similar population not treated with Neurontin®.

Tumorigenic Potential

In standard preclinical *in vivo* lifetime carcinogenicity studies, an unexpectedly high incidence of pancreatic acinar adenocarcinomas was identified in male, but not female, rats. (See PRECAUTIONS: Carcinogenesis, Mutagenesis, Impairment of Fertility.) The clinical significance of this finding is unknown. Clinical experience during gabapentin's premarketing development provides no direct means to assess its potential for inducing tumors in humans.

In clinical studies comprising 2085 patient-years of exposure in patients >12 years of age, new tumors were reported in 10 patients (2 breast, 3 brain, 2 lung, 1 adrenal, 1 non-Hodgkin's lymphoma, 1 endometrial carcinoma *in situ*), and preexisting tumors worsened in 11 patients (9 brain, 1 breast, 1 prostate) during or up to 2 years following discontinuation of Neurontin®. Without knowledge of the background incidence and recurrence in a similar population not treated with Neurontin®, it is impossible to know whether the incidence seen in this cohort is or is not affected by treatment.

Sudden and Unexplained Deaths

During the course of premarketing development of Neurontin®, 8 sudden and unexplained deaths were recorded among a cohort of 2203 patients treated (2103 patient-years of exposure).

Some of these could represent seizure-related deaths in which the seizure was not observed, e.g., at night. This represents an incidence of 0.0038 deaths per patient-year. Although this rate exceeds that expected in a healthy population matched for age and sex, it is within the range of estimates for the incidence of sudden unexplained deaths in patients with epilepsy not receiving Neurontin® (ranging from 0.0005 for the general population of epileptics to 0.003 for a clinical trial population similar to that in the Neurontin® program, to 0.005 for patients with refractory epilepsy). Consequently, whether these figures are reassuring or raise further concern depends on comparability of the populations reported upon to the Neurontin® cohort and the accuracy of the estimates provided.

PRECAUTIONS

Information for Patients

Patients should be instructed to take Neurontin® only as prescribed.

Patients should be advised that Neurontin® may cause dizziness, somnolence and other symptoms and signs of CNS depression. Accordingly, they should be advised neither to drive a car nor to operate other complex machinery until they have gained sufficient experience on Neurontin® to gauge whether or not it affects their mental and/or motor performance adversely.

Laboratory Tests

Clinical trials data do not indicate that routine monitoring of clinical laboratory parameters is necessary for the safe use of Neurontin®. The value of monitoring Neurontin® blood concentrations has not been established. Neurontin® may be used in combination with other antiepileptic drugs without concern for alteration of the blood concentrations of gabapentin or of other antiepileptic drugs.

Drug Interactions

Gabapentin is not appreciably metabolized nor does it interfere with the metabolism of commonly coadministered antiepileptic drugs.

The drug interaction data described in this section were obtained from studies involving healthy adults and adult patients with epilepsy.

Phenytoin: In a single and multiple dose study of Neurontin® (400 mg T.I.D.) in epileptic patients (N=8) maintained on phenytoin monotherapy for at least 2 months, gabapentin had no effect on the steady-state trough plasma concentrations of phenytoin and phenytoin had no effect on gabapentin pharmacokinetics.

Carbamazepine: Steady-state trough plasma carbamazepine and carbamazepine 10, 11 epoxide concentrations were not affected by concomitant gabapentin (400 mg T.I.D.; N=12) administration. Likewise, gabapentin pharmacokinetics were unaltered by carbamazepine administration.

Valproic Acid: The mean steady-state trough serum valproic acid concentrations prior to and during concomitant gabapentin administration (400 mg T.I.D.; N=17) were not different and neither were gabapentin pharmacokinetic parameters affected by valproic acid.

Phenobarbital: Estimates of steady-state pharmacokinetic parameters for phenobarbital or gabapentin (300 mg T.I.D.; N=12) are identical whether the drugs are administered alone or together.

Cimetidine: In the presence of cimetidine at 300 mg Q.I.D. (N=12) the mean apparent oral clearance of gabapentin fell by 14% and creatinine clearance fell by 10%. Thus cimetidine appeared to alter the renal excretion of both gabapentin and creatinine, an endogenous marker of renal function. This small decrease in excretion of gabapentin by cimetidine is not expected to be of clinical importance. The effect of gabapentin on cimetidine was not evaluated.

Oral Contraceptive: Based on AUC and half-life, multiple-dose pharmacokinetic profiles of norethindrone and ethinyl estradiol following administration of tablets containing 2.5 mg of norethindrone acetate and 50 mcg of ethinyl estradiol were similar with and without coadministration of gabapentin (400 mg T.I.D.; N=13). The Cmax of norethindrone was 13% higher when it was coadministered with gabapentin; this interaction is not expected to be of clinical importance.

Antacid (Maalox®): Maalox reduced the bioavailability of gabapentin (N=16) by about 20%. This decrease in bioavailability was about 5% when gabapentin was administered 2 hours after Maalox. It is recommended that gabapentin be taken at least 2 hours following Maalox administration.

Effect of Probenecid: Probenecid is a blocker of renal tubular secretion. Gabapentin pharmacokinetic parameters without and with probenecid were comparable. This indicates that gabapentin does not undergo renal tubular secretion by the pathway that is blocked by probenecid.

Drug/Laboratory Tests Interactions

Because false positive readings were reported with the Ames N-Multistix SG® dipstick test for urinary protein when gabapentin was added to other antiepileptic drugs, the more specific sulfosalicylic acid precipitation procedure is recommended to determine the presence of urine protein.

Carcinogenesis, Mutagenesis, Impairment of Fertility

Gabapentin was given in the diet to mice at 200, 600, and 2000 mg/kg/day and to rats at 250, 1000, and 2000 mg/kg/day for 2 years. A statistically significant increase in the incidence of pancreatic acinar cell adenomas and carcinomas was found in male rats receiving the high dose; the no-effect dose for the occurrence of carcinomas was 1000 mg/kg/day. Peak plasma concentrations of gabapentin in rats receiving the high dose of 2000 mg/kg were 10 times higher than plasma concentrations in humans receiving 3600 mg per day, and in rats receiving 1000 mg/kg/day peak plasma concentrations were 6.5 times higher than in humans receiving 3600 mg/day. The pancreatic acinar cell carcinomas did not affect survival, did not metastasize and were not locally invasive. The relevance of this finding to carcinogenic risk in humans is unclear.

Studies designed to investigate the mechanism of gabapentin-induced pancreatic carcinogenesis in rats indicate that gabapentin stimulates DNA synthesis in rat pancreatic acinar cells *in vitro* and, thus, may be acting as a tumor promoter by enhancing mitogenic activity. It is not known whether gabapentin has the ability to increase cell proliferation in other cell types or in other species, including humans.

Gabapentin did not demonstrate mutagenic or genotoxic potential in three *in vitro* and four *in vivo* assays. It was negative in the Ames test and the *in vitro* HGPRT forward mutation assay in Chinese hamster lung cells; it did not produce significant increases in chromosomal aberrations in the *in vitro* Chinese hamster lung cell assay; it was negative in the *in vivo* chromosomal aberration assay and in the *in vivo* micronucleus test in Chinese hamster bone marrow; it was negative in the *in vivo* mouse micronucleus assay; and it did not induce unscheduled DNA synthesis in hepatocytes from rats given gabapentin.

No adverse effects on fertility or reproduction were observed in rats at doses up to 2000 mg/kg (approximately 5 times the maximum recommended human dose on an mg/m^2 basis).

Pregnancy

Pregnancy Category C: Gabapentin has been shown to be fetotoxic in rodents, causing delayed ossification of several bones in the skull, vertebrae, forelimbs, and hindlimbs. These effects occurred when pregnant mice received oral doses of 1000 or 3000 mg/kg/day during the period of organogenesis, or approximately 1 to 4 times the maximum dose of 3600 mg/day given to epileptic patients on a mg/m^2 basis. The no-effect level was 500 mg/kg/day or approximately ½ of the human dose on a mg/m^2 basis.

When rats were dosed prior to and during mating, and throughout gestation, pups from all dose groups (500, 1000 and 2000 mg/kg/day) were affected. These doses are equivalent to less than approximately 1 to 5 times the maximum

Continued on next page

Neurontin—Cont.

human dose on a mg/m² basis. There was an increased incidence of hydroureter and/or hydronephrosis in rats in a study of fertility and general reproductive performance at 2000 mg/kg/day with no effect at 1000 mg/kg/day, in a teratology study at 1500 mg/kg/day with no effect at 300 mg/kg/day, and in a perinatal and postnatal study at all doses studied (500, 1000 and 2000 mg/kg/day). The doses at which the effects occurred are approximately 1 to 5 times the maximum human dose of 3600 mg/day on a mg/m² basis; the no-effect doses were approximately 3 times (Fertility and General Reproductive Performance study) and approximately equal to (Teratogenicity study) the maximum human dose on a mg/m² basis. Other than hydroureter and hydronephrosis, the etiologies of which are unclear, the incidence of malformations was not increased compared to controls in offspring of mice, rats, or rabbits given doses up to 50 times (mice), 30 times (rats), and 25 times (rabbits) the human daily dose on a mg/kg basis, or 4 times (mice), 5 times (rats), or 8 times (rabbits) the human daily dose on a mg/m² basis.

In a teratology study in rabbits, an increased incidence of postimplantation fetal loss occurred in dams exposed to 60, 300 and 1500 mg/kg/day, or less than approximately ¼ to 8 times the maximum human dose on a mg/m² basis. There are no adequate and well-controlled studies in pregnant women. Because animal reproduction studies are not always predictive of human response, this drug should be used during pregnancy only if the potential benefit justifies the potential risk to the fetus.

Use in Nursing Mothers

Gabapentin is secreted into human milk following oral administration. A nursed infant could be exposed to a maximum dose of approximately 1 mg/kg/day of gabapentin. Because the effect on the nursing infant is unknown, Neurontin® should be used in women who are nursing only if the benefits clearly outweigh the risks.

Pediatric Use

Effectiveness in pediatric patients below the age of 3 years has not been established (see CLINICAL PHARMACOLOGY, Clinical Studies).

Geriatric Use

Clinical studies of Neurontin did not include sufficient numbers of subjects aged 65 and over to determine whether they responded differently from younger subjects. Other reported clinical experience has not identified differences in responses between the elderly and younger patients. In general, dose selection for an elderly patient should be cautious, usually starting at the low end of the dosing range, reflecting the greater frequency of decreased hepatic, renal, or cardiac function, and of concomitant disease or other drug therapy.

This drug is known to be substantially excreted by the kidney, and the risk of toxic reactions to this drug may be greater in patients with impaired renal function. Because elderly patients are more likely to have decreased renal function, care should be taken in dose selection, and it may be useful to monitor renal function (see CLINICAL PHARMACOLOGY, ADVERSE REACTIONS, and DOSAGE AND ADMINISTRATION sections).

ADVERSE REACTIONS

The most commonly observed adverse events associated with the use of Neurontin® in combination with other antiepileptic drugs in patients >12 years of age, not seen at an equivalent frequency among placebo-treated patients, were somnolence, dizziness, ataxia, fatigue, and nystagmus. The most commonly observed adverse events reported with the use of Neurontin in combination with other antiepileptic drugs in pediatric patients 3 to 12 years of age, not seen at an equal frequency among placebo-treated patients, were viral infection, fever, nausea and/or vomiting, somnolence, and hostility (see WARNINGS, Neuropsychiatric Adverse Events).

Approximately 7% of the 2074 patients >12 years of age and approximately 7% of the 449 pediatric patients 3 to 12 years of age who received Neurontin® in premarketing clinical trials discontinued treatment because of an adverse event. The adverse events most commonly associated with withdrawal in patients >12 years of age were somnolence (1.2%), ataxia (0.8%), fatigue (0.6%), nausea and/or vomiting (0.6%), and dizziness (0.6%). The adverse events most commonly associated with withdrawal in pediatric patients were emotional lability (1.6%), hostility (1.3%), and hyperkinesia (1.1%).

Incidence in Controlled Clinical Trials

Table 1 lists treatment-emergent signs and symptoms that occurred in at least 1% of Neurontin®-treated patients >12 years of age with epilepsy participating in placebo-controlled trials and were numerically more common in the Neurontin® group. In these studies, either Neurontin® or placebo was added to the patient's current antiepileptic drug therapy. Adverse events were usually mild to moderate in intensity.

The prescriber should be aware that these figures, obtained when Neurontin® was added to concurrent antiepileptic drug therapy, cannot be used to predict the frequency of adverse events in the course of usual medical practice where patient characteristics and other factors may differ from those prevailing during clinical studies. Similarly, the cited frequencies cannot be directly compared with figures obtained from other clinical investigations involving different treatments, uses, or investigators. An inspection of these frequencies, however, does provide the prescribing physician with one basis to estimate the relative contribution of drug and nondrug factors to the adverse event incidences in the population studied.

TABLE 1. Treatment-Emergent Adverse Event Incidence in Controlled Add-On Trials In Patients >12 years of age (Events in at least 1% of Neurontin patients and numerically more frequent than in the placebo group)

Body System/Adverse Event	Neurontin®[a] N=543 %	Placebo[a] N=378 %
Body As A Whole		
Fatigue	11.0	5.0
Weight Increase	2.9	1.6
Back Pain	1.8	0.5
Peripheral Edema	1.7	0.5
Cardiovascular		
Vasodilatation	1.1	0.3
Digestive System		
Dyspepsia	2.2	0.5
Mouth or Throat Dry	1.7	0.5
Constipation	1.5	0.8
Dental Abnormalities	1.5	0.3
Increased Appetite	1.1	0.8
Hematologic and Lymphatic Systems		
Leukopenia	1.1	0.5
Musculoskeletal System		
Myalgia	2.0	1.9
Fracture	1.1	0.8
Nervous System		
Somnolence	19.3	8.7
Dizziness	17.1	6.9
Ataxia	12.5	5.6
Nystagmus	8.3	4.0
Tremor	6.8	3.2
Nervousness	2.4	1.9
Dysarthria	2.4	0.5
Amnesia	2.2	0.0
Depression	1.8	1.1
Thinking Abnormal	1.7	1.3
Twitching	1.3	0.5
Coordination Abnormal	1.1	0.3
Respiratory System		
Rhinitis	4.1	3.7
Pharyngitis	2.8	1.6
Coughing	1.8	1.3
Skin and Appendages		
Abrasion	1.3	0.0
Pruritus	1.3	0.5
Urogenital System		
Impotence	1.5	1.1
Special Senses		
Diplopia	5.9	1.9
Amblyopia[b]	4.2	1.1
Laboratory Deviations		
WBC Decreased	1.1	0.5

[a]Plus background antiepileptic drug therapy
[b]Amblyopia was often described as blurred vision.

Other events in more than 1% of patients >12 years of age but equally or more frequent in the placebo group included: headache, viral infection, fever, nausea and/or vomiting, abdominal pain, diarrhea, convulsions, confusion, insomnia, emotional lability, rash, acne.

Among the treatment-emergent adverse events occurring at an incidence of at least 10% of Neurontin-treated patients, somnolence and ataxia appeared to exhibit a positive dose-response relationship.

The overall incidence of adverse events and the types of adverse events seen were similar among men and women treated with Neurontin®. The incidence of adverse events increased slightly with increasing age in patients treated with either Neurontin® or placebo. Because only 3% of patients (28/921) in placebo-controlled studies were identified as nonwhite (black or other), there are insufficient data to support a statement regarding the distribution of adverse events by race.

Table 2 lists treatment-emergent signs and symptoms that occurred in at least 2% of Neurontin-treated patients age 3 to 12 years of age with epilepsy participating in placebo-controlled trials and were numerically more common in the Neurontin group. Adverse events were usually mild to moderate in intensity.

TABLE 2. Treatment-Emergent Adverse Event Incidence in Pediatric Patients Age 3 to 12 Years in a Controlled Add-On Trial (Events in at least 2% of Neurontin patients and numerically more frequent than in the placebo group)

Body System/Adverse Event	Neurontin[a] N=119 %	Placebo[a] N=128 %
Body As A Whole		
Viral Infection	10.9	3.1
Fever	10.1	3.1
Weight Increase	3.4	0.8
Fatigue	3.4	1.6
Digestive System		
Nausea and/or Vomiting	8.4	7.0
Nervous System		
Somnolence	8.4	4.7
Hostility	7.6	2.3
Emotional Lability	4.2	1.6
Dizziness	2.5	1.6
Hyperkinesia	2.5	0.8
Respiratory System		
Bronchitis	3.4	0.8
Respiratory Infection	2.5	0.8

[a]Plus background antiepileptic drug therapy

Other events in more than 2% of pediatric patients 3 to 12 years of age but equally or more frequent in the placebo group included: pharyngitis, upper respiratory infection, headache, rhinitis, convulsions, diarrhea, anorexia, coughing, and otitis media.

Other Adverse Events Observed During All Clinical Trials

Neurontin® has been administered to 2074 patients >12 years of age during all clinical trials, only some of which were placebo-controlled. During these trials, all adverse events were recorded by the clinical investigators using terminology of their own choosing. To provide a meaningful estimate of the proportion of individuals having adverse events, similar types of events were grouped into a smaller number of standardized categories using modified COSTART dictionary terminology. These categories are used in the listing below. The frequencies presented represent the proportion of the 2074 patients >12 years of age exposed to Neurontin® who experienced an event of the type cited on at least one occasion while receiving Neurontin®. All reported events are included except those already listed in the previous table, those too general to be informative, and those not reasonably associated with the use of the drug.

Events are further classified within body system categories and enumerated in order of decreasing frequency using the following definitions: frequent adverse events are defined as those occurring in at least 1/100 patients; infrequent adverse events are those occurring in 1/100 to 1/1000 patients; rare events are those occurring in fewer than 1/1000 patients.

Body As A Whole: *Frequent:* asthenia, malaise, face edema; *Infrequent:* allergy, generalized edema, weight decrease, chill; *Rare:* strange feelings, lassitude, alcohol intolerance, hangover effect.

Cardiovascular System: *Frequent:* hypertension; *Infrequent:* hypotension, angina pectoris, peripheral vascular disorder, palpitation, tachycardia, migraine, murmur; *Rare:* atrial fibrillation, heart failure, thrombophlebitis, deep thrombophlebitis, myocardial infarction, cerebrovascular accident, pulmonary thrombosis, ventricular extrasystoles, bradycardia, premature atrial contraction, pericardial rub, heart block, pulmonary embolus, hyperlipidemia, hypercholesterolemia, pericardial effusion, pericarditis.

Digestive System: *Frequent:* anorexia, flatulence, gingivitis; *Infrequent:* glossitis, gum hemorrhage, thirst, stomatitis, increased salivation, gastroenteritis, hemorrhoids, bloody stools, fecal incontinence, hepatomegaly; *Rare:* dysphagia, eructation, pancreatitis, peptic ulcer, colitis, blisters in mouth, tooth discolor, perlèche, salivary gland enlarged, lip hemorrhage, esophagitis, hiatal hernia, hematemesis, proctitis, irritable bowel syndrome, rectal hemorrhage, esophageal spasm.

Endocrine System: *Rare:* hyperthyroid, hypothyroid, goiter, hypoestrogen, ovarian failure, epididymitis, swollen testicle, cushingoid appearance.

Hematologic and Lymphatic System: *Frequent:* purpura most often described as bruises resulting from physical trauma; *Infrequent:* anemia, thrombocytopenia, lymphadenopathy; *Rare:* WBC count increased, lymphocytosis, non-Hodgkin's lymphoma, bleeding time increased.

Musculoskeletal System: *Frequent:* arthralgia; *Infrequent:* tendinitis, arthritis, joint stiffness, joint swelling, positive Romberg test; *Rare:* costochondritis, osteoporosis, bursitis, contracture.

Nervous System: *Frequent:* vertigo, hyperkinesia, paresthesia, decreased or absent reflexes, increased reflexes, anxiety, hostility; *Infrequent:* CNS tumors, syncope, dreaming abnormal, aphasia, hypesthesia, intracranial hemorrhage, hypotonia, dysesthesia, paresis, dystonia, hemiplegia, facial paralysis, stupor, cerebellar dysfunction, positive Babinski sign, decreased position sense, subdural hematoma, apathy, hallucination, decrease or loss of libido, agitation, paranoia, depersonalization, euphoria, feeling high, doped-up sensation, suicidal, psychosis; *Rare:* choreoathetosis, orofacial dyskinesia, encephalopathy, nerve palsy, personality disorder, increased libido, subdued temperament, apraxia, fine motor control disorder, meningismus, local myoclonus, hyperesthesia, hypokinesia, mania, neurosis, hysteria, antisocial reaction, suicide gesture.

Respiratory System: *Frequent:* pneumonia; *Infrequent:* epistaxis, dyspnea, apnea; *Rare:* mucositis, aspiration pneumonia, hyperventilation, hiccup, laryngitis, nasal obstruction, snoring, bronchospasm, hypoventilation, lung edema.

Dermatological: *Infrequent:* alopecia, eczema, dry skin, increased sweating, urticaria, hirsutism, seborrhea, cyst, herpes simplex; *Rare:* herpes zoster, skin discolor, skin papules, photosensitive reaction, leg ulcer, scalp seborrhea, psoriasis, desquamation, maceration, skin nodules, subcutaneous nodule, melanosis, skin necrosis, local swelling.

Urogenital System: *Infrequent:* hematuria, dysuria, urination frequency, cystitis, urinary retention, urinary incontinence, vaginal hemorrhage, amenorrhea, dysmenorrhea, menorrhagia, breast cancer, unable to climax, ejaculation abnormal; *Rare:* kidney pain, leukorrhea, pruritus genital, renal stone, acute renal failure, anuria, glycosuria, nephrosis, nocturia, pyuria, urination urgency, vaginal pain, breast pain, testicle pain.

Special Senses: *Frequent:* abnormal vision; *Infrequent:* cataract, conjunctivitis, eyes dry, eye pain, visual field defect, photophobia, bilateral or unilateral ptosis, eye hemorrhage, hordeolum, hearing loss, earache, tinnitus, inner ear infection, otitis, taste loss, unusual taste, eye twitching, ear fullness; *Rare:* eye itching, abnormal accommodation, perforated ear drum, sensitivity to noise, eye focusing problem, watery eyes, retinopathy, glaucoma, iritis, corneal disorders, lacrimal dysfunction, degenerative eye changes, blindness, retinal degeneration, miosis, chorioretinitis, strabismus, eustachian tube dysfunction, labyrinthitis, otitis externa, odd smell.

Adverse events occurring during clinical trials in 449 pediatric patients 3 to 12 years of age treated with gabapentin that were not reported in adjunctive trials in adults are:

Body as a Whole: dehydration, infectious mononucleosis
Digestive System: hepatitis
Hemic and Lymphatic System: coagulation defect
Nervous System: aura disappeared, occipital neuralgia
Psychobiologic Function: sleepwalking
Respiratory System: pseudocroup, hoarseness

Postmarketing and Other Experience

In addition to the adverse experiences reported during clinical testing of Neurontin®, the following adverse experiences have been reported in patients receiving marketed Neurontin®. These adverse experiences have not been listed above and data are insufficient to support an estimate of their incidence or to establish causation. The listing is alphabetized: angioedema, blood glucose fluctuation, erythema multiforme, elevated liver function tests, fever, hyponatremia, jaundice, Stevens-Johnson syndrome.

DRUG ABUSE AND DEPENDENCE

The abuse and dependence potential of Neurontin® has not been evaluated in human studies.

OVERDOSAGE

A lethal dose of gabapentin was not identified in mice and rats receiving single oral doses as high as 8000 mg/kg. Signs of acute toxicity in animals included ataxia, labored breathing, ptosis, sedation, hypoactivity, or excitation.

Acute oral overdoses of Neurontin® up to 49 grams have been reported. In these cases, double vision, slurred speech, drowsiness, lethargy and diarrhea were observed. All patients recovered with supportive care.

Gabapentin can be removed by hemodialysis. Although hemodialysis has not been performed in the few overdose cases reported, it may be indicated by the patient's clinical state or in patients with significant renal impairment.

DOSAGE AND ADMINISTRATION

Neurontin® is recommended for add-on therapy in patients 3 years of age and older. Effectiveness in pediatric patients below the age of 3 years has not been established.

Neurontin® is given orally with or without food.

Patients >12 years of age: The effective dose of Neurontin® is 900 to 1800 mg/day and given in divided doses (three times a day) using 300 or 400 mg capsules, or 600 or 800 mg tablets. The starting dose is 300 mg three times a day. If necessary, the dose may be increased using 300 or 400 mg capsules, or 600 or 800 mg tablets three times a day up to 1800 mg/day. Dosages up to 2400 mg/day have been well tolerated in long-term clinical studies. Doses of 3600 mg/day have also been administered to a small number of patients for a relatively short duration, and have been well tolerated. The maximum time between doses in the T.I.D. schedule should not exceed 12 hours.

Pediatric Patients Age 3–12 years: The starting dose should range from 10–15 mg/kg/day in 3 divided doses, and the effective dose reached by upward titration over a period of approximately 3 days. The effective dose of Neurontin in patients 5 years of age and older is 25–35 mg/kg/day and given in divided doses (three times a day). The effective dose in pediatric patients ages 3 and 4 years is 40 mg/kg/day and given in divided doses (three times a day). (See CLINICAL PHARMACOLOGY, Pediatrics.) Neurontin® may be administered as the oral solution, capsule, or tablet, or using combinations of these formulations. Dosages up to 50 mg/kg/day have been well-tolerated in a long-term clinical study. The maximum time interval between doses should not exceed 12 hours.

It is not necessary to monitor gabapentin plasma concentrations to optimize Neurontin® therapy. Further, because there are no significant pharmacokinetic interactions among Neurontin® and other commonly used antiepileptic drugs, the addition of Neurontin® does not alter the plasma levels of these drugs appreciably.

If Neurontin® is discontinued and/or an alternate anticonvulsant medication is added to the therapy, this should be done gradually over a minimum of 1 week.

Creatinine clearance is difficult to measure in outpatients. In patients with stable renal function, creatinine clearance (C_{Cr}) can be reasonably well estimated using the equation of Cockcroft and Gault:

for females $C_{Cr}=(0.85)(140\text{-age})(\text{weight})/[(72)(S_{Cr})]$

for males $C_{Cr}=(140\text{-age})(\text{weight})/[(72)(S_{Cr})]$

where age is in years, weight is in kilograms and S_{Cr} is serum creatinine in mg/dL.

Dosage adjustment in patients ≥12 years of age with compromised renal function or undergoing hemodialysis is recommended as follows:

TABLE 3. Neurontin® Dosage Based on Renal Function

Renal Function Creatinine Clearance (mL/min)	Total Daily Dose (mg/day)	Dose Regimen (mg)
>60	1200	400 T.I.D.
30–60	600	300 B.I.D.
15–30	300	300 Q.D.
<15	150	300 Q.O.D.[a]
Hemodialysis	—	200–300[b]

[a] Every other day

[b] Loading dose of 300 to 400 mg in patients who have never received Neurontin®, then 200 to 300 mg Neurontin® following each 4 hours of hemodialysis.

The use of Neurontin® in patients <12 years of age with compromised renal function has not been studied.

HOW SUPPLIED

Neurontin® (gabapentin) capsules, tablets and oral solution are supplied as follows:

100 mg capsules;
White hard gelatin capsules printed with "PD" on one side and "Neurontin®/100 mg" on the other; available in:
Bottles of 100: N 0071-0803-24
Unit dose 50's: N 0071-0803-40

300 mg capsules;
Yellow hard gelatin capsules printed with "PD" on one side and "Neurontin®/300 mg" on the other; available in:
Bottles of 100: N 0071-0805-24
Unit dose 50's: N 0071-0805-40

400 mg capsules;
Orange hard gelatin capsules printed with "PD" on one side and "Neurontin®/400 mg" on the other; available in:
Bottles of 100: N 0071-0806-24
Unit dose 50's: N 0071-0806-40

600 mg tablets;
White elliptical film-coated tablets printed in black ink with "Neurontin® 600" on one side; available in:
Bottles of 100: N 0071-0416-24
Bottles of 500: N 0071-0416-30
Unit dose 50's: N 0071-0416-40

800 mg tablets;
White elliptical film-coated tablets printed in orange with "Neurontin® 800" on one side; available in:
Bottles of 100: N 0071-0426-24
Bottles of 500: N 0071-0426-30
Unit dose 50's: N 0071-0426-40

250 mg/5 mL oral solution;
Clear colorless to slightly yellow solution; each 5 mL of oral solution contains 250 mg of gabapentin; available in:
Bottles containing 470 mL: N0071-2012-23

Storage (Capsules)

Store at Controlled Room Temperature 15°–30°C (59°–86°F).

Storage (Tablets)

Store at 25°C (77°F); excursions permitted to 15°–30°C (59°–86°F) [see USP Controlled Room Temperature].

Storage (Oral Solution)

Store refrigerated, 2°–8°C (36°–46°F)

Rx only

Revised November 2000

Capsules and Tablets:
Manufactured by:
Parke Davis Pharmaceuticals, Ltd.
Vega Baja, PR 00694

Oral Solution:
Manufactured for:
Parke Davis Pharmaceuticals, Ltd.
Vega Baja, PR 00694

Distributed by:
PARKE-DAVIS
Div of Warner-Lambert Co
Morris Plains, NJ 07950 USA

0416G641

To keep your **PDR** up to date throughout the year, note these revisions on the corresponding pages of the annual volume. Simply write **"See Supplement A"** next to the product heading.

Pfizer Inc.

235 EAST 42ND STREET
NEW YORK, NY 10017–5755

For Medical Information Contact:
(800) 438-1985
24 hours a day, seven days a week.

CARDURA® ℞

[kar' dŭr ə]
(doxazosin mesylate)
Tablets

Prescribing information for this product, which appears on pages 2668–2671 of the 2002 PDR, has been completely revised as follows. Please write "See Supplement A" next to the product heading.

DESCRIPTION

CARDURA® (doxazosin mesylate) is a quinazoline compound that is a selective inhibitor of the $alpha_1$ subtype of alpha adrenergic receptors. The chemical name of doxazosin mesylate is 1-(4-amino-6,7-dimethoxy-2-quinazolinyl)-4-(1,4-benzodioxan-2-ylcarbonyl) piperazine methanesulfonate. The empirical formula for doxazosin mesylate is $C_{23}H_{25}N_5O_5 \bullet CH_4O_3S$ and the molecular weight is 547.6. It has the following structure:

CARDURA® (doxazosin mesylate) is freely soluble in dimethylsulfoxide, soluble in dimethylformamide, slightly soluble in methanol, ethanol, and water (0.8% at 25°C), and very slightly soluble in acetone and methylene chloride. CARDURA® is available as colored tablets for oral use and contains 1 mg (white), 2 mg (yellow), 4 mg (orange) and 8 mg (green) of doxazosin as the free base.

The inactive ingredients for all tablets are: microcrystalline cellulose, lactose, sodium starch glycolate, magnesium stearate and sodium lauryl sulfate. The 2 mg tablet contains D & C yellow 10 and FD & C yellow 6; the 4 mg tablet contains FD & C yellow 6; the 8 mg tablet contains FD & C blue 10 and D & C yellow 10.

CLINICAL PHARMACOLOGY

Pharmacodynamics

A. Benign Prostatic Hyperplasia (BPH)

Benign prostatic hyperplasia (BPH) is a common cause of urinary outflow obstruction in aging males. Severe BPH may lead to urinary retention and renal damage. A static and a dynamic component contribute to the symptoms and reduced urinary flow rate associated with BPH. The static component is related to an increase in prostate size caused, in part, by a proliferation of smooth muscle cells in the prostatic stroma. However, the severity of BPH symptoms and the degree of urethral obstruction do not correlate well with the size of the prostate. The dynamic component of BPH is associated with an increase in smooth muscle tone in the prostate and bladder neck. The degree of tone in this area is mediated by the $alpha_1$ adrenoceptor, which is present in high density in the prostatic stroma, prostatic capsule and bladder neck. Blockade of the $alpha_1$ receptor decreases urethral resistance and may relieve the obstruction and BPH symptoms. In the human prostate, CARDURA® antagonizes phenylephrine ($alpha_1$ agonist)-induced contractions, *in vitro*, and binds with high affinity to the $alpha_{1c}$ adrenoceptor. The receptor subtype is thought to be the predominant functional type in the prostate. CARDURA® acts within 1–2 weeks to decrease the severity of BPH symptoms and improve urinary flow rate. Since $alpha_1$ adrenoceptors are of low density in the urinary bladder (apart from the bladder neck), CARDURA® should maintain bladder contractility.

The efficacy of CARDURA® was evaluated extensively in over 900 patients with BPH in double-blind, placebo-controlled trials. CARDURA® treatment was superior to placebo in improving patient symptoms and urinary flow rate. Significant relief with CARDURA® was seen as early as one week into the treatment regimen, with CARDURA® treated patients (N=173) showing a significant (p<0.01) increase in maximum flow rate of 0.8 mL/sec compared to a decrease of 0.5 mL/sec in the placebo group (N=41). In long-term studies improvement was maintained for up to 2 years of treatment. In 66–71% of patients, improvements above baseline were seen in both symptoms and maximum urinary flow rate.

In three placebo-controlled studies of 14–16 weeks duration obstructive symptoms (hesitation, intermittency, dribbling, weak urinary stream, incomplete emptying of the bladder) and irritative symptoms (nocturia, daytime frequency, urgency, burning) of BPH were evaluated at each visit by patient-assessed symptom questionnaires. The bothersomeness of symptoms was measured with a modified Boyarsky questionnaire. Symptom severity/frequency was assessed

Continued on next page

Cardura—Cont.

using a modified Boyarsky questionnaire or an AUA-based questionnaire. Uroflowmetric evaluations were performed at times of peak (2–6 hours post-dose) and/or trough (24 hours post-dose) plasma concentrations of CARDURA®. The results from the three placebo-controlled studies (N=609) showing significant efficacy with 4 mg and 8 mg doxazosin are summarized in Table 1. In all three studies, CARDURA® resulted in statistically significant relief of obstructive and irritative symptoms compared to placebo. Statistically significant improvements of 2.3–3.3 mL/sec in maximum flow rate were seen with CARDURA® in Studies 1 and 2, compared to 0.1–0.7 mL/sec with placebo.
[See table 1 above]
In one fixed dose study (Study 2) CARDURA® (doxazosin mesylate) therapy (4–8 mg, once daily) resulted in a significant and sustained improvement in maximum urinary flow rate of 2.3–3.3 mL/sec (Table 1) compared to placebo (0.1 mL/sec). In this study, the only study in which weekly evaluations were made, significant improvement with CARDURA® vs. placebo was seen after one week. The proportion of patients who responded with a maximum flow rate improvement of ≥3 mL/sec was significantly larger with CARDURA® (34–42%) than placebo (13–17%). A significantly greater improvement was also seen in average flow rate with CARDURA® (1.6 mL/sec) than with placebo (0.2 mL/sec). The onset and time course of symptom relief and increased urinary flow from Study 1 are illustrated in Figure 1.

TABLE 1
SUMMARY OF EFFECTIVENESS DATA IN PLACEBO-CONTROLLED TRIALS

	SYMPTOM SCORE[a]			MAXIMUM FLOW RATE (mL/sec)		
	N	MEAN BASELINE	MEAN[b] CHANGE	N	MEAN BASELINE	MEAN[c] CHANGE
STUDY 1 (Titration to maximum dose of 8 mg)[e]						
Placebo	47	15.6	-2.3	41	9.7	+0.7
CARDURA	49	14.5	-4.9**	41	9.8	+2.9**
STUDY 2 (Titration to fixed dose–14 weeks)[d]						
Placebo	37	20.7	-2.5	30	10.6	+0.1
CARDURA 4 mg	38	21.2	-5.0**	32	9.8	+2.3*
CARDURA 8 mg	42	19.9	-4.2*	36	10.5	+3.3**
STUDY 3 (Titration to fixed dose–12 weeks)						
Placebo	47	14.9	-4.7	44	9.9	+2.1
CARDURA 4 mg	46	16.6	-6.1*	46	9.6	+2.6

[a] AUA questionnaire (range 0-30) in studies 1 and 3. Modified Boyarsky Questionnaire (range 7-39) in study 2.
[b] Change is to endpoint.
[c] Change is to fixed-dose efficacy phase, 22-26 hours post-dose for studies 1 and 3 and 2-6 hours post-dose for study 2.
[d] Study in hypertensives with BPH
[e] 36 patients received a dose of 8 mg CARDURA*
*(**) p < 0.05 (0.01) compared to placebo mean change.

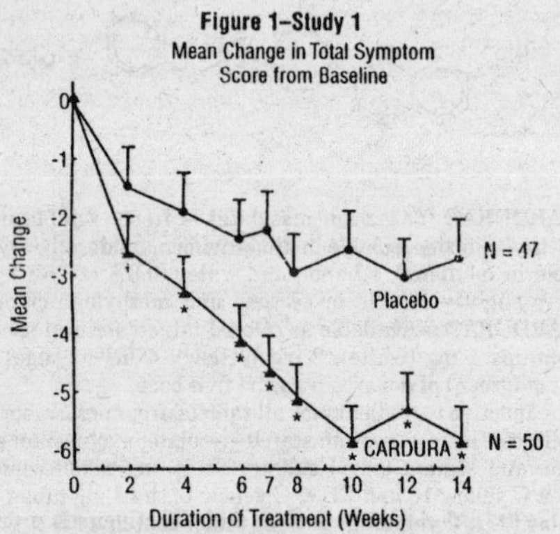

Figure 1–Study 1
Mean Change in Total Symptom Score from Baseline

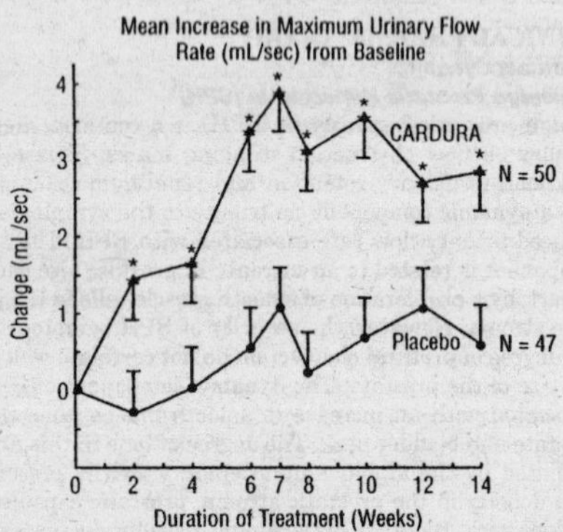

Mean Increase in Maximum Urinary Flow Rate (mL/sec) from Baseline

*p <0.05 Compared to Placebo; †p <0.05 Compared to Baseline; Doxazosin Titration to Maximum of 8 mg.

In BPH patients (N=450) treated for up to 2 years in open-label studies, CARDURA® therapy resulted in significant improvement above baseline in urinary flow rates and BPH symptoms. The significant effects of CARDURA® were maintained over the entire treatment period.
Although blockade of alpha$_1$ adrenoceptors also lowers blood pressure in hypertensive patients with increased peripheral vascular resistance, CARDURA® treatment of normotensive men with BPH did not result in a clinically significant blood pressure lowering effect (Table 2). The proportion of normotensive patients with a sitting systolic blood pressure less than 90 mmHg and/or diastolic blood pressure less than 60 mmHg at any time during treatment with CARDURA® 1–8 mg once daily was 6.7% with doxazosin and not significantly different (statistically) from that with placebo (5%).
[See table 2 above]

TABLE 2
Mean Changes in Blood Pressure from Baseline to the Mean of the Final Efficacy Phase in Normotensives (Diastolic BP <90 mmHg) in Two Double-blind, Placebo-controlled U.S. Studies with CARDURA® 1–8 mg once daily.

	PLACEBO (N=85)		CARDURA® (N=183)	
Sitting BP (mmHg)	**Baseline**	**Change**	**Baseline**	**Change**
Systolic	128.4	−1.4	128.8	−4.9*
Diastolic	79.2	−1.2	79.6	−2.4*
Standing BP (mmHg)	**Baseline**	**Change**	**Baseline**	**Change**
Systolic	128.5	−0.6	128.5	−5.3*
Diastolic	80.5	−0.7	80.4	−2.6*

*p ≤0.05 compared to placebo

B. *Hypertension*
The mechanism of action of CARDURA® (doxazosin mesylate) is selective blockade of the alpha$_1$ (postjunctional) subtype of adrenergic receptors. Studies in normal human subjects have shown that doxazosin competitively antagonized the pressor effects of phenylephrine (an alpha$_1$ agonist) and the systolic pressor effect of norepinephrine. Doxazosin and prazosin have similar abilities to antagonize phenylephrine. The antihypertensive effect of CARDURA® results from a decrease in systemic vascular resistance. The parent compound doxazosin is primarily responsible for the antihypertensive activity. The low plasma concentrations of known active and inactive metabolites of doxazosin (2-piperazinyl, 6′- and 7′-hydroxy and 6- and 7-O-desmethyl compounds) compared to parent drug indicate that the contribution of even the most potent compound (6′-hydroxy) to the antihypertensive effect of doxazosin in man is probably small. The 6′- and 7′-hydroxy metabolites have demonstrated antioxidant properties at concentrations of 5 μM, *in vitro*.
Administration of CARDURA® results in a reduction in systemic vascular resistance. In patients with hypertension there is little change in cardiac output. Maximum reductions in blood pressure usually occur 2–6 hours after dosing and are associated with a small increase in standing heart rate. Like other alpha$_1$-adrenergic blocking agents, doxazosin has a greater effect on blood pressure and heart rate in the standing position.
In a pooled analysis of placebo-controlled hypertension studies with about 300 hypertensive patients per treatment group, doxazosin, at doses of 1–16 mg given once daily, lowered blood pressure at 24 hours by about 10/8 mmHg compared to placebo in the standing position and about 9/5 mmHg in the supine position. Peak blood pressure effects (1–6 hours) were larger by about 50–75% (i.e., trough values were about 55–70% of peak effect), with the larger peak-trough differences seen in systolic pressures. There was no apparent difference in the blood pressure response of Caucasians and blacks or of patients above and below age 65. In these predominantly normocholesterolemic patients doxazosin produced small reductions in total serum cholesterol (2–3%), LDL cholesterol (4%), and a similarly small increase in HDL/total cholesterol ratio (4%). The clinical significance of these findings is uncertain. In the same patient population, patients receiving CARDURA® gained a mean of 0.6 kg compared to a mean loss of 0.1 kg for placebo patients.

Pharmacokinetics
After oral administration of therapeutic doses, peak plasma levels of CARDURA® (doxazosin mesylate) occur at about 2–3 hours. Bioavailability is approximately 65%, reflecting first pass metabolism of doxazosin by the liver. The effect of food on the pharmacokinetics of CARDURA® was examined in a crossover study with twelve hypertensive subjects. Reductions of 18% in mean maximum plasma concentration and 12% in the area under the concentration-time curve occurred when CARDURA® was administered with food. Neither of these differences was statistically or clinically significant.
CARDURA® is extensively metabolized in the liver, mainly by O-demethylation of the quinazoline nucleus or hydroxylation of the benzodioxan moiety. Although several active metabolites of doxazosin have been identified, the pharmacokinetics of these metabolites have not been characterized. In a study of two subjects administered radiolabelled doxazosin 2 mg orally and 1 mg intravenously on two separate occasions, approximately 63% of the dose was eliminated in the feces and 9% of the dose was found in the urine. On average only 4.8% of the dose was excreted as unchanged drug in the feces and only a trace of the total radioactivity in the urine was attributed to unchanged drug. At the plasma concentrations achieved by therapeutic doses approximately 98% of the circulating drug is bound to plasma proteins.
Plasma elimination of doxazosin is biphasic, with a terminal elimination half-life of about 22 hours. Steady-state studies in hypertensive patients given doxazosin doses of 2–16 mg once daily showed linear kinetics and dose proportionality. In two studies, following the administration of 2 mg orally once daily, the mean accumulation ratios (steady-state AUC vs. first dose AUC) were 1.2 and 1.7. Enterohepatic recycling is suggested by secondary peaking of plasma doxazosin concentrations.
In a crossover study in 24 normotensive subjects, the pharmacokinetics and safety of doxazosin were shown to be similar with morning and evening dosing regimens. The area under the curve after morning dosing was, however, 11% less than that after evening dosing and the time to peak concentration after evening dosing occurred significantly later than that after morning dosing (5.6 hr vs. 3.5 hr).
The pharmacokinetics of CARDURA® (doxazosin mesylate) in young (<65 years) and elderly (≥65 years) subjects were similar for plasma half-life values and oral clearance. Pharmacokinetic studies in elderly patients and patients with renal impairment have shown no significant alterations compared to younger patients with normal renal function. Administration of a single 2 mg dose to patients with cirrhosis (Child-Pugh Class A) showed a 40% increase in exposure to doxazosin. There are only limited data on the effects of drugs known to influence the hepatic metabolism of doxazosin [e.g., cimetidine (see PRECAUTIONS)]. As with any drug wholly metabolized by the liver, use of CARDURA® in patients with altered liver function should be undertaken with caution.
In two placebo-controlled studies, of normotensive and hypertensive BPH patients, in which doxazosin was administered in the morning and the titration interval was two weeks and one week, respectively, trough plasma concentrations of CARDURA® were similar in the two populations. Linear kinetics and dose proportionality were observed.

INDICATIONS AND USAGE

A. ***Benign Prostatic Hyperplasia (BPH).*** CARDURA® is indicated for the treatment of both the urinary outflow obstruction and obstructive and irritative symptoms associated with BPH: obstructive symptoms (hesitation, intermittency, dribbling, weak urinary stream, incomplete emptying of the bladder) and irritative symptoms (nocturia, daytime frequency, urgency, burning). CARDURA® may be used in all BPH patients whether hypertensive or normotensive. In patients with hypertension and BPH, both conditions were effectively treated with CARDURA® monotherapy. CARDURA® provides rapid improvement in symptoms and urinary flow rate in 66–71% of patients. Sustained improvements with CARDURA® were seen in patients treated for up to 14 weeks in double-blind studies and up to 2 years in open-label studies.

B. ***Hypertension.*** CARDURA® (doxazosin mesylate) is also indicated for the treatment of hypertension. CARDURA® may be used alone or in combination with diuretics, beta-adrenergic blocking agents, calcium channel blockers or angiotensin-converting enzyme inhibitors.

CONTRAINDICATIONS

CARDURA® is contraindicated in patients with a known sensitivity to quinazolines (e.g., prazosin, terazosin), doxazosin, or any of the inert ingredients.

WARNINGS

Syncope and "First-dose" Effect: Doxazosin, like other alpha-adrenergic blocking agents, can cause marked hypotension, especially in the upright position, with syncope and other postural symptoms such as dizziness. Marked orthostatic effects are most common with the first dose but can also occur when there is a dosage increase, or if therapy is interrupted for more than a few days. To decrease the likelihood of excessive hypotension and syncope, it is essential that treatment be initiated with the 1 mg dose. The 2, 4, and 8 mg tablets are not for initial therapy. Dosage should then be adjusted slowly (see DOSAGE AND ADMINISTRATION section) with evaluations and increases in dose every two weeks to the recommended dose. Additional antihypertensive agents should be added with caution.

Patients being titrated with doxazosin should be cautioned to avoid situations where injury could result should syncope occur, during both the day and night.

In an early investigational study of the safety and tolerance of increasing daily doses of doxazosin in normotensives beginning at 1 mg/day, only 2 of 6 subjects could tolerate more than 2 mg/day without experiencing symptomatic postural hypotension. In another study of 24 healthy normotensive male subjects receiving initial doses of 2 mg/day of doxazosin, seven (29%) of the subjects experienced symptomatic postural hypotension between 0.5 and 6 hours after the first dose necessitating termination of the study. In this study, 2 of the normotensive subjects experienced syncope. Subsequent trials in hypertensive patients always began doxazosin dosing at 1 mg/day resulting in a 4% incidence of postural side effects at 1 mg/day with no cases of syncope.

In multiple dose clinical trials in hypertension involving over 1500 hypertensive patients with dose titration every one to two weeks, syncope was reported in 0.7% of patients. None of these events occurred at the starting dose of 1 mg and 1.2% (8/664) occurred at 16 mg/day.

In placebo-controlled, clinical trials in BPH, 3 out of 665 patients (0.5%) taking doxazosin reported syncope. Two of the patients were taking 1 mg doxazosin, while one patient was taking 2 mg doxazosin when syncope occurred. In the open-label, long-term extension follow-up of approximately 450 BPH patients, there were 3 reports of syncope (0.7%). One patient was taking 2 mg, one patient was taking 8 mg and one patient was taking 12 mg when syncope occurred. In a clinical pharmacology study, one subject receiving 2 mg experienced syncope.

If syncope occurs, the patient should be placed in a recumbent position and treated supportively as necessary.

Priapism: Rarely (probably less frequently than once in every several thousand patients), alpha$_1$ antagonists, including doxazosin, have been associated with priapism (painful penile erection, sustained for hours and unrelieved by sexual intercourse or masturbation). Because this condition can lead to permanent impotence if not promptly treated, patients must be advised about the seriousness of the condition (see **PRECAUTIONS: Information for Patients**).

PRECAUTIONS

General:

Prostate Cancer: Carcinoma of the prostate causes many of the symptoms associated with BPH and the two disorders frequently co-exist. Carcinoma of the prostate should therefore be ruled out prior to commencing therapy with CARDURA®.

Orthostatic Hypotension: While syncope is the most severe orthostatic effect of CARDURA®, other symptoms of lowered blood pressure, such as dizziness, lightheadedness, or vertigo can occur, especially at initiation of therapy or at the time of dose increases.

a) Hypertension

These symptoms were common in clinical trials in hypertension, occurring in up to 23% of all patients treated and causing discontinuation of therapy in about 2%.

In placebo-controlled titration trials in hypertension, orthostatic effects were minimized by beginning therapy at 1 mg per day and titrating every two weeks to 2, 4, or 8 mg per day. There was an increased frequency of orthostatic effects in patients given 8 mg or more, 10%, compared to 5% at 1–4 mg and 3% in the placebo group.

b) Benign Prostatic Hyperplasia

In placebo-controlled trials in BPH, the incidence of orthostatic hypotension with doxazosin was 0.3% and did not increase with increasing dosage (to 8 mg/day). The incidence of discontinuations due to hypotensive or orthostatic symptoms was 3.3% with doxazosin and 1% with placebo. The titration interval in these studies was one to two weeks.

Patients in occupations in which orthostatic hypotension could be dangerous should be treated with particular caution. As alpha$_1$ antagonists can cause orthostatic effects, it is important to evaluate standing blood pressure two minutes after standing and patients should be advised to exercise care when arising from a supine or sitting position.

If hypotension occurs, the patient should be placed in the supine position and, if this measure is inadequate, volume expansion with intravenous fluids or vasopressor therapy may be used. A transient hypotensive response is not a contraindication to further doses of CARDURA® (doxazosin mesylate).

Information for Patients *(See patient package insert)*: Patients should be made aware of the possibility of syncopal and orthostatic symptoms, especially at the initiation of therapy, and urged to avoid driving or hazardous tasks for 24 hours after the first dose, after a dosage increase, and after interruption of therapy when treatment is resumed. They should be cautioned to avoid situations where injury could result should syncope occur during initiation of doxazosin therapy. They should also be advised of the need to sit or lie down when symptoms of lowered blood pressure occur, although these symptoms are not always orthostatic, and to be careful when rising from a sitting or lying position. If dizziness, lightheadedness, or palpitations are bothersome they should be reported to the physician, so that dose adjustment can be considered. Patients should also be told that drowsiness or somnolence can occur with CARDURA® (doxazosin mesylate) or any selective alpha$_1$ adrenoceptor antagonist, requiring caution in people who must drive or operate heavy machinery.

Patients should be advised about the possibility of priapism as a result of treatment with alpha$_1$ antagonists. Patients should know that this adverse event is very rare. If they experience priapism, it should be brought to immediate medical attention for if not treated promptly it can lead to permanent erectile dysfunction (impotence).

Drug/Laboratory Test Interactions: CARDURA® does not affect the plasma concentration of prostate specific antigen in patients treated for up to 3 years. Both doxazosin, an alpha$_1$ inhibitor, and finasteride, a 5-alpha reductase inhibitor, are highly protein bound and hepatically metabolized. There is no definitive controlled clinical experience on the concomitant use of alpha$_1$ inhibitors and 5-alpha reductase inhibitors at this time.

Impaired Liver Function: CARDURA® should be administered with caution to patients with evidence of impaired hepatic function or to patients receiving drugs known to influence hepatic metabolism (see CLINICAL PHARMACOLOGY).

Leukopenia/Neutropenia: Analysis of hematologic data from hypertensive patients receiving CARDURA® in controlled hypertension clinical trials showed that the mean WBC (N=474) and mean neutrophil counts (N=419) were decreased by 2.4% and 1.0%, respectively, compared to placebo, a phenomenon seen with other alpha blocking drugs. In BPH patients the incidence of clinically significant WBC abnormalities was 0.4% (2/459) with CARDURA® and 0% (0/147) with placebo, with no statistically significant difference between the two treatment groups. A search through a data base of 2400 hypertensive patients and 665 BPH patients revealed 4 hypertensives in which drug-related neutropenia could not be ruled out and one BPH patient in which drug related leukopenia could not be ruled out. Two hypertensives had a single low value on the last day of treatment. Two hypertensives had stable, non-progressive neutrophil counts in the 1000/mm^3 range over periods of 20 and 40 weeks. One BPH patient had a decrease from a WBC count of 4800/mm^3 to 2700/mm^3 at the end of the study; there was no evidence of clinical impairment. In cases where follow-up was available the WBCs and neutrophil counts returned to normal after discontinuation of CARDURA®. No patients became symptomatic as a result of the low WBC or neutrophil counts.

Drug Interactions: Most (98%) of plasma doxazosin is protein bound. *In vitro* data in human plasma indicate that CARDURA® has no effect on protein binding of digoxin, warfarin, phenytoin or indomethacin. There is no information on the effect of other highly plasma protein bound drugs on doxazosin binding. CARDURA® has been administered without any evidence of an adverse drug interaction to patients receiving thiazide diuretics, beta-blocking agents, and nonsteroidal anti-inflammatory drugs. In a placebo-controlled trial in normal volunteers, the administration of a single 1 mg dose of doxazosin on day 1 of a four-day regimen of oral cimetidine (400 mg twice daily) resulted in a 10% increase in mean AUC of doxazosin (p=0.006), and a slight but not statistically significant increase in mean C_{max} and mean half-life of doxazosin. The clinical significance of this increase in doxazosin AUC is unknown.

In clinical trials, CARDURA® tablets have been administered to patients on a variety of concomitant medications; while no formal interaction studies have been conducted, no interactions were observed. CARDURA® tablets have been used with the following drugs or drug classes: 1) analgesic/anti-inflammatory (e.g., acetaminophen, aspirin, codeine and codeine combinations, ibuprofen, indomethacin); 2) antibiotics (e.g., erythromycin, trimethoprim and sulfamethoxazole, amoxicillin); 3) antihistamines (e.g., chlorpheniramine); 4) cardiovascular agents (e.g., atenolol, hydrochlorothiazide, propranolol); 5) corticosteroids; 6) gastrointestinal agents (e.g., antacids); 7) hypoglycemics and endocrine drugs; 8) sedatives and tranquilizers (e.g., diazepam); 9) cold and flu remedies.

Cardiac Toxicity in Animals: An increased incidence of myocardial necrosis or fibrosis was displayed by Sprague-Dawley rats after 6 months of dietary administration at concentrations calculated to provide 80 mg doxazosin/kg/day and after 12 months of dietary administration at concentrations calculated to provide 40 mg doxazosin/kg/day (AUC exposure in rats 8 times the human AUC exposure with a 12 mg/day therapeutic dose). Myocardial fibrosis was observed in both rats and mice treated in the same manner with 40 mg doxazosin/kg/day for 18 months (exposure 8 times human AUC exposure in rats and somewhat equivalent to human C_{max} exposure in mice). No cardiotoxicity was observed at lower doses (up to 10 or 20 mg/kg/day, depending on the study) in either species. These lesions were not observed after 12 months of oral dosing in dogs at maximum doses of 20 mg/kg/day [maximum plasma concentrations (C_{max}) in dogs 14 times the C_{max} exposure in humans receiving a 12 mg/day therapeutic dose] and in Wistar rats at doses of 100 mg/kg/day (C_{max} exposures 15 times human C_{max} exposure with a 12 mg/day therapeutic dose). There is no evidence that similar lesions occur in humans.

Carcinogenesis, Mutagenesis, Impairment of Fertility: Chronic dietary administration (up to 24 months) of doxazosin mesylate at maximally tolerated doses of 40 mg/kg/day in rats and 120 mg/kg/day in mice revealed no evidence of carcinogenic potential. The highest doses evaluated in the rat and mouse studies are associated with AUCs (a measure of systemic exposure) that are 8 times and 4 times, respectively, the human AUC at a dose of 16 mg/day. Mutagenicity studies revealed no drug- or metabolite-related effects at either chromosomal or subchromosomal levels.

Studies in rats showed reduced fertility in males treated with doxazosin at oral doses of 20 (but not 5 or 10) mg/kg/day, about 4 times the AUC exposures obtained with a 12 mg/day human dose. This effect was reversible within two weeks of drug withdrawal. There have been no reports of any effects of doxazosin on male fertility in humans.

Pregnancy: Teratogenic Effects, Pregnancy Category C. Studies in pregnant rabbits and rats at daily oral doses of up to 41 and 20 mg/kg, respectively (plasma drug concentrations 10 and 4 times human C_{max} and AUC exposures with a 12 mg/day therapeutic dose), have revealed no evidence of harm to the fetus. A dosage regimen of 82 mg/kg/day in the rabbit was associated with reduced fetal survival. There are no adequate and well-controlled studies in pregnant women. Because animal reproduction studies are not always predictive of human response, CARDURA® should be used during pregnancy only if clearly needed.

Radioactivity was found to cross the placenta following oral administration of labelled doxazosin to pregnant rats.

Nonteratogenic Effects: In peri-postnatal studies in rats, postnatal development at maternal doses of 40 or 50 mg/kg/day of doxazosin (8 times human AUC exposure with a 12 mg/day therapeutic dose) was delayed as evidenced by slower body weight gain and slightly later appearance of anatomical features and reflexes.

Nursing Mothers: Studies in lactating rats given a single oral dose of 1 mg/kg of [2-^{14}C]-CARDURA® indicate that doxazosin accumulates in rat breast milk with a maximum concentration about 20 times greater than the maternal plasma concentration. It is not known whether this drug is excreted in human milk. Because many drugs are excreted in human milk, caution should be exercised when CARDURA® is administered to a nursing mother.

Pediatric Use: The safety and effectiveness of CARDURA® as an antihypertensive agent have not been established in children.

Use in Elderly: The safety and effectiveness profile of CARDURA® in BPH was similar in the elderly (age ≥65 years) and younger (age <65 years) patients.

ADVERSE REACTIONS

A. Benign Prostatic Hyperplasia

The incidence of adverse events has been ascertained from worldwide clinical trials in 965 BPH patients. The incidence rates presented below (Table 3) are based on combined data from seven placebo-controlled trials involving once daily administration of CARDURA® (doxazosin mesylate) in doses of 1–16 mg in hypertensives and 0.5–8 mg in normotensives. The adverse events when the incidence in the CARDURA® group was at least 1% are summarized in Table 3. No significant difference in the incidence of adverse events compared to placebo was seen except for dizziness, fatigue, hypotension, edema and dyspnea. Dizziness and dyspnea appeared to be dose-related.

TABLE 3
ADVERSE REACTIONS DURING PLACEBO-CONTROLLED STUDIES
BENIGN PROSTATIC HYPERPLASIA

Body System	CARDURA® (N=665)	PLACEBO (N=300)
BODY AS A WHOLE		
Back pain	1.8%	2.0%
Chest pain	1.2%	0.7%
Fatigue	8.0%*	1.7%
Headache	9.9%	9.0%
Influenza-like symptoms	1.1%	1.0%
Pain	2.0%	1.0%
CARDIOVASCULAR SYSTEM		
Hypotension	1.7%*	0.0%
Palpitation	1.2%	0.3%
DIGESTIVE SYSTEM		
Abdominal Pain	2.4%	2.0%
Diarrhea	2.3%	2.0%
Dyspepsia	1.7%	1.7%
Nausea	1.5%	0.7%
METABOLIC AND NUTRITIONAL DISORDERS		
Edema	2.7%*	0.7%
NERVOUS SYSTEM		
Dizziness†	15.6%*	9.0%
Mouth Dry	1.4%	0.3%
Somnolence	3.0%	1.0%

Continued on next page

Cardura—Cont.

RESPIRATORY SYSTEM		
Dyspnea	2.6%*	0.3%
Respiratory Disorder	1.1%	0.7%
SPECIAL SENSES		
Vision Abnormal	1.4%	0.7%
UROGENITAL SYSTEM		
Impotence	1.1%	1.0%
Urinary Tract Infection	1.4%	2.3%
SKIN & APPENDAGES		
Sweating Increased	1.1%	1.0%
PSYCHIATRIC DISORDERS		
Anxiety	1.1%	0.3%
Insomnia	1.2%	0.3%

*p ≤0.05 for treatment differences
†Includes vertigo

In these placebo-controlled studies of 665 CARDURA® patients, treated for a mean of 85 days, additional adverse reactions have been reported. These are less than 1% and not distinguishable from those that occurred in the placebo group. Adverse reactions with an incidence of less than 1% but of clinical interest are (CARDURA® vs. placebo): *Cardiovascular System:* angina pectoris (0.6% vs. 0.7%), postural hypotension (0.3% vs. 0.3%), syncope (0.5% vs. 0.0%), tachycardia (0.9% vs. 0.0%); *Urogenital System:* dysuria (0.5% vs. 1.3%), and *Psychiatric Disorders:* libido decreased (0.8% vs. 0.3%). The safety profile in patients treated for up to three years was similar to that in the placebo-controlled studies.
The majority of adverse experiences with CARDURA® were mild.

B. *Hypertension*
CARDURA® has been administered to approximately 4000 hypertensive patients, of whom 1679 were included in the hypertension clinical development program. In that program, minor adverse effects were frequent, but led to discontinuation of treatment in only 7% of patients. In placebo-controlled studies adverse effects occurred in 49% and 40% of patients in the doxazosin and placebo groups, respectively, and led to discontinuation in 2% of patients in each group. The major reasons for discontinuation were postural effects (2%), edema, malaise/fatigue, and some heart rate disturbance, each about 0.7%.
In controlled hypertension clinical trials directly comparing CARDURA® to placebo there was no significant difference in the incidence of side effects, except for dizziness (including postural), weight gain, somnolence and fatigue/malaise. Postural effects and edema appeared to be dose related. The prevalence rates presented below are based on combined data from placebo-controlled studies involving once daily administration of doxazosin at doses ranging from 1–16 mg. Table 4 summarizes those adverse experiences (possibly/probably related) reported for patients in these hypertension studies where the prevalence rate in the doxazosin group was at least 0.5% or where the reaction is of particular interest.

TABLE 4
ADVERSE REACTIONS DURING PLACEBO-CONTROLLED STUDIES

	HYPERTENSION	
	DOXAZOSIN (N=339)	PLACEBO (N=336)
CARDIOVASCULAR SYSTEM		
Dizziness	19%	9%
Vertigo	2%	1%
Postural Hypotension	0.3%	0%
Edema	4%	3%
Palpitation	2%	3%
Arrhythmia	1%	0%
Hypotension	1%	0%
Tachycardia	0.3%	1%
Peripheral Ischemia	0.3%	0%
SKIN & APPENDAGES		
Rash	1%	1%
Pruritus	1%	1%
MUSCULOSKELETAL SYSTEM		
Arthralgia/Arthritis	1%	0%
Muscle Weakness	1%	0%
Myalgia	1%	0%
CENTRAL & PERIPHERAL N.S.		
Headache	14%	16%
Paresthesia	1%	1%
Kinetic Disorders	1%	0%
Ataxia	1%	0%
Hypertonia	1%	0%
Muscle Cramps	1%	0%
AUTONOMIC		
Mouth Dry	2%	2%
Flushing	1%	0%
SPECIAL SENSES		
Vision Abnormal	2%	1%
Conjunctivitis/Eye Pain	1%	1%
Tinnitus	1%	0.3%
PSYCHIATRIC		
Somnolence	5%	1%
Nervousness	2%	2%
Depression	1%	1%
Insomnia	1%	1%
Sexual Dysfunction	2%	1%
GASTROINTESTINAL		
Nausea	3%	4%
Diarrhea	2%	3%
Constipation	1%	1%
Dyspepsia	1%	1%
Flatulence	1%	1%
Abdominal Pain	0%	2%
Vomiting	0%	1%
RESPIRATORY		
Rhinitis	3%	1%
Dyspnea	1%	1%
Epistaxis	1%	0%
URINARY		
Polyuria	2%	0%
Urinary Incontience	1%	0%
Micturition Frequency	0%	2%
GENERAL		
Fatigue/Malaise	12%	6%
Chest Pain	2%	2%
Asthenia	1%	1%
Face Edema	1%	0%
Pain	2%	2%

Additional adverse reactions have been reported, but these are, in general, not distinguishable from symptoms that might have occurred in the absence of exposure to doxazosin. The following adverse reactions occurred with a frequency of between 0.5% and 1%: syncope, hypoesthesia, increased sweating, agitation, increased weight. The following additional adverse reactions were reported by <0.5% of 3960 patients who received doxazosin in controlled or open, short- or long-term clinical studies, including international studies. *Cardiovascular System:* angina pectoris, myocardial infarction, cerebrovascular accident; *Autonomic Nervous System:* pallor; *Metabolic:* thirst, gout, hypokalemia; *Hematopoietic:* lymphadenopathy, purpura; *Reproductive System:* breast pain; *Skin Disorders:* alopecia, dry skin, eczema; *Central Nervous System:* paresis, tremor, twitching, confusion, migraine, impaired concentration; *Psychiatric:* paroniria, amnesia, emotional lability, abnormal thinking, depersonalization; *Special Senses:* parosmia, earache, taste perversion, photophobia, abnormal lacrimation; *Gastrointestinal System:* increased appetite, anorexia, fecal incontinence, gastroenteritis; *Respiratory System:* bronchospasm, sinusitis, coughing, pharyngitis; *Urinary System:* renal calculus; *General Body System:* hot flushes, back pain, infection, fever/rigors, decreased weight, influenza-like symptoms.
CARDURA® has not been associated with any clinically significant changes in routine biochemical tests. No clinically relevant adverse effects were noted on serum potassium, serum glucose, uric acid, blood urea nitrogen, creatinine or liver function tests. CARDURA® has been associated with decreases in white blood cell counts (see PRECAUTIONS).
In post-marketing experience the following additional adverse reactions have been reported: *Autonomic Nervous System:* priapism; *Central Nervous System:* hypoesthesia; *Endocrine System:* gynecomastia; *Gastrointestinal System:* vomiting; *General Body System:* allergic reaction; *Heart Rate/Rhythm:* bradycardia; *Hematopoietic:* leukopenia, thrombocytopenia; *Liver/Biliary System:* hepatitis, hepatitis cholestatic; *Respiratory System:* bronchospasm aggravated; *Skin Disorders:* urticaria; *Urinary System:* hematuria, micturition disorder, micturition frequency, nocturia.

OVERDOSAGE

Experience with CARDURA® overdosage is limited. Two adolescents who each intentionally ingested 40 mg CARDURA® with diclofenac or paracetamol, were treated with gastric lavage with activated charcoal and made full recoveries. A two-year-old child who accidently ingested 4 mg CARDURA® was treated with gastric lavage and remained normotensive during the five-hour emergency room observation period. A six-month-old child accidentally received a crushed 1 mg tablet of CARDURA® and was reported to have been drowsy. A 32-year-old female with chronic renal failure, epilepsy and depression intentionally ingested 60 mg CARDURA® (blood level 0.9 μg/mL; normal values in hypertensives=0.02 μg/mL); death was attributed to a grand mal seizure resulting from hypotension. A 39-year-old female who ingested 70 mg CARDURA®, alcohol and Dalmane® (flurazepam) developed hypotension which responded to fluid therapy.
The oral LD_{50} of doxazosin is greater than 1000 mg/kg in mice and rats. The most likely manifestation of overdosage would be hypotension, for which the usual treatment would be intravenous infusion of fluid. As doxazosin is highly protein bound, dialysis would not be indicated.

DOSAGE AND ADMINISTRATION

DOSAGE MUST BE INDIVIDUALIZED. The initial dosage of CARDURA® in patients with hypertension and/or BPH is 1 mg given once daily in the a.m. or p.m. This starting dose is intended to minimize the frequency of postural hypotension and first dose syncope associated with CARDURA®. Postural effects are most likely to occur between 2 and 6 hours after a dose. Therefore blood pressure measurements should be taken during this time period after the first dose and with each increase in dose. If CARDURA® administration is discontinued for several days, therapy should be restarted using the initial dosing regimen.

A. *BENIGN PROSTATIC HYPERPLASIA 1–8 mg once daily.* The initial dosage of CARDURA® is 1 mg, given once daily in the a.m. or p.m. Depending on the individual patient's urodynamics and BPH symptomatology, dosage may then be increased to 2 mg and thereafter to 4 mg and 8 mg once daily, the maximum recommended dose for BPH. The recommended titration interval is 1–2 weeks. Blood pressure should be evaluated routinely in these patients.

B. *HYPERTENSION 1–16 mg once daily.* The initial dosage of CARDURA® is 1 mg given once daily. Depending on the individual patient's standing blood pressure response (based on measurements taken at 2–6 hours post-dose and 24 hours post-dose), dosage may then be increased to 2 mg and thereafter if necessary to 4 mg, 8 mg and 16 mg to achieve the desired reduction in blood pressure. **Increases in dose beyond 4 mg increase the likelihood of excessive postural effects including syncope, postural dizziness/vertigo and postural hypotension. At a titrated dose of 16 mg once daily the frequency of postural effects is about 12% compared to 3% for placebo.**

HOW SUPPLIED

CARDURA® (doxazosin mesylate) is available as colored tablets for oral administration. Each tablet contains doxazosin mesylate equivalent to 1 mg (white), 2 mg (yellow), 4 mg (orange) or 8 mg (green) of the active constituent, doxazosin.
CARDURA® TABLETS (doxazosin mesylate) are available as 1 mg (white), 2 mg (yellow), 4 mg (orange) and 8 mg (green) scored tablets.

Bottles of 100:	1 mg (NDC 0049-2750-66)
	2 mg (NDC 0049-2760-66)
	4 mg (NDC 0049-2770-66)
	8 mg (NDC 0049-2780-66)
Unit Dose Packages of 100:	1 mg (NDC 0049-2750-41)
	2 mg (NDC 0049-2760-41)
	4 mg (NDC 0049-2770-41)
	8 mg (NDC 0049-2780-41)

Recommended Storage: Store below 86°F (30°C).
RX only

Pfizer Roerig
Division of Pfizer Inc, NY, NY 10017
70-4538-00-8
Printed in U.S.A.
Revised October 2001

CELEBREX® ℞
(celecoxib capsules)
[*sĕlă brəks'*]

Prescribing information for this product, which appears on pages 2676–2680 of the 2002 PDR, has been completely revised as follows. Please write "See Supplement A" next to the product heading.

DESCRIPTION

CELEBREX (celecoxib) is chemically designated as 4-[5-(4-methylphenyl)-3-(trifluoromethyl)-1H-pyrazol-1-yl] benzenesulfonamide and is a diaryl substituted pyrazole. It has the following chemical structure:

The empirical formula for celecoxib is $C_{17}H_{14}F_3N_3O_2S$, and the molecular weight is 381.38.
CELEBREX oral capsules contain 100 mg and 200 mg of celecoxib.
The inactive ingredients in CELEBREX capsules include: croscarmellose sodium, edible inks, gelatin, lactose monohydrate, magnesium stearate, povidone, sodium lauryl sulfate and titanium dioxide.

CLINICAL PHARMACOLOGY

Mechanism of Action: CELEBREX is a nonsteroidal anti-inflammatory drug that exhibits anti-inflammatory, analgesic, and antipyretic activities in animal models. The mechanism of action of CELEBREX is believed to be due to inhibition of prostaglandin synthesis, primarily via inhibition of cyclooxygenase-2 (COX-2), and at therapeutic concentrations in humans, CELEBREX does not inhibit the cyclooxygenase-1 (COX-1) isoenzyme. In animal colon tumor models, celecoxib reduced the incidence and multiplicity of tumors.
Pharmacokinetics:
Absorption
Peak plasma levels of celecoxib occur approximately 3 hrs after an oral dose. Under fasting conditions, both peak plasma levels (C_{max}) and area under the curve (AUC) are

Table 1: Summary of Single Dose (200 mg) Disposition Kinetics of Celecoxib in Healthy Subjects[1]

Mean (%CV) PK Parameter Values				
C_{max}, ng/mL	T_{max}, hr	Effective $t_{1/2}$, hr	V_{ss}/F, L	CL/F, L/hr
705 (38)	2.8 (37)	11.2 (31)	429 (34)	27.7 (28)

[1]Subjects under fasting conditions (n=36, 19–52 yrs.)

roughly dose proportional up to 200 mg BID; at higher doses there are less than proportional increases in C_{max} and AUC (see Food Effects). Absolute bioavailability studies have not been conducted. With multiple dosing, steady state conditions are reached on or before day 5.
The pharmacokinetic parameters of celecoxib in a group of healthy subjects are shown in Table 1.
[See table 1 above]

Food Effects
When CELEBREX capsules were taken with a high fat meal, peak plasma levels were delayed for about 1 to 2 hours with an increase in total absorption (AUC) of 10% to 20%. Under fasting conditions, at doses above 200 mg, there is less than a proportional increase in C_{max} and AUC, which is thought to be due to the low solubility of the drug in aqueous media. Coadministration of CELEBREX with an aluminum- and magnesium-containing antacid resulted in a reduction in plasma celecoxib concentrations with a decrease of 37% in C_{max} and 10% in AUC. CELEBREX, at doses up to 200 mg BID can be administered without regard to the timing of meals. Higher doses (400 mg BID) should be administered with food to improve absorption.

Distribution
In healthy subjects, celecoxib is highly protein bound (~97%) within the clinical dose range. *In vitro* studies indicate that celecoxib binds primarily to albumin and, to a lesser extent, α_1-acid glycoprotein. The apparent volume of distribution at steady state (V_{ss}/F) is approximately 400 L, suggesting extensive distribution into the tissues. Celecoxib is not preferentially bound to red blood cells.

Metabolism
Celecoxib metabolism is primarily mediated via cytochrome P450 2C9. Three metabolites, a primary alcohol, the corresponding carboxylic acid and its glucuronide conjugate, have been identified in human plasma. These metabolites are inactive as COX-1 or COX-2 inhibitors. Patients who are known or suspected to be P450 2C9 poor metabolizers based on a previous history should be administered celecoxib with caution as they may have abnormally high plasma levels due to reduced metabolic clearance.

Excretion
Celecoxib is eliminated predominantly by hepatic metabolism with little (<3%) unchanged drug recovered in the urine and feces. Following a single oral dose of radiolabeled drug, approximately 57% of the dose was excreted in the feces and 27% was excreted into the urine. The primary metabolite in both urine and feces was the carboxylic acid metabolite (73% of dose) with low amounts of the glucuronide also appearing in the urine. It appears that the low solubility of the drug prolongs the absorption process making terminal half-life ($t_{1/2}$) determinations more variable. The effective half-life is approximately 11 hours under fasted conditions. The apparent plasma clearance (CL/F) is about 500 mL/min.

Special Populations
Geriatric: At steady state, elderly subjects (over 65 years old) had a 40% higher C_{max} and a 50% higher AUC compared to the young subjects. In elderly females, celecoxib C_{max} and AUC are higher than those for elderly males, but these increases are predominantly due to lower body weight in elderly females. Dose adjustment in the elderly is not generally necessary. However, for patients of less than 50 kg in body weight, initiate therapy at the lowest recommended dose.
Pediatric: CELEBREX capsules have not been investigated in pediatric patients below 18 years of age.
Race: Meta-analysis of pharmacokinetic studies has suggested an approximately 40% higher AUC of celecoxib in Blacks compared to Caucasians. The cause and clinical significance of this finding is unknown.
Hepatic Insufficiency: A pharmacokinetic study in subjects with mild (Child-Pugh Class I) and moderate (Child-Pugh Class II) hepatic impairment has shown that steady-state celecoxib AUC is increased about 40% and 180%, respectively, above that seen in healthy control subjects. Therefore, the daily recommended dose of CELEBREX capsules should be reduced by approximately 50% in patients with moderate (Child-Pugh Class II) hepatic impairment. Patients with severe hepatic impairment have not been studied. The use of CELEBREX in patients with severe hepatic impairment is not recommended.
Renal Insufficiency: In a cross-study comparison, celecoxib AUC was approximately 40% lower in patients with chronic renal insufficiency (GFR 35-60 mL/min) than that seen in subjects with normal renal function. No significant relationship was found between GFR and celecoxib clearance. Patients with severe renal insufficiency have not been studied.

Drug Interactions
Also see **PRECAUTIONS—Drug Interactions.**
General: Significant interactions may occur when celecoxib is administered together with drugs that inhibit P450 2C9. *In vitro* studies indicate that celecoxib is not an inhibitor of cytochrome P450 2C9, 2C19 or 3A4.
Clinical studies with celecoxib have identified potentially significant interactions with fluconazole and lithium. Experience with nonsteroidal anti-inflammatory drugs (NSAIDs) suggests the potential for interactions with furosemide and ACE inhibitors. The effects of celecoxib on the pharmacokinetics and/or pharmacodynamics of glyburide, ketoconazole, methotrexate, phenytoin, and tolbutamide have been studied *in vivo* and clinically important interactions have not been found.

CLINICAL STUDIES

Osteoarthritis (OA): CELEBREX has demonstrated significant reduction in joint pain compared to placebo. CELEBREX was evaluated for treatment of the signs and the symptoms of OA of the knee and hip in approximately 4,200 patients in placebo- and active-controlled clinical trials of up to 12 weeks duration. In patients with OA, treatment with CELEBREX 100 mg BID or 200 mg QD resulted in improvement in WOMAC (Western Ontario and McMaster Universities) osteoarthritis index, a composite of pain, stiffness, and functional measures in OA. In three 12-week studies of pain accompanying OA flare, CELEBREX doses of 100 mg BID and 200 mg BID provided significant reduction of pain within 24–48 hours of initiation of dosing. At doses of 100 mg BID or 200 mg BID the effectiveness of CELEBREX was shown to be similar to that of naproxen 500 mg BID. Doses of 200 mg BID provided no additional benefit above that seen with 100 mg BID. A total daily dose of 200 mg has been shown to be equally effective whether administered as 100 mg BID or 200 mg QD.
Rheumatoid Arthritis (RA): CELEBREX has demonstrated significant reduction in joint tenderness/pain and joint swelling compared to placebo. CELEBREX was evaluated for treatment of the signs and symptoms of RA in approximately 2,100 patients in placebo- and active-controlled clinical trials of up to 24 weeks in duration. CELEBREX was shown to be superior to placebo in these studies, using the ACR20 Responder Index, a composite of clinical, laboratory, and functional measures in RA. CELEBREX doses of 100 mg BID and 200 mg BID were similar in effectiveness and both were comparable to naproxen 500 mg BID.
Although CELEBREX 100 mg BID and 200 mg BID provided similar overall effectiveness, some patients derived additional benefit from the 200 mg BID dose. Doses of 400 mg BID provided no additional benefit above that seen with 100–200 mg BID.
Analgesia, including primary dysmenorrhea: In acute analgesic models of post-oral surgery pain, post-orthopedic surgical pain, and primary dysmenorrhea, CELEBREX relieved pain that was rated by patients as moderate to severe. Single doses (see DOSAGE AND ADMINISTRATION) of CELEBREX provided pain relief within 60 minutes.
Familial Adenomatous Polyposis (FAP): CELEBREX was evaluated to reduce the number of adenomatous colorectal polyps. A randomized double-blind placebo-controlled study was conducted in 83 patients with FAP. The study population included 58 patients with a prior subtotal or total colectomy and 25 patients with an intact colon. Thirteen patients had the attenuated FAP phenotype.
One area in the rectum and up to four areas in the colon were identified at baseline for specific follow-up, and polyps were counted at baseline and following six months of treatment. The mean reduction in the number of colorectal polyps was 28% for CELEBREX 400 mg BID, 12% for CELEBREX 100 mg BID and 5% for placebo. The reduction in polyps observed with CELEBREX 400 mg BID was statistically superior to placebo at the six-month timepoint (p=0.003). (See Figure 1.)

Figure 1
Percent Change from Baseline in Number of Colorectal Polyps (FAP Patients)

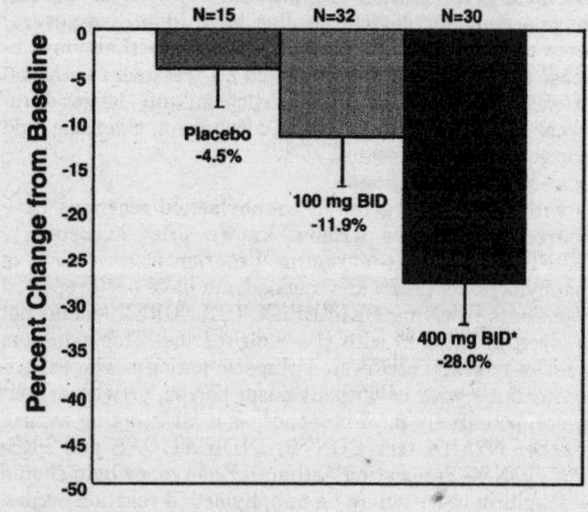

*p=0.003 versus placebo

Special Studies
Gastrointestinal: Scheduled upper GI endoscopic evaluations were performed in over 4,500 arthritis patients who were enrolled in five controlled randomized 12–24 week trials using active comparators, two of which also included placebo controls. Twelve-week endoscopic ulcer data are available on approximately 1,400 patients and 24 week endoscopic ulcer data are available on 184 patients on CELEBREX at doses ranging from 50–400 mg BID. In all three studies that included naproxen 500 mg BID, and in the study that included ibuprofen 800 mg TID, CELEBREX was associated with a statistically significantly lower incidence of endoscopic ulcers over the study period. Two studies compared CELEBREX with diclofenac 75 mg BID; one study revealed a statistically significantly higher prevalence of endoscopic ulcers in the diclofenac group at the study endpoint (6 months on treatment), and one study revealed no statistically significant difference between cumulative endoscopic ulcer incidence rates in the diclofenac and CELEBREX groups after 1, 2, and 3 months of treatment. There was no consistent relationship between the incidence of gastroduodenal ulcers and the dose of CELEBREX over the range studied.
Figure 2 and Table 2 summarize the incidence of endoscopic ulcers in two 12-week studies that enrolled patients in whom baseline endoscopies revealed no ulcers.

Figure 2
Incidence of Endoscopically Observed Gastroduodenal Ulcers after Twelve Weeks of Treatment

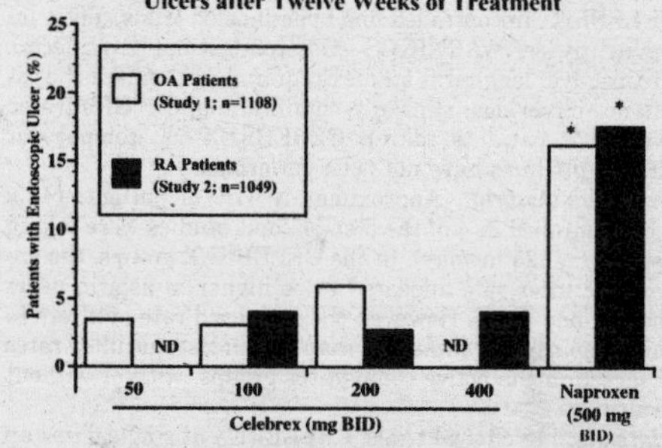

ND= Not Done
* Significantly different from all other treatments: p<0.05.
Celebrex 100 mg BID and 200 mg QD, BID are the recommended doses.
These studies were not powered to compare the endoscopic ulcer rates of Celebrex vs placebo.
Study 1: placebo ulcer rate = 2.3%
Study 2: placebo ulcer rate = 2.0%

[See table 2 at top of next page]
Figure 3 and Table 3 summarize data from two 12-week studies that enrolled patients in whom baseline endoscopies revealed no ulcers. Patients underwent interval endoscopies every 4 weeks to give information on ulcer risk over time.

Figure 3
Cumulative Incidence of Gastroduodenal Ulcers Based on 4 Serial Endoscopies over 12 Weeks

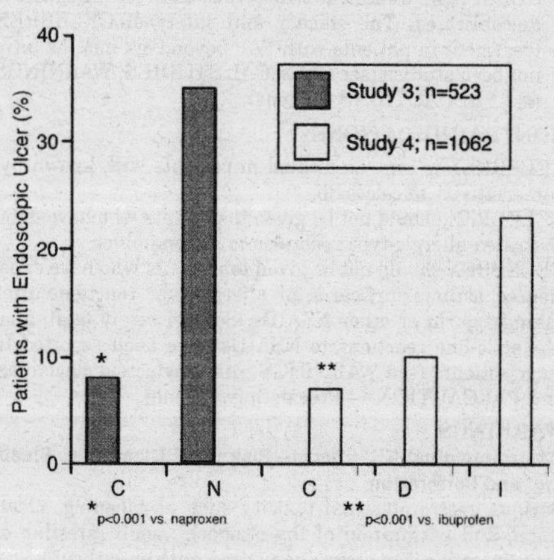

C= Celecoxib 200 mg BID D= Diclofenac 75 mg BID
N= Naproxen 500 mg BID I= Ibuprofen 800 mg TID

[See table 3 at top of next page]
One randomized and double-blinded 6-month study in 430 RA patients was conducted in which an endoscopic examination was performed at 6 months. The results are shown in Figure 4.
[See figure at top of next column]
The correlation between findings of endoscopic studies, and the relative incidence of clinically serious upper GI events that may be observed with different products, has not been fully established. Serious clinically significant upper GI

Continued on next page

Celebrex—Cont.

Figure 4

Prevalence of Endoscopically Observed Gastroduodenal Ulcers after Six Months of Treatment in Patients with Rheumatoid Arthritis

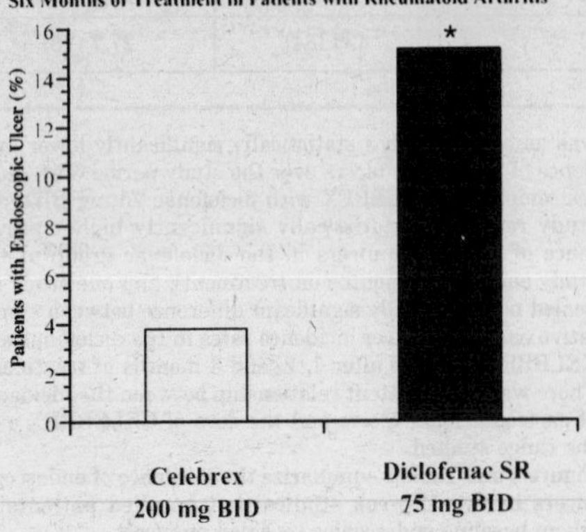

* Significantly different from Celebrex; p<0.001

bleeding has been observed in patients receiving CELEBREX in controlled and open-labeled trials, albeit infrequently (see WARNINGS—Gastrointestinal [GI] Effects). Prospective, long-term studies required to compare the incidence of serious, clinically significant upper GI adverse events in patients taking CELEBREX vs. comparator NSAID products have not been performed.

Use with Aspirin: Approximately 11% of patients (440/4,000) enrolled in 4 of the 5 endoscopic studies were taking aspirin (≤ 325 mg/day). In the CELEBREX groups, the endoscopic ulcer rate appeared to be higher in aspirin users than in non-users. However, the increased rate of ulcers in these aspirin users was less than the endoscopic ulcer rates observed in the active comparator groups, with or without aspirin.

Platelets: In clinical trials, CELEBREX at single doses up to 800 mg and multiple doses of 600 mg BID for up to 7 days duration (higher than recommended therapeutic doses) had no effect on platelet aggregation and bleeding time. Comparators (naproxen 500 mg BID, ibuprofen 800 mg TID, diclofenac 75 mg BID) significantly reduced platelet aggregation and prolonged bleeding time.

INDICATIONS AND USAGE

CELEBREX is indicated:

1) For relief of the signs and symptoms of osteoarthritis.
2) For relief of the signs and symptoms of rheumatoid arthritis in adults.
3) For the management of acute pain in adults (see CLINICAL STUDIES).
4) For the treatment of primary dysmenorrhea.
5) To reduce the number of adenomatous colorectal polyps in familial adenomatous polyposis (FAP), as an adjunct to usual care (e.g., endoscopic surveillance, surgery). It is not known whether there is a clinical benefit from a reduction in the number of colorectal polyps in FAP patients. It is also not known whether the effects of CELEBREX treatment will persist after CELEBREX is discontinued. The efficacy and safety of CELEBREX treatment in patients with FAP beyond six months have not been studied (see CLINICAL STUDIES, WARNINGS and PRECAUTIONS sections).

CONTRAINDICATIONS

CELEBREX is contraindicated in patients with known hypersensitivity to celecoxib.

CELEBREX should not be given to patients who have demonstrated allergic-type reactions to sulfonamides.

CELEBREX should not be given to patients who have experienced asthma, urticaria, or allergic-type reactions after taking aspirin or other NSAIDs. Severe, rarely fatal, anaphylactic-like reactions to NSAIDs have been reported in such patients (see WARNINGS—Anaphylactoid Reactions, and PRECAUTIONS—Preexisting Asthma).

WARNINGS

Gastrointestinal (GI) Effects—Risk of GI Ulceration, Bleeding, and Perforation

Serious gastrointestinal toxicity such as bleeding, ulceration, and perforation of the stomach, small intestine or large intestine, can occur at any time, with or without warning symptoms, in patients treated with nonsteroidal anti-inflammatory drugs (NSAIDs). Minor upper gastrointestinal problems, such as dyspepsia, are common and may also occur at any time during NSAID therapy. Therefore, physicians and patients should remain alert for ulceration and bleeding, even in the absence of previous GI tract symptoms. Patients should be informed about the signs and/or symptoms of serious GI toxicity and the steps to take if they occur. The utility of periodic laboratory monitoring has not been demonstrated, nor has it been adequately assessed. Only one in five patients who develop a serious upper GI adverse event on NSAID therapy is symptomatic. It has been demonstrated that upper GI ulcers, gross bleeding or perforation, caused by NSAIDs, appear to occur in approximately 1% of patients treated for 3–6 months, and in about 2–4% of patients treated for one year. These trends continue thus, increasing the likelihood of developing a serious GI event at some time during the course of therapy. However, even short-term therapy is not without risk.

Table 2
Incidence of Gastroduodenal Ulcers from Endoscopic Studies in OA and RA Patients

	3 Month Studies	
	Study 1 (n=1108)	**Study 2 (n=1049)**
Placebo	2.3% (5/217)	2.0% (4/200)
Celebrex 50 mg BID	3.4% (8/233)	—
Celebrex 100 mg BID	3.1% (7/227)	4.0% (9/223)
Celebrex 200 mg BID	5.9% (13/221)	2.7% (6/219)
Celebrex 400 mg BID	—	4.1% (8/197)
Naproxen 500 mg BID	16.2% (34/210)*	17.6% (37/210)*

*p≤0.05 vs all other treatments

Table 3
Incidence of Gastroduodenal Ulcers from 3-Month Serial Endoscopy Studies in OA and RA Patients

	Week 4	Week 8	Week 12	Final
Study 3 (n=523)				
Celebrex 200 mg BID	4.0% (10/252)*	2.2% (5/227)*	1.5% (3/196)*	7.5% (20/266)*
Naproxen 500 mg BID	19.0% (47/247)	14.2% (26/182)	9.9% (14/141)	34.6% (89/257)
Study 4 (n=1062)				
Celebrex 200 mg BID	3.9% (13/337)†	2.4% (7/296)†	1.8% (5/274)†	7.0% (25/356)†
Diclofenac 75 mg BID	5.1% (18/350)	3.3% (10/306)	2.9% (8/278)	9.7% (36/372)
Ibuprofen 800 mg TID	13.0% (42/323)	6.2% (15/241)	9.6% (21/219)	23.3% (78/334)

*p≤0.05 Celebrex vs. naproxen based on interval and cumulative analyses
†p≤0.05 Celebrex vs. ibuprofen based on interval and cumulative analyses

It is unclear, at the present time, how the above rates apply to CELEBREX (see CLINICAL STUDIES—Special Studies). Among 5,285 patients who received CELEBREX in controlled clinical trials of 1 to 6 months duration (most were 3 month studies) at a daily dose of 200 mg or more, 2 (0.04%) experienced significant upper GI bleeding, at 14 and 22 days after initiation of dosing. Approximately 40% of these 5,285 patients were in studies that required them to be free of ulcers by endoscopy at study entry. Thus it is unclear if this study population is representative of the general population. Prospective, long-term studies required to compare the incidence of serious, clinically significant upper GI adverse events in patients taking CELEBREX vs. comparator NSAID products have not been performed.

NSAIDs should be prescribed with extreme caution in patients with a prior history of ulcer disease or gastrointestinal bleeding. Most spontaneous reports of fatal GI events are in elderly or debilitated patients and therefore special care should be taken in treating this population. **To minimize the potential risk for an adverse GI event, the lowest effective dose should be used for the shortest possible duration.** For high risk patients, alternate therapies that do not involve NSAIDs should be considered.

Studies have shown that patients with a *prior history of peptic ulcer disease and/or gastrointestinal bleeding* and who use NSAIDs, have a greater than 10-fold higher risk for developing a GI bleed than patients with neither of these risk factors. In addition to a past history of ulcer disease, pharmacoepidemiological studies have identified several other co-therapies or co-morbid conditions that may increase the risk for GI bleeding such as: treatment with oral corticosteroids, treatment with anticoagulants, longer duration of NSAID therapy, smoking, alcoholism, older age, and poor general health status.

Anaphylactoid Reactions

As with NSAIDs in general, anaphylactoid reactions have occurred in patients without known prior exposure to CELEBREX. In post-marketing experience, rare cases of anaphylactic reactions and angioedema have been reported in patients receiving CELEBREX. CELEBREX should not be given to patients with the aspirin triad. This symptom complex typically occurs in asthmatic patients who experience rhinitis with or without nasal polyps, or who exhibit severe, potentially fatal bronchospasm after taking aspirin or other NSAIDs (see CONTRAINDICATIONS and PRECAUTIONS—Preexisting Asthma). Emergency help should be sought in cases where an anaphylactoid reaction occurs.

Advanced Renal Disease

No information is available regarding the use of CELEBREX in patients with advanced kidney disease. Therefore, treatment with CELEBREX is not recommended in these patients. If CELEBREX therapy must be initiated, close monitoring of the patient's kidney function is advisable (see PRECAUTIONS—Renal Effects).

Pregnancy

In late pregnancy CELEBREX should be avoided because it may cause premature closure of the ductus arteriosus.

Familial Adenomatous Polyposis (FAP): Treatment with CELEBREX in FAP has not been shown to reduce the risk of gastrointestinal cancer or the need for prophylactic colectomy or other FAP-related surgeries. Therefore, the usual care of FAP patients should not be altered because of the concurrent administration of CELEBREX. In particular, the frequency of routine endoscopic surveillance should not be decreased and prophylactic colectomy or other FAP-related surgeries should not be delayed.

PRECAUTIONS

General: CELEBREX cannot be expected to substitute for corticosteroids or to treat corticosteroid insufficiency. Abrupt discontinuation of corticosteroids may lead to exacerbation of corticosteroid-responsive illness. Patients on prolonged corticosteroid therapy should have their therapy tapered slowly if a decision is made to discontinue corticosteroids.

The pharmacological activity of CELEBREX in reducing inflammation, and possibly fever, may diminish the utility of these diagnostic signs in detecting infectious complications of presumed noninfectious, painful conditions.

Hepatic Effects: Borderline elevations of one or more liver tests may occur in up to 15% of patients taking NSAIDs, and notable elevations of ALT or AST (approximately three or more times the upper limit of normal) have been reported in approximately 1% of patients in clinical trials with NSAIDs. These laboratory abnormalities may progress, may remain unchanged, or may be transient with continuing therapy. Rare cases of severe hepatic reactions, including jaundice and fatal fulminant hepatitis, liver necrosis and hepatic failure (some with fatal outcome) have been reported with NSAIDs, including CELEBREX. (See ADVERSE REACTIONS—post-marketing experience.) In controlled clinical trials of CELEBREX, the incidence of borderline elevations of liver tests was 6% for CELEBREX and 5% for placebo, and approximately 0.2% of patients taking CELEBREX and 0.3% of patients taking placebo had notable elevations of ALT and AST.

A patient with symptoms and/or signs suggesting liver dysfunction, or in whom an abnormal liver test has occurred, should be monitored carefully for evidence of the development of a more severe hepatic reaction while on therapy with CELEBREX. If clinical signs and symptoms consistent with liver disease develop, or if systemic manifestations occur (e.g., eosinophilia, rash, etc.), CELEBREX should be discontinued.

Renal Effects: Long-term administration of NSAIDs has resulted in renal papillary necrosis and other renal injury. Renal toxicity has also been seen in patients in whom renal prostaglandins have a compensatory role in the maintenance of renal perfusion. In these patients, administration of a nonsteroidal anti-inflammatory drug may cause a dose-dependent reduction in prostaglandin formation and, secondarily, in renal blood flow, which may precipitate overt renal decompensation. Patients at greatest risk of this reaction are those with impaired renal function, heart failure, liver dysfunction, those taking diuretics and ACE inhibitors, and the elderly. Discontinuation of NSAID therapy is usually followed by recovery to the pretreatment state. Clinical trials with CELEBREX have shown renal effects similar to those observed with comparator NSAIDs.

Caution should be used when initiating treatment with CELEBREX in patients with considerable dehydration. It is advisable to rehydrate patients first and then start therapy with CELEBREX. Caution is also recommended in patients with preexisting kidney disease (see WARNINGS—Advanced Renal Disease).

Hematological Effects: Anemia is sometimes seen in patients receiving CELEBREX. In controlled clinical trials the incidence of anemia was 0.6% with CELEBREX and 0.4% with placebo. Patients on long-term treatment with CELEBREX should have their hemoglobin or hematocrit checked if they exhibit any signs or symptoms of anemia or blood loss. CELEBREX does not generally affect platelet counts, prothrombin time (PT), or partial thromboplastin time (PTT), and does not appear to inhibit platelet aggregation at indicated dosages (See CLINICAL STUDIES—Special Studies—Platelets).

Fluid Retention and Edema: Fluid retention and edema have been observed in some patients taking CELEBREX (see ADVERSE REACTIONS). Therefore, CELEBREX should be used with caution in patients with fluid retention, hypertension, or heart failure.

Preexisting Asthma: Patients with asthma may have aspirin-sensitive asthma. The use of aspirin in patients with aspirin-sensitive asthma has been associated with severe bronchospasm which can be fatal. Since cross reactivity, including bronchospasm, between aspirin and other nonsteroidal anti-inflammatory drugs has been reported in such aspirin-sensitive patients, CELEBREX should not be administered to patients with this form of aspirin sensitivity and should be used with caution in patients with preexisting asthma.

Information for Patients: CELEBREX can cause discomfort and, rarely, more serious side effects, such as gastrointestinal bleeding, which may result in hospitalization and even fatal outcomes. Although serious GI tract ulcerations and bleeding can occur without warning symptoms, patients should be alert for the signs and symptoms of ulcerations and bleeding, and should ask for medical advice when observing any indicative signs or symptoms. Patients should be apprised of the importance of this follow-up (see WARNINGS—Risk of Gastrointestinal Ulceration, Bleeding and Perforation).

Patients should promptly report signs or symptoms of gastrointestinal ulceration or bleeding, skin rash, unexplained weight gain, or edema to their physicians.

Patients should be informed of the warning signs and symptoms of hepatotoxicity (e.g., nausea, fatigue, lethargy, pruritus, jaundice, right upper quadrant tenderness, and "flu-like" symptoms). If these occur, patients should be instructed to stop therapy and seek immediate medical therapy.

Patients should also be instructed to seek immediate emergency help in the case of an anaphylactoid reaction (see WARNINGS).

In late pregnancy CELEBREX should be avoided because it may cause premature closure of the ductus arteriosus.

Patients with familial adenomatous polyposis (FAP) should be informed that CELEBREX has not been shown to reduce colorectal, duodenal or other FAP-related cancers, or the need for endoscopic surveillance, prophylactic or other FAP-related surgery. Therefore, all patients with FAP should be instructed to continue their usual care while receiving CELEBREX.

Laboratory Tests: Because serious GI tract ulcerations and bleeding can occur without warning symptoms, physicians should monitor for signs or symptoms of GI bleeding. During the controlled clinical trials, there was an increased incidence of hyperchloremia in patients receiving celecoxib compared with patients on placebo. Other laboratory abnormalities that occurred more frequently in the patients receiving celecoxib included hypophosphatemia, and elevated BUN. These laboratory abnormalities were also seen in patients who received comparator NSAIDs in these studies. The clinical significance of these abnormalities has not been established.

Drug Interactions

General: Celecoxib metabolism is predominantly mediated via cytochrome P450 2C9 in the liver. Co-administration of celecoxib with drugs that are known to inhibit 2C9 should be done with caution.

In vitro studies indicate that celecoxib, although not a substrate, is an inhibitor of cytochrome P450 2D6. Therefore, there is a potential for an *in vivo* drug interaction with drugs that are metabolized by P450 2D6.

ACE-inhibitors: Reports suggest that NSAIDs may diminish the antihypertensive effect of Angiotensin Converting Enzyme (ACE) inhibitors. This interaction should be given consideration in patients taking CELEBREX concomitantly with ACE-inhibitors.

Furosemide: Clinical studies, as well as post marketing observations, have shown that NSAIDs can reduce the natriuretic effect of furosemide and thiazides in some patients. This response has been attributed to inhibition of renal prostaglandin synthesis.

Aspirin: CELEBREX can be used with low dose aspirin. However, concomitant administration of aspirin with CELEBREX may result in an increased rate of GI ulceration or other complications, compared to use of CELEBREX alone (see CLINICAL STUDIES—Special Studies—Gastrointestinal). Because of its lack of platelet effects, CELEBREX is not a substitute for aspirin for cardiovascular prophylaxis.

Fluconazole: Concomitant administration of fluconazole at 200 mg QD resulted in a two-fold increase in celecoxib plasma concentration. This increase is due to the inhibition of celecoxib metabolism via P450 2C9 by fluconazole (see Pharmacokinetics—Metabolism). CELEBREX should be introduced at the lowest recommended dose in patients receiving fluconazole.

Table 4
Adverse Events Occurring in ≥2% of Celebrex Patients From Controlled Arthritis Trials

	Celebrex (100–200 mg BID or 200 mg QD) (N=4146)	Placebo (N=1864)	Naproxen 500 mg BID (N=1366)	Diclofenac 75 mg BID (N=387)	Ibuprofen 800 mg TID (N=345)
Gastrointestinal					
Abdominal pain	4.1%	2.8%	7.7%	9.0%	9.0%
Diarrhea	5.6%	3.8%	5.3%	9.3%	5.8%
Dyspepsia	8.8%	6.2%	12.2%	10.9%	12.8%
Flatulence	2.2%	1.0%	3.6%	4.1%	3.5%
Nausea	3.5%	4.2%	6.0%	3.4%	6.7%
Body as a whole					
Back pain	2.8%	3.6%	2.2%	2.6%	0.9%
Peripheral edema	2.1%	1.1%	2.1%	1.0%	3.5%
Injury-accidental	2.9%	2.3%	3.0%	2.6%	3.2%
Central and peripheral nervous system					
Dizziness	2.0%	1.7%	2.6%	1.3%	2.3%
Headache	15.8%	20.2%	14.5%	15.5%	15.4%
Psychiatric					
Insomnia	2.3%	2.3%	2.9%	1.3%	1.4%
Respiratory					
Pharyngitis	2.3%	1.1%	1.7%	1.6%	2.6%
Rhinitis	2.0%	1.3%	2.4%	2.3%	0.6%
Sinusitis	5.0%	4.3%	4.0%	5.4%	5.8%
Upper respiratory tract infection	8.1%	6.7%	9.9%	9.8%	9.9%
Skin					
Rash	2.2%	2.1%	2.1%	1.3%	1.2%

	Celebrex (100–200 mg BID or 200 mg QD)
Gastrointestinal:	Constipation, diverticulitis, dysphagia, eructation, esophagitis, gastritis, gastroenteritis, gastroesophageal reflux, hemorrhoids, hiatal hernia, melena, dry mouth, stomatitis, tenesmus, tooth disorder, vomiting
Cardiovascular:	Aggravated hypertension, angina pectoris, coronary artery disorder, myocardial infarction
General:	Allergy aggravated, allergic reaction, asthenia, chest pain, cyst NOS, edema generalized, face edema, fatigue, fever, hot flushes, influenza-like symptoms, pain, peripheral pain
Resistance mechanism disorders:	Herpes simplex, herpes zoster, infection bacterial, infection fungal, infection soft tissue, infection viral, moniliasis, moniliasis genital, otitis media
Central, peripheral nervous system:	Leg cramps, hypertonia, hypoesthesia, migraine, neuralgia, neuropathy, paresthesia, vertigo
Female reproductive:	Breast fibroadenosis, breast neoplasm, breast pain, dysmenorrhea, menstrual disorder, vaginal hemorrhage, vaginitis
Male reproductive:	Prostatic disorder
Hearing and vestibular:	Deafness, ear abnormality, earache, tinnitus
Heart rate and rhythm:	Palpitation, tachycardia
Liver and biliary system:	Hepatic function abnormal, SGOT increased, SGPT increased
Metabolic and nutritional:	BUN increased, CPK increased, diabetes mellitus, hypercholesterolemia, hyperglycemia, hypokalemia, NPN increase, creatinine increased, alkaline phosphatase increased, weight increase
Musculoskeletal:	Arthralgia, arthrosis, bone disorder, fracture accidental, myalgia, neck stiffness, synovitis, tendinitis
Platelets (bleeding or clotting):	Ecchymosis, epistaxis, thrombocythemia
Psychiatric:	Anorexia, anxiety, appetite increased, depression, nervousness, somnolence
Hemic:	Anemia
Respiratory:	Bronchitis, bronchospasm, bronchospasm aggravated, coughing, dyspnea, laryngitis, pneumonia
Skin and appendages:	Alopecia, dermatitis, nail disorder, photosensitivity reaction, pruritus, rash erythematous, rash maculopapular, skin disorder, skin dry, sweating increased, urticaria
Application site disorders:	Cellulitis, dermatitis contact, injection site reaction, skin nodule
Special senses:	Taste perversion
Urinary system:	Albuminuria, cystitis, dysuria, hematuria, micturition frequency, renal calculus, urinary incontinence, urinary tract infection
Vision:	Blurred vision, cataract, conjunctivitis, eye pain, glaucoma

Cardiovascular:	Syncope, congestive heart failure, ventricular fibrillation, pulmonary embolism, cerebrovascular accident, peripheral gangrene, thrombophlebitis, *vasculitis*
Gastrointestinal:	Intestinal obstruction, intestinal perforation, gastrointestinal bleeding, colitis with bleeding, esophageal perforation, pancreatitis, ileus
Liver and biliary system:	Cholelithiasis, *hepatitis, jaundice, liver failure*
Hemic and lymphatic:	Thrombocytopenia, *agranulocytosis, aplastic anemia, pancytopenia, leukopenia*
Metabolic:	*Hypoglycemia*
Nervous system:	Ataxia, suicide
Renal:	Acute renal failure, *interstitial nephritis*
Skin:	*Erythema multiforme, exfoliative dermatitis, Stevens-Johnson syndrome, toxic epidermal necrolysis*
General:	Sepsis, sudden death, *anaphylactoid reaction, angioedema*

Lithium: In a study conducted in healthy subjects, mean steady-state lithium plasma levels increased approximately 17% in subjects receiving lithium 450 mg BID with CELEBREX 200 mg BID as compared to subjects receiving lithium alone. Patients on lithium treatment should be closely monitored when CELEBREX is introduced or withdrawn.

Methotrexate: In an interaction study of rheumatoid arthritis patients taking methotrexate, CELEBREX did not have a significant effect on the pharmacokinetics of methotrexate.

Warfarin: Anticoagulant activity should be monitored, particularly in the first few days, after initiating or changing CELEBREX therapy in patients receiving warfarin or similar agents, since these patients are at an increased risk of bleeding complications. The effect of celecoxib on the anticoagulant effect of warfarin was studied in a group of healthy subjects receiving daily doses of 2–5 mg of warfarin. In these subjects, celecoxib did not alter the anticoagulant effect of warfarin as determined by prothrombin time. However, in post-marketing experience, bleeding events have been reported, predominantly in the elderly, in association with increases in prothrombin time in patients receiving CELEBREX concurrently with warfarin.

Carcinogenesis, mutagenesis, impairment of fertility: Celecoxib was not carcinogenic in rats given oral doses up to 200 mg/kg for males and 10 mg/kg for females (approximately 2- to 4-fold the human exposure as measured by the AUC_{0-24} at 200 mg BID) or in mice given oral doses up to 25 mg/kg for males and 50 mg/kg for females (approximately equal to human exposure as measured by the AUC_{0-24} at 200 mg BID) for two years.

Celecoxib was not mutagenic in an Ames test and a mutation assay in Chinese hamster ovary (CHO) cells, nor clastogenic in a chromosome aberration assay in CHO cells and an *in vivo* micronucleus test in rat bone marrow.

Celecoxib did not impair male and female fertility in rats at oral doses up to 600 mg/kg/day (approximately 11-fold human exposure at 200 mg BID based on the AUC_{0-24}).

Continued on next page

Celebrex—Cont.

Pregnancy

Teratogenic effects: Pregnancy Category C. Celecoxib at oral doses ≥150 mg/kg/day (approximately 2-fold human exposure at 200 mg BID as measured by AUC_{0-24}), caused an increased incidence of ventricular septal defects, a rare event, and fetal alterations, such as ribs fused, sternebrae fused and sternebrae misshapen when rabbits were treated throughout organogenesis. A dose-dependent increase in diaphragmatic hernias was observed when rats were given celecoxib at oral doses ≥30 mg/kg/day (approximately 6-fold human exposure based on the AUC_{0-24} at 200 mg BID) throughout organogenesis. There are no studies in pregnant women. CELEBREX should be used during pregnancy only if the potential benefit justifies the potential risk to the fetus.

Nonteratogenic effects: Celecoxib produced pre-implantation and post-implantation losses and reduced embryo/fetal survival in rats at oral dosages ≥50 mg/kg/day (approximately 6-fold human exposure based on the AUC_{0-24} at 200 mg BID). These changes are expected with inhibition of prostaglandin synthesis and are not the result of permanent alteration of female reproductive function, nor are they expected at clinical exposures. No studies have been conducted to evaluate the effect of celecoxib on the closure of the ductus arteriosus in humans. Therefore, use of CELEBREX during the third trimester of pregnancy should be avoided.

Labor and delivery: Celecoxib produced no evidence of delayed labor or parturition at oral doses up to 100 mg/kg in rats (approximately 7-fold human exposure as measured by the AUC_{0-24} at 200 mg BID). The effects of CELEBREX on labor and delivery in pregnant women are unknown.

Nursing mothers: Celecoxib is excreted in the milk of lactating rats at concentrations similar to those in plasma. It is not known whether this drug is excreted in human milk. Because many drugs are excreted in human milk and because of the potential for serious adverse reactions in nursing infants from CELEBREX, a decision should be made whether to discontinue nursing or to discontinue the drug, taking into account the importance of the drug to the mother.

Pediatric Use

Safety and effectiveness in pediatric patients below the age of 18 years have not been evaluated.

Geriatric Use

Of the total number of patients who received CELEBREX in clinical trials, more than 2,100 were 65–74 years of age, while approximately 800 additional patients were 75 years and over. While the incidence of adverse experiences tended to be higher in elderly patients, no substantial differences in safety and effectiveness were observed between these subjects and younger subjects. Other reported clinical experience has not identified differences in response between the elderly and younger patients, but greater sensitivity of some older individuals cannot be ruled out.

In clinical studies comparing renal function as measured by the GFR, BUN and creatinine, and platelet function as measured by bleeding time and platelet aggregation, the results were not different between elderly and young volunteers.

ADVERSE REACTIONS

Of the CELEBREX treated patients in controlled trials, approximately 4,250 were patients with OA, approximately 2,100 were patients with RA, and approximately 1,050 were patients with post-surgical pain. More than 8,500 patients have received a total daily dose of CELEBREX of 200 mg (100 mg BID or 200 mg QD) or more, including more than 400 treated at 800 mg (400 mg BID). Approximately 3,900 patients have received CELEBREX at these doses for 6 months or more; approximately 2,300 of these have received it for 1 year or more and 124 of these have received it for 2 years or more.

Adverse events from controlled arthritis trials: Table 4 lists all adverse events, regardless of causality, occurring in ≥2% of patients receiving CELEBREX from 12 controlled studies conducted in patients with OA or RA that included a placebo and/or a positive control group.

[See table 4 at top of previous page]

In placebo- or active-controlled clinical trials, the discontinuation rate due to adverse events was 7.1% for patients receiving CELEBREX and 6.1% for patients receiving placebo. Among the most common reasons for discontinuation due to adverse events in the CELEBREX treatment groups were dyspepsia and abdominal pain (cited as reasons for discontinuation in 0.8% and 0.7% of CELEBREX patients, respectively). Among patients receiving placebo, 0.6% discontinued due to dyspepsia and 0.6% withdrew due to abdominal pain.

The following adverse events occurred in 0.1–1.9% of patients regardless of causality.

[See second table at top of previous page]

Other serious adverse reactions which occur rarely (estimated <0.1%), regardless of causality: The following serious adverse events have occurred rarely in patients, taking CELEBREX. Cases reported only in the post-marketing experience are indicated in italics.

[See third table at top of previous page]

Adverse events from analgesia and dysmenorrhea studies: Approximately 1,700 patients were treated with CELEBREX in analgesia and dysmenorrhea studies. All patients in post-oral surgery pain studies received a single dose of study medication. Doses up to 600 mg/day of CELEBREX were studied in primary dysmenorrhea and post-orthopedic surgery pain studies.

The types of adverse events in the analgesia and dysmenorrhea studies were similar to those reported in arthritis studies. The only additional adverse event reported was post-dental extraction alveolar osteitis (dry socket) in the post-oral surgery pain studies.

In approximately 700 patients treated with CELEBREX in the post-general and orthopedic surgery pain studies, the most commonly reported adverse events were nausea, vomiting, headache, dizziness and fever.

Adverse events from the controlled trial in familial adenomatous polyposis: The adverse event profile reported for the 83 patients with familial adenomatous polyposis enrolled in the randomized, controlled clinical trial was similar to that reported for patients in the arthritis controlled trials. Intestinal anastomotic ulceration was the only new adverse event reported in the FAP trial, regardless of causality, and was observed in 3 of 58 patients (one at 100 mg BID, and two at 400 mg BID) who had prior intestinal surgery.

OVERDOSAGE

Symptoms following acute NSAID overdoses are usually limited to lethargy, drowsiness, nausea, vomiting, and epigastric pain, which are generally reversible with supportive care. Gastrointestinal bleeding can occur. Hypertension, acute renal failure, respiratory depression and coma may occur, but are rare. Anaphylactoid reactions have been reported with therapeutic ingestion of NSAIDs, and may occur following an overdose.

Patients should be managed by symptomatic and supportive care following an NSAID overdose. There are no specific antidotes. No information is available regarding the removal of celecoxib by hemodialysis, but based on its high degree of plasma protein binding (>97%) dialysis is unlikely to be useful in overdose. Emesis and/or activated charcoal (60 to 100 g in adults, 1 to 2 g/kg in children) and/or osmotic cathartic may be indicated in patients seen within 4 hours of ingestion with symptoms or following a large overdose. Forced diuresis, alkalinization of urine, hemodialysis, or hemoperfusion may not be useful due to high protein binding.

DOSAGE AND ADMINISTRATION

For osteoarthritis and rheumatoid arthritis, the lowest dose of CELEBREX should be sought for each patient. These doses can be given without regard to timing of meals.

Osteoarthritis: For relief of the signs and symptoms of osteoarthritis the recommended oral dose is 200 mg per day administered as a single dose or as 100 mg twice per day.

Rheumatoid arthritis: For relief of the signs and symptoms of rheumatoid arthritis the recommended oral dose is 100 to 200 mg twice per day.

Management of Acute Pain and Treatment of Primary Dysmenorrhea: The recommended dose of CELEBREX is 400 mg initially, followed by an additional 200 mg dose if needed on the first day. On subsequent days, the recommended dose is 200 mg twice daily as needed.

Familial adenomatous polyposis (FAP): Usual medical care for FAP patients should be continued while on CELEBREX. To reduce the number of adenomatous colorectal polyps in patients with FAP, the recommended oral dose is 400 mg (2 × 200 mg capsules) twice per day to be taken with food.

Special Populations

Hepatic Insufficiency: The daily recommended dose of CELEBREX capsules in patients with moderate hepatic impairment (Child-Pugh Class II) should be reduced by approximately 50% (see CLINICAL PHARMACOLOGY—Special Populations).

HOW SUPPLIED

CELEBREX 100-mg capsules are white, reverse printed white on blue band of body and cap with markings of 7767 on the cap and 100 on the body, supplied as:

NDC Number	Size
0025-1520-31	bottle of 100
0025-1520-51	bottle of 500
0025-1520-34	carton of 100 unit dose

CELEBREX 200-mg capsules are white, with reverse printed white on gold band with markings of 7767 on the cap and 200 on the body, supplied as:

NDC Number	Size
0025-1525-31	bottle of 100
0025-1525-51	bottle of 500
0025-1525-34	carton of 100 unit dose

Store at 25°C (77°F); excursions permitted to 15–30°C (59–86°F) [See USP Controlled Room Temperature]

Rx only Revised: October 2001

Manufactured for:
G.D. Searle LLC
A subsidiary of Pharmacia Corporation
Chicago IL 60680 USA
Pfizer Inc
New York, NY 10017, USA
by:
Searle Ltd.
Caguas, PR 00725
PHARMACIA
CELEBREX®
celecoxib capsules
A05264-7

GEODON™ ℞

[*jē'-ō dän*]

(ziprasidone HCl)

Prescribing information for this product, which appears on pages 2688–2692 of the 2002 PDR, has been completely revised as follows. Please write "See Supplement A" next to the product heading.

DESCRIPTION

GEODON™ is available as GEODON Capsules (ziprasidone hydrochloride) for oral administration. Ziprasidone is an antipsychotic agent that is chemically unrelated to phenothiazine or butyrophenone antipsychotic agents. It has a molecular weight of 412.94 (free base), with the following chemical name: 5-[2-[4-(1,2-benzisothiazol-3-yl)-1-piperazinyl]ethyl]-6-chloro-1,3-dihydro-2*H*-indol-2-one. The empirical formula of $C_{21}H_{21}ClN_4OS$ (free base of ziprasidone) represents the following structural formula:

GEODON Capsules contain a monohydrochloride, monohydrate salt of ziprasidone. Chemically, ziprasidone hydrochloride monohydrate is 5-[2-[4-(1,2-benzisothiazol-3-yl)-1-piperazinyl]ethyl]-6-chloro-1, 3-dihydro-2*H*-indol-2-one, monohydrochloride, monohydrate. The empirical formula is $C_{21}H_{21}ClN_4OS \cdot HCl \cdot H_2O$ and its molecular weight is 467.42. Ziprasidone hydrochloride monohydrate is a white to slightly pink powder.

GEODON Capsules are supplied for oral administration in 20 mg (blue/white), 40 mg (blue/blue), 60 mg (white/white), and 80 mg (blue/white) capsules. GEODON Capsules contain ziprasidone hydrochloride monohydrate, lactose, pregelatinized starch, and magnesium stearate.

CLINICAL PHARMACOLOGY

Pharmacodynamics

Ziprasidone exhibited high *in vitro* binding affinity for the dopamine D_2 and D_3, the serotonin $5HT_{2A}$, $5HT_{2C}$, $5HT_{1A}$, $5HT_{1D}$, and α_1-adrenergic receptors (K_i's of 4.8, 7.2, 0.4, 1.3, 3.4, 2, and 10 nM, respectively), and moderate affinity for the histamine H_1 receptor (K_i=47 nM). Ziprasidone functioned as an antagonist at the D_2, $5HT_{2A}$, and $5HT_{1D}$ receptors, and as an agonist at the $5HT_{1A}$ receptor. Ziprasidone inhibited synaptic reuptake of serotonin and norepinephrine. No appreciable affinity was exhibited for other receptor/binding sites tested, including the cholinergic muscarinic receptor (IC_{50} >1 μM).

The mechanism of action of ziprasidone, as with other drugs having efficacy in schizophrenia, is unknown. However, it has been proposed that this drug's efficacy in schizophrenia is mediated through a combination of dopamine type 2 (D_2) and serotonin type 2 ($5HT_2$) antagonism. Antagonism at receptors other than dopamine and $5HT_2$ with similar receptor affinities may explain some of the other therapeutic and side effects of ziprasidone.

Ziprasidone's antagonism of histamine H_1 receptors may explain the somnolence observed with this drug.

Ziprasidone's antagonism of α_1-adrenergic receptors may explain the orthostatic hypotension observed with this drug.

Pharmacokinetics

Ziprasidone's activity is primarily due to the parent drug. The multiple-dose pharmacokinetics of ziprasidone are dose-proportional within the proposed clinical dose range, and ziprasidone accumulation is predictable with multiple dosing. Elimination of ziprasidone is mainly via hepatic metabolism with a mean terminal half-life of about 7 hours within the proposed clinical dose range. Steady-state concentrations are achieved within one to three days of dosing. The mean apparent systemic clearance is 7.5 mL/min/kg. Ziprasidone is unlikely to interfere with the metabolism of drugs metabolized by cytochrome P450 enzymes.

Absorption: Ziprasidone is well absorbed after oral administration, reaching peak plasma concentrations in 6 to 8 hours. The absolute bioavailability of a 20 mg dose under fed conditions is approximately 60%. The absorption of ziprasidone is increased up to two-fold in the presence of food.

Distribution: Ziprasidone has a mean apparent volume of distribution of 1.5 L/kg. It is greater than 99% bound to plasma proteins, binding primarily to albumin and α_1-acid glycoprotein. The *in vitro* plasma protein binding of ziprasidone was not altered by warfarin or propranolol, two highly protein-bound drugs, nor did ziprasidone alter the binding of these drugs in human plasma. Thus, the potential for drug interactions with ziprasidone due to displacement is minimal.

Metabolism and Elimination: Ziprasidone is extensively metabolized after oral administration with only a small amount excreted in the urine (<1%) or feces (<4%) as unchanged drug. Ziprasidone is primarily cleared via three metabolic routes to yield four major circulating metabolites, benzisothiazole (BITP) sulphoxide, BITP-sulphone, ziprasidone sulphoxide, and S-methyl-dihydroziprasidone. Approximately 20% of the dose is excreted in the urine, with approximately 66% being eliminated in the feces. Unchanged ziprasidone represents about 44% of total drug-related material in serum. *In vitro* studies using human liver subcellular fractions indicate that S-methyl-dihydroziprasidone is generated in two steps. The data indicate that the reduction reaction is mediated by aldehyde oxidase and the subsequent methylation is mediated by thiol methyltransferase. *In vitro* studies using human liver microsomes and recombinant enzymes indicate that CYP3A4 is the major CYP contributing to the oxidative metabolism of ziprasidone. CYP1A2 may contribute to a much lesser extent. Based on *in vivo* abundance of excretory metabolites, less than one-third of ziprasidone metabolic clearance is mediated by cytochrome P450 catalyzed oxidation and approximately two-thirds via reduction by aldehyde oxidase. There are no known clinically relevant inhibitors or inducers of aldehyde oxidase.

Special Populations

Age and Gender Effects—In a multiple-dose (8 days of treatment) study involving 32 subjects, there was no difference in the pharmacokinetics of ziprasidone between men and women or between elderly (>65 years) and young (18 to 45 years) subjects. Additionally, population pharmacokinetic evaluation of patients in controlled trials has revealed no evidence of clinically significant age or gender-related differences in the pharmacokinetics of ziprasidone. Dosage modifications for age or gender are, therefore, not recommended.

Race—No specific pharmacokinetic study was conducted to investigate the effects of race. Population pharmacokinetic evaluation has revealed no evidence of clinically significant race-related differences in the pharmacokinetics of ziprasidone. Dosage modifications for race are, therefore, not recommended.

Smoking—Based on *in vitro* studies utilizing human liver enzymes, ziprasidone is not a substrate for CYP1A2; smoking should therefore not have an effect on the pharmacokinetics of ziprasidone. Consistent with these *in vitro* results, population pharmacokinetic evaluation has not revealed any significant pharmacokinetic differences between smokers and nonsmokers.

Renal Impairment—Because ziprasidone is highly metabolized, with less than 1% of the drug excreted unchanged, renal impairment alone is unlikely to have a major impact on the pharmacokinetics of ziprasidone. The pharmacokinetics of ziprasidone following 8 days of 20 mg BID dosing were similar among subjects with varying degrees of renal impairment (n=27), and subjects with normal renal function, indicating that dosage adjustment based upon the degree of renal impairment is not required. Ziprasidone is not removed by hemodialysis.

Hepatic Impairment—As ziprasidone is cleared substantially by the liver, the presence of hepatic impairment would be expected to increase the AUC of ziprasidone; a multiple-dose study at 20 mg BID for 5 days in subjects (n=13) with clinically significant (Childs-Pugh Class A and B) cirrhosis revealed an increase in AUC $_{0-12}$ of 13% and 34% in Childs-Pugh Class A and B, respectively, compared to a matched control group (n=14). A half-life of 7.1 hours was observed in subjects with cirrhosis compared to 4.8 hours in the control group.

Drug-Drug Interactions

An *in vitro* enzyme inhibition study utilizing human liver microsomes showed that ziprasidone had little inhibitory effect on CYP1A2, CYP2C9, CYP2C19, CYP2D6 and CYP3A4, and thus would not likely interfere with the metabolism of drugs primarily metabolized by these enzymes. *In vivo* studies have revealed no effect of ziprasidone on the pharmacokinetics of dextromethorphan, estrogen, progesterone, or lithium (see **Drug Interactions** under **PRECAUTIONS**).

In vivo studies have revealed an approximately 35% decrease in ziprasidone AUC by concomitantly administered carbamazepine, an approximately 35–40% increase in ziprasidone AUC by concomitantly administered ketoconazole, but no effect on ziprasidone's pharmacokinetics by cimetidine or antacid (see **Drug Interactions** under **PRECAUTIONS**).

Clinical Trials

The efficacy of ziprasidone in the treatment of schizophrenia was evaluated in 5 placebo-controlled studies, 4 short-term (4- and 6-week) trials and one long-term (52-week) trial. All trials were in inpatients, most of whom met DSM III-R criteria for schizophrenia. Each study included 2 to 3 fixed doses of ziprasidone as well as placebo. Four of the 5 trials were able to distinguish ziprasidone from placebo; one short-term study did not. Although a single fixed-dose haloperidol arm was included as a comparative treatment in one of the three short-term trials, this single study was inadequate to provide a reliable and valid comparison of ziprasidone and haloperidol.

Several instruments were used for assessing psychiatric signs and symptoms in these studies. The Brief Psychiatric Rating Scale (BPRS) and the Positive and Negative Syndrome Scale (PANSS) are both multi-item inventories of general psychopathology usually used to evaluate the effects of drug treatment in schizophrenia. The BPRS psychosis cluster (conceptual disorganization, hallucinatory behavior, suspiciousness, and unusual thought content) is considered a particularly useful subset for assessing actively psychotic schizophrenic patients. A second widely used assessment, the Clinical Global Impression (CGI), reflects the impression of a skilled observer, fully familiar with the manifestations of schizophrenia, about the overall clinical state of the patient. In addition, the Scale for Assessing Negative Symptoms (SANS) was employed for assessing negative symptoms in one trial.

The results of the trials follow:

(1) In a 4-week, placebo-controlled trial (n=139) comparing 2 fixed doses of ziprasidone (20 and 60 mg BID) with placebo, only the 60 mg BID dose was superior to placebo on the BPRS total score and the CGI severity score. This higher dose group was not superior to placebo on the BPRS psychosis cluster or on the SANS.

(2) In a 6-week, placebo-controlled trial (n=302) comparing 2 fixed doses of ziprasidone (40 and 80 mg BID) with placebo, both dose groups were superior to placebo on the BPRS total score, the BPRS psychosis cluster, the CGI severity score and the PANSS total and negative subscale scores. Although 80 mg BID had a numerically greater effect than 40 mg BID, the difference was not statistically significant.

(3) In a 6-week, placebo-controlled trial (n=419) comparing 3 fixed doses of ziprasidone (20, 60, and 100 mg BID) with placebo, all three dose groups were superior to placebo on the PANSS total score, the BPRS total score, the BPRS psychosis cluster, and the CGI severity score. Only the 100 mg BID dose group was superior to placebo on the PANSS negative subscale score. There was no clear evidence for a dose-response relationship within the 20 mg BID to 100 mg BID dose range.

(4) In a 4-week, placebo-controlled trial (n=200) comparing 3 fixed doses of ziprasidone (5, 20 and 40 mg BID), none of the dose groups was statistically superior to placebo on any outcome of interest.

(5) A study was conducted in chronic, symptomatically stable schizophrenic inpatients (n=294) randomized to 3 fixed doses of ziprasidone (20, 40, or 80 mg BID) or placebo and followed for 52 weeks. Patients were observed for "impending psychotic relapse", defined as CGI-improvement score of ≥6 (much worse or very much worse) and/or scores ≥6 (moderately severe) on the hostility or uncooperativeness items of the PANSS on two consecutive days. Ziprasidone was significantly superior to placebo in both time to relapse and rate of relapse, with no significant difference between the different dose groups.

There were insufficient data to examine population subsets based on age and race. Examination of population subsets based on gender did not reveal any differential responsiveness.

INDICATIONS AND USAGE

Ziprasidone is indicated for the treatment of schizophrenia. When deciding among the alternative treatments available for this condition, the prescriber should consider the finding of ziprasidone's greater capacity to prolong the QT/QTc interval compared to several other antipsychotic drugs (see **WARNINGS**). Prolongation of the QTc interval is associated in some other drugs with the ability to cause torsade de pointes-type arrhythmia, a potentially fatal polymorphic ventricular tachycardia, and sudden death. In many cases this would lead to the conclusion that other drugs should be tried first. Whether ziprasidone will cause torsade de pointes or increase the rate of sudden death is not yet known (see **WARNINGS**).

The efficacy of ziprasidone was established in short-term (4- and 6-week) controlled trials of schizophrenic inpatients (see **CLINICAL PHARMACOLOGY**).

In a placebo-controlled trial involving the follow-up for up to 52 weeks of stable schizophrenic inpatients, GEODON was demonstrated to delay the time to and rate of relapse. The physician who elects to use GEODON for extended periods should periodically re-evaluate the long-term usefulness of the drug for the individual patient.

CONTRAINDICATIONS

QT Prolongation

Because of ziprasidone's dose-related prolongation of the QT interval and the known association of fatal arrhythmias with QT prolongation by some other drugs, ziprasidone is contraindicated in patients with a known history of QT prolongation (including congenital long QT syndrome), with recent acute myocardial infarction, or with uncompensated heart failure (see **WARNINGS**).

Pharmacokinetic/pharmacodynamic studies between ziprasidone and other drugs that prolong the QT interval have not been performed. An additive effect of ziprasidone and other drugs that prolong the QT interval cannot be excluded. Therefore, ziprasidone should not be given with dofetilide, sotalol, quinidine, other Class Ia and III anti-arrhythmics, mesoridazine, thioridazine, chlorpromazine, droperidol, pimozide, sparfloxacin, gatifloxacin, moxifloxacin, halofantrine, mefloquine, pentamidine, arsenic trioxide, levomethadyl acetate, dolasetron mesylate, probucol or tacrolimus. Ziprasidone is also contraindicated with drugs that have demonstrated QT prolongation as one of their pharmacodynamic effects and have this effect described in the full prescribing information as a contraindication or a boxed or bolded warning (see **WARNINGS**).

Hypersensitivity

Ziprasidone is contraindicated in individuals with a known hypersensitivity to the product.

WARNINGS

QT Prolongation and Risk of Sudden Death

Ziprasidone use should be avoided in combination with other drugs that are known to prolong the QTc interval (see CONTRAINDICATIONS, and see Drug Interactions under PRECAUTIONS). Additionally, clinicians should be alert to the identification of other drugs that have been consistently observed to prolong the QTc interval. Such drugs should not be prescribed with ziprasidone. Ziprasidone should also be avoided in patients with congenital long QT syndrome and in patients with a history of cardiac arrhythmias (see CONTRAINDICATIONS).

A study directly comparing the QT/QTc prolonging effect of ziprasidone with several other drugs effective in the treatment of schizophrenia was conducted in patient volunteers. In the first phase of the trial, ECGs were obtained at the time of maximum plasma concentration when the drug was administered alone. In the second phase of the trial, ECGs were obtained at the time of maximum plasma concentration while the drug was coadministered with an inhibitor of the CYP4503A4 metabolism of the drug.

In the first phase of the study, the mean change in QTc from baseline was calculated for each drug, using a sample-based correction that removes the effect of heart rate on the QT interval. The mean increase in QTc from baseline for ziprasidone ranged from approximately 9 to 14 msec greater than for four of the comparator drugs (risperidone, olanzapine, quetiapine, and haloperidol), but was approximately 14 msec less than the prolongation observed for thioridazine.

In the second phase of the study, the effect of ziprasidone on QTc length was not augmented by the presence of a metabolic inhibitor (ketoconazole 200 mg BID).

In placebo-controlled trials, ziprasidone increased the QTc interval compared to placebo by approximately 10 msec at the highest recommended daily dose of 160 mg. In clinical trials with ziprasidone, the electrocardiograms of 2/2988 (0.06%) patients who received GEODON and 1/440 (0.23%) patients who received placebo revealed QTc intervals exceeding the potentially clinically relevant threshold of 500 msec. In the ziprasidone-treated patients, neither case suggested a role of ziprasidone. One patient had a history of prolonged QTc and a screening measurement of 489 msec; QTc was 503 msec during ziprasidone treatment. The other patient had a QTc of 391 msec at the end of treatment with ziprasidone and upon switching to thioridazine experienced QTc measurements of 518 and 593 msec.

Some drugs that prolong the QT/QTc interval have been associated with the occurrence of torsade de pointes and with sudden unexplained death. The relationship of QT prolongation to torsade de pointes is clearest for larger increases (20 msec and greater) but it is possible that smaller QT/QTc prolongations may also increase risk, or increase it in susceptible individuals, such as those with hypokalemia, hypomagnesemia, or genetic predisposition. Although torsade de pointes has not been observed in association with the use of ziprasidone at recommended doses in premarketing studies, experience is too limited to rule out an increased risk.

As with other antipsychotic drugs and placebo, sudden unexplained deaths have been reported in patients taking ziprasidone at recommended doses. The premarketing experience for ziprasidone did not reveal an excess risk of mortality for ziprasidone compared to other antipsychotic drugs or placebo, but the extent of exposure was limited, especially for the drugs used as active controls and placebo. Nevertheless, ziprasidone's larger prolongation of QTc length compared to several other antipsychotic drugs raises the possibility that the risk of sudden death may be greater for ziprasidone than for other available drugs for treating schizophrenia. This possibility needs to be considered in deciding among alternative drug products (see INDICATIONS AND USAGE).

Certain circumstances may increase the risk of the occurrence of torsade de pointes and/or sudden death in association with the use of drugs that prolong the QTc interval, including (1) bradycardia; (2) hypokalemia or hypomagnesemia; (3) concomitant use of other drugs that prolong the QTc interval; and (4) presence of congenital prolongation of the QT interval. It is recommended that patients being considered for ziprasidone treatment who are at risk for significant electrolyte disturbances, hypokalemia in particular, have baseline serum potassium and magnesium measurements. Hypokalemia (and/or hypomagnesemia) may increase the risk of QT prolongation and arrhythmia. Hypokalemia may result from diuretic therapy, diarrhea, and other causes. Patients with low serum potassium and/or magnesium should be repleted with those electrolytes before proceeding with treatment. It is essential to periodically monitor serum electrolytes in patients for whom diuretic therapy is introduced during ziprasidone treatment. Persistently prolonged QTc intervals may also increase the risk of further prolongation and arrhythmia, but it is not clear that routine screening ECG measures are effective in detecting such patients. Rather, ziprasidone should be avoided in patients with histories of significant cardiovascular illness, e.g., QT prolongation, recent acute myocardial infarction, uncompensated heart failure, or cardiac arrhythmia. Ziprasidone should be discontinued in patients who are found to have persistent QTc measurements >500 msec.

For patients taking ziprasidone who experience symptoms that could indicate the occurrence of torsade de pointes, e.g., dizziness, palpitations, or syncope, the prescriber should initiate further evaluation, e.g., Holter monitoring may be useful.

Neuroleptic Malignant Syndrome (NMS)

A potentially fatal symptom complex sometimes referred to as Neuroleptic Malignant Syndrome (NMS) has been reported in association with administration of antipsychotic drugs. Clinical manifestations of NMS are hyperpyrexia,

Continued on next page

Geodon—Cont.

muscle rigidity, altered mental status and evidence of autonomic instability (irregular pulse or blood pressure, tachycardia, diaphoresis, and cardiac dysrhythmia). Additional signs may include elevated creatinine phosphokinase, myoglobinuria (rhabdomyolysis), and acute renal failure.

The diagnostic evaluation of patients with this syndrome is complicated. In arriving at a diagnosis, it is important to exclude cases where the clinical presentation includes both serious medical illness (e.g., pneumonia, systemic infection, etc.) and untreated or inadequately treated extrapyramidal signs and symptoms (EPS). Other important considerations in the differential diagnosis include central anticholinergic toxicity, heat stroke, drug fever, and primary central nervous system (CNS) pathology.

The management of NMS should include: (1) immediate discontinuation of antipsychotic drugs and other drugs not essential to concurrent therapy; (2) intensive symptomatic treatment and medical monitoring; and (3) treatment of any concomitant serious medical problems for which specific treatments are available. There is no general agreement about specific pharmacological treatment regimens for NMS.

If a patient requires antipsychotic drug treatment after recovery from NMS, the potential reintroduction of drug therapy should be carefully considered. The patient should be carefully monitored, since recurrences of NMS have been reported.

Tardive Dyskinesia

A syndrome of potentially irreversible, involuntary, dyskinetic movements may develop in patients undergoing treatment with antipsychotic drugs. Although the prevalence of the syndrome appears to be highest among the elderly, especially elderly women, it is impossible to rely upon prevalence estimates to predict, at the inception of antipsychotic treatment, which patients are likely to develop the syndrome. Whether antipsychotic drug products differ in their potential to cause tardive dyskinesia is unknown.

The risk of developing tardive dyskinesia and the likelihood that it will become irreversible are believed to increase as the duration of treatment and the total cumulative dose of antipsychotic drugs administered to the patient increase. However, the syndrome can develop, although much less commonly, after relatively brief treatment periods at low doses.

There is no known treatment for established cases of tardive dyskinesia, although the syndrome may remit, partially or completely, if antipsychotic treatment is withdrawn. Antipsychotic treatment itself, however, may suppress (or partially suppress) the signs and symptoms of the syndrome and thereby may possibly mask the underlying process. The effect that symptomatic suppression has upon the long-term course of the syndrome is unknown.

Given these considerations, ziprasidone should be prescribed in a manner that is most likely to minimize the occurrence of tardive dyskinesia. Chronic antipsychotic treatment should generally be reserved for patients who suffer from a chronic illness that (1) is known to respond to antipsychotic drugs, and (2) for whom alternative, equally effective, but potentially less harmful treatments are not available or appropriate. In patients who do require chronic treatment, the smallest dose and the shortest duration of treatment producing a satisfactory clinical response should be sought. The need for continued treatment should be reassessed periodically.

If signs and symptoms of tardive dyskinesia appear in a patient on ziprasidone, drug discontinuation should be considered. However, some patients may require treatment with ziprasidone despite the presence of the syndrome.

PRECAUTIONS

General

Rash—In premarketing trials with ziprasidone, about 5% of patients developed rash and/or urticaria, with discontinuation of treament in about one-sixth of these cases. The occurrence of rash was related to dose of ziprasidone, although the finding might also be explained by the longer exposure time in the higher dose patients. Several patients with rash had signs and symptoms of associated systemic illness, e.g., elevated WBCs. Most patients improved promptly with adjunctive treatment with antihistamines or steroids and/or upon discontinuation of ziprasidone, and all patients experiencing these events were reported to recover completely. Upon appearance of rash for which an alternative etiology cannot be identified, ziprasidone should be discontinued.

Orthostatic Hypotension—Ziprasidone may induce orthostatic hypotension associated with dizziness, tachycardia, and, in some patients, syncope, especially during the initial dose-titration period, probably reflecting its α_1-adrenergic antagonist properties. Syncope was reported in 0.6% of the patients treated with ziprasidone.

Ziprasidone should be used with particular caution in patients with known cardiovascular disease (history of myocardial infarction or ischemic heart disease, heart failure or conduction abnormalities), cerebrovascular disease or conditions which would predispose patients to hypotension (dehydration, hypovolemia, and treatment with antihypertensive medications).

Seizures—During clinical trials, seizures occurred in 0.4% of patients treated with ziprasidone. There were confounding factors that may have contributed to the occurrence of seizures in many of these cases. As with other antipsychotic drugs, ziprasidone should be used cautiously in patients with a history of seizures or with conditions that potentially lower the seizure threshold, e.g., Alzheimer's dementia. Conditions that lower the seizure threshold may be more prevalent in a population of 65 years or older.

Hyperprolactinemia—As with other drugs that antagonize dopamine D_2 receptors, ziprasidone elevates prolactin levels in humans. Increased prolactin levels were also observed in animal studies with this compound, and were associated with an increase in mammary gland neoplasia in mice; a similar effect was not observed in rats (see **Carcinogenesis**). Tissue culture experiments indicate that approximately one-third of human breast cancers are prolactin-dependent *in vitro*, a factor of potential importance if the prescription of these drugs is contemplated in a patient with previously detected breast cancer. Although disturbances such as galactorrhea, amenorrhea, gynecomastia, and impotence have been reported with prolactin-elevating compounds, the clinical significance of elevated serum prolactin levels is unknown for most patients. Neither clinical studies nor epidemiologic studies conducted to date have shown an association between chronic administration of this class of drugs and tumorigenesis in humans; the available evidence is considered too limited to be conclusive at this time.

Potential for Cognitive and Motor Impairment—Somnolence was a commonly reported adverse event in patients treated with ziprasidone. In the 4- and 6-week placebo-controlled trials, somnolence was reported in 14% of patients on ziprasidone compared to 7% of placebo patients. Somnolence led to discontinuation in 0.3% of patients in short-term clinical trials. Since ziprasidone has the potential to impair judgment, thinking, or motor skills, patients should be cautioned about performing activities requiring mental alertness, such as operating a motor vehicle (including automobiles) or operating hazardous machinery until they are reasonably certain that ziprasidone therapy does not affect them adversely.

Priapism—One case of priapism was reported in the premarketing database. While the relationship of the event to ziprasidone use has not been established, other drugs with alpha-adrenergic blocking effects have been reported to induce priapism, and it is possible that ziprasidone may share this capacity. Severe priapism may require surgical intervention.

Body Temperature Regulation—Although not reported with ziprasidone in premarketing trials, disruption of the body's ability to reduce core body temperature has been attributed to antipsychotic agents. Appropriate care is advised when prescribing ziprasidone for patients who will be experiencing conditions which may contribute to an elevation in core body temperature, e.g., exercising strenuously, exposure to extreme heat, receiving concomitant medication with anticholinergic activity, or being subject to dehydration.

Dysphagia—Esophageal dysmotility and aspiration have been associated with antipsychotic drug use. Aspiration pneumonia is a common cause of morbidity and mortality in elderly patients, in particular those with advanced Alzheimer's dementia. Ziprasidone and other antipsychotic drugs should be used cautiously in patients at risk for aspiration pneumonia.

Suicide—The possibility of a suicide attempt is inherent in psychotic illness and close supervision of high-risk patients should accompany drug therapy. Prescriptions for ziprasidone should be written for the smallest quantity of capsules consistent with good patient management in order to reduce the risk of overdose.

Use in Patients with Concomitant Illness—Clinical experience with ziprasidone in patients with certain concomitant systemic illnesses (see **Renal Impairment** and **Hepatic Impairment** under **CLINICAL PHARMACOLOGY, Special Populations**) is limited.

Ziprasidone has not been evaluated or used to any appreciable extent in patients with a recent history of myocardial infarction or unstable heart disease. Patients with these diagnoses were excluded from premarketing clinical studies. Because of the risk of QTc prolongation and orthostatic hypotension with ziprasidone, caution should be observed in cardiac patients (see **QTc Prolongation** under **WARNINGS** and **Orthostatic Hypotension** under **PRECAUTIONS**).

Information for Patients

Please refer to the patient package insert. To assure safe and effective use of GEODON, the information and instructions provided in the patient information should be discussed with patients.

Laboratory Tests

Patients being considered for ziprasidone treatment that are at risk of significant electrolyte disturbances should have baseline serum potassium and magnesium measurements. Low serum potassium and magnesium should be repleted before proceeding with treatment. Patients who are started on diuretics during ziprasidone therapy need periodic monitoring of serum potassium and magnesium. Ziprasidone should be discontinued in patients who are found to have persistent QTc measurements >500 msec (see **WARNINGS**).

Drug Interactions

Drug-drug interactions can be pharmacodynamic (combined pharmacologic effects) or pharmacokinetic (alteration of plasma levels). The risks of using ziprasidone in combination with other drugs have been evaluated as described below. Based upon the pharmacodynamic and pharmacokinetic profile of ziprasidone, possible interactions could be anticipated:

Pharmacodynamic Interactions

(1) Ziprasidone should not be used with any drug that prolongs the QT interval (**see CONTRAINDICATIONS**).

(2) Given the primary CNS effects of ziprasidone, caution should be used when it is taken in combination with other centrally acting drugs.

(3) Because of its potential for inducing hypotension, ziprasidone may enhance the effects of certain antihypertensive agents.

(4) Ziprasidone may antagonize the effects of levodopa and dopamine agonists.

Pharmacokinetic Interactions

The Effect of Other Drugs on Ziprasidone

Carbamazepine—Carbamazepine is an inducer of CYP3A4; administration of 200 mg BID for 21 days resulted in a decrease of approximately 35% in the AUC of ziprasidone. This effect may be greater when higher doses of carbamazepine are administered.

Ketoconazole—Ketoconazole, a potent inhibitor of CYP3A4, at a dose of 400 mg QD for 5 days, increased the AUC and Cmax of ziprasidone by about 35–40%. Other inhibitors of CYP3A4 would be expected to have similar effects.

Cimetidine—Cimetidine at a dose of 800 mg QD for 2 days did not affect ziprasidone pharmacokinetics.

Antacid—The coadministration of 30 mL of MAALOX with ziprasidone did not affect the pharmacokinetics of ziprasidone.

In addition, population pharmacokinetic analysis of schizophrenic patients enrolled in controlled clinical trials has not revealed evidence of any clinically significant pharmacokinetic interactions with benztropine, propranolol, or lorazepam.

Effect of Ziprasidone on Other Drugs

In vitro studies revealed little potential for ziprasidone to interfere with the metabolism of drugs cleared primarily by CYP1A2, CYP2C9, CYP2C19, CYP2D6, and CYP3A4, and little potential for drug interactions with ziprasidone due to displacement (see **CLINICAL PHARMACOLOGY, Pharmacokinetics**).

Lithium—Ziprasidone at a dose of 40 mg BID administered concomitantly with lithium at a dose of 450 mg BID for 7 days did not affect the steady-state level or renal clearance of lithium.

Oral Contraceptives—Ziprasidone at a dose of 20 mg BID did not affect the pharmacokinetics of concomitantly administered oral contraceptives, ethinylestradiol (0.03 mg) and levonorgestrel (0.15 mg).

Dextromethorphan—Consistent with *in vitro* results, a study in normal healthy volunteers showed that ziprasidone did not alter the metabolism of dextromethorphan, a CYP2D6 model substrate, to its major metabolite, dextrorphan. There was no statistically significant change in the urinary dextromethorphan/dextrorphan ratio.

Carcinogenesis, Mutagenesis, Impairment of Fertility

Carcinogenesis—Lifetime carcinogenicity studies were conducted with ziprasidone in Long Evans rats and CD-1 mice. Ziprasidone was administered for 24 months in the diet at doses of 2, 6, or 12 mg/kg/day to rats, and 50, 100, or 200 mg/kg/day to mice (0.1 to 0.6 and 1 to 5 times the maximum recommended human dose [MRHD] of 200 mg/day on a mg/m^2 basis, respectively). In the rat study, there was no evidence of an increased incidence of tumors compared to controls. In male mice, there was no increase in incidence of tumors relative to controls. In female mice, there were dose-related increases in the incidences of pituitary gland adenoma and carcinoma, and mammary gland adenocarcinoma at all doses tested (50 to 200 mg/kg/day or 1 to 5 times the MRHD on a mg/m^2 basis). Proliferative changes in the pituitary and mammary glands of rodents have been observed following chronic administration of other antipsychotic agents and are considered to be prolactin-mediated. Increases in serum prolactin were observed in a 1-month dietary study in female, but not male, mice at 100 and 200 mg/kg/day (or 2.5 and 5 times the MRHD on a mg/m^2 basis). Ziprasidone had no effect on serum prolactin in rats in a 5-week dietary study at the doses that were used in the carcinogenicity study. The relevance for human risk of the findings of prolactin-mediated endocrine tumors in rodents is unknown (see **Hyperprolactinemia** under **PRECAUTIONS, General**).

Mutagenesis—Ziprasidone was tested in the Ames bacterial mutation assay, the *in vitro* mammalian cell gene mutation mouse lymphoma assay, the *in vitro* chromosomal aberration assay in human lymphocytes, and the *in vivo* chromosomal aberration assay in mouse bone marrow. There was a reproducible mutagenic response in the Ames assay in one strain of *S. typhimurium* in the absence of metabolic activation. Positive results were obtained in both the *in vitro* mammalian cell gene mutation assay and the *in vitro* chromosomal aberration assay in human lymphocytes.

Impairment of Fertility—Ziprasidone was shown to increase time to copulation in Sprague-Dawley rats in two fertility and early embryonic development studies at doses of 10 to 160 mg/kg/day (0.5 to 8 times the MRHD of 200 mg/day on a mg/m^2 basis). Fertility rate was reduced at 160 mg/kg/day (8 times the MRHD on a mg/m^2 basis). There was no effect on fertility at 40 mg/kg/day (2 times the MRHD on a mg/m^2 basis). The effect on fertility appeared to be in the female since fertility was not impaired when males given 160 mg/kg/day (8 times the MRHD on a mg/m^2 basis) were mated with untreated females. In a 6-month study in male rats given 200 mg/kg/day (10 times the MRHD on a mg/m^2 basis) there were no treatment-related findings observed in the testes.

Pregnancy—Pregnancy Category C—In animal studies ziprasidone demonstrated developmental toxicity, including possible teratogenic effects at doses similar to human therapeutic doses. When ziprasidone was administered to preg-

GEODON™ Capsules

Package Configuration	Capsule Strength (mg)	NDC Code	Imprint
Bottles of 60	20	NDC-0049-3960-60	396
Bottles of 60	40	NDC-0049-3970-60	397
Bottles of 60	60	NDC-0049-3980-60	398
Bottles of 60	80	NDC-0049-3990-60	399
Unit dose/80	20	NDC-0049-3960-41	396
Unit dose/80	40	NDC-0049-3970-41	397
Unit dose/80	60	NDC-0049-3980-41	398
Unit dose/80	80	NDC-0049-3990-41	399

nant rabbits during the period of organogenesis, an increased incidence of fetal structural abnormalities (ventricular septal defects and other cardiovascular malformations and kidney alterations) was observed at a dose of 30 mg/kg/day (3 times the MRHD of 200 mg/day on a mg/m^2 basis). There was no evidence to suggest that these developmental effects were secondary to maternal toxicity. The developmental no-effect dose was 10 mg/kg/day (equivalent to the MRHD on a mg/m^2 basis). In rats, embryofetal toxicity (decreased fetal weights, delayed skeletal ossification) was observed following administration of 10 to 160 mg/kg/day (0.5 to 8 times the MRHD on a mg/m^2 basis) during organogenesis or throughout gestation, but there was no evidence of teratogenicity. Doses of 40 and 160 mg/kg/day (2 and 8 times the MRHD on a mg/m^2 basis) were associated with maternal toxicity. The developmental no-effect dose was 5 mg/kg/day (0.2 times the MRHD on a mg/m^2 basis).

There was an increase in the number of pups born dead and a decrease in postnatal survival through the first 4 days of lactation among the offspring of female rats treated during gestation and lactation with doses of 10 mg/kg/day (0.5 times the MRHD on a mg/m^2 basis) or greater. Offspring developmental delays and neurobehavioral functional impairment were observed at doses of 5 mg/kg/day (0.2 times the MRHD on a mg/m^2 basis) or greater. A no-effect level was not established for these effects.

There are no adequate and well-controlled studies in pregnant women. Ziprasidone should be used during pregnancy only if the potential benefit justifies the potential risk to the fetus.

Labor and Delivery—The effect of ziprasidone on labor and delivery in humans is unknown.

Nursing Mothers—It is not known whether, and if so in what amount, ziprasidone or its metabolites are excreted in human milk. It is recommended that women receiving ziprasidone should not breast feed.

Pediatric Use—The safety and effectiveness of ziprasidone in pediatric patients have not been established.

Geriatric Use—Of the approximately 4500 patients treated with ziprasidone in clinical studies, 2.4% (109) were 65 years of age or over. In general, there was no indication of any different tolerability of ziprasidone or for reduced clearance of ziprasidone in the elderly compared to younger adults. Nevertheless, the presence of multiple factors that might increase the pharmacodynamic response to ziprasidone, or cause poorer tolerance or orthostasis, should lead to consideration of a lower starting dose, slower titration, and careful monitoring during the initial dosing period for some elderly patients.

ADVERSE REACTIONS

The premarketing development program for ziprasidone included over 5400 patients and/or normal subjects exposed to one or more doses of ziprasidone. Of these 5400 subjects, over 4500 were patients who participated in multiple-dose effectiveness trials, and their experience corresponded to approximately 1733 patient years. The conditions and duration of treatment with ziprasidone included open-label and double-blind studies, inpatient and outpatient studies, and short-term and longer-term exposure.

Adverse events during exposure were obtained by collecting voluntarily reported adverse experiences, as well as results of physical examinations, vital signs, weights, laboratory analyses, ECGs, and results of ophthalmologic examinations. Adverse experiences were recorded by clinical investigators using terminology of their own choosing. Consequently, it is not possible to provide a meaningful estimate of the proportion of individuals experiencing adverse events without first grouping similar types of events into a smaller number of standardized event categories. In the table and tabulations that follow, standard COSTART dictionary terminology has been used to classify reported adverse events. The stated frequencies of adverse events represent the proportion of individuals who experienced, at least once, a treatment-emergent adverse event of the type listed. An event was considered treatment emergent if it occurred for the first time or worsened while receiving therapy following baseline evaluation.

Adverse Findings Observed in Short-Term, Placebo-Controlled Trials

The following findings are based on a pool of two 6-week, and two 4-week placebo-controlled trials in which ziprasidone was administered in doses ranging from 10 to 200 mg/day.

Adverse Events Associated with Discontinuation of Treatment in Short-Term, Placebo-Controlled Trials

Approximately 4.1% (29/702) of ziprasidone-treated patients in short-term, placebo-controlled studies discontinued treatment due to an adverse event, compared with about 2.2% (6/273) on placebo. The most common event associated with dropout was rash, including 7 dropouts for rash among ziprasidone patients (1%) compared to no placebo patients (see **PRECAUTIONS**).

Adverse Events Occurring at an Incidence of 1% or More Among Ziprasidone-Treated Patients in Short-Term, Placebo-Controlled Trials

Table 1 enumerates the incidence, rounded to the nearest percent, of treatment-emergent adverse events that occurred during acute therapy (up to 6 weeks) in predominantly schizophrenic patients, including only those events that occurred in 1% or more of patients treated with ziprasidone and for which the incidence in patients treated with ziprasidone was greater than the incidence in placebo-treated patients.

The prescriber should be aware that these figures cannot be used to predict the incidence of side effects in the course of usual medical practice where patient characteristics and other factors differ from those which prevailed in the clinical trials. Similarly, the cited frequencies cannot be compared with figures obtained from other clinical investigations involving different treatments, uses, and investigators. The cited figures, however, do provide the prescribing physician with some basis for estimating the relative contribution of drug and non-drug factors to the side effect incidence rate in the population studied.

In these studies, the most commonly observed adverse events associated with the use of ziprasidone (incidence of 5% or greater) and observed at a rate on ziprasidone at least twice that of placebo were somnolence (14%), extrapyramidal syndrome (5%), and respiratory disorder (8%).

Table 1. Treatment-Emergent Adverse Event Incidence In Short-Term Placebo-Controlled Trials

	Percentage of Patients Reporting Event	
Body System/Adverse Event	Ziprasidone (N=702)	Placebo (N=273)
Body as a Whole		
Asthenia	5	3
Accidental Injury	4	2
Cardiovascular		
Tachycardia	2	1
Postural Hypotension	1	0
Digestive		
Nausea	10	7
Constipation	9	8
Dyspepsia	8	7
Diarrhea	5	4
Dry Mouth	4	2
Anorexia	2	1
Musculoskeletal		
Myalgia	1	0
Nervous		
Somnolence	14	7
Akathisia	8	7
Dizziness	8	6
Extrapyramidal Syndrome	5	1
Dystonia	4	2
Hypertonia	3	2
Respiratory		
Respiratory Disorder*	8	3
Rhinitis	4	2
Cough Increased	3	1
Skin and Appendages		
Rash	4	3
Fungal Dermatitis	2	1
Special Senses		
Abnormal Vision	3	2

*Cold symptoms and upper respiratory infection account for >90% of investigator terms pointing to "respiratory disorder".

Explorations for interactions on the basis of gender did not reveal any clinically meaningful differences in the adverse event occurrence on the basis of this demographic factor.

Dose Dependency of Adverse Events in Short-Term, Placebo-Controlled Trials

An analysis for dose response in this 4-study pool revealed an apparent relation of adverse event to dose for the following events: asthenia, postural hypotension, anorexia, dry mouth, increased salivation, arthralgia, anxiety, dizziness, dystonia, hypertonia, somnolence, tremor, rhinitis, rash, and abnormal vision.

Extrapyramidal Symptoms (EPS)—The incidence of reported EPS for ziprasidone-treated patients in the short-term, placebo-controlled trials was 5% vs. 1% for placebo. Objectively collected data from those trials on the Simpson Angus Rating Scale (for EPS) and the Barnes Akathisia Scale (for akathisia) did not generally show a difference between ziprasidone and placebo.

Vital Sign Changes—Ziprasidone is associated with orthostatic hypotension (see **PRECAUTIONS**).

Weight Gain—The proportions of patients meeting a weight gain criterion of ≥7% of body weight were compared in a pool of four 4- and 6- week placebo-controlled clinical trials, revealing a statistically significantly greater incidence of weight gain for ziprasidone (10%) compared to placebo (4%). A median weight gain of 0.5 kg was observed in ziprasidone patients compared to no median weight change in placebo patients. In this set of clinical trials, weight gain was reported as an adverse event in 0.4% and 0.4% of ziprasidone and placebo patients, respectively. During long-term therapy with ziprasidone, a categorization of patients at baseline on the basis of body mass index (BMI) revealed the greatest mean weight gain and highest incidence of clinically significant weight gain (>7% of body weight) in patients with low BMI (<23) compared to normal (23–27) or overweight patients (>27). There was a mean weight gain of 1.4 kg for those patients with a "low" baseline BMI, no mean change for patients with a "normal" BMI, and a 1.3 kg mean weight loss for patients who entered the program with a "high" BMI.

ECG Changes—Ziprasidone is associated with an increase in the QTc interval (see **WARNINGS**). Ziprasidone was associated with a mean increase in heart rate of 1.4 beats per minute compared to a 0.2 beats per minute decrease among placebo patients.

Other Adverse Events Observed During the Premarketing Evaluation of Ziprasidone

Following is a list of COSTART terms that reflect treatment-emergent adverse events as defined in the introduction to the **ADVERSE REACTIONS** section reported by patients treated with ziprasidone at multiple doses >4 mg/day within the database of 3834 patients. All reported events are included except those already listed in Table 1 or elsewhere in labeling, those event terms that were so general as to be uninformative, events reported only once and that did not have a substantial probability of being acutely life-threatening, events that are part of the illness being treated or are otherwise common as background events, and events considered unlikely to be drug-related. It is important to emphasize that, although the events reported occurred during treatment with ziprasidone, they were not necessarily caused by it.

Events are further categorized by body system and listed in order of decreasing frequency according to the following definitions: frequent adverse events are those occurring in at least 1/100 patients (only those not already listed in the tabulated results from placebo-controlled trials appear in this listing); infrequent adverse events are those occurring in 1/100 to 1/1000 patients; rare events are those occurring in fewer than 1/1000 patients.

Body as a Whole: *Frequent:* abdominal pain, flu syndrome, fever, accidental fall, face edema, chills, photosensitivity reaction, flank pain, hypothermia, motor vehicle accident.

Cardiovascular System: *Frequent:* hypertension; *Infrequent:* bradycardia, angina pectoris, atrial fibrillation; *Rare:* first degree AV block, bundle branch block, phlebitis, pulmo-

Continued on next page

Geodon—Cont.

nary embolus, cardiomegaly, cerebral infarct, cerebrovascular accident, deep thrombophlebitis, myocarditis, thrombophlebitis.

Digestive System: *Frequent:* vomiting; *Infrequent:* rectal hemorrhage, dysphagia, tongue edema; *Rare:* gum hemorrhage, jaundice, fecal impaction, gamma glutamyl transpeptidase increased, hematemesis, cholestatic jaundice, hepatitis, hepatomegaly, leukoplakia of mouth, fatty liver deposit, melena.

Endocrine: *Rare:* hypothyroidism, hyperthyroidism, thyroiditis.

Hemic and Lymphatic System: *Infrequent:* anemia, ecchymosis, leukocytosis, leukopenia, eosinophilia, lymphadenopathy; *Rare:* thrombocytopenia, hypochromic anemia, lymphocytosis, monocytosis, basophilia, lymphedema, polycythemia, thrombocythemia.

Metabolic and Nutritional Disorders: *Infrequent:* thirst, transaminase increased, peripheral edema, hyperglycemia, creatine phosphokinase increased, alkaline phosphatase increased, hypercholesteremia, dehydration, lactic dehydrogenase increased, albuminuria, hypokalemia; *Rare:* BUN increased, creatinine increased, hyperlipemia, hypocholesteremia, hyperkalemia, hypochloremia, hypoglycemia, hyponatremia, hypoproteinemia, glucose tolerance decreased, gout, hyperchloremia, hyperuricemia, hypocalcemia, hypoglycemic reaction, hypomagnesemia, ketosis, respiratory alkalosis.

Musculoskeletal System: *Infrequent:* tenosynovitis; *Rare:* myopathy.

Nervous System: *Frequent:* agitation, tremor, dyskinesia, hostility, paresthesia, confusion, vertigo, hypokinesia, hyperkinesia, abnormal gait, oculogyric crisis, hypesthesia, ataxia, amnesia, cogwheel rigidity, delirium, hypotonia, akinesia, dysarthria, withdrawal syndrome, buccoglossal syndrome, choreoathetosis, diplopia, incoordination, neuropathy; *Rare:* myoclonus, nystagmus, torticollis, circumoral paresthesia, opisthotonos, reflexes increased, trismus.

Respiratory System: *Frequent:* dyspnea; *Infrequent:* pneumonia, epistaxis; Rare: hemoptysis, laryngismus.

Skin and Appendages: *Infrequent:* maculopapular rash, urticaria, alopecia, eczema, exfoliative dermatitis, contact dermatitis, vesiculobullous rash.

Special Senses: *Infrequent:* conjunctivitis, dry eyes, tinnitus, blepharitis, cataract, photophobia; *Rare:* eye hemorrhage, visual field defect, keratitis, keratoconjunctivitis.

Urogenital System: *Infrequent:* impotence, abnormal ejaculation, amenorrhea, hematuria, menorrhagia, female lactation, polyuria, urinary retention, metrorrhagia, male sexual dysfunction, anorgasmia, glycosuria; *Rare:* gynecomastia, vaginal hemorrhage, nocturia, oliguria, female sexual dysfunction, uterine hemorrhage.

DRUG ABUSE AND DEPENDENCE

Controlled Substance Class—Ziprasidone is not a controlled substance.

Physical and Psychological Dependence—Ziprasidone has not been systematically studied, in animals or humans, for its potential for abuse, tolerance, or physical dependence. While the clinical trials did not reveal any tendency for drug-seeking behavior, these observations were not systematic and it is not possible to predict on the basis of this limited experience the extent to which ziprasidone will be misused, diverted, and/or abused once marketed. Consequently, patients should be evaluated carefully for a history of drug abuse, and such patients should be observed closely for signs of ziprasidone misuse or abuse (e.g., development of tolerance, increases in dose, drug-seeking behavior).

OVERDOSAGE

Human Experience—In premarketing trials involving more than 5400 patients and/or normal subjects, accidental or intentional overdosage of ziprasidone was documented in 10 patients. All of these patients survived without sequelae. In the patient taking the largest confirmed amount, 3240 mg, the only symptoms reported were minimal sedation, slurring of speech, and transitory hypertension (200/95).

Management of Overdosage—In case of acute overdosage, establish and maintain an airway and ensure adequate oxygenation and ventilation. Intravenous access should be established and gastric lavage (after intubation, if patient is unconscious) and administration of activated charcoal together with a laxative should be considered. The possibility of obtundation, seizure, or dystonic reaction of the head and neck following overdose may create a risk of aspiration with induced emesis.

Cardiovascular monitoring should commence immediately and should include continuous electrocardiographic monitoring to detect possible arrhythmias. If antiarrhythmic therapy is administered, disopyramide, procainamide, and quinidine carry a theoretical hazard of additive QT-prolonging effects that might be additive to those of ziprasidone.

Hypotension and circulatory collapse should be treated with appropriate measures such as intravenous fluids. If sympathomimetic agents are used for vascular support, epinephrine and dopamine should not be used, since beta stimulation combined with α_1 antagonism associated with ziprasidone may worsen hypotension. Similarly, it is reasonable to expect that the alpha-adrenergic-blocking properties of bretylium might be additive to those of ziprasidone, resulting in problematic hypotension.

In cases of severe extrapyramidal symptoms, anticholinergic medication should be administered. There is no specific antidote to ziprasidone, and it is not dialyzable. The possibility of multiple drug involvement should be considered. Close medical supervision and monitoring should continue until the patient recovers.

DOSAGE AND ADMINISTRATION

When deciding among the alternative treatments available for schizophrenia, the prescriber should consider the finding of ziprasidone's greater capacity to prolong the QT/QTc interval compared to several other antipsychotic drugs (see **WARNINGS**).

Initial Treatment

GEODON Capsules should be administered at an initial daily dose of 20 mg BID with food. In some patients, daily dosage may subsequently be adjusted on the basis of individual clinical status up to 80 mg BID. Dosage adjustments, if indicated, should generally occur at intervals of not less than 2 days, as steady-state is achieved within 1 to 3 days. In order to ensure use of the lowest effective dose, ordinarily patients should be observed for improvement for several weeks before upward dosage adjustment.

Efficacy in schizophrenia was demonstrated in a dose range of 20 to 100 mg BID in short-term, placebo-controlled clinical trials. There were trends toward dose response within the range of 20 to 80 mg BID, but results were not consistent. An increase to a dose greater than 80 mg BID is not generally recommended. The safety of doses above 100 mg BID has not been systematically evaluated in clinical trials.

Dosing in Special Populations

Dosage adjustments are generally not required on the basis of age, gender, race, or renal or hepatic impairment.

Maintenance Treatment

While there is no body of evidence available to answer the question of how long a patient treated with ziprasidone should remain on it, systematic evaluation of ziprasidone has shown that its efficacy in schizophrenia is maintained for periods of up to 52 weeks at a dose of 20 to 80 mg BID (see **CLINICAL PHARMACOLOGY**). No additional benefit was demonstrated for doses above 20 mg BID. Patients should be periodically reassessed to determine the need for maintenance treatment.

HOW SUPPLIED

GEODON™ Capsules are differentiated by capsule color/size and are imprinted in black ink with "Pfizer" and a unique number. GEODON Capsules are supplied for oral administration in 20 mg (blue/white), 40 mg (blue/blue), 60 mg (white/white), and 80 mg (blue/white) capsules. They are supplied in the following strengths and package configurations:

[See first table at top of previous page]

Storage and Handling—GEODON Capsules should be stored at controlled room temperature, 15°–30°C (59°–86°F).

Rx only

Distributed by
Pfizer Roerig
Division of Pfizer Inc, NY, NY 10017
69-5770-00-2 Revised February 2002

GLUCOTROL XL® ℞

[*glū' cō-trōl*]
(glipizide)
Extended Release Tablets
For Oral Use

Prescribing information for this product, which appears on pages 2693–2696 of the 2002 PDR, has been completely revised as follows. Please write "See Supplement A" next to the product heading.

DESCRIPTION

Glipizide is an oral blood-glucose-lowering drug of the sulfonylurea class.

The Chemical Abstracts name of glipizide is 1-cyclohexyl-3-[[p-[2-(5-methylpyrazinecarboxamido)ethyl] phenyl]sulfonyl]urea. The molecular formula is $C_{21}H_{27}N_5O_4S$; the molecular weight is 445.55; the structural formula is shown below:

Glipizide is a whitish, odorless powder with a pKa of 5.9. It is insoluble in water and alcohols, but soluble in 0.1 *N* NaOH; it is freely soluble in dimethylformamide. GLUCOTROL XL® is a registered trademark for glipizide GITS. Glipizide GITS (Gastrointestinal Therapeutic System) is formulated as a once-a-day controlled release tablet for oral use and is designed to deliver 2.5, 5, or 10 mg of glipizide.

Inert ingredients in the 2.5 mg, 5 mg and 10 mg formulations are: polyethylene oxide, hydroxypropyl methylcellulose, magnesium stearate, sodium chloride, red ferric oxide, cellulose acetate, polyethylene glycol, opadry blue (OY-LS-20921)(2.5 mg tablets), opadry white (YS-2-7063)(5 mg and 10 mg tablet) and black ink (S-1-8106).

System Components and Performance

GLUCOTROL XL Extended Release Tablet is similar in appearance to a conventional tablet. It consists, however, of an osmotically active drug core surrounded by a semipermeable membrane. The core itself is divided into two layers: an "active" layer containing the drug, and a "push" layer containing pharmacologically inert (but osmotically active) components. The membrane surrounding the tablet is permeable to water but not to drug or osmotic excipients. As water from the gastrointestinal tract enters the tablet, pressure increases in the osmotic layer and "pushes" against the drug layer, resulting in the release of drug through a small, laser-drilled orifice in the membrane on the drug side of the tablet.

The GLUCOTROL XL Extended Release Tablet is designed to provide a controlled rate of delivery of glipizide into the gastrointestinal lumen which is independent of pH or gastrointestinal motility. The function of the GLUCOTROL XL Extended Release Tablet depends upon the existence of an osmotic gradient between the contents of the bi-layer core and fluid in the GI tract. Drug delivery is essentially constant as long as the osmotic gradient remains constant, and then gradually falls to zero. The biologically inert components of the tablet remain intact during GI transit and are eliminated in the feces as an insoluble shell.

CLINICAL PHARMACOLOGY

Mechanism of Action: Glipizide appears to lower blood glucose acutely by stimulating the release of insulin from the pancreas, an effect dependent upon functioning beta cells in the pancreatic islets. Extrapancreatic effects also may play a part in the mechanism of action of oral sulfonylurea hypoglycemic drugs. Two extrapancreatic effects shown to be important in the action of glipizide are an increase in insulin sensitivity and a decrease in hepatic glucose production. However, the mechanism by which glipizide lowers blood glucose during long-term administration has not been clearly established. Stimulation of insulin secretion by glipizide in response to a meal is of major importance. The insulinotropic response to a meal is enhanced with GLUCOTROL XL administration in diabetic patients. The postprandial insulin and C-peptide responses continue to be enhanced after at least 6 months of treatment. In 2 randomized, double-blind, dose-response studies comprising a total of 347 patients, there was no significant increase in fasting insulin in all GLUCOTROL XL-treated patients combined compared to placebo, although minor elevations were observed at some doses. There was no increase in fasting insulin over the long term.

Some patients fail to respond initially, or gradually lose their responsiveness to sulfonylurea drugs, including glipizide. Alternatively, glipizide may be effective in some patients who have not responded or have ceased to respond to other sulfonylureas.

Effects on Blood Glucose

The effectiveness of GLUCOTROL XL Extended Release Tablets in type 2 diabetes at doses from 5–60 mg once daily has been evaluated in 4 therapeutic clinical trials each with long-term open extensions involving a total of 598 patients. Once daily administration of 5, 10 and 20 mg produced statistically significant reductions from placebo in hemoglobin A_{1C}, fasting plasma glucose and postprandial glucose in patients with mild to severe type 2 diabetes. In a pooled analysis of the patients treated with 5 mg and 20 mg, the relationship between dose and GLUCOTROL XL's effect of reducing hemoglobin A_{1C} was not established. However, in the case of fasting plasma glucose patients treated with 20 mg had a statistically significant reduction of fasting plasma glucose compared to the 5 mg-treated group.

The reductions in hemoglobin A_{1C} and fasting plasma glucose were similar in younger and older patients. Efficacy of GLUCOTROL XL was not affected by gender, race or weight (as assessed by body mass index). In long term extension trials, efficacy of GLUCOTROL XL was maintained in 81% of patients for up to 12 months.

In an open, two-way crossover study 132 patients were randomly assigned to either GLUCOTROL XL or Glucotrol® for 8 weeks and then crossed over to the other drug for an additional 8 weeks. GLUCOTROL XL administration resulted in significantly lower fasting plasma glucose levels and equivalent hemoglobin A_{1C} levels, as compared to Glucotrol.

Other Effects: It has been shown that GLUCOTROL XL therapy is effective in controlling blood glucose without deleterious changes in the plasma lipoprotein profiles of patients treated for type 2 diabetes.

In a placebo-controlled, crossover study in normal volunteers, glipizide had no antidiuretic activity, and, in fact, led to a slight increase in free water clearance.

Pharmacokinetics and Metabolism: Glipizide is rapidly and completely absorbed following oral administration in an immediate release dosage form. The absolute bioavailability of glipizide was 100% after single oral doses in patients with type 2 diabetes. Beginning 2 to 3 hours after administration of GLUCOTROL XL Extended Release Tablets, plasma drug concentrations gradually rise reaching maximum concentrations within 6 to 12 hours after dosing. With subsequent once daily dosing of GLUCOTROL XL Extended Release Tablets, effective plasma glipizide concentrations are maintained throughout the 24 hour dosing interval with less peak to trough fluctuation than that observed with twice daily dosing of immediate release glipizide. The mean relative bioavailability of glipizide in 21 males with type 2 diabetes after administration of 20 mg GLUCOTROL XL Extended Release Tablets, compared to immediate release Glucotrol (10 mg given twice daily), was 90% at steady-state. Steady-state plasma concentrations were achieved by at least the fifth day of dosing with GLUCOTROL XL Extended Release Tablets in 21 males with type 2 diabetes and patients younger than 65 years. Approximately 1 to 2 days longer were required to reach steady-state in 24 elderly (≥65 years) males and females with type 2 diabetes. No accumulation of drug was observed in patients with type 2 diabetes during chronic dosing with GLUCOTROL XL Extended Release Tablets. Administration of GLUCOTROL XL with food has no effect on the 2 to 3 hour lag time in drug absorption. In a single dose, food effect study in 21 healthy male subjects, the administration of GLUCOTROL XL immediately before a high fat breakfast resulted in a 40% increase in the glipizide mean Cmax value, which was significant, but the effect on the AUC was not significant. There was no change in glucose response between the fed and fasting state. Markedly reduced GI retention times of the GLUCOTROL XL tablets over prolonged periods (e.g., short bowel syndrome) may influence the pharmacokinetic profile of the drug and potentially result in lower plasma concentrations. In a multiple dose study in 26 males with type 2 diabetes, the pharmacokinetics of glipizide were linear over the dose range of 5 to 60 mg of GLUCOTROL XL in that the plasma drug concentrations increased proportionately with dose. In a single dose study in 24 healthy subjects, four 5 mg, two 10 mg, and one 20 mg GLUCOTROL XL Extended Release Tablets were bioequivalent. In a separate single dose study in 36 healthy subjects, four 2.5-mg GLUCOTROL XL Extended Release Tablets were bioequivalent to one 10-mg GLUCOTROL XL Extended Release Tablet.

Glipizide is eliminated primarily by hepatic biotransformation: less than 10% of a dose is excreted as unchanged drug in urine and feces; approximately 90% of a dose is excreted as biotransformation products in urine (80%) and feces (10%). The major metabolites of glipizide are products of aromatic hydroxylation and have no hypoglycemic activity. A minor metabolite which accounts for less than 2% of a dose, an acetylamino-ethyl benzene derivative, is reported to have 1/10 to 1/3 as much hypoglycemic activity as the parent compound. The mean total body clearance of glipizide was approximately 3 liters per hour after single intravenous doses in patients with type 2 diabetes. The mean apparent volume of distribution was approximately 10 liters. Glipizide is 98–99% bound to serum proteins, primarily to albumin. The mean terminal elimination half-life of glipizide ranged from 2 to 5 hours after single or multiple doses in patients with type 2 diabetes. There were no significant differences in the pharmacokinetics of glipizide after single dose administration to older diabetic subjects compared to younger healthy subjects. There is only limited information regarding the effects of renal impairment on the disposition of glipizide, and no information regarding the effects of hepatic disease. However, since glipizide is highly protein bound and hepatic biotransformation is the predominant route of elimination, the pharmacokinetics and/or pharmacodynamics of glipizide may be altered in patients with renal or hepatic impairment.

In mice no glipizide or metabolites were detectable autoradiographically in the brain or spinal cord of males or females, nor in the fetuses of pregnant females. In another study, however, very small amounts of radioactivity were detected in the fetuses of rats given labelled drug.

INDICATIONS AND USAGE

GLUCOTROL XL is indicated as an adjunct to diet for the control of hyperglycemia and its associated symptomatology in patients with type 2 diabetes formerly known as non-insulin-dependent diabetes mellitus (NIDDM) or maturity-onset diabetes, after an adequate trial of dietary therapy has proved unsatisfactory. GLUCOTROL XL is indicated when diet alone has been unsuccessful in correcting hyperglycemia, but even after the introduction of the drug in the patient's regimen, dietary measures should continue to be considered as important. In 12 week, well-controlled studies there was a maximal average net reduction in hemoglobin A_{1C} of 1.7% in absolute units between placebo-treated and GLUCOTROL XL-treated patients.

In initiating treatment for type 2 diabetes, diet should be emphasized as the primary form of treatment. Caloric restriction and weight loss are essential in the obese diabetic patient. Proper dietary management alone may be effective in controlling blood glucose and symptoms of hyperglycemia. The importance of regular physical activity should also be stressed, cardiovascular risk factors should be identified, and corrective measures taken where possible.

If this treatment program fails to reduce symptoms and/or blood glucose, the use of an oral sulfonylurea should be considered. If additional reduction of symptoms and/or blood glucose is required, the addition of insulin to the treatment regimen should be considered. Use of GLUCOTROL XL must be viewed by both the physician and patient as a treatment in addition to diet, and not as a substitute for diet or as a convenient mechanism for avoiding dietary restraint. Furthermore, loss of blood-glucose control on diet alone also may be transient, thus requiring only short-term administration of glipizide.

Some patients fail to respond initially or gradually lose their responsiveness to sulfonylurea drugs, including GLUCOTROL XL. In these cases, concomitant use of GLUCOTROL XL with other oral blood-glucose-lowering agents can be considered. Other approaches that can be considered include substitution of GLUCOTROL XL therapy with that of another oral blood-glucose-lowering agent or insulin. GLUCOTROL XL should be discontinued if it no longer contributes to glucose lowering. Judgment of response to therapy should be based on regular clinical and laboratory evaluations.

In considering the use of GLUCOTROL XL in asymptomatic patients, it should be recognized that controlling blood glucose in type 2 diabetes has not been definitely established to be effective in preventing the long-term cardiovascular or neural complications of diabetes. However, in insulin-dependent diabetes mellitus controlling blood glucose has been effective in slowing the progression of diabetic retinopathy, nephropathy, and neuropathy.

CONTRAINDICATIONS

Glipizide is contraindicated in patients with:

1. Known hypersensitivity to the drug.
2. Diabetic ketoacidosis, with or without coma. This condition should be treated with insulin.

WARNINGS

SPECIAL WARNING ON INCREASED RISK OF CARDIOVASCULAR MORTALITY: The administration of oral hypoglycemic drugs has been reported to be associated with increased cardiovascular mortality as compared to treatment with diet alone or diet plus insulin. This warning is based on the study conducted by the University Group Diabetes Program (UGDP), a long-term prospective clinical trial designed to evaluate the effectiveness of glucose-lowering drugs in preventing or delaying vascular complications in patients with type 2 diabetes. The study involved 823 patients who were randomly assigned to one of four treatment groups (*Diabetes*, 19, SUPP. 2: 747–830, 1970).

UGDP reported that patients treated for 5 to 8 years with diet plus a fixed dose of tolbutamide (1.5 grams per day) had a rate of cardiovascular mortality approximately 2½ times that of patients treated with diet alone. A significant increase in total mortality was not observed, but the use of tolbutamide was discontinued based on the increase in cardiovascular mortality, thus limiting the opportunity for the study to show an increase in overall mortality. Despite controversy regarding the interpretation of these results, the findings of the UGDP study provide an adequate basis for this warning. The patient should be informed of the potential risks and advantages of glipizide and of alternative modes of therapy.

Although only one drug in the sulfonylurea class (tolbutamide) was included in this study, it is prudent from a safety standpoint to consider that this warning may also apply to other oral hypoglycemic drugs in this class, in view of their close similarities in mode of action and chemical structure.

As with any other non-deformable material, caution should be used when administering GLUCOTROL XL Extended Release Tablets in patients with preexisting severe gastrointestinal narrowing (pathologic or iatrogenic). There have been rare reports of obstructive symptoms in patients with known strictures in association with the ingestion of another drug in this non-deformable sustained release formulation.

PRECAUTIONS

General

Renal and Hepatic Disease: The pharmacokinetics and/or pharmacodynamics of glipizide may be affected in patients with impaired renal or hepatic function. If hypoglycemia should occur in such patients, it may be prolonged and appropriate management should be instituted.

GI Disease: Markedly reduced GI retention times of the GLUCOTROL XL Extended Release Tablets may influence the pharmacokinetic profile and hence the clinical efficacy of the drug.

Hypoglycemia: All sulfonylurea drugs are capable of producing severe hypoglycemia. Proper patient selection, dosage, and instructions are important to avoid hypoglycemic episodes. Renal or hepatic insufficiency may affect the disposition of glipizide and the latter may also diminish gluconeogenic capacity, both of which increase the risk of serious hypoglycemic reactions. Elderly, debilitated or malnourished patients, and those with adrenal or pituitary insufficiency are particularly susceptible to the hypoglycemic action of glucose-lowering drugs. Hypoglycemia may be difficult to recognize in the elderly, and in people who are taking beta-adrenergic blocking drugs. Hypoglycemia is more likely to occur when caloric intake is deficient, after severe or prolonged exercise, when alcohol is ingested, or when more than one glucose-lowering drug is used. Therapy with a combination of glucose-lowering agents may increase the potential for hypoglycemia.

Loss of Control of Blood Glucose: When a patient stabilized on any diabetic regimen is exposed to stress such as fever, trauma, infection, or surgery, a loss of control may occur. At such times, it may be necessary to discontinue glipizide and administer insulin.

The effectiveness of any oral hypoglycemic drug, including glipizide, in lowering blood glucose to a desired level decreases in many patients over a period of time, which may be due to progression of the severity of the diabetes or to diminished responsiveness to the drug. This phenomenon is known as secondary failure, to distinguish it from primary failure in which the drug is ineffective in an individual patient when first given. Adequate adjustment of dose and adherence to diet should be assessed before classifying a patient as a secondary failure.

Laboratory Tests: Blood and urine glucose should be monitored periodically. Measurement of hemoglobin A_{1C} may be useful.

Information for Patients: Patients should be informed that GLUCOTROL XL Extended Release Tablets should be swallowed whole. Patients should not chew, divide or crush tablets. Patients should not be concerned if they occasionally notice in their stool something that looks like a tablet. In the GLUCOTROL XL Extended Release Tablet, the medication is contained within a nonabsorbable shell that has been specially designed to slowly release the drug so the body can absorb it. When this process is completed, the empty tablet is eliminated from the body.

Patients should be informed of the potential risks and advantages of GLUCOTROL XL and of alternative modes of therapy. They should also be informed about the importance of adhering to dietary instructions, of a regular exercise program, and of regular testing of urine and/or blood glucose. The risks of hypoglycemia, its symptoms and treatment, and conditions that predispose to its development should be explained to patients and responsible family members. Primary and secondary failure also should be explained.

Drug Interactions: The hypoglycemic action of sulfonylureas may be potentiated by certain drugs including nonsteroidal anti-inflammatory agents and other drugs that are highly protein bound, salicylates, sulfonamides, chloramphenicol, probenecid, coumarins, monoamine oxidase inhibitors, and beta-adrenergic blocking agents. When such drugs are administered to a patient receiving glipizide, the patient should be observed closely for hypoglycemia. When such drugs are withdrawn from a patient receiving glipizide, the patient should be observed closely for loss of control. *In vitro* binding studies with human serum proteins indicate that glipizide binds differently than tolbutamide and does not interact with salicylate or dicumarol. However, caution must be exercised in extrapolating these findings to the clinical situation and in the use of glipizide with these drugs.

Certain drugs tend to produce hyperglycemia and may lead to loss of control. These drugs include the thiazides and other diuretics, corticosteroids, phenothiazines, thyroid products, estrogens, oral contraceptives, phenytoin, nicotinic acid, sympathomimetics, calcium channel blocking drugs, and isoniazid. When such drugs are administered to a patient receiving glipizide, the patient should be closely observed for loss of control. When such drugs are withdrawn from a patient receiving glipizide, the patient should be observed closely for hypoglycemia.

A potential interaction between oral miconazole and oral hypoglycemic agents leading to severe hypoglycemia has been reported. Whether this interaction also occurs with the intravenous, topical, or vaginal preparations of miconazole is not known. The effect of concomitant administration of Diflucan® (fluconazole) and Glucotrol has been demonstrated in a placebo-controlled crossover study in normal volunteers. All subjects received Glucotrol alone and following treatment with 100 mg of Diflucan® as a single daily oral dose for 7 days. The mean percentage increase in the Glucotrol AUC after fluconazole administration was 56.9% (range: 35 to 81%).

Carcinogenesis, Mutagenesis, Impairment of Fertility: A twenty month study in rats and an eighteen month study in mice at doses up to 75 times the maximum human dose revealed no evidence of drug-related carcinogenicity. Bacterial and *in vivo* mutagenicity tests were uniformly negative. Studies in rats of both sexes at doses up to 75 times the human dose showed no effects on fertility.

Pregnancy: Pregnancy Category C: Glipizide was found to be mildly fetotoxic in rat reproductive studies at all dose levels (5–50 mg/kg). This fetotoxicity has been similarly noted with other sulfonylureas, such as tolbutamide and tolazamide. The effect is perinatal and believed to be directly related to the pharmacologic (hypoglycemic) action of glipizide. In studies in rats and rabbits no teratogenic effects were found. There are no adequate and well controlled studies in pregnant women. Glipizide should be used during pregnancy only if the potential benefit justifies the potential risk to the fetus.

Because recent information suggests that abnormal blood-glucose levels during pregnancy are associated with a higher incidence of congenital abnormalities, many experts recommend that insulin be used during pregnancy to maintain blood-glucose levels as close to normal as possible.

Nonteratogenic Effects: Prolonged severe hypoglycemia (4 to 10 days) has been reported in neonates born to mothers who were receiving a sulfonylurea drug at the time of delivery. This has been reported more frequently with the use of agents with prolonged half-lives. If glipizide is used during pregnancy, it should be discontinued at least one month before the expected delivery date.

Nursing Mothers: Although it is not known whether glipizide is excreted in human milk, some sulfonylurea drugs are known to be excreted in human milk. Because the potential for hypoglycemia in nursing infants may exist, a decision should be made whether to discontinue nursing or to discontinue the drug, taking into account the importance of the drug to the mother. If the drug is discontinued and if diet alone is inadequate for controlling blood glucose, insulin therapy should be considered.

Pediatric Use: Safety and effectiveness in children have not been established.

Geriatric Use: Of the total number of patients in clinical studies of GLUCOTROL XL, 33 percent were 65 and over. No overall differences in effectiveness or safety were observed between these patients and younger patients, but greater sensitivity of some individuals cannot be ruled out. Approximately 1–2 days longer were required to reach

Continued on next page

Glucotrol XL—Cont.

steady-state in the elderly. (See CLINICAL PHARMACOLOGY and DOSAGE AND ADMINISTRATION.)

ADVERSE REACTIONS

In U.S. controlled studies the frequency of serious adverse experiences reported was very low and causal relationship has not been established.

The 580 patients from 31 to 87 years of age who received GLUCOTROL XL Extended Release Tablets in doses from 5 mg to 60 mg in both controlled and open trials were included in the evaluation of adverse experiences. All adverse experiences reported were tabulated independently of their possible causal relation to medication.

Hypoglycemia: See PRECAUTIONS and OVERDOSAGE sections.

Only 3.4% of patients receiving GLUCOTROL XL Extended Release Tablets had hypoglycemia documented by a blood-glucose measurement <60 mg/dL and/or symptoms believed to be associated with hypoglycemia. In a comparative efficacy study of GLUCOTROL XL and Glucotrol, hypoglycemia occurred rarely with an incidence of less than 1% with both drugs.

In double-blind, placebo-controlled studies the adverse experiences reported with an incidence of 3% or more in GLUCOTROL XL-treated patients include:

Adverse Effect	GLUCOTROL XL (%) (N=278)	Placebo (%) (N=69)
Asthenia	10.1	13.0
Headache	8.6	8.7
Dizziness	6.8	5.8
Nervousness	3.6	2.9
Tremor	3.6	0.0
Diarrhea	5.4	0.0
Flatulence	3.2	1.4

The following adverse experiences occurred with an incidence of less than 3% in GLUCOTROL XL-treated patients:

- Body as a whole–pain
- Nervous system–insomnia, paresthesia, anxiety, depression and hypesthesia
- Gastrointestinal–nausea, dyspepsia, constipation and vomiting
- Metabolic–hypoglycemia
- Musculoskeletal–arthralgia, leg cramps and myalgia
- Cardiovascular–syncope
- Skin–sweating and pruritus
- Respiratory–rhinitis
- Special senses–blurred vision
- Urogenital–polyuria

Other adverse experiences occurred with an incidence of less than 1% in GLUCOTROL XL-treated patients:

- Body as a whole–chills
- Nervous system–hypertonia, confusion, vertigo, somnolence, gait abnormality and decreased libido
- Gastrointestinal–anorexia and trace blood in stool
- Metabolic–thirst and edema
- Cardiovascular–arrhythmia, migraine, flushing and hypertension
- Skin–rash and urticaria
- Respiratory–pharyngitis and dyspnea
- Special senses–pain in the eye, conjunctivitis and retinal hemorrhage
- Urogenital–dysuria

Although these adverse experiences occurred in patients treated with GLUCOTROL XL, a causal relationship to the medication has not been established in all cases.

There have been rare reports of gastrointestinal irritation and gastrointestinal bleeding with use of another drug in this non-deformable sustained release formulation, although causal relationship to the drug is uncertain.

The following are adverse experiences reported with immediate release glipizide and other sulfonylureas, but have not been observed with GLUCOTROL XL:

Hematologic: Leukopenia, agranulocytosis, thrombocytopenia, hemolytic anemia, aplastic anemia, and pancytopenia have been reported with sulfonylureas.

Metabolic: Hepatic porphyria and disulfiram-like reactions have been reported with sulfonylureas. In the mouse, glipizide pretreatment did not cause an accumulation of acetaldehyde after ethanol administration. Clinical experience to date has shown that glipizide has an extremely low incidence of disulfiram-like alcohol reactions.

Endocrine Reactions: Cases of hyponatremia and the syndrome of inappropriate antidiuretic hormone (SIADH) secretion have been reported with glipizide and other sulfonylureas.

Laboratory Tests: The pattern of laboratory test abnormalities observed with glipizide was similar to that for other sulfonylureas. Occasional mild to moderate elevations of SGOT, LDH, alkaline phosphatase, BUN and creatinine were noted. One case of jaundice was reported. The relationship of these abnormalities to glipizide is uncertain, and they have rarely been associated with clinical symptoms.

OVERDOSAGE

There is no well-documented experience with GLUCOTROL XL overdosage in humans. There have been no known suicide attempts associated with purposeful overdosing with GLUCOTROL XL. In nonclinical studies the acute oral toxicity of glipizide was extremely low in all species tested (LD_{50} greater than 4 g/kg). Overdosage of sulfonylureas including glipizide can produce hypoglycemia. Mild hypoglycemic symptoms without loss of consciousness or neurologic findings should be treated aggressively with oral glucose and adjustments in drug dosage and/or meal patterns. Close monitoring should continue until the physician is assured that the patient is out of danger. Severe hypoglycemic reactions with coma, seizure, or other neurological impairment occur infrequently, but constitute medical emergencies requiring immediate hospitalization. If hypoglycemic coma is diagnosed or suspected, the patient should be given rapid intravenous injection of concentrated (50%) glucose solution. This should be followed by a continuous infusion of a more dilute (10%) glucose solution at a rate that will maintain the blood glucose at a level above 100 mg/dL. Patients should be closely monitored for a minimum of 24 to 48 hours since hypoglycemia may recur after apparent clinical recovery. Clearance of glipizide from plasma may be prolonged in persons with liver disease. Because of the extensive protein binding of glipizide, dialysis is unlikely to be of benefit.

DOSAGE AND ADMINISTRATION

There is no fixed dosage regimen for the management of diabetes mellitus with GLUCOTROL XL Extended Release Tablet or any other hypoglycemic agent. Glycemic control should be monitored with hemoglobin A_{1C} and/or blood-glucose levels to determine the minimum effective dose for the patient; to detect primary failure, i.e., inadequate lowering of blood glucose at the maximum recommended dose of medication; and to detect secondary failure, i.e., loss of an adequate blood-glucose-lowering response after an initial period of effectiveness. Home blood-glucose monitoring may also provide useful information to the patient and physician. Short-term administration of GLUCOTROL XL Extended Release Tablet may be sufficient during periods of transient loss of control in patients usually controlled on diet.

In general, GLUCOTROL XL should be given with breakfast.

Recommended Dosing: The usual starting dose of GLUCOTROL XL as initial therapy is 5 mg per day, given with breakfast. Those patients who may be more sensitive to hypoglycemic drugs may be started at a lower dose.

Dosage adjustment should be based on laboratory measures of glycemic control. While fasting blood-glucose levels generally reach steady-state following initiation or change in GLUCOTROL XL dosage, a single fasting glucose determination may not accurately reflect the response to therapy. In most cases, hemoglobin A_{1C} level measured at three month intervals is the preferred means of monitoring response to therapy.

Hemoglobin A_{1C} should be measured as GLUCOTROL XL therapy is initiated and repeated approximately three months later. If the result of this test suggests that glycemic control over the preceding three months was inadequate, the GLUCOTROL XL dose may be increased.

Subsequent dosage adjustments should be made on the basis of hemoglobin A_{1C} levels measured at three month intervals. If no improvement is seen after three months of therapy with a higher dose, the previous dose should be resumed. Decisions which utilize fasting blood glucose to adjust GLUCOTROL XL therapy should be based on at least two or more similar, consecutive values obtained seven days or more after the previous dose adjustment.

Most patients will be controlled with 5 mg to 10 mg taken once daily. However, some patients may require up to the maximum recommended daily dose of 20 mg. While the glycemic control of selected patients may improve with doses which exceed 10 mg, clinical studies conducted to date have not demonstrated an additional group average reduction of hemoglobin A_{1C} beyond what was achieved with the 10 mg dose.

Based on the results of a randomized crossover study, patients receiving immediate release glipizide may be switched safely to GLUCOTROL XL Extended Release Tablets once-a-day at the nearest equivalent total daily dose. Patients receiving immediate release Glucotrol also may be titrated to the appropriate dose of GLUCOTROL XL starting with 5 mg once daily. The decision to switch to the nearest equivalent dose or to titrate should be based on clinical judgment.

In elderly patients, debilitated or malnourished patients, and patients with impaired renal or hepatic function, the initial and maintenance dosing should be conservative to avoid hypoglycemic reactions (see PRECAUTIONS section).

Combination Use:

When adding other blood-glucose-lowering agents to GLUCOTROL XL for combination therapy, the agent should be initiated at the lowest recommended dose, and patients should be observed carefully for hypoglycemia. Refer to the product information supplied with the oral agent for additional information.

When adding GLUCOTROL XL to other blood-glucose-lowering agents, GLUCOTROL XL can be initiated at 5 mg. Those patients who may be more sensitive to hypoglycemic drugs may be started at a lower dose. Titration should be based on clinical judgment.

Patients Receiving Insulin: As with other sulfonylurea-class hypoglycemics, many patients with stable type 2 diabetes receiving insulin may be transferred safely to treatment with GLUCOTROL XL Extended Release Tablets. When transferring patients from insulin to GLUCOTROL XL, the following general guidelines should be considered:

For patients whose daily insulin requirement is 20 units or less, insulin may be discontinued and GLUCOTROL XL therapy may begin at usual dosages. Several days should elapse between titration steps.

For patients whose daily insulin requirement is greater than 20 units, the insulin dose should be reduced by 50% and GLUCOTROL XL therapy may begin at usual dosages. Subsequent reductions in insulin dosage should depend on individual patient response. Several days should elapse between titration steps.

During the insulin withdrawal period, the patient should test urine samples for sugar and ketone bodies at least three times daily. Patients should be instructed to contact the prescriber immediately if these tests are abnormal. In some cases, especially when the patient has been receiving greater than 40 units of insulin daily, it may be advisable to consider hospitalization during the transition period.

Patients Receiving Other Oral Hypoglycemic Agents: As with other sulfonylurea-class hypoglycemics, no transition period is necessary when transferring patients to GLUCOTROL XL Extended Release Tablets. Patients should be observed carefully (1–2 weeks) for hypoglycemia when being transferred from longer half-life sulfonylureas (e.g., chlorpropamide) to GLUCOTROL XL due to potential overlapping of drug effect.

HOW SUPPLIED

GLUCOTROL XL® (glipizide) Extended Release Tablets are supplied as 2.5 mg, 5 mg, and 10 mg round, biconvex tablets and imprinted with black ink as follows:

2.5 mg tablets are blue and imprinted with "GLUCOTROL XL 2.5" on one side.
Bottles of 30: NDC 0049-1620-30

5 mg tablets are white and imprinted with "GLUCOTROL XL 5" on one side.
Bottles of 100: NDC 0049-1550-66
Bottles of 500: NDC 0049-1550-73

10 mg tablets are white and imprinted with "GLUCOTROL XL 10" on one side.
Bottles of 100: NDC 0049-1560-66
Bottles of 500: NDC 0049-1560-73

Recommended Storage: The tablets should be protected from moisture and humidity and stored at controlled room temperature, 59° to 86°F (15° to 30°C).

Rx only

Pfizer U.S. Pharmaceuticals
Pfizer Inc, NY, NY 10017

Printed in U.S.A.
69-4951-00-6 Revised April 2001

LIPITOR® ℞
(Atorvastatin Calcium) Tablets

Prescribing information for this product, which appears on pages 2696–2699 of the 2002 PDR, has been completely revised as follows. Please write "See Supplement A" next to the product heading.

DESCRIPTION

Lipitor® (atorvastatin calcium) is a synthetic lipid-lowering agent. Atorvastatin is an inhibitor of 3-hydroxy-3-methylglutaryl-coenzyme A (HMG-CoA) reductase. This enzyme catalyzes the conversion of HMG-CoA to mevalonate, an early and rate-limiting step in cholesterol biosynthesis.

Atorvastatin calcium is [R-(R*, R*)]-2-(4-fluorophenyl)-β, δ-dihydroxy-5-(1-methylethyl)-3-phenyl-4-[(phenylamino) carbonyl]-1H-pyrrole-1-heptanoic acid, calcium salt (2:1) trihydrate. The empirical formula of atorvastatin calcium is $(C_{33}H_{34}FN_2O_5)_2Ca \cdot 3H_2O$ and its molecular weight is 1209.42. Its structural formula is:

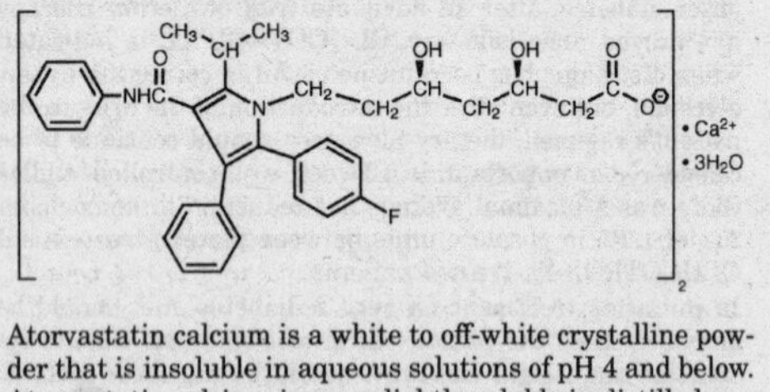

Atorvastatin calcium is a white to off-white crystalline powder that is insoluble in aqueous solutions of pH 4 and below. Atorvastatin calcium is very slightly soluble in distilled water, pH 7.4 phosphate buffer, and acetonitrile, slightly soluble in ethanol, and freely soluble in methanol.

Lipitor tablets for oral administration contain 10, 20, 40 or 80 mg atorvastatin and the following inactive ingredients: calcium carbonate, USP; candelilla wax, FCC; croscarmellose sodium, NF; hydroxypropyl cellulose, NF; lactose monohydrate, NF; magnesium stearate, NF; microcrystalline cellulose, NF; Opadry White YS-1-7040 (hydroxypropylmethylcellulose, polyethylene glycol, talc, titanium dioxide); polysorbate 80, NF; simethicone emulsion.

CLINICAL PHARMACOLOGY

Mechanism of Action

Atorvastatin is a selective, competitive inhibitor of HMG-CoA reductase, the rate-limiting enzyme that converts 3-hydroxy-3-methylglutaryl-coenzyme A to mevalonate, a precursor of sterols, including cholesterol. Cholesterol and triglycerides circulate in the bloodstream as part of lipoprotein complexes. With ultracentrifugation, these complexes separate into HDL (high-density lipoprotein), IDL (intermediate-density lipoprotein), LDL (low-density lipoprotein), and VLDL (very-low-density lipoprotein) fractions. Triglycerides (TG) and cholesterol in the liver are incorporated into VLDL and released into the plasma for delivery to peripheral tissues. LDL is formed from VLDL and is catabolized primarily through the high-affinity LDL receptor. Clinical and pathologic studies show that elevated plasma levels of total cholesterol (total-C), LDL-cholesterol (LDL-C), and apolipoprotein B (apo B) promote human atherosclerosis and are risk factors for developing cardiovascular disease, while increased levels of HDL-C are associated with a decreased cardiovascular risk.

In animal models, Lipitor lowers plasma cholesterol and lipoprotein levels by inhibiting HMG-CoA reductase and cholesterol synthesis in the liver and by increasing the number of hepatic LDL receptors on the cell-surface to enhance uptake and catabolism of LDL; Lipitor also reduces LDL production and the number of LDL particles. Lipitor reduces LDL-C in some patients with homozygous familial hypercholesterolemia (FH), a population that rarely responds to other lipid-lowering medication(s).

A variety of clinical studies have demonstrated that elevated levels of total-C, LDL-C, and apo B (a membrane complex for LDL-C) promote human atherosclerosis. Similarly, decreased levels of HDL-C (and its transport complex, apo A) are associated with the development of atherosclerosis. Epidemiologic investigations have established that cardiovascular morbidity and mortality vary directly with the level of total-C and LDL-C, and inversely with the level of HDL-C.

Lipitor reduces total-C, LDL-C, and apo B in patients with homozygous and heterozygous FH, nonfamilial forms of hypercholesterolemia, and mixed dyslipidemia. Lipitor also reduces VLDL-C and TG and produces variable increases in HDL-C and apolipoprotein A-1. Lipitor reduces total-C, LDL-C, VLDL-C, apo B, TG, and non-HDL-C, and increases HDL-C in patients with isolated hypertriglyceridemia. Lipitor reduces intermediate density lipoprotein cholesterol (IDL-C) in patients with dysbetalipoproteinemia. The effect of Lipitor on cardiovascular morbidity and mortality has not been determined.

Like LDL, cholesterol-enriched triglyceride-rich lipoproteins, including VLDL, intermediate density lipoprotein (IDL), and remnants, can also promote atherosclerosis. Elevated plasma triglycerides are frequently found in a triad with low HDL-C levels and small LDL particles, as well as in association with non-lipid metabolic risk factors for coronary heart disease. As such, total plasma TG has not consistently been shown to be an independent risk factor for CHD. Furthermore, the independent effect of raising HDL or lowering TG on the risk of coronary and cardiovascular morbidity and mortality has not been determined.

Pharmacodynamics

Atorvastatin as well as some of its metabolites are pharmacologically active in humans. The liver is the primary site of action and the principal site of cholesterol synthesis and LDL clearance. Drug dosage rather than systemic drug concentration correlates better with LDL-C reduction. Individualization of drug dosage should be based on therapeutic response (see DOSAGE AND ADMINISTRATION).

Pharmacokinetics and Drug Metabolism

Absorption: Atorvastatin is rapidly absorbed after oral administration; maximum plasma concentrations occur within 1 to 2 hours. Extent of absorption increases in proportion to atorvastatin dose. The absolute bioavailability of atorvastatin (parent drug) is approximately 14% and the systemic availability of HMG-CoA reductase inhibitory activity is approximately 30%. The low systemic availability is attributed to presystemic clearance in gastrointestinal mucosa and/or hepatic first-pass metabolism. Although food decreases the rate and extent of drug absorption by approximately 25% and 9%, respectively, as assessed by Cmax and AUC, LDL-C reduction is similar whether atorvastatin is given with or without food. Plasma atorvastatin concentrations are lower (approximately 30% for Cmax and AUC) following evening drug administration compared with morning. However, LDL-C reduction is the same regardless of the time of day of drug administration (see DOSAGE AND ADMINISTRATION).

Distribution: Mean volume of distribution of atorvastatin is approximately 381 liters. Atorvastatin is ≥98% bound to plasma proteins. A blood/plasma ratio of approximately 0.25 indicates poor drug penetration into red blood cells. Based on observations in rats, atorvastatin is likely to be secreted in human milk (see CONTRAINDICATIONS, Pregnancy and Lactation, and PRECAUTIONS, Nursing Mothers).

Metabolism: Atorvastatin is extensively metabolized to ortho- and parahydroxylated derivatives and various beta-oxidation products. *In vitro* inhibition of HMG-CoA reductase by ortho- and parahydroxylated metabolites is equivalent to that of atorvastatin. Approximately 70% of circulating inhibitory activity for HMG-CoA reductase is attributed to active metabolites. *In vitro* studies suggest the importance of atorvastatin metabolism by cytochrome P450 3A4, consistent with increased plasma concentrations of atorvastatin in humans following coadministration with erythromycin, a known inhibitor of this isozyme (see PRECAUTIONS, Drug Interactions). In animals, the ortho-hydroxy metabolite undergoes further glucuronidation.

Excretion: Atorvastatin and its metabolites are eliminated primarily in bile following hepatic and/or extra-hepatic metabolism; however, the drug does not appear to undergo enterohepatic recirculation. Mean plasma elimination half-life of atorvastatin in humans is approximately 14 hours, but the half-life of inhibitory activity for HMG-CoA reductase is 20 to 30 hours due to the contribution of active metabolites. Less than 2% of a dose of atorvastatin is recovered in urine following oral administration.

TABLE 1. Dose-Response in Patients With Primary Hypercholesterolemia (Adjusted Mean % Change From Baseline)[a]

Dose	N	TC	LDL-C	Apo B	TG	HDL-C	Non-HDL-C/ HDL-C
Placebo	21	4	4	3	10	-3	7
10	22	-29	-39	-32	-19	6	-34
20	20	-33	-43	-35	-26	9	-41
40	21	-37	-50	-42	-29	6	-45
80	23	-45	-60	-50	-37	5	-53

[a]Results are pooled from 2 dose-response studies

TABLE 2. Mean Percent Change From Baseline at End Point (Double-Blind, Randomized, Active-Controlled Trials)

Treatment (Daily Dose)	N	Total-C	LDL-C	Apo B	TG	HDL-C	Non-HDL-C/ HDL-C
Study 1							
Atorvastatin 10 mg	707	-27[a]	-36[a]	-28[a]	-17[a]	+7	-37[a]
Lovastatin 20 mg	191	-19	-27	-20	-6	+7	-28
95% CI for Diff[1]		-9.2, -6.5	-10.7, -7.1	-10.0, -6.5	-15.2, -7.1	-1.7, 2.0	-11.1, -7.1
Study 2							
Atorvastatin 10 mg	222	-25[b]	-35[b]	-27[b]	-17[b]	+6	-36[b]
Pravastatin 20 mg	77	-17	-23	-17	-9	+8	-28
95% CI for Diff[1]		-10.8, -6.1	-14.5, -8.2	-13.4, -7.4	-14.1, -0.7	-4.9, 1.6	-11.5, -4.1
Study 3							
Atorvastatin 10 mg	132	-29[c]	-37[c]	-34[c]	-23[c]	+7	-39[c]
Simvastatin 10 mg	45	-24	-30	-30	-15	+7	-33
95% CI for Diff[1]		-8.7, -2.7	-10.1, -2.6	-8.0, -1.1	-15.1, -0.7	-4.3, 3.9	-9.6, -1.9

[1] A negative value for the 95% CI for the difference between treatments favors atorvastatin for all except HDL-C, for which a positive value favors atorvastatin. If the range does not include 0, this indicates a statistically significant difference.
[a] Significantly different from lovastatin, ANCOVA, p ≤0.05
[b] Significantly different from pravastatin, ANCOVA, p ≤0.05
[c] Significantly different from simvastatin, ANCOVA, p ≤0.05

TABLE 3. Combined Patients With Isolated Elevated TG; Median (min, max) Percent Changes From Baseline

	Placebo (N=12)	Atorvastatin 10 mg (N=37)	Atorvastatin 20 mg (N=13)	Atorvastatin 80 mg (N=14)
Triglycerides	-12.4 (-36.6, 82.7)	-41.0 (-76.2, 49.4)	-38.7 (-62.7, 29.5)	-51.8 (-82.8, 41.3)
Total-C	-2.3 (-15.5, 24.4)	-28.2 (-44.9, -6.8)	-34.9 (-49.6, -15.2)	-44.4 (-63.5, -3.8)
LDL-C	3.6 (-31.3, 31.6)	-26.5 (-57.7, 9.8)	-30.4 (-53.9, 0.3)	-40.5 (-60.6, -13.8)
HDL-C	3.8 (-18.6, 13.4)	13.8 (-9.7, 61.5)	11.0 (-3.2, 25.2)	7.5 (-10.8, 37.2)
VLDL-C	-1.0 (-31.9, 53.2)	-48.8 (-85.8, 57.3)	-44.6 (-62.2, -10.8)	-62.0 (-88.2, 37.6)
non-HDL-C	-2.8 (-17.6, 30.0)	-33.0 (-52.1, -13.3)	-42.7 (-53.7, -17.4)	-51.5 (-72.9, -4.3)

Special Populations

Geriatric: Plasma concentrations of atorvastatin are higher (approximately 40% for Cmax and 30% for AUC) in healthy elderly subjects (age ≥65 years) than in young adults. Clinical data suggest a greater degree of LDL-lowering at any dose of drug in the elderly patient population compared to younger adults (see PRECAUTIONS section; Geriatric Use subsection).

Pediatric: Pharmacokinetic data in the pediatric population are not available.

Gender: Plasma concentrations of atorvastatin in women differ from those in men (approximately 20% higher for Cmax and 10% lower for AUC); however, there is no clinically significant difference in LDL-C reduction with Lipitor between men and women.

Renal Insufficiency: Renal disease has no influence on the plasma concentrations or LDL-C reduction of atorvastatin; thus, dose adjustment in patients with renal dysfunction is not necessary (see DOSAGE AND ADMINISTRATION).

Hemodialysis: While studies have not been conducted in patients with end-stage renal disease, hemodialysis is not expected to significantly enhance clearance of atorvastatin since the drug is extensively bound to plasma proteins.

Hepatic Insufficiency: In patients with chronic alcoholic liver disease, plasma concentrations of atorvastatin are markedly increased. Cmax and AUC are each 4-fold greater in patients with Childs-Pugh A disease. Cmax and AUC are approximately 16-fold and 11-fold increased, respectively, in patients with Childs-Pugh B disease (see CONTRAINDICATIONS).

Clinical Studies

Hypercholesterolemia (Heterozygous Familial and Nonfamilial) and Mixed Dyslipidemia (*Fredrickson* Types IIa and IIb)

Lipitor reduces total-C, LDL-C, VLDL-C, apo B, and TG, and increases HDL-C in patients with hypercholesterolemia and mixed dyslipidemia. Therapeutic response is seen within 2 weeks, and maximum response is usually achieved within 4 weeks and maintained during chronic therapy.

Lipitor is effective in a wide variety of patient populations with hypercholesterolemia, with and without hypertriglyceridemia, in men and women, and in the elderly. Experience in pediatric patients has been limited to patients with homozygous FH.

In two multicenter, placebo-controlled, dose-response studies in patients with hypercholesterolemia, Lipitor given as a single dose over 6 weeks significantly reduced total-C, LDL-C, apo B, and TG (Pooled results are provided in Table 1).

[See table 1 above]

In patients with *Fredrickson* Types IIa and IIb hyperlipoproteinemia pooled from 24 controlled trials, the median (25th and 75th percentile) percent changes from baseline in HDL-C for atorvastatin 10, 20, 40, and 80 mg were 6.4 (-1.4, 14), 8.7(0, 17), 7.8(0, 16), and 5.1 (-2.7, 15), respectively. Additionally, analysis of the pooled data demonstrated consistent and significant decrease in total-C, LDL-C, TG, total-C/HDL-C, and LDL-C/HDL-C.

In three multicenter, double-blind studies in patients with hypercholesterolemia, Lipitor was compared to other HMG-CoA reductase inhibitors. After randomization, patients were treated for 16 weeks with either Lipitor 10 mg per day or a fixed dose of the comparative agent (Table 2).

[See table 2 above]

The impact on clinical outcomes of the differences in lipid-altering effects between treatments shown in Table 2 is not known. Table 2 does not contain data comparing the effects of atorvastatin 10 mg and higher doses of lovastatin, pravastatin, and simvastatin. The drugs compared in the studies summarized in the table are not necessarily interchangeable.

Hypertriglyceridemia (*Fredrickson* Type IV)

The response to Lipitor in 64 patients with isolated hypertriglyceridemia treated across several clinical trials is shown in the table below. For the atorvastatin-treated patients, median (min, max) baseline TG level was 565 (267-1502).

[See table 3 above]

Dysbetalipoproteinemia (*Fredrickson* Type III)

The results of an open-label crossover study of 16 patients (genotypes: 14 apo E2/E2 and 2 apo E3/E2) with dysbetalipoproteinemia (*Fredrickson* Type III) are shown in the table below.

[See table 4 at top of next page]

Homozygous Familial Hypercholesterolemia

In a study without a concurrent control group, 29 patients ages 6 to 37 years with homozygous FH received maximum daily doses of 20 to 80 mg of Lipitor. The mean LDL-C reduction in this study was 18%. Twenty-five patients with a

Continued on next page

Lipitor—Cont.

reduction in LDL-C had a mean response of 20% (range of 7% to 53%, median of 24%); the remaining 4 patients had 7% to 24% increases in LDL-C. Five of the 29 patients had absent LDL-receptor function. Of these, 2 patients also had a portacaval shunt and had no significant reduction in LDL-C. The remaining 3 receptor-negative patients had a mean LDL-C reduction of 22%.

INDICATIONS AND USAGE

Lipitor is indicated:

1. as an adjunct to diet to reduce elevated total-C, LDL-C, apo B, and TG levels and to increase HDL-C in patients with primary hypercholesterolemia (heterozygous familial and nonfamilial) and mixed dyslipidemia (*Fredrickson* Types IIa and IIb);
2. as an adjunct to diet for the treatment of patients with elevated serum TG levels (*Fredrickson* Type IV);
3. for the treatment of patients with primary dysbetalipoproteinemia (*Fredrickson* Type III) who do not respond adequately to diet;
4. to reduce total-C and LDL-C in patients with homozygous familial hypercholesterolemia as an adjunct to other lipid-lowering treatments (eg, LDL apheresis) or if such treatments are unavailable.

Therapy with lipid-altering agents should be a component of multiple-risk-factor intervention in individuals at increased risk for atherosclerotic vascular disease due to hypercholesterolemia. Lipid-altering agents should be used in addition to a diet restricted in saturated fat and cholesterol only when the response to diet and other nonpharmacological measures has been inadequate (see *National Cholesterol Education Program (NCEP) Guidelines*, summarized in Table 5).

[See table 5 above]

After the LDL-C goal has been achieved, if the TG is still ≥200 mg/dL, non HDL-C (total-C minus HDL-C) becomes a secondary target of therapy. Non-HDL-C goals are set 30 mg/dL higher than LDL-C goals for each risk category.

Prior to initiating therapy with Lipitor, secondary causes for hypercholesterolemia (eg, poorly controlled diabetes mellitus, hypothyroidism, nephrotic syndrome, dysproteinemias, obstructive liver disease, other drug therapy, and alcoholism) should be excluded, and a lipid profile performed to measure total-C, LDL-C, HDL-C, and TG. For patients with TG <400 mg/dL (<4.5 mmol/L), LDL-C can be estimated using the following equation: LDL-C = total-C - (0.20 × [TG] + HDL-C). For TG levels >400 mg/dL (>4.5 mmol/L), this equation is less accurate and LDL-C concentrations should be determined by ultracentrifugation.

Lipitor has not been studied in conditions where the major lipoprotein abnormality is elevation of chylomicrons (*Fredrickson* Types I and V).

CONTRAINDICATIONS

Active liver disease or unexplained persistent elevations of serum transaminases.

Hypersensitivity to any component of this medication.

Pregnancy and Lactation

Atherosclerosis is a chronic process and discontinuation of lipid-lowering drugs during pregnancy should have little impact on the outcome of long-term therapy of primary hypercholesterolemia. Cholesterol and other products of cholesterol biosynthesis are essential components for fetal development (including synthesis of steroids and cell membranes). Since HMG-CoA reductase inhibitors decrease cholesterol synthesis and possibly the synthesis of other biologically active substances derived from cholesterol, they may cause fetal harm when administered to pregnant women. Therefore, HMG-CoA reductase inhibitors are contraindicated during pregnancy and in nursing mothers. ATORVASTATIN SHOULD BE ADMINISTERED TO WOMEN OF CHILDBEARING AGE ONLY WHEN SUCH PATIENTS ARE HIGHLY UNLIKELY TO CONCEIVE AND HAVE BEEN INFORMED OF THE POTENTIAL HAZARDS. If the patient becomes pregnant while taking this drug, therapy should be discontinued and the patient apprised of the potential hazard to the fetus.

WARNINGS

Liver Dysfunction

HMG-CoA reductase inhibitors, like some other lipid-lowering therapies, have been associated with biochemical abnormalities of liver function. **Persistent elevations (>3 times the upper limit of normal [ULN] occurring on 2 or more occasions) in serum transaminases occurred in 0.7% of patients who received atorvastatin in clinical trials. The incidence of these abnormalities was 0.2%, 0.2%, 0.6%, and 2.3% for 10, 20, 40, and 80 mg, respectively.**

One patient in clinical trials developed jaundice. Increases in liver function tests (LFT) in other patients were not associated with jaundice or other clinical signs or symptoms. Upon dose reduction, drug interruption, or discontinuation, transaminase levels returned to or near pretreatment levels without sequelae. Eighteen of 30 patients with persistent LFT elevations continued treatment with a reduced dose of atorvastatin.

It is recommended that liver function tests be performed prior to and at 12 weeks following both the initiation of therapy and any elevation of dose, and periodically (eg, semiannually) thereafter. Liver enzyme changes generally occur in the first 3 months of treatment with atorvastatin. Patients who develop increased transaminase levels should

TABLE 4. Open-Label Crossover Study of 16 Patients With Dysbetalipoproteinemia (*Fredrickson* Type III)

	Median (min, max) at Baseline (mg/dL)	Median % Change (min, max)	
		Atorvastatin 10 mg	Atorvastatin 80 mg
Total-C	442 (225, 1320)	-37 (-85, 17)	-58 (-90, -31)
Triglycerides	678 (273, 5990)	-39 (-92, -8)	-53 (-95, -30)
IDL-C + VLDL-C	215 (111, 613)	-32 (-76, 9)	-63 (-90, -8)
non-HDL-C	411 (218, 1272)	-43 (-87, -19)	-64 (-92, -36)

TABLE 5: NCEP Treatment Guidelines: LDL-C Goals and Cutpoints for Therapeutic Lifestyle Changes and Drug Therapy in Different Risk Categories

Risk Category	LDL Goal (mg/dL)	LDL Level at Which to Initiate Therapeutic Lifestyle Changes (mg/dL)	LDL Level at Which to Consider Drug Therapy (mg/dL)
CHD[a] or CHD risk equivalents (10-year risk >20%)	<100	≥100	≥130 (100-129: drug optional)[b]
2+ Risk Factors (10-year risk ≤20%)	<130	≥130	10-year risk 10%-20%: ≥130 10-year risk <10%: ≥ 160
0-1 Risk factor[c]	<160	≥160	≥190 (160-189: LDL-lowering drug optional)

[a] CHD, coronary heart disease

[b] Some authorities recommend use of LDL-lowering drugs in this category if an LDL-C level of <100 mg/dL cannot be achieved by therapeutic lifestyle changes. Others prefer use of drugs that primarily modify triglycerides and HDL-C, e.g., nicotinic acid or fibrate. Clinical judgment also may call for deferring drug therapy in this subcategory.

[c] Almost all people with 0-1 risk factor have 10-year risk <10%; thus, 10-year risk assessment in people with 0-1 risk factor is not necessary.

be monitored until the abnormalities resolve. Should an increase in ALT or AST of >3 times ULN persist, reduction of dose or withdrawal of atorvastatin is recommended.

Atorvastatin should be used with caution in patients who consume substantial quantities of alcohol and/or have a history of liver disease. Active liver disease or unexplained persistent transaminase elevations are contraindications to the use of atorvastatin (see CONTRAINDICATIONS).

Skeletal Muscle

Rare cases of rhabdomyolysis with acute renal failure secondary to myoglobinuria have been reported with atorvastatin and with other drugs in this class.

Uncomplicated myalgia has been reported in atorvastatin-treated patients (see ADVERSE REACTIONS). Myopathy, defined as muscle aches or muscle weakness in conjunction with increases in creatine phosphokinase (CPK) values >10 times ULN, should be considered in any patient with diffuse myalgias, muscle tenderness or weakness, and/or marked elevation of CPK. Patients should be advised to report promptly unexplained muscle pain, tenderness or weakness, particularly if accompanied by malaise or fever. Atorvastatin therapy should be discontinued if markedly elevated CPK levels occur or myopathy is diagnosed or suspected.

The risk of myopathy during treatment with drugs in this class is increased with concurrent administration of cyclosporine, fibric acid derivatives, erythromycin, niacin, or azole antifungals. Physicians considering combined therapy with atorvastatin and fibric acid derivatives, erythromycin, immunosuppressive drugs, azole antifungals, or lipid-lowering doses of niacin should carefully weigh the potential benefits and risks and should carefully monitor patients for any signs or symptoms of muscle pain, tenderness, or weakness, particularly during the initial months of therapy and during any periods of upward dosage titration of either drug. Periodic creatine phosphokinase (CPK) determinations may be considered in such situations, but there is no assurance that such monitoring will prevent the occurrence of severe myopathy.

Atorvastatin therapy should be temporarily withheld or discontinued in any patient with an acute, serious condition suggestive of a myopathy or having a risk factor predisposing to the development of renal failure secondary to rhabdomyolysis (eg, severe acute infection, hypotension, major surgery, trauma, severe metabolic, endocrine and electrolyte disorders, and uncontrolled seizures).

PRECAUTIONS

General

Before instituting therapy with atorvastatin, an attempt should be made to control hypercholesterolemia with appropriate diet, exercise, and weight reduction in obese patients, and to treat other underlying medical problems (see INDICATIONS AND USAGE).

Information for Patients

Patients should be advised to report promptly unexplained muscle pain, tenderness, or weakness, particularly if accompanied by malaise or fever.

Drug Interactions

The risk of myopathy during treatment with drugs of this class is increased with concurrent administration of cyclosporine, fibric acid derivatives, niacin (nicotinic acid), erythromycin, azole antifungals (see WARNINGS, Skeletal Muscle).

Antacid: When atorvastatin and Maalox® TC suspension were coadministered, plasma concentrations of atorvastatin decreased approximately 35%. However, LDL-C reduction was not altered.

Antipyrine: Because atorvastatin does not affect the pharmacokinetics of antipyrine, interactions with other drugs metabolized via the same cytochrome isozymes are not expected.

Colestipol: Plasma concentrations of atorvastatin decreased approximately 25% when colestipol and atorvastatin were coadministered. However, LDL-C reduction was greater when atorvastatin and colestipol were coadministered than when either drug was given alone.

Cimetidine: Atorvastatin plasma concentrations and LDL-C reduction were not altered by coadministration of cimetidine.

Digoxin: When multiple doses of atorvastatin and digoxin were coadministered, steady-state plasma digoxin concentrations increased by approximately 20%. Patients taking digoxin should be monitored appropriately.

Erythromycin: In healthy individuals, plasma concentrations of atorvastatin increased approximately 40% with coadministration of atorvastatin and erythromycin, a known inhibitor of cytochrome P450 3A4 (see WARNINGS, Skeletal Muscle).

Oral Contraceptives: Coadministration of atorvastatin and an oral contraceptive increased AUC values for norethindrone and ethinyl estradiol by approximately 30% and 20%. These increases should be considered when selecting an oral contraceptive for a woman taking atorvastatin.

Warfarin: Atorvastatin had no clinically significant effect on prothrombin time when administered to patients receiving chronic warfarin treatment.

Endocrine Function

HMG-CoA reductase inhibitors interfere with cholesterol synthesis and theoretically might blunt adrenal and/or gonadal steroid production. Clinical studies have shown that atorvastatin does not reduce basal plasma cortisol concentration or impair adrenal reserve. The effects of HMG-CoA reductase inhibitors on male fertility have not been studied in adequate numbers of patients. The effects, if any, on the pituitary-gonadal axis in premenopausal women are unknown. Caution should be exercised if an HMG-CoA reductase inhibitor is administered concomitantly with drugs that may decrease the levels or activity of endogenous steroid hormones, such as ketoconazole, spironolactone, and cimetidine.

CNS Toxicity

Brain hemorrhage was seen in a female dog treated for 3 months at 120 mg/kg/day. Brain hemorrhage and optic nerve vacuolation were seen in another female dog that was sacrificed in moribund condition after 11 weeks of escalating doses up to 280 mg/kg/day. The 120 mg/kg dose resulted in a systemic exposure approximately 16 times the human plasma area-under-the-curve (AUC, 0-24 hours) based on the maximum human dose of 80 mg/day. A single tonic convulsion was seen in each of 2 male dogs (one treated at 10 mg/kg/day and one at 120 mg/kg/day) in a 2-year study. No CNS lesions have been observed in mice after chronic treatment for up to 2 years at doses up to 400 mg/kg/day or in rats at doses up to 100 mg/kg/day. These doses were 6 to 11 times (mouse) and 8 to 16 times (rat) the human AUC (0-24) based on the maximum recommended human dose of 80 mg/day.

TABLE 6. Adverse Events in Placebo-Controlled Studies (% of Patients)

BODY SYSTEM/ Adverse Event	Placebo N = 270	Atorvastatin 10 mg N = 863	Atorvastatin 20 mg N = 36	Atorvastatin 40 mg N = 79	Atorvastatin 80 mg N = 94
BODY AS A WHOLE					
Infection	10.0	10.3	2.8	10.1	7.4
Headache	7.0	5.4	16.7	2.5	6.4
Accidental Injury	3.7	4.2	0.0	1.3	3.2
Flu Syndrome	1.9	2.2	0.0	2.5	3.2
Abdominal Pain	0.7	2.8	0.0	3.8	2.1
Back Pain	3.0	2.8	0.0	3.8	1.1
Allergic Reaction	2.6	0.9	2.8	1.3	0.0
Asthenia	1.9	2.2	0.0	3.8	0.0
DIGESTIVE SYSTEM					
Constipation	1.8	2.1	0.0	2.5	1.1
Diarrhea	1.5	2.7	0.0	3.8	5.3
Dyspepsia	4.1	2.3	2.8	1.3	2.1
Flatulence	3.3	2.1	2.8	1.3	1.1
RESPIRATORY SYSTEM					
Sinusitis	2.6	2.8	0.0	2.5	6.4
Pharyngitis	1.5	2.5	0.0	1.3	2.1
SKIN AND APPENDAGES					
Rash	0.7	3.9	2.8	3.8	1.1
MUSCULOSKELETAL SYSTEM					
Arthralgia	1.5	2.0	0.0	5.1	0.0
Myalgia	1.1	3.2	5.6	1.3	0.0

CNS vascular lesions, characterized by perivascular hemorrhages, edema, and mononuclear cell infiltration of perivascular spaces, have been observed in dogs treated with other members of this class. A chemically similar drug in this class produced optic nerve degeneration (Wallerian degeneration of retinogeniculate fibers) in clinically normal dogs in a dose-dependent fashion at a dose that produced plasma drug levels about 30 times higher than the mean drug level in humans taking the highest recommended dose.

Carcinogenesis, Mutagenesis, Impairment of Fertility

In a 2-year carcinogenicity study in rats at dose levels of 10, 30, and 100 mg/kg/day, 2 rare tumors were found in muscle in high-dose females: in one, there was a rhabdomyosarcoma and, in another, there was a fibrosarcoma. This dose represents a plasma AUC (0-24) value of approximately 16 times the mean human plasma drug exposure after an 80 mg oral dose.

A 2-year carcinogenicity study in mice given 100, 200, or 400 mg/kg/day resulted in a significant increase in liver adenomas in high-dose males and liver carcinomas in high-dose females. These findings occurred at plasma AUC (0-24) values of approximately 6 times the mean human plasma drug exposure after an 80 mg oral dose.

In vitro, atorvastatin was not mutagenic or clastogenic in the following tests with and without metabolic activation: the Ames test with *Salmonella typhimurium* and *Escherichia coli*, the HGPRT forward mutation assay in Chinese hamster lung cells, and the chromosomal aberration assay in Chinese hamster lung cells. Atorvastatin was negative in the *in vivo* mouse micronucleus test.

Studies in rats performed at doses up to 175 mg/kg (15 times the human exposure) produced no changes in fertility. There was aplasia and aspermia in the epididymis of 2 of 10 rats treated with 100 mg/kg/day of atorvastatin for 3 months (16 times the human AUC at the 80 mg dose); testis weights were significantly lower at 30 and 100 mg/kg and epididymal weight was lower at 100 mg/kg. Male rats given 100 mg/kg/day for 11 weeks prior to mating had decreased sperm motility, spermatid head concentration, and increased abnormal sperm. Atorvastatin caused no adverse effects on semen parameters, or reproductive organ histopathology in dogs given doses of 10, 40, or 120 mg/kg for two years.

Pregnancy

Pregnancy Category X

See CONTRAINDICATIONS

Safety in pregnant women has not been established. Atorvastatin crosses the rat placenta and reaches a level in fetal liver equivalent to that of maternal plasma. Atorvastatin was not teratogenic in rats at doses up to 300 mg/kg/day or in rabbits at doses up to 100 mg/kg/day. These doses resulted in multiples of about 30 times (rat) or 20 times (rabbit) the human exposure based on surface area (mg/m^2).

In a study in rats given 20, 100, or 225 mg/kg/day, from gestation day 7 through to lactation day 21 (weaning), there was decreased pup survival at birth, neonate, weaning, and maturity in pups of mothers dosed with 225 mg/kg/day. Body weight was decreased on days 4 and 21 in pups of mothers dosed at 100 mg/kg/day; pup body weight was decreased at birth and at days 4, 21, and 91 at 225 mg/kg/day. Pup development was delayed (rotorod performance at 100 mg/kg/day and acoustic startle at 225 mg/kg/day; pinnae detachment and eye opening at 225 mg/kg/day). These doses correspond to 6 times (100 mg/kg) and 22 times (225 mg/kg) the human AUC at 80 mg/day. Rare reports of congenital anomalies have been received following intrauterine exposure to HMG-CoA reductase inhibitors. There has been one report of severe congenital bony deformity, tracheo-esophageal fistula, and anal atresia (VATER association) in a baby born to a woman who took lovastatin with dextroamphetamine sulfate during the first trimester of pregnancy. Lipitor should be administered to women of child-bearing potential only when such patients are highly unlikely to conceive and have been informed of the potential hazards. If the woman becomes pregnant while taking Lipitor, it should be discontinued and the patient advised again as to the potential hazards to the fetus.

Nursing Mothers

Nursing rat pups had plasma and liver drug levels of 50% and 40%, respectively, of that in their mother's milk. Because of the potential for adverse reactions in nursing infants, women taking Lipitor should not breast-feed (see CONTRAINDICATIONS).

Pediatric Use

Treatment experience in a pediatric population is limited to doses of Lipitor up to 80 mg/day for 1 year in 8 patients with homozygous FH. No clinical or biochemical abnormalities were reported in these patients. None of these patients was below 9 years of age.

Geriatric Use

The safety and efficacy of atorvastatin (10-80 mg) in the geriatric population (≥65 years of age) was evaluated in the ACCESS study. In this 54-week open-label trial 1,958 patients initiated therapy with atorvastatin 10 mg. Of these, 835 were elderly (≥65 years) and 1,123 were non-elderly. The mean change in LDL-C from baseline after 6 weeks of treatment with atorvastatin 10 mg was −38.2% in the elderly patients versus −34.6% in the non-elderly group.

The rates of discontinuation due to adverse events were similar between the two age groups. There were no differences in clinically relevant laboratory abnormalities between the age groups.

ADVERSE REACTIONS

Lipitor is generally well-tolerated. Adverse reactions have usually been mild and transient. In controlled clinical studies of 2502 patients, <2% of patients were discontinued due to adverse experiences attributable to atorvastatin. The most frequent adverse events thought to be related to atorvastatin were constipation, flatulence, dyspepsia, and abdominal pain.

Clinical Adverse Experiences

Adverse experiences reported in ≥2% of patients in placebo-controlled clinical studies of atorvastatin, regardless of causality assessment, are shown in Table 6.

[See table 6 above]

The following adverse events were reported, regardless of causality assessment in patients treated with atorvastatin in clinical trials. The events in italics occurred in ≥2% of patients and the events in plain type occurred in <2% of patients.

Body as a Whole: *Chest pain*, face edema, fever, neck rigidity, malaise, photosensitivity reaction, generalized edema.

Digestive System: *Nausea*, gastroenteritis, liver function tests abnormal, colitis, vomiting, gastritis, dry mouth, rectal hemorrhage, esophagitis, eructation, glossitis, mouth ulceration, anorexia, increased appetite, stomatitis, biliary pain, cheilitis, duodenal ulcer, dysphagia, enteritis, melena, gum hemorrhage, stomach ulcer, tenesmus, ulcerative stomatitis, hepatitis, pancreatitis, cholestatic jaundice.

Respiratory System: *Bronchitis, rhinitis*, pneumonia, dyspnea, asthma, epistaxis.

Nervous System: *Insomnia, dizziness*, paresthesia, somnolence, amnesia, abnormal dreams, libido decreased, emotional lability, incoordination, peripheral neuropathy, torticollis, facial paralysis, hyperkinesia, depression, hypesthesia, hypertonia.

Musculoskeletal System: *Arthritis*, leg cramps, bursitis, tenosynovitis, myasthenia, tendinous contracture, myositis.

Skin and Appendages: Pruritus, contact dermatitis, alopecia, dry skin, sweating, acne, urticaria, eczema, seborrhea, skin ulcer.

Urogenital System: *Urinary tract infection*, urinary frequency, cystitis, hematuria, impotence, dysuria, kidney calculus, nocturia, epididymitis, fibrocystic breast, vaginal hemorrhage, albuminuria, breast enlargement, metrorrhagia, nephritis, urinary incontinence, urinary retention, urinary urgency, abnormal ejaculation, uterine hemorrhage.

Special Senses: Amblyopia, tinnitus, dry eyes, refraction disorder, eye hemorrhage, deafness, glaucoma, parosmia, taste loss, taste perversion.

Cardiovascular System: Palpitation, vasodilatation, syncope, migraine, postural hypotension, phlebitis, arrhythmia, angina pectoris, hypertension.

Metabolic and Nutritional Disorders: *Peripheral edema*, hyperglycemia, creatine phosphokinase increased, gout, weight gain, hypoglycemia.

Hemic and Lymphatic System: Ecchymosis, anemia, lymphadenopathy, thrombocytopenia, petechia.

Postintroduction Reports

Adverse events associated with Lipitor therapy reported since market introduction, that are not listed above, regardless of causality assessment, include the following: anaphylaxis, angioneurotic edema, bullous rashes (including erythema multiforme, Stevens-Johnson syndrome, and toxic epidermal necrolysis), and rhabdomyolysis.

OVERDOSAGE

There is no specific treatment for atorvastatin overdosage. In the event of an overdose, the patient should be treated symptomatically, and supportive measures instituted as required. Due to extensive drug binding to plasma proteins, hemodialysis is not expected to significantly enhance atorvastatin clearance.

DOSAGE AND ADMINISTRATION

The patient should be placed on a standard cholesterol-lowering diet before receiving Lipitor and should continue on this diet during treatment with Lipitor.

Hypercholesterolemia (Heterozygous Familial and Nonfamilial) and Mixed Dyslipidemia (*Fredrickson* Types IIa and IIb)

The recommended starting dose of Lipitor is 10 or 20 mg once daily. Patients who require a large reduction in LDL-C (more than 45%) may be started at 40 mg once daily. The dosage range is 10 to 80 mg once daily. Lipitor can be administered as a single dose at any time of the day, with or without food. The starting dose and maintenance doses of Lipitor should be individualized according to patient characteristics such as goal of therapy and response (see *NCEP Guidelines*, summarized in Table 5). After initiation and/or upon titration of Lipitor, lipid levels should be analyzed within 2 to 4 weeks and dosage adjusted accordingly.

Since the goal of treatment is to lower LDL-C, the NCEP recommends that LDL-C levels be used to initiate and assess treatment response. Only if LDL-C levels are not available, should total-C be used to monitor therapy.

Homozygous Familial Hypercholesterolemia

The dosage of Lipitor in patients with homozygous FH is 10 to 80 mg daily. Lipitor should be used as an adjunct to other lipid-lowering treatments (eg, LDL apheresis) in these patients or if such treatments are unavailable.

Concomitant Therapy

Atorvastatin may be used in combination with a bile acid binding resin for additive effect. The combination of HMG-CoA reductase inhibitors and fibrates should generally be avoided (see WARNINGS, Skeletal Muscle, and PRECAUTIONS, Drug Interactions for other drug-drug interactions).

Dosage in Patients With Renal Insufficiency

Renal disease does not affect the plasma concentrations nor LDL-C reduction of atorvastatin; thus, dosage adjustment in patients with renal dysfunction is not necessary (see CLINICAL PHARMACOLOGY, Pharmacokinetics).

HOW SUPPLIED

Lipitor is supplied as white, elliptical, film-coated tablets of atorvastatin calcium containing 10, 20, 40 and 80 mg atorvastatin.

10 mg tablets: coded "PD 155" on one side and "10" on the other.
N0071-0155-23 bottles of 90
N0071-0155-34 bottles of 5000
N0071-0155-40 10 × 10 unit dose blisters

20 mg tablets: coded "PD 156" on one side and "20" on the other.
N0071-0156-23 bottles of 90
N0071-0156-40 10 × 10 unit dose blisters

40 mg tablets: coded "PD 157" on one side and "40" on the other.
N0071-0157-23 bottles of 90

80 mg tablets: coded "PD 158" on one side and "80" on the other.
N0071-0158-23 bottles of 90

Storage

Store at controlled room temperature 20°C to 25°C (68°F to 77°F) [see USP].

Rx only

Manufactured by:
Pfizer Ireland Pharmaceuticals
Dublin, Ireland
Distributed by:
PFIZER/PARKE-DAVIS
Division of **PFIZER** Inc, NY, NY 10017
MADE IN PUERTO RICO
69-5884-00-1 Revised April 2002

NAVANE® ℞
[*nah 'vān*]
(thiothixene) CAPSULES
NAVANE® ℞
(thiothixene hydrochloride) CONCENTRATE

Prescribing information for this product, which appears on pages 2701–2703 of the 2002 PDR, has been completely revised as follows. Please write "See Supplement A" next to the product heading.

Continued on next page

Navane—Cont.

DESCRIPTION

Navane® (thiothixene) is a thioxanthene derivative. Specifically, it is the *cis* isomer of N,N-dimethyl-9-[3-(4-methyl-1-piperazinyl)-propylidene] thioxanthene-2-sulfonamide.

The thioxanthenes differ from the phenothiazines by the replacement of nitrogen in the central ring with a carbon-linked side chain fixed in space in a rigid structural configuration. An N,N-dimethyl sulfonamide functional group is bonded to the thioxanthene nucleus.
Inert ingredients for the capsule formulations are: hard gelatin capsules (which contain gelatin and titanium dioxide; may contain Yellow 10, Yellow 6, Blue 1, Green 3, Red 3, and other inert ingredients); lactose; magnesium stearate; sodium lauryl sulfate; starch.
Inert ingredients for the oral concentrate formulation are: alcohol; cherry flavor; dextrose; passion fruit flavor; sorbitol solution; water.

ACTIONS

Navane is an antipsychotic of the thioxanthene series. Navane possesses certain chemical and pharmacological similarities to the piperazine phenothiazines and differences from the aliphatic group of phenothiazines.

INDICATIONS

Navane is effective in the management of schizophrenia. Navane has not been evaluated in the management of behavioral complications in patients with mental retardation.

CONTRAINDICATIONS

Navane is contraindicated in patients with circulatory collapse, comatose states, central nervous system depression due to any cause, and blood dyscrasias. Navane is contraindicated in individuals who have shown hypersensitivity to the drug. It is not known whether there is a cross sensitivity between the thioxanthenes and the phenothiazine derivatives, but this possibility should be considered.

WARNINGS

Tardive Dyskinesia—Tardive dyskinesia, a syndrome consisting of potentially irreversible, involuntary, dyskinetic movements may develop in patients treated with antipsychotic drugs. Although the prevalence of the syndrome appears to be highest among the elderly, especially elderly women, it is impossible to rely upon prevalence estimates to predict, at the inception of antipsychotic treatment, which patients are likely to develop the syndrome. Whether antipsychotic drug products differ in their potential to cause tardive dyskinesia is unknown.
Both the risk of developing the syndrome and the likelihood that it will become irreversible are believed to increase as the duration of treatment and the total cumulative dose of antipsychotic drugs administered to the patient increase. However, the syndrome can develop, although much less commonly, after relatively brief treatment periods at low doses.
There is no known treatment for established cases of tardive dyskinesia, although the syndrome may remit, partially or completely, if antipsychotic treatment is withdrawn. Antipsychotic treatment, itself, however, may suppress (or partially suppress) the signs and symptoms of the syndrome and thereby may possibly mask the underlying disease process. The effect that symptomatic suppression has upon the long-term course of the syndrome is unknown.
Given these considerations, antipsychotics should be prescribed in a manner that is most likely to minimize the occurrence of tardive dyskinesia. Chronic antipsychotic treatment should generally be reserved for patients who suffer from a chronic illness that, 1) is known to respond to antipsychotic drugs, and, 2) for whom alternative, equally effective, but potentially less harmful treatments are *not* available or appropriate. In patients who do require chronic treatment, the smallest dose and the shortest duration of treatment producing a satisfactory clinical response should be sought. The need for continued treatment should be reassessed periodically.
If signs and symptoms of tardive dyskinesia appear in a patient on antipsychotics, drug discontinuation should be considered. However, some patients may require treatment despite the presence of the syndrome.
(For further information about the description of tardive dyskinesia and its clinical detection, please refer to "Information for Patients" in the PRECAUTIONS section, and to the ADVERSE REACTIONS section.)
Neuroleptic Malignant Syndrome (NMS)—A potentially fatal symptom complex sometimes referred to as Neuroleptic Malignant Syndrome (NMS) has been reported in association with antipsychotic drugs. Clinical manifestations of NMS are hyperpyrexia, muscle rigidity, altered mental status and evidence of autonomic instability (irregular pulse or blood pressure, tachycardia, diaphoresis, and cardiac dysrhythmias).
The diagnostic evaluation of patients with this syndrome is complicated. In arriving at a diagnosis, it is important to identify cases where the clinical presentation includes both serious medical illness (e.g., pneumonia, systemic infection, etc.) and untreated or inadequately treated extrapyramidal signs and symptoms (EPS). Other important considerations in the differential diagnosis include central anticholinergic toxicity, heat stroke, drug fever and primary central nervous system (CNS) pathology.
The management of NMS should include 1) immediate discontinuation of antipsychotic drugs and other drugs not essential to concurrent therapy, 2) intensive symptomatic treatment and medical monitoring, and 3) treatment of any concomitant serious medical problems for which specific treatments are available. There is no general agreement about specific pharmacological treatment regimens for uncomplicated NMS.
If a patient requires antipsychotic drug treatment after recovery from NMS, the potential reintroduction of drug therapy should be carefully considered. The patient should be carefully monitored, since recurrences of NMS have been reported.
Usage in Pregnancy—Safe use of Navane during pregnancy has not been established. Therefore, this drug should be given to pregnant patients only when, in the judgment of the physician, the expected benefits from the treatment exceed the possible risks to mother and fetus. Animal reproduction studies and clinical experience to date have not demonstrated any teratogenic effects.
In the animal reproduction studies with Navane, there was some decrease in conception rate and litter size, and an increase in resorption rate in rats and rabbits. Similar findings have been reported with other psychotropic agents. After repeated oral administration of Navane to rats (5 to 15 mg/kg/day), rabbits (3 to 50 mg/kg/day), and monkeys (1 to 3 mg/kg/day) before and during gestation, no teratogenic effects were seen.
Usage in Children—The use of Navane in children under 12 years of age is not recommended because safe conditions for its use have not been established.
As is true with many CNS drugs, Navane may impair the mental and/or physical abilities required for the performance of potentially hazardous tasks such as driving a car or operating machinery, especially during the first few days of therapy. Therefore, the patient should be cautioned accordingly.
As in the case of other CNS-acting drugs, patients receiving Navane (thiothixene) should be cautioned about the possible additive effects (which may include hypotension) with CNS depressants and with alcohol.

PRECAUTIONS

An antiemetic effect was observed in animal studies with Navane; since this effect may also occur in man, it is possible that Navane may mask signs of overdosage of toxic drugs and may obscure conditions such as intestinal obstruction and brain tumor.
In consideration of the known capability of Navane and certain other psychotropic drugs to precipitate convulsions, extreme caution should be used in patients with a history of convulsive disorders or those in a state of alcohol withdrawal, since it may lower the convulsive threshold. Although Navane potentiates the actions of the barbiturates, the dosage of the anticonvulsant therapy should not be reduced when Navane is administered concurrently.
Though exhibiting rather weak anticholinergic properties, Navane should be used with caution in patients who might be exposed to extreme heat or who are receiving atropine or related drugs.
Use with caution in patients with cardiovascular disease.
Caution as well as careful adjustment of the dosages is indicated when Navane is used in conjunction with other CNS depressants.
Also, careful observation should be made for pigmentary retinopathy and lenticular pigmentation (fine lenticular pigmentation has been noted in a small number of patients treated with Navane for prolonged periods). Blood dyscrasias (agranulocytosis, pancytopenia, thrombocytopenic purpura), and liver damage (jaundice, biliary stasis) have been reported with related drugs.
Antipsychotic drugs elevate prolactin levels; the elevation persists during chronic administration. Tissue culture experiments indicate that approximately one-third of human breast cancers are prolactin dependent *in vitro*, a factor of potential importance if the prescription of these drugs is contemplated in a patient with a previously detected breast cancer. Although disturbances such as galactorrhea, amenorrhea, gynecomastia, and impotence have been reported, the clinical significance of elevated serum prolactin levels is unknown for most patients. An increase in mammary neoplasms has been found in rodents after chronic administration of antipsychotic drugs. Neither clinical studies nor epidemiologic studies conducted to date, however, have shown an association between chronic administration of these drugs and mammary tumorigenesis; the available evidence is considered too limited to be conclusive at this time.
Information for Patients: Given the likelihood that some patients exposed chronically to antipsychotics will develop tardive dyskinesia, it is advised that all patients in whom chronic use is contemplated be given, if possible, full information about this risk. The decision to inform patients and/or their guardians must obviously take into account the clinical circumstances and the competency of the patient to understand the information provided.

ADVERSE REACTIONS

NOTE: Not all of the following adverse reactions have been reported with Navane. However, since Navane has certain chemical and pharmacologic similarities to the phenothiazines, all of the known side effects and toxicity associated with phenothiazine therapy should be borne in mind when Navane is used.
Cardiovascular Effects: Tachycardia, hypotension, lightheadedness, and syncope. In the event hypotension occurs, epinephrine should not be used as a pressor agent since a paradoxical further lowering of blood pressure may result. Nonspecific EKG changes have been observed in some patients receiving Navane. These changes are usually reversible and frequently disappear on continued Navane therapy. The incidence of these changes is lower than that observed with some phenothiazines. The clinical significance of these changes is not known.
CNS Effects: Drowsiness, usually mild, may occur although it usually subsides with continuation of Navane therapy. The incidence of sedation appears similar to that of the piperazine group of phenothiazines but less than that of certain aliphatic phenothiazines. Restlessness, agitation and insomnia have been noted with Navane. Seizures and paradoxical exacerbation of psychotic symptoms have occurred with Navane infrequently.
Hyperreflexia has been reported in infants delivered from mothers having received structurally related drugs.
In addition, phenothiazine derivatives have been associated with cerebral edema and cerebrospinal fluid abnormalities.
Extrapyramidal symptoms, such as pseudoparkinsonism, akathisia and dystonia have been reported. Management of these extra-pyramidal symptoms depends upon the type and severity. Rapid relief of acute symptoms may require the use of an injectable antiparkinson agent. More slowly emerging symptoms may be managed by reducing the dosage of Navane and/or administering an oral antiparkinson agent.
Persistent Tardive Dyskinesia: As with all antipsychotic agents, tardive dyskinesia may appear in some patients on long-term therapy or may occur after drug therapy has been discontinued. The syndrome is characterized by rhythmical involuntary movements of the tongue, face, mouth or jaw (e.g., protrusion of tongue, puffing of cheeks, puckering of mouth, chewing movements). Sometimes these may be accompanied by involuntary movements of extremities.
Since early detection of tardive dyskinesia is important, patients should be monitored on an ongoing basis. It has been reported that fine vermicular movement of the tongue may be an early sign of the syndrome. If this or any other presentation of the syndrome is observed, the clinician should consider possible discontinuation of antipsychotic medication. (See WARNINGS section.)
Hepatic Effects: Elevations of serum transaminase and alkaline phosphatase, usually transient, have been infrequently observed in some patients. No clinically confirmed cases of jaundice attributable to Navane (thiothixene) have been reported.
Hematologic Effects: As is true with certain other psychotropic drugs, leukopenia and leucocytosis, which are usually transient, can occur occasionally with Navane. Other antipsychotic drugs have been associated with agranulocytosis, eosinophilia, hemolytic anemia, thrombocytopenia and pancytopenia.
Allergic Reactions: Rash, pruritus, urticaria, photosensitivity and rare cases of anaphylaxis have been reported with Navane. Undue exposure to sunlight should be avoided. Although not experienced with Navane, exfoliative dermatitis and contact dermatitis (in nursing personnel) have been reported with certain phenothiazines.
Endocrine Disorders: Lactation, moderate breast enlargement and amenorrhea have occurred in a small percentage of females receiving Navane. If persistent, this may necessitate a reduction in dosage or the discontinuation of therapy. Phenothiazines have been associated with false positive pregnancy tests, gynecomastia, hypoglycemia, hyperglycemia and glycosuria.
Autonomic Effects: Dry mouth, blurred vision, nasal congestion, constipation, increased sweating, increased salivation and impotence have occurred infrequently with Navane therapy. Phenothiazines have been associated with miosis, mydriasis, and adynamic ileus.
Other Adverse Reactions: Hyperpyrexia, anorexia, nausea, vomiting, diarrhea, increase in appetite and weight, weakness or fatigue, polydipsia, and peripheral edema.
Although not reported with Navane, evidence indicates there is a relationship between phenothiazine therapy and the occurrence of a systemic lupus erythematosus-like syndrome.
Neuroleptic Malignant Syndrome (NMS): Please refer to the text regarding NMS in the WARNINGS section.
NOTE: Sudden deaths have occasionally been reported in patients who have received certain phenothiazine derivatives. In some cases the cause of death was apparently cardiac arrest or asphyxia due to failure of the cough reflex. In others, the cause could not be determined nor could it be established that death was due to phenothiazine administration.

DOSAGE AND ADMINISTRATION

Dosage of Navane should be individually adjusted depending on the chronicity and severity of the symptoms of schizophrenia. In general, small doses should be used initially and gradually increased to the optimal effective level, based on patient response.
Some patients have been successfully maintained on once-a-day Navane therapy.
The use of Navane in children under 12 years of age is not recommended because safe conditions for its use have not been established.

In milder conditions, an initial dose of 2 mg three times daily. If indicated, a subsequent increase to 15 mg/day total daily dose is often effective.

In more severe conditions, an initial dose of 5 mg twice daily.

The usual optimal dose is 20 to 30 mg daily. If indicated, an increase to 60 mg/day total daily dose is often effective. Exceeding a total daily dose of 60 mg rarely increases the beneficial response.

OVERDOSAGE

Manifestations include muscular twitching, drowsiness and dizziness. Symptoms of gross overdosage may include CNS depression, rigidity, weakness, torticollis, tremor, salivation, dysphagia, hypotension, disturbances of gait, or coma.

Treatment: Essentially symptomatic and supportive. Early gastric lavage is helpful. Keep patient under careful observation and maintain an open airway, since involvement of the extrapyramidal system may produce dysphagia and respiratory difficulty in severe overdosage. If hypotension occurs, the standard measures for managing circulatory shock should be used (I.V. fluids and/or vasoconstrictors).

If a vasoconstrictor is needed, levarterenol and phenylephrine are the most suitable drugs. Other pressor agents, including epinephrine, are not recommended, since phenothiazine derivatives may reverse the usual pressor action of these agents and cause further lowering of blood pressure.

If CNS depression is marked, symptomatic treatment is indicated. Extrapyramidal symptoms may be treated with antiparkinson drugs.

There are no data on the use of peritoneal or hemodialysis, but they are known to be of little value in phenothiazine intoxication.

HOW SUPPLIED

Navane® (thiothixene) Capsules

Bottles of 100's:	
	1 mg (NDC 0049-5710-66)
	2 mg (NDC 0049-5720-66)
	5 mg (NDC 0049-5730-66)
	10 mg (NDC 0049-5740-66)
	20 mg (NDC 0049-5770-66)

RX Only

Pfizer Roerig

Division of Pfizer Inc, NY, NY 10017

Printed in U.S.A. Revised May 2001

69-1655-00-9

VIBRAMYCIN® Calcium ℞

[*vī-brə 'mīs-ᵊn*]

(doxycycline calcium)

oral syspension

SYRUP

VIBRAMYCIN® Hyclate

[*vī-brə 'mīs-ᵊn*]

(doxycycline hyclate)

CAPSULES

VIBRAMYCIN® Monohydrate

[*vī-brə 'mīs-ᵊn*]

(doxycycline monohydrate)

for ORAL SUSPENSION

VIBRA-TABS®

[*vī-brə 'tăbs*]

(doxycycline hyclate)

FILM COATED TABLETS

Prescribing information for this product, which appears on pages 2735–2737 of the 2002 PDR, has been completely revised as follows. Please write "See Supplement A" next to the product heading.

DESCRIPTION

Vibramycin® is a broad-spectrum antibiotic synthetically derived from oxytetracycline, and is available as Vibramycin Monohydrate (doxycycline monohydrate); Vibramycin Hyclate and Vibra-Tabs (doxycycline hydrochloride hemiethanolate hemihydrate); and Vibramycin Calcium (doxycycline calcium) for oral administration.

The structural formula of doxycycline monohydrate is

with a molecular formula of $C_{22}H_{24}N_2O_8 \bullet H_2O$ and a molecular weight of 462.46. The chemical designation for doxycycline is 4-(Dimethylamino)-1, 4, 4a, 5, 5a, 6, 11, 12a-octahydro-3, 5, 10, 12, 12a-pentahydroxy-6-methyl-1, 11-dioxo-2-naphthacenecarboxamide monohydrate. The molecular formula for doxycycline hydrochloride hemiethanolate hemihydrate is $(C_{22}H_{24}N_2O_8 \bullet HCl)_2 \bullet C_2H_6O \bullet H_2O$ and the molecular weight is 1025.89. Doxycycline is a light-yellow crystalline powder. Doxycycline hyclate is soluble in water, while doxycycline monohydrate is very slightly soluble in water.

Doxycycline has a high degree of lipoid solubility and a low affinity for calcium binding. It is highly stable in normal human serum. Doxycycline will not degrade into an epianhydro form.

Inert ingredients in the syrup formulation are: apple flavor; butylparaben; calcium chloride; carmine; glycerin; hydrochloric acid; magnesium aluminum silicate; povidone; propylene glycol; propylparaben; raspberry flavor; simethicone emulsion; sodium hydroxide; sodium metabisulfite; sorbitol solution; water.

Inert ingredients in the capsule formulations are: hard gelatin capsules (which may contain Blue 1 and other inert ingredients); magnesium stearate; microcrystalline cellulose; sodium lauryl sulfate.

Inert ingredients for the oral suspension formulation are: carboxymethylcellulose sodium; Blue 1; methylparaben; microcrystalline cellulose; propylparaben; raspberry flavor; Red 28; simethicone emulsion; sucrose.

Inert ingredients for the tablet formulation are: ethylcellulose; hydroxypropyl methylcellulose; magnesium stearate; microcrystalline cellulose; propylene glycol; sodium lauryl sulfate; talc; titanium dioxide; Yellow 6 Lake.

CLINICAL PHARMACOLOGY

Tetracyclines are readily absorbed and are bound to plasma proteins in varying degree. They are concentrated by the liver in the bile, and excreted in the urine and feces at high concentrations and in a biologically active form. Doxycycline is virtually completely absorbed after oral administration.

Following a 200 mg dose, normal adult volunteers averaged peak serum levels of 2.6 mcg/mL of doxycycline at 2 hours decreasing to 1.45 mcg/mL at 24 hours. Excretion of doxycycline by the kidney is about 40%/72 hours in individuals with normal function (creatinine clearance about 75 mL/min.). This percentage excretion may fall as low as 1–5%/72 hours in individuals with severe renal insufficiency (creatinine clearance below 10 mL/min.). Studies have shown no significant difference in serum half-life of doxycycline (range 18–22 hours) in individuals with normal and severely impaired renal function.

Hemodialysis does not alter serum half-life.

Results of animal studies indicate that tetracyclines cross the placenta and are found in fetal tissues.

Microbiology

The tetracyclines are primarily bacteriostatic and are thought to exert their antimicrobial effect by the inhibition of protein synthesis. The tetracyclines, including doxycycline, have a similar antimicrobial spectrum of activity against a wide range of gram-positive and gram-negative organisms. Cross-resistance of these organisms to tetracyclines is common.

Gram-Negative Bacteria

Neisseria gonorrhoeae
Calymmatobacterium granulomatis
Haemophilus ducreyi
Haemophilus influenzae
Yersinia pestis (formerly *Pasteurella pestis*)
Francisella tularensis (formerly *Pasteurella tularensis*)
Vibrio cholerae (formerly *Vibrio comma*)
Bartonella bacilliformis
Brucella species

Because many strains of the following groups of gram-negative microorganisms have been shown to be resistant to tetracyclines, culture and susceptibility testing are recommended:

Escherichia coli
Klebsiella species
Enterobacter aerogenes
Shigella species
Acinetobacter species (formerly *Mima* species and *Herellea* species)
Bacteroides species

Gram-Positive Bacteria

Because many strains of the following groups of gram-positive microorganisms have been shown to be resistant to tetracycline, culture and susceptibility testing are recommended. Up to 44 percent of strains of *Streptococcus pyogenes* and 74 percent of *Streptococcus faecalis* have been found to be resistant to tetracycline drugs. Therefore, tetracycline should not be used for streptococcal disease unless the organism has been demonstrated to be susceptible.

Streptococcus pyogenes
Streptococcus pneumoniae
Enterococcus group (*Streptococcus faecalis* and *Streptococcus faecium*)
Alpha-hemolytic streptococci (viridans group)

Other Microorganisms

Rickettsiae
Chlamydia psittaci
Chlamydia trachomatis
Mycoplasma pneumoniae
Ureaplasma urealyticum
Borrelia recurrentis
Treponema pallidum
Treponema pertenue
Clostridium species
Fusobacterium fusiforme
Actinomyces species
Bacillus anthracis
Propionibacterium acnes
Entamoeba species
Balantidium coli
Plasmodium falciparum

Doxycycline has been found to be active against the asexual erythrocytic forms of *Plasmodium falciparum* but not against the gametocytes of *P. falciparum*. The precise mechanism of action of the drug is not known.

Susceptibility tests: Diffusion techniques: Quantitative methods that require measurement of zone diameters give the most precise estimate of the susceptibility of bacteria to antimicrobial agents. One such standard procedure[1] which has been recommended for use with disks to test susceptibility of organisms to doxycycline uses the 30-mcg tetracycline-class disk or the 30-mcg doxycycline disk. Interpretation involves the correlation of the diameter obtained in the disk test with the minimum inhibitory concentration (MIC) for tetracycline or doxycycline, respectively.

Reports from the laboratory giving results of the standard single-disk susceptibility test with a 30-mcg tetracycline-class disk or the 30-mcg doxycycline disk should be interpreted according to the following criteria:

Zone Diameter (mm)		Interpretation
tetracycline	doxycycline	
≥19	≥16	Susceptible
15–18	13–15	Intermediate
≤14	≤12	Resistant

A report of "Susceptible" indicates that the pathogen is likely to be inhibited by generally achievable blood levels. A report of "Intermediate" suggests that the organism would be susceptible if a high dosage is used or if the infection is confined to tissues and fluids in which high antimicrobial levels are attained. A report of "Resistant" indicates that achievable concentrations are unlikely to be inhibitory, and other therapy should be selected.

Standardized procedures require the use of laboratory control organisms. The 30-mcg tetracycline-class disk or the 30-mcg doxycycline disk should give the following zone diameters:

Organism	Zone Diameter (mm)	
	tetracycline	doxycycline
E. coli ATCC 25922	18–25	18–24
S. aureus ATCC 25923	19–28	23–29

Dilution techniques: Use a standardized dilution method[2] (broth, agar, microdilution) or equivalent with tetracycline powder. The MIC values obtained should be interpreted according to the following criteria:

MIC (mcg/mL)	Interpretation
≤4	Susceptible
8	Intermediate
≥16	Resistant

As with standard diffusion techniques, dilution methods require the use of laboratory control organisms. Standard tetracycline powder should provide the following MIC values:

Organism	MIC (mcg/mL)
E. coli ATCC 25922	1.0–4.0
S. aureus ATCC 29213	0.25–1.0
E. faecalis ATCC 29212	8–32
P. aeruginosa ATCC 27853	8–32

INDICATIONS AND USAGE

Treatment:

Doxycycline is indicated for the treatment of the following infections:

- Rocky Mountain spotted fever, typhus fever and the typhus group, Q fever, rickettsialpox, and tick fevers caused by Rickettsiae.
- Respiratory tract infections caused by *Mycoplasma pneumoniae.*
- Lymphogranuloma venereum caused by *Chlamydia trachomatis.*
- Psittacosis (ornithosis) caused by *Chlamydia psittaci.*
- Trachoma caused by *Chlamydia trachomatis*, although the infectious agent is not always eliminated as judged by immunofluorescence.
- Inclusion conjunctivitis caused by *Chlamydia trachomatis.*
- Uncomplicated urethral, endocervical or rectal infections in adults caused by *Chlamydia trachomatis.*
- Nongonococcal urethritis caused by *Ureaplasma urealyticum.*
- Relapsing fever due to *Borrelia recurrentis.*

Doxycycline is also indicated for the treatment of infections caused by the following gram-negative microorganisms:

- Chancroid caused by *Haemophilus ducreyi.*
- Plague due to *Yersinia pestis* (formerly *Pasteurella pestis*).
- Tularemia due to *Francisella tularensis* (formerly *Pasteurella tularensis*).
- Cholera caused by *Vibrio cholerae* (formerly *Vibrio comma*).
- Campylobacter fetus infections caused by *Campylobacter fetus* (formerly *Vibrio fetus*).
- Brucellosis due to *Brucella* species (in conjunction with streptomycin).
- Bartonellosis due to *Bartonella bacilliformis.*
- Granuloma inguinale caused by *Calymmatobacterium granulomatis.*

Because many strains of the following groups of microorganisms have been shown to be resistant to doxycycline, culture and susceptibility testing are recommended.

Doxycycline is indicated for treatment of infections caused by the following gram-negative microorganisms, when bacteriologic testing indicates appropriate susceptibility to the drug:

Escherichia coli.
Enterobacter aerogenes (formerly *Aerobacter aerogenes*).
Shigella species.
Acinetobacter species (formerly *Mima* species and *Herellea* species).

Continued on next page

Vibramycin—Cont.

Respiratory tract infections caused by *Haemophilus influenzae*.

Respiratory tract and urinary tract infections caused by *Klebsiella* species.

Doxycycline is indicated for treatment of infections caused by the following gram-positive microorganisms when bacteriologic testing indicates appropriate susceptibility to the drug:

Upper respiratory infections caused by *Streptococcus pneumoniae* (formerly *Diplococcus pneumoniae*).

Anthrax due to *Bacillus anthracis*, including inhalational anthrax (post-exposure): to reduce the incidence or progression of disease following exposure to aerosolized *Bacillus anthracis*.

When penicillin is contraindicated, doxycycline is an alternative drug in the treatment of the following infections:

Uncomplicated gonorrhea caused by *Neisseria gonorrhoeae*.

Syphilis caused by *Treponema pallidum*.

Yaws caused by *Treponema pertenue*.

Listeriosis due to *Listeria monocytogenes*.

Vincent's infection caused by *Fusobacterium fusiforme*.

Actinomycosis caused by *Actinomyces israelii*.

Infections caused by *Clostridium* species.

In acute intestinal amebiasis, doxycycline may be a useful adjunct to amebicides.

In severe acne, doxycycline may be useful adjunctive therapy.

Prophylaxis:

Doxycycline is indicated for the prophylaxis of malaria due to *Plasmodium falciparum* in short-term travelers (<4 months) to areas with chloroquine and/or pyrimethamine-sulfadoxine resistant strains. See DOSAGE AND ADMINISTRATION section and Information for Patients subsection of the PRECAUTIONS section.

CONTRAINDICATIONS

This drug is contraindicated in persons who have shown hypersensitivity to any of the tetracyclines.

WARNINGS

THE USE OF DRUGS OF THE TETRACYCLINE CLASS DURING TOOTH DEVELOPMENT (LAST HALF OF PREGNANCY, INFANCY AND CHILDHOOD TO THE AGE OF 8 YEARS) MAY CAUSE PERMANENT DISCOLORATION OF THE TEETH (YELLOW-GRAY-BROWN). This adverse reaction is more common during long-term use of the drugs, but it has been observed following repeated short-term courses. Enamel hypoplasia has also been reported. TETRACYCLINE DRUGS, THEREFORE, SHOULD NOT BE USED IN THIS AGE GROUP, EXCEPT FOR ANTHRAX, INCLUDING INHALATIONAL ANTHRAX (POST-EXPOSURE), UNLESS OTHER DRUGS ARE NOT LIKELY TO BE EFFECTIVE OR ARE CONTRAINDICATED.

All tetracyclines form a stable calcium complex in any bone-forming tissue. A decrease in fibula growth rate has been observed in prematures given oral tetracycline in doses of 25 mg/kg every 6 hours. This reaction was shown to be reversible when the drug was discontinued.

Results of animal studies indicate that tetracyclines cross the placenta, are found in fetal tissues, and can have toxic effects on the developing fetus (often related to retardation of skeletal development). Evidence of embryotoxicity has also been noted in animals treated early in pregnancy. If any tetracycline is used during pregnancy or if the patient becomes pregnant while taking this drug, the patient should be apprised of the potential hazard to the fetus.

The antianabolic action of the tetracyclines may cause an increase in BUN. Studies to date indicate that this does not occur with the use of doxycycline in patients with impaired renal function.

Photosensitivity manifested by an exaggerated sunburn reaction has been observed in some individuals taking tetracyclines. Patients apt to be exposed to direct sunlight or ultraviolet light should be advised that this reaction can occur with tetracycline drugs, and treatment should be discontinued at the first evidence of skin erythema.

Vibramycin Syrup contains sodium metabisulfite, a sulfite that may cause allergic-type reactions, including anaphylactic symptoms and life-threatening or less severe asthmatic episodes in certain susceptible people. The overall prevalence of sulfite sensitivity in the general population is unknown and probably low. Sulfite sensitivity is seen more frequently in asthmatic than in non-asthmatic people.

PRECAUTIONS

General

As with other antibiotic preparations, use of this drug may result in overgrowth of nonsusceptible organisms, including fungi. If superinfection occurs, the antibiotic should be discontinued and appropriate therapy instituted.

Bulging fontanels in infants and benign intracranial hypertension in adults have been reported in individuals receiving tetracyclines. These conditions disappeared when the drug was discontinued.

Incision and drainage or other surgical procedures should be performed in conjunction with antibiotic therapy, when indicated.

Doxycycline offers substantial but not complete suppression of the asexual blood stages of *Plasmodium* strains.

Doxycycline does not suppress *P. falciparum*'s sexual blood stage gametocytes. Subjects completing this prophylactic regimen may still transmit the infection to mosquitoes outside endemic areas.

Information for Patients

Patients taking doxycycline for malaria prophylaxis should be advised:

— that no present-day antimalarial agent, including doxycycline, guarantees protection against malaria.

— to avoid being bitten by mosquitoes by using personal protective measures that help avoid contact with mosquitoes, especially from dusk to dawn (e.g., staying in well-screened areas, using mosquito nets, covering the body with clothing, and using an effective insect repellent).

— that doxycycline prophylaxis:

— should begin 1–2 days before travel to the malarious area,

— should be continued daily while in the malarious area and after leaving the malarious area,

— should be continued for 4 further weeks to avoid development of malaria after returning from an endemic area,

— should not exceed 4 months.

All patients taking doxycycline should be advised:

— to avoid excessive sunlight or artificial ultraviolet light while receiving doxycycline and to discontinue therapy if phototoxicity (e.g., skin eruption, etc.) occurs. Sunscreen or sunblock should be considered (See WARNINGS.)

— to drink fluids liberally along with doxycycline to reduce the risk of esophageal irritation and ulceration. (See ADVERSE REACTIONS.)

— that the absorption of tetracyclines is reduced when taken with foods, especially those which contain calcium. However, the absorption of doxycycline is not markedly influenced by simultaneous ingestion of food or milk. (See DRUG INTERACTIONS.)

— that the absorption of tetracyclines is reduced when taking bismuth subsalicylate (See DRUG INTERACTIONS.)

— that the use of doxycycline might increase the incidence of vaginal candidiasis.

Laboratory Tests

In venereal disease, when co-existent syphilis is suspected, dark field examinations should be done before treatment is started and the blood serology repeated monthly for at least 4 months.

In long-term therapy, periodic laboratory evaluation of organ systems, including hematopoietic, renal, and hepatic studies, should be performed.

Drug Interactions

Because tetracyclines have been shown to depress plasma prothrombin activity, patients who are on anticoagulant therapy may require downward adjustment of their anticoagulant dosage.

Since bacteriostatic drugs may interfere with the bactericidal action of penicillin, it is advisable to avoid giving tetracyclines in conjunction with penicillin.

Absorption of tetracyclines is impaired by antacids containing aluminum, calcium, or magnesium, and iron-containing preparations.

Absorption of tetracyclines is impaired by bismuth subsalicylate.

Barbiturates, carbamazepine, and phenytoin decrease the half-life of doxycycline.

The concurrent use of tetracycline and Penthrane® (methoxyflurane) has been reported to result in fatal renal toxicity.

Concurrent use of tetracycline may render oral contraceptives less effective.

Drug/Laboratory Test Interactions

False elevations of urinary catecholamine levels may occur due to interference with the fluorescence test.

Carcinogenesis, Mutagenesis, Impairment of Fertility

Long-term studies in animals to evaluate carcinogenic potential of doxycycline have not been conducted. However, there has been evidence of oncogenic activity in rats in studies with the related antibiotics, oxytetracycline (adrenal and pituitary tumors), and minocycline (thyroid tumors).

Likewise, although mutagenicity studies of doxycycline have not been conducted, positive results in *in vitro* mammalian cell assays have been reported for related antibiotics (tetracycline, oxytetracycline).

Doxycycline administered orally at dosage levels as high as 250 mg/kg/day had no apparent effect on the fertility of female rats. Effect on male fertility has not been studied.

Pregnancy Category

Teratogenic effects: Category "D"—(See WARNINGS).

Nonteratogenic effects: (See WARNINGS).

Labor and Delivery

The effect of tetracyclines on labor and delivery is unknown.

Nursing Mothers

Tetracyclines are excreted in human milk. Because of the potential for serious adverse reactions in nursing infants from doxycycline, a decision should be made whether to discontinue nursing or to discontinue the drug, taking into account the importance of the drug to the mother. (See WARNINGS.)

Pediatric Use

See WARNINGS and DOSAGE AND ADMINISTRATION.

ADVERSE REACTIONS

Due to oral doxycycline's virtually complete absorption, side effects of the lower bowel, particularly diarrhea, have been infrequent. The following adverse reactions have been observed in patients receiving tetracyclines:

Gastrointestinal: anorexia, nausea, vomiting, diarrhea, glossitis, dysphagia, enterocolitis, and inflammatory lesions (with monilial overgrowth) in the anogenital region. Hepatotoxicity has been reported rarely. These reactions have been caused by both the oral and parenteral administration of tetracyclines. Rare instances of esophagitis and esophageal ulcerations have been reported in patients receiving capsule and tablet forms of the drugs in the tetracycline class. Most of these patients took medications immediately before going to bed. (See DOSAGE AND ADMINISTRATION.)

Skin: maculopapular and erythematous rashes. Exfoliative dermatitis has been reported but is uncommon. Photosensitivity is discussed above. (See WARNINGS.)

Renal toxicity: Rise in BUN has been reported and is apparently dose related. (See WARNINGS.)

Hypersensitivity reactions: urticaria, angioneurotic edema, anaphylaxis, anaphylactoid purpura, serum sickness, pericarditis, and exacerbation of systemic lupus erythematosus.

Blood: Hemolytic anemia, thrombocytopenia, neutropenia, and eosinophilia have been reported.

Other: bulging fontanels in infants and intracranial hypertension in adults. (See PRECAUTIONS—General.)

When given over prolonged periods, tetracyclines have been reported to produce brown-black microscopic discoloration of the thyroid gland. No abnormalities of thyroid function studies are known to occur.

OVERDOSAGE

In case of overdosage, discontinue medication, treat symptomatically and institute supportive measures. Dialysis does not alter serum half-life and thus would not be of benefit in treating cases of overdosage.

DOSAGE AND ADMINISTRATION

THE USUAL DOSAGE AND FREQUENCY OF ADMINISTRATION OF DOXYCYCLINE DIFFERS FROM THAT OF THE OTHER TETRACYCLINES. EXCEEDING THE RECOMMENDED DOSAGE MAY RESULT IN AN INCREASED INCIDENCE OF SIDE EFFECTS. Adults: The usual dose of oral doxycycline is 200 mg on the first day of treatment (administered 100 mg every 12 hours) followed by a maintenance dose of 100 mg/day. The maintenance dose may be administered as a single dose or as 50 mg every 12 hours.

In the management of more severe infections (particularly chronic infections of the urinary tract), 100 mg every 12 hours is recommended.

For children above eight years of age: The recommended dosage schedule for children weighing 100 pounds or less is 2 mg/lb of body weight divided into two doses on the first day of treatment, followed by 1 mg/lb of body weight given as a single daily dose or divided into two doses, on subsequent days. For more severe infections up to 2 mg/lb of body weight may be used. For children over 100 lb the usual adult dose should be used.

The therapeutic antibacterial serum activity will usually persist for 24 hours following recommended dosage.

When used in streptococcal infections, therapy should be continued for 10 days.

Administration of adequate amounts of fluid along with capsule and tablet forms of drugs in the tetracycline class is recommended to wash down the drugs and reduce the risk of esophageal irritation and ulceration. (See ADVERSE REACTIONS.)

If gastric irritation occurs, it is recommended that doxycycline be given with food or milk. The absorption of doxycycline is not markedly influenced by simultaneous ingestion of food or milk.

Studies to date have indicated that administration of doxycycline at the usual recommended doses does not lead to excessive accumulation of the antibiotic in patients with renal impairment.

Uncomplicated gonococcal infections in adults (except anorectal infections in men): 100 mg, by mouth, twice a day for 7 days. As an alternate single visit dose, administer 300 mg stat followed in one hour by a second 300 mg dose. The dose may be administered with food, including milk or carbonated beverage, as required.

Uncomplicated urethral, endocervical, or rectal infection in adults caused by *Chlamydia trachomatis:* 100 mg by mouth twice a day for 7 days.

Nongonococcal urethritis (NGU) caused by *C. trachomatis* or *U. urealyticum:* 100 mg by mouth twice a day for 7 days.

Syphilis — early: Patients who are allergic to penicillin should be treated with doxycycline 100 mg by mouth twice a day for 2 weeks.

Syphilis of more than one year's duration: Patients who are allergic to penicillin should be treated with doxycycline 100 mg by mouth twice a day for 4 weeks.

Acute epididymo-orchitis caused by *N. gonorrhoeae:* 100 mg, by mouth, twice a day for at least 10 days.

Acute epididymo-orchitis caused by *C. trachomatis:* 100 mg, by mouth, twice a day for at least 10 days.

For prophylaxis of malaria: For adults, the recommended dose is 100 mg daily. For children over 8 years of age, the recommended dose is 2 mg/kg given once daily up to the adult dose. Prophylaxis should begin 1–2 days before travel to the malarious area. Prophylaxis should be continued daily during travel in the malarious area and for 4 weeks after the traveler leaves the malarious area.

Inhalational anthrax (post-exposure):

ADULTS: 100 mg of doxycycline, by mouth, twice a day for 60 days.

CHILDREN: weighing less than 100 lb (45 kg); 1 mg/lb (2.2 mg/kg) of body weight, by mouth, twice a day for 60 days. Children weighing 100 lb or more should receive the adult dose.

HOW SUPPLIED

Vibramycin® Hyclate (doxycycline hyclate) is available in capsules containing doxycycline hyclate equivalent to:

50 mg doxycycline
bottles of 50 (NDC 0069-0940-50)

The capsules are white and light blue and are imprinted with "VIBRA" on one half and "PFIZER 094" on the other half.

100 mg doxycycline
bottles of 50 (NDC 0069-0950-50)

The capsules are light blue and are imprinted with "VIBRA" on one half and "PFIZER 095" on the other half.

Vibra-Tabs® (doxycycline hyclate) is available in salmon colored film-coated tablets containing doxycycline hyclate equivalent to:

100 mg doxycycline
bottles of 50 (NDC 0069-0990-50)

The tablets are imprinted on one side with "VIBRA-TABS" and "PFIZER 099" on the other side.

Vibramycin® Calcium Syrup (doxycycline calcium) oral suspension is available as a raspberry-apple flavored oral suspension. Each teaspoonful (5 mL) contains doxycycline calcium equivalent to 50 mg of doxycycline: 1 pint (473 mL) bottles (NDC 0069-0971-93).

Vibramycin® Monohydrate (doxycycline monohydrate) for Oral Suspension is available as a raspberry-flavored, dry powder for oral suspension. When reconstituted, each teaspoonful (5 mL) contains doxycycline monohydrate equivalent to 25 mg of doxycycline: 2 oz (60 mL) bottles (NDC 0069-0970-65).

All products are to be stored below 86°F (30°C) and dispensed in tight, light-resistant containers (USP).

ANIMAL PHARMACOLOGY AND ANIMAL TOXICOLOGY

Hyperpigmentation of the thyroid has been produced by members of the tetracycline class in the following species: in rats by oxytetracycline, doxycycline, tetracycline PO_4, and methacycline; in minipigs by doxycycline, minocycline, tetracycline PO_4, and methacycline; in dogs by doxycycline and minocycline; in monkeys by minocycline.

Minocycline, tetracycline PO_4, methacycline, doxycycline, tetracycline base, oxytetracycline HCl, and tetracycline HCl were goitrogenic in rats fed a low iodine diet. This goitrogenic effect was accompanied by high radioactive iodine uptake. Administration of minocycline also produced a large goiter with high radioiodine uptake in rats fed a relatively high iodine diet.

Treatment of various animal species with this class of drugs has also resulted in the induction of thyroid hyperplasia in the following: in rats and dogs (minocycline); in chickens (chlortetracycline); and in rats and mice (oxytetracycline). Adrenal gland hyperplasia has been observed in goats and rats treated with oxytetracycline.

REFERENCES

1. National Committee for Clinical Laboratory Standards, *Performance Standards for Antimicrobial Disk Susceptibility Tests*, Fourth Edition. Approved Standard NCCLS Document M2-A4, Vol. 10, No. 7 NCCLS, Villanova, PA, April 1990.

2. National Committee for Clinical Laboratory Standards, *Methods for Dilution Antimicrobial Susceptibility Tests for Bacteria that Grow Aerobically*, Second Edition. Approved Standard NCCLS Document M7-A2, Vol. 10, No. 8 NCCLS, Villanova, PA, April 1990.

Rx only

Pfizer Labs
Division of Pfizer Inc, NY, NY 10017
69-1680-32-6 Revised November 2001

VIBRAMYCIN® Hyclate ℞

[*vī "bra-mī 'sin*]

doxycycline hyclate for injection
INTRAVENOUS
FOR INTRAVENOUS USE ONLY

Prescribing information for this product, which appears on pages 2737–2738 of the 2002 PDR, has been completely revised as follows. Please write "See Supplement A" next to the product heading.

DESCRIPTION

Vibramycin (doxycycline hyclate for injection) Intravenous is a broad-spectrum antibiotic synthetically derived from oxytetracycline, and is available as Vibramycin Hyclate (doxycycline hydrochloride hemiethanolate hemihydrate). The chemical designation of this light-yellow crystalline powder is alpha-6-deoxy-5-oxytetracycline. Doxycycline has a high degree of lipoid solubility and a low affinity for calcium binding. It is highly stable in normal human serum.

ACTIONS

Doxycycline is primarily bacteriostatic and thought to exert its antimicrobial effect by the inhibition of protein synthesis. Doxycycline is active against a wide range of gram-positive and gram-negative organisms.

The drugs in the tetracycline class have closely similar antimicrobial spectra and cross resistance among them is common. Microorganisms may be considered susceptible to doxycycline (likely to respond to doxycycline therapy) if the minimum inhibitory concentration (M.I.C.) is not more than 4.0 mcg/mL. Microorganisms may be considered intermediate (harboring partial resistance) if the M.I.C. is 4.0 to 12.5 mcg/mL and resistant (not likely to respond to therapy) if the M.I.C. is greater than 12.5 mcg/mL.

Susceptibility plate testing: If the Kirby-Bauer method of disc susceptibility testing is used, a 30 mcg doxycycline disc should give a zone of at least 16 mm when tested against a doxycycline-susceptible bacterial strain. A tetracycline disc may be used to determine microbial susceptibility. If the Kirby-Bauer method of disc susceptibility testing is used, a 30 mcg tetracycline disc should give a zone of at least 19 mm when tested against a tetracycline-susceptible bacterial strain.

Tetracyclines are readily absorbed and are bound to plasma proteins in varying degree. They are concentrated by the liver in the bile, and excreted in the urine and feces at high concentrations and in a biologically active form.

Following a single 100 mg dose administered in a concentration of 0.4 mg/mL in a one-hour infusion, normal adult volunteers average a peak of 2.5 mcg/mL, while 200 mg of a concentration of 0.4 mg/mL administered over two hours averaged a peak of 3.6 mcg/mL. Excretion of doxycycline by the kidney is about 40 percent/72 hours in individuals with normal function (creatinine clearance about 75 mL/min.). This percentage excretion may fall as low as 1–5 percent/72 hours in individuals with severe renal insufficiency (creatinine clearance below 10 mL/min.). Studies have shown no significant difference in serum half-life of doxycycline (range 18–22 hours) in individuals with normal and severely impaired renal function.

Hemodialysis does not alter this serum half-life of doxycycline.

INDICATIONS

Doxycycline is indicated in infections caused by the following microorganisms:

Rickettsiae (Rocky Mountain spotted fever, typhus fever, and the typhus group, Q fever, rickettsialpox and tick fevers).

Mycoplasma pneumoniae (PPLO, Eaton Agent).

Agents of psittacosis and ornithosis.

Agents of lymphogranuloma venereum and granuloma inguinale.

The spirochetal agent of relapsing fever (*Borrelia recurrentis*).

The following gram-negative microorganisms:

Haemophilus ducreyi (chancroid),
Pasteurella pestis and *Pasteurella tularensis*,
Bartonella bacilliformis,
Bacteroides species,
Vibrio comma and *Vibrio fetus*,
Brucella species (in conjunction with streptomycin).

Because many strains of the following groups of microorganisms have been shown to be resistant to tetracyclines, culture and susceptibility testing are recommended.

Doxycycline is indicated for treatment of infections caused by the following gram-negative microorganisms when bacteriologic testing indicates appropriate susceptibility to the drug:

Escherichia coli,
Enterobacter aerogenes (formerly *Aerobacter aerogenes*),
Shigella species,
Mima species and *Herellea* species,
Haemophilus influenzae (respiratory infections),
Klebsiella species (respiratory and urinary infections).

Doxycycline is indicated for treatment of infections caused by the following gram-positive microorganisms when bacteriologic testing indicates appropriate susceptibility to the drug:

Streptococcus species:

Up to 44 percent of strains of *Streptococcus pyogenes* and 74 percent of *Streptococcus faecalis* have been found to be resistant to tetracycline drugs. Therefore, tetracyclines should not be used for streptococcal disease unless the organism has been demonstrated to be sensitive.

For upper respiratory infections due to group A beta-hemolytic streptococci, penicillin is the usual drug of choice, including prophylaxis of rheumatic fever.

Diplococcus pneumoniae,

Staphylococcus aureus, respiratory skin and soft tissue infections. Tetracyclines are not the drugs of choice in the treatment of any type of staphylococcal infections.

Anthrax due to *Bacillus anthracis*, including inhalational anthrax (post-exposure): to reduce the incidence or progression of disease following exposure to aerosolized *Bacillus anthracis*.

When penicillin is contraindicated, doxycycline is an alternative drug in the treatment of infections due to:

Neisseria gonorrhoeae and *N. meningitidis*,
Treponema pallidum and *Treponema pertenue* (syphilis and yaws),
Listeria monocytogenes,
Clostridium species,
Fusobacterium fusiforme (Vincent's infection),
Actinomyces species.

In acute intestinal amebiasis, doxycycline may be a useful adjunct to amebicides.

Doxycycline is indicated in the treatment of trachoma, although the infectious agent is not always eliminated, as judged by immunofluorescence.

CONTRAINDICATIONS

This drug is contraindicated in persons who have shown hypersensitivity to any of the tetracyclines.

WARNINGS

THE USE OF DRUGS OF THE TETRACYCLINE CLASS DURING TOOTH DEVELOPMENT (LAST HALF OF PREGNANCY, INFANCY AND CHILDHOOD TO THE AGE OF 8 YEARS) MAY CAUSE PERMANENT DISCOLORATION OF THE TEETH (YELLOW-GRAY-BROWN). This adverse reaction is more common during long-term use of the drugs but has been observed following repeated short-term courses. Enamel hypoplasia has also been reported. TETRACYCLINE DRUGS, THEREFORE, SHOULD NOT BE USED IN THIS AGE GROUP, EXCEPT FOR ANTHRAX, INCLUDING INHALATIONAL ANTHRAX (POST-EXPOSURE), UNLESS OTHER DRUGS ARE NOT LIKELY TO BE EFFECTIVE OR ARE CONTRAINDICATED.

Photosensitivity manifested by an exaggerated sunburn reaction has been observed in some individuals taking tetracyclines. Patients apt to be exposed to direct sunlight or ultraviolet light, should be advised that this reaction can occur with tetracycline drugs, and treatment should be discontinued at the first evidence of skin erythema. The antianabolic action of the tetracyclines may cause an increase in BUN. Studies to date indicate that this does not occur with the use of doxycycline in patients with impaired renal function.

Usage in Pregnancy

(See above WARNINGS about use during tooth development.)

Vibramycin Intravenous has not been studied in pregnant patients. It should not be used in pregnant women unless, in the judgment of the physician, it is essential for the welfare of the patient.

Results of animal studies indicate that tetracyclines cross the placenta, are found in fetal tissues and can have toxic effects on the developing fetus (often related to retardation of skeletal development). Evidence of embryotoxicity has also been noted in animals treated early in pregnancy.

Usage in Children

The use of Vibramycin Intravenous in children under 8 years is not recommended because safe conditions for its use have not been established.

(See above WARNINGS about use during tooth development.)

As with other tetracyclines, doxycycline forms a stable calcium complex in any bone-forming tissue. A decrease in the fibula growth rate has been observed in prematures given oral tetracycline in doses of 25 mg/kg every 6 hours. This reaction was shown to be reversible when the drug was discontinued.

Tetracyclines are present in the milk of lactating women who are taking a drug in this class.

PRECAUTIONS

As with other antibiotic preparations, use of this drug may result in overgrowth of nonsusceptible organisms, including fungi. If superinfection occurs, the antibiotic should be discontinued and appropriate therapy instituted.

In venereal diseases when coexistent syphilis is suspected, a dark field examination should be done before treatment is started and the blood serology repeated monthly for at least 4 months.

Because tetracyclines have been shown to depress plasma prothrombin activity, patients who are on anticoagulant therapy may require downward adjustment of their anticoagulant dosage.

In long-term therapy, periodic laboratory evaluation of organ systems, including hematopoietic, renal, and hepatic studies should be performed. All infections due to group A beta-hemolytic streptococci should be treated for at least 10 days.

Since bacteriostatic drugs may interfere with the bactericidal action of penicillin, it is advisable to avoid giving tetracycline in conjunction with penicillin.

ADVERSE REACTIONS

Gastrointestinal: anorexia, nausea, vomiting, diarrhea, glossitis, dysphagia, enterocolitis, and inflammatory lesions (with monilial overgrowth) in the anogenital region. Hepatotoxicity has been reported rarely. These reactions have been caused by both the oral and parenteral administration of tetracyclines.

Skin: maculopapular and erythematous rashes. Exfoliative dermatitis has been reported but is uncommon. Photosensitivity is discussed above. (See WARNINGS.)

Renal toxicity: Rise in BUN has been reported and is apparently dose related. (See WARNINGS.)

Hypersensitivity reactions: urticaria, angioneurotic edema, anaphylaxis, anaphylactoid purpura, pericarditis and exacerbation of systemic lupus erythematosus.

Bulging fontanels in infants and benign intracranial hypertension in adults have been reported in individuals receiving full therapeutic dosages. These conditions disappeared rapidly when the drug was discontinued.

Blood: Hemolytic anemia, thrombocytopenia, neutropenia and eosinophilia have been reported.

When given over prolonged periods, tetracyclines have been reported to produce brown-black microscopic discoloration of thyroid glands. No abnormalities of thyroid function studies are known to occur.

Continued on next page

Vibramycin Hyclate—Cont.

DOSAGE AND ADMINISTRATION

Note: Rapid administration is to be avoided. Parenteral therapy is indicated only when oral therapy is not indicated. Oral therapy should be instituted as soon as possible. If intravenous therapy is given over prolonged periods of time, thrombophlebitis may result.

THE USUAL DOSAGE AND FREQUENCY OF ADMINISTRATION OF VIBRAMYCIN I.V. (100-200 MG/DAY) DIFFERS FROM THAT OF THE OTHER TETRACYCLINES (1-2 G/DAY). EXCEEDING THE RECOMMENDED DOSAGE MAY RESULT IN AN INCREASED INCIDENCE OF SIDE EFFECTS.

Studies to date have indicated that Vibramycin at the usual recommended doses does not lead to excessive accumulation of the antibiotic in patients with renal impairment.

Adults: The usual dosage of Vibramycin I.V. is 200 mg on the first day of treatment administered in one or two infusions. Subsequent daily dosage is 100 to 200 mg depending upon the severity of infection, with 200 mg administered in one or two infusions.

In the treatment of primary and secondary syphilis, the recommended dosage is 300 mg daily for at least 10 days.

In the treatment of inhalational anthrax (post-exposure) the recommended dose is 100 mg of doxycycline, twice a day. Parenteral therapy is only indicated when oral therapy is not indicated and should not be continued over a prolonged period of time. Oral therapy should be instituted as soon as possible. Therapy must continue for a total of 60 days.

For children above eight years of age: The recommended dosage schedule for children weighing 100 pounds or less is 2 mg/lb of body weight on the first day of treatment, administered in one or two infusions. Subsequent daily dosage is 1 to 2 mg/lb of body weight given as one or two infusions, depending on the severity of the infection. For children over 100 pounds the usual adult dose should be used. (See WARNINGS Section for Usage in Children.)

In the treatment of inhalational anthrax (post-exposure) the recommended dose is 1 mg/lb (2.2 mg/kg) of body weight, twice a day in children weighing less than 100 lb (45 kg). Parenteral therapy is only indicated when oral therapy is not indicated and should not be continued over a prolonged period of time. Oral therapy should be instituted as soon as possible. Therapy must continue for a total of 60 days.

General: The duration of infusion may vary with the dose (100 to 200 mg per day), but is usually one to four hours. A recommended minimum infusion time for 100 mg of a 0.5 mg/mL solution is one hour. Therapy should be continued for at least 24-48 hours after symptoms and fever have subsided. The therapeutic antibacterial serum activity will usually persist for 24 hours following recommended dosage.

Intravenous solutions should not be injected intramuscularly or subcutaneously. Caution should be taken to avoid the inadvertent introduction of the intravenous solution into the adjacent soft tissue.

PREPARATION OF SOLUTION

To prepare a solution containing 10 mg/mL, the contents of the vial should be reconstituted with 10 mL (for the 100 mg/vial container) or 20 mL (for the 200 mg/vial container) of Sterile Water for Injection or any of the ten intravenous infusion solutions listed below. Each 100 mg of Vibramycin (i.e., withdraw entire solution from the 100 mg vial) is further diluted with 100 mL to 1000 mL of the intravenous solutions listed below. Each 200 mg of Vibramycin (i.e., withdraw entire solution from the 200 mg vial) is further diluted with 200 mL to 2000 mL of the following intravenous solutions:

1. Sodium Chloride Injection, USP
2. 5% Dextrose Injection, USP
3. Ringer's Injection, USP
4. Invert Sugar, 10% in Water
5. Lactated Ringer's Injection, USP
6. Dextrose 5% in Lactated Ringer's
7. Normosol-M® in D5-W (Abbott)
8. Normosol-R® in D5-W (Abbott)
9. Plasma-Lyte® 56 in 5% Dextrose (Travenol)
10. Plasma-Lyte® 148 in 5% Dextrose (Travenol)

This will result in desired concentrations of 0.1 to 1.0 mg/mL. Concentrations lower than 0.1 mg/mL or higher than 1.0 mg/mL are not recommended.

Stability

Vibramycin IV is stable for 48 hours in solution when diluted with Sodium Chloride Injection, USP, or 5% Dextrose Injection, USP, to concentrations between 1.0 mg/mL and 0.1 mg/mL and stored at 25°C. Vibramycin IV in these solutions is stable under fluorescent light for 48 hours, but must be protected from direct sunlight during storage and infusion. Reconstituted solutions (1.0 to 0.1 mg/mL) may be stored up to 72 hours prior to start of infusion if refrigerated and protected from sunlight and artificial light. Infusion must then be completed within 12 hours. Solutions must be used within these time periods or discarded.

Vibramycin IV, when diluted with Ringer's Injection, USP, or Invert Sugar, 10% in Water, or Normosol-M® in D5-W (Abbott), or Normosol-R® in D5-W (Abbott), or Plasma-Lyte® 56 in 5% Dextrose (Travenol), or Plasma-Lyte® 148 in 5% Dextrose (Travenol) to a concentration between 1.0 mg/mL and 0.1 mg/mL, must be completely infused within 12 hours after reconstitution to ensure adequate stability. During infusion, the solution must be protected from direct sunlight. Reconstituted solutions (1.0 to 0.1 mg/mL) may be stored up to 72 hours prior to start of infusion if refrigerated and protected from sunlight and artificial light. Infusion must then be completed within 12 hours. Solutions must be used within these time periods or discarded.

When diluted with Lactated Ringer's Injection, USP, or Dextrose 5% in Lactated Ringer's, infusion of the solution (ca. 1.0 mg/mL) or lower concentrations (not less than 0.1 mg/mL) must be completed within six hours after reconstitution to ensure adequate stability. During infusion, the solution must be protected from direct sunlight. Solutions must be used within this time period or discarded.

Solutions of Vibramycin (doxycycline hyclate for injection) at a concentration of 10 mg/mL in Sterile Water for Injection, when frozen immediately after reconstitution are stable for 8 weeks when stored at −20°C. If the product is warmed, care should be taken to avoid heating it after the thawing is complete. Once thawed the solution should not be refrozen.

HOW SUPPLIED

Vibramycin (doxycycline hyclate for injection) Intravenous is available as a sterile powder in a vial containing doxycycline hyclate equivalent to 100 mg of doxycycline with 480 mg of ascorbic acid; packages of 5 (0049-0960-77), and in individually packaged vials containing doxycycline hyclate equivalent to 200 mg of doxycycline with 960 mg of ascorbic acid (0049-0980-81).

Rx only

Pfizer Roerig
Division of Pfizer Inc, NY, NY 10017
69-1940-00-3 Revised November 2001

ZITHROMAX® ℞

[zi' thrō-max]
(azithromycin tablets)
and
(azithromycin for oral suspension)

Prescribing information for this product, which appears on pages 2739–2743 of the 2002 PDR, has been completely revised as follows. Please write "See Supplement A" next to the product heading.

DESCRIPTION

ZITHROMAX® (azithromycin tablets and azithromycin for oral suspension) contain the active ingredient azithromycin, an azalide, a subclass of macrolide antibiotics, for oral administration. Azithromycin has the chemical name (*2R,3S,4R,5R,8R,10R,11R,12S,13S,14R*)-13-[(2,6-dideoxy-3-*C*-methyl-3-*O*-methyl-α-*L*-*ribo*-hexopyranosyl) oxy]-2-ethyl-3,4,10-trihydroxy-3,5,6,8,10,12,14-heptamethyl-11-[[3,4,6-trideoxy-3-(dimethylamino)-β-*D*-*xylo*-hexopyranosyl]oxy]-1-oxa-6-azacyclopentadecan-15-one. Azithromycin is derived from erythromycin; however, it differs chemically from erythromycin in that a methyl-substituted nitrogen atom is incorporated into the lactone ring. Its molecular formula is $C_{38}H_{72}N_2O_{12}$, and its molecular weight is 749.00. Azithromycin has the following structural formula:

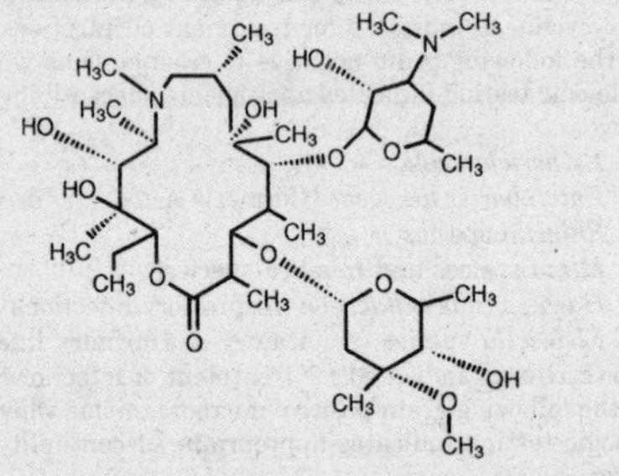

Azithromycin, as the dihydrate, is a white crystalline powder with a molecular formula of $C_{38}H_{72}N_2O_{12}•2H_2O$ and a molecular weight of 785.0.

ZITHROMAX® is supplied for oral administration as film-coated, modified capsular shaped tablets containing azithromycin dihydrate equivalent to 250 mg azithromycin and the following inactive ingredients: dibasic calcium phosphate anhydrous, pregelatinized starch, sodium croscarmellose, magnesium stearate, sodium lauryl sulfate, hydroxypropyl methylcellulose, lactose, titanium dioxide, triacetin and D&C Red #30 aluminum lake.

ZITHROMAX® for oral suspension is supplied in bottles containing azithromycin dihydrate powder equivalent to 300 mg, 600 mg, 900 mg, or 1200 mg azithromycin per bottle and the following inactive ingredients: sucrose; sodium phosphate, tribasic, anhydrous; hydroxypropyl cellulose; xanthan gum; FD&C Red #40; and spray dried artificial cherry, creme de vanilla and banana flavors. After constitution, each 5 mL of suspension contains 100 mg or 200 mg of azithromycin.

CLINICAL PHARMACOLOGY

Adult Pharmacokinetics: Following oral administration, azithromycin is rapidly absorbed and widely distributed throughout the body. Rapid distribution of azithromycin into tissues and high concentration within cells result in significantly higher azithromycin concentrations in tissues than in plasma or serum.

The pharmacokinetic parameters of azithromycin capsules in plasma after a loading dose of 500 mg (2–250 mg capsules) on Day one followed by 250 mg (1–250 mg capsule) q.d. on Days 2 through 5 in healthy young adults (age 18–40 years old) are portrayed in the following chart:

Pharmacokinetic Parameters (Mean)	Total n=12 Day 1	Day 5
C_{max} (μg/mL)	0.41	0.24
T_{max} (h)	2.5	3.2
AUC_{0-24} (μg•h/mL)	2.6	2.1
C_{min} (μg/mL)	0.05	0.05
Urinary Excret. (% dose)	4.5	6.5

In this study, there was no significant difference in the disposition of azithromycin between male and female subjects. Plasma concentrations of azithromycin following single 500 mg oral and i.v. doses declined in a polyphasic pattern resulting in an average terminal half-life of 68 hours. With a regimen of 500 mg on Day 1 and 250 mg/day on Days 2–5, C_{min} and C_{max} remained essentially unchanged from Day 2 through Day 5 of therapy. However, without a loading dose, azithromycin C_{min} concentrations required 5 to 7 days to reach steady-state.

When two 250 mg tablets were administered to 36 fasted healthy male volunteers, the mean (SD) pharmacokinetic parameters were AUC_{0-72} = 4.3 (1.2) μg•h/mL; C_{max} = 0.5 (0.2) μg/mL; T_{max} = 2.2 (0.9) hours. Azithromycin 250 mg tablets are bioequivalent to 250 mg capsules in the fasted state.

In an open label, randomized, two-way crossover study in 12 healthy subjects to assess the effect of a high fat standard meal on the serum concentrations of azithromycin resulting from the oral administration of two 250-mg film-coated tablets, it was shown that food increased C_{max} by 23% while there was no change in AUC.

When azithromycin suspension was administered with food to 28 adult healthy male subjects, C_{max} increased by 56% and AUC was unchanged.

The AUC of azithromycin was unaffected by co-administration of an antacid containing aluminum and magnesium hydroxide with azithromycin capsules; however, the C_{max} was reduced by 24%. Administration of cimetidine (800 mg) two hours prior to azithromycin had no effect on azithromycin absorption.

When studied in healthy elderly subjects aged 65 to 85 years, the pharmacokinetic parameters of azithromycin in elderly men were similar to those in young adults; however, in elderly women, although higher peak concentrations (increased by 30 to 50%) were observed, no significant accumulation occurred.

The high values in adults for apparent steady-state volume of distribution (31.1 L/kg) and plasma clearance (630 mL/min) suggest that the prolonged half-life is due to extensive uptake and subsequent release of drug from tissues.

The serum protein binding of azithromycin is variable in the concentration range approximating human exposure, decreasing from 51% at 0.02 μg/mL to 7% at 2 μg/mL.

Biliary excretion of azithromycin, predominantly as unchanged drug, is a major route of elimination. Over the course of a week, approximately 6% of the administered dose appears as unchanged drug in urine.

There are no pharmacokinetic data available from studies in hepatically- or renally-impaired individuals.

The effect of azithromycin on the plasma concentrations or pharmacokinetics of theophylline administered in multiple doses adequate to reach therapeutic steady-state is not known. (See **PRECAUTIONS.**)

Selected tissue (or fluid) concentration and tissue (or fluid) to plasma/serum concentration ratios are shown in the following table:

[See first table at top of next page]

The extensive tissue distribution was confirmed by examination of additional tissues and fluids (bone, ejaculum, prostate, ovary, uterus, salpinx, stomach, liver, and gallbladder). As there are no data from adequate and well-controlled studies of azithromycin treatment of infections in these additional body sites, the clinical importance of these tissue concentration data is unknown.

Following a regimen of 500 mg on the first day and 250 mg daily for 4 days, only very low concentrations were noted in cerebrospinal fluid (less than 0.01 μg/mL) in the presence of non-inflamed meninges.

Pediatric Pharmacokinetics:

In two clinical studies, azithromycin for oral suspension was dosed at 10 mg/kg on Day 1, followed by 5 mg/kg on Days 2 through 5 to two groups of children (aged 1–5 years and 5–15 years, respectively). The mean pharmacokinetic parameters at Day 5 were C_{max}=0.216 μg/mL, T_{max}=1.9 hours, and AUC_{0-24}=1.822 μg•hr/mL for the 1- to 5-year-old group and were C_{max}=0.383 μg/mL, T_{max}=2.4 hours, and AUC_{0-24}=3.109 μg•hr/mL for the 5- to 15-year-old group.

Two clinical studies were conducted in 68 children aged 3–16 years to determine the pharmacokinetics and safety of azithromycin for oral suspension in children.

Azithromycin was administered following a low-fat breakfast.

The first study consisted of 35 pediatric patients treated with 20 mg/kg/day (maximum daily dose 500 mg) for 3 days of whom 34 patients were evaluated for pharmacokinetics.

In the second study, 33 pediatric patients received doses of 12 mg/kg/day (maximum daily dose 500 mg) for 5 days of whom 31 patients were evaluated for pharmacokinetics.

In both studies, azithromycin concentrations were determined over a 24 hour period following the last daily dose. Patients weighing above 25.0 kg in the 3-day study or 41.7 kg in the 5-day study received the maximum adult daily dose of 500 mg. Eleven patients (weighing 25.0 kg or less) in the first study and 17 patients (weighing 41.7 kg or less) in the second study received a total dose of 60 mg/kg. The following table shows pharmacokinetic data in the subset of children who received a total dose of 60 mg/kg.

	3-Day Regimen (20 mg/kg × 3 days)	5-Day Regimen (12 mg/kg × 5 days)
n	11	17
C_{max} (μg/mL)	1.1 (0.4)[a]	0.5 (0.4)[a]
T_{max} (hr)	2.7 (1.9)[a]	2.2 (0.8)[a]
AUC_{0-24}(μg•hr/mL)	7.9 (2.9)[a]	3.9 (1.9)[a]

[a]Mean (SD)

The similarity of the overall exposure ($AUC_{0-\infty}$) between the 3-day and 5-day regimens is unknown.

Single dose pharmacokinetics in children given doses of 30 mg/kg have not been studied.

Microbiology: Azithromycin acts by binding to the 50S ribosomal subunit of susceptible microorganisms and, thus, interfering with microbial protein synthesis. Nucleic acid synthesis is not affected.

Azithromycin concentrates in phagocytes and fibroblasts as demonstrated by *in vitro* incubation techniques. Using such methodology, the ratio of intracellular to extracellular concentration was >30 after one hour incubation. *In vivo* studies suggest that concentration in phagocytes may contribute to drug distribution to inflamed tissues.

Azithromycin has been shown to be active against most isolates of the following microorganisms, both *in vitro* and in clinical infections as described in the **INDICATIONS AND USAGE** section.

Aerobic and facultative gram-positive microorganisms

Staphylococcus aureus
Streptococcus agalactiae
Streptococcus pneumoniae
Streptococcus pyogenes

NOTE: Azithromycin demonstrates cross-resistance with erythromycin-resistant gram-positive strains. Most strains of *Enterococcus faecalis* and methicillin-resistant staphylococci are resistant to azithromycin.

Aerobic and facultative gram-negative microorganisms

Haemophilus ducreyi
Haemophilus influenzae
Moraxella catarrhalis
Neisseria gonorrhoeae

"Other" microorganisms

Chlamydia pneumoniae
Chlamydia trachomatis
Mycoplasma pneumoniae

Beta-lactamase production should have no effect on azithromycin activity.

The following *in vitro* data are available, **but their clinical significance is unknown.**

At least 90% of the following microorganisms exhibit an *in vitro* minimum inhibitory concentration (MIC) less than or equal to the susceptible breakpoints for azithromycin. However, the safety and effectiveness of azithromycin in treating clinical infections due to these microorganisms have not been established in adequate and well-controlled trials.

Aerobic and facultative gram-positive microorganisms

Streptococci (Groups C, F, G)
Viridans group streptococci

Aerobic and facultative gram-negative microorganisms

Bordetella pertussis
Legionella pneumophila

Anaerobic microorganisms

Peptostreptococcus species
Prevotella bivia

"Other" microorganisms

Ureaplasma urealyticum

Susceptibility Testing Methods: When available, the results of *in vitro* susceptibility test results for antimicrobial drugs used in resident hospitals should be provided to the physician as periodic reports which describe the susceptibility profile of nosocomial and community-acquired pathogens. These reports may differ from susceptibility data obtained from outpatient use, but could aid the physician in selecting the most effective antimicrobial.

Dilution techniques:

Quantitative methods are used to determine antimicrobial minimum inhibitory concentrations (MICs). These MICs provide estimates of the susceptibility of bacteria to antimicrobial compounds. The MICs should be determined using a standardized procedure. Standardized procedures are based on a dilution method[1,3] (broth or agar) or equivalent with standardized inoculum concentrations and standardized concentrations of azithromycin powder. The MIC values should be interpreted according to criteria provided in Table 1.

Diffusion techniques:

Quantitative methods that require measurement of zone diameters also provide reproducible estimates of the susceptibility of bacteria to antimicrobial compounds. One such standardized procedure[2,3] requires the use of standardized inoculum concentrations. This procedure uses paper disks impregnated with 15-μg azithromycin to test the susceptibility of microorganisms to azithromycin. The disk diffusion interpretive criteria are provided in Table 1.

[See table 1 above]

No interpretive criteria have been established for testing *Neisseria gonorrhoeae*. This species is not usually tested.

A report of "susceptible" indicates that the pathogen is likely to be inhibited if the antimicrobial compound reaches the concentrations usually achievable. A report of "intermediate" indicates that the result should be considered equivocal, and, if the microorganism is not fully susceptible to alternative, clinically feasible drugs, the test should be repeated. This category implies possible clinical applicability in body sites where the drug is physiologically concentrated or in situations where high dosage of drug can be used. This category also provides a buffer zone which prevents small uncontrolled technical factors from causing major discrepancies in interpretation. A report of "resistant" indicates that the pathogen is not likely to be inhibited if the antimicrobial compound reaches the concentrations usually achievable; other therapy should be selected.

QUALITY CONTROL:

Standardized susceptibility test procedures require the use of quality control microorganisms to control the technical aspects of the test procedures. Standard azithromycin powder should provide the following range of values noted in Table 2. Quality control microorganisms are specific strains of organisms with intrinsic biological properties. QC strains are very stable strains which will give a standard and repeatable susceptibility pattern. The specific strains used for microbiological quality control are not clinically significant.

[See table 2 above]

AZITHROMYCIN CONCENTRATIONS FOLLOWING ADMINISTRATION OF TWO 250 mg (500 mg) CAPSULES IN ADULTS[1]

TISSUE OR FLUID	TIME AFTER DOSE (h)	TISSUE OR FLUID CONCENTRATION (μg/g or μg/mL)[2]	CORRESPONDING PLASMA OR SERUM LEVEL (μg/mL)	TISSUE (FLUID) PLASMA (SERUM) RATIO[2]
SKIN	72–96	0.4	0.012	35
LUNG	72–96	4.0	0.012	>100
SPUTUM*	2–4	1.0	0.64	2
SPUTUM**	10–12	2.9	0.1	30
TONSIL***	9–18	4.5	0.03	>100
TONSIL***	180	0.9	0.006	>100
CERVIX****	19	2.8	0.04	70

[1] Azithromycin tissue concentrations were originally determined using 250 mg capsules, which are bioequivalent to 250 mg tablets. (See **HOW SUPPLIED.**)

[2] High tissue concentrations should not be interpreted to be quantitatively related to clinical efficacy. The antimicrobial activity of azithromycin is pH related. Azithromycin is concentrated in cell lysosomes which have a low intraorganelle pH, at which the drug's activity is reduced. However, the extensive distribution of drug to tissues may be relevant to clinical activity.

* Sample was obtained 2–4 hours after the first dose.

** Sample was obtained 10–12 hours after the first dose.

*** Dosing regimen of two doses of 250 mg each, separated by 12 hours.

**** Sample was obtained 19 hours after a single 500 mg dose.

Table 1. Susceptibility Interpretive Criteria for Azithromycin
Susceptibility Test Result Interpretive Criteria

Pathogen	Minimum Inhibitory Concentrations (μg/mL)			Disk Diffusion (zone diameters in mm)		
	S	I	R[a]	S	I	R[a]
Haemophilus spp.	≤ 4	—	—	≥ 12	—	—
Staphylococcus aureus	≤ 2	4	≥ 8	≥ 18	14–17	≤ 13
Streptococci including *S. pneumoniae*	≤ 0.5	1	≥ 2	≥ 18	14–17	≤ 13

[a]The current absence of data on resistant strains precludes defining any category other than "susceptible." If strains yield MIC results other than susceptible, they should be submitted to a reference laboratory for further testing.

Table 2. Acceptable Quality Control Ranges for Azithromycin

QC Strain	Minimum Inhibitory Concentrations (μg/mL)	Disk Diffusion (zone diameters in mm)
Haemophilus influenzae ATCC 49247	1.0–4.0	13–21
Staphylococcus aureus ATCC 29213	0.5–2.0	
Staphylococcus aureus ATCC 25923		21–26
Streptococcus pneumoniae ATCC 49619	0.06–0.25	19–25

INDICATIONS AND USAGE

ZITHROMAX® (azithromycin) is indicated for the treatment of patients with mild to moderate infections (pneumonia: see **WARNINGS**) caused by susceptible strains of the designated microorganisms in the specific conditions listed below. As recommended dosages, durations of therapy and applicable patient populations vary among these infections, please see **DOSAGE AND ADMINISTRATION** for specific dosing recommendations.

Adults:

Acute bacterial exacerbations of chronic obstructive pulmonary disease due to *Haemophilus influenzae, Moraxella catarrhalis* or *Streptococcus pneumoniae.*

Community-acquired pneumonia due to *Chlamydia pneumoniae, Haemophilus influenzae, Mycoplasma pneumoniae* or *Streptococcus pneumoniae* in patients appropriate for oral therapy.

NOTE: Azithromycin should not be used in patients with pneumonia who are judged to be inappropriate for oral therapy because of moderate to severe illness or risk factors such as any of the following:

patients with cystic fibrosis,
patients with nosocomially acquired infections,
patients with known or suspected bacteremia,
patients requiring hospitalization,
elderly or debilitated patients, or
patients with significant underlying health problems that may compromise their ability to respond to their illness (including immunodeficiency or functional asplenia).

Pharyngitis/tonsillitis caused by *Streptococcus pyogenes* as an alternative to first-line therapy in individuals who cannot use first-line therapy.

NOTE: Penicillin by the intramuscular route is the usual drug of choice in the treatment of *Streptococcus pyogenes* infection and the prophylaxis of rheumatic fever. ZITHROMAX® is often effective in the eradication of susceptible strains of *Streptococcus pyogenes* from the nasopharynx. Because some strains are resistant to ZITHROMAX®, susceptibility tests should be performed when patients are treated with ZITHROMAX®. Data establishing efficacy of azithromycin in subsequent prevention of rheumatic fever are not available.

Uncomplicated skin and skin structure infections due to *Staphylococcus aureus, Streptococcus pyogenes,* or *Streptococcus agalactiae.* Abscesses usually require surgical drainage.

Urethritis and cervicitis due to *Chlamydia trachomatis* or *Neisseria gonorrhoeae.*

Genital ulcer disease in men due to *Haemophilus ducreyi* (chancroid). Due to the small number of women included in clinical trials, the efficacy of azithromycin in the treatment of chancroid in women has not been established.

ZITHROMAX®, at the recommended dose, should not be relied upon to treat syphilis. Antimicrobial agents used in

Continued on next page

Zithromax Tabs/O.S.—Cont.

high doses for short periods of time to treat non-gonococcal urethritis may mask or delay the symptoms of incubating syphilis. All patients with sexually-transmitted urethritis or cervicitis should have a serologic test for syphilis and appropriate cultures for gonorrhea performed at the time of diagnosis. Appropriate antimicrobial therapy and follow-up tests for these diseases should be initiated if infection is confirmed.

Appropriate culture and susceptibility tests should be performed before treatment to determine the causative organism and its susceptibility to azithromycin. Therapy with ZITHROMAX® may be initiated before results of these tests are known; once the results become available, antimicrobial therapy should be adjusted accordingly.

Children: (See **PRECAUTIONS—Pediatric Use** and **CLINICAL STUDIES IN PEDIATRIC PATIENTS.**)

Acute otitis media caused by *Haemophilus influenzae, Moraxella catarrhalis* or *Streptococcus pneumoniae*. (For specific dosage recommendation, see **DOSAGE AND ADMINISTRATION.**)

Community-acquired pneumonia due to *Chlamydia pneumoniae, Haemophilus influenzae, Mycoplasma pneumoniae* or *Streptococcus pneumoniae* in patients appropriate for oral therapy. (For specific dosage recommendation, see **DOSAGE AND ADMINISTRATION.**)

NOTE: Azithromycin should not be used in pediatric patients with pneumonia who are judged to be inappropriate for oral therapy because of moderate to severe illness or risk factors such as any of the following:

- **patients with cystic fibrosis,**
- **patients with nosocomially acquired infections,**
- **patients with known or suspected bacteremia,**
- **patients requiring hospitalization, or**
- **patients with significant underlying health problems that may compromise their ability to respond to their illness (including immunodeficiency or functional asplenia).**

Pharyngitis/tonsillitis caused by *Streptococcus pyogenes* as an alternative to first-line therapy in individuals who cannot use first-line therapy. (For specific dosage recommendation, see **DOSAGE AND ADMINISTRATION.**)

NOTE: Penicillin by the intramuscular route is the usual drug of choice in the treatment of *Streptococcus pyogenes* infection and the prophylaxis of rheumatic fever. ZITHROMAX® is often effective in the eradication of susceptible strains of *Streptococcus pyogenes* from the nasopharynx. Because some strains are resistant to ZITHROMAX®, susceptibility tests should be performed when patients are treated with ZITHROMAX®. Data establishing efficacy of azithromycin in subsequent prevention of rheumatic fever are not available.

Appropriate culture and susceptibility tests should be performed before treatment to determine the causative organism and its susceptibility to azithromycin. Therapy with ZITHROMAX® may be initiated before results of these tests are known; once the results become available, antimicrobial therapy should be adjusted accordingly.

CONTRAINDICATIONS

ZITHROMAX® is contraindicated in patients with known hypersensitivity to azithromycin, erythromycin or any macrolide antibiotic.

WARNINGS

Serious allergic reactions, including angioedema, anaphylaxis, and dermatologic reactions including Stevens Johnson Syndrome and toxic epidermal necrolysis have been reported rarely in patients on azithromycin therapy. Although rare, fatalities have been reported. (See **CONTRAINDICATIONS.**) Despite initially successful symptomatic treatment of the allergic symptoms, when symptomatic therapy was discontinued, the allergic symptoms **recurred soon thereafter in some patients without further azithromycin exposure.** These patients required prolonged periods of observation and symptomatic treatment. The relationship of these episodes to the long tissue half-life of azithromycin and subsequent prolonged exposure to antigen is unknown at present.

If an allergic reaction occurs, the drug should be discontinued and appropriate therapy should be instituted. Physicians should be aware that reappearance of the allergic symptoms may occur when symptomatic therapy is discontinued.

In the treatment of pneumonia, azithromycin has only been shown to be safe and effective in the treatment of community-acquired pneumonia due to *Chlamydia pneumoniae, Haemophilus influenzae, Mycoplasma pneumoniae* or *Streptococcus pneumoniae* in patients appropriate for oral therapy. Azithromycin should not be used in patients with pneumonia who are judged to be inappropriate for oral therapy because of moderate to severe illness or risk factors such as any of the following: patients with cystic fibrosis, patients with nosocomially acquired infections, patients with known or suspected bacteremia, patients requiring hospitalization, elderly or debilitated patients, or patients with significant underlying health problems that may compromise their ability to respond to their illness (including immunodeficiency or functional asplenia).

Pseudomembranous colitis has been reported with nearly all antibacterial agents and may range in severity from mild to life-threatening. Therefore, it is important to consider this diagnosis in patients who present with diarrhea subsequent to the administration of antibacterial agents.

Treatment with antibacterial agents alters the normal flora of the colon and may permit overgrowth of clostridia. Studies indicate that a toxin produced by *Clostridium difficile* is a primary cause of "antibiotic-associated colitis."

After the diagnosis of pseudomembranous colitis has been established, therapeutic measures should be initiated. Mild cases of pseudomembranous colitis usually respond to discontinuation of the drug alone. In moderate to severe cases, consideration should be given to management with fluids and electrolytes, protein supplementation, and treatment with an antibacterial drug clinically effective against *Clostridium difficile* colitis.

PRECAUTIONS

General: Because azithromycin is principally eliminated via the liver, caution should be exercised when azithromycin is administered to patients with impaired hepatic function. There are no data regarding azithromycin usage in patients with renal impairment; thus, caution should be exercised when prescribing azithromycin in these patients.

The following adverse events have been reported with macrolide products: ventricular arrhythmias, including ventricular tachycardia and *torsade de pointes*, in individuals with prolonged QT intervals.

There has been a spontaneous report from the post-marketing experience of a patient with previous history of arrhythmias who experienced *torsade de pointes* and subsequent myocardial infarction following a course of azithromycin therapy.

Information for Patients:

ZITHROMAX® tablets and oral suspension can be taken with or without food.

Patients should also be cautioned not to take aluminum- and magnesium-containing antacids and azithromycin simultaneously.

The patient should be directed to discontinue azithromycin immediately and contact a physician if any signs of an allergic reaction occur.

Drug Interactions: Aluminum- and magnesium-containing antacids reduce the peak serum concentrations (rate) but not the AUC (extent) of azithromycin absorption.

Administration of cimetidine (800 mg) two hours prior to azithromycin had no effect on azithromycin absorption.

Azithromycin did not affect the plasma concentrations or pharmacokinetics of theophylline administered as a single intravenous dose. The effect of azithromycin on the plasma concentrations or pharmacokinetics of theophylline administered in multiple doses resulting in therapeutic steady-state concentrations of theophylline is not known. However, concurrent use of macrolides and theophylline has been associated with increases in the serum concentrations of theophylline. Therefore, until further data are available, prudent medical practice dictates careful monitoring of plasma theophylline concentrations in patients receiving azithromycin and theophylline concomitantly.

Azithromycin did not affect the prothrombin time response to a single dose of warfarin. However, prudent medical practice dictates careful monitoring of prothrombin time in all patients treated with azithromycin and warfarin concomitantly. Concurrent use of macrolides and warfarin in clinical practice has been associated with increased anticoagulant effects.

The following drug interactions have not been reported in clinical trials with azithromycin; however, no specific drug interaction studies have been performed to evaluate potential drug-drug interaction. Nonetheless, they have been observed with macrolide products. Until further data are developed regarding drug interactions when azithromycin and these drugs are used concomitantly, careful monitoring of patients is advised:

Digoxin—elevated digoxin concentrations.

Ergotamine or dihydroergotamine—acute ergot toxicity characterized by severe peripheral vasospasm and dysesthesia.

Triazolam—decrease the clearance of triazolam and thus may increase the pharmacologic effect of triazolam.

Drugs metabolized by the cytochrome P450 system—elevations of serum carbamazepine, terfenadine, cyclosporine, hexobarbital, and phenytoin concentrations.

Laboratory Test Interactions: There are no reported laboratory test interactions.

Carcinogenesis, Mutagenesis, Impairment of Fertility: Long-term studies in animals have not been performed to evaluate carcinogenic potential. Azithromycin has shown no mutagenic potential in standard laboratory tests: mouse lymphoma assay, human lymphocyte clastogenic assay, and mouse bone marrow clastogenic assay. No evidence of impaired fertility due to azithromycin was found.

Pregnancy: Teratogenic Effects. Pregnancy Category B: Reproduction studies have been performed in rats and mice at doses up to moderately maternally toxic dose concentrations (i.e., 200 mg/kg/day). These doses, based on a mg/m^2 basis, are estimated to be 4 and 2 times, respectively, the human daily dose of 500 mg. In the animal studies, no evidence of harm to the fetus due to azithromycin was found. There are, however, no adequate and well-controlled studies in pregnant women. Because animal reproduction studies are not always predictive of human response, azithromycin should be used during pregnancy only if clearly needed.

Nursing Mothers: It is not known whether azithromycin is excreted in human milk. Because many drugs are excreted in human milk, caution should be exercised when azithromycin is administered to a nursing woman.

Pediatric Use: (See **CLINICAL PHARMACOLOGY, INDICATIONS AND USAGE,** and **DOSAGE AND ADMINISTRATION.**)

Acute Otitis Media (total dosage regimen: 30 mg/kg, see **DOSAGE AND ADMINISTRATION**): Safety and effectiveness in the treatment of children with otitis media under 6 months of age have not been established.

Community-Acquired Pneumonia (dosage regimen: 10 mg/kg on Day 1 followed by 5 mg/kg on Days 2–5): Safety and effectiveness in the treatment of children with community-acquired pneumonia under 6 months of age have not been established. Safety and effectiveness for pneumonia due to *Chlamydia pneumoniae* and *Mycoplasma pneumoniae* were documented in pediatric clinical trials. Safety and effectiveness for pneumonia due to *Haemophilus influenzae* and *Streptococcus pneumoniae* were not documented bacteriologically in the pediatric clinical trial due to difficulty in obtaining specimens. Use of azithromycin for these two microorganisms is supported, however, by evidence from adequate and well-controlled studies in adults.

Pharyngitis/Tonsillitis (dosage regimen: 12 mg/kg on Days 1–5): Safety and effectiveness in the treatment of children with pharyngitis/tonsillitis under 2 years of age have not been established.

Studies evaluating the use of repeated courses of therapy have not been conducted. (See CLINICAL PHARMACOLOGY and ANIMAL TOXICOLOGY.)

Geriatric Use: Pharmacokinetic parameters in older volunteers (65–85 years old) were similar to those in younger volunteers (18–40 years old) for the 5-day therapeutic regimen. Dosage adjustment does not appear to be necessary for older patients with normal renal and hepatic function receiving treatment with this dosage regimen. (See **CLINICAL PHARMACOLOGY.**)

ADVERSE REACTIONS

In clinical trials, most of the reported side effects were mild to moderate in severity and were reversible upon discontinuation of the drug. Potentially serious side effects of angioedema and cholestatic jaundice were reported rarely. Approximately 0.7% of the patients (adults and children) from the 5-day multiple-dose clinical trials discontinued ZITHROMAX® (azithromycin) therapy because of treatment-related side effects. In clinical trials in children given 30 mg/kg, either as a single dose or over 3 days, discontinuation from the trials due to treatment-related side effects was approximately 1%. (See **DOSAGE AND ADMINISTRATION.**) Most of the side effects leading to discontinuation were related to the gastrointestinal tract, e.g., nausea, vomiting, diarrhea, or abdominal pain. (See **CLINICAL STUDIES IN PEDIATRIC PATIENTS.**)

Clinical:

Adults:

Multiple-dose regimen: Overall, the most common side effects in adult patients receiving a multiple-dose regimen of ZITHROMAX® were related to the gastrointestinal system with diarrhea/loose stools (5%), nausea (3%), and abdominal pain (3%) being the most frequently reported.

No other side effects occurred in patients on the multiple-dose regimen of ZITHROMAX® with a frequency greater than 1%. Side effects that occurred with a frequency of 1% or less included the following:

Cardiovascular: Palpitations, chest pain.

Gastrointestinal: Dyspepsia, flatulence, vomiting, melena and cholestatic jaundice.

Genitourinary: Monilia, vaginitis and nephritis.

Nervous System: Dizziness, headache, vertigo and somnolence.

General: Fatigue.

Allergic: Rash, photosensitivity and angioedema.

Single 1-gram dose regimen: Overall, the most common side effects in patients receiving a single-dose regimen of 1 gram of ZITHROMAX® were related to the gastrointestinal system and were more frequently reported than in patients receiving the multiple-dose regimen.

Side effects that occurred in patients on the single one-gram dosing regimen of ZITHROMAX® with a frequency of 1% or greater included diarrhea/loose stools (7%), nausea (5%), abdominal pain (5%), vomiting (2%), dyspepsia (1%) and vaginitis (1%).

Single 2-gram dose regimen: Overall, the most common side effects in patients receiving a single 2-gram dose of ZITHROMAX® were related to the gastrointestinal system. Side effects that occurred in patients in this study with a frequency of 1% or greater included nausea (18%), diarrhea/loose stools (14%), vomiting (7%), abdominal pain (7%), vaginitis (2%), dyspepsia (1%) and dizziness (1%). The majority of these complaints were mild in nature.

Children:

Single and Multiple-dose regimens: The types of side effects in children were comparable to those seen in adults, with different incidence rates for the dosage regimens recommended in children.

Acute Otitis Media: For the recommended total dosage regimen of 30 mg/kg, the most frequent side effects (≥1%) attributed to treatment were diarrhea, abdominal pain, vomiting, nausea and rash. (See **DOSAGE AND ADMINISTRATION** and **CLINICAL STUDIES IN PEDIATRIC PATIENTS.**)

The incidence, based on dosing regimen, is described in the table below:

[See first table at top of next page]

Community-Acquired Pneumonia: For the recommended dosage regimen of 10 mg/kg on Day 1 followed by 5 mg/kg on

Days 2–5, the most frequent side effects attributed to treatment were diarrhea/loose stools, abdominal pain, vomiting, nausea and rash.

The incidence is described in the table below:

[See second table above]

Pharyngitis/tonsillitis: For the recommended dosage regimen of 12 mg/kg on Days 1–5, the most frequent side effects attributed to treatment were diarrhea, vomiting, abdominal pain, nausea and headache.

The incidence is described in the table below:

[See third table above]

With any of the treatment regimens, no other treatment-related side effects occurred in children treated with ZITHROMAX® with a frequency greater than 1%. Side effects that occurred with a frequency of 1% or less included the following:

Cardiovascular: Chest pain.

Gastrointestinal: Dyspepsia, constipation, anorexia, enteritis, flatulence, gastritis, jaundice, loose stools and oral moniliasis.

Hematologic and Lymphatic: Anemia and leukopenia.

Nervous System: Headache (otitis media dosage), hyperkinesia, dizziness, agitation, nervousness and insomnia.

General: Fever, face edema, fatigue, fungal infection, malaise and pain.

Allergic: Rash and allergic reaction.

Respiratory: Cough increased, pharyngitis, pleural effusion and rhinitis.

Skin and Appendages: Eczema, fungal dermatitis, pruritus, sweating, urticaria and vesiculobullous rash.

Special Senses: Conjunctivitis.

Post-Marketing Experience:

Adverse events reported with azithromycin during the post-marketing period in adult and/or pediatric patients for which a causal relationship may not be established include:

Allergic: Arthralgia, edema, urticaria and angioedema.

Cardiovascular: Arrhythmias including ventricular tachycardia and hypotension.

Gastrointestinal: Anorexia, constipation, dyspepsia, flatulence, vomiting/diarrhea rarely resulting in dehydration, pseudomembranous colitis, pancreatitis, oral candidiasis and rare reports of tongue discoloration.

General: Asthenia, paresthesia, fatigue, malaise and anaphylaxis (rarely fatal).

Genitourinary: Interstitial nephritis and acute renal failure and vaginitis.

Hematopoietic: Thrombocytopenia.

Liver/Biliary: Abnormal liver function including hepatitis and cholestatic jaundice, as well as rare cases of hepatic necrosis and hepatic failure, some of which have resulted in death.

Nervous System: Convulsions, dizziness/vertigo, headache, somnolence, hyperactivity, nervousness, agitation and syncope.

Psychiatric: Aggressive reaction and anxiety.

Skin/Appendages: Pruritus, rarely serious skin reactions including erythema multiforme, Stevens-Johnson syndrome, and toxic epidermal necrolysis.

Special Senses: Hearing disturbances including hearing loss, deafness and/or tinnitus and rare reports of taste perversion.

Laboratory Abnormalities:

Adults:

Significant abnormalities (irrespective of drug relationship) occurring during the clinical trials were reported as follows: with an incidence of 1–2%, elevated serum creatine phosphokinase, potassium, ALT (SGPT), GGT, and AST (SGOT); with an incidence of less than 1%, leukopenia, neutropenia, decreased platelet count, elevated serum alkaline phosphatase, bilirubin, BUN, creatinine, blood glucose, LDH and phosphate.

When follow-up was provided, changes in laboratory tests appeared to be reversible.

In multiple-dose clinical trials involving more than 3000 patients, three patients discontinued therapy because of treatment-related liver enzyme abnormalities and one because of a renal function abnormality.

Children:

One, Three and Five Day Regimens

Laboratory data collected from comparative clinical trials employing two 3-day regimens (30 mg/kg or 60 mg/kg in divided doses over 3 days), or two 5-day regimens (30 mg/kg or 60 mg/kg in divided doses over 5 days) were similar for regimens of azithromycin and all comparators combined, with most clinically significant laboratory abnormalities occurring at incidences of 1–5%. Laboratory data for patients receiving 30 mg/kg as a single dose were collected in one single center trial. In that trial, an absolute neutrophil count between 500–1500 cells/mm^3 was observed in 10/64 patients receiving 30 mg/kg as a single dose, 9/62 patients receiving 30 mg/kg given over 3 days, and 8/63 comparator patients. No patient had an absolute neutrophil count <500 cells/mm^3. (See **DOSAGE AND ADMINISTRATION.**)

In multiple-dose clinical trials involving approximately 4700 pediatric patients, no patients discontinued therapy because of treatment-related laboratory abnormalities.

DOSAGE AND ADMINISTRATION

(See **INDICATIONS AND USAGE** and **CLINICAL PHARMACOLOGY.**)

Adults:

The recommended dose of ZITHROMAX® for the treatment of mild to moderate acute bacterial exacerbations of chronic obstructive pulmonary disease, community-acquired pneumonia of mild severity, pharyngitis/tonsillitis (as second-line therapy), and uncomplicated skin and skin structure infections due to the indicated organisms is: 500 mg as a single dose on the first day followed by 250 mg once daily on Days 2 through 5.

ZITHROMAX® tablets can be taken with or without food.

The recommended dose of ZITHROMAX® for the treatment of genital ulcer disease due to *Haemophilus ducreyi* (chancroid), non-gonococcal urethritis and cervicitis due to *C. trachomatis* is: a single 1 gram (1000 mg) dose of ZITHROMAX®.

The recommended dose of ZITHROMAX® for the treatment of urethritis and cervicitis due to *Neisseria gonorrhoeae* is a single 2 gram (2000 mg) dose of ZITHROMAX®.

Children:

ZITHROMAX® for oral suspension can be taken with or without food.

Acute Otitis Media: The recommended dose of ZITHROMAX® for oral suspension for the treatment of children with acute otitis media is 30 mg/kg given as a single dose or 10 mg/kg once daily for 3 days or 10 mg/kg as a single dose on the first day followed by 5 mg/kg/day on Days 2 through 5. (See chart below.)

Community-Acquired Pneumonia: The recommended dose of ZITHROMAX® for oral suspension for the treatment of children with community-acquired pneumonia is 10 mg/kg as a single dose on the first day followed by 5 mg/kg on Days 2 through 5. (See chart below.)

[See fourth table above]

[See fifth table above]

[See first table at top of next page]

The safety of re-dosing azithromycin in children who vomit after receiving 30 mg/kg as a single dose has not been established. In clinical studies involving 487 patients with acute otitis media given a single 30 mg/kg dose of azithromycin, eight patients who vomited within 30 minutes of dosing were re-dosed at the same total dose.

Pharyngitis/Tonsillitis: The recommended dose of ZITHROMAX® for children with pharyngitis/tonsillitis is 12 mg/kg once daily for 5 days. (See chart below.)

[See second table at top of next page]

Constituting instructions for ZITHROMAX® Oral Suspension, 300, 600, 900, 1200 mg bottles. The table below indicates the volume of water to be used for constitution:

[See third table at top of next page]

Following constitution, and for use with the oral syringe, the supplied Press in Bottle Adapter should be inserted into the neck of the bottle then sealed with the original closure. Shake well before each use. Oversized bottle provides shake space. Keep tightly closed.

Use only the dosing device provided to measure the correct amount of suspension. (See **HOW SUPPLIED.**) The dosing device may need to be filled multiple times to provide the complete dose prescribed. Rinse the device with water after the complete daily dose has been administered.

Continued on next page

Dosage Regimen	Diarrhea, %	Abdominal Pain, %	Vomiting, %	Nausea, %	Rash, %
1-day	4.3%	1.4%	4.9%	1.0%	1.0%
3-day	2.6%	1.7%	2.3%	0.4%	0.6%
5-day	1.8%	1.2%	1.1%	0.5%	0.4%

Dosage Regimen	Diarrhea/Loose stools, %	Abdominal Pain, %	Vomiting, %	Nausea, %	Rash, %
5-day	5.8%	1.9%	1.9%	1.9%	1.6%

Dosage Regimen	Diarrhea, %	Vomiting, %	Abdominal Pain, %	Nausea, %	Rash, %	Headache, %
5-day	5.4%	5.6%	3.4%	1.8%	0.7%	1.1%

PEDIATRIC DOSAGE GUIDELINES FOR OTITIS MEDIA AND COMMUNITY-ACQUIRED PNEUMONIA
(Age 6 months and above, see PRECAUTIONS—Pediatric Use.)
Based on Body Weight

OTITIS MEDIA AND COMMUNITY-ACQUIRED PNEUMONIA: 5-Day Regimen*

Dosing Calculated on 10 mg/kg/day Day 1 and 5 mg/kg/day Days 2 to 5.

Weight		100 mg/5 mL		200 mg/5 mL		Total mL per Treatment Course	Total mg per Treatment Course
Kg	Lbs.	Day 1	Days 2–5	Day 1	Days 2–5		
5	11	2.5 mL (1/2 tsp)	1.25 mL (1/4 tsp)			7.5 mL	150 mg
10	22	5 mL (1 tsp)	2.5 mL (1/2 tsp)			15 mL	300 mg
20	44			5 mL (1 tsp)	2.5 mL (1/2 tsp)	15 mL	600 mg
30	66			7.5 mL (1 1/2tsp)	3.75 mL (3/4tsp)	22.5 mL	900 mg
40	88			10 mL (2 tsp)	5 mL (1 tsp)	30 mL	1200 mg
50 and above	110 and above			12.5 mL (2 1/2 tsp)	6.25 mL (1 1/4 tsp)	37.5 mL	1500 mg

*Effectiveness of the 3-day or 1-day regimen in children with community-acquired pneumonia has not been established.

OTITIS MEDIA: (3-Day Regimen)

Dosing Calculated on 10 mg/kg/day

Weight		100 mg/5 mL	200 mg/5 mL	Total mL per Treatment Course	Total mg per Treatment Course
Kg	Lbs.	Day 1–3	Day 1–3		
5	11	2.5 mL (1/2 tsp)		7.5 mL	150 mg
10	22	5 mL (1 tsp)		15 mL	300 mg
20	44		5 mL (1 tsp)	15 mL	600 mg
30	66		7.5 mL (1 1/2 tsp)	22.5 mL	900 mg
40	88		10 mL (2 tsp)	30 mL	1200 mg
50 and above	110 and above		12.5 mL (2 1/2 tsp)	37.5 mL	1500 mg

Zithromax Tabs/O.S.—Cont.

After mixing, store suspension at 5° to 30°C (41° to 86°F) and use within 10 days. Discard after full dosing is completed.

HOW SUPPLIED

ZITHROMAX® tablets are supplied as pink modified capsular shaped, engraved, film-coated tablets containing azithromycin dihydrate equivalent to 250 mg of azithromycin.

ZITHROMAX® tablets are engraved with "PFIZER" on one side and "306" on the other. These are packaged in bottles and blister cards of 6 tablets (Z-PAKS®) as follows:

Bottles of 30	NDC 0069-3060-30
Boxes of 3 (Z-PAKS® of 6)	NDC 0069-3060-75
Unit Dose package of 50	NDC 0069-3060-86

ZITHROMAX® tablets should be stored between 15° to 30°C (59° to 86°F).

ZITHROMAX® for oral suspension after constitution contains a flavored suspension.

ZITHROMAX® for oral suspension is supplied to provide 100 mg/5 mL or 200 mg/5 mL suspension in bottles with accompanying calibrated dosing device as follows:

Azithromycin contents per bottle	NDC
300 mg	0069-3110-19
600 mg	0069-3120-19
900 mg	0069-3130-19
1200 mg	0069-3140-19

See **DOSAGE AND ADMINISTRATION** for constitution instructions with each bottle type.

Storage: Store dry powder below 30°C (86°F). Store constituted suspension between 5° to 30°C (41° to 86°F) and discard when full dosing is completed.

CLINICAL STUDIES IN PEDIATRIC PATIENTS

(See **INDICATIONS AND USAGE** and **Pediatric Use.**)

From the perspective of evaluating pediatric clinical trials, Days 11–14 were considered on-therapy evaluations because of the extended half-life of azithromycin. Day 11–14 data are provided for clinical guidance. Day 24–32 evaluations were considered the primary test of cure endpoint.

Acute Otitis Media

Safety and efficacy using azithromycin 30 mg/kg given over 5 days

Protocol 1

In a double-blind, controlled clinical study of acute otitis media performed in the United States, azithromycin (10 mg/kg on Day 1 followed by 5 mg/kg on Days 2–5) was compared to amoxicillin/clavulanate potassium (4:1). For the 553 patients who were evaluated for clinical efficacy, the clinical success rate (i.e., cure plus improvement) at the Day 11 visit was 88% for azithromycin and 88% for the control agent. For the 521 patients who were evaluated at the Day 30 visit, the clinical success rate was 73% for azithromycin and 71% for the control agent.

In the safety analysis of the above study, the incidence of treatment-related adverse events, primarily gastrointestinal, in all patients treated was 9% with azithromycin and 31% with the control agent. The most common side effects were diarrhea/loose stools (4% azithromycin vs. 20% control), vomiting (2% azithromycin vs. 7% control), and abdominal pain (2% azithromycin vs. 5% control).

Protocol 2

In a non-comparative clinical and microbiologic trial performed in the United States, where significant rates of beta-lactamase producing organisms (35%) were found, 131 patients were evaluable for clinical efficacy. The combined clinical success rate (i.e., cure and improvement) at the Day 11 visit was 84% for azithromycin. For the 122 patients who were evaluated at the Day 30 visit, the clinical success rate was 70% for azithromycin.

Microbiologic determinations were made at the pre-treatment visit. Microbiology was not reassessed at later visits. The following presumptive bacterial/clinical cure outcomes (i.e., clinical success) were obtained from the evaluable group:

[See fourth table above]

In the safety analysis of this study, the incidence of treatment-related adverse events, primarily gastrointestinal, in all patients treated was 9%. The most common side effect was diarrhea (4%).

Protocol 3

In another controlled comparative clinical and microbiologic study of otitis media performed in the United States, azithromycin was compared to amoxicillin/clavulanate potassium (4:1). This study utilized two of the same investigators as Protocol 2 (above), and these two investigators enrolled 90% of the patients in Protocol 3. For this reason, Protocol 3 was not considered to be an independent study. Significant rates of beta-lactamase producing organisms (20%) were found. Ninety-two (92) patients were evaluable for clinical and microbiologic efficacy. The combined clinical success rate (i.e., cure and improvement) of those patients with a baseline pathogen at the Day 11 visit was 88% for azithromycin vs. 100% for control; at the Day 30 visit, the clinical success rate was 82% for azithromycin vs. 80% for control.

Microbiologic determinations were made at the pre-treatment visit. Microbiology was not reassessed at later visits. At the Day 11 and Day 30 visits, the following presumptive bacterial/clinical cure outcomes (i.e., clinical success) were obtained from the evaluable group:

OTITIS MEDIA: (1-Day Regimen)

Dosing Calculated on 30 mg/kg as a single dose

Weight Kg	Weight Lbs.	200 mg/5 mL Day 1	Total mL per Treatment Course	Total mg per Treatment Course
5	11	3.75 mL (3/4 tsp)	3.75 mL	150 mg
10	22	7.5 mL ($1^1/_2$ tsp)	7.5 mL	300 mg
20	44	15 mL (3 tsp)	15 mL	600 mg
30	66	22.5 mL ($4^1/_2$ tsp)	22.5 mL	900 mg
40	88	30 mL (6 tsp)	30 mL	1200 mg
50 and above	110 and above	37.5 mL ($7^1/_2$ tsp)	37.5 mL	1500 mg

PEDIATRIC DOSAGE GUIDELINES FOR PHARYNGITIS/TONSILLITIS
(Age 2 years and above, see PRECAUTIONS—Pediatric Use.)
Based on Body Weight

PHARYNGITIS/TONSILLITIS: (5-Day Regimen)

Dosing Calculated on 12 mg/kg/day for 5 days.

Weight Kg	Weight Lbs.	200 mg/5 mL Day 1–5	Total mL per Treatment Course	Total mg per Treatment Course
8	18	2.5 mL ($^1/_2$ tsp)	12.5 mL	500 mg
17	37	5 mL (1 tsp)	25 mL	1000 mg
25	55	7.5 mL ($1^1/_2$ tsp)	37.5 mL	1500 mg
33	73	10 mL (2 tsp)	50 mL	2000 mg
40	88	12.5 mL ($2^1/_2$ tsp)	62.5 mL	2500 mg

Amount of water to be added	Total volume after constitution (azithromycin content)	Azithromycin concentration after constitution
9 mL (300 mg)	15 mL (300 mg)	100 mg/5 mL
9 mL (600 mg)	15 mL (600 mg)	200 mg/5 mL
12 mL (900 mg)	22.5 mL (900 mg)	200 mg/5 mL
15 mL (1200 mg)	30 mL (1200 mg)	200 mg/5 mL

Presumed Bacteriologic Eradication

	Day 11 Azithromycin	Day 30 Azithromycin
S. pneumoniae	61/74 (82%)	40/56 (71%)
H. influenzae	43/54 (80%)	30/47 (64%)
M. catarrhalis	28/35 (80%)	19/26 (73%)
S. pyogenes	11/11 (100%)	7/7
Overall	177/217 (82%)	97/137 (73%)

Presumed Bacteriologic Eradication

	Day 11 Azithromycin	Day 11 Control	Day 30 Azithromycin	Day 30 Control
S. pneumoniae	25/29 (86%)	26/26 (100%)	22/28 (79%)	18/22 (82%)
H. influenzae	9/11 (82%)	9/9	8/10 (80%)	6/8
M. catarrhalis	7/7	5/5	5/5	2/3
S. pyogenes	2/2	5/5	2/2	4/4
Overall	43/49 (88%)	45/45 (100%)	37/45 (82%)	30/37 (81%)

[See fifth table above]

In the safety analysis of the above study, the incidence of treatment-related adverse events, primarily gastrointestinal, in all patients treated was 4% with azithromycin and 31% with the control agent. The most common side effect was diarrhea/loose stools (2% azithromycin vs. 29% control).

Safety and efficacy using azithromycin 30 mg/kg given over 3 days

Protocol 4

In a double-blind, controlled, randomized clinical study of acute otitis media in children from 6 months to 12 years of age, azithromycin (10 mg/kg per day for 3 days) was compared to amoxicillin/clavulanate potassium (7:1) in divided doses q12h for 10 days. Each child received active drug and placebo matched for the comparator.

For the 373 patients who were evaluated for clinical efficacy, the clinical success rate (i.e., cure plus improvement) at the Day 12 visit was 83% for azithromycin and 88% for the control agent. For the 362 patients who were evaluated at the Day 24–28 visit, the clinical success rate was 74% for azithromycin and 69% for the control agent.

In the safety analysis of the above study, the incidence of treatment-related adverse events, primarily gastrointestinal, in all patients treated was 10.6% with azithromycin and 20.0% with the control agent. The most common side effects were diarrhea/loose stools (5.9% azithromycin vs. 14.6% control), vomiting (2.1% azithromycin vs. 1.1% control), and rash (0.0% azithromycin vs. 4.3% control).

Safety and efficacy using azithromycin 30 mg/kg given as a single dose

Protocol 5

A double blind, controlled, randomized trial was performed at nine clinical centers. Infants and children from 6 months to 12 years of age were randomized 1:1 to treatment with either azithromycin (given at 30 mg/kg as a single dose on Day 1) or amoxicillin/clavulanate potassium (7:1), divided q12h for 10 days. Each child received active drug, and placebo matched for the comparator.

Clinical response (Cure, Improvement, Failure) was evaluated at End of Therapy (Day 12–16) and Test of Cure (Day 28–32). Safety was evaluated throughout the trial for all treated subjects. For the 321 subjects who were evaluated at End of Treatment, the clinical success rate (cure plus improvement) was 87% for azithromycin, and 88% for the comparator. For the 305 subjects who were evaluated at Test of Cure, the clinical success rate was 75% for both azithromycin and the comparator.

In the safety analysis, the incidence of treatment-related adverse events, primarily gastrointestinal, was 16.8% with

Presumed Bacteriologic Eradication		
	Day 10	Day 24–28
S. pneumoniae	70/76 (92%)	67/76 (88%)
H. influenzae	30/42 (71%)	28/44 (64%)
M. catarrhalis	10/10 (100%)	10/10 (100%)
Overall	110/128 (86%)	105/130 (81%)

Three U.S. Streptococcal Pharyngitis Studies
Azithromycin vs. Penicillin V
EFFICACY RESULTS

	Day 14	Day 30
Bacteriologic Eradication:		
Azithromycin	323/340 (95%)	255/330 (77%)
Penicillin V	242/332 (73%)	206/325 (63%)
Clinical Success (Cure plus improvement):		
Azithromycin	336/343 (98%)	310/330 (94%)
Penicillin V	284/338 (84%)	241/325 (74%)

azithromycin, and 22.5% with the comparator. The most common side effects were diarrhea (6.4% with azithromycin vs. 12.7% with the comparator), vomiting (4% with each agent), rash (1.7% with azithromycin vs. 5.2% with the comparator) and nausea (1.7% with azithromycin vs. 1.2% with the comparator).

Protocol 6

In a non-comparative clinical and microbiological trial, 248 patients from 6 months to 12 years of age with documented acute otitis media were dosed with a single oral dose of azithromycin (30 mg/kg on Day 1).

For the 240 patients who were evaluable for clinical modified Intent-to-Treat (MITT) analysis, the clinical success rate (i.e., cure plus improvement) at Day 10 was 89% and for the 242 patients evaluable at Day 24–28, the clinical success rate (cure) was 85%.

[See table above]

In the safety analysis of this study, the incidence of treatment-related adverse events, primarily gastrointestinal, in all the subjects treated was 12.1%. The most common side effects were vomiting (5.6%), diarrhea (3.2%), and abdominal pain (1.6%).

Pharyngitis/Tonsillitis

In three double-blind controlled studies, conducted in the United States, azithromycin (12 mg/kg once a day for 5 days) was compared to penicillin V (250 mg three times a day for 10 days) in the treatment of pharyngitis due to documented Group A β-hemolytic streptococci (GABHS or *S. pyogenes*). Azithromycin was clinically and microbiologically statistically superior to penicillin at Day 14 and Day 30 with the following clinical success (i.e., cure and improvement) and bacteriologic efficacy rates (for the combined evaluable patient with documented GABHS):

[See table above]

Approximately 1% of azithromycin-susceptible *S. pyogenes* isolates were resistant to azithromycin following therapy.

The incidence of treatment-related adverse events, primarily gastrointestinal, in all patients treated was 18% on azithromycin and 13% on penicillin. The most common side effects were diarrhea/loose stools (6% azithromycin vs. 2% penicillin), vomiting (6% azithromycin vs. 4% penicillin), and abdominal pain (3% azithromycin vs. 1% penicillin).

ANIMAL TOXICOLOGY

Phospholipidosis (intracellular phospholipid accumulation) has been observed in some tissues of mice, rats, and dogs given multiple doses of azithromycin. It has been demonstrated in numerous organ systems (e.g., eye, dorsal root ganglia, liver, gallbladder, kidney, spleen, and pancreas) in dogs treated with azithromycin at doses which, expressed on a mg/kg basis, are only two times greater than the recommended adult human dose and in rats at doses comparable to the recommended adult human dose. This effect has been reversible after cessation of azithromycin treatment. Phospholipidosis has been observed to a similar extent in the tissues of neonatal rats and dogs given daily doses of azithromycin ranging from 10 days to 30 days. Based on the pharmacokinetic data, phospholipidosis has been seen in the rat (30 mg/kg dose) at observed C_{max} value of 1.3 μg/mL (six times greater than the observed C_{max} of 0.216 μg/mL at the pediatric dose of 10 mg/kg). Similarly, it has been shown in the dog (10 mg/kg dose) at observed C_{max} value of 1.5 μg/mL (seven times greater than the observed same C_{max} and drug dose in the studied pediatric population). On a mg/m^2 basis, 30 mg/kg dose in the rat (135 mg/m^2) and 10 mg/kg dose in the dog (79 mg/m^2) are approximately 0.4 and 0.6 times, respectively, the recommended dose in the pediatric patients with an average body weight of 25 kg. This effect, similar to that seen in the adult animals, is reversible after cessation of azithromycin treatment. The significance of these findings for animals and for humans is unknown.

REFERENCES:

1. National Committee for Clinical Laboratory Standards, *Methods for Dilution Antimicrobial Susceptibility Tests for Bacteria That Grow Aerobically*—Fifth Edition. Approved Standard NCCLS, Document M7-A5, Vol. 20, No. 2 (ISBN 1-56238-394-9). NCCLS, 940 West Valley Road, Suite 1400, Wayne, PA 19087-1898, January, 2000.
2. National Committee for Clinical Laboratory Standards, *Performance Standards for Antimicrobial Disk Susceptibility Tests*—Seventh Edition. Approved Standard NCCLS Document, M2-A7, Vol. 20, No. 1 (ISBN 1-56238-393-0). NCCLS, 940 West Valley Road, Suite 1400, Wayne, PA 19087-1898, January, 2000.
3. National Committee for Clinical Laboratory Standards. *Performance Standards for Antimicrobial Susceptibility Testing*—Eleventh Informational Supplement. NCCLS Document M100-S11, Vol. 21, No. 1 (ISBN 1-56238-426-0). NCCLS, 940 West Valley Road, Suite 1400, Wayne, PA 19087-1898, January, 2001.

Rx only

Licensed from Pliva

Distributed by:
Pfizer Labs
Division of Pfizer Inc, NY, NY 10017
Printed in U.S.A.
70-5179-00-9 Revised January 2002

ZITHROMAX® ℞

[*zi' thrō-max*]

(azithromycin capsules)
(azithromycin tablets)
and
(azithromycin for oral suspension)

Prescribing information for this product, which appears on pages 2743–2748 of the 2002 PDR, has been completely revised as follows. Please write "See Supplement A" next to the product heading.

DESCRIPTION

ZITHROMAX® (azithromycin capsules, azithromycin tablets and azithromycin for oral suspension) contain the active ingredient azithromycin, an azalide, a subclass of macrolide antibiotics, for oral administration. Azithromycin has the chemical name (*2R,3S,4R,5R,8R,10R,11R,12S,13S,14R*)-13-[(2,6-dideoxy-3-*C*-methyl-3-*O*-methyl-α-*L*-*ribo*-hexopyranosyl)oxy]-2-ethyl-3,4,10-trihydroxy-3,5,6,8,10,12,14-heptamethyl-11-[[3,4,6-trideoxy-3-(dimethylamino)-β-*D*-*xylo*-hexopyranosyl]oxy]-1-oxa-6-azacyclopentadecan-15-one. Azithromycin is derived from erythromycin; however, it differs chemically from erythromycin in that a methyl-substituted nitrogen atom is incorporated into the lactone ring. Its molecular formula is $C_{38}H_{72}N_2O_{12}$, and its molecular weight is 749.0. Azithromycin has the following structural formula:

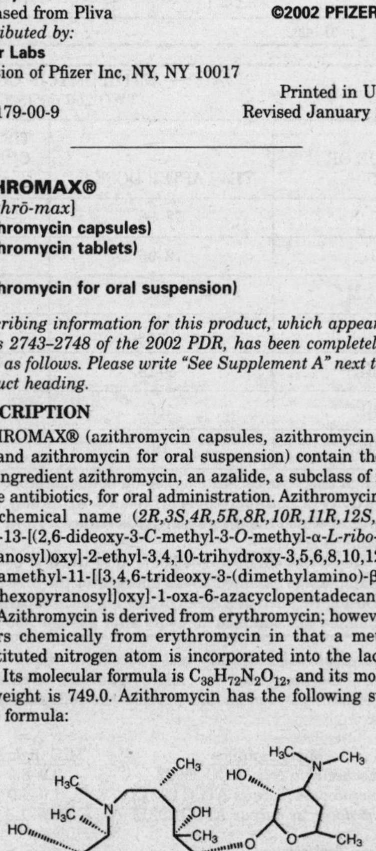

Azithromycin, as the dihydrate, is a white crystalline powder with a molecular formula of $C_{38}H_{72}N_2O_{12}•2H_2O$ and a molecular weight of 785.0.

ZITHROMAX® capsules contain azithromycin dihydrate equivalent to 250 mg of azithromycin. The capsules are supplied in red opaque hard-gelatin capsules (containing FD&C Red #40). They also contain the following inactive ingredients: anhydrous lactose, corn starch, magnesium stearate, and sodium lauryl sulfate.

ZITHROMAX® tablets contain azithromycin dihydrate equivalent to 600 mg azithromycin. The tablets are supplied as white, modified oval-shaped, film-coated tablets. They also contain the following inactive ingredients: dibasic calcium phosphate anhydrous, pregelatinized starch, sodium croscarmellose, magnesium stearate, sodium lauryl sulfate and an aqueous film coat consisting of hydroxypropyl methyl cellulose, titanium dioxide, lactose and triacetin.

ZITHROMAX® for oral suspension is supplied in a single dose packet containing azithromycin dihydrate equivalent to 1 g azithromycin. It also contains the following inactive ingredients: colloidal silicon dioxide, sodium phosphate tribasic, anhydrous; spray dried artificial banana flavor, spray dried artificial cherry flavor, and sucrose.

CLINICAL PHARMACOLOGY

Pharmacokinetics: Following oral administration, azithromycin is rapidly absorbed and widely distributed throughout the body. Rapid distribution of azithromycin into tissues and high concentration within cells result in significantly higher azithromycin concentrations in tissues than in plasma or serum. The 1 g single dose packet is bioequivalent to four 250 mg capsules.

The pharmacokinetic parameters of azithromycin in plasma after dosing as per labeled recommendations in healthy young adults and asymptomatic HIV-seropositive adults (age 18–40 years old) are portrayed in the following chart:

[See first table at top of next page]

In these studies (500 mg Day 1, 250 mg Days 2–5), there was no significant difference in the disposition of azithromycin between male and female subjects. Plasma concentrations of azithromycin following single 500 mg oral and i.v. doses declined in a polyphasic pattern resulting in an average terminal half-life of 68 hours. With a regimen of 500 mg on Day 1 and 250 mg/day on Days 2–5, C_{min} and C_{max} remained essentially unchanged from Day 2 through Day 5 of therapy. However, without a loading dose, azithromycin C_{min} levels required 5 to 7 days to reach steady-state.

In asymptomatic HIV-seropositive adult subjects receiving 600-mg ZITHROMAX® tablets once daily for 22 days, steady state azithromycin serum levels were achieved by Day 15 of dosing.

When azithromycin capsules were administered with food, the rate of absorption (C_{max}) of azithromycin was reduced by 52% and the extent of absorption (AUC) by 43%.

When the oral suspension of azithromycin was administered with food, the C_{max} increased by 46% and the AUC by 14%.

The absolute bioavailability of two 600 mg tablets was 34% (CV=56%). Administration of two 600 mg tablets with food increased C_{max} by 31% (CV=43%) while the extent of absorption (AUC) was unchanged (mean ratio of AUCs=1.00; CV=55%).

The AUC of azithromycin in 250 mg capsules was unaffected by coadministration of an antacid containing aluminum and magnesium hydroxide with ZITHROMAX® (azithromycin); however, the C_{max} was reduced by 24%. Administration of cimetidine (800 mg) two hours prior to azithromycin had no effect on azithromycin absorption.

When studied in healthy elderly subjects from age 65 to 85 years, the pharmacokinetic parameters of azithromycin (500 mg Day 1, 250 mg Days 2–5) in elderly men were similar to those in young adults; however, in elderly women, although higher peak concentrations (increased by 30 to 50%) were observed, no significant accumulation occurred.

The high values in adults for apparent steady-state volume of distribution (31.1 L/kg) and plasma clearance (630 mL/min) suggest that the prolonged half-life is due to extensive uptake and subsequent release of drug from tissues. Selected tissue (or fluid) concentration and tissue (or fluid) to plasma/serum concentration ratios are shown in the following table:

[See second table at top of next page]

The extensive tissue distribution was confirmed by examination of additional tissues and fluids (bone, ejaculum, prostate, ovary, uterus, salpinx, stomach, liver, and gallbladder). As there are no data from adequate and well-controlled studies of azithromycin treatment of infections in these additional body sites, the clinical significance of these tissue concentration data is unknown.

Following a regimen of 500 mg on the first day and 250 mg daily for 4 days, only very low concentrations were noted in cerebrospinal fluid (less than 0.01 μg/mL) in the presence of non-inflamed meninges.

Following oral administration of a single 1200 mg dose (two 600 mg tablets), the mean maximum concentration in peripheral leukocytes was 140 μg/mL. Concentrations remained above 32 μg/mL for approximately 60 hr. The mean half-lives for 6 males and 6 females were 34 hr and 57 hr, respectively. Leukocyte to plasma C_{max} ratios for males and females were 258 (±77%) and 175 (±60%), respectively, and the AUC ratios were 804 (±31%) and 541 (±28%), respectively. The clinical relevance of these findings is unknown.

Following oral administration of multiple daily doses of 600 mg (1 tablet/day) to asymptomatic HIV-seropositive adults, mean maximum concentration in peripheral leukocytes was 252 μg/mL (±49%). Trough concentrations in peripheral leukocytes at steady-state averaged 146 μg/mL (±33%). The mean leukocyte to serum C_{max} ratio was 456 (±38%) and the mean leukocyte to serum AUC ratio was 816 (±31%). The clinical relevance of these findings is unknown.

The serum protein binding of azithromycin is variable in the concentration range approximating human exposure, decreasing from 51% at 0.02 μg/mL to 7% at 2 μg/mL. Biliary excretion of azithromycin, predominantly as unchanged drug, is a major route of elimination. Over the course of a week, approximately 6% of the administered dose appears as unchanged drug in urine.

There are no pharmacokinetic data available from studies in hepatically- or renally-impaired individuals.

The effect of azithromycin on the plasma levels or pharmacokinetics of theophylline administered in multiple doses adequate to reach therapeutic steady-state plasma levels is not known. (See PRECAUTIONS.)

Mechanism of Action: Azithromycin acts by binding to the 50S ribosomal subunit of susceptible microorganisms and, thus, interfering with microbial protein synthesis. Nucleic acid synthesis is not affected.

Continued on next page

Zithromax Caps/Tabs/O.S.—Cont.

Azithromycin concentrates in phagocytes and fibroblasts as demonstrated by *in vitro* incubation techniques. Using such methodology, the ratio of intracellular to extracellular concentration was >30 after one hour incubation. *In vivo* studies suggest that concentration in phagocytes may contribute to drug distribution to inflamed tissues.

MEAN (CV%) PK PARAMETER

DOSE/DOSAGE FORM (serum, except as indicated)	Subjects	Day No.	C_{max} (μg/mL)	T_{max} (hr)	C_{24} (μg/mL)	AUC (μg•hr/mL)	$T_{½}$ (hr)	Urinary Excretion (% of dose)
500 mg/250 mg capsule	12	Day 1	0.41	2.5	0.05	2.6[a]	—	4.5
and 250 mg on Days 2–5	12	Day 5	0.24	3.2	0.05	2.1[a]	—	6.5
1200 mg/600 mg tablets	12	Day 1	0.66	2.5	0.074	6.8[b]	40	—
%CV			(62%)	(79%)	(49%)	(64%)	(33%)	
600 mg tablet/day	7	1	0.33	2.0	0.039	2.4[a]		
%CV			25%	(50%)	(36%)	(19%)		
	7	22	0.55	2.1	0.14	5.8[a]	84.5	—
%CV			(18%)	(52%)	(26%)	(25%)		—
600 mg tablet/day (leukocytes)	7	22	252	10.9	146	4763[a]	82.8	—
%CV			(49%)	(28%)	(33%)	(42%)	—	—

[a]AUC_{0-24}; [b]0-last.

AZITHROMYCIN CONCENTRATIONS FOLLOWING TWO 250 mg (500 mg) CAPSULES IN ADULTS

TISSUE OR FLUID	TIME AFTER DOSE (h)	TISSUE OR FLUID CONCENTRATION (μg/g or μg/mL)[1]	CORRESPONDING PLASMA OR SERUM LEVEL (μg/mL)	TISSUE (FLUID) PLASMA (SERUM) RATIO[1]
SKIN	72–96	0.4	0.012	35
LUNG	72–96	4.0	0.012	>100
SPUTUM*	2–4	1.0	0.64	2
SPUTUM**	10–12	2.9	0.1	30
TONSIL***	9–18	4.5	0.03	>100
TONSIL***	180	0.9	0.006	>100
CERVIX****	19	2.8	0.04	70

[1] High tissue concentrations should not be interpreted to be quantitatively related to clinical efficacy. The antimicrobial activity of azithromycin is pH related. Azithromycin is concentrated in cell lysosomes which have a low intraorganelle pH, at which the drug's activity is reduced. However, the extensive distribution of drug to tissues may be relevant to clinical activity.

* Sample was obtained 2–4 hours after the first dose.
** Sample was obtained 10–12 hours after the first dose.
*** Dosing regimen of 2 doses of 250 mg each, separated by 12 hours.
**** Sample was obtained 19 hours after a single 500 mg dose.

Microbiology:
Azithromycin has been shown to be active against most strains of the following microorganisms, both *in vitro* and in clinical infections as described in the INDICATIONS AND USAGE section.

Aerobic Gram-Positive Microorganisms
Staphylococcus aureus
Streptococcus agalactiae
Streptococcus pneumoniae
Streptococcus pyogenes

NOTE: Azithromycin demonstrates cross-resistance with erythromycin-resistant gram-positive strains. Most strains of *Enterococcus faecalis* and methicillin-resistant staphylococci are resistant to azithromycin.

Aerobic Gram-Negative Microorganisms
Haemophilus influenzae
Moraxella catarrhalis

"Other" Microorganisms
Chlamydia trachomatis

Beta-lactamase production should have no effect on azithromycin activity.

Azithromycin has been shown to be active *in vitro* and in the prevention and treatment of disease caused by the following microorganisms:

Mycobacteria
Mycobacterium avium complex (MAC) consisting of:
Mycobacterium avium
Mycobacterium intracellulare.

The following *in vitro* data are available, *but their clinical significance is unknown.*

Azithromycin exhibits *in vitro* minimal inhibitory concentrations (MICs) of 2.0 μg/mL or less against most (≥90%) strains of the following microorganisms; however, the safety and effectiveness of azithromycin in treating clinical infections due to these microorganisms have not been established in adequate and well-controlled trials.

Aerobic Gram-Positive Microorganisms
Streptococci (Groups C, F, G)
Viridans group streptococci

Aerobic Gram-Negative Microorganisms
Bordetella pertussis
Campylobacter jejuni
Haemophilus ducreyi
Legionella pneumophila

Anaerobic Microorganisms
Bacteroides bivius
Clostridium perfringens
Peptostreptococcus species

"Other" Microorganisms
Borrelia burgdorferi
Mycoplasma pneumoniae
Treponema pallidum
Ureaplasma urealyticum

Susceptibility Testing of Bacteria Excluding Mycobacteria
The *in vitro* potency of azithromycin is markedly affected by the pH of the microbiological growth medium during incubation. Incubation in a 10% CO_2 atmosphere will result in lowering of media pH (7.2 to 6.6) within 18 hours and in an apparent reduction of the *in vitro* potency of azithromycin. Thus, the initial pH of the growth medium should be 7.2–7.4, and the CO_2 content of the incubation atmosphere should be as low as practical.

Azithromycin can be solubilized for *in vitro* susceptibility testing by dissolving in a minimum amount of 95% ethanol and diluting to working concentration with water.

Dilution Techniques:
Quantitative methods are used to determine minimal inhibitory concentrations that provide reproducible estimates of the susceptibility of bacteria to antimicrobial compounds. One such standardized procedure uses a standardized dilution method[1] (broth, agar or microdilution) or equivalent with azithromycin powder. The MIC values should be interpreted according to the following criteria:

MIC (μg/mL)	Interpretation
≤ 2	Susceptible (S)
4	Intermediate (I)
≥ 8	Resistant (R)

A report of "Susceptible" indicates that the pathogen is likely to respond to monotherapy with azithromycin. A report of "Intermediate" indicates that the result should be considered equivocal, and, if the microorganism is not fully susceptible to alternative, clinically feasible drugs, the test should be repeated. This category also provides a buffer zone which prevents small uncontrolled technical factors from causing major discrepancies in interpretation. A report of "Resistant" indicates that usually achievable drug concentrations are unlikely to be inhibitory and that other therapy should be selected.

Measurement of MIC or MBC and achieved antimicrobial compound concentrations may be appropriate to guide therapy in some infections. (See CLINICAL PHARMACOLOGY section for further information on drug concentrations achieved in infected body sites and other pharmacokinetic properties of this antimicrobial drug product.)

Standardized susceptibility test procedures require the use of laboratory control microorganisms. Standard azithromycin powder should provide the following MIC values:

Microorganism	MIC (μg/mL)
Escherichia coli ATCC 25922	2.0–8.0
Enterococcus faecalis ATCC 29212	1.0–4.0
Staphylococcus aureus ATCC 29213	0.25–1.0

Diffusion Techniques:
Quantitative methods that require measurement of zone diameters also provide reproducible estimates of the susceptibility of bacteria to antimicrobial compounds. One such standardized procedure[2] that has been recommended for use with disks to test the susceptibility of microorganisms to azithromycin uses the 15-μg azithromycin disk. Interpretation involves the correlation of the diameter obtained in the disk test with the minimal inhibitory concentration (MIC) for azithromycin.

Reports from the laboratory providing results of the standard single-disk susceptibility test with a 15 μg azithromycin disk should be interpreted according to the following criteria:

Zone Diameter (mm)	Interpretation
≥ 18	(S) Susceptible
14–17	(I) Intermediate
≤ 13	(R) Resistant

Interpretation should be as stated above for results using dilution techniques.

As with standardized dilution techniques, diffusion methods require the use of laboratory control microorganisms. The 15-μg azithromycin disk should provide the following zone diameters in these laboratory test quality control strains:

Microorganism	Zone Diameter (mm)
Staphylococcus aureus ATCC 25923	21–26

***In Vitro* Activity of Azithromycin Against Mycobacteria.**
Azithromycin has demonstrated *in vitro* activity against *Mycobacterium avium* complex (MAC) organisms. While gene probe techniques may be used to distinguish between *M. avium* and *M. intracellulare*, many studies only reported results on *M. avium* complex (MAC) isolates. Azithromycin has also been shown to be active against phagocytized *M. avium* complex (MAC) organisms in mouse and human macrophage cell cultures as well as in the beige mouse infection model.

Various *in vitro* methodologies employing broth or solid media at different pHs, with and without oleic acid-albumin dextrose-catalase (OADC), have been used to determine azithromycin MIC values for *Mycobacterium avium* complex strains. In general, azithromycin MIC values decreased 4 to 8 fold as the pH of Middlebrook 7H11 agar media increased from 6.6 to 7.4. At pH 7.4, azithromycin MIC values determined with Mueller-Hinton agar were 4 fold higher than that observed with Middlebrook 7H12 media at the same pH. Utilization of oleic acid-albumin-dextrose-catalase (OADC) in these assays has been shown to further alter MIC values. The relationship between azithromycin and clarithromycin MIC values has not been established. In general, azithromycin MIC values were observed to be 2 to 32 fold higher than clarithromycin independent of the susceptibility method employed.

The ability to correlate MIC values and plasma drug levels is difficult as azithromycin concentrates in macrophages and tissues. (See CLINICAL PHARMACOLOGY)

Drug Resistance:
Complete cross-resistance between azithromycin and clarithromycin has been observed with *Mycobacterium avium* complex (MAC) isolates. In most isolates, a single point mutation at a position that is homologous to the *Escherichia coli* positions 2058 or 2059 on the 23S rRNA gene is the mechanism producing this cross-resistance pattern.[3,4] *Mycobacterium avium* complex (MAC) isolates exhibiting cross-resistance show an increase in azithromycin MICs to ≥128 μg/mL with clarithromycin MICs increasing to ≥32 μg/mL. These MIC values were determined employing the radiometric broth dilution susceptibility testing method with Middlebrook 7H12 medium. The clinical significance of azithromycin and clarithromycin cross-resistance is not fully understood at this time but preclinical data suggest that reduced activity to both agents will occur after *M. avium* complex strains produce the 23S rRNA mutation.

Susceptibility testing for *Mycobacterium avium* complex (MAC):
The disk diffusion techniques and dilution methods for susceptibility testing against Gram-positive and Gram-negative bacteria should not be used for determining azithromycin MIC values against mycobacteria. *In vitro*

susceptibility testing methods and diagnostic products currently available for determining minimal inhibitory concentration (MIC) values against *Mycobacterium avium* complex (MAC) organisms have not been standardized or validated. Azithromycin MIC values will vary depending on the susceptibility testing method employed, composition and pH of media and the utilization of nutritional supplements. Breakpoints to determine whether clinical isolates of *M. avium* or *M. intracellulare* are susceptible or resistant to azithromycin have not been established.

The clinical relevance of azithromycin *in vitro* susceptibility test results for other mycobacterial species, including *Mycobacterium tuberculosis*, using any susceptibility testing method has not been determined.

INDICATIONS AND USAGE

ZITHROMAX® (azithromycin) is indicated for the treatment of patients with mild to moderate infections (pneumonia: see WARNINGS) caused by susceptible strains of the designated microorganisms in the specific conditions listed below.

Lower Respiratory Tract:

Acute bacterial exacerbations of chronic obstructive pulmonary disease due to *Haemophilus influenzae, Moraxella catarrhalis*, or *Streptococcus pneumoniae*.

Community-acquired pneumonia of mild severity due to *Streptococcus pneumoniae* or *Haemophilus influenzae* in patients appropriate for outpatient oral therapy.

NOTE: Azithromycin should not be used in patients with pneumonia who are judged to be inappropriate for outpatient oral therapy because of moderate to severe illness or risk factors such as any of the following:

patients with nosocomially acquired infections,
patients with known or suspected bacteremia,
patients requiring hospitalization,
elderly or debilitated patients, or
patients with significant underlying health problems that may compromise their ability to respond to their illness (including immunodeficiency or functional asplenia).

Upper Respiratory Tract:

Streptococcal pharyngitis/tonsillitis—As an alternative to first line therapy of acute pharyngitis/tonsillitis due to *Streptococcus pyogenes* occurring in individuals who cannot use first line therapy.

NOTE: Penicillin is the usual drug of choice in the treatment of *Streptococcus pyogenes* infection and the prophylaxis of rheumatic fever. ZITHROMAX® is often effective in the eradication of susceptible strains of *Streptococcus pyogenes* from the nasopharynx. Data establishing efficacy of azithromycin in subsequent prevention of rheumatic fever are not available.

Skin and Skin Structure

Uncomplicated skin and skin structure infections due to *Staphylococcus aureus, Streptococcus pyogenes*, or *Streptococcus agalactiae*. Abscesses usually require surgical drainage.

Sexually Transmitted Diseases

Non-gonococcal urethritis and cervicitis due to *Chlamydia trachomatis*.

ZITHROMAX®, at the recommended dose, should not be relied upon to treat gonorrhea or syphilis. Antimicrobial agents used in high doses for short periods of time to treat non-gonococcal urethritis may mask or delay the symptoms of incubating gonorrhea or syphilis. All patients with sexually-transmitted urethritis or cervicitis should have a serologic test for syphilis and appropriate cultures for gonorrhea performed at the time of diagnosis. Appropriate antimicrobial therapy and follow-up tests for these diseases should be initiated if infection is confirmed.

Appropriate culture and susceptibility tests should be performed before treatment to determine the causative organism and its susceptibility to azithromycin. Therapy with ZITHROMAX® may be initiated before results of these tests are known; once the results become available, antimicrobial therapy should be adjusted accordingly.

Mycobacterial Infections

Prophylaxis of Disseminated *Mycobacterium avium* complex (MAC) Disease

ZITHROMAX®, taken alone or in combination with rifabutin at its approved dose, is indicated for the prevention of disseminated *Mycobacterium avium* complex (MAC) disease in persons with advanced HIV infection. (See DOSAGE AND ADMINISTRATION, CLINICAL STUDIES)

Treatment of Disseminated *Mycobacterium avium* complex (MAC) Disease

ZITHROMAX®, taken in combination with ethambutol, is indicated for the treatment of disseminated MAC infections in persons with advanced HIV infection. (See DOSAGE AND ADMINISTRATION, CLINICAL STUDIES)

CONTRAINDICATIONS

ZITHROMAX® is contraindicated in patients with known hypersensitivity to azithromycin, erythromycin, or any macrolide antibiotic.

WARNINGS

Rare serious allergic reactions, including angioedema and anaphylaxis, have been reported rarely in patients on azithromycin therapy. (See **CONTRAINDICATIONS.**) Despite initially successful symptomatic treatment of the allergic symptoms, when symptomatic therapy was discontinued, the allergic symptoms **recurred soon thereafter in some patients without further azithromycin exposure.** These patients required prolonged periods of observation and symptomatic treatment. The relationship of these episodes to the long tissue half-life of azithromycin and subsequent prolonged exposure to antigen is unknown at present. If an allergic reaction occurs, the drug should be discontinued and appropriate therapy should be instituted. Physicians should be aware that reappearance of the allergic symptoms may occur when symptomatic therapy is discontinued.

In the treatment of pneumonia, azithromycin has only been shown to be safe and effective in the treatment of community-acquired pneumonia of mild severity due to *Streptococcus pneumoniae* or *Haemophilus influenzae* in patients appropriate for outpatient oral therapy. Azithromycin should not be used in patients with pneumonia who are judged to be inappropriate for outpatient oral therapy because of moderate to severe illness or risk factors such as any of the following: patients with nosocomially acquired infections, patients with known or suspected bacteremia, patients requiring hospitalization, elderly or debilitated patients, or patients with significant underlying health problems that may compromise their ability to respond to their illness (including immunodeficiency or functional asplenia).

Pseudomembranous colitis has been reported with nearly all antibacterial agents and may range in severity from mild to life-threatening. Therefore, it is important to consider this diagnosis in patients who present with diarrhea subsequent to the administration of antibacterial agents.

Treatment with antibacterial agents alters the normal flora of the colon and may permit overgrowth of clostridia. Studies indicate that a toxin produced by *Clostridium difficile* is a primary cause of "antibiotic-associated colitis."

After the diagnosis of pseudomembranous colitis has been established, therapeutic measures should be initiated. Mild cases of pseudomembranous colitis usually respond to discontinuation of the drug alone. In moderate to severe cases, consideration should be given to management with fluids and electrolytes, protein supplementation, and treatment with an antibacterial drug clinically effective against *Clostridium difficile* colitis.

PRECAUTIONS

General: Because azithromycin is principally eliminated via the liver, caution should be exercised when azithromycin is administered to patients with impaired hepatic function. There are no data regarding azithromycin usage in patients with renal impairment; thus, caution should be exercised when prescribing azithromycin in these patients.

The following adverse events have been reported with macrolide products: ventricular arrhythmias, including ventricular tachycardia and *torsades de pointes*, in individuals with prolonged QT intervals.

There has been a spontaneous report from the post-marketing experience of a patient with previous history of arrhythmias who experienced *torsades de pointes* and subsequent myocardial infarction following a course of azithromycin therapy.

Information for Patients:

Patients should be cautioned to take ZITHROMAX® capsules at least one hour prior to a meal or at least two hours after a meal. Azithromycin capsules should not be taken with food.

ZITHROMAX® tablets may be taken with or without food. However, increased tolerability has been observed when tablets are taken with food.

ZITHROMAX® for oral suspension in single 1 g packets can be taken with or without food after constitution.

Patients should also be cautioned not to take aluminum- and magnesium-containing antacids and azithromycin simultaneously.

The patient should be directed to discontinue azithromycin immediately and contact a physician if any signs of an allergic reaction occur.

Drug Interactions: Aluminum- and magnesium-containing antacids reduce the peak serum levels (rate) but not the AUC (extent) of azithromycin (500 mg) absorption.

Administration of cimetidine (800 mg) two hours prior to azithromycin had no effect on azithromycin (500 mg) absorption.

A single oral dose of 1200 mg azithromycin (2 × 600 mg ZITHROMAX® tablets) did not alter the pharmacokinetics of a single 800 mg oral dose of fluconazole in healthy adult subjects.

Total exposure (AUC) and half-life of azithromycin following the single oral tablet dose of 1200 mg were unchanged and the reduction in Cmax was not significant (mean decrease of 18%) by coadministration with 800 mg fluconazole.

A single oral dose of 1200 mg azithromycin (2 × 600 mg ZITHROMAX® tablets) had no significant effect on the pharmacokinetics of indinavir (800 mg indinavir tid for 5 days) in healthy adult subjects.

Coadministration of a single oral dose of 1200 mg azithromycin (2 × 600 mg ZITHROMAX® tablets) with steady-state nelfinavir (750 mg tid) to healthy adult subjects produced a decrease of approximately 15% in mean AUC_{0-8} of nelfinavir and its M8 metabolite. Mean Cmax of nelfinavir and its M8 metabolite were not significantly affected. No dosage adjustment of nelfinavir is required when nelfinavir is coadministered with azithromycin.

Coadministration of nelfinavir (750 mg tid) at steady state with a single oral dose of 1200 mg azithromycin increased the mean $AUC_{0-\infty}$ of azithromycin by approximately a factor of 2-times (range of up to 4 times) of that when azithromycin was given alone. The mean Cmax of azithromycin was also increased by approximately a factor of 2-times (range of up to 5 times) of that when azithromycin was given alone. Dose adjustment of azithromycin is not recommended. However, when administered in conjunction with nelfinavir, close monitoring for known side effects of azithromycin, such as liver enzyme abnormalities and hearing impairment, is warranted. (See ADVERSE REACTIONS.)

Following administration of trimethoprim/sulfamethoxazole DS (160 mg/800 mg) for 7 days to healthy adult subjects, coadministration of 1200 mg azithromycin (2 × 600 mg ZITHROMAX® tablets) on the 7th day had no significant effects on peak concentrations (C_{max}), total exposure (AUC), and the urinary excretion of either trimethoprim or sulfamethoxazole.

Coadministration of trimethoprim/sulfamethoxazole DS for 7 days had no significant effect on the peak concentration (C_{max}) and total exposure (AUC) of azithromycin following administration of the single 1200 mg tablet dose to healthy adult subjects.

Administration of a 600 mg single oral dose of azithromycin had no effect on the pharmacokinetics of efavirenz given at 400 mg doses for 7 days to healthy adult subjects.

Efavirenz, when administered at a dose of 400 mg for seven days produced a 22% increase in the C_{max} of azithromycin administered as a 600 mg single oral dose, while the AUC of azithromycin was not affected.

Azithromycin (500 mg Day 1, 250 mg Days 2–5) did not affect the plasma levels or pharmacokinetics of theophylline administered as a single intravenous dose. The effect of azithromycin on the plasma levels or pharmacokinetics of theophylline administered in multiple doses resulting in therapeutic steady-state levels of theophylline is not known. However, concurrent use of macrolides and theophylline has been associated with increases in the serum concentrations of theophylline. Therefore, until further data are available, prudent medical practice dictates careful monitoring of plasma theophylline levels in patients receiving azithromycin and theophylline concomitantly.

Azithromycin (500 mg Day 1, 250 mg Days 2–5) did not affect the prothrombin time response to a single dose of warfarin. However, prudent medical practice dictates careful monitoring of prothrombin time in all patients treated with azithromycin and warfarin concomitantly. Concurrent use of macrolides and warfarin in clinical practice has been associated with increased anticoagulant effects.

Dose adjustments are not indicated when azithromycin and zidovudine are coadministered. When zidovudine (100 mg q3h ×5) was coadministered with daily azithromycin (600 mg, n=5 or 1200 mg, n=7), mean C_{max}, AUC and Clr increased by 26% (CV 54%), 10% (CV 26%) and 38% (CV 114%), respectively. The mean AUC of phosphorylated zidovudine increased by 75% (CV 95%), while zidovudine glucuronide C_{max} and AUC increased by less than 10%. In another study, addition of 1 gram azithromycin per week to a regimen of 10 mg/kg daily zidovudine resulted in 25% (CV 70%) and 13% (CV 37%) increases in zidovudine C_{max} and AUC, respectively. Zidovudine glucuronide mean C_{max} and AUC increased by 16% (CV 61%) and 8.0% (CV 32%), respectively.

Doses of 1200 mg/day azithromycin for 14 days in 6 subjects increased C_{max} of concurrently administered didanosine (200 mg *q*.12h) by 44% (54% CV) and AUC by 14% (23% CV). However, none of these changes were significantly different from those produced in a parallel placebo control group of subjects.

Preliminary data suggest that coadministration of azithromycin and rifabutin did not markedly affect the mean serum concentrations of either drug. Administration of 250 mg azithromycin daily for 10 days (500 mg on the first day) produced mean concentrations of azithromycin 1 day after the last dose of 53 ng/mL when coadministered with 300 mg daily rifabutin and 49 mg/mL when coadministered with placebo. Mean concentrations 5 days after the last dose were 23 ng/mL and 21 ng/mL in the two groups of subjects. Administration of 300 mg rifabutin for 10 days produced mean concentrations of rifabutin one half day after the last dose of 60 mg/ml when coadministered with daily 250 mg azithromycin and 71 ng/mL when coadministered with placebo. Mean concentrations 5 days after the last dose were 8.1 ng/mL and 9.2 ng/mL in the two groups of subjects.

The following drug interactions have not been reported in clinical trials with azithromycin; however, no specific drug interaction studies have been performed to evaluate potential drug-drug interaction. Nonetheless, they have been observed with macrolide products. Until further data are developed regarding drug interactions when azithromycin and these drugs are used concomitantly, careful monitoring of patients is advised:

Digoxin—elevated digoxin levels.

Ergotamine or dihydroergotamine—acute ergot toxicity characterized by severe peripheral vasospasm and dysesthesia.

Triazolam—decrease the clearance of triazolam and thus may increase the pharmacologic effect of triazolam.

Drugs metabolized by the cytochrome P^{450} system—elevations of serum carbamazepine, cyclosporine, hexobarbital, and phenytoin levels.

Laboratory Test Interactions: There are no reported laboratory test interactions.

Carcinogenesis, Mutagenesis, Impairment of Fertility: Long-term studies in animals have not been performed to

Continued on next page

Zithromax Caps/Tabs/O.S.—Cont.

evaluate carcinogenic potential. Azithromycin has shown no mutagenic potential in standard laboratory tests: mouse lymphoma assay, human lymphocyte clastogenic assay, and mouse bone marrow clastogenic assay.

Pregnancy: Teratogenic Effects. Pregnancy Category B: Reproduction studies have been performed in rats and mice at doses up to moderately maternally toxic dose levels (i.e., 200 mg/kg/day). These doses, based on a mg/m^2 basis, are estimated to be 4 and 2 times, respectively, the human daily dose of 500 mg.

With regard to the MAC treatment dose of 600 mg daily, on a mg/m^2/day basis, the doses in rats and mice are approximately 3.3 and 1.7 times the human dose, respectively.

With regard to the MAC prophylaxis dose of 1200 mg weekly, on a mg/m^2/day basis, the doses in rats and mice are approximately 2 and 1 times the human dose, respectively. No evidence of impaired fertility or harm to the fetus due to azithromycin was found. There are, however, no adequate and well-controlled studies in pregnant women. Because animal reproduction studies are not always predictive of human response, azithromycin should be used during pregnancy only if clearly needed.

Nursing Mothers: It is not known whether azithromycin is excreted in human milk. Because many drugs are excreted in human milk, caution should be exercised when azithromycin is administered to a nursing woman.

Pediatric Use:

In controlled clinical studies, azithromycin has been administered to pediatric patients ranging in age from 6 months to 12 years. For information regarding the use of ZITHROMAX (azithromycin for oral suspension) in the treatment of pediatric patients, please refer to the INDICATIONS AND USAGE and DOSAGE AND ADMINISTRATION sections of the prescribing information for ZITHROMAX (azithromycin for oral suspension) 100 mg/5 mL and 200 mg/5 mL bottles.

Safety in HIV-Infected Pediatric Patients: Safety and efficacy of azithromycin for the prevention or treatment of MAC in HIV-infected children have not been established. Safety data are available for 72 children 5 months to 18 years of age (mean 7 years) who received azithromycin for treatment of opportunistic infections. The mean duration of therapy was 242 days (range 3–2004 days) at doses of <1 to 52 mg/kg/day (mean 12 mg/kg/day). Adverse events were similar to those observed in the adult population, most of which involved the gastrointestinal tract. Treatment related reversible hearing impairment in children was observed in 4 subjects (5.6%). Two (2.8%) children prematurely discontinued treatment due to side effects: one due to back pain and one due to abdominal pain, hot and cold flushes, dizziness, headache, and numbness. A third child discontinued due to a laboratory abnormality (eosinophilia). The protocols upon which these data are based specified a daily dose of 10–20 mg/kg/day (oral and/or i.v.) of azithromycin.

Geriatric Use: Pharmacokinetic parameters in older volunteers (65–85 years old) were similar to those in younger volunteers (18–40 years old) for the 5-day therapeutic regimen. Dosage adjustment does not appear to be necessary for older patients with normal renal and hepatic function receiving treatment with this dosage regimen. (See CLINICAL PHARMACOLOGY.)

Geriatric Patients with Opportunistic Infections, Including *Mycobacterium avium* complex (MAC) Disease: Safety data are available for 30 patients (65–94 years old) treated with azithromycin at doses >300 mg/day for a mean of 207 days. These patients were treated for a variety of opportunistic infections, including MAC. The side effect profile was generally similar to that seen in younger patients, except for a higher incidence of side effects relating to the gastrointestinal system and to reversible impairment of hearing. (See DOSAGE AND ADMINISTRATION.)

Cumulative Incidence Rate, %: Placebo (n=89)

Month	MAC Free and Alive	MAC	Adverse Experience	Lost to Follow-up
6	69.7	13.5	6.7	10.1
12	47.2	19.1	15.7	18.0
18	37.1	22.5	18.0	22.5

Cumulative Incidence Rate, %: Azithromycin (n=85)

Month	MAC Free and Alive	MAC	Adverse Experience	Lost to Follow-up
6	84.7	3.5	9.4	2.4
12	63.5	8.2	16.5	11.8
18	44.7	11.8	25.9	17.6

Cumulative Incidence Rate, %: Rifabutin (n=223)

Month	MAC Free and Alive	MAC	Adverse Experience	Lost to Follow-up
6	83.4	7.2	8.1	1.3
12	60.1	15.2	16.1	8.5
18	40.8	21.5	24.2	13.5

Cumulative Incidence Rate, %: Azithromycin (n=223)

Month	MAC Free and Alive	MAC	Adverse Experience	Lost to Follow-up
6	85.2	3.6	5.8	5.4
12	65.5	7.6	16.1	10.8
18	45.3	12.1	23.8	18.8

Cumulative Incidence Rate, %: Azithromycin/Rifabutin Combination (n=218)

Month	MAC Free and Alive	MAC	Adverse Experience	Lost to Follow-up
6	89.4	1.8	5.5	3.2
12	71.6	2.8	15.1	10.6
18	49.1	6.4	29.4	15.1

ADVERSE REACTIONS

In clinical trials, most of the reported side effects were mild to moderate in severity and were reversible upon discontinuation of the drug. Approximately 0.7% of the patients from the multiple-dose clinical trials discontinued ZITHROMAX® (azithromycin) therapy because of treatment-related side effects. Most of the side effects leading to discontinuation were related to the gastrointestinal tract, e.g., nausea, vomiting, diarrhea, or abdominal pain. Rarely but potentially serious side effects were angioedema and cholestatic jaundice.

Clinical:

Multiple-dose regimen:

Overall, the most common side effects in adult patients receiving a multiple-dose regimen of ZITHROMAX® were related to the gastrointestinal system with diarrhea/loose stools (5%), nausea (3%), and abdominal pain (3%) being the most frequently reported.

No other side effects occurred in patients on the multiple-dose regimen of ZITHROMAX® with a frequency greater than 1%. Side effects that occurred with a frequency of 1% or less included the following:

Cardiovascular: Palpitations, chest pain.

Gastrointestinal: Dyspepsia, flatulence, vomiting, melena, and cholestatic jaundice.

Genitourinary: Monilia, vaginitis, and nephritis.

Nervous System: Dizziness, headache, vertigo, and somnolence.

General: Fatigue.

Allergic: Rash, photosensitivity, and angioedema.

Chronic therapy with 1200 mg weekly regimen: The nature of side effects seen with the 1200 mg weekly dosing regimen for the prevention of *Mycobacterium avium* infection in severely immunocompromised HIV-infected patients were similar to those seen with short term dosing regimens. (See CLINICAL STUDIES.)

Chronic therapy with 600 mg daily regimen combined with ethambutol: The nature of side effects seen with the 600 mg daily dosing regimen for the treatment of *Mycobacterium avium* complex infection in severely immunocompromised HIV-infected patients were similar to those seen with short term dosing regimens. Five percent of patients experienced reversible hearing impairment in the pivotal clinical trial for the treatment of disseminated MAC in patients with AIDS. Hearing impairment has been reported with macrolide antibiotics, especially at higher doses. Other treatment related side effects occurring in >5% of subjects and seen at any time during a median of 87.5 days of therapy include: abdominal pain (14%), nausea (14%), vomiting (13%), diarrhea (12%), flatulence (5%), headache (5%) and abnormal vision (5%). Discontinuations from treatment due to laboratory abnormalities or side effects considered related to study drug occurred in 8/88 (9.1%) of subjects.

Single 1-gram dose regimen: Overall, the most common side effects in patients receiving a single-dose regimen of 1 gram of ZITHROMAX® were related to the gastrointestinal system and were more frequently reported than in patients receiving the multiple-dose regimen.

Side effects that occurred in patients on the single one-gram dosing regimen of ZITHROMAX® with a frequency of 1% or greater included diarrhea/loose stools (7%), nausea (5%), abdominal pain (5%), vomiting (2%), dyspepsia (1%), and vaginitis (1%).

Post-Marketing Experience:

Adverse events reported with azithromycin during the post-marketing period in adult and/or pediatric patients for which a causal relationship may not be established include:

Allergic: Arthralgia, edema, urticaria, angioedema.

Cardiovascular: Arrhythmias including ventricular tachycardia, hypotension.

Gastrointestinal: Anorexia, constipation, dyspepsia, flatulence, vomiting/diarrhea rarely resulting in dehydration, pseudomembranous colitis, pancreatitis, oral candidiasis and rare reports of tongue discoloration.

General: Asthenia, paresthesia, fatigue, malaise and anaphylaxis (rarely fatal).

Genitourinary: Interstitial nephritis and acute renal failure, vaginitis.

Hematopoietic: Thrombocytopenia.

Liver/Biliary: Abnormal liver function including hepatitis and cholestatic jaundice, as well as rare cases of hepatic necrosis and hepatic failure, some of which have resulted in death.

Nervous System: Convulsions, dizziness/vertigo, headache, somnolence, hyperactivity, nervousness, agitation and syncope.

Psychiatric: Aggressive reaction and anxiety.

Skin/Appendages: Pruritus, rarely serious skin reactions including erythema multiforme, Stevens Johnson Syndrome, and toxic epidermal necrolysis.

Special Senses: Hearing disturbances including hearing loss, deafness, and/or tinnitus, rare reports of taste perversion.

Laboratory Abnormalities:

Significant abnormalities (irrespective of drug relationship) occurring during the clinical trials were reported as follows: With an incidence of 1–2%, elevated serum creatine phosphokinase, potassium, ALT (SGPT), GGT, and AST (SGOT). With an incidence of less than 1%, leukopenia, neutropenia, decreased platelet count, elevated serum alkaline phosphatase, bilirubin, BUN, creatinine, blood glucose, LDH, and phosphate.

When follow-up was provided, changes in laboratory tests appeared to be reversible.

In multiple-dose clinical trials involving more than 3000 patients, 3 patients discontinued therapy because of treatment-related liver enzyme abnormalities and 1 because of a renal function abnormality.

In a phase I drug interaction study performed in normal volunteers, 1 of 6 subjects given the combination of azithromycin and rifabutin, 1 of 7 given rifabutin alone and 0 of 6 given azithromycin alone developed a clinically significant neutropenia (<500 cells/mm^3).

Laboratory abnormalities seen in clinical trials for the prevention of disseminated *Mycobacterium avium* disease in severely immunocompromised HIV-infected patients are presented in the CLINICAL STUDIES section.

Chronic therapy (median duration: 87.5 days, range: 1–229 days) that resulted in laboratory abnormalities in >5% subjects with normal baseline values in the pivotal trial for treatment of disseminated MAC in severely immunocompromised HIV infected patients treated with azithromycin 600 mg daily in combination with ethambutol include: a reduction in absolute neutrophils to <50% of the lower limit of normal (10/52, 19%) and an increase to five times the upper limit of normal in alkaline phosphatase (3/35, 9%). These findings in subjects with normal baseline values are similar when compared to all subjects for analyses of neutrophil reductions (22/75 [29%]) and elevated alkaline phosphatase (16/80 [20%]). Causality of these laboratory abnormalities due to the use of study drug has not been established.

DOSAGE AND ADMINISTRATION

(See INDICATIONS AND USAGE.)

ZITHROMAX® capsules should be given at least 1 hour before or 2 hours after a meal.

ZITHROMAX® capsules should not be mixed with or taken with food.

ZITHROMAX® for oral suspension (single dose 1 g packet) can be taken with or without food after constitution. Not for pediatric use. For pediatric suspension, please refer to the INDICATIONS AND USAGE and DOSAGE AND ADMINISTRATION sections of the prescribing information for ZITHROMAX (azithromycin for oral suspension) 100 mg/5 mL and 200 mg/5 mL bottles.

ZITHROMAX® tablets may be taken without regard to food. However, increased tolerability has been observed when tablets are taken with food.

The recommended dose of ZITHROMAX® or the treatment of individuals 16 years of age and older with mild to moderate acute bacterial exacerbations of chronic obstructive pulmonary disease, pneumonia, pharyngitis/tonsillitis (as second line therapy), and uncomplicated skin and skin structure infections due to the indicated organisms is: 500 mg as a single dose on the first day followed by 250 mg once daily on Days 2 through 5 for a total dose of 1.5 grams of ZITHROMAX®.

The recommended dose of ZITHROMAX® for the treatment of non-gonococcal urethritis and cervicitis due to *C. trachomatis* is: a single 1 gram (1000 mg) dose of ZITHROMAX®. This dose can be administered as four 250 mg capsules or as one single dose packet (1 g).

Prevention of Disseminated MAC Infections

The recommended dose of ZITHROMAX® for the prevention of disseminated *Mycobacterium avium* complex (MAC) disease is: 1200 mg taken once weekly. This dose of ZITHROMAX® may be combined with the approved dosage regimen of rifabutin.

Treatment of Disseminated MAC Infections

ZITHROMAX® should be taken at a daily dose of 600 mg, in combination with ethambutol at the recommended daily dose of 15 mg/kg. Other antimycobacterial drugs that have shown *in vitro* activity against MAC may be added to the regimen of azithromycin plus ethambutol at the discretion of the physician or health care provider.

DIRECTIONS FOR ADMINISTRATION OF ZITHROMAX® for oral suspension in the single dose packet (1 g): The entire contents of the packet should be mixed thoroughly with two ounces (approximately 60 mL) of water. Drink the entire contents immediately; add an additional two ounces of water, mix, and drink to assure complete consumption of dosage. **The single dose packet should not be used to administer doses other than 1000 mg of azithromycin. This packet not for pediatric use.**

HOW SUPPLIED

ZITHROMAX® capsules (imprinted with "Pfizer 305") are supplied in red opaque hard-gelatin capsules containing azithromycin dihydrate equivalent to 250 mg of azithromycin. These are packaged in bottles and blister cards of 6 capsules (Z-PAKS®) as follows:

Bottles of 50	NDC 0069-3050-50
Boxes of 3 (Z-PAKS® of 6)	NDC 0069-3050-34
Unit Dose package of 50	NDC 0069-3050-86

Store capsules below 30°C (86°F).

ZITHROMAX® 600 mg tablets (engraved on front with "PFIZER" and on back with "308") are supplied as white, modified oval-shaped, film-coated tablets containing azithromycin dihydrate equivalent to 600 mg azithromycin. These are packaged in bottles of 30 tablets. ZITHROMAX® tablets are supplied as follows:

Bottles of 30	NDC 0069-3080-30

Tablets should be stored at or below 30°C (86°F).

ZITHROMAX® for oral suspension is supplied in single dose packets containing azithromycin dihydrate equivalent to 1 gram of azithromycin as follows:

Boxes of 10 Single Dose Packets (1 g)	NDC 0069-3051-07
Boxes of 3 Single Dose Packets (1 g)	NDC 0069-3051-75

Store single dose packets between 5° and 30°C (41° and 86°F).

CLINICAL STUDIES IN PATIENTS WITH ADVANCED HIV INFECTION FOR THE PREVENTION AND TREATMENT OF DISEASE DUE TO DISSEMINATED *MYCOBACTERIUM AVIUM* COMPLEX (MAC) (See INDICATIONS AND USAGE):

Prevention of Disseminated MAC Disease

Two randomized, double blind clinical trials were performed in patients with CD4 counts <100 cells/μL. The first study (155) compared azithromycin (1200 mg once weekly) to placebo and enrolled 182 patients with a mean CD4 count of 35 cells/μL. The second study (174) randomized 723 patients to either azithromycin (1200 mg once weekly), rifabutin (300 mg daily) or the combination of both. The mean CD4 count was 51 cells/μL. The primary endpoint in these studies was disseminated MAC disease. Other endpoints included the incidence of clinically significant MAC disease and discontinuations from therapy for drug-related side effects.

MAC bacteremia

In trial 155, 85 patients randomized to receive azithromycin and 89 patients randomized to receive placebo met study entrance criteria. Cumulative incidences at 6, 12 and 18 months of the possible outcomes are in the following table:

[See table at top of previous page]

The difference in the one year cumulative incidence rates of disseminated MAC disease (placebo-azithromycin) is 10.9%. This difference is statistically significant (p=0.037) with a 95% confidence interval for this difference of (0.8%, 20.9%). The comparable number of patients experiencing adverse events and the fewer number of patients lost to follow-up on azithromycin should be taken into account when interpreting the significance of this difference.

INCIDENCE OF ONE OR MORE TREATMENT RELATED* ADVERSE EVENTS IN HIV INFECTED PATIENTS RECEIVING PROPHYLAXIS FOR DISSEMINATED MAC OVER APPROXIMATELY 1 YEAR**

	Study 155		Study 174		
	Placebo (N=91)	Azithromycin 1200 mg weekly (N=89)	Azithromycin 1200 mg weekly (N=233)	Rifabutin 300 mg daily (N=236)	Azithromycin + Rifabutin (N=224)
Mean Duration of Therapy (days)	303.8	402.9	315	296.1	344.4
Discontinuation of Therapy	2.3	8.2	13.5	15.9	22.7
Autonomic Nervous System					
Mouth Dry	0	0	0	3.0	2.7
Central Nervous System					
Dizziness	0	1.1	3.9	1.7	0.4
Headache	0	0	3.0	5.5	4.5
Gastrointestinal					
Diarrhea	15.4	52.8	50.2	19.1	50.9
Loose Stools	6.6	19.1	12.9	3.0	9.4
Abdominal Pain	6.6	27	32.2	12.3	31.7
Dyspepsia	1.1	9	4.7	1.7	1.8
Flatulence	4.4	9	10.7	5.1	5.8
Nausea	11	32.6	27.0	16.5	28.1
Vomiting	1.1	6.7	9.0	3.8	5.8
General					
Fever	1.1	0	2.1	4.2	4.9
Fatigue	0	2.2	3.9	2.1	3.1
Malaise	0	1.1	0.4	0	2.2
Musculoskeletal					
Arthralgia	0	0	3.0	4.2	7.1
Psychiatric					
Anorexia	1.1	0	2.1	2.1	3.1
Skin & Appendages					
Pruritus	3.3	0	3.9	3.4	7.6
Rash	3.2	3.4	8.1	9.4	11.1
Skin discoloration	0	0	0	2.1	2.2
Special Senses					
Tinnitus	4.4	3.4	0.9	1.3	0.9
Hearing Decreased	2.2	1.1	0.9	0.4	0
Uveitis	0	0	0.4	1.3	1.8
Taste Perversion	0	0	1.3	2.5	1.3

* Includes those events considered possibly or probably related to study drug
** >2% adverse event rates for any group (except uveitis).

Prophylaxis Against Disseminated MAC Abnormal Laboratory Values*

		Placebo	Azithromycin 1200 mg weekly	Rifabutin 300 mg daily	Azithromycin & Rifabutin
Hemoglobin	<8 g/dl	1/51 2%	4/170 2%	4/114 4%	8/107 8%
Platelet Count	$<50 \times 10^3/mm^3$	1/71 1%	4/260 2%	2/182 1%	6/181 3%
WBC Count	$<1 \times 10^3/mm^3$	0/8 0%	2/70 3%	2/47 4%	0/43 0%
Neutrophils	$<500/mm^3$	0/26 0%	4/106 4%	3/82 4%	2/78 3%
SGOT	>5 × ULN[a]	1/41 2%	8/158 5%	3/121 3%	6/114 5%
SGPT	>5 × ULN	0/49 0%	8/166 5%	3/130 2%	5/117 4%
Alk Phos	>5 × ULN	1/80 1%	4/247 2%	2/172 1%	3/164 2%

[a]=Upper Limit of Normal
*excludes subjects outside of the relevant normal range at baseline

Response to therapy of patients taking ethambutol and either azithromycin 600 mg qd or clarithromycin 500 mg bid

	Azithromycin 600 mg qd	Clarithromycin 500 mg bid	**95.1% CI on difference
Patients with positive culture at baseline	68	57	
Week 24			
Two consecutive negative blood cultures*	31/68 (46%)	32/57 (56%)	[−28, 7]
Mortality	16/68 (24%)	15/57 (26%)	[−18, 13]

* Primary endpoint

** [95% confidence interval] on difference in rates (azithromycin-clarithromycin)

In trial 174, 223 patients randomized to receive rifabutin, 223 patients randomized to receive azithromycin, and 218 patients randomized to receive both rifabutin and azithromycin met study entrance criteria. Cumulative incidences at 6, 12 and 18 months of the possible outcomes are recorded in the following table:

[See table at top of previous page]

Comparing the cumulative one year incidence rates, azithromycin monotherapy is at least as effective as rifabutin monotherapy. The difference (rifabutin-azithromycin) in the one year rates (7.6%) is statistically significant (p=0.022) with an adjusted 95% confidence interval (0.9%, 14.3%). Additionally, azithromycin/rifabutin combination therapy is more effective than rifabutin alone. The difference (rifabutin-azithromycin/rifabutin) in the cumulative one year incidence rates (12.5%) is statistically significant (p<0.001) with an adjusted 95% confidence interval of (6.6%, 18.4%). The comparable number of patients experiencing adverse events and the fewer number of patients lost to follow-up on rifabutin should be taken into account when interpreting the significance of this difference.

In Study 174, sensitivity testing[5] was performed on all available MAC isolates from subjects randomized to either azithromycin, rifabutin or the combination. The distribution of MIC values for azithromycin from susceptibility testing of the breakthrough isolates was similar between study arms. As the efficacy of azithromycin in the treatment of disseminated MAC has not been established, the clinical relevance of these *in vitro* MICs as an indicator of susceptibility or resistance is not known.

Clinically Significant Disseminated MAC Disease

In association with the decreased incidence of bacteremia, patients in the groups randomized to either azithromycin alone or azithromycin in combination with rifabutin showed reductions in the signs and symptoms of disseminated MAC disease, including fever or night sweats, weight loss and anemia.

Discontinuations From Therapy For Drug-Related Side Effects

In Study 155, discontinuations for drug-related toxicity occurred in 8.2% of subjects treated with azithromycin and

Continued on next page

Zithromax Caps/Tabs/O.S.—Cont.

2.3% of those given placebo (p=0.121). In Study 174, more subjects discontinued from the combination of azithromycin and rifabutin (22.7%) than from azithromycin alone (13.5%; p=0.026) or rifabutin alone (15.9%; p=0.209).

Safety

As these patients with advanced HIV disease were taking multiple concomitant medications and experienced a variety of intercurrent illnesses, it was often difficult to attribute adverse events to study medication. Overall, the nature of side effects seen on the weekly dosage regimen of azithromycin over a period of approximately one year in patients with advanced HIV disease was similar to that previously reported for shorter course therapies.

[See first table at top of previous page]

Side effects related to the gastrointestinal tract were seen more frequently in patients receiving azithromycin than in those receiving placebo or rifabutin. In Study 174, 86% of diarrheal episodes were mild to moderate in nature with discontinuation of therapy for this reason occurring in only 9/233 (3.8%) of patients.

Changes in Laboratory Values

In these immunocompromised patients with advanced HIV infection, it was necessary to assess laboratory abnormalities developing on study with additional criteria if baseline values were outside the relevant normal range.

[See second table at top of previous page]

Treatment of Disseminated MAC Disease

One randomized, double blind clinical trial (Study 189) was performed in patients with disseminated MAC. In this trial, 246 HIV infected patients with disseminated MAC received either azithromycin 250 mg qd (N=65), azithromycin 600 mg qd (N=91) or clarithromycin 500 mg bid (N=90), each administered with ethambutol 15 mg/kg qd, for 24 weeks. Patients were cultured and clinically assessed every 3 weeks through week 12 and monthly thereafter through week 24. After week 24, patients were switched to any open label therapy at the discretion of the investigator and followed every 3 months through the last follow up visit of the trial. Patients were followed from the baseline visit for a period of up to 3.7 years (median: 9 months). MAC isolates recovered during study treatment or post-treatment were obtained whenever possible.

The primary endpoint was sterilization by week 24. Sterilization was based on data from the central laboratory, and was defined as two consecutive observed negative blood cultures for MAC, independent of missing culture data between the two negative observations. Analyses were performed on all randomized patients who had a positive baseline culture for MAC.

The azithromycin 250 mg arm was discontinued after an interim analysis at 12 weeks showed a significantly lower clearance of bacteremia compared to clarithromycin 500 mg bid.

Efficacy results for the azithromycin 600 mg qd and clarithromycin 500 mg bid treatment regimens are described in the following table:

[See third table at top of previous page]

The primary endpoint, rate of sterilization of blood cultures (two consecutive negative cultures) at 24 weeks, was lower in the azithromycin 600 mg qd group than in the clarithromycin 500 mg bid group.

Sterilization by Baseline Colony Count

Within both treatment groups, the sterilization rates at week 24 decreased as the range of MAC cfu/mL increased.

	Azithromycin 600 mg (N=68)	Clarithromycin 500 mg bid (N=57)
Groups Stratified by MAC Colony Counts at Baseline	No. (%) Subjects in Stratified Group Sterile at Week 24	No. (%) Subjects in Stratified Group Sterile at Week 24
≤ 10 cfu/mL	10/15 (66.7%)	12/17 (70.6%)
11–100 cfu/mL	13/28 (46.4%)	13/19 (68.4%)
101–1,000 cfu/mL	7/19 (36.8%)	5/13 (38.5%)
1,001–10,000 cfu/mL	1/5 (20.0%)	1/5 (20%)
>10,000 cfu/mL	0/1 (0.0%)	1/3 (33.3%)

Susceptibility Pattern of MAC Isolates:

Susceptibility testing was performed on MAC isolates recovered at baseline, at the time of breakthrough on therapy or during post-therapy follow-up. The T100 radiometric broth method was employed to determine azithromycin and clarithromycin MIC values. Azithromycin MIC values ranged from <4 to >256 μg/mL and clarithromycin MICs ranged from <1 to >32 μg/mL. The individual MAC susceptibility results demonstrated that azithromycin MIC values could be 4 to 32 fold higher than clarithromycin MIC values. During study treatment and post-treatment follow up for up to 3.7 years (median: 9 months) in study 189, a total of 6/68 (9%) and 6/57 (11%) of the patients randomized to azithromycin 600 mg daily and clarithromycin 500 mg bid, respectively, developed MAC blood culture isolates that had a sharp increase in MIC values. All twelve MAC isolates had azithromycin MIC's ≥256 μg/mL and clarithromycin MIC's >32 μg/mL. These high MIC values suggest development of drug resistance. However, at this time, specific breakpoints for separating susceptible and resistant MAC isolates have not been established for either macrolide.

ANIMAL TOXICOLOGY

Phospholipidosis (intracellular phospholipid binding) has been observed in some tissues of mice, rats, and dogs given multiple doses of azithromycin. It has been demonstrated in numerous organ systems (e.g., eye, dorsal root ganglia, liver, gallbladder, kidney, spleen, and pancreas) in dogs administered doses which, based on pharmacokinetics, are as low as 2 times greater than the recommended adult human dose and in rats at doses comparable to the recommended adult human dose. This effect has been reversible after cessation of azithromycin treatment. The significance of these findings for humans is unknown.

REFERENCES:

1. National Committee for Clinical Laboratory Standards. Methods for Dilution Antimicrobial Susceptibility Tests for Bacteria that Grow Aerobically—Third Edition. Approved Standard NCCLS Document M7-A3, Vol. 13, No. 25, NCCLS, Villanova, PA, December 1993
2. National Committee for Clinical Laboratory Standards. Performance Standards for Antimicrobial Disk Susceptibility Tests—Fifth Edition. Approved Standard NCCLS Document M2-A5, Vol. 13, No. 24, NCCLS, Villanova, PA, December 1993.
3. Dunne MW, Foulds G, Retsema JA. Rationale for the use of azithromycin as *Mycobacterium avium* chemoprophylaxis. *American J Medicine* 1997; 102(5C):37–49.
4. Meier A, Kirshner P, Springer B, et al,. Identification of mutations in 23S rRNA gene of clarithromycin-resistant *Mycobacterium intracellulare. Antimicrob Agents Chemother*. 1994;38:381–384.
5. Methodology per Inderlied CB, et al. Determination of *In Vitro* Susceptibility of *Mycobacterium avium* Complex Isolates to Antimicrobial Agents by Various Methods. *Antimicrob Agents Chemother* 1987; 31:1697–1702.

Rx only

Licensed from Pliva

Distributed by
Pfizer Labs
Division of Pfizer Inc, NY, NY 10017
69-4763-00-6 Printed in U.S.A.
Revised December 2001

ZOLOFT® ℞

(sertraline hydrochloride)
Tablets and Oral Concentrate

Prescribing information for this product, which appears on pages 2751–2756 of the 2002 PDR, has been completely revised as follows. Please write "See Supplement A" next to the product heading.

DESCRIPTION

ZOLOFT® (sertraline hydrochloride) is a selective serotonin reuptake inhibitor (SSRI) for oral administration. It has a molecular weight of 342.7. Sertraline hydrochloride has the following chemical name: (1S-cis)-4-(3,4-dichlorophenyl)-1,2,3,4-tetrahydro-N-methyl-1-naphthalenamine hydrochloride. The empirical formula $C_{17}H_{17}NCl_2 \bullet HCl$ is represented by the following structural formula:

NHCH₃•HCl

Cl

Cl

Sertraline hydrochloride is a white crystalline powder that is slightly soluble in water and isopropyl alcohol, and sparingly soluble in ethanol.

ZOLOFT is supplied for oral administration as scored tablets containing sertraline hydrochloride equivalent to 25, 50 and 100 mg of sertraline and the following inactive ingredients: dibasic calcium phosphate dihydrate, D & C Yellow #10 aluminum lake (in 25 mg tablet), FD & C Blue #1 aluminum lake (in 25 mg tablet), FD & C Red #40 aluminum lake (in 25 mg tablet), FD & C Blue #2 aluminum lake (in 50 mg tablet), hydroxypropyl cellulose, hydroxypropyl methylcellulose, magnesium stearate, microcrystalline cellulose, polyethylene glycol, polysorbate 80, sodium starch glycolate, synthetic yellow iron oxide (in 100 mg tablet), and titanium dioxide.

ZOLOFT oral concentrate is available in a multidose 60 mL bottle. Each mL of solution contains sertraline hydrochloride equivalent to 20 mg of sertraline. The solution contains the following inactive ingredients: glycerin, alcohol (12%), menthol, butylated hydroxytoluene (BHT). The oral concentrate must be diluted prior to administration (see PRECAUTIONS, Information for Patients and DOSAGE AND ADMINISTRATION).

CLINICAL PHARMACOLOGY

Pharmacodynamics

The mechanism of action of sertraline is presumed to be linked to its inhibition of CNS neuronal uptake of serotonin (5HT). Studies at clinically relevant doses in man have demonstrated that sertraline blocks the uptake of serotonin into human platelets. *In vitro* studies in animals also suggest that sertraline is a potent and selective inhibitor of neuronal serotonin reuptake and has only very weak effects on norepinephrine and dopamine neuronal reuptake. *In vitro* studies have shown that sertraline has no significant affinity for adrenergic (alpha$_1$, alpha$_2$, beta), cholinergic, GABA, dopaminergic, histaminergic, serotonergic ($5HT_{1A}$, $5HT_{1B}$, $5HT_2$), or benzodiazepine receptors; antagonism of such receptors has been hypothesized to be associated with various anticholinergic, sedative, and cardiovascular effects for other psychotropic drugs. The chronic administration of sertraline was found in animals to downregulate brain norepinephrine receptors, as has been observed with other drugs effective in the treatment of major depressive disorder. Sertraline does not inhibit monoamine oxidase.

Pharmacokinetics

Systemic Bioavailability—In man, following oral once-daily dosing over the range of 50 to 200 mg for 14 days, mean peak plasma concentrations (Cmax) of sertraline occurred between 4.5 to 8.4 hours post-dosing. The average terminal elimination half-life of plasma sertraline is about 26 hours. Based on this pharmacokinetic parameter, steady-state sertraline plasma levels should be achieved after approximately one week of once-daily dosing. Linear dose-proportional pharmacokinetics were demonstrated in a single dose study in which the Cmax and area under the plasma concentration time curve (AUC) of sertraline were proportional to dose over a range of 50 to 200 mg. Consistent with the terminal elimination half-life, there is an approximately two-fold accumulation, compared to a single dose, of sertraline with repeated dosing over a 50 to 200 mg dose range. The single dose bioavailability of sertraline tablets is approximately equal to an equivalent dose of solution.

In a relative bioavailability study comparing the pharmacokinetics of 100 mg sertraline as the oral solution to a 100 mg sertraline tablet in 16 healthy adults, the solution to tablet ratio of geometric mean AUC and Cmax values were 114.8% and 120.6%, respectively. 90% confidence intervals (CI) were within the range of 80–125% with the exception of the upper 90% CI limit for Cmax which was 126.5%.

The effects of food on the bioavailability of the sertraline tablet and oral concentrate were studied in subjects administered a single dose with and without food. For the tablet, AUC was slightly increased when drug was administered with food but the Cmax was 25% greater, while the time to reach peak plasma concentration (Tmax) decreased from 8 hours post-dosing to 5.5 hours. For the oral concentrate, Tmax was slightly prolonged from 5.9 hours to 7.0 hours with food.

Metabolism—Sertraline undergoes extensive first pass metabolism. The principal initial pathway of metabolism for sertraline is N-demethylation. N-desmethylsertraline has a plasma terminal elimination half-life of 62 to 104 hours. Both *in vitro* biochemical and *in vivo* pharmacological testing have shown N-desmethylsertraline to be substantially less active than sertraline. Both sertraline and N-desmethylsertraline undergo oxidative deamination and subsequent reduction, hydroxylation, and glucuronide conjugation. In a study of radiolabeled sertraline involving two healthy male subjects, sertraline accounted for less than 5% of the plasma radioactivity. About 40–45% of the administered radioactivity was recovered in urine in 9 days. Unchanged sertraline was not detectable in the urine. For the same period, about 40–45% of the administered radioactivity was accounted for in feces, including 12–14% unchanged sertraline.

Desmethylsertraline exhibits time-related, dose dependent increases in AUC (0–24 hour), Cmax and Cmin, with about a 5–9 fold increase in these pharmacokinetic parameters between day 1 and day 14.

Protein Binding—*In vitro* protein binding studies performed with radiolabeled ^{3}H-sertraline showed that sertraline is highly bound to serum proteins (98%) in the range of 20 to 500 ng/mL. However, at up to 300 and 200 ng/mL concentrations, respectively, sertraline and N-desmethylsertraline did not alter the plasma protein binding of two other highly protein bound drugs, viz., warfarin and propranolol (see PRECAUTIONS).

Pediatric Pharmacokinetics—Sertraline pharmacokinetics were evaluated in a group of 61 pediatric patients (29 aged 6–12 years, 32 aged 13–17 years) with a DSM-III-R diagnosis of major depressive disorder or obsessive-compulsive disorder. Patients included both males (N=28) and females (N=33). During 42 days of chronic sertraline dosing, sertraline was titrated up to 200 mg/day and maintained at that dose for a minimum of 11 days. On the final day of sertraline 200 mg/day, the 6–12 year old group exhibited a mean sertraline AUC (0–24 hr) of 3107 ng-hr/mL, mean Cmax of 165 ng/mL, and mean half-life of 26.2 hr. The 13–17 year old group exhibited a mean sertraline AUC (0–24 hr) of 2296 ng-hr/mL, mean Cmax of 123 ng/mL, and mean half-life of 27.8 hr. Higher plasma levels in the 6–12 year old group were largely attributable to patients with lower body weights. No gender associated differences were observed. By comparison, a group of 22 separately studied adults between 18 and 45 years of age (11 male, 11 female) received 30 days of 200 mg/day sertraline and exhibited a mean sertraline AUC (0–24 hr) of 2570 ng-hr/mL, mean Cmax of 142 ng/mL, and mean half-life of 27.2 hr. Relative to the adults, both the 6–12 year olds and the 13–17 year olds showed about 22% lower AUC (0–24 hr) and Cmax values when plasma concentration was adjusted for weight. These data suggest that pediatric patients metabolize sertraline with slightly greater efficiency than adults. Nevertheless, lower doses may be advisable for pediatric patients given their lower body weights, especially in very young patients, in order to avoid excessive plasma levels (see DOSAGE AND ADMINISTRATION).

Age—Sertraline plasma clearance in a group of 16 (8 male, 8 female) elderly patients treated for 14 days at a dose of 100 mg/day was approximately 40% lower than in a similarly studied group of younger (25 to 32 y.o.) individuals. Steady-state, therefore, should be achieved after 2 to 3 weeks in older patients. The same study showed a decreased clearance of desmethylsertraline in older males, but not in older females.

Liver Disease—As might be predicted from its primary site of metabolism, liver impairment can affect the elimination of sertraline. In patients with chronic mild liver impairment (N=10, 8 patients with Child-Pugh scores of 5–6 and 2 patients with Child-Pugh scores of 7–8) who received 50 mg sertraline per day maintained for 21 days, sertraline clearance was reduced, resulting in approximately 3-fold greater exposure compared to age-matched volunteers with no hepatic impairment (N=10). The exposure to desmethylsertraline was approximately 2-fold greater compared to age-matched volunteers with no hepatic impairment. There were no significant differences in plasma protein binding observed between the two groups. The effects of sertraline in patients with moderate and severe hepatic impairment have not been studied. The results suggest that the use of sertraline in patients with liver disease must be approached with caution. If sertraline is administered to patients with liver impairment, a lower or less frequent dose should be used (see PRECAUTIONS and DOSAGE AND ADMINISTRATION).

Renal Disease—Sertraline is extensively metabolized and excretion of unchanged drug in urine is a minor route of elimination. In volunteers with mild to moderate (CLcr=30–60 mL/min), moderate to severe (CLcr=10–29 mL/min) or severe (receiving hemodialysis) renal impairment (N=10 each group), the pharmacokinetics and protein binding of 200 mg sertraline per day maintained for 21 days were not altered compared to age-matched volunteers (N=12) with no renal impairment. Thus sertraline multiple dose pharmacokinetics appear to be unaffected by renal impairment (see PRECAUTIONS).

Clinical Trials

Major Depressive Disorder—The efficacy of ZOLOFT as a treatment for major depressive disorder was established in two placebo-controlled studies in adult outpatients meeting DSM-III criteria for major depressive disorder. Study 1 was an 8-week study with flexible dosing of ZOLOFT in a range of 50 to 200 mg/day; the mean dose for completers was 145 mg/day. Study 2 was a 6-week fixed-dose study, including ZOLOFT doses of 50, 100, and 200 mg/day. Overall, these studies demonstrated ZOLOFT to be superior to placebo on the Hamilton Depression Rating Scale and the Clinical Global Impression Severity and Improvement scales. Study 2 was not readily interpretable regarding a dose response relationship for effectiveness.

Study 3 involved depressed outpatients who had responded by the end of an initial 8-week open treatment phase on ZOLOFT 50–200 mg/day. These patients (N=295) were randomized to continuation for 44 weeks on double-blind ZOLOFT 50-200 mg/day or placebo. A statistically significantly lower relapse rate was observed for patients taking ZOLOFT compared to those on placebo. The mean dose for completers was 70 mg/day.

Analyses for gender effects on outcome did not suggest any differential responsiveness on the basis of sex.

Obsessive-Compulsive Disorder (OCD)—The effectiveness of ZOLOFT in the treatment of OCD was demonstrated in three multicenter placebo-controlled studies of adult outpatients (Studies 1–3). Patients in all studies had moderate to severe OCD (DSM-III or DSM-III-R) with mean baseline ratings on the Yale Brown Obsessive-Compulsive Scale (YBOCS) total score ranging from 23 to 25.

Study 1 was an 8-week study with flexible dosing of ZOLOFT in a range of 50 to 200 mg/day; the mean dose for completers was 186 mg/day. Patients receiving ZOLOFT experienced a mean reduction of approximately 4 points on the YBOCS total score which was significantly greater than the mean reduction of 2 points in placebo-treated patients.

Study 2 was a 12-week fixed-dose study, including ZOLOFT doses of 50, 100, and 200 mg/day. Patients receiving ZOLOFT doses of 50 and 200 mg/day experienced mean reductions of approximately 6 points on the YBOCS total score which were significantly greater than the approximately 3 point reduction in placebo-treated patients.

Study 3 was a 12-week study with flexible dosing of ZOLOFT in a range of 50 to 200 mg/day; the mean dose for completers was 185 mg/day. Patients receiving ZOLOFT experienced a mean reduction of approximately 7 points on the YBOCS total score which was significantly greater than the mean reduction of approximately 4 points in placebo-treated patients.

Analyses for age and gender effects on outcome did not suggest any differential responsiveness on the basis of age or sex.

The effectiveness of ZOLOFT for the treatment of OCD was also demonstrated in a 12-week, multicenter, placebo-controlled, parallel group study in a pediatric outpatient population (children and adolescents, ages 6–17). Patients receiving ZOLOFT in this study were initiated at doses of either 25 mg/day (children, ages 6–12) or 50 mg/day (adolescents, ages 13–17), and then titrated over the next four weeks to a maximum dose of 200 mg/day, as tolerated. The mean dose for completers was 178 mg/day. Dosing was once a day in the morning or evening. Patients in this study had moderate to severe OCD (DSM-III-R) with mean baseline ratings on the Children's Yale-Brown Obsessive-Compulsive Scale (CYBOCS) total score of 22. Patients receiving sertraline experienced a mean reduction of approximately 7 points on the CYBOCS total score which was significantly greater than the 3 point reduction for placebo patients. Analyses for age and gender effects on outcome did not suggest any differential responsiveness on the basis of age or sex.

Panic Disorder—The effectiveness of ZOLOFT in the treatment of panic disorder was demonstrated in three double-blind, placebo-controlled studies (Studies 1–3) of adult outpatients who had a primary diagnosis of panic disorder (DSM-III-R), with or without agoraphobia.

Studies 1 and 2 were 10-week flexible dose studies. ZOLOFT was initiated at 25 mg/day for the first week, and then patients were dosed in a range of 50–200 mg/day on the basis of clinical response and toleration. The mean ZOLOFT doses for completers to 10 weeks were 131 mg/day and 144 mg/day, respectively, for Studies 1 and 2. In these studies, ZOLOFT was shown to be significantly more effective than placebo on change from baseline in panic attack frequency and on the Clinical Global Impression Severity of Illness and Global Improvement scores. The difference between ZOLOFT and placebo in reduction from baseline in the number of full panic attacks was approximately 2 panic attacks per week in both studies.

Study 3 was a 12-week fixed-dose study, including ZOLOFT doses of 50, 100, and 200 mg/day. Patients receiving ZOLOFT experienced a significantly greater reduction in panic attack frequency than patients receiving placebo. Study 3 was not readily interpretable regarding a dose response relationship for effectiveness.

Subgroup analyses did not indicate that there were any differences in treatment outcomes as a function of age, race, or gender.

Posttraumatic Stress Disorder (PTSD)—The effectiveness of ZOLOFT in the treatment of PTSD was established in two multicenter placebo-controlled studies (Studies 1–2) of adult outpatients who met DSM-III-R criteria for PTSD. The mean duration of PTSD for these patients was 12 years (Studies 1 and 2 combined) and 44% of patients (169 of the 385 patients treated) had secondary depressive disorder.

Studies 1 and 2 were 12-week flexible dose studies. ZOLOFT was initiated at 25 mg/day for the first week, and patients were then dosed in the range of 50–200 mg/day on the basis of clinical response and toleration. The mean ZOLOFT dose for completers was 146 mg/day and 151 mg/day, respectively for Studies 1 and 2. Study outcome was assessed by the Clinician-Administered PTSD Scale Part 2 (CAPS) which is a multi-item instrument that measures the three PTSD diagnostic symptom clusters of reexperiencing/intrusion, avoidance/numbing, and hyperarousal as well as the patient-rated Impact of Event Scale (IES) which measures intrusion and avoidance symptoms. ZOLOFT was shown to be significantly more effective than placebo on change from baseline to endpoint on the CAPS, IES and on the Clinical Global Impressions (CGI) Severity of Illness and Global Improvement scores. In two additional placebo-controlled PTSD trials, the difference in response to treatment between patients receiving ZOLOFT and patients receiving placebo was not statistically significant. One of these additional studies was conducted in patients similar to those recruited for Studies 1 and 2, while the second additional study was conducted in predominantly male veterans.

As PTSD is a more common disorder in women than men, the majority (76%) of patients in these trials were women (152 and 139 women on sertraline and placebo versus 39 and 55 men on sertraline and placebo; Studies 1 and 2 combined). Post hoc exploratory analyses revealed a significant difference between ZOLOFT and placebo on the CAPS, IES and CGI in women, regardless of baseline diagnosis of comorbid major depressive disorder, but essentially no effect in the relatively smaller number of men in these studies. The clinical significance of this apparent gender interaction is unknown at this time. There was insufficient information to determine the effect of race or age on outcome.

In a longer-term study, patients meeting DSM-III-R criteria for PTSD who had responded during a 24-week open trial on ZOLOFT 50–200 mg/day (n=96) were randomized to continuation of ZOLOFT or to substitution of placebo for up to 28 weeks of observation for relapse. Response during the open phase was defined as a CGI-I of 1 (very much improved) or 2 (much improved), and a decrease in the CAPS-2 score of > 30% compared to baseline. Relapse during the double-blind phase was defined as the following conditions being met on two consecutive visits: (1) CGI-I ≥ 3; (2) CAPS-2 score increased by ≥ 30% and by ≥ 15 points relative to baseline; and (3) worsening of the patient's condition in the investigator's judgment. Patients receiving continued ZOLOFT treatment experienced significantly lower relapse rates over the subsequent 28 weeks compared to those receiving placebo. This pattern was demonstrated in male and female subjects.

INDICATIONS AND USAGE

Major Depressive Disorder—ZOLOFT® (sertraline hydrochloride) is indicated for the treatment of major depressive disorder.

The efficacy of ZOLOFT in the treatment of a major depressive episode was established in six to eight week controlled trials of outpatients whose diagnoses corresponded most closely to the DSM-III category of major depressive disorder (see Clinical Trials under CLINICAL PHARMACOLOGY).

A major depressive episode implies a prominent and relatively persistent depressed or dysphoric mood that usually interferes with daily functioning (nearly every day for at least 2 weeks); it should include at least 4 of the following 8 symptoms: change in appetite, change in sleep, psychomotor agitation or retardation, loss of interest in usual activities or decrease in sexual drive, increased fatigue, feelings of guilt or worthlessness, slowed thinking or impaired concentration, and a suicide attempt or suicidal ideation.

The antidepressant action of ZOLOFT in hospitalized depressed patients has not been adequately studied.

The efficacy of ZOLOFT in maintaining an antidepressant response for up to 44 weeks following 8 weeks of open-label acute treatment (52 weeks total) was demonstrated in a placebo-controlled trial. The usefulness of the drug in patients receiving ZOLOFT for extended periods should be reevaluated periodically (see Clinical Trials under CLINICAL PHARMACOLOGY).

Obsessive-Compulsive Disorder—ZOLOFT is indicated for the treatment of obsessions and compulsions in patients with obsessive-compulsive disorder (OCD), as defined in the DSM-III-R; i.e., the obsessions or compulsions cause marked distress, are time-consuming, or significantly interfere with social or occupational functioning.

The efficacy of ZOLOFT was established in 12-week trials with obsessive-compulsive outpatients having diagnoses of obsessive-compulsive disorder as defined according to DSM-III or DSM-III-R criteria (see Clinical Trials under CLINICAL PHARMACOLOGY).

Obsessive-compulsive disorder is characterized by recurrent and persistent ideas, thoughts, impulses, or images (obsessions) that are ego-dystonic and/or repetitive, purposeful, and intentional behaviors (compulsions) that are recognized by the person as excessive or unreasonable.

The effectiveness of ZOLOFT in long-term use for OCD, i.e., for more than 12 weeks, has not been systematically evaluated in placebo-controlled trials. Therefore, the physician who elects to use ZOLOFT for extended periods should periodically reevaluate the long-term usefulness of the drug for the individual patient (see DOSAGE AND ADMINISTRATION).

Panic Disorder—ZOLOFT is indicated for the treatment of panic disorder, with or without agoraphobia, as defined in DSM-IV. Panic disorder is characterized by the occurrence of unexpected panic attacks and associated concern about having additional attacks, worry about the implications or consequences of the attacks, and/or a significant change in behavior related to the attacks.

The efficacy of ZOLOFT was established in three 10–12 week trials in panic disorder patients whose diagnoses corresponded to the DSM-III-R category of panic disorder (see Clinical Trials under CLINICAL PHARMACOLOGY).

Panic disorder (DSM-IV) is characterized by recurrent unexpected panic attacks, i.e., a discrete period of intense fear or discomfort in which four (or more) of the following symptoms develop abruptly and reach a peak within 10 minutes: (1) palpitations, pounding heart, or accelerated heart rate; (2) sweating; (3) trembling or shaking; (4) sensations of shortness of breath or smothering; (5) feeling of choking; (6) chest pain or discomfort; (7) nausea or abdominal distress; (8) feeling dizzy, unsteady, lightheaded, or faint; (9) derealization (feelings of unreality) or depersonalization (being detached from oneself); (10) fear of losing control; (11) fear of dying; (12) paresthesias (numbness or tingling sensations); (13) chills or hot flushes.

The effectiveness of ZOLOFT® (sertraline hydrochloride) in long-term use, that is, for more than 12 weeks, has not been systematically evaluated in controlled trials. Therefore, the physician who elects to use ZOLOFT for extended periods should periodically re-evaluate the long-term usefulness of the drug for the individual patient (see DOSAGE AND ADMINISTRATION).

Posttraumatic Stress Disorder (PTSD)—ZOLOFT (sertraline hydrochloride) is indicated for the treatment of posttraumatic stress disorder.

The efficacy of ZOLOFT in the treatment of PTSD was established in two 12-week placebo-controlled trials of outpatients whose diagnosis met criteria for the DSM-III-R category of PTSD (see Clinical Trials under CLINICAL PHARMACOLOGY).

PTSD, as defined by DSM-III-R/IV, requires exposure to a traumatic event that involved actual or threatened death or serious injury, or threat to the physical integrity of self or others, and a response which involves intense fear, helplessness, or horror. Symptoms that occur as a result of exposure to the traumatic event include reexperiencing of the event in the form of intrusive thoughts, flashbacks or dreams, and intense psychological distress and physiological reactivity on exposure to cues to the event; avoidance of situations reminiscent of the traumatic event, inability to recall details of the event, and/or numbing of general responsiveness manifested as diminished interest in significant activities, estrangement from others, restricted range of affect, or sense of foreshortened future; and symptoms of autonomic arousal including hypervigilance, exaggerated startle response, sleep disturbance, impaired concentration, and irritability or outbursts of anger. A PTSD diagnosis requires that the symptoms are present for at least a month and that they cause clinically significant distress or impairment in social, occupational, or other important areas of functioning.

The efficacy of ZOLOFT in maintaining a response in patients with PTSD for up to 28 weeks following 24 weeks of

Continued on next page

Zoloft—Cont.

open-label treatment was demonstrated in a placebo-controlled trial. Nevertheless, the physician who elects to use ZOLOFT for extended periods should periodically re-evaluate the long-term usefulness of the drug for the individual patient (see Clinical Trials under CLINICAL PHARMACOLOGY).

CONTRAINDICATIONS

All Dosage Forms of ZOLOFT:
Concomitant use in patients taking monoamine oxidase inhibitors (MAOIs) is contraindicated (see WARNINGS).
Oral Concentrate:
ZOLOFT oral concentrate is contraindicated with ANTABUSE (disulfiram) due to the alcohol content of the concentrate.

WARNINGS

Cases of serious sometimes fatal reactions have been reported in patients receiving ZOLOFT® (sertraline hydrochloride), a selective serotonin reuptake inhibitor (SSRI), in combination with a monoamine oxidase inhibitor (MAOI). Symptoms of a drug interaction between an SSRI and an MAOI include: hyperthermia, rigidity, myoclonus, autonomic instability with possible rapid fluctuations of vital signs, mental status changes that include confusion, irritability, and extreme agitation progressing to delirium and coma. These reactions have also been reported in patients who have recently discontinued an SSRI and have been started on an MAOI. Some cases presented with features resembling neuroleptic malignant syndrome. Therefore, ZOLOFT should not be used in combination with an MAOI, or within 14 days of discontinuing treatment with an MAOI. Similarly, at least 14 days should be allowed after stopping ZOLOFT before starting an MAOI.

PRECAUTIONS

General

Activation of Mania/Hypomania—During premarketing testing, hypomania or mania occurred in approximately 0.4% of ZOLOFT® (sertraline hydrochloride) treated patients.

Weight Loss—Significant weight loss may be an undesirable result of treatment with sertraline for some patients, but on average, patients in controlled trials had minimal, 1 to 2 pound weight loss, versus smaller changes on placebo. Only rarely have sertraline patients been discontinued for weight loss.

Seizure—ZOLOFT has not been evaluated in patients with a seizure disorder. These patients were excluded from clinical studies during the product's premarket testing. No seizures were observed among approximately 3000 patients treated with ZOLOFT in the development program for major depressive disorder. However, 4 patients out of approximately 1800 (220<18 years of age) exposed during the development program for obsessive-compulsive disorder experienced seizures, representing a crude incidence of 0.2%. Three of these patients were adolescents, two with a seizure disorder and one with a family history of seizure disorder, none of whom were receiving anticonvulsant medication. Accordingly, ZOLOFT should be introduced with care in patients with a seizure disorder.

Suicide—The possibility of a suicide attempt is inherent in major depressive disorder and may persist until significant remission occurs. Close supervision of high risk patients should accompany initial drug therapy. Prescriptions for ZOLOFT should be written for the smallest quantity of tablets consistent with good patient management, in order to reduce the risk of overdose.

Because of the well-established comorbidity between OCD and major depressive disorder, panic disorder and major depressive disorder, and PTSD and major depressive disorder, the same precautions observed when treating patients with major depressive disorder should be observed when treating patients with OCD, panic disorder or PTSD.

Weak Uricosuric Effect—ZOLOFT® (sertraline hydrochloride) is associated with a mean decrease in serum uric acid of approximately 7%. The clinical significance of this weak uricosuric effect is unknown.

Use in Patients with Concomitant Illness—Clinical experience with ZOLOFT in patients with certain concomitant systemic illness is limited. Caution is advisable in using ZOLOFT in patients with diseases or conditions that could affect metabolism or hemodynamic responses.

ZOLOFT has not been evaluated or used to any appreciable extent in patients with a recent history of myocardial infarction or unstable heart disease. Patients with these diagnoses were excluded from clinical studies during the product's premarket testing. However, the electrocardiograms of 774 patients who received ZOLOFT in double-blind trials were evaluated and the data indicate that ZOLOFT is not associated with the development of significant ECG abnormalities.

ZOLOFT is extensively metabolized by the liver. In patients with chronic mild liver impairment, sertraline clearance was reduced, resulting in increased AUC, Cmax and elimination half-life. The effects of sertraline in patients with moderate and severe hepatic impairment have not been studied. The use of sertraline in patients with liver disease must be approached with caution. If sertraline is administered to patients with liver impairment, a lower or less frequent dose should be used (see CLINICAL PHARMACOLOGY and DOSAGE AND ADMINISTRATION).

Since ZOLOFT is extensively metabolized, excretion of unchanged drug in urine is a minor route of elimination. A clinical study comparing sertraline pharmacokinetics in healthy volunteers to that in patients with renal impairment ranging from mild to severe (requiring dialysis) indicated that the pharmacokinetics and protein binding are unaffected by renal disease. Based on the pharmacokinetic results, there is no need for dosage adjustment in patients with renal impairment (see CLINICAL PHARMACOLOGY).

Interference with Cognitive and Motor Performance—In controlled studies, ZOLOFT did not cause sedation and did not interfere with psychomotor performance. (See **Information for Patients.**)

Hyponatremia—Several cases of hyponatremia have been reported and appeared to be reversible when ZOLOFT was discontinued. Some cases were possibly due to the syndrome of inappropriate antidiuretic hormone secretion. The majority of these occurrences have been in elderly individuals, some in patients taking diuretics or who were otherwise volume depleted.

Platelet Function—There have been rare reports of altered platelet function and/or abnormal results from laboratory studies in patients taking ZOLOFT. While there have been reports of abnormal bleeding or purpura in several patients taking ZOLOFT, it is unclear whether ZOLOFT had a causative role.

Information for Patients

Physicians are advised to discuss the following issues with patients for whom they prescribe ZOLOFT:

Patients should be told that although ZOLOFT has not been shown to impair the ability of normal subjects to perform tasks requiring complex motor and mental skills in laboratory experiments, drugs that act upon the central nervous system may affect some individuals adversely. Therefore, patients should be told that until they learn how they respond to ZOLOFT they should be careful doing activities when they need to be alert, such as driving a car or operating machinery.

Patients should be told that although ZOLOFT has not been shown in experiments with normal subjects to increase the mental and motor skill impairments caused by alcohol, the concomitant use of ZOLOFT and alcohol is not advised.

Patients should be told that while no adverse interaction of ZOLOFT with over-the-counter (OTC) drug products is known to occur, the potential for interaction exists. Thus, the use of any OTC product should be initiated cautiously according to the directions of use given for the OTC product.

Patients should be advised to notify their physician if they become pregnant or intend to become pregnant during therapy.

Patients should be advised to notify their physician if they are breast feeding an infant.

ZOLOFT oral concentrate is contraindicated with ANTABUSE (disulfiram) due to the alcohol content of the concentrate.

ZOLOFT Oral Concentrate contains 20 mg/mL of sertraline (as the hydrochloride) as the active ingredient and 12% alcohol. ZOLOFT Oral Concentrate must be diluted before use. Just before taking, use the dropper provided to remove the required amount of ZOLOFT Oral Concentrate and mix with 4 oz (1/2 cup) of water, ginger ale, lemon/lime soda, lemonade or orange juice ONLY. Do not mix ZOLOFT Oral Concentrate with anything other than the liquids listed. The dose should be taken immediately after mixing. Do not mix in advance. At times, a slight haze may appear after mixing; this is normal. Note that caution should be exercised for persons with latex sensitivity, as the dropper dispenser contains dry natural rubber.

Laboratory Tests

None.

Drug Interactions

Potential Effects of Coadministration of Drugs Highly Bound to Plasma Proteins—Because sertraline is tightly bound to plasma protein, the administration of ZOLOFT® (sertraline hydrochloride) to a patient taking another drug which is tightly bound to protein (e.g., warfarin, digitoxin) may cause a shift in plasma concentrations potentially resulting in an adverse effect. Conversely, adverse effects may result from displacement of protein bound ZOLOFT by other tightly bound drugs.

In a study comparing prothrombin time AUC (0–120 hr) following dosing with warfarin (0.75 mg/kg) before and after 21 days of dosing with either ZOLOFT (50–200 mg/day) or placebo, there was a mean increase in prothrombin time of 8% relative to baseline for ZOLOFT compared to a 1% decrease for placebo ($p<0.02$). The normalization of prothrombin time for the ZOLOFT group was delayed compared to the placebo group. The clinical significance of this change is unknown. Accordingly, prothrombin time should be carefully monitored when ZOLOFT therapy is initiated or stopped.

Cimetidine—In a study assessing disposition of ZOLOFT (100 mg) on the second of 8 days of cimetidine administration (800 mg daily), there were significant increases in ZOLOFT mean AUC (50%), Cmax (24%) and half-life (26%) compared to the placebo group. The clinical significance of these changes is unknown.

CNS Active Drugs—In a study comparing the disposition of intravenously administered diazepam before and after 21 days of dosing with either ZOLOFT (50 to 200 mg/day escalating dose) or placebo, there was a 32% decrease relative to baseline in diazepam clearance for the ZOLOFT group compared to a 19% decrease relative to baseline for the placebo group ($p<0.03$). There was a 23% increase in Tmax for desmethyldiazepam in the ZOLOFT group compared to a 20% decrease in the placebo group ($p<0.03$). The clinical significance of these changes is unknown.

In a placebo-controlled trial in normal volunteers, the administration of two doses of ZOLOFT did not significantly alter steady-state lithium levels or the renal clearance of lithium.

Nonetheless, at this time, it is recommended that plasma lithium levels be monitored following initiation of ZOLOFT therapy with appropriate adjustments to the lithium dose.

The risk of using ZOLOFT in combination with other CNS active drugs has not been systematically evaluated. Consequently, caution is advised if the concomitant administration of ZOLOFT and such drugs is required.

There is limited controlled experience regarding the optimal timing of switching from other drugs effective in the treatment of major depressive disorder, obsessive-compulsive disorder, panic disorder, and posttraumatic stress disorder to ZOLOFT. Care and prudent medical judgment should be exercised when switching, particularly from long-acting agents. The duration of an appropriate washout period which should intervene before switching from one selective serotonin reuptake inhibitor (SSRI) to another has not been established.

Monoamine Oxidase Inhibitors—See CONTRAINDICATIONS and WARNINGS.

Drugs Metabolized by P450 3A4—In two separate *in vivo* interaction studies, sertraline was co-administered with cytochrome P450 3A4 substrates, terfenadine or carbamazepine, under steady-state conditions. The results of these studies demonstrated that sertraline co-administration did not increase plasma concentrations of terfenadine or carbamazepine. These data suggest that sertraline's extent of inhibition of P450 3A4 activity is not likely to be of clinical significance.

Drugs Metabolized by P450 2D6—Many drugs effective in the treatment of major depressive disorder, e.g., the SSRIs, including sertraline, and most tricyclic antidepressant drugs effective in the treatment of major depressive disorder inhibit the biochemical activity of the drug metabolizing isozyme cytochrome P450 2D6 (debrisoquin hydroxylase), and, thus, may increase the plasma concentrations of co-administered drugs that are metabolized by P450 2D6. The drugs for which this potential interaction is of greatest concern are those metabolized primarily by 2D6 and which have a narrow therapeutic index, e.g., the tricyclic antidepressant drugs effective in the treatment of major depressive disorder and the Type 1C antiarrhythmics propafenone and flecainide. The extent to which this interaction is an important clinical problem depends on the extent of the inhibition of P450 2D6 by the antidepressant and the therapeutic index of the co-administered drug. There is variability among the drugs effective in the treatment of major depressive disorder in the extent of clinically important 2D6 inhibition, and in fact sertraline at lower doses has a less prominent inhibitory effect on 2D6 than some others in the class. Nevertheless, even sertraline has the potential for clinically important 2D6 inhibition. Consequently, concomitant use of a drug metabolized by P450 2D6 with ZOLOFT may require lower doses than usually prescribed for the other drug. Furthermore, whenever ZOLOFT is withdrawn from co-therapy, an increased dose of the co-administered drug may be required (see Tricyclic Antidepressant Drugs Effective in the Treatment of Major Depressive Disorder under PRECAUTIONS).

Sumatriptan—There have been rare postmarketing reports describing patients with weakness, hyperreflexia, and incoordination following the use of a selective serotonin reuptake inhibitor (SSRI) and sumatriptan. If concomitant treatment with sumatriptan and an SSRI (e.g., citalopram, fluoxetine, fluvoxamine, paroxetine, sertraline) is clinically warranted, appropriate observation of the patient is advised.

Tricyclic Antidepressant Drugs Effective in the Treatment of Major Depressive Disorder (TCAs)—The extent to which SSRI–TCA interactions may pose clinical problems will depend on the degree of inhibition and the pharmacokinetics of the SSRI involved. Nevertheless, caution is indicated in the co-administration of TCAs with ZOLOFT, because sertraline may inhibit TCA metabolism. Plasma TCA concentrations may need to be monitored, and the dose of TCA may need to be reduced, if a TCA is co-administered with ZOLOFT (see Drugs Metabolized by P450 2D6 under PRECAUTIONS).

Hypoglycemic Drugs—In a placebo-controlled trial in normal volunteers, administration of ZOLOFT for 22 days (including 200 mg/day for the final 13 days) caused a statistically significant 16% decrease from baseline in the clearance of tolbutamide following an intravenous 1000 mg dose. ZOLOFT administration did not noticeably change either the plasma protein binding or the apparent volume of distribution of tolbutamide, suggesting that the decreased clearance was due to a change in the metabolism of the drug. The clinical significance of this decrease in tolbutamide clearance is unknown.

Atenolol—ZOLOFT (100 mg) when administered to 10 healthy male subjects had no effect on the beta-adrenergic blocking ability of atenolol.

Digoxin—In a placebo-controlled trial in normal volunteers, administration of ZOLOFT for 17 days (including 200 mg/day for the last 10 days) did not change serum digoxin levels or digoxin renal clearance.

Microsomal Enzyme Induction—Preclinical studies have shown ZOLOFT to induce hepatic microsomal enzymes. In clinical studies, ZOLOFT was shown to induce hepatic enzymes minimally as determined by a small (5%) but statistically significant decrease in antipyrine half-life following administration of 200 mg/day for 21 days. This small change in antipyrine half-life reflects a clinically insignificant change in hepatic metabolism.

Electroconvulsive Therapy—There are no clinical studies establishing the risks or benefits of the combined use of electroconvulsive therapy (ECT) and ZOLOFT.

Alcohol—Although ZOLOFT did not potentiate the cognitive and psychomotor effects of alcohol in experiments with normal subjects, the concomitant use of ZOLOFT and alcohol is not recommended.

Carcinogenesis—Lifetime carcinogenicity studies were carried out in CD-1 mice and Long-Evans rats at doses up to 40 mg/kg/day. These doses correspond to 1 times (mice) and 2 times (rats) the maximum recommended human dose (MRHD) on a mg/m^2 basis. There was a dose-related increase of liver adenomas in male mice receiving sertraline at 10–40 mg/kg (0.25–1.0 times the MRHD on a mg/m^2 basis). No increase was seen in female mice or in rats of either sex receiving the same treatments, nor was there an increase in hepatocellular carcinomas. Liver adenomas have a variable rate of spontaneous occurrence in the CD-1 mouse and are of unknown significance to humans. There was an increase in follicular adenomas of the thyroid in female rats receiving sertraline at 40 mg/kg (2 times the MRHD on a mg/m^2 basis); this was not accompanied by thyroid hyperplasia. While there was an increase in uterine adenocarcinomas in rats receiving sertraline at 10–40 mg/kg (0.5–2.0 times the MRHD on a mg/m^2 basis) compared to placebo controls, this effect was not clearly drug related.

Mutagenesis—Sertraline had no genotoxic effects, with or without metabolic activation, based on the following assays: bacterial mutation assay; mouse lymphoma mutation assay; and tests for cytogenetic aberrations *in vivo* in mouse bone marrow and *in vitro* in human lymphocytes.

Impairment of Fertility—A decrease in fertility was seen in one of two rat studies at a dose of 80 mg/kg (4 times the maximum recommended human dose on a mg/m^2 basis).

Pregnancy-Pregnancy Category C—Reproduction studies have been performed in rats and rabbits at doses up to 80 mg/kg/day and 40 mg/kg/day, respectively. These doses correspond to approximately 4 times the maximum recommended human dose (MRHD) on a mg/m^2 basis. There was no evidence of teratogenicity at any dose level. When pregnant rats and rabbits were given sertraline during the period of organogenesis, delayed ossification was observed in fetuses at doses of 10 mg/kg (0.5 times the MRHD on a mg/m^2 basis) in rats and 40 mg/kg (4 times the MRHD on a mg/m^2 basis) in rabbits. When female rats received sertraline during the last third of gestation and throughout lactation, there was an increase in the number of stillborn pups and in the number of pups dying during the first 4 days after birth. Pup body weights were also decreased during the first four days after birth. These effects occurred at a dose of 20 mg/kg (1 times the MRHD on a mg/m^2 basis). The no effect dose for rat pup mortality was 10 mg/kg (0.5 times the MRHD on a mg/m^2 basis). The decrease in pup survival was shown to be due to *in utero* exposure to sertraline. The clinical significance of these effects is unknown. There are no adequate and well-controlled studies in pregnant women. ZOLOFT® (sertraline hydrochloride) should be used during pregnancy only if the potential benefit justifies the potential risk to the fetus.

Labor and Delivery—The effect of ZOLOFT on labor and delivery in humans is unknown.

Nursing Mothers—It is not known whether, and if so in what amount, sertraline or its metabolites are excreted in human milk. Because many drugs are excreted in human milk, caution should be exercised when ZOLOFT is administered to a nursing woman.

Pediatric Use—The efficacy of ZOLOFT for the treatment of obsessive-compulsive disorder was demonstrated in a 12-week, multicenter, placebo-controlled study with 187 outpatients ages 6–17 (see Clinical Trials under CLINICAL PHARMACOLOGY). The efficacy of ZOLOFT in pediatric patients with major depressive disorder, panic disorder or PTSD has not been systematically evaluated.

The safety of ZOLOFT use in children and adolescents, ages 6–18, was evaluated in a 12-week, multicenter, placebo-controlled study with 187 outpatients, ages 6–17, and in a flexible dose, 52 week open extension study of 137 patients, ages 6–18, who had completed the initial 12-week, double-blind, placebo-controlled study. ZOLOFT was administered at doses of either 25 mg/day (children, ages 6–12) or 50 mg/day (adolescents, ages 13–18) and then titrated in weekly 25 mg/day or 50 mg/day increments, respectively, to a maximum dose of 200 mg/day based upon clinical response. The mean dose for completers was 157 mg/day. In the acute 12 week pediatric study and in the 52 week study, ZOLOFT had an adverse event profile generally similar to that observed in adults.

Sertraline pharmacokinetics were evaluated in 61 pediatric patients between 6 and 18 years of age with major depressive disorder and/or OCD and revealed similar drug exposures to those of adults when plasma concentration was adjusted for weight (see Pharmacokinetics under CLINICAL PHARMACOLOGY).

More than 250 patients with major depressive disorder and/or OCD between 6 and 18 years of age have received ZOLOFT in clinical trials. The adverse event profile observed in these patients was generally similar to that observed in adult studies with ZOLOFT (see ADVERSE REACTIONS). As with other SSRIs, decreased appetite and weight loss have been observed in association with the use of ZOLOFT. Consequently, regular monitoring of weight and growth is recommended if treatment of a child with an SSRI is to be continued long term. Safety and effectiveness in pediatric patients below the age of 6 have not been established.

The risks, if any, that may be associated with the use of ZOLOFT beyond 1 year in children and adolescents with OCD have not been systematically assessed. The prescriber should be mindful that the evidence relied upon to conclude that sertraline is safe for use in children and adolescents derives from clinical studies that were 12 to 52 weeks in duration and from the extrapolation of experience gained with adult patients. In particular, there are no studies that directly evaluate the effects of long-term sertraline use on the growth, development, and maturation of children and adolescents. Although there is no affirmative finding to suggest that sertraline possesses a capacity to adversely affect growth, development or maturation, the absence of such findings is not compelling evidence of the absence of the potential of sertraline to have adverse effects in chronic use.

Geriatric Use—U.S. geriatric clinical studies of ZOLOFT in major depressive disorder included 663 ZOLOFT-treated subjects ≥ 65 years of age, of those, 180 were ≥ 75 years of age. No overall differences in the pattern of adverse reactions were observed in the geriatric clinical trial subjects relative to those reported in younger subjects (see ADVERSE REACTIONS), and other reported experience has not identified differences in safety patterns between the elderly and younger subjects. As with all medications, greater sensitivity of some older individuals cannot be ruled out. There were 947 subjects in placebo-controlled geriatric clinical studies of ZOLOFT in major depressive disorder. No overall differences in the pattern of efficacy were observed in the geriatric clinical trial subjects relative to those reported in younger subjects.

Other Adverse Events in Geriatric Patients. In 354 geriatric subjects treated with ZOLOFT in placebo-controlled trials, the overall profile of adverse events was generally similar to that shown in Tables 1 and 2. Urinary tract infection was the only adverse event not appearing in Tables 1 and 2 and reported at an incidence of at least 2% and at a rate greater than placebo in placebo-controlled trials.

As with other SSRIs, ZOLOFT has been associated with cases of clinically significant hyponatremia in elderly patients (see Hyponatremia under PRECAUTIONS).

ADVERSE REACTIONS

During its premarketing assessment, multiple doses of ZOLOFT were administered to over 4000 adult subjects as of February 26, 1998. The conditions and duration of exposure to ZOLOFT varied greatly, and included (in overlapping categories) clinical pharmacology studies, open and double-blind studies, uncontrolled and controlled studies, inpatient and outpatient studies, fixed-dose and titration studies, and studies for multiple indications, including major depressive disorder, OCD, panic disorder and PTSD.

Untoward events associated with this exposure were recorded by clinical investigators using terminology of their own choosing. Consequently, it is not possible to provide a meaningful estimate of the proportion of individuals experiencing adverse events without first grouping similar types of untoward events into a smaller number of standardized event categories.

In the tabulations that follow, a World Health Organization dictionary of terminology has been used to classify reported adverse events. The frequencies presented, therefore, represent the proportion of the over 4000 adult individuals exposed to multiple doses of ZOLOFT who experienced a treatment-emergent adverse event of the type cited on at least one occasion while receiving ZOLOFT. An event was considered treatment-emergent if it occurred for the first time or worsened while receiving therapy following baseline evaluation. It is important to emphasize that events reported during therapy were not necessarily caused by it.

The prescriber should be aware that the figures in the tables and tabulations cannot be used to predict the incidence of side effects in the course of usual medical practice where patient characteristics and other factors differ from those that prevailed in the clinical trials. Similarly, the cited frequencies cannot be compared with figures obtained from other clinical investigations involving different treatments, uses, and investigators. The cited figures, however, do provide the prescribing physician with some basis for estimating the relative contribution of drug and nondrug factors to the side effect incidence rate in the population studied.

Incidence in Placebo-Controlled Trials—Table 1 enumerates the most common treatment-emergent adverse events associated with the use of ZOLOFT (incidence of at least 5% for ZOLOFT and at least twice that for placebo within at least one of the indications) for the treatment of adult patients with major depressive disorder/other*, OCD, panic disorder and PTSD in placebo-controlled clinical trials. Most patients received doses of 50 to 200 mg/day. Table 2 enumerates treatment-emergent adverse events that occurred in 2% or more of adult patients treated with ZOLOFT and with incidence greater than placebo who participated in controlled clinical trials comparing ZOLOFT with placebo in

TABLE 1
MOST COMMON TREATMENT-EMERGENT ADVERSE EVENTS: INCIDENCE IN PLACEBO-CONTROLLED CLINICAL TRIALS

	Percentage of Patients Reporting Event							
	Major Depressive Disorder/Other*		OCD		Panic Disorder		PTSD	
Body System/Adverse Event	ZOLOFT (N=861)	Placebo (N=853)	ZOLOFT (N=533)	Placebo (N=373)	ZOLOFT (N=430)	Placebo (N=275)	ZOLOFT (N=374)	Placebo (N=376)
Autonomic Nervous System Disorders								
Ejaculation Failure[(1)]	7	<1	17	2	19	1	11	1
Mouth Dry	16	9	14	9	15	10	11	6
Sweating Increased	8	3	6	1	5	1	4	2
Centr. & Periph. Nerv. System Disorders								
Somnolence	13	6	15	8	15	9	13	9
Tremor	11	3	8	1	5	1	5	1
General								
Fatigue	11	8	14	10	11	6	10	5
Gastrointestinal Disorders								
Anorexia	3	2	11	2	7	2	8	2
Constipation	8	6	6	4	7	3	3	3
Diarrhea/Loose Stools	18	9	24	10	20	9	24	15
Dyspepsia	6	3	10	4	10	8	6	6
Nausea	26	12	30	11	29	18	21	11
Psychiatric Disorders								
Agitation	6	4	6	3	6	2	5	5
Insomnia	16	9	28	12	25	18	20	11
Libido Decreased	1	<1	11	2	7	1	7	2

[(1)]Primarily ejaculatory delay. Denominator used was for male patients only (N=271 ZOLOFT major depressive disorder/other*; N=271 placebo major depressive disorder/other*; N=296 ZOLOFT OCD; N=219 placebo OCD; N=216 ZOLOFT panic disorder; N=134 placebo panic disorder; N=130 ZOLOFT PTSD; N=149 placebo PTSD).
*Major depressive disorder and other premarketing controlled trials.

Continued on next page

Zoloft—Cont.

the treatment of major depressive disorder/other*, OCD, panic disorder and PTSD. Table 2 provides combined data for the pool of studies that are provided separately by indication in Table 1.

[See table 1 at top of previous page]

TABLE 2
TREATMENT-EMERGENT ADVERSE EVENTS: INCIDENCE IN PLACEBO-CONTROLLED CLINICAL TRIALS
Percentage of Patients Reporting Event
Major Depressive Disorder/Other*, OCD, Panic Disorder and PTSD combined

Body System/Adverse Event**	ZOLOFT (N=2198)	Placebo (N=1877)
Autonomic Nervous System Disorders		
Ejaculation Failure[(1)]	14	1
Mouth Dry	15	9
Sweating Increased	6	2
Centr. & Periph. Nerv. System Disorders		
Somnolence	14	7
Dizziness	12	7
Headache	26	24
Paresthesia	3	2
Tremor	8	2
Disorders of Skin and Appendages		
Rash	3	2
Gastrointestinal Disorders		
Anorexia	6	2
Constipation	7	5
Diarrhea/Loose Stools	21	11
Dyspepsia	8	4
Flatulence	4	3
Nausea	27	13
Vomiting	4	2
General		
Fatigue	11	7
Hot Flushes	2	1
Psychiatric Disorders		
Agitation	6	4
Anxiety	4	3
Insomnia	22	11
Libido Decreased	6	1
Nervousness	6	4
Special Senses		
Vision Abnormal	4	2

[(1)]Primarily ejaculatory delay. Denominator used was for male patients only (N=913 ZOLOFT; N=773 placebo).
*Major depressive disorder and other premarketing controlled trials.
**Included are events reported by at least 2% of patients taking ZOLOFT except the following events, which had an incidence on placebo greater than or equal to ZOLOFT: abdominal pain and pharyngitis.

Associated with Discontinuation in Placebo-Controlled Clinical Trials
Table 3 lists the adverse events associated with discontinuation of ZOLOFT® (sertraline hydrochloride) treatment (incidence at least twice that for placebo and at least 1% for ZOLOFT in clinical trials) in major depressive disorder/other*, OCD, panic disorder and PTSD.

[See table 3 above]

TABLE 3
MOST COMMON ADVERSE EVENTS ASSOCIATED WITH DISCONTINUATION IN PLACEBO-CONTROLLED CLINICAL TRIALS

Adverse Event	Major Depressive Disorder/Other*, OCD, Panic Disorder and PTSD combined (N=2198)	Major Depressive Disorder/Other* (N=861)	OCD (N=533)	Panic Disorder (N=430)	PTSD (N=374)
Agitation	1%	1%	—	2%	—
Diarrhea	2%	2%	2%	1%	—
Dizziness	1%	—	1%	—	—
Dry Mouth	—	1%	—	—	—
Dyspepsia	—	—	—	1%	—
Ejaculation Failure[(1)]	1%	1%	1%	2%	—
Headache	1%	2%	—	—	1%
Insomnia	2%	1%	3%	2%	—
Nausea	3%	4%	3%	3%	2%
Nervousness	—	—	—	2%	—
Somnolence	2%	1%	2%	2%	—
Tremor	—	2%	—	—	—

[(1)]Primarily ejaculatory delay. Denominator used was for male patients only (N=271 major depressive disorder/other*; N=296 OCD; N=216 panic disorder; N=130 PTSD).
*Major depressive disorder and other premarketing controlled trials.

TABLE 4

Treatment	Ejaculation failure (primarily delayed ejaculation)		Decreased libido	
	N (males only)	Incidence	N (males and females)	Incidence
ZOLOFT	913	14%	2198	6%
Placebo	773	1%	1877	1%

Male and Female Sexual Dysfunction with SSRIs
Although changes in sexual desire, sexual performance and sexual satisfaction often occur as manifestations of a psychiatric disorder, they may also be a consequence of pharmacologic treatment. In particular, some evidence suggests that selective serotonin reuptake inhibitors (SSRIs) can cause such untoward sexual experiences. Reliable estimates of the incidence and severity of untoward experiences involving sexual desire, performance and satisfaction are difficult to obtain, however, in part because patients and physicians may be reluctant to discuss them. Accordingly, estimates of the incidence of untoward sexual experience and performance cited in product labeling, are likely to underestimate their actual incidence.
Table 4 below displays the incidence of sexual side effects reported by at least 2% of patients taking ZOLOFT in placebo-controlled trials.

[See table 4 above]

There are no adequate and well-controlled studies examining sexual dysfunction with sertraline treatment.
Priapism has been reported with all SSRIs.
While it is difficult to know the precise risk of sexual dysfunction associated with the use of SSRIs, physicians should routinely inquire about such possible side effects.

Other Adverse Events in Pediatric Patients—In approximately N=250 pediatric patients treated with ZOLOFT, the overall profile of adverse events was generally similar to that seen in adult studies, as shown in Tables 1 and 2. However, the following adverse events, not appearing in Tables 1 and 2, were reported at an incidence of at least 2% and occurred at a rate of at least twice the placebo rate in a controlled trial (N=187): hyperkinesia, twitching, fever, malaise, purpura, weight decrease, concentration impaired, manic reaction, emotional lability, thinking abnormal, and epistaxis.

Other Events Observed During the Premarketing Evaluation of ZOLOFT® (sertraline hydrochloride)—Following is a list of treatment-emergent adverse events reported during premarketing assessment of ZOLOFT in clinical trials (over 4000 adult subjects) except those already listed in the previous tables or elsewhere in labeling.
In the tabulations that follow, a World Health Organization dictionary of terminology has been used to classify reported adverse events. The frequencies presented, therefore, represent the proportion of the over 4000 adult individuals exposed to multiple doses of ZOLOFT who experienced an event of the type cited on at least one occasion while receiving ZOLOFT. All events are included except those already listed in the previous tables or elsewhere in labeling and those reported in terms so general as to be uninformative and those for which a causal relationship to ZOLOFT treatment seemed remote. It is important to emphasize that although the events reported occurred during treatment with ZOLOFT, they were not necessarily caused by it.
Events are further categorized by body system and listed in order of decreasing frequency according to the following definitions: frequent adverse events are those occurring on one or more occasions in at least 1/100 patients; infrequent adverse events are those occurring in 1/100 to 1/1000 patients; rare events are those occurring in fewer than 1/1000 patients. Events of major clinical importance are also described in the PRECAUTIONS section.

Autonomic Nervous System Disorders—*Frequent:* impotence; *Infrequent:* flushing, increased saliva, cold clammy skin, mydriasis; *Rare:* pallor, glaucoma, priapism, vasodilation.

Body as a Whole–General Disorders—*Rare:* allergic reaction, allergy.

Cardiovascular—*Frequent:* palpitations, chest pain; *Infrequent:* hypertension, tachycardia, postural dizziness, postural hypotension, periorbital edema, peripheral edema, hypotension, peripheral ischemia, syncope, edema, dependent edema; *Rare:* precordial chest pain, substernal chest pain, aggravated hypertension, myocardial infarction, cerebrovascular disorder.

Central and Peripheral Nervous System Disorders—*Frequent:* hypertonia, hypoesthesia; *Infrequent:* twitching, confusion, hyperkinesia, vertigo, ataxia, migraine, abnormal coordination, hyperesthesia, leg cramps, abnormal gait, nystagmus, hypokinesia; *Rare:* dysphonia, coma, dyskinesia, hypotonia, ptosis, choreoathetosis, hyporeflexia.

Disorders of Skin and Appendages—*Infrequent:* pruritus, acne, urticaria, alopecia, dry skin, erythematous rash, photosensitivity reaction, maculopapular rash; *Rare:* follicular rash, eczema, dermatitis, contact dermatitis, bullous eruption, hypertrichosis, skin discoloration, pustular rash.

Endocrine Disorders—*Rare:* exophthalmos, gynecomastia.

Gastrointestinal Disorders—*Frequent:* appetite increased; *Infrequent:* dysphagia, tooth caries aggravated, eructation, esophagitis, gastroenteritis; *Rare:* melena, glossitis, gum hyperplasia, hiccup, stomatitis, tenesmus, colitis, diverticulitis, fecal incontinence, gastritis, rectum hemorrhage, hemorrhagic peptic ulcer, proctitis, ulcerative stomatitis, tongue edema, tongue ulceration.

General—*Frequent:* back pain, asthenia, malaise, weight increase; *Infrequent:* fever, rigors, generalized edema; *Rare:* face edema, aphthous stomatitis.

Hearing and Vestibular Disorders—*Rare:* hyperacusis, labyrinthine disorder.

Hematopoietic and Lymphatic—*Rare:* anemia, anterior chamber eye hemorrhage.

Liver and Biliary System Disorders—*Rare:* abnormal hepatic function.

Metabolic and Nutritional Disorders—*Infrequent:* thirst; *Rare:* hypoglycemia, hypoglycemia reaction.

Musculoskeletal System Disorders—*Frequent:* myalgia; *Infrequent:* arthralgia, dystonia, arthrosis, muscle cramps, muscle weakness.

Psychiatric Disorders—*Frequent:* yawning, other male sexual dysfunction, other female sexual dysfunction; *Infrequent:* depression, amnesia, paroniria, teeth-grinding, emotional lability, apathy, abnormal dreams, euphoria, paranoid reaction, hallucination, aggressive reaction, aggravated depression, delusions; *Rare:* withdrawal syn-

drome, suicide ideation, libido increased, somnambulism, illusion.
Reproductive—*Infrequent:* menstrual disorder, dysmenorrhea, intermenstrual bleeding, vaginal hemorrhage, amenorrhea, leukorrhea; *Rare:* female breast pain, menorrhagia, balanoposthitis, breast enlargement, atrophic vaginitis, acute female mastitis.
Respiratory System Disorders—*Frequent:* rhinitis; *Infrequent:* coughing, dyspnea, upper respiratory tract infection, epistaxis, bronchospasm, sinusitis; *Rare:* hyperventilation, bradypnea, stridor, apnea, bronchitis, hemoptysis, hypoventilation, laryngismus, laryngitis.
Special Senses—*Frequent:* tinnitus; *Infrequent:* conjunctivitis, earache, eye pain, abnormal accommodation; *Rare:* xerophthalmia, photophobia, diplopia, abnormal lacrimation, scotoma, visual field defect.
Urinary System Disorders—*Infrequent:* micturition frequency, polyuria, urinary retention, dysuria, nocturia, urinary incontinence; *Rare:* cystitis, oliguria, pyelonephritis, hematuria, renal pain, strangury.
Laboratory Tests—In man, asymptomatic elevations in serum transaminases (SGOT [or AST] and SGPT [or ALT]) have been reported infrequently (approximately 0.8%) in association with ZOLOFT® (sertraline hydrochloride) administration. These hepatic enzyme elevations usually occurred within the first 1 to 9 weeks of drug treatment and promptly diminished upon drug discontinuation.
ZOLOFT therapy was associated with small mean increases in total cholesterol (approximately 3%) and triglycerides (approximately 5%), and a small mean decrease in serum uric acid (approximately 7%) of no apparent clinical importance.
The safety profile observed with ZOLOFT treatment in patients with major depressive disorder, OCD, panic disorder and PTSD is similar.
Other Events Observed During the Postmarketing Evaluation of ZOLOFT—Reports of adverse events temporally associated with ZOLOFT that have been received since market introduction, that are not listed above and that may have no causal relationship with the drug, include the following: acute renal failure, anaphylactoid reaction, angioedema, blindness, optic neuritis, cataract, increased coagulation times, bradycardia, AV block, atrial arrhythmias, QT-interval prolongation, ventricular tachycardia (including torsade de pointes-type arrhythmias), hypothyroidism, agranulocytosis, aplastic anemia and pancytopenia, leukopenia, thrombocytopenia, lupus-like syndrome, serum sickness, hyperglycemia, galactorrhea, hyperprolactinemia, neuroleptic malignant syndrome-like events, extrapyramidal symptoms, oculogyric crisis, serotonin syndrome, psychosis, pulmonary hypertension, severe skin reactions, which potentially can be fatal, such as Stevens-Johnson syndrome, vasculitis, photosensitivity and other severe cutaneous disorders, rare reports of pancreatitis, and liver events—clinical features (which in the majority of cases appeared to be reversible with discontinuation of ZOLOFT) occurring in one or more patients include: elevated enzymes, increased bilirubin, hepatomegaly, hepatitis, jaundice, abdominal pain, vomiting, liver failure and death.

DRUG ABUSE AND DEPENDENCE
Controlled Substance Class—ZOLOFT® (sertraline hydrochloride) is not a controlled substance.
Physical and Psychological Dependence—In a placebo-controlled, double-blind, randomized study of the comparative abuse liability of ZOLOFT, alprazolam, and d-amphetamine in humans, ZOLOFT did not produce the positive subjective effects indicative of abuse potential, such as euphoria or drug liking, that were observed with the other two drugs. Premarketing clinical experience with ZOLOFT did not reveal any tendency for a withdrawal syndrome or any drug-seeking behavior. In animal studies ZOLOFT does not demonstrate stimulant or barbiturate-like (depressant) abuse potential. As with any CNS active drug, however, physicians should carefully evaluate patients for history of drug abuse and follow such patients closely, observing them for signs of ZOLOFT misuse or abuse (e.g., development of tolerance, incrementation of dose, drug-seeking behavior).

OVERDOSAGE
Human Experience—Of 1,027 cases of overdose involving sertraline hydrochloride worldwide, alone or with other drugs, there were 72 deaths (circa 1999).
Among 634 overdoses in which sertraline hydrochloride was the only drug ingested, 8 resulted in fatal outcome, 75 completely recovered, and 27 patients experienced sequelae after overdosage to include alopecia, decreased libido, diarrhea, ejaculation disorder, fatigue, insomnia, somnolence and serotonin syndrome. The remaining 524 cases had an unknown outcome. The most common signs and symptoms associated with non-fatal sertraline hydrochloride overdosage were somnolence, vomiting, tachycardia, nausea, dizziness, agitation and tremor.
The largest known ingestion was 13.5 grams in a patient who took sertraline hydrochloride alone and subsequently recovered. However, another patient who took 2.5 grams of sertraline hydrochloride alone experienced a fatal outcome. Other important adverse events reported with sertraline hydrochloride overdose (single or multiple drugs) include bradycardia, bundle branch block, coma, convulsions, delirium, hallucinations, hypertension, hypotension, manic reaction, pancreatitis, QT-interval prolongation, serotonin syndrome, stupor and syncope.
Overdose Management—Treatment should consist of those general measures employed in the management of overdosage with any antidepressant.
Ensure an adequate airway, oxygenation and ventilation. Monitor cardiac rhythm and vital signs. General supportive and symptomatic measures are also recommended. Induction of emesis is not recommended. Gastric lavage with a large-bore orogastric tube with appropriate airway protection, if needed, may be indicated if performed soon after ingestion, or in symptomatic patients.
Activated charcoal should be administered. Due to large volume of distribution of this drug, forced diuresis, dialysis, hemoperfusion and exchange transfusion are unlikely to be of benefit. No specific antidotes for sertraline are known.
In managing overdosage, consider the possibility of multiple drug involvement. The physician should consider contacting a poison control center on the treatment of any overdose. Telephone numbers for certified poison control centers are listed in the *Physicians' Desk Reference*® (PDR®).

DOSAGE AND ADMINISTRATION
Initial Treatment
Dosage for Adults
Major Depressive Disorder and Obsessive-Compulsive Disorder—ZOLOFT treatment should be administered at a dose of 50 mg once daily.
Panic Disorder and Posttraumatic Stress Disorder—ZOLOFT treatment should be initiated with a dose of 25 mg once daily. After one week, the dose should be increased to 50 mg once daily.
While a relationship between dose and effect has not been established for major depressive disorder, OCD, panic disorder or PTSD, patients were dosed in a range of 50–200 mg/day in the clinical trials demonstrating the effectiveness of ZOLOFT for the treatment of these indications. Consequently, a dose of 50 mg, administered once daily, is recommended as the initial dose. Patients not responding to a 50 mg dose may benefit from dose increases up to a maximum of 200 mg/day. Given the 24 hour elimination half-life of ZOLOFT, dose changes should not occur at intervals of less than 1 week.
ZOLOFT should be administered once daily, either in the morning or evening.
Dosage for Pediatric Population (Children and Adolescents)
Obsessive-Compulsive Disorder—ZOLOFT treatment should be initiated with a dose of 25 mg once daily in children (ages 6–12) and at a dose of 50 mg once daily in adolescents (ages 13–17).
While a relationship between dose and effect has not been established for OCD, patients were dosed in a range of 25–200 mg/day in the clinical trials demonstrating the effectiveness of ZOLOFT for pediatric patients (6–17 years) with OCD. Patients not responding to an initial dose of 25 or 50 mg/day may benefit from dose increases up to a maximum of 200 mg/day. For children with OCD, their generally lower body weights compared to adults should be taken into consideration in advancing the dose, in order to avoid excess dosing. Given the 24 hour elimination half-life of ZOLOFT, dose changes should not occur at intervals of less than 1 week.
ZOLOFT should be administered once daily, either in the morning or evening.
Dosage for Hepatically Impaired Patients
The use of sertraline in patients with liver disease should be approached with caution. The effects of sertraline in patients with moderate and severe hepatic impairment have not been studied. If sertraline is administered to patients with liver impairment, a lower or less frequent dose should be used (see CLINICAL PHARMACOLOGY and PRECAUTIONS).
Maintenance/Continuation/Extended Treatment
Major Depressive Disorder—It is generally agreed that acute episodes of major depressive disorder require several months or longer of sustained pharmacologic therapy beyond response to the acute episode. Systematic evaluation of ZOLOFT has demonstrated that its antidepressant efficacy is maintained for periods of up to 44 weeks following 8 weeks of initial treatment at a dose of 50–200 mg/day (mean dose of 70 mg/day) (see Clinical Trials under CLINICAL PHARMACOLOGY). It is not known whether the dose of ZOLOFT needed for maintenance treatment is identical to the dose needed to achieve an initial response. Patients should be periodically reassessed to determine the need for maintenance treatment.
Posttraumatic Stress Disorder—It is generally agreed that PTSD requires several months or longer of sustained pharmacological therapy beyond response to initial treatment. Systematic evaluation of ZOLOFT has demonstrated that its efficacy in PTSD is maintained for periods of up to 28 weeks following 24 weeks of treatment at a dose of 50–200 mg/day (see Clinical Trials under CLINICAL PHARMACOLOGY). It is not known whether the dose of ZOLOFT needed for maintenance treatment is identical to the dose needed to achieve an initial response. Patients should be periodically reassessed to determine the need for maintenance treatment.
Obsessive-Compulsive Disorder and Panic Disorder—Although the efficacy of ZOLOFT beyond 10–12 weeks of dosing for OCD and Panic Disorder has not been systematically demonstrated in controlled trials, both are chronic conditions, and it is reasonable to consider continuation of a responding patient. Dosage adjustments may be needed to maintain the patient on the lowest effective dosage and patients should be periodically reassessed to determine the need for continued treatment.
Switching Patients to or from a Monoamine Oxidase Inhibitor—At least 14 days should elapse between discontinuation of an MAOI and initiation of therapy with ZOLOFT. In addition, at least 14 days should be allowed after stopping ZOLOFT before starting an MAOI (see CONTRAINDICATIONS and WARNINGS).
ZOLOFT Oral Concentrate
ZOLOFT Oral Concentrate contains 20 mg/mL of sertraline (as the hydrochloride) as the active ingredient and 12% alcohol. ZOLOFT Oral Concentrate must be diluted before use. Just before taking, use the dropper provided to remove the required amount of ZOLOFT Oral Concentrate and mix with 4 oz (1/2 cup) of water, ginger ale, lemon/lime soda, lemonade or orange juice ONLY. Do not mix ZOLOFT Oral Concentrate with anything other than the liquids listed. The dose should be taken immediately after mixing. Do not mix in advance. At times, a slight haze may appear after mixing; this is normal. Note that caution should be exercised for patients with latex sensitivity, as the dropper dispenser contains dry natural rubber.
ZOLOFT oral concentrate is contraindicated with ANTABUSE (disulfiram) due to the alcohol content of the concentrate.

HOW SUPPLIED
ZOLOFT® (sertraline hydrochloride) capsular-shaped scored tablets, containing sertraline hydrochloride equivalent to 25, 50 and 100 mg of sertraline, are packaged in bottles.
ZOLOFT® 25 mg Tablets: light green film coated tablets engraved on one side with ZOLOFT and on the other side scored and engraved with 25 mg.

NDC 0049-4960-50	Bottles of 50

ZOLOFT® 50 mg Tablets: light blue film coated tablets engraved on one side with ZOLOFT and on the other side scored and engraved with 50 mg.

NDC 0049-4900-66	Bottles of 100
NDC 0049-4900-73	Bottles of 500
NDC 0049-4900-94	Bottles of 5000
NDC 0049-4900-41	Unit Dose Packages of 100

ZOLOFT® 100 mg Tablets: light yellow film coated tablets engraved on one side with ZOLOFT and on the other side scored and engraved with 100 mg.

NDC 0049-4910-66	Bottles of 100
NDC 0049-4910-73	Bottles of 500
NDC 0049-4910-94	Bottles of 5000
NDC 0049-4910-41	Unit Dose Packages of 100

Store at controlled room temperature, 59° to 86°F (15° to 30°C).
ZOLOFT® Oral Concentrate: ZOLOFT Oral Concentrate is a clear, colorless solution with a menthol scent containing sertraline hydrochloride equivalent to 20 mg of sertraline per mL and 12% alcohol. It is supplied as a 60 mL bottle with an accompanying calibrated dropper.

NDC 0049-4940-23	Bottles of 60 mL

Store at controlled room temperature, 59° to 86°F (15° to 30°C).
Rx only
Distributed by
Pfizer
Roerig
Division of Pfizer Inc, NY, NY 10017
Printed in U.S.A.
Revised November 2000
69-4721-00-1

The Purdue Frederick Company
ONE STAMFORD FORUM
STAMFORD, CT 06901-3431

For Medical Information Contact:
888-726-7535
Adverse Drug Experiences:
888-726-7535
Customer Service:
800-877-5666
FAX 800-877-3210

MSIR® Ⓒ℞
[em 'es ī "ahr]
Oral Solution
(morphine sulfate)
MSIR® Ⓒ℞
Oral Solution Concentrate*
(morphine sulfate)
MSIR® Ⓒ℞
Immediate-Release Oral Tablets
(morphine sulfate)
MSIR® Ⓒ℞
Immediate-Release Oral Capsules
(morphine sulfate)

***This product contains dry natural rubber**

Prescribing information for this product, which appears on pages 2898–2900 of the 2002 PDR, has been revised as follows. Please write "See Supplement A" next to the product heading.
Add the following sentence, as the first sentence, under the heading DOSAGE AND ADMINISTRATION:
WARNING: DRUG CONCENTRATE-CHECK DOSAGE AND MEASURE ACCURATELY.

Continued on next page

UNIPHYL® ℞
[ū 'nĭ-fĭl]
400 mg and 600 mg Tablets
(theophylline)
UNICONTIN® Controlled-Release System

Prescribing information for this product, which appears on pages 2903–2908 of the 2002 PDR, has been revised as follows. Please write "See Supplement A" next to the product heading.
The following Drug Interaction was added to Table II:

TABLE II. Clinically significant drug interactions with theophylline*

Hypericum perforatum (St. John's Wort)	**Increases theophylline clearance by induction of microsomal enzyme activity**	**Higher doses of theophylline may be required to achieve desired effect. Stopping St. John's Wort may result in theophylline toxicity.**

The following 4th sentence was added to the **Geriatric Use** *subsection:*
Geriatric Use
Elderly patients also appear to be more sensitive to the toxic effects of theophylline after chronic overdosage than younger patients.

Purdue Pharma L.P.
ONE STAMFORD FORUM
STAMFORD, CT 06901-3431

For Medical Inquiries:
888-726-7535
Adverse Drug Experiences:
888-726-7535
Customer Service:
800-877-5666
FAX 800-877-3210

CHIROCAINE® (Levobupivacaine Injection) ℞
[kī'-rō-kān]

Prescribing information for this product, which appears on pages 2909–2912 of the 2002 PDR, has been revised as follows. Please write "See Supplement A" next to the product heading.
The **Dosage Recommendations** *chart was revised as follows:*
[See table below]
November 27, 2001

OXYCONTIN® Ⓒ ℞
(OXYCODONE HCl CONTROLLED-RELEASE) TABLETS
10 mg 20 mg 40 mg 80 mg* 160 mg*

***80 mg and 160 mg for use in opioid-tolerant patients only**

Prescribing information for this product, which appears on pages 2912–2916 of the 2002 PDR, has been revised as follows. Please write "See Supplement A" next to the product heading.

The following patient information was added to the end of the insert:

PATIENT INFORMATION
OXYCONTIN® Schedule II
(Oxycodone HCl Controlled-Release) Tablets
OxyContin® Tablets, 10 mg
OxyContin® Tablets, 20 mg
OxyContin® Tablets, 40 mg
OxyContin® Tablets, 80 mg
OxyContin® Tablets, 160 mg

Read this information carefully before you take OxyContin® (ox-e-CON-tin) tablets. Also read the information you get with your refills. There may be something new. This information does not take the place of talking with your doctor about your medical condition or your treatment. Only you and your doctor can decide if OxyContin is right for you. Share the important information in this leaflet with members of your household.

What Is The Most Important Information I Should Know About OxyContin®?
- **Use OxyContin the way your doctor tells you to.**
- **Use OxyContin only for the condition for which it was prescribed.**
- **OxyContin is not for occasional ("as needed") use.**
- **Swallow the tablets whole.** Do not break, crush, dissolve, or chew them before swallowing. OxyContin® works properly over 12 hours only when swallowed whole. **If a tablet is broken, crushed, dissolved, or chewed, the entire 12 hour dose will be absorbed into your body all at once. This can be dangerous, causing an overdose, and possibly death.**
- **Keep OxyContin® out of the reach of children.** Accidental overdose by a child is dangerous and may result in death.
- **Prevent theft and misuse.** OxyContin contains a narcotic painkiller that can be a target for people who abuse prescription medicines. Therefore, keep your tablets in a secure place, to protect them from theft. Never give them to anyone else. Selling or giving away this medicine is dangerous and against the law.

What Is OxyContin®?
OxyContin® is a tablet that comes in several strengths and contains the medicine oxycodone (ox-e-KOE-done). This medicine is a painkiller like morphine. OxyContin treats moderate to severe pain that is expected to last for an extended period of time. Use OxyContin regularly during treatment. It contains enough medicine to last for up to twelve hours.

Who Should Not Take OxyContin®?
Do not take OxyContin® if
- your doctor did not prescribe OxyContin® for you.
- your pain is mild or will go away in a few days.
- your pain can be controlled by occasional use of other painkillers.
- you have severe asthma or severe lung problems.
- you have had a severe allergic reaction to codeine, hydrocodone, dihydrocodeine, or oxycodone (such as Tylox, Tylenol with Codeine, or Vicodin). A severe allergic reaction includes a severe rash, hives, breathing problems, or dizziness.
- you had surgery less than 12–24 hours ago and you were not taking OxyContin just before surgery.

Your doctor should know about all your medical conditions before deciding if OxyContin is right for you and what dose is best. Tell your doctor about all of your medical problems, especially the ones listed below:
- trouble breathing or lung problems
- head injury
- liver or kidney problems
- adrenal gland problems, such as Addison's disease
- convulsions or seizures
- alcoholism
- hallucinations or other severe mental problems
- past or present substance abuse or drug addiction

If any of these conditions apply to you, and you haven't told your doctor, then you should tell your doctor before taking OxyContin.
If you are pregnant or plan to become pregnant, talk with your doctor. OxyContin may not be right for you. **Tell your doctor if you are breast feeding.** OxyContin will pass through the milk and may harm the baby.
Tell your doctor about all the medicines you take, including prescription and non-prescription medicines, vitamins, and herbal supplements. They may cause serious medical problems when taken with OxyContin, especially if they cause drowsiness.

How Should I Take OxyContin®?
- **Follow your doctor's directions exactly.** Your doctor may change your dose based on your reactions to the medicine. Do not change your dose unless your doctor tells you to change it. Do not take OxyContin more often than prescribed.
- **Swallow the tablets whole. Do not break, crush, dissolve, or chew before swallowing. If the tablets are not whole, your body will absorb too much medicine at one time. This can lead to serious problems, including overdose and death.**
- **If you miss a dose,** take it as soon as possible. If it is almost time for your next dose, skip the missed dose and go back to your regular dosing schedule. Do not take 2 doses at once unless your doctor tells you to.
- **If case of overdose,** call your local emergency number or poison control center right away.
- **Review your pain regularly with your doctor** to determine if you still need OxyContin®.
- **You may see tablets in your stools (bowel movements).** Do not be concerned. Your body has already absorbed the medicine.

If you continue to have pain or bothersome side effects, call your doctor.
Stopping OxyContin®. Consult your doctor for instructions on how to stop this medicine slowly to avoid uncomfortable symptoms. You should not stop taking OxyContin all at once if you have been taking it for more than a few days.
After you stop taking OxyContin, flush the unused tablets down the toilet.

What Should I Avoid While Taking OxyContin®?
- **Do not drive, operate heavy machinery, or participate in any other possibly dangerous activities** until you know how you react to this medicine. OxyContin can make you sleepy.
- **Do not drink alcohol while using OxyContin. It may increase the chance of getting dangerous side effects.**
- **Do not take other medicines without your doctor's approval.** Other medicines include prescription and non-prescription medicines, vitamins, and supplements. Be especially careful about products that make you sleepy.

What are the Possible Side Effects of OxyContin®?
Call your doctor or get medical help right away if
- your breathing slows down
- you feel faint, dizzy, confused, or have any other unusual symptoms

Some of the common side effects of OxyContin® are nausea, vomiting, dizziness, drowsiness, constipation, itching, dry mouth, sweating, weakness, and headache. Some of these side effects may decrease with continued use.
There is a risk of abuse or addiction with narcotic painkillers. If you have abused drugs in the past, you may have a higher chance of developing abuse or addiction again while using OxyContin. We do not know how often patients with continuing (chronic) pain become addicted to narcotics, but the risk has been reported to be small.
These are not all the possible side effects of OxyContin. For a complete list, ask your doctor or pharmacist.

General Advice About OxyContin®
- Do not use OxyContin for conditions for which it was not prescribed.
- Do not give OxyContin to other people, even if they have the same symptoms you have. Sharing is illegal and may cause severe medical problems, including death.

This leaflet summarizes the most important information about OxyContin. If you would like more information, talk with your doctor. Also, you can ask your pharmacist or doctor for information about OxyContin that is written for health professionals.
Rx Only
Purdue Pharma L.P.
Stamford, CT 06901-3431

January 25, 2002
OT00367A
300514-0A-001

Dosage Recommendations

	% Concentration	Dose mL	Dose mg	Motor Block
Surgical Anesthesia				
Epidural for surgery	0.5–0.75	10–20	50–150	Moderate to complete
Epidural for Cesarean Section	0.5	20–30	100–150	Moderate to complete
Peripheral Nerve	0.25–0.5	30 0.4 mL/kg	75–150 1–2 mg/kg	Moderate to complete
Ophthalmic	0.75	5–15	37.5–112.5	Moderate to complete
Local Infiltration	0.25	60	150	Not Applicable
Pain Management[a]				
Labor Analgesia (epidural bolus)	0.25	10–20	25–50	Minimal to moderate
Post-operative pain (epidural infusion)	0.125[b,c]–0.25[c]	4–10 mL/h	5–25 mg/h	Minimal to moderate

[a] In pain management Chirocaine® can be used epidurally with fentanyl or clonidine.
[b] 0.125% is to be used only as adjunct therapy in combination with fentanyl or clonidine.
[c] Dilutions of Chirocaine standard solutions should be made with preservative free 0.9% saline according to standard hospital procedures for sterility.

To keep your **PDR** up to date throughout the year, note these revisions on the corresponding pages of the annual volume. Simply write **"See Supplement A"** next to the product heading.

A. H. Robins Company

1407 CUMMINGS DRIVE
RICHMOND, VA 23220

Direct General Inquiries to:
(610) 688-4400

For Emergency Medical Information Contact:
Day: (800) 934-5556 8:30 AM to 4:30 PM (Eastern Standard Time), Weekdays only
Night: (610) 688-4400 (Emergencies only; non-emergencies should wait until the next day)

For Medical/Pharmacy Inquiries on Marketed Products Call:
Medical Affairs, (800) 934-5556 8:30 AM to 4:30 PM (Eastern Standard Time), Weekdays only

QUINIDEX EXTENTABS® Tablets ℞

[*kwĭn' ĭ" dĕks ĕks"tĕn'tăbs*]
(quinidine sulfate extended-release tablets, USP)

Prescribing information for this product, which appears on pages 2933–2935 of the 2002 PDR, has been revised as follows. Please write "See Supplement A" next to the product heading.

The subheading **Drug Interactions** in the **PRECAUTIONS** *section should be changed to* **Drug and Diet Interactions.**

The words "(P450 3A4)" *should be added to the end of the first sentence of the third paragraph under the subheading "Altered pharmacokinetics of quinidine" under* **Drug Interactions** *in the* **PRECAUTIONS** *section.*

The word "$P_{450}IIIA_4$" *should be changed to* "P450 2D6" *wherever it appears in the* **Drug Interactions** *subsection in the* **PRECAUTIONS** *section.*

The following paragraphs should be added as the last two paragraphs under the subheading "Altered pharmacokinetics of quinidine" under **Drug Interactions** *in the* **PRECAUTIONS** *section:*

Grapefruit juice inhibits P450 3A4-mediated metabolism of quinidine to 3-hydroxyquinidine. Although the clinical significance of this interaction is unknown, grapefruit juice should be avoided.

The rate and extent of quinidine absorption may be affected by changes in **dietary salt** intake; a decrease in dietary salt intake may lead to an increase in plasma quinidine concentrations.

The paragraph under the heading **Geriatric Use** *in the* **PRECAUTIONS** *should be deleted and replaced with the following two paragraphs:*

Clinical studies of quinidine generally were not adequate to determine if significant safety or efficacy differences exist between elderly patients (65 years or older) and younger patients.

Quinidine clearance is apparently independent of age (see **CLINICAL PHARMACOLOGY—Pharmacokinetics**). However, renal or hepatic dysfunction causes the elimination of quinidine to be slowed (see **WARNINGS—Pharmacokinetic Considerations**), and since these conditions are more common in the elderly, appropriate dosing reductions should be considered in these individuals.

The following paragraph should be added as the second paragraph under the heading **OVERDOSAGE:**

A case of tablet ingestion by a 16-month-old infant has been reported in which a concretion or bezoar was formed in the stomach, resulting in nondeclining toxic levels of quinidine. The mass was only dimly visible on plain radiographs, but a gastric aspirate revealed quinidine levels approximately 50 times higher than those in the plasma. In cases of massive overdose with prolonged high plasma levels, diagnostic/therapeutic endoscopy may be appropriate.

In the storage information that appears after the **HOW SUPPLIED** *section, the word* **"tablets"** *should be inserted after the word* **"Store."**

Under the storage information, the sentence "Caution: Federal law prohibits dispensing without prescription." *should be deleted and replaced with* "Rx only."

CI 4675-3 Revised September 28, 2000

ROBINUL® INJECTABLE ℞

[*rō'bĭ-nūl*]
(glycopyrrolate injection, USP)

Prescribing information for this product, which appears on pages 2940–2942 of the 2002 PDR, has been revised as follows. Please write "See Supplement A" next to the product heading.

The following paragraph should be added as the third paragraph under the **CONTRAINDICATIONS** *section:*

There have been reports of fatal 'gasping syndrome' in neonates following the administrations of intravenous solutions containing the preservative benzyl alcohol. Symptoms include a striking onset of gasping respiration, hypotension, bradycardia, and cardiovascular collapse.

CI6387-2 Issued September 2001

Roche Pharmaceuticals

Roche Laboratories Inc.
340 Kingsland Street
Nutley, NJ 07110-1199

For Medical Information:
(Including routine inquiries, adverse drug events and product complaints)
Call: (800) 526-6367
In Emergencies: 24-hour service
For the Medical Needs Program:
Call: (800) 285-4484
Write: Professional Product Information

EC-NAPROSYN® (naproxen) ℞
Delayed-Release Tablets
NAPROSYN® (naproxen) Tablets
ANAPROX®/ANAPROX® DS
(naproxen sodium) Tablets
NAPROSYN® (naproxen) Suspension

Prescribing information for these products, which appear on pages 2967–2970 of the 2002 PDR has been revised as follows. Please write "See Supplement A" next to the product heading.

Replace the HOW SUPPLIED *section with the following:*

HOW SUPPLIED

NAPROSYN Tablets: 250 mg: round, yellow, biconvex, engraved with NPR LE 250 on one side and scored on the other. Packaged in light-resistant bottles of 100.
100's (bottle): NDC 0004-6313-01.

375 mg: pink, biconvex oval, engraved with NPR LE 375 on one side. Packaged in light-resistant bottles of 100 and 500.
100's (bottle): NDC 0004-6314-01; 500's (bottle): NDC 0004-6314-14.

500 mg: yellow, capsule-shaped, engraved with NPR LE 500 on one side and scored on the other. Packaged in light-resistant bottles of 100 and 500.
100's (bottle): NDC 0004-6316-01; 500's (bottle): NDC 0004-6316-14.

Store at 15° to 30°C (59° to 86°F) in well-closed containers; dispense in light-resistant containers.

NAPROSYN Suspension: 125 mg/5 mL (contains 39 mg sodium, about 1.5 mEq/teaspoon): Available in 1 pint (473 mL) light-resistant bottles (NDC 0004-0028-28).

Store at 15° to 30°C (59° to 86°F); avoid excessive heat, above 40°C (104°F). Dispense in light-resistant containers.

EC-NAPROSYN Delayed-Release Tablets:
375 mg: white, capsule-shaped, imprinted with EC-NAPROSYN on one side and 375 on the other.
Packaged in light-resistant bottles of 100.
100's (bottle): NDC 0004-6415-01.

500 mg: white, capsule-shaped, imprinted with EC-NAPROSYN on one side and 500 on the other.
Packaged in light-resistant bottles of 100.
100's (bottle): NDC 0004-6416-01.

Store at 15° to 30°C (59° to 86°F) in well-closed containers; dispense in light-resistant containers.

ANAPROX Tablets: Naproxen sodium 275 mg: light blue, oval-shaped, engraved with NPS-275 on one side. Packaged in bottles of 100.
100's (bottle): NDC 0004-6202-01.

Store at 15° to 30°C (59° to 86°F) in well-closed containers.

ANAPROX DS Tablets: Naproxen sodium 550 mg: dark blue, oblong-shaped, engraved with NPS 550 on one side and scored on both sides. Packaged in bottles of 100 and 500.
100's (bottle): NDC 0004-6203-01; 500's (bottle): NDC 0004-6203-14.

Store at 15° to 30°C (59° to 86°F) in well-closed containers.

Revised: May 2001

XELODA® ℞
(capecitabine)
TABLETS

Prescribing information for this product, which appears on pages 3039–3043 of the 2002 PDR has been revised as follows. Please write "See Supplement A" next to the product heading.

WARNING

XELODA Warfarin Interaction: Patients receiving concomitant capecitabine and oral coumarin-derivative anticoagulant therapy should have their anticoagulant response (INR or prothrombin time) monitored frequently in order to adjust the anticoagulant dose accordingly. A clinically important XELODA-Warfarin drug interaction was demonstrated in a clinical pharmacology trial (see CLINICAL PHARMACOLOGY and PRECAUTIONS). Altered coagulation parameters and/or bleeding, including death, have been reported in patients taking XELODA concomitantly with coumarin-derivative anticoagulants such as warfarin and phenprocoumon. Postmarketing reports have shown clinically significant increases in prothrombin time (PT) and INR in patients who were stabilized on anticoagulants at the time XELODA was introduced. These events occurred within several days and up to several months after initiating XELODA therapy and, in a few cases, within one month after stopping XELODA. These events occurred in patients with and without liver metastases. Age greater than 60 and a diagnosis of cancer independently predispose patients to an increased risk of coagulopathy.

DESCRIPTION

XELODA (capecitabine) is a fluoropyrimidine carbamate with antineoplastic activity. It is an orally administered systemic prodrug of 5'-deoxy-5-fluorouridine (5'-DFUR) which is converted to 5-fluorouracil.

The chemical name for capecitabine is 5'-deoxy-5-fluoro-N-[(pentyloxy) carbonyl]-cytidine and has a molecular weight of 359.35. Capecitabine has the following structural formula:

Capecitabine is a white to off-white crystalline powder with an aqueous solubility of 26 mg/mL at 20°C.

XELODA is supplied as biconvex, oblong film-coated tablets for oral administration. Each light peach-colored tablet contains 150 mg capecitabine and each peach-colored tablet contains 500 mg capecitabine. The inactive ingredients in XELODA include: anhydrous lactose, croscarmellose sodium, hydroxypropyl methylcellulose, microcrystalline cellulose, magnesium stearate and purified water. The peach or light peach film coating contains hydroxypropyl methylcellulose, talc, titanium dioxide, and synthetic yellow and red iron oxides.

CLINICAL PHARMACOLOGY

XELODA is relatively non-cytotoxic in vitro. This drug is enzymatically converted to 5-fluorouracil (5-FU) in vivo.

Bioactivation: Capecitabine is readily absorbed from the gastrointestinal tract. In the liver, a 60 kDa carboxylesterase hydrolyzes much of the compound to 5'-deoxy-5-fluorocytidine (5'-DFCR). Cytidine deaminase, an enzyme found in most tissues, including tumors, subsequently converts 5'-DFCR to 5'-deoxy-5-fluorouridine (5'-DFUR). The enzyme, thymidine phosphorylase (dThdPase), then hydrolyzes 5'-DFUR to the active drug 5-FU. Many tissues throughout the body express thymidine phosphorylase. Some human carcinomas express this enzyme in higher concentrations than surrounding normal tissues.

Metabolic Pathway of capecitabine to 5-FU

Capecitabine → (Carboxylesterase) → 5'-DFCR → (Cyd deaminase) → 5'-DFUR → (dThdPase) → 5-FU

Mechanism of Action: Both normal and tumor cells metabolize 5-FU to 5-fluoro-2'-deoxyuridine monophosphate (FdUMP) and 5-fluorouridine triphosphate (FUTP). These metabolites cause cell injury by two different mechanisms. First, FdUMP and the folate cofactor, N^{5-10}-methylenetetrahydrofolate, bind to thymidylate synthase (TS) to form a covalently bound ternary complex. This binding inhibits the formation of thymidylate from 2'-deoxyuridylate. Thymidylate is the necessary precursor of thymidine triphosphate, which is essential for the synthesis of DNA, so that a deficiency of this compound can inhibit cell division. Second, nuclear transcriptional enzymes can mistakenly incorporate FUTP in place of uridine triphosphate (UTP) during the synthesis of RNA. This metabolic error can interfere with RNA processing and protein synthesis.

Pharmacokinetics in Colorectal Tumors and Adjacent Healthy Tissue: Following oral administration of XELODA 7 days before surgery in patients with colorectal cancer, the median ratio of 5-FU concentration in colorectal tumors to adjacent tissues was 2.9 (range from 0.9 to 8.0). These ratios have not been evaluated in breast cancer patients or compared to 5-FU infusion.

Human Pharmacokinetics: The pharmacokinetics of XELODA and its metabolites have been evaluated in about 200 cancer patients over a dosage range of 500 to 3500 mg/m²/day. Over this range, the pharmacokinetics of XELODA and its metabolite, 5'-DFCR were dose proportional and did not change over time. The increases in the AUCs of 5'-DFUR and 5-FU, however, were greater than proportional to the increase in dose and the AUC of 5-FU

Continued on next page

Xeloda—Cont.

was 34% higher on day 14 than on day 1. The elimination half-life of both parent capecitabine and 5-FU was about 3/4 of an hour. The inter-patient variability in the C_{max} and AUC of 5-FU was greater than 85%.

Absorption, Distribution, Metabolism and Excretion: Capecitabine reached peak blood levels in about 1.5 hours (T_{max}) with peak 5-FU levels occurring slightly later, at 2 hours. Food reduced both the rate and extent of absorption of capecitabine with mean C_{max} and $AUC_{0-\infty}$ decreased by 60% and 35%, respectively. The C_{max} and $AUC_{0-\infty}$ of 5-FU were also reduced by food by 43% and 21%, respectively. Food delayed T_{max} of both parent and 5-FU by 1.5 hours (see PRECAUTIONS and DOSAGE AND ADMINISTRATION).

Plasma protein binding of capecitabine and its metabolites is less than 60% and is not concentration-dependent. Capecitabine was primarily bound to human albumin (approximately 35%).

Capecitabine is extensively metabolized enzymatically to 5-FU. The enzyme dihydropyrimidine dehydrogenase hydrogenates 5-FU, the product of capecitabine metabolism, to the much less toxic 5-fluoro-5, 6-dihydro-fluorouracil (FUH_2). Dihydropyrimidinase cleaves the pyrimidine ring to yield 5-fluoro-ureido-propionic acid (FUPA). Finally, β-ureido-propionase cleaves FUPA to α-fluoro-β-alanine (FBAL) which is cleared in the urine.

Capecitabine and its metabolites are predominantly excreted in urine; 95.5% of administered capecitabine dose is recovered in urine. Fecal excretion is minimal (2.6%). The major metabolite excreted in urine is FBAL which represents 57% of the administered dose. About 3% of the administered dose is excreted in urine as unchanged drug.

A clinical phase 1 study evaluating the effect of XELODA on the pharmacokinetics of docetaxel (Taxotere®) and the effect of docetaxel on the pharmacokinetics of XELODA was conducted in 26 patients with solid tumors. XELODA was found to have no effect on the pharmacokinetics of docetaxel (C_{max} and AUC) and docetaxel has no effect on the pharmacokinetics of capecitabine and the 5-FU precursor 5′-DFUR.

Special Populations:

A population analysis of pooled data from the two large controlled studies in patients with colorectal cancer (n=505) who were administered XELODA at 1250 mg/m^2 twice a day indicated that gender (202 females and 303 males) and race (455 white/caucasian patients, 22 black patients, and 28 patients of other race) have no influence on the pharmacokinetics of 5′-DFUR, 5-FU and FBAL. Age has no significant influence on the pharmacokinetics of 5′-DFUR and 5-FU over the range of 27 to 86 years. A 20% increase in age results in a 15% increase in AUC of FBAL (see WARNINGS and DOSAGE AND ADMINISTRATION).

Hepatic Insufficiency: XELODA has been evaluated in 13 patients with mild to moderate hepatic dysfunction due to liver metastases defined by a composite score including bilirubin, AST/ALT and alkaline phosphatase following a single 1255 mg/m^2 dose of XELODA. Both $AUC_{0-\infty}$ and C_{max} of capecitabine increased by 60% in patients with hepatic dysfunction compared to patients with normal hepatic function (n=14). The $AUC_{0-\infty}$ and C_{max} of 5-FU were not affected. In patients with mild to moderate hepatic dysfunction due to liver metastases, caution should be exercised when XELODA is administered. The effect of severe hepatic dysfunction on XELODA is not known (see PRECAUTIONS and DOSAGE AND ADMINISTRATION).

Renal Insufficiency: Following oral administration of 1250 mg/m^2 capecitabine twice a day to cancer patients with varying degrees of renal impairment, patients with moderate (creatinine clearance=30–50 mL/min) and severe (creatinine clearance <30 mL/min) renal impairment showed 85% and 258% higher systemic exposure to FBAL on day 1 compared to normal renal function patients (creatinine clearance >80 mL/min). Systemic exposure to 5′-DFUR was 42% and 71% greater in moderately and severely renal impaired patients, respectively, than in normal patients. Systemic exposure to capecitabine was about 25% greater in both moderately and severely renal impaired patients (see CONTRAINDICATIONS, WARNINGS, and DOSAGE AND ADMINISTRATION).

Drug-Drug Interactions:

Anticoagulants: In four patients with cancer, chronic administration of capecitabine (1250 mg/m^2 bid) with a single 20 mg dose of warfarin increased the mean AUC of S-warfarin by 57% and decreased its clearance by 37%. Baseline corrected AUC of INR in these 4 patients increased by 2.8 fold, and the maximum observed mean INR value was increased by 91% (see Boxed WARNING and PRECAUTIONS: *Drug-Drug Interactions*).

Drugs Metabolized by Cytochrome P450 Enzymes: In vitro enzymatic studies with human liver microsomes indicated that capecitabine and its metabolites (5′-DFUR, 5′-DFCR, 5-FU, and FBAL) had no inhibitory effects on substrates of cytochrome P450 for the major isoenzymes such as 1A2, 2A6, 3A4, 2C9, 2C19, 2D6, and 2E1.

Antacid: When Maalox® (20 mL), an aluminum hydroxide- and magnesium hydroxide-containing antacid, was administered immediately after XELODA (1250 mg/m^2, n=12 cancer patients), AUC and C_{max} increased by 16% and 35%, respectively, for capecitabine and by 18% and 22%, respectively, for 5′-DFCR. No effect was observed on the other three major metabolites (5′-DFUR, 5-FU, FBAL) of XELODA.

XELODA has a low potential for pharmacokinetic interactions related to plasma protein binding.

Table 1. Baseline Demographics of Controlled Colorectal Trials

	Study 1		Study 2	
	XELODA (n=302)	**5-FU/LV (n=303)**	**XELODA (n=301)**	**5-FU/LV (n=301)**
Age (median, years) Range	64 (23–86)	63 (24–87)	64 (29–84)	64 (36–86)
Gender Male (%) Female (%)	 181 (60) 121 (40)	 197 (65) 106 (35)	 172 (57) 129 (43)	 173 (57) 128 (43)
Karnofsky PS (median) Range	90 (70–100)	90 (70–100)	90 (70–100)	90 (70–100)
Colon (%) Rectum (%)	222 (74) 79 (26)	232 (77) 70 (23)	199 (66) 101 (34)	196 (65) 105 (35)
Prior radiation therapy (%)	52 (17)	62 (21)	42 (14)	42 (14)
Prior adjuvant 5-FU (%)	84 (28)	110 (36)	56 (19)	41 (14)

Table 2. Efficacy of XELODA vs 5-FU/LV in Colorectal Cancer (Study 1)

	XELODA (n=302)	5-FU/LV (n=303)
Overall Response Rate (%, 95% C.I.)	21 (16–26)	11 (8–15)
(*p*-value)	0.0014	
Time to Progression (Median, days, 95% C.I.)	128 (120–136)	131 (105–153)
Hazard Ratio (XELODA/5-FU/LV) 95% C.I. for Hazard Ratio	0.99 (0.84.–1.17)	
Survival (Median, days)	380 (321–434)	407 (366–446)
Hazard Ratio (XELODA/5-FU/LV) 95% C.I. for Hazard Ratio	1.00 0.84–1.18	

Table 3. Efficacy of XELODA vs 5-FU/LV in Colorectal Cancer (Study 2)

	XELODA (n=301)	5-FU/LV (n=301)
Overall Response Rate (%, 95% C.I.)	21 (16–26)	14 (10–18)
(*p*-value)	0.027	
Time to Progression (Median, days, 95% C.I.)	137 (128–165)	131 (102–156)
Hazard Ratio (XELODA/5-FU/LV) 95% C.I. for Hazard Ratio	0.97 0.82–1.14	
Survival (Median, days, 95% C.I.)	404 (367–452)	369 (338–430)
Hazard Ratio (XELODA/5-FU/LV) 95% C.I. for Hazard Ratio	0.92 0.78–1.09	

CLINICAL STUDIES

Colorectal Carcinoma: The recommended dose of XELODA was determined in an open-label, randomized clinical study, exploring the efficacy and safety of continuous therapy with capecitabine (1331 mg/m^2/day in two divided doses, n=39), intermittent therapy with capecitabine (2510 mg/m^2/day in two divided doses, n=34), and intermittent therapy with capecitabine in combination with oral leucovorin (LV) (capecitabine 1657 mg/m^2/day in two divided doses, n=35; leucovorin 60 mg/day) in patients with advanced and/or metastatic colorectal carcinoma in the first-line metastatic setting. There was no apparent advantage in response rate to adding leucovorin to XELODA; however, toxicity was increased. XELODA, 1250 mg/m^2 twice daily for 14 days followed by a 1-week rest, was selected for further clinical development based on the overall safety and efficacy profile of the three schedules studied.

Data from 2 open-label, multicenter, randomized, controlled clinical trials involving 1207 patients support the use of XELODA in the first-line treatment of patients with metastatic colorectal carcinoma. The two clinical studies were identical in design and were conducted in 120 centers in different countries. Study 1 was conducted in the US, Canada, Mexico, and Brazil; Study 2 was conducted in Europe, Israel, Australia, New Zealand, and Taiwan. Altogether, in both trials, 603 patients were randomized to treatment with XELODA at a dose of 1250 mg/m^2 twice daily for 2 weeks followed by a 1-week rest period and given as 3-week cycles; 604 patients were randomized to treatment with 5-FU and leucovorin (20 mg/m^2 leucovorin IV followed by 425 mg/m^2 IV bolus 5-FU, on days 1 to 5, every 28 days).

In both trials, overall survival, time to progression and response rate (complete plus partial responses) were assessed. Responses were defined by the World Health Organization criteria and submitted to a blinded independent review committee (IRC). Differences in assessments between the investigator and IRC were reconciled by the sponsor, blinded to treatment arm, according to a specified algorithm. Survival was assessed based on a non-inferiority analysis.

The baseline demographics for XELODA and 5-FU/LV patients are shown in Table 1.

[See table 1 above]

The efficacy endpoints for the two phase 3 trials are shown in Tables 2 and 3.

[See table 2 above]

[See table 3 above]

Figure 1. Kaplan-Meier Curve for Overall Survival of Pooled Data (Studies 1 and 2)

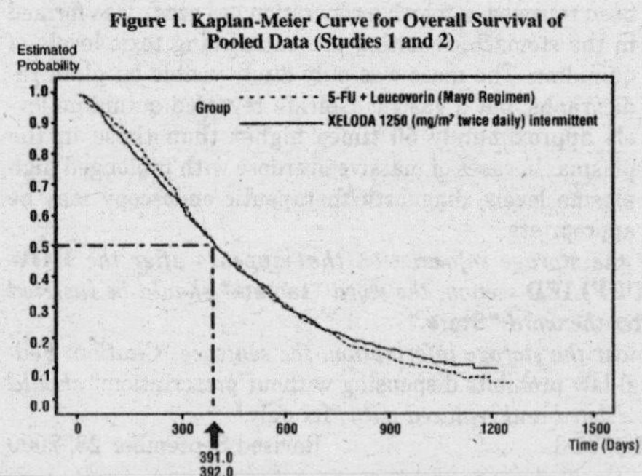

XELODA was superior to 5-FU/LV for objective response rate in Study 1 and Study 2. The similarity of XELODA and 5-FU/LV in these studies was assessed by examining the potential difference between the two treatments. In order to assure that XELODA has a clinically meaningful survival effect, statistical analyses were performed to determine the percent of the survival effect of 5-FU/LV that was retained by XELODA. The estimate of the survival effect of 5-FU/LV was derived from a meta-analysis of ten randomized studies from the published literature comparing 5-FU to regimens of 5-FU/LV that were similar to the control arms used in these Studies 1 and 2. The method for comparing the treatments was to examine the worst case (95% confidence upper bound) for the difference between 5-FU/LV and XELODA, and to show that loss of more than 50% of the 5-FU/LV survival effect was ruled out. It was demonstrated that the percent of the survival effect of 5-FU/LV maintained was at least 61% for Study 2 and 10% for Study 1. The pooled result is consistent with a retention of at least 50% of the ef-

Table 4. Baseline Demographics and Clinical Characteristics XELODA and Docetaxel Combination vs Docetaxel in Breast Cancer Trial

	XELODA + Docetaxel (n=255)	Docetaxel (n=256)
Age (median, years)	52	51
Karnofsky PS (median)	90	90
Site of Disease		
Lymph nodes	121 (47%)	125 (49%)
Liver	116 (45%)	122 (48%)
Bone	107 (42%)	119 (46%)
Lung	95 (37%)	99 (39%)
Skin	73 (29%)	73 (29%)
Prior Chemotherapy		
Anthracycline[1]	255 (100%)	256 (100%)
5-FU	196 (77%)	189 (74%)
Paclitaxel	25 (10%)	22 (9%)
Resistance to an Anthracycline		
No resistance	19 (7%)	19 (7%)
Progression on anthracycline therapy	65 (26%)	73 (29%)
Stable disease after 4 cycles of anthracycline therapy	41 (16%)	40 (16%)
Relapsed within 2 years of completion of anthracycline-adjuvant therapy	78 (31%)	74 (29%)
Experienced a brief response to anthracycline therapy, with subsequent progression while on therapy or within 12 months after last dose	51 (20%)	50 (20%)
No. of Prior Chemotherapy Regimens for Treatment of Metastatic Disease		
0	89 (35%)	80 (31%)
1	123 (48%)	135 (53%)
2	43 (17%)	39 (15%)
3	0 (0%)	2 (1%)

[1]Includes 10 patients in combination and 18 patients in monotherapy arms treated with an anthracenedione

Table 5. Efficacy of XELODA and Docetaxel Combination vs Docetaxel Monotherapy

Efficacy Parameter	Combination Therapy	Monotherapy	p-value	Hazard Ratio
Time to Disease Progression				
Median Days	186	128	0.0001	0.643
95% C.I.	(165–198)	(105–136)		
Overall Survival				
Median Days	442	352	0.0126	0.775
95% C.I.	(375–497)	(298–387)		
Response Rate[1]	32%	22%	0.009	NA[2]

[1] The response rate reported represents a reconciliation of the investigator and IRC assessments performed by the sponsor according to a predefined algorithm.
[2] NA = Not Applicable

Table 6. Baseline Demographics and Clinical Characteristics—Single Arm Breast Cancer Trial

	Patients With Measurable Disease (n=135)	All Patients (n=162)
Age (median, years)	55	56
Karnofsky PS	90	90
No. Disease Sites		
1–2	43 (32%)	60 (37%)
3–4	63 (46%)	69 (43%)
>5	29 (22%)	34 (21%)
Dominant Site of Disease		
Visceral[1]	101 (75%)	110 (68%)
Soft Tissue	30 (22%)	35 (22%)
Bone	4 (3%)	17 (10%)
Prior Chemotherapy		
Paclitaxel	135 (100%)	162 (100%)
Anthracycline[2]	122 (90%)	147 (91%)
5-FU	110 (81%)	133 (82%)
Resistance to Paclitaxel	103 (76%)	124 (77%)
Resistance to an Anthracycline[2]	55 (41%)	67 (41%)
Resistance to both Paclitaxel and an Anthracycline[2]	43 (32%)	51 (31%)

[1]Lung, pleura, liver, peritoneum
[2]Includes 2 patients treated with an anthracenedione

fect of 5-FU/LV. It should be noted that these values for preserved effect are based on the upper bound of the 5-FU/LV vs XELODA difference. These results do not exclude the possibility of true equivalence of XELODA to 5-FU/LV (see Tables 2 and 3 and Kaplan-Meier Figure 1).

Breast Carcinoma: XELODA has been evaluated in clinical trials in combination with docetaxel (Taxotere®) and as monotherapy.

Breast Cancer Combination Therapy: The dose of XELODA used in phase 3 clinical trial in combination with docetaxel was based on the results of a phase 1 study, where a range of doses of docetaxel administered in 3-week cycles in combination with an intermittent regimen of XELODA (14 days of treatment, followed by a 7-day rest period) were evaluated. The combination dose regimen was selected based on the tolerability profile of the 75 mg/m^2 administered in 3-week cycles of docetaxel in combination with 1250 mg/m^2 twice daily for 14 days of XELODA administered in 3-week cycles. The approved dose of 100 mg/m^2 of docetaxel administered in 3-week cycles was the control arm of the phase 3 study.

XELODA in combination with docetaxel was assessed in an open-label, multicenter, randomized trial in 75 centers in Europe, North America, South America, Asia, and Australia. A total of 511 patients with metastatic breast cancer resistant to, or recurring during or after an anthracycline-containing therapy, or relapsing during or recurring within two years of completing an anthracycline-containing adjuvant therapy were enrolled. Two hundred and fifty-five (255) patients were randomized to receive XELODA 1250 mg/m^2 twice daily for 14 days followed by one week without treatment and docetaxel 75 mg/m^2 as a 1-hour intravenous infusion administered in 3-week cycles. In the monotherapy arm, 256 patients received docetaxel 100 mg/m^2 as a 1-hour intravenous infusion administered in 3-week cycles. Patient demographics are provided in Table 4.

[See table 4 above]

XELODA in combination with docetaxel resulted in statistically significant improvement in time to disease progression, overall survival and objective response rate compared to monotherapy with docetaxel as shown in Table 5 and Figures 2 and 3.

[See table 5 above]

Figure 2. Kaplan-Meier Estimates for Time to Disease Progression – XELODA and Docetaxel vs Docetaxel

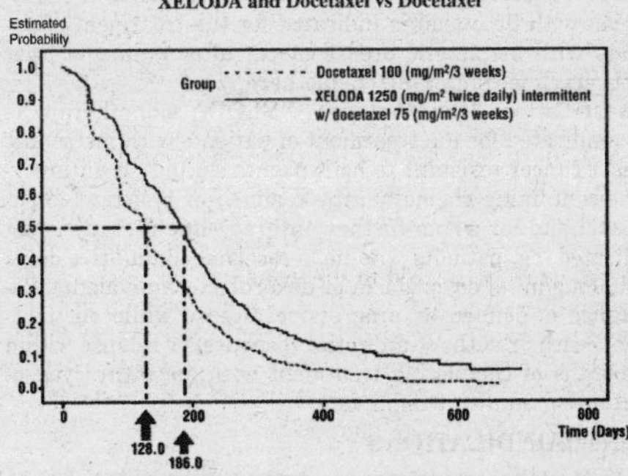

Figure 3. Kaplan-Meier Estimates of Survival – XELODA and Docetaxel vs Docetaxel

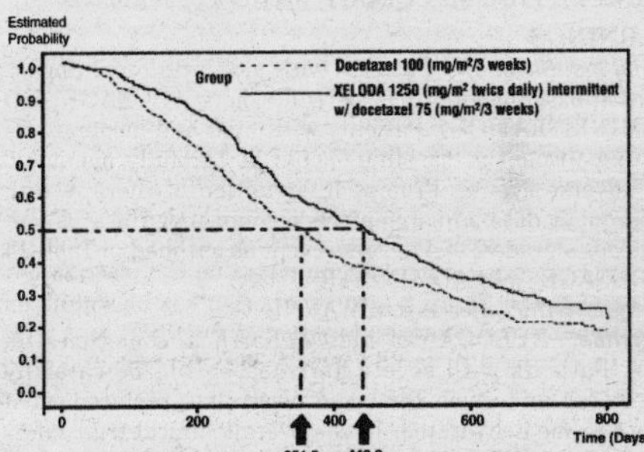

Breast Cancer Monotherapy: The antitumor activity of XELODA as a monotherapy was evaluated in an open-label single-arm trial conducted in 24 centers in the US and Canada. A total of 162 patients with stage IV breast cancer were enrolled. The primary endpoint was tumor response rate in patients with measurable disease, with response defined as a ≥50% decrease in sum of the products of the perpendicular diameters of bidimensionally measurable disease for at least 1 month. XELODA was administered at a dose of 1255 mg/m^2 twice daily for 2 weeks followed by a 1-week rest period and given as 3-week cycles. The baseline demographics and clinical characteristics for all patients (n=162) and those with measurable disease (n=135) are shown in Table 6. Resistance was defined as progressive disease while on treatment, with or without an initial response, or relapse within 6 months of completing treatment with an anthracycline-containing adjuvant chemotherapy regimen.

[See table 6 above]

Antitumor responses for patients with disease resistant to both paclitaxel and an anthracycline are shown in Table 7.

Table 7. Response Rates in Doubly-Resistant Patients—Single Arm Breast Cancer Trial

	Resistance to Both Paclitaxel and an Anthracycline (n=43)
CR	0
PR[1]	11
CR + PR[1]	11
Response Rate[1] (95% C.I.)	25.6% (13.5, 41.2)
Duration of Response,[1] Median in days[2] (Range)	154 (63 to 233)

[1]Includes 2 patients treated with an anthracenedione
[2]From date of first response

For the subgroup of 43 patients who were doubly resistant, the median time to progression was 102 days and the median survival was 255 days. The objective response rate in this population was supported by a response rate of 18.5%

Continued on next page

Xeloda—Cont.

(1 CR, 24 PRs) in the overall population of 135 patients with measurable disease, who were less resistant to chemotherapy (see Table 6). The median time to progression was 90 days and the median survival was 306 days.

INDICATIONS AND USAGE

Colorectal Cancer: XELODA is indicated as first-line treatment of patients with metastatic colorectal carcinoma when treatment with fluoropyrimidine therapy alone is preferred. Combination chemotherapy has shown a survival benefit compared to 5-FU/LV alone. A survival benefit over 5-FU/LV has not been demonstrated with XELODA monotherapy. Use of XELODA instead of 5-FU/LV in combinations has not been adequately studied to assure safety or preservation of the survival advantage.

Breast Cancer Combination Therapy: XELODA in combination with docetaxel is indicated for the treatment of patients with metastatic breast cancer after failure of prior anthracycline-containing chemotherapy.

Breast Cancer Monotherapy: XELODA monotherapy is also indicated for the treatment of patients with metastatic breast cancer resistant to both paclitaxel and an anthracycline-containing chemotherapy regimen or resistant to paclitaxel and for whom further anthracycline therapy is not indicated, eg, patients who have received cumulative doses of 400 mg/m^2 of doxorubicin or doxorubicin equivalents. Resistance is defined as progressive disease while on treatment, with or without an initial response, or relapse within 6 months of completing treatment with an anthracycline-containing adjuvant regimen.

CONTRAINDICATIONS

XELODA is contraindicated in patients who have a known hypersensitivity to 5-fluorouracil. XELODA is also contraindicated in patients with severe renal impairment (creatinine clearance below 30 mL/min [Cockroft and Gault]) (see CLINICAL PHARMACOLOGY: *Special Populations*).

WARNINGS

Renal Insufficiency: Patients with moderate renal impairment at baseline require dose reduction (see DOSAGE AND ADMINISTRATION). Patients with mild and moderate renal impairment at baseline should be carefully monitored for adverse events. Prompt interruption of therapy with subsequent dose adjustments is recommended if a patient develops a grade 2 to 4 adverse event as outlined in Table 14 in DOSAGE AND ADMINISTRATION.

Coagulopathy: See Boxed WARNING.

Diarrhea: XELODA can induce diarrhea, sometimes severe. Patients with severe diarrhea should be carefully monitored and given fluid and electrolyte replacement if they become dehydrated. In the overall clinical trial safety database of XELODA monotherapy (N=875), the median time to first occurrence of grade 2 to 4 diarrhea was 34 days (range from 1 to 369 days). The median duration of grade 3 to 4 diarrhea was 5 days. National Cancer Institute of Canada (NCIC) grade 2 diarrhea is defined as an increase of 4 to 6 stools/day or nocturnal stools, grade 3 diarrhea as an increase of 7 to 9 stools/day or incontinence and malabsorption, and grade 4 diarrhea as an increase of ≥10 stools/day or grossly bloody diarrhea or the need for parenteral support. If grade 2, 3 or 4 diarrhea occurs, administration of XELODA should be immediately interrupted until the diarrhea resolves or decreases in intensity to grade 1. Following a reoccurrence of grade 2 diarrhea or occurrence of any grade 3 or 4 diarrhea, subsequent doses of XELODA should be decreased (see DOSAGE AND ADMINISTRATION). Standard antidiarrheal treatments (eg, loperamide) are recommended.

Necrotizing enterocolitis (typhlitis) has been reported.

Geriatric Patients: Patients ≥80 years old may experience a greater incidence of grade 3 or 4 adverse events (see PRECAUTIONS: *Geriatric Use*). In the overall clinical trial safety database of XELODA monotherapy (N=875), 62% of the 21 patients ≥80 years of age treated with XELODA experienced a treatment-related grade 3 or 4 adverse event: diarrhea in 6 (28.6%), nausea in 3 (14.3%), hand-and-foot syndrome in 3 (14.3%), and vomiting in 2 (9.5%) patients. Among the 10 patients 70 years of age and greater (no patients were >80 years of age) treated with XELODA in combination with docetaxel, 30% (3 out of 10) of patients experienced grade 3 or 4 diarrhea and stomatitis, and 40% (4 out of 10) experienced grade 3 hand-and-foot syndrome.

Among the 67 patients ≥60 years of age receiving XELODA in combination with docetaxel, the incidence of grade 3 or 4 treatment-related adverse events, treatment-related serious adverse events, withdrawals due to adverse events, treatment discontinuations due to adverse events and treatment discontinuations within the first two treatment cycles was higher then in the <60 years of age patient group.

Pregnancy: XELODA may cause fetal harm when given to a pregnant woman. Capecitabine at doses of 198 mg/kg/day during organogenesis caused malformations and embryo death in mice. In separate pharmacokinetic studies, this dose in mice produced 5′-DFUR AUC values about 0.2 times the corresponding values in patients administered the recommended daily dose. Malformations in mice included cleft palate, anophthalmia, microphthalmia, oligodactyly, polydactyly, syndactyly, kinky tail and dilation of cerebral ventricles. At doses of 90 mg/kg/day, capecitabine given to pregnant monkeys during organogenesis caused fetal death. This dose produced 5′-DFUR AUC values about 0.6 times the corresponding values in patients administered the recommended daily dose. There are no adequate and well-controlled studies in pregnant women using XELODA. If the drug is used during pregnancy, or if the patient becomes pregnant while receiving this drug, the patient should be apprised of the potential hazard to the fetus. Women of childbearing potential should be advised to avoid becoming pregnant while receiving treatment with XELODA.

Table 8. Pooled Phase 3 Colorectal Trials: Percent Incidence of Adverse Events Related or Unrelated to Treatment in ≥5% of Patients

	XELODA (n=596)			5-FU/LV (n=593)		
	Total %	Grade 3 %	Grade 4 %	Total %	Grade 3 %	Grade 4 %
Number of Patients With > One Adverse Event	96	52	9	94	45	9
Body System/Adverse Event						
GI						
Diarrhea	55	13	2	61	10	2
Nausea	43	4	–	51	3	<1
Vomiting	27	4	<1	30	4	<1
Stomatitis	25	2	<1	62	14	1
Abdominal Pain	35	9	<1	31	5	–
Gastrointestinal Motility Disorder	10	<1	–	7	<1	–
Constipation	14	1	<1	17	1	–
Oral Discomfort	10	–	–	10	–	–
Upper GI Inflammatory Disorders	8	<1	–	10	1	–
Gastrointestinal Hemorrhage	6	1	<1	3	1	–
Ileus	6	4	1	5	2	1
Skin and Subcutaneous						
Hand-and-Foot Syndrome	54	17	NA	6	1	NA
Dermatitis	27	1	–	26	1	–
Skin Discoloration	7	<1	–	5	–	–
Alopecia	6	–	–	21	<1	–
General						
Fatigue/Weakness	42	4	–	46	4	–
Pyrexia	18	1	–	21	2	–
Edema	15	1	–	9	1	–
Pain	12	1	–	10	1	–
Chest Pain	6	1	–	6	1	<1
Neurological						
Peripheral Sensory Neuropathy	10	–	–	4	–	–
Headache	10	1	–	7	–	–
Dizziness*	8	<1	–	8	<1	–
Insomnia	7	–	–	7	–	–
Taste Disturbance	6	1	–	11	<1	1
Metabolism						
Appetite Decreased	26	3	<1	31	2	<1
Dehydration	7	2	<1	8	3	1
Eye						
Eye Irritation	13	–	–	10	<1	–
Vision Abnormal	5	–	–	2	–	–
Respiratory						
Dyspnea	14	1	–	10	<1	1
Cough	7	<1	1	8	–	–
Pharyngeal Disorder	5	–	–	5	–	–
Epistaxis	3	<1	–	6	–	–
Sore Throat	2	–	–	6	–	–
Musculoskeletal						
Back Pain	10	2	—	9	<1	–
Arthralgia	8	1	—	6	1	–
Vascular						
Venous Thrombosis	8	3	<1	6	2	–
Psychiatric						
Mood Alteration	5	–	–	6	<1	–
Depression	5	–	–	4	<1	–
Infections						
Viral	5	<1	–	5	<1	–
Blood and Lymphatic						
Anemia	80	2	<1	79	1	<1
Neutropenia	13	1	2	46	8	13
Hepatobiliary						
Hyperbilirubinemia	48	18	5	17	3	3

– Not observed
* Excluding vertigo
NA = Not Applicable

PRECAUTIONS

General: Patients receiving therapy with XELODA should be monitored by a physician experienced in the use of cancer chemotherapeutic agents. Most adverse events are reversible and do not need to result in discontinuation, although doses may need to be withheld or reduced (see DOSAGE AND ADMINISTRATION).

Combination With Other Drugs: Use of XELODA in combination with irinotecan has not been adequately studied.

Hand-and-Foot Syndrome: Hand-and-foot syndrome (palmar-plantar erythrodysesthesia or chemotherapy-induced acral erythema) is a cutaneous toxicity (median time to onset of 79 days, range from 11 to 360 days) with a severity range of grades 1 to 3. Grade 1 is characterized by any of the following: numbness, dysesthesia/paresthesia, tingling, painless swelling or erythema of the hands and/or feet and/or discomfort which does not disrupt normal activities. Grade 2 hand-and-foot syndrome is defined as painful erythema and swelling of the hands and/or feet and/or discomfort affecting the patient's activities of daily living. Grade 3 hand-and-foot syndrome is defined as moist desquamation, ulceration, blistering or severe pain of the hands and/or feet and/or severe discomfort that causes the patient to be unable to work or perform activities of daily living. If grade 2 or 3 hand-and-foot syndrome occurs, administration of XELODA should be interrupted until the event resolves or decreases in intensity to grade 1. Following grade 3 hand-and-foot syndrome, subsequent doses of XELODA should be decreased (see DOSAGE AND ADMINISTRATION).

Cardiotoxicity: The cardiotoxicity observed with XELODA includes myocardial infarction/ischemia, angina, dysrhythmias, cardiac arrest, cardiac failure, sudden death, electrocardiographic changes, and cardiomyopathy. These adverse events may be more common in patients with a prior history of coronary artery disease.

Hepatic Insufficiency: Patients with mild to moderate hepatic dysfunction due to liver metastases should be carefully monitored when XELODA is administered. The effect of severe hepatic dysfunction on the disposition of XELODA is not known (see CLINICAL PHARMACOLOGY and DOSAGE AND ADMINISTRATION).

Hyperbilirubinemia: In the overall clinical trial safety database of XELODA monotherapy (N=875), grade 3 (1.5–3 × ULN) hyperbilirubinemia occurred in 15.2% (n=133) and grade 4 (>3 × ULN) hyperbilirubinemia occurred in 3.9% (n=34) of 875 patients with either metastatic breast or colorectal cancer who received at least one dose of XELODA 1250 mg/m^2 twice daily as monotherapy for 2 weeks followed by a 1-week rest period. Of 566 patients who had hepatic metastases at baseline and 309 patients without hepatic metastases at baseline, grade 3 or 4 hyperbilirubinemia occurred in 22.8% and 12.3%, respectively. Of the 167 patients with grade 3 or 4 hyperbilirubinemia, 18.6% (n=31) also had postbaseline elevations (grades 1 to 4, without elevations at baseline) in alkaline phosphatase and 27.5% (n=46) had postbaseline elevations in transaminases at any time (not necessarily concurrent). The majority of these patients, 64.5% (n=20) and 71.7% (n=33), had liver metastases at baseline. In addition, 57.5% (n=96) and 35.3% (n=59) of the 167 patients had elevations (grades 1 to 4) at both prebaseline and postbaseline in alkaline phosphatase or transaminases, respectively. Only 7.8% (n=13) and 3.0% (n=5) had grade 3 or 4 elevations in alkaline phosphatase or transaminases.

In the 596 patients treated with XELODA as first-line therapy for metastatic colorectal cancer, the incidence of grade 3 or 4 hyperbilirubinemia was similar to the overall clinical trial safety database of XELODA monotherapy. The median time to onset for grade 3 or 4 hyperbilirubinemia in the colorectal cancer population was 64 days and median total bilirubin increased from 8 μm/L at baseline to 13 μm/L during treatment with XELODA. Of the 136 colorectal cancer patients with grade 3 or 4 hyperbilirubinemia, 49 patients had grade 3 or 4 hyperbilirubinemia as their last measured value, of which 46 had liver metastases at baseline.

In 251 patients with metastatic breast cancer who received a combination of XELODA and docetaxel, grade 3 (1.5–3 × ULN) hyperbilirubinemia occurred in 7% (n=17) and grade 4 (>3 × ULN) hyperbilirubinemia occurred in 2% (n=5).

If drug-related grade 2 to 4 elevations in bilirubin occur, administration of XELODA should be immediately interrupted until the hyperbilirubinemia resolves or decreases in intensity to grade 1. NCIC grade 2 hyperbilirubinemia is defined as 1.5 × normal, grade 3 hyperbilirubinemia as 1.5–3 × normal and grade 4 hyperbilirubinemia as >3 × normal. (See recommended dose modifications under DOSAGE AND ADMINISTRATION.)

Hematologic: In 875 patients with either metastatic breast or colorectal cancer who received a dose of 1250 mg/m^2 administered twice daily as monotherapy for 2 weeks followed by a 1-week rest period, 3.2%, 1.7%, and 2.4% of patients had grade 3 or 4 neutropenia, thrombocytopenia or decreases in hemoglobin, respectively. In 251 patients with metastatic breast cancer who received a dose of XELODA in combination with docetaxel, 68% had grade 3 or 4 neutropenia, 2.8% had grade 3 or 4 thrombocytopenia, and 9.6% had grade 3 or 4 anemia.

Carcinogenesis, Mutagenesis and Impairment of Fertility: Adequate studies investigating the carcinogenic potential of XELODA have not been conducted. Capecitabine was not mutagenic in vitro to bacteria (Ames test) or mammalian cells (Chinese hamster V79/HPRT gene mutation assay). Capecitabine was clastogenic in vitro to human peripheral blood lymphocytes but not clastogenic in vivo to mouse bone marrow (micronucleus test). Fluorouracil causes mutations in bacteria and yeast. Fluorouracil also causes chromosomal abnormalities in the mouse micronucleus test in vivo.

Impairment of Fertility: In studies of fertility and general reproductive performance in mice, oral capecitabine doses of 760 mg/kg/day disturbed estrus and consequently caused a decrease in fertility. In mice that became pregnant, no fetuses survived this dose. The disturbance in estrus was reversible. In males, this dose caused degenerative changes in the testes, including decreases in the number of spermatocytes and spermatids. In separate pharmacokinetic studies, this dose in mice produced 5′-DFUR AUC values about 0.7 times the corresponding values in patients administered the recommended daily dose.

Information for Patients (see Patient Package Insert): Patients and patients' caregivers should be informed of the expected adverse effects of XELODA, particularly nausea, vomiting, diarrhea, and hand-and-foot syndrome, and should be made aware that patient-specific dose adaptations during therapy are expected and necessary (see DOSAGE AND ADMINISTRATION). Patients should be encouraged to recognize the common grade 2 toxicities associated with XELODA treatment.

Diarrhea: Patients experiencing grade 2 diarrhea (an increase of 4 to 6 stools/day or nocturnal stools) or greater should be instructed to stop taking XELODA immediately. Standard antidiarrheal treatments (eg, loperamide) are recommended.

Nausea: Patients experiencing grade 2 nausea (food intake significantly decreased but able to eat intermittently) or greater should be instructed to stop taking XELODA immediately. Initiation of symptomatic treatment is recommended.

Vomiting: Patients experiencing grade 2 vomiting (2 to 5 episodes in a 24-hour period) or greater should be instructed to stop taking XELODA immediately. Initiation of symptomatic treatment is recommended.

Hand-and-Foot Syndrome: Patients experiencing grade 2 hand-and-foot syndrome (painful erythema and swelling of the hands and/or feet and/or discomfort affecting the patients' activities of daily living) or greater should be instructed to stop taking XELODA immediately.

Stomatitis: Patients experiencing grade 2 stomatitis (painful erythema, edema or ulcers of the mouth or tongue, but able to eat) or greater should be instructed to stop taking XELODA immediately. Initiation of symptomatic treatment is recommended (see DOSAGE AND ADMINISTRATION).

Fever and Neutropenia: Patients who develop a fever of 100.5°F or greater or other evidence of potential infection should be instructed to call their physician.

Drug-Food Interaction: In all clinical trials, patients were instructed to administer XELODA within 30 minutes after a meal. Since current safety and efficacy data are based upon administration with food, it is recommended that XELODA be administered with food (see DOSAGE AND ADMINISTRATION).

Table 9. Percent Incidence of Adverse Events Considered Related or Unrelated to Treatment in ≥5% of Patients Participating in the XELODA and Docetaxel Combination vs Docetaxel Monotherapy Study

Adverse Event	XELODA 1250 mg/m^2/bid With Docetaxel 75 mg/m^2/3 weeks (n=251)			Docetaxel 100 mg/m^2/3 weeks (n=255)		
	Total %	Grade 3 %	Grade 4 %	Total %	Grade 3 %	Grade 4 %
Number of Patients With at Least One Adverse Event	99	76.5	29.1	97	57.6	31.8
Body System/Adverse Event						
GI						
Diarrhea	67	14	<1	48	5	<1
Stomatitis	67	17	<1	43	5	–
Nausea	45	7	–	36	2	–
Vomiting	35	4	1	24	2	–
Constipation	20	2	–	18	–	–
Abdominal Pain	30	<3	<1	24	2	–
Dyspepsia	14	–	–	8	1	–
Dry Mouth	6	<1	–	5	–	–
Skin and Subcutaneous						
Hand-and-Foot Syndrome	63	24	NA	8	1	NA
Alopecia	41	6	–	42	7	–
Nail Disorder	14	2	–	15	–	–
Dermatitis	8	–	–	11	1	–
Rash Erythematous	9	<1	–	5	–	–
Nail Discoloration	6	–	–	4	<1	–
Onycholysis	5	1	–	5	1	–
Pruritus	4	–	–	5	–	–
General						
Pyrexia	28	2	–	34	2	–
Asthenia	26	4	<1	25	6	–
Fatigue	22	4	–	27	6	–
Weakness	16	2	–	11	2	–
Pain in Limb	13	<1	–	13	2	–
Lethargy	7	–	–	6	2	–
Pain	7	<1	–	5	1	–
Chest Pain (non-cardiac)	4	<1	–	6	2	–
Influenza-like Illness	5	–	–	5	–	–
Neurological						
Taste Disturbance	16	<1	–	14	<1	–
Headache	15	3	–	15	2	–
Paresthesia	12	<1	–	16	1	–
Dizziness	12	–	–	8	<1	–
Insomnia	8	–	–	10	<1	–
Peripheral Neuropathy	6	–	–	10	1	–
Hypoaesthesia	4	<1	–	8	<1	–
Metabolism						
Anorexia	13	1	–	11	<1	–
Appetite Decreased	10	–	–	5	–	–
Weight Decreased	7	–	–	5	–	–
Dehydration	10	2	–	7	<1	<1
Eye						
Lacrimation Increased	12	–	–	7	<1	–
Conjunctivitis	5	–	–	4	–	–
Eye Irritation	5	–	–	1	–	–
Musculoskeletal						
Arthralgia	15	2	–	24	3	–
Myalgia	15	2	–	25	2	–
Back Pain	12	<1	–	11	3	–
Bone Pain	8	<1	–	10	2	–
Cardiac						
Edema	33	<2	–	34	<3	1
Blood						
Neutropenic Fever	16	3	13	21	5	16
Respiratory						
Dyspnea	14	2	<1	16	2	–
Cough	13	1	–	22	<1	–
Sore Throat	12	2	–	11	<1	–
Epistaxis	7	<1	–	6	–	–
Rhinorrhea	5	–	–	3	–	–
Pleural Effusion	2	1	–	7	4	–
Infection						
Oral Candidiasis	7	<1	–	8	<1	–
Urinary Tract Infection	6	<1	–	4	–	–
Upper Respiratory Tract	4	–	–	5	1	–
Vascular						
Flushing	5	–	–	5	–	–
Lymphoedema	3	<1	–	5	1	–
Psychiatric						
Depression	5	–	–	5	1	–

–Not observed
NA = Not Applicable

Drug-Drug Interactions:

Antacid: The effect of an aluminum hydroxide- and magnesium hydroxide-containing antacid (Maalox) on the pharmacokinetics of XELODA was investigated in 12 cancer patients. There was a small increase in plasma concentrations of XELODA and one metabolite (5′-DFCR); there was no effect on the 3 major metabolites (5′-DFUR, 5-FU and FBAL).

Anticoagulants: Patients receiving concomitant capecitabine and oral coumarin-derivative anticoagulant therapy should have their anticoagulant response (INR or prothrombin time) monitored closely with great frequency and the anticoagulant dose should be adjusted accordingly (see Boxed WARNING and CLINICAL PHARMACOLOGY). Altered coagulation parameters and/or bleeding have been reported in patients taking XELODA concomitantly with coumarin-derivative anticoagulants such as warfarin and phenprocoumon. These events occurred within several days and up to several months after initiating XELODA therapy and, in a few cases, within one month after stopping XELODA. These events occurred in patients with and without liver metastases. In a drug interaction study with single dose warfarin administration, there was a significant increase in the mean AUC of S-warfarin. The maximum observed INR value increased by 91%. This interaction is probably due to an inhibition of cytochrome P450 2C9 by capecitabine and/or its metabolites (see CLINICAL PHARMACOLOGY).

CYP2C9 substrates: Other than warfarin, no formal drug-drug interaction studies between XELODA and other CYP2C9 substrates have been conducted. Care should be

Continued on next page

Xeloda—Cont.

exercised when XELODA is co-administered with CYP2C9 substrates.

Phenytoin: The level of phenytoin should be carefully monitored in patients taking XELODA and phenytoin dose may need to be reduced (see DOSAGE AND ADMINISTRATION: *Dose Modification Guidelines*). Postmarketing reports indicate that some patients receiving XELODA and phenytoin had toxicity associated with elevated phenytoin levels. Formal drug-drug interaction studies with phenytoin have not been conducted, but the mechanism of interaction is presumed to be inhibition of the CYP2C9 isoenzyme by capecitabine and/or its metabolites (see PRECAUTIONS: *Drug-Drug Interactions: Anticoagulants*).

Leucovorin: The concentration of 5-fluorouracil is increased and its toxicity may be enhanced by leucovorin. Deaths from severe enterocolitis, diarrhea, and dehydration have been reported in elderly patients receiving weekly leucovorin and fluorouracil.

Pregnancy: Teratogenic Effects: Category D (see WARNINGS). Women of childbearing potential should be advised to avoid becoming pregnant while receiving treatment with XELODA.

Nursing Women: Lactating mice given a single oral dose of capecitabine excreted significant amounts of capecitabine metabolites into the milk. Because of the potential for serious adverse reactions in nursing infants from capecitabine, it is recommended that nursing be discontinued when receiving XELODA therapy.

Pediatric Use: The safety and effectiveness of XELODA in persons <18 years of age have not been established.

Geriatric Use: Physicians should pay particular attention to monitoring the adverse effects of XELODA in the elderly (see WARNINGS: *Geriatric Patients*).

ADVERSE REACTIONS

Colorectal Cancer: Table 8 shows the adverse events occurring in ≥5% of patients from pooling the two phase 3 trials in colorectal cancer. Rates are rounded to the nearest whole number. A total of 596 patients with metastatic colorectal cancer were treated with 1250 mg/m^2 twice a day of XELODA administered for 2 weeks followed by a 1-week rest period, and 593 patients were administered 5-FU and leucovorin in the Mayo regimen (20 mg/m^2 leucovorin IV followed by 425 mg/m^2 IV bolus 5-FU, on days 1–5, every 28 days). In the pooled colorectal database the median duration of treatment was 139 days for capecitabine-treated patients and 140 days for 5-FU/LV-treated patients. A total of 78 (13%) and 63 (11%) capecitabine and 5-FU/LV-treated patients, respectively, discontinued treatment because of adverse events/intercurrent illness. A total of 82 deaths due to all causes occurred either on study or within 28 days of receiving study drug: 50 (8.4%) patients randomized to XELODA and 32 (5.4%) randomized to 5-FU/LV.

[See table 8 at top of page 300]

Breast Cancer Combination: The following data are shown for the combination study with XELODA and docetaxel in patients with metastatic breast cancer in Table 9. In the XELODA and docetaxel combination arm the treatment was XELODA administered orally 1250 mg/m^2 twice daily as intermittent therapy (2 weeks of treatment followed by one week without treatment) for at least 6 weeks and docetaxel administered as a 1-hour intravenous infusion at a dose of 75 mg/m^2 on the first day of each 3-week cycle for at least 6 weeks. In the monotherapy arm docetaxel was administered as a 1-hour intravenous infusion at a dose of 100 mg/m^2 on the first day of each 3-week cycle for at least 6 weeks. The mean duration of treatment was 129 days in the combination arm and 98 days in the monotherapy arm. A total of 66 patients (26%) in the combination arm and 49 (19%) in the monotherapy arm withdrew from the study because of adverse events. The percentage of patients requiring dose reductions due to adverse events were 65% in the combination arm and 36% in the monotherapy arm. The percentage of patients requiring treatment interruptions due to adverse events in the combination arm was 79%. Treatment interruptions were part of the dose modification scheme for the combination therapy arm but not for the docetaxel monotherapy-treated patients.

[See table 9 at top of previous page]

[See table 10 above]

Breast Cancer XELODA Monotherapy: The following data are shown for the study in stage IV breast cancer patients who received a dose of 1250 mg/m^2 administered twice daily for 2 weeks followed by a 1-week rest period. The mean duration of treatment was 114 days. A total of 13 out of 162 patients (8%) discontinued treatment because of adverse events/intercurrent illness.

[See table 11 above]

OTHER ADVERSE EVENTS:

XELODA and Docetaxel in Combination: Shown below by body system are the clinically relevant adverse events in <5% of patients in the overall clinical trial safety database of 251 patients (Study Details) reported as related to the administration of XELODA in combination with docetaxel and that were clinically at least remotely relevant. In parentheses is the incidence of grade 3 and 4 occurrences of each adverse event.

It is anticipated that the same types of adverse events observed in the XELODA monotherapy studies may be observed in patients treated with the combination of XELODA plus docetaxel.

Table 10. Percent of Patients With Laboratory Abnormalities Participating in the XELODA and Docetaxel Combination vs Docetaxel Monotherapy Study

Adverse Event	XELODA 1250 mg/m^2/bid With Docetaxel 75 mg/m^2/3 weeks (n=251)			Docetaxel 100 mg/m^2/3 weeks (n=255)		
Body System/Adverse Event	**Total %**	**Grade 3 %**	**Grade 4 %**	**Total %**	**Grade 3 %**	**Grade 4 %**
Hematologic						
Leukopenia	91	37	24	88	42	33
Neutropenia/Granulocytopenia	86	20	49	87	10	66
Thrombocytopenia	41	2	1	23	1	2
Anemia	80	7	3	83	5	<1
Lymphocytopenia	99	48	41	98	44	40
Hepatobiliary						
Hyperbilirubinemia	20	7	2	6	2	2

Table 11. Percent Incidence of Adverse Events Considered Remotely, Possibly or Probably Related to Treatment in ≥5% of Patients Participating in the Single Arm Trial in Stage IV Breast Cancer

Adverse Event	Phase 2 Trial in Stage IV Breast Cancer (n=162)		
Body System/Adverse Event	**Total**	**Grade 3**	**Grade 4**
GI			
Diarrhea	57	12	3
Nausea	53	4	–
Vomiting	37	4	–
Stomatitis	24	7	–
Abdominal Pain	20	4	–
Constipation	15	1	–
Dyspepsia	8	–	–
Skin and Subcutaneous			
Hand-and-Foot Syndrome	57	11	N/A
Dermatitis	37	1	–
Nail Disorder	7	–	–
General			
Fatigue	41	8	–
Pyrexia	12	1	–
Pain in Limb	6	1	–
Neurological			
Paresthesia	21	1	–
Headache	9	1	–
Dizziness	8	–	–
Insomnia	8	–	–
Metabolism			
Anorexia	23	3	–
Dehydration	7	4	1
Eye			
Eye Irritation	15	–	–
Musculoskeletal			
Myalgia	9	–	–
Cardiac			
Edema	9	1	–
Blood			
Neutropenia	26	2	2
Thrombocytopenia	24	3	1
Anemia	72	3	1
Lymphopenia	94	44	15
Hepatobiliary			
Hyperbilirubinemia	22	9	2

–Not observed or applicable
NA = Not Applicable

Table 12. XELODA Dose Calculation According to Body Surface Area

Dose Level 1250 mg/m^2 Twice a Day		Number of Tablets to be Taken at Each Dose (Morning and Evening)	
Surface Area (m^2)	**Total Daily* Dose (mg)**	**150 mg**	**500 mg**
≤ 1.25	3000	0	3
1.26–1.37	3300	1	3
1.38–1.51	3600	2	3
1.52–1.65	4000	0	4
1.66–1.77	4300	1	4
1.78–1.91	4600	2	4
1.92–2.05	5000	0	5
2.06–2.17	5300	1	5
≥ 2.18	5600	2	5

*Total Daily Dose divided by 2 to allow equal morning and evening doses

Gastrointestinal: ileus (0.39), necrotizing enterocolitis (0.39), esophageal ulcer (0.39), hemorrhagic diarrhea (0.80)
Neurological: ataxia (0.39), syncope (1.20), taste loss (0.80), polyneuropathy (0.39), migraine (0.39)
Cardiac: supraventricular tachycardia (0.39)
Infection: neutropenic sepsis (2.39), sepsis (0.39), bronchopneumonia (0.39)
Blood and Lymphatic: agranulocytosis (0.39), prothrombin decreased (0.39)
Vascular: hypotension (1.20), venous phlebitis and thrombophlebitis (0.39), postural hypotension (0.80)
Renal: renal failure (0.39)
Hepatobiliary: jaundice (0.39), abnormal liver function tests (0.39), hepatic failure (0.39), hepatic coma (0.39), hepatotoxicity (0.39)
Immune System: hypersensitivity (1.20)

XELODA Monotherapy: Shown below by body system are the clinically relevant adverse events in <5% of patients in

the overall clinical trial safety database of 875 patients (phase 3 colorectal studies – 596 patients, phase 2 colorectal study – 34 patients, phase 2 breast cancer studies – 245 patients) reported as related to the administration of XELODA and that were clinically at least remotely relevant. In parentheses is the incidence of grade 3 or 4 occurrences of each adverse event.
Gastrointestinal: abdominal distension, dysphagia, proctalgia, ascites (0.1), gastric ulcer (0.1), ileus (0.3), toxic dilation of intestine, gastroenteritis (0.1)
Skin and Subcutaneous: nail disorder (0.1), sweating increased (0.1), photosensitivity reaction (0.1), skin ulceration, pruritus, radiation recall syndrome (0.2)
General: chest pain (0.2), influenza-like illness, hot flushes, pain (0.1), hoarseness, irritability, difficulty in walking, thirst, chest mass, collapse, fibrosis (0.1), hemorrhage, edema, sedation
Neurological: insomnia, ataxia (0.5), tremor, dysphasia, encephalopathy (0.1), abnormal coordination, dysarthria, loss of consciousness (0.2), impaired balance
Metabolism: increased weight, cachexia (0.4), hypertriglyceridemia (0.1), hypokalemia, hypomagnesemia
Eye: conjunctivitis
Respiratory: cough (0.1), epistaxis (0.1), asthma (0.2), hemoptysis, respiratory distress (0.1), dyspnea
Cardiac: tachycardia (0.1), bradycardia, atrial fibrillation, ventricular extrasystoles, extrasystoles, myocarditis (0.1), pericardial effusion
Infections: laryngitis (1.0), bronchitis (0.2), pneumonia (0.2), bronchopneumonia (0.2), keratoconjunctivitis, sepsis (0.3), fungal infections (including candidiasis) (0.2)
Musculoskeletal: myalgia, bone pain (0.1), arthritis (0.1), muscle weakness
Blood and Lymphatic: leukopenia (0.2), coagulation disorder (0.1), bone marrow depression (0.1), idiopathic thrombocytopenia purpura (1.0), pancytopenia (0.1)
Vascular: hypotension (0.2), hypertension (0.1), lymphoedema (0.1), pulmonary embolism (0.2), cerebrovascular accident (0.1)
Psychiatric: depression, confusion (0.1)
Renal: renal impairment (0.6)
Ear: vertigo
Hepatobiliary: hepatic fibrosis (0.1), hepatitis (0.1), cholestatic hepatitis (0.1), abnormal liver function tests
Immune System: drug hypersensitivity (0.1)
Postmarketing: hepatic failure

OVERDOSAGE

The manifestations of acute overdose would include nausea, vomiting, diarrhea, gastrointestinal irritation and bleeding, and bone marrow depression. Medical management of overdose should include customary supportive medical interventions aimed at correcting the presenting clinical manifestations. Although no clinical experience using dialysis as a treatment for XELODA overdose has been reported, dialysis may be of benefit in reducing circulating concentrations of 5′-DFUR, a low-molecular weight metabolite of the parent compound.
Single doses of XELODA were not lethal to mice, rats, and monkeys at doses up to 2000 mg/kg (2.4, 4.8, and 9.6 times the recommended human daily dose on a mg/m^2 basis).

DOSAGE AND ADMINISTRATION

The recommended dose of XELODA is 1250 mg/m^2 administered orally twice daily (morning and evening; equivalent to 2500 mg/m^2 total daily dose) for 2 weeks followed by a 1-week rest period given as 3-week cycles. XELODA tablets should be swallowed with water within 30 minutes after a meal. Table 12 displays the total daily dose by body surface area and the number of tablets to be taken at each dose.
[See table 12 at top of previous page]
Dose Modification Guidelines: Patients should be carefully monitored for toxicity. Toxicity due to XELODA administration may be managed by symptomatic treatment, dose interruptions and adjustment of XELODA dose. Once the dose has been reduced it should not be increased at a later time.
The dose of phenytoin and the dose of a coumarin-derivative anticoagulants may need to be reduced when either drug is administered concomitantly with XELODA (see PRECAUTIONS: *Drug-Drug Interactions*).
Dose modification for the use of XELODA and docetaxel in combination are shown in Table 13.
[See table 13 above]
Dose modification for the use of XELODA as monotherapy is shown in Table 14.
[See table 14 at top of next page]
Dosage modifications are not recommended for grade 1 events. Therapy with XELODA should be interrupted upon the occurrence of a grade 2 or 3 adverse experience. Once the adverse event has resolved or decreased in intensity to grade 1, then XELODA therapy may be restarted at full dose or as adjusted according to the above table. If a grade 4 experience occurs, therapy should be discontinued or interrupted until resolved or decreased to grade 1, and therapy should be restarted at 50% of the original dose. Doses of XELODA omitted for toxicity are not replaced or restored; instead the patient should resume the planned treatment cycles.

Adjustment of Starting Dose in Special Populations:
Hepatic Impairment: In patients with mild to moderate hepatic dysfunction due to liver metastases, no starting dose adjustment is necessary; however, patients should be carefully monitored. Patients with severe hepatic dysfunction have not been studied.

Table 13. XELODA in Combination With Docetaxel Dose Reduction Schedule

Toxicity NCIC Grades*	Grade 2	Grade 3	Grade 4
1st appearance	Grade 2 occurring during the 14 days of XELODA treatment: interrupt XELODA treatment until resolved to grade 0–1. Treatment may be resumed during the cycle at the same dose of XELODA. Doses of XELODA missed during a treatment cycle are not to be replaced. Prophylaxis for toxicities should be implemented where possible. Grade 2 persisting at the time the next XELODA/docetaxel treatment is due: delay treatment until resolved to grade 0–1, then continue at 100% of the original XELODA and docetaxel dose. Prophylaxis for toxicities should be implemented where possible.	Grade 3 occurring during the 14 days of XELODA treatment: interrupt the XELODA treatment until resolved to grade 0–1. Treatment may be resumed during the cycle at 75% of the XELODA dose. Doses of XELODA missed during a treatment cycle are not to be replaced. Prophylaxis for toxicities should be implemented where possible. Grade 3 persisting at the time the next XELODA/docetaxel treatment is due: delay treatment until resolved to grade 0–1. For patients developing grade 3 toxicity at any time during the treatment cycle, upon resolution to grade 0–1, subsequent treatment cycles should be continued at 75% of the original XELODA dose and at 55 mg/m^2 of docetaxel. Prophylaxis for toxicities should be implemented where possible.	Discontinue treatment unless treating physician considers it to be in the best interest of the patient to continue with XELODA at 50% of original dose.
2nd appearance of same toxicity	Grade 2 occurring during the 14 days of XELODA treatment: interrupt XELODA treatment until resolved to grade 0–1. Treatment may be resumed during the cycle at 75% of original XELODA dose. Doses of XELODA missed during a treatment cycle are not to be replaced. Prophylaxis for toxicities should be implemented where possible. Grade 2 persisting at the time the next XELODA/docetaxel treatment is due: delay treatment until resolved to grade 0–1. For patients developing 2nd occurrence of grade 2 toxicity at any time during the treatment cycle, upon resolution to grade 0–1, subsequent treatment cycles should be continued at 75% of the original XELODA dose and at 55 mg/m^{2}of docetaxel. Prophylaxis for toxicities should be implemented where possible.	Grade 3 occurring during the 14 days of XELODA treatment: interrput the XELODA treatment until resolved to grade 0–1. Treatment may be resumed during the cycle at 50% of the XELODA dose. Doses of XELODA missed during a treatment cycle are not to be replaced. Prophylaxis for toxicities should be implemented where possible. Grade 3 persisting at the time the next XELODA/docetaxel treatment is due: delay treatment until resolved to grade 0–1 For patients developing grade 3 toxicity at any time during the treatment cycle, upon resolution to grade 0–1, subsequent treatment cycles should be continued at 50% of the original XELODA dose and the docetaxel discontinued. Prophylaxis for toxicities should be implemented where possible.	Discontinue treatment
3rd appearance of same toxicity	Grade 2 occurring during the 14 days of XELODA treatment: interrupt XELODA treatment until resolved to grade 0–1. Treatment may be resumed during the cycle at 50% of the original XELODA dose. Doses of XELODA missed during a treatment cycle are not to be replaced. Prophylaxis for toxicities should be implemented where possible. Grade 2 persisting at the time the next XELODA/docetaxel treatment is due: delay treatment until resolved to grade 0–1. For patients developing 3rd occurrence of grade 2 toxicity at any time during the treatment cycle, upon resolution to grade 0–1, subsequent treatment cycles should be continued at 50% of the original XELODA dose and the docetaxel discontinued. Prophylaxis for toxicities should be implemented where possible.	Discontinue treatment.	
4th appearance of same toxicity	Discontinue treatment.		

*National Cancer Institute of Canada Common Toxicity Criteria were used except for hand-and-foot syndrome (see PRECAUTIONS).

Renal Impairment: No adjustment to the starting dose of XELODA is recommended in patients with mild renal impairment (creatinine clearance=51–80 mL/min [Cockroft and Gault, as shown below]). In patients with moderate renal impairment (baseline creatinine clearance= 30–50 mL/min), a dose reduction to 75% of the XELODA starting dose when used as monotherapy or in combination with docetaxel (from 1250 mg/m^2 to 950 mg/m^2 twice daily)

Continued on next page

Xeloda—Cont.

is recommended (see CLINICAL PHARMACOLOGY: *Special Populations*). Subsequent dose adjustment is recommended as outlined in Table 14 if a patient develops a grade 2 to 4 adverse event (see WARNINGS).
[See table above]
Geriatrics: Physicians should exercise caution in monitoring the effects of XELODA in the elderly. Insufficient data are available to provide a dosage recommendation.

HOW SUPPLIED

XELODA is supplied as biconvex, oblong film-coated tablets, available in bottles as follows:
150 mg
color: light peach
engraving: XELODA on one side, 150 on the other
150 mg tablets packaged in bottles of 120 (NDC 0004-1100-51)
500 mg
color: peach
engraving: XELODA on one side, 500 on the other
500 mg tablets packaged in bottles of 240 (NDC 0004-1101-16)
Storage Conditions: Store at 25°C (77°F); excursions permitted to 15° to 30°C (59° to 86°F), keep tightly closed. [See USP Controlled Room Temperature]
Maalox is a registered trademark of Novartis.
Taxotere is a registered trademark of Aventis Pharmaceuticals Products Inc.
For full Taxotere prescribing information, please refer to Taxotere Package Insert.

Table 14. Recommended Dose Modifications

Toxicity NCIC Grades*	During a Course of Therapy	Dose Adjustment for Next Cycle (% of starting dose)
• *Grade 1*	Maintain dose level	Maintain dose level
• *Grade 2*		
-1st appearance	Interrupt until resolved to grade 0–1	100%
-2nd appearance	Interrupt until resolved to grade 0–1	75%
-3rd appearance	Interrupt until resolved to grade 0–1	50%
-4th appearance	Discontinue treatment permanently	
• *Grade 3*		
-1st appearance	Interrupt until resolved to grade 0–1	75%
-2nd appearance	Interrupt until resolved to grade 0–1	50%
-3rd appearance	Discontinue treatment permanently	
• *Grade 4*		
-1st appearance	Discontinue permanently *or* If physician deems it to be in the patient's best interest to continue, interrupt until resolved to grade 0–1	50%

*National Cancer Institute of Canada Common Toxicity Criteria were used except for hand-and-foot syndrome (see PRECAUTIONS).

Cockroft and Gault Equation:

$$\text{Creatinine clearance for males} = \frac{(140 - \text{age [yrs]})\ (\text{body wt [kg]})}{(72)\ (\text{serum creatinine [mg/dL]})}$$

$$\text{Creatinine clearance for females} = 0.85 \times \text{male value}$$

Patient Information

XELODA® (capecitabine) Tablets

Read this leaflet before you start taking XELODA® [zeh-LOE-duh] and each time you renew your prescription. It contains important information. However, this information does not take the place of talking with your doctor. This information cannot cover all possible risks and benefits of XELODA. Your doctor should always be your first choice for detailed information about your medical condition and this medicine.

What is XELODA?

XELODA is a medicine you take by mouth (orally) that is used to treat:

- cancer of the colon or rectum that has spread to other parts of the body (metastatic colorectal cancer) when fluoropyrimidine therapy alone is preferred. Patients and physicians should note that combination chemotherapy has shown a survival benefit compared to 5-FU/LV alone. A survival benefit over 5-FU/LV has not been demonstrated with XELODA monotherapy.
- breast cancer that has spread to other parts of the body and has not responded to treatment with certain other medicines. These medicines include paclitaxel (Taxol®) and anthracycline-containing therapy such as Adriamycin® and doxorubicin.

XELODA is changed in the body to the substance 5-fluorouracil. In some patients with colon, rectum or breast cancer, this substance stops cancer cells from growing and decreases the size of the tumor.

Who should not take XELODA?

1. DO NOT TAKE XELODA IF YOU

- are nursing a baby. Tell your doctor if you are nursing. XELODA may pass to the baby in your milk and harm the baby.
- are allergic to 5-fluorouracil.

2. TELL YOUR DOCTOR IF YOU

- **take a blood thinner such as warfarin (Coumadin®). This is very important because XELODA may increase the effect of the blood thinner. If you are taking blood thinners and XELODA, your doctor needs to check how fast your blood clots more frequently and adjust the dose of the blood thinner, if needed.**
- take phenytoin (Dilantin®). Your doctor needs to test the levels of phenytoin in your blood more often or change your dose of phenytoin.
- are pregnant. XELODA may not be right for you.
- have kidney problems. Your doctor may prescribe a different medicine or reduce the XELODA dose.
- have liver problems. You may need to be checked for liver problems while you take XELODA.
- take the vitamin folic acid. It may affect how XELODA works.

How should I take XELODA?

Your doctor will prescribe a dose and treatment plan that is right for *you*. Your doctor may want you to take a combination of 150 mg and 500 mg tablets for each dose. If a combination of tablets is prescribed, you must correctly identify the tablets. Taking the wrong tablets could cause an overdose (too much medicine) or underdose (too little medicine). The 150 mg tablets are light peach in color and have 150 engraved on one side. The 500 mg tablets are peach in color and have 500 engraved on one side. Your doctor may change the amount of medicine you take during your treatment. Your doctor may prescribe XELODA Tablets in combination with Taxotere® or docetaxel injection.

- Take the tablets in the combination prescribed by your doctor for your **morning and evening** doses.
- Take the tablets **within 30 minutes after the end of a meal** (breakfast and dinner).
- **Swallow XELODA with water.**
- If you miss a dose of XELODA, do not take the missed dose at all and do not double the next one. Instead, continue your regular dosing schedule and check with your doctor.
- It is recommended that XELODA be taken for 14 days followed by a 7-day rest period (no drug), given as a 21-day cycle. Your doctor will tell you how many cycles of treatment you will need.
- In case of accidental swallowing, or if you suspect that too much medicine has been taken, contact your doctor or local poison control center or emergency room **right away.**

What should I avoid while taking XELODA?

- Women should not become pregnant while taking XELODA. XELODA may harm your unborn child. Use effective birth control while taking XELODA. Tell your doctor if you become pregnant.
- Men should practice birth control measures while taking XELODA.
- Do not breast-feed. XELODA may pass through your milk and harm the baby.

What are the most common side effects of XELODA?

The most common side effects of XELODA are:

- diarrhea, nausea, vomiting, stomatitis (sores in mouth and throat), abdominal (stomach area) pain, upset stomach, constipation, loss of appetite, and dehydration (too much water loss from the body). These side effects are more common in patients age 80 and older.
- hand-and-foot syndrome (palms of the hands or soles of the feet tingle, become numb, painful, swollen or red), rash, dry, itchy or discolored skin, nail problems, and hair loss.
- tiredness, weakness, dizziness, headache, fever, pain (including chest, back, joint, and muscle pain), trouble sleeping, and taste problems.

These side effects may differ when taking XELODA in combination with Taxotere. Please consult your doctor for possible side effects that may be caused by taking XELODA with Taxotere.

If you are concerned about these or any other side effects while taking XELODA, talk to your doctor.

Contact your doctor right away if you have the side effects listed below. Your doctor can help reduce the chance that the side effects will continue or become serious. Your doctor may tell you to decrease the dose or stop XELODA treatment for a while.

Contact your doctor right away if you have:

- ***Diarrhea:*** if you have more than 4 bowel movements each day or any diarrhea at night
- ***Vomiting:*** if you vomit more than once in a 24-hour time period
- ***Nausea:*** if you lose your appetite, and the amount of food you eat each day is much less than usual
- ***Stomatitis:*** if you have pain, redness, swelling or sores in your mouth
- ***Hand-and-Foot Syndrome:*** if you have pain and swelling or redness of your hands or feet that prevents normal activity
- ***Fever or Infection:*** if you have a temperature of 100.5°F or greater, or other signs of infection

If caught early, most of these side effects usually improve after you stop taking XELODA. If they do not improve within 2 to 3 days, call your doctor again. After side effects have improved, your doctor will tell you whether to start taking XELODA again and what dose to use.

How should I store and use XELODA?

- **Never share XELODA with anyone.**
- **XELODA should be stored at normal room temperature (about 65° to 85°F).**
- **Keep this and all other medications out of the reach of children.**
- **In case of accidental ingestion or if you suspect that more than the prescribed dose of this medication has been taken, contact your doctor or local poison control center or emergency room IMMEDIATELY.**

General advice about prescription medicines:

Medicines are sometimes prescribed for conditions that are not mentioned in patient information leaflets. Do not use XELODA for a condition for which it was not prescribed. Do not give XELODA to other people, even if they have the same symptoms you have. It may harm them.

This leaflet summarizes the most important information about XELODA. If you would like more information, talk with your doctor. You can ask your pharmacist or doctor for information about XELODA that is written for health professionals.

Adriamycin is a registered trademark of Pharmacia & Upjohn Company.
Coumadin is a registered trademark of DuPont Pharma.
Dilantin is a registered trademark of Parke-Davis.
Taxol is a registered trademark of Bristol-Myers Squibb Company.
Taxotere is a registered trademark of Aventis Pharmaceuticals Products Inc.
Rx only

Revised: September 2001
Printed in USA

In the PDR annual,
the **Brand and Generic Name Index**
(PINK section)
alphabetizes drugs under both
brand and generic names.

Sanofi-Synthelabo Inc.
90 PARK AVENUE
NEW YORK, NY 10016

Direct Inquiries to:
(212) 551-4000

For Medical Information Contact:
Product Information Services
(800) 446-6267

Sales and Ordering:
East Coast: (800) 223-1062
West Coast: (800) 223-5511

PLAVIX® ℞
[pla' vĭcks]
clopidogrel bisulfate tablets

Prescribing information for this product, which appears on pages 3084–3086 of the 2002 PDR, has been completely revised as follows. Please write "See Supplement A" next to the product heading.

DESCRIPTION

PLAVIX (clopidogrel bisulfate) is an inhibitor of ADP-induced platelet aggregation acting by direct inhibition of adenosine diphosphate (ADP) binding to its receptor and of the subsequent ADP-mediated activation of the glycoprotein GPIIb/IIIa complex. Chemically it is methyl (+)-(*S*)-α-(2-chlorophenyl)-6,7-dihydrothieno[3,2-c]pyridine-5(4*H*)-acetate sulfate (1:1). The empirical formula of clopidogrel bisulfate is $C_{16}H_{16}Cl\ NO_2S{\bullet}H_2SO_4$ and its molecular weight is 419.9.

The structural formula is as follows:

Clopidogrel bisulfate is a white to off-white powder. It is practically insoluble in water at neutral pH but freely soluble at pH 1. It also dissolves freely in methanol, dissolves sparingly in methylene chloride, and is practically insoluble in ethyl ether. It has a specific optical rotation of about +56°.

PLAVIX for oral administration is provided as pink, round, biconvex, debossed film-coated tablets containing 97.875 mg of clopidogrel bisulfate which is the molar equivalent of 75 mg of clopidogrel base.

Each tablet contains hydrogenated castor oil, hydroxypropylcellulose, mannitol, microcrystalline cellulose and polyethylene glycol 6000 as inactive ingredients. The pink film coating contains ferric oxide, hydroxypropyl methylcellulose 2910, lactose monohydrate, titanium dioxide and triacetin. The tablets are polished with Carnauba wax.

CLINICAL PHARMACOLOGY

Mechanism of Action

Clopidogrel is an inhibitor of platelet aggregation. A variety of drugs that inhibit platelet function have been shown to decrease morbid events in people with established atherosclerotic disease as evidenced by stroke or transient ischemic attacks, myocardial infarction, unstable angina or the need for vascular bypass or angioplasty. This indicates that platelets participate in the initiation and/or evolution of these events and that inhibiting them can reduce the event rate.

Pharmacodynamic Properties

Clopidogrel selectively inhibits the binding of adenosine diphosphate (ADP) to its platelet receptor and the subsequent ADP-mediated activation of the glycoprotein GPIIb/IIIa complex, thereby inhibiting platelet aggregation. Biotransformation of clopidogrel is necessary to produce inhibition of platelet aggregation, but an active metabolite responsible for the activity of the drug has not been isolated. Clopidogrel also inhibits platelet aggregation induced by agonists other than ADP by blocking the amplification of platelet activation by released ADP. Clopidogrel does not inhibit phosphodiesterase activity.

Clopidogrel acts by irreversibly modifying the platelet ADP receptor. Consequently, platelets exposed to clopidogrel are affected for the remainder of their lifespan.

Dose dependent inhibition of platelet aggregation can be seen 2 hours after single oral doses of PLAVIX. Repeated doses of 75 mg PLAVIX per day inhibit ADP-induced platelet aggregation on the first day, and inhibition reaches steady state between Day 3 and Day 7. At steady state, the average inhibition level observed with a dose of 75 mg PLAVIX per day was between 40% and 60%. Platelet aggregation and bleeding time gradually return to baseline values after treatment is discontinued, generally in about 5 days.

Pharmacokinetics and Metabolism

After repeated 75-mg oral doses of clopidogrel (base), plasma concentrations of the parent compound, which has no platelet inhibiting effect, are very low and are generally below the quantification limit (0.00025 mg/L) beyond 2 hours after dosing. Clopidogrel is extensively metabolized by the liver. The main circulating metabolite is the carboxylic acid derivative, and it too has no effect on platelet aggregation. It represents about 85% of the circulating drug-related compounds in plasma.

Following an oral dose of ^{14}C-labeled clopidogrel in humans, approximately 50% was excreted in the urine and approximately 46% in the feces in the 5 days after dosing. The elimination half-life of the main circulating metabolite was 8 hours after single and repeated administration. Covalent binding to platelets accounted for 2% of radiolabel with a half-life of 11 days.

Effect of Food: Administration of PLAVIX (clopidogrel bisulfate) with meals did not significantly modify the bioavailability of clopidogrel as assessed by the pharmacokinetics of the main circulating metabolite.

Absorption and Distribution: Clopidogrel is rapidly absorbed after oral administration of repeated doses of 75 mg clopidogrel (base), with peak plasma levels (≅3 mg/L) of the main circulating metabolite occurring approximately 1 hour after dosing. The pharmacokinetics of the main circulating metabolite are linear (plasma concentrations increased in proportion to dose) in the dose range of 50 to 150 mg of clopidogrel. Absorption is at least 50% based on urinary excretion of clopidogrel-related metabolites.

Clopidogrel and the main circulating metabolite bind reversibly *in vitro* to human plasma proteins (98% and 94%, respectively). The binding is nonsaturable *in vitro* up to a concentration of 100 µg/mL.

Metabolism and Elimination: In vitro and *in vivo*, clopidogrel undergoes rapid hydrolysis into its carboxylic acid derivative. In plasma and urine, the glucuronide of the carboxylic acid derivative is also observed.

Special Populations

Geriatric Patients: Plasma concentrations of the main circulating metabolite are significantly higher in elderly (≥75 years) compared to young healthy volunteers but these higher plasma levels were not associated with differences in platelet aggregation and bleeding time. No dosage adjustment is needed for the elderly.

Renally Impaired Patients: After repeated doses of 75 mg PLAVIX per day, plasma levels of the main circulating metabolite were lower in patients with severe renal impairment (creatinine clearance from 5 to 15 mL/min) compared to subjects with moderate renal impairment (creatinine clearance 30 to 60 mL/min) or healthy subjects. Although inhibition of ADP-induced platelet aggregation was lower (25%) than that observed in healthy volunteers, the prolongation of bleeding time was similar to healthy volunteers receiving 75 mg of PLAVIX per day. No dosage adjustment is needed in renally impaired patients.

Gender: No significant difference was observed in the plasma levels of the main circulating metabolite between males and females. In a small study comparing men and women, less inhibition of ADP-induced platelet aggregation was observed in women, but there was no difference in prolongation of bleeding time. In the large, controlled clinical study (Clopidogrel vs. Aspirin in Patients at Risk of Ischemic Events; CAPRIE), the incidence of clinical outcome events, other adverse clinical events, and abnormal clinical laboratory parameters was similar in men and women.

Race: Pharmacokinetic differences due to race have not been studied.

CLINICAL STUDIES

The clinical evidence for the efficacy of PLAVIX is derived from two double-blind trials: the CAPRIE study (Clopidogrel vs. Aspirin in Patients at Risk of Ischemic Events), a comparison of PLAVIX to aspirin, and the CURE study (Clopidogrel in Unstable Angina to Prevent Recurrent Ischemic Events), a comparison of PLAVIX to placebo, both given in combination with aspirin and other standard therapy.

The CAPRIE trial was a 19,185-patient, 304-center, international, randomized, double-blind, parallel-group study comparing PLAVIX (75 mg daily) to aspirin (325 mg daily). The patients randomized had: 1) recent histories of myocardial infarction (within 35 days); 2) recent histories of ischemic stroke (within 6 months) with at least a week of residual neurological signs; or 3) objectively established peripheral arterial disease. Patients received randomized treatment for an average of 1.6 years (maximum of 3 years).

The trial's primary outcome was the time to first occurrence of new ischemic stroke (fatal or not), new myocardial infarction (fatal or not), or other vascular death. Deaths not easily attributable to nonvascular causes were all classified as vascular.

Table 1: Outcome Events in the CAPRIE Primary Analysis

Patients	PLAVIX 9599	apririn 9586
IS (fatal or not)	438 (4.6%)	461 (4.8%)
MI (fatal or not)	275 (2.9%)	333 (3.5%)
Other vascular death	226 (2.4%)	226 (2.4%)
Total	939 (9.8%)	1020 (10.6%)

As shown in the table, PLAVIX (clopidogrel bisulfate) was associated with a lower incidence of outcome events of every kind. The overall risk reduction (9.78% vs. 10.64%) was 8.7%, P=0.045. Similar results were obtained when all-cause mortality and all-cause strokes were counted instead of vascular mortality and ischemic strokes (risk reduction 6.9%). In patients who survived an on-study stroke or myocardial infarction, the incidence of subsequent events was again lower in the PLAVIX group.

The curves showing the overall event rate are shown in Figure 1. The event curves separated early and continued to diverge over the 3-year follow-up period.

Figure 1: Fatal or Non-Fatal Vascular Events in the CAPRIE Study

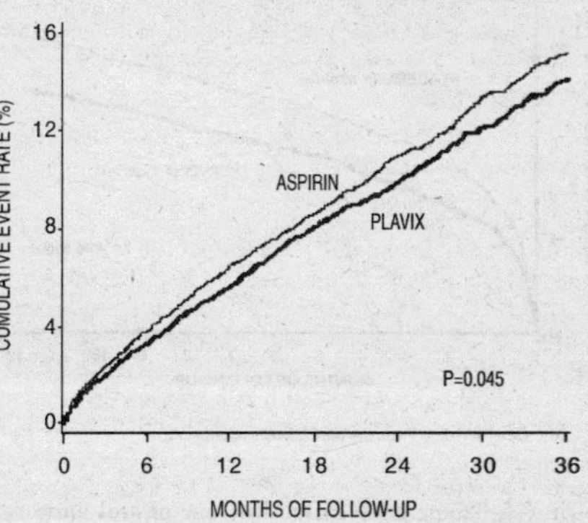

Although the statistical significance favoring PLAVIX over aspirin was marginal (P=0.045), and represents the result of a single trial that has not been replicated, the comparator drug, aspirin, is itself effective (vs. placebo) in reducing cardiovascular events in patients with recent myocardial infarction or stroke. Thus, the difference between PLAVIX and placebo, although not measured directly, is substantial.

The CAPRIE trial included a population that was randomized on the basis of 3 entry criteria. The efficacy of PLAVIX relative to aspirin was heterogeneous across the randomized subgroups (P=0.043). It is not clear whether this difference is real or a chance occurrence. Although the CAPRIE trial was not designed to evaluate the relative benefit of PLAVIX over aspirin in the individual patient subgroups, the benefit appeared to be strongest in patients who were enrolled because of peripheral vascular disease (especially those who also had a history of myocardial infarction) and weaker in stroke patients. In patients who were enrolled in the trial on the sole basis of a recent myocardial infarction, PLAVIX was not numerically superior to aspirin.

In the meta-analyses of studies of aspirin vs. placebo in patients similar to those in CAPRIE, aspirin was associated with a reduced incidence of atherothrombotic events. There was a suggestion of heterogeneity in these studies too, with the effect strongest in patients with a history of myocardial infarction, weaker in patients with a history of stroke, and not discernible in patients with a history of peripheral vascular disease. With respect to the inferred comparison of PLAVIX to placebo, there is no indication of heterogeneity.

The CURE study included 12,562 patients with acute coronary syndrome without ST segment elevation (unstable angina or non-Q-wave myocardial infarction) and presenting within 24 hours of onset of the most recent episode of chest pain or symptoms consistent with ischemia. Patients were required to have either ECG changes compatible with new ischemia (without ST segment elevation) or elevated cardiac enzymes or troponin I or T to at least twice the upper limit of normal. The patient population was largely Caucasian (82%) and included 38% women, and 52% patients ≥65 years of age.

Patients were randomized to receive PLAVIX (300 mg loading dose followed by 75 mg/day) or placebo, and were treated for up to a year. Patients also received aspirin (75–325 mg once daily) and other standard therapies such as heparin. The use of GPIIb/IIIa inhibitors was not permitted for three days prior to randomization.

The number of patients experiencing the primary outcome (CV death, MI, or stroke) was 582 (9.30%) in the PLAVIX-treated group and 719 (11.41%) in the placebo-treated group, a 20% relative risk reduction (95% CI of 10%-28%; p=0.00009) for the PLAVIX-treated group (see Table 2).

At the end of 12 months, the number of patients experiencing the co-primary outcome (CV death, MI, stroke or refractory ischemia) was 1035 (16.54%) in the PLAVIX-treated group and 1187 (18.83%) in the placebo-treated group, a 14% relative risk reduction (95% CI of 6%-21%, p=0.0005) for the PLAVIX-treated group (see Table 2).

In the PLAVIX-treated group, each component of the two primary endpoints (CV death, MI, stroke, refractory ischemia) occurred less frequently than in the placebo-treated group.

[See table 2 at top of next page]

The benefits of PLAVIX were maintained throughout the course of the trial (up to 12 months).

[See figure at top of next column]

In CURE, the use of PLAVIX was associated with a lower incidence of CV death, MI or stroke in patient populations with different characteristics, as shown in Figure 3. The benefits associated with PLAVIX were independent of the use of other acute and long-term cardiovascular therapies, including heparin/LMWH (low molecular weight heparin), IV glycoprotein IIb/IIIa (GPIIb/IIIa) inhibitors, lipid-lowering drugs, beta-blockers, and ACE-inhibitors. The efficacy of PLAVIX was observed independently of the dose of

Continued on next page

Plavix—Cont.

Figure 2. Cardiovascular Death, Myocardial Infarction, and Stroke in the CURE Study

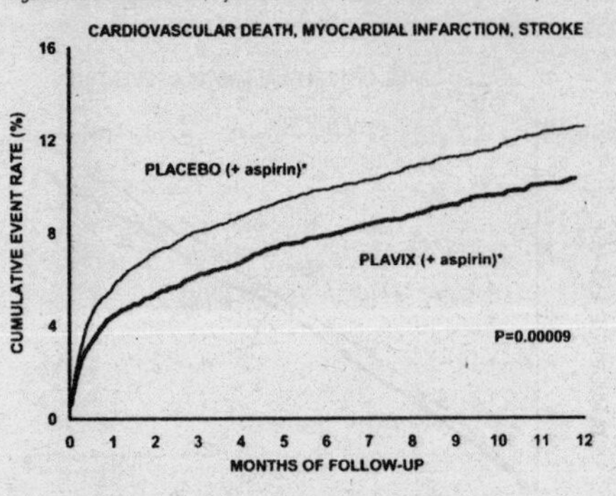

*Other standard therapies were used as appropriate

aspirin (75–325mg once daily). The use of oral anticoagulants, non-study anti-platelet drugs and chronic NSAIDs was not allowed in CURE.

Figure 3. Hazard Ratio for Patient Baseline Characteristics and On-Study Concomitant Medications/Interventions for the CURE Study

Baseline Characteristics		N	Percent Events PLAVIX (+aspirin)*	Percent Events Placebo (+aspirin)*
Overall		12562	9.3	11.4
Diagnosis	Non-Q-W	3295	12.7	15.5
	Unst Ang	8298	7.3	8.7
	Other	968	15.1	19.7
Elev Card Enzy	No	9381	8.8	10.9
	Yes	3176	10.7	13.0
ST Depr >1.0mm	No	7273	7.5	8.9
	Yes	5288	11.8	14.8
Diabetes	No	9721	7.9	9.9
	Yes	2840	14.2	16.7
Previous MI	No	8517	7.8	9.5
	Yes	4044	12.5	15.4
Previous Stroke	No	12055	8.9	11.0
	Yes	506	17.9	22.4
Concomitant Medication / Therapy				
Heparin/LMWH	No	951	4.9	7.7
	Yes	11611	9.7	11.7
Aspirin	<100mg	1927	8.5	9.7
	100-200mg	7428	9.2	10.9
	>200mg	3201	9.9	13.7
GPIIb/IIIa Antag	No	11739	8.9	10.8
	Yes	823	15.7	19.2
Beta-Blocker	No	2032	9.9	12.0
	Yes	10530	9.2	11.3
ACEI	No	4813	6.3	8.1
	Yes	7749	11.2	13.5
Lipid-Lowering	No	4461	10.9	13.1
	Yes	8101	8.4	10.5
PTCA/CABG	No	7977	8.1	10.0
	Yes	4585	11.4	13.8

*Other standard therapies were used as appropriate

The use of PLAVIX in CURE was associated with a decrease in the use of thrombolytic therapy (71 patients [1.1%] in the PLAVIX group, 126 patients [2.0%] in the placebo group; relative risk reduction of 43%, P=0.0001), and GPIIb/IIIa inhibitors (369 patients [5.9%] in the PLAVIX group, 454 patients [7.2%] in the placebo group; relative risk reduction of 18%, P=0.003). The use of PLAVIX in CURE did not impact the number of patients treated with CABG or PCI (with or without stenting), (2253 patients [36.0%] in the PLAVIX group, 2324 patients [36.9%] in the placebo group; relative risk reduction of 4.0%, P=0.1658).

INDICATIONS AND USAGE

PLAVIX (clopidogrel bisulfate) is indicated for the reduction of atherosclerotic events as follows:

- **Recent MI, Recent Stroke or Established Peripheral Arterial Disease**

  For patients with a history of recent myocardial infarction (MI), recent stroke, or established peripheral arterial disease, PLAVIX has been shown to reduce the rate of a combined endpoint of new ischemic stroke (fatal or not), new MI (fatal or not), and other vascular death.

- **Acute Coronary Syndrome**

  For patients with acute coronary syndrome (unstable angina/non-Q-wave MI), including patients who are to be managed medically and those who are to be managed with percutaneous coronary intervention (with or without stent) or CABG, PLAVIX has been shown to decrease the rate of a combined endpoint of cardiovascular death, MI, or stroke as well as the rate of a combined endpoint of cardiovascular death, MI, stroke, or refractory ischemia.

CONTRAINDICATIONS

The use of PLAVIX is contraindicated in the following conditions:

Hypersensitivity to the drug substance or any component of the product.

Active pathological bleeding such as peptic ulcer or intracranial hemorrhage.

WARNINGS

Thrombotic thrombocytopenic purpura (TTP): TTP has been reported rarely following use of PLAVIX, sometimes after a short exposure (<2 weeks). TTP is a serious condition requiring prompt treatment. It is characterized by thrombocytopenia, microangiopathic hemolytic anemia (schistocytes [fragmented RBCs] seen on peripheral smear), neurological findings, renal dysfunction, and fever. TTP was not seen during clopidogrel's clinical trials, which included over 17,500 clopidogrel-treated patients. In world-wide postmarketing experience, however, TTP has been reported at a rate of about four cases per million patients exposed, or about 11 cases per million patient-years. The background

Table 2: Outcome Events in the CURE Primary Analysis

Outcome	PLAVIX (+ aspirin)* (n=6259)		Placebo (+ aspirin)* (n=6303)		Relative Risk Reduction (%) (95% CI)
Primary outcome (Cardiovascular death, MI, Stroke)	582	(9.3%)	719	(11.4%)	20% (10.3, 27.9) P=0.00009
Co-primary outcome (Cardiovascular death, MI, Stroke, Refractory Ischemia)	1035	(16.5%)	1187	(18.8%)	14% (6.2, 20.6) P=0.00052
All Individual Outcome Events:†					
CV death	318	(5.1%)	345	(5.5%)	7% (−7.7, 20.6)
MI	324	(5.2%)	419	(6.6%)	23% (11.0, 33.4)
Stroke	75	(1.2%)	87	(1.4%)	14% (−17.7, 36.6)
Refractory ischemia	544	(8.7%)	587	(9.3%)	7% (−4.0, 18.0)

*Other standard therapies were used as appropriate.
†The individual components do not represent a breakdown of the primary and co-primary outcomes, but rather the total number of subjects experiencing an event during the course of the study.

Table 3: CURE Incidence of bleeding complications (% patients)

Event	PLAVIX (+ aspirin)* (n=6259)	Placebo (+ aspirin)* (n=6303)	P-value
Major bleeding†	3.7‡	2.7§	0.001
Life-threatening bleeding	2.2	1.8	0.13
Fatal	0.2	0.2	
5 g/dL hemoglobin drop	0.9	0.9	
Requiring surgical intervention	0.7	0.7	
Hemorrhagic strokes	0.1	0.1	
Requiring inotropes	0.5	0.5	
Requiring transfusion (≥4 units)	1.2	1.0	
Other major bleeding	1.6	1.0	0.005
Significantly disabling	0.4	0.3	
Intraocular bleeding with significant loss of vision	0.05	0.03	
Requiring 2–3 units of blood	1.3	0.9	
Minor bleeding ¶	5.1	2.4	< 0.001

* Other standard therapies were used as appropriate.
† Life threatening and other major bleeding.
‡ Major bleeding event rate for PLAVIX + aspirin was dose-dependent on aspirin: <100mg=2.6%; 100–200mg=3.5%; >200mg=4.9%
§ Major bleeding event rate for placebo + aspirin was dose-dependent on aspirin: <100mg=2.0%; 100–200mg=2.3%; >200mg=4.0%
¶ Led to interruption of study medication.

rate is thought to be about four cases per million person-years.

PRECAUTIONS

General

As with other antiplatelet agents, PLAVIX should be used with caution in patients who may be at risk of increased bleeding from trauma, surgery, or other pathological conditions. If a patient is to undergo elective surgery and an antiplatelet effect is not desired, PLAVIX should be discontinued 5 days prior to surgery.

GI Bleeding: PLAVIX prolongs the bleeding time. In CAPRIE, PLAVIX was associated with a rate of gastrointestinal bleeding of 2.0%, vs. 2.7% on aspirin. In CURE, the incidence of major gastrointestinal bleeding was 1.3% vs 0.7% (PLAVIX + aspirin vs placebo + aspirin, respectively.) PLAVIX should be used with caution in patients who have lesions with a propensity to bleed (such as ulcers). Drugs that might induce such lesions should be used with caution in patients taking PLAVIX.

Use in Hepatically Impaired Patients: Experience is limited in patients with severe hepatic disease, who may have bleeding diatheses. PLAVIX should be used with caution in this population.

Information for Patients

Patients should be told that it may take them longer than usual to stop bleeding when they take PLAVIX, and that they should report any unusual bleeding to their physician. Patients should inform physicians and dentists that they are taking PLAVIX before any surgery is scheduled and before any new drug is taken.

Drug Interactions

Study of specific drug interactions yielded the following results:

Aspirin: Aspirin did not modify the clopidogrel-mediated inhibition of ADP-induced platelet aggregation. Concomitant administration of 500 mg of aspirin twice a day for 1 day did not significantly increase the prolongation of bleeding time induced by PLAVIX. PLAVIX potentiated the effect of aspirin on collagen-induced platelet aggregation. PLAVIX and aspirin have been administered together for up to one year.

Heparin: In a study in healthy volunteers, PLAVIX did not necessitate modification of the heparin dose or alter the effect of heparin on coagulation. Coadministration of heparin had no effect on inhibition of platelet aggregation induced by PLAVIX.

Nonsteroidal Anti-Inflammatory Drugs (NSAIDs): In healthy volunteers receiving naproxen, concomitant administration of PLAVIX was associated with increased occult gastrointestinal blood loss. NSAIDs and PLAVIX should be coadministered with caution.

Warfarin: The safety of the coadministration of PLAVIX with warfarin has not been established. Consequently, concomitant administration of these two agents should be undertaken with caution. (See **Precautions—General.**)

Other Concomitant Therapy: No clinically significant pharmacodynamic interactions were observed when PLAVIX was coadministered with **atenolol, nifedipine,** or both atenolol and nifedipine. The pharmacodynamic activity of PLAVIX was also not significantly influenced by the coadministration of **phenobarbital, cimetidine** or **estrogen.**

The pharmacokinetics of **digoxin** or **theophylline** were not modified by the coadministration of PLAVIX (clopidogrel bisulfate).

At high concentrations *in vitro*, clopidogrel inhibits P_{450} (2C9). Accordingly, PLAVIX may interfere with the metabolism of **phenytoin, tamoxifen, tolbutamide, warfarin, torsemide, fluvastatin,** and many **non-steroidal anti-inflammatory agents,** but there are no data with which to predict the magnitude of these interactions. Caution should be used when any of these drugs is coadministered with PLAVIX.

In addition to the above specific interaction studies, patients entered into clinical trials with PLAVIX received a variety of concomitant medications including **diuretics, beta-blocking agents, angiotensin converting enzyme inhibitors, calcium antagonists, cholesterol lowering agents, coronary vasodilators, antidiabetic agents** (including **insulin**), **antiepileptic agents, hormone replacement therapy, heparins** (unfractionated and LMWH) and **GPIIb/IIIa antagonists** without evidence of clinically significant adverse interactions. The use of oral anticoagulants, non-study antiplatelet drug and chronic NSAIDS was not allowed in CURE and there are no data on their concomitant use with clopidogrel.

Drug/Laboratory Test Interactions

None known.

Carcinogenesis, Mutagenesis, Impairment of Fertility

There was no evidence of tumorigenicity when clopidogrel was administered for 78 weeks to mice and 104 weeks to rats at dosages up to 77 mg/kg per day, which afforded plasma exposures >25 times that in humans at the recommended daily dose of 75 mg.

Clopidogrel was not genotoxic in four *in vitro* tests (Ames test, DNA-repair test in rat hepatocytes, gene mutation assay in Chinese hamster fibroblasts, and metaphase chromosome analysis of human lymphocytes) and in one *in vivo* test (micronucleus test by oral route in mice).

Clopidogrel was found to have no effect on fertility of male and female rats at oral doses up to 400 mg/kg per day (52 times the recommended human dose on a mg/m^2 basis).

Pregnancy

Pregnancy Category B. Reproduction studies performed in rats and rabbits at doses up to 500 and 300 mg/kg/day (respectively, 65 and 78 times the recommended daily human dose on a mg/m^2 basis), revealed no evidence of impaired fertility or fetotoxicity due to clopidogrel. There are, however, no adequate and well-controlled studies in pregnant women. Because animal reproduction studies are not always predictive of a human response, PLAVIX should be used during pregnancy only if clearly needed.

Nursing Mothers

Studies in rats have shown that clopidogrel and/or its metabolites are excreted in the milk. It is not known whether this drug is excreted in human milk. Because many drugs are excreted in human milk and because of the potential for serious adverse reactions in nursing infants, a decision should be made whether to discontinue nursing or to discontinue the drug, taking into account the importance of the drug to the nursing woman.

Pediatric Use

Safety and effectiveness in the pediatric population have not been established.

ADVERSE REACTIONS

PLAVIX has been evaluated for safety in more than 17,500 patients, including over 9,000 patients treated for 1 year or more. The overall tolerability of PLAVIX in CAPRIE was similar to that of aspirin regardless of age, gender and race, with an approximately equal incidence (13%) of patients withdrawing from treatment because of adverse reactions. The clinically important adverse events observed in CAPRIE and CURE are discussed below.

Hemorrhagic: In CAPRIE patients receiving PLAVIX, gastrointestinal hemorrhage occurred at a rate of 2.0%, and required hospitalization in 0.7%. In patients receiving aspirin, the corresponding rates were 2.7% and 1.1%, respectively. The incidence of intracranial hemorrhage was 0.4% for PLAVIX compared to 0.5% for aspirin.

In CURE, PLAVIX use with aspirin was associated with an increase in bleeding compared to placebo with aspirin (see Table 3). There was an excess in major bleeding in patients receiving PLAVIX plus aspirin compared with placebo plus aspirin, primarily gastrointestinal and at puncture sites. The incidence of intracranial hemorrhage (0.1%), and fatal bleeding (0.2%), was the same in both groups.

In patients receiving both PLAVIX and aspirin in CURE, the incidence of bleeding is described in Table 3.

[See table 3 at top of previous page]

Ninety-two percent (92%) of the patients in the CURE study received heparin/LMWH, and the rate of bleeding in these patients was similar to the overall results.

There was no excess in major bleeds within seven days after coronary bypass graft surgery in patients who stopped therapy more than five days prior to surgery (event rate 4.4% PLAVIX + aspirin; 5.3% placebo + aspirin). In patients who remained on therapy within five days of bypass graft surgery, the event rate was 9.6% for PLAVIX + aspirin, and 6.3% for placebo + aspirin.

Neutropenia / agranulocytosis: Ticlopidine, a drug chemically similar to PLAVIX, is associated with a 0.8% rate of severe neutropenia (less than 450 neutrophils/μL). In CAPRIE severe neutropenia was observed in six patients, four on PLAVIX and two on aspirin. Two of the 9599 patients who received PLAVIX and none of the 9586 patients who received aspirin had neutrophil counts of zero. One of the four PLAVIX patients in CAPRIE was receiving cytotoxic chemotherapy, and another recovered and returned to the trial after only temporarily interrupting treatment with PLAVIX (clopidogrel bisulfate). In CURE, the numbers of patients with thrombocytopenia (19 PLAVIX+ aspirin vs 24 placebo + aspirin) or neutropenia (3 vs 3) were similar.

Although the risk of myelotoxicity with PLAVIX thus appears to be quite low, this possibility should be considered when a patient receiving PLAVIX demonstrates fever or other sign of infection.

Gastrointestinal: Overall, the incidence of gastrointestinal events (e.g. abdominal pain, dyspepsia, gastritis and constipation) in patients receiving PLAVIX (clopidogrel bisulfate) was 27.1%, compared to 29.8% in those receiving aspirin in the CAPRIE trial. In the CURE trial the incidence of these gastrointestinal events for patients receiving PLAVIX + aspirin was 11.7% compared to 12.5% for those receiving placebo + aspirin.

In the CAPRIE trial, the incidence of peptic, gastric or duodenal ulcers was 0.7% for PLAVIX and 1.2% for aspirin. In the CURE trial the incidence of peptic, gastric or duodenal ulcers was 0.4% for PLAVIX + aspirin and 0.3% for placebo + aspirin.

Cases of diarrhea were reported in the CAPRIE trial in 4.5% of patients in the PLAVIX group compared to 3.4% in the aspirin group. However, these were rarely severe (PLAVIX=0.2% and aspirin=0.1%). In the CURE trial, the incidence of diarrhea for patients receiving PLAVIX + aspirin was 2.1% compared to 2.2% for those receiving placebo + aspirin.

In the CAPRIE trial, the incidence of patients withdrawing from treatment because of gastrointestinal adverse reactions was 3.2% for PLAVIX and 4.0% for aspirin. In the CURE trial, the incidence of patients withdrawing from treatment because of gastrointestinal adverse reactions was 0.9% for PLAVIX + aspirin compared with 0.8% for placebo + aspirin.

Rash and Other Skin Disorders: In the CAPRIE trial, the incidence of skin and appendage disorders in patients receiving PLAVIX was 15.8% (0.7% serious); the corresponding rate in aspirin patients was 13.1% (0.5% serious). In the CURE trial the incidence of rash or other skin disorders in patients receiving PLAVIX + aspirin was 4.0% compared to 3.5% for those receiving placebo + aspirin.

In the CAPRIE trial, the overall incidence of patients withdrawing from treatment because of skin and appendage disorders adverse reactions was 1.5% for PLAVIX and 0.8% for aspirin. In the CURE trial, the incidence of patients withdrawing because of skin and appendage disorders adverse reactions was 0.7% for PLAVIX + aspirin compared with 0.3% for placebo + aspirin.

Adverse events occurring in ≥2.5% of patients on PLAVIX in the CAPRIE controlled clinical trial are shown below regardless of relationship to PLAVIX. The median duration of therapy was 20 months, with a maximum of 3 years.

[See table 4 above]

Table 4: Adverse Events Occurring in ≥2.5% of PLAVIX Patients in CAPRIE

Body System / Event	PLAVIX [n=9599] % Incidence	(% Discontinuation)	Aspirin [n=9586] % Incidence	(% Discontinuation)
Body as a Whole—general disorders				
Chest Pain	8.3	(0.2)	8.3	(0.3)
Accidental/Inflicted Injury	7.9	(0.1)	7.3	(0.1)
Influenza-like symptoms	7.5	(<0.1)	7.0	(<0.1)
Pain	6.4	(0.1)	6.3	(0.1)
Fatigue	3.3	(0.1)	3.4	(0.1)
Cardiovascular disorders, general				
Edema	4.1	(<0.1)	4.5	(<0.1)
Hypertension	4.3	(<0.1)	5.1	(<0.1)
Central & peripheral nervous system disorders				
Headache	7.6	(0.3)	7.2	(0.2)
Dizziness	6.2	(0.2)	6.7	(0.3)
Gastrointestinal system disorders				
Abdominal pain	5.6	(0.7)	7.1	(1.0)
Dyspepsia	5.2	(0.6)	6.1	(0.7)
Diarrhea	4.5	(0.4)	3.4	(0.3)
Nausea	3.4	(0.5)	3.8	(0.4)
Metabolic & nutritional disorders				
Hypercholesterolemia	4.0	(0)	4.4	(<0.1)
Musculo-skeletal system disorders				
Arthralgia	6.3	(0.1)	6.2	(0.1)
Back Pain	5.8	(0.1)	5.3	(<0.1)
Platelet, bleeding, & clotting disorders				
Purpura/Bruise	5.3	(0.3)	3.7	(0.1)
Epistaxis	2.9	(0.2)	2.5	(0.1)
Psychiatric disorders				
Depression	3.6	(0.1)	3.9	(0.2)
Respiratory system disorders				
Upper resp tract infection	8.7	(<0.1)	8.3	(<0.1)
Dyspnea	4.5	(0.1)	4.7	(0.1)
Rhinitis	4.2	(0.1)	4.2	(<0.1)
Bronchitis	3.7	(0.1)	3.7	(0)
Coughing	3.1	(<0.1)	2.7	(<0.1)
Skin & appendage disorders				
Rash	4.2	(0.5)	3.5	(0.2)
Pruritus	3.3	(0.3)	1.6	(0.1)
Urinary system disorders				
Urinary tract infection	3.1	(0)	3.5	(0.1)

Incidence of discontinuation, regardless of relationship to therapy, is shown in parentheses.

Adverse events occurring in ≥2.0% of patients on PLAVIX in the CURE controlled clinical trial are shown below regardless of relationship to PLAVIX.

[See table 5 above]

Table 5: Adverse Events Occurring in ≥2.0% of PLAVIX Patients in CURE

Body System / Event	PLAVIX (+ aspirin)* [n=6259] % Incidence	(% Discontinuation)	Placebo (+ aspirin)* [n=6303] % Incidence	(% Discontinuation)
Body as a Whole—general disorders				
Chest Pain	2.7	(<0.1)	2.8	(0.0)
Central & peripheral nervous system disorders				
Headache	3.1	(0.1)	3.2	(0.1)
Dizziness	2.4	(0.1)	2.0	(<0.1)
Gastrointestinal system disorders				
Abdominal pain	2.3	(0.3)	2.8	(0.3)
Dyspepsia	2.0	(0.1)	1.9	(<0.1)
Diarrhea	2.1	(0.1)	2.2	(0.1)

*Other standard therapies were used as appropriate.

Other adverse experiences of potential importance occurring in 1% to 2.5% of patients receiving PLAVIX (clopidogrel bisulfate) in the CAPRIE or CURE controlled clinical trials are listed below regardless of relationship to PLAVIX. In general, the incidence of these events was similar to that in patients receiving aspirin (in CAPRIE) or placebo + aspirin (in CURE).

Autonomic Nervous System Disorders: Syncope, Palpitation. *Body as a Whole—general disorders:* Asthenia, Fever, Hernia. *Cardiovascular disorders:* Cardiac failure. *Central and peripheral nervous system disorders:* Cramps legs, Hypoaesthesia, Neuralgia, Paraesthesia, Vertigo. *Gastrointestinal system disorders:* Constipation, Vomiting. *Heart rate and rhythm disorders:* Fibrillation atrial. *Liver and biliary system disorders:* Hepatic enzymes increased. *Metabolic*

Continued on next page

Plavix—Cont.

and nutritional disorders: Gout, hyperuricemia, non-protein nitrogen (NPN) increased. *Musculo-skeletal system disorders:* Arthritis, Arthrosis. *Platelet, bleeding & clotting disorders:* GI hemorrhage, hematoma, platelets decreased. *Psychiatric disorders:* Anxiety, Insomnia. *Red blood cell disorders:* Anemia. *Respiratory system disorders:* Pneumonia, Sinusitis. *Skin and appendage disorders:* Eczema, Skin ulceration. *Urinary system disorders:* Cystitis. *Vision disorders:* Cataract, Conjunctivitis.

Other potentially serious adverse events which may be of clinical interest but were rarely reported (<1%) in patients who received PLAVIX in the CAPRIE or CURE controlled clinical trials are listed below regardless of relationship to PLAVIX. In general, the incidence of these events was similar to that in patients receiving aspirin (in CAPRIE) or placebo + aspirin (in CURE).

Body as a whole: Allergic reaction, necrosis ischemic. *Cardiovascular disorders:* Edema generalized. *Gastrointestinal system disorders:* Gastric ulcer perforated, gastritis hemorrhagic, upper GI ulcer hemorrhagic. *Liver and Biliary system disorders:* Bilirubinemia, hepatitis infectious, liver fatty. *Platelet, bleeding and clotting disorders:* hemarthrosis, hematuria, hemoptysis, hemorrhage intracranial, hemorrhage retroperitoneal, hemorrhage of operative wound, ocular hemorrhage, pulmonary hemorrhage, purpura allergic, Thrombocytopenia. *Red blood cell disorders:* Anemia aplastic, anemia hypochromic. *Reproductive disorders, female:* Menorrhagia. Hemothorax. *Skin and appendage disorders:* Bullous eruption, rash erythematous, rash maculopapular, urticaria. *Urinary system disorders:* Abnormal renal function, acute renal failure. *White cell and reticuloendothelial system disorders:* Agranulocytosis, granulocytopenia, leukemia, leukopenia, neutrophils decreased.

Postmarketing Experience

The following events have been reported spontaneously from worldwide postmarketing experience: fever, very rare cases of hypersensitivity reactions including angioedema, bronchospasms, and anaphylactoid reactions. Suspected thrombotic thrombocytopenic purpura (TTP) has been reported as part of the world-wide postmarketing experience, see **WARNINGS**.

OVERDOSAGE

One case of deliberate overdosage with PLAVIX was reported in the large, CAPRIE controlled clinical study. A 34-year-old woman took a single 1,050-mg dose of PLAVIX (equivalent to 14 standard 75-mg tablets). There were no associated adverse events. No special therapy was instituted, and she recovered without sequelae.

No adverse events were reported after single oral administration of 600 mg (equivalent to 8 standard 75-mg tablets) of PLAVIX in healthy volunteers. The bleeding time was prolonged by a factor of 1.7, which is similar to that typically observed with the therapeutic dose of 75 mg of PLAVIX per day.

A single oral dose of clopidogrel at 1500 or 2000 mg/kg was lethal to mice and to rats and at 3000 mg/kg to baboons. Symptoms of acute toxicity were vomiting (in baboons), prostration, difficult breathing, and gastrointestinal hemorrhage in all species.

Recommendations About Specific Treatment:

Based on biological plausibility, platelet transfusion may be appropriate to reverse the pharmacological effects of PLAVIX if quick reversal is required.

DOSAGE AND ADMINISTRATION

Recent MI, Recent Stroke or Established Peripheral Arterial Disease

The recommended daily dose of PLAVIX is 75 mg once daily.

Acute Coronary Syndrome

For patients with acute coronary syndrome (unstable angina/non-Q-wave MI), PLAVIX should be initiated with a single 300 mg loading dose and then continued at 75 mg once daily. Aspirin (75 mg-325 mg once daily) should be initiated and continued in combination with PLAVIX. In CURE, most patients with Acute Coronary Syndrome also received heparin acutely (see **CLINICAL STUDIES**).

PLAVIX can be administered with or without food.

No dosage adjustment is necessary for elderly patients or patients with renal disease. (See **Clinical Pharmacology: Special Populations.**)

HOW SUPPLIED

PLAVIX (clopidogrel bisulfate) is available as a pink, round, biconvex, film-coated tablet debossed with <<75>> on one side and <<1171>> on the other. Tablets are provided as follows:

NDC 63653-1171-6 bottles of 30
NDC 63653-1171-1 bottles of 90
NDC 63653-1171-5 bottles of 500
NDC 63653-1171-3 blisters of 100

Storage

Store at 25° C (77° F); excursions permitted to 15°–30° C (59°–86° F) [See USP Controlled Room Temperature]

Distributed by:

Bristol-Myers Squibb/Sanofi Pharmaceuticals Partnership
New York, NY 10016

sanofi~synthelabo
Bristol-Myers
Squibb Company

PLAVIX® is a registered trademark of Sanofi-Synthelabo.

Schering Corporation

a wholly-owned subsidiary of Schering-Plough Corporation
GALLOPING HILL ROAD
KENILWORTH, NJ 07033

Direct Inquiries to:
(908) 298-4000
CUSTOMER SERVICE:
(800) 222-7579
FAX: (908) 820-6400

For Medical Information Contact:
Schering Laboratories
Drug Information Services
2000 Galloping Hill Road
Kenilworth, NJ 07033
(800) 526-4099
FAX: (908) 298-2188

DIPROLENE® AF ℞

brand of augmented betamethasone dipropionate*
Cream, 0.05%
(potency expressed as betamethasone)
*Vehicle augments the penetration of the steroid.
For Dermatologic Use Only—Not for Ophthalmic Use

Prescribing information for this product, which appears on pages 3106–3107 of the 2002 PDR, has been completely revised as follows. Please write "See Supplement A" next to the product heading.

DESCRIPTION

DIPROLENE® AF Cream 0.05% contains betamethasone dipropionate, USP, a synthetic adrenocorticosteroid, for dermatologic use in an emollient base. Betamethasone, an analog of prednisolone, has a high degree of corticosteroid activity and a slight degree of mineralocorticoid activity. Betamethasone dipropionate is the 17, 21-dipropionate ester of betamethasone.

Chemically, betamethasone dipropionate is 9-fluoro-11β,17,21-trihydroxy-16 β-methylpregna-1,4-diene-3,20-dione 17,21-dipropionate, with the empirical formula $C_{28}H_{37}FO_7$, a molecular weight of 504.6, and the following structural formula:

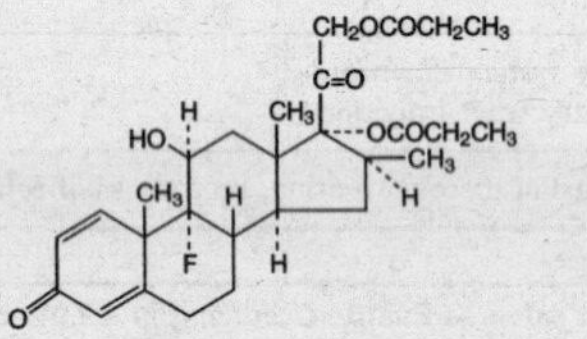

Betamethasone dipropionate is a white to creamy white, odorless crystalline powder, insoluble in water.

Each gram of DIPROLENE AF Cream 0.05% contains: 0.643 mg betamethasone dipropionate, USP (equivalent to 0.5 mg betamethasone) in an emollient cream base of purified water, USP; chlorocresol; propylene glycol, USP; white petrolatum, USP; white wax, NF; cyclomethicone; sorbitol solution, USP; glyceryl oleate/propylene glycol; ceteareth-30; carbomer 940, NF; and sodium hydroxide R.

CLINICAL PHARMACOLOGY

The corticosteroids are a class of compounds comprising steroid hormones secreted by the adrenal cortex and their synthetic analogs. In pharmacologic doses, corticosteroids are used primarily for their anti-inflammatory and/or immunosuppressive effects.

Topical corticosteroids, such as betamethasone dipropionate, are effective in the treatment of corticosteroid-responsive dermatoses primarily because of their anti-inflammatory, antipruritic, and vasoconstrictive actions. However, while the physiologic, pharmacologic, and clinical effects of the corticosteroids are well known, the exact mechanisms of their actions in each disease are uncertain. Betamethasone dipropionate, a corticosteroid, has been shown to have topical (dermatologic) and systemic pharmacologic and metabolic effects characteristic of this class of drugs.

Pharmacokinetics: The extent of percutaneous absorption of topical corticosteroids is determined by many factors including the vehicle, the integrity of the epidermal barrier, and the use of occlusive dressings. (See **DOSAGE AND ADMINISTRATION** section.)

Topical corticosteroids can be absorbed through normal intact skin. Inflammation and/or other disease processes in the skin may increase percutaneous absorption. Occlusive dressings substantially increase the percutaneous absorption of topical corticosteroids. (See **DOSAGE AND ADMINISTRATION** section.)

Once absorbed through the skin, topical corticosteroids enter pharmacokinetic pathways similar to systemically administered corticosteroids. Corticosteroids are bound to plasma proteins in varying degrees, are metabolized primarily in the liver and excreted by the kidneys. Some of the topical corticosteroids and their metabolites are also excreted into the bile.

DIPROLENE AF Cream 0.05% was applied once daily at 7 grams per day for 1 week to diseased skin, in adult patients with psoriasis or atopic dermatitis, to study its effects on the hypothalamic-pituitary-adrenal (HPA) axis. The results suggested that the drug caused a slight lowering of adrenal corticosteroid secretion, although in no case did plasma cortisol levels go below the lower limit of the normal range.

Sixty-seven pediatric patients ages 1 to 12 years, with atopic dermatitis, were enrolled in an openlabel, hypothalamic-pituitary-adrenal (HPA) axis safety study. DIPROLENE AF Cream 0.05% was applied twice daily for 2 to 3 weeks over a mean body surface area of 58% (range 35% to 95%). In 19 of 60 (32%) evaluable patients, adrenal suppression was indicated by either a ≤ 5 mcg/dL pre-stimulation cortisol, or a cosyntropin post-stimulation cortisol ≤ 18 mcg/dL and/or an increase of < 7 mcg/dL from the baseline cortisol. Studies performed with DIPROLENE AF Cream 0.05% indicate that it is in the high range of potency as compared with other topical corticosteroids.

INDICATIONS AND USAGE

DIPROLENE AF Cream 0.05% is a high-potency corticosteroid indicated for relief of the inflammatory and pruritic manifestations of corticosteroid-responsive dermatoses in patients 13 years and older.

CONTRAINDICATIONS

DIPROLENE AF Cream 0.05% is contraindicated in patients who are hypersensitive to betamethasone dipropionate, to other corticosteroids, or to any ingredient in this preparation.

PRECAUTIONS

General: Systemic absorption of topical corticosteroids has produced reversible HPA axis suppression, manifestations of Cushing's syndrome, hyperglycemia, and glucosuria in some patients.

Conditions which augment systemic absorption include the application of the more potent corticosteroids, use over large surface areas, prolonged use, and the addition of occlusive dressings. Use of more than one corticosteroid-containing product at the same time may increase total systemic glucocorticoid exposure. (See **DOSAGE AND ADMINISTRATION** section.)

Therefore, patients receiving a large dose of a potent topical steroid applied to a large surface area should be evaluated periodically for evidence of HPA axis suppression by using the urinary free cortisol and ACTH stimulation tests. If HPA axis suppression is noted, an attempt should be made to withdraw the drug, to reduce the frequency of application, or to substitute a less potent steroid.

Recovery of HPA axis function is generally prompt and complete upon discontinuation of the drug. In an open-label pediatric study of 60 evaluable patients, of the 19 who showed evidence of suppression, 4 patients were tested 2 weeks after discontinuation of DIPROLENE AF Cream 0.05%, and 3 of the 4 (75%) had complete recovery of HPA axis function. Infrequently, signs and symptoms of steroid withdrawal may occur, requiring supplemental systemic corticosteroids.

Children may absorb proportionally larger amounts of topical corticosteroids and thus be more susceptible to systemic toxicity. (See **PRECAUTIONS—Pediatric Use.**)

If irritation develops, topical corticosteroids should be discontinued and appropriate therapy instituted.

In the presence of dermatological infections, the use of an appropriate antifungal or antibacterial agent should be instituted. If a favorable response does not occur promptly, the corticosteroid should be discontinued until the infection has been adequately controlled.

Information for Patients: Patients using topical corticosteroids should receive the following information and instructions. This information is intended to aid in the safe and effective use of this medication. It is not a disclosure of all possible adverse or intended effects.

1. This medication is to be used as directed by the physician and should not be used longer than the prescribed time period. It is for external use only. Avoid contact with the eyes.
2. Patients should be advised not to use this medication for any disorder other than that for which it was prescribed.
3. The treated skin area should not be bandaged or otherwise covered or wrapped as to be occlusive. (See **DOSAGE AND ADMINISTRATION** section.)
4. Patients should report any signs of local adverse reactions.
5. Other corticosteroid-containing products should not be used with DIPROLENE AF Cream 0.05% without first talking to your physician.

Laboratory Tests: The following tests may be helpful in evaluating HPA axis suppression:

Urinary free cortisol test
ACTH stimulation test

Carcinogenesis, Mutagenesis, and Impairment of Fertility: Long-term animal studies have not been performed to evaluate the carcinogenic potential of betamethasone dipropionate.

Betamethasone was negative in the bacterial mutagenicity assay (*Salmonella typhimurium* and *Escherichia coli*), and in the mammalian cell mutagenicity assay (CHO/HGPRT). It was positive in the *in vitro* human lymphocyte chromosome aberration assay, and equivocal in the *in vivo* mouse bone marrow micronucleus assay. This pattern of response is similar to that of dexamethasone and hydrocortisone.

Reproductive studies with betamethasone dipropionate carried out in rabbits at doses of 1.0 mg/kg by the intramuscular route and in mice up to 33 mg/kg by the intramuscular route indicated no impairment of fertility except for dose-related increases in fetal resorption rates in both species. These doses are approximately 5- and 38-fold the human dose based on a mg/m^2 comparison, respectively.

Pregnancy: Teratogenic Effects: Pregnancy Category C: Corticosteroids are generally teratogenic in laboratory animals when administered systemically at relatively low dosage levels.

Betamethasone dipropionate has been shown to be teratogenic in rabbits when given by the intramuscular route at doses of 0.05 mg/kg. This dose is approximately 0.2-fold the maximum human dose based on a mg/m^2 comparison. The abnormalities observed included umbilical hernias, cephalocele and cleft palates.

Some corticosteroids have been shown to be teratogenic after dermal application in laboratory animals. There are no adequate and well-controlled studies in pregnant women on teratogenic effects from topically applied corticosteroids. Therefore, topical corticosteroids should be used during pregnancy only if the potential benefit justifies the potential risk to the fetus. Drugs of this class should not be used extensively on pregnant patients, in large amounts, or for prolonged periods of time.

Nursing Mothers: It is not known whether topical administration of corticosteroids can result in sufficient systemic absorption to produce detectable quantities in breast milk. Systemically administered corticosteroids are secreted into breast milk in quantities not likely to have a deleterious effect on the infant. Nevertheless, a decision should be made whether to discontinue nursing or to discontinue the drug, taking into account the importance of the drug to the mother.

Pediatric Use: Use of DIPROLENE AF Cream 0.05% in pediatric patients 12 years of age and younger is not recommended. (See **CLINICAL PHARMACOLOGY** and **ADVERSE REACTIONS** sections.) In an open-label study, 19 of 60 (32%) evaluable pediatric patients (aged 3 months–12 years old) using DIPROLENE AF Cream 0.05% for treatment of atopic dermatitis demonstrated HPA axis suppression. The proportion of patients with adrenal suppression in this study was progressively greater, the younger the age group. (See **CLINICAL PHARMACOLOGY Pharmacokinetics.**)

Pediatric patients may demonstrate greater susceptibility to topical corticosteroid-induced HPA axis suppression and Cushing's syndrome than mature patients because of a larger skin surface area to body weight ratio. The study described above supports this premise, as adrenal suppression in 9–12 year olds, 6-8 year olds, 2–5 year olds, and 3 months–1 year old was 17%, 32%, 38% and 50% respectively.

Hypothalamic-pituitary-adrenal (HPA) axis suppression, Cushing's syndrome, and intracranial hypertension have been reported in children receiving topical corticosteroids. Manifestations of adrenal suppression in children include linear growth retardation, delayed weight gain, low plasma cortisol levels, and absence of response to ACTH stimulation. Manifestations of intracranial hypertension include bulging fontanelles, headaches, and bilateral papilledema. Chronic corticosteroid therapy may interfere with the growth and development of children.

ADVERSE REACTIONS

The only local adverse reaction reported to be possibly or probably related to treatment with DIPROLENE AF Cream 0.05% during adult, controlled clinical studies was stinging. It occurred in 1 patient, 0.4%, of the 242 patients or subjects involved in the studies.

Adverse reactions reported to be possibly or probably related to treatment with DIPROLENE AF Cream 0.05% during a pediatric clinical study include signs of skin atrophy (telangiectasia, bruising, shininess). Skin atrophy occurred in 7 of 67 (10%) patients, involving all age groups from 3 months–12 years of age.

The following local adverse reactions are reported infrequently when topical corticosteroids are used as recommended. These reactions are listed in an approximate decreasing order of occurrence: burning, itching, irritation, dryness, folliculitis, hypertrichosis, acneiform eruptions, hypopigmentation, perioral dermatitis, allergic contact dermatitis, maceration of the skin, secondary infection, skin atrophy, striae, miliaria.

Systemic absorption of topical corticosteroids has produced reversible hypothalamic-pituitary-adrenal (HPA) axis suppression, manifestations of Cushing's syndrome, hyperglycemia, and glucosuria in some patients.

OVERDOSAGE

Topically applied corticosteroids can be absorbed in sufficient amounts to produce systemic effects. (See **PRECAUTIONS.**)

DOSAGE AND ADMINISTRATION

Apply a thin film of DIPROLENE AF Cream to the affected skin areas once or twice daily. Treatment with DIPROLENE AF Cream 0.05% should be limited to 45 g per week.

DIPROLENE AF Cream 0.05% is not to be used with occlusive dressings.

HOW SUPPLIED

DIPROLENE AF Cream 0.05% is supplied in 15-g (NDC 0085-0517-01) and 50-g (NDC 0085-0517-04) tubes; boxes of one.

Store between 2° and 30°C (36° and 86°F).

DIPROLENE® AF
brand of augmented betamethasone dipropionate*
Cream, 0.05%
(potency expressed as betamethasone)
*Vehicle augments the penetration of the steroid.
For Dermatologic Use Only-
Not for Ophthalmic Use
Schering Corporation
Kenilworth, NJ 07033 USA
Rev. 10/01 B-17968645
18670330T

DIPROSONE® ℞

[dī' prō-sōn]
brand of betamethasone
dipropionate
Cream, USP 0.05%
(potency expressed as betamethasone)
For Dermatologic Use Only—
Not for Ophthalmic Use

Prescribing information for this product, which appears on pages 3109–3110 of the 2002 PDR, has been completely revised as follows. Please write "See Supplement A" next to the product heading.

DESCRIPTION

DIPROSONE Cream 0.05% contains betamethasone dipropionate, USP, a synthetic adrenocorticosteroid, for dermatologic use. Betamethasone, an analog of prednisolone, has high corticosteroid activity and slight mineralocorticoid activity. Betamethasone dipropionate is the 17, 21-dipropionate ester of betamethasone.

Chemically, betamethasone dipropionate is 9-Fluoro-11β,17,21-trihydroxy-16β-methyl-pregna-1,4-diene-3,20-dione 17,21-dipropionate, with the empirical formula $C_{28}H_{37}FO_7$, a molecular weight of 504.6, and the following structural formula:

Betamethasone dipropionate is a white to creamy white, odorless crystalline powder, insoluble in water.

Each gram of DIPROSONE Cream 0.05% contains: 0.643 mg betamethasone dipropionate, USP (equivalent to 0.5 mg betamethasone) in a hydrophilic emollient cream consisting of purified water, USP; mineral oil, USP; white petrolatum, USP; ceteareth-30; cetearyl alcohol 70/30 (7.2%); sodium phosphate monobasic monohydrate R; and phosphoric acid, NF; chlorocresol and propylene glycol, USP as preservatives. May also contain sodium hydroxide R to adjust pH to approximately 5.0.

CLINICAL PHARMACOLOGY

The corticosteroids are a class of compounds comprising steroid hormones secreted by the adrenal cortex and their synthetic analogs. In pharmacologic doses corticosteroids are used primarily for their anti-inflammatory and/or immunosuppressive effects.

Topical corticosteroids, such as betamethasone dipropionate, are effective in the treatment of corticosteroid-responsive dermatoses primarily because of their anti-inflammatory, antipruritic, and vasoconstrictive actions. However, while the physiologic, pharmacologic, and clinical effects of the corticosteroids are well known, the exact mechanisms of their actions in each disease are uncertain. Betamethasone dipropionate, a corticosteroid, has been shown to have topical (dermatologic) and systemic pharmacologic and metabolic effects characteristic of this class of drugs.

Pharmacokinetics The extent of percutaneous absorption of topical corticosteroids is determined by many factors including the vehicle, the integrity of the epidermal barrier, and the use of occlusive dressings. (See **DOSAGE AND ADMINISTRATION.**)

Topical corticosteroids can be absorbed from normal intact skin. Inflammation and/or other disease processes in the skin increase percutaneous absorption. Occlusive dressings substantially increase the percutaneous absorption of topical corticosteroids. (See **DOSAGE AND ADMINISTRATION.**)

Once absorbed through the skin, topical corticosteroids are handled through pharmacokinetic pathways similar to systemically administered corticosteroids. Corticosteroids are bound to plasma proteins in varying degrees. Corticosteroids are metabolized primarily in the liver and are then excreted by the kidneys. Some of the topical corticosteroids and their metabolites are also excreted into the bile.

Sixty-three pediatric patients ages 1 to 12 years, with atopic dermatitis, were enrolled in an open-label, hypothalamic-pituitary-adrenal (HPA) axis safety study. DIPROSONE Cream 0.05% was applied twice daily for 2 to 3 weeks over a mean body surface area of 40% (range 35% to 90%). In 10 of 43 (23%) evaluable patients, adrenal suppression was indicated by either a ≤ 5 mcg/dL pre-stimulation cortisol, or a cosyntropin post-stimulation cortisol ≤ 18 mcg/dL and/or an increase of < 7 mcg/dL from the baseline cortisol. Studies performed with DIPROSONE Cream 0.05% indicate that it is in the medium range of potency as compared with other topical corticosteroids.

INDICATIONS AND USAGE

DIPROSONE Cream 0.05% is a medium-potency corticosteroid indicated for relief of the inflammatory and pruritic manifestations of corticosteroid-responsive dermatoses in patients 13 years and older.

CONTRAINDICATIONS

DIPROSONE Cream 0.05% is contraindicated in patients who are hypersensitive to betamethasone dipropionate, to other corticosteroids, or to any ingredient in these preparations.

PRECAUTIONS

General: Systemic absorption of topical corticosteroids has produced reversible hypothalamic-pituitary-adrenal (HPA) axis suppression, manifestations of Cushing's syndrome, hyperglycemia, and glucosuria in some patients.

Conditions which augment systemic absorption include the application of the more potent steroids, use over large surface areas, prolonged use, and the addition of occlusive dressings. Use of more than one corticosteroid-containing product at the same time may increase total systemic glucocorticoid exposure. (See **DOSAGE AND ADMINISTRATION.**)

Therefore, patients receiving a large dose of a potent topical steroid applied to a large surface area should be evaluated periodically for evidence of HPA axis suppression by using the urinary-free cortisol and ACTH stimulation tests. If HPA axis suppression is noted, an attempt should be made to withdraw the drug, to reduce the frequency of application, or to substitute a less potent steroid.

Recovery of HPA axis function is generally prompt and complete upon discontinuation of the drug. In an open-label pediatric study of 43 evaluable patients, of the 10 patients who showed evidence of suppression, 2 patients were tested 2 weeks after discontinuation of DIPROSONE Cream, 0.05%, and 1 of the 2 (50%) had complete recovery of HPA axis function. Infrequently, signs and symptoms of steroid withdrawal may occur, requiring supplemental systemic corticosteroids.

Pediatric patients may absorb proportionally larger amounts of topical corticosteroids and thus be more susceptible to systemic toxicity. (See **PRECAUTIONS—Pediatric Use.**)

If irritation develops, topical corticosteroids should be discontinued and appropriate therapy instituted.

In the presence of dermatological infections, the use of an appropriate antifungal or antibacterial agent should be instituted. If a favorable response does not occur promptly, the corticosteroid should be discontinued until the infection has been adequately controlled.

Information for Patients This information is intended to aid in the safe and effective use of this medication. It is not a disclosure of all possible adverse or intended effects.

Patients using topical corticosteroids should receive the following information and instructions:

1. This medication is to be used as directed by the physician. It is for external use only. Avoid contact with the eyes.
2. Patients should be advised not to use this medication for any disorder other than that for which it was prescribed.
3. The treated skin area should not be bandaged or otherwise covered or wrapped as to be occlusive. (See **DOSAGE AND ADMINISTRATION.**)
4. Patients should report any signs of local adverse reactions.
5. Other corticosteroid-containing products should not be used with DIPROSONE Cream 0.05% without first talking to your physician.

Laboratory Tests The following tests may be helpful in evaluating HPA axis suppression:

Urinary-free cortisol test
ACTH stimulation test

Carcinogenesis, Mutagenesis, and Impairment of Fertility Long-term animal studies have not been performed to evaluate the carcinogenic potential of betamethasone dipropionate.

Betamethasone was negative in the bacterial mutagenicity assay (*Salmonella typhimurium* and *Escherichia coli*), and in the mammalian cell mutagenicity assay (CHO/HGPRT). It was positive in the *in vitro* human lymphocyte chromosome aberration assay, and equivocal in the *in vivo* mouse bone marrow micronucleus assay. This pattern of response is similar to that of dexamethasone and hydrocortisone.

Reproductive studies with betamethasone dipropionate carried out in rabbits at doses of 1.0 mg/kg by the intramuscular route and in mice up to 33 mg/kg by the intramuscular route indicated no impairment of fertility except for dose-related increases in fetal reabsorption rates in both species. These doses are approximately 0.5 and 4-fold the estimated maximum human dose based on a mg/m^2 comparison, respectively.

Continued on next page

Diprosone Cream—Cont.

Pregnancy: Teratogenic Effects: Pregnancy Category C Corticosteroids are generally teratogenic in laboratory animals when administered systemically at relatively low dosage levels. Betamethasone dipropionate has been shown to be teratogenic in rabbits when given by the intramuscular route at doses of 0.05 mg/kg. This dose is approximately 0.03-fold the estimated maximum human dose based on a mg/m^2 comparison. The abnormalities observed included umbilical hernias, cephalocele and cleft palates. The more potent corticosteroids have been shown to be teratogenic after dermal application in laboratory animals. There are no adequate and well-controlled studies in pregnant women on teratogenic effects from topically applied corticosteroids. Therefore, topical corticosteroids should be used during pregnancy only if the potential benefit justifies the potential risk to the fetus. Drugs of this class should not be used extensively on pregnant patients, in large amounts, or for prolonged periods of time.

Nursing Mothers It is not known whether topical administration of corticosteroids could result in sufficient systemic absorption to produce detectable quantities in breast milk. Systemically administered corticosteroids are secreted into breast milk in quantities not likely to have a deleterious effect on the infant. Nevertheless, caution should be exercised when topical corticosteroids are prescribed for a nursing woman.

Pediatric Use Use of DIPROSONE Cream, 0.05% in pediatric patients 12 years of age and younger is not recommended. (See **CLINICAL PHARMACOLOGY** and **ADVERSE REACTIONS**).

In an open-label study, 10 of 43 (23%) evaluable pediatric patients (aged 2 years–12 years old) using DIPROSONE Cream 0.05% for treatment of atopic dermatitis for 2–3 weeks demonstrated HPA axis suppression. The proportion of patients with adrenal suppression in this study was progressively greater, the younger the age group. (See **CLINICAL PHARMACOLOGY—Pharmacokinetics.**)

Pediatric patients may demonstrate greater susceptibility to topical corticosteroid-induced HPA axis suppression and Cushing's syndrome than mature patients because of a larger skin surface area to body weight ratio. The study described above supports this premise, as suppression in 9–12 year olds, 6–8 year olds, and 2–5 year olds was 14%, 23% and 30% respectively.

Hypothalamic-pituitary-adrenal (HPA) axis suppression, Cushing's syndrome, and intracranial hypertension have been reported in pediatric patients receiving topical corticosteroids. Manifestations of adrenal suppression in pediatric patients include linear growth retardation, delayed weight gain, low plasma cortisol levels, and absence of response to ACTH stimulation. Manifestations of intracranial hypertension include bulging fontanelles, headaches, and bilateral papilledema.

Administration of topical corticosteroids to pediatric patients should be limited to the least amount compatible with an effective therapeutic regimen. Chronic corticosteroid therapy may interfere with the growth and development of pediatric patients.

ADVERSE REACTIONS

The following local adverse reactions are reported infrequently when DIPROSONE Cream 0.05% is used as recommended in the **DOSAGE AND ADMINISTRATION** section. These reactions are listed in an approximate decreasing order of occurrence: burning, itching, irritation, dryness, folliculitis, hypertrichosis, acneiform eruptions, hypopigmentation, perioral dermatitis, allergic contact dermatitis, maceration of the skin, secondary infection, skin atrophy, striae, miliaria.

Adverse reactions reported to be possibly or probably related to treatment with DIPROSONE Cream 0.05% during a pediatric clinical study include signs of skin atrophy (bruising, shininess). Skin atrophy occurred in 3 of 63 (5%) patients, a 3-year old, a 5-year old, and a 7-year old.

Systemic absorption of topical corticosteroids has produced reversible hypothalamic-pituitary-adrenal (HPA) axis suppression, manifestations of Cushing's syndrome, hyperglycemia, and glucosuria in some patients.

OVERDOSAGE

Topically applied corticosteroids can be absorbed in sufficient amounts to produce systemic effects. (See **PRECAUTIONS.**)

DOSAGE AND ADMINISTRATION

Apply a thin film of DIPROSONE Cream 0.05% to the affected skin areas once daily. In some cases, a twice-daily dosage may be necessary.

DIPROSONE Cream 0.05% is not to be used with occlusive dressings.

HOW SUPPLIED

DIPROSONE Cream 0.05% is supplied in 15-g (NDC 0085-0853-02) and 45-g (NDC 0085-0853-03) tubes; boxes of one.

Store DIPROSONE Cream 0.05% between 2° and 30°C (36° and 86°F).

Schering Corporation
Kenilworth, NJ 07033 USA

10/01 B-25604601
25604504T

DIPROSONE® ℞

[dī' prō-sōn]
brand of betamethasone dipropionate
Lotion, USP 0.05% w/w
(potency expressed as betamethasone)

For Dermatologic Use Only—
Not for Ophthalmic Use

Prescribing information for this product, which appears on pages 3109–3110 of the 2002 PDR, has been completely revised as follows. Please write "See Supplement A" next to the product heading.

DESCRIPTION

DIPROSONE Lotion contains betamethasone dipropionate, USP, a synthetic adrenocorticosteroid, for dermatologic use. Betamethasone, an analog of prednisolone, has high corticosteroid activity and slight mineralocorticoid activity. Betamethasone dipropionate is the 17, 21-dipropionate ester of betamethasone.

Chemically, betamethasone dipropionate is 9-Fluoro-11β,17,21-trihydroxy-16β-methyl-pregna-1,4-diene-3,20-dione 17,21-dipropionate, with the empirical formula $C_{28}H_{37}FO_7$, a molecular weight of 504.6, and the following structural formula:

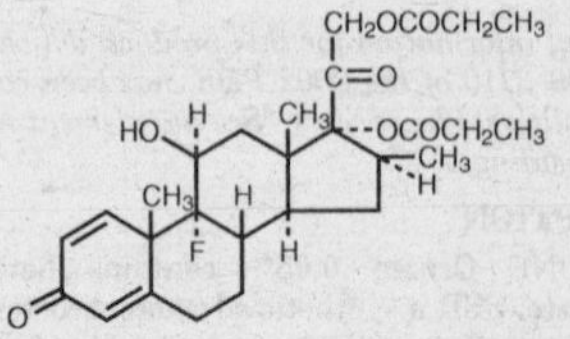

Betamethasone dipropionate is a white to creamy white, odorless crystalline powder, insoluble in water.

Each gram of DIPROSONE Lotion 0.05% w/w contains: 0.643 mg betamethasone dipropionate, USP (equivalent to 0.5 mg betamethasone) in a lotion base of isopropyl alcohol, USP (39.25%) and purified water, USP; slightly thickened with carbomer 974P; the pH is adjusted to approximately 4.7 with sodium hydroxide R.

CLINICAL PHARMACOLOGY

The corticosteroids are a class of compounds comprising steroid hormones secreted by the adrenal cortex and their synthetic analogs. In pharmacologic doses corticosteroids are used primarily for their anti-inflammatory and/or immunosuppressive effects.

Topical corticosteroids, such as betamethasone dipropionate, are effective in the treatment of corticosteroid-responsive dermatoses primarily because of their anti-inflammatory, antipruritic, and vasoconstrictive actions. However, while the physiologic, pharmacologic, and clinical effects of the corticosteroids are well known, the exact mechanisms of their actions in each disease are uncertain. Betamethasone dipropionate, a corticosteroid, has been shown to have topical (dermatologic) and systemic pharmacologic and metabolic effects characteristic of this class of drugs.

Pharmacokinetics The extent of percutaneous absorption of topical corticosteroids is determined by many factors including the vehicle, the integrity of the epidermal barrier, and the use of occlusive dressings. (See **DOSAGE AND ADMINISTRATION.**)

Topical corticosteroids can be absorbed from normal intact skin. Inflammation and/or other disease processes in the skin increase percutaneous absorption. Occlusive dressings substantially increase the percutaneous absorption of topical corticosteroids. (See **DOSAGE AND ADMINISTRATION.**)

Once absorbed through the skin, topical corticosteroids are handled through pharmacokinetic pathways similar to systemically administered corticosteroids. Corticosteroids are bound to plasma proteins in varying degrees. Corticosteroids are metabolized primarily in the liver and are then excreted by the kidneys. Some of the topical corticosteroids and their metabolites are also excreted into the bile.

Twenty-five pediatric patients ages 6 to 12 years, with atopic dermatitis, were enrolled in an open-label, hypothalamic-pituitary-adrenal (HPA) axis safety study. DIPROSONE Lotion 0.05% was applied twice daily for 2 to 3 weeks over a mean body surface area of 45% (range 35% to 72%). In 11 of 15 (73%) evaluable patients, adrenal suppression was indicated by either a ≤ 5 mcg/dL pre-stimulation cortisol, or a cosyntropin post-stimulation cortisol ≤ 18 mcg/dL and/or an increase of < 7 mcg/dL from the baseline cortisol. Studies performed with DIPROSONE Lotion 0.05% indicate that it is in the medium range of potency as compared with other topical corticosteroids.

INDICATIONS AND USAGE

DIPROSONE Lotion 0.05% is a medium-potency corticosteroid indicated for relief of the inflammatory and pruritic manifestations of corticosteroid-responsive dermatoses in patients 13 years and older.

CONTRAINDICATIONS

DIPROSONE Lotion 0.05% is contraindicated in patients who are hypersensitive to betamethasone dipropionate, to other corticosteroids, or to any ingredient in these preparations.

PRECAUTIONS

General: Systemic absorption of topical corticosteroids has produced reversible hypothalamic-pituitary-adrenal (HPA) axis suppression, manifestations of Cushing's syndrome, hyperglycemia, and glucosuria in some patients.

Conditions which augment systemic absorption include the application of the more potent steroids, use over large surface areas, prolonged use, and the addition of occlusive dressings. Use of more than one corticosteroid-containing product at the same time may increase total systemic glucocortoid exposure. (See **DOSAGE AND ADMINISTRATION.**)

Therefore, patients receiving a large dose of a potent topical steroid applied to a large surface area should be evaluated periodically for evidence of HPA axis suppression by using the urinary-free cortisol and ACTH stimulation tests. If HPA axis suppression is noted, an attempt should be made to withdraw the drug, to reduce the frequency of application, or to substitute a less potent steroid.

Recovery of HPA axis function is generally prompt and complete upon discontinuation of the drug. In an open-label pediatric study of 15 evaluable patients, of the 11 patients who showed evidence of suppression, 6 patients were tested 2 weeks after discontinuation of DIPROSONE Lotion, 0.05%, and 4 of the 6 patients (67%) had complete recovery of HPA axis function. Infrequently, signs and symptoms of steroid withdrawal may occur, requiring supplemental systemic corticosteroids.

Pediatric patients may absorb proportionally larger amounts of topical corticosteroids and thus be more susceptible to systemic toxicity. (See **PRECAUTIONS—Pediatric Use.**)

If irritation develops, topical corticosteroids should be discontinued and appropriate therapy instituted.

In the presence of dermatological infections, the use of an appropriate antifungal or antibacterial agent should be instituted. If a favorable response does not occur promptly, the corticosteroid should be discontinued until the infection has been adequately controlled.

Information for Patients This information is intended to aid in the safe and effective use of this medication. It is not a disclosure of all possible adverse or intended effects.

Patients using topical corticosteroids should receive the following information and instructions:

1. This medication is to be used as directed by the physician. It is for external use only. Avoid contact with the eyes.
2. Patients should be advised not to use this medication for any disorder other than that for which it was prescribed.
3. The treated skin area should not be bandaged or otherwise covered or wrapped as to be occlusive. (See **DOSAGE AND ADMINISTRATION.**)
4. Patients should report any signs of local adverse reactions.
5. Other corticosteroid-containing products should not be used with DIPROSONE Lotion 0.05% without first talking to your physician. (See **DOSAGE AND ADMINISTRATION.**)

Laboratory Tests The following tests may be helpful in evaluating HPA axis suppression:

Urinary-free cortisol test
ACTH stimulation test

Carcinogenesis, Mutagenesis, and Impairment of Fertility Long-term animal studies have not been performed to evaluate the carcinogenic potential of betamethasone dipropionate.

Betamethasone was negative in the bacterial mutagenicity assay (*Salmonella typhimurium* and *Escherichia coli*), and in the mammalian cell mutagenicity assay (CHO/HGPRT). It was positive in the *in vitro* human lymphocyte chromosome aberration assay, and equivocal in the *in vivo* mouse bone marrow micronucleus assay. This pattern of response is similar to that of dexamethasone and hydrocortisone.

Reproductive studies with betamethasone dipropionate carried out in rabbits at doses of 1.0 mg/kg by the intramuscular route and in mice up to 33 mg/kg by the intramuscular route indicated no impairment of fertility except for dose-related increases in fetal resorption rates in both species. These doses are approximately 0.5 and 4-fold the maximum human dose based on a mg/m^2 comparison, respectively.

Pregnancy: Teratogenic Effects: Pregnancy Category C Corticosteroids are generally teratogenic in laboratory animals when administered systemically at relatively low dosage levels.

Betamethasone dipropionate has been shown to be teratogenic in rabbits when given by the intramuscular route at doses of 0.05 mg/kg. This dose is approximately 0.03-fold the human dose based on a mg/m^2 comparison. The abnormalities observed included umbilical hernias, cephalocele and cleft palates.

Some corticosteroids have been shown to be teratogenic after dermal application in laboratory animals. There are no adequate and well-controlled studies in pregnant women on teratogenic effects from topically applied corticosteroids. Therefore, topical corticosteroids should be used during pregnancy only if the potential benefit justifies the potential risk to the fetus. Drugs of this class should not be used extensively on pregnant patients, in large amounts, or for prolonged periods of time.

Nursing Mothers It is not known whether topical administration of corticosteroids could result in sufficient systemic absorption to produce detectable quantities in breast milk. Systemically administered corticosteroids are secreted into breast milk in quantities not likely to have a deleterious effect on the infant. Nevertheless, caution should be exercised when topical corticosteroids are prescribed for a nursing woman.

Pediatric Use Use of DIPROSONE Lotion, 0.05% in pediatric patients 12 years of age and younger is not recommended. (See **CLINICAL PHARMACOLOGY** and **ADVERSE REACTIONS.**)
In an open-label study, 11 of 15 (73%) evaluable pediatric patients (aged 6 years–12 years old) using DIPROSONE Lotion for treatment of atopic dermatitis for 2–3 weeks demonstrated adrenal suppression. (See **CLINICAL PHARMACOLOGY—Pharmacokinetics.**)
Pediatric patients may demonstrate greater susceptibility to topical corticosteroid-induced HPA axis suppression and Cushing's syndrome than mature patients because of a larger skin surface area to body weight ratio.
Hypothalamic-pituitary-adrenal (HPA) axis suppression, Cushing's syndrome, and intracranial hypertension have been reported in pediatric patients receiving topical corticosteroids. Manifestations of adrenal suppression in pediatric patients include linear growth retardation, delayed weight gain, low plasma cortisol levels, and absence of response to ACTH stimulation. Manifestations of intracranial hypertension include bulging fontanelles, headaches, and bilateral papilledema.
Administration of topical corticosteroids to pediatric patients should be limited to the least amount compatible with an effective therapeutic regimen. Chronic corticosteroid therapy may interfere with the growth and development of pediatric patients.

ADVERSE REACTIONS

The following local adverse reactions are reported infrequently when DIPROSONE Lotion 0.05% is used as recommended in the **DOSAGE AND ADMINISTRATION** section. These reactions are listed in an approximate decreasing order of occurrence: burning, itching, irritation, dryness, folliculitis, hypertrichosis, acneiform eruptions, hypopigmentation, perioral dermatitis, allergic contact dermatitis, maceration of the skin, secondary infection, skin atrophy, striae, miliaria.
Adverse reactions reported to be possibly or probably related to treatment with DIPROSONE Lotion 0.05% during a pediatric study include: paresthesia (burning), erythema, erythematous rash, and dry skin. These adverse reactions each occurred in a different patient; 4% of the 25 patient population, respectively. An adverse reaction reported to be possibly or probably related to treatment in 2 different patients, 8%, of the 25 patients is pruritis.
Systemic absorption of topical corticosteroids has produced reversible hypothalamic-pituitary-adrenal (HPA) axis suppression, manifestations of Cushing's syndrome, hyperglycemia, and glucosuria in some patients.

OVERDOSAGE

Topically applied corticosteroids can be absorbed in sufficient amounts to produce systemic effects. (See **PRECAUTIONS.**)

DOSAGE AND ADMINISTRATION

Apply a few drops of DIPROSONE Lotion 0.05% to the affected area and massage lightly until it disappears. Apply twice daily, in the morning and at night. For the most effective and economical use, apply nozzle very close to affected area and gently squeeze bottle.
DIPROSONE Lotion 0.05% is not to be used with occlusive dressings.

HOW SUPPLIED

DIPROSONE Lotion 0.05% w/w is available in 20-mL (18.7-g) (NDC 0085-0028-04) and 60-mL (56.2-g) (NDC 0085-0028-06) plastic squeeze bottles; boxes of one. **Protect from light. Store in carton until contents are used.**
Store DIPROSONE Lotion between 2° and 30°C (36° and 86°F).
Schering Corporation
Kenilworth, NJ 07033 USA
10/01 B-25604709
 25604407T

LOTRISONE® CREAM
LOTRISONE® LOTION ℞

(clotrimazole and betamethasone dipropionate)
[lō' tri-sōn]

Prescribing information for this product, which appears on pages 3129–3131 of the 2002 PDR, has been completely revised as follows. Please write "See Supplement A" next to the product heading.

FOR TOPICAL USE ONLY. NOT FOR OPHTHALMIC, ORAL, OR INTRAVAGINAL USE. NOT RECOMMENDED FOR PATIENTS UNDER THE AGE OF 17 YEARS AND NOT RECOMMENDED FOR DIAPER DERMATITIS.

DESCRIPTION

LOTRISONE Cream and Lotion contain combinations of clotrimazole, a synthetic antifungal agent, and betamethasone dipropionate, a synthetic corticosteroid, for dermatologic use.
Chemically, clotrimazole is 1-(o-chloro-α,α-diphenylbenzyl) imidazole, with the empirical formula $C_{22}H_{17}ClN_2$, a molecular weight of 344.84, and the following structural formula:
[See chemical structure at top of next column]
Clotrimazole is an odorless, white crystalline powder, insoluble in water and soluble in ethanol.
Betamethasone dipropionate has the chemical name 9-fluoro-11β,17,21-trihydroxy-16β-methylpregna-1,4-diene-3,20-dione 17,21-dipropionate, with the empirical formula

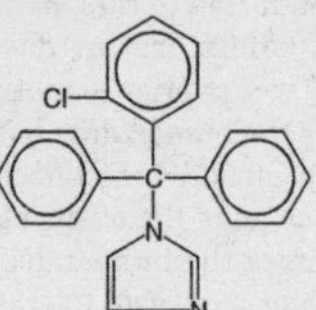

$C_{28}H_{37}FO_7$, a molecular weight of 504.59, and the following structural formula:

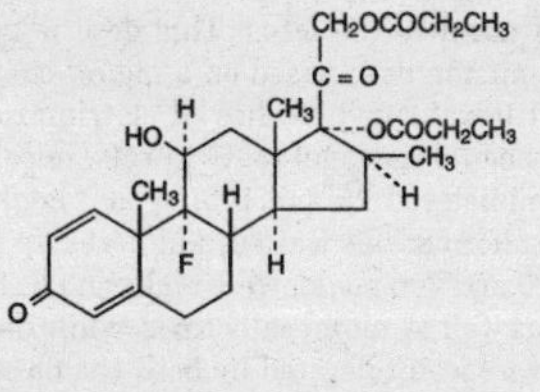

Betamethasone dipropionate is a white to creamy white, odorless crystalline powder, insoluble in water.
Each gram of LOTRISONE Cream contains 10 mg clotrimazole and 0.643 mg betamethasone dipropionate (equivalent to 0.5 mg betamethasone), in a hydrophilic cream consisting of purified water, mineral oil, white petrolatum, cetearyl alcohol 70/30, ceteareth-30, propylene glycol, sodium phosphate monobasic monohydrate, and phosphoric acid; benzyl alcohol as preservative.
LOTRISONE Cream is smooth, uniform, and white to off-white in color.
Each gram of LOTRISONE Lotion contains 10 mg clotrimazole and 0.643 mg betamethasone dipropionate (equivalent to 0.5 mg betamethasone), in a hydrophilic base of purified water, mineral oil, white petrolatum, cetearyl alcohol 70/30, ceteareth-30, propylene glycol, sodium phosphate monobasic monohydrate, and phosphoric acid; benzyl alcohol as a preservative.
LOTRISONE Lotion may contain sodium hydroxide. LOTRISONE Lotion is opaque and white in color.

CLINICAL PHARMACOLOGY

Clotrimazole and Betamethasone Dipropionate
LOTRISONE Cream has been shown to be least as effective as clotrimazole alone in a different cream vehicle. No comparative studies have been conducted with LOTRISONE Lotion and clotrimazole alone. Use of corticosteroids in the treatment of a fungal infection may lead to suppression of host inflammation leading to worsening or decreased cure rate.
Clotrimazole
Skin penetration and systemic absorption of clotrimazole following topical application of LOTRISONE Cream or Lotion have not been studied. The following information was obtained using 1% clotrimazole cream and solution formulations. Six hours after the application of radioactive clotrimazole 1% cream and 1% solution onto intact and acutely inflamed skin, the concentration of clotrimazole varied from 100 mcg/cm^3 in the stratum corneum, to 0.5 to 1 mcg/cm^3 in the reticular dermis, and 0.1 mcg/cm^3 in the subcutis. No measurable amount of radioactivity (<0.001 mcg/mL) was found in the serum within 48 hours after application under occlusive dressing of 0.5 mL of the solution or 0.8 g of the cream. Only 0.5% or less of the applied radioactivity was excreted in the urine.
Microbiology: Mechanism of Action: Clotrimazole is an imidazole antifungal agent. Imidazoles inhibit 14-α-demethylation of lanosterol in fungi by binding to one of the cytochrome P-450 enzymes. This leads to the accumulation of 14-α-methylsterols and reduced concentrations of ergosterol, a sterol essential for a normal fungal cytoplasmic membrane. The methylsterols may affect the electron transport system, thereby inhibiting growth of fungi.
Activity *In Vivo:* Clotrimazole has been shown to be active against most strains of the following dermatophytes, both *in vitro* and in clinical infections as described in the **INDICATIONS AND USAGE** section: *Epidermophyton floccosum, Trichophyton mentagrophytes,* and *Trichophyton rubrum.*
Activity *In Vitro: In vitro,* clotrimazole has been shown to have activity against many dermatophytes, **but the clinical significance of this information is unknown.**
Drug Resistance: Strains of dermatophytes having a natural resistance to clotrimazole have not been reported. Resistance to azoles including clotrimazole has been reported in some *Candida* species.
No single-step or multiple-step resistance to clotrimazole has developed during successive passages of *Trichophyton mentagrophytes.*
Betamethasone Dipropionate
Betamethasone dipropionate, a corticosteroid, has been shown to have topical (dermatologic) and systemic pharmacologic and metabolic effects characteristic of this class of drugs.
Pharmacokinetics: The extent of percutaneous absorption of topical corticosteroids is determined by many factors, including the vehicle, the integrity of the epidermal barrier and the use of occlusive dressings. (See **DOSAGE AND ADMINISTRATION** section.) Topical corticosteroids can be absorbed from normal intact skin. Inflammation and/or other disease processes in the skin may increase percutaneous absorption of topical corticosteroids. Occlusive dressings substantially increase the percutaneous absorption of topical corticosteroids. (See **DOSAGE AND ADMINISTRATION** section.)
Once absorbed through the skin, the pharmacokinetics of topical corticosteroids are similar to systemically administered corticosteroids. Corticosteroids are bound to plasma proteins in varying degrees. Corticosteroids are metabolized primarily in the liver and are then excreted by the kidneys. Some of the topical corticosteroids and their metabolites are also excreted into the bile.
Studies performed with LOTRISONE Cream and Lotion indicate that these topical combination antifungal/corticosteroids may have vasoconstrictor potencies in a range that is comparable to high potency topical corticosteroids. Therefore, use is not recommended in patients less than 17 years of age, in diaper dermatitis, and under occlusion.

CLINICAL STUDIES (LOTRISONE Cream)

In clinical studies of tinea corporis, tinea cruris, and tinea pedis, patients treated with LOTRISONE Cream showed a better clinical response at the first return visit than patients treated with clotrimazole cream. In tinea corporis and tinea cruris, the patient returned 3 to 5 days after starting treatment, and in tinea pedis, after 1 week. Mycological cure rates observed in patients treated with LOTRISONE Cream were as good as or better than in those patients treated with clotrimazole cream. In these same clinical studies, patients treated with LOTRISONE Cream showed better clinical responses and mycological cure rates when compared with patients treated with betamethasone dipropionate cream.

CLINICAL STUDIES (LOTRISONE Lotion)
In the treatment of tinea pedis twice daily for 4 weeks, LOTRISONE Lotion was shown to be superior to vehicle in relieving symptoms of erythema, scaling, pruritus, and maceration at week 2. LOTRISONE Lotion was also shown to have a superior mycological cure rate compared to vehicle 2 weeks after discontinuation of treatment. It is unclear if the relief of symptoms at 2 weeks in this clinical study with LOTRISONE Lotion was due to the contribution of betamethasone dipropionate, clotrimazole, or both.
In the treatment of tinea cruris twice daily for 2 weeks, LOTRISONE Lotion was shown to be superior to vehicle in the relief of symptoms of erythema, scaling, and pruritus after 3 days. It is unclear if the relief of symptoms after 3 days in this clinical study with LOTRISONE Lotion was due to the contribution of betamethasone dipropionate, clotrimazole, or both.
The comparative efficacy and safety of LOTRISONE Lotion versus clotrimazole alone in a lotion vehicle have not been studied in the treatment of tinea pedis or tinea cruris or tinea corporis. The comparative efficacy and safety of LOTRISONE Lotion and LOTRISONE Cream have also not been studied.

INDICATIONS AND USAGE

LOTRISONE Cream and Lotion are indicated in patients 17 years and older for the topical treatment of symptomatic inflammatory tinea pedis, tinea cruris, and tinea corporis due to *Epidermophyton floccosum, Trichophyton mentagrophytes,* and *Trichophyton rubrum.* Effective treatment without the risks associated with topical corticosteroid use may be obtained using a topical antifungal agent that does not contain a corticosteroid, especially for noninflammatory tinea infections. The efficacy of LOTRISONE Cream or Lotion for the treatment of infections caused by zoophilic dermatophytes (eg, *Microsporum canis*) has not been established. Several cases of treatment failure of LOTRISONE Cream in the treatment of infections caused by *Microsporum canis* have been reported.

CONTRAINDICATIONS

LOTRISONE Cream or Lotion is contraindicated in patients who are sensitive to clotrimazole, betamethasone dipropionate, other corticosteroids or imidazoles, or to any ingredient in these preparations.

PRECAUTIONS

General: Systemic absorption of topical corticosteroids can produce reversible hypothalamic-pituitary-adrenal (HPA) axis suppression with the potential for glucocorticosteroid insufficiency after withdrawal of treatment. Manifestations of Cushing's syndrome, hyperglycemia, and glucosuria can also be produced in some patients by systemic absorption of topical corticosteroids while on treatment.
Conditions which augment systemic absorption include use over large surface areas, prolonged use, and use under occlusive dressings. Use of more than one corticosteroid-containing product at the same time may increase total systemic glucocorticoid exposure. Patients applying LOTRISONE Cream or Lotion to a large surface area or to areas under occlusion should be evaluated periodically for evidence of HPA axis suppression. This may be done by using the ACTH stimulation, morning plasma cortisol, and urinary free cortisol tests.
If HPA axis suppression is noted, an attempt should be made to withdraw the drug, to reduce the frequency of application, or to substitute a less potent corticosteroid. Recovery of HPA axis function is generally prompt upon discon-

Continued on next page

Lotrisone—Cont.

tinuation of topical corticosteroids. Infrequently, signs and symptoms of glucocorticosteroid insufficiency may occur, requiring supplemental systemic corticosteroids.

In a small study, LOTRISONE Cream was applied using large dosages, 7 g daily for 14 days (BID) to the crural area of normal adult subjects. Three of the eight normal subjects on whom LOTRISONE Cream was applied exhibited low morning plasma cortisol levels during treatment. One of these subjects had an abnormal Cortrosyn test. The effect on morning plasma cortisol was transient and subjects recovered one week after discontinuing dosing. In addition, two separate studies in pediatric patients demonstrated adrenal suppression as determined by cosyntropin testing (See **PRECAUTIONS—Pediatric Use** section).

Pediatric patients may be more susceptible to systemic toxicity from equivalent doses due to their larger skin surface to body mass ratios. (See **PRECAUTIONS—Pediatric Use** section.)

If irritation develops, LOTRISONE Cream or Lotion should be discontinued and appropriate therapy instituted.

THE SAFETY OF LOTRISONE CREAM OR LOTION HAS NOT BEEN DEMONSTRATED IN THE TREATMENT OF DIAPER DERMATITIS. ADVERSE EVENTS CONSISTENT WITH CORTICOSTEROID USE HAVE BEEN OBSERVED IN PATIENTS TREATED WITH LOTRISONE CREAM FOR DIAPER DERMATITIS. THE USE OF LOTRISONE CREAM OR LOTION IN THE TREATMENT OF DIAPER DERMATITIS IS NOT RECOMMENDED.

Information for Patients: Patients using LOTRISONE Cream or Lotion should receive the following information and instructions:

1. The medication is to be used as directed by the physician and is not recommended for use longer than the prescribed time period. It is for external use only. Avoid contact with the eyes, the mouth, or intravaginally.
2. This medication is to be used for the full prescribed treatment time, even though the symptoms may have improved. Notify the physician if there is no improvement after 1 week of treatment for tinea cruris or tinea corporis, or after 2 weeks for tinea pedis.
3. This medication should only be used for the disorder for which it was prescribed.
4. Other corticosteroid-containing products should not be used with LOTRISONE without first talking with your physician.
5. The treated skin area should not be bandaged, covered, or wrapped so as to be occluded. (See **DOSAGE AND ADMINISTRATION** section.)
6. Any signs of local adverse reactions should be reported to your physician.
7. Patients should avoid sources of infection or reinfection.
8. When using LOTRISONE Cream or Lotion in the groin area, patients should use the medication for 2 weeks only, and apply the cream or lotion sparingly. Patients should wear loose-fitting clothing. Notify the physician if the condition persists after 2 weeks.
9. The safety of LOTRISONE Cream or Lotion has not been demonstrated in the treatment of diaper dermatitis. Adverse events consistent with corticosteroid use have been observed in patients treated with LOTRISONE Cream for diaper dermatitis. The use of LOTRISONE Cream or Lotion in the treatment of diaper dermatitis is not recommended.

Laboratory Tests: If there is a lack of response to LOTRISONE Cream or Lotion, appropriate confirmation of the diagnosis, including possible mycological studies, is indicated before instituting another course of therapy.

The following tests may be helpful in evaluating HPA-axis suppression due to the corticosteroid components:

Urinary free cortisol test
Morning plasma cortisol test
ACTH (cosyntropin) stimulation test

Carcinogenesis, Mutagenesis, Impairment of Fertility: There are no laboratory animal studies with either the combination of clotrimazole and betamethasone dipropionate or with either component individually to evaluate carcinogenesis.

Betamethasone was negative in the bacterial mutagenicity assay (*Salmonella typhimurium* and *Escherichia coli*), and in the mammalian cell mutagenicity assay (CHO/HGPRT). It was positive in the *in vitro* human lymphocyte chromosome aberration assay, and equivocal in the *in vivo* mouse bone marrow micronucleus assay. This pattern of response is similar to that of dexamethasone and hydrocortisone.

In genotoxicity testing of clotrimazole, chromosomes of the spermatophores of Chinese hamsters, which had been exposed to five daily oral clotrimazole doses of 100 mg/kg body weight, were examined for structural changes during the metaphase. The results of this study showed that clotrimazole had no mutagenic effect.

Reproductive studies with betamethasone dipropionate carried out in rabbits at doses of 1.0 mg/kg by the intramuscular route and in mice up to 33 mg/kg by the intramuscular route indicated no impairment of fertility except for dose-related increases in fetal resorption rates in both species. These doses are approximately 5- and 38-fold the human dose based on a mg/m^2 comparison, respectively.

Oral doses of clotrimazole in mice resulted in decreased litter size at doses of 120 mg/kg and higher. This dose is approximately 10-fold the human dose based on a mg/m^2 comparison.

A Segment I (fertility and general reproduction) study of clotrimazole was conducted in rats. Males and females were dosed orally (diet admixture) at doses of 5, 10, 25, or 50 mg/kg/day for 10 weeks prior to mating. At 50 mg/kg (approximately 8 times the human dose based on a mg/m^2 comparison), there was an adverse effect on maternal body weight gain and rearing of the offspring. Doses of 25 mg/kg (approximately 4 times the human dose based on a mg/m^2 comparison) and lower were well tolerated and produced no adverse effects on fertility or reproduction.

Pregnancy Category C: There have been no teratogenic studies performed in animals or humans with the combination of clotrimazole and betamethasone dipropionate. Corticosteroids are generally teratogenic in laboratory animals when administered at relatively low dosage levels.

A Segment II (teratology) study in pregnant rats with intravaginal doses up to 100 mg/kg clotrimazole have revealed no evidence of harm to the fetus. This dose is approximately 17-fold the human dose based on a mg/m^2 comparison.

Segment II (teratology) studies of clotrimazole were conducted by the oral (gavage) route in rats, mice, and rabbits. In rats administered 25, 50, 100, or 200 mg/kg/day, no increase in malformations was seen at doses up to 200 mg/kg. Doses of 100 and 200 mg/kg were embryotoxic (increased resorptions) as well as maternally toxic, while doses of 25 and 50 mg/kg were well tolerated by both the dams and the fetuses. These doses were approximately 4-, 8-, 17-, and 34-fold the human dose based on a mg/m^2 comparison, respectively.

In pregnant mice, clotrimazole at oral doses of 25, 50, 100, or 200 mg/kg/day was not teratogenic and was well tolerated by both the dams and the fetuses. These doses were approximately 2-, 4-, 8-, and 17-fold the human dose based on a mg/m^2 comparison, respectively.

No evidence of maternal toxicity or embryotoxicity was seen in pregnant rabbits dosed orally with 60, 120, or 180 mg/kg/day. These doses were approximately 20-, 40-, and 61-fold the human dose based on a mg/m^2 comparison, respectively.

Betamethasone dipropionate has been shown to be teratogenic in rabbits when given by the intramuscular route at doses of 0.05 mg/kg. This dose is approximately one-fifth the human dose based on a mg/m^2 comparison. The abnormalities observed included umbilical hernias, cephalocele and cleft palates.

Betamethasone dipropionate has not been tested for teratogenic potential by the dermal route of administration. Some corticosteroids have been shown to be teratogenic after dermal application to laboratory animals.

Nursing Mothers: Systemically administered corticosteroids appear in human milk and could suppress growth, interfere with endogenous corticosteroid production, or cause other untoward effects. It is not known whether topical administration of corticosteroids could result in sufficient systemic absorption to produce detectable quantities in human milk. Because many drugs are excreted in human milk, caution should be exercised when LOTRISONE Cream or Lotion is administered to a nursing woman.

Pediatric Use: Adverse events consistent with corticosteroid use have been observed in patients under 12 years of age treated with LOTRISONE Cream. In open-label studies, 17 of 43 (39.5%) evaluable pediatric patients (aged 12 to 16 years old) using LOTRISONE Cream for treatment of tinea pedis demonstrated adrenal suppression as determined by cosyntropin testing. In another open-label study, 8 of 17 (47.1%) evaluable pediatric patients (aged 12 to 16 years old) using LOTRISONE Cream for treatment of tinea cruris demonstrated adrenal suppression as determined by cosyntropin testing. **THE USE OF LOTRISONE CREAM OR LOTION IN THE TREATMENT OF PATIENTS UNDER 17 YEARS OF AGE OR PATIENTS WITH DIAPER DERMATITIS IS NOT RECOMMENDED.**

Because of higher ratio of skin surface area to body mass, pediatric patients under the age of 12 years are at a higher risk with LOTRISONE Cream or Lotion. The studies described above suggest that pediatric patients under the age of 17 years may also have this risk. They are at increased risk of developing Cushing's syndrome while on treatment and adrenal insufficiency after withdrawal of treatment. Adverse effects, including striae and growth retardation, have been reported with inappropriate use of LOTRISONE Cream in infants and children. (See **PRECAUTIONS** and **ADVERSE REACTIONS** sections.)

Hypothalamic-pituitary-adrenal (HPA) axis suppression, Cushing's syndrome, linear growth retardation, delayed weight gain and intracranial hypertension have been reported in children receiving topical corticosteroids. Manifestations of adrenal suppression in children include low plasma cortisol levels and absence of response to ACTH stimulation. Manifestations of intracranial hypertension include bulging fontanelles, headaches, and bilateral papilledema.

Geriatric Use: Clinical studies of LOTRISONE Cream and Lotion did not include sufficient numbers of subjects aged 65 and over to determine whether they respond differently from younger subjects. Postmarket adverse event reporting for LOTRISONE Cream in patients aged 65 and above includes reports of skin atrophy and rare reports of skin ulceration. Caution should be exercised with the use of these corticosteroid-containing topical products on thinning skin. **THE USE OF LOTRISONE CREAM OR LOTION UNDER OCCLUSION, SUCH AS IN DIAPER DERMATITIS, IS NOT RECOMMENDED.**

ADVERSE REACTIONS

Adverse reactions reported for LOTRISONE Cream in clinical trials were paresthesia in 1.9% of patients, and rash, edema, and secondary infection, each in less than 1% of patients.

Adverse reactions reported for LOTRISONE Lotion in clinical trials were burning and dry skin in 1.6% of patients and stinging in less than 1% of patients.

The following local adverse reactions have been reported with topical corticosteroids and may occur more frequently with the use of occlusive dressings. These reactions are listed in an approximate decreasing order of occurrence: itching, irritation, dryness, folliculitis, hypertrichosis, acneiform eruptions, hypopigmentation, perioral dermatitis, allergic contact dermatitis, maceration of the skin, secondary infection, skin atrophy, striae, and miliaria. In the pediatric population, reported adverse events for LOTRISONE Cream include growth retardation, benign intracranial hypertension, Cushing's syndrome (HPA axis suppression), and local cutaneous reactions, including skin atrophy.

Systemic absorption of topical corticosteroids has produced reversible hypothalamic-piuitary-adrenal (HPA) axis suppression, manifestations of Cushing's syndrome, hyperglycemia, and glucosuria in some patients.

Adverse reactions reported with the use of clotrimazole are as follows: erythema, stinging, blistering, peeling, edema, pruritus, urticaria and general irritation of the skin.

OVERDOSAGE

Amounts greater than 45 g/week of LOTRISONE Cream or 45 mL/week of LOTRISONE Lotion should not be used. Acute overdosage with topical application of LOTRISONE Cream or Lotion is unlikely and would not be expected to lead to a life-threatening situation. LOTRISONE Cream or Lotion should not be used for longer than the prescribed time period.

Topically applied corticosteroids, such as the one contained in LOTRISONE Cream or Lotion can be absorbed in sufficient amounts to produce systemic effects. (See **PRECAUTIONS** section.)

DOSAGE AND ADMINISTRATION

Gently massage sufficient LOTRISONE Cream or Lotion into the affected skin areas twice a day, in the morning and evening.

LOTRISONE Cream or Lotion should not be used longer than 2 weeks in the treatment of tinea corporis or tinea cruris, and amounts greater than 45 g per week of LOTRISONE Cream or amounts greater than 45 mL per week of LOTRISONE Lotion should not be used. If a patient with tinea corporis or tinea cruris shows no clinical improvement after 1 week of treatment with LOTRISONE Cream or Lotion, the diagnosis should be reviewed.

LOTRISONE Cream or Lotion should not be used longer than 4 weeks in the treatment of tinea pedis and amounts greater than 45 g per week of LOTRISONE Cream or amounts greater than 45 mL per week of LOTRISONE Lotion should not be used. If a patient with tinea pedis shows no clinical improvement after 2 weeks of treatment with LOTRISONE Cream or Lotion, the diagnosis should be reviewed.

LOTRISONE Cream or Lotion should not be used with occlusive dressings.

HOW SUPPLIED

LOTRISONE Cream is supplied in 15-g (NDC 0085-0924-01) and 45-g tubes (NDC 0085-0924-02); boxes of one. **Store between 2°C and 30°C (36°F and 86°F).**

LOTRISONE Lotion is supplied in 30-mL bottles (NDC 0085-0809-01), box of one. **Store at 25°C (77°F) in the upright position only; excursions permitted between 15°C and 30°C (59°F and 86°F).**

SHAKE WELL BEFORE EACH USE.

Rx only

Schering Corporation/Key Pharmaceuticals, Inc.
Kenilworth, NJ 07033 USA
Rev. 10/01 B-25218213

 24441911T

Patient's Instructions for Use

SHAKE WELL BEFORE EACH USE

LOTRISONE® Cream

LOTRISONE® Lotion

(clotrimazole and betamethasone dipropionate)

Patient Information Leaflet

What is LOTRISONE Cream or Lotion?

LOTRISONE Cream and Lotion are medications used on the skin to treat fungal infections of the feet, groin and body, as diagnosed by your doctor. LOTRISONE Cream or Lotion should be used for fungal infections that are inflamed and have symptoms of redness and/or itching. Talk to your doctor if your fungal infection does not have these symptoms. LOTRISONE Cream and Lotion contain a corticosteroid. Notify your doctor if you notice side effects with the use of LOTRISONE Cream or Lotion (see **"What are the possible side effects of LOTRISONE Cream and Lotion?"** below). LOTRISONE Cream or Lotion is not to be used in the eyes, in the mouth, or in the vagina.

How do LOTRISONE Cream and Lotion work?

LOTRISONE Cream and Lotion are combinations of an antifungal agent (clotrimazole) and a corticosteroid (betamethasone dipropionate). Clotrimazole works against fungus. Betamethasone dipropionate, a corticosteroid, is used to help relieve redness, swelling, itching, and other discomforts of fungal infections.

Who should NOT use LOTRISONE Cream or Lotion?
LOTRISONE Cream and Lotion are not recommended for use in patients under the age of 17 years. LOTRISONE Cream or Lotion is not recommended for use in diaper rash. Patients who are sensitive to clotrimazole and betamethasone dipropionate, other corticosteroids or imidazoles, or any ingredients in the preparation should not use LOTRISONE Cream and Lotion.

How should I use LOTRISONE Cream or Lotion?
Gently massage sufficient LOTRISONE Cream or Lotion into the affected and surrounding skin areas twice a day, in the morning and evening. Treatment for 2 weeks on the groin or on the body, and for 4 weeks on the feet is recommended. The use of LOTRISONE Cream or Lotion for longer than 4 weeks is not recommended for any condition. Prolonged use of LOTRISONE Cream or Lotion may lead to unwanted side effects.

What other important information should I know about LOTRISONE Cream and Lotion?

1. This medication is to be used for the full prescribed treatment time, even though the symptoms may have improved. Notify your doctor if there is no improvement after 1 week of treatment on the groin or body or after 2 weeks on the feet.
2. This medication should only be used for the disorder for which it was prescribed.
3. The treated skin area should not be bandaged or otherwise covered or wrapped.
4. Other corticosteroid-containing products should not be used with LOTRISONE without first talking with your physician.
5. Any signs of side effects where LOTRISONE Cream or Lotion is applied should be reported to your doctor.
6. When using LOTRISONE Cream or Lotion in the groin area, it is especially important to use the medication for 2 weeks only, and to apply the cream or lotion sparingly. You should tell your doctor if your problem persists after 2 weeks. You should also wear loosefitting clothing so as to avoid tightly covering the area where LOTRISONE Cream or Lotion is applied.
7. This medication is not recommended for use in diaper rash.

What are the possible side effects of LOTRISONE Cream and Lotion?
The following side effects have been reported with topical corticosteroid medications: itching, irritation, dryness, infection of the hair follicles, increased hair, acne, change in skin color, allergic skin reaction, skin thinning, and stretch marks. In children, reported adverse events for LOTRISONE Cream include slower growth, Cushing's syndrome (a type of hormone imbalance that can be very serious), and local skin reactions, including thinning skin and stretch marks. Hormone imbalance (adrenal suppression) was demonstrated in clinical studies in children.

Can LOTRISONE Cream or Lotion be used if I am pregnant or plan to become pregnant or if I am nursing?
Before using LOTRISONE Cream or Lotion, tell your doctor if you are pregnant or plan to become pregnant. Also, tell your doctor if you are nursing.

How should LOTRISONE Cream or Lotion be stored?
LOTRISONE Cream should be stored between 2°C and 30°C (36°F and 86°F).
LOTRISONE Lotion should only be stored in an upright position between 15°C and 30°C (59°F and 86°F). Shake well before using LOTRISONE Lotion.

General advice about prescription medicines
This medicine was prescribed for your particular condition. Only use LOTRISONE Cream or Lotion to treat the condition for which your doctor has prescribed. Do not give LOTRISONE Cream or Lotion to other people. It may harm them.
This leaflet summarizes the most important information about LOTRISONE Cream and Lotion. If you would like more information, talk with your doctor. You can ask your pharmacist or doctor for information about LOTRISONE Cream and Lotion that is written for health professionals.

Rx only
Schering Corporation/
Key Pharmaceuticals, Inc.
Kenilworth, NJ 07033 USA

Rev. 10/01 25218213
24441911T

NORMODYNE® ℞

[*nor'-mō-dīn*]
brand of
labetalol hydrochloride
Tablets, USP

Prescribing information for this product, which appears on pages 3137–3140 of the 2002 PDR, has been completely revised as follows. Please write "See Supplement A" next to the product heading.

DESCRIPTION

NORMODYNE (labetalol HCl) is an adrenergic receptor blocking agent that has both selective alpha$_1$- and nonselective beta-adrenergic receptor blocking actions in a single substance.

Labetalol HCl is a racemate, chemically designated as 5-[1-hydroxy-2-[(1-methyl-3-phenylpropyl) amino] ethyl]salicylamide monohydrochloride, and has the following structure:

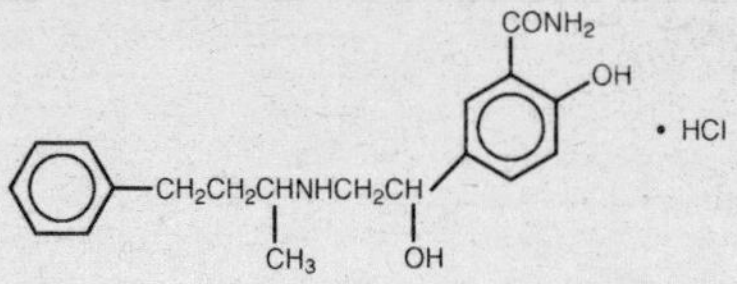

Labetalol HCl has the empirical formula $C_{19}H_{24}N_2O_3$•HCl and a molecular weight of 364.9. It has two asymmetric centers and therefore exists as a molecular complex of two diastereoisomeric pairs. Dilevalol, the R,R' stereoisomer, makes up 25% of racemic labetalol.

Labetalol HCl is a white or off-white crystalline powder, soluble in water.

NORMODYNE Tablets contain 100 mg, 200 mg, or 300 mg labetalol HCl, USP and are taken orally.

The inactive ingredients for NORMODYNE Tablets, 100 mg, include: corn starch, Opaspray Light Brown K-1-2630, hydroxypropyl methylcellulose, lactose, magnesium stearate, methylparaben, PEG, and propylparaben. May also contain: potato starch and wheat starch.

The inactive ingredients for NORMODYNE Tablets, 200 mg, include: corn starch, hydroxypropyl methylcellulose, lactose, magnesium stearate, methylparaben, PEG, propylparaben, and Opaspray White K-1-7000. May also contain: potato starch and wheat starch.

The inactive ingredients for NORMODYNE Tablets, 300 mg, include: corn starch, Opaspray Blue K-1-4212, hydroxypropyl methylcellulose, lactose, magnesium stearate, methylparaben, PEG, and propylparaben. May also contain: potato starch and wheat starch.

CLINICAL PHARMACOLOGY

NORMODYNE (labetalol HCl) combines both selective, competitive alpha$_1$-adrenergic blocking and nonselective, competitive beta-adrenergic blocking activity in a single substance. In man, the ratios of alpha- to beta-blockade have been estimated to be approximately 1:3 and 1:7 following oral and intravenous administration, respectively. Beta$_2$-agonist activity has been demonstrated in animals with minimal beta$_1$-agonist (ISA) activity detected. In animals, at doses greater than those required for alpha- or beta-adrenergic blockade, a membrane-stabilizing effect has been demonstrated.

Pharmacodynamics: The capacity of labetalol HCl to block alpha receptors in man has been demonstrated by attenuation of the pressor effect of phenylephrine and by a significant reduction of the pressor response caused by immersing the hand in ice-cold water ("cold-pressor test"). Labetalol HCl's beta$_1$-receptor blockade in man was demonstrated by a small decrease in the resting heart rate, attenuation of tachycardia produced by isoproterenol or exercise, and by attenuation of the reflex tachycardia to the hypotension produced by amyl nitrite. Beta$_2$-receptor blockade was demonstrated by inhibition of the isoproterenol-induced fall in diastolic blood pressure. Both the alpha- and beta-blocking actions of orally administered labetalol HCl contribute to a decrease in blood pressure in hypertensive patients. Labetalol HCl consistently, in dose-related fashion, blunted increases in exercise-induced blood pressure and heart rate, and in their double product. The pulmonary circulation during exercise was not affected by labetalol HCl dosing.

Single oral doses of labetalol HCl administered in patients with coronary artery disease had no significant effect on sinus rate, intraventricular conduction, or QRS duration. The AV conduction time was modestly prolonged in 2 of 7 patients. In another study, intravenous labetalol HCl slightly prolonged AV nodal conduction time and atrial effective refractory period with only small changes in heart rate. The effects on AV nodal refractoriness were inconsistent.

Labetalol HCl produces dose-related falls in blood pressure without reflex tachycardia and without significant reduction in heart rate, presumably through a mixture of its alpha-blocking and beta-blocking effects. Hemodynamic effects are variable with small nonsignificant changes in cardiac output seen in some studies but not others, and small decreases in total peripheral resistance. Elevated plasma renins are reduced.

Doses of labetalol HCl that controlled hypertension did not affect renal function in mild to severe hypertensive patients with normal renal function.

Due to the alpha$_1$-receptor blocking activity of labetalol HCl, blood pressure is lowered more in the standing than in the supine position, and symptoms of postural hypotension (2%), including rare instances of syncope, can occur. Following oral administration, when postural hypotension has occurred, it has been transient and is uncommon when the recommended starting dose and titration increments are closely followed (see **DOSAGE AND ADMINISTRATION**). Symptomatic postural hypotension is most likely to occur 2 to 4 hours after a dose, especially following the use of large initial doses or upon large changes in dose.

The peak effects of single oral doses of labetalol HCl occur within 2 to 4 hours. The duration of effect depends upon dose, lasting at least 8 hours following single oral doses of 100 mg and more than 12 hours following single oral doses of 300 mg. The maximum, steady-state blood pressure response upon oral, twice-a-day dosing occurs within 24 to 72 hours.

The antihypertensive effect of labetalol has a linear correlation with the logarithm of labetalol plasma concentration, and there is also a linear correlation between the reduction in exercise-induced tachycardia occurring at 2 hours after oral administration of labetalol HCl and the logarithm of the plasma concentration.

About 70% of the maximum beta-blocking effect is present for 5 hours after the administration of a single oral dose of 400 mg, with suggestion that about 40% remains at 8 hours. The anti-anginal efficacy of labetalol HCl has not been studied. In 37 patients with hypertension and coronary artery disease, labetalol HCl did not increase the incidence or severity of angina attacks.

Exacerbation of angina and, in some cases, myocardial infarction and ventricular dysrhythmias have been reported after abrupt discontinuation of therapy with beta-adrenergic blocking agents in patients with coronary artery disease. Abrupt withdrawal of these agents in patients without coronary artery disease has resulted in transient symptoms, including tremulousness, sweating, palpitation, headache, and malaise. Several mechanisms have been proposed to explain these phenomena, among them increased sensitivity to catecholamines because of increased numbers of beta receptors.

Although beta-adrenergic receptor blockade is useful in the treatment of angina and hypertension, there are also situations in which sympathetic stimulation is vital. For example, in patients with severely damaged hearts, adequate ventricular function may depend on sympathetic drive. Beta-adrenergic blockade may worsen AV block by preventing the necessary facilitating effects of sympathetic activity on conduction. Beta$_2$-adrenergic blockade results in passive bronchial constriction by interfering with endogenous adrenergic bronchodilator activity in patients subject to bronchospasm and may also interfere with exogenous bronchodilators in such patients.

Pharmacokinetics and Metabolism: Labetalol HCl is completely absorbed from the gastrointestinal tract with peak plasma levels occurring 1 to 2 hours after oral administration. The relative bioavailability of labetalol HCl tablets compared to an oral solution is 100%. The absolute bioavailability (fraction of drug reaching systemic circulation) of labetalol when compared to an intravenous infusion is 25%; this is due to extensive "first-pass" metabolism. Despite "first-pass" metabolism there is a linear relationship between oral doses of 100 to 3000 mg and peak plasma levels. The absolute bioavailability of labetalol is increased when administered with food.

The plasma half-life of labetalol following oral administration is about 6 to 8 hours. Steady-state plasma levels of labetalol during repetitive dosing are reached by about the third day of dosing. In patients with decreased hepatic or renal function, the elimination half-life of labetalol is not altered; however, the relative bioavailability in hepatically impaired patients is increased due to decreased "first-pass" metabolism.

The metabolism of labetalol is mainly through conjugation to glucuronide metabolites. These metabolites are present in plasma and are excreted in the urine and, via the bile, into the feces. Approximately 55% to 60% of a dose appears in the urine as conjugates or unchanged labetalol within the first 24 hours of dosing.

Labetalol has been shown to cross the placental barrier in humans. Only negligible amounts of the drug crossed the blood-brain barrier in animal studies. Labetalol is approximately 50% protein bound. Neither hemodialysis nor peritoneal dialysis removes a significant amount of labetalol HCl from the general circulation (<1%).

INDICATIONS AND USAGE

NORMODYNE (labetalol HCl) Tablets are indicated in the management of hypertension. NORMODYNE Tablets may be used alone or in combination with other antihypertensive agents, especially thiazide and loop diuretics.

CONTRAINDICATIONS

NORMODYNE (labetalol HCl) Tablets are contraindicated in bronchial asthma, overt cardiac failure, greater than first degree heart block, cardiogenic shock, severe bradycardia, other conditions associated with severe and prolonged hypotension, and in patients with a history of hypersensitivity to any component of the product (see **WARNINGS**). Beta-blockers, even those with apparent cardioselectivity, should not be used in patients with a history of obstructive airway disease, including asthma.

WARNINGS

Hepatic Injury: Severe hepatocellular injury, confirmed by rechallenge in at least one case, occurs rarely with labetalol therapy. The hepatic injury is usually reversible, but hepatic necrosis and death have been reported. Injury has occurred after both short- and long-term treatment and may be slowly progressive despite minimal symptomatology. Similar hepatic events have been reported with a related compound, dilevalol HCl, including two deaths. Dilevalol HCl is one of the four isomers of labetalol HCl. Thus, for patients taking labetalol, periodic determination of suitable hepatic laboratory tests would be appropriate. Laboratory testing should also be done at the very first symptom or sign of liver dysfunction (eg, pruritus, dark urine, persistent anorexia, jaundice, right upper quadrant tenderness, or unexplained "flu-like" symptoms). If the patient has jaundice or laboratory evidence of liver injury, labetalol HCl should be stopped and not restarted.

Continued on next page

Normodyne—Cont.

Cardiac Failure: Sympathetic stimulation is a vital component supporting circulatory function in congestive heart failure. Beta blockade carries a potential hazard of further depressing myocardial contractility and precipitating more severe failure. Although beta-blockers should be avoided in overt congestive heart failure, if necessary, labetalol HCl can be used with caution in patients with a history of heart failure who are well-compensated. Congestive heart failure has been observed in patients receiving labetalol HCl. Labetalol HCl does not abolish the inotropic action of digitalis on heart muscle.

In Patients Without a History of Cardiac Failure: In patients with latent cardiac insufficiency, continued depression of the myocardium with beta-blocking agents over a period of time can, in some cases, lead to cardiac failure. At the first sign or symptom of impending cardiac failure, patients should be fully digitalized and/or be given a diuretic, and the response observed closely. If cardiac failure continues, despite adequate digitalization and diuretic, NORMODYNE (labetalol HCl) therapy should be withdrawn (gradually if possible).

Exacerbation of Ischemic Heart Disease Following Abrupt Withdrawal: Angina pectoris has not been reported upon labetalol HCl discontinuation. However, hypersensitivity to catecholamines has been observed in patients withdrawn from beta-blocker therapy; exacerbation of angina and, in some cases, myocardial infarction have occurred after *abrupt* discontinuation of such therapy. When discontinuing chronically administered NORMODYNE (labetalol HCl), particularly in patients with ischemic heart disease, the dosage should be gradually reduced over a period of 1 to 2 weeks and the patient should be carefully monitored. If angina markedly worsens or acute coronary insufficiency develops, NORMODYNE (labetalol HCl) administration should be reinstituted promptly, at least temporarily, and other measures appropriate for the management of unstable angina should be taken. Patients should be warned against interruption or discontinuation of therapy without the physician's advice. Because coronary artery disease is common and may be unrecognized, it may be prudent not to discontinue NORMODYNE (labetalol HCl) therapy abruptly even in patients treated only for hypertension.

Nonallergic bronchospasm (eg, chronic bronchitis and emphysema) patients with bronchospastic disease should, in general, not receive beta-blockers. NORMODYNE (labetalol HCl) may be used with caution, however, in patients who do not respond to, or cannot tolerate, other antihypertensive agents. It is prudent, if NORMODYNE (labetalol HCl) is used, to use the smallest effective dose, so that inhibition of endogenous or exogenous beta-agonists is minimized.

Pheochromocytoma: Labetalol HCl has been shown to be effective in lowering the blood pressure and relieving symptoms in patients with pheochromocytoma. However, paradoxical hypertensive responses have been reported in a few patients with this tumor; therefore, use caution when administering labetalol HCl to patients with pheochromocytoma.

Diabetes Mellitus and Hypoglycemia: Beta-adrenergic blockade may prevent the appearance of premonitory signs and symptoms (eg, tachycardia) of acute hypoglycemia. This is especially important with labile diabetics. Beta-blockade also reduces the release of insulin in response to hyperglycemia; it may therefore be necessary to adjust the dose of antidiabetic drugs.

Major Surgery: The necessity or desirability of withdrawing beta-blocking therapy prior to major surgery is controversial. Protracted severe hypotension and difficulty in restarting or maintaining a heartbeat have been reported with beta-blockers. The effect of labetalol HCl's alpha-adrenergic activity has not been evaluated in this setting.

A synergism between labetalol HCl and halothane anesthesia has been shown (see **PRECAUTIONS—Drug Interactions**).

PRECAUTIONS

General: *Impaired Hepatic Function:* NORMODYNE (labetalol HCl) Tablets should be used with caution in patients with impaired hepatic function since metabolism of the drug may be diminished.

Jaundice or Hepatic Dysfunction: (See **WARNINGS**.)

Information for Patients: As with all drugs with beta-blocking activity, certain advice to patients being treated with labetalol HCl is warranted. This information is intended to aid in the safe and effective use of this medication. It is not a disclosure of all possible adverse or intended effects. While no incident of the abrupt withdrawal phenomenon (exacerbation of angina pectoris) has been reported with labetalol HCl, dosing with NORMODYNE (labetalol HCl) Tablets should not be interrupted or discontinued without a physician's advice. Patients being treated with NORMODYNE (labetalol HCl) Tablets should consult a physician at any signs or symptoms of impending cardiac failure or hepatic dysfunction (see **WARNINGS**). Also, transient scalp tingling may occur, usually when treatment with NORMODYNE (labetalol HCl) Tablets is initiated (see **ADVERSE REACTIONS**).

Laboratory Tests: As with any new drug given over prolonged periods, laboratory parameters should be observed over regular intervals. In patients with concomitant illnesses, such as impaired renal function, appropriate tests should be done to monitor these conditions.

	Labetalol HCl (N=227) %	Placebo (N=98) %	Propranolol (N=84) %	Metoprolol (N=49) %
Body as a whole				
fatigue	5	0	12	12
asthenia	1	1	1	0
headache	2	1	1	2
Gastrointestinal				
nausea	6	1	1	2
vomiting	<1	0	0	0
dyspepsia	3	1	1	0
abdominal pain	0	0	1	2
diarrhea	<1	0	2	0
taste distortion	1	0	0	0
Central and Peripheral Nervous Systems				
dizziness	11	3	4	4
paresthesias	<1	0	0	0
drowsiness	<1	2	2	2
Autonomic Nervous System				
nasal stuffiness	3	0	0	0
ejaculation failure	2	0	0	0
impotence	1	0	1	3
increased sweating	<1	0	0	0
Cardiovascular				
edema	1	0	0	0
postural hypotension	1	0	0	0
bradycardia	0	0	5	12
Respiratory				
dyspnea	2	0	1	2
Skin				
rash	1	0	0	0
Special Senses				
vision abnormality	1	0	0	0
vertigo	2	1	0	0

Labetalol HCl Daily Dose (mg)	**200**	**300**	**400**	**600**	**800**	**900**	**1200**	**1600**	**2400**
Number of patients	522	181	606	608	503	117	411	242	175
Dizziness (%)	2	3	3	3	5	1	9	13	16
Fatigue	2	1	4	4	5	3	7	6	10
Nausea	<1	0	1	2	4	0	7	11	19
Vomiting	0	0	<1	<1	<1	0	1	2	3
Dyspepsia	1	0	2	1	1	0	2	2	4
Paresthesias	2	0	2	2	1	1	2	5	5
Nasal Stuffiness	1	1	2	2	2	2	4	5	6
Ejaculation Failure	0	2	1	2	3	0	4	3	5
Impotence	1	1	1	1	2	4	3	4	3
Edema	1	0	1	1	1	0	1	2	2

Drug Interactions: In one survey, 2.3% of patients taking labetalol HCl in combination with tricyclic antidepressants experienced tremor as compared to 0.7% reported to occur with labetalol HCl alone. The contribution of each of the treatments to this adverse reaction is unknown but the possibility of a drug interaction cannot be excluded.

Drugs possessing beta-blocking properties can blunt the bronchodilator effect of beta-receptor agonist drugs in patients with bronchospasm; therefore, doses greater than the normal anti-asthmatic dose of beta-agonist bronchodilator drugs may be required.

Cimetidine has been shown to increase the bioavailability of labetalol HCl. Since this could be explained either by enhanced absorption or by an alteration of hepatic metabolism of labetalol HCl, special care should be used in establishing the dose required for blood pressure control in such patients.

Synergism has been shown between halothane anesthesia and intravenously administered labetalol HCl. During controlled hypotensive anesthesia using labetalol HCl in association with halothane, high concentrations (3% or above) of halothane should not be used because the degree of hypotension will be increased and because of the possibility of a large reduction in cardiac output and an increase in central venous pressure. The anesthesiologist should be informed when a patient is receiving labetalol HCl.

Labetalol HCl blunts the reflex tachycardia produced by nitroglycerin without preventing its hypotensive effect. If labetalol HCl is used with nitroglycerin in patients with angina pectoris, additional antihypertensive effects may occur. Care should be taken if labetalol HCl is used concomitantly with calcium antagonists of the verapamil type.

Risk of Anaphylactic Reaction: While taking beta-blockers, patients with a history of severe anaphylactic reaction to a variety of allergens may be more reactive to repeated challenge, either accidental, diagnostic, or therapeutic. Such patients may be unresponsive to the usual doses of epinephrine used to treat allergic reaction.

Drug/Laboratory Test Interactions: The presence of labetalol metabolites in the urine may result in falsely elevated levels of urinary catecholamines, metanephrine, normetanephrine, and vanillylmandelic acid (VMA) when measured by fluorimetric or photometric methods. In screening patients suspected of having a pheochromocytoma and being treated with labetalol HCl, a specific method, such as a high performance liquid chromatographic assay with solid phase extraction (eg, *J Chromatogr* 385:241,1987) should be employed in determining levels of catecholamines.

Labetalol HCl has also been reported to produce a false-positive test for amphetamine when screening urine for the presence of drugs using the commercially available assay methods Toxi-Lab A® (thin-layer chromatographic assay) and Emit-d.a.u.® (radioenzymatic assay). When patients being treated with labetalol HCl have a positive urine test for amphetamine using these techniques, confirmation should be made by using more specific methods, such as a gas chromatographic-mass spectrometer technique.

Carcinogenesis, Mutagenesis, Impairment of Fertility: Long-term oral dosing studies with labetalol HCl for 18 months in mice and for 2 years in rats showed no evidence of carcinogenesis. Studies with labetalol HCl, using dominant lethal assays in rats and mice, and exposing microorganisms according to modified Ames tests, showed no evidence of mutagenesis.

Pregnancy Category C: Teratogenic studies have been performed with labetalol HCl in rats and rabbits at oral doses up to approximately 6 and 4 times the maximum recommended human dose (MRHD), respectively. No reproducible evidence of fetal malformations was observed. Increased fetal resorptions were seen in both species at doses approximating the MRHD. A teratology study performed with labetalol HCl in rabbits at intravenous doses up to 1.7 times the MRHD revealed no evidence of drug-related harm to the fetus. There are no adequate and well-controlled studies in pregnant women. Labetalol HCl should be used during pregnancy only if the potential benefit justifies the potential risk to the fetus.

Nonteratogenic Effects: Hypotension, bradycardia, hypoglycemia, and respiratory depression have been reported in infants of mothers who were treated with labetalol HCl for hypertension during pregnancy. Oral administration of labetalol to rats during late gestation through weaning at doses of 2 to 4 times the MRHD caused a decrease in neonatal survival.

Labor and Delivery: Labetalol HCl given to pregnant women with hypertension did not appear to affect the usual course of labor and delivery.

Nursing Mothers: Small amounts of labetalol (approximately 0.004% of the maternal dose) are excreted in human milk. Caution should be exercised when NORMODYNE (labetalol HCl) Tablets are administered to a nursing woman.

Pediatric Use: Safety and effectiveness in pediatric patients have not been established.

ADVERSE REACTIONS

Most adverse effects are mild, transient and occur early in the course of treatment. In controlled clinical trials of 3 to 4 months duration, discontinuation of NORMODYNE (labetalol HCl) Tablets due to one or more adverse effects was required in 7% of all patients. In these same trials, beta-blocker control agents led to discontinuation in 8% to 10% of patients, and a centrally acting alpha-agonist in 30% of patients.

The incidence rates of adverse reactions listed in the following table were derived from multicenter controlled clinical trials, comparing labetalol HCl, placebo, metoprolol, and propranolol, over treatment periods of 3 and 4 months. Where the frequency of adverse effects for labetalol HCl and placebo is similar, causal relationship is uncertain. The rates are based on adverse reactions considered probably drug related by the investigator. If all reports are considered, the rates are somewhat higher (eg, dizziness 20%, nausea 14%, fatigue 11%), but the overall conclusions are unchanged.

[See first table at top of previous page]

The adverse effects were reported spontaneously and are representative of the incidence of adverse effects that may be observed in a properly selected hypertensive patient population, ie, a group excluding patients with bronchospastic disease, overt congestive heart failure, or other contraindications to beta-blocker therapy.

Clinical trials also included studies utilizing daily doses up to 2400 mg in more severely hypertensive patients. Certain of the side effects increased with increasing dose as shown in the table below which depicts the entire U.S. therapeutic trials data base for adverse reactions that are clearly or possibly drug related.

[See second table at top of previous page]

In addition, a number of other less common adverse events have been reported:

Body as a Whole: Fever.

Cardiovascular: Hypotension, and rarely, syncope, bradycardia, heart block.

Central and Peripheral Nervous Systems: Paresthesias, most frequently described as scalp tingling. In most cases, it was mild, transient and usually occurred at the beginning of treatment.

Collagen Disorders: Systemic lupus erythematosus; positive antinuclear factor (ANF).

Eyes: Dry eyes.

Immunological System: Antimitochondrial antibodies.

Liver and Biliary System: Hepatic necrosis; hepatitis; cholestatic jaundice; elevated liver function tests.

Musculoskeletal System: Muscle cramps; toxic myopathy.

Respiratory System: Bronchospasm.

Skin and Appendages: Rashes of various types, such as generalized maculopapular; lichenoid; urticarial; bullous lichen planus; psoriaform; facial erythema; Peyronie's disease; reversible alopecia.

Urinary System: Difficulty in micturition, including acute urinary bladder retention.

Hypersensitivity: Rare reports of hypersensitivity (eg, rash, urticaria, pruritus, angioedema, dyspnea) and anaphylactoid reactions.

Following approval for marketing in the United Kingdom, a monitored release survey involving approximately 6,800 patients was conducted for further safety and efficacy evaluation of this product. Results of this survey indicate that the type, severity, and incidence of adverse effects were comparable to those cited above.

Potential Adverse Effects: In addition, other adverse effects not listed above have been reported with other beta-adrenergic blocking agents.

Central Nervous System: Reversible mental depression progressing to catatonia; an acute reversible syndrome characterized by disorientation for time and place, short-term memory loss, emotional lability, slightly clouded sensorium, and decreased performance on neuropsychometrics.

Cardiovascular: Intensification of AV block (see **CONTRAINDICATIONS**).

Allergic: Fever combined with aching and sore throat; laryngospasm; respiratory distress.

Hematologic: Agranulocytosis; thrombocytopenic or nonthrombocytopenic purpura.

Gastrointestinal: Mesenteric artery thrombosis; ischemic colitis.

The oculomucocutaneous syndrome associated with the beta-blocker practolol has not been reported with labetalol HCl.

Clinical Laboratory Tests: There have been reversible increases of serum transaminases in 4% of patients treated with labetalol HCl and tested, and more rarely, reversible increases in blood urea.

OVERDOSAGE

Overdosage with NORMODYNE (labetalol HCl) Tablets causes excessive hypotension that is posture sensitive, and sometimes, excessive bradycardia. Patients should be placed supine and their legs raised if necessary to improve the blood supply to the brain. If overdosage with labetalol HCl follows oral ingestion, gastric lavage or pharmacologically induced emesis (using syrup of ipecac) may be useful for removal of the drug shortly after ingestion. The following additional measures should be employed if necessary: *Excessive bradycardia*—administer atropine or epinephrine. *Cardiac failure*—administer a digitalis glycoside and a diuretic. Dopamine or dobutamine may also be useful. *Hypotension*—administer vasopressors, eg, norepinephrine. There is pharmacological evidence that norepinephrine may be the drug of choice. *Bronchospasm*—administer epinephrine and/or an aerosolized beta$_2$-agonist. *Seizures*—administer diazepam.

In severe beta-blocker overdose resulting in hypotension and/or bradycardia, glucagon has been shown to be effective when administered in large doses (5 to 10 mg rapidly over 30 seconds, followed by continuous infusion of 5 mg/hr that can be reduced as the patient improves).

Neither hemodialysis nor peritoneal dialysis removes a significant amount of labetalol HCl from the general circulation (<1%).

The oral LD$_{50}$ value of labetalol HCl in the mouse is approximately 600 mg/kg and in the rat is greater than 2 g/kg. The intravenous LD$_{50}$ in these species is 50 to 60 mg/kg.

DOSAGE AND ADMINISTRATION

DOSAGE MUST BE INDIVIDUALIZED. The recommended initial dose is 100 mg twice daily whether used alone or added to a diuretic regimen. After 2 or 3 days, using standing blood pressure as an indicator, dosage may be titrated in increments of 100 mg b.i.d. every 2 or 3 days. The usual maintenance dosage of labetalol HCl is between 200 and 400 mg twice daily.

Since the full antihypertensive effect of labetalol HCl is usually seen within the first 1 to 3 hours of the initial dose or dose increment, the assurance of a lack of an exaggerated hypotensive response can be clinically established in the office setting. The antihypertensive effects of continued dosing can be measured at subsequent visits, approximately 12 hours after a dose, to determine whether further titration is necessary.

Patients with severe hypertension may require from 1200 mg to 2400 mg per day, with or without thiazide diuretics. Should side effects (principally nausea or dizziness) occur with these doses administered b.i.d., the same total daily dose administered t.i.d. may improve tolerability and facilitate further titration. Titration increments should not exceed 200 mg b.i.d.

When a diuretic is added, an additive antihypertensive effect can be expected. In some cases this may necessitate a labetalol HCl dosage adjustment. As with most antihypertensive drugs, optimal dosages of NORMODYNE (labetalol HCl) Tablets are usually lower in patients also receiving a diuretic.

When transferring patients from other antihypertensive drugs, NORMODYNE (labetalol HCl) Tablets should be introduced as recommended and the dosage of the existing therapy progressively decreased.

HOW SUPPLIED

NORMODYNE (labetalol HCl) Tablets, 100 mg, light brown, round, scored, film-coated tablets engraved on one side with Schering and product identification numbers 244, and on the other side the number 100 for the strength and "NORMODYNE"; bottles of 100 (NDC-0085-0244-04), bottles of 500 (NDC-0085-0244-05), and box of 100 for unit-dose dispensing (NDC-0085-0244-08).

NORMODYNE (labetalol HCl) Tablets, 200 mg, white, round, scored, film-coated tablets engraved on one side with Schering and product identification numbers 752, and on the other side the number 200 for the strength and "NORMODYNE"; bottles of 100 (NDC-0085-0752-04), bottles of 500 (NDC-0085-0752-05), and box of 100 for unit-dose dispensing (NDC-0085-0752-08).

NORMODYNE (labetalol HCl) Tablets, 300 mg, blue, round, film-coated tablets engraved on one side with Schering and product identification numbers 438, and on the other side the number 300 for the strength and "NORMODYNE"; bottles of 100 (NDC-0085-0438-03), bottles of 500 (NDC-0085-0438-05), and box of 100 for unit-dose dispensing (NDC-0085-0438-06).

NORMODYNE (labetalol HCl) Tablets should be stored between 2° and 30°C (36° and 86°F).

NORMODYNE (labetalol HCl) Tablets in the unit-dose boxes should be protected from excessive moisture.

Key Pharmaceuticals, Inc.
Kenilworth, NJ 07033 USA
Rev. 5/00 B-16833541
23116715T

PEG-Intron™ ℞
(Peginterferon alfa-2b)
Powder for Injection

Prescribing information for this product, which appears on pages 3140–3142 of the 2002 PDR, has been completely revised as follows. Please write "See Supplement A" next to the product heading.

Alpha interferons, including PEG-Intron, cause or aggravate fatal or life-threatening neuropsychiatric, autoimmune, ischemic, and infectious disorders. Patients should be monitored closely with periodic clinical and laboratory evaluations. Patients with persistently severe or worsening signs or symptoms of these conditions should be withdrawn from therapy. In many but not all cases these disorders resolve after stopping PEG-Intron therapy. See WARNINGS, ADVERSE REACTIONS.

Use with Ribavirin. Ribavirin may cause birth defects and/or death of the unborn child. Extreme care must be taken to avoid pregnancy in female patients and in female partners of male patients. Ribavirin causes hemolytic anemia. The anemia associated with REBETOL therapy may result in a worsening of cardiac disease. Ribavirin is genotoxic and mutagenic and should be considered a potential carcinogen. (See REBETOL package insert for additional information and other warnings).

DESCRIPTION

PEG-Intron™, peginterferon alfa-2b Powder for Injection, is a covalent conjugate of recombinant alfa-2b interferon with monomethoxy polyethylene glycol (PEG). The average molecular weight of the PEG portion of the molecule is 12,000 daltons. The average molecular weight of the PEG-Intron molecule is approximately 31,000 daltons. The specific activity of peginterferon alfa-2b is approximately 0.7 x 10^8 IU/mg protein.

Interferon alfa-2b, is a water-soluble protein with a molecular weight of 19,271 daltons produced by recombinant DNA techniques. It is obtained from the bacterial fermentation of a strain of *Escherichia coli* bearing a genetically engineered plasmid containing an interferon gene from human leukocytes.

PEG-Intron is a white to off-white lyophilized powder supplied in 2-mL vials for subcutaneous use. Each vial contains either 74 µg, 118.4 µg, 177.6 µg, or 222 µg of PEG-Intron, and 1.11 mg dibasic sodium phosphate anhydrous, 1.11 mg monobasic sodium phosphate dihydrate, 59.2 mg sucrose and 0.074 mg polysorbate 80. Following reconstitution with 0.7 mL of the supplied diluent (Sterile Water for Injection, USP), each vial contains PEG-Intron at strengths of either 50 µg per 0.5 mL, 80 µg per .05 mL, 120 µg per 0.5 mL, or 150 µg per 0.5 mL.

CLINICAL PHARMACOLOGY

General: The biological activity of PEG-Intron is derived from its interferon alfa-2b moiety. Interferons exert their cellular activities by binding to specific membrane receptors on the cell surface and initiate a complex sequence of intracellular events. These include the induction of certain enzymes, suppression of cell proliferation, immunomodulating activities such as enhancement of the phagocytic activity of macrophages and augmentation of the specific cytotoxicity of lymphocytes for target cells, and inhibition of virus replication in virus-infected cells. Interferon alfa upregulates the Th1 T-helper cell subset in *in vitro* studies. The clinical relevance of these findings is not known.

Pharmacodynamics: PEG-Intron raises concentrations of effector proteins such as serum neopterin and 2′5′ oligoadenylate synthetase, raises body temperature, and causes reversible decreases in leukocyte and platelet counts. The correlation between the *in vitro* and *in vivo* pharmacologic and pharmacodynamic and clinical effects is unknown.

Pharmacokinetics: Following a single subcutaneous (SC) dose of PEG-Intron, the mean absorption half-life ($t_{1/2}\ k_a$) was 4.6 hours. Maximal serum concentrations (C_{max}) occur between 15–44 hours post-dose, and are sustained for up to 48–72 hours. The C_{max} and AUC measurements of PEG-Intron increase in a dose-related manner. After multiple dosing, there is an increase in bioavailability of PEG-Intron. Week 48 mean trough concentrations (320 pg/mL; range 0, 2960) are approximately 3-fold higher than Week 4 mean trough concentrations (94 pg/mL; range 0, 416). The mean PEG-Intron elimination half-life is approximately 40 hours (range 22 to 60 hours) in patients with HCV infection. The apparent clearance of PEG-Intron is estimated to be approximately 22.0 mL/hr•kg. Renal elimination accounts for 30% of the clearance. Single dose peginterferon alfa-2b pharmacokinetics following a subcutaneous 1.0 µg/kg dose suggest the clearance of peginterferon alfa-2b is reduced by approximately half in subjects with impaired renal function (creatinine clearance <50 mL/minute).

Pegylation of interferon alfa-2b produces a product (PEG-Intron) whose clearance is lower than that of non-pegylated interferon alfa-2b. When compared to INTRON A, PEG-Intron (1.0 µg/kg) has approximately a seven-fold lower mean apparent clearance and a five-fold greater mean half-life permitting a reduced dosing frequency. At effective therapeutic doses, PEG-Intron has approximately ten-fold greater C_{max} and 50-fold greater AUC than interferon alfa-2b.

The pharmacokinetics of geriatric subjects (> 65 years of age) treated with a single subcutaneous dose of 1.0 µg/kg of PEG-Intron were similar in C_{max}, AUC, clearance, or elimination half-life as compared to younger subjects (28 to 44 years of age).

During the 48 week treatment period with PEG-Intron, no differences in the pharmacokinetic profiles were observed between male and female patients with chronic hepatitis C infection.

Effect of Food on Absorption of Ribavirin Both AUC_{tf} and C_{max} increased by 70% when REBETOL Capsules were administered with a high-fat meal (841 kcal, 53.8 g fat, 31.6 g protein, and 57.4 g carbohydrate) in a single-dose pharmacokinetic study. (See **DOSAGE AND ADMINISTRATION**).

Drug Interactions: It is not known if PEG-Intron therapy causes clinically significant drug-drug interactions with drugs metabolized by the liver in patients with hepatitis C. In 12 healthy subjects known to be CYP2D6 extensive metabolizers, a single subcutaneous dose of 1 µg/kg PEG-Intron did not inhibit CYP1A2, 2C8/9, 2D6, hepatic 3A4 or N-acetyltransferase; the effects of PEG-Intron on CYP2C19 were not assessed.

CLINICAL STUDIES

PEG-Intron Monotherapy-Study 1

A randomized study compared treatment with PEG-Intron (0.5, 1.0, or 1.5 µg/kg once weekly SC) to treatment with INTRON A, (3 million units three times weekly SC) in 1219 adults with chronic hepatitis from HCV infection. The patients were not previously treated with interferon alfa, had

Continued on next page

PEG-Intron—Cont.

compensated liver disease, detectable HCV RNA, elevated ALT, and liver histopathology consistent with chronic hepatitis. Patients were treated for 48 weeks and were followed for 24 weeks post-treatment. Seventy percent of all patients were infected with HCV genotype 1, and 74 percent of all patients had high baseline levels of HCV RNA (more than 2 million copies per mL of serum), two factors known to predict poor response to treatment.

Response to treatment was defined as undetectable HCV RNA and normalization of ALT at 24 weeks post-treatment. The response rates to the 1.0 and 1.5 μg/kg PEG-Intron doses were similar (approximately 24%) to each other and were both higher than the response rate to INTRON A (12%). (See Table 1)

[See table 1 above]

TABLE 1. Rates of Response to Treatment-Study 1

	A PEG-Intron 0.5 μg/kg (N=315)	B PEG-Intron 1.0 μg/kg (N=298)	C INTRON A 3 MIU TIW (N=307)	B-C (95% CI) Difference between PEG-Intron 1.0 μg/kg and INTRON A
Treatment Response (Combined Virologic Response and ALT Normalization)	17%	24%	12%	11 (5, 18)
Virologic Response[a]	18%	25%	12%	12 (6, 19)
ALT Normalization	24%	29%	18%	11 (5, 18)

[a]Serum HCV is measured by a research-based quantitative polymerase chain reaction assay by a central laboratory.

Patients with both viral genotype 1 and high serum levels of HCV RNA at baseline were less likely to respond to treatment with PEG-Intron. Among patients with the two unfavorable prognostic variables, 8% (12/157) responded to PEG-Intron treatment and 2% (4/169) responded to INTRON A. Doses of PEG-Intron higher than the recommended dose did not result in higher response rates in these patients.

Patients receiving PEG-Intron with viral genotype 1 had a response rate of 14% (28/199) while patients with other viral genotypes had a 45% (43/96) response rate.

Ninety-six percent of the responders in the PEG-Intron groups and 100% of responders in the INTRON A group first cleared their viral RNA by week-24 of treatment. See **DOSAGE AND ADMINISTRATION**.

The treatment response rates were similar in men and women. Response rates were lower in African American and Hispanic patients and higher in Asians compared to Caucasians. Although African Americans had a higher proportion of poor prognostic factors compared to Caucasians the number of non-Caucasians studied (9% of the total) was insufficient to allow meaningful conclusions about differences in response rates after adjusting for prognostic factors.

Liver biopsies were obtained before and after treatment in 60% of patients. A modest reduction in inflammation compared to baseline that was similar in all four treatment groups was observed.

PEG-Intron/REBETOL Combination Therapy-Study 2

A randomized study compared treatment with two PEG-Intron/REBETOL regimens [PEG-Intron 1.5 μg/kg SC once weekly (QW)/REBETOL 800 mg PO daily (in divided doses); PEG-Intron 1.5 μg/kg SC QW for 4 weeks then 0.5 μg/kg SC QW for 44 weeks/REBETOL 1000/1200 mg PO daily (in divided doses)] with INTRON A (3 MIU SC thrice weekly (TIW)/REBETOL 1000/1200 mg PO daily (in divided doses) in 1530 adults with chronic hepatitis C. Interferon naïve patients were treated for 48 weeks and followed for 24 weeks post-treatment. Eligible patients had compensated liver disease, detectable HCV RNA, elevated ALT, and liver histopathology consistent with chronic hepatitis.

Response to treatment was defined as undetectable HCV RNA at 24 weeks post-treatment. The response rate to the PEG-Intron 1.5 μg/kg plus ribavirin 800 mg dose was higher than the response rate to INTRON A/REBETOL (See **Table 2**). The response rate to PEG-Intron 1.5→0.5g/kg/ REBETOL was essentially the same as the response to INTRON A/REBETOL (data not shown).

[See table 2 above]

TABLE 2. Rates of Response to Treatment-Study 2

	PEG-Intron 1.5 μg/kg QW REBETOL 800 mg QD	INTRON A 3 MIU TIW REBETOL 1000/1200 mg QD
Overall[1,2] response	52% (264/511)	46% (231/505)
Genotype 1	41% (141/348)	33% (112/343)
Genotype 2–6	75% (123/163)	73% (119/162)

[1]Serum HCV RNA is measured with a research-based quantitative polymerase chain reaction assay by a central laboratory.
[2]Difference in overall treatment response (PEG-Intron/REBETOL vs. INTRON A/REBETOL) is 6% with 95% confidence interval of (0.18, 11.63) adjusted for viral genotype and presence of cirrhosis at baseline.

Patients with viral genotype 1, regardless of viral load, had a lower response rate to PEG-Intron (1.5 μg/kg)/REBETOL compared to patients with other viral genotypes. Patients with both poor prognostic factors (genotype 1 and high viral load) had a response rate of 30% (78/256) compared to a response rate of 29% (71/247) with INTRON A/REBETOL.

Patients with lower body weight tended to have higher adverse event rates (see **ADVERSE REACTIONS**) and higher response rates than patients with higher body weights. Differences in response rates between treatment arms did not substantially vary with body weight.

Treatment response rates with PEG-Intron/REBETOL were 49% in men and 56% in women. Response rates were lower in African American and Hispanic patients and higher in Asians compared to Caucasians. Although African Americans had a higher proportion of poor prognostic factors compared to Caucasians the number of non-Caucasians studied (11% of the total) was insufficient to allow meaningful conclusions about differences in response rates after adjusting for prognostic factors.

Liver biopsies were obtained before and after treatment in 68% of patients. Compared to baseline approximately 2/3 of patients in all treatment groups were observed to have a modest reduction in inflammation.

INDICATIONS AND USAGE

PEG-Intron, peginterferon alfa-2b, is indicated for use alone or in combination with REBETOL (ribavirin, USP) for the treatment of chronic hepatitis C in patients with compensated liver disease who have not been previously treated with interferon alpha and are at least 18 years of age.

CONTRAINDICATIONS

PEG-Intron is contraindicated in patients with:

- hypersensitivity to PEG-Intron or any other component of the product
- autoimmune hepatitis
- decompensated liver disease

PEG-Intron/REBETOL combination therapy is additionally contraindicated in:

- patients with hypersensitivity to ribavirin or any other component of the product
- women who are pregnant
- men whose female partners are pregnant
- patients with hemoglobinopathies (e.g., thalassemia major, sickle-cell anemia)

WARNINGS

Patients should be monitored for the following serious conditions, some of which may become life threatening. Patients with persistently severe or worsening signs or symptoms should be withdrawn from therapy.

Neuropsychiatric events

Life-threatening or fatal neuropsychiatric events, including suicide, suicidal and homicidal ideation, depression, relapse of drug addiction/overdose, and aggressive behavior have occurred in patients with and without a previous psychiatric disorder during PEG-Intron treatment and follow-up. Psychoses, hallucinations, bipolar disorders, and mania have been observed in patients treated with alpha interferons. PEG-Intron should be used with extreme caution in patients with a history of psychiatric disorders. Patients should be advised to report immediately any symptoms of depression and/or suicidal ideation to their prescribing physicians. Physicians should monitor all patients for evidence of depression and other psychiatric symptoms. In severe cases, PEG-Intron should be stopped immediately and psychiatric intervention instituted. (See **DOSAGE AND ADMINISTRATION: Dose Reduction.**)

Bone marrow toxicity

PEG-Intron suppresses bone marrow function, sometimes resulting in severe cytopenias. PEG-Intron should be discontinued in patients who develop severe decreases in neutrophil or platelet counts. (See **DOSAGE AND ADMINISTRATION: Dose Reduction**). Ribavirin may potentiate the neutropenia induced by interferon alpha. Very rarely alpha interferons may be associated with aplastic anemia.

Endocrine disorders

PEG-Intron causes or aggravates hypothyroidism and hyperthyroidism. Hyperglycemia has been observed in patients treated with PEG-Intron. Diabetes mellitus has been observed in patients treated with alpha interferons. Patients with these conditions who cannot be effectively treated by medication should not begin PEG-Intron therapy. Patients who develop these conditions during treatment and cannot be controlled with medication should not continue PEG-Intron therapy.

Cardiovascular events

Cardiovascular events, which include hypotension, arrhythmia, tachycardia, cardiomyopathy, angina pectoris, and myocardial infarction, have been observed in patients treated with PEG-Intron. PEG-Intron should be used cautiously in patients with cardiovascular disease. Patients with a history of myocardial infarction and arrhythmic disorder who require PEG-Intron therapy should be closely monitored (see **Laboratory Tests**). Patients with a history of significant or unstable cardiac disease should not be treated with PEG-Intron/REBETOL combination therapy. [See **REBETOL package insert.**]

Pulmonary disorders

Dyspnea, pulmonary infiltrates, pneumonia, bronchiolitis obliterans, interstitial pneumonitis and sarcoidosis some resulting in respiratory failure and/or patient deaths, may be induced or aggravated by PEG-Intron or alpha interferon therapy. Recurrence of respiratory failure has been observed with interferon rechallenge. PEG-Intron combination treatment should be suspended in patients who develop pulmonary infiltrates or pulmonary function impairment. Patients who resume interferon treatment should be closely monitored.

Colitis

Fatal and nonfatal ulcerative or hemorrhagic/ischemic colitis have been observed within 12 weeks of the start of alpha interferon treatment. Abdominal pain, bloody diarrhea, and fever are the typical manifestations. PEG-Intron treatment should be discontinued immediately in patients who develop these symptoms and signs. The colitis usually resolves within 1–3 weeks of discontinuation of alpha interferons.

Pancreatitis

Fatal and nonfatal pancreatitis has been observed in patients treated with alpha interferon. PEG-Intron therapy should be suspended in patients with signs and symptoms suggestive of pancreatitis and discontinued in patients diagnosed with pancreatitis.

Autoimmune disorders

Development or exacerbation of autoimmune disorders (e.g. thyroiditis, thrombocytopenia, rheumatoid arthritis, interstitial nephritis, systemic lupus erythematosus, psoriasis) have been observed in patients receiving PEG-Intron. PEG-Intron should be used with caution in patients with autoimmune disorders.

Ophthalmologic disorders

Decrease or loss of vision, retinal artery or vein thrombosis, retinal hemorrhages and cotton wool spots, optic neuritis, and papilledema are induced or aggravated by treatment with PEG-Intron or other alpha interferons. All patients should receive an eye examination at baseline. Patients with preexisting ophthalmologic disorders (e.g. diabetic or hypertensive retinopathy) should receive periodic ophthalmologic exams during interferon alpha treatment. Any patient who develops ocular symptoms should receive a prompt and complete eye examination. PEG-interferon treatment should be discontinued in patients who develop new or worsening ophthalmologic disorders.

Hypersensitivity

Serious, acute hypersensitivity reactions (e.g., urticaria, angioedema, bronchoconstriction, anaphylaxis) have been rarely observed during alpha interferon therapy. If such a reaction develops during treatment with PEG-Intron, discontinue treatment and institute appropriate medical therapy immediately. Transient rashes do not necessitate interruption of treatment.

Use with Ribavirin-(See also REBETOL Package Insert)

REBETOL may cause birth defects and/or death of the unborn child. REBETOL therapy should not be started until a report of a negative pregnancy test has been obtained immediately prior to planned initiation of therapy. Patients should use at least two forms of contraception and have monthly pregnancy tests (See BOXED WARNING, CONTRAINDICATIONS and PRECAUTIONS: Information for Patients and REBETOL package insert).

Anemia

Ribavirin caused hemolytic anemia in 10% of PEG-Intron/ REBETOL treated patients within 1-4 weeks of initiation of therapy. Complete blood counts should be obtained pretreatment and at week 2 and week 4 of therapy or more frequently if clinically indicated. Anemia associated with REBETOL therapy may result in a worsening of cardiac disease. Decrease in dosage or discontinuation of REBETOL may be necessary. (See **DOSAGE AND ADMINISTRATION: Dose Reduction.**)

PRECAUTIONS

- PEG-Intron alone or in combination with REBETOL has not been studied in patients who have failed other alpha interferon treatments.

- **The safety and efficacy of PEG-Intron alone or in combination with REBETOL for the treatment of hepatitis C in liver or other organ transplant recipients have not been studied.**
- **The safety and efficacy of PEG-Intron/REBETOL for the treatment of patients with HCV co-infected with HIV or HBV have not been established.**

Patients with renal failure: Patients with impairment of renal function should be closely monitored for signs and symptoms of interferon toxicity and doses of PEG-Intron should be adjusted accordingly. PEG-Intron should be used with caution in patients with creatinine clearance <50 mL/min. See **DOSAGE AND ADMINISTRATION: Dose Modification.**

Immunogenicity: Approximately 2% of patients receiving PEG-Intron (32/1759) or INTRON A (11/728) with or without REBETOL developed low-titer (≤160) neutralizing antibodies to PEG-Intron or INTRON A. The clinical and pathological significance of the appearance of serum neutralizing antibodies is unknown. No apparent correlation of antibody development to clinical response or adverse events was observed. The incidence of post-treatment binding antibody ranged from 8 to 15 percent. The data reflect the percentage of patients whose test results were considered positive for antibodies to PEG-Intron in a Biacore assay that is used to measure binding antibodies, and in an antiviral neutralization assay, which measures serum-neutralizing antibodies. The percentage of patients whose test results were considered positive for antibodies is highly dependent on the sensitivity and specificity of the assays. Additionally the observed incidence of antibody positivity in these assays may be influenced by several factors including sample timing and handling, concomitant medications, and underlying disease. For these reasons, comparison of the incidence of antibodies to PEG-Intron with the incidence of antibodies to other products may be misleading.

Laboratory Tests: PEG-Intron alone or in combination with ribavirin may cause severe decreases in neutrophil and platelet counts, and hematologic, endocrine (e.g. TSH) and hepatic abnormalities. Transient elevations in ALT (2–5 fold above baseline) were observed in 10% of patients treated with PEG-Intron, and was not associated with deterioration of other liver functions.

Patients on PEG-Intron or PEG-Intron/REBETOL combination therapy should have hematology and blood chemistry testing before the start of treatment and then periodically thereafter. In the clinical trial CBC (including hemoglobin, neutrophil and platelet counts) and chemistries (including AST, ALT, bilirubin, and uric acid) were measured during the treatment period at weeks 2, 4, 8, 12, and then at 6-week intervals or more frequently if abnormalities developed. TSH levels were measured every 12 weeks during the treatment period.

HCV RNA should be measured at 6 months of treatment. PEG-Intron or PEG-Intron/REBETOL combination therapy should be discontinued in patients with persistent high viral levels.

Patients who have pre-existing cardiac abnormalities should have electrocardiograms administered before treatment with PEG-Intron/REBETOL.

Information for Patients: Patients receiving PEG-Intron alone or in combination with REBETOL should be directed in its appropriate use, informed of the benefits and risks associated with treatment, and referred to the **MEDICATION GUIDES for PEG-Intron and, if applicable, REBETOL (ribavirin, USP).**

Patients must be informed that REBETOL may cause birth defects and/or death of the unborn child. Extreme care must be taken to avoid pregnancy in female patients and in female partners of male patients taking combination PEG-Intron/REBETOL therapy. Combination PEG-Intron/REBETOL therapy should not be initiated until a report of a negative pregnancy test has been obtained immediately prior to initiation of therapy. It is recommended that patients undergo monthly pregnancy tests during therapy and for 6 months post-therapy. (**See CONTRAINDICATIONS and REBETOL package insert).**

A puncture-resistant container for the disposal of used syringes and needles should be supplied to the patient for at home use. Patients should be thoroughly instructed in the importance of proper disposal and cautioned against any reuse of needles and syringes. The full container should be disposed of according to the directions provided by the physician (see **MEDICATION GUIDE**).

Patients should be informed that there are no data regarding whether PEG-Intron therapy will prevent transmission of HCV infection to others. Also, it is not known if treatment with PEG-Intron will cure hepatitis C or prevent cirrhosis, liver failure, or liver cancer that may be the result of infection with the hepatitis C virus.

Patients should be advised that laboratory evaluations are required before starting therapy and periodically thereafter (see **Laboratory Tests**). It is advised that patients be well-hydrated, especially during the initial stages of treatment. "Flu-like" symptoms associated with administration of PEG-Intron may be minimized by bedtime administration of PEG-Intron or by use of antipyretics.

Carcinogenesis, Mutagenesis, and Impairment of Fertility

Carcinogenesis and Mutagenesis: PEG-Intron has not been tested for its carcinogenic potential. Neither PEG-Intron, nor its components interferon or methoxypolyethylene glycol caused damage to DNA when tested in the standard battery of mutagenesis assays, in the presence and absence of metabolic activation.

Use with Ribavirin: Ribavirin is genotoxic and mutagenic and should be considered a potential carcinogen. See REBETOL package insert for additional warnings relevant to PEG-Intron therapy in combination with ribavirin.

TABLE 3. Adverse Events Occurring in >5% of Patients

	*Percentage of Patients Reporting Adverse Events**			
	Study 1		**Study 2**	
Adverse Events	**PEG-Intron 1.0 µg/kg (n=297)**	**INTRON A 3 MIU (n=303)**	**PEG-Intron 1.5 µg/kg/ REBETOL (n=511)**	**INTRON A/ REBETOL (n=505)**
Application Site				
Injection Site Inflammation/Reaction	47	20	75	49
Autonomic Nervous Sys.				
Mouth Dry	6	7	12	8
Sweating Increased	6	7	11	7
Flushing	6	3	4	3
Body as a Whole				
Fatigue/Asthenia	52	54	66	63
Headache	56	52	62	58
Rigors	23	19	48	41
Fever	22	12	46	33
Weight Decrease	11	13	29	20
RUQ Pain	8	8	12	6
Chest Pain	6	4	8	7
Malaise	7	6	4	6
Central/Periph. Nerv. Sys.				
Dizziness	12	10	21	17
Endocrine Disorders				
Hypothyroidism	5	3	5	4
Gastrointestinal				
Nausea	26	20	43	33
Anorexia	20	17	32	27
Diarrhea	18	16	22	17
Vomiting	7	6	14	12
Abdominal Pain	15	11	13	13
Dyspepsia	6	7	9	8
Constipation	1	3	5	5
Hematologic Disorders				
Neutropenia	6	2	26	14
Anemia	0	0	12	17
Leukopenia	<1	0	6	5
Thrombocytopenia	7	<1	5	2
Liver and Biliary System Disorders				
Hepatomegaly	6	5	4	4
Musculoskeletal				
Myalgia	54	53	56	50
Arthralgia	23	27	34	28
Musculoskeletal Pain	28	22	21	19
Psychiatric				
Insomnia	23	23	40	41
Depression	29	25	31	34
Anxiety/Emotional Lability/Irritability	28	34	47	47
Concentration Impaired	10	8	17	21
Agitation	2	2	8	5
Nervousness	4	3	6	6
Reproductive, Female				
Menstrual Disorder	4	3	7	6
Resistance Mechanism				
Infection Viral	11	10	12	12
Infection Fungal	<1	3	6	1
Respiratory System				
Dyspnea	4	2	26	24
Coughing	8	5	23	16
Pharyngitis	10	7	12	13
Rhinitis	2	2	8	6
Sinusitis	7	7	6	5
Skin and Appendages				
Alopecia	22	22	36	32
Pruritis	12	8	29	28
Rash	6	7	24	23
Skin Dry	11	9	24	23
Special Senses Other,				
Taste Perversion	<1	2	9	4
Vision Disorders				
Vision blurred	2	3	5	6
Conjunctivitis	4	2	4	5

*Patients reporting one or more adverse events. A patient may have reported more than one adverse event within a body system/organ class category.

Impairment of Fertility: PEG-Intron may impair human fertility. Irregular menstrual cycles were observed in female cynomolgus monkeys given subcutaneous injections of 4239 µg/m² PEG-Intron alone every other day for one month, (approximately 345 times the recommended weekly human dose based upon body surface area). These effects included transiently decreased serum levels of estradiol and progesterone, suggestive of anovulation. Normal menstrual cycles and serum hormone levels resumed in these animals 2 to 3 months following cessation of PEG-Intron treatment. Every other day dosing with 262 µg/m² (approximately 21 times the weekly human dose) had no effects on cycle duration or reproductive hormone status. The effects of PEG-Intron on male fertility have not been studied.

Pregnancy Category C: PEG-Intron monotherapy: Nonpegylated Interferon alfa-2b, has been shown to have abortifacient effects in *Macaca mulatta* (rhesus monkeys) at 15 and 30 million IU/kg (estimated human equivalent of 5 and

Continued on next page

PEG-Intron—Cont.

10 million IU/kg, based on body surface area adjustment for a 60 kg adult). PEG-Intron should be assumed to also have abortifacient potential. There are no adequate and well-controlled studies in pregnant women. PEG-Intron therapy is to be used during pregnancy only if the potential benefit justifies the potential risk to the fetus. Therefore, PEG-Intron is recommended for use in fertile women only when they are using effective contraception during the treatment period.

Pregnancy Category X : Use with Ribavirin

Significant teratogenic and/or embryocidal effects have been demonstrated in all animal species exposed to ribavirin. REBETOL therapy is contraindicated in women who are pregnant and in the male partners of women who are pregnant. See CONTRAINDICATIONS and the REBETOL Package Insert.

If pregnancy occurs in a patient or partner of a patient during treatment with PEG-Intron and REBETOL during the 6 months after treatment cessation, physicians should report such cases by calling (800) 727-7064.

Pediatric. Safety and effectiveness in pediatric patients below the age of 18 years have not been established.

Geriatric. In general, younger patients tend to respond better than older patients to interferon-based therapies. Clinical studies of PEG-Intron alone or in combination with REBETOL did not include sufficient numbers of subjects aged 65 and over, however, to determine whether they respond differently than younger subjects. Treatment with alpha interferons, including PEG-Intron, is associated with neuropsychiatric, cardiac, pulmonary, GI and systemic (flu-like) adverse effects. Because these adverse reactions may be more severe in the elderly, caution should be exercised in use of PEG-Intron in this population. This drug is known to be substantially excreted by the kidney. Because elderly patients are more likely to have decreased renal function, the risk of toxic reactions to this drug may be greater in patients with impaired renal function. REBETOL should not be used in patients with creatinine clearance <50 mL/min. When using PEG-Intron/REBETOL therapy, refer also to the REBETOL Medication Guide.

ADVERSE REACTIONS

Nearly all study patients in clinical trials experienced one or more adverse events. In the PEG monotherapy trial the incidence of serious adverse events was similar (about 12%) in all treatment groups. In the PEG-Intron/REBETOL combination trial the incidence of serious adverse events was 17% in the PEG-Intron/REBETOL groups compared to 14% in the INTRON A/REBETOL group.

In many but not all cases, adverse events resolved after dose reduction or discontinuation of therapy. Some patients experienced ongoing or new serious adverse events during the 6-month follow-up period. In the PEG-Intron/REBETOL trial 13 patients experienced life-threatening psychiatric events (suicidal ideation or attempt) and one patient accomplished suicide.

There have been five patient deaths which occurred in clinical trials: one suicide in a patient receiving PEG-Intron monotherapy and one suicide in a patient receiving PEG-Intron/REBETOL combination therapy; two deaths among patients receiving INTRON A monotherapy (1 murder/suicide and 1 sudden death) and one patient death in the INTRON A/REBETOL group (motor vehicle accident).

Overall 10–14% of patients receiving PEG-Intron, alone or in combination with REBETOL, discontinued therapy compared with 6% treated with INTRON A alone and 13% treated with INTRON A in combination with REBETOL. The most common reasons for discontinuation of therapy were related to psychiatric, systemic (e.g. fatigue, headache), or gastrointestinal adverse events.

In the combination therapy trial, dose reductions due to adverse reactions occurred in 42% of patients receiving PEG-Intron (1.5 µg/kg)/REBETOL and in 34% of those receiving INTRON A/REBETOL. The majority of patients (57%) weighing 60 kg or less receiving PEG-Intron (1.5 µg/kg)/REBETOL required dose reduction. Reduction of interferon was dose related (PEG-Intron 1.5 µg/kg > PEG-Intron 0.5 µg/kg or INTRON A), 40%, 27%, 28%, respectively. Dose reduction for REBETOL was similar across all three groups, 33–35%. The most common reasons for dose modifications were neutropenia (18%), or anemia (9%). (See **Laboratory Values**). Other common reasons included depression, fatigue, nausea, and thrombocytopenia.

In the PEG-Intron/REBETOL combination trial the most common adverse events were psychiatric which occurred among 77% of patients and included most commonly depression, irritability, and insomnia, each reported by approximately 30–40% of subjects in all treatment groups. Suicidal behavior (ideation, attempts, and suicides) occurred in 2% of all patients during treatment or during follow-up after treatment cessation (see **WARNINGS**).

PEG-Intron induced fatigue or headache in approximately two-thirds of patients, and induced fever or rigors in approximately half of the patients. The severity of some of these systemic symptoms (e.g. fever and headache) tended to decrease as treatment continues. The incidence tends to be higher with PEG-Intron than with INTRON A therapy alone or in combination with REBETOL.

Application site inflammation and reaction (e.g. bruise, itchiness, irritation) occurred at approximately twice the incidence with PEG-Intron therapies (in up to 75% of patients)

TABLE 4. Recommended PEG-Intron Monotherapy Dosing

Body weight (kg)	PEG-Intron Vial Strength	Amount of PEG-Intron (µg) to Administer	Volume (mL)* of PEG-Intron to Administer
≤45	50 µg per 0.5 mL	40	0.4
46–56		50	0.5
57–72	80 µg per 0.5 mL	64	0.4
73–88		80	0.5
89–106	120 µg per 0.5 mL	96	0.4
107–136		120	0.5
137–160	150 µg per 0.5 mL	150	0.5

*When reconstituted as directed

TABLE 5. Recommended PEG-Intron Combination Therapy Dosing

Body weight (kg)	PEG-Intron Vial Strength	Amount of PEG-Intron (µg) to Administer	Volume (mL) of PEG-Intron to Administer
<40	50 µg per 0.5 mL	50	0.5
40–50	80 µg per 0.5 mL	64	0.4
51–60		80	0.5
61–75	120 µg per 0.5 mL	96	0.4
76–85		120	0.5
>85	150 µg per 0.5 mL	150	0.5

TABLE 6. Guidelines for Modification or Discontinuation of PEG-Intron or PEG-Intron/REBETOL and for Scheduling Visits for Patients with Depression

Depression Severity[1]	Initial Management (4–8 wks)		Depression		
	Dose modification	Visit schedule	Remains stable	Improves	Worsens
Mild	No change	Evaluate once weekly by visit and/or phone.	Continue weekly visit schedule.	Resume normal visit schedule.	(See moderate or severe depression)
Moderate	Decrease IFN dose 50%	Evaluate once weekly (office visit at least every other week).	Consider psychiatric consultation. Continue reduced dosing.	If symptoms improve and are stable for 4 wks, may resume normal visit schedule. Continue reducing dosing or return to normal dose.	(See severe depression)
Severe	Discontinue IFN/R permanently.	Obtain immediate psychiatric consultation.	Psychiatric therapy necessary		

[1]See DSM-IV for definitions

TABLE 7. Guidelines for Dose Modification and Discontinuation of PEG-Intron or PEG-Intron/REBETOL for Hematologic Toxicity

Laboratory Values		PEG-Intron	REBETOL
Hgb*	<10.0 g/dL <8.5 g/dL	--------------------- Permanently discontinue	Decrease by 200 mg/day Permanently discontinue
WBC	$<1.5 \times 10^9$/L $<1.0 \times 10^9$/L	Reduce dose by 50% Permanently discontinue	--------------------- Permanently discontinue
Neutrophils	$<0.75 \times 10^9$/L $<0.5 \times 10^9$/L	Reduce dose by 50% Permanently discontinue	--------------------- Permanently discontinue
Platelets	$<80 \times 10^9$/L $<50 \times 10^9$/L	Reduce dose by 50% Permanently discontinue	--------------------- Permanently discontinue

*For patients with a history of stable cardiac disease receiving PEG-Intron in combination with ribavirin, the PEG-Intron dose should be reduced by half and the ribavirin dose by 200 mg/day if a >2g/dL decrease in hemoglobin is observed during any 4 week period. Both PEG-Intron and ribavirin should be permanently discontinued if patients have hemoglobin levels <12 g/dL after this ribavirin dose reduction.

compared with INTRON A. However injection site pain was infrequent (2–3%) in all groups.

Other common adverse events in the PEG-Intron/REBETOL group included myalgia (56%), arthralgia (34%), nausea (43%), anorexia (32%), weight loss (29%), alopecia (36%), and pruritus (29%).

In the PEG-Intron monotherapy trial the incidence of severe adverse events was 13% in the INTRON A group and 17% in the PEG-Intron groups. In the PEG-Intron/REBETOL combination therapy trial the incidence of severe adverse events was 23% in the INTRON A/REBETOL group and 31–34% in the PEG-Intron/ REBETOL groups. The incidence of life-threatening adverse events was ≤1% across all groups in the monotherapy and combination therapy trials.

Adverse events that occurred in the clinical trial at >5% incidence are provided in **Table 3** by treatment group. Due to potential differences in ascertainment procedures, adverse event rate comparisons across studies should not be made. [See table at top of previous page]

Many patients continued to experience adverse events several months after discontinuation of therapy. By the end of the 6-month follow-up period the incidence of ongoing adverse events by body class in the PEG-Intron 1.5/REBETOL

Each PEG-Intron Package Contains:	
A box containing one 50 µg per 0.5 mL vial of PEG-Intron Powder for Injection and one 5 mL vial of Diluent (Sterile Water for Injection, USP), 2 Safety-Lok* syringes with a safety sleeve and 2 alcohol swabs.	(NDC 0085-1368-01)
A box containing one 80 µg per 0.5 mL vial of PEG-Intron Powder for Injection and one 5 mL vial of Diluent (Sterile Water for Injection, USP), 2 Safety-Lok* syringes with a safety sleeve and 2 alcohol swabs.	(NDC 0085-1291-01)
A box containing one 120 µg per 0.5 mL vial of PEG-Intron Powder for Injection and one 5 mL vial of Diluent (Sterile Water for Injection, USP), 2 Safety-Lok* syringes with a safety sleeve and 2 alcohol swabs.	(NDC 0085-1304-01)
A box containing one 150 µg per 0.5 mL vial of PEG-Intron Powder for Injection and one 5 mL vial of Diluent (Sterile Water for Injection, USP), 2 Safety-Lok* syringes with a safety sleeve and 2 alcohol swabs.	(NDC 0085-1279-01)

group was 33% (psychiatric), 20% (musculoskeletal), and 10% (for endocrine and for GI). In approximately 10–15% of patients weight loss, fatigue and headache had not resolved. Individual serious adverse events occurred at a frequency ≤1% and included suicide attempt, suicidal ideation, severe depression; psychosis, aggressive reaction, relapse of drug addiction/overdose; nerve palsy (facial, oculomotor); cardiomyopathy, myocardial infarction, angina, pericardial effusion, retinal ischemia, retinal artery or vein thrombosis, blindness, decreased visual acuity, optic neuritis, transient ischemic attack, supraventricular arrhythmias, loss of consciousness; neutropenia, infection (sepsis, pneumonia, abscess, cellulitis); emphysema, bronchiolitis obliterans, pleural effusion, gastroenteritis, pancreatitis, gout, hyperglycemia, hyperthyroidism and hypothyroidism, autoimmune thrombocytopenia with or without purpura, rheumatoid arthritis, interstitial nephritis, lupus-like syndrome, sarcoidosis, aggravated psoriasis; urticaria, injection-site necrosis, vasculitis, phototoxicity.

Laboratory Values

Changes in selected laboratory values during treatment with PEG-Intron alone or in combination with REBETOL treatment are described below. **Decreases in hemoglobin, neutrophils, and platelets may require dose reduction or permanent discontinuation from therapy. (See DOSAGE AND ADMINISTRATION- Dose Reduction)**

Hemoglobin. REBETOL induced a decrease in hemoglobin levels in approximately two thirds of patients. Hemoglobin levels decreased to <11g/dL in about 30% of patients. Severe anemia (<8 g/dL) occurred in <1% of patients. Dose modification was required in 9 and 13% of patients in the PEG-Intron/REBETOL and INTRON A/REBETOL groups. Hemoglobin levels become stable by treatment week 4–6 on average. Hemoglobin levels return to baseline between 4 and 12 weeks posttreatment. In the PEG-Intron monotherapy trial hemoglobin decreases were generally mild and dose modifications were rarely necessary. **(See DOSAGE AND ADMINISTRATION: Dose Modification).**

Neutrophils. Decreases in neutrophil counts were observed in a majority of patients treated with PEG-Intron alone (70%) or as combination therapy with REBETOL (85%) and INTRON A/REBETOL (60%). Severe potentially life-threatening neutropenia ($<0.5 \times 10^9$/L) occurred in 1% of patients treated with PEG-Intron monotherapy, 2% of patients treated with INTRON A/REBETOL and in 4% of patients treated with PEG-Intron/REBETOL. Two percent of patients receiving PEG-Intron monotherapy and 18% of patients receiving PEG-Intron /REBETOL required modification of interferon dosage. Few patients (≤1%) required permanent discontinuation of treatment. Neutrophil counts generally return to pre-treatment levels within 4 weeks of cessation of therapy. **(See DOSAGE AND ADMINISTRATION: Dose Modification).**

Platelets. Platelet counts decrease in approximately 20% of patients treated with PEG-Intron alone or with REBETOL and in 6% of patients treated with INTRON A/REBETOL. Severe decreases in platelet counts (<50,000/mm^3) occur in <1% of patients. Patients may require discontinuation or dose modification as a result of platelet decreases. **(See DOSAGE AND ADMINISTRATION: Dose Modification).** In the PEG-Intron/REBETOL combination therapy trial 1% or 3% of patients required dose modification of INTRON A or PEG-Intron respectively. Platelet counts generally returned to pretreatment levels within 4 weeks of the cessation of therapy.

Thyroid Function. Development of TSH abnormalities, with and without clinical manifestations, are associated with interferon therapies. Clinically apparent thyroid disorders occur among patients treated with either INTRON A or PEG-Intron (with or without REBETOL) at a similar incidence (5% for hypothyroidism and 3% for hyperthyroidism). Subjects developed new onset TSH abnormalities while on treatment and during the follow-up period. At the end of the follow-up period 7% of subjects still had abnormal TSH values.

Bilirubin and uric acid. In the PEG-Intron/REBETOL trial 10–14% of patients developed hyperbilirubinemia and 33–38% developed hyperuricemia in association with hemolysis. Six patients developed mild to moderate gout.

OVERDOSAGE

There is limited experience with overdosage. In the clinical studies, a few patients accidentally received a dose greater than that prescribed. There were no instances in which a participant in the monotherapy or combination therapy trials received more than 10.5 times the intended dose of PEG-Intron. The maximum dose received by any patient was 3.45 µg/kg weekly over a period of approximately 12 weeks. The maximum known overdosage of REBETOL was an intentional ingestion of 10 g (fifty 200 mg capsules). There were no serious reactions attributed to these overdosages. In cases of overdosing, symptomatic treatment and close observation of the patient are recommended.

DOSAGE AND ADMINISTRATION

There are no safety and efficacy data on treatment for longer than one year. A patient should self-inject PEG-Intron only if the physician determines that it is appropriate and the patient agrees to medical follow-up as necessary and training in proper injection technique has been given to him/her. (See illustrated **MEDICATION GUIDE** for instructions.)

It is recommended that patients receiving PEG-Intron, alone or in combination with ribavirin, be discontinued from therapy if HCV viral levels remain high after 6 months of therapy.

PEG-Intron Monotherapy

The recommended dose of PEG-Intron regimen is 1.0 µg/kg/week for one year.

The volume of PEG-Intron to be injected depends on the vial strength used and the patient's weight (see **Table 4 below**).

[See table 4 at top of previous page]

PEG-Intron/REBETOL Combination Therapy

When administered in combination with REBETOL, the recommended dose of PEG-Intron is 1.5 micrograms/kg/week. The volume of PEG-Intron to be injected depends on the vial strength of PEG-Intron and patient's body weight. (See **Table 5** below).

[See table 5 at top of previous page]

The recommended dose of REBETOL is 800 mg/day in 2 divided doses: two capsules (400 mg) with breakfast and two capsules (400 mg) with dinner. REBETOL should not be used in patients with creatinine clearance <50 mL/min.

Dose Reduction

If a serious adverse reaction develops during the course of treatment (See **WARNINGS**) discontinue or modify the dosage of PEG-Intron and/or REBETOL until the adverse event abates or decreases in severity. If persistent or recurrent serious adverse events develop despite adequate dosage adjustment, discontinue treatment. For guidelines for dose modifications and discontinuation based on laboratory parameters, see **Tables 6 and 7**. In the combination therapy trial dose reductions occurred among 42% of patients receiving PEG-Intron 1.5 µg/kg/REBETOL 800 mg daily including 57% of those patients weighing 60 kg or less (see **ADVERSE REACTIONS**).

[See table 6 at top of previous page]
[See table 7 at top of previous page]

Preparation and Administration

Two Safety-Lok* syringes are provided in the package; one syringe is for the reconstitution steps and one for the patient injection. There is a plastic safety sleeve to be pulled over the needle after use. The syringe locks with an audible click when the green stripe on the safety sleeve covers the red stripe on the needle. Brief instructions for the preparation and administration of PEG-Intron Powder for Injection are provided below. Please refer to the Medication Guide for detailed, step-by-step instructions.

Reconstitute the PEG-Intron lyophilized product with only 0.7 mL of supplied diluent (Sterile Water for Injection, USP). **The diluent vial is for single use only. The remaining diluent should be discarded.** No other medications should be added to solutions containing PEG-Intron, and PEG-Intron should not be reconstituted with other diluents. Swirl gently to hasten complete dissolution of the powder. The reconstituted solution should be clear and colorless. Visually inspect the solution for particulate matter and discoloration prior to administration. The solution should not be used if discolored or cloudy, or if particulates are present (see **MEDICATION GUIDE** for detailed instructions).

The reconstituted solution should be used immediately and cannot be stored for more than 24 hours at 2°–8°C (See **Storage**). The appropriate PEG-Intron dose should be withdrawn and injected subcutaneously. (See **MEDICATION GUIDE** for detailed instructions). The PEG-Intron vial is a single use vial and does not contain a preservative. **DO NOT REENTER VIAL. DISCARD UNUSED PORTION.** Once the dose from a single dose vial has been withdrawn, the sterility of any remaining product can no longer be guaranteed. Pooling of unused portions of some medications has been linked to bacterial contamination and morbidity.

After preparation and administration of the PEG-Intron injection, it is essential to follow the procedure for proper disposal of syringes and needles. A puncture-resistant container should be used for disposal of syringes. Patients should be instructed in the technique and importance of proper syringe disposal and be cautioned against reuse of these items (See **MEDICATION GUIDE** for detailed instructions.)

Storage

PEG-Intron should be stored at 25°C (77°F): excursions permitted to 15°–30°C (59°–86°F)[see USP Controlled Room Temperature]. After reconstitution with supplied Diluent the solution should be used immediately, but may be stored up to 24 hours at 2° to 8°C (36° to 46°F). The reconstituted solution contains no preservative, is clear and colorless. **Do not freeze.**

HOW SUPPLIED

PEG-Intron is a white to off-white lyophilized powder supplied in 2-mL vials. The PEG-Intron Powder for Injection should be reconstituted with 0.7 mL of the supplied Diluent (Sterile Water for Injection, USP) prior to use.

[See table above]

Schering Corporation
Kenilworth, NJ 07033 USA

Rev. 8/01 B-24564720

*Safety-Lok is a trademark of Becton Dickinson and Company.

TEMODAR® ℞
[*tĕm-ō-dăr*]
(temozolomide)
CAPSULES

Prescribing information for this product, which appears on pages 3157–3160 of the 2002 PDR, has been completely revised as follows. Please write "See Supplement A" next to the product heading.

DESCRIPTION

TEMODAR Capsules for oral administration contain temozolomide, an imidazotetrazine derivative. The chemical name of temozolomide is 3, 4-dihydro-3-methyl-4-oxoimidazo[5,1-d]-*as*-tetrazine-8-carboxamide. The structural formula is:

The material is a white to light tan/light pink powder with a molecular formula of $C_6H_6N_6O_2$ and a molecular weight of 194.15. The molecule is stable at acidic pH (<5), and labile at pH >7, hence can be administered orally. The prodrug, temozolomide, is rapidly hydrolysed to the active 5-(3-methyltriazen-1-yl)imidazole-4-carboxamide (MTIC) at neutral and alkaline pH values, with hydrolysis taking place even faster at alkaline pH.

Each capsule contains either 5 mg, 20 mg, 100 mg, or 250 mg of temozolomide. The inactive ingredients for TEMODAR Capsules are lactose anhydrous, colloidal silicon dioxide, sodium starch glycolate, tartaric acid, and stearic acid. Gelatin capsule shells contain titanium dioxide. The capsules are imprinted with pharmaceutical ink.

TEMODAR 5 mg: green imprint contains pharmaceutical grade shellac, anhydrous ethyl alcohol, isopropyl alcohol, n-butyl alcohol, propylene glycol, ammonium hydroxide, titanium dioxide, yellow iron oxide, and FD&C Blue #2 aluminum lake.

TEMODAR 20 mg: brown imprint also contains pharmaceutical grade shellac, anhydrous ethyl alcohol, isopropyl alcohol, n-butyl alcohol, propylene glycol, purified water, ammonium hydroxide, potassium hydroxide, titanium dioxide, black iron oxide, yellow iron oxide, brown iron oxide, and red iron oxide.

TEMODAR 100 mg: blue imprint contains pharmaceutical glaze (modified) in an ethanol/shellac mixture, isopropyl alcohol, n-butyl alcohol, propylene glycol, titanium dioxide, and FD&C Blue #2 aluminum lake.

TEMODAR 250 mg: black imprint contains pharmaceutical grade shellac, anhydrous ethyl alcohol, isopropyl alcohol, n-butyl alcohol, propylene glycol, purified water, ammonium hydroxide, potassium hydroxide, and black iron oxide.

CLINICAL PHARMACOLOGY

Mechanism of Action: Temozolomide is not directly active but undergoes rapid nonenzymatic conversion at physiologic pH to the reactive compound MTIC. The cytotoxicity of MTIC is thought to be primarily due to alkylation of DNA. Alkylation (methylation) occurs mainly at the O^6 and N^7 positions of guanine.

Pharmacokinetics: Temozolomide is rapidly and completely absorbed after oral administration; peak plasma concentrations occur in 1 hour. Food reduces the rate and extent of temozolomide absorption. Mean peak plasma concentration and AUC decreased by 32% and 9%, respectively, and T_{max} increased 2-fold (from 1.1 to 2.25 hours) when temozolomide was administered after a modified high-fat breakfast. Temozolomide is rapidly eliminated with a mean elimination half-life of 1.8 hours and exhibits linear kinetics over the therapeutic dosing range. Temozolomide has a mean apparent volume of distribution of 0.4 L/kg (%CV=13%). It is weakly bound to human plasma proteins; the mean percent bound of drug-related total radioactivity is 15%.

Continued on next page

Temodar—Cont.

Metabolism and Elimination: Temozolomide is spontaneously hydrolyzed at physiologic pH to the active species, 3-methyl-(triazen-1-yl)imidazole-4-carboxamide (MTIC) and to temozolomide acid metabolite. MTIC is further hydrolyzed to 5-amino-imidazole-4-carboxamide (AIC) which is known to be an intermediate in purine and nucleic acid biosynthesis and to methylhydrazine, which is believed to be the active alkylating species. Cytochrome P450 enzymes play only a minor role in the metabolism of temozolomide and MTIC. Relative to the AUC of temozolomide, the exposure to MTIC and AIC is 2.4% and 23%, respectively. About 38% of the administered temozolomide total radioactive dose is recovered over 7 days; 37.7% in urine and 0.8% in feces. The majority of the recovery of radioactivity in urine is as unchanged temozolomide (5.6%), AIC (12%), temozolomide acid metabolite (2.3%), and unidentified polar metabolite(s) (17%). Overall clearance of temozolomide is about 5.5 L/hr/m^2.

Special Populations: *Age* Population pharmacokinetic analysis indicates that age (range 19 to 78 years) has no influence on the pharmacokinetics of temozolomide. In the anaplastic astrocytoma study population, patients 70 years of age or older had a higher incidence of Grade 4 neutropenia and Grade 4 thrombocytopenia in the first cycle of therapy than patients under 70 years of age (see **PRECAUTIONS**). In the entire safety database, however, there did not appear to be a higher incidence in patients 70 years of age or older (see **ADVERSE REACTIONS**).

Gender Population pharmacokinetic analysis indicates that women have an approximately 5% lower clearance (adjusted for body surface area) for temozolomide than men. Women have higher incidences of Grade 4 neutropenia and thrombocytopenia in the first cycle of therapy than men (see **ADVERSE REACTIONS**).

Race The effect of race on the pharmacokinetics of temozolomide has not been studied.

Tobacco Use Population pharmacokinetic analysis indicates that the oral clearance of temozolomide is similar in smokers and nonsmokers.

Creatinine Clearance Population pharmacokinetic analysis indicates that creatinine clearance over the range of 36–130 mL/min/m^2 has no effect on the clearance of temozolomide after oral administration. The pharmacokinetics of temozolomide have not been studied in patients with severely impaired renal function (CLcr < 36 mL/min/m^2). Caution should be exercised when TEMODAR is administered to patients with severe renal impairment. TEMODAR has not been studied in patients on dialysis.

Hepatically Impaired Patients In a pharmacokinetic study, the pharmacokinetics of temozolomide in patients with mild-to-moderate hepatic impairment (Child's-Pugh Class I–II) were similar to those observed in patients with normal hepatic function. Caution should be exercised when temozolomide is administered to patients with severe hepatic impairment.

Pediatrics Pediatric patients (3 to 17 years of age) and adult patients have similar clearance and half-life values for temozolomide. There is no clinical experience with the use of TEMODAR in children under the age of 3 years.

Drug-Drug Interactions In a multiple-dose study, administration of TEMODAR with ranitidine did not change the C_{max} or AUC values for temozolomide or MTIC.

Population analysis indicates that administration of valproic acid decreases the clearance of temozolomide by about 5% (see **PRECAUTIONS**).

Population analysis failed to demonstrate any influence of coadministered dexamethasone, prochlorperazine, phenytoin, carbamazepine, ondansetron, H_2-receptor antagonists, or phenobarbital on the clearance of orally administered temozolomide.

Clinical Studies A single-arm, multicenter study was conducted in 162 patients who had anaplastic astrocytoma at first relapse and who had a baseline Karnofsky performance status of 70 or greater. Patients had previously received radiation therapy and may also have previously received a nitrosourea with or without other chemotherapy. Fifty-four patients had disease progression on prior therapy with both a nitrosourea and procarbazine and their malignancy was considered refractory to chemotherapy (refractory anaplastic astrocytoma population). Median age of this subgroup of 54 patients was 42 years (19 to 76). Sixty-five percent were male. Seventy-two percent of patients had a KPS of ≥80. Sixty-three percent of patients had surgery other than a biopsy at the time of initial diagnosis. Of those patients undergoing resection, 73% underwent a subtotal resection and 27% underwent a gross total resection. Eighteen percent of patients had surgery at the time of first relapse. The median time from initial diagnosis to first relapse was 13.8 months (4.2 to 75.4).

TEMODAR was given for the first 5 consecutive days of a 28-day cycle at a starting dose of 150 mg/m^2/day. If the nadir and day of dosing (Day 29, Day 1 of next cycle) absolute neutrophil count was ≥1.5 × 10^9/L (1,500/µL) and the nadir and Day 29, Day 1 of next cycle, platelet count was ≥100 × 10^9/L (100,000/µL), the TEMODAR dose was increased to 200 mg/m^2/day for the first 5 consecutive days of a 28-day cycle.

In the refractory anaplastic astrocytoma population the overall tumor response rate (CR + PR) was 22% (12/54 patients) and the complete response rate was 9% (5/54 patients). The median duration of all responses was 50 weeks (range of 16 to 114 weeks) and the median duration of complete responses was 64 weeks (range of 52 to 114 weeks). In this population, progression-free survival at 6 months was 45% (95% confidence interval 31% to 58%) and progression-free survival at 12 months was 29% (95% confidence interval 16% to 42%). Median progression-free survival was 4.4 months. Overall survival at 6 months was 74% (95% confidence interval 62% to 86%) and 12-month overall survival was 65% (95% confidence interval 52% to 78%). Median overall survival was 15.9 months.

INDICATIONS AND USAGE

TEMODAR (temozolomide) Capsules are indicated for the treatment of adult patients with refractory anaplastic astrocytoma, ie, patients at first relapse who have experienced disease progression on a drug regimen containing a nitrosourea and procarbazine.

This indication is based on the response rate in the indicated population. No results are available from randomized controlled trials in recurrent anaplastic astrocytoma that demonstrate a clinical benefit resulting from treatment, such as improvement in disease-related symptoms, delayed disease progression, or improved survival.

CONTRAINDICATIONS

TEMODAR (temozolomide) Capsules are contraindicated in patients who have a history of hypersensitivity reaction to any of its components. TEMODAR is also contraindicated in patients who have a history of hypersensitivity to DTIC, since both drugs are metabolized to MTIC.

WARNINGS

Patients treated with TEMODAR may experience myelosuppression. Prior to dosing, patients must have an absolute neutrophil count (ANC) ≥1.5 × 10^9/L and a platelet count ≥100 × 10^9/L. A complete blood count should be obtained on Day 22 (21 days after the first dose) or within 48 hours of that day, and weekly until the ANC is above 1.5 × 10^9/L and platelet count exceeds 100 × 10^9/L. In the clinical trials, if the ANC fell to <1.0 × 10^9/L or the platelet count was <50 × 10^9/L during any cycle, the next cycle was reduced by 50 mg/m^2, but not below 100 mg/m^2. Patients who do not tolerate 100 mg/m^2 should not receive TEMODAR. Geriatric patients and women have been shown in clinical trials to have a higher risk of developing myelosuppression. Myelosuppression generally occurred late in the treatment cycle. The median nadirs occurred at 26 days for platelets (range 21 to 40 days) and 28 days for neutrophils (range 1 to 44 days). Only 14% (22/158) of patients had a neutrophil nadir and 20% (32/158) of patients had a platelet nadir which may have delayed the start of the next cycle. Neutrophil and platelet counts returned to normal, on average, within 14 days of nadir counts (see **PRECAUTIONS**).

Pregnancy: Temozolomide may cause fetal harm when administered to a pregnant woman. Five consecutive days of oral administration of 75 mg/m^2/day in rats and 150 mg/m^2/day in rabbits during the period of organogenesis (3/8 and 3/4 the maximum recommended human dose, respectively) caused numerous malformations of the external organs, soft tissues, and skeleton in both species. Doses of 150 mg/m^2/day in rats and rabbits also caused embryolethality as indicated by increased resorptions. There are no adequate and well-controlled studies in pregnant women. If this drug is used during pregnancy, or if the patient becomes pregnant while taking this drug, the patient should be apprised of the potential hazard to the fetus. Women of childbearing potential should be advised to avoid becoming pregnant during therapy with TEMODAR.

PRECAUTIONS

Information for Patients: In clinical trials, the most frequently occurring adverse effects were nausea and vomiting. These were usually either self-limiting or readily controlled with standard antiemetic therapy. Capsules should not be opened. If capsules are accidentally opened or damaged, rigorous precautions should be taken with the capsule contents to avoid inhalation or contact with the skin or mucous membranes. The medication should be kept away from children and pets.

Drug Interaction: Administration of valproic acid decreases oral clearance of temozolomide by about 5%. The clinical implication of this effect is not known.

Patients with Severe Hepatic or Renal Impairment: Caution should be exercised when TEMODAR is administered to patients with severe hepatic or renal impairment (see **Special Populations**).

Geriatrics: Clinical studies of temozolomide did not include sufficient numbers of subjects aged 65 and over to determine whether they responded differently from younger subjects. Other reported clinical experience has not identified differences in responses between the elderly and younger patients. Caution should be exercised when treating elderly patients.

In the anaplastic astrocytoma study population, patients 70 years of age or older had a higher incidence of Grade 4 neutropenia and Grade 4 thrombocytopenia (2/8; 25%, p=.31 and 2/10; 20%, p=.09, respectively) in the first cycle of therapy than patients under 70 years of age (see **ADVERSE REACTIONS**).

Laboratory Tests: A complete blood count should be obtained on Day 22 (21 days after the first dose). Blood counts should be performed weekly until recovery if the ANC falls below 1.5 × 10^9/L and the platelet count falls below 100 × 10^9/L.

Carcinogenesis, Mutagenesis, and Impairment of Fertility: Standard carcinogenicity studies were not conducted with temozolomide. In rats treated with 200 mg/m^2 temozolomide (equivalent to the maximum recommended daily human dose) on 5 consecutive days every 28 days for 3 cycles, mammary carcinomas were found in both males and females. With 6 cycles of treatment at 25, 50, and 125 mg/m^2 (about 1/8 to 1/2 the maximum recommended daily human dose), mammary carcinomas were observed at all doses and fibrosarcomas of the heart, eye, seminal vesicles, salivary glands, abdominal cavity, uterus, and prostate; carcinoma of the seminal vesicles, schwannoma of the heart, optic nerve, and harderian gland; and adenomas of the skin, lung, pituitary, and thyroid were observed at the high dose.

Temozolomide was mutagenic *in vitro* in bacteria (Ames assay) and clastogenic in mammalian cells (human peripheral blood lymphocyte assays).

Reproductive function studies have not been conducted with temozolomide. However, multicycle toxicology studies in rats and dogs have demonstrated testicular toxicity (syncytial cells/immature sperm, testicular atrophy) at doses of 50 mg/m^2 in rats and 125 mg/m^2 in dogs (1/4 and 5/8, respectively, of the maximum recommended human dose on a body surface area basis).

Pregnancy Category D: See **WARNINGS** section.

Nursing Mothers: It is not known whether this drug is excreted in human milk. Because many drugs are excreted in human milk and because of the potential for serious adverse reactions in nursing infants from TEMODAR, patients receiving TEMODAR should discontinue nursing.

Pediatric Use: Safety and effectiveness in pediatric patients have not been established.

ADVERSE REACTIONS

Tables 1 and **2** show the incidence of adverse events in the 158 patients in the anaplastic astrocytoma study for whom data are available. In the absence of a control group, it is not clear in many cases whether these events should be attributed to temozolomide or the patients' underlying conditions, but nausea, vomiting, fatigue, and hematologic effects appear to be clearly drug related. The most frequently occurring side effects were nausea, vomiting, headache, and fatigue. The adverse events were usually NCI Common Toxicity Criteria (CTC) Grade 1 or 2 (mild to moderate in severity) and were self-limiting, with nausea and vomiting readily controlled with antiemetics. The incidence of severe nausea and vomiting (CTC Grade 3 or 4) was 10% and 6%, respectively. Myelosuppression (thrombocytopenia and neutropenia) was the dose-limiting adverse event. It usually occurred within the first few cycles of therapy and was not cumulative.

Myelosuppression occurred late in the treatment cycle and returned to normal, on average, within 14 days of nadir counts. The median nadirs occurred at 26 days for platelets (range 21 to 40 days) and 28 days for neutrophils (range 1 to 44 days). Only 14% (22/158) of patients had a neutrophil nadir and 20% (32/158) of patients had a platelet nadir which may have delayed the start of the next cycle (see **WARNINGS**). Less than 10% of patients required hospitalization, blood transfusion, or discontinuation of therapy due to myelosuppression.

In clinical trial experience with 110 to 111 women and 169 to 174 men (depending on measurements), there were higher rates of Grade 4 neutropenia (ANC < 500 cells/µL) and thrombocytopenia (< 20,000 cells/µL) in women than men in the first cycle of therapy: (12% versus 5% and 9% versus 3%, respectively).

In the entire safety database for which hematologic data exist (N=932), 7% (4/61) and 9.5% (6/63) of patients over age 70 experienced Grade 4 neutropenia or thrombocytopenia in the first cycle, respectively. For patients less than or equal to age 70, 7% (62/871) and 5.5% (48/879) experienced Grade 4 neutropenia or thrombocytopenia in the first cycle, respectively. Pancytopenia, leukopenia, and anemia have also been reported.

In addition, the following spontaneous adverse experiences have been reported during the marketing surveillance of TEMODAR Capsules: allergic reactions including rare cases of anaphylaxis. Rare cases of erythema multiforme have been reported which resolved after discontinuation of TEMODAR and, in some cases, recurred upon rechallenge.

Table 1
Adverse Events in the Anaplastic Astrocytoma Trial (≥5%)

	No. (%) of TEMODAR Patients (N=158)	
	All Events	**Grade 3/4**
Any Adverse Event	153 (97)	79 (50)
Body as a Whole		
Headache	65 (41)	10 (6)
Fatigue	54 (34)	7 (4)
Asthenia	20 (13)	9 (6)
Fever	21 (13)	3 (2)
Back pain	12 (8)	4 (3)
Cardiovascular		
Edema peripheral	17 (11)	1 (1)
Central and Peripheral Nervous System		
Convulsions	36 (23)	8 (5)
Hemiparesis	29 (18)	10 (6)
Dizziness	19 (12)	1 (1)

Coordination abnormal	17 (11)	2 (1)
Amnesia	16 (10)	6 (4)
Insomnia	16 (10)	0
Paresthesia	15 (9)	1 (1)
Somnolence	15 (9)	5 (3)
Paresis	13 (8)	4 (3)
Urinary incontinence	13 (8)	3 (2)
Ataxia	12 (8)	3 (2)
Dysphasia	11 (7)	1 (1)
Convulsions local	9 (6)	0
Gait abnormal	9 (6)	1 (1)
Confusion	8 (5)	0
Endocrine		
Adrenal hypercorticism	13 (8)	0
Gastrointestinal System		
Nausea	84 (53)	16 (10)
Vomiting	66 (42)	10 (6)
Constipation	52 (33)	1 (1)
Diarrhea	25 (16)	3 (2)
Abdominal pain	14 (9)	2 (1)
Anorexia	14 (9)	1 (1)
Metabolic		
Weight increase	8 (5)	0
Musculoskeletal System		
Myalgia	8 (5)	
Psychiatric Disorders		
Anxiety	11 (7)	1 (1)
Depression	10 (6)	0
Reproductive Disorders		
Breast pain, female	4 (6)	
Resistance Mechanism Disorders		
Infection viral	17 (11)	0
Respiratory System		
Upper respiratory tract infection	13 (8)	0
Pharyngitis	12 (8)	0
Sinusitis	10 (6)	0
Coughing	8 (5)	0
Skin and Appendages		
Rash	13 (8)	0
Pruritus	12 (8)	2 (1)
Urinary System		
Urinary tract infection	12 (8)	0
Micturition increased frequency	9 (6)	0
Vision		
Diplopia	8 (5)	0
Vision Abnormal*	8 (5)	

*Blurred vision, visual deficit, vision changes, vision troubles.

Table 2
Adverse Hematologic Effects (Grade 3 to 4) in the Anaplastic Astrocytoma Trial

	TEMODAR[a]
Hemoglobin	7/158 (4%)
Neutrophils	20/142 (14%)
Platelets	29/156 (19%)
WBC	18/158 (11%)

[a]Change from Grade 0 to 2 at baseline to Grade 3 or 4 during treatment.

OVERDOSAGE

Doses of 500, 750, 1,000, and 1,250 mg/m^2 (total dose per cycle over 5 days) have been evaluated clinically in patients. Dose-limiting toxicity was hematologic and was reported at 1,000 mg/m^2 and at 1,250 mg/m^2. Up to 1,000 mg/m^2 has been taken as a single dose, with only the expected effects of neutropenia and thrombocytopenia resulting. In the event of an overdose, hematologic evaluation is needed. Supportive measures should be provided as necessary.

DOSAGE AND ADMINISTRATION

Dosage of TEMODAR must be adjusted according to nadir neutrophil and platelet counts in the previous cycle and neutrophil and platelet counts at the time of initiating the next cycle. The initial dose is 150 mg/m^2 orally once daily for 5 consecutive days per 28-day treatment cycle. If both the nadir and day of dosing (Day 29, Day 1 of next cycle) absolute neutrophil counts (ANC) are $\geq 1.5 \times 10^9$/L (1,500/μL) and both the nadir and Day 29, Day 1 of next cycle platelet counts are $\geq 100 \times 10^9$/L (100,000/μL), the TEMODAR dose may be increased to 200 mg/m^2/day for 5 consecutive days per 28-day treatment cycle. During treatment, a complete blood count should be obtained on Day 22 (21 days after the first dose) or within 48 hours of that day, and weekly until the ANC is above 1.5×10^9/L (1,500/μL) and the platelet count exceeds 100×10^9/L (100,000/μL). The next cycle of TEMODAR should not be started until the ANC and platelet count exceed these levels. If the ANC falls to $<1.0 \times 10^9$/L (1,000/μL) or the platelet count is $<50 \times 10^9$/L (50,000/μL) during any cycle, the next cycle should be reduced by 50 mg/m^2, but not below 100 mg/m^2, the lowest recommended dose (see **Table 3**) (see **WARNINGS**).
TEMODAR therapy can be continued until disease progression. In the clinical trial, treatment could be continued for a maximum of 2 years; but the optimum duration of therapy is not known. For TEMODAR dosage calculations based on body surface area (BSA), see **Table 4**. For suggested capsule combinations based on daily dose, see **Table 5**.

Table 3 Dosing Modification Table

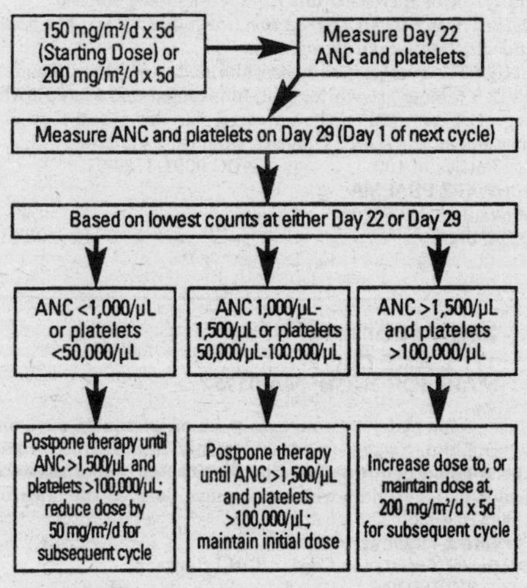

Table 4
Daily Dose Calculations by Body Surface Area (BSA) for 5 consecutive days per 28-day treatment cycle for the initial chemotherapy cycle (150 mg/m^2) and for subsequent chemotherapy cycles (200 mg/m^2) for patients whose nadir and day of dosing (Day 29, Day 1 of next cycle) absolute neutrophil count (ANC) is >1.5 $\times 10^9$/L (1,500/μL) and whose nadir and Day 29, Day 1 of next cycle platelet count is >100$\times 10^9$/L (100,000/μL).

Total BSA (m^2)	150 mg/m^2 (mg daily)	200 mg/m^2 (mg daily)
0.5	75	100
0.6	90	120
0.7	105	140
0.8	120	160
0.9	135	180
1.0	150	200
1.1	165	220
1.2	180	240
1.3	195	260
1.4	210	280
1.5	225	300
1.6	240	320
1.7	255	340
1.8	270	360
1.9	285	380
2.0	300	400
2.1	315	420
2.2	330	440
2.3	345	460
2.4	360	480
2.5	375	500

Table 5

Suggested Capsule Combinations Based on Daily Dose

	Number of Daily Capsules by Strength (mg)			
Total Daily Dose (mg)	250	100	20	5
200	0	2	0	0
205	0	2	0	1
210	0	2	0	2
215	0	2	0	3
220	0	2	1	0
225	0	2	1	1
230	0	2	1	2
235	0	2	1	3
240	0	2	2	0
245	0	2	2	1
250	1	0	0	0
255	1	0	0	1
260	1	0	0	2
265	1	0	0	3
270	1	0	1	0
275	1	0	1	1
280	1	0	1	2
285	1	0	1	3
290	1	0	2	0
295	1	0	2	1
300	0	3	0	0
305	0	3	0	1
310	0	3	0	2
315	0	3	0	3
320	0	3	1	0
325	0	3	1	1
330	1	0	4	0
335	1	0	4	1
340	0	3	2	0
345	0	3	2	1
350	1	1	0	0
355	1	1	0	1
360	1	1	0	2
365	1	1	0	3
370	1	1	1	0
375	1	1	1	1
380	1	1	1	2
385	1	1	1	3
390	1	1	2	0
395	1	1	2	1
400	0	4	0	0
405	0	4	0	1
410	0	4	0	2
415	0	4	0	3
420	0	4	1	0
425	0	4	1	1
430	1	1	4	0
435	0	4	1	3
440	0	4	2	0
445	0	4	2	1
450	1	2	0	0
455	1	2	0	1
460	1	2	0	2
465	1	2	0	3
470	1	2	1	0
475	1	2	1	1
480	1	2	1	2
485	1	2	1	3
490	1	2	2	0
495	1	2	2	1
500	2	0	0	0

In the clinical trial, TEMODAR was administered under both fasting and nonfasting conditions; however, absorption is affected by food (see **CLINICAL PHARMACOLOGY**) and consistency of administration with respect to food is recommended. There are no dietary restrictions with temozolomide. To reduce nausea and vomiting, temozolomide should be taken on an empty stomach. Bedtime administration may be advised. Antiemetic therapy may be administered prior to and/or following administration of TEMODAR.
TEMODAR (temozolomide) Capsules should not be opened or chewed. They should be swallowed whole with a glass of water.
Handling and Disposal: Temozolomide causes the rapid appearance of malignant tumors in rats. Capsules should not be opened. If capsules are accidentally opened or damaged, rigorous precautions should be taken with the capsule contents to avoid inhalation or contact with the skin or mucous membranes. Procedures for proper handling and disposal of anticancer drugs should be considered.[1-7] Several guidelines on this subject have been published. There is no general agreement that all of the procedures recommended in the guidelines are necessary or appropriate.

HOW SUPPLIED

TEMODAR (temozolomide) Capsules are supplied in amber glass bottles with child-resistant polypropylene caps containing the following capsule strengths:
TEMODAR (temozolomide) Capsules 5 mg: 5 and 20 capsule bottles.
5 count—NDC 0085-1248-01
20 count—NDC 0085-1248-02
TEMODAR (temozolomide) Capsules 20 mg: 5 and 20 capsule bottles.
5 count—NDC 0085-1244-01
20 count—NDC 0085-1244-02
TEMODAR (temozolomide) Capsules 100 mg: 5 and 20 capsule bottles.
5 count—NDC 0085-1259-01
20 count—NDC 0085-1259-02
TEMODAR (temozolomide) Capsules 250 mg: 5 and 20 capsule bottles.
5 count—NDC 0085-1252-01
20 count—NDC 0085-1252-02
Store at 25°C (77°F); excursions permitted to 15°–30°C (59°–86°F).

Continued on next page

Temodar—Cont.

[See USP Controlled Room Temperature]

REFERENCES

1. Recommendations for the Safe Handling of Parenteral Antineoplastic Drugs, NIH Publication No. 83-2621. For sale by the Superintendent of Documents, U.S. Government Printing Office, Washington, DC 20402.
2. AMA Council Report, Guidelines for Handling Parenteral Antineoplastics. *JAMA*. 1985;2.53(11):1590–1592.
3. National Study Commission on Cytotoxic Exposure—Recommendations for Handling Cytotoxic Agents. Available from Louis P. Jeffrey, ScD., Chairman, National Study Commission on Cytotoxic Exposure, Massachusetts College of Pharmacy and Allied Health Sciences, 179 Longwood Avenue, Boston, Massachusetts 02115.
4. Clinical Oncological Society of Australia, Guidelines and Recommendations for Safe Handling of Antineoplastic Agents. *Med J Australia*. 1983;1:426–428.
5. Jones RB, et al. Safe Handling Of Chemotherapeutic Agents: A Report from the Mount Sinai Medical Center. CA—*A Cancer Journal for Clinicians*. 1983;(Sept/Oct):258–263.
6. American Society of Hospital Pharmacists Technical Assistance Bulletin on Handling Cytotoxic and Hazardous Drugs. *Am J Hosp Pharm*. 1990;47:1033–1049.
7. Controlling Occupational Exposure to Hazardous Drugs. (OSHA Work-Practice Guidelines), *Am J Health-Syst Pharm*. 1996;53:1669–1685.

Schering Corporation
Kenilworth, NJ 07033 USA
Rev. 11/01 22487825

Schwarz Pharma, Inc.

6140 W. EXECUTIVE DRIVE
MEQUON, WI 53092

For Medical Information Contact:
Schwarz Pharma, Inc.
Professional Services
(262) 238-9994
(800) 558-5114

UNIRETIC™ ℞

[*yü-nə-retic*]
(moexipril hydrochloride/hydrochlorothiazide)
Tablets
7.5 mg/12.5 mg
15 mg/25 mg
Rx only

Prescribing information for this product, which appears on pages 3178–3181 of the 2002 PDR, has been revised as follows. Please write "See Supplement A" next to the product heading.

In the **Product Name** *listing:* **UNIRETIC™** *delete the ™ and replace it with* **®** *and insert* **15 mg/12.5 mg** *in between the "7.5 mg/12.5 mg" and "15 mg/25 mg".*

In the **DESCRIPTION** *section, the third paragraph that begins* "UNIRETIC is available for oral administration..." *has been revised as follows:*

UNIRETIC® is available for oral administration in three tablet strengths. The inactive ingredients in all strengths are lactose, magnesium oxide, crospovidone, magnesium stearate and gelatin. The film coating in all strengths contains hydroxypropyl methylcellulose, hydroxypropyl cellulose, polyethylene glycol 6000, magnesium stearate and titanium dioxide. In addition, the film coating for UNIRETIC® 7.5/12.5 and UNIRETIC® 15/25 contains ferric oxide.

In the **CLINICAL PHARMACOLOGY** *section, under the* **Pharmacodynamics and Clinical Effect/Moexipril-Hydrochlorothiazide** *heading, in the second paragraph, the second sentence that begins* "In UNIRETIC controlled clinical trials..." *has been revised as follows:*

In UNIRETIC® controlled clinical trials, the average change in serum potassium was near zero in subjects who received 3.75/6.25 mg or 7.5/12.5 mg, but subjects who received 15/12.5 mg or 15/25 mg experienced a mild decrease in serum potassium, similar to that experienced by subjects who received the same dose of hydrochlorothiazide monotherapy.

In the **PRECAUTIONS** *section, under the* **Drug Interactions** *heading, the first paragraph that begins "Potassium Supplements and Potassium-Sparing Diuretics..." has been revised as follows:*

Potassium Supplements and Potassium-Sparing Diuretics: As noted above (*Serum Electrolyte Imbalances*), the net effect of UNIRETIC® may be to elevate a patient's serum potassium, to reduce it, or to leave it unchanged. Potassium-sparing diuretics (spironolactone, amiloride, triamterene) or potassium supplements can increase the risk of hyperkalemia. If concomitant use of such agents is indicated, they should be given with caution, and the patient's serum potassium should be monitored.

In the **PRECAUTIONS** *section, under the* **Geriatric Use** *heading, in the second paragraph, the first sentence that begins "This drug is..." has been revised as follows:*

Hydrochlorothiazide is known to be substantially excreted by the kidney, and the risk of toxic reactions to this drug may be greater in patients with impaired renal function.

In the **DOSAGE AND ADMINISTRATION** *section, in the second paragraph, the third sentence that begins* "In UNIRETIC controlled clinical trials, ..." *has been revised as follows:*

In UNIRETIC® controlled clinical trials, the average change in serum potassium was near zero in subjects who received 3.75/6.25 mg or 7.5/12.5 mg, but subjects who received 15/12.5 mg or 15/25 mg experienced a mild decrease in serum potassium, similar to that experienced by subjects who received the same dose of hydrochlorothiazide monotherapy.

In the **DOSAGE AND ADMINISTRATION** *section, the third paragraph that begins* "Dose Titration Guided by Clinical Effect..." *has been revised as follows:*

Dose Titration Guided by Clinical Effect: A patient whose blood pressure is not adequately controlled with either moexipril or hydrochlorothiazide monotherapy may be given UNIRETIC® 7.5/12.5, UNIRETIC® 15/12.5 or UNIRETIC® 15/25 one hour before a meal. Further increases of moexipril, hydrochlorothiazide or both depend on clinical response. The hydrochlorothiazide dose should generally not be increased until 2–3 weeks have elapsed.

In the **HOW SUPPLIED** *section, the following text has been added as the second paragraph:*

UNIRETIC® (moexipril hydrochloride/hydrochlorothiazide) 15/12.5 tablets are white, oval, film-coated and scored with engraved code 720 on the unscored side and S and P on either side of the score. They are supplied as follows:

Bottles of 100 NDC 0091-3720-01

SCHWARZ PHARMA
Milwaukee, WI 53201
PC2459D Rev. 05/01

Sepracor Inc.

111 LOCKE DRIVE
MARLBOROUGH, MA 01752

For Medical Information for Healthcare Professionals Contact:
1-800-739-0565
For Direct Inquiries to the Customer Assistance Center (CAC) Contact:
1-877-SEPRACOR
FAX 1-508-357-7589
or write to Sepracor CAC at the address above.

XOPENEX® ℞

[*zō' pə-neks"*]
(levalbuterol HCl) Inhalation Solution,
0.31 mg*, 0.63 mg*, 1.25 mg*
***Potency expressed as levalbuterol**

Prescribing information for this product, which appears on pages 3207–3209 of the 2002 PDR, has been completely revised as follows. Please write "See Supplement A" next to the product heading.

PRESCRIBING INFORMATION

DESCRIPTION

Xopenex (levalbuterol HCl) Inhalation Solution is a sterile, clear, colorless, preservative-free solution of the hydrochloride salt of levalbuterol, the (R)-enantiomer of the drug substance racemic albuterol. Levalbuterol HCl is a relatively selective beta$_2$-adrenergic receptor agonist (see **CLINICAL PHARMACOLOGY**). The chemical name for levalbuterol HCl is (R)-α^1-[[(1,1-dimethylethyl)amino]methyl]-4-hydroxy-1,3-benzenedimethanol hydrochloride, and its established chemical structure is as follows:

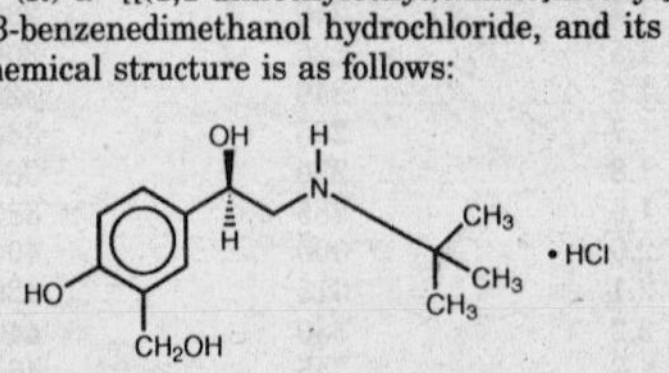

The molecular weight of levalbuterol HCl is 275.8, and its empirical formula is $C_{13}H_{21}NO_3 \bullet HCl$. It is a white to off-white, crystalline solid, with a melting point of approximately 187°C and solubility of approximately 180 mg/mL in water.

Levalbuterol HCl is the USAN modified name for (R)-albuterol HCl in the United States.

Xopenex (levalbuterol HCl) Inhalation Solution is supplied in unit-dose vials and requires no dilution before administration by nebulization. Each 3 mL unit-dose vial contains either 0.31 mg of levalbuterol (as 0.36 mg of levalbuterol HCl) or 0.63 mg of levalbuterol (as 0.73 mg of levalbuterol HCl) or 1.25 mg of levalbuterol (as 1.44 mg of levalbuterol HCl), sodium chloride to adjust tonicity, and sulfuric acid to adjust the pH to 4.0 (3.3 to 4.5).

CLINICAL PHARMACOLOGY

Activation of beta$_2$-adrenergic receptors on airway smooth muscle leads to the activation of adenylcyclase and to an increase in the intracellular concentration of cyclic-3′, 5′-adenosine monophosphate (cyclic AMP). This increase in cyclic AMP leads to the activation of protein kinase A, which inhibits the phosphorylation of myosin and lowers intracellular ionic calcium concentrations, resulting in relaxation. Levalbuterol relaxes the smooth muscles of all airways, from the trachea to the terminal bronchioles. Levalbuterol acts as a functional antagonist to relax the airway irrespective of the spasmogen involved, thus protecting against all bronchoconstrictor challenges. Increased cyclic AMP concentrations are also associated with the inhibition of release of mediators from mast cells in the airway.

While it is recognized that beta$_2$-adrenergic receptors are the predominant receptors on bronchial smooth muscle, data indicate that there is a population of beta$_2$-receptors in the human heart that comprise between 10% and 50% of cardiac beta-adrenergic receptors. The precise function of these receptors has not been established (see **WARNINGS**). However, all beta-adrenergic agonist drugs can produce a significant cardiovascular effect in some patients, as measured by pulse rate, blood pressure, symptoms, and/or electrocardiographic changes.

Preclinical Studies

Results from an *in vitro* study of binding to human beta-adrenergic receptors demonstrated that levalbuterol has approximately 2-fold greater binding affinity than racemic albuterol and approximately 100-fold greater binding affinity than (S)-albuterol. In guinea pig airways, levalbuterol HCl and racemic albuterol decreased the response to spasmogens (e.g., acetylcholine and histamine), whereas (S)-albuterol was ineffective. These results suggest that most of the bronchodilatory effect of racemic albuterol is due to the (R)-enantiomer.

Intravenous studies in rats with racemic albuterol sulfate have demonstrated that albuterol crosses the blood-brain barrier and reaches brain concentrations amounting to approximately 5.0% of the plasma concentrations. In structures outside the blood-brain barrier (pineal and pituitary glands), albuterol concentrations were found to be 100 times those in the whole brain.

Studies in laboratory animals (minipigs, rodents, and dogs) have demonstrated the occurrence of cardiac arrhythmias and sudden death (with histologic evidence of myocardial necrosis) when beta-agonists and methylxanthines are administered concurrently. The clinical significance of these findings is unknown.

Pharmacokinetics (Adults and Adolescents ≥12 years old)

The inhalation pharmacokinetics of Xopenex Inhalation Solution were investigated in a randomized cross-over study in 30 healthy adults following administration of a single dose of 1.25 mg and a cumulative dose of 5 mg of Xopenex Inhalation Solution and a single dose of 2.5 mg and a cumulative dose of 10 mg of racemic albuterol sulfate inhalation solution by nebulization using a PARI LC Jet™ nebulizer with a Dura-Neb® 2000 compressor.

Following administration of a single 1.25 mg dose of Xopenex Inhalation Solution, exposure to (R)-albuterol (AUC of 3.3 ng•hr/mL) was approximately 2-fold higher than following administration of a single 2.5 mg dose of racemic albuterol inhalation solution (AUC of 1.7 ng•hr/mL) (see **Table 1**). Following administration of a cumulative 5 mg dose of Xopenex Inhalation Solution (1.25 mg given every 30 minutes for a total of four doses) or a cumulative 10 mg dose of racemic albuterol inhalation solution (2.5 mg given every 30 minutes for a total of four doses), C_{max} and AUC of (R)-albuterol were comparable (see **Table 1**).

[See table 1 at top of next page]

Pharmacokinetics (Children 6–11 years old)

The pharmacokinetic parameters of (R)- and (S)-albuterol in children with asthma were obtained using population pharmacokinetic analysis. These data are presented in Table 2. For comparison, adult data obtained by conventional pharmacokinetic analysis from a different study are also presented in Table 2.

In children, AUC and C_{max} of (R)-albuterol following administration of 0.63 mg Xopenex Inhalation Solution were comparable to that following administration of 1.25 mg racemic albuterol sulfate inhalation solution.

Given the same dose of 0.63 mg of Xopenex to children and adults, the predicted C_{max} of (R)-albuterol in children was similar to that in adults (0.52 vs. 0.56 ng/mL), while predicted AUC in children (2.55 ng·hr/mL) was about 1.5-fold higher than that in adults (1.65 ng·hr/mL). These data support lower doses for children 6–11 years old compared to the adult doses (see **Dosage and Administration**).

[See table 2 at top of next page]

Pharmacodynamics

(Adults and Adolescents ≥12 years old)

In a randomized, double-blind, placebo-controlled, crossover study, 20 adults with mild-to-moderate asthma received single doses of Xopenex Inhalation Solution (0.31, 0.63, and 1.25 mg) and racemic albuterol sulfate inhalation solution (2.5 mg). All doses of active treatment produced a significantly greater degree of bronchodilation (as measured by percent change from pre-dose in mean FEV_1) than placebo, and there were no significant differences between any of the active treatment arms. The bronchodilator responses to 1.25 mg of Xopenex Inhalation Solution and 2.5 mg of racemic albuterol sulfate inhalation solution were clinically comparable over the 6-hour evaluation period, except for a slightly longer duration of action (>15% increase in FEV_1 from baseline) after administration of 1.25 mg of Xopenex Inhalation Solution. Systemic beta-adrenergic adverse effects were observed with all active doses and were generally dose-related for (R)-albuterol. Xopenex Inhalation Solution at a dose of 1.25 mg produced a slightly higher rate of systemic beta-adrenergic adverse effects than the 2.5 mg dose of racemic albuterol sulfate inhalation solution.

In a randomized, double-blind, placebo-controlled, crossover study, 12 adults with mild-to-moderate asthma were challenged with inhaled methacholine chloride 20 and 180 minutes following administration of a single dose of either 2.5 mg of racemic albuterol sulfate, 1.25 mg of Xopenex, 1.25 mg of (S)-albuterol, or placebo using a PARI LC Jet™ nebulizer. Racemic albuterol sulfate, Xopenex, and (S)-albuterol had a protective effect against methacholine-induced bronchoconstriction 20 minutes after administration, although the effect of (S)-albuterol was minimal. At 180 minutes after administration, the bronchoprotective effect of 1.25 mg of Xopenex was comparable to that of 2.5 mg of racemic albuterol sulfate. At 180 minutes after administration, 1.25 mg of (S)-albuterol had no bronchoprotective effect.

In a clinical study in adults with mild-to-moderate asthma, comparable efficacy (as measured by change from baseline in FEV_1) and safety (as measured by heart rate, blood pressure, ECG, serum potassium, and tremor) were demonstrated after a cumulative dose of 5 mg of Xopenex Inhalation Solution (four consecutive doses of 1.25 mg administered every 30 minutes) and 10 mg of racemic albuterol sulfate inhalation solution (four consecutive doses of 2.5 mg administered every 30 minutes).

Clinical Trials (Adults and Adolescents ≥12 years old)

The safety and efficacy of Xopenex Inhalation Solution were evaluated in a 4-week, multicenter, randomized, double-blind, placebo-controlled, parallel group study in 362 adult and adolescent patients 12 years of age and older, with mild-to-moderate asthma (mean baseline FEV_1 60% of predicted). Approximately half of the patients were also receiving inhaled corticosteroids. Patients were randomized to receive Xopenex 0.63 mg, Xopenex 1.25 mg, racemic albuterol sulfate 1.25 mg, racemic albuterol sulfate 2.5 mg, or placebo three times a day administered via a PARI LC Plus™ nebulizer and a Dura-Neb® portable compressor. Racemic albuterol delivered by a chlorofluorocarbon (CFC) metered dose inhaler (MDI) was used on an as-needed basis as the rescue medication.

Efficacy, as measured by the mean percent change from baseline in FEV_1, was demonstrated for all active treatment regimens compared with placebo on day 1 and day 29. On both day 1 (see **Figure 1**) and day 29 (see **Figure 2**), 1.25 mg of Xopenex demonstrated the largest mean percent change from baseline in FEV_1 compared to the other active treatments. A dose of 0.63 mg of Xopenex and 2.5 mg of racemic albuterol sulfate produced a clinically comparable mean percent change from baseline in FEV_1 on both day 1 and day 29.

Figure 1: Mean Percent Change from Baseline FEV_1 on Day 1, Adults and Adolescents ≥ 12 years old

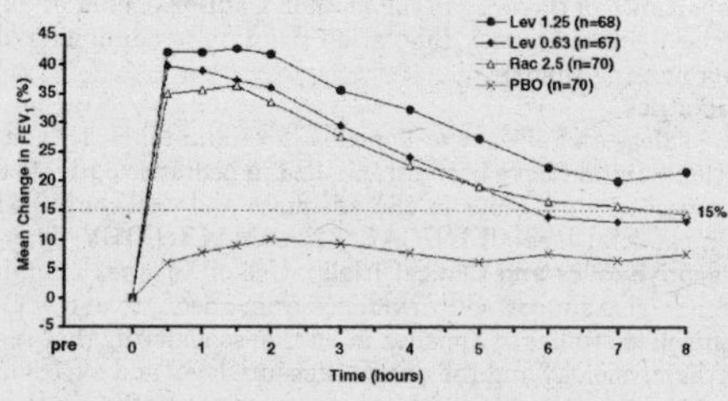

Figure 2: Mean Percent Change from Baseline FEV_1 on Day 29, Adults and Adolescents ≥ 12 years old

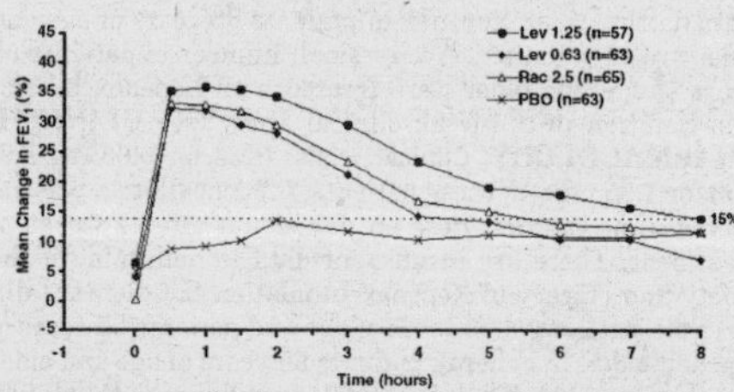

The mean time to onset of a 15% increase in FEV_1 over baseline for levalbuterol at doses of 0.63 mg and 1.25 mg was approximately 17 minutes and 10 minutes, respectively, and the mean time to peak effect for both doses was approximately 1.5 hours after 4 weeks of treatment. The mean duration of effect, as measured by a >15% increase from baseline in FEV_1, was approximately 5 hours after administration of 0.63 mg of levalbuterol and approximately 6 hours after administration of 1.25 mg of levalbuterol after 4 weeks of treatment. In some patients, the duration of effect was as long as 8 hours.

Clinical Trials (Children 6–11 years old)

A multi-center, randomized, double-blind, placebo- and active-controlled study was conducted in children with mild-to-moderate asthma (mean baseline FEV_1 73% of predicted) (n =316). Following a one week placebo run-in, subjects were randomized to Xopenex (0.31 or 0.63 mg), racemic albuterol (1.25 or 2.5 mg), or placebo, which were delivered three times a day for three weeks using a PARI LC Plus™ nebulizer and a Dura-Neb® 3000 compressor.

Efficacy, as measured by mean peak percent change from baseline in FEV_1, was demonstrated for all active treatment regimens compared with placebo on day 1 and day 21. Time profile FEV_1 curves for day 1 and day 21 are shown in Figure 3 and Figure 4, respectively. The onset of effect (time to a 15% increase in FEV_1 over test day baseline) and duration of effect (maintenance of a >15% increase in FEV_1 over test day baseline) of levalbuterol were clinically comparable to those of racemic albuterol.

Table 1: Mean (SD) Values for Pharmacokinetic Parameters in Healthy Adults

	Single Dose		Cumulative Dose	
	Xopenex 1.25 mg	Racemic albuterol sulfate 2.5 mg	Xopenex 5 mg	Racemic albuterol sulfate 10 mg
C_{max} (ng/mL) (R)-albuterol	1.1 (0.45)	0.8 (0.41)**	4.5 (2.20)	4.2 (1.51)**
T_{max} (h)$^{\gamma}$ (R)-albuterol	0.2 (0.17, 0.37)	0.2 (0.17, 1.50)	0.2 (−0.18*, 1.25)	0.2 (−0.28*, 1.00)
AUC (ng•h/mL) (R)-albuterol	3.3 (1.58)	1.7 (0.99)**	17.4 (8.56)	16.0 (7.12)**
$T_{½}$ (h) (R)-albuterol	3.3 (2.48)	1.5 (0.61)	4.0 (1.05)	4.1 (0.97)

$^{\gamma}$ Median (Min, Max) reported for T_{max}.
* A negative T_{max} indicates C_{max} occurred between first and last nebulizations.
**Values reflect only (R)-albuterol and do not include (S)-albuterol.

Table 2: (R)-Albuterol Exposure in Adults and Pediatric Subjects (6–11 years)

	Children 6–11 years				Adults ≥12 years	
Treatment	Xopenex 0.31 mg	Xopenex 0.63 mg	Racemic albuterol 1.25 mg	Racemic albuterol 2.5 mg	Xopenex 0.63 mg	Xopenex 1.25 mg
$AUC_{0-\infty}$ (ng·hr/mL) [c]	1.36	2.55	2.65	5.02	1.65 [a]	3.3 [b]
C_{max} (ng/mL) [d]	0.303	0.521	0.553	1.08	0.56 [a]	1.1 [b]

[a] The values are predicted by assuming linear pharmacokinetics
[b] The data obtained from Table 1
[c] Area under the plasma concentration curve from time 0 to infinity
[d] Maximum plasma concentration

Figure 3: Mean Percent Change from Baseline FEV_1 on Day 1, Children 6-11 Years of Age

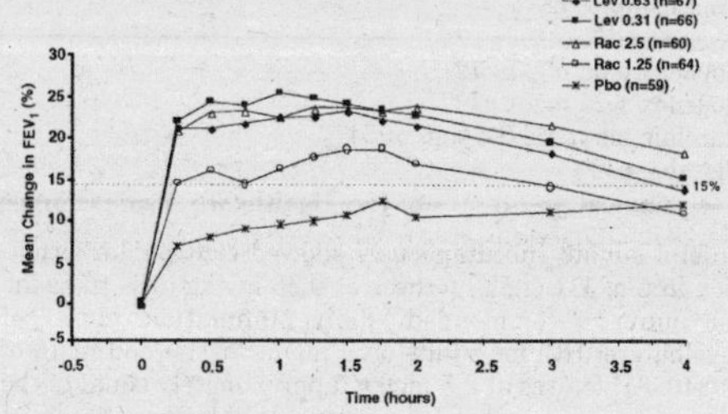

Figure 4: Mean Percent Change from Baseline FEV_1 on Day 21, Children 6-11 Years of Age

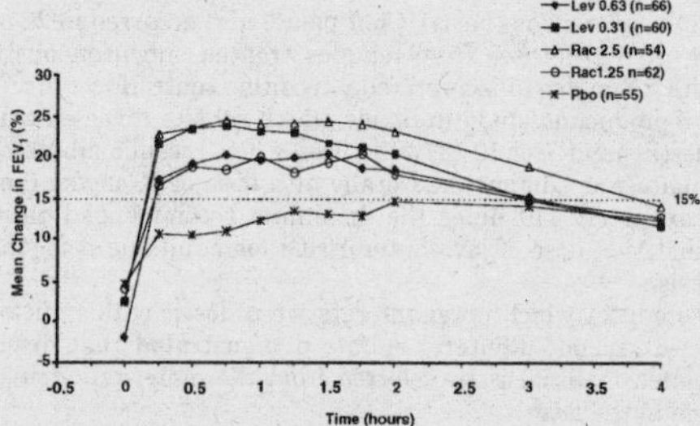

INDICATIONS AND USAGE

Xopenex (levalbuterol HCl) Inhalation Solution is indicated for the treatment or prevention of bronchospasm in adults, adolescents and children 6 years of age and older with reversible obstructive airway disease.

CONTRAINDICATIONS

Xopenex (levalbuterol HCl) Inhalation Solution is contraindicated in patients with a history of hypersensitivity to levalbuterol HCl or racemic albuterol.

WARNINGS

1. Paradoxical Bronchospasm: Like other inhaled beta-adrenergic agonists, Xopenex Inhalation Solution can produce paradoxical bronchospasm, which may be life threatening. If paradoxical bronchospasm occurs, Xopenex Inhalation Solution should be discontinued immediately and alternative therapy instituted. It should be recognized that paradoxical bronchospasm, when associated with inhaled formulations, frequently occurs with the first use of a new canister or vial.
2. Deterioration of Asthma: Asthma may deteriorate acutely over a period of hours or chronically over several days or longer. If the patient needs more doses of Xopenex Inhalation Solution than usual, this may be a marker of destabilization of asthma and requires reevaluation of the patient and treatment regimen, giving special consideration to the possible need for anti-inflammatory treatment, e.g., corticosteroids.
3. Use of Anti-Inflammatory Agents: The use of beta-adrenergic agonist bronchodilators alone may not be adequate to control asthma in many patients. Early consideration should be given to adding anti-inflammatory agents, e.g., corticosteroids, to the therapeutic regimen.
4. Cardiovascular Effects: Xopenex Inhalation Solution, like all other beta-adrenergic agonists, can produce a clinically significant cardiovascular effect in some patients, as measured by pulse rate, blood pressure, and/or symptoms. Although such effects are uncommon after administration of Xopenex Inhalation Solution at recommended doses, if they occur, the drug may need to be discontinued. In addition, beta-agonists have been reported to produce ECG changes, such as flattening of the T wave, prolongation of the QTc interval, and ST segment depression. The clinical significance of these findings is unknown. Therefore, Xopenex Inhalation Solution, like all sympathomimetic amines, should be used with caution in patients with cardiovascular disorders, especially coronary insufficiency, cardiac arrhythmias, and hypertension.
5. Do Not Exceed Recommended Dose: Fatalities have been reported in association with excessive use of inhaled sympathomimetic drugs in patients with asthma. The exact cause of death is unknown, but cardiac arrest following an unexpected development of a severe acute asthmatic crisis and subsequent hypoxia is suspected.
6. Immediate Hypersensitivity Reactions: Immediate hypersensitivity reactions may occur after administration of racemic albuterol, as demonstrated by rare cases of urticaria, angioedema, rash, bronchospasm, anaphylaxis, and oropharyngeal edema. The potential for hypersensitivity must be considered in the clinical evaluation of patients who experience immediate hypersensitivity reactions while receiving Xopenex Inhalation Solution.

PRECAUTIONS

General

Levalbuterol HCl, like all sympathomimetic amines, should be used with caution in patients with cardiovascular disorders, especially coronary insufficiency, hypertension, and cardiac arrhythmias; in patients with convulsive disorders, hyperthyroidism, or diabetes mellitus; and in patients who are unusually responsive to sympathomimetic amines. Clinically significant changes in systolic and diastolic blood pressure have been seen in individual patients and could be expected to occur in some patients after the use of any beta-adrenergic bronchodilator.

Large doses of intravenous racemic albuterol have been reported to aggravate preexisting diabetes mellitus and ketoacidosis. As with other beta-adrenergic agonist medications, levalbuterol may produce significant hypokalemia in some patients, possibly through intracellular shunting, which has the potential to produce adverse cardiovascular effects. The decrease is usually transient, not requiring supplementation.

Information for Patients

See illustrated Patient's Instructions for Use.

The action of Xopenex (levalbuterol HCl) Inhalation Solution may last up to 8 hours. Xopenex Inhalation Solution should not be used more frequently than recommended. Do not increase the dose or frequency of dosing of Xopenex Inhalation Solution without consulting your physician. If you find that treatment with Xopenex Inhalation Solution becomes less effective for symptomatic relief, your symptoms become worse, and/or you need to use the product more frequently than usual, you should seek medical attention immediately. While you are taking Xopenex Inhalation Solution, other inhaled drugs and asthma medications should be taken only as directed by your physician. Common adverse effects include palpitations, chest pain, rapid heart rate, headache, dizziness, and tremor or nervousness. If you are pregnant or nursing, contact your physician about the use of Xopenex Inhalation Solution.

Continued on next page

Xopenex—Cont.

Effective and safe use of Xopenex Inhalation Solution requires consideration of the following information in addition to that provided under Patient's Instructions for Use:
Xopenex Inhalation Solution single-use low-density polyethylene (LDPE) vials should be protected from light and excessive heat. Store in the protective foil pouch between 20°C and 25°C (68°F and 77°F) [see USP Controlled Room Temperature]. Do not use after the expiration date stamped on the container. Unused vials should be stored in the protective foil pouch. Once the foil pouch is opened, the vials should be used within two weeks. Vials removed from the pouch, if not used immediately, should be protected from light and used within one week. Discard any vial if the solution is not colorless.
The drug compatibility (physical and chemical), efficacy, and safety of Xopenex Inhalation Solution when mixed with other drugs in a nebulizer have not been established.

Drug Interactions

Other short-acting sympathomimetic aerosol bronchodilators or epinephrine should be used with caution with levalbuterol. If additional adrenergic drugs are to be administered by any route, they should be used with caution to avoid deleterious cardiovascular effects.

1. Beta-blockers: Beta-adrenergic receptor blocking agents not only block the pulmonary effect of beta-agonists such as Xopenex (levalbuterol HCl) Inhalation Solution, but may also produce severe bronchospasm in asthmatic patients. Therefore, patients with asthma should not normally be treated with beta-blockers. However, under certain circumstances, e.g., as prophylaxis after myocardial infarction, there may be no acceptable alternatives to the use of beta-adrenergic blocking agents in patients with asthma. In this setting, cardioselective beta-blockers could be considered, although they should be administered with caution.
2. Diuretics: The ECG changes and/or hypokalemia that may result from the administration of non-potassium sparing diuretics (such as loop or thiazide diuretics) can be acutely worsened by beta-agonists, especially when the recommended dose of the beta-agonist is exceeded. Although the clinical significance of these effects is not known, caution is advised in the coadministration of beta-agonists with non-potassium sparing diuretics.
3. Digoxin: Mean decreases of 16% and 22% in serum digoxin levels were demonstrated after single-dose intravenous and oral administration of racemic albuterol, respectively, to normal volunteers who had received digoxin for 10 days. The clinical significance of these findings for patients with obstructive airway disease who are receiving levalbuterol HCl and digoxin on a chronic basis is unclear. Nevertheless, it would be prudent to carefully evaluate the serum digoxin levels in patients who are currently receiving digoxin and Xopenex Inhalation Solution.
4. Monoamine Oxidase Inhibitors or Tricyclic Antidepressants: Xopenex Inhalation Solution should be administered with extreme caution to patients being treated with monoamine oxidase inhibitors or tricyclic antidepressants, or within 2 weeks of discontinuation of such agents, because the action of levalbuterol HCl on the vascular system may be potentiated.

Carcinogenesis, Mutagenesis, and Impairment of Fertility

No carcinogenesis or impairment of fertility studies have been carried out with levalbuterol HCl alone. However, racemic albuterol sulfate has been evaluated for its carcinogenic potential and ability to impair fertility.
In a 2-year study in Sprague-Dawley rats, racemic albuterol sulfate caused a significant dose-related increase in the incidence of benign leiomyomas of the mesovarium at and above dietary doses of 2 mg/kg (approximately 2 times the maximum recommended daily inhalation dose of levalbuterol HCl for adults and children on a mg/m^2 basis). In another study, this effect was blocked by the coadministration of propranolol, a nonselective beta-adrenergic antagonist. In an 18-month study in CD-1 mice, racemic albuterol sulfate showed no evidence of tumorigenicity at dietary doses up to 500 mg/kg (approximately 260 times the maximum recommended daily inhalation dose of levalbuterol HCl for adults and children on a mg/m^2 basis). In a 22-month study in the Golden hamster, racemic albuterol sulfate showed no evidence of tumorigenicity at dietary doses up to 50 mg/kg (approximately 35 times the maximum recommended daily inhalation dose of levalbuterol HCl for adults and children on a mg/m^2 basis).
Levalbuterol HCl was not mutagenic in the Ames test or the CHO/HPRT Mammalian Forward Gene Mutation Assay. Although levalbuterol HCl has not been tested for clastogenicity, racemic albuterol sulfate was not clastogenic in a human peripheral lymphocyte assay or in an AH1 strain mouse micronucleus assay. Reproduction studies in rats using racemic albuterol sulfate demonstrated no evidence of impaired fertility at oral doses up to 50 mg/kg (approximately 55 times the maximum recommended daily inhalation dose of levalbuterol HCl for adults on a mg/m^2 basis).

Teratogenic Effects—Pregnancy Category C

A reproduction study in New Zealand White rabbits demonstrated that levalbuterol HCl was not teratogenic when administered orally at doses up to 25 mg/kg (approximately 110 times the maximum recommended daily inhalation dose of levalbuterol HCl for adults on a mg/m^2 basis). However, racemic albuterol sulfate has been shown to be teratogenic in mice and rabbits. A study in CD-1 mice given racemic albuterol sulfate subcutaneously showed cleft palate formation in 5 of 111 (4.5%) fetuses at 0.25 mg/kg (less than the maximum recommended daily inhalation dose of levalbuterol HCl for adults on a mg/m^2 basis) and in 10 of 108 (9.3%) fetuses at 2.5 mg/kg (approximately equal to the maximum recommended daily inhalation dose of levalbuterol HCl for adults on a mg/m^2 basis). The drug did not induce cleft palate formation when administered subcutaneously at a dose of 0.025 mg/kg (less than the maximum recommended daily inhalation dose of levalbuterol HCl for adults on a mg/m^2 basis). Cleft palate also occurred in 22 of 72 (30.5%) fetuses from females treated subcutaneously with 2.5 mg/kg of isoproterenol (positive control).
A reproduction study in Stride Dutch rabbits revealed cranioschisis in 7 of 19 (37%) fetuses when racemic albuterol sulfate was administered orally at a dose of 50 mg/kg (approximately 110 times the maximum recommended daily inhalation dose of levalbuterol HCl for adults on a mg/m^2 basis).
A study in which pregnant rats were dosed with radiolabeled racemic albuterol sulfate demonstrated that drug-related material is transferred from the maternal circulation to the fetus.
There are no adequate and well-controlled studies of Xopenex Inhalation Solution in pregnant women. Because animal reproduction studies are not always predictive of human response, Xopenex Inhalation Solution should be used during pregnancy only if the potential benefit justifies the potential risk to the fetus.
During marketing experience of racemic albuterol, various congenital anomalies, including cleft palate and limb defects, have been rarely reported in the offspring of patients being treated with racemic albuterol. Some of the mothers were taking multiple medications during their pregnancies. No consistent pattern of defects can be discerned, and a relationship between racemic albuterol use and congenital anomalies has not been established.

Use in Labor and Delivery

Because of the potential for beta-adrenergic agonists to interfere with uterine contractility, the use of Xopenex Inhalation Solution for the treatment of bronchospasm during labor should be restricted to those patients in whom the benefits clearly outweigh the risk.

Tocolysis

Levalbuterol HCl has not been approved for the management of preterm labor. The benefit:risk ratio when levalbuterol HCl is administered for tocolysis has not been established. Serious adverse reactions, including maternal pulmonary edema, have been reported during or following treatment of premature labor with beta$_2$-agonists, including racemic albuterol.

Nursing Mothers

Plasma levels of levalbuterol after inhalation of therapeutic doses are very low in humans, but it is not known whether levalbuterol is excreted in human milk.
Because of the potential for tumorigenicity shown for racemic albuterol in animal studies and the lack of experience with the use of Xopenex Inhalation Solution by nursing mothers, a decision should be made whether to discontinue nursing or to discontinue the drug, taking into account the importance of the drug to the mother. Caution should be exercised when Xopenex Inhalation Solution is administered to a nursing woman.

Pediatrics

The safety and efficacy of Xopenex (levalbuterol HCl) Inhalation Solution have been established in pediatric patients 6 years of age and older in one adequate and well-controlled clinical trial (see **CLINICAL PHARMACOLOGY; Pharmacodynamics and Clinical Trials**). Use of Xopenex in children is also supported by evidence from adequate and well-controlled studies of Xopenex in adults, considering that the pathophysiology and the drug's exposure level and effects in pediatric and adult patients are substantially similar. Safety and effectiveness of Xopenex in pediatric patients below the age of 6 years have not been established.

Geriatrics

Data on the use of Xopenex in patients 65 years of age and older are very limited. A very small number of patients 65 years of age and older were treated with Xopenex Inhalation Solution in a 4-week clinical study (see **CLINICAL PHARMACOLOGY; Clinical Trials**) (n=2 for 0.63 mg and n=3 for 1.25 mg). In these patients, bronchodilation was observed after the first dose on day 1 and after 4 weeks of treatment. There are insufficient data to determine if the safety and efficacy of Xopenex Inhalation Solution are different in patients < 65 years of age and patients 65 years of age and older. In general, patients 65 years of age and older should be started at a dose of 0.63 mg of Xopenex Inhalation Solution. If clinically warranted due to insufficient bronchodilator response, the dose of Xopenex Inhalation Solution may be increased in elderly patients as tolerated, in conjunction with frequent clinical and laboratory monitoring, to the maximum recommended daily dose (see **DOSAGE AND ADMINISTRATION**).

ADVERSE REACTIONS

(Adults and Adolescents ≥12 years old)

Adverse events reported in ≥2% of patients receiving Xopenex Inhalation Solution or racemic albuterol and more frequently than in patients receiving placebo in a 4-week, controlled clinical trial are listed in **Table 4**.
[See table 4 above]
The incidence of certain systemic beta-adrenergic adverse effects (e.g., tremor, nervousness) was slightly less in the Xopenex 0.63 mg group as compared to the other active treatment groups. The clinical significance of these small differences is unknown.
Changes in heart rate 15 minutes after drug administration and in plasma glucose and potassium one hour after drug administration on day 1 and day 29 were clinically comparable in the Xopenex 1.25 mg and the racemic albuterol 2.5 mg groups (see **Table 5**). Changes in heart rate and plasma glucose were slightly less in the Xopenex 0.63 mg group compared to the other active treatment groups (see

Table 4: Adverse Events Reported in a 4-Week, Controlled Clinical Trial in Adults and Adolescents ≥12 years old

	Percent of Patients			
Body System Preferred Term	Placebo (n=75)	Xopenex 1.25 mg (n=73)	Xopenex 0.63 mg (n=72)	Racemic albuterol 2.5 mg (n=74)
Body as a Whole				
Allergic reaction	1.3	0	0	2.7
Flu syndrome	0	1.4	4.2	2.7
Accidental injury	0	2.7	0	0
Pain	1.3	1.4	2.8	2.7
Back pain	0	0	0	2.7
Cardiovascular System				
Tachycardia	0	2.7	2.8	2.7
Migraine	0	2.7	0	0
Digestive System				
Dyspepsia	1.3	2.7	1.4	1.4
Musculoskeletal System				
Leg cramps	1.3	2.7	0	1.4
Central Nervous System				
Dizziness	1.3	2.7	1.4	0
Hypertonia	0	0	0	2.7
Nervousness	0	9.6	2.8	8.1
Tremor	0	6.8	0	2.7
Anxiety	0	2.7	0	0
Respiratory System				
Cough increased	2.7	4.1	1.4	2.7
Infection viral	9.3	12.3	6.9	12.2
Rhinitis	2.7	2.7	11.1	6.8
Sinusitis	2.7	1.4	4.2	2.7
Turbinate edema	0	1.4	2.8	0

Table 5: Mean Changes from Baseline in Heart Rate at 15 Minutes and in Glucose and Potassium at 1 Hour after First Dose (Day 1) in Adults and Adolescents ≥12 years old

	Mean Changes (day 1)		
Treatment	Heart Rate (bpm)	Glucose (mg/dL)	Potassium (mEq/L)
Xopenex 0.63 mg, n=72	2.4	4.6	−0.2
Xopenex 1.25 mg, n=73	6.9	10.3	−0.3
Racemic albuterol 2.5 mg, n=74	5.7	8.2	−0.3
Placebo, n=75	−2.8	−0.2	−0.2

Table 6: Most Frequently Reported Adverse Events (≥2% in Any Treatment Group) and More Frequently Than Placebo During the Double-Blind Period (ITT Population, 6–11 Years Old)

Body System Preferred Term	Percent of Patients Placebo (n=59)	 Xopenex 0.31 mg (n=66)	 Xopenex 0.63 mg (n=67)	 Racemic albuterol 1.25 mg (n=64)	 Racemic albuterol 2.5 mg (n=60)
Body as a Whole					
Abdominal pain	3.4	0	1.5	3.1	6.7
Accidental injury	3.4	6.1	4.5	3.1	5.0
Asthenia	0	3.0	3.0	1.6	1.7
Fever	5.1	9.1	3.0	1.6	6.7
Headache	8.5	7.6	11.9	9.4	3.3
Pain	3.4	3.0	1.5	4.7	6.7
Viral Infection	5.1	7.6	9.0	4.7	8.3
Digestive System					
Diarrhea	0	1.5	6.0	1.6	0
Hemic and Lymphatic					
Lymphadenopathy	0	3.0	0	1.6	0
Musculoskeletal System					
Myalgia	0	0	1.5	1.6	3.3
Respiratory System					
Asthma	5.1	9.1	9.0	6.3	10.0
Pharyngitis	6.8	3.0	10.4	0	6.7
Rhinitis	1.7	6.1	10.4	3.1	5.0
Skin and Appendages					
Eczema	0	0	0	0	3.3
Rash	0	0	7.5	1.6	0
Urticaria	0	0	3.0	0	0
Special Senses					
Otitis Media	1.7	0	0	0	3.3

Note: Subjects may have more than one adverse event per body system and preferred term.

Table 7: Mean Changes from Baseline in Heart Rate at 30 Minutes and in Glucose and Potassium at 1 Hour after First Dose (Day 1) and Last Dose (Day 21) in Children 6–11 years old

Treatment	Mean Changes (Day 1) Heart Rate (bpm)	 Glucose (mg/dL)	 Potassium (mEq/L)
Xopenex 0.31 mg, n=66	0.8	4.9	−0.31
Xopenex 0.63 mg, n=67	6.7	5.2	−0.36
Racemic albuterol 1.25 mg, n=64	6.4	8.0	−0.27
Racemic albuterol 2.5 mg, n=60	10.9	10.8	−0.56
Placebo, n=59	−1.8	0.6	−0.05
	Mean Changes (Day 21) Heart Rate (bpm)	 Glucose (mg/dL)	 Potassium (mEq/L)
Xopenex 0.31 mg, n=60	0	2.6	−0.32
Xopenex 0.63 mg, n=66	3.8	5.8	−0.34
Racemic albuterol 1.25 mg, n=62	5.8	1.7	−0.18
Racemic albuterol 2.5 mg, n=54	5.7	11.8	−0.26
Placebo, n=55	−1.7	1.1	−0.04

Table 5). The clinical significance of these small differences is unknown. After 4 weeks, effects on heart rate, plasma glucose, and plasma potassium were generally diminished compared with day 1 in all active treatment groups.

[See table 5 at top of previous page]

No other clinically relevant laboratory abnormalities related to administration of Xopenex Inhalation Solution were observed in this study.

In the clinical trials, a slightly greater number of serious adverse events, discontinuations due to adverse events, and clinically significant ECG changes were reported in patients who received Xopenex 1.25 mg compared to the other active treatment groups.

The following adverse events, considered potentially related to Xopenex, occurred in less than 2% of the 292 subjects who received Xopenex and more frequently than in patients who received placebo in any clinical trial:

Body as a Whole:	chills, pain, chest pain
Cardiovascular System:	ECG abnormal, ECG change, hypertension, hypotension, syncope
Digestive System:	diarrhea, dry mouth, dry throat, dyspepsia, gastroenteritis, nausea
Hemic and Lymphatic System:	lymphadenopathy
Musculoskeletal System:	leg cramps, myalgia
Nervous System:	anxiety, hypesthesia of the hand, insomnia, paresthesia, tremor
Special Senses:	eye itch

The following events, considered potentially related to Xopenex, occurred in less than 2% of the treated subjects but at a frequency less than in patients who received placebo: asthma exacerbation, cough increased, wheezing, sweating, and vomiting.

ADVERSE REACTIONS (Children 6-11 years old)

Adverse events reported in ≥2% of patients in any treatment group and more frequently than in patients receiving placebo in a 3-week, controlled clinical trial are listed in Table 6.

[See table 6 above]

Changes in heart rate, plasma glucose, and serum potassium are shown in Table 7. The clinical significance of these small differences is unknown.

[See table 7 above]

OVERDOSAGE

The expected symptoms with overdosage are those of excessive beta-adrenergic receptor stimulation and/or occurrence or exaggeration of any of the symptoms listed under **ADVERSE REACTIONS**, e.g., seizures, angina, hypertension or hypotension, tachycardia with rates up to 200 beats/min., arrhythmias, nervousness, headache, tremor, dry mouth, palpitation, nausea, dizziness, fatigue, malaise, and sleeplessness. Hypokalemia also may occur. As with all sympathomimetic medications, cardiac arrest and even death may be associated with the abuse of Xopenex Inhalation Solution. Treatment consists of discontinuation of Xopenex Inhalation Solution together with appropriate symptomatic therapy. The judicious use of a cardioselective beta-receptor blocker may be considered, bearing in mind that such medication can produce bronchospasm. There is insufficient evidence to determine if dialysis is beneficial for overdosage of Xopenex Inhalation Solution.

The intravenous median lethal dose of levalbuterol HCl in mice is approximately 66 mg/kg (approximately 70 times the maximum recommended daily inhalation dose of levalbuterol HCl for adults and children on a mg/m^2 basis). The inhalation median lethal dose has not been determined in animals.

DOSAGE AND ADMINISTRATION

Children 6–11 years old: The recommended dosage of Xopenex (levalbuterol HCl) Inhalation Solution for patients 6–11 years old is 0.31 mg administered three times a day, by nebulization. Routine dosing should not exceed 0.63 mg three times a day.

Adults and Adolescents ≥12 years old: The recommended starting dosage of Xopenex (levalbuterol HCl) Inhalation Solution for patients 12 years of age and older is 0.63 mg administered three times a day, every 6 to 8 hours, by nebulization.

Patients 12 years of age and older with more severe asthma or patients who do not respond adequately to a dose of 0.63 mg of Xopenex Inhalation Solution may benefit from a dosage of 1.25 mg three times a day.

Patients receiving the highest dose of Xopenex Inhalation Solution should be monitored closely for adverse systemic effects, and the risks of such effects should be balanced against the potential for improved efficacy.

The use of Xopenex Inhalation Solution can be continued as medically indicated to control recurring bouts of bronchospasm. During this time, most patients gain optimal benefit from regular use of the inhalation solution.

If a previously effective dosage regimen fails to provide the expected relief, medical advice should be sought immediately, since this is often a sign of seriously worsening asthma that would require reassessment of therapy.

The drug compatibility (physical and chemical), efficacy, and safety of Xopenex Inhalation Solution when mixed with other drugs in a nebulizer have not been established.

The safety and efficacy of Xopenex Inhalation Solution have been established in clinical trials when administered using the PARI LC Jet™ and the PARI LC Plus™ nebulizers, and the PARI Master® Dura-Neb® 2000 and Dura-Neb® 3000 compressors. The safety and efficacy of Xopenex Inhalation Solution when administered using other nebulizer systems have not been established.

HOW SUPPLIED

Xopenex (levalbuterol HCl) Inhalation Solution is supplied in 3 mL unit-dose, low-density polyethylene (LDPE) vials as a clear, colorless, sterile, preservative-free, aqueous solution in three different strengths of levalbuterol (0.31 mg, 0.63 mg, 1.25 mg). Each strength of Xopenex Inhalation Solution is available in a shelf-carton containing one or more foil pouches, each containing 12 unit-dose LDPE vials.

Xopenex (levalbuterol HCl) Inhalation Solution, 0.31 mg *(foil pouch label color green)* contains 0.31 mg of levalbuterol (as 0.36 mg of levalbuterol HCl) and is available in cartons of 24 unit-dose LDPE vials (NDC 63402-511-24).

Xopenex (levalbuterol HCl) Inhalation Solution, 0.63 mg *(foil pouch label color yellow)* contains 0.63 mg of levalbuterol (as 0.73 mg of levalbuterol HCl) and is available in cartons of 24 unit-dose LDPE vials (NDC 63402-512-24).

Xopenex (levalbuterol HCl) Inhalation Solution, 1.25 mg *(foil pouch label color red)* contains 1.25 mg of levalbuterol (as 1.44 mg of levalbuterol HCl) and is available in cartons of 24 unit-dose LDPE vials (NDC 63402-513-24).

CAUTION

Federal law (U.S.) prohibits dispensing without prescription.

Store the Xopenex (levalbuterol HCl) Inhalation Solution in the protective foil pouch at 20–25°C (68–77°F) [see USP Controlled Room Temperature]. Protect from light and excessive heat. Keep unopened vials in the foil pouch. Once the foil pouch is opened, the vials should be used within two weeks. Vials removed from the pouch, if not used immediately, should be protected from light and used within one week. Discard any vial if the solution is not colorless.

Manufactured for:
Sepracor Inc.
Marlborough, MA 01752 USA
by Automatic Liquid Packaging, Woodstock, IL 60098 USA
1-877-SEPRACOR
To report adverse events, call 1-877-737-7226.
For medical information, call 1-800-739-0565.
January 2002
400437-R2

PHARMACIST—DETACH HERE AND GIVE INSTRUCTIONS TO PATIENT

Patient's Instructions for Use

Xopenex® (levalbuterol HCl) Inhalation Solution; 0.31 mg*, 0.63 mg*, 1.25 mg*; 3 mL Unit-Dose Vials

***Potency expressed as levalbuterol**

Read complete instructions carefully before using.

1. Open the foil pouch by tearing on the serrated edge along the seam of the pouch. Remove one unit-dose vial for immediate use. Keep the rest of the unused unit-dose vials in the foil pouch to protect them from light.
2. Carefully twist open the top of one unit-dose vial (**Figure 1**) and squeeze the entire contents into the nebulizer reservoir.

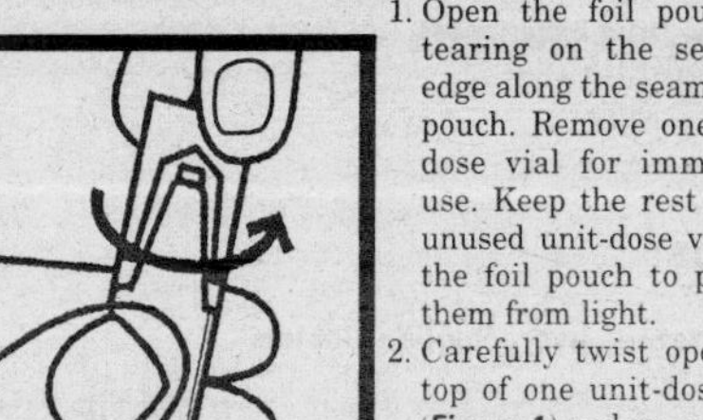

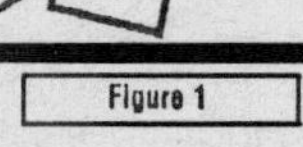
Figure 1

Continued on next page

Xopenex—Cont.

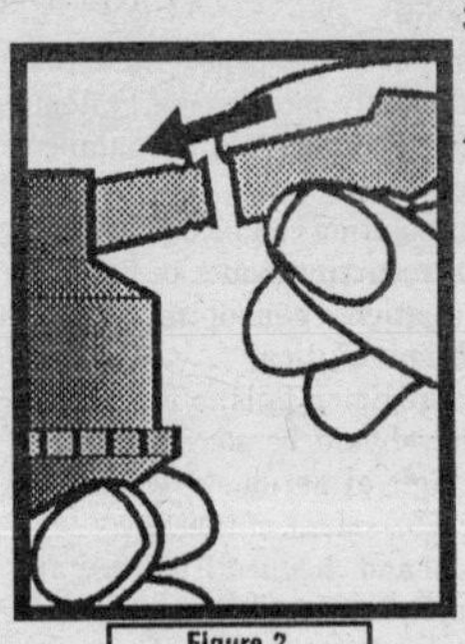

Figure 2

3. Connect the nebulizer reservoir to the mouthpiece or face mask (**Figure 2**).
4. Connect the nebulizer to the compressor.

Figure 3

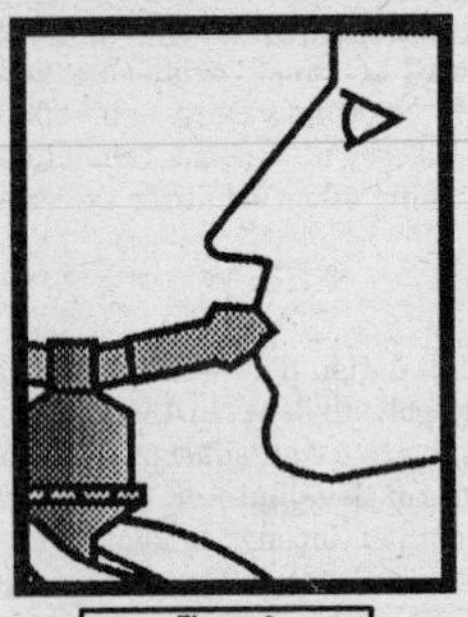

5. Sit in a comfortable, upright position. Place the mouthpiece in your mouth (**Figure 3**) (or put on the face mask) and turn on the compressor.
6. Breathe as calmly, deeply, and evenly as possible until no more mist is formed in the nebulizer reservoir (about 5 to 15 minutes). At this point, the treatment is finished.
7. Clean the nebulizer (see manufacturer's instructions).

Note: Xopenex (levalbuterol HCl) Inhalation Solution should be used in a nebulizer only under the direction of a physician. More frequent administration or higher doses are not recommended without first discussing with your doctor. This solution should not be injected or administered orally. Protect from light and excessive heat. Store in the protective foil pouch at 20–25°C (68–77°F) [see USP Controlled Room Temperature]. Keep unopened vials in the foil pouch. Once the foil pouch is opened, the vials should be used within two weeks. Vials removed from the pouch, if not used immediately, should be protected from light and used within one week. Discard any vial if the solution is not colorless.
The safety and effectiveness of Xopenex Inhalation Solution have not been determined when one or more drugs are mixed with it in a nebulizer. Check with your doctor before mixing any medications in your nebulizer.
Manufactured for:
Sepracor Inc.
Marlborough, MA 01752 USA
by Automatic Liquid Packaging, Woodstock, IL 60098 USA
1-877-SEPRACOR
To report adverse events, call 1-877-737-7226.
For medical information, call 1-800-739-0565.
January 2002
400437-R2

Takeda Pharmaceuticals America, Inc.

475 HALF DAY ROAD, SUITE 500
LINCOLNSHIRE, IL 60069

Direct Inquiries to:
Sales and Ordering:
Customer Service
(877) 5 TAKEDA
(877) 582-5332

For Medical Information Contact:
Generally:
(877) TAKEDA 7
(877) 825-3327

Adverse Drug Experiences:
(877) TAKEDA 7
(877) 825-3327

ACTOS® ℞

[*act-ōs*]
(pioglitazone hydrochloride) Tablets

Prescribing information for this product, which appears on pages 3275–3279 of the 2002 PDR, has been completely revised as follows. Please write "See Supplement A" next to the product heading.

DESCRIPTION

ACTOS (pioglitazone hydrochloride) is an oral antidiabetic agent that acts primarily by decreasing insulin resistance. ACTOS is used in the management of type 2 diabetes mellitus (also known as non-insulin-dependent diabetes mellitus [NIDDM] or adult-onset diabetes). Pharmacological studies indicate that ACTOS improves sensitivity to insulin in muscle and adipose tissue and inhibits hepatic gluconeogenesis. ACTOS improves glycemic control while reducing circulating insulin levels.
Pioglitazone [(±)-5-[[4-[2-(5-ethyl-2-pyridinyl)ethoxy]phenyl]methyl]-2,4-] thiazolidinedione monohydrochloride belongs to a different chemical class and has a different pharmacological action than the sulfonylureas, metformin, or the α-glucosidase inhibitors. The molecule contains one asymmetric carbon, and the compound is synthesized and used as the racemic mixture. The two enantiomers of pioglitazone inter-convert in vivo. No differences were found in the pharmacologic activity between the two enantiomers.
The structural formula is as shown:

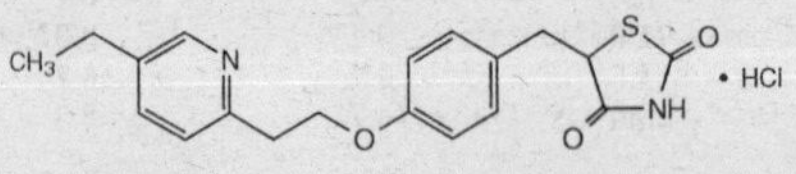

Pioglitazone hydrochloride is an odorless white crystalline powder that has a molecular formula of $C_{19}H_{20}N_2O_3S \bullet HCl$ and a molecular weight of 392.90 daltons. It is soluble in N,N-dimethylformamide, slightly soluble in anhydrous ethanol, very slightly soluble in acetone and acetonitrile, practically insoluble in water, and insoluble in ether.
ACTOS is available as a tablet for oral administration containing 15 mg, 30 mg, or 45 mg of pioglitazone (as the base) formulated with the following excipients: lactose monohydrate NF, hydroxypropylcellulose NF, carboxymethylcellulose calcium NF, and magnesium stearate NF.

CLINICAL PHARMACOLOGY

Mechanism of Action
ACTOS is a thiazolidinedione antidiabetic agent that depends on the presence of insulin for its mechanism of action. ACTOS decreases insulin resistance in the periphery and in the liver resulting in increased insulin-dependent glucose disposal and decreased hepatic glucose output. Unlike sulfonylureas, pioglitazone is not an insulin secretagogue. Pioglitazone is a potent and highly selective agonist for peroxisome proliferator-activated receptor-gamma (PPARγ). PPAR receptors are found in tissues important for insulin action such as adipose tissue, skeletal muscle, and liver. Activation of PPARγ nuclear receptors modulates the transcription of a number of insulin responsive genes involved in the control of glucose and lipid metabolism.
In animal models of diabetes, pioglitazone reduces the hyperglycemia, hyperinsulinemia, and hypertriglyceridemia characteristic of insulin-resistant states such as type 2 diabetes. The metabolic changes produced by pioglitazone result in increased responsiveness of insulin-dependent tissues and are observed in numerous animal models of insulin resistance.
Since pioglitazone enhances the effects of circulating insulin (by decreasing insulin resistance), it does not lower blood glucose in animal models that lack endogenous insulin.

Pharmacokinetics and Drug Metabolism
Serum concentrations of total pioglitazone (pioglitazone plus active metabolites) remain elevated 24 hours after once daily dosing. Steady-state serum concentrations of both pioglitazone and total pioglitazone are achieved within 7 days. At steady-state, two of the pharmacologically active metabolites of pioglitazone, Metabolites III (M-III) and IV (M-IV), reach serum concentrations equal to or greater than pioglitazone. In both healthy volunteers and in patients with type 2 diabetes, pioglitazone comprises approximately 30% to 50% of the peak total pioglitazone serum concentrations and 20% to 25% of the total area under the serum concentration-time curve (AUC).
Maximum serum concentration (C_{max}), AUC, and trough serum concentrations (C_{min}) for both pioglitazone and total pioglitazone increase proportionally at doses of 15 mg and 30 mg per day. There is a slightly less than proportional increase for pioglitazone and total pioglitazone at a dose of 60 mg per day.
Absorption: Following oral administration, in the fasting state, pioglitazone is first measurable in serum within 30 minutes, with peak concentrations observed within 2 hours. Food slightly delays the time to peak serum concentration to 3 to 4 hours, but does not alter the extent of absorption.
Distribution: The mean apparent volume of distribution (Vd/F) of pioglitazone following single-dose administration is 0.63 ± 0.41 (mean ± SD) L/kg of body weight. Pioglitazone is extensively protein bound (> 99%) in human serum, principally to serum albumin. Pioglitazone also binds to other serum proteins, but with lower affinity. Metabolites M-III and M-IV also are extensively bound (> 98%) to serum albumin.
Metabolism: Pioglitazone is extensively metabolized by hydroxylation and oxidation; the metabolites also partly convert to glucuronide or sulfate conjugates. Metabolites M-II and M-IV (hydroxy derivatives of pioglitazone) and M-III (keto derivative of pioglitazone) are pharmacologically active in animal models of type 2 diabetes. In addition to pioglitazone, M-III and M-IV are the principal drug-related species found in human serum following multiple dosing. At steady-state, in both healthy volunteers and in patients with type 2 diabetes, pioglitazone comprises approximately 30% to 50% of the total peak serum concentrations and 20% to 25% of the total AUC.
Pioglitazone incubated with expressed human P450 or human liver microsomes results in the formation of M-IV and to a much lesser degree, M-II. The major cytochrome P450 isoforms involved in the hepatic metabolism of pioglitazone are CYP2C8 and CYP3A4 with contributions from a variety of other isoforms including the mainly extrahepatic CYP1A1. Ketoconazole inhibited up to 85% of hepatic pioglitazone metabolism in vitro at a concentration equal molar to pioglitazone. Pioglitazone did not inhibit P450 activity when incubated with human P450 liver microsomes. In vivo human studies have not been performed to investigate any induction of CYP3A4 by pioglitazone.
Excretion and Elimination: Following oral administration, approximately 15% to 30% of the pioglitazone dose is recovered in the urine. Renal elimination of pioglitazone is negligible, and the drug is excreted primarily as metabolites and their conjugates. It is presumed that most of the oral dose is excreted into the bile either unchanged or as metabolites and eliminated in the feces.
The mean serum half-life of pioglitazone and total pioglitazone ranges from 3 to 7 hours and 16 to 24 hours, respectively. Pioglitazone has an apparent clearance, CL/F, calculated to be 5 to 7 L/hr.

Special Populations
Renal Insufficiency: The serum elimination half-life of pioglitazone, M-III, and M-IV remains unchanged in patients with moderate (creatinine clearance 30 to 60 mL/min) to severe (creatinine clearance < 30 mL/min) renal impairment when compared to normal subjects. No dose adjustment in patients with renal dysfunction is recommended (see DOSAGE AND ADMINISTRATION).
Hepatic Insufficiency: Compared with normal controls, subjects with impaired hepatic function (Child-Pugh Grade B/C) have an approximate 45% reduction in pioglitazone and total pioglitazone mean peak concentrations but no change in the mean AUC values.
ACTOS therapy should not be initiated if the patient exhibits clinical evidence of active liver disease or serum transaminase levels (ALT) exceed 2.5 times the upper limit of normal (see PRECAUTIONS, Hepatic Effects).
Elderly: In healthy elderly subjects, peak serum concentrations of pioglitazone and total pioglitazone are not significantly different, but AUC values are slightly higher and the terminal half-life values slightly longer than for younger subjects. These changes were not of a magnitude that would be considered clinically relevant.
Pediatrics: Pharmacokinetic data in the pediatric population are not available.
Gender: The mean C_{max} and AUC values were increased 20% to 60% in females. As monotherapy and in combination with sulfonylurea, metformin, or insulin, ACTOS improved glycemic control in both males and females. In controlled clinical trials, hemoglobin A_{1c} (HbA_{1c}) decreases from baseline were generally greater for females than for males (average mean difference in HbA_{1c} 0.5%). Since therapy should be individualized for each patient to achieve glycemic control, no dose adjustment is recommended based on gender alone.
Ethnicity: Pharmacokinetic data among various ethnic groups are not available.

Pharmacodynamics and Clinical Effects
Clinical studies demonstrate that ACTOS improves insulin sensitivity in insulin-resistant patients. ACTOS enhances cellular responsiveness to insulin, increases insulin-dependent glucose disposal, improves hepatic sensitivity to insulin, and improves dysfunctional glucose homeostasis. In patients with type 2 diabetes, the decreased insulin resistance produced by ACTOS results in lower blood glucose concentrations, lower plasma insulin levels, and lower HbA_{1c} values. Based on results from an open-label extension study, the glucose lowering effects of ACTOS appear to persist for at least one year. In controlled clinical trials, ACTOS in combination with sulfonylurea, metformin, or insulin had an additive effect on glycemic control.
Patients with lipid abnormalities were included in clinical trials with ACTOS. Overall, patients treated with ACTOS had mean decreases in triglycerides, mean increases in HDL cholesterol, and no consistent mean changes in LDL and total cholesterol.
In a 26-week, placebo-controlled, dose-ranging study, mean triglyceride levels decreased in the 15 mg, 30 mg, and 45 mg ACTOS dose groups compared to a mean increase in the placebo group. Mean HDL levels increased to a greater extent in patients treated with ACTOS than in the placebo-treated patients. There were no consistent differences for LDL and total cholesterol in patients treated with ACTOS compared to placebo (Table 1).
[See table 1 at top of next page]
In the two other monotherapy studies (24 weeks and 16 weeks) and in combination therapy studies with sulfonylurea (16 weeks) and metformin (16 weeks), the results were generally consistent with the data above. For patients treated with ACTOS, the placebo-corrected mean changes from baseline decreased 5% to 26% for triglycerides and increased 6% to 13% for HDL cholesterol.
In the combination therapy study with insulin (16 weeks), the placebo-corrected mean percent change from baseline in triglyceride values for patients treated with ACTOS was also decreased. A placebo-corrected mean change from baseline in LDL cholesterol of 7% was observed for the 15 mg dose group. Similar results to those noted above for HDL and total cholesterol were observed.

CLINICAL STUDIES

Monotherapy
In the U.S., three randomized, double-blind, placebo-controlled trials with durations from 16 to 26 weeks were conducted to evaluate the use of ACTOS as monotherapy in patients with type 2 diabetes. These studies examined ACTOS at doses up to 45 mg or placebo once daily in 865 patients.
In a 26-week dose-ranging study, 408 patients with type 2 diabetes were randomized to receive 7.5 mg, 15 mg, 30 mg, or 45 mg of ACTOS, or placebo once daily. Therapy with any

previous antidiabetic agent was discontinued 8 weeks prior to the double-blind period. Treatment with 15 mg, 30 mg, and 45 mg of ACTOS produced statistically significant improvements in HbA_{1c} and fasting blood glucose (FBG) at endpoint compared to placebo (see Figure 1, Table 2).

Figure 1 shows the time course for changes in FBG and HbA_{1c} for the entire study population in this 26-week study.

[See figure 1 above]

Table 2 shows HbA_{1c} and FBG values for the entire study population.

[See table 2 above]

The study population included patients not previously treated with antidiabetic medication (naïve; 31%) and patients who were receiving antidiabetic medication at the time of study enrollment (previously treated; 69%). The data for the naïve and previously treated patient subsets are shown in Table 3. All patients entered an 8 week washout/run-in period prior to double-blind treatment. This run-in period was associated with little change in HbA_{1c} and FBG values from screening to baseline for the naïve patients; however, for the previously-treated group, washout from previous antidiabetic medication resulted in deterioration of glycemic control and increases in HbA_{1c} and FBG. Although most patients in the previously-treated group had a decrease from baseline in HbA_{1c} and FBG with ACTOS, in many cases the values did not return to screening levels by the end of the study. The study design did not permit the evaluation of patients who switched directly to ACTOS from another antidiabetic agent.

[See table 3 above]

In a 24-week study, 260 patients with type 2 diabetes were randomized to one of two forced-titration ACTOS treatment groups or a mock titration placebo group. Therapy with any previous antidiabetic agent was discontinued 6 weeks prior to the double-blind period. In one ACTOS treatment group, patients received an initial dose of 7.5 mg once daily. After four weeks, the dose was increased to 15 mg once daily and after another four weeks, the dose was increased to 30 mg once daily for the remainder of the study (16 weeks). In the second ACTOS treatment group, patients received an initial dose of 15 mg once daily and were titrated to 30 mg once daily and 45 mg once daily in a similar manner. Treatment with ACTOS, as described, produced statistically significant improvements in HbA_{1c} and FBG at endpoint compared to placebo (see Table 4).

[See table 4 at top of next page]

For patients who had not been previously treated with antidiabetic medication (24%), mean values at screening were 10.1% for HbA_{1c} and 238 mg/dL for FBG. At baseline, mean HbA_{1c} was 10.2% and mean FBG was 243 mg/dL. Compared with placebo, treatment with ACTOS titrated to a final dose of 30 mg and 45 mg resulted in reductions from baseline in mean HbA_{1c} of 2.3% and 2.6% and mean FBG of 63 mg/dL and 95 mg/dL, respectively. For patients who had been previously treated with antidiabetic medication (76%), this medication was discontinued at screening. Mean values at screening were 9.4% for HbA_{1c} and 216 mg/dL for FBG. At baseline, mean HbA_{1c} was 10.7% and mean FBG was 290 mg/dL. Compared with placebo, treatment with ACTOS titrated to a final dose of 30 mg and 45 mg resulted in reductions from baseline in mean HbA_{1c} of 1.3% and 1.4% and mean FBG of 55 mg/dL and 60 mg/dL, respectively. For many previously-treated patients, HbA_{1c} and FBG had not returned to screening levels by the end of the study.

In a 16-week study, 197 patients with type 2 diabetes were randomized to treatment with 30 mg of ACTOS or placebo once daily. Therapy with any previous antidiabetic agent was discontinued 6 weeks prior to the double-blind period. Treatment with 30 mg of ACTOS produced statistically significant improvements in HbA_{1c} and FBG at endpoint compared to placebo (see Table 5).

[See table 5 at top of next page]

For patients who had not been previously treated with antidiabetic medication (40%), mean values at screening were 10.3% for HbA_{1c} and 240 mg/dL for FBG. At baseline, mean HbA_{1c} was 10.4% and mean FBG was 254 mg/dL. Compared with placebo, treatment with ACTOS 30 mg resulted in reductions from baseline in mean HbA_{1c} of 1.0% and mean FBG of 62 mg/dL. For patients who had been previously treated with antidiabetic medication (60%), this medication was discontinued at screening. Mean values at screening were 9.4% for HbA_{1c} and 216 mg/dL for FBG. At baseline, mean HbA_{1c} was 10.6% and mean FBG was 287 mg/dL. Compared with placebo, treatment with ACTOS 30 mg resulted in reductions from baseline in mean HbA_{1c} of 1.3% and mean FBG of 46 mg/dL. For many previously-treated patients, HbA_{1c} and FBG had not returned to screening levels by the end of the study.

Combination Therapy

Three 16-week, randomized, double-blind, placebo-controlled clinical studies were conducted to evaluate the effects of ACTOS on glycemic control in patients with type 2 diabetes who were inadequately controlled ($HbA_{1c} \geq 8\%$) despite current therapy with a sulfonylurea, metformin, or insulin. Previous diabetes treatment may have been monotherapy or combination therapy.

In one combination study, 560 patients with type 2 diabetes on a sulfonylurea, either alone or combined with another antidiabetic agent, were randomized to receive 15 mg or 30 mg of ACTOS or placebo once daily in addition to their current sulfonylurea regimen. Any other antidiabetic agent was withdrawn. Compared with placebo, the addition of ACTOS to the sulfonylurea significantly reduced the mean HbA_{1c} by 0.9% and 1.3% for the 15 mg and 30 mg doses, respectively. Compared with placebo, mean FBG decreased by 39 mg/dL (15 mg dose) and 58 mg/dL (30 mg dose). The therapeutic effect of ACTOS in combination with sulfonylurea was observed in patients regardless of whether the patients were receiving low, medium, or high doses of sulfonylurea (< 50%, 50%, or > 50% of the recommended maximum daily dose).

In a second combination study, 328 patients with type 2 diabetes on metformin either alone or combined with another antidiabetic agent, were randomized to receive either 30 mg of ACTOS or placebo once daily in addition to their metformin. Any other antidiabetic agent was withdrawn. Compared to placebo, the addition of ACTOS to metformin significantly reduced the mean HbA_{1c} by 0.8% and decreased the mean FBG by 38 mg/dL. The therapeutic effect of

Continued on next page

Table 1 **Lipids in a 26-Week Placebo-Controlled Dose-Ranging Study**

	Placebo	ACTOS 15 mg Once Daily	ACTOS 30 mg Once Daily	ACTOS 45 mg Once Daily
Triglycerides (mg/dL)	N=79	N=79	N=84	N=77
Baseline (mean)	262.8	283.8	261.1	259.7
Percent change from baseline (mean)	4.8%	−9.0%	−9.6%	−9.3%
HDL Cholesterol (mg/dL)	N=79	N=79	N=83	N=77
Baseline (mean)	41.7	40.4	40.8	40.7
Percent change from baseline (mean)	8.1%	14.1%	12.2%	19.1%
LDL Cholesterol (mg/dL)	N=65	N=63	N=74	N=62
Baseline (mean)	138.8	131.9	135.6	126.8
Percent change from baseline (mean)	4.8%	7.2%	5.2%	6.0%
Total Cholesterol (mg/dL)	N=79	N=79	N=84	N=77
Baseline (mean)	224.6	220.0	222.7	213.7
Percent change from baseline (mean)	4.4%	4.6%	3.3%	6.4%

Figure 1: Mean Change from Baseline for FBG and HbA_{1c} in a 26-Week Placebo-Controlled Dose-Ranging Study

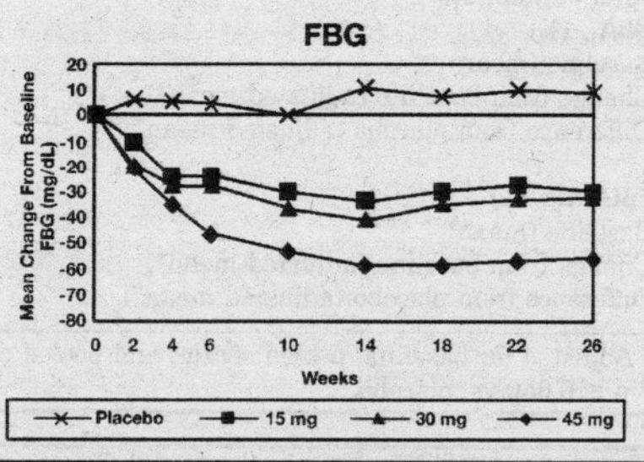

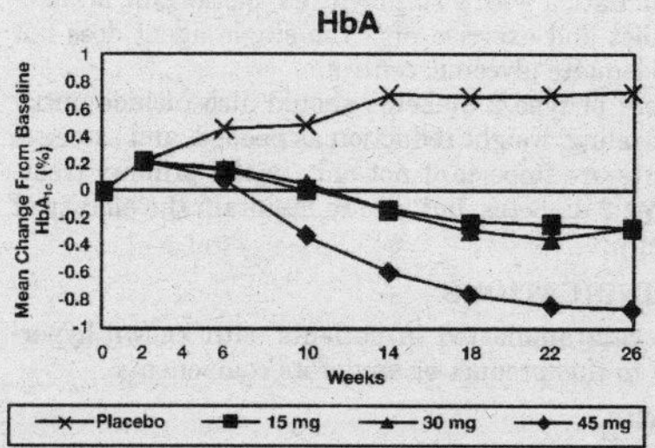

Table 2 **Glycemic Parameters in a 26-Week Placebo-Controlled Dose-Ranging Study**

	Placebo	ACTOS 15 mg Once Daily	ACTOS 30 mg Once Daily	ACTOS 45 mg Once Daily
Total Population				
HbA_{1c} (%)	N=79	N=79	N=85	N=76
Baseline (mean)	10.4	10.2	10.2	10.3
Change from baseline (adjusted mean⁺)	0.7	−0.3	−0.3	−0.9
Difference from placebo (adjusted mean⁺)		−1.0*	−1.0*	−1.6*
FBG (mg/dL)	N=79	N=79	N=84	N=77
Baseline (mean)	268	267	269	276
Change from baseline (adjusted mean⁺)	9	−30	−32	−56
Difference from placebo (adjusted mean⁺)		−39*	−41*	−65*

⁺ Adjusted for baseline, pooled center, and pooled center by treatment interaction
* $p \leq 0.050$ vs. placebo

Table 3 **Glycemic Parameters in a 26-Week Placebo-Controlled Dose-Ranging Study**

	Placebo	ACTOS 15 mg Once Daily	ACTOS 30 mg Once Daily	ACTOS 45 mg Once Daily
Naïve to Therapy				
HbA_{1c} (%)	N=25	N=26	N=26	N=21
Screening (mean)	9.3	10.0	9.5	9.8
Baseline (mean)	9.0	9.9	9.3	10.0
Change from baseline (adjusted mean*)	0.6	−0.8	−0.6	−1.9
Difference from placebo (adjusted mean*)		−1.4	−1.3	−2.6
FBG (mg/dL)	N=25	N=26	N=26	N=21
Screening (mean)	223	245	239	239
Baseline (mean)	229	251	225	235
Change from baseline (adjusted mean*)	16	−37	−41	−64
Difference from placebo (adjusted mean*)		−52	−56	−80
Previously Treated				
HbA_{1c} (%)	N=54	N=53	N=59	N=55
Screening (mean)	9.3	9.0	9.1	9.0
Baseline (mean)	10.9	10.4	10.4	10.6
Change from baseline (adjusted mean*)	0.8	−0.1	−0.0	−0.6
Difference from placebo (adjusted mean*)		−1.0	−0.9	−1.4
FBG (mg/dL)	N=54	N=53	N=58	N=56
Screening (mean)	222	209	230	215
Baseline (mean)	285	275	286	292
Change from baseline (adjusted mean*)	4	−32	−27	−55
Difference from placebo (adjusted mean*)		−36	−31	−59

* Adjusted for baseline and pooled center

Actos—Cont.

ACTOS in combination with metformin was observed in patients regardless of whether the patients were receiving lower or higher doses of metformin (< 2000 mg per day or ≥ 2000 mg per day).

In a third combination study, 566 patients with type 2 diabetes receiving a median of 60.5 units per day of insulin, either alone or combined with another antidiabetic agent, were randomized to receive either 15 mg or 30 mg of ACTOS or placebo once daily in addition to their insulin. Any other antidiabetic agent was discontinued. Compared to placebo, treatment with ACTOS in addition to insulin significantly reduced both HbA_{1c} (0.7% for the 15 mg dose and 1.0% for the 30 mg dose) and FBG (35 mg/dL for the 15 mg dose and 49 mg/dL for the 30 mg dose). The therapeutic effect of ACTOS in combination with insulin was observed in patients regardless of whether the patients were receiving lower or higher doses of insulin (< 60.5 units per day or ≥ 60.5 units per day).

INDICATIONS AND USAGE

ACTOS is indicated as an adjunct to diet and exercise to improve glycemic control in patients with type 2 diabetes (non-insulin-dependent diabetes mellitus, NIDDM). ACTOS is indicated for monotherapy. ACTOS is also indicated for use in combination with a sulfonylurea, metformin, or insulin when diet and exercise plus the single agent does not result in adequate glycemic control.

Management of type 2 diabetes should also include nutritional counseling, weight reduction as needed, and exercise. These efforts are important not only in the primary treatment of type 2 diabetes, but also to maintain the efficacy of drug therapy.

CONTRAINDICATIONS

ACTOS is contraindicated in patients with known hypersensitivity to this product or any of its components.

WARNINGS

Cardiac Failure and Other Cardiac Effects

ACTOS, like other thiazolidinediones, can cause fluid retention when used alone or in combination with other antidiabetic agents, including insulin. Fluid retention may lead to or exacerbate heart failure. Patients should be observed for signs and symptoms of heart failure (see Information for Patients). ACTOS should be discontinued if any deterioration in cardiac status occurs. Patients with New York Heart Association (NYHA) Class III and IV cardiac status were not studied during clinical trials; therefore, ACTOS is not recommended in these patients (see PRECAUTIONS, Cardiovascular).

In one 16-week U.S. double-blind, placebo-controlled clinical trial involving 566 patients with type 2 diabetes, ACTOS at doses of 15 mg and 30 mg in combination with insulin were compared to insulin therapy alone. This trial included patients with long-standing diabetes and a high prevalence of pre-existing medical conditions as follows: arterial hypertension (57.2%), peripheral neuropathy (22.6%), coronary heart disease (19.6%), retinopathy (13.1%), myocardial infarction (8.8%), vascular disease (6.4%), angina pectoris (4.4%), stroke and/or transient ischemic attack (4.1%), and congestive heart failure (2.3%).

In this study two of the 191 patients receiving 15 mg ACTOS plus insulin (1.1%) and two of the 188 patients receiving 30 mg ACTOS plus insulin (1.1%) developed congestive heart failure compared with none of the 187 patients on insulin therapy alone. All four of these patients had previous histories of cardiovascular conditions including coronary artery disease, previous CABG procedures, and myocardial infarction.

Analysis of data from this study did not identify specific factors that predict increased risk of congestive heart failure on combination therapy with insulin.

PRECAUTIONS

General

ACTOS exerts its antihyperglycemic effect only in the presence of insulin. Therefore, ACTOS should not be used in patients with type 1 diabetes or for the treatment of diabetic ketoacidosis.

Hypoglycemia: Patients receiving ACTOS in combination with insulin or oral hypoglycemic agents may be at risk for hypoglycemia, and a reduction in the dose of the concomitant agent may be necessary.

Cardiovascular: In U.S. placebo-controlled clinical trials that excluded patients with New York Heart Association (NYHA) Class III and IV cardiac status, the incidence of serious cardiac adverse events related to volume expansion was not increased in patients treated with ACTOS as monotherapy or in combination with sulfonylureas or metformin vs. placebo-treated patients. In insulin combination studies, a small number of patients with a history of previously existing cardiac disease developed congestive heart failure when treated with ACTOS in combination with insulin (see WARNINGS). Patients with NYHA Class III and IV cardiac status were not studied in ACTOS clinical trials. ACTOS is not indicated in patients with NYHA Class III or IV cardiac status.

In postmarketing experience with ACTOS, cases of congestive heart failure have been reported in patients both with and without previously known heart disease.

Edema: ACTOS should be used with caution in patients with edema. In all U.S. clinical trials, edema was reported more frequently in patients treated with ACTOS than in placebo-treated patients (see ADVERSE REACTIONS). In postmarketing experience, reports of initiation or worsening of edema have been received.

Weight Gain: Dose related weight gain was seen with ACTOS alone and in combination with other hypoglycemic agents (Table 6). The mechanism of weight gain is unclear but probably involves a combination of fluid retention and fat accumulation.

[See table 6 above]

Table 4 Glycemic Parameters in a 24-Week Placebo-Controlled Forced-Titration Study

	Placebo	ACTOS 30 mg⁺ Once Daily	ACTOS 45 mg⁺ Once Daily
Total Population			
HbA_{1c} (%)	N=83	N=85	N=85
Baseline (mean)	10.8	10.3	10.8
Change from baseline (adjusted mean⁺⁺)	0.9	−0.6	−0.6
Difference from placebo (adjusted mean⁺⁺)		−1.5*	−1.5*
FBG (mg/dL)	N=78	N=82	N=85
Baseline (mean)	279	268	281
Change from baseline (adjusted mean⁺⁺)	18	−44	−50
Difference from placebo (adjusted mean⁺⁺)		−62*	−68*

⁺ Final dose in forced titration
⁺⁺ Adjusted for baseline, pooled center, and pooled center by treatment interaction
* $p \leq 0.050$ vs. placebo

Table 5 Glycemic Parameters in a 16-Week Placebo-Controlled Study

	Placebo	ACTOS 30 mg Once Daily
Total Population		
HbA_{1c} (%)	N=93	N=100
Baseline (mean)	10.3	10.5
Change from baseline (adjusted mean⁺)	0.8	−0.6
Difference from placebo (adjusted mean⁺)		−1.4*
FBG (mg/dL)	N=91	N=99
Baseline (mean)	270	273
Change from baseline (adjusted mean⁺)	8	−50
Difference from placebo (adjusted mean⁺)		−58*

⁺ Adjusted for baseline, pooled center, and pooled center by treatment interaction
* $p \leq 0.050$ vs. placebo

Table 6 Weight Changes (kg) from Baseline during Double-Blind Clinical Trials with ACTOS

		Control Group (Placebo)	ACTOS 15 mg	ACTOS 30 mg	ACTOS 45 mg
		Median (25th / 75th percentile)	Median (25th / 75th percentile)	Median (25th / 75th percentile)	Median (25th / 75th percentile)
Monotherapy		−1.4 (−2.7/0.0) n=256	0.9 (−0.5/3.4) n=79	1.0 (−0.9/3.4) n=188	2.6 (0.2/5.4) n=79
Combination Therapy	Sulfonylurea	−0.5 (−1.8/0.7) n=187	2.0 (0.2/3.2) n=183	2.7 (1.1/4.5) n=186	N/A
	Metformin	−1.4 (−3.2/0.3) n=160	N/A	1.4 (−0.9/3.0) n=167	N/A
	Insulin	0.2 (−1.4/1.4) n=182	2.3 (0.5/4.3) n=190	3.6 (1.4/5.9) n=188	N/A

Ovulation: Therapy with ACTOS, like other thiazolidinediones, may result in ovulation in some premenopausal anovulatory women. As a result, these patients may be at an increased risk for pregnancy while taking ACTOS. Thus, adequate contraception in premenopausal women should be recommended. This possible effect has not been investigated in clinical studies so the frequency of this occurrence is not known.

Hematologic: ACTOS may cause decreases in hemoglobin and hematocrit. Across all clinical studies, mean hemoglobin values declined by 2% to 4% in patients treated with ACTOS. These changes primarily occurred within the first 4 to 12 weeks of therapy and remained relatively constant thereafter. These changes may be related to increased plasma volume and have not been associated with any significant hematologic clinical effects (see ADVERSE REACTIONS, Laboratory Abnormalities).

Hepatic Effects: Another drug of the thiazolidinedione class, troglitazone, has been associated with idiosyncratic hepatotoxicity, and very rare cases of liver failure, liver transplants, and death have been reported during postmarketing clinical use. In pre-approval controlled clinical trials in patients with type 2 diabetes, troglitazone was more frequently associated with clinically significant elevations of hepatic enzymes (ALT > 3 times the upper limit of normal) compared to placebo, and very rare cases of reversible jaundice were reported.

In pre-approval clinical studies worldwide, over 4500 subjects were treated with ACTOS. In U.S. clinical studies, over 2500 patients with type 2 diabetes received ACTOS. There was no evidence of drug-induced hepatotoxicity or elevation of ALT levels in the clinical studies.

During pre-approval placebo-controlled clinical trials in the U.S., a total of 4 of 1526 (0.26%) patients treated with ACTOS and 2 of 793 (0.25%) placebo-treated patients had ALT values ≥ 3 times the upper limit of normal. The ALT elevations in patients treated with ACTOS were reversible and were not clearly related to therapy with ACTOS.

In postmarketing experience with ACTOS, reports of hepatitis and of hepatic enzyme elevations to 3 or more times the upper limit of normal have been received. Very rarely, these reports have involved hepatic failure with and without fatal outcome, although causality has not been established.

Pioglitazone is structurally related to troglitazone, a thiazolidinedione no longer marketed in the United States, which was associated with idiosyncratic hepatotoxicity and rare cases of liver failure, liver transplants and death during postmarketing clinical use.

Pending the availability of the results of additional large, long-term controlled clinical trials and additional postmarketing safety data, it is recommended that patients treated with ACTOS undergo periodic monitoring of liver enzymes.

Serum ALT (alanine aminotransferase) levels should be evaluated prior to the initiation of therapy with ACTOS in all patients, every two months for the first year of therapy, and periodically thereafter. Liver function tests should also be obtained for patients if symptoms suggestive of hepatic dysfunction occur, e.g., nausea, vomiting, abdominal pain, fatigue, anorexia, dark urine. The decision whether to continue the patient on therapy with ACTOS should be guided by clinical judgement pending laboratory evaluations. If jaundice is observed, drug therapy should be discontinued.

Therapy with ACTOS should not be initiated if the patient exhibits clinical evidence of active liver disease or the ALT levels exceed 2.5 times the upper limit of normal. Patients with mildly elevated liver enzymes (ALT levels at 1 to 2.5 times the upper limit of normal) at baseline or any time during therapy with ACTOS should be evaluated to determine the cause of the liver enzyme elevation. Initiation or continuation of therapy with ACTOS in patients with mildly elevated liver enzymes should proceed with caution and include appropriate clinical follow-up which may include more frequent liver enzyme monitoring. If serum transaminase levels are increased (ALT > 2.5 times the upper limit of normal), liver function tests should be evaluated more frequently until the levels return to normal or pretreatment values. If ALT levels exceed 3 times the upper limit of normal, the test should be repeated as soon as possible. If ALT levels remain > 3 times the upper limit of normal or if the patient is jaundiced, ACTOS therapy should be discontinued.

There are no data available to evaluate the safety of ACTOS in patients who experienced liver abnormalities, hepatic dysfunction, or jaundice while on troglitazone. ACTOS should not be used in patients who experienced jaundice while taking troglitazone.

Laboratory Tests

FBG and HbA_{1c} measurements should be performed periodically to monitor glycemic control and the therapeutic response to ACTOS.

Liver enzyme monitoring is recommended prior to initiation of therapy with ACTOS in all patients and periodically thereafter (see PRECAUTIONS, General, Hepatic Effects and ADVERSE REACTIONS, Serum Transaminase Levels).

Information for Patients

It is important to instruct patients to adhere to dietary instructions and to have blood glucose and glycosylated hemoglobin tested regularly. During periods of stress such as fever, trauma, infection, or surgery, medication requirements may change and patients should be reminded to seek medical advice promptly.

Patients who experience an unusually rapid increase in weight or edema or who develop shortness of breath or other symptoms of heart failure while on ACTOS should immediately report these symptoms to their physician.

Patients should be told that blood tests for liver function will be performed prior to the start of therapy, every two months for the first year, and periodically thereafter. Patients should be told to seek immediate medical advice for unexplained nausea, vomiting, abdominal pain, fatigue, anorexia, or dark urine.

Patients should be told to take ACTOS once daily. ACTOS can be taken with or without meals. If a dose is missed on one day, the dose should not be doubled the following day.

When using combination therapy with insulin or oral hypoglycemic agents, the risks of hypoglycemia, its symptoms and treatment, and conditions that predispose to its development should be explained to patients and their family members.

Therapy with ACTOS, like other thiazolidinediones, may result in ovulation in some premenopausal anovulatory women. As a result, these patients may be at an increased risk for pregnancy while taking ACTOS. Thus, adequate contraception in premenopausal women should be recommended. This possible effect has not been investigated in clinical studies so the frequency of this occurrence is not known.

Drug Interactions

Oral Contraceptives: Administration of another thiazolidinedione with an oral contraceptive containing ethinyl estradiol and norethindrone reduced the plasma concentrations of both hormones by approximately 30%, which could result in loss of contraception. The pharmacokinetics of coadministration of ACTOS and oral contraceptives have not been evaluated in patients receiving ACTOS and an oral contraceptive. Therefore, additional caution regarding contraception should be exercised in patients receiving ACTOS and an oral contraceptive.

Glipizide: In healthy volunteers, coadministration of ACTOS (45 mg once daily) and glipizide (5.0 mg once daily) for seven days did not alter the steady-state pharmacokinetics of glipizide.

Digoxin: In healthy volunteers, coadministration of ACTOS (45 mg once daily) with digoxin (0.25 mg once daily) for seven days did not alter the steady-state pharmacokinetics of digoxin.

Warfarin: In healthy volunteers, coadministration of ACTOS (45 mg once daily) for seven days with warfarin did not alter the steady-state pharmacokinetics of warfarin. In addition, ACTOS has no clinically significant effect on prothrombin time when administered to patients receiving chronic warfarin therapy.

Metformin: In healthy volunteers, coadministration of metformin (1000 mg) and ACTOS (45 mg) after seven days of ACTOS (45 mg once daily) did not alter the pharmacokinetics of the single dose of metformin.

The cytochrome P450 isoform CYP3A4 is partially responsible for the metabolism of pioglitazone. Specific formal pharmacokinetic interaction studies have not been conducted with ACTOS and other drugs metabolized by this enzyme such as: erythromycin, astemizole, calcium channel blockers, cisapride, corticosteroids, cyclosporine, HMG-CoA reductase inhibitors, tacrolimus, triazolam, and trimetrexate, as well as inhibitory drugs such as ketoconazole and itraconazole. In vitro, ketoconazole appears to significantly inhibit the metabolism of pioglitazone (see CLINICAL PHARMACOLOGY, Metabolism). Pending the availability of additional data, patients receiving ketoconazole concomitantly with ACTOS should be evaluated more frequently with respect to glycemic control.

Carcinogenesis, Mutagenesis, Impairment of Fertility

A two-year carcinogenicity study was conducted in male and female rats at oral doses up to 63 mg/kg (approximately 14 times the maximum recommended human oral dose of 45 mg based on mg/m^2). Drug-induced tumors were not observed in any organ except for the urinary bladder. Benign and/or malignant transitional cell neoplasms were observed in male rats at 4 mg/kg/day and above (approximately equal to the maximum recommended human oral dose based on mg/m^2). The relationship of these findings in male rats to humans is unclear. A two-year carcinogenicity study was conducted in male and female mice at oral doses up to 100 mg/kg/day (approximately 11 times the maximum recommended human oral dose based on mg/m^2). No drug-induced tumors were observed in any organ.

During prospective evaluation of urinary cytology involving more than 1800 patients receiving ACTOS in clinical trials up to one year in duration, no new cases of bladder tumors were identified. Occasionally, abnormal urinary cytology results indicating possible malignancy were observed in both patients treated with ACTOS (0.72%) and patients treated with placebo (0.88%).

Pioglitazone HCl was not mutagenic in a battery of genetic toxicology studies, including the Ames bacterial assay, a mammalian cell forward gene mutation assay (CHO/HPRT and AS52/XPRT), an in vitro cytogenetics assay using CHL cells, an unscheduled DNA synthesis assay, and an in vivo micronucleus assay.

No adverse effects upon fertility were observed in male and female rats at oral doses up to 40 mg/kg pioglitazone HCl daily prior to and throughout mating and gestation (approximately 9 times the maximum recommended human oral dose based on mg/m^2).

Animal Toxicology

Heart enlargement has been observed in mice (100 mg/kg), rats (4 mg/kg and above) and dogs (3 mg/kg) treated orally with pioglitazone HCl (approximately 11, 1, and 2 times the maximum recommended human oral dose for mice, rats, and dogs, respectively, based on mg/m^2). In a one-year rat study, drug-related early death due to apparent heart dysfunction occurred at an oral dose of 160 mg/kg/day (approximately 35 times the maximum recommended human oral dose based on mg/m^2). Heart enlargement was seen in a 13-week study in monkeys at oral doses of 8.9 mg/kg and above (approximately 4 times the maximum recommended human oral dose based on mg/m^2), but not in a 52-week study at oral doses up to 32 mg/kg (approximately 13 times the maximum recommended human oral dose based on mg/m^2).

Pregnancy

Pregnancy Category C. Pioglitazone was not teratogenic in rats at oral doses up to 80 mg/kg or in rabbits given up to 160 mg/kg during organogenesis (approximately 17 and 40 times the maximum recommended human oral dose based on mg/m^2, respectively). Delayed parturition and embryotoxicity (as evidenced by increased postimplantation losses, delayed development and reduced fetal weights) were observed in rats at oral doses of 40 mg/kg/day and above (approximately 10 times the maximum recommended human oral dose based on mg/m^2). No functional or behavioral toxicity was observed in offspring of rats. In rabbits, embryotoxicity was observed at an oral dose of 160 mg/kg (approximately 40 times the maximum recommended human oral dose based on mg/m^2). Delayed postnatal development, attributed to decreased body weight, was observed in offspring of rats at oral doses of 10 mg/kg and above during late gestation and lactation periods (approximately 2 times the maximum recommended human oral dose based on mg/m^2).

There are no adequate and well-controlled studies in pregnant women. ACTOS should be used during pregnancy only if the potential benefit justifies the potential risk to the fetus.

Because current information strongly suggests that abnormal blood glucose levels during pregnancy are associated with a higher incidence of congenital anomalies, as well as increased neonatal morbidity and mortality, most experts recommend that insulin be used during pregnancy to maintain blood glucose levels as close to normal as possible.

Nursing Mothers

Pioglitazone is secreted in the milk of lactating rats. It is not known whether ACTOS is secreted in human milk. Because many drugs are excreted in human milk, ACTOS should not be administered to a breast-feeding woman.

Pediatric Use

Safety and effectiveness of ACTOS in pediatric patients have not been established.

Elderly Use

Approximately 500 patients in placebo-controlled clinical trials of ACTOS were 65 and over. No significant differences in effectiveness and safety were observed between these patients and younger patients.

ADVERSE REACTIONS

In worldwide clinical trials, over 3700 patients with type 2 diabetes have been treated with ACTOS. In U.S. clinical trials, over 2500 patients have received ACTOS, over 1100 patients have been treated for 6 months or longer, and over 450 patients for one year or longer.

The overall incidence and types of adverse events reported in placebo-controlled clinical trials of ACTOS monotherapy at doses of 7.5 mg, 15 mg, 30 mg, or 45 mg once daily are shown in Table 7.

Placebo-Controlled Clinical Studies at ACTOS Monotherapy: Adverse Events Reported at a Frequency ≥ 5% of Patients Treated with ACTOS

(% of Patients)

	Placebo N=259	ACTOS N=806
Upper Respiratory Tract Infection	8.5	13.2
Headache	6.9	9.1
Sinusitis	4.6	6.3
Myalgia	2.7	5.4
Tooth Disorder	2.3	5.3
Diabetes Mellitus Aggravated	8.1	5.1
Pharyngitis	0.8	5.1

For most clinical adverse events the incidence was similar for groups treated with ACTOS monotherapy and those treated in combination with sulfonylureas, metformin, and insulin. There was an increase in the occurrence of edema in the patients treated with ACTOS and insulin compared to insulin alone.

In the ACTOS plus insulin trial (n=379), 10 patients treated with ACTOS plus insulin developed dyspnea and also, at some point during their therapy, developed either weight change or edema. Seven of these 10 patients received diuretics to treat these symptoms. This was not reported in the insulin plus placebo group.

The incidence of withdrawals from clinical trials due to an adverse event other than hyperglycemia was similar for patients treated with placebo (2.8%) or ACTOS (3.3%).

Mild to moderate hypoglycemia was reported during combination therapy with sulfonylurea or insulin. Hypoglycemia was reported for 1% of placebo-treated patients and 2% of patients when ACTOS was used in combination with a sulfonylurea. In combination with insulin, hypoglycemia was reported for 5% of placebo-treated patients, 8% for patients treated with 15 mg of ACTOS, and 15% for patients treated with 30 mg of ACTOS (see PRECAUTIONS, General, Hypoglycemia).

In U.S. double-blind studies, anemia was reported for 1.0% of patients treated with ACTOS and 0.0% of placebo-treated patients in monotherapy studies. Anemia was reported for 1.6% of patients treated with ACTOS and 1.6% of placebo-treated patients in combination with insulin. Anemia was reported for 0.3% of patients treated with ACTOS and 1.6% of placebo-treated patients in combination with sulfonylurea. Anemia was reported for 1.2% of patients treated with ACTOS and 0.0% of placebo-treated patients in combination with metformin.

In monotherapy studies, edema was reported for 4.8% of patients treated with ACTOS versus 1.2% of placebo-treated patients. In combination therapy studies, edema was reported for 7.2% of patients treated with ACTOS and sulfonylureas compared to 2.1% of patients on sulfonylureas alone. In combination therapy studies with metformin, edema was reported in 6.0% of patients on combination therapy compared to 2.5% of patients on metformin alone. In combination therapy studies with insulin, edema was reported in 15.3% of patients on combination therapy compared to 7.0% of patients on insulin alone. Most of these events were considered mild or moderate in intensity (see PRECAUTIONS, General, Edema).

In one 16-week clinical trial of insulin plus ACTOS combination therapy, more patients developed congestive heart failure on combination therapy (1.1%) compared to none on insulin alone (see WARNINGS, Cardiac Failure and Other Cardiac Effects).

Laboratory Abnormalities

Hematologic: ACTOS may cause decreases in hemoglobin and hematocrit. Across all clinical studies, mean hemoglobin values declined by 2% to 4% in patients treated with ACTOS. These changes generally occurred within the first 4 to 12 weeks of therapy and remained relatively stable thereafter. These changes may be related to increased plasma volume associated with ACTOS therapy and have not been associated with any significant hematologic clinical effects.

Serum Transaminase Levels: During placebo-controlled clinical trials in the U.S., a total of 4 of 1526 (0.26%) patients treated with ACTOS and 2 of 793 (0.25%) placebo-treated patients had ALT values ≥ 3 times the upper limit of normal. During all clinical studies in the U.S., 11 of 2561 (0.43%) patients treated with ACTOS had ALT values ≥ 3 times the upper limit of normal. All patients with follow-up values had reversible elevations in ALT. In the population of patients treated with ACTOS, mean values for bilirubin, AST, ALT, alkaline phosphatase, and GGT were decreased at the final visit compared with baseline. Fewer than 0.12% of patients treated with ACTOS were withdrawn from clinical trials in the U.S. due to abnormal liver function tests. In pre-approval clinical trials, there were no cases of idiosyncratic drug reactions leading to hepatic failure (see PRECAUTIONS, Hepatic Effects).

CPK Levels: During required laboratory testing in clinical trials, sporadic, transient elevations in creatine phosphokinase levels (CPK) were observed. A single, isolated elevation to greater than 10 times the upper limit of normal (values of 2150 to 8610) was noted in 7 patients. Five of these patients continued to receive ACTOS and the other two patients had completed receiving study medication at the time of the elevated value. These elevations resolved without any apparent clinical sequelae. The relationship of these events to ACTOS therapy is unknown.

OVERDOSAGE

During controlled clinical trials, one case of overdose with ACTOS was reported. A male patient took 120 mg per day for four days, then 180 mg per day for seven days. The patient denied any clinical symptoms during this period.

Continued on next page

Actos—Cont.

In the event of overdosage, appropriate supportive treatment should be initiated according to patient's clinical signs and symptoms.

DOSAGE AND ADMINISTRATION

ACTOS should be taken once daily without regard to meals. The management of antidiabetic therapy should be individualized. Ideally, the response to therapy should be evaluated using HbA_{1c} which is a better indicator of long-term glycemic control than FBG alone. HbA_{1c} reflects glycemia over the past two to three months. In clinical use, it is recommended that patients be treated with ACTOS for a period of time adequate to evaluate change in HbA_{1c} (three months) unless glycemic control deteriorates.

Monotherapy

ACTOS monotherapy in patients not adequately controlled with diet and exercise may be initiated at 15 mg or 30 mg once daily. For patients who respond inadequately to the initial dose of ACTOS, the dose can be increased in increments up to 45 mg once daily. For patients not responding adequately to monotherapy, combination therapy should be considered.

Combination Therapy

Sulfonylureas: ACTOS in combination with a sulfonylurea may be initiated at 15 mg or 30 mg once daily. The current sulfonylurea dose can be continued upon initiation of ACTOS therapy. If patients report hypoglycemia, the dose of the sulfonylurea should be decreased.

Metformin: ACTOS in combination with metformin may be initiated at 15 mg or 30 mg once daily. The current metformin dose can be continued upon initiation of ACTOS therapy. It is unlikely that the dose of metformin will require adjustment due to hypoglycemia during combination therapy with ACTOS.

Insulin: ACTOS in combination with insulin may be initiated at 15 mg or 30 mg once daily. The current insulin dose can be continued upon initiation of ACTOS therapy. In patients receiving ACTOS and insulin, the insulin dose can be decreased by 10% to 25% if the patient reports hypoglycemia or if plasma glucose concentrations decrease to less than 100 mg/dL. Further adjustments should be individualized based on glucose-lowering response.

Maximum Recommended Dose

The dose of ACTOS should not exceed 45 mg once daily since doses higher than 45 mg once daily have not been studied in placebo-controlled clinical studies. No placebo-controlled clinical studies of more than 30 mg once daily have been conducted in combination therapy.

Dose adjustment in patients with renal insufficiency is not recommended (see CLINICAL PHARMACOLOGY, Pharmacokinetics and Drug Metabolism).

Therapy with ACTOS should not be initiated if the patient exhibits clinical evidence of active liver disease or increased serum transaminase levels (ALT greater than 2.5 times the upper limit of normal) at start of therapy (see PRECAUTIONS, General, Hepatic Effects and CLINICAL PHARMACOLOGY, Special Populations, Hepatic Insufficiency). Liver enzyme monitoring is recommended in all patients prior to initiation of therapy with ACTOS and periodically thereafter (see PRECAUTIONS, General, Hepatic Effects).

There are no data on the use of ACTOS in patients under 18 years of age; therefore, use of ACTOS in pediatric patients is not recommended. No data are available on the use of ACTOS in combination with another thiazolidinedione.

HOW SUPPLIED

ACTOS is available in 15 mg, 30 mg, and 45 mg tablets as follows:

15 mg Tablet: white to off-white, round, convex, non-scored tablet with "ACTOS" on one side, and "15" on the other, available in:
NDC 64764-151-04 Bottle of 30
NDC 64764-151-05 Bottle of 90
NDC 64764-151-06 Bottle of 500

30 mg Tablet: white to off-white, round, flat, non-scored tablet with "ACTOS" on one side, and "30" on the other, available in:
NDC 64764-301-14 Bottle of 30
NDC 64764-301-15 Bottle of 90
NDC 64764-301-16 Bottle of 500

45 mg Tablet: white to off-white, round, flat, non-scored tablet with "ACTOS" on one side, and "45" on the other, available in:
NDC 64764-451-24 Bottle of 30
NDC 64764-451-25 Bottle of 90
NDC 64764-451-26 Bottle of 500

STORAGE

Store at 25°C (77°F); excursions permitted to 15–30°C (59–86°F) [see USP Controlled Room Temperature]. Keep container tightly closed, and protect from moisture and humidity.

Rx only

Manufactured by:
Takeda Chemical Industries, Ltd.
Osaka, Japan
Marketed by:
Takeda Pharmaceuticals America, Inc.
475 Half Day Road, Suite 500
Lincolnshire, IL 60069
and
Eli Lilly and Company
Lilly Corporate Center
Indianapolis, IN 46285

5012100-04 Revised: January 2002

TAP Pharmaceuticals Inc.
LAKE FOREST, IL 60045

For Medical Information Contact:
Medical Department
(800) 622-2011 (LUPRON)
(800) 478-9526 (PREVACID)
In Emergencies:
(800) 622-2011 (LUPRON)
(800) 478-9526 (PREVACID)

This is combined labeling. Examples of different fonts appear below.

- General information
- Information on endometriosis
- **Information on uterine fibroids**

LUPRON DEPOT® 3.75 mg ℞
(leuprolide acetate for depot suspension)

Prescribing information for this product, which appears on pages 3281–3284 of the 2002 PDR, has been completely revised as follows. Please write "See Supplement A" next to the product heading.

DESCRIPTION

Leuprolide acetate is a synthetic nonapeptide analog of naturally occurring gonadotropin-releasing hormone (GnRH or LH-RH). The analog possesses greater potency than the natural hormone. The chemical name is 5-oxo-L-prolyl-L-histidyl-L-tryptophyl-L-seryl-L-tyrosyl-D-leucyl-L-leucyl-L-arginyl-N-ethyl-L-prolinamide acetate (salt) with the following structural formula:

[See chemical structure below]

LUPRON DEPOT is available in a prefilled dual-chamber syringe containing sterile lyophilized microspheres which, when mixed with diluent, become a suspension intended as a monthly intramuscular injection.

The front chamber of LUPRON DEPOT 3.75 mg prefilled dual-chamber syringe contains leuprolide acetate (3.75 mg), purified gelatin (0.65 mg), DL-lactic and glycolic acids copolymer (33.1 mg), and D-mannitol (6.6 mg). The second chamber of diluent contains carboxymethylcellulose sodium (5 mg), D-mannitol (50 mg), polysorbate 80 (1 mg), water for injection, USP, and glacial acetic acid, USP to control pH.

During the manufacture of LUPRON DEPOT 3.75 mg, acetic acid is lost, leaving the peptide.

CLINICAL PHARMACOLOGY

Leuprolide acetate is a long-acting GnRH analog. A single monthly injection of LUPRON DEPOT 3.75 mg results in an initial stimulation followed by a prolonged suppression of pituitary gonadotropins. Repeated dosing at monthly intervals results in decreased secretion of gonadal steroids; consequently, tissues and functions that depend on gonadal steroids for their maintenance become quiescent. This effect is reversible on discontinuation of drug therapy.

Leuprolide acetate is not active when given orally. Intramuscular injection of the depot formulation provides plasma concentrations of leuprolide over a period of one month.

Pharmacokinetics

Absorption A single dose of LUPRON DEPOT 3.75 mg was administered by intramuscular injection to healthy female volunteers. The absorption of leuprolide was characterized by an initial increase in plasma concentration, with peak concentration ranging from 4.6 to 10.2 ng/mL at four hours postdosing. However, intact leuprolide and an inactive metabolite could not be distinguished by the assay used in the study. Following the initial rise, leuprolide concentrations started to plateau within two days after dosing and remained relatively stable for about four to five weeks with plasma concentrations of about 0.30 ng/mL.

Distribution The mean steady-state volume of distribution of leuprolide following intravenous bolus administration to healthy male volunteers was 27 L. *In vitro* binding to human plasma proteins ranged from 43% to 49%.

Metabolism In healthy male volunteers, a 1 mg bolus of leuprolide administered intravenously revealed that the mean systemic clearance was 7.6 L/h, with a terminal elimination half-life of approximately 3 hours based on a two compartment model.

In rats and dogs, administration of ^{14}C-labeled leuprolide was shown to be metabolized to smaller inactive peptides, a pentapeptide (Metabolite I), tripeptides (Metabolites II and III) and a dipeptide (Metabolite IV). These fragments may be further catabolized.

The major metabolite (M-I) plasma concentrations measured in 5 prostate cancer patients reached maximum concentration 2 to 6 hours after dosing and were approximately 6% of the peak parent drug concentration. One week after dosing, mean plasma M-I concentrations were approximately 20% of mean leuprolide concentrations.

Excretion Following administration of LUPRON DEPOT 3.75 mg to 3 patients, less than 5% of the dose was recovered as parent and M-I metabolite in the urine.

Special Populations The pharmacokinetics of the drug in hepatically and renally impaired patients have not been determined.

CLINICAL STUDIES

Endometriosis: In controlled clinical studies, LUPRON DEPOT 3.75 mg monthly for six months was shown to be comparable to danazol 800 mg/day in relieving the clinical sign/symptoms of endometriosis (pelvic pain, dysmenorrhea, dyspareunia, pelvic tenderness, and induration) and in reducing the size of endometrial implants as evidenced by laparoscopy. The clinical significance of a decrease in endometriotic lesions is not known at this time, and in addition laparoscopic staging of endometriosis does not necessarily correlate with the severity of symptoms.

LUPRON DEPOT 3.75 mg monthly induced amenorrhea in 74% and 98% of the patients after the first and second treatment months respectively. Most of the remaining patients reported episodes of only light bleeding or spotting. In the first, second and third post-treatment months, normal menstrual cycles resumed in 7%, 71% and 95% of patients, respectively, excluding those who became pregnant.

Figure 1 illustrates the percent of patients with symptoms at baseline, final treatment visit and sustained relief at 6 and 12 months following discontinuation of treatment for the various symptoms evaluated during the study. This included all patients at end of treatment and those who elected to participate in the follow-up period. This might provide a slight bias in the results at follow-up as 75% of the original patients entered the follow-up study, and 36% were evaluated at 6 months and 26% at 12 months.

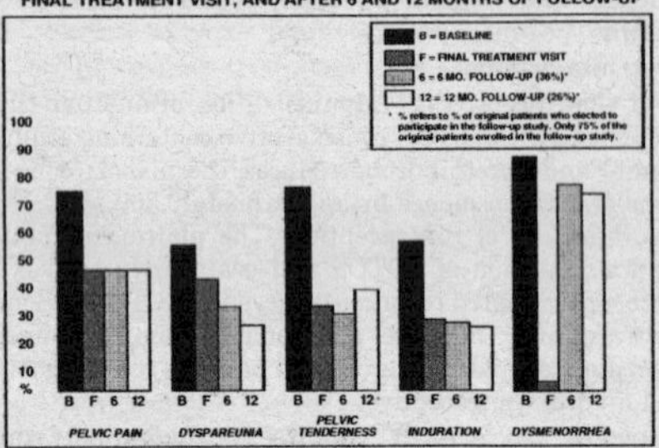

FIGURE 1–PERCENT OF PATIENTS WITH SIGN/SYMPTOMS AT BASELINE, FINAL TREATMENT VISIT, AND AFTER 6 AND 12 MONTHS OF FOLLOW-UP

Hormonal replacement therapy: Two clinical studies with a treatment duration of 12 months indicate that concurrent hormonal therapy (norethindrone acetate 5 mg daily) is effective in significantly reducing the loss of bone mineral density associated with LUPRON, without compromising the efficacy of LUPRON in relieving symptoms of endometriosis. (All patients in these studies received calcium supplementation with 1000 mg elemental calcium). One controlled, randomized and double-blind study included 51 women treated with LUPRON DEPOT alone and 55 women treated with LUPRON plus norethindrone acetate 5 mg daily. The second study was an open label study in which 136 women were treated with LUPRON plus norethindrone acetate 5 mg daily. This study confirmed the reduction in loss of bone mineral density that was observed in the controlled study. Suppression of menses was maintained throughout treatment in 84% and 73% of patients receiving LD/N in the controlled study and open label study, respectively. The median time for menses resumption after treatment with LD/N was 8 weeks.

Figure 2 illustrates the mean pain scores for the LD/N group from the controlled study.

[See figure at top of next column]

Uterine Leiomyomata (Fibroids): **In controlled clinical trials, administration of LUPRON DEPOT 3.75 mg for a period of three or six months was shown to decrease uterine and fibroid volume, thus allowing for relief of clinical symptoms (abdominal bloating, pelvic pain, and pressure). Excessive vaginal bleeding (menorrhagia and men-**

Figure 2
Treatment Period Mean Pain Scores for LD/N* Patients

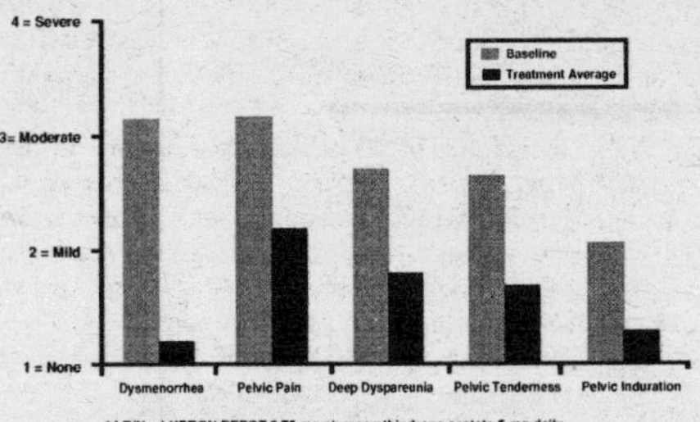

* LD/N = LUPRON DEPOT 3.75 mg plus norethindrone acetate 5 mg daily

ometrorrhagia) decreased, resulting in improvement in hematologic parameters.

In three clinical trials, enrollment was not based on hematologic status. Mean uterine volume decreased by 41% and myoma volume decreased by 37% at final visit as evidenced by ultrasound or MRI. These patients also experienced a decrease in symptoms including excessive vaginal bleeding and pelvic discomfort. Benefit occurred by three months of therapy, but additional gain was observed with an additional three months of LUPRON DEPOT 3.75 mg. Ninety-five percent of these patients became amenorrheic with 61%, 25%, and 4% experiencing amenorrhea during the first, second, and third treatment months respectively.

Post-treatment follow-up was carried out for a small percentage of LUPRON DEPOT 3.75 mg patients among the 77% who demonstrated a ≥25% decrease in uterine volume while on therapy. Menses usually returned within two months of cessation of therapy. Mean time to return to pretreatment uterine size was 8.3 months. Regrowth did not appear to be related to pretreatment uterine volume.

In another controlled clinical study, enrollment was based on hematocrit ≤30% and/or hemoglobin ≤10.2 g/dL. Administration of LUPRON DEPOT 3.75 mg, concomitantly with iron, produced an increase of ≥6% hematocrit and ≥2 g/dL hemoglobin in 77% of patients at three months of therapy. The mean change in hematocrit was 10.1% and the mean change in hemoglobin was 4.2 g/dL. Clinical response was judged to be a hematocrit of ≥36% and hemoglobin of ≥12 g/dL, thus allowing for autologous blood donation prior to surgery. At three months, 75% of patients met this criterion.

At three months, 80% of patients experienced relief from either menorrhagia or menometrorrhagia. As with the previous studies, episodes of spotting and menstrual-like bleeding were noted in some patients.

In this same study, a decrease of ≥25% was seen in uterine and myoma volumes in 60% and 54% of patients respectively. LUPRON DEPOT 3.75 mg was found to relieve symptoms of bloating, pelvic pain, and pressure.

There is no evidence that pregnancy rates are enhanced or adversely affected by the use of LUPRON DEPOT 3.75 mg.

INDICATIONS AND USAGE

Endometriosis:

LUPRON DEPOT 3.75 mg is indicated for management of endometriosis, including pain relief and reduction of endometriotic lesions. LUPRON DEPOT monthly with norethindrone acetate 5 mg daily is also indicated for initial management of endometriosis and for management of recurrence of symptoms. (Refer also to norethindrone acetate prescribing information for WARNINGS, PRECAUTIONS, CONTRAINDICATIONS and ADVERSE REACTIONS associated with norethindrone acetate) Duration of initial treatment or retreatment should be limited to 6 months.

Uterine Leiomyomata (Fibroids):

LUPRON DEPOT 3.75 mg concomitantly with iron therapy is indicated for the preoperative hematologic improvement of patients with anemia caused by uterine leiomyomata. The clinician may wish to consider a one-month trial period on iron alone inasmuch as some of the patients will respond to iron alone. (See Table 1.) LUPRON may be added if the response to iron alone is considered inadequate. Recommended duration of therapy with LUPRON DEPOT 3.75 mg is up to three months.

Experience with LUPRON DEPOT in females has been limited to women 18 years of age and older.

Table 1
PERCENT OF PATIENTS ACHIEVING HEMOGLOBIN ≥ 12 GM/DL

Treatment Group	Week 4	Week 8	Week 12
LUPRON DEPOT 3.75 mg with Iron	41*	71**	79*
Iron Alone	17	40	56

* P-Value < 0.01
** P-Value < 0.001

CONTRAINDICATIONS

1. Hypersensitivity to GnRH, GnRH agonist analogs or any of the excipients in LUPRON DEPOT.
2. Undiagnosed abnormal vaginal bleeding.
3. LUPRON DEPOT is contraindicated in women who are or may become pregnant while receiving the drug. LUPRON DEPOT may cause fetal harm when administered to a pregnant woman. Major fetal abnormalities were observed in rabbits but not in rats after administration of LUPRON DEPOT throughout gestation. There was increased fetal mortality and decreased fetal weights in rats and rabbits. (See **Pregnancy** section.) The effects on fetal mortality are expected consequences of the alterations in hormonal levels brought about by the drug. If this drug is used during pregnancy, or if the patient becomes pregnant while taking this drug, the patient should be apprised of the potential hazard to the fetus.
4. Use in women who are breast-feeding. (See **Nursing Mothers** section.)
5. Norethindrone acetate is contraindicated in women with the following conditions:
   — Thrombophlebitis, thromboembolic disorders, cerebral apoplexy, or a past history of these conditions
   — Markedly impaired liver function or liver disease
   — Known or suspected carcinoma of the breast

WARNINGS

Safe use of leuprolide acetate or norethindrone acetate in pregnancy has not been established clinically. Before starting treatment with LUPRON DEPOT, pregnancy must be excluded.

When used monthly at the recommended dose, LUPRON DEPOT usually inhibits ovulation and stops menstruation. Contraception is not insured, however, by taking LUPRON DEPOT. Therefore, patients should use non-hormonal methods of contraception. Patients should be advised to see their physician if they believe they may be pregnant. If a patient becomes pregnant during treatment, the drug must be discontinued and the patient must be apprised of the potential risk to the fetus.

During the early phase of therapy, sex steroids temporarily rise above baseline because of the physiologic effect of the drug. Therefore, an increase in clinical signs and symptoms may be observed during the initial days of therapy, but these will dissipate with continued therapy.

Symptoms consistent with an anaphylactoid or asthmatic process have been rarely reported post-marketing.

The following applies to co-treatment with LUPRON and norethindrone acetate:

Norethindrone acetate treatment should be discontinued if there is a sudden partial or complete loss of vision or if there is sudden onset of proptosis, diplopia, or migraine. If examination reveals papilledema or retinal vascular lesions, medication should be withdrawn.

Because of the occasional occurrence of thrombophlebitis and pulmonary embolism in patients taking progestogens, the physician should be alert to the earliest manifestations of the disease in women taking norethindrone acetate.

Assessment and management of risk factors for cardiovascular disease is recommended prior to initiation of add-back therapy with norethindrone acetate. Norethindrone acetate should be used with caution in women with risk factors, including lipid abnormalities or cigarette smoking.

PRECAUTIONS

Information for Patients An information pamphlet for patients is included with the product. Patients should be aware of the following information:

1. Since menstruation should stop with effective doses of LUPRON DEPOT, the patient should notify her physician if regular menstruation persists. Patients missing successive doses of LUPRON DEPOT may experience breakthrough bleeding.
2. Patients should not use LUPRON DEPOT if they are pregnant, breast feeding, have undiagnosed abnormal vaginal bleeding, or are allergic to any of the ingredients in LUPRON DEPOT.
3. Safe use of the drug in pregnancy has not been established clinically. Therefore, a non-hormonal method of contraception should be used during treatment. Patients should be advised that if they miss successive doses of LUPRON DEPOT, breakthrough bleeding or ovulation may occur with the potential for conception. If a patient becomes pregnant during treatment, she should discontinue treatment and consult her physician.
4. Adverse events occurring in clinical studies with LUPRON DEPOT that are associated with hypoestrogenism include: hot flashes, headaches, emotional lability, decreased libido, acne, myalgia, reduction in breast size, and vaginal dryness. Estrogen levels returned to normal after treatment was discontinued.
5. Patients should be counseled on the possibility of the development or worsening of depression and the occurrence of memory disorders.
6. The induced hypoestrogenic state **also** results in a loss in bone density over the course of treatment, some of which may not be reversible. For a period up to six months, this bone loss should not be clinically significant. Clinical studies show that concurrent hormonal therapy with norethindrone acetate 5 mg daily is effective in reducing loss of bone mineral density that occurs with LUPRON. (All patients received calcium supplementation with 1000 mg elemental calcium.) (See ***Changes in Bone Density*** section).
7. If the symptoms of endometriosis recur after a course of therapy, retreatment with a six-month course of LUPRON DEPOT and norethindrone acetate 5 mg daily may be considered. Retreatment beyond this one six month course cannot be recommended. It is recommended that bone density be assessed before retreatment begins to ensure that values are within normal limits. Retreatment with LUPRON DEPOT alone is not recommended.
8. In patients with major risk factors for decreased bone mineral content such as chronic alcohol and/or tobacco use, strong family history of osteoporosis, or chronic use of drugs that can reduce bone mass such as anticonvulsants or corticosteroids, LUPRON DEPOT therapy may pose an additional risk. In these patients, the risks and benefits must be weighed carefully before therapy with LUPRON DEPOT alone is instituted, and concomitant treatment with norethindrone acetate 5 mg daily should be considered. Retreatment with gonadotropin-releasing hormone analogs, including LUPRON is not advisable in patients with major risk factors for loss of bone mineral content.
9. Because norethindrone acetate may cause some degree of fluid retention, conditions which might be influenced by this factor, such as epilepsy, migraine, asthma, cardiac or renal dysfunctions require careful observation during norethindrone acetate add-back therapy.
10. Patients who have a history of depression should be carefully observed during treatment with norethindrone acetate and norethindrone acetate should be discontinued if severe depression occurs.

Laboratory Tests See **ADVERSE REACTIONS** section.

Drug Interactions No pharmacokinetic-based drug-drug interaction studies have been conducted with LUPRON DEPOT. However, because leuprolide acetate is a peptide that is primarily degraded by peptidase and not by cytochrome P-450 enzymes as noted in specific studies, and the drug is only about 46% bound to plasma proteins, drug interactions would not be expected to occur.

Drug/Laboratory Test Interactions Administration of LUPRON DEPOT in therapeutic doses results in suppression of the pituitary-gonadal system. Normal function is usually restored within three months after treatment is discontinued. Therefore, diagnostic tests of pituitary gonadotropic and gonadal functions conducted during treatment and for up to three months after discontinuation of LUPRON DEPOT may be misleading.

Carcinogenesis, Mutagenesis, Impairment of Fertility A two-year carcinogenicity study was conducted in rats and mice. In rats, a dose-related increase of benign pituitary hyperplasia and benign pituitary adenomas was noted at 24 months when the drug was administered subcutaneously at high daily doses (0.6 to 4 mg/kg). There was a significant but not dose-related increase of pancreatic islet-cell adenomas in females and of testicular interstitial cell adenomas in males (highest incidence in the low dose group). In mice, no leuprolide acetate-induced tumors or pituitary abnormalities were observed at a dose as high as 60 mg/kg for two years. Patients have been treated with leuprolide acetate for up to three years with doses as high as 10 mg/day and for two years with doses as high as 20 mg/day without demonstrable pituitary abnormalities.

Mutagenicity studies have been performed with leuprolide acetate using bacterial and mammalian systems. These studies provided no evidence of a mutagenic potential.

Clinical and pharmacologic studies in adults (>18 years) with leuprolide acetate and similar analogs have shown reversibility of fertility suppression when the drug is discontinued after continuous administration for periods of up to 24 weeks. Although no clinical studies have been completed in children to assess the full reversibility of fertility suppression, animal studies (prepubertal and adult rats and monkeys) with leuprolide acetate and other GnRH analogs have shown functional recovery.

Pregnancy, Teratogenic Effects Pregnancy Category X. (See **CONTRAINDICATIONS** section.) When administered on day 6 of pregnancy at test dosages of 0.00024, 0.0024, and 0.024 mg/kg (1/300 to 1/3 of the human dose) to rabbits, LUPRON DEPOT produced a dose-related increase in major fetal abnormalities. Similar studies in rats failed to demonstrate an increase in fetal malformations. There was increased fetal mortality and decreased fetal weights with the two higher doses of LUPRON DEPOT in rabbits and with the highest dose (0.024 mg/kg) in rats.

Nursing Mothers It is not known whether LUPRON DEPOT is excreted in human milk. Because many drugs are excreted in human milk, and because the effects of LUPRON DEPOT on lactation and/or the breast-fed child have not been determined, LUPRON DEPOT should not be used by nursing mothers.

Pediatric Use Experience with LUPRON DEPOT 3.75 mg for treatment of endometriosis has been limited to women 18 years of age and older. See LUPRON DEPOT-PED® (leuprolide acetate for depot suspension) labeling for the safety and effectiveness in children with central precocious puberty.

Geriatric Use This product has not been studied in women over 65 years of age and is not indicated in this population.

ADVERSE REACTIONS

Clinical Trials

Estradiol levels may increase during the first weeks following the initial injection of LUPRON, but then decline to menopausal levels. This transient increase in estradiol can be associated with a temporary worsening of signs and symptoms. (See **WARNINGS** section.)

As would be expected with a drug that lowers serum estradiol levels, the most frequently reported adverse reactions were those related to hypoestrogenism.

Endometriosis: In controlled studies comparing LUPRON DEPOT 3.75 mg monthly and danazol (800 mg/day) or placebo, adverse

Continued on next page

Lupron Depot 3.75 mg—Cont.

reactions most frequently reported and thought to be possibly or probably drug-related are shown in Figure 3.

[See figure above]

In these same studies, other symptoms reported included: *Cardiovascular System* - Palpitations, Syncope, Tachycardia; *Gastrointestinal System* - Appetite changes, Dry mouth, Thirst; *Central/Peripheral Nervous System* - Anxiety*, Delusions, Memory disorder, Personality disorder; *Integumentary System* - Alopecia, Ecchymosis, Hair disorder; *Urogenital System* - Dysuria,* Lactation; *Miscellaneous* - Lymphadenopathy, Ophthalmologic disorders.*

*Possible effect of decreased estrogen

Table 2 lists the potentially drug-related adverse events observed in at least 5 % of patients in any treatment group during the first 6 months of treatment in the add-back clinical studies.

[See table 2 above]

In the controlled clinical trial, 50 of 51 (98%) patients in the LD group and 48 of 55 (87%) patients in the LD/N group reported experiencing hot flashes on one or more occasions during treatment. During Month 6 of treatment, 32 of 37 (86%) patients in the LD group and 22 of 38 (58%) patients in the LD/N group reported having experienced hot flashes. The mean number of days on which hot flashes were reported during this month of treatment was 19 and 7 in the LD and LD/N treatment groups, respectively. The mean maximum number of hot flashes in a day during this month of treatment was 5.8 and 1.9 in the LD and LD/N treatment groups, respectively.

Uterine Leiomyomata (Fibroids): **In controlled clinical trials comparing LUPRON DEPOT 3.75 mg and placebo, adverse events reported in >5% of patients and thought to be potentially related to drug are noted in Table 3.**

Table 3
ADVERSE EVENTS OBSERVED IN > 5% OF PATIENTS AND THOUGHT TO BE POTENTIALLY RELATED TO DRUG

	LUPRON DEPOT 3.75 mg		Placebo	
	N=166	(%)	N=163	(%)
Body as a Whole				
Asthenia	14	(8.4)	8	(4.9)
General pain	14	(8.4)	10	(6.1)
Headache*	43	(25.9)	29	(17.8)
Cardiovascular System				
Hot flashes/sweats*	121	(72.9)	29	(17.8)
Metabolic and Nutritional Disorders				
Edema	9	(5.4)	2	(1.2)
Musculoskeletal System				
Joint disorder*	13	(7.8)	5	(3.1)
Nervous System				
Depression/ emotional lability*	18	(10.8)	7	(4.3)
Urogenital System				
Vaginitis*	19	(11.4)	3	(1.8)

Symptoms reported in < 5% of patients included: *Body as Whole* - Body odor, Flu syndrome, Injection site reactions; *Cardiovascular System* - Tachycardia; *Digestive System* - Appetite changes, Dry mouth, GI disturbances, Nausea/vomiting; *Metabolic and Nutritional Disorders* - Weight changes; *Musculoskeletal System* - Myalgia; *Nervous System* - Anxiety, Decreased libido,* Dizziness, Insomnia, Nervousness,* Neuromuscular disorders,* Paresthesias; *Respiratory System* - Rhinitis; *Integumentary System* - Androgen-like effects, Nail disorder, Skin reactions; *Special Senses* - Conjunctivitis, Taste perversion; *Urogenital System* - Breast changes,* Menstrual disorders.

*** = Possible effect of decreased estrogen.**

In one controlled clinical trial, patients received a higher dose (7.5 mg) of LUPRON DEPOT. Events seen with this dose that were thought to be potentially related to drug and were not seen at the lower dose included palpitations, syncope, glossitis, ecchymosis, hypesthesia, confusion, lactation, pyelonephritis, and urinary disorders. Generally, a higher incidence of hypoestrogenic effects was observed at the higher dose.

Changes in Bone Density

In controlled clinical studies, patients with endometriosis (six months of therapy) or uterine fibroids (three months of therapy) were treated with LUPRON DEPOT 3.75 mg. In endometriosis patients, vertebral bone density as measured by dual energy x-ray absorptiometry (DEXA) decreased by an average of 3.2% at six months compared with the pretreatment value. Clinical studies demonstrate that concurrent hormonal therapy (norethindrone acetate 5 mg daily) and calcium supplementation is effective in significantly reducing the loss of bone mineral density that occurs with LUPRON treatment, without compromising the efficacy of LUPRON in relieving symptoms of endometriosis.

LUPRON DEPOT 3.75 mg plus norethindrone acetate 5 mg daily was evaluated in two clinical trials. The results from this regimen were similar in both studies. LUPRON DEPOT 3.75 mg was used as a control group in one study. The bone mineral density data of the lumbar spine from these two studies are presented in Table 4.

[See table 4 above]

When LUPRON DEPOT 3.75 mg was administered for three months in uterine fibroid patients, vertebral trabecular bone mineral density as assessed by quantitative digital radiography (QDR) revealed a mean decrease of 2.7% compared with baseline. Six months after discontinuation of therapy, a trend toward recovery was observed. Use of LUPRON DEPOT for longer than three months (uterine fibroids) or six months (endometriosis) or in the presence of other known risk factors for decreased bone mineral content may cause additional bone loss **and is not recommended.**

Changes in Laboratory Values During **Treatment**

Plasma Enzymes

Endometriosis: During early clinical trials with LUPRON DEPOT 3.75 mg, regular laboratory monitoring revealed that AST levels were more than twice the upper limit of normal in only one patient. There was no clinical or other laboratory evidence of abnormal liver function.

In two other clinical trials, 6 of 191 patients receiving LUPRON DEPOT 3.75 mg plus norethindrone acetate 5 mg daily for up to 12 months developed an elevated (at least twice the upper limit of normal) SGPT or GGT. Five of the 6 increases were observed beyond 6 months of treatment. None were associated with elevated bilirubin concentration.

Uterine Leiomyomata (Fibroids): **In clinical trials with LUPRON DEPOT 3.75 mg, five (3%) patients had a post-treatment transaminase value that was at least twice the**

FIGURE 3–ADVERSE EVENTS REPORTED DURING 6 MONTHS OF TREATMENT WITH LUPRON DEPOT 3.75 MG

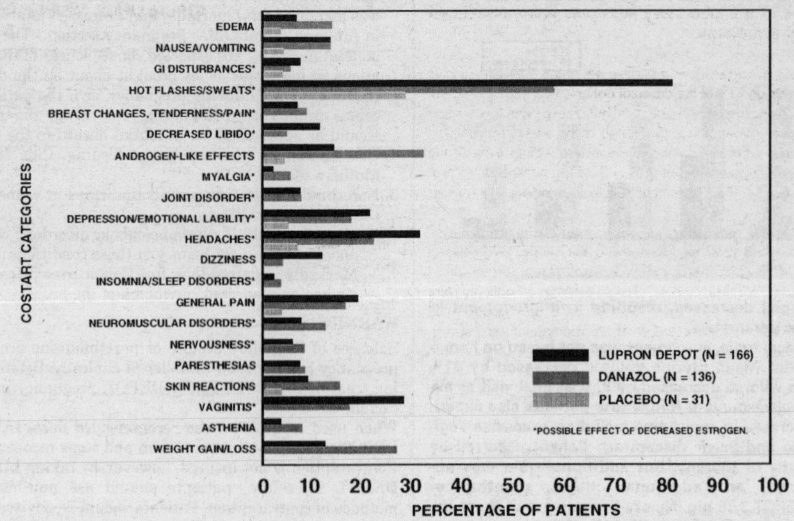

Table 2
TREATMENT-RELATED ADVERSE EVENTS OCCURRING IN ≥ 5% OF PATIENTS

	Controlled Study				Open Label Study	
	LD-Only[1] N=51		LD/N[2] N=55		LD/N[2] N=136	
Adverse Events	**N**	**(%)**	**N**	**(%)**	**N**	**(%)**
Any Adverse Event	50	(98)	53	(96)	126	(93)
Body as a Whole						
Asthenia	9	(18)	10	(18)	15	(11)
Headache/Migraine	33	(65)	28	(51)	63	(46)
Injection Site Reaction	1	(2)	5	(9)	4	(3)
Pain	12	(24)	16	(29)	29	(21)
Cardiovascular System						
Hot flashes/Sweats	50	(98)	48	(87)	78	(57)
Digestive System						
Altered Bowel Function	7	(14)	8	(15)	14	(10)
Changes in Appetite	2	(4)	0	(0)	8	(6)
GI Disturbance	2	(4)	4	(7)	6	(4)
Nausea/Vomiting	13	(25)	16	(29)	17	(13)
Metabolic and Nutritional Disorders						
Edema	0	(0)	5	(9)	9	(7)
Weight Changes	6	(12)	7	(13)	6	(4)
Nervous System						
Anxiety	3	(6)	0	(0)	11	(8)
Depression/Emotional Lability	16	(31)	15	(27)	46	(34)
Dizziness/Vertigo	8	(16)	6	(11)	10	(7)
Insomnia/Sleep Disorders	16	(31)	7	(13)	20	(15)
Libido Changes	5	(10)	2	(4)	10	(7)
Memory Disorder	3	(6)	1	(2)	6	(4)
Nervousness	4	(8)	2	(4)	15	(11)
Neuromuscular Disorder	1	(2)	5	(9)	4	(3)
Skin and Appendages						
Alopecia	0	(0)	5	(9)	4	(3)
Androgen-Like Effects	2	(4)	3	(5)	24	(18)
Skin/Mucous Membrane Reaction	2	(4)	5	(9)	15	(11)
Urogential System						
Breast Changes/Pain/Tenderness	3	(6)	7	(13)	11	(8)
Menstrual Disorders	1	(2)	0	(0)	7	(5)
Vaginitis	10	(20)	8	(15)	11	(8)

1 LD-Only = LUPRON DEPOT 3.75 mg
2 LD/N = LUPRON DEPOT 3.75 mg plus norethindrone acetate 5mg

Table 4
MEAN PERCENT CHANGE FROM BASELINE IN BONE MINERAL DENSITY OF LUMBAR SPINE

	LUPRON DEPOT 3.75mg		LUPRON DEPOT 3.75 mg plus norethindrone acetate 5 mg daily			
	Controlled Study		Controlled Study		Open Label Study	
	N	Change	N	Change	N	Change
Week 24[1]	41	−3.2%	42	−0.3%	115	−0.2%
Week 52[2]	29	−6.3%	32	−1.0%	84	−1.1%

1 Includes on-treatment measurements that fell within 2-252 days after the first day of treatment.
2 Includes on-treatment measurements >252 days after the first day of treatment.

baseline value and above the upper limit of the normal range. None of the laboratory increases were associated with clinical symptoms.

Lipids

Endometriosis: In earlier clinical studies, 4% of the LUPRON DEPOT 3.75 mg patients and 1% of the danazol patients had total cholesterol values above the normal range at enrollment. These patients also had cholesterol values above the normal range at the end of treatment. Of those patients whose pretreatment cholesterol values were in the normal range, 7% of the LUPRON DEPOT 3.75 mg patients and 9% of the danazol patients had post-treatment values above the normal range.

The mean (±SEM) pretreatment values for total cholesterol from all patients were 178.8 (2.9) mg/dL in the LUPRON DEPOT 3.75 mg groups and 175.3 (3.0) mg/dL in the danazol group. At the end of treatment, the mean values for total cholesterol from all patients were 193.3 mg/dL in the LUPRON DEPOT 3.75 mg group and 194.4 mg/dL in the danazol group. These increases from the pretreatment values were statistically significant ($p<0.03$) in both groups.

Triglycerides were increased above the upper limit of normal in 12% of the patients who received LUPRON DEPOT 3.75 mg and in 6% of the patients who received danazol.

At the end of treatment, HDL cholesterol fractions decreased below the lower limit of the normal range in 2% of the LUPRON DEPOT 3.75 mg patients compared with 54% of those receiving danazol. LDL cholesterol fractions increased above the upper limit of the normal range in 6% of the patients receiving LUPRON DEPOT 3.75 mg compared with 23% of those receiving danazol. There was no increase in the LDL/HDL ratio in patients receiving LUPRON DEPOT 3.75 mg but there was approximately a two-fold increase in the LDL/HDL ratio in patients receiving danazol.

In two other clinical trials, LUPRON DEPOT 3.75 mg plus norethindrone acetate 5 mg daily was evaluated for 12 months of treatment. LUPRON DEPOT 3.75 mg was used as a control group in one study. Percent changes from baseline for serum lipids and percentages of patients with serum lipid values outside of the normal range in the two studies are summarized in the tables below.

[See table 5 above]

Changes from baseline tended to be greater at Week 52. After treatment, mean serum lipid levels from patients with follow up data returned to pretreatment values.

[See table 6 above]

Low HDL-cholesterol (<40 mg/dL) and elevated LDL-cholesterol (> 160 mg/dL) are recognized risk factors for cardiovascular disease. The long-term significance of the observed treatment-related changes in serum lipids in women with endometriosis is unknown. Therefore assessment of cardiovascular risk factors should be considered prior to initiation of concurrent treatment with LUPRON and norethindrone acetate.

Uterine Leiomyomata (Fibroids): **In patients receiving LUPRON DEPOT 3.75 mg, mean changes in cholesterol (+11 mg/dL to +29 mg/dL), LDL cholesterol (+8 mg/dL to +22 mg/dL), HDL cholesterol (0 to +6 mg/dL), and the LDL/HDL ratio (−0.1 to +0.5) were observed across studies. In the one study in which triglycerides were determined, the mean increase from baseline was 32 mg/dL.**

Other Changes

Endometriosis: The following changes were seen in approximately 5% to 8% of patients. In the earlier comparative studies, LUPRON DEPOT 3.75 mg was associated with elevations of LDH and phosphorus, and decreases in WBC counts. Danazol therapy was associated with increases in hematocrit, platelet count, and LDH. In the hormonal add-back studies LUPRON DEPOT in combination with norethindrone acetate was associated with elevations of GGT and SGPT.

Uterine Leiomyomata (Fibroids):

Hematology: (See CLINICAL STUDIES section.) In LUPRON DEPOT 3.75 mg treated patients, although there were statistically significant mean decreases in platelet counts from baseline to final visit, the last mean platelet counts were within the normal range. Decreases in total WBC count and neutrophils were observed, but were not clinically significant.

Chemistry: Slight to moderate mean increases were noted for glucose, uric acid, BUN, creatinine, total protein, albumin, bilirubin, alkaline phosphatase, LDH, calcium, and phosphorus. None of these increases were clinically significant.

Postmarketing

During postmarketing surveillance, the following adverse events were reported. Like other drugs in this class, mood swings, including depression, have been reported as a physiologic effect of decreased sex steroids. There have been rare reports of suicidal ideation and attempt. Many, but not all, of these patients had a history of depression or other psychiatric illness. Patients should be counseled on the possibility of development or worsening of depression during treatment with LUPRON.

Symptoms consistent with an anaphylactoid or asthmatic process have been rarely reported. Rash, urticaria, and photosensitivity reactions have also been reported.

Localized reactions including induration and abscess have been reported at the site of injection. Symptoms consistent with fibromyalgia (eg: joint and muscle pain, headaches, sleep disorder, gastrointestinal distress, and shortness of breath) have been reported individually and collectively.

Other events reported are:

Cardiovascular System - Hypotension; *Hemic and Lymphatic System* - Decreased WBC; *Central/Peripheral Nervous System* - Peripheral neuropathy, Spinal fracture/paralysis; *Musculoskeletal System* - Tenosynovitis-like symptoms; *Urogenital System* - Prostate pain.

See other LUPRON DEPOT and LUPRON Injection package inserts for other events reported in different patient populations.

Table 5
SERUM LIPIDS: MEAN PERCENT CHANGES FROM BASELINE VALUES AT TREATMENT WEEK 24

	LUPRON		LUPRON plus norethindrone acetate 5 mg daily			
	Controlled Study (n = 39)		Controlled Study (n = 41)		Open Label Study (n = 117)	
	Baseline Value *	Wk 24 % Change	Baseline Value *	Wk 24 % Change	Baseline Value *	Wk 24 % Change
Total Cholesterol	170.5	9.2%	179.3	0.2%	181.2	2.8%
HDL Cholesterol	52.4	7.4%	51.8	−18.8%	51.0	−14.6%
LDL Cholesterol	96.6	10.9%	101.5	14.1%	109.1	13.1%
LDL/HDL Ratio	2.0**	5.0%	2.1**	43.4%	2.3**	39.4%
Triglycerides	107.8	17.5%	130.2	9.5%	105.4	13.8%

* mg/dL
** ratio

Table 6
PERCENTAGE OF PATIENTS WITH SERUM LIPID VALUES OUTSIDE OF THE NORMAL RANGE

	LUPRON		LUPRON plus norethindrone acetate 5 mg daily			
	Controlled Study (n = 39)		Controlled Study (n = 41)		Open Label Study (n = 117)	
	Wk 0	Wk 24*	Wk 0	Wk 24*	Wk 0	Wk 24*
Total Cholesterol (>240 mg/dL)	15%	23%	15%	20%	6%	7%
HDL Cholesterol (<40 mg/dL)	15%	10%	15%	44%	15%	41%
LDL Cholesterol (>160 mg/dL)	0%	8%	5%	7%	9%	11%
LDL/HDL Ratio (>4.0)	0%	3%	2%	15%	7%	21%
Triglycerides (>200 mg/dL)	13%	13%	12%	10%	5%	9%

* Includes all patients regardless of baseline value.

OVERDOSAGE

In rats subcutaneous administration of 250 to 500 times the recommended human dose, expressed on a per body weight basis, resulted in dyspnea, decreased activity, and local irritation at the injection site. There is no evidence that there is a clinical counterpart of this phenomenon. In early clinical trials using daily subcutaneous leuprolide acetate in patients with prostate cancer, doses as high as 20 mg/day for up to two years caused no adverse effects differing from those observed with the 1 mg/day dose.

DOSAGE AND ADMINISTRATION

LUPRON DEPOT Must Be Administered Under The Supervision Of A Physician.

The recommended dose of LUPRON DEPOT is 3.75 mg, incorporated in a depot formulation. The lyophilized microspheres are to be reconstituted and administered monthly as a single intramuscular injection, in accord with the following directions:

1. To prepare for injection, screw the white plunger into the end stopper until the stopper begins to turn.
2. Remove and discard the tab around the base of the needle.
3. Holding the syringe upright, release the diluent by SLOWLY PUSHING the plunger until the first stopper is at the blue line in the middle of the barrel.
4. Gently shake the syringe to thoroughly mix the particles to form a uniform suspension. The suspension will appear milky.
5. If the microspheres (particles) adhere to the stopper, tap the syringe against your finger.
6. Then remove the needle guard and advance the plunger to expel the air from the syringe.
7. At the time of reconstitution, inject the entire contents of the syringe intramuscularly as you would for a normal injection. The suspension settles very quickly following reconstitution; therefore, it is preferable that LUPRON DEPOT 3.75 mg be mixed and used immediately. Reshake suspension if settling occurs.

Since the product does not contain a preservative, the suspension should be discarded if not used immediately.

Endometriosis: The recommended duration of treatment with LUPRON DEPOT 3.75 mg alone or in combination with norethindrone acetate is six months. The choice of LUPRON alone or LUPRON plus norethindrone acetate therapy for initial management of the symptoms and signs of endometriosis should be made by the health care professional in consultation with the patient and should take into consideration the risks and benefits of the addition of norethindrone to LUPRON alone.

If the symptoms of endometriosis recur after a course of therapy, retreatment with a six-month course of LUPRON DEPOT monthly and norethindrone acetate 5 mg daily may be considered. Retreatment beyond this one six-month course cannot be recommended. It is recommended that bone density be assessed before retreatment begins to ensure that values are within normal limits. LUPRON DEPOT alone is not recommended for retreatment. If norethindrone acetate is contraindicated for the individual patient, then retreatment is not recommended.

An assessment of cardiovascular risk and management of risk factors such as cigarette smoking is recommended before beginning treatment with LUPRON and norethindrone acetate.

Uterine Leiomyomata (Fibroids): **Recommended duration of therapy with LUPRON DEPOT 3.75 mg is up to 3 months. The symptoms associated with uterine leiomyomata will recur following discontinuation of therapy. If additional treatment with LUPRON DEPOT 3.75 mg is contemplated, bone density should be assessed prior to initiation of therapy to ensure that values are within normal limits.**

As with other drugs administered by injection, the injection site should be varied periodically.

HOW SUPPLIED

LUPRON DEPOT 3.75 mg is packaged as follows:

Kit with prefilled dual-chamber syringe NDC 0300-3641-01

Each syringe contains sterile lyophilized microspheres, which is leuprolide incorporated in a biodegradable copolymer of lactic and glycolic acids. When mixed with diluent, LUPRON DEPOT 3.75 mg is administered as a single monthly IM injection.

Store at 25°C (77°F); excursions permitted to 15–30°C (59–86°F) [See USP Controlled Room Temperature]

Rx only

U.S. Patent Nos. 4,652,441; 4,677,191; 4,728,721; 4,849,228; 4,917,893; 4,954,298; 5,330,767; 5,476,663; 5,575,987; 5,631,020; 5,631,021; and 5,716,640.

Manufactured for
TAP Pharmaceuticals Inc.
Lake Forest, IL 60045, U.S.A.
by Takeda Chemical Industries, Ltd.
Osaka, JAPAN 541
®—Registered Trademark
(No. 3641)
03-5160-R14; Revised: October, 2001

This is combined labeling. Examples of different fonts appear below.

- General information
- *Information on endometriosis*
- **Information on uterine fibroids**

LUPRON DEPOT®-3 Month 11.25 mg ℞
(leuprolide acetate for depot suspension)
3-MONTH FORMULATION

Prescribing information for this product, which appears on pages 3285–3288 of the 2002 PDR, has been completely revised as follows. Please write "See Supplement A" next to the product heading.

DESCRIPTION

Leuprolide acetate is a synthetic nonapeptide analog of naturally occurring gonadotropin-releasing hormone (GnRH or LH-RH). The analog possesses greater potency than the natural hormone. The chemical name is 5-oxo-L-prolyl-L-histidyl-L-tryptophyl-L-seryl-L-tyrosyl-D-leucyl-L-leucyl-L-arginyl-N-ethyl-L-prolinamide acetate (salt) with the following structural formula:

[See chemical structure at top of next page]

LUPRON DEPOT–3 Month 11.25 mg is available in a prefilled dual-chamber syringe containing sterile lyophilized microspheres which, when mixed with diluent, become a suspension intended as an intramuscular injection to be given **ONCE EVERY THREE MONTHS.**

The front chamber of LUPRON DEPOT–3 Month 11.25 mg prefilled dual-chamber syringe contains leuprolide acetate

Continued on next page

Lupron Depot-3 Month—Cont.

(11.25 mg), polylactic acid (99.3 mg) and D-mannitol (19.45 mg). The second chamber of diluent contains carboxymethylcellulose sodium (7.5 mg), D-mannitol (75.0 mg), polysorbate 80 (1.5 mg), water for injection, USP, and glacial acetic acid, USP to control pH.

During the manufacture of LUPRON DEPOT–3 Month 11.25 mg, acetic acid is lost, leaving the peptide.

CLINICAL PHARMACOLOGY

Leuprolide acetate is a long-acting GnRH analog. A single injection of LUPRON DEPOT–3 Month 11.25 mg will result in an initial stimulation followed by a prolonged suppression of pituitary gonadotropins. Repeated dosing at quarterly (LUPRON DEPOT–3 Month 11.25 mg) intervals results in decreased secretion of gonadal steroids; consequently, tissues and functions that depend on gonadal steroids for their maintenance become quiescent. This effect is reversible on discontinuation of drug therapy.

Leuprolide acetate is not active when given orally.

Pharmacokinetics

Absorption Following a single injection of the three month formulation of LUPRON DEPOT–3 Month 11.25 mg in female subjects, a mean plasma leuprolide concentration of 36.3 ng/mL was observed at 4 hours. Leuprolide appeared to be released at a constant rate following the onset of steady-state levels during the third week after dosing and mean levels then declined gradually to near the lower limit of detection by 12 weeks. The mean (± standard deviation) leuprolide concentration from 3 to 12 weeks was 0.23 ± 0.09 ng/mL. However, intact leuprolide and an inactive major metabolite could not be distinguished by the assay which was employed in the study. The initial burst, followed by the rapid decline to a steady-state level, was similar to the release pattern seen with the monthly formulation.

Distribution The mean steady-state volume of distribution of leuprolide following intravenous bolus administration to healthy male volunteers was 27 L. *In vitro* binding to human plasma proteins ranged from 43% to 49%.

Metabolism In healthy male volunteers, a 1 mg bolus of leuprolide administered intravenously revealed that the mean systemic clearance was 7.6 L/h, with a terminal elimination half-life of approximately 3 hours based on a two compartment model.

In rats and dogs, administration of ^{14}C-labeled leuprolide was shown to be metabolized to smaller inactive peptides, a pentapeptide (Metabolite I), tripeptides (Metabolites II and III) and a dipeptide (Metabolite IV). These fragments may be further catabolized.

In a pharmacokinetic/pharmacodynamic study of endometriosis patients, intramuscular 11.25 mg LUPRON DEPOT (n=19) every 12 weeks or intramuscular 3.75 mg LUPRON DEPOT (n=15) every 4 weeks was administered for 24 weeks. There was no statistically significant difference in changes of serum estradiol concentration from baseline between the 2 treatment groups.

M-I plasma concentrations measured in 5 prostate cancer patients reached maximum concentration 2 to 6 hours after dosing and were approximately 6% of the peak parent drug concentration. One week after dosing, mean plasma M-I concentrations were approximately 20% of mean leuprolide concentrations.

Excretion Following administration of LUPRON DEPOT 3.75 mg to 3 patients, less than 5% of the dose was recovered as parent and M-I metabolite in the urine.

Special Populations The pharmacokinetics of the drug in hepatically and renally impaired patients have not been determined.

Drug Interactions No pharmacokinetic-based drug-drug interaction studies have been conducted with LUPRON DEPOT. However, because leuprolide acetate is a peptide that is primarily degraded by peptidase and not by cytochrome P-450 enzymes as noted in specific studies, and the drug is only about 46% bound to plasma proteins, drug interactions would not be expected to occur.

CLINICAL STUDIES

In a pharmacokinetic/pharmacodynamic study of healthy female subjects (N=20), the onset of estradiol suppression was observed for individual subjects between day 4 and week 4 after dosing. By the third week following the injection, the mean estradiol concentration (8 pg/mL) was in the menopausal range. Throughout the remainder of the dosing period, mean serum estradiol levels ranged from the menopausal to the early follicular range.

Serum estradiol was suppressed to ≤20 pg/mL in all subjects within four weeks and remained suppressed (≤40 pg/mL) in 80% of subjects until the end of the 12-week dosing interval, at which time two of these subjects had a value between 40 and 50 pg/mL. Four additional subjects had at least two consecutive elevations of estradiol (range 43–240 pg/mL) levels during the 12-week dosing interval, but there was no indication of luteal function for any of the subjects during this period.

LUPRON DEPOT–3 Month 11.25 mg induced amenorrhea in 85% (N=17) of subjects during the initial month and 100% during the second month following the injection. All subjects remained amenorrheic through the remainder of the 12-week dosing interval. Episodes of light bleeding and spotting were reported by a majority of subjects during the first month after the injection and in a few subjects at later time-points. Menses resumed on average 12 weeks (range 2.9 to 20.4 weeks) following the end of the 12-week dosing interval.

LUPRON DEPOT–3 Month 11.25 mg produced similar pharmacodynamic effects in terms of hormonal and menstrual suppression to those achieved with monthly injections of LUPRON DEPOT 3.75 mg during the controlled clinical trials for the management of endometriosis and the anemia caused by uterine fibroids.

Endometriosis: In a Phase IV pharmacokinetic/pharmacodynamic study of patients, LUPRON DEPOT–3 Month 11.25 mg (N=21) was shown to be comparable to monthly LUPRON DEPOT 3.75 mg (N=20) in relieving the clinical signs/symptoms of endometriosis (dysmenorrhea, non-menstrual pelvic pain, pelvic tenderness and pelvic induration). In both treatment groups, suppression of menses was achieved in 100% of the patients who remained in the study for at least 60 days. Suppression is defined as no new menses for at least 60 consecutive days.

In controlled clinical studies, LUPRON DEPOT 3.75 mg monthly for six months was shown to be comparable to danazol 800 mg/day in relieving the clinical sign/symptoms of endometriosis (pelvic pain, dysmenorrhea, dyspareunia, pelvic tenderness, and induration) and in reducing the size of endometrial implants as evidenced by laparoscopy.

The clinical significance of a decrease in endometriotic lesions is not known at this time, and in addition laparoscopic staging of endometriosis does not necessarily correlate with the severity of symptoms.

LUPRON DEPOT 3.75 mg monthly induced amenorrhea in 74% and 98% of the patients after the first and second treatment months respectively. Most of the remaining patients reported episodes of only light bleeding or spotting. In the first, second and third post-treatment months, normal menstrual cycles resumed in 7%, 71% and 95% of patients, respectively, excluding those who became pregnant.

Figure 1 illustrates the percent of patients with symptoms at baseline, final treatment visit and sustained relief at 6 and 12 months following discontinuation of treatment for the various symptoms evaluated during the two controlled clinical studies. A total of 166 patients received LUPRON DEPOT 3.75 mg. Seventy-five percent (N=125) of these elected to participate in the follow-up period. Of these patients, 36% and 24% are included in the 6 month and 12 month follow-up analysis, respectively. All the patients who had a pain evaluation at baseline and at a minimum of one treatment visit, are included in the Baseline (B) and final treatment visit (F) analysis.

FIGURE 1 – PERCENT OF PATIENTS WITH SIGN/SYMPTOMS OF ENDOMETRIOSIS AT BASELINE, FINAL TREATMENT VISIT, AND AFTER 6 AND 12 MONTHS OF FOLLOW-UP

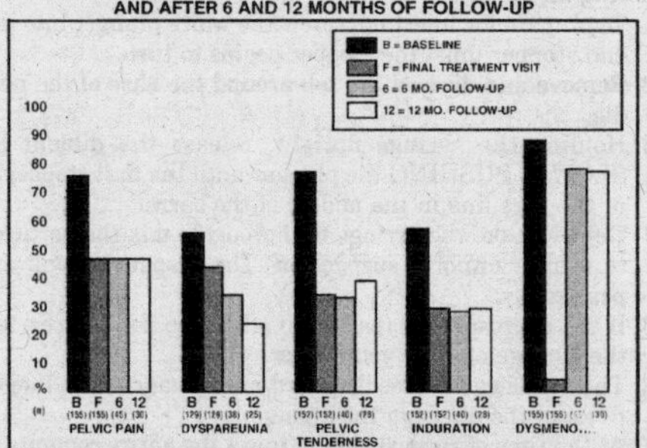

Hormonal add-back therapy: Two clinical studies with a treatment duration of 12 months indicate that concurrent hormonal therapy (norethindrone acetate 5 mg daily) is effective in significantly reducing the loss of bone mineral density associated with LUPRON, without compromising the efficacy of LUPRON in relieving symptoms of endometriosis. (All patients in these studies received calcium supplementation with 1000 mg elemental calcium). One controlled, randomized and double-blind study included 51 women treated with LUPRON DEPOT 3.75 mg alone and 55 women treated with LUPRON DEPOT 3.75 mg plus norethindrone acetate 5 mg (LD/N) daily. The second study was an open label study in which 136 women were treated with monthly LUPRON DEPOT 3.75 mg plus norethindrone acetate 5 mg daily. This study confirmed the reduction in loss of bone mineral density th was observed in the controlled study. Suppression of menses was maintained throughout treatment in 84% and 73% of patients receiving LD/N, in the controlled study and open label study, respectively. The median time for menses resumption after treatment with LD/N was 8 weeks.

Figure 2 illustrates the mean pain scores for the LD/N groups from the controlled study.

[See figure at top of next column]

Uterine Leiomyomata (Fibroids): **LUPRON DEPOT 3.75 mg for a period of three to six months was studied in four controlled clinical trials.**

In one of these clinical studies, enrollment was based on hematocrit ≤30% and/or hemoglobin ≤10.2 g/dL. Administration of LUPRON DEPOT 3.75 mg, concomitantly with iron, produced an increase of ≥6% hematocrit and ≥2 g/dL hemoglobin in 77% of patients at three months of therapy. The mean change in hematocrit was 10.1% and the mean change in hemoglobin was 4.2 g/dL. Clinical response was judged to be a hematocrit of ≥36% and hemoglobin of ≥12 g/dL, thus allowing for autologous blood donation prior to surgery. At two and three months respectively, 71% and 75% of patients met this criterion (Table 1). These data suggest however, that some patients may benefit from iron alone or 1 to 2 months of LUPRON DEPOT 3.75 mg.

Figure 2
Treatment Period Mean Pain Scores for LD/N* Patients

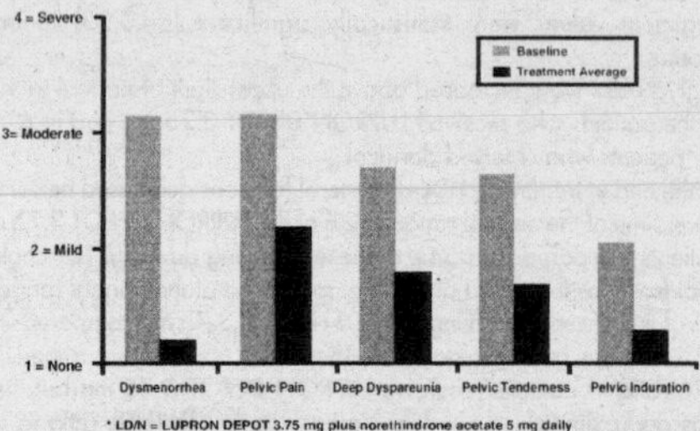

* LD/N = LUPRON DEPOT 3.75 mg plus norethindrone acetate 5 mg daily

Table 1
PERCENT OF PATIENTS ACHIEVING HEMATOCRIT ≥36% AND HEMOGLOBIN ≥12 GM/DL

Treatment Group	Week 4	Week 8	Week 12
LUPRON DEPOT 3.75 mg with Iron (N=104)	40*	71**	75*
Iron Alone (N=98)	17	39	49

* P-Value < 0.01
** P-Value < 0.001

Excessive vaginal bleeding (menorrhagia or menometrorrhagia) decreased in 80% of patients at three months. Episodes of spotting and menstrual-like bleeding were noted in 16% of patients at final visit.

In this same study, a decrease of ≥25% was seen in uterine and myoma volumes in 60% and 54% of patients respectively. The mean fibroid diameter was 6.3 cm at pretreatment and decreased to 5.6 cm at the end of treatment. LUPRON DEPOT 3.75 mg was found to relieve symptoms of bloating, pelvic pain, and pressure.

In three other controlled clinical trials, enrollment was not based on hematologic status. Mean uterine volume decreased by 41% and myoma volume decreased by 37% at final visit as evidenced by ultrasound or MRI. The mean fibroid diameter was 5.6 cm at pretreatment and decreased to 4.7 cm at the end of treatment. These patients also experienced a decrease in symptoms including excessive vaginal bleeding and pelvic discomfort. Ninety-five percent of these patients became amenorrheic with 61%, 25%, and 4% experiencing amenorrhea during the first, second, and third treatment months respectively.

In addition, posttreatment follow-up was carried out in one clinical trial for a small percentage of LUPRON DEPOT 3.75 mg patients (N=46) among the 77% who demonstrated a ≥25% decrease in uterine volume while on therapy. Menses usually returned within two months of cessation of therapy. Mean time to return to pretreatment uterine size was 8.3 months. Regrowth did not appear to be related to pretreatment uterine volume.

There is no evidence that pregnancy rates are enhanced or adversely affected by the use of LUPRON DEPOT.

INDICATIONS AND USAGE

Endometriosis: LUPRON DEPOT–3 Month 11.25 mg is indicated for management of endometriosis, including pain relief and reduction of endometriotic lesions. LUPRON DEPOT with norethindrone acetate 5 mg daily is also indicated for initial management of endometriosis and for management of recurrence of symptoms. (Refer also to norethindrone acetate prescribing information for WARNINGS, PRECAUTIONS, CONTRAINDICATIONS and ADVERSE REACTIONS associated with norethindrone acetate). Duration of initial treatment or retreatment should be limited to 6 months.

Uterine Leiomyomata (Fibroids): **LUPRON DEPOT–3 Month 11.25 mg concomitantly with iron therapy is indicated for the preoperative hematologic improvement of patients with anemia caused by uterine leiomyomata. The clinician may wish to consider a one-month trial period on iron alone inasmuch as some of the patients will respond to iron alone. (See Table 1, CLINICAL STUDIES section.) LUPRON may be added if the response to iron alone is considered inadequate. Recommended therapy is a single injection of LUPRON DEPOT–3 Month 11.25 mg. This dosage form is indicated only for women for whom three months of hormonal suppression is deemed necessary.**

Experience with LUPRON DEPOT in females has been limited to women 18 years of age and older treated for no more than 6 months.

CONTRAINDICATIONS

1. Hypersensitivity to GnRH, GnRH agonist analogs or any of the excipients in LUPRON DEPOT.
2. Undiagnosed abnormal vaginal bleeding.
3. LUPRON DEPOT is contraindicated in women who are or may become pregnant while receiving the drug. LUPRON DEPOT may cause fetal harm when administered to a pregnant woman. Major fetal abnormalities were observed in rabbits but not in rats after administration of LUPRON DEPOT throughout gestation. There was increased fetal mortality and decreased fetal weights in rats and rabbits. (See **Pregnancy** section.) The effects on fetal mortality are expected consequences of the alterations in hormonal levels brought about by the drug. If this drug is used during pregnancy or if the patient becomes pregnant while taking this drug, the patient should be apprised of the potential hazard to the fetus.
4. Use in women who are breast-feeding. (See **Nursing Mothers** section.)
5. Norethindrone acetate is contraindicated in women with the following conditions:
   — Thrombophlebitis, thromboembolic disorders, cerebral apoplexy, or a past history of these conditions
   — Markedly impaired liver function or liver disease
   — Known or suspected carcinoma of the breast

WARNINGS

1. As the effects of LUPRON DEPOT–3 Month 11.25 mg are present throughout the course of therapy, the drug should only be used in patients who require hormonal suppression for at least three months.
2. Experience with LUPRON DEPOT in females has been limited to six months; therefore, exposure should be limited to six months of therapy.
3. Safe use of leuprolide acetate or norethindrone acetate in pregnancy has not been established clinically. Before starting treatment with LUPRON DEPOT pregnancy must be excluded.
4. When used at the recommended dose and dosing interval, LUPRON DEPOT usually inhibits ovulation and stops menstruation. Contraception is not insured, however, by taking LUPRON DEPOT. Therefore, patients should use non-hormonal methods of contraception. Patients should be advised to see their physician if they believe they may be pregnant. If a patient becomes pregnant during treatment, the drug must be discontinued and the patient must be apprised of the potential risk to the fetus. (See **CONTRAINDICATIONS** section.)
5. During the early phase of therapy, sex steroids temporarily rise above baseline because of the physiologic effect of the drug. Therefore, an increase in clinical signs and symptoms may be observed during the initial days of therapy, but these will dissipate with continued therapy.
6. Symptoms consistent with an anaphylactoid or asthmatic process have been rarely reported post-marketing.
7. The following applies to co-treatment with LUPRON and norethindrone acetate:
   Norethindrone acetate treatment should be discontinued if there is a sudden partial or complete loss of vision or if there is sudden onset of proptosis, diplopia, or migraine. If examination reveals papilledema or retinal vascular lesions, medication should be withdrawn.
   Because of the occasional occurrence of thrombophlebitis and pulmonary embolism in patients taking progestogens, the physician should be alert to the earliest manifestations of the disease in women taking norethindrone acetate.
   Assessment and management of risk factors for cardiovascular disease is recommended prior to initiation of add-back therapy with norethindrone acetate. Norethindrone acetate should be used with caution in women with risk factors, including lipid abnormalities or cigarette smoking.

PRECAUTIONS

Information for Patients An information pamphlet for patients is included with the product. Patients should be aware of the following information:

1. Since menstruation should stop with effective doses of LUPRON DEPOT, the patient should notify her physician if regular menstruation persists. Patients missing successive doses of LUPRON DEPOT may experience breakthrough bleeding.
2. Patients should not use LUPRON DEPOT if they are pregnant, breast feeding, have undiagnosed abnormal vaginal bleeding, or are allergic to any of the ingredients in LUPRON DEPOT.
3. LUPRON DEPOT is contraindicated for use during pregnancy. Therefore, a non-hormonal method of contraception should be used during treatment. Patients should be advised that if they miss successive doses of LUPRON DEPOT, breakthrough bleeding or ovulation may occur with the potential for conception. If a patient becomes pregnant during treatment, she should discontinue treatment and consult her physician.
4. Adverse events occurring in clinical studies with LUPRON DEPOT that are associated with hypoestrogenism include: hot flashes, headaches, emotional lability, decreased libido, acne, myalgia, reduction in breast size, and vaginal dryness. Estrogen levels returned to normal after treatment was discontinued.

Table 2
ADVERSE EVENTS REPORTED TO BE CAUSALLY RELATED TO DRUG IN ≥ 5% OF PATIENTS

	Endometriosis (2 Studies)						**Uterine Fibroids (4 Studies)**			
	LUPRON DEPOT 3.75 mg N=166		Danazol N=136		Placebo N=31		**LUPRON DEPOT 3.75 mg N=166**		**Placebo N=163**	
	N	(%)	N	(%)	N	(%)	**N**	**(%)**	**N**	**(%)**
Body as a Whole										
Asthenia	5	(3)	9	(7)	0	(0)	**14**	**(8.4)**	**8**	**(4.9)**
General pain	31	(19)	22	(16)	1	(3)	**14**	**(8.4)**	**10**	**(6.1)**
Headache*	53	(32)	30	(22)	2	(6)	**43**	**(25.9)**	**29**	**(17.8)**
Cardiovascular System										
Hot flashes/sweats*	139	(84)	77	(57)	9	(29)	**121**	**(72.9)**	**29**	**(17.8)**
Gastrointestinal System										
Nausea/vomiting	21	(13)	17	(13)	1	(3)	**8**	**(4.8)**	**6**	**(3.7)**
GI disturbances*	11	(7)	8	(6)	1	(3)	**5**	**(3.0)**	**2**	**(1.2)**
Metabolic and Nutritional Disorders										
Edema	12	(7)	17	(13)	1	(3)	**9**	**(5.4)**	**2**	**(1.2)**
Weight gain/loss	22	(13)	36	(26)	0	(0)	**5**	**(3.0)**	**2**	**(1.2)**
Endocrine System										
Acne	17	(10)	27	(20)	0	(0)	**0**	**(0)**	**0**	**(0)**
Hirsutism	2	(1)	9	(7)	1	(3)	**1**	**(0.6)**	**0**	**(0)**
Musculoskeletal System										
Joint disorder*	14	(8)	11	(8)	0	(0)	**13**	**(7.8)**	**5**	**(3.1)**
Myalgia*	1	(1)	7	(5)	0	(0)	**1**	**(0.6)**	**0**	**(0)**
Nervous System										
Decreased libido*	19	(11)	6	(4)	0	(0)	**3**	**(1.8)**	**0**	**(0)**
Depression/emotional lability*	36	(22)	27	(20)	1	(3)	**18**	**(10.8)**	**7**	**(4.3)**
Dizziness	19	(11)	4	(3)	0	(0)	**3**	**(1.8)**	**6**	**(3.7)**
Nervousness*	8	(5)	11	(8)	0	(0)	**8**	**(4.8)**	**1**	**(0.6)**
Neuromuscular disorders*	11	(7)	17	(13)	0	(0)	**3**	**(1.8)**	**0**	**(0)**
Paresthesias	12	(7)	11	(8)	0	(0)	**2**	**(1.2)**	**1**	**(0.6)**
Skin and Appendages										
Skin reactions	17	(10)	20	(15)	1	(3)	**5**	**(3.0)**	**2**	**(1.2)**
Urogenital System										
Breast changes/tenderness/pain*	10	(6)	12	(9)	0	(0)	**3**	**(1.8)**	**7**	**(4.3)**
Vaginitis*	46	(28)	23	(17)	0	(0)	**19**	**(11.4)**	**3**	**(1.8)**

5. Patients should be counseled on the possibility of the development or worsening of depression and the occurrence of memory disorders.
6. The induced hypoestrogenic state **also** results in a loss in bone density over the course of treatment, some of which may not be reversible. For a period up to six months, this bone loss should not be clinically significant. Clinical studies show that concurrent hormonal therapy with norethindrone acetate 5 mg daily is effective in reducing loss of bone mineral density that occurs with LUPRON. (All patients received calcium supplementation with 1000 mg elemental calcium.) (See ***Changes in Bone Density*** section).
7. If the symptoms of endometriosis recur after a course of therapy, retreatment with a six-month course of LUPRON DEPOT and norethindrone acetate 5 mg daily may be considered. Retreatment beyond this one six-month course cannot be recommended. It is recommended that bone density be assessed before retreatment begins to ensure that values are within normal limits. Retreatment with LUPRON DEPOT alone is not recommended.
8. In patients with major risk factors for decreased bone mineral content such as chronic alcohol and/or tobacco use, strong family history of osteoporosis, or chronic use of drugs that can reduce bone mass such as anticonvulsants or corticosteroids, LUPRON DEPOT therapy may pose an additional risk. In these patients, the risks and benefits must be weighed carefully before therapy with LUPRON DEPOT alone is instituted, and concomitant treatment with norethindrone acetate 5 mg daily should be considered. Retreatment with gonadotropin-releasing hormone analogs, including LUPRON is not advisable in patients with major risk factors for loss of bone mineral content.
9. Because norethindrone acetate may cause some degree of fluid retention, conditions which might be influenced by this factor, such as epilepsy, migraine, asthma, cardiac or renal dysfunctions require careful observation during norethindrone acetate add-back therapy.
10. Patients who have a history of depression should be carefully observed during treatment with norethindrone acetate and norethindrone acetate should be discontinued if severe depression occurs.

Laboratory Tests See **ADVERSE REACTIONS** section.

Drug Interactions No pharmacokinetic-based drug-drug interaction studies have been conducted with LUPRON DEPOT. However, because leuprolide acetate is a peptide that is primarily degraded by peptidase and not by cytochrome P-450 enzymes as noted in specific studies, and the drug is only about 46% bound to plasma proteins, drug interactions would not be expected to occur.

Drug/Laboratory Test Interactions Administration of LUPRON DEPOT in therapeutic doses results in suppression of the pituitary-gonadal system. Normal function is usually restored within three months after treatment is discontinued. Therefore, diagnostic tests of pituitary gonadotropic and gonadal functions conducted during treatment and for up to three months after discontinuation of LUPRON DEPOT may be misleading.

Carcinogenesis, Mutagenesis, Impairment of Fertility A two-year carcinogenicity study was conducted in rats and mice. In rats, a dose-related increase of benign pituitary hyperplasia and benign pituitary adenomas was noted at 24 months when the drug was administered subcutaneously at high daily doses (0.6 to 4 mg/kg). There was a significant but not dose-related increase of pancreatic islet-cell adenomas in females and of testicular interstitial cell adenomas in males (highest incidence in the low dose group). In mice, no leuprolide acetate-induced tumors or pituitary abnormalities were observed at a dose as high as 60 mg/kg for two years. Patients have been treated with leuprolide acetate for up to three years with doses as high as 10 mg/day and for two years with doses as high as 20 mg/day without demonstrable pituitary abnormalities.

Mutagenicity studies have been performed with leuprolide acetate using bacterial and mammalian systems. These studies provided no evidence of a mutagenic potential.

Clinical and pharmacologic studies in adults (>18 years) with leuprolide acetate and similar analogs have shown reversibility of fertility suppression when the drug is discontinued after continuous administration for periods of up to 24 weeks. Although no clinical studies have been completed in children to assess the full reversibility of fertility suppression, animal studies (prepubertal and adult rats and monkeys) with leuprolide acetate and other GnRH analogs have shown functional recovery.

Pregnancy, Teratogenic Effects Pregnancy Category X. (See **CONTRAINDICATIONS** section.) When administered on day 6 of pregnancy at test dosages of 0.00024, 0.0024, and 0.024 mg/kg (1/300 to 1/3 of the human dose) to rabbits, LUPRON DEPOT produced a dose-related increase in major fetal abnormalities. Similar studies in rats failed to demonstrate an increase in fetal malformations. There was increased fetal mortality and decreased fetal weights with the two higher doses of LUPRON DEPOT in rabbits and with the highest dose (0.024 mg/kg) in rats.

Nursing Mothers It is not known whether LUPRON DEPOT is excreted in human milk. Because many drugs are excreted in human milk, and because the effects of LUPRON DEPOT on lactation and/or the breast-fed child have not been determined, LUPRON DEPOT should not be used by nursing mothers.

Pediatric Use Safety and effectiveness of LUPRON DEPOT–3 Month 11.25 mg have not been established in pediatric patients. Experience with LUPRON DEPOT for treatment of endometriosis has been limited to women 18 years of age and older. See LUPRON DEPOT-PED® (leuprolide acetate for depot suspension) labeling for the safety and effectiveness in children with central precocious puberty.

Geriatric Use This product has not been studied in women over 65 years of age and is not indicated in this population.

ADVERSE REACTIONS

Clinical Trials

The **monthly formulation of LUPRON DEPOT 3.75 mg** was utilized in controlled clinical trials that studied the drug in 166 endometriosis and 166 uterine fibroids patients. Adverse events reported in ≥5% of patients in either of these populations and thought to be potentially related to drug are noted in the following table.

[See table above]

In these same studies, symptoms reported in <5% of patients included: *Body as a Whole* – Body odor, Flu syndrome,

Continued on next page

Lupron Depot-3 Month—Cont.

Injection site reactions; *Cardiovascular System* – Palpitations, Syncope, Tachycardia; *Digestive System* – Appetite changes, Dry mouth, Thirst; *Endocrine System* – Androgen-like effects; *Hemic and Lymphatic System* – Ecchymosis, Lymphadenopathy; *Nervous System* – Anxiety,* Insomnia/Sleep disorders,* Delusions, Memory disorder, Personality disorder; *Respiratory System* – Rhinitis; *Skin and Appendages* – Alopecia, Hair disorder, Nail disorder; *Special Senses* – Conjunctivitis, Ophthalmologic disorders,* Taste perversion; *Urogenital System* – Dysuria,* Lactation, Menstrual disorders.

* = Possible effect of decreased estrogen.

In one controlled clinical trial utilizing the monthly formulation of LUPRON DEPOT, patients diagnosed with uterine fibroids received a higher dose (7.5 mg) of LUPRON DEPOT. Events seen with this dose that were thought to be potentially related to drug and were not seen at the lower dose included glossitis, hypesthesia, lactation, pyelonephritis, and urinary disorders. Generally, a higher incidence of hypoestrogenic effects was observed at the higher dose.

In a pharmacokinetic trial involving 20 healthy female subjects receiving LUPRON DEPOT–3 Month 11.25 mg, a few adverse events were reported with this formulation that were not reported previously. These included face edema, agitation, laryngitis, and ear pain.

In a Phase IV study involving endometriosis patients receiving LUPRON DEPOT 3.75 mg (N=20) or LUPRON DEPOT–3 Month 11.25 mg (N=21), similar adverse events were reported by the two groups of patients. In general the safety profiles of the two formulations were comparable in this study.

Table 3 lists the potentially drug-related adverse events observed in at least 5% of patients in any treatment group, during the first 6 months of treatment in the add-back clinical studies, in which patients were treated with monthly LUPRON DEPOT 3.75 mg with or without norethindrone acetate co-treatment.

[See table 3 above]

In the controlled clinical trial, 50 of 51 (98%) patients in the LD group (LUPRON DEPOT 3.75 mg) and 48 of 55 (87%) patients in the LD/N group (LUPRON DEPOT 3.75 mg plus norethindrone acetate 5 mg daily) reported experiencing hot flashes on one or more occasions during treatment. During Month 6 of treatment, 32 of 37 (86%) patients in the LD group and 22 of 38 (58%) patients in the LD/N group reported having experienced hot flashes. The mean number of days on which hot flashes were reported during this month of treatment was 19 and 7 in the LD and LD/N treatment groups, respectively. The mean maximum number of hot flashes in a day during this month of treatment was 5.8 and 1.9 in the LD and LD/N treatment groups, respectively.

Changes in Bone Density

In controlled clinical studies, patients with endometriosis (six months of therapy) or uterine fibroids (three months of therapy) were treated with LUPRON DEPOT 3.75 mg. In endometriosis patients, vertebral bone density as measured by dual energy x-ray absorptiometry (DEXA) decreased by an average of 3.2% at six months compared with the pretreatment value. Clinical studies demonstrate that concurrent hormonal therapy (norethindrone acetate 5 mg daily) and calcium supplementation is effective in significantly reducing the loss of bone mineral density that occurs with LUPRON treatment, without compromising the efficacy of LUPRON in relieving symptoms of endometriosis. LUPRON DEPOT 3.75 mg plus norethindrone acetate 5 mg daily was evaluated in two clinical trials. The results from this regimen were similar in both studies. LUPRON DEPOT 3.75 mg was used as a control group in one study. The bone mineral density data of the lumbar spine from these two studies are presented in Table 4.

[See table 4 above]

In the Phase IV, six-month pharmacokinetic/pharmacodynamic study in endometriosis patients who were treated with LUPRON DEPOT 3.75 mg or LUPRON DEPOT–3 Month 11.25 mg, vertebral bone density measured by DEXA decreased compared with baseline by an average of 3.0% and 2.8% at six months for the two groups, respectively.

When LUPRON DEPOT 3.75 mg was administered for three months in uterine fibroid patients, vertebral trabecular bone mineral density as assessed by quantitative digital radiography (QDR) revealed a mean decrease of 2.7% compared with baseline. Six months after discontinuation of therapy, a trend toward recovery was observed. Use of LUPRON DEPOT for longer than three months (uterine fibroids) or six months (endometriosis) or in the presence of other known risk factors for decreased bone mineral content may cause additional bone loss **and is not recommended.**

Changes in Laboratory Values During Treatment

Liver Enzymes

Three percent of uterine fibroid patients treated with LUPRON DEPOT 3.75 mg, manifested posttreatment transaminase values that were at least twice the baseline value and above the upper limit of the normal range. None of the laboratory increases were associated with clinical symptoms.

In two other clinical trials, 6 of 191 patients receiving LUPRON DEPOT 3.75 mg plus norethindrone acetate 5 mg daily for up to 12 months developed an elevated (at least twice the upper limit of normal) SGPT or GGT. Five of the 6 increases were observed beyond 6 months of treatment. None were associated with an elevated bilirubin concentration.

Lipids

Triglycerides were increased above the upper limit of normal in 12% of the endometriosis patients who received LUPRON DEPOT 3.75 mg and in 32% of the subjects receiving LUPRON DEPOT–3 Month 11.25 mg.

Of those endometriosis and uterine fibroid patients whose pretreatment cholesterol values were in the normal range, mean change following therapy was +16 mg/dL to +17 mg/dL in endometriosis patients and +11 mg/dL to +29 mg/dL in uterine fibroid patients. In the endometriosis treated patients, increases from the pretreatment values were statistically significant ($p<0.03$). There was essentially no increase in the LDL/HDL ratio in patients from either population receiving LUPRON DEPOT 3.75 mg.

In two other clinical trials, LUPRON DEPOT 3.75 mg plus norethindrone acetate 5 mg daily were evaluated for 12 months of treatment. LUPRON DEPOT 3.75 mg was used as a control group in one study. Percent changes from baseline for serum lipids and percentages of patients with serum lipid values outside of the normal range in the two studies are summarized in the tables below.

[See table 5 above]

Changes from baseline tended to be greater at Week 52. After treatment, mean serum lipid levels from patients with follow up data returned to pretreatment values.

[See table at top of next page]

Low HDL-cholesterol (<40 mg/dL) and elevated LDL-cholesterol (> 160 mg/dL) are recognized risk factors for cardiovascular disease. The long-term significance of the observed treatment-related changes in serum lipids in women with endometriosis is unknown. Therefore assessment of cardiovascular risk factors should be considered prior to initiation of concurrent treatment with LUPRON and norethindrone acetate.

Table 3
TREATMENT-RELATED ADVERSE EVENTS OCCURRING IN ≥ 5% OF PATIENTS

	Controlled Study				Open Label Study	
	LD-Only[1] N=51		LD/N[2] N=55		LD/N[2] N=136	
Adverse Events	N	(%)	N	(%)	N	(%)
Any Adverse Event	50	(98)	53	(96)	126	(93)
Body as a Whole						
Asthenia	9	(18)	10	(18)	15	(11)
Headache/Migraine	33	(65)	28	(51)	63	(46)
Injection Site Reaction	1	(2)	5	(9)	4	(3)
Pain	12	(24)	16	(29)	29	(21)
Cardiovascular System						
Hot flashes/Sweats	50	(98)	48	(87)	78	(57)
Digestive System						
Altered Bowel Function	7	(14)	8	(15)	14	(10)
Changes in Appetite	2	(4)	0	(0)	8	(6)
GI Disturbance	2	(4)	4	(7)	6	(4)
Nausea/Vomiting	13	(25)	16	(29)	17	(13)
Metabolic and Nutritional Disorders						
Edema	0	(0)	5	(9)	9	(7)
Weight Changes	6	(12)	7	(13)	6	(4)
Nervous System						
Anxiety	3	(6)	0	(0)	11	(8)
Depression/Emotional Lability	16	(31)	15	(27)	46	(34)
Dizziness/Vertigo	8	(16)	6	(11)	10	(7)
Insomnia/Sleep Disorder	16	(31)	7	(13)	20	(15)
Libido Changes	5	(10)	2	(4)	10	(7)
Memory Disorder	3	(6)	1	(2)	6	(4)
Nervousness	4	(8)	2	(4)	15	(11)
Neuromuscular Disorder	1	(2)	5	(9)	4	(3)
Skin and Appendages						
Alopecia	0	(0)	5	(9)	4	(3)
Androgen-Like Effects	2	(4)	3	(5)	24	(18)
Skin/Mucous Membrane Reaction	2	(4)	5	(9)	15	(11)
Urogenital System						
Breast Changes/Pain/Tenderness	3	(6)	7	(13)	11	(8)
Menstrual Disorders	1	(2)	0	(0)	7	(5)
Vaginitis	10	(20)	8	(15)	11	(8)

[1] LD-Only = LUPRON DEPOT 3.75 mg
[2] LD/N = LUPRON DEPOT 3.75 mg plus norethindrone acetate 5 mg

Table 4
MEAN PERCENT CHANGE FROM BASELINE IN BONE MINERAL DENSITY OF LUMBAR SPINE

	LUPRON DEPOT 3.75 mg		LUPRON DEPOT 3.75 mg plus norethindrone acetate 5 mg daily			
	Controlled Study		Controlled Study		Open Label Study	
	N	Change	N	Change	N	Change
Week 24[1]	41	−3.2%	42	−0.3%	115	−0.2%
Week 52[2]	29	−6.3%	32	−1.0%	84	−1.1%

[1] Includes on-treatment measurements that fell within 2–252 days after the first day of treatment.
[2] Includes on-treatment measurements >252 days after the first day of treatment.

Table 5
SERUM LIPIDS: MEAN PERCENT CHANGES FROM BASELINE VALUES AT TREATMENT WEEK 24

	LUPRON DEPOT 3.75 mg		LUPRON DEPOT 3.75 mg plus norethindrone acetate 5 mg daily			
	Controlled Study (n=39)		Controlled Study (n=41)		Open Label Study (n=117)	
	Baseline Value*	Wk 24 % Change	Baseline Value*	Wk 24 % Change	Baseline Value*	Wk 24 % Change
Total Cholesterol	170.5	9.2%	179.3	0.2%	181.2	2.8%
HDL Cholesterol	52.4	7.4%	51.8	−18.8%	51.0	−14.6%
LDL Cholesterol	96.6	10.9%	101.5	14.1%	109.1	13.1%
LDL/HDL Ratio	2.0**	5.0%	2.1**	43.4%	2.3**	39.4%
Triglycerides	107.8	17.5%	130.2	9.5%	105.4	13.8%

* mg/dL
** ratio

Table 6
PERCENTAGE OF PATIENTS WITH SERUM LIPID VALUES OUTSIDE OF THE NORMAL RANGE

	LUPRON DEPOT 3.75 mg		LUPRON DEPOT 3.75 mg plus norethindrone acetate 5 mg daily			
	Controlled Study (n = 39)		Controlled Study (n = 41)		Open Label Study (n = 117)	
	Wk 0	Wk 24*	Wk 0	Wk 24*	Wk 0	Wk 24*
Total Cholesterol (>240 mg/dL)	15%	23%	15%	20%	6%	7%
HDL Cholesterol (<40 mg/dL)	15%	10%	15%	44%	15%	41%
LDL Cholesterol (>160 mg/dL)	0%	8%	5%	7%	9%	11%
LDL/HDL Ratio (>4.0)	0%	3%	2%	15%	7%	21%
Triglycerides (>200 mg/dL)	13%	13%	12%	10%	5%	9%

* Includes all patients regardless of baseline value.

Chemistry
Slight to moderate mean increases were noted for glucose, uric acid, BUN, creatinine, total protein, albumin, bilirubin, alkaline phosphatase, LDH, calcium, and phosphorus. None of these increases were clinically significant. In the hormonal add-back studies LUPRON DEPOT in combination with norethindrone acetate was associated with elevations of GGT and SGPT in 6% to 7% of patients.

Postmarketing
During postmarketing surveillance with other dosage forms and in the same and/or different populations, the following adverse events were reported. Like other drugs in this class, mood swings, including depression, have been reported. There have been very rare reports of suicidal ideation and attempt. Many, but not all, of these patients had a history of depression or other psychiatric illness. Patients should be counseled on the possibility of development or worsening of depression during treatment with LUPRON.
Symptoms consistent with an anaphylactoid or asthmatic process have been reported. Rash, urticaria, and photosensitivity reactions have also been reported.
Localized reactions including induration and abscess have been reported at the site of injection.
Symptoms consistent with fibromyalgia (eg: joint and muscle pain, headaches, sleep disorders, gastrointestinal distress, and shortness of breath) have been reported individually and collectively.
Other events reported are:
Cardiovascular System – Hypotension, Pulmonary embolism; *Hemic and Lymphatic System* – Decreased WBC; *Central/Peripheral Nervous System* – Peripheral neuropathy, Spinal fracture/paralysis; *Musculoskeletal System* – Tenosynovitis-like symptoms; *Urogenital System* – Prostate pain.
See other LUPRON DEPOT and LUPRON Injection package inserts for other events reported in the same and different patient populations.

OVERDOSAGE

In clinical trials using daily subcutaneous leuprolide acetate in patients with prostate cancer, doses as high as 20 mg/day for up to two years caused no adverse effects differing from those observed with the 1 mg/day dose.

DOSAGE AND ADMINISTRATION

LUPRON DEPOT Must Be Administered Under the Supervision of a Physician.

Endometriosis: The recommended duration of treatment with LUPRON DEPOT–3 Month 11.25 mg alone or in combination with norethindrone acetate is six months. The choice of LUPRON alone or LUPRON plus norethindrone acetate therapy for initial management of the symptoms and signs of endometriosis should be made by the health care professional in consultation with the patient and should take into consideration the risks and benefits of the addition of norethindrone to LUPRON alone.
If the symptoms of endometriosis recur after a course of therapy, retreatment with a six-month course of LUPRON DEPOT and norethindrone acetate 5 mg daily may be considered. Retreatment beyond this one six-month course cannot be recommended. It is recommended that bone density be assessed before retreatment begins to ensure that values are within normal limits. LUPRON DEPOT alone is not recommended for retreatment. If norethindrone acetate is contraindicated for the individual patient, then retreatment is not recommended.
An assessment of cardiovascular risk and management of risk factors such as cigarette smoking is recommended before beginning treatment with LUPRON and norethindrone acetate.

Uterine Leiomyomata (Fibroids): **The recommended dose of LUPRON DEPOT–3 Month 11.25 mg is one injection. The symptoms associated with uterine leiomyomata will recur following discontinuation of therapy. If additional treatment with LUPRON DEPOT–3 Month 11.25 mg is contemplated, bone density should be assessed prior to initiation of therapy to ensure that values are within normal limits.**

Due to different release characteristics, a fractional dose of the 3-month depot formulation is not equivalent to the same dose of the monthly formulation and should not be given.

Incorporated in a depot formulation, the lyophilized microspheres are to be reconstituted and administered as a single intramuscular injection, in accord with the following directions:

1. To prepare for injection, screw the white plunger into the end stopper until the stopper begins to turn.
2. Remove and discard the tab around the base of the needle.
3. Holding the syringe upright, release the diluent by SLOWLY PUSHING the plunger until the first stopper is at the blue line in the middle of the barrel.
4. Gently shake the syringe to thoroughly mix the particles to form a uniform suspension. The suspension will appear milky.
5. If the microspheres (particles) adhere to the stopper, tap the syringe against your finger.
6. Then remove the needle guard and advance the plunger to expel the air from the syringe.
7. At the time of reconstitution, inject the entire contents of the syringe intramuscularly as you would for a normal injection. The suspension settles very quickly following reconstitution; therefore, it is preferable that LUPRON DEPOT–3 Month 11.25 mg be mixed and used immediately. Reshake suspension if settling occurs.

Since the product does not contain a preservative, the suspension should be discarded if not used immediately.
As with other drugs administered by injection, the injection site should be varied periodically.

HOW SUPPLIED

LUPRON DEPOT–3 Month 11.25 mg is packaged as follows:
Kit with prefilled dual-chamber syringe NDC 0300-3663-01

Each syringe contains sterile lyophilized microspheres which are leuprolide acetate incorporated in a biodegradable polymer of polylactic acid. When mixed with 1.5 mL of the diluent, LUPRON DEPOT–3 Month 11.25 mg is administered as a single IM injection **EVERY THREE MONTHS.**
Store at 25°C (77°F); excursions permitted to 15–30°C (59–86°F) [See USP Controlled Room Temperature]
Rx only
U.S. Patent Nos. 4,652,441; 4,728,721; 4,849,228; 4,917,893; 4,954,298; 5,330,767; 5,476,663; 5,480,656; 5,575,987; 5,631,020; 5,631,021; 5,643,607; and 5,716,640.
Manufactured for
TAP Pharmaceuticals Inc.
Lake Forest, IL 60045, U.S.A.
by Takeda Chemical Industries, Ltd.
Osaka, JAPAN 541
®—Registered Trademark
(No. 3663)
03-5159-R9; Revised: October, 2001

PREVACID® ℞
[prĕ-va-sĭd]
(lansoprazole)
Delayed-Release Capsules

PREVACID®
(lansoprazole)
For Delayed-Release Oral Suspension

Prescribing information for this product, which appears on pages 3292–3298 of the 2002 PDR, has been completely revised as follows. Please write "See Supplement A" next to the product heading.

DESCRIPTION

The active ingredient in PREVACID (lansoprazole) Delayed-Release Capsules and PREVACID (lansoprazole) for Delayed-Release Oral Suspension is a substituted benzimidazole, 2-[[[3-methyl-4-(2,2,2-trifluoroethoxy)-2-pyridyl] methyl] sulfinyl] benzimidazole, a compound that inhibits gastric acid secretion. Its empirical formula is $C_{16}H_{14}F_3N_3O_2S$ with a molecular weight of 369.37. The structural formula is:

Lansoprazole is a white to brownish-white odorless crystalline powder which melts with decomposition at approximately 166°C. Lansoprazole is freely soluble in dimethylformamide; soluble in methanol; sparingly soluble in ethanol; slightly soluble in ethyl acetate, dichloromethane and acetonitrile; very slightly soluble in ether; and practically insoluble in hexane and water.
Lansoprazole is stable when exposed to light for up to two months. The compound degrades in aqueous solution, the rate of degradation increasing with decreasing pH. At 25°C the $t_{1/2}$ is approximately 0.5 hour at pH 5.0 and approximately 18 hours at pH 7.0.
PREVACID is supplied in delayed-release capsules for oral administration and in a packet for delayed-release oral suspension.
The delayed-release capsules contain the active ingredient, lansoprazole, in the form of enteric-coated granules and are available in two dosage strengths: 15 mg and 30 mg of lansoprazole per capsule. Each delayed-release capsule contains enteric-coated granules consisting of lansoprazole, hydroxypropyl cellulose, low substituted hydroxypropyl cellulose, colloidal silicon dioxide, magnesium carbonate, methacrylic acid copolymer, starch, talc, sugar sphere, sucrose, polyethylene glycol, polysorbate 80, and titanium dioxide. Components of the gelatin capsule include gelatin, titanium dioxide, D&C Red No. 28, FD&C Blue No. 1, FD&C Green No. 3*, and FD&C Red No. 40.
PREVACID for Delayed-Release Oral Suspension is composed of the active ingredient, lansoprazole, in the form of enteric-coated granules and also contains inactive granules. The packets contain lansoprazole granules which are identical to those contained in PREVACID Delayed-Release Capsules and are available in 15 mg and 30 mg strengths. Inactive granules are composed of the following ingredients: confectioner's sugar, mannitol, docusate sodium, ferric oxide, colloidal silicon dioxide, xanthan gum, crospovidone, citric acid, sodium citrate, magnesium stearate, and artificial strawberry flavor. The lansoprazole granules and inactive granules, present in unit dose packets, are constituted with water to form a suspension and consumed orally.

* PREVACID 15-mg capsules only.

CLINICAL PHARMACOLOGY

Pharmacokinetics and Metabolism
PREVACID Delayed-Release Capsules and PREVACID for Delayed-Release Oral Suspension contain an enteric-coated granule formulation of lansoprazole. Absorption of lansoprazole begins only after the granules leave the stomach. Absorption is rapid, with mean peak plasma levels of lansoprazole occurring after approximately 1.7 hours. Peak plasma concentrations of lansoprazole (C_{max}) and the area under the plasma concentration curve (AUC) of lansoprazole are approximately proportional in doses from 15 mg to 60 mg after single-oral administration. Lansoprazole does not accumulate and its pharmacokinetics are unaltered by multiple dosing.

Absorption
The absorption of lansoprazole is rapid, with mean C_{max} occurring approximately 1.7 hours after oral dosing, and relatively complete with absolute bioavailability over 80%. In healthy subjects, the mean (±SD) plasma half-life was 1.5 (±1.0) hours. Both C_{max} and AUC are diminished by about 50% if the drug is given 30 minutes after food as opposed to the fasting condition. There is no significant food effect if the drug is given before meals.

Distribution
Lansoprazole is 97% bound to plasma proteins. Plasma protein binding is constant over the concentration range of 0.05 to 5.0 µg/mL.

Metabolism
Lansoprazole is extensively metabolized in the liver. Two metabolites have been identified in measurable quantities in plasma (the hydroxylated sulfinyl and sulfone derivatives of lansoprazole). These metabolites have very little or no antisecretory activity. Lansoprazole is thought to be transformed into two active species which inhibit acid secretion by (H^+,K^+)-ATPase within the parietal cell canaliculus, but are not present in the systemic circulation. The plasma elimination half-life of lansoprazole does not reflect its duration of suppression of gastric acid secretion. Thus, the plasma elimination half-life is less than two hours, while the acid inhibitory effect lasts more than 24 hours.

Elimination
Following single-dose oral administration of lansoprazole, virtually no unchanged lansoprazole was excreted in the urine. In one study, after a single oral dose of ^{14}C-lansoprazole, approximately one-third of the administered radiation was excreted in the urine and two-thirds was recovered in the feces. This implies a significant biliary excretion of the metabolites of lansoprazole.

Special Populations
Geriatric
The clearance of lansoprazole is decreased in the elderly, with elimination half-life increased approximately 50% to 100%. Because the mean half-life in the elderly remains between 1.9 to 2.9 hours, repeated once daily dosing does not result in accumulation of lansoprazole. Peak plasma levels were not increased in the elderly.
Pediatric
The pharmacokinetics of lansoprazole has not been investigated in patients <18 years of age.
Gender
In a study comparing 12 male and 6 female human subjects, no gender differences were found in pharmacokinetics and intragastric pH results. (Also see **Use in Women.**)

Continued on next page

Prevacid—Cont.

Renal Insufficiency
In patients with severe renal insufficiency, plasma protein binding decreased by 1.0%–1.5% after administration of 60 mg of lansoprazole. Patients with renal insufficiency had a shortened elimination half-life and decreased total AUC (free and bound). AUC for free lansoprazole in plasma, however, was not related to the degree of renal impairment, and C_{max} and T_{max} were not different from subjects with healthy kidneys.
Hepatic Insufficiency
In patients with various degrees of chronic hepatic disease, the mean plasma half-life of the drug was prolonged from 1.5 hours to 3.2–7.2 hours. An increase in mean AUC of up to 500% was observed at steady state in hepatically-impaired patients compared to healthy subjects. Dose reduction in patients with severe hepatic disease should be considered.
Race
The pooled mean pharmacokinetic parameters of lansoprazole from twelve U.S. Phase 1 studies (N=513) were compared to the mean pharmacokinetic parameters from two Asian studies (N=20). The mean AUCs of lansoprazole in Asian subjects were approximately twice those seen in pooled U.S. data; however, the inter-individual variability was high. The C_{max} values were comparable.
Pharmacodynamics
Mechanism of Action
Lansoprazole belongs to a class of antisecretory compounds, the substituted benzimidazoles, that do not exhibit anticholinergic or histamine H_2-receptor antagonist properties, but that suppress gastric acid secretion by specific inhibition of the (H^+,K^+)-ATPase enzyme system at the secretory surface of the gastric parietal cell. Because this enzyme system is regarded as the acid (proton) pump within the parietal cell, lansoprazole has been characterized as a gastric acid-pump inhibitor, in that it blocks the final step of acid production. This effect is dose-related and leads to inhibition of both basal and stimulated gastric acid secretion irrespective of the stimulus.
Antisecretory Activity
After oral administration, lansoprazole was shown to significantly decrease the basal acid output and significantly increase the mean gastric pH and percent of time the gastric pH was >3 and >4. Lansoprazole also significantly reduced meal-stimulated gastric acid output and secretion volume, as well as pentagastrin-stimulated acid output. In patients with hypersecretion of acid, lansoprazole significantly reduced basal and pentagastrin-stimulated gastric acid secretion. Lansoprazole inhibited the normal increases in secretion volume, acidity and acid output induced by insulin.
In a crossover study that included lansoprazole 15 and 30 mg for five days, the following effects on intragastric pH were noted:
[See first table above]
After the initial dose in this study, increased gastric pH was seen within 1–2 hours with lansoprazole 30 mg and 2–3 hours with lansoprazole 15 mg. After multiple daily dosing, increased gastric pH was seen within the first hour postdosing with lansoprazole 30 mg and within 1–2 hours postdosing with lansoprazole 15 mg.
Acid suppression may enhance the effect of antimicrobials in eradicating *Helicobacter pylori (H. pylori)*. The percentage of time gastric pH was elevated above 5 and 6 was evaluated in a crossover study of PREVACID given q.d., b.i.d. and t.i.d.
[See second table above]
The inhibition of gastric acid secretion as measured by intragastric pH returns gradually to normal over two to four days after multiple doses. There is no indication of rebound gastric acidity.
Enterochromaffin-like (ECL) Cell Effects
During lifetime exposure of rats with up to 150 mg/kg/day of lansoprazole dosed seven days per week, marked hypergastrinemia was observed followed by ECL cell proliferation and formation of carcinoid tumors, especially in female rats. (See **PRECAUTIONS, Carcinogenesis, Mutagenesis, Impairment of Fertility.**)
Gastric biopsy specimens from the body of the stomach from approximately 150 patients treated continuously with lansoprazole for at least one year did not show evidence of ECL cell effects similar to those seen in rat studies. Longer term data are needed to rule out the possibility of an increased risk of the development of gastric tumors in patients receiving long-term therapy with lansoprazole.
Other Gastric Effects in Humans
Lansoprazole did not significantly affect mucosal blood flow in the fundus of the stomach. Due to the normal physiologic effect caused by the inhibition of gastric acid secretion, a decrease of about 17% in blood flow in the antrum, pylorus, and duodenal bulb was seen. Lansoprazole significantly slowed the gastric emptying of digestible solids. Lansoprazole increased serum pepsinogen levels and decreased pepsin activity under basal conditions and in response to meal stimulation or insulin injection. As with other agents that elevate intragastric pH, increases in gastric pH were associated with increases in nitrate-reducing bacteria and elevation of nitrite concentration in gastric juice in patients with gastric ulcer. No significant increase in nitrosamine concentrations was observed.
Serum Gastrin Effects
In over 2100 patients, median fasting serum gastrin levels increased 50% to 100% from baseline but remained within normal range after treatment with lansoprazole given

Mean Antisecretory Effects After Single and Multiple Daily Dosing

		PREVACID			
		15 mg		30 mg	
Parameter	Baseline Value	Day 1	Day 5	Day 1	Day 5
Mean 24-Hour pH	2.1	2.7+	4.0+	3.6*	4.9*
Mean Nighttime pH	1.9	2.4	3.0+	2.6	3.8*
% Time Gastric pH>3	18	33+	59+	51*	72*
% Time Gastric pH>4	12	22+	49+	41*	66*

NOTE: An intragastric pH of >4 reflects a reduction in gastric acid by 99%.
*(p<0.05) versus baseline and lansoprazole 15 mg.
+(p<0.05) versus baseline only.

Mean Antisecretory Effects After 5 Days of b.i.d. and t.i.d. Dosing

	PREVACID			
Parameter	30 mg q.d.	15 mg b.i.d.	30 mg b.i.d.	30 mg t.i.d.
% Time Gastric pH>5	43	47	59+	77*
% Time Gastric pH>6	20	23	28	45*

+(p<0.05) versus PREVACID 30 mg q.d.
*(p<0.05) versus PREVACID 30 mg q.d., 15 mg b.i.d. and 30 mg b.i.d.

Clarithromycin Susceptibility Test Results and Clinical/Bacteriological Outcomes[a]

Clarithromycin Pretreatment Results		Clarithromycin Post-treatment Results				
		H. pylori negative–eradicated	*H. pylori* positive–not eradicated			
			Post-treatment susceptibility results			
			S[b]	I[b]	R[b]	No MIC
Triple Therapy 14-Day (lansoprazole 30 mg b.i.d./amoxicillin 1 gm b.i.d./clarithromycin 500 mg b.i.d.) (M95-399, M93-131, M95-392)						
Susceptible[b]	112	105				7
Intermediate[b]	3	3				
Resistant[b]	17	6			7	4
Triple Therapy 10-Day (lansoprazole 30 mg b.i.d./amoxicillin 1 gm b.i.d./clarithromycin 500 mg b.i.d.) (M95-399)						
Susceptible[b]	42	40	1		1	
Intermediate[b]						
Resistant[b]	4	1			3	

[a] Includes only patients with pretreatment clarithromycin susceptibility test results
[b] Susceptible (S) MIC ≤0.25 µg/mL, Intermediate (I) MIC 0.5–1.0 µg/mL, Resistant (R) MIC ≥2 µg/mL

orally in doses of 15 mg to 60 mg. These elevations reached a plateau within two months of therapy and returned to pretreatment levels within four weeks after discontinuation of therapy.
Endocrine Effects
Human studies for up to one year have not detected any clinically significant effects on the endocrine system. Hormones studied include testosterone, luteinizing hormone (LH), follicle stimulating hormone (FSH), sex hormone binding globulin (SHBG), dehydroepiandrosterone sulfate (DHEA-S), prolactin, cortisol, estradiol, insulin, aldosterone, parathormone, glucagon, thyroid stimulating hormone (TSH), triiodothyronine (T_3), thyroxine (T_4), and somatotropic hormone (STH). Lansoprazole in oral doses of 15 to 60 mg for up to one year had no clinically significant effect on sexual function. In addition, lansoprazole in oral doses of 15 to 60 mg for two to eight weeks had no clinically significant effect on thyroid function.
In 24-month carcinogenicity studies in Sprague-Dawley rats with daily dosages up to 150 mg/kg, proliferative changes in the Leydig cells of the testes, including benign neoplasm, were increased compared to control rates.
Other Effects
No systemic effects of lansoprazole on the central nervous system, lymphoid, hematopoietic, renal, hepatic, cardiovascular or respiratory systems have been found in humans. No visual toxicity was observed among 56 patients who had extensive baseline eye evaluations, were treated with up to 180 mg/day of lansoprazole and were observed for up to 58 months. Other rat-specific findings after lifetime exposure included focal pancreatic atrophy, diffuse lymphoid hyperplasia in the thymus, and spontaneous retinal atrophy.
Microbiology
Lansoprazole, clarithromycin and/or amoxicillin have been shown to be active against most strains of *Helicobacter pylori in vitro* and in clinical infections as described in the **INDICATIONS AND USAGE** section.
Helicobacter
Helicobacter pylori
Pretreatment Resistance
Clarithromycin pretreatment resistance (≥2.0 µg/mL) was 9.5% (91/960) by E-test and 11.3% (12/106) by agar dilution in the dual and triple therapy clinical trials (M93-125, M93-130, M93-131, M95-392, and M95-399).
Amoxicillin pretreatment susceptible isolates (≤0.25 µg/mL) occurred in 97.8% (936/957) and 98.0% (98/100) of the patients in the dual and triple therapy clinical trials by E-test and agar dilution, respectively. Twenty-one of 957 patients (2.2%) by E-test and 2 of 100 patients (2.0%) by agar dilution had amoxicillin pretreatment MICs of >0.25 µg/mL. One patient on the 14-day triple therapy regimen had an unconfirmed pretreatment amoxicillin minimum inhibitory concentration (MIC) of >256 µg/mL by E-test and the patient was eradicated of *H. pylori*.
[See third table above]
Patients not eradicated of *H. pylori* following lansoprazole/amoxicillin/clarithromycin triple therapy will likely have clarithromycin resistant *H. pylori*. Therefore, for those patients who fail therapy, clarithromycin susceptibility testing should be done when possible. Patients with clarithromycin resistant *H. pylori* should not be treated with lansoprazole/amoxicillin/clarithromycin triple therapy or with regimens which include clarithromycin as the sole antimicrobial agent.
Amoxicillin Susceptibility Test Results and Clinical/Bacteriological Outcomes
In the dual and triple therapy clinical trials, 82.6% (195/236) of the patients that had pretreatment amoxicillin susceptible MICs (≤0.25 µg/mL) were eradicated of *H. pylori*. Of those with pretreatment amoxicillin MICs of >0.25 µg/mL, three of six had the *H. pylori* eradicated. A total of 30% (21/70) of the patients failed lansoprazole 30 mg t.i.d./amoxicillin 1 gm t.i.d. dual therapy and a total of 12.8% (22/172) of the patients failed the 10- and 14-day triple therapy regimens. Post-treatment susceptibility results were not obtained on 11 of the patients who failed therapy. Nine of the 11 patients with amoxicillin post-treatment MICs that failed the triple therapy regimen also had clarithromycin resistant *H. pylori* isolates.
Susceptibility Test for *Helicobacter pylori*
The reference methodology for susceptibility testing of *H. pylori* is agar dilution MICs.[1] One to three microliters of an inoculum equivalent to a No. 2 McFarland standard ($1 \times 10^7 - 1 \times 10^8$ CFU/mL for *H. pylori*) are inoculated directly onto freshly prepared antimicrobial-containing Mueller-Hinton agar plates with 5% aged defibrinated sheep blood (≥ 2 weeks old). The agar dilution plates are incubated at 35°C in a microaerobic environment produced by a gas generating system suitable for campylobacters. After 3 days of incubation, the MICs are recorded as the lowest concentration of antimicrobial agent required to inhibit growth of the organism. The clarithromycin and amoxicillin MIC values should be interpreted according to the following criteria:

Clarithromycin MIC (μg/mL)[a]	Interpretation
≤0.25	Susceptible (S)
0.5–1.0	Intermediate (I)
≥2.0	Resistant (R)

Amoxicillin MIC (μg/mL)[b]	Interpretation
≤0.25	Susceptible (S)

[a] These are tentative breakpoints for the agar dilution methodology and they should not be used to interpret results obtained using alternative methods.
[b] There were not enough organisms with MICs >0.25 μg/mL to determine a resistance breakpoint.

Standardized susceptibility test procedures require the use of laboratory control microorganisms to control the technical aspects of the laboratory procedures. Standard clarithromycin and amoxicillin powders should provide the following MIC values:
[See first table above]

REFERENCE

1. National Committee for Clinical Laboratory Standards. Summary Minutes, Subcommittee on Antimicrobial Susceptibility Testing, Tampa, FL, January 11–13, 1998.

CLINICAL STUDIES

Duodenal Ulcer

In a U.S. multicenter, double-blind, placebo-controlled, dose-response (15, 30, and 60 mg of PREVACID once daily) study of 284 patients with endoscopically documented duodenal ulcer, the percentage of patients healed after two and four weeks was significantly higher with all doses of PREVACID than with placebo. There was no evidence of a greater or earlier response with the two higher doses compared with PREVACID 15 mg. Based on this study and the second study described below, the recommended dose of PREVACID in duodenal ulcer is 15 mg per day.
[See second table above]
PREVACID 15 mg was significantly more effective than placebo in relieving day and nighttime abdominal pain and in decreasing the amount of antacid taken per day.
In a second U.S. multicenter study, also double-blind, placebo-controlled, dose-comparison (15 and 30 mg of PREVACID once daily), and including a comparison with ranitidine, in 280 patients with endoscopically documented duodenal ulcer, the percentage of patients healed after four weeks was significantly higher with both doses of PREVACID than with placebo. There was no evidence of a greater or earlier response with the higher dose of PREVACID. Although the 15 mg dose of PREVACID was superior to ranitidine at 4 weeks, the lack of significant difference at 2 weeks and the absence of a difference between 30 mg of PREVACID and ranitidine leaves the comparative effectiveness of the two agents undetermined.
[See third table above]

H. pylori Eradication to Reduce the Risk of Duodenal Ulcer Recurrence

Randomized, double-blind clinical studies performed in the U.S. in patients with *H. pylori* and duodenal ulcer disease (defined as an active ulcer or history of an ulcer within one year) evaluated the efficacy of PREVACID in combination with amoxicillin capsules and clarithromycin tablets as triple 14-day therapy or in combination with amoxicillin capsules as dual 14-day therapy for the eradication of *H. pylori*. Based on the results of these studies, the safety and efficacy of two different eradication regimens were established:

Triple therapy: PREVACID 30 mg b.i.d./
amoxicillin 1 gm b.i.d./
clarithromycin 500 mg b.i.d.
Dual therapy: PREVACID 30 mg t.i.d./
amoxicillin 1 gm t.i.d.

All treatments were for 14 days. *H. pylori* eradication was defined as two negative tests (culture and histology) at 4–6 weeks following the end of treatment.
Triple therapy was shown to be more effective than all possible dual therapy combinations. Dual therapy was shown to be more effective than both monotherapies. Eradication of *H. pylori* has been shown to reduce the risk of duodenal ulcer recurrence.
A randomized, double-blind clinical study performed in the U.S. in patients with *H. pylori* and duodenal ulcer disease (defined as an active ulcer or history of an ulcer within one year) compared the efficacy of PREVACID triple therapy for 10 and 14 days. This study established that the 10-day triple therapy was equivalent to the 14-day triple therapy in eradicating *H. pylori*.
[See fourth table above]
[See fifth table above]

Long-Term Maintenance Treatment of Duodenal Ulcers

PREVACID has been shown to prevent the recurrence of duodenal ulcers. Two independent, double-blind, multicenter, controlled trials were conducted in patients with endoscopically confirmed healed duodenal ulcers. Patients remained healed significantly longer and the number of recurrences of duodenal ulcers was significantly less in patients treated with PREVACID than in patients treated with placebo over a 12-month period.
[See first table at top of next page]
In trial #2, no significant difference was noted between PREVACID 15 mg and 30 mg in maintaining remission.

Gastric Ulcer

In a U.S. multicenter, double-blind, placebo-controlled study of 253 patients with endoscopically documented gastric ulcer, the percentage of patients healed at four and eight weeks was significantly higher with PREVACID 15 mg and 30 mg once a day than with placebo.
[See second table at top of next page]
Patients treated with any PREVACID dose reported significantly less day and night abdominal pain along with fewer days of antacid use and fewer antacid tablets used per day than the placebo group.
Independent substantiation of the effectiveness of PREVACID 30 mg was provided by a meta-analysis of published and unpublished data.

Healing of NSAID-Associated Gastric Ulcer

In two U.S. and Canadian multicenter, double-blind, active-controlled studies in patients with endoscopically confirmed

Continued on next page

Microorganism	Antimicrobial Agent	MIC (μg/mL)[a]
H. pylori ATCC 43504	Clarithromycin	0.015–0.12 μg/mL
H. pylori ATCC 43504	Amoxicillin	0.015–0.12 μg/mL

[a] These are quality control ranges for the agar dilution methodology and they should not be used to control test results obtained using alternative methods.

Duodenal Ulcer Healing Rates

	PREVACID			Placebo
Week	15 mg q.d. (N=68)	30 mg q.d. (N=74)	60 mg q.d. (N=70)	(N=72)
2	42.4%*	35.6%*	39.1%*	11.3%
4	89.4%*	91.7%*	89.9%*	46.1%

*($p \leq 0.001$) versus placebo.

Duodenal Ulcer Healing Rates

	PREVACID		Ranitidine	Placebo
Week	15 mg q.d. (N=80)	30 mg q.d. (N=77)	300 mg h.s. (N=82)	(N=41)
2	35.0%	44.2%	30.5%	34.2%
4	92.3%**	80.3%*	70.5%*	47.5%

* ($p \leq 0.05$) versus placebo.
**($p \leq 0.05$) versus placebo and ranitidine.

***H. pylori* Eradication Rates—Triple Therapy**
(PREVACID/amoxicillin/clarithromycin)
Percent of Patients Cured
[95% Confidence Interval]
(Number of Patients)

Study	Duration	Triple Therapy Evaluable Analysis*	Triple Therapy Intent-to-Treat Analysis#
M93-131	14 days	92† [80.0–97.7] (N=48)	86† [73.3–93.5] (N=55)
M95-392	14 days	86‡ [75.7–93.6] (N=66)	83‡ [72.0–90.8] (N=70)
M95-399+	14 days	85 [77.0–91.0] (N=113)	82 [73.9–88.1] (N=126)
	10 days	84 [76.0–89.8] (N=123)	81 [73.9–87.6] (N=135)

* Based on evaluable patients with confirmed duodenal ulcer (active or within one year) and *H. pylori* infection at baseline defined as at least two of three positive endoscopic tests from CLOtest®, histology and/or culture. Patients were included in the analysis if they completed the study. Additionally, if patients dropped out of the study due to an adverse event related to the study drug, they were included in the evaluable analysis as failures of therapy.
\# Patients were included in the analysis if they had documented *H. pylori* infection at baseline as defined above and had a confirmed duodenal ulcer (active or within one year). All dropouts were included as failures of therapy.
† ($p<0.05$) versus PREVACID/amoxicillin and PREVACID/clarithromycin dual therapy
‡ ($p<0.05$) versus clarithromcyin/amoxicillin dual therapy
\+ The 95% confidence interval for the difference in eradication rates, 10-day minus 14-day is (−10.5, 8.1) in the evaluable analysis and (−9.7, 9.1) in the intent-to-treat analysis.

***H. pylori* Eradication Rates—14-Day Dual Therapy**
(PREVACID/amoxicillin)
Percent of Patients Cured
[95% Confidence Interval]
(Number of patients)

Study	Dual Therapy Evaluable Analysis*	Dual Therapy Intent-to-Treat Analysis#
M93-131	77† [62.5–87.2] (N=51)	70† [56.8–81.2] (N=60)
M93-125	66‡ [51.9–77.5] (N=58)	61‡ [48.5–72.9] (N=67)

* Based on evaluable patients with confirmed duodenal ulcer (active or within one year) and *H. pylori* infection at baseline defined as at least two of three positive endoscopic tests from CLOtest®, histology and/or culture. Patients were included in the analysis if they completed the study. Additionally, if patients dropped out of the study due to an adverse event related to the study drug, they were included in the analysis as failures of therapy.
\# Patients were included in the analysis if they had documented *H. pylori* infection at baseline as defined above and had a confirmed duodenal ulcer (active or within one year). All dropouts were included as failures of therapy.
† ($p<0.05$) versus PREVACID alone.
‡ ($p<0.05$) versus PREVACID alone or amoxicillin alone.

Prevacid—Cont.

NSAID-associated gastric ulcer who continued their NSAID use, the percentage of patients healed after 8 weeks was statistically significantly higher with 30 mg of PREVACID than with the active control. A total of 711 patients were enrolled in the study, and 701 patients were treated. Patients ranged in age from 18 to 88 years (median age 59 years), with 67% female patients and 33% male patients. Race was distributed as follows: 87% Caucasian, 8% Black, 5% other. There was no statistically significant difference between PREVACID 30 mg q.d. and the active control on symptom relief (i.e., abdominal pain).

[See third table above]

Risk Reduction of NSAID-Associated Gastric Ulcer

In one large U.S., multicenter, double-blind, placebo- and misoprostol-controlled (misoprostol blinded only to the endoscopist) study in patients who required chronic use of an NSAID and who had a history of an endoscopically documented gastric ulcer, the proportion of patients remaining free from gastric ulcer at 4, 8, and 12 weeks was significantly higher with 15 or 30 mg of PREVACID than placebo. A total of 537 patients were enrolled in the study, and 535 patients were treated. Patients ranged in age from 23 to 89 years (median age 60 years), with 65% female patients and 35% male patients. Race was distributed as follows: 90% Caucasian, 6% Black, 4% other. The 30 mg dose of PREVACID demonstrated no additional benefit in risk reduction of the NSAID-associated gastric ulcer than the 15 mg dose.

[See fourth table above]

Gastroesophageal Reflux Disease (GERD)

Symptomatic GERD

In a U.S. multicenter, double-blind, placebo-controlled study of 214 patients with frequent GERD symptoms, but no esophageal erosions by endoscopy, significantly greater relief of heartburn associated with GERD was observed with the administration of lansoprazole 15 mg once daily up to 8 weeks than with placebo. No significant additional benefit from lansoprazole 30 mg once daily was observed.

The intent-to-treat analyses demonstrated significant reduction in frequency and severity of day and night heartburn. Data for frequency and severity for the 8-week treatment period were as follows:

[See fifth table above]

Figure 1

Mean Severity of Day Heartburn By Study Day For Evaluable Patients (3=Severe, 2=Moderate, 1=Mild, 0=None)

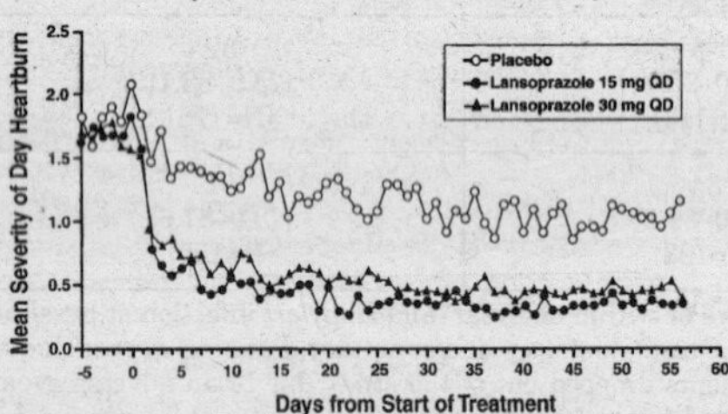

Figure 2

Mean Severity of Night Heartburn By Study Day For Evaluable Patients (3=Severe, 2=Moderate, 1=Mild, 0=None)

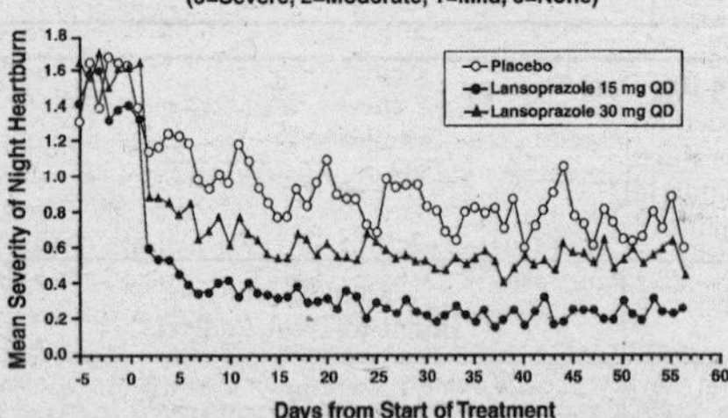

In two U.S., multicenter double-blind, ranitidine-controlled studies of 925 total patients with frequent GERD symptoms, but no esophageal erosions by endoscopy, lansoprazole 15 mg was superior to ranitidine 150 mg (b.i.d.) in decreasing the frequency and severity of day and night heartburn associated with GERD for the 8-week treatment period. No significant additional benefit from lansoprazole 30 mg once daily was observed.

Erosive Esophagitis

In a U.S. multicenter, double-blind, placebo-controlled study of 269 patients entering with an endoscopic diagnosis of esophagitis with mucosal grading of 2 or more and grades 3 and 4 signifying erosive disease, the percentages of patients with healing were as follows:

[See first table at top of next page]

In this study, all PREVACID groups reported significantly greater relief of heartburn and less day and night abdominal pain along with fewer days of antacid use and fewer antacid tablets taken per day than the placebo group.

Although all doses were effective, the earlier healing in the higher two doses suggests 30 mg q.d. as the recommended dose.

PREVACID was also compared in a U.S. multicenter, double-blind study to a low dose of ranitidine in 242 patients with erosive reflux esophagitis. PREVACID at a dose of 30 mg was significantly more effective than ranitidine 150 mg b.i.d. as shown below.

Endoscopic Remission Rates

Trial	Drug	No. of Pts.	Percent in Endoscopic Remission 0–3 mo.	0–6 mo.	0–12 mo.
#1	PREVACID 15 mg q.d.	86	90%*	87%*	84%*
	Placebo	83	49%	41%	39%
#2	PREVACID 30 mg q.d.	18	94%*	94%*	85%*
	PREVACID 15 mg q.d.	15	87%*	79%*	70%*
	Placebo	15	33%	0%	0%

%=Life Table Estimate
* (p≤0.001) versus placebo.

Gastric Ulcer Healing Rates

Week	PREVACID 15 mg q.d. (N=65)	PREVACID 30 mg q.d. (N=63)	PREVACID 60 mg q.d. (N=61)	Placebo (N=64)
4	64.6%*	58.1%*	53.3%*	37.5%
8	92.2%*	96.8%*	93.2%*	76.7%

* (p≤0.05) versus placebo.

NSAID-Associated Gastric Ulcer Healing Rates[1]

Study #1

	PREVACID 30 mg q.d.	Active Control[2]
Week 4	60% (53/88)[3]	28% (23/83)
Week 8	79% (62/79)[3]	55% (41/74)

Study #2

	PREVACID 30 mg q.d.	Active Control[2]
Week 4	53% (40/75)	38% (31/82)
Week 8	77% (47/61)[3]	50% (33/66)

[1] Actual observed ulcer(s) healed at time points ± 2 days
[2] Dose for healing of gastric ulcer
[3] (p≤0.05) versus the active control

NSAID-Associated Gastric Ulcer Risk Reduction Rates

% of Patients Remaining Gastric Ulcer-Free[1]

Week	PREVACID 15 mg q.d. (N=121)	PREVACID 30 mg q.d. (N=116)	Misoprostol 200 µg q.i.d. (N=106)	Placebo (N=112)
4	90%	92%	96%	66%
8	86%	88%	95%	60%
12	80%	82%	93%	51%

[1] %=Life Table Estimate
(p<0.001) PREVACID 15 mg q.d. versus placebo; PREVACID 30 mg q.d. versus placebo; and misoprostol 200 µg q.i.d. versus placebo.
(p<0.05) Misoprostol 200 µg q.i.d. versus PREVACID 15 mg q.d.; and misoprostol 200 µg q.i.d. versus PREVACID 30 mg q.d.

Frequency of Heartburn

Variable	Placebo (n=43)	PREVACID 15 mg (n=80)	PREVACID 30 mg (n=86)
	Median		
% of Days without Hearburn			
Week 1	0%	71%*	46%*
Week 4	11%	81%*	76%*
Week 8	13%	84%*	82%*
% of Nights without Heartburn			
Week 1	17%	86%*	57%*
Week 4	25%	89%*	73%*
Week 8	36%	92%*	80%*

* (p<0.01) versus placebo.

Erosive Esophagitis Healing Rates

Week	PREVACID 30 mg q.d. (N=115)	Ranitidine 150 mg b.i.d. (N=127)
2	66.7%*	38.7%
4	82.5%*	52.0%
6	93.0%*	67.8%
8	92.1%*	69.9%

* (p≤0.001) versus ranitidine.

In addition, patients treated with PREVACID reported less day and nighttime heartburn and took less antacid tablets for fewer days than patients taking ranitidine 150 mg b.i.d. Although this study demonstrates effectiveness of PREVACID in healing erosive esophagitis, it does not represent an adequate comparison with ranitidine because the recommended ranitidine dose for esophagitis is 150 mg q.i.d., twice the dose used in this study.

In the two trials described and in several smaller studies involving patients with moderate to severe erosive esophagitis, PREVACID produced healing rates similar to those shown above.

In a U.S. multicenter, double-blind, active-controlled study, 30 mg of PREVACID was compared with ranitidine 150 mg b.i.d. in 151 patients with erosive reflux esophagitis that was poorly responsive to a minimum of 12 weeks of treatment with at least one H_2-receptor antagonist given at the dose indicated for symptom relief or greater, namely, cimetidine 800 mg/day, ranitidine 300 mg/day, famotidine 40 mg/day or nizatidine 300 mg/day. PREVACID 30 mg was more effective than ranitidine 150 mg b.i.d. in healing reflux esophagitis, and the percentage of patients with healing were as follows. This study does not constitute a comparison of the effectiveness of histamine H_2-receptor antagonists with PREVACID, as all patients had demonstrated unresponsiveness to the histamine H_2-receptor antagonist mode of treatment. It does indicate, however, that PREVACID may be useful in patients failing on a histamine H_2-receptor antagonist.

Reflux Esophagitis Healing Rates in Patients Poorly Responsive to Histamine H_2-Receptor Antagonist Therapy

Week	PREVACID 30 mg q.d. (N=100)	Ranitidine 150 mg b.i.d. (N=51)
4	74.7%*	42.6%
8	83.7%*	32.0%

* (p≤0.001) versus ranitidine.

Long-Term Maintenance Treatment of Erosive Esophagitis
Two independent, double-blind, multicenter, controlled trials were conducted in patients with endoscopically confirmed healed esophagitis. Patients remained in remission significantly longer and the number of recurrences of erosive esophagitis was significantly less in patients treated with PREVACID than in patients treated with placebo over a 12-month period.
[See second table above]
Regardless of initial grade of erosive esophagitis, PREVACID 15 mg and 30 mg were similar in maintaining remission.
In a U.S., randomized, double-blind, study, PREVACID 15 mg q.d. (n = 100) was compared with ranitidine 150 mg b.i.d (n = 106), at the recommended dosage, in patients with endoscopically-proven healed erosive esophagitis over a 12-month period. Treatment with PREVACID resulted in patients remaining healed (Grade 0 lesions) of erosive esophagitis for significantly longer periods of time than those treated with ranitidine (p<0.001). In addition, PREVACID was significantly more effective than ranitidine in providing complete relief of both daytime and nighttime heartburn. Patients treated with PREVACID remained asymptomatic for a significantly longer period of time than patients treated with ranitidine.

Pathological Hypersecretory Conditions Including Zollinger-Ellison Syndrome
In open studies of 57 patients with pathological hypersecretory conditions, such as Zollinger-Ellison (ZE) syndrome with or without multiple endocrine adenomas, PREVACID significantly inhibited gastric acid secretion and controlled associated symptoms of diarrhea, anorexia and pain. Doses ranging from 15 mg every other day to 180 mg per day maintained basal acid secretion below 10 mEq/hr in patients without prior gastric surgery and below 5 mEq/hr in patients with prior gastric surgery.
Initial doses were titrated to the individual patient need, and adjustments were necessary with time in some patients. (See **DOSAGE AND ADMINISTRATION**.) PREVACID was well tolerated at these high dose levels for prolonged periods (greater than four years in some patients). In most ZE patients, serum gastrin levels were not modified by PREVACID. However, in some patients, serum gastrin increased to levels greater than those present prior to initiation of lansoprazole therapy.

Erosive Esophagitis Healing Rates

Week	PREVACID 15 mg q.d. (N=69)	PREVACID 30 mg q.d. (N=65)	PREVACID 60 mg q.d. (N=72)	Placebo (N=63)
4	67.6%*	81.3%**	80.6%**	32.8%
6	87.7%*	95.4%*	94.3%*	52.5%
8	90.9%*	95.4%*	94.4%*	52.5%

* (p≤0.001) versus placebo.
** (p≤0.05) versus PREVACID 15 mg and placebo.

Endoscopic Remission Rates

Trial	Drug	No. of Pts.	Percent in Endoscopic Remission 0–3 mo.	0–6 mo.	0–12 mo.
#1	PREVACID 15 mg q.d.	59	83%*	81%*	79%*
	PREVACID 30 mg q.d.	56	93%*	93%*	90%*
	Placebo	55	31%	27%	24%
#2	PREVACID 15 mg q.d.	50	74%*	72%*	67%*
	PREVACID 30 mg q.d.	49	75%*	72%*	55%*
	Placebo	47	16%	13%	13%

%=Life Table Estimate
* (p≤0.001) versus placebo.

INDICATIONS AND USAGE

Short-Term Treatment of Active Duodenal Ulcer
PREVACID Delayed-Release Capsules and PREVACID for Delayed-Release Oral Suspension are indicated for short-term treatment (up to 4 weeks) for healing and symptom relief of active duodenal ulcer.

***H. pylori* Eradication to Reduce the Risk of Duodenal Ulcer Recurrence**
Triple Therapy: PREVACID/amoxicillin/clarithromycin
PREVACID Delayed-Release Capsules and PREVACID for Delayed-Release Oral Suspension, in combination with amoxicillin plus clarithromycin as triple therapy, are indicated for the treatment of patients with *H. pylori* infection and duodenal ulcer disease (active or one-year history of a duodenal ulcer) to eradicate *H. pylori*. Eradication of *H. pylori* has been shown to reduce the risk of duodenal ulcer recurrence. (See **CLINICAL STUDIES** and **DOSAGE AND ADMINISTRATION**.)
Dual Therapy: PREVACID/amoxicillin
PREVACID Delayed-Release Capsules and PREVACID for Delayed-Release Oral Suspension, in combination with amoxicillin as dual therapy, are indicated for the treatment of patients with *H. pylori* infection and duodenal ulcer disease (active or one-year history of a duodenal ulcer) **who are either allergic or intolerant to clarithromycin or in whom resistance to clarithromycin is known or suspected.** (See the clarithromycin package insert, **MICROBIOLOGY** section.) Eradication of *H. pylori* has been shown to reduce the risk of duodenal ulcer recurrence. (See **CLINICAL STUDIES** and **DOSAGE AND ADMINISTRATION**.)

Maintenance of Healed Duodenal Ulcers
PREVACID Delayed-Release Capsules and PREVACID for Delayed-Release Oral Suspension are indicated to maintain healing of duodenal ulcers. Controlled studies do not extend beyond 12 months.

Short-Term Treatment of Active Benign Gastric Ulcer
PREVACID Delayed-Release Capsules and PREVACID for Delayed-Release Oral Suspension are indicated for short-term treatment (up to 8 weeks) for healing and symptom relief of active benign gastric ulcer.

Healing of NSAID-Associated Gastric Ulcer
PREVACID Delayed-Release Capsules and PREVACID for Delayed-Release Oral Suspension are indicated for the treatment of NSAID-associated gastric ulcer in patients who continue NSAID use. Controlled studies did not extend beyond 8 weeks.

Risk Reduction of NSAID-Associated Gastric Ulcer
PREVACID Delayed-Release Capsules and PREVACID for Delayed-Release Oral Suspension are indicated for reducing the risk of NSAID-associated gastric ulcers in patients with a history of a documented gastric ulcer who require the use of an NSAID. Controlled studies did not extend beyond 12 weeks.

Gastroesophageal Reflux Disease (GERD)
Short-Term Treatment of Symptomatic GERD
PREVACID Delayed-Release Capsules and PREVACID for Delayed-Release Oral Suspension are indicated for the treatment of heartburn and other symptoms associated with GERD.
Short-Term Treatment of Erosive Esophagitis
PREVACID Delayed-Release Capsules and PREVACID for Delayed-Release Oral Suspension are indicated for short-term treatment (up to 8 weeks) for healing and symptom relief of all grades of erosive esophagitis.
For patients who do not heal with PREVACID for 8 weeks (5–10%), it may be helpful to give an additional 8 weeks of treatment.
If there is a recurrence of erosive esophagitis an additional 8-week course of PREVACID may be considered.

Maintenance of Healing of Erosive Esophagitis
PREVACID Delayed-Release Capsules and PREVACID for Delayed-Release Oral Suspension are indicated to maintain healing of erosive esophagitis. Controlled studies did not extend beyond 12 months.

Pathological Hypersecretory Conditions Including Zollinger-Ellison Syndrome
PREVACID Delayed-Release Capsules and PREVACID for Delayed-Release Oral Suspension are indicated for the long-term treatment of pathological hypersecretory conditions, including Zollinger-Ellison syndrome.

CONTRAINDICATIONS

PREVACID Delayed-Release Capsules and PREVACID for Delayed-Release Oral Suspension are contraindicated in patients with known hypersensitivity to any component of the formulations.
Amoxicillin is contraindicated in patients with a known hypersensitivity to any penicillin. (Please refer to full prescribing information for amoxicillin before prescribing.)
Clarithromycin is contraindicated in patients with a known hypersensitivity to any macrolide antibiotic, and in patients receiving terfenadine therapy who have preexisting cardiac abnormalities or electrolyte disturbances. (Please refer to full prescribing information for clarithromycin before prescribing.)

WARNINGS

CLARITHROMYCIN SHOULD NOT BE USED IN PREGNANT WOMEN EXCEPT IN CLINICAL CIRCUMSTANCES WHERE NO ALTERNATIVE THERAPY IS APPROPRIATE. IF PREGNANCY OCCURS WHILE TAKING CLARITHROMYCIN, THE PATIENT SHOULD BE APPRISED OF THE POTENTIAL HAZARD TO THE FETUS. (SEE **WARNINGS** IN PRESCRIBING INFORMATION FOR CLARITHROMYCIN.)
Pseudomembranous colitis has been reported with nearly all antibacterial agents, including clarithromycin and amoxicillin, and may range in severity from mild to life threatening. Therefore, it is important to consider this diagnosis in patients who present with diarrhea subsequent to the administration of antibacterial agents.
Treatment with antibacterial agents alters the normal flora of the colon and may permit overgrowth of clostridia. Studies indicate that a toxin produced by *Clostridium difficile* is a primary cause of "antibiotic-associated colitis."
After the diagnosis of pseudomembranous colitis has been established, therapeutic measures should be initiated. Mild cases of pseudomembranous colitis usually respond to discontinuation of the drug alone. In moderate to severe cases, consideration should be given to management with fluids and electrolytes, protein supplementation, and treatment with an antibacterial drug clinically effective against *Clostridium difficile* colitis.
Serious and occasionally fatal hypersensitivity (anaphylactic) reactions have been reported in patients on penicillin therapy. These reactions are more apt to occur in individuals with a history of penicillin hypersensitivity and/or a history of sensitivity to multiple allergens.
There have been well-documented reports of individuals with a history of penicillin hypersensitivity reactions who have experienced severe hypersensitivity reactions when treated with a cephalosporin. Before initiating therapy with any penicillin, careful inquiry should be made concerning previous hypersensitivity reactions to penicillins, cephalosporins, and other allergens. If an allergic reaction occurs, amoxicillin should be discontinued and the appropriate therapy instituted.
SERIOUS ANAPHYLACTIC REACTIONS REQUIRE IMMEDIATE EMERGENCY TREATMENT WITH EPINEPHRINE. OXYGEN, INTRAVENOUS STEROIDS, AND AIRWAY MANAGEMENT, INCLUDING INTUBATION, SHOULD ALSO BE ADMINISTERED AS INDICATED.

PRECAUTIONS

General
Symptomatic response to therapy with lansoprazole does not preclude the presence of gastric malignancy.

Information for Patients
PREVACID Delayed-Release Capsules and PREVACID for Delayed-Release Oral Suspension should be taken before eating.
Alternative Administration Options
PREVACID Delayed-Release Capsules
For patients who have difficulty swallowing capsules, PREVACID Delayed-Release Capsules can be opened, and the intact granules contained within can be sprinkled on one tablespoon of either applesauce, ENSURE® pudding, cottage cheese, yogurt, or strained pears and swallowed immediately. The granules should not be chewed or crushed. Alternatively, PREVACID Delayed-Release Capsules may be emptied into a small volume of either orange juice or tomato juice (60 mL – approximately 2 ounces), mixed briefly and swallowed immediately. To insure complete delivery of the dose, the glass should be rinsed with two or more volumes of juice and the contents swallowed immediately. The granules have also been shown *in vitro* to remain intact when exposed to apple, cranberry, grape, orange, pineapple, prune, tomato, and V-8® vegetable juice and stored for up to 30 minutes.
PREVACID for Delayed-Release Oral Suspension
In addition, for patients who have difficulty swallowing capsules, PREVACID for Delayed-Release Oral Suspension is available in strengths of 15 mg and 30 mg. Directions for use: Empty packet contents into a container containing 2 tablespoons of **WATER**. DO NOT USE OTHER LIQUIDS OR FOODS. Stir well, and drink immediately. DO NOT CRUSH OR CHEW THE GRANULES. If any material remains after drinking, add more water, stir, and drink immediately.

Drug Interactions
Lansoprazole is metabolized through the cytochrome P_{450} system, specifically through the CYP3A and CYP2C19 isozymes. Studies have shown that lansoprazole does not have clinically significant interactions with other drugs metabolized by the cytochrome P_{450} system, such as warfarin, antipyrine, indomethacin, ibuprofen, phenytoin, propranolol, prednisone, diazepam, clarithromycin, or terfenadine in healthy subjects. These compounds are metabolized through various cytochrome P_{450} isozymes including CYP1A2, CYP2C9, CYP2C19, CYP2D6, and CYP3A. When lansoprazole was administered concomitantly with theophylline (CYP1A2, CYP3A), a minor increase (10%) in the clearance of theophylline was seen. Because of the small magnitude and the direction of the effect on theophylline clearance, this interaction is unlikely to be of clinical concern. Nonetheless, individual patients may require additional titration of their theophylline dosage when lansoprazole is started or stopped to ensure clinically effective blood levels.

Continued on next page

Prevacid—Cont.

Lansoprazole has also been shown to have no clinically significant interaction with amoxicillin.
In a single-dose crossover study examining lansoprazole 30 mg and omeprazole 20 mg each administered alone and concomitantly with sucralfate 1 gram, absorption of the proton pump inhibitors was delayed and their bioavailability was reduced by 17% and 16%, respectively, when administered concomitantly with sucralfate. Therefore, proton pump inhibitors should be taken at least 30 minutes prior to sucralfate. In clinical trials, antacids were administered concomitantly with PREVACID Delayed-Release Capsules; this did not interfere with its effect.
Lansoprazole causes a profound and long-lasting inhibition of gastric acid secretion; therefore, it is theoretically possible that lansoprazole may interfere with the absorption of drugs where gastric pH is an important determinant of bioavailability (e.g., ketoconazole, ampicillin esters, iron salts, digoxin).

Carcinogenesis, Mutagenesis, Impairment of Fertility
In two 24-month carcinogenicity studies, Sprague-Dawley rats were treated orally with doses of 5 to 150 mg/kg/day, about 1 to 40 times the exposure on a body surface (mg/m^2) basis, of a 50-kg person of average height (1.46 m^2 body surface area) given the recommended human dose of 30 mg/day (22.2 mg/m^2). Lansoprazole produced dose-related gastric enterochromaffin-like (ECL) cell hyperplasia and ECL cell carcinoids in both male and female rats. It also increased the incidence of intestinal metaplasia of the gastric epithelium in both sexes. In male rats, lansoprazole produced a dose-related increase of testicular interstitial cell adenomas. The incidence of these adenomas in rats receiving doses of 15 to 150 mg/kg/day (4 to 40 times the recommended human dose based on body surface area) exceeded the low background incidence (range = 1.4 to 10%) for this strain of rat. Testicular interstitial cell adenoma also occurred in 1 of 30 rats treated with 50 mg/kg/day (13 times the recommended human dose based on body surface area) in a 1-year toxicity study.
In a 24-month carcinogenicity study, CD-1 mice were treated orally with doses of 15 to 600 mg/kg/day, 2 to 80 times the recommended human dose based on body surface area. Lansoprazole produced a dose-related increased incidence of gastric ECL cell hyperplasia. It also produced an increased incidence of liver tumors (hepatocellular adenoma plus carcinoma). The tumor incidences in male mice treated with 300 and 600 mg/kg/day (40 to 80 times the recommended human dose based on body surface area) and female mice treated with 150 to 600 mg/kg/day (20 to 80 times the recommended human dose based on body surface area) exceeded the ranges of background incidences in historical controls for this strain of mice. Lansoprazole treatment produced adenoma of rete testis in male mice receiving 75 to 600 mg/kg/day (10 to 80 times the recommended human dose based on body surface area).
Lansoprazole was not genotoxic in the Ames test, the *ex vivo* rat hepatocyte unscheduled DNA synthesis (UDS) test, the *in vivo* mouse micronucleus test or the rat bone marrow cell chromosomal aberration test. It was positive in *in vitro* human lymphocyte chromosomal aberration assays.
Lansoprazole at oral doses up to 150 mg/kg/day (40 times the recommended human dose based on body surface area) was found to have no effect on fertility and reproductive performance of male and female rats.

Pregnancy: Teratogenic Effects.
Pregnancy Category B
Lansoprazole
Teratology studies have been performed in pregnant rats at oral doses up to 150 mg/kg/day (40 times the recommended human dose based on body surface area) and pregnant rabbits at oral doses up to 30 mg/kg/day (16 times the recommended human dose based on body surface area) and have revealed no evidence of impaired fertility or harm to the fetus due to lansoprazole.
There are, however, no adequate or well-controlled studies in pregnant women. Because animal reproduction studies are not always predictive of human response, this drug should be used during pregnancy only if clearly needed.
Pregnancy Category C
Clarithromycin
See **WARNINGS** (above) and full prescribing information for clarithromycin before using in pregnant women.

Nursing Mothers
Lansoprazole or its metabolites are excreted in the milk of rats. It is not known whether lansoprazole is excreted in human milk. Because many drugs are excreted in human milk, because of the potential for serious adverse reactions in nursing infants from lansoprazole, and because of the potential for tumorigenicity shown for lansoprazole in rat carcinogenicity studies, a decision should be made whether to discontinue nursing or to discontinue the drug, taking into account the importance of the drug to the mother.

Pediatric Use
Safety and effectiveness in pediatric patients have not been established.

Use in Women
Over 4,000 women were treated with lansoprazole. Ulcer healing rates in females were similar to those in males. The incidence rates of adverse events were also similar to those seen in males.

Use in Geriatric Patients
Ulcer healing rates in elderly patients are similar to those in a younger age group. The incidence rates of adverse events and laboratory test abnormalities are also similar to those seen in younger patients. For elderly patients, dosage and administration of lansoprazole need not be altered for a particular indication.

Incidence of Possibly or Probably Treatment-Related Adverse Events in Short-Term, Placebo-Controlled Studies

Body System/Adverse Event	PREVACID (N=2768) %	Placebo (N=1023) %
Body as a Whole		
Abdominal Pain	2.1	1.2
Digestive System		
Constipation	1.0	0.4
Diarrhea	3.8	2.3
Nausea	1.3	1.2

Indication	Dose	Frequency
Duedenal Ulcers		
Short-Term Treatment	15 mg	Once daily for 4 weeks
Maintenance of Healed	15 mg	Once daily
***H. pylori* Eradication to Reduce the Risk of Duodenal Ulcer Recurrence**		
Triple Therapy:		
PREVACID	30 mg	Twice daily (q12h) for 10 or 14 days
Amoxicillin	1 gram	Twice daily (q12h) for 10 or 14 days
Clarithromycin	500 mg	Twice daily (q12h) for 10 or 14 days
Dual Therapy:		
PREVACID	30 mg	Three times daily (q8h) for 14 days
Amoxicillin	1 gram	Three times daily (q8h) for 14 days
Benign Gastric Ulcer		
Short-Term Treatment	30 mg	Once daily for up to 8 weeks
NSAID-associated Gastric Ulcer		
Healing	30 mg	Once daily for up to 8 weeks*
Risk Reduction	15 mg	Once daily for up to 12 weeks*
Gastroesophageal Reflux Disease (GERD)		
Short-Term Treatment of Symptomatic GERD	15 mg	Once daily for up to 8 weeks
Short-Term Treatment of Erosive Esophagitis	30 mg	Once daily for up to 8 weeks**
Maintenance of Healing of Erosive Esophagitis	15 mg	Once daily
Zollinger-Ellison Syndrome (and other Pathological hypersecretory condition)	60 mg	Once daily***

NOTE: Additional information is available in CLINICAL STUDIES and/or INDICATIONS AND USAGE.
* Controlled studies did not extend beyond indicated duration.
** For patients who do not heal with PREVACID for 8 weeks (5–10%), it may be helpful to give an additional 8 weeks of treatment. If there is a recurrence of erosive esophagitis an additional 8 week course of PREVACID may be considered.
*** Dosages up to 90 mg b.i.d. have been administered. Daily dosage of greater than 120 mg should be administered in divided doses.

ADVERSE REACTIONS

Clinical
Worldwide, over 10,000 patients have been treated with lansoprazole in Phase 2–3 clinical trials involving various dosages and durations of treatment. The adverse reaction profiles for PREVACID Delayed-Release Capsules and PREVACID for Delayed-Release Oral Suspension are similar. In general, lansoprazole treatment has been well-tolerated in both short-term and long-term trials.
The following adverse events were reported by the treating physician to have a possible or probable relationship to drug in 1% or more of PREVACID-treated patients and occurred at a greater rate in PREVACID-treated patients than placebo-treated patients:
[See first table above]
Headache was also seen at greater than 1% incidence but was more common on placebo. The incidence of diarrhea was similar between patients who received placebo and patients who received lansoprazole 15 mg and 30 mg, but higher in the patients who received lansoprazole 60 mg (2.9%, 1.4%, 4.2%, and 7.4%, respectively).
The most commonly reported possibly or probably treatment-related adverse event during maintenance therapy was diarrhea.
In the risk reduction study of PREVACID for NSAID-associated gastric ulcers, the incidence of diarrhea for patients treated with PREVACID was 5%, misoprostol 22%, and placebo 3%.
Additional adverse experiences occurring in <1% of patients or subjects in domestic trials are shown below. Refer to **Postmarketing** for adverse reactions occurring since the drug was marketed.
Body as a Whole—abdomen enlarged, allergic reaction, asthenia, back pain, candidiasis, carcinoma, chest pain (not otherwise specified), chills, edema, fever, flu syndrome, halitosis, infection (not otherwise specified), malaise, neck pain, neck rigidity, pain, pelvic pain; *Cardiovascular System*—angina, arrhythmia, bradycardia, cerebrovascular accident/cerebral infarction, hypertension/hypotension, migraine, myocardial infarction, palpitations, shock (circulatory failure), syncope, tachycardia, vasodilation; *Digestive System*—abnormal stools, anorexia, bezoar, cardiospasm, cholelithiasis, colitis, dry mouth, dyspepsia, dysphagia, enteritis, eructation, esophageal stenosis, esophageal ulcer, esophagitis, fecal discoloration, flatulence, gastric nodules/fundic gland polyps, gastritis, gastroenteritis, gastrointestinal anomaly, gastrointestinal disorder, gastrointestinal hemorrhage, glossitis, gum hemorrhage, hematemesis, increased appetite, increased salivation, melena, mouth ulceration, nausea and vomiting, nausea and vomiting and diarrhea, oral moniliasis, rectal disorder, rectal hemorrhage, stomatitis, tenesmus, thirst, tongue disorder, ulcerative colitis, ulcerative stomatitis; *Endocrine System*—diabetes mellitus, goiter, hypothyroidism; *Hemic and Lymphatic System*—anemia, hemolysis, lymphadenopathy; *Metabolic and Nutritional Disorders*—gout, dehydration, hyperglycemia/hypoglycemia, peripheral edema, weight gain/loss; *Musculoskeletal System*—arthralgia, arthritis, bone disorder, joint disorder, leg cramps, musculoskeletal pain, myalgia, myasthenia, synovitis; *Nervous System*—abnormal dreams, agitation, amnesia, anxiety, apathy, confusion, convulsion, depersonalization, depression, diplopia, dizziness, emotional lability, hallucinations, hemiplegia, hostility aggravated, hyperkinesia, hypertonia, hypesthesia, insomnia, libido decreased/increased, nervousness, neurosis, paresthesia, sleep disorder, somnolence, thinking abnormality, tremor, vertigo; *Respiratory System*—asthma, bronchitis, cough increased, dyspnea, epistaxis, hemoptysis, hiccup, laryngeal neoplasia, pharyngitis, pleural disorder, pneumonia, respiratory disorder, upper respiratory inflammation/infection, rhinitis, sinusitis, stridor; *Skin and Appendages*—acne, alopecia, contact dermatitis, dry skin, fixed eruption, hair disorder, maculopapular rash, nail disorder, pruritus, rash, skin carcinoma, skin disorder, sweating, urticaria; *Special Senses*—abnormal vision, blurred vision, conjunctivitis, deafness, dry eyes, ear disorder, eye pain, otitis media, parosmia, photophobia, retinal degeneration, taste loss, taste perversion, tinnitus, visual field defect; *Urogenital System*—abnormal menses, breast enlargement, breast pain, breast tenderness, dysmenorrhea, dysuria, gynecomastia, impotence, kidney calculus, kidney pain, leukorrhea, menorrhagia, menstrual disorder, penis disorder, polyuria, testis disorder, urethral pain, urinary frequency, urinary tract infection, urinary urgency, urination impaired, vaginitis.

Postmarketing
On-going Safety Surveillance: Additional adverse experiences have been reported since lansoprazole has been marketed. The majority of these cases are foreign-sourced and a relationship to lansoprazole has not been established. Be-

cause these events were reported voluntarily from a population of unknown size, estimates of frequency cannot be made. These events are listed below by COSTART body system.

Body as a Whole—anaphylactoid-like reaction; *Digestive System*—hepatotoxicity, vomiting; *Hemic and Lymphatic System*—agranulocytosis, aplastic anemia, hemolytic anemia, leukopenia, neutropenia, pancytopenia, thrombocytopenia, and thrombotic thrombocytopenic purpura; *Special Senses*—speech disorder; *Urogenital System*—urinary retention.

Combination Therapy with Amoxicillin and Clarithromycin

In clinical trials using combination therapy with PREVACID plus amoxicillin and clarithromycin, and PREVACID plus amoxicillin, no adverse reactions peculiar to these drug combinations were observed. Adverse reactions that have occurred have been limited to those that had been previously reported with PREVACID, amoxicillin, or clarithromycin.

Triple Therapy: PREVACID/amoxicillin/clarithromycin

The most frequently reported adverse events for patients who received triple therapy for 14 days were diarrhea (7%), headache (6%), and taste perversion (5%). There were no statistically significant differences in the frequency of reported adverse events between the 10- and 14-day triple therapy regimens. No treatment-emergent adverse events were observed at significantly higher rates with triple therapy than with any dual therapy regimen.

Dual Therapy: PREVACID/amoxicillin

The most frequently reported adverse events for patients who received PREVACID t.i.d. plus amoxicillin t.i.d. dual therapy were diarrhea (8%) and headache (7%). No treatment-emergent adverse events were observed at significantly higher rates with PREVACID t.i.d. plus amoxicillin t.i.d. dual therapy than with PREVACID alone.

For more information on adverse reactions with amoxicillin or clarithromycin, refer to their package inserts, **ADVERSE REACTIONS** sections.

Laboratory Values

The following changes in laboratory parameters for lansoprazole were reported as adverse events:

Abnormal liver function tests, increased SGOT (AST), increased SGPT (ALT), increased creatinine, increased alkaline phosphatase, increased globulins, increased GGTP, increased/decreased/abnormal WBC, abnormal AG ratio, abnormal RBC, bilirubinemia, eosinophilia, hyperlipemia, increased/decreased electrolytes, increased/decreased cholesterol, increased glucocorticoids, increased LDH, increased/decreased/abnormal platelets, and increased gastrin levels. Urine abnormalities such as albuminuria, glycosuria, and hematuria were also reported. Additional isolated laboratory abnormalities were reported.

In the placebo controlled studies, when SGOT (AST) and SGPT (ALT) were evaluated, 0.4% (4/978) placebo patients and 0.4% (11/2677) lansoprazole patients had enzyme elevations greater than three times the upper limit of normal range at the final treatment visit. None of these lansoprazole patients reported jaundice at any time during the study.

In clinical trials using combination therapy with PREVACID plus amoxicillin and clarithromycin, and PREVACID plus amoxicillin, no increased laboratory abnormalities particular to these drug combinations were observed.

For more information on laboratory value changes with amoxicillin or clarithromycin, refer to their package inserts, **ADVERSE REACTIONS** section.

OVERDOSAGE

Oral doses up to 5000 mg/kg in rats (approximately 1300 times the recommended human dose based on body surface area) and mice (about 675.7 times the recommended human dose based on body surface area) did not produce deaths or any clinical signs.

Lansoprazole is not removed from the circulation by hemodialysis. In one reported case of overdose, the patient consumed 600 mg of lansoprazole with no adverse reaction.

DOSAGE AND ADMINISTRATION

[See second table at top of previous page]

Alternative Administration Options

PREVACID Delayed-Release Capsules

For patients who have difficulty swallowing capsules, PREVACID Delayed-Release Capsules can be opened, and the intact granules contained within can be sprinkled on one tablespoon of either applesauce, ENSURE® pudding, cottage cheese, yogurt, or strained pears and swallowed immediately. The granules should not be chewed or crushed. Alternatively, PREVACID Delayed-Release Capsules may be emptied into a small volume of either orange juice or tomato juice (60 mL–approximately 2 ounces), mixed briefly and swallowed immediately. To insure complete delivery of the dose, the glass should be rinsed with two or more volumes of juice and the contents swallowed immediately. The granules have also been shown *in vitro* to remain intact when exposed to apple, cranberry, grape, orange, pineapple, prune, tomato, and V-8® vegetable juice and stored for up to 30 minutes.

For patients who have a nasogastric tube in place, PREVACID Delayed-Release Capsules can be opened and the intact granules mixed in 40 mL of apple juice and injected through the nasogastric tube into the stomach. After administering the granules, the nasogastric tube should be flushed with additional apple juice to clear the tube.

PREVACID for Delayed-Release Oral Suspension

In addition, for patients who have difficulty swallowing capsules, PREVACID for Delayed-Release Oral Suspension is available in strengths of 15 mg and 30 mg. Directions for use: Empty packet contents into a container containing 2 tablespoons of **WATER**. DO NOT USE OTHER LIQUIDS OR FOODS. Stir well, and drink immediately. DO NOT CRUSH OR CHEW THE GRANULES. If any material remains after drinking, add more water, stir, and drink immediately.

HOW SUPPLIED

PREVACID Delayed-Release Capsules, 15 mg, are opaque, hard gelatin, colored pink and green with the TAP logo and "PREVACID 15" imprinted on the capsules. The 30 mg capsules are opaque, hard gelatin, colored pink and black with the TAP logo and "PREVACID 30" imprinted on the capsules. They are available as follows:

NDC 0300-1541-30 Unit of use bottles of 30: 15-mg capsules
NDC 0300-1541-19 Bottles of 1000: 15-mg capsules
NDC 0300-1541-11 Unit dose package of 100: 15-mg capsules
NDC 0300-3046-13 Bottles of 100: 30-mg capsules
NDC 0300-3046-19 Bottles of 1000: 30-mg capsules
NDC 0300-3046-11 Unit dose package of 100: 30-mg capsules

PREVACID for Delayed-Release Oral Suspension contains white to pale brownish lansoprazole granules and inactive pink granules in a unit dose packet. They are available as follows:

NDC 0300-7309-30 Unit dose carton of 30: 15-mg packets
NDC 0300-7311-30 Unit dose carton of 30: 30-mg packets

Storage: Store between 15°C and 30°C (59°F and 86°F). Store in a tight container protected from moisture.

Rx only

U.S. Patent Nos. 4,628,098; 4,689,333; 5,013,743; 5,026,560 and 5,045,321.

Manufactured for
TAP Pharmaceuticals Inc.
Lake Forest, IL 60045, U.S.A.
by Takeda Chemical Industries Limited
Osaka, Japan 541

ENSURE® is a registered trademark of Abbott Laboratories.
V-8® is a registered trademark of the Campbell Soup Company.
CLOtest® is a registered trademark of Delta West Ltd., Bentley, Australia.

03-5133-R17-Rev. September, 2001
IN-5080/S

PREVPAC® ℞

(lansoprazole 30-mg capsules, amoxicillin 500-mg capsules, USP, and clarithromycin 500-mg tablets, USP)

Prescribing information for this product, which appears on pages 3298–3302 of the 2002 PDR, has been completely revised as follows. Please write "See Supplement A" next to the product heading.

THESE PRODUCTS ARE INTENDED ONLY FOR USE AS DESCRIBED. The individual products contained in this package should not be used alone or in combination for other purposes. The information described in this labeling concerns only the use of these products as indicated in this daily administration pack. For information on use of the individual components when dispensed as individual medications outside this combined use for treating *Helicobacter pylori (H. pylori)*, please see the package inserts for each individual product.

DESCRIPTION

PREVPAC consists of a daily administration pack containing two PREVACID 30-mg capsules, four amoxicillin 500-mg capsules, USP, and two clarithromycin 500-mg tablets, USP, for oral administration.

PREVACID® (lansoprazole) Delayed-Release Capsules

The active ingredient in PREVACID capsules is a substituted benzimidazole, 2-[[[3-methyl-4-(2,2,2-trifluoroethoxy)-2-pyridyl]methyl] sulfinyl] benzimidazole, a compound that inhibits gastric acid secretion. Its empirical formula is $C_{16}H_{14}F_3N_3O_2S$ with a molecular weight of 369.37. The structural formula is:

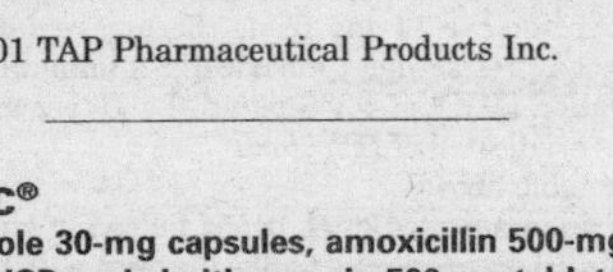

Lansoprazole is a white to brownish-white odorless crystalline powder which melts with decomposition at approximately 166°C. Lansoprazole is freely soluble in dimethylformamide; soluble in methanol; sparingly soluble in ethanol; slightly soluble in ethyl acetate, dichloromethane and acetonitrile; very slightly soluble in ether; and practically insoluble in hexane and water.

Each delayed-release capsule contains enteric-coated granules consisting of lansoprazole (30 mg), hydroxypropyl cellulose, low substituted hydroxypropyl cellulose, colloidal silicon dioxide, magnesium carbonate, methacrylic acid copolymer, starch, talc, sugar sphere, sucrose, polyethylene glycol, polysorbate 80, and titanium dioxide. Components of the gelatin capsule include gelatin, titanium dioxide, D&C Red No. 28, FD&C Blue No. 1, and FD&C Red No. 40.

TRIMOX® (amoxicillin, USP)

Amoxicillin, USP, (2*S*,5*R*,6*R*)-6-[(*R*)-(–)-2-Amino-2-(*p*-hydroxyphenyl) acetamido]-3,3-dimethyl-7-oxo-4-thia-1-azabicyclo[3.2.0] heptane-2-carboxylic acid trihydrate, is a semisynthetic penicillin, an analogue of ampicillin. It has the following chemical structure:

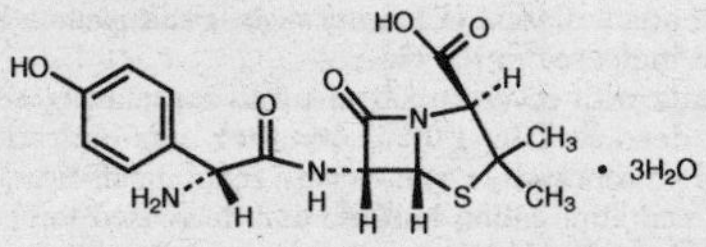

The empirical formula is $C_{16}H_{19}N_3O_5S \cdot 3H_2O$, and the molecular weight is 419.45.

The maroon and light-pink capsules contain amoxicillin trihydrate equivalent to 500 mg of amoxicillin. The inactive ingredient in the capsules is magnesium stearate.

BIAXIN® Filmtab® (clarithromycin tablets, USP)

Clarithromycin is a semi-synthetic macrolide antibiotic. Chemically, it is 6-*0*-methylerythromycin. The molecular formula is $C_{38}H_{69}NO_{13}$, and the molecular weight is 747.96. The structural formula is:

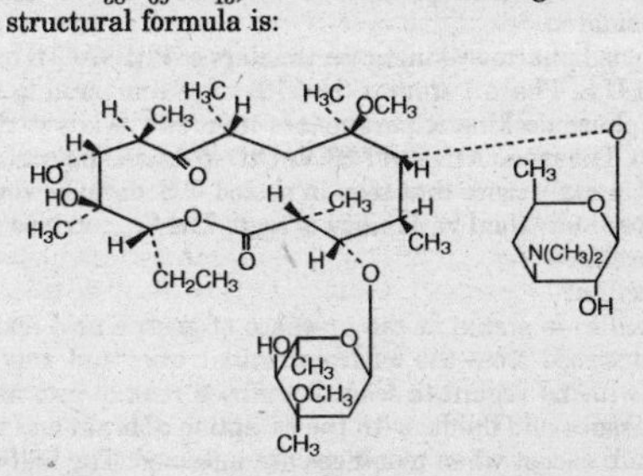

Clarithromycin is a white to off-white crystalline powder. It is soluble in acetone, slightly soluble in methanol, ethanol, and acetonitrile, and practically insoluble in water.

Each yellow oval film-coated immediate-release tablet contains 500 mg of clarithromycin and the following inactive ingredients: hydroxypropyl methylcellulose, hydroxypropyl cellulose, colloidal silicon dioxide, croscarmellose sodium, D&C Yellow No. 10, magnesium stearate, microcrystalline cellulose, povidone, propylene glycol, sorbic acid, sorbitan monooleate, titanium dioxide, and vanillin.

CLINICAL PHARMACOLOGY

Pharmacokinetics

Pharmacokinetics when all three of the PREVPAC components (PREVACID capsules, amoxicillin capsules, clarithromycin tablets) were coadministered has not been studied. Studies have shown no clinically significant interactions of PREVACID and amoxicillin or PREVACID and clarithromycin when administered together. There is no information about the gastric mucosal concentrations of PREVACID, amoxicillin and clarithromycin after administration of these agents concomitantly. The systemic pharmacokinetic information presented below is based on studies in which each product was administered alone.

PREVACID:

PREVACID capsules contain an enteric-coated granule formulation of lansoprazole. Absorption of lansoprazole begins only after the granules leave the stomach. Absorption is rapid, with mean peak plasma levels of lansoprazole occurring after approximately 1.7 hours. Peak plasma concentrations of lansoprazole (C_{max}) and the area under the plasma concentration curve (AUC) of lansoprazole are approximately proportional in doses from 15 mg to 60 mg after single-dose oral administration. Lansoprazole does not accumulate and its pharmacokinetics are unaltered by multiple dosing.

The absorption of lansoprazole is rapid, with mean C_{max} occurring approximately 1.7 hours after oral dosing, and relatively complete with absolute bioavailability over 80%. In healthy subjects, the mean (± SD) plasma half-life was 1.5 (± 1.0) hours. Both C_{max} and AUC are diminished by about 50% if the drug is given 30 minutes after food as opposed to the fasting condition. There is no significant food effect if the drug is given before meals.

Lansoprazole is 97% bound to plasma proteins. Plasma protein binding is consistent over the concentration range of 0.05 to 5.0 mcg/mL.

Lansoprazole is extensively metabolized in the liver. Two metabolites have been identified in measurable quantities in plasma (the hydroxylated sulfinyl and sulfone derivatives of lansoprazole). These metabolites have very little or no antisecretory activity. Lansoprazole is thought to be transformed into two active species which inhibit acid secretion by (H^+,K^+)-ATPase within the parietal cell canaliculus, but are not present in the systemic circulation. The plasma elimination half-life of lansoprazole does not reflect its duration of suppression of gastric acid secretion. Thus, the plasma elimination half-life is less than two hours while the acid inhibitory effect lasts more than 24 hours.

Following single-dose oral administration of PREVACID, virtually no unchanged lansoprazole was excreted in the urine. In one study, after a single oral dose of ^{14}C-lansoprazole, approximately one-third of the administered radiation was excreted in the urine and two-thirds was recovered in the feces. This implies a significant biliary excretion of the metabolites of lansoprazole.

Continued on next page

PREVPAC—Cont.

The clearance of lansoprazole is decreased in the elderly, with elimination half-life increased approximately 50% to 100%. Because the mean half-life in the elderly remains between 1.9 to 2.9 hours, repeated once daily dosing does not result in accumulation of lansoprazole. Peak plasma levels were not increased in the elderly.

In patients with severe renal insufficiency, plasma protein binding decreased by 1.0%–1.5% after administration of 60 mg of lansoprazole. Patients with renal insufficiency had a shortened elimination half-life and decreased total AUC (free and bound). AUC for free lansoprazole in plasma, however, was not related to the degree of renal impairment, and C_{max} and T_{max} were not different from subjects with healthy kidneys.

In patients with various degrees of chronic hepatic disease, the mean plasma half-life of the drug was prolonged from 1.5 hours to 3.2–7.2 hours. An increase in mean AUC of up to 500% was observed at steady state in hepatically-impaired patients compared to healthy subjects. Dose reduction in patients with severe hepatic disease should be considered.

The pooled pharmacokinetic parameters of PREVACID from twelve U.S. Phase I studies (N=513) were compared to the mean pharmacokinetic parameters from two Asian studies (N=20). The mean AUCs of PREVACID in Asian subjects are approximately twice that seen in pooled U.S. data; however, the inter-individual variability is high. The C_{max} values are comparable.

Amoxicillin:

Amoxicillin is stable in the presence of gastric acid and is well absorbed from the gastrointestinal tract and may be given with no regard to food. It diffuses readily into most body tissues and fluids, with the exception of brain and spinal fluid, except when meninges are inflamed. The half-life of amoxicillin is 61.3 minutes. Most of the amoxicillin is excreted unchanged in the urine; its excretion can be delayed by concurrent administration of probenecid. Amoxicillin is not highly protein-bound. In blood serum, amoxicillin is approximately 20% protein-bound as compared to 60% for penicillin G.

Orally administered doses of 500-mg amoxicillin capsules result in average peak blood levels 1 to 2 hours after administration in the range of 5.5 to 7.5 μg/mL.

Detectable serum levels are observed up to eight hours after an orally administered dose of amoxicillin. Approximately 60% of an orally administered dose of amoxicillin is excreted in the urine within 6 to 8 hours.

Clarithromycin:

Clarithromycin is rapidly absorbed from the gastrointestinal tract after oral administration. The absolute bioavailability of 250 mg clarithromycin tablets was approximately 50%. Food slightly delays both the onset of clarithromycin absorption and the formation of the antimicrobially active metabolite, 14-OH clarithromycin, but does not affect the extent of bioavailability. Therefore, clarithromycin tablets may be given without regard to food.

In fasting healthy human subjects, peak serum concentrations were attained within two hours after oral dosing. Steady-state peak serum clarithromycin concentrations were attained in two to three days and were approximately 2 to 3 μg/mL with a 500-mg dose administered every 12 hours. The elimination half-life of clarithromycin was 5 to 7 hours with 500 mg administered every 8 to 12 hours. The nonlinearity of clarithromycin pharmacokinetics is slight at the recommended dose of 500 mg administered every 12 hours. With a 500-mg dose every 8 to 12 hours, the peak steady-state concentration of 14-OH clarithromycin, the principal metabolite, is up to 1 μg/mL and its elimination half-life is about 7 to 9 hours. The steady-state concentration of this metabolite is generally attained within 2 to 3 days.

After a 500-mg tablet every 12 hours, the urinary excretion of clarithromycin is approximately 30%. The renal clearance of clarithromycin approximates the normal glomerular filtration rate. The major metabolite found in urine is 14-OH clarithromycin, which accounts for an additional 10% to 15% of the dose with a 500-mg tablet administered every 12 hours.

The steady-state concentrations of clarithromycin in subjects with impaired hepatic function did not differ from those in normal subjects; however, the 14-OH clarithromycin concentrations were lower in the hepatically impaired subjects. The decreased formation of 14-OH clarithromycin was at least partially offset by an increase in renal clearance of clarithromycin in the subjects with impaired hepatic function when compared to healthy subjects.

The pharmacokinetics of clarithromycin was also altered in subjects with impaired renal function. (See **PRECAUTIONS** and **DOSAGE AND ADMINISTRATION**.)

Pharmacodynamics

MICROBIOLOGY

Lansoprazole, clarithromycin and/or amoxicillin have been shown to be active against most strains of *Helicobacter pylori in vitro* and in clinical infections as described in the **INDICATIONS AND USAGE** section.

Helicobacter

Helicobacter pylori

Pretreatment Resistance

Clarithromycin pretreatment resistance (≥2.0 μg/mL) was 9.5% (91/960) by E-test and 11.3% (12/106) by agar dilution in the dual and triple therapy clinical trials (M93-125, M93-130, M93-131, M95-392, and M95-399).

Clarithromycin Susceptibility Test Results and Clinical/Bacteriological Outcomes[a]

Clarithromycin Pretreatment Results		Clarithromycin Post-treatment Results				
		H. pylori negative-eradicated	*H. pylori* positive - not eradicated Post-treatment susceptibility results S[b]	I[b]	R[b]	No MIC
Triple Therapy 14-Day (lansoprazole 30 mg b.i.d./amoxicillin 1 gm b.i.d./clarithromycin 500 mg b.i.d.) (M95-399, M93-131, M95-392)						
Susceptible[b]	112	105				7
Intermediate[b]	3	3				
Resistant[b]	17	6			7	4
Triple Therapy 10-Day (lansoprazole 30 mg b.i.d./amoxicillin 1 gm b.i.d./clarithromycin 500 mg b.i.d.) (M95-399)						
Susceptible[b]	42	40	1		1	
Intermediate[b]						
Resistant[b]	4	1			3	

[a] Includes only patients with pretreatment clarithromycin susceptibility test results

[b] Susceptible (S) MIC ≤0.25 μg/mL, Intermediate (I) MIC 0.5–1.0 μg/mL, Resistant (R) MIC ≥2 μg/mL

Mean Antisecretory Effects after Single and Multiple Daily Dosing

Parameter	Baseline Value	PREVACID 15 mg Day 1	PREVACID 15 mg Day 5	PREVACID 30 mg Day 1	PREVACID 30 mg Day 5
Mean 24-Hour pH	2.1	2.7^+	4.0^+	3.6^*	4.9^*
Mean Nighttime pH	1.9	2.4	3.0^+	2.6	3.8^*
% Time Gastric pH>3	18	33^+	59^+	51^*	72^*
% Time Gastric pH>4	12	22^+	49^+	41^*	66^*

NOTE: An intragastric pH of >4 reflects a reduction in gastric acid by 99%.

* ($p<0.05$) versus baseline and lansoprazole 15 mg.

$^+$ ($p<0.05$) versus baseline only.

Amoxicillin pretreatment susceptible isolates (≤0.25 μg/mL) occurred in 97.8% (936/957) and 98.0% (98/100) of the patients in the dual and triple therapy clinical trials by E-test and agar dilution, respectively. Twenty-one of 957 patients (2.2%) by E-test and 2 of 100 patients (2.0%) by agar dilution had amoxicillin pretreatment MICs of >0.25 μg/mL. One patient on the 14-day triple therapy regimen had an unconfirmed pretreatment amoxicillin minimum inhibitory concentration (MIC) of >256 μg/mL by E-test and the patient was eradicated of *H. pylori*.

[See first table above]

Patients not eradicated of *H. pylori* following lansoprazole/amoxicillin/clarithromycin triple therapy will likely have clarithromycin resistant *H. pylori*. Therefore, for those patients who fail therapy, clarithromycin susceptibility testing should be done when possible. Patients with clarithromycin resistant *H. pylori* should not be treated with lansoprazole/amoxicillin/clarithromycin triple therapy or with regimens which include clarithromycin as the sole antimicrobial agent.

Amoxicillin Susceptibility Test Results and Clinical/Bacteriological Outcomes

In the dual and triple therapy clinical trials, 82.6% (195/236) of the patients that had pretreatment amoxicillin susceptible MICs (≤0.25 μg/mL) were eradicated of *H. pylori*. Of those with pretreatment amoxicillin MICs of >0.25 μg/mL, three of six had the *H. pylori* eradicated. A total of 30% (21/70) of the patients failed lansoprazole 30 mg t.i.d./amoxicillin 1 gm t.i.d. dual therapy and a total of 12.8% (22/172) of the patients failed the 10- and 14-day triple therapy regimens. Post-treatment susceptibility results were not obtained on 11 of the patients who failed therapy. Nine of the 11 patients with amoxicillin post-treatment MICs that failed the triple therapy regimen also had clarithromycin resistant *H. pylori* isolates.

Susceptibility Test for *Helicobacter pylori*

The reference methodology for susceptibility testing of *H. pylori* is agar dilution MICs.[1] One to three microliters of an inoculum equivalent to a No. 2 McFarland standard (1×10^7 - 1×10^8 CFU/mL for *H. pylori*) are inoculated directly onto freshly prepared antimicrobial containing Mueller-Hinton agar plates with 5% aged defibrinated sheep blood (≥2 weeks old). The agar dilution plates are incubated at 35°C in a microaerobic environment produced by a gas generating system suitable for campylobacters. After 3 days of incubation, the MICs are recorded as the lowest concentration of antimicrobial agent required to inhibit growth of the organism. The clarithromycin and amoxicillin MIC values should be interpreted according to the following criteria:

Clarithromycin MIC (μg/mL)[a]	Interpretation
≤0.25	Susceptible (S)
0.5–1.0	Intermediate (I)
≥2.0	Resistant (R)

Amoxicillin MIC (μg/mL)[b]	Interpretation
≤0.25	Susceptible (S)

[a] These are tentative breakpoints for the agar dilution methodology and they should not be used to interpret results obtained using alternative methods.

[b] There were not enough organisms with MICs >0.25 μg/mL to determine a resistance breakpoint.

Standardized susceptibility test procedures require the use of laboratory control microorganisms to control the technical aspects of the laboratory procedures. Standard clarithromycin and amoxicillin powders should provide the following MIC values:

Microorganisms	Antimicrobial Agent	MIC (μg/mL)[a]
H. pylori ATCC 43504	Clarithromycin	0.015–0.12 mcg/mL
H. pylori ATCC 43504	Amoxicillin	0.015–0.12 mcg/mL

[a] These are quality control ranges for the agar dilution methodology and they should not be used to control test results obtained using alternative methods.

Reference

1. National Committee for Clinical Laboratory Standards. Summary Minutes, Subcommittee on Antimicrobial Susceptibility Testing, Tampa, FL, January 11–13, 1998.

Antisecretory activity

After oral administration, lansoprazole was shown to significantly decrease the basal acid output and significantly increase the mean gastric pH and percent of time the gastric pH was >3 and >4. Lansoprazole also significantly reduced meal-stimulated gastric acid output and secretion volume, as well as pentagastrin-stimulated acid output. In patients with hypersecretion of acid, lansoprazole significantly reduced basal and pentagastrin-stimulated gastric acid secretion. Lansoprazole inhibited the normal increases in secretion volume, acidity and acid output induced by insulin.

In a crossover study that included lansoprazole 15 and 30 mg for five days, the following effects on intragastric pH were noted:

[See second table above]

After the initial dose in this study, increased gastric pH was seen within 1–2 hours with lansoprazole 30 mg and 2–3 hours with lansoprazole 15 mg. After multiple daily dosing, increased gastric pH was seen within the first hour postdosing with lansoprazole 30 mg and within 1–2 hours postdosing with lansoprazole 15 mg.

The percentage of time gastric pH was elevated above 5 and 6 was evaluated in a crossover study of PREVACID given q.d., b.i.d. and t.i.d.

[See first table at top of next page]

The inhibition of gastric acid secretion as measured by intragastric pH returns gradually to normal over two to four days after multiple doses. There is no indication of rebound gastric acidity.

CLINICAL STUDIES

***H. pylori* Eradication to Reduce the Risk of Duodenal Ulcer Recurrence**

Randomized, double-blind clinical studies performed in the U.S. in patients with *H. pylori* and duodenal ulcer disease (defined as an active ulcer or history of an ulcer within one year) evaluated the efficacy of PREVPAC as triple 14-day therapy for the eradication of *H. pylori*. The triple therapy regimen (PREVACID 30 mg BID plus amoxicillin 1 gm BID plus clarithromycin 500 mg BID) produced statistically significantly higher eradication rates than PREVACID plus amoxicillin, PREVACID plus clarithromycin, and amoxicillin plus clarithromycin dual therapies.

H. pylori eradication was defined as two negative tests (culture and histology) at 4 to 6 weeks following the end of treatment.

Triple therapy was shown to be more effective than all possible dual therapy combinations. The combination of PREVACID plus amoxicillin and clarithromycin as triple therapy was effective in eradicating *H. pylori*. Eradication of *H. pylori* has been shown to reduce the risk of duodenal ulcer recurrence.

A randomized, double-blind clinical study performed in the U.S. in patients with *H. pylori* and duodenal ulcer disease (defined as an active ulcer or history of an ulcer within one year) compared the efficacy of PREVACID triple therapy for 10 and 14 days. This study established that the 10-day triple therapy was equivalent to the 14-day triple therapy in eradicating *H. pylori*.

[See second table above]

INDICATIONS AND USAGE

***H. pylori* Eradication to Reduce the Risk of Duodenal Ulcer Recurrence**

The components in PREVPAC (PREVACID, amoxicillin, and clarithromycin) are indicated for the treatment of patients with *H. pylori* infection and duodenal ulcer disease (active or one-year history of a duodenal ulcer) to eradicate *H. pylori*. Eradication of *H. pylori* has been shown to reduce the risk of duodenal ulcer recurrence (See **CLINICAL STUDIES** and **DOSAGE AND ADMINISTRATION**).

CONTRAINDICATIONS

PREVPAC is contraindicated in patients with known hypersensitivity to any component of the formulation of PREVACID, any macrolide antibiotic, or any penicillin.

Concomitant administration of PREVPAC with cisapride, pimozide, or terfenadine is contraindicated. There have been postmarketing reports of drug interactions when clarithromycin and/or erythromycin are co-administered with cisapride, pimozide, or terfenadine resulting in cardiac arrhythmias (QT prolongation, ventricular tachycardia, ventricular fibrillation, and torsades de pointes) most likely due to inhibition of hepatic metabolism of these drugs by erythromycin and clarithromycin. Fatalities have been reported.

WARNINGS

Amoxicillin:

Serious and occasionally fatal hypersensitivity (anaphylactoid) reactions have been reported in patients on penicillin therapy. Although anaphylaxis is more frequent following parenteral therapy, it has occurred in patients on oral penicillins. These reactions are more apt to occur in individuals with a history of penicillin hypersensitivity and/or a history of sensitivity to multiple allergens.

There have been well documented reports of individuals with a history of penicillin hypersensitivity reactions who have experienced severe hypersensitivity reactions when treated with a cephalosporin. Before initiating therapy with any penicillin, careful inquiry should be made concerning previous hypersensitivity reactions to penicillins, cephalosporins, and other allergens. If an allergic reaction occurs, amoxicillin should be discontinued and the appropriate therapy instituted.

SERIOUS ANAPHYLACTOID REACTIONS REQUIRE IMMEDIATE EMERGENCY TREATMENT WITH EPINEPHRINE. OXYGEN, INTRAVENOUS STEROIDS, AND AIRWAY MANAGEMENT, INCLUDING INTUBATION, SHOULD ALSO BE ADMINISTERED AS INDICATED.

Clarithromycin:

CLARITHROMYCIN SHOULD NOT BE USED IN PREGNANT WOMEN EXCEPT IN CLINICAL CIRCUMSTANCES WHERE NO ALTERNATIVE THERAPY IS APPROPRIATE. IF PREGNANCY OCCURS WHILE TAKING CLARITHROMYCIN, THE PATIENT SHOULD BE APPRISED OF THE POTENTIAL HAZARD TO THE FETUS. CLARITHROMYCIN HAS DEMONSTRATED ADVERSE EFFECTS OF PREGNANCY OUTCOME AND/OR EMBRYO-FETAL DEVELOPMENT IN MONKEYS, RATS, MICE, AND RABBITS AT DOSES THAT PRODUCED PLASMA LEVELS 2 TO 17 TIMES THE SERUM LEVELS ACHIEVED IN HUMANS TREATED AT THE MAXIMUM RECOMMENDED HUMAN DOSES. (See PRECAUTIONS—Pregnancy.)

Pseudomembranous colitis has been reported with nearly all antibacterial agents, including clarithromycin, and may range in severity from mild to life threatening. Therefore, it is important to consider this diagnosis in patients who present with diarrhea subsequent to the administration of antibacterial agents.

Treatment with antibacterial agents alters the normal flora of the colon and may permit overgrowth of clostridia. Studies indicate that a toxin produced by *Clostridium difficile* is a primary cause of "antibiotic-associated colitis."

After the diagnosis of pseudomembranous colitis has been established, therapeutic measures should be initiated. Mild cases of pseudomembranous colitis usually respond to discontinuation of the drug alone. In moderate to severe cases, consideration should be given to management with fluids and electrolytes, protein supplementation, and treatment with an antibacterial drug clinically effective against *Clostridium difficile* colitis.

PRECAUTIONS

Clarithromycin is principally excreted via the liver and kidney. Clarithromycin may be administered without dosage adjustment to patients with hepatic impairment and normal renal function. However, in the presence of severe renal impairment with or without coexisting hepatic impairment, decreased dosage or prolonged dosing intervals may be appropriate.

Mean Antisecretory Effects After 5 Days of b.i.d. and t.i.d. Dosing

	PREVACID			
Parameter	30 mg q.d.	15 mg b.i.d.	30 mg b.i.d.	30 mg t.i.d.
% Time Gastric pH>5	43	47	59+	77*
% Time Gastric pH>6	20	23	28	45*

+ ($p<0.05$) versus PREVACID 30 mg q.d.

* ($p<0.05$) versus PREVACID 30 mg q.d., 15 mg b.i.d. and 30 mg b.i.d.

***H. pylori* Eradication Rates—Triple Therapy**
(PREVACID/amoxicillin/clarithromycin)
Percent of Patients Cured
[95% Confidence Interval]
(Number of patients)

Study	Duration	Triple Therapy Evaluable Analysis*	Triple Therapy Intent-to-Treat Analysis#
M93-131	14 days	92† [80.0–97.7] (N=48)	86† [73.3–93.5] (N=55)
M95-392	14 days	86‡ [75.7–93.6] (N=66)	83‡ [72.0–90.8] (N=70)
M95-399+	14 days	85 [77.0–91.0] (N=113)	82 [73.9–88.1] (N=126)
	10 days	84 [76.0–89.8] (N=123)	81 [73.9–87.6] (N=135)

* Based on evaluable patients with confirmed duodenal ulcer (active or within one year) and *H. pylori* infection at baseline defined as at least two of three positive endoscopic tests from CLOtest® (Delta West Ltd., Bentley, Australia), histology and/or culture. Patients were included in the analysis if they completed the study. Additionally, if patients dropped out of the study due to an adverse event related to the study drug, they were included in the evaluable analysis as failures of therapy.

Patients were included in the analysis if they had documented *H. pylori* infection at baseline as defined above and had a confirmed duodenal ulcer (active or within one year). All dropouts were included as failures of therapy.

† ($p<0.05$) versus PREVACID/amoxicillin and PREVACID/clarithromycin dual therapy

‡ ($p<0.05$) versus clarithromycin/amoxicillin dual therapy

+ The 95% confidence interval for the difference in eradication rates, 10-day minus 14-day is (−10.5, 8.1) in the evaluable analysis and (−9.7, 9.1) in the intent-to-treat analysis.

The possibility of superinfections with mycotic organisms or bacterial pathogens should be kept in mind during therapy. In such cases, discontinue PREVPAC and substitute appropriate treatment.

Symptomatic response to therapy with PREVACID does not preclude the presence of gastric malignancy.

Information for Patients: Each dose of PREVPAC contains four pills: one pink and black capsule (PREVACID), two maroon and light-pink capsules (amoxicillin) and one yellow tablet (clarithromycin). Each dose should be taken twice per day before eating. Patients should be instructed to swallow each pill whole.

Drug Interactions

PREVACID:

PREVACID is metabolized through the cytochrome P_{450} system, specifically through the CYP3A and CYP2C19 isozymes. Studies have shown that PREVACID does not have clinically significant interactions with other drugs metabolized by the cytochrome P_{450} system, such as warfarin, antipyrine, indomethacin, ibuprofen, phenytoin, propranolol, prednisone, diazepam, clarithromycin, or terfenadine in healthy subjects. These compounds are metabolized through various cytochrome P_{450} isozymes including CYP1A2, CYP2C9, CYP2C19, CYP2D6, and CYP3A. When PREVACID was administered concomitantly with theophylline (CYP1A2, CYP3A), a minor increase (10%) in the clearance of theophylline was seen. Because of the small magnitude and the direction of the effect on theophylline clearance, this interaction is unlikely to be of clinical concern. Nonetheless, individual patients may require additional titration of their theophylline dosage when PREVACID is started or stopped to ensure clinically effective blood levels.

PREVACID has also been shown to have no clinically significant interaction with amoxicillin.

In a single-dose crossover study examining PREVACID 30 mg and omeprazole 20 mg each administered alone and concomitantly with sucralfate 1 gram, absorption of the proton pump inhibitors was delayed and their bioavailability was reduced by 17% and 16%, respectively, when administered concomitantly with sucralfate. Therefore, proton pump inhibitors should be taken at least 30 minutes prior to sucralfate. In clinical trials, antacids were administered concomitantly with PREVACID Delayed-Release Capsules; this did not interfere with its effect.

PREVACID causes a profound and long-lasting inhibition of gastric acid secretion; therefore, it is theoretically possible that PREVACID may interfere with the absorption of drugs where gastric pH is an important determinant of bioavailability (e.g., ketoconazole, ampicillin esters, iron salts, digoxin).

Clarithromycin:

Clarithromycin use in patients who are receiving theophylline may be associated with an increase of serum theophylline concentrations. Monitoring of serum theophylline concentrations should be considered for patients receiving high doses of theophylline or with baseline concentrations in the upper therapeutic range. In two studies in which theophylline was administered with clarithromycin (a theophylline sustained-release formulation was dosed at either 6.5 mg/kg or 12 mg/kg together with 250 or 500 mg q12h clarithromycin), the steady-state levels of C_{max}, C_{min}, and the area under the serum concentration time curve (AUC) of theophylline increased about 20%.

Concomitant administration of single doses of clarithromycin and carbamazepine has been shown to result in increased plasma concentrations of carbamazepine. Blood level monitoring of carbamazepine may be considered.

When clarithromycin and terfenadine were coadministered, plasma concentrations of the active acid metabolite of terfenadine were threefold higher, on average, than the values observed when terfenadine was administered alone. The pharmacokinetics of clarithromycin and the 14-hydroxy-clarithromycin were not significantly affected by coadministration of terfenadine once clarithromycin reached steady-state conditions. Concomitant administration of clarithromycin with terfenadine is contraindicated. (See **CONTRAINDICATIONS.**)

Spontaneous reports in the postmarketing period suggest that concomitant administration of clarithromycin and oral anticoagulants may potentiate the effects of the oral anticoagulants. Prothrombin times should be carefully monitored while patients are receiving clarithromycin and oral anticoagulants simultaneously.

Elevated digoxin serum concentrations in patients receiving clarithromycin and digoxin concomitantly have also been reported in postmarketing surveillance. Some patients have shown clinical signs consistent with digoxin toxicity, including potentially fatal arrhythmias. Serum digoxin levels should be carefully monitored while patients are receiving digoxin and clarithromycin simultaneously.

For information on interactions between clarithromycin in combination with other drugs which may be administered to HIV-infected patients, see the BIAXIN package insert, Drug Interactions, under the **PRECAUTIONS** section.

The following drug interactions, other than increased serum concentrations of carbamazepine and active acid metabolite of terfenadine, have not been reported in clinical trials with clarithromycin; however, they have been observed with erythromycin products and/or with clarithromycin in postmarketing experience.

Concurrent use of erythromycin or clarithromycin and ergotamine or dihydroergotamine has been associated in some patients with acute ergot toxicity characterized by severe peripheral vasospasm and dysesthesia.

Erythromycin has been reported to decrease the clearance of triazolam and, thus, may increase the pharmacologic effect of triazolam. There have been postmarketing reports of drug interactions and CNS effects (e.g., somnolence and confusion) with the concomitant use of clarithromycin and triazolam.

Continued on next page

PREVPAC—Cont.

There have been reports of an interaction between erythromycin and astemizole resulting in QT prolongation and torsades de pointes. Concomitant administration of erythromycin and astemizole is contraindicated. Because clarithromycin is also metabolized by cytochrome P_{450}, concomitant administration of clarithromycin with astemizole is not recommended.
As with other macrolides, clarithromycin has been reported to increase concentrations of HMG-CoA reductase inhibitors (e.g., lovastatin and simvastatin), through inhibition of cytochrome P_{450} metabolism of these drugs. Rare reports of rhabdomyolysis have been reported in patients taking these drugs concomitantly.
The use of erythromycin and clarithromycin in patients concurrently taking drugs metabolized by the cytochrome P_{450} system may be associated with elevations in serum levels of these other drugs. There have been reports of interactions of erythromycin and/or clarithromycin with carbamazepine, cyclosporine, tacrolimus, hexobarbital, phenytoin, alfentanil, disopyramide, lovastatin, bromocriptine, valproate, terfenadine, cisapride, pimozide, rifabutin, and astemizole. Serum concentrations of drugs metabolized by the cytochrome P_{450} system should be monitored closely in patients concurrently receiving these drugs.

Carcinogenesis, Mutagenesis, Impairment of Fertility

PREVACID:
In two 24-month carcinogenicity studies, Sprague-Dawley rats were treated orally with doses of 5 to 150 mg/kg/day, about 1 to 40 times the exposure on a body surface (mg/m^2) basis, of a 50-kg person of average height (1.46 m^2 body surface area) given the recommended human dose of 30 mg/day (22.2 mg/m^2). Lansoprazole produced dose-related gastric enterochromaffin-like (ECL) cell hyperplasia and ECL cell carcinoids in both male and female rats. It also increased the incidence of intestinal metaplasia of the gastric epithelium in both sexes. In male rats, lansoprazole produced a dose-related increase of testicular interstitial cell adenomas. The incidence of these adenomas in rats receiving doses of 15 to 150 mg/kg/day (4 to 40 times the recommended human dose based on body surface area) exceeded the low background incidence (range = 1.4 to 10%) for this strain of rat. Testicular interstitial cell adenoma also occurred in 1 of 30 rats treated with 50 mg/kg/day (13 times the recommended human dose based on body surface area) in a 1-year toxicity study.
In a 24-month carcinogenicity study, CD-1 mice were treated orally with doses of 15 to 600 mg/kg/day, 2 to 80 times the recommended human dose based on body surface area. Lansoprazole produced a dose-related increased incidence of gastric ECL cell hyperplasia. It also produced an increased incidence of liver tumors (hepatocellular adenoma plus carcinoma). The tumor incidences in male mice treated with 300 and 600 mg/kg/day (40 to 80 times the recommended human dose based on body surface area) and female mice treated with 150 to 600 mg/kg/day (20 to 80 times the recommended human dose based on body surface area) exceeded the ranges of background incidences in historical controls for this strain of mice. Lansoprazole treatment produced adenoma of rete testis in male mice receiving 75 to 600 mg/kg/day (10 to 80 times the recommended human dose based on body surface area).
Lansoprazole was not genotoxic in the Ames test, the *ex vivo* rat hepatocyte unscheduled DNA synthesis (UDS) test, the *in vivo* mouse micronucleus test or the rat bone marrow cell chromosomal aberration test. It was positive in *in vitro* human lymphocyte chromosomal aberration assays.
Lansoprazole at oral doses up to 150 mg/kg/day (40 times the recommended human dose based on body surface area) was found to have no effect on fertility and reproductive performance of male and female rats.

Amoxicillin:
Long-term studies in animals have not been performed with amoxicillin.

Clarithromycin:
The following *in vitro* mutagenicity tests have been conducted with clarithromycin:

Salmonella/Mammalian Microsomes Test
Bacterial Induced Mutation Frequency Test
In Vitro Chromosome Aberration Test
Rat Hepatocyte DNA Synthesis Assay
Mouse Lymphoma Assay
Mouse Dominant Lethal Study
Mouse Micronucleus Test

All tests had negative results except the *In Vitro* Chromosome Aberration Test which was weakly positive in one test and negative in another.
In addition, a Bacterial Reverse-Mutation Test (Ames Test) has been performed on clarithromycin metabolites with negative results.
Fertility and reproduction studies have shown that daily doses of up to 160 mg/kg/day (1.3 times the recommended maximum human dose based on mg/m^2) to male and female rats caused no adverse effects on the estrous cycle, fertility, parturition, or number and viability of offspring. Plasma levels in rats after 150 mg/kg/day were 2 times the human serum levels.
In the 150 mg/kg/day monkey studies, plasma levels were 3 times the human serum levels. When given orally at 150 mg/kg/day (2.4 times the recommended maximum human dose based on mg/m^2), clarithromycin was shown to produce embryonic loss in monkeys. This effect has been attributed to marked maternal toxicity of the drug at this high dose.
In rabbits, *in utero* fetal loss occurred at an intravenous dose of 33 mg/m^2, which is 17 times less than the maximum proposed human oral daily dose of 618 mg/m^2.
Long-term studies in animals have not been performed to evaluate the carcinogenic potential of clarithromycin.

Pregnancy

Teratogenic Effects. Pregnancy Category C

Category C is based on the pregnancy category for clarithromycin.
Four teratogenicity studies in rats (three with oral doses and one with intravenous doses up to 160 mg/kg/day administered during the period of major organogenesis) and two in rabbits at oral doses up to 125 mg/kg/day (approximately 2 times the recommended maximum human dose based on mg/m^2) or intravenous doses of 30 mg/kg/day administered during gestation days 6 to 18 failed to demonstrate any teratogenicity from clarithromycin. Two additional oral studies in a different rat strain at similar doses and similar conditions demonstrated a low incidence of cardiovascular anomalies at doses of 150 mg/kg/day administered during gestation days 6 to 15. Plasma levels after 150 mg/kg/day were 2 times the human serum levels. Four studies in mice revealed a variable incidence of cleft palate following oral doses of 1000 mg/kg/day (2 and 4 times the recommended maximum human dose based on mg/m^2, respectively) during gestation days 6 to 15. Cleft palate was also seen at 500 mg/kg/day. The 1000 mg/kg/day exposure resulted in plasma levels 17 times the human serum levels. In monkeys, an oral dose of 70 mg/kg/day (an approximate equidose of the recommended maximum human dose based on mg/m^2) produced fetal growth retardation at plasma levels that were 2 times the human serum levels.
There were no adequate and well-controlled studies of PREVPAC in pregnant women. PREVPAC should be used during pregnancy only if the potential benefit justifies the potential risk to the fetus. (See **WARNINGS**.)

Labor and Delivery

Oral ampicillin-class antibiotics are poorly absorbed during labor. Studies in guinea pigs showed that intravenous administration of ampicillin slightly decreased the uterine tone and frequency of contractions, but moderately increased the height and duration of contractions. However, it is not known whether use of these drugs in humans during labor or delivery has immediate or delayed adverse effects on the fetus, prolongs the duration of labor, or increases the likelihood that forceps delivery or other obstetrical intervention or resuscitation of the newborn will be necessary.

Nursing Mothers

Amoxicillin is excreted in human milk in very small amounts. Because of the potential for serious adverse reactions in nursing infants from PREVPAC, a decision should be made whether to discontinue nursing or to discontinue the drug therapy, taking into account the importance of the therapy to the mother.

Pediatric Use

Safety and effectiveness of PREVPAC in pediatric patients infected with *H. pylori* have not been established. (See **CONTRAINDICATIONS** and **WARNINGS**.)

Use in Geriatric Patients

Elderly patients may suffer from asymptomatic renal and hepatic dysfunction. Care should be taken when administering PREVPAC to this patient population.

ADVERSE REACTIONS

The most common adverse reactions (≥3%) reported in clinical trials when all three components of this therapy were given concomitantly for 14 days are listed in the table below.

Adverse Reactions Most Frequently Reported in Clinical Trials (≥ 3%)

Adverse Reaction	Triple Therapy n=138 (%)
Diarrhea	7.0
Headache	6.0
Taste Perversion	5.0

The additional adverse reactions which were reported as possibly or probably related to treatment (<3%) in clinical trials when all three components of this therapy were given concomitantly are listed below and divided by body system: *Body as a Whole*—abdominal pain; *Digestive System*—dark stools, dry mouth/thirst, glossitis, rectal itching, nausea, oral moniliasis, stomatitis, tongue discoloration, tongue disorder, vomiting; *Musculoskeletal System*—myalgia; *Nervous System*—confusion, dizziness; *Respiratory System*—respiratory disorders; *Skin and Appendages*—skin reactions; *Urogenital System*—vaginitis, vaginal moniliasis. There were no statistically significant differences in the frequency of reported adverse events between the 10- and 14-day triple therapy regimens.

PREVACID:
The following adverse reactions from the labeling for lansoprazole are provided for information.
Worldwide, over 10,000 patients have been treated with lansoprazole in Phase 2–3 clinical trials involving various dosages and durations of treatment. In general, lansoprazole treatment has been well tolerated in both short-term and long-term trials.

Incidence in Clinical Trials

The following adverse events were reported by the treating physician to have a possible or probable relationship to drug in 1% or more of patients treated with PREVACID capsules and occurred at a greater rate in patients treated with PREVACID capsules than placebo-treated patients:

Incidence of Possibly or Probably Treatment-Related Adverse Events in Short-term, Placebo-Controlled Studies

Body System/Adverse Event	PREVACID (N=2768) %	Placebo (N=1023) %
Body as a Whole		
Abdominal Pain	2.1	1.2
Digestive System		
Constipation	1.0	0.4
Diarrhea	3.8	2.3
Nausea	1.3	1.2

Headache was also seen at greater than 1% incidence but was more common on placebo. The incidence of diarrhea is similar between placebo and lansoprazole 15 mg and 30 mg patients, but higher in the lansoprazole 60 mg patients (2.9%, 1.4%, 4.2%, and 7.4%, respectively).
The most commonly reported possibly or probably treatment-related adverse event during maintenance therapy was diarrhea.
Additional adverse experiences occurring in <1% of patients or subjects in domestic trials are shown below.
Refer to ***Postmarketing*** for adverse reactions occurring since the drug was marketed.
Body as a Whole—abdomen enlarged, allergic reaction, asthenia, back pain, candidiasis, carcinoma, chest pain (not otherwise specified), chills, edema, fever, flu syndrome, halitosis, infection (not otherwise specified), malaise, neck pain, neck rigidity, pain, pelvic pain; *Cardiovascular System*—angina, arrhythmia, bradycardia, cerebrovascular accident/cerebral infarction, hypertension/hypotension, migraine, myocardial infarction, palpitations, shock (circulatory failure), syncope, tachycardia, vasodilation; *Digestive System*—abnormal stools, anorexia, bezoar, cardiospasm, cholelithiasis, colitis, dry mouth, dyspepsia, dysphagia, enteritis, eructation, esophageal stenosis, esophageal ulcer, esophagitis, fecal discoloration, flatulence, gastric nodules/fundic gland polyps, gastritis, gastroenteritis, gastrointestinal anomaly, gastrointestinal disorder, gastrointestinal hemorrhage, glossitis, gum hemorrhage, hematemesis, increased appetite, increased salivation, melena, mouth ulceration, nausea and vomiting, nausea and vomiting and diarrhea, oral moniliasis, rectal disorder, rectal hemorrhage, stomatitis, tenesmus, thirst, tongue disorder, ulcerative colitis, ulcerative stomatitis; *Endocrine System*—diabetes mellitus, goiter, hypothyroidism; *Hemic and Lymphatic System*—anemia, hemolysis, lymphadenopathy; *Metabolic and Nutritional Disorders*—gout, dehydration, hyperglycemia/hypoglycemia, peripheral edema, weight gain/loss; *Musculoskeletal System*—arthralgia, arthritis, bone disorder, joint disorder, leg cramps, musculoskeletal pain, myalgia, myasthenia, synovitis; *Nervous System*—abnormal dreams, agitation, amnesia, anxiety, apathy, confusion, convulsion, depersonalization, depression, diplopia, dizziness, emotional lability, hallucinations, hemiplegia, hostility aggravated, hyperkinesia, hypertonia, hypesthesia, insomnia, libido decreased/increased, nervousness, neurosis, paresthesia, sleep disorder, somnolence, thinking abnormality, tremor, vertigo; 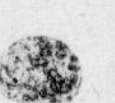 *Respiratory System*—asthma, bronchitis, cough increased, dyspnea, epistaxis, hemoptysis, hiccup, laryngeal neoplasia, pharyngitis, pleural disorder, pneumonia, respiratory disorder, upper respiratory inflammation/infection, rhinitis, sinusitis, stridor; *Skin and Appendages*—acne, alopecia, contact dermatitis, dry skin, fixed eruption, hair disorder, maculopapular rash, nail disorder, pruritus, rash, skin carcinoma, skin disorder, sweating, urticaria; *Special Senses*—abnormal vision, blurred vision, conjunctivitis, deafness, dry eyes, ear disorder, eye pain, otitis media, parosmia, photophobia, retinal degeneration, taste loss, taste perversion, tinnitus, visual field defect; *Urogenital System*—abnormal menses, breast enlargement, breast pain, breast tenderness, dysmenorrhea, dysuria, gynecomastia, impotence, kidney calculus, kidney pain, leukorrhea, menorrhagia, menstrual disorder, penis disorder, polyuria, testis disorder, urethral pain, urinary frequency, urinary tract infection, urinary urgency, urination impaired, vaginitis.

Postmarketing

Ongoing Safety Surveillance: Additional adverse experiences have been reported since lansoprazole has been marketed. The majority of these cases are foreign-sourced and a relationship to lansoprazole has not been established. Because these events were reported voluntarily from a population of unknown size, estimates of frequency cannot be made. These events are listed below by COSTART body system.
Body as a Whole—anaphylactoid-like reaction; *Digestive System*—hepatotoxicity, vomiting; *Hemic and Lymphatic System*—agranulocytosis, aplastic anemia, hemolytic anemia, leukopenia, neutropenia, pancytopenia, thrombocytopenia, and thrombotic thrombocytopenic purpura; *Special Senses*—speech disorder; *Urogenital System*—urinary retention.

Laboratory Values

The following changes in laboratory parameters were reported as adverse events.

Abnormal liver function tests, increased SGOT (AST), increased SGPT (ALT), increased creatinine, increased alkaline phosphatase, increased globulins, increased GGTP, increased/decreased/abnormal WBC, abnormal AG ratio, abnormal RBC, bilirubinemia, eosinophilia, hyperlipemia, increased/decreased electrolytes, increased/decreased cholesterol, increased glucocorticoids, increased LDH, increased/decreased/abnormal platelets, and increased gastrin levels. Urine abnormalities such as albuminuria, glycosuria, and hematuria were also reported. Additional isolated laboratory abnormalities were reported.

In the placebo-controlled studies, when SGOT (AST) and SGPT (ALT) were evaluated, 0.4% (4/978) placebo patients and 0.4% (11/2677) lansoprazole patients had enzyme elevations greater than three times the upper limit of normal range at the final treatment visit. None of these lansoprazole patients reported jaundice at any time during the study.

Amoxicillin:

The following adverse reactions from the labeling for amoxicillin are provided for information.

As with other penicillins, it may be expected that untoward reactions will be essentially limited to sensitivity phenomena. They are more likely to occur in individuals who have previously demonstrated hypersensitivity to penicillins and in those with a history of allergy, asthma, hay fever, or urticaria.

The following adverse reactions have been reported as associated with the use of penicillin:

Gastrointestinal—Glossitis, stomatitis, black "hairy" tongue, nausea, vomiting, and diarrhea. (These reactions are usually associated with oral dosage forms.)

Hypersensitivity Reactions—Skin rashes and urticaria have been reported frequently. A few cases of exfoliative dermatitis and erythema multiforme have been reported. Anaphylaxis is the most serious reaction experienced and has usually been associated with the parenteral dosage form. **Note:** Urticaria, other skin rashes, and serum sickness-like reactions may be controlled with antihistamines and, if necessary, systemic corticosteroids. Whenever such reactions occur, penicillin should be discontinued unless, in the opinion of the physician, the condition being treated is life threatening and amenable only to penicillin therapy. Serious anaphylactic reactions require the immediate use of epinephrine, oxygen, and intravenous steroids.

Liver—A moderate rise in serum glutamic oxaloacetic transaminase (SGOT) has been noted, particularly in infants, but the significance of this finding is unknown.

Hemic and Lymphatic Systems— Anemia, thrombocytopenia, thrombocytopenic purpura, eosinophilia, leukopenia, and agranulocytosis have been reported during therapy with the penicillins. These reactions are usually reversible on discontinuation of therapy and are believed to be hypersensitivity phenomena.

Clarithromycin:

The following adverse reactions from the labeling for clarithromycin are provided for information.

The majority of side effects observed in clinical trials were of a mild and transient nature. Fewer than 3% of adult patients without mycobacterial infections discontinued therapy because of drug-related side effects.

The most frequently reported events in adults were diarrhea (3%), nausea (3%), abnormal taste (3%), dyspepsia (2%), abdominal pain/discomfort (2%), and headache (2%). Most of these events were described as mild or moderate in severity. Of the reported adverse events, only 1% was described as severe.

Postmarketing Experience:

Allergic reactions ranging from urticaria and mild skin eruptions to rare cases of anaphylaxis, Stevens-Johnson syndrome, and toxic epidermal necrolysis have occurred. Other spontaneously reported adverse events include glossitis, stomatitis, oral moniliasis, anorexia, vomiting, tongue discoloration, thrombocytopenia, leukopenia, neutropenia, and dizziness. There have been reports of tooth discoloration in patients treated with clarithromycin. Tooth discoloration is usually reversible with professional dental cleaning. There have been isolated reports of hearing loss, which is usually reversible, occurring chiefly in elderly women. Reports of alterations of the sense of smell, usually in conjunction with taste perversion or taste loss have also been reported.

Transient CNS events including anxiety, behavioral changes, confusional states, depersonalization, disorientation, hallucinations, insomnia, manic behavior, nightmares, psychosis, tinnitus, tremor, and vertigo have been reported during postmarketing surveillance. Events usually resolve with discontinuation of the drug.

Hepatic dysfunction, including increased liver enzymes and hepatocellular and/or cholestatic hepatitis, with or without jaundice, has been infrequently reported with clarithromycin. This hepatic dysfunction may be severe and is usually reversible. In very rare instances, hepatic failure with fatal outcome has been reported and generally has been associated with serious underlying diseases and/or concomitant medications.

There have been rare reports of hypoglycemia, some of which have occurred in patients taking oral hypoglycemic agents or insulin.

As with other macrolides, clarithromycin has been associated with QT prolongation and ventricular arrhythmias, including ventricular tachycardia and torsades de pointes.

Changes in Laboratory Values: Changes in laboratory values with possible clinical significance were as follows: *Hepatic*—elevated SGPT (ALT) < 1%, SGOT (AST) < 1%, GGT < 1%, alkaline phosphatase < 1%, LDH < 1%, total bilirubin < 1%; *Hematologic*—decreased WBC < 1%, elevated prothrombin time 1%; *Renal*— elevated BUN 4%, elevated serum creatinine < 1%. GGT, alkaline phosphatase, and prothrombin time are from adult studies only.

OVERDOSAGE

In case of an overdose, patients should contact a physician, poison control center, or emergency room. There is neither a pharmacologic basis nor data suggesting an increased toxicity of the combination compared to individual components.

Lansoprazole:

Oral doses up to 5000 mg/kg in rats (approximately 1300 times the 30 mg human dose based on body surface area) and mice (about 675.7 times the 30 mg human dose based on body surface area) did not produce deaths or any clinical signs.

Lansoprazole is not removed from the circulation by hemodialysis. In one reported case of overdose, the patient consumed 600 mg of lansoprazole with no adverse reaction.

Amoxicillin:

In case of overdosage, discontinue medication, treat symptomatically and institute supportive measures as required. Amoxicillin can be removed from circulation by hemodialysis.

DOSAGE AND ADMINISTRATION

***H. pylori* Eradication to Reduce the Risk of Duodenal Ulcer Recurrence**

The recommended adult oral dose is 30 mg PREVACID, 1 g amoxicillin, and 500 mg clarithromycin administered together twice daily (morning and evening) for 10 or 14 days. (See **INDICATIONS AND USAGE**.)

PREVPAC is not recommended in patients with creatinine clearance less than 30 mL/min.

HOW SUPPLIED

PREVPAC is supplied as an individual daily administration pack, each containing:

PREVACID:

— two opaque, hard gelatin, black and pink PREVACID 30-mg capsules, with the TAP logo and "PREVACID 30" imprinted on the capsules.

TRIMOX:

— four maroon and light pink amoxicillin 500-mg capsules, USP, with "BRISTOL 7279" imprinted on the capsules.

BIAXIN Filmtab:

— two yellow oval film-coated clarithromycin 500-mg tablets, USP, debossed with the Abbott logo on one side and "KL" on the other side of the tablets.

NDC 0300-3702-01 Daily administration pack
NDC 0300-3702-11 Daily administration card

Storage: Protect from light and moisture.

Store at a controlled room temperature between 20°C and 25°C (68°F and 77°F).

Rx only

U.S. Patent No. 5,013,743

PREVPAC is distributed by TAP Pharmaceuticals Inc.
PREVACID® (lansoprazole) Delayed-Release Capsules
Manufactured for TAP Pharmaceuticals Inc.
Lake Forest, Illinois 60045, U.S.A.
by Takeda Chemical Industries Limited
Osaka, Japan 541
TRIMOX® (amoxicillin, USP)
Manufactured by APOTHECON®
A Bristol-Myers Squibb Company
Princeton, NJ 08540, U.S.A.
BIAXIN® Filmtab® (clarithromycin tablets, USP)
Manufactured by Abbott Laboratories
North Chicago, IL 60064, U.S.A.
03-5145-R4-Rev. September, 2001

Wyeth-Ayerst Pharmaceuticals

Division of American Home Products Corporation
P.O. BOX 8299
PHILADELPHIA, PA 19101

Direct General Inquiries to:
(610) 688-4400

For Medical Information Contact:
Medical Affairs
Day: (800) 934-5556
8:30 AM to 4:30 PM (Eastern Standard Time),
Weekdays only

In Emergencies:
Day: (800) 934-5556
Night: (610) 688-4400
(Emergencies only;
non-emergencies should wait until the next day)

ALESSE®-21 ℞

[ă'lĕs]

(levonorgestrel and ethinyl estradiol tablets)

Prescribing information for this product, which appears on pages 3468–3473 of the 2002 PDR, has been revised as follows. Please write "See Supplement A" next to the product heading.

The **CONTRAINDICATIONS** *section should be deleted and replaced with the following:*

Combination oral contraceptives should not be used in women with any of the following conditions:
Thrombophlebitis or thromboembolic disorders
A past history of deep-vein thrombophlebitis or thromboembolic disorders
Cerebrovascular or coronary artery disease
Thrombogenic valvulopathies
Thrombogenic rhythm disorders
Diabetes with vascular involvement
Uncontrolled hypertension
Known or suspected carcinoma of the breast
Carcinoma of the endometrium or other known or suspected estrogen-dependent neoplasia
Undiagnosed abnormal genital bleeding
Cholestatic jaundice of pregnancy or jaundice with prior pill use
Hepatic adenomas or carcinomas, or active liver disease, as long as liver function has not returned to normal
Known or suspected pregnancy
Hypersensitivity to any of the components of Alesse.

The boxed warning under the **WARNINGS** *heading should be deleted and replaced with the following:*

Cigarette smoking increases the risk of serious cardiovascular side effects from oral-contraceptive use. This risk increases with age and with the extent of smoking (in epidemiologic studies, 15 or more cigarettes per day was associated with a significantly increased risk) and is quite marked in women over 35 years of age. Women who use oral contraceptives should be strongly advised not to smoke.

The paragraph under the boxed warning under the **WARNINGS** *heading should be deleted and replaced with the following paragraph:*

The use of oral contraceptives is associated with increased risks of several serious conditions including venous and arterial thrombotic and thromboembolic events (such as myocardial infarction, thromboembolism, and stroke), hepatic neoplasia, gallbladder disease, and hypertension, although the risk of serious morbidity or mortality is very small in healthy women without underlying risk factors. The risk of morbidity and mortality increases significantly in the presence of other underlying risk factors such as certain inherited or acquired thrombophilias, hypertension, hyperlipidemias, obesity and diabetes. Practitioners prescribing oral contraceptives should be familiar with the following information relating to these risks.

The first paragraph following the subheading "b. Thromboembolism" under "1. THROMBOEMBOLIC DISORDERS AND OTHER VASCULAR PROBLEMS" *in the* **WARNINGS** *section should be deleted and replaced with the following paragraph:*

An increased risk of venous thromboembolic and thrombotic disease associated with the use of oral contraceptives is well established. Case control studies have found the relative risk of users compared to non-users to be 3 for the first episode of superficial venous thrombosis, 4 to 11 for deep-vein thrombosis or pulmonary embolism, and 1.5 to 6 for women with predisposing conditions for venous thromboembolic disease. Cohort studies have shown the relative risk to be somewhat lower, about 3 for new cases and about 4.5 for new cases requiring hospitalization. The approximate incidence of deep-vein thrombosis and pulmonary embolism in users of low dose (<50µg ethinyl estradiol) combination oral contraceptives is up to 4 per 10,000 woman-years compared to 0.5–3 per 10,000 woman-years for non-users. However, the incidence is substantially less than that associated with pregnancy (6 per 10,000 woman-years). The risk of thromboembolic disease due to oral contraceptives is not related to length of use and disappears after pill use is stopped.

The following sentence should be added to the end of the second paragraph following the subheading "c. Cerebrovascular diseases" under "1. THROMBOEMBOLIC DISORDERS AND OTHER VASCULAR PROBLEMS" *in the* **WARNINGS** *section:*

Oral contraceptives also increase the risk for stroke in women with other underlying risk factors such as certain inherited or acquired thrombophilias, hyperlipidemias, and obesity.

In the paragraph under "3. CARCINOMA REPRODUCTIVE ORGANS" *in the* **WARNINGS** *section, the word "invasive" should be inserted before the word* "cervical" *in the sentence that starts* "Some studies suggest...."

The paragraph under "5. OCULAR LESIONS" *in the* **WARNINGS** *section should be deleted and replaced with the following paragraph:*

There have been clinical case reports of retinal thrombosis associated with the use of oral contraceptives that may lead to partial or complete loss of vision. Oral contraceptives should be discontinued if there is unexplained partial or complete loss of vision; onset of proptosis or diplopia; papilledema; or retinal vascular lesions. Appropriate diagnostic and therapeutic measures should be undertaken immediately.

The paragraph under "11. BLEEDING IRREGULARITIES" *in the* **WARNINGS** *section should be deleted and replaced with the following paragraph:*

11. BLEEDING IRREGULARITIES

Breakthrough bleeding and spotting are sometimes encountered in patients on oral contraceptives, especially during the first three months of use. The type and dose of proges-

Continued on next page

Alesse-21—Cont.

togen may be important. If bleeding persists or recurs, nonhormonal causes should be considered and adequate diagnostic measures taken to rule out malignancy or pregnancy in the event of breakthrough bleeding, as in the case of any abnormal vaginal bleeding. If pathology has been excluded, time or a change to another formulation may solve the problem. In the event of amenorrhea, pregnancy should be ruled out if the oral contraceptive has not been taken according to directions prior to the first missed withdrawal bleed or if two consecutive withdrawal bleeds have been missed.

Some women may encounter post-pill amenorrhea or oligomenorrhea (possibly with anovulation), especially when such a consition was preexistent.

The entire **PRECAUTIONS** *section should be deleted and replaced with the following:*

Precautions

1. GENERAL

Patients should be counseled that this product does not protect against HIV infection (AIDS) and other sexually transmitted diseases.

2. PHYSICAL EXAMINATION AND FOLLOW-UP

A periodic personal and family medical history and complete physical examination are appropriate for all women, including women using oral contraceptives. The physical examination, however, may be deferred until after initiation of oral contraceptives if requested by the woman and judged appropriate by the clinician. The physical examination should include special reference to blood pressure, breasts, abdomen and pelvic organs, including cervical cytology, and relevant laboratory tests. In case of undiagnosed, persistent or recurrent abnormal vaginal bleeding, appropriate diagnostic measures should be conducted to rule out malignancy. Women with a strong family history of breast cancer or who have breast nodules should be monitored with particular care.

3. LIPID DISORDERS

Women who are being treated for hyperlipidemias should be followed closely if they elect to use oral contraceptives. Some progestogens may elevate LDL levels and may render the control of hyperlipidemias more difficult. (See "**Warnings**," 1d.)

In patients with familial defects of lipoprotein metabolism receiving estrogen-containing preparations, there have been case reports of significant elevations of plasma triglycerides leading to pancreatitis.

4. LIVER FUNCTION

If jaundice develops in any woman receiving such drugs, the medication should be discontinued. Steroid hormones may be poorly metabolized in patients with impaired liver function.

5. FLUID RETENTION

Oral contraceptives may cause some degree of fluid retention. They should be prescribed with caution, and only with careful monitoring, in patients with conditions which might be aggravated by fluid retention.

6. EMOTIONAL DISORDERS

Patients becoming significantly depressed while taking oral contraceptives should stop the medication and use an alternate method of contraception in an attempt to determine whether the symptoms is drug related. Women with a history of depression should be carefully observed and the drug discontinued if depression recurs to a serious degree.

7. CONTACT LENSES

Contact-lens wearers who develop visual changes or changes in lens tolerance should be assessed by an opthalmologist.

8. GASTROINTESTINAL MOTILITY

Diarrhea and/or vomiting may reduce hormone absorption.

9. DRUG INTERACTIONS

Interactions between ethinyl estradiol and other substances may lead to decreased or increased serum ethinyl estradiol concentrations.

Decreased ethinyl estradiol plasma concentrations may cause an increased incidence of breakthrough bleeding and menstrual irregularities and may possibly reduce efficacy of the combination oral contraceptive.

Reduced ethinyl estradiol concentrations have been associated with concomitant use of substances that induce hepatic microsomal enzymes, such as rifampin, rifabutin, barbiturates, phenylbutazone, phenytoin, griseofulvin, topiramate, some protease inhibitors, modafinil, and possibly St. John's wort.

Substances that may decrease plasma ethinyl estradiol concentrations by other mechanisms include any substance that reduces gut transit time and certain antibiotics (e.g. ampicillin and other penicillins, tetracyclines) by a decrease of enterohepatic circulation of estrogens.

During concomitant use of ethinyl estradiol containing products and substances that may lead to decreased plasma steroid hormone concentrations, it is recommended that a nonhormonal back-up method of birth control be used in addition to the regular intake of Alesse (levonorgestrel and ethinyl estradiol tablets). If the use of a substance which leads to decreased ethinyl estradiol plasma concentrations is required for a prolonged period of time, combination oral contraceptives should not be considered the primary contraceptive. After discontinuation of substances that may lead to decreased ethinyl estradiol plasma concentrations, use of a nonhormonal back-up method of birth control is recommended for 7 days. Longer use of a back-up method is advisable after discontinuation of substances that have led to induction of hepatic microsomal enzymes, resulting in decreased ethinyl estradiol concentrations. It may take several weeks until enzyme induction has completely subsided, depending on dosage, duration of use, and rate of elimination of the inducing substance.

Some substances may increase plasma ethinyl estradiol concentrations. These include:

- Competitive inhibitors for sulfation of ethinyl estradiol in the gastrointestinal wall, such as ascorbic acid (vitamin C) and acetaminophen.
- Substances that inhibit cytochrome P450 3A4 isoenzymes such as indinavir, fluconazole, and troleandomycin. Troleandomycin may increase the risk of intrahepatic cholestasis during coadministration with combination oral contraceptives.
- Atorvastatin (unknown mechanism)

Ethinyl estradiol may interfere with the mechanism of other drugs by inhibiting hepatic microsomal enzymes, or by inducing hepatic drug conjugation, particularly glucuronidation. Accordingly, tissue concentrations may be either increased (e.g. cyclosporine, theophylline, corticosteroids) or decreased. The prescribing information of concomitant medications should be consulted to identify potential interactions:

10. INTERACTIONS WITH LABORATORY TESTS

Certain endocrine- and liver-function tests and blood components may be affected by oral contraceptives:

a. Increased prothrombin and factors VII, VIII, IX, and X; decreased antithrombin 3; increased norephinephrine-induced platelet aggregability.

b. Increased thyroid-binding globulin (TBG) leading to increased circulating total thyroid hormone, as measured by protein-bound iodine (PBI), T4 by column or by radioimmunoassay. Free T3 resin uptake is decreased, reflecting the elevated TBG; free T4 concentration is unaltered.

c. Other binding proteins may be elevated in serum.

d. Sex-hormone binding globulins are increased and result in elevated levels of total circulating sex steroids; however, free or biologically active levels remain unchanged.

e. Triglycerides may be increased.

f. Glucose tolerance may be decreased.

g. Serum folate levels may be depressed by oral-contraceptive therapy. This may be of clinical significance if a woman becomes pregnant shortly after discontinuing oral contraceptives.

11. CARCINOGENESIS

See "**Warnings**" section.

12. PREGNANCY

Pregnancy Category X. See "**Contraindications**" and "**Warnings**" sections.

13. NURSING MOTHERS

Small amounts of oral-contraceptive steroids and/or metabolites have been identified in the milk of nursing mothers, and a few adverse effects on the child have been reported, including jaundice and breast enlargement. In addition, combination oral contraceptives given in the postpartum period may interfere with lactation by decreasing the quantity and quality of breast milk. If possible, the nursing mother should be advised not to use combination oral contraceptives but to use other forms of contraception until she has completely weaned her child.

14. PEDIATRIC USE

Safety and efficacy of Alesse have been established in women of reproductive age. Safety and efficacy are expected to be the same for postpubertal adolescents under the age of 16 and users 16 and older. Use of this product before menarche is not indicated.

INFORMATION FOR THE PATIENT

See Patient Labeling Printed Below.

The entire **ADVERSE REACTIONS** *section should be deleted and replaced with the following:*

An increased risk of the following serious adverse reactions [see "**Warnings**" section for additional information] has been associated with the use of oral contraceptives:

Thromboembolic disorders and other vascular problems (including thrombophlebitis, arterial thromboembolism, pulmonary embolism, myocardial infarction, cerebral hemorrhage, cerebral thrombosis), carcinoma of the reproductive organs, hepatic neoplasia (including hepatic adenomas or benign liver tumors), ocular lesions (including retinal vascular thrombosis), gallbladder disease, carbohydrate and lipid effects, elevated blood pressure, and headache.

The following adverse reactions have been reported in patients receiving oral contraceptives and are believed to be drug related:

Nausea
Vomiting
Gastrointestinal symptoms (such as abdominal pain, cramps and bloating)
Breakthrough bleeding
Spotting
Change in menstrual flow
Amenorrhea
Temporary infertility after discontinuation of treatment
Edema/fluid retention
Melasma/chloasma which may persist
Breast changes: tenderness, pain, enlargement, secretion
Change in weight or appetite (increase or decrease)
Change in cervical erosion and secretion
Diminution in lactation when given immediately postpartum
Cholestatic jaundice
Rash (allergic)
Mood changes, including depression
Vaginitis, including candidiasis
Change in corneal curvature (steepening)
Intolerance to contact lenses
Mesenteric thrombosis
Decrease in serum folate levels
Exacerbation of systemic lupus erythematosus
Exacerbation of porphyria
Exacerbation of chorea
Aggravation of varicose veins
Anaphylactic/anaphylactoid reactions, including urticaria, angioedema, and severe reactions with respiratory and circulatory symptoms

The following adverse reactions have been reported in users of oral contraceptives and the association has been neither confirmed nor refuted:

Premenstrual syndrome
Cataracts
Optic neuritis, which may lead to partial or complete loss of vision
Cystitis-like syndrome
Nervousness
Dizziness
Hirsutism
Loss of scalp hair
Erythema multiforme
Erythema nodosum
Hemorrhagic eruption
Impaired renal function
Hemolytic uremic syndrome
Budd-Chiari syndrome
Acne
Changes in libido
Colitis
Pancreatitis
Dysmenorrhea

The entire **DOSAGE AND ADMINISTRATION** *section should be deleted and replaced with the following:*

To achieve maximum contraceptive effectiveness, Alesse® (levonorgestrel and ethinyl estradiol tablets) must be taken exactly as directed and at intervals not exceeding 24 hours. The dispenser should be kept in the wallet supplied to avoid possible fading of the pills. If the pills fade, patients should continue to take them as directed.

The dosage of Alesse-21 is one pink tablet daily for 21 consecutive days, followed by 7 days when no tablets are taken. It is recommended that Alesse-21 tablets be taken at the same time each day.

Sunday start:

During the first cycle of medication, the patient is instructed to begin taking Alesse-21 on the first Sunday after the onset of menstruation. If menstruation begins on a Sunday, the first tablet (pink) is taken that day. One pink tablet should be taken daily for 21 consecutive days, followed by seven days when no tablet is taken. Withdrawal bleeding should usually occur within three days following discontinuation of pink tablets and may not have finished before the next pack is started. During the first cycle, contraceptive reliance should not be placed on Alesse-21 until a pink tablet has been taken daily for 7 consecutive days and a nonhormonal back-up method of birth control should be used during those 7 days. The possibility of ovulation and conception prior to initiation of medication should be considered.

The patient begins her next and all subsequent 21-day courses of tablets on the same day of the week (Sunday) on which she began her first course, following the same schedule: 21 days on pink tablets—7 days when no tablets are taken. If in any cycle the patient starts tablets later than the proper day, she should protect herself against pregnancy by using another method of birth control until she has taken a pink tablet daily for 7 consecutive days.

Day 1 start:

During the first cycle of medication, the patient is instructed to begin taking Alesse-21 during the first 24 hours of her period (day one of her menstrual cycle). One pink tablet should be taken daily for 21 consecutive days. Withdrawal bleeding should usually occur within three days following discontinuation of pink tablets and may not have finished before the next pack is started. If medication is begun on day one of the menstrual cycle, no back-up contraception is necessary. If Alesse-21 tablets are started later than day one of the first menstrual cycle or postpartum, contraceptive reliance should not be placed on Alesse-21 tablets until after the first 7 consecutive days of administration and a nonhormonal back-up method of birth control should be used during those 7 days. The possibility of ovulation and conception prior to initiation of medication should be considered.

When the patient is switching from a 21-day regimen of tablets, she should wait 7 days after her last tablet before she starts Alesse. She will probably experience withdrawal bleeding during that week. She should be sure that no more than 7 days pass after her previous 21-day regimen. When the patient is switching from a 28-day regimen of tablets, she should start her first pack of Alesse on the day after her last tablet. She should not wait any days between packs. The patient may switch any day from a progestin-only pill and should begin Alesse the next day. If switching from an implant or injection, the patient should start Alesse on the day of implant removal or, if using an injection, the day the next injection would be due. In switching from a progestin-only pill, injection or implant, the patient should be advised to use a nonhormonal back-up method of birth control for the first 7 days of tablet-taking.

If spotting or breakthrough bleeding occur, the patient is instructed to continue on the same regimen. This type of bleeding is usually transient and without significance; however, if the bleeding is persistent or prolonged, the patient is advised to consult her physician. While there is little likelihood of ovulation occurring if only one or two pink tablets are missed, the possibility of ovulation increases with each successive day that scheduled pink tablets are missed. Although the occurrence of pregnancy is unlikely if Alesse is taken according to directions, if withdrawal bleeding does not occur, the possibility of pregnancy must be considered. If the patient has not adhered to the prescribed schedule (missed one or more tablets or started taking them on a day later than she should have), the probability of pregnancy should be considered at the time of the first missed period and appropriate diagnostic measures taken before the medication is resumed. If the patient has adhered to the prescribed regimen and misses two consecutive periods, pregnancy should be ruled out before continuing the contraceptive regimen.

The risk of pregnancy increases with each active (pink) tablet missed. For additional patient instructions regarding missed tablets, see the "WHAT TO DO IF YOU MISS PILLS" section in the **DETAILED PATIENT LABELING** below.

Alesse may be initiated no earlier than day 28 postpartum in the nonlactating mother or after a second-trimester abortion, due to the increased risk for thromboembolism (see **"Contraindications"**, **"Warnings"**, and **"Precautions"** concerning thromboembolic disease). The patient should be advised to use a nonhormonal back-up method for the first 7 days of tablet-taking. However, if intercourse has already occurred, pregnancy should be excluded before the start of combined oral contraceptive use or the patient must wait for her first menstrual period.

In the case of first-trimester abortion, if the patient starts Alesse immediately, additional contraceptive measures are not needed.

The second paragraph under the heading **Brief Summary Patient Package Insert** *should be deleted and replaced with the following paragraph:*

Oral contraceptives, also known as "birth-control pills" or "the pill", are taken to prevent pregnancy, and when taken correctly, have a failure rate of less than 1.0% per year when used without missing any pills. The average failure rate of large numbers of pill users is 5% per year when women who miss pills are included. For most women oral contraceptives are also free of serious or unpleasant side effects. However, forgetting to take pills considerably increases the chances of pregnancy.

The boxed warning in the **Brief Summary Patient Package Insert** *should be deleted and replaced with the following:*

Cigarette smoking increases the risk of serious adverse effects on the heart and blood vessels from oral-contraceptive use. This risk increases with age and with the amount of smoking (15 or more cigarettes per day has been associated with a significantly increased risk) and is quite marked in women over 35 years of age. Women who use oral contraceptives should not smoke.

In the last sentence of the first paragraph under "3. High blood pressure, although blood pressure usually returns to normal when the pill is stopped.", *the words* "and possibly St. John's wort" *should be inserted after* "some antibiotics".

In the first paragraph under the subheading "EFFECTIVENESS OF ORAL CONTRACEPTIVES" *under* **DETAILED PATIENT LABELING,** *the sentence* "Typical failure rates are less than 3% per year." *should be deleted and replaced with* "Average failure rates are 5% per year."

In the first sentence of the second paragraph under the subheading "EFFECTIVENESS OF ORAL CONTRACEPTIVES" *under* **DETAILED PATIENT LABELING,** *the word* "typical" *should be deleted and replaced with the word* "average."

The boxed warning under the subheading WHO SHOULD NOT TAKE ORAL CONTRACEPTIVES *under* **DETAILED PATIENT LABELING** *should be deleted and replaced with the following:*

Cigarette smoking increases the risk of serious adverse effects on the heart and blood vessels from oral-contraceptive use. This risk increases with age and with the amount of smoking (15 or more cigarettes per day has been associated with a significantly increased risk) and is quite marked in women over 35 years of age. Women who use oral contraceptives should not smoke.

The following should be inserted under "•Known or suspected pregnancy." *under the subheading* WHO SHOULD NOT TAKE ORAL CONTRACEPTIVES *under* **DETAILED PATIENT LABELING:**

- Heart valve or heart rhythm disorders that may be associated with formation of blood clots.
- Diabetes affecting your circulation.
- Uncontrolled high blood pressure.
- Active liver disease with abnormal liver function tests.

The paragraph under "5. Other side effects" under SIDE EFFECTS OF ORAL CONTRACEPTIVES *in the* **DETAILED PATIENT LABELING** *section should be deleted and replaced with the following paragraph:*

Other side effects may include nausea, breast tenderness, change in appetite, headache, nervousness, depression, dizziness, loss of scalp hair, rash, vaginal infections, inflammation of the pancreas, and allergic reactions.

The two paragraphs under "4. Drug interactions" under GENERAL PRECAUTIONS *in the* **DETAILED PATIENT LABELING** *section should be deleted and replaced with the following three paragraphs:*

Certain drugs may interact with birth-control pills to make them less effective in preventing pregnancy or cause an increase in breakthrough bleeding. Such drugs include rifampin, drugs used for epilepsy such as barbiturates (for example, phenobarbital) and phenytoin (Dilantin® is one brand of this drug), primidone (Mysoline®), topiramate (Topamax®), phenylbutazone (Butazolidin® is one brand), some drugs used for HIV such as ritonavir (Norvir®), modafinil (Provigil®) and possibly certain antibiotics (such as ampicillin and other penicillins, and tetracyclines) and St. John's wort. You may need to use an additional method of contraception during any cycle in which you take drugs that can make oral contraceptives less effective.

You may be at higher risk of a specific type of liver dysfunction if you take troleandomycin and oral contraceptives at the same time.

You should inform your healthcare provider about all medicines you are taking, including nonprescription products.

The following should be added to the end of the section GENERAL PRECAUTIONS *in the* **DETAILED PATIENT LABELING:**

5. *Sexually transmitted diseases*

This product (like all oral contraceptives) is intended to prevent pregnancy. It does not protect against transmission of HIV (AIDS) and other sexually transmitted diseases such as chlamydia, genital herpes, genital warts, gonorrhea, hepatitis B, and syphilis.

The first paragraph under the subheading HOW TO TAKE THE PILL *in the* **DETAILED PATIENT LABELING** *should be deleted.*

The paragraph after the number 5 under **IMPORTANT POINTS TO REMEMBER** *in the* **DETAILED PATIENT LABELING** *should be deleted and replaced with the following:*

5. IF YOU HAVE VOMITING (within 3 to 4 hours after you take your pill), you should follow the instructions for WHAT TO DO IF YOU MISS PILLS. IF YOU HAVE DIARRHEA or IF YOU TAKE SOME MEDICINES, including some antibiotics, your pills may not work as well.

Use a back-up method (such as condoms, spermicide, or sponge) until you check with your doctor or clinic.

The words "(such as condoms or foam)" *should be deleted and replaced with the words* "(such as condoms, spermicide, or sponge)" *wherever they appear in the* **DETAILED PATIENT LABELING.**

Under the subheading "Pregnancy due to pill failure" in the **DETAILED PATIENT LABELING** *section,* "typical failure rates are less than 3%" *should be deleted and replaced with* "average failure rates are 5%."

CI 6157-3 Revised August 28, 2001

CORDARONE® Tablets ℞

[*kŏr'dă-rōn*]

(amiodarone HCl)

Prescribing information for this product, which appears on pages 3487–3491 of the 2002 PDR, has been revised as follows. Please write "See Supplement A" next to the product heading.

The following paragraph should be added after the first paragraph under the subheading **Worsening Arrhythmias** *in the* **WARNINGS** *section:*

The need to co-administer amiodarone with any other drug known to prolong the QTc interval must be based on a careful assessment of the potential risks and benefits of doing so for each patient. A careful assessment of the potential risks and benefits of administering Cordarone must be made in patients with thyroid dysfunction due to the possibility of arrhythmia breakthrough or exacerbation of arrhythmia in these patients.

The words ", which may result in death" *should be added to the end of the second sentence of the fourth paragraph under the subheading* **Thyroid Abnormalities** *in the* **PRECAUTIONS** *section.*

The **Drug Interactions** *section in the* **PRECAUTIONS** *section should be deleted and replaced with the following:*

Drug Interactions

Amiodarone is metabolized to desethylamiodarone by the cytochrome P450 (CYP450) enzyme group, specifically cytochrome P450 3A4 (CYP3A4). This isoenzyme is present in both the liver and intestines (see **"CLINICAL PHARMACOLOGY, Pharmacokinetics and Metabolism"**). Amiodarone is also known to be an inhibitor of CYP3A4. Therefore, amiodarone has the **potential** for interactions with drugs or substances that may be substrates, inhibitors or inducers of CYP3A4. While only a limited number of *in vivo* drug-drug interactions with amiodarone have been reported, the potential for other interactions should be anticipated. This is especially important for drugs associated with serious toxicity, such as other antiarrhythmics. If such drugs are needed, their dose should be reassessed and, where appropriate, plasma concentration measured.

In view of the long and variable half-life of amiodarone, potential for drug interactions exists not only with concomitant medication but also with drugs administered after discontinuation of amiodarone.

Since amiodarone is a substrate for CYP3A4, drugs/substances that inhibit CYP3A4 may decrease the metabolism and increase serum concentrations of amiodarone, with the potential for toxic effects. Reported examples of this interaction include the following:

Protease Inhibitors:

Protease inhibitors are known to inhibit CYP3A4 to varying degrees. Inhibition of CYP3A4 by **indinavir** has been reported to result in increased serum concentrations of amiodarone. Monitoring for amiodarone toxicity and serial measurement of amiodarone serum concentration during concomitant protease inhibitor therapy should be considered.

Histamine H_2 antagonists:

Cimetidine inhibits CYP3A4 and can increase serum amiodarone levels.

Other substances:

Grapefruit juice inhibits CYP3A4-mediated metabolism of oral amiodarone in the intestinal mucosa, resulting in increased plasma levels of amiodarone; therefore, grapefruit juice should not be taken during treatment with oral amiodarone (see **"DOSAGE AND ADMINISTRATION"**).

Amiodarone may suppress certain CYP450 enzymes (enzyme inhibition). This can result in unexpectedly high plasma levels of other drugs which are metabolized by those CYP450 enzymes and may lead to toxic effects. Reported examples of this interaction include the following:

Immunosuppressives:

Cyclosporine (CYP3A4 substrate) administered in combination with oral amiodarone has been reported to produce persistently elevated plasma concentrations of cyclosporine resulting in elevated creatinine, despite reduction in dose of cyclosporine.

Cardiovasculars:

Cardiac glycosides: In patients receiving **digoxin** therapy, administration of oral amiodarone regularly results in an increase in the serum digoxin concentration that may reach toxic levels with resultant clinical toxicity. Amiodarone taken concomitantly with digoxin increases the serum digoxin concentration by 70% after one day. **On initiation of oral amiodarone, the need for digitalis therapy should be reviewed and the dose reduced by approximately 50% or discontinued.** If digitalis treatment is continued, serum levels should be closely monitored and patients observed for clinical evidence of toxicity. These precautions probably should apply to digitoxin administration as well.

Antiarrhythmics:

Other antiarrhythmic drugs, such as **quinidine, procainamide, disopyramide,** and **phenytoin,** have been used concurrently with oral amiodarone.

There have been case reports of increased steady-state levels of quinidine, procainamide, and phenytoin during concomitant therapy with amiodarone. Phenytoin decreases serum amiodarone levels. Amiodarone taken concomitantly with quinidine increases quinidine serum concentration by 33% after two days. Amiodarone taken concomitantly with procainamide for less than seven days increases plasma concentrations of procainamide and n-acetyl procainamide by 55% and 33%, respectively. Quinidine and procainamide doses should be reduced by one-third when either is administered with amiodarone. Plasma levels of **flecainide** have been reported to increase in the presence of oral amiodarone; because of this, the dosage of flecainide should be adjusted when these drugs are administered concomitantly. In general, any added antiarrhythmic drug should be initiated at a lower than usual dose with careful monitoring.

Combination of amiodarone with other antiarrhythmic therapy should be reserved for patients with life-threatening ventricular arrhythmias who are incompletely responsive to a single agent or incompletely responsive to amiodarone.

During transfer to amiodarone the dose levels of previously administered agents should be reduced by 30 to 50% several days after the addition of amiodarone, when arrhythmia suppression should be beginning. The continued need for the other antiarrhythmic agent should be reviewed after the effects of amiodarone have been established, and discontinuation ordinarily should be attempted. If the treatment is continued, these patients should be particularly carefully monitored for adverse effects, especially conduction disturbances and exacerbation of tachyarrhythmias, as amiodarone is continued. In amiodarone-treated patients who require additional antiarrhythmic therapy, the initial dose of such agents should be approximately half of the usual recommended dose.

Antihypertensives:

Amiodarone should be used with caution in patients receiving **β-receptor blocking agents** (e.g., propranolol, a CYP3A4 inhibitor) or **calcium channel antagonists** (e.g., verapamil, a CYP3A4 substrate, and diltiazem, a CYP3A4 inhibitor) because of the possible potentiation of bradycardia, sinus arrest, and AV block; if necessary, amiodarone can continue to be used after insertion of a pacemaker in patients with severe bradycardia or sinus arrest.

Anticoagulants:

Potentiation of **warfarin**-type (CYP2C9 and CYP3A4 substrate) anticoagulant response is almost always seen in patients receiving amiodarone and can result in serious or fatal bleeding. Since the concomitant administration of warfarin with amiodarone increases the prothrombin time by 100% after 3 to 4 days, **the dose of the anticoagulant should be reduced by one-third to one-half, and prothrombin times should be monitored closely.**

Some drugs/substances are known to accelerate the metabolism of amiodarone by stimulating the synthesis of

Continued on next page

Cordarone Tablets—Cont.

CYP3A4 (enzyme induction). This may lead to low amiodarone serum levels and potential decrease in efficacy. Reported examples of this interaction include the following:

Antibiotics:

Rifampin is a potent inducer of CYP3A4. Administration of rifampin concomitantly with oral amiodarone has been shown to result in decreases in serum concentrations of amiodarone and desethylamiodarone.

Other substances, including herbal preparations:

St. John's Wort (Hypericum perforatum) induces CYP3A4. Since amiodarone is a substrate for CYP3A4, there is the potential that the use of St. John's Wort in patients receiving amiodarone could result in reduced amiodarone levels.

Other reported interactions with amiodarone:

Fetanyl (CYP3A4 substrate) in combination with amiodarone may cause hypotension, bradycardia, decreased cardiac output.

Sinus bradycardia has been reported with oral amiodarone in combination with **lidocaine** (CYP3A4 substrate) given for local anesthesia. Seizure, associated with increased lidocaine concentrations, has been reported with concomitant administration of intravenous amiodarone.

Dextromethorphan is a substrate for both CYP2D6 and CYP3A4. Amiodarone inhibits CYP2D6.

Cholestyramine increases enterohepatic elimination of amiodarone and may reduce serum levels and $t_{1/2}$.

Disopyramide increases QT prolongation which could cause arrhythmia.

Hemodynamic and electrophysiologic interactions have also been observed after concomitant administration with **propranolol, diltiazem,** and **verapamil.**

Volatile Anesthetic Agents (See **"PRECAUTIONS, Surgery,** *Volatile Anesthetic Agents.*")

In addition to the interactions noted above, chronic (> 2 weeks) ***oral*** Cordarone administration impairs metabolism of phenytoin, dextromethorphan, and methotrexate.

The following sentence should be added to the end of the paragraph under the subheading **Electrolyte Disturbances** *in the* **PRECAUTIONS** *section:*

Use caution when coadministering Cordarone with drugs which may induce hypokalemia and/or hypomagnesemia.

The following subsection should be added to the end of the **ADVERSE REACTIONS** *section:*

Postmarketing Reports

In postmarketing surveillance, sinus arrest, hepatitis, cholestatic hepatitis, cirrhosis, epididymitis, impotence, vasculitis, pseudotumor cerebri, thrombocytopenia, angioedema, bronchiolitis obliterans organizing pneumonia (possibly fatal), bronchospasm, pleuritis, pancreatitis, toxic epidermal necrolysis, myopathy, hemolytic anemia, aplastic anemia, pancytopenia, neutropenia, erythema multiforme, Stevens-Johnson syndrome, and exfoliative dermatitis, also have been reported in patients receiving Cordarone.

The paragraph under the heading **OVERDOSAGE** *should be deleted and replaced with the following:*

There have been cases, some fatal, of Cordarone overdose. In addition to general supportive measures, the patient's cardiac rhythm and blood pressure should be monitored, and if bradycardia ensues, a β-adrenergic agonist or a pacemaker may be used. Hypotension with inadequate tissue perfusion should be treated with positive inotropic and/or vasopressor agents. Neither Cordarone nor its metabolite is dialyzable.

The acute LD_{50} of amiodarone HCl in mice and rats is greater than 3,000 mg/kg.

The following paragraph should be added as the fourth paragraph of the **DOSAGE AND ADMINISTRATION** *section:*

Since grapefruit juice is known to inhibit CYP3A4-mediated metabolism of oral amiodarone in the intestinal mucosa, resulting in increased levels of amiodarone; grapefruit juice should not be taken during treatment with oral amiodarone (see **"PRECAUTIONS, Drug Interactions"**).

CI 6036-3 Revised August 20, 2001

CORDARONE® INTRAVENOUS ℞

[*kŏr 'dă-rōn*]

(amiodarone hydrochloride)

Rx only

Prescribing information for this product, which appears on pages 3491–3494 of the 2002 PDR, has been revised as follows. Please write "See Supplement A" next to the product heading.

The second paragraph under the subheading **Liver Enzyme Elevations** *in the* **PRECAUTIONS** *should be deleted and replaced with the following paragraph:*

Rare cases of fatal hepatocellular necrosis after treatment with Cordarone I.V. have been reported. Two patients, one 28 years of age and the other 60 years of age, were treated for atrial arrhythmias with an initial infusion of 1500 mg over 5 hours, a rate much higher than recommended. Both patients developed hepatic and renal failure within 24 hours after the start of Cordarone I.V. treatment and died on day 14 and day 4, respectively. Because these episodes of hepatic necrosis may have been due to the rapid rate of infusion with possible rate-related hypotension, ***the initial rate of infusion should be monitored closely and should not exceed that prescribed in*** **DOSAGE AND ADMINISTRATION.**

The following should be added after the first paragraph under the subheading **Proarrhythmia** *in the* **PRECAUTIONS** *section:*

Combination of amiodarone with other antiarrhythmic therapy that prolongs the QTc should be reserved for patients with life-threatening ventricular arrhythmias who are incompletely responsive to a single agent.

The need to co-administer amiodarone with any other drug known to prolong the QTc interval must be based on a careful assessment of the potential risks and benefits of doing so for each patient.

A careful assessment of the potential risks and benefits of administering Cordarone I.V. must be made in patients with thyroid dysfunction due to the possibility of arrhythmia breakthrough or exacerbation of arrhythmia, which may result in death, in these patients.

The **Drug Interactions** *section in the* **PRECAUTIONS** *section should be deleted and replaced with the following:*

Amiodarone is metabolized to desethylamiodarone by the cytochrome P450 (CYP450) enzyme group, specifically cytochrome P450 3A4 (CYP3A4). This isoenzyme is present in both the liver and intestines (see **CLINICAL PHARMACOLOGY, Pharmacokinetics and Metabolism**). Amiodarone is also known to be an inhibitor of CYP3A4. Therefore, amiodarone has the **potential** for interactions with drugs or substances that may be substrates, inhibitors or inducers of CYP3A4. While only a limited number of *in vivo* drug-drug interactions with amiodarone have been reported, chiefly with the oral formulation, the potential for other interactions should be anticipated. This is especially important for drugs associated with serious toxicity, such as other antiarrhythmics. If such drugs are needed, their dose should be reassessed and, where appropriate, plasma concentration measured. In view of the long and variable half-life of amiodarone, potential for drug interactions exists not only with concomitant medication but also with drugs administered after discontinuation of amiodarone.

Since amiodarone is a substrate for CYP3A4, drugs/substances that inhibit CYP3A4 may decrease the metabolism and increase serum concentrations of amiodarone, with the potential for toxic effects. Reported examples of this interaction include the following:

Protease Inhibitors:

Protease inhibitors are known to inhibit CYP3A4 to varying degrees. Inhibition of CYP3A4 by **indinavir** has been reported to result in increased serum concentrations of amiodarone. Monitoring for amiodarone toxicity and serial measurement of amiodarone serum concentration during concomitant protease inhibitor therapy should be considered.

Histamine H_2 antagonists:

Cimetidine inhibits CYP3A4 and can increase serum amiodarone levels.

Other substances:

Grapefruit juice inhibits CYP3A4-mediated metabolism of oral amiodarone in the intestinal mucosa, resulting in increased plasma levels of amiodarone; therefore, grapefruit juice should not be taken during treatment with oral amiodarone. This information should be considered when changing from intravenous amiodarone to oral amiodarone (see **DOSAGE AND ADMINISTRATION, Intravenous to Oral Transition**).

Amiodarone may suppress certain CYP450 enzymes (enzyme inhibition). This can result in unexpectedly high plasma levels of other drugs which are metabolized by those CYP450 enzymes and may lead to toxic effects. Reported examples of this interaction include the following:

Immunosuppressives:

Cyclosporine (CYP3A4 substrate) administered in combination with oral amiodarone has been reported to produce persistently elevated plasma concentrations of cyclosporine resulting in elevated creatinine, despite reduction in dose of cyclosporine.

Cardiovasculars:

Cardiac glycosides: In patients receiving **digoxin** therapy, administration of oral amiodarone regularly results in an increase in serum digoxin concentration that may reach toxic levels with resultant clinical toxicity. Amiodarone taken concomitantly with digoxin increases the serum digoxin concentration by 70% after one day. **On administration of oral amiodarone, the need for digitalis therapy should be reviewed and the dose reduced by approximately 50% or discontinued.** If digitalis treatment is continued, serum levels should be closely monitored and patients observed for clinical evidence of toxicity. These precautions probably should apply to digitoxin administration as well.

Antiarrhythmics: Other antiarrhythmic drugs, such as **quinidine, procainamide, disopyramide,** and **phenytoin,** have been used concurrently with amiodarone. There have been case reports of increased steady-state levels of quinidine, procainamide, and phenytoin during concomitant therapy with amiodarone. Phenytoin decreases serum amiodarone levels. Amiodarone taken concomitantly with quinidine increases quinidine serum concentration by 33% after two days. Amiodarone taken concomitantly with procainamide for less than seven days increases plasma concentrations of procainamide and n-acetyl procainamide by 55% and 33%, respectively. Quinidine and procainamide doses should be reduced by one-third when either is administered with amiodarone. Plasma levels of **flecainide** have been reported to increase in the presence of oral amiodarone; because of this, the dosage of flecainide should be adjusted when these drugs are administered concomitantly. In general, any added antiarrhythmic drug should be initiated at a lower than usual dose with careful monitoring. Combination of amiodarone with other antiarrhythmic therapy should be reserved for patients with life-threatening ventricular arrhythmias who are incompletely responsive to a single agent or incompletely responsive to amiodarone. During transfer to oral amiodarone, the dose levels of previously administered agents should be reduced by 30 to 50% several days after the addition of oral amiodarone (see **DOSAGE AND ADMINISTRATION, Intravenous to Oral Transition**). The continued need for the other antiarrhythmic agent should be reviewed after the effects of amiodarone have been established, and discontinuation ordinarily should be attempted. If the treatment is continued, these patients should be particularly carefully monitored for adverse effects, especially conduction disturbances and exacerbation of tachyarrhythmias, as amiodarone is continued. In amiodarone-treated patients who require additional antiarrhythmic therapy, the initial dose of such agents should be approximately half of the usual recommended dose.

Antihypertensives: Amiodarone should be used with caution in patients receiving **β-receptor blocking agents** (e.g., propanolol, a CYP3A4 inhibitor) or **calcium channel antagonists** (e.g., verapamil, a CYP3A4 substrate, and diltiazem, a CYP3A4 inhibitor) because of the possible potentiation of bradycardia, sinus arrest, and AV block; if necessary, amiodarone can continue to be used after insertion of a pacemaker in patients with severe bradycardia or sinus arrest.

Anticoagulants: Potentiation of **warfarin**-type (CYP2C9 and CYP3A4 substrate) anticoagulant response is almost always seen in patients receiving amiodarone and can result in serious or fatal bleeding. Since the concomitant administration of warfarin with amiodarone increases the prothrombin time by 100% after 3 to 4 days, **the dose of the anticoagulant should be reduced by one-third to one-half, and prothrombin times should be monitored closely.**

Some drugs/substances are known to accelerate the metabolism of amiodarone by stimulating the synthesis of CYP3A4 (enzyme induction). This may lead to low amiodarone serum levels and potential decrease in efficacy. Reported examples of this interaction include the following:

Antibiotics:

Rifampin is a potent inducer of CYP3A4. Administration of rifampin concomitantly with oral amiodarone has been shown to result in decreases in serum concentrations of amiodarone and desethylamiodarone.

Other substances, including herbal preparations:

St. John's Wort (Hypericum perforatum) induces CYP3A4. Since amiodarone is a substrate for CYP3A4, there is the potential that the use of St. John's Wort in patients receiving amiodarone could result in reduced amiodarone levels.

Other reported interactions with amiodarone:

Fentanyl (CYP3A4 substrate) in combination with amiodarone may cause hypotension, bradycardia, decreased cardiac output.

Sinus bradycardia has been reported with oral amiodarone in combination with **lidocaine** (CYP3A4 substrate) given for local anesthesia. Seizure, associated with increased lidocaine concentrations, has been reported with concomitant administration of intravenous amiodarone.

Dextromethorphan is a substrate for both CYP2D6 and CYP3A4. Amiodarone inhibits CYP2D6.

Cholestyramine increases enterohepatic elimination of amiodarone and may reduce serum levels and $t_{1/2}$.

Disopyramide increases QT prolongation which could cause arrhythmia.

Hemodynamic and electrophysiologic interactions have also been observed after concomitant administration with **propranolol, diltiazem, and verapamil.**

Volatile Anesthetic Agents: (see **PRECAUTIONS, Surgery**).

In addition to the interactions noted above, chronic (> 2 weeks) ***oral*** Cordarone administration impairs metabolism of phenytoin, dextromethorphan, and methotrexate.

The paragraph under the subheading **Electrolyte Disturbances** *should be deleted and replaced with the following:*

Patients with hypokalemia or hypomagnesemia should have the condition corrected whenever possible before being treated with Cordarone I.V., as these disorders can exaggerate the degree of QTc prolongation and increase the potential for torsades de pointes. Special attention should be given to electrolyte and acid-base balance in patients experiencing severe or prolonged diarrhea or in patients receiving concomitant diuretics.

The following should be added to the end of the **ADVERSE REACTIONS** *section:*

Postmarketing Reports

In postmarketing surveillance, sinus arrest, pseudotumor cerebri, toxic epidermal necrolysis, exfoliative dermatitis, pancytopenia, neutropenia, erythema multiforme, angioedema, bronchospasm, and anaphylactic shock also have been reported with amiodarone therapy.

The first sentence of the **OVERDOSAGE** *section should be deleted and replaced with the following:*

There have been cases, some fatal, of amiodarone overdose. Effects of an inadvertent overdose of Cordarone I.V. included hypotension, cardiogenic shock, bradycardia, AV block, and hepatotoxicity.

The following two paragraphs should be added after the first paragraph under the subheading **Intravenous to Oral Transition** *in the* **DOSAGE AND ADMINISTRATION** *section:*

Since there are some differences between the safety and efficacy profiles of the intravenous and oral formulations, the prescriber is advised to review the package insert for oral amiodarone when switching from intravenous to oral amiodarone therapy.

Since grapefruit juice is known to inhibit CYP3A4-mediated metabolism of oral amiodarone in the intestinal mucosa, resulting in increased plasma levels of amiodarone: grapefruit juice should not be taken during treatment with oral amiodarone (see **PRECAUTIONS, Drug Interactions**).

CI 5032-5 Revised August 20, 2001

EFFEXOR® ℞

[ĕf-fĕks 'ŏr]

(venlafaxine hydrochloride)
Tablets
Rx only

Prescribing information for this product, which appears on pages 3495–3499 of the 2002 PDR, has been revised as follows. Please write "See Supplement A" next to the product heading.

The subheading "Skin and Mucous Membrane Bleeding" and the paragraph under it in the **General** *subheading under the* **PRECAUTIONS** *section should be deleted and replaced with the following:*

Abnormal Bleeding

There have been reports of abnormal bleeding (most commonly ecchymosis) associated with venlafaxine treatment. While a causal relationship to venlafaxine is unclear, impaired platelet aggregation may result from platelet serotonin depletion and contribute to such occurrences.

In the first paragraph under the subheading "Concomitant Medication" under **General** *in the* **PRECAUTIONS** *section, the words* ",including herbal preparations," *should be inserted after the words* "over-the-counter-drugs."

The following changes should be made to the lists of adverse reactions under the heading **Other Events Observed During the Premarketing Evaluation of Venlafaxine** *in the* **ADVERSE REACTIONS** *section:*

Under "Body as a whole", "bacteremia" *should be added after* "appendicitis" *in the list of reactions following* **"Rare"**; *under* "Cardiovascular system", *in the list of adverse reactions following* **"Rare"**, *the words* "aortic aneurysm" *should be added right after the word* **"Rare"** *and the words* "capillary fragility" *should be added after* "bundle branch block"; *under* "Metabolic and nutritional", *the words* "healing abnormal" *should be inserted after the word* "gout" *in the list of adverse reactions following* **"Rare"**; *and under* "Urogenital system", *the words* "breast discharge" *should be inserted after the word* "anuria" *in the list of adverse reactions following* **"Rare"**.

In the list of adverse reactions under the subheading **Postmarketing Reports**, *the following changes should be made:*

The words "(such as atrial fibrillation, supraventricular tachycardia, ventricular extrasystoles, ventricular tachycardia)" *should be deleted and replaced with* "such as QT prolongation; cardiac arrhythmias including atrial fibrillation, supraventricular tachycardia, ventricular extrasystoles, and rare reports of ventricular fibrillation and ventricular tachycardia, including torsade de pointes"; *the word* "fatigue" *should be deleted; and the words* "night sweats" *should be inserted just before* "pancreatitis."

The paragraph under **Maintenance/Continuation/Extended Treatment** *in the* **DOSAGE AND ADMINISTRATION** *section should be deleted and replaced with the following:*

It is generally agreed that acute episodes of depression require several months or longer of sustained pharmacological therapy beyond response to the acute episode. In one study, in which patients responding during 8 weeks of acute treatment with Effexor XR were assigned randomly to placebo or to the same dose of Effexor XR (75, 150, or 225 mg/day, qAM) during 26 weeks of maintenance treatment as they had received during the acute stabilization phase, longer-term efficacy has demonstrated the efficacy of Effexor in maintaining an antidepressant response in patients with recurrent depression who had responded and continued to be improved during an initial 26 weeks of treatment and were randomly assigned to placebo or Effexor for period of up to 52 weeks on the same dose (100 to 200 mg/day, on a b.i.d. schedule) (see **CLINICAL TRIALS**). Based on these limited data, it is not known whether or not the dose of Effexor/Effexor XR needed for maintenance treatment is identical to the dose needed to achieve an initial response. Patients should be periodically reassessed to determine the need for maintenance treatment and the appropriate dose for such treatment.

CI 6027-6 Revised August 17, 2001

EFFEXOR® XR ℞

[ĕf-fĕks' ŏr XR]

(venlafaxine hydrochloride)
Extended-Release Capsules
℞ only

Prescribing information for this product, which appears on pages 3499–3504 of the 2002 PDR, has been completely revised as follows. Please write "See Supplement A" next to the product heading.

DESCRIPTION

Effexor XR is an extended-release capsule for oral administration that contains venlafaxine hydrochloride, a structurally novel antidepressant. Venlafaxine hydrochloride is chemically unrelated to tricyclic, tetracyclic, and other available antidepressants and to other agents used to treat Generalized Anxiety Disorder. It is designated (R/S)-1-[2-(dimethylamino)-1-(4-methoxyphenyl)ethyl] cyclohexanol hydrochloride or (±)-1-[α- [(dimethylamino)methyl]-p-methoxybenzyl] cyclohexanol hydrochloride and has the empirical formula of $C_{17}H_{27}NO_2$ hydrochloride. Its molecular weight is 313.87. The structural formula is shown below.

$N(CH_3)_2$ OH C H •HCl H_3CO

venlafaxine hydrochloride

Venlafaxine hydrochloride is a white to off-white crystalline solid with a solubility of 572 mg/mL in water (adjusted to ionic strength of 0.2 M with sodium chloride). Its octanol:water (0.2 M sodium chloride) partition coefficient is 0.43.

Effexor XR is formulated as an extended-release capsule for once-a-day oral administration. Drug release is controlled by diffusion through the coating membrane on the spheroids and is not pH dependent. Capsules contain venlafaxine hydrochloride equivalent to 37.5 mg, 75 mg, or 150 mg venlafaxine. Inactive ingredients consist of cellulose, ethylcellulose, gelatin, hydroxypropyl methylcellulose, iron oxide, and titanium dioxide. The 37.5 mg capsule also contains D&C Red #28, D&C Yellow #10, and FD&C Blue #1.

CLINICAL PHARMACOLOGY

Pharmacodynamics

The mechanism of the antidepressant action of venlafaxine in humans is believed to be associated with its potentiation of neurotransmitter activity in the CNS. Preclinical studies have shown that venlafaxine and its active metabolite, O-desmethylvenlafaxine (ODV), are potent inhibitors of neuronal serotonin and norepinephrine reuptake and weak inhibitors of dopamine reuptake. Venlafaxine and ODV have no significant affinity for muscarinic cholinergic, H_1-histaminergic, or α_1-adrenergic receptors in vitro. Pharmacologic activity at these receptors is hypothesized to be associated with the various anticholinergic, sedative, and cardiovascular effects seen with other psychotropic drugs. Venlafaxine and ODV do not possess monoamine oxidase (MAO) inhibitory activity.

Pharmacokinetics

Steady-state concentrations of venlafaxine and ODV in plasma are attained within 3 days of oral multiple dose therapy. Venlafaxine and ODV exhibited linear kinetics over the dose range of 75 to 450 mg/day. Mean±SD steady-state plasma clearance of venlafaxine and ODV is 1.3±0.6 and 0.4±0.2 L/h/kg, respectively; apparent elimination half-life is 5±2 and 11±2 hours, respectively; and apparent (steady-state) volume of distribution is 7.5±3.7 and 5.7±1.8 L/kg, respectively. Venlafaxine and ODV are minimally bound at therapeutic concentrations to plasma proteins (27% and 30%, respectively).

Absorption

Venlafaxine is well absorbed and extensively metabolized in the liver. O-desmethylvenlafaxine (ODV) is the only major active metabolite. On the basis of mass balance studies, at least 92% of a single oral dose of venlafaxine is absorbed. The absolute bioavailability of venlafaxine is about 45%.

Administration of Effexor XR (150 mg q24 hours) generally resulted in lower C_{max} (150 ng/mL for venlafaxine and 260 ng/mL for ODV) and later T_{max} (5.5 hours for venlafaxine and 9 hours for ODV) than for immediate release venlafaxine tablets (C_{max}'s for immediate release 75 mg q12 hours were 225 ng/mL for venlafaxine and 290 ng/mL for ODV; T_{max}'s were 2 hours for venlafaxine and 3 hours for ODV). When equal daily doses of venlafaxine were administered as either an immediate release tablet or the extended-release capsule, the exposure to both venlafaxine and ODV was similar for the two treatments, and the fluctuation in plasma concentrations was slightly lower with the Effexor XR capsule. Effexor XR, therefore, provides a slower rate of absorption, but the same extent of absorption compared with the immediate release tablet.

Food did not affect the bioavailability of venlafaxine or its active metabolite, ODV. Time of administration (AM vs PM) did not affect the pharmacokinetics of venlafaxine and ODV from the 75 mg Effexor XR capsule.

Metabolism and Excretion

Following absorption, venlafaxine undergoes extensive presystemic metabolism in the liver, primarily to ODV, but also to N-desmethylvenlafaxine, N,O-didesmethylvenlafaxine, and other minor metabolites. In vitro studies indicate that the formation of ODV is catalyzed by CYP2D6; this has been confirmed in a clinical study showing that patients with low CYP2D6 levels ("poor metabolizers") had increased levels of venlafaxine and reduced levels of ODV compared to people with normal CYP2D6 ("extensive metabolizers"). The differences between the CYP2D6 poor and extensive metabolizers, however, are not expected to be clinically important because the sum of venlafaxine and ODV is similar in the two groups and venlafaxine and ODV are pharmacologically approximately equiactive and equipotent.

Approximately 87% of a venlafaxine dose is recovered in the urine within 48 hours as unchanged venlafaxine (5%), unconjugated ODV (29%), conjugated ODV (26%), or other minor inactive metabolites (27%). Renal elimination of venlafaxine and its metabolites is thus the primary route of excretion.

Special Populations

Age and Gender: A population pharmacokinetic analysis of 404 venlafaxine-treated patients from two studies involving both b.i.d. and t.i.d. regimens showed that dose-normalized trough plasma levels of either venlafaxine or ODV were unaltered by age or gender differences. Dosage adjustment based on the age or gender of a patient is generally not necessary (see **DOSAGE AND ADMINISTRATION**).

Extensive/Poor Metabolizers: Plasma concentrations of venlafaxine were higher in CYP2D6 poor metabolizers than extensive metabolizers. Because the total exposure (AUC) of venlafaxine and ODV was similar in poor and extensive metabolizer groups, however, there is no need for different venlafaxine dosing regimens for these two groups.

Liver Disease: In 9 patients with hepatic cirrhosis, the pharmacokinetic disposition of both venlafaxine and ODV was significantly altered after oral administration of venlafaxine. Venlafaxine elimination half-life was prolonged by about 30%, and clearance decreased by about 50% in cirrhotic patients compared to normal subjects. ODV elimination half-life was prolonged by about 60%, and clearance decreased by about 30% in cirrhotic patients compared to normal subjects. A large degree of intersubject variability was noted. Three patients with more severe cirrhosis had a more substantial decrease in venlafaxine clearance (about 90%) compared to normal subjects. Dosage adjustment is necessary in these patients (see **DOSAGE AND ADMINISTRATION**).

Renal Disease: In a renal impairment study, venlafaxine elimination half-life after oral administration was prolonged by about 50% and clearance was reduced by about 24% in renally impaired patients (GFR=10 to 70 mL/min), compared to normal subjects. In dialysis patients, venlafaxine elimination half-life was prolonged by about 180% and clearance was reduced by about 57% compared to normal subjects. Similarly, ODV elimination half-life was prolonged by about 40% although clearance was unchanged in patients with renal impairment (GFR=10 to 70 mL/min) compared to normal subjects. In dialysis patients, ODV elimination half-life was prolonged by about 142% and clearance was reduced by about 56% compared to normal subjects. A large degree of intersubject variability was noted. Dosage adjustment is necessary in these patients (see **DOSAGE AND ADMINISTRATION**).

Clinical Trials

Depression

The efficacy of Effexor XR (venlafaxine hydrochloride) extended-release capsules as a treatment for depression was established in two placebo-controlled, short-term, flexible-dose studies in adult outpatients meeting DSM-III-R or DSM-IV criteria for major depression.

A 12-week study utilizing Effexor XR doses in a range 75 to 150 mg/day (mean dose for completers was 136 mg/day) and an 8-week study utilizing Effexor XR doses in a range 75 to 225 mg/day (mean dose for completers was 177 mg/day) both demonstrated superiority of Effexor XR over placebo on the HAM-D total score, HAM-D Depressed Mood Item, the MADRS total score, the Clinical Global Impressions (CGI) Severity of Illness item, and the CGI Global Improvement item. In both studies, Effexor XR was also significantly better than placebo for certain factors of the HAM-D, including the anxiety/somatization factor, the cognitive disturbance factor, and the retardation factor, as well as for the psychic anxiety score.

A 4-week study of inpatients meeting DSM-III-R criteria for major depression with melancholia utilizing Effexor (the immediate release form of venlafaxine) in a range of 150 to 375 mg/day (t.i.d. schedule) demonstrated superiority of Effexor over placebo. The mean dose in completers was 350 mg/day.

Examination of gender subsets of the population studied did not reveal any differential responsiveness on the basis of gender.

In one longer-term study, outpatients meeting DSM-IV criteria for major depressive disorder who had responded during an 8-week open trial on Effexor XR (75, 150, or 225 mg, qAM) were randomized to continuation of their same Effexor XR dose or to placebo, for up to 26 weeks of observation for relapse. Response during the open phase was defined as a CGI Severity of Illness item score of ≤3 and a HAM-D-21 total score of ≤10 at the day 56 evaluation. Relapse during the double-blind phase was defined as follows: (1) a reappearance of major depressive disorder as defined by DSM-IV criteria and a CGI Severity of Illness item score of ≥4 (moderately ill), (2) 2 consecutive CGI Severity of Illness item scores of ≥4, or (3) a final CGI Severity of Illness

Continued on next page

Effexor XR—Cont.

item score of ≥4 for any patient who withdrew from the study for any reason. Patients receiving continued Effexor XR treatment experienced significantly lower relapse rates over the subsequent 26 weeks compared with those receiving placebo.

In a second longer-term trial, outpatients meeting DSM-III-R criteria for major depressive disorder, recurrent type, who had responded (HAM-D-21 total score ≤12 at the day 56 evaluation) and continued to be improved [defined as the following criteria being met for days 56 through 180: (1) no HAM-D-21 total score 20; (2) no more than 2 HAM-D-21 total scores >10, and (3) no single CGI Severity of Illness item score ≥4 (moderately ill)] during an initial 26 weeks of treatment on Effexor (100 to 200 mg/day, on a b.i.d. schedule) were randomized to continuation of their same Effexor dose or to placebo. The follow-up period to observe patients for relapse, defined as a CGI Severity of Illness item score ≥4, was for up to 52 weeks. Patients receiving continued Effexor treatment experienced significantly lower relapse rates over the subsequent 52 weeks compared with those receiving placebo.

Generalized Anxiety Disorder

The efficacy of Effexor XR capsules as a treatment for Generalized Anxiety Disorder (GAD) was established in two 8-week, placebo-controlled, fixed-dose studies, one 6-month, placebo-controlled, fixed-dose study, and one 6-month, placebo-controlled, flexible-dose study in outpatients meeting DSM-IV criteria for GAD.

One 8-week study evaluating Effexor XR doses of 75, 150, and 225 mg/day, and placebo showed that the 225 mg/day dose was more effective than placebo on the Hamilton Rating Scale for Anxiety (HAM-A) total score, both the HAM-A anxiety and tension items, and the Clinical Global Impressions (CGI) scale. While there was also evidence for superiority over placebo for the 75 and 150 mg/day doses, these doses were not as consistently effective as the highest dose.

A second 8-week study evaluating Effexor XR doses of 75 and 150 mg/day and placebo showed that both doses were more effective than placebo on some of these same outcomes; however, the 75 mg/day dose was more consistently effective than the 150 mg/day dose. A dose-response relationship for effectiveness in GAD was not clearly established in the 75 to 225 mg/day dose range utilized in these two studies.

Two 6-month studies, one evaluating Effexor XR doses of 37.5, 75, and 150 mg/day and the other evaluating Effexor XR doses of 75 to 225 mg/day, showed that daily doses of 75 mg or higher were more effective than placebo on the HAM-A total, both the HAM-A anxiety and tension items, and the CGI scale during 6 months of treatment. While there was also evidence for superiority over placebo for the 37.5 mg/day dose, this dose was not as consistently effective as the higher doses.

Examination of gender subsets of the population studied did not reveal any differential responsiveness on the basis of gender.

INDICATIONS AND USAGE

Depression

Effexor XR (venlafaxine hydrochloride) extended-release capsules is indicated for the treatment of depression.

The efficacy of Effexor XR in the treatment of depression was established in 8- and 12-week controlled trials of outpatients whose diagnoses corresponded most closely to the DSM-III-R or DSM-IV category of major depressive disorder (see **Clinical Trials**).

A major depressive episode (DSM-IV) implies a prominent and relatively persistent (nearly every day for at least 2 weeks) depressed mood or the loss of interest or pleasure in nearly all activities, representing a change from previous functioning, and includes the presence of at least five of the following nine symptoms during the same two-week period: depressed mood, markedly diminished interest or pleasure in usual activities, significant change in weight and/or appetite, insomnia or hypersomnia, psychomotor agitation or retardation, increased fatigue, feelings of guilt or worthlessness, slowed thinking or impaired concentration, a suicide attempt or suicidal ideation.

The efficacy of Effexor (the immediate release form of venlafaxine) in the treatment of depression in inpatients meeting diagnostic criteria for major depressive disorder with melancholia was established in a 4-week controlled trial (see **Clinical Trials**). The safety and efficacy of Effexor XR in hospitalized depressed patients have not been adequately studied.

The efficacy of Effexor XR in maintaining an antidepressant response for up to 26 weeks following 8 weeks of acute treatment was demonstrated in a placebo-controlled trial. The efficacy of Effexor in maintaining an antidepressant response in patients with recurrent depression who had responded and continued to be improved during an initial 26 weeks of treatment and were then followed for a period of up to 52 weeks was demonstrated in a second placebo-controlled trial (see **Clinical Trials**). Nevertheless, the physician who elects to use Effexor/Effexor XR for extended periods should periodically re-evaluate the long-term usefulness of the drug for the individual patient (see **DOSAGE AND ADMINISTRATION**).

Generalized Anxiety Disorder

Effexor XR is indicated for the treatment of Generalized Anxiety Disorder (GAD) as defined in DSM-IV. Anxiety or tension associated with the stress of everyday life usually does not require treatment with an anxiolytic.

The efficacy of Effexor XR in the treatment of GAD was established in 8-week and 6-month placebo-controlled trials in outpatients diagnosed with GAD according to DSM-IV criteria (see **Clinical Trials**).

Generalized Anxiety Disorder (DSM-IV) is characterized by excessive anxiety and worry (apprehensive expectation) that is persistent for at least 6 months and which the person finds difficult to control. It must be associated with at least 3 of the following 6 symptoms: restlessness or feeling keyed up or on edge, being easily fatigued, difficulty concentrating or mind going blank, irritability, muscle tension, sleep disturbance.

Although the effectiveness of Effexor XR has been demonstrated in 6-month clinical trials in patients with GAD, the physician who elects to use Effexor XR for extended periods should periodically re-evaluate the long-term usefulness of the drug for the individual patient (see **DOSAGE AND ADMINISTRATION**).

CONTRAINDICATIONS

Hypersensitivity to venlafaxine hydrochloride or to any excipients in the formulation.

Concomitant use in patients taking monoamine oxidase inhibitors (MAOIs) is contraindicated (see **WARNINGS**).

WARNINGS

Potential for Interaction with Monoamine Oxidase Inhibitors

Adverse reactions, some of which were serious, have been reported in patients who have recently been discontinued from a monoamine oxidase inhibitor (MAOI) and started on venlafaxine, or who have recently had venlafaxine therapy discontinued prior to initiation of an MAOI. These reactions have included tremor, myoclonus, diaphoresis, nausea, vomiting, flushing, dizziness, hyperthermia with features resembling neuroleptic malignant syndrome, seizures, and death. In patients receiving antidepressants with pharmacological properties similar to venlafaxine in combination with an MAOI, there have also been reports of serious, sometimes fatal, reactions. For a selective serotonin reuptake inhibitor, these reactions have included hyperthermia, rigidity, myoclonus, autonomic instability with possible rapid fluctuations of vital signs, and mental status changes that include extreme agitation progressing to delirium and coma. Some cases presented with features resembling neuroleptic malignant syndrome. Severe hyperthermia and seizures, sometimes fatal, have been reported in association with the combined use of tricyclic antidepressants and MAOIs. These reactions have also been reported in patients who have recently discontinued these drugs and have been started on an MAOI. The effects of combined use of venlafaxine and MAOIs have not been evaluated in humans or animals. Therefore, because venlafaxine is an inhibitor of both norepinephrine and serotonin reuptake, it is recommended that Effexor XR (venlafaxine hydrochloride) extended-release capsules not be used in combination with an MAOI, or within at least 14 days of discontinuing treatment with an MAOI. Based on the half-life of venlafaxine, at least 7 days should be allowed after stopping venlafaxine before starting an MAOI.

Sustained Hypertension

Venlafaxine treatment is associated with sustained increases in blood pressure in some patients. Among patients treated with 75 to 375 mg per day of Effexor XR in premarketing depression studies, 3% (19/705) experienced sustained hypertension [defined as treatment-emergent supine diastolic blood pressure (SDBP) ≥ 90 mm Hg and ≥ 10 mm Hg above baseline for 3 consecutive on-therapy visits]. Among patients treated with 37.5 to 225 mg per day of Effexor XR in premarketing GAD studies, 0.5% (5/1011) experienced sustained hypertension. Experience with the immediate-release venlafaxine showed that sustained hypertension was dose-related, increasing from 3 to 7% at 100 to 300 mg per day to 13% at doses above 300 mg per day. An insufficient number of patients received mean doses of Effexor XR over 300 mg/day to fully evaluate the incidence of sustained increases in blood pressure at these higher doses.

In placebo-controlled premarketing depression studies with Effexor XR 75 to 225 mg/day, a final on-drug mean increase in supine diastolic blood pressure (SDBP) of 1.2 mm Hg was observed for Effexor XR-treated patients compared with a mean decrease of 0.2 mm Hg for placebo-treated patients. In placebo-controlled premarketing GAD studies with Effexor XR 37.5 to 225 mg/day, up to 8 weeks or up to 6 months, a final on-drug mean increase in SDBP of 0.3 mm Hg was observed for Effexor XR-treated patients compared with a mean decrease of 0.9 and 0.8 mm Hg, respectively, for placebo-treated patients.

In premarketing depression studies, 0.7% (5/705) of the Effexor XR-treated patients discontinued treatment because of elevated blood pressure. Among these patients, most of the blood pressure increases were in a modest range (12 to 16 mm Hg, SDBP). In premarketing GAD studies up to 8 weeks and up to 6 months, 0.7% (10/1381) and 1.3% (7/535) of the Effexor XR-treated patients, respectively, discontinued treatment because of elevated blood pressure. Among these patients, most of the blood pressure increases were in a modest range (12 to 25 mm Hg, SDBP up to 8 weeks; 8 to 28 mm Hg up to 6 months).

Sustained increases of SDBP could have adverse consequences. Therefore, it is recommended that patients receiving Effexor XR have regular monitoring of blood pressure. For patients who experience a sustained increase in blood pressure while receiving venlafaxine, either dose reduction or discontinuation should be considered.

PRECAUTIONS

General

Insomnia and Nervousness

Treatment-emergent insomnia and nervousness were more commonly reported for patients treated with Effexor XR (venlafaxine hydrochloride) extended-release capsules than with placebo in pooled analyses of short-term depression and GAD studies, as shown in Table 1.

[See table below]

Insomnia and nervousness each led to drug discontinuation in 0.9% of the patients treated with Effexor XR in Phase 3 depression studies.

In Phase 3 GAD trials, insomnia and nervousness led to drug discontinuation in 3% and 2%, respectively, of the patients treated with Effexor XR up to 8 weeks and 2% and 0.7%, respectively, of the patients treated with Effexor XR up to 6 months.

Changes in Appetite and Weight

Treatment-emergent anorexia was more commonly reported for Effexor XR-treated (8%) than placebo-treated patients (4%) in the pool of short-term depression studies. Significant weight loss, especially in underweight depressed patients, may be an undesirable result of Effexor XR treatment. A loss of 5% or more of body weight occurred in 7% of Effexor XR-treated and 2% of placebo-treated patients in placebo-controlled depression trials. Discontinuation rates for anorexia and weight loss associated with Effexor XR were low (1.0% and 0.1%, respectively, of Effexor XR-treated patients in Phase 3 depression studies).

In the pool of GAD studies, treatment-emergent anorexia was reported in 8% and 2% of patients receiving Effexor XR and placebo up to 8 weeks, respectively. A loss of 7% or more of body weight occurred in 3% of the Effexor XR-treated and 1% of the placebo-treated patients up to 6 months in these trials. Discontinuation rates for anorexia and weight loss were low for patients receiving Effexor XR up to 8 weeks (0.9% and 0.3%, respectively).

Activation of Mania/Hypomania

During premarketing depression studies, mania or hypomania occurred in 0.3% of Effexor XR-treated patients and 0.0% placebo patients. In premarketing GAD studies, 0.0% of Effexor XR-treated patients and 0.2% of placebo-treated patients experienced mania or hypomania. In all premarketing depression trials with Effexor, mania or hypomania occurred in 0.5% of venlafaxine-treated patients compared with 0% of placebo patients. Mania/hypomania has also been reported in a small proportion of patients with mood disorders who were treated with other marketed antidepressants. As with all antidepressants, Effexor XR should be used cautiously in patients with a history of mania.

Hyponatremia

Hyponatremia and/or the syndrome of inappropriate antidiuretic hormone secretion (SIADH) may occur with venlafaxine. This should be taken into consideration in patients who are, for example, volume-depleted, elderly, or taking diuretics.

Mydriasis

Mydriasis has been reported in association with venlafaxine; therefore patients with raised intraocular pressure or those at risk of acute narrow-angle glaucoma should be monitored.

Seizures

During premarketing experience, no seizures occurred among 705 Effexor XR-treated patients in the depression studies or among 1381 Effexor XR-treated patients in GAD studies. In all premarketing depression trials with Effexor, seizures were reported at various doses in 0.3% (8/3082) of venlafaxine-treated patients. Effexor XR, like many antidepressants, should be used cautiously in patients with a history of seizures and should be discontinued in any patient who develops seizures.

Abnormal Bleeding

There have been reports of abnormal bleeding (most commonly ecchymosis) associated with venlafaxine treatment. While a causal relationship to venlafaxine is unclear, impaired platelet aggregation may result from platelet serotonin depletion and contribute to such occurrences.

Suicide

The possibility of a suicide attempt is inherent in depression and may persist until significant remission occurs. Close supervision of high-risk patients should accompany initial drug therapy. Prescriptions for Effexor XR should be

Table 1
Incidence of Insomnia and Nervousness in Placebo-Controlled Depression and GAD Trials

	Depression		GAD	
Symptom	Effexor XR n = 357	Placebo n = 285	Effexor XR n = 1381	Placebo n = 555
Insomnia	17%	11%	15%	10%
Nervousness	10%	5%	6%	4%

written for the smallest quantity of capsules consistent with good patient management in order to reduce the risk of overdose.

The same precautions observed when treating patients with depression should be observed when treating patients with GAD.

Use in Patients With Concomitant Illness

Premarketing experience with venlafaxine in patients with concomitant systemic illness is limited. Caution is advised in administering Effexor XR to patients with diseases or conditions that could affect hemodynamic responses or metabolism.

Venlafaxine has not been evaluated or used to any appreciable extent in patients with a recent history of myocardial infarction or unstable heart disease. Patients with these diagnoses were systematically excluded from many clinical studies during venlafaxine's premarketing testing. The electrocardiograms for 357 patients who received Effexor XR and 285 patients who received placebo in 8- to 12-week double-blind, placebo-controlled trials in depression and the electrocardiograms for 610 patients who received Effexor XR and 298 patients who received placebo in 8-week double-blind, placebo-controlled trials in GAD were analyzed. The mean change from baseline in corrected QT interval (QTc) for Effexor XR-treated patients in depression studies was increased relative to that for placebo-treated patients (increase of 4.7 msec for Effexor XR and decrease of 1.9 msec for placebo). The mean change from baseline in corrected QT interval (QTc) for Effexor XR-treated patients in the GAD studies did not differ significantly from that with placebo.

In these same trials, the mean change from baseline in heart rate for Effexor XR-treated patients in the depression studies was significantly higher than that for placebo (a mean increase of 4 beats per minute for Effexor XR and 1 beat per minute for placebo). The mean change from baseline in heart rate for Effexor XR-treated patients in the GAD studies was significantly higher than that for placebo (a mean increase of 3 beats per minute for Effexor XR and no change for placebo).

In a flexible-dose study, with Effexor doses in the range of 200 to 375 mg/day and mean dose greater than 300 mg/day, Effexor-treated patients had a mean increase in heart rate of 8.5 beats per minute compared with 1.7 beats per minute in the placebo group.

As increases in heart rate were observed, caution should be exercised in patients whose underlying medical conditions might be compromised by increases in heart rate (eg, patients with hyperthyroidism, heart failure, or recent myocardial infarction), particularly when using doses of Effexor above 200 mg/day.

Evaluation of the electrocardiograms for 769 patients who received immediate release Effexor in 4- to 6-week double-blind, placebo-controlled trials showed that the incidence of trial-emergent conduction abnormalities did not differ from that with placebo. In patients with renal impairment (GFR=10 to 70 mL/min) or cirrhosis of the liver, the clearances of venlafaxine and its active metabolites were decreased, thus prolonging the elimination half-lives of these substances. A lower dose may be necessary (see **DOSAGE AND ADMINISTRATION**). Effexor XR, like all antidepressants, should be used with caution in such patients.

Information for Patients

Physicians are advised to discuss the following issues with patients for whom they prescribe Effexor XR (venlafaxine hydrochloride) extended-release capsules:

Interference with Cognitive and Motor Performance

Clinical studies were performed to examine the effects of venlafaxine on behavioral performance of healthy individuals. The results revealed no clinically significant impairment of psychomotor, cognitive, or complex behavior performance. However, since any psychoactive drug may impair judgment, thinking, or motor skills, patients should be cautioned about operating hazardous machinery, including automobiles, until they are reasonably certain that venlafaxine therapy does not adversely affect their ability to engage in such activities.

Concomitant Medication

Patients should be advised to inform their physicians if they are taking, or plan to take, any prescription or over-the-counter drugs, including herbal preparations, since there is a potential for interactions.

Alcohol

Although venlafaxine has not been shown to increase the impairment of mental and motor skills caused by alcohol, patients should be advised to avoid alcohol while taking venlafaxine.

Allergic Reactions

Patients should be advised to notify their physician if they develop a rash, hives, or a related allergic phenomenon.

Pregnancy

Patients should be advised to notify their physician if they become pregnant or intend to become pregnant during therapy.

Nursing

Patients should be advised to notify their physician if they are breast-feeding an infant.

Laboratory Tests

There are no specific laboratory tests recommended.

Drug Interactions

As with all drugs, the potential for interaction by a variety of mechanisms is a possibility.

Alcohol

A single dose of ethanol (0.5 g/kg) had no effect on the pharmacokinetics of venlafaxine or O-desmethylvenlafaxine (ODV) when venlafaxine was administered at 150 mg/day in 15 healthy male subjects. Additionally, administration of venlafaxine in a stable regimen did not exaggerate the psychomotor and psychometric effects induced by ethanol in these same subjects when they were not receiving venlafaxine.

Cimetidine

Concomitant administration of cimetidine and venlafaxine in a steady-state study for both drugs resulted in inhibition of first-pass metabolism of venlafaxine in 18 healthy subjects. The oral clearance of venlafaxine was reduced by about 43%, and the exposure (AUC) and maximum concentration (C_{max}) of the drug were increased by about 60%. However, co-administration of cimetidine had no apparent effect on the pharmacokinetics of ODV, which is present in much greater quantity in the circulation than venlafaxine. The overall pharmacological activity of venlafaxine plus ODV is expected to increase only slightly, and no dosage adjustment should be necessary for most normal adults. However, for patients with pre-existing hypertension, and for elderly patients or patients with hepatic dysfunction, the interaction associated with the concomitant use of venlafaxine and cimetidine is not known and potentially could be more pronounced. Therefore, caution is advised with such patients.

Diazepam

Under steady-state conditions for venlafaxine administered at 150 mg/day, a single 10 mg dose of diazepam did not appear to affect the pharmacokinetics of either venlafaxine or ODV in 18 healthy male subjects. Venlafaxine also did not have any effect on the pharmacokinetics of diazepam or its active metabolite, desmethyldiazepam, or affect the psychomotor and psychometric effects induced by diazepam.

Haloperidol

Venlafaxine administered under steady-state conditions at 150 mg/day in 24 healthy subjects decreased total oral-dose clearance (Cl/F) of a single 2 mg dose of haloperidol by 42%, which resulted in a 70% increase in haloperidol AUC. In addition, the haloperidol C_{max} increased 88% when coadministered with venlafaxine, but the haloperidol elimination half-life ($t_{1/2}$) was unchanged. The mechanism explaining this finding is unknown.

Lithium

The steady-state pharmacokinetics of venlafaxine administered at 150 mg/day were not affected when a single 600 mg oral dose of lithium was administered to 12 healthy male subjects. ODV also was unaffected. Venlafaxine had no effect on the pharmacokinetics of lithium.

Drugs Highly Bound to Plasma Proteins

Venlafaxine is not highly bound to plasma proteins; therefore, administration of Effexor XR to a patient taking another drug that is highly protein bound should not cause increased free concentrations of the other drug.

Drugs that Inhibit Cytochrome P450 Isoenzymes

CYP2D6 Inhibitors: In vitro and in vivo studies indicate that venlafaxine is metabolized to its active metabolite, ODV, by CYP2D6, the isoenzyme that is responsible for the genetic polymorphism seen in the metabolism of many antidepressants. Therefore, the potential exists for a drug interaction between drugs that inhibit CYP2D6-mediated metabolism of venlafaxine, reducing the metabolism of venlafaxine to ODV, resulting in increased plasma concentrations of venlafaxine and decreased concentrations of the active metabolite. CYP2D6 inhibitors such as quinidine would be expected to do this, but the effect would be similar to what is seen in patients who are genetically CYP2D6 poor metabolizers (see *Metabolism and Excretion* under **CLINICAL PHARMACOLOGY**). Therefore, no dosage adjustment is required when venlafaxine is coadministered with a CYP2D6 inhibitor.

The concomitant use of venlafaxine with drug treatment(s) that potentially inhibits both CYP2D6 and CYP3A4, the primary metabolizing enzymes for venlafaxine, has not been studied. Therefore, caution is advised should a patient's therapy include venlafaxine and any agent(s) that produce simultaneous inhibition of these two enzymes systems.

Drugs Metabolized by Cytochrome P450 Isoenzymes

CYP2D6: In vitro studies indicate that venlafaxine is a relatively weak inhibitor of CYP2D6. These findings have been confirmed in a clinical drug interaction study comparing the effect of venlafaxine with that of fluoxetine on the CYP2D6-mediated metabolism of dextromethorphan to dextrorphan.

Imipramine—Venlafaxine did not affect the pharmacokinetics of imipramine and 2-OH-imipramine. However, desipramine AUC, C_{max}, and C_{min} increased by about 35% in the presence of venlafaxine. The 2-OH-desipramine AUC's increased by at least 2.5 fold (with venlafaxine 37.5 mg q12h) and by 4.5 fold (with venlafaxine 75 mg q12h). Imipramine did not affect the pharmacokinetics of venlafaxine and ODV. The clinical significance of elevated 2-OH-desipramine levels is unknown.

Risperidone—Venlafaxine administered under steady-state conditions at 150 mg/day slightly inhibited the CYP2D6-mediated metabolism of risperidone (administered as a single 1 mg oral dose) to its active metabolite, 9-hydroxyrisperidone, resulting in an approximate 32% increase in risperidone AUC. However, venlafaxine coadministration did not significantly alter the pharmacokinetic profile of the total active moiety (risperidone plus 9-hydroxyrisperidone.)

CYP3A4: Venlafaxine did not inhibit CYP3A4 in vitro. This finding was confirmed in vivo by clinical drug interaction studies in which venlafaxine did not inhibit the metabolism of several CYP3A4 substrates, including alprazolam, diazepam, and terfenadine.

Indinavir—In a study of 9 healthy volunteers, venlafaxine administered under steady-state conditions at 150 mg/day resulted in a 28% decrease in the AUC of a single 800 mg oral dose of indinavir and a 36% decrease in indinavir C_{max}. Indinavir did not affect the pharmacokinetics of venlafaxine and ODV. The clinical significance of this finding is unknown.

CYP1A2: Venlafaxine did not inhibit CYP1A2 in vitro. This finding was confirmed in vivo by a clinical drug interaction study in which venlafaxine did not inhibit the metabolism of caffeine, a CYP1A2 substrate.

CYP2C9: Venlafaxine did not inhibit CYP2C9 in vitro. The clinical significance of this finding is unknown.

CYP2C19: Venlafaxine did not inhibit the metabolism of diazepam, which is partially metabolized by CYP2C19 (see *Diazepam* above.)

Monoamine Oxidase Inhibitors

See **CONTRAINDICATIONS** and **WARNINGS**.

CNS-Active Drugs

The risk of using venlafaxine in combination with other CNS-active drugs has not been systematically evaluated (except in the case of those CNS-active drugs noted above). Consequently, caution is advised if the concomitant administration of venlafaxine and such drugs is required.

Electroconvulsive Therapy

There are no clinical data establishing the benefit of electroconvulsive therapy combined with Effexor XR (venlafaxine hydrochloride) extended-release capsules treatment.

Postmarketing Spontaneous Drug Interaction Reports

See **ADVERSE REACTIONS, Postmarketing Reports.**

Carcinogenesis, Mutagenesis, Impairment of Fertility

Carcinogenesis

Venlafaxine was given by oral gavage to mice for 18 months at doses up to 120 mg/kg per day, which was 1.7 times the maximum recommended human dose on a mg/m^2 basis. Venlafaxine was also given to rats by oral gavage for 24 months at doses up to 120 mg/kg per day. In rats receiving the 120 mg/kg dose, plasma concentrations of venlafaxine at necropsy were 1 times (male rats) and 6 times (female rats) the plasma concentrations of patients receiving the maximum recommended human dose. Plasma levels of the O-desmethyl metabolite were lower in rats than in patients receiving the maximum recommended dose. Tumors were not increased by venlafaxine treatment in mice or rats.

Mutagenesis

Venlafaxine and the major human metabolite, O-desmethylvenlafaxine (ODV), were not mutagenic in the Ames reverse mutation assay in Salmonella bacteria or the Chinese hamster ovary/HGPRT mammalian cell forward gene mutation assay. Venlafaxine was also not mutagenic or clastogenic in the in vitro BALB/c-3T3 mouse cell transformation assay, the sister chromatid exchange assay in cultured Chinese hamster ovary cells, or in the in vivo chromosomal aberration assay in rat bone marrow. ODV was not clastogenic in the in vitro Chinese hamster ovary cell chromosomal aberration assay, but elicited a clastogenic response in the in vivo chromosomal aberration assay in rat bone marrow.

Impairment of Fertility

Reproduction and fertility studies in rats showed no effects on male or female fertility at oral doses of up to 2 times the maximum recommended human dose on a mg/m^2 basis.

Pregnancy

Teratogenic Effects—Pregnancy Category C

Venlafaxine did not cause malformations in offspring of rats or rabbits given doses up to 2.5 times (rat) or 4 times (rabbit) the maximum recommended human daily dose on a mg/m^2 basis. However, in rats, there was a decrease in pup weight, an increase in stillborn pups, and an increase in pup deaths during the first 5 days of lactation, when dosing began during pregnancy and continued until weaning. The cause of these deaths is not known. These effects occurred at 2.5 times (mg/m^2) the maximum human daily dose. The no effect dose for rat pup mortality was 0.25 times the human dose on a mg/m^2 basis. There are no adequate and well-controlled studies in pregnant women. Because animal reproduction studies are not always predictive of human response, this drug should be used during pregnancy only if clearly needed.

Non-teratogenic Effects

If venlafaxine is used until or shortly before birth, discontinuation effects in the newborn should be considered.

Labor and Delivery

The effect of venlafaxine on labor and delivery in humans is unknown.

Nursing Mothers

Venlafaxine and ODV have been reported to be excreted in human milk. Because of the potential for serious adverse reactions in nursing infants from Effexor XR, a decision should be made whether to discontinue nursing or to discontinue the drug, taking into account the importance of the drug to the mother.

Pediatric Use

Safety and effectiveness in pediatric patients have not been established.

Geriatric Use

Approximately 4% (14/357) and 6% (77/1381) of Effexor XR-treated patients in placebo-controlled premarketing depres-

Continued on next page

Effexor XR—Cont.

sion and GAD trials, respectively, were 65 years of age or over. Of 2,897 Effexor-treated patients in premarketing phase depression studies, 12% (357) were 65 years of age or over. No overall differences in effectiveness or safety were observed between geriatric patients and younger patients, and other reported clinical experience generally has not identified differences in response between the elderly and younger patients. However, greater sensitivity of some older individuals cannot be ruled out. As with other antidepressants, several cases of hyponatremia and syndrome of inappropriate antidiuretic hormone secretion (SIADH) have been reported, usually in the elderly.

The pharmacokinetics of venlafaxine and ODV are not substantially altered in the elderly (see **CLINICAL PHARMACOLOGY**). No dose adjustment is recommended for the elderly on the basis of age alone, although other clinical circumstances, some of which may be more common in the elderly, such as renal or hepatic impairment, may warrant a dose reduction (see **DOSAGE AND ADMINISTRATION**).

ADVERSE REACTIONS

The information included in the Adverse Findings Observed in Short-Term, Placebo-Controlled Studies with Effexor XR subsection is based on data from a pool of three 8- and 12-week controlled clinical trials in depression (includes two U.S. trials and one European trial) and on data up to 8 weeks from a pool of five controlled clinical trials in GAD with Effexor XR®. Information on additional adverse events associated with Effexor XR in the entire development program for the formulation and with Effexor (the immediate release formulation of venlafaxine) is included in the **Other Adverse Events Observed During the Premarketing Evaluation of Effexor and Effexor XR** subsection (see also **WARNINGS** and **PRECAUTIONS**).

Adverse Findings Observed in Short-Term, Placebo-Controlled Studies with Effexor XR

Adverse Events Associated with Discontinuation of Treatment

Approximately 11% of the 357 patients who received Effexor® XR (venlafaxine hydrochloride) extended-release capsules in placebo-controlled clinical trials for depression discontinued treatment due to an adverse experience, compared with 6% of the 285 placebo-treated patients in those studies. Approximately 18% of the 1381 patients who received Effexor XR capsules in placebo-controlled clinical trials for GAD discontinued treatment due to an adverse experience, compared with 12% of the 555 placebo-treated patients in those studies. The most common events leading to discontinuation and considered to be drug-related (ie, leading to discontinuation in at least 1% of the Effexor XR-treated patients at a rate at least twice that of placebo for either indication) are shown in Table 2.

[See table above]

Table 2
Common Adverse Events Leading to Discontinuation of Treatment in Placebo-Controlled Trials[1]

Adverse Event	Percentage of Patients Discontinuing Due to Adverse Event: Depression Indication[2] Effexor XR n=357	Depression Indication[2] Placebo n=285	GAD Indication[3,4] Effexor XR n=1381	GAD Indication[3,4] Placebo n=555
Body as a Whole				
Asthenia	—	—	3%	<1%
Digestive System				
Nausea	4%	<1%	8%	<1%
Anorexia	1%	<1%	—	—
Dry Mouth	1%	0%	2%	<1%
Vomiting	—	—	1%	<1%
Nervous System				
Dizziness	2%	1%	—	—
Insomnia	1%	<1%	3%	<1%
Somnolence	2%	<1%	3%	<1%
Nervousness	—	—	2%	<1%
Tremor	—	—	1%	0%
Skin				
Sweating	—	—	2%	<1%

[1] Two of the depression studies were flexible dose and one was fixed dose. Four of the GAD studies were fixed dose and one was flexible dose.

[2] In U.S. placebo-controlled trials for depression, the following were also common events leading to discontinuation and were considered to be drug-related for Effexor XR-treated patients (% Effexor XR [n = 192], % Placebo [n = 202]: hypertension (1%, <1%); diarrhea (1%, 0%); paresthesia (1%, 0%); tremor (1%, 0%); abnormal vision, mostly blurred vision (1%, 0%); and abnormal, mostly delayed, ejaculation (1%, 0%).

[3] In two short-term U.S. placebo-controlled trials for GAD, the following were also common events leading to discontinuation and were considered to be drug-related for Effexor XR-treated patients (% Effexor XR [n = 476]), % Placebo [n = 201]: headache (4%, <1%); vasodilatation (1%, 0%); anorexia (2%, <1%); dizziness (4%, 1%); thinking abnormal (1%, 0%); and abnormal vision (1%, 0%).

[4] In long-term placebo-controlled trials for GAD, the following was also a common event leading to discontinuation and was considered to be drug-related for Effexor XR-treated patients (% Effexor XR [n = 535], % Placebo [n = 257]): decreased libido (1%, 0%).

Adverse Events Occurring at an Incidence of 2% or More Among Effexor XR-Treated Patients

Tables 3 and 4 enumerate the incidence, rounded to the nearest percent, of treatment-emergent adverse events that occurred during acute therapy of depression (up to 12 weeks; dose range of 75 to 225 mg/day) and of GAD (up to 8 weeks; dose range of 37.5 to 225 mg/day), respectively, in 2% or more of patients treated with Effexor XR (venlafaxine hydrochloride) where the incidence in patients treated with Effexor XR was greater than the incidence for the respective placebo-treated patients. The table shows the percentage of patients in each group who had at least one episode of an event at some time during their treatment. Reported adverse events were classified using a standard COSTART-based Dictionary terminology.

The prescriber should be aware that these figures cannot be used to predict the incidence of side effects in the course of usual medical practice where patient characteristics and other factors differ from those which prevailed in the clinical trials. Similarly, the cited frequencies cannot be compared with figures obtained from other clinical investigations involving different treatments, uses and investigators. The cited figures, however, do provide the prescribing physician with some basis for estimating the relative contribution of drug and nondrug factors to the side effect incidence rate in the population studied.

Commonly Observed Adverse Events from Tables 3 and 4:

Depression

Note in particular the following adverse events that occurred in at least 5% of the Effexor XR patients and at a rate at least twice that of the placebo group for all placebo-controlled trials for the depression indication (Table 3): Abnormal ejaculation, gastrointestinal complaints (nausea, dry mouth, and anorexia), CNS complaints (dizziness, somnolence, and abnormal dreams), and sweating. In the two U.S. placebo-controlled trials, the following additional events occurred in at least 5% of Effexor XR-treated patients (n = 192) and at a rate at least twice that of the placebo group: Abnormalities of sexual function (impotence in men, anorgasmia in women, and libido decreased), gastrointestinal complaints (constipation and flatulence), CNS complaints (insomnia, nervousness, and tremor), problems of special senses (abnormal vision), cardiovascular effects (hypertension and vasodilatation), and yawning.

Generalized Anxiety Disorder

Note in particular the following adverse events that occurred in at least 5% of the Effexor XR patients and at a rate at least twice that of the placebo group for all placebo-controlled trials for the GAD indication (Table 4): Abnormalities of sexual function (abnormal ejaculation and impotence), gastrointestinal complaints (nausea, dry mouth, anorexia, and constipation), problems of special senses (abnormal vision), and sweating.

Table 3
Treatment-Emergent Adverse Event Incidence in Short-Term Placebo-Controlled Effexor XR Clinical Trials in Depressed Patients[1,2]

Body System / Preferred Term	% Reporting Event: Effexor XR (n=357)	Placebo (n=285)
Body as a Whole		
Asthenia	8%	7%
Cardiovascular System		
Vasodilatation[3]	4%	2%
Hypertension	4%	1%
Digestive System		
Nausea	31%	12%
Constipation	8%	5%
Anorexia	8%	4%
Vomiting	4%	2%
Flatulence	4%	3%
Metabolic/Nutritional		
Weight Loss	3%	0%
Nervous System		
Dizziness	20%	9%
Somnolence	17%	8%
Insomnia	17%	11%
Dry Mouth	12%	6%
Nervousness	10%	5%
Abnormal Dreams[4]	7%	2%
Tremor	5%	2%
Depression	3%	<1%
Paresthesia	3%	1%
Libido Decreased	3%	<1%
Agitation	3%	1%
Respiratory System		
Pharyngitis	7%	6%
Yawn	3%	0%
Skin		
Sweating	14%	3%
Special Senses		
Abnormal Vision[5]	4%	<1%
Urogenital System		
Abnormal Ejaculation (male)[6,7]	16%	<1%
Impotence[7]	4%	<1%
Anorgasmia (female)[8,9]	3%	<1%

[1] Incidence, rounded to the nearest %, for events reported by at least 2% of patients treated with Effexor XR, except the following events which had an incidence equal to or less than placebo: abdominal pain, accidental injury, anxiety, back pain, bronchitis, diarrhea, dysmenorrhea, dyspepsia, flu syndrome, headache, infection, pain, palpitation, rhinitis, and sinusitis.

[2] <1% indicates an incidence greater than zero but less than 1%.

[3] Mostly "hot flashes."

[4] Mostly "vivid dreams," "nightmares," and "increased dreaming."

[5] Mostly "blurred vision" and "difficulty focusing eyes."

[6] Mostly "delayed ejaculation."

[7] Incidence is based on the number of male patients.

[8] Mostly "delayed orgasm" or "anorgasmia."

[9] Incidence is based on the number of female patients.

Table 4
Treatment-Emergent Adverse Event Incidence in Short-Term Placebo-Controlled Effexor XR Clinical Trials in GAD Patients[1,2]

Body System / Preferred Term	% Reporting Event: Effexor XR (n=1381)	Placebo (n=555)
Body as a Whole		
Asthenia	12%	8%
Cardiovascular System		
Vasodilatation[3]	4%	2%
Digestive System		
Nausea	35%	12%
Constipation	10%	4%
Anorexia	8%	2%
Vomiting	5%	3%
Nervous System		
Dizziness	16%	11%
Dry Mouth	16%	6%
Insomnia	15%	10%
Somnolence	14%	8%
Nervousness	6%	4%
Libido Decreased	4%	2%
Tremor	4%	<1%
Abnormal Dreams[4]	3%	2%
Hypertonia	3%	2%
Paresthesia	2%	1%
Respiratory System		
Yawn	3%	<1%
Skin		
Sweating	10%	3%
Special Senses		
Abnormal Vision[5]	5%	<1%
Urogenital System		
Abnormal Ejaculation[6,7]	11%	<1%
Impotence[7]	5%	<1%
Orgasmic Dysfunction (female)[8,9]	2%	0%

[1] Adverse events for which the Effexor XR reporting rate was less than or equal to the placebo rate are not included. These events are: abdominal pain, accidental injury, anxiety, back pain, diarrhea, dysmenorrhea, dyspepsia, flu syndrome, headache, infection, myalgia, pain, palpitation, pharyngitis, rhinitis, tinnitus, and urinary frequency.

[2] <1% means greater than zero but less than 1%.

[3] Mostly "hot flashes."

[4] Mostly "vivid dreams," "nightmares," and "increased dreaming."

[5] Mostly "blurred vision" and "difficulty focusing eyes."

[6] Includes "delayed ejaculation," and "anorgasmia."

[7] Percentage based on the number of males (Effexor XR=525, placebo=220).

[8] Includes "delayed orgasm," "abnormal orgasm," and "anorgasmia."

[9] Percentage based on the number of females (Effexor XR=856, placebo=335).

Vital Sign Changes

Effexor XR (venlafaxine hydrochloride) extended-release capsules treatment for up to 12 weeks in premarketing placebo-controlled depression trials was associated with a mean final on-therapy increase in pulse rate of approximately 2 beats per minute, compared with 1 beat per minute for placebo. Effexor XR treatment for up to 8 weeks in premarketing placebo-controlled GAD trials was associated with a mean final on-therapy increase in pulse rate of approximately 2 beats per minute, compared with less than 1 beat per minute for placebo. (See the **Sustained Hypertension** section of **WARNINGS** for effects on blood pressure). In a flexible-dose study, with Effexor doses in the range of 200 to 375 mg/day and mean dose greater than 300 mg/day, the mean pulse was increased by about 2 beats per minute compared with a decrease of about 1 beat per minute for placebo.

Laboratory Changes

Effexor XR (venlafaxine hydrochloride) extended-release capsules treatment for up to 12 weeks in premarketing placebo-controlled depression trials was associated with a mean final on-therapy increase in serum cholesterol concentration of approximately 1.5 mg/dL. Effexor XR treatment for up to 8 weeks and up to 6 months in premarketing placebo-controlled GAD trials was associated with mean final on-therapy increases in serum cholesterol concentration of approximately 1.0 mg/dL and 2.3 mg/dL, respectively.

Patients treated with Effexor tablets (the immediate-release form of venlafaxine) for at least 3 months in placebo-controlled 12-month extension trials had a mean final on-therapy increase in total cholesterol of 9.1 mg/dL. This increase was duration dependent over the 12-month study period and tended to be greater with higher doses. An increase in serum cholesterol from baseline by ≥50 mg/dL and to values >260 mg/dL, at any time after baseline, has been recorded in 8.1% of patients.

ECG Changes

In a flexible-dose study, with Effexor doses in the range of 200 to 375 mg/day and mean dose greater than 300 mg/day, the mean change in heart rate was 8.5 beats per minute compared with 1.7 beats per minute for placebo. (See the *Use in Patients with Concomitant Illnesses* section of **PRECAUTIONS**).

Other Adverse Events Observed During the Premarketing Evaluation of Effexor and Effexor XR

During its premarketing assessment, multiple doses of Effexor XR were administered to 705 patients in Phase 3 depression studies and Effexor was administered to 96 patients. During its premarketing assessment, multiple doses of Effexor XR were administered to 1381 patients in Phase 3 GAD studies. In addition, in premarketing assessment of Effexor, multiple doses were administered to 2897 patients in Phase 2 and Phase 3 depression studies. The conditions and duration of exposure to venlafaxine in both development programs varied greatly, and included (in overlapping categories) open and double-blind studies, uncontrolled and controlled studies, inpatient (Effexor only) and outpatient studies, fixed-dose, and titration studies. Untoward events associated with this exposure were recorded by clinical investigators using terminology of their own choosing. Consequently, it is not possible to provide a meaningful estimate of the proportion of individuals experiencing adverse events without first grouping similar types of untoward events into a smaller number of standardized event categories.

In the tabulations that follow, reported adverse events were classified using a standard COSTART-based Dictionary terminology. The frequencies presented, therefore, represent the proportion of the 5079 patients exposed to multiple doses of either formulation of venlafaxine who experienced an event of the type cited on at least one occasion while receiving venlafaxine. All reported events are included except those already listed in Tables 3 and 4 and those events for which a drug cause was remote. If the COSTART term for an event was so general as to be uninformative, it was replaced with a more informative term. It is important to emphasize that, although the events reported occurred during treatment with venlafaxine, they were not necessarily caused by it.

Events are further categorized by body system and listed in order of decreasing frequency using the following definitions: **frequent** adverse events are defined as those occurring on one or more occasions in at least 1/100 patients; **infrequent** adverse events are those occurring in 1/100 to 1/1000 patients; **rare** events are those occurring in fewer than 1/1000 patients.

Body as a whole—**Frequent**: chest pain substernal, chills, fever, neck pain; **Infrequent**: face edema, intentional injury, malaise, moniliasis, neck rigidity, pelvic pain, photosensitivity reaction, suicide attempt, withdrawal syndrome; **Rare**: appendicitis, bacteremia, carcinoma, cellulitis.

Cardiovascular system—**Frequent**: migraine, postural hypotension, tachycardia; **Infrequent**: angina pectoris, arrhythmia, extrasystoles, hypotension, peripheral vascular disorder (mainly cold feet and/or cold hands), syncope, thrombophlebitis; **Rare**: aortic aneurysm, arteritis, first-degree atrioventricular block, bigeminy, bradycardia, bundle branch block, capillary fragility, cerebral ischemia, coronary artery disease, congestive heart failure, heart arrest, cardiovascular disorder (mitral valve and circulatory disturbance), mucocutaneous hemorrhage, myocardial infarct, pallor.

Digestive system—**Frequent**: eructation, increased appetite; **Infrequent**: bruxism, colitis, dysphagia, tongue edema, esophagitis, gastritis, gastroenteritis, gastrointestinal ulcer, gingivitis, glossitis, rectal hemorrhage, hemorrhoids, melena, oral moniliasis, stomatitis, mouth ulceration; **Rare**: cheilitis, cholecystitis, cholelithiasis, esophageal spasms, duodenitis, hematemesis, gastrointestinal hemorrhage, gum hemorrhage, hepatitis, ileitis, jaundice, intestinal obstruction, parotitis, proctitis, increased salivation, soft stools, tongue discoloration.

Endocrine system—**Rare**: goiter, hyperthyroidism, hypothyroidism, thyroid nodule, thyroiditis.

Hemic and lymphatic system—**Frequent**: ecchymosis; **Infrequent**: anemia, leukocytosis, leukopenia, lymphadenopathy, thrombocythemia, thrombocytopenia; **Rare**: basophilia, bleeding time increased, cyanosis, eosinophilia, lymphocytosis, multiple myeloma, purpura.

Metabolic and nutritional—**Frequent**: edema, weight gain; **Infrequent**: alkaline phosphatase increased, dehydration, hypercholesteremia, hyperglycemia, hyperlipemia, hypokalemia, SGOT increased, SGPT increased, thirst; **Rare**: alcohol intolerance, bilirubinemia, BUN increased, creatinine increased, diabetes mellitus, glycosuria, gout, healing abnormal, hemochromatosis, hypercalcinuria, hyperkalemia, hyperphosphatemia, hyperuricemia, hypocholesteremia, hypoglycemia, hyponatremia, hypophosphatemia, hypoproteinemia, uremia.

Musculoskeletal system—**Frequent**: arthralgia; **Infrequent**: arthritis, arthrosis, bone pain, bone spurs, bursitis, leg cramps, myasthenia, tenosynovitis; **Rare**: pathological fracture, myopathy, osteoporosis, osteosclerosis, rheumatoid arthritis, tendon rupture.

Nervous system—**Frequent**: amnesia, confusion, depersonalization, emotional lability, hypesthesia, thinking abnormal, trismus, vertigo; **Infrequent**: apathy, ataxia, circumoral paresthesia, CNS stimulation, euphoria, hallucinations, hostility, hyperesthesia, hyperkinesia, hypotonia, incoordination, manic reaction, myoclonus, neuralgia, neuropathy, psychosis, seizure, abnormal speech, stupor, twitching; **Rare**: akathisia, akinesia, alcohol abuse, aphasia, bradykinesia, buccoglossal syndrome, cerebrovascular accident, loss of consciousness, delusions, dementia, dystonia, facial paralysis, abnormal gait, Guillain-Barre Syndrome, hyperchlohydria, hypokinesia, impulse control difficulties, libido increased, neuritis, nystagmus, paranoid reaction, paresis, psychotic depression, reflexes decreased, reflexes increased, suicidal ideation, torticollis.

Respiratory system—**Frequent**: cough increased, dyspnea; **Infrequent**: asthma, chest congestion, epistaxis, hyperventilation, laryngismus, laryngitis, pneumonia, voice alteration; **Rare**: atelectasis, hemoptysis, hypoventilation, hypoxia, larynx edema, pleurisy, pulmonary embolus, sleep apnea.

Skin and appendages—**Frequent**: rash, pruritus; **Infrequent**: acne, alopecia, brittle nails, contact dermatitis, dry skin, eczema, skin hypertrophy, maculopapular rash, psoriasis, urticaria; **Rare**: erythema nodosum, exfoliative dermatitis, lichenoid dermatitis, hair discoloration, skin discoloration, furunculosis, hirsutism, leukoderma, petechial rash, pustular rash, vesiculobullous rash, seborrhea, skin atrophy, skin striae.

Special senses—**Frequent**: abnormality of accommodation, mydriasis, taste perversion; **Infrequent**: cataract, conjunctivitis, corneal lesion, diplopia, dry eyes, eye pain, hyperacusis, otitis media, parosmia, photophobia, taste loss, visual field defect; **Rare**: blepharitis, chromatopsia, conjunctival edema, deafness, exophthalmos, glaucoma, retinal hemorrhage, subconjunctival hemorrhage, keratitis, labyrinthitis, miosis, papilledema, decreased pupillary reflex, otitis externa, scleritis, uveitis.

Urogenital system—**Frequent**: dysuria, metrorrhagia,* prostatic disorder (prostatitis and enlarged prostate),* urination impaired, vaginitis*; **Infrequent**: albuminuria, amenorrhea,* cystitis, hematuria, leukorrhea,* menorrhagia,* nocturia, bladder pain, breast pain, polyuria, pyuria, urinary incontinence, urinary retention, urinary urgency, vaginal hemorrhage*; **Rare**: abortion,* anuria, breast discharge, breast engorgement, balanitis,* breast enlargement, endometriosis,* female lactation,* fibrocystic breast, calcium crystalluria, cervicitis,* orchitis,* ovarian cyst,* prolonged erection,* gynecomastia (male),* hypomenorrhea,* kidney calculus, kidney pain, kidney function abnormal, mastitis, menopause,* pyelonephritis, oliguria, salpingitis,* urolithiasis, uterine hemorrhage,* uterine spasm.*

*Based on the number of men and women as appropriate.

Postmarketing Reports

Voluntary reports of other adverse events temporally associated with the use of venlafaxine that have been received since market introduction and that may have no causal relationship with the use of venlafaxine include the following: agranulocytosis, anaphylaxis, aplastic anemia, catatonia, congenital anomalies, CPK increased, deep vein thrombophlebitis, delirium, EKG abnormalities such as QT prolongation; cardiac arrhythmias including atrial fibrillation, supraventricular tachycardia, ventricular extrasystoles, and rare reports of ventricular fibrillation and ventricular tachycardia, including torsade de pointes; epidermal necrosis/Stevens-Johnson Syndrome, erythema multiforme, extrapyramidal symptoms (including tardive dyskinesia), hemorrhage (including eye and gastrointestinal bleeding), hepatic events (including GGT elevation; abnormalities of unspecified liver function tests; liver damage, necrosis, or failure; and fatty liver), involuntary movements, LDH increased, neuroleptic malignant syndrome-like events (including a case of a 10-year-old who may have been taking methylphenidate, was treated and recovered), neutropenia, night sweats, pancreatitis, pancytopenia, panic, prolactin increased, renal failure, serotonin syndrome, shock-like electrical sensations (in some cases, subsequent to the discontinuation of venlafaxine or tapering of dose), and syndrome of inappropriate antidiuretic hormone secretion (usually in the elderly).

There have been reports of elevated clozapine levels that were temporally associated with adverse events, including seizures, following the addition of venlafaxine. There have been reports of increases in prothrombin time, partial thromboplastin time, or INR when venlafaxine was given to patients receiving warfarin therapy.

DRUG ABUSE AND DEPENDENCE

Controlled Substance Class

Effexor XR (venlafaxine hydrochloride) extended-release capsules is not a controlled substance.

Physical and Psychological Dependence

In vitro studies revealed that venlafaxine has virtually no affinity for opiate, benzodiazepine, phencyclidine (PCP), or N-methyl-D-aspartic acid (NMDA) receptors.

Venlafaxine was not found to have any significant CNS stimulant activity in rodents. In primate drug discrimination studies, venlafaxine showed no significant stimulant or depressant abuse liability.

Discontinuation effects have been reported in patients receiving venlafaxine (see **DOSAGE AND ADMINISTRATION**).

While venlafaxine has not been systematically studied in clinical trials for its potential for abuse, there was no indication of drug-seeking behavior in the clinical trials. However, it is not possible to predict on the basis of premarketing experience the extent to which a CNS active drug will be misused, diverted, and/or abused once marketed. Consequently, physicians should carefully evaluate patients for history of drug abuse and follow such patients closely, observing them for signs of misuse or abuse of venlafaxine (eg, development of tolerance, incrementation of dose, drug-seeking behavior).

OVERDOSAGE

Human Experience

Among the patients included in the premarketing evaluation of Effexor XR, there were 2 reports of acute overdosage with Effexor XR in depression trials, either alone or in combination with other drugs. One patient took a combination of 6 g of Effexor XR and 2.5 mg of lorazepam. This patient was hospitalized, treated symptomatically, and recovered without any untoward effects. The other patient took 2.85 g of Effexor XR. This patient reported paresthesia of all four limbs but recovered without sequelae.

There were 2 reports of acute overdose with Effexor XR in GAD trials. One patient took a combination of 0.75 g of Effexor XR and 200 mg of paroxetine and 50 mg of zolpidem. This patient was described as being alert, able to communicate, and a little sleepy. This patient was hospitalized, treated with activated charcoal, and recovered without any untoward effects. The other patient took 1.2 g of Effexor XR. This patient recovered and no other specific problems were found. The patient had moderate dizziness, nausea, numb hands and feet, and hot-cold spells 5 days after the overdose. These symptoms resolved over the next week.

Among the patients included in the premarketing evaluation with Effexor, there were 14 reports of acute overdose with venlafaxine, either alone or in combination with other drugs and/or alcohol. The majority of the reports involved ingestion in which the total dose of venlafaxine taken was estimated to be no more than several-fold higher than the usual therapeutic dose. The 3 patients who took the highest doses were estimated to have ingested approximately 6.75 g, 2.75 g, and 2.5 g. The resultant peak plasma levels of venlafaxine for the latter 2 patients were 6.24 and 2.35 µg/mL, respectively, and the peak plasma levels of O-desmethylvenlafaxine were 3.37 and 1.30 µg/mL, respectively. Plasma venlafaxine levels were not obtained for the patient who ingested 6.75 g of venlafaxine. All 14 patients recovered without sequelae. Most patients reported no symptoms. Among the remaining patients, somnolence was the most commonly reported symptom. The patient who ingested 2.75 g of venlafaxine was observed to have 2 generalized convulsions and a prolongation of QTc to 500 msec, compared with 405 msec at baseline. Mild sinus tachycardia was reported in 2 of the other patients.

In postmarketing experience, overdose with venlafaxine has occurred predominantly in combination with alcohol and/or other drugs. Electrocardiogram changes (eg, prolongation of QT interval, bundle branch block, QRS prolongation), sinus and ventricular tachycardia, bradycardia, hypotension, altered level of consciousness (ranging from somnolence to coma), seizures, vertigo, and death have been reported.

Management of Overdosage

Treatment should consist of those general measures employed in the management of overdosage with any antidepressant.

Ensure an adequate airway, oxygenation, and ventilation. Monitor cardiac rhythm and vital signs. General supportive and symptomatic measures are also recommended. Induction of emesis is not recommended. Gastric lavage with a large bore orogastric tube with appropriate airway protection, if needed, may be indicated if performed soon after ingestion or in symptomatic patients.

Activated charcoal should be administered. Due to the large volume of distribution of this drug, forced diuresis, dialysis, hemoperfusion, and exchange transfusion are unlikely to be of benefit. No specific antidotes for venlafaxine are known.

In managing overdosage, consider the possibility of multiple drug involvement. The physician should consider contacting a poison control center for additional information on the

Continued on next page

Effexor XR—Cont.

treatment of any overdose. Telephone numbers for certified poison control centers are listed in the *Physicians' Desk Reference (PDR)*.

DOSAGE AND ADMINISTRATION

Effexor XR should be administered in a single dose with food either in the morning or in the evening at approximately the same time each day. Each capsule should be swallowed whole with fluid and not divided, crushed, chewed, or placed in water.

Initial Treatment

Depression

For most patients, the recommended starting dose for Effexor XR is 75 mg/day, administered in a single dose. In the clinical trials establishing the efficacy of Effexor XR in moderately depressed outpatients, the initial dose of venlafaxine was 75 mg/day. For some patients, it may be desirable to start at 37.5 mg/day for 4 to 7 days, to allow new patients to adjust to the medication before increasing to 75 mg/day. While the relationship between dose and antidepressant response for Effexor XR has not been adequately explored, patients not responding to the initial 75 mg/day dose may benefit from dose increases to a maximum of approximately 225 mg/day. Dose increases should be in increments of up to 75 mg/day, as needed, and should be made at intervals of not less than 4 days, since steady state plasma levels of venlafaxine and its major metabolites are achieved in most patients by day 4. In the clinical trials establishing efficacy, upward titration was permitted at intervals of 2 weeks or more; the average doses were about 140 to 180 mg/day (see **Clinical Trials** under **CLINICAL PHARMACOLOGY**).

It should be noted that, while the maximum recommended dose for moderately depressed outpatients is also 225 mg/day for Effexor (the immediate release form of venlafaxine), more severely depressed inpatients in one study of the development program for that product responded to a mean dose of 350 mg/day (range of 150 to 375 mg/day). Whether or not higher doses of Effexor XR are needed for more severely depressed patients is unknown; however, the experience with Effexor XR doses higher than 225 mg/day is very limited.

Generalized Anxiety Disorder

For most patients, the recommended starting dose for Effexor XR is 75 mg/day, administered in a single dose. In clinical trials establishing the efficacy of Effexor XR in outpatients with Generalized Anxiety Disorder (GAD), the initial dose of venlafaxine was 75 mg/day. For some patients, it may be desirable to start at 37.5 mg/day for 4 to 7 days, to allow new patients to adjust to the medication before increasing to 75 mg/day. Although a dose-response relationship for effectiveness in GAD was not clearly established in fixed-dose studies, certain patients not responding to the initial 75 mg/day dose may benefit from dose increases to a maximum of approximately 225 mg/day. Dose increases should be in increments of up to 75 mg/day, as needed, and should be made at intervals of not less than 4 days. (see the "*Use in Patients with Concomitant Illnesses*" section of **PRECAUTIONS**).

Switching Patients from Effexor Tablets

Depressed patients who are currently being treated at a therapeutic dose with Effexor may be switched to Effexor XR at the nearest equivalent dose (mg/day), eg, 37.5 mg venlafaxine two-times-a-day to 75 mg Effexor XR once daily. However, individual dosage adjustments may be necessary.

Patients with Hepatic Impairment

Given the decrease in clearance and increase in elimination half-life for both venlafaxine and ODV that is observed in patients with hepatic cirrhosis compared with normal subjects (see **CLINICAL PHARMACOLOGY**), it is recommended that the starting dose be reduced by 50% in patients with moderate hepatic impairment. Because there was much individual variability in clearance between patients with cirrhosis, individualization of dosage may be desirable in some patients.

Patients with Renal Impairment

Given the decrease in clearance for venlafaxine and the increase in elimination half-life for both venlafaxine and ODV that is observed in patients with renal impairment (GFR = 10 to 70 mL/min) compared with normal subjects (see **CLINICAL PHARMACOLOGY**), it is recommended that the total daily dose be reduced by 25% to 50%. In patients undergoing hemodialysis, it is recommended that the total daily dose be reduced by 50% and that the dose be withheld until the dialysis treatment is completed (4 hrs). Because there was much individual variability in clearance between patients with renal impairment, individualization of dosage may be desirable in some patients.

Elderly Patients

No dose adjustment is recommended for elderly patients solely on the basis of age. As with any drug for the treatment of depression or generalized anxiety disorder, however, caution should be exercised in treating the elderly. When individualizing the dosage, extra care should be taken when increasing the dose.

Maintenance/Extended Treatment

There is no body of evidence available from controlled trials to indicate how long patients with depression or generalized anxiety disorder should be treated with Effexor XR.

It is generally agreed that acute episodes of depression require several months or longer of sustained pharmacological therapy beyond response to the acute episode. In one study, in which patients responding during 8 weeks of acute treatment with Effexor XR were assigned randomly to placebo or to the same dose of Effexor XR (75, 150, or 225 mg/day, qAM) during 26 weeks of maintenance treatment as they had received during the acute stabilization phase, longer-term efficacy was demonstrated. A second longer-term study has demonstrated the efficacy of Effexor in maintaining an antidepressant response in patients with recurrent depression who had responded and continued to be improved during an initial 26 weeks of treatment and were then randomly assigned to placebo or Effexor for period of up to 52 weeks on the same dose (100 to 200 mg/day, on a b.i.d. schedule) (see Clinical Trials under CLINICAL PHARMACOLOGY). Based on these limited data, it is not known whether or not the dose of Effexor/Effexor XR needed for maintenance treatment is identical to the dose needed to achieve an initial response. Patients should be periodically reassessed to determine the need for maintenance treatment and the appropriate dose for such treatment. In patients with Generalized Anxiety Disorder, Effexor XR has been shown to be effective in 6-month clinical trials. The need for continuing medication in patients with GAD who improve with Effexor XR treatment should be periodically reassessed.

Discontinuing Effexor XR

When discontinuing Effexor XR after more than 1 week of therapy, it is generally recommended that the dose be tapered to minimize the risk of discontinuation symptoms. Patients who have received Effexor XR for 6 weeks or more should have their dose tapered over at least a 2-week period. In clinical trials with Effexor XR, tapering was achieved by reducing the daily dose by 75 mg at 1 week intervals. Individualization of tapering may be necessary.

Discontinuation symptoms have been systematically evaluated in patients taking venlafaxine, to include prospective analyses of clinical trials in Generalized Anxiety Disorder and retrospective surveys of trials in depression. Abrupt discontinuation or dose reduction of venlafaxine at various doses has been found to be associated with the appearance of new symptoms, the frequency of which increased with increased dose level and with longer duration of treatment. Reported symptoms include agitation, anorexia, anxiety, confusion, coordination impaired, diarrhea, dizziness, dry mouth, dysphoric mood, fasciculation, fatigue, headaches, hypomania, insomnia, nausea, nervousness, nightmares, sensory disturbances (including shock-like electrical sensations), somnolence, sweating, tremor, vertigo, and vomiting. It is therefore recommended that the dosage of Effexor XR be tapered gradually and the patient monitored. The period required for tapering may depend on the dose, duration of therapy and the individual patient. Discontinuation effects are well known to occur with antidepressants.

Switching Patients To or From a Monoamine Oxidase Inhibitor

At least 14 days should elapse between discontinuation of an MAOI and initiation of therapy with Effexor XR. In addition, at least 7 days should be allowed after stopping Effexor XR before starting an MAOI (see **CONTRAINDICATIONS** and **WARNINGS**).

HOW SUPPLIED

Effexor® XR (venlafaxine hydrochloride) extended-release capsules are available as follows:

37.5 mg, grey cap/peach body with "W" and "Effexor XR" on the cap and "37.5" on the body.

NDC 0008-0837-01, bottle of 100 capsules. NDC 0008-0837-03, carton of 10 Redipak® blister strips of 10 capsules each.

Store at controlled room temperature, 20°C to 25°C (68°F to 77°F).

Bottles: Protect from light. Dispense in light-resistant container.

Blisters: Protect from light. Use blister carton to protect contents from light.

75 mg, peach cap and body with "W" and "Effexor XR" on the cap and "75" on the body.

NDC 0008-0833-01, bottle of 100 capsules. NDC 0008-0833-03, carton of 10 Redipak® blister strips of 10 capsules each.

Store at controlled room temperature, 20°C to 25°C (68°F to 77°F).

150 mg, dark orange cap and body with "W" and "Effexor XR" on the cap and "150" on the body.

NDC 0008-0836-01, bottle of 100 capsules. NDC 0008-0836-03, carton of 10 Redipak® blister strips of 10 capsules each.

Store at controlled room temperature, 20°C to 25°C (68°F to 77°F).

The appearance of these capsules is a trademark of Wyeth-Ayerst Laboratories.

Wyeth Laboratories
A Wyeth-Ayerst Company
Philadelphia, PA 19101
CI 7509-3 Revised February 21, 2002

ENBREL® ℞

[ĕn' brĕl]

etanercept

Prescribing information for this product, which appears on pages 3504–3507 of the 2002 PDR, has been revised as follows. Please write "See Supplement A" next to the product heading.

The third sentence of the first paragraph under the subheading **General** *in the* **CLINICAL PHARMACOLOGY** *section should be deleted and replaced with the following:*

Elevated levels of TNF are found in synovial fluid of RA patients and in both the synovium and psoriatic plaques of patients with psoriatic arthritis.[3,4]

The following should be added after the third sentence of the third paragraph under the subheading **Adult Rheumatoid Arthritis** *in the* **CLINICAL STUDIES** *section:*

The study was unblended after all patients had completed at least 12 months (and a median of 17.3 months) of therapy. The majority of patients remained in the study on the treatment to which they were randomized through 2 years.

The word "below" in the fourth sentence of the third paragraph under the subheading **Adult Rheumatoid Arthritis** *in the* **CLINICAL STUDIES** *section should be deleted and replaced with* "Table 1."

The fourth paragraph under the subheading **Clinical Response** *in the* **CLINICAL STUDIES** *section should be deleted and replaced with the following:*

In Study III, ACR response rates and improvement in all the individual ACR response criteria were maintained through 24 months of ENBREL therapy. Over the 2-year study, 23% of ENBREL patients achieved a major clinical response, defined as maintenance of an ACR 70 response over a 6-month period.

The last sentence of the fifth paragraph under the subheading **Clinical Response** *in the* **CLINICAL STUDIES** *section should be deleted and replaced with the following:*

Similar results were observed for ENBREL-treated patients in Studies II and III.

The paragraph under the subheading **Radiographic Response** *in the* **CLINICAL STUDIES** *section should be deleted and replaced with the following two paragraphs:*

In Study III, structural joint damage was assessed radiographically and expressed as change in total Sharp score (TSS) and its components, the erosion score and joint space narrowing (JSN) score. Radiographs of hands/wrists and forefeet were obtained at baseline, 6 months, 12 months, and 24 months and scored by readers who were unaware of treatment group. The results are shown in Table 3. A significant difference for change in erosion score was observed at 6 months and maintained at 12 months.

Patients continued on the therapy to which they were randomized for the second year of Study III. Seventy-two percent of patients had x-rays obtained at 24 months. Compared to the patients in the MTX group, patients randomized to ENBREL experienced less change in TSS, erosion score, and JSN at 24 months.

The entire paragraph under the subheading **Immunogenicity** *as well as the subheading in the* **CLINICAL STUDIES** *section should be deleted.*

The following subsection should be added to the end of the **CLINICAL STUDIES** *section:*

Psoriatic Arthritis

The safety and efficacy of ENBREL were assessed in a randomized, double-blind, placebo-controlled study in 205 patients with psoriatic arthritis. Patients were between 18 and 70 years of age and had active psoriatic arthritis (≥3 swollen joints and ≥3 tender joints) in one or more of the following forms: (1) distal interphalangeal (DIP) involvement (n = 104); (2) polyarticular arthritis (absence of rheumatoid nodules and presence of psoriasis; n = 173); (3) arthritis mutilans (n = 3); (4) asymmetric psoriatic arthritis (n = 81); or (5) ankylosing spondylitis-like (n = 7). Patients also had plaque psoriasis with a qualifying target lesion ≥2 cm in diameter. Patients currently on MTX therapy (stable for ≥2 months) could continue at a stable dose of ≤25 mg/week MTX. Doses of 25 mg ENBREL or placebo were administered SC twice a week for 6 months. Compared to placebo, treatment with ENBREL resulted in significant improvements in measures of disease activity (Table 4).

[See table 4 at top of next page]

Among patients with psoriatic arthritis who received ENBREL, the clinical responses were apparent at the time of the first visit (4 weeks) and were maintained through 6 months of therapy. Responses were similar in patients who were or were not receiving concomitant methotrexate therapy at baseline. At 6 months, the ACR 20/50/70 responses were achieved by 50%, 37%, and 9%, respectively, of patients receiving ENBREL, compared to 13%, 4%, and 1%, respectively, of patients receiving placebo. Similar responses were seen in patients with each of the subtypes of psoriatic arthritis, although few patients were enrolled with the arthritis mutilans and ankylosing spondylitis-like subtypes. The results of this study were similar to those seen in an earlier single-center, randomized, placebo-controlled study of 60 patients with psoriatic arthritis.[13]

The skin lesions of psoriasis were also improved with ENBREL, relative to placebo, as measured by percentages of patients achieving improvements in the psoriasis area and severity index (PASI).[14] Responses increased over time, and at 6 months, the proportions of patients achieving a 50% or 75% improvement in the PASI were 47% and 23%, respectively, in the ENBREL group (n = 66), compared to 18% and 3%, respectively, in the placebo group (n = 62). Responses were similar in patients who were or were not receiving concomitant methotrexate therapy at baseline.

The following should be added to the end of the **INDICATIONS AND USAGE** *section:*

ENBREL is indicated for reducing signs and symptoms of active arthritis in patients with psoriatic arthritis.

ENBREL can be used in combination with methotrexate in patients who do not respond adequately to methotrexate alone.

The following sentence should be added to the end of the paragraph under the subheading **Information to Patients** *in the* **PRECAUTIONS** *section:*

If the product is intended for multiple use, additional syringes, needles, and alcohol swabs will be required.

The paragraph under the subheading **Immunosuppression** *in the* **PRECAUTIONS** *section should be deleted and replaced with the following:*

Anti-TNF therapies, including ENBREL, affect host defenses against infections and malignancies since TNF mediates inflammation and modulates cellular immune responses. In a study of 49 patients with RA treated with ENBREL, there was no evidence of depression of delayed-type hypersensitivity, depression of immunoglobulin levels, or change in enumeration of effector cell populations. The impact of treatment with ENBREL on the development and course of malignancies, as well as active and/or chronic infections, is not fully understood (see **WARNINGS, ADVERSE REACTIONS, Infections** and **Malignancies**). The safety and efficacy of ENBREL in patients with immunosuppression or chronic infections have not been evaluated.

The two paragraphs under the subheading **Immunizations** *in the* **PRECAUTIONS** *section should be deleted and replaced with the following:*

Most psoriatic arthritis patients receiving ENBREL were able to mount effective B-cell immune responses to pneumococcal polysaccharide vaccine, but titers in aggregate were moderately lower and fewer patients had two-fold rises in titers compared to patients not receiving ENBREL. The clinical significance of this is unknown. Patients receiving ENBREL may receive concurrent vaccinations, except for live vaccines. No data are available on the secondary transmission of infection by live vaccines in patients receiving ENBREL (see **PRECAUTIONS, Immunosuppression**).

It is recommended that JRA patients, if possible, be brought up to date with all immunizations in agreement with current immunization guidelines prior to initiating ENBREL therapy. Patients with a significant exposure to varicella virus should temporarily discontinue ENBREL therapy and be considered for prophylactic treatment with Varicella Zoster Immune Globulin.

The **ADVERSE REACTIONS** *should be deleted and replaced with the following:*

Adverse Reactions in Adult Patients with RA or Psoriatic Arthritis

ENBREL has been studied in approximately 1200 patients with RA followed for up to 36 months, and in 157 patients with psoriatic arthritis for 6 months. The proportion of patients who discontinued treatment due to adverse events was approximately 4% in both ENBREL- and placebo-treated patients. The vast majority of these patients were treated with the recommended dose of 25 mg SC twice weekly.

Injection Site Reactions

In controlled trials, approximately 37% of patients treated with ENBREL developed injection site reactions. All injection site reactions were described as mild to moderate (erythema and/or itching, pain, or swelling) and generally did not necessitate drug discontinuation. Injection site reactions generally occurred in the first month and subsequently decreased in frequency. The mean duration of injection site reactions was 3 to 5 days. Seven percent of patients experienced redness at a previous injection site when subsequent injections were given. In post-marketing experience, injection site bleeding and bruising have also been observed in conjunction with ENBREL therapy.

Infections

In controlled trials, there were no differences in rates of infection among RA and psoriatic arthritis patients treated with ENBREL and those treated with placebo or MTX. The most common type of infection was upper respiratory infection, which occurred at a rate of approximately 20% among both ENBREL- and placebo-treated patients.

In placebo-controlled trials in RA and psoriatic arthritis, no increase in the incidence of serious infections was observed (approximately 1% in both placebo- and ENBREL-treated groups). In all clinical trials in RA, 50 of 1197 subjects exposed to ENBREL for up to 36 months experienced serious infections, including pyelonephritis, bronchitis, septic arthritis, abdominal abscess, cellulitis, osteomyelitis, wound infection, pneumonia, foot abscess, leg ulcer, diarrhea, sinusitis, and sepsis. Serious infections, including sepsis and death, have also been reported during post-marketing use of ENBREL. Some have occurred within a few weeks after initiating treatment with ENBREL. Many of the patients had underlying conditions (e.g., diabetes, congestive heart failure, history of active or chronic infections) in addition to their rheumatoid arthritis (see **WARNINGS**). Data from a sepsis clinical trial not specifically in patients with RA suggest that ENBREL treatment may increase mortality in patients with established sepsis.[17]

In post-marketing experience, infections have been observed with various pathogens including viral, bacterial, fungal, and protozoal organisms. Infections have been noted in all organ systems and have been reported in patients receiving ENBREL alone or in combination with immunosuppressive agents.

Malignancies

Seventeen malignancies of various types were observed in 1197 RA patients treated in clinical trials with ENBREL for up to 36 months. The observed rates and incidences were similar to those expected for the population studied.

Table 4: Components of Disease Activity in Psoriatic Arthritis

	Placebo N = 104		ENBREL[a] N = 101	
Parameter (median)	Baseline	6 Months	Baseline	6 Months
Number of tender joints[b]	17.0	13.0	18.0	5.0
Number of swollen joints[c]	12.5	9.5	13.0	5.0
Physician global assessment[d]	3.0	3.0	3.0	1.0
Patient global assessment[d]	3.0	3.0	3.0	1.0
Morning stiffness (minutes)	60	60	60	15
Pain[e]	3.0	3.0	3.0	1.0
Disability index[f]	1.0	0.9	1.1	0.3
CRP (mg/dL)[g]	1.1	1.1	1.6	0.2

a. $p < 0.001$ for all comparisons between ENBREL and placebo at 6 months.
b. Scale 0–78.
c. Scale 0–76.
d. Likert scale; 0 = best, 5 = worst.
e. Visual analog scale; 0 = best, 10 = worst.
f. Health assessment questionnaire; 0 = best, 3 = worst; includes eight categories: dressing and grooming, arising, eating, walking, hygiene, reach, grip, and activities.
g. Normal range: 0–0.79 mg/dL.

Table 5: Percent of RA Patients Reporting Adverse Events in Controlled Clinical Trials*

	Placebo Controlled		Active Controlled (Study III)	
	Percent of patients		Percent of patients	
Event	Placebo† (n = 152)	ENBREL (n = 349)	MTX (n = 217)	ENBREL (n = 415)
Injection site reaction	10	37	7	34
Infection (total)**	32	35	72	64
Non-upper respiratory infection (non-URI)**	32	38	60	51
Upper respiratory infection (URI)**	16	29	39	31
Headache	13	17	27	24
Nausea	10	9	29	15
Rhinitis	8	12	14	16
Dizziness	5	7	11	8
Pharyngitis	5	7	9	6
Cough	3	6	6	5
Asthenia	3	5	12	11
Abdominal Pain	3	5	10	10
Rash	3	5	23	14
Peripheral edema	3	2	4	8
Respiratory disorder	1	5	NA	NA
Dyspepsia	1	4	10	11
Sinusitis	2	3	3	5
Vomiting	—	3	8	5
Mouth ulcer	1	2	14	6
Alopecia	1	1	12	6
Pneumonitis ("MTX lung")	—	—	2	0

* *Includes data from the 6-month study in which patients received concurrent MTX therapy.*
† *The duration of exposure for patients receiving placebo was less than the ENBREL-treated patients.*
***Infection (total) includes data from all three placebo-controlled trials. Non-URI and URI include data only from the two placebo-controlled trials where infections were collected separately from adverse events (placebo n = 110, ENBREL n = 213).*

Immunogenicity

Patients with RA or psoriatic arthritis were tested at multiple timepoints for antibodies to ENBREL. Antibodies to the TNF receptor portion or other protein components of the ENBREL drug product, all non-neutralizing, were detected at least once in sera of <5% of adult patients with rheumatoid arthritis or psoriatic arthritis. No apparent correlation of antibody development to clinical response or adverse events was observed. Results from JRA patients were similar to those seen in adult RA patients treated with ENBREL. The long-term immunogenicity of ENBREL is unknown.

The data reflect the percentage of patients whose test results were considered positive for antibodies to ENBREL in an ELISA assay, and are highly dependent on the sensitivity and specificity of the assay. Additionally, the observed incidence of antibody positivity in an assay may be influenced by several factors including sample handling, concomitant medications, and underlying disease. For these reasons, comparison of the incidence of antibodies to ENBREL with the incidence of antibodies to other products may be misleading.

Autoantibodies

Patients had serum samples tested for autoantibodies at multiple timepoints. In Studies I and II, the percentage of patients evaluated for antinuclear antibodies (ANA) who developed new positive ANA (titer ≥ 1:40) was higher in patients treated with ENBREL (11%) than in placebo-treated patients (5%). The percentage of patients who developed new positive anti-double-stranded DNA antibodies was also higher by radioimmunoassay (15% of patients treated with ENBREL compared to 4% of placebo-treated patients) and by crithidia lucilae assay (3% of patients treated with ENBREL compared to none of placebo-treated patients). The proportion of patients treated with ENBREL who developed anticardiolipin antibodies was similarly increased compared to placebo-treated patients. In Study III, no pattern of increased autoantibody development was seen in ENBREL patients compared to MTX patients.

No patients in placebo- and active-controlled trials developed clinical signs suggestive of a lupus-like syndrome. The impact of long-term treatement with ENBREL on the development of autoimmune diseases is unknown. In post-marketing experience, very rare spontaneous adverse event reports have described patients with rheumatoid factor positive and/or erosive RA who have developed additional autoantibodies in conjunction with rash after ENBREL therapy.

Other Adverse Reactions

Table 5 summarizes events reported in at least 3% of all patients with higher incidence in patients treated with ENBREL compared to controls in placebo-controlled RA trials (including the combination methotrexate trial) and relevant events from Study III. Adverse events in the psoriatic arthritis trial were similar to those reported in RA clinical trials.

[See table 5 above]

In controlled trials of RA and psoriatic arthritis, rates of serious adverse events were seen at a frequency of approximately 5% among ENBREL- and control-treated patients. Among patients with RA in placebo-controlled, active-controlled, and open-label trials of ENBREL, malignancies (see **ADVERSE REACTIONS, Malignancies**) and infections (see **ADVERSE REACTIONS, Infections**) were the most common serious adverse events observed. Other infrequent serious adverse events observed in RA and psoriatic arthritis clinical trials are listed by body system below:

Cardiovascular:	heart failure, myocardial infarction, myocardial ischemia, hypertension, hypotension, deep vein thrombosis, thrombophlebitis
Digestive:	cholecystitis, pancreatitis, gastrointestinal hemorrhage
Musculoskeletal:	bursitis, polymyositis
Nervous:	cerebral ischemia, depression, multiple sclerosis (see **WARNINGS**)
Respiratory:	dyspnea, pulmonary embolism
Urogenital:	membranous glomerulonephropathy

In a randomized controlled trial in which 51 patients with RA received ENBREL 50 mg twice weekly and 25 patients received ENBREL 25 mg twice weekly, the following serious adverse events were observed in the 50 mg twice weekly arm: gastrointestinal bleeding, normal pressure hydrocephalus, seizure, and stroke. No serious adverse events were observed in the 25 mg arm.

Continued on next page

Enbrel—Cont.

Adverse Reactions in Patients with JRA
In general, the adverse events in pediatric patients were similar in frequency and type as those seen in adult patients (see **WARNINGS** and other sections under **ADVERSE REACTIONS**). Differences from adults and other special considerations are discussed in the following paragraphs.
Severe adverse reactions reported in 69 JRA patients ages 4 to 17 years included varicella (see also **PRECAUTIONS, Immunizations**), gastroenteritis, depression/personality disorder, cutaneous ulcer, esophagitis/gastritis, group A streptococcal septic shock, type I diabetes mellitus, and soft tissue and post-operative wound infection.
Forty-three of 69 (62%) children with JRA experienced an infection while receiving ENBREL during three months of study (part 1 open-label), and the frequency and severity of infections was similar in 58 patients completing 12 months of open-label extension therapy. The types of infections reported in JRA patients were generally mild and consistent with those commonly seen in outpatient pediatric populations. Two JRA patients developed varicella infection and signs and symptoms of aseptic meningitis which resolved without sequelae.
The following adverse events were reported more commonly in 69 JRA patients receiving 3 months of ENBREL compared to the 349 adult RA patients in placebo-controlled trials. These included headache (19% of patients, 1.7 events per patient-year), nausea (9%, 1.0 events per patient-year), abdominal pain (19%, 0.74 events per patient-year), and vomiting (13%, 0.74 events per patient-year).
In post-marketing experience, the following additional serious adverse events have been reported in pediatric patients: abscess with bacteremia, optic neuritis, pancytopenia, seizures, tuberculous arthritis, urinary tract infection (see **WARNINGS**), coagulopathy, cutaneous vasculitis, and transaminase elevations. The frequency of these events and their causal relationship to ENBREL therapy are unknown.
Adverse Reaction Information from Spontaneous Reports
Adverse events have been reported during post-approval use of ENBREL. Because these events are reported voluntarily from a population of uncertain size, it is not always possible to reliably estimate their frequency or establish a causal relationship to ENBREL exposure.
Additional adverse events are listed by body system below:

Body as a whole:	angioedema, fatigue, fever, flu syndrome, generalized pain, weight gain
Cardiovascular:	chest pain, vasodilation (flushing)
Digestive:	altered sense of taste, anorexia, diarrhea, dry mouth, intestinal perforation
Hematologic/Lymphatic:	adenopathy, anemia, aplastic anemia, leukopenia, pancytopenia, thrombocytopenia (see **WARNINGS**)
Musculoskeletal:	joint pain
Nervous:	paresthesias, stroke, seizures and central nervous system events suggestive of multiple sclerosis or isolated demyelinating conditions such as transverse myelitis or optic neuritis (see **WARNINGS**)
Ocular:	dry eyes, ocular inflammation
Respiratory:	dyspnea, interstitial lung disease, pulmonary disease, worsening of prior lung disorder
Skin:	cutaneous vasculitis, pruritis, subcutaneous nodules, urticaria

In the text, the references numbers should be renumbered in the following way:
Reference numbers 4, 5, 6, 7, 8, 9, 10, 11, should be renumbered as 5, 6, 7, 8, 9, 10, 11, 12, respectively, and numbers 12, 13, 14 should be renumbered as 15, 16, 17, respectively.
The following should be added as new references 13 and 14:

13. Mease PJ, Goffe BS, Metz J, Vanderstoep A, Finck B, Burge DJ. Etanercept in the treatment of psoriatic arthritis and psoriasis: a randomized trial. Lancet 2000;356:385.
14. Fredriksson T, Petersson U. Severe psoriasis—oral therapy with a new retinoid. Dermatologica 1978;157:238.

10662-10SP Issue Date 1/2002

INDERIDE® ℞
[ĭn' dĕ-rīd]
(propranolol hydrochloride [INDERAL®] and hydrochlorothiazide)

Prescribing information for this product, which appears on pages 3517–3519 of the 2002 PDR, has been revised as follows. Please write "See Supplement A" next to the product heading.
The words "Rx only." *should be inserted above the* **DESCRIPTION** *section.*
The following new section should be inserted at the end of the **PRECAUTIONS** *section:*
Geriatric Use
Clinical studies of Inderide did not include sufficient numbers of subjects aged 65 and over to determine whether they respond differently from younger subjects. Other reported clinical experience has not identified differences in responses between the elderly and younger patients.
In general, dose selection for an elderly patient should be cautious, usually starting at the low end of the dosing range, reflecting the greater frequency of decreased hepatic, renal, or cardiac function, and of concomitant disease or other drug therapy.
CI 4982-3 Revised May 8, 2001

INDERIDE® LA ℞
[ĭn 'dă-rīde]
(propranolol hydrochloride and hydrochlorothiazide) Long-Acting Capsules

Prescribing information for this product, which appears on pages 3519–3521 of the 2002 PDR, has been revised as follows. Please write "See Supplement A" next to the product heading.
The words "Rx only." *should be inserted above the* **DESCRIPTION** *section, just after the capsule descriptions.*
The following new section should be inserted at the end of the **PRECAUTIONS** *section:*
Geriatric Use
Clinical studies of Inderide LA did not include sufficient numbers of subjects aged 65 and over to determine whether they respond differently from younger subjects. Other reported clinical experience has not identified differences in responses between the elderly and younger patients.
In general, dose selection for an elderly patient should be cautious, usually starting at the low end of the dosing range, reflecting the greater frequency of decreased hepatic, renal, or cardiac function, and of concomitant disease or other drug therapy.
CI 7439-1 Issued May 8, 2001

ISORDIL® ℞
[ī 'sŏr-dĭl]
(isosorbide dinitrate) Sublingual Tablets

Prescribing information for this product, which appears on pages 3525–3526 of the 2002 PDR, has been revised as follows. Please write "See Supplement A" next to the product heading.
The words "Rx only." *should be inserted above the* **DESCRIPTION** *section.*
The following new section should be inserted at the end of the **PRECAUTIONS** *section:*
Geriatric Use
Clinical studies of Isordil (isosorbide dinitrate) Sublingual did not include sufficient numbers of subjects aged 65 and over to determine whether they respond differently from younger subjects. Other reported clinical experience has not identified differences in responses between the elderly and younger patients. In general, dose selection for an elderly patient should be cautious, usually starting at the low end of the dosing range, reflecting the greater frequency of decreased hepatic, renal, or cardiac function, and of concomitant disease or other drug therapy.
CI 4370-3 Revised July 18, 2001

ISORDIL® TITRADOSE® ℞
[ī 'sŏr-dĭl]
(isosorbide dinitrate) Tablets

Prescribing information for this product, which appears on pages 3526–3528 of the 2002 PDR, has been revised as follows. Please write "See Supplement A" next to the product heading.
The words "Rx only." *should be inserted above the* **DESCRIPTION** *section.*
The following new section should be inserted at the end of the **PRECAUTIONS** *section:*
Geriatric Use
Clinical studies of Isordil (isosorbide dinitrate) Titradose® did not include sufficient numbers of subjects aged 65 and over to determine whether they respond differently from younger subjects. Other reported clinical experience has not identified differences in responses between the elderly and younger patients. In general, dose selection for an elderly patient should be cautious, usually starting at the low end of the dosing range, reflecting the greater frequency of decreased hepatic, renal, or cardiac function, and of concomitant disease or other drug therapy.
CI 5182-2 Revised July 18, 2001

NORPLANT® SYSTEM ℞
[nŏr'plănt]
(levonorgestrel implants)

Prescribing information for this product, which appears on pages 3543–3548 of the 2002 PDR, has been revised as follows. Please write "See Supplement A" next to the product heading.
The paragraph following the subheading "1. Cigarette Smoking" under **B. Warnings Based on Experience with Combination (Progestin plus Estrogen) Oral Contraceptives** *should be deleted and replaced with the following paragraph:*
Cigarette smoking increases the risk of serious cardiovascular side effects from the use of combination oral contraceptives. This risk increases with age and with the extent of smoking (in epidemiologic studies, 15 or more cigarettes per day was associated with a significantly increased risk) and is quite marked in women over 35 years old. While this is believed to be an estrogen-related effect, it is not known whether a similar risk exists with progestin-only methods such as the NORPLANT SYSTEM; however, women who use the NORPLANT SYSTEM should be advised not to smoke.
The three paragraphs following the subheading "3. Carcinoma" under **B. Warnings Based on Experience with Combination (Progestin plus Estrogen) Oral Contraceptives** *should be deleted and replaced with the following three paragraphs:*
A meta-analysis from 54 epidemiological studies reported that there is a slightly increased relative risk (RR=1.24) of having breast cancer diagnosed in women who are currently using combination oral contraceptives compared to never-users. The increased risk gradually disappears during the course of the 10 years after cessation of combination oral contraceptive use. These studies do not provide evidence for causation. The observed pattern of increased risk of breast cancer diagnosis may be due to earlier detection of breast cancer in combination oral contraceptive users, the biological effects of combination oral contraceptives, or a combination of both. Because breast cancer is rare in women under 40 years of age, the excess number of breast cancer diagnoses in current and recent combination oral contraceptive users is small in relation to the lifetime risk of breast cancer. Breast cancers diagnosed in ever-users tend to be less advanced clinically than the cancers diagnosed in never-users. Although the results were broadly similar for progestin-only oral contraceptives, the data are based on much smaller numbers of progestin-only oral contraceptive users and therefore are less conclusive than for combination oral contraceptives. This information should be considered when prescribing the NORPLANT SYSTEM.
Some studies suggest that combination oral-contraceptive use has been associated with an increase in the risk of cervical intraepithelial neoplasia or invasive cervical cancer in some populations of women. However; there continues to be controversy about the extent to which such findings may be due to differences in sexual behavior and other factors. In spite of many studies of the relationship between combination oral-contraceptive use and breast and cervical cancers, a cause-and-effect relationship has not been established.
Evidence indicates that combination oral contraceptives may decrease the risk of ovarian and endometrial cancer. Irregular bleeding patterns associated with the NORPLANT SYSTEM could mask symptoms of cervical or endometrial cancer.
The paragraph following the heading "5. Ocular Lesions" under **B. Warnings Based on Experience with Combination (Progestin plus Estrogen) Oral Contraceptives** *should be deleted and replaced with the following paragraph:*
There have been clinical case reports of retinal thrombosis associated with the use of oral contraceptives that may lead to partial or complete loss of vision. Although it is believed that this adverse reaction is related to the estrogen component of oral contraceptives, the NORPLANT SYSTEM capsules should be removed if there is unexplained partial or complete loss of vision; onset of proptosis or diplopia; papilledema; or retinal vascular lesions. Appropriate diagnostic and therapeutic measures should be undertaken immediately.
CI 7502-1 Issued October 12, 2001

PHENERGAN® ℞
[fĕn 'ĕr-găn]
(promethazine HCl) INJECTION

Prescribing information for this product, which appears on pages 3553–3554 of the 2002 PDR, has been revised as follows. Please write "See Supplement A" next to the product heading.
The subheading **Sulfite Sensitivity** *and the paragraph under it in the* **WARNINGS** *section should be deleted.*
The paragraph under the subheading **CNS Depression** *in the* **WARNINGS** *section should be deleted and replaced with the following:*
Phenergan Injection may impair the mental and/or physical abilities required for the performance of potentially hazardous tasks; such as driving a vehicle or operating machinery. The impairment may be amplified by concomitant use of other central-nervous-system depressants such as alcohol, sedative/hypnotics (including barbiturates), general anesthetics, narcotics, narcotic analgesics, tricyclic antidepressants, and tranquilizers; therefore such agents should either be eliminated or given in reduced dosage in the presence of promethazine hydrochloride (see **PRECAUTIONS—Information for Patients**).

The following subheading and subsection should be added after the subsection under the subheading **CNS Depression** *in the* **WARNINGS** *section:*

Respiratory Depression

Phenergan Injection may lead to potentially fatal respiratory depression.

Use of Phenergan Injection in patients with compromised respiratory function (e.g. COPD, sleep apnea) should be avoided.

The following should be added after the subsection under the subheading **Bone-Marrow Depression** *in the* **WARNINGS** *section:*

Neuroleptic Malignant Syndrome

A potentially fatal symptom complex sometimes referred to as Neuroleptic Malignant Syndrome (NMS) has been reported in association with promethazine HCl alone or in combination with antipsychotic drugs. Clinical manifestations of NMS are hyperpyrexia, muscle rigidity, altered mental status and evidence of autonomic instability (irregular pulse or blood pressure, tachycardia, diaphoresis and cardiac dysrhythmias).

The diagnostic evaluation of patients with this syndrome is complicated. In arriving at a diagnosis, it is important to identify cases where the clinical presentation includes both serious medical illness (e.g., pneumonia, systemic infection, etc.) and untreated or inadequately treated extrapyramidal signs and symptoms (EPS). Other important considerations in the differential diagnosis include central anticholinergic toxicity, heat stroke, drug fever and primary central nervous system (CNS) pathology.

The management of NMS should include 1) immediate discontinuation of promethazine HCl, antipsychotic drugs, if any, and other drugs not essential to concurrent therapy, 2) intensive symptomatic treatment and medical monitoring, and 3) treatment of any concomitant serious medical problems for which specific treatments are available. There is no general agreement about specific pharmacological treatment regimens for uncomplicated NMS.

Since recurrences of NMS have been reported with phenothiazines, the reintroduction of promethazine HCl should be carefully considered.

The first sentence under the subheading **Other Considerations** *in the* **WARNINGS** *section should be deleted.*

The subheading **Laboratory Test Interactions** *in the* **PRECAUTIONS** *should be changed to* **Drugs/Laboratory Test Interactions.**

The **ADVERSE REACTIONS** *section should be deleted and replaced with the following:*

ADVERSE REACTIONS

Central Nervous System

Drowsiness is the most prominent CNS effect of this drug. Sedation, somnolence, blurred vision, dizziness; confusion, disorientation, and extrapyramidal symptoms such as oculogyric crisis, torticollis, and tongue protrusion; lassitude, tinnitus, incoordination, fatigue, euphoria, nervousness, diplopia, insomnia, tremors, convulsive seizures, excitation, catatonic-like states, hysteria. Hallucinations have also been reported.

Cardiovascular

Increased or decreased blood pressure, tachycardia, bradycardia, faintness. Venous thrombosis at the injection site has been reported. INTRA-ARTERIAL INJECTION MAY RESULT IN GANGRENE OF THE AFFECTED EXTREMITY (see **WARNINGS—Inadvertent Intra-arterial Injection**).

Dermatologic

Dermatitis, photosensitivity, urticaria.

Hematologic

Leukopenia, thrombocytopenia, thrombocytopenic purpura, agranulocytosis.

Gastrointestinal

Dry mouth, nausea, vomiting, jaundice.

Respiratory

Asthma, nasal stuffiness, respiratory depression (potentially fatal) and apnea (potentially fatal). (See **WARNINGS—Respiratory Depression.**)

Other

Angioneurotic edema. Neuroleptic malignant syndrome (potentially fatal) has also been reported. (See **WARNINGS—Neuroleptic Malignant Syndrome**). Subcutaneous injection has resulted in tissue necrosis.

The first paragraph of the **OVERDOSAGE** *section should be deleted and replaced with the following:*

Signs and symptoms of overdosage range from mild depression of the central nervous system and cardiovascular system to profound hypotension, respiratory depression, unconsciousness, and sudden death. Other reported reactions include hyperreflexia, hypertonia, ataxia, athetosis, and extensor-plantar reflexes (babinski reflex).

CI 3727-9 Revised May 25, 2001

PREMARIN® INTRAVENOUS ℞

[*prem' ă rĭn*]

(conjugated estrogens, USP)
for injection
Specially prepared for Intravenous & Intramuscular use

℞ only

Prescribing information for this product, which appears on pages 3563–3566 of the 2002 PDR, has been revised as follows. Please write "See Supplement A" next to the product heading.

Paragraphs 2–7 under the subheading "2. Cardiovascular risk." under the heading "A. GENERAL" in the **PRECAUTIONS** *section should be deleted and replaced with the following two paragraphs:*

From a large ongoing randomized placebo-controlled trial, preliminary observations suggest that there is a small increase in the number of heart attacks, stroke and VTE in women without established CHD on estrogen alone or estrogen plus progestin compared to those on placebo.

Physicians are advised to weigh the potential benefits and risks of therapy for each individual patient.

The following paragraph should be added after the first paragraph under the subheading "Cardiovascular Disease" under the heading **Risks of Estrogens** *in the* **INFORMATION FOR THE PATIENT** *section:*

In a large, ongoing, long-term study in predominantly healthy postmenopausal women, preliminary information from the study suggests that women without coronary heart disease may have a small increase in the number of heart attacks, strokes, and blood clots with estrogen or estrogen/progestin therapy. Talk to your doctor about the potential risks of estrogen/progestin therapy.

CI 7412-2 Revised September 11, 2001

PREMARIN® ℞

[*prĕm 'ă-rĭn*]

(conjugated estrogens tablets, USP)

Rx only

Prescribing information for this product, which appears on pages 3566–3570 of the 2002 PDR, has been revised as follows. Please write "See Supplement A" next to the product heading.

In the **PRECAUTIONS** *section, under the subheading* **"A. General,"** *paragraphs 2–7 under the subheading "2. Cardiovascular risk" should be deleted.*

The following two paragraphs should be added after the first paragraph following the subheading "2. Cardiovascular risk" under the subheading **"A. GENERAL"** *in the* **PRECAUTIONS** *section:*

From a large ongoing randomized placebo-controlled trial, preliminary observations suggest that there is a small increase in the number of heart attacks, stroke and VTE in women without established CHD on estrogen alone or estrogen plus progestin compared to those on placebo.

Physicians are advised to weigh the potential benefits and risks of therapy for each individual patient.

The following paragraph should be added after the first paragraph under the subheading "Cardiovasular disease" under the heading **"Risks of Estrogens"** *in the* **INFORMATION FOR THE PATIENT** *section:*

In a large ongoing, long-term study in predominantly healthy postmenopausal women, preliminary information from the study suggests that women without coronary heart disease may have a small increase in the number of heart attacks, strokes, and blood clots with estrogen or estrogen/progestin therapy. Talk to your doctor about the potential risks of estrogen/progestin therapy.

CI 6032-7 Revised October 16, 2001

PREMARIN® (conjugated estrogens) ℞

[*prem' ă rĭn*]

Vaginal Cream in a nonliquefying base

Rx only

Prescribing information for this product, which appears on pages 3570–3572 of the 2002 PDR, has been revised as follows. Please write "See Supplement A" next to the product heading.

The following two paragraphs should be added after the first paragraph under the subheading "A. GENERAL" *in the* **PRECAUTIONS** *section:*

From a large ongoing randomized placebo-controlled trial, preliminary observations suggest that there is a small increase in the number of heart attacks, stroke and VTE in women without established CHD on estrogen alone or estrogen plus progestin compared to those on placebo.

Physicians are advised to weigh the potential benefits and risks of therapy for each individual patient.

The following paragraph should be added after the first paragraph under the subheading "7. Cardiovascular Disease" under the heading **RISKS OF ESTROGENS** *in the* **INFORMATION FOR THE PATIENT** *section:*

In a large, ongoing, long-term study in predominantly healthy postmenopausal women, preliminary information from the study suggests that women without coronary heart disease may have a small increase in the number of heart attacks, strokes, and blood clots with estrogen or estrogen/progestin therapy. Talk to your doctor about the potential risks of estrogen/progestin therapy.

CI 7415-3 Revised September 11, 2001

PREMPRO™ ℞

[*prĕm' prō*]

(conjugated estrogens/medroxyprogesterone acetate tablets)

PREMPHASE® ℞

[*prĕm' fāz*]

(conjugated estrogens/medroxyprogesterone acetate tablets)

Rx only

Prescribing information for this product, which appears on pages 3572–3577 of the 2002 PDR, has been revised as follows. Please write "See Supplement A" next to the product heading.

The entire section following the subheading "1. Cardiovascular Risk." under the subheading "GENERAL" in the **PRECAUTIONS** *section should be deleted and replaced with the following paragraphs:*

1. *Cardiovascular Risk.* The effects of estrogen replacement on the risk of cardiovascular disease have not been adequately studied. However, data from the Heart and Estrogen/Progestin Replacement Study (HERS), a controlled clinical trial of secondary prevention of 2,763 postmenopausal women with documented heart disease, demonstrated no benefit. During an average follow-up of 4.1 years, treatment with oral conjugated estrogen plus medroxyprogesterone acetate did not reduce the overall rate of coronary heart disease (CHD) events in postmenopausal women with established coronary disease. These were more CHD events in the hormone treated group than in the placebo group in year 1, but fewer events in years 3 through 5.

   From a large ongoing randomized placebo-controlled trial, preliminary observations suggest that there is a small increase in the number of heart attacks, stroke and VTE in women without established CHD on estrogen alone or estrogen plus progestin compared to those on placebo.

   Physicians are advised to weigh the potential benefits and risks of therapy for each individual patient.

The following paragraph should be added after the first paragraph under the subheading "Heart Disease" under the heading **RISKS OF ESTROGENS AND/OR PROGESTINS** *in the* **INFORMATION FOR THE PATIENT** *section:*

In a large, ongoing, long-term study in predominantly healthy postmenopausal women, preliminary information from the study suggests that women without coronary heart disease may have a small increase in the number of heart attacks, strokes, and blood clots with estrogen or estrogen/progestin therapy. Talk to your doctor about the potential risks of estrogen or estrogen/progestin therapy.

CI 6096-4 Revised October 5, 2001

PROTONIX® ℞

[*prō 'tŏn-ĭks*]

(pantoprazole sodium)
Delayed-Release Tablets

Prescribing information for this product, which appears on pages 3577–3580 of the 2002 PDR, has been completely revised as follows. Please write "See Supplement A" next to the product heading.

DESCRIPTION

The active ingredient in PROTONIX® (pantoprazole sodium) Delayed-Release Tablets is a substituted benzimidazole, sodium 5-(difluoromethoxy)-2-[[(3,4-dimethoxy-2-pyridinyl)methyl] sulfinyl]-1*H*-benzimidazole sesquihydrate, a compound that inhibits gastric acid secretion. Its empirical formula is $C_{16}H_{14}F_2N_3NaO_4S \times 1.5\ H_2O$, with a molecular weight of 432.4. The structural formula is:

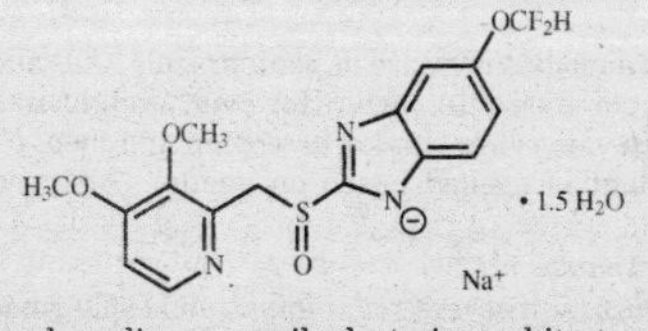

Pantoprazole sodium sesquihydrate is a white to off-white crystalline powder and is racemic. Pantoprazole has weakly basic and acidic properties. Pantoprazole sodium sesquihydrate is freely soluble in water, very slightly soluble in phosphate buffer at pH 7.4, and practically insoluble in n-hexane.

The stability of the compound in aqueous solution is pH-dependent. The rate of degradation increases with decreasing pH. At ambient temperature, the degradation half-life is approximately 2.8 hours at pH 5.0 and approximately 220 hours at pH 7.8.

PROTONIX is supplied as a delayed-release tablet for oral administration, available in 2 strengths. Each delayed-release tablet contains 45.1 mg or 22.6 mg of pantoprazole sodium sesquihydrate (equivalent to 40 mg or 20 mg pantoprazole, respectively) with the following inactive ingredients: calcium stearate, crospovidone, hydroxypropyl methylcellulose, iron oxide, mannitol, methacrylic acid copolymer, polysorbate 80, povidone, propylene glycol, sodium carbonate, sodium lauryl sulfate, titanium dioxide, and triethyl citrate.

Continued on next page

Protonix—Cont.

CLINICAL PHARMACOLOGY

Pharmacokinetics

PROTONIX is prepared as an enteric-coated tablet so that absorption of pantoprazole begins only after the tablet leaves the stomach. Peak serum concentration (C_{max}) and area under the serum concentration time curve (AUC) increase in a manner proportional to oral and intravenous doses from 10 mg to 80 mg. Pantoprazole does not accumulate and its pharmacokinetics are unaltered with multiple daily dosing. Following oral or intravenous administration, the serum concentration of pantoprazole declines biexponentially with a terminal elimination half-life of approximately one hour. In extensive metabolizers (see Metabolism section) with normal liver function receiving an oral dose of the enteric-coated 40 mg pantoprazole tablet, the peak concentration (C_{max}) is 2.5 μg/mL, the time to reach the peak concentration (t_{max}) is 2.5 h and the total area under the plasma concentration versus time curve (AUC) is 4.8 μg·hr/mL. When pantoprazole is given with food, its t_{max} is highly variable and may increase significantly. Following intravenous administration of pantoprazole to extensive metabolizers, its total clearance is 7.6–14.0 L/h and its apparent volume of distribution is 11.0–23.6L.

Absorption

The absorption of pantoprazole is rapid, with a C_{max} of 2.5 μg/mL that occurs approximately 2.5 hours after single or multiple oral 40-mg doses. Pantoprazole is well absorbed; it undergoes little first-pass metabolism resulting in an absolute bioavailability of approximately 77%. Pantoprazole absorption is not affected by concomitant administration of antacids. Administration of pantoprazole with food may delay its absorption up to 2 hours or longer; however, the C_{max} and the extent of pantoprazole absorption (AUC) are not altered. Thus, pantoprazole may be taken without regard to timing of meals.

Distribution

The apparent volume of distribution of pantoprazole is approximately 11.0–23.6L, distributing mainly in extracellular fluid. The serum protein binding of pantoprazole is about 98%, primarily to albumin.

Metabolism

Pantoprazole is extensively metabolized in the liver through the cytochrome P450 (CYP) system. Pantoprazole metabolism is independent of the route of administration (intravenous or oral). The main metabolic pathway is demethylation, by CYP2C19, with subsequent sulfation; other metabolic pathways include oxidation by CYP3A4. There is no evidence that any of the pantoprazole metabolites have significant pharmacologic activity. CYP2C19 displays a known genetic polymorphism due to its deficiency in some sub-populations (e.g. 3% of Caucasians and African-Americans and 17–23% of Asians). Although these sub-populations of slow pantoprazole metabolizers have elimination half-life values of 3.5 to 10.0 hours, they still have minimal accumulation (≤ 23%) with once daily dosing.

Elimination

After a single oral or intravenous dose of ^{14}C-labeled pantoprazole to healthy, normal metabolizer volunteers, approximately 71% of the dose was excreted in the urine with 18% excreted in the feces through biliary excretion. There was no renal excretion of unchanged pantoprazole.

Special Populations

Geriatric

Only slight to moderate increases in pantoprazole AUC (43%) and C_{max} (26%) were found in elderly volunteers (64 to 76 years of age) after repeated oral administration, compared with younger subjects. No dosage adjustment is recommended based on age.

Pediatric

The pharmacokinetics of pantoprazole have not been investigated in patients <18 years of age.

Gender

There is a modest increase in pantoprazole AUC and C_{max} in women compared to men. However, weight-normalized clearance values are similar in women and men. No dosage adjustment is needed based on gender (Also see Use in Women).

Renal Impairment

In patients with severe renal impairment, pharmacokinetic parameters for pantoprazole were similar to those of healthy subjects. No dosage adjustment is necessary in patients with renal impairment or in patients undergoing hemodialysis.

Hepatic Impairment

In patients with mild to severe hepatic impairment, maximum pantoprazole concentrations increased only slightly (1.5-fold) relative to healthy subjects. Although serum half-life values increased to 7–9 hours and AUC values increased by 5- to 7-fold in hepatic-impaired patients, these increases were no greater than those observed in slow CYP2C19 metabolizers, where no dosage frequency adjustment is warranted. These pharmacokinetic changes in hepatic-impaired patients result in minimal drug accumulation following once daily multiple-dose administration. No dosage adjustment is needed in patients with mild to severe hepatic impairment.

Drug-Drug Interactions

Pantoprazole is metabolized mainly by CYP2C19 and to minor extents by CYPs 3A4, 2D6 and 2C9. In *in vivo* drug-drug interaction studies with CYP2C19 substrates (diazepam [also a CYP3A4 substrate] and phenytoin [also a CYP3A4 inducer]), nifedipine, midazolam, and clarithromycin (CYP3A4 substrates), metoprolol (a CYP2D6 substrate), diclofenac (a CYP2C9 substrate) and theophylline (a CYP1A2 substrate) in healthy subjects, the pharmacokinetics of pantoprazole were not significantly altered. It is, therefore, expected that other drugs metabolized by CYPs 2C19, 3A4, 2D6, 2C9 and 1A2 would not significantly affect the pharmacokinetics of pantoprazole. *In vivo* studies also suggest that pantoprazole does not significantly affect the kinetics of other drugs (theophylline, diazepam [and its active metabolite, desmethyldiazepam], phenytoin, warfarin, metoprolol, nifedipine, carbamazepine, midazolam, clarithromycin, and oral contraceptives) metabolized by CYPs 2C19, 3A4, 2C9, 2D6 and 1A2. Therefore, it is expected that pantoprazole would not significantly affect the pharmacokinetics of other drugs metabolized by these isozymes. Dosage adjustment of such drugs is not necessary when they are co-administered with pantoprazole. In other *in vivo* studies, digoxin, ethanol, glyburide, antipyrine, caffeine, metronidazole, and amoxicillin had no clinically relevant interactions with pantoprazole.

Pharmacodynamics

Mechanism of Action

Pantoprazole is a proton pump inhibitor (PPI) that suppresses the final step in gastric acid production by forming a covalent bond to two sites of the (H^+,K^+)-ATPase enzyme system at the secretory surface of the gastric parietal cell. This effect is dose-related and leads to inhibition of both basal and stimulated gastric acid secretion irrespective of the stimulus. The binding to the (H^+,K^+)-ATPase results in a duration of antisecretory effect that persists longer than 24 hours.

Antisecretory Activity

Under maximal acid stimulatory conditions using pentagastrin, a dose-dependent decrease in gastric acid output occurs after a single dose of oral (20–80 mg) or a single dose of intravenous (20–120 mg) pantoprazole in healthy volunteers. Pantoprazole given once daily results in increasing inhibition of gastric acid secretion. Following the initial oral dose of 40 mg pantoprazole, a 51% mean inhibition was achieved by 2.5 hours. With once a day dosing for 7 days the mean inhibition was increased to 85%. Pantoprazole suppressed acid secretion in excess of 95% in half of the subjects. Acid secretion had returned to normal within a week after the last dose of pantoprazole; there was no evidence of rebound hypersecretion.

In a series of dose-response studies pantoprazole, at oral doses ranging from 20 to 120 mg, caused dose-related increases in median basal gastric pH and in the percent of time gastric pH was > 3 and > 4. Treatment with 40 mg of pantoprazole produced optimal increases in gastric pH which were significantly greater than the 20-mg dose. Doses higher than 40 mg (60, 80, 120 mg) did not result in further significant increases in median gastric pH. The effects of pantoprazole on median pH from one double-blind crossover study are shown below.

[See first table above]

Effect of Single Daily Doses of Oral Pantoprazole on Intragastric pH

Time	Median pH on day 7: Placebo	20 mg	40 mg	80 mg
8 a.m.–8 a.m. (24 hours)	1.3	2.9*	3.8*#	3.9*#
8 a.m.–10 p.m. (Daytime)	1.6	3.2*	4.4*#	4.8*#
10 p.m.–8 a.m. (Nighttime)	1.2	2.1*	3.0*	2.6*

* Significantly different from placebo
# Significantly different from 20 mg

Serum Gastrin Effects

Fasting serum gastrin levels were assessed in two double-blind studies of the acute healing of erosive esophagitis (EE) in which 682 patients with gastroesophageal reflux disease (GERD) received 10, 20, or 40 mg of PROTONIX for up to 8 weeks. At 4 weeks of treatment there was an increase in mean gastrin levels of 7%, 35%, and 72% over pretreatment values in the 10, 20, and 40 mg treatment groups, respectively. A similar increase in serum gastrin levels was noted at the 8 week visit with mean increases of 3%, 26%, and 84% for the three pantoprazole dose groups. Median serum gastrin levels remained within normal limits during maintenance therapy with PROTONIX (pantoprazole sodium) Delayed-Release Tablets.

In long-term international studies involving over 800 patients, a 2- to 3-fold mean increase from the pretreatment fasting serum gastrin level was observed in the initial months of treatment with pantoprazole at doses of 40 mg per day during GERD maintenance studies and 40 mg or higher per day in patients with refractory GERD. Fasting serum gastrin levels generally remained at approximately 2 to 3 times baseline for up to 4 years of periodic follow-up in clinical trials.

Following healing of gastric or duodenal ulcers with pantoprazole treatment, elevated gastrin levels return to normal by at least 3 months.

Enterochromaffin-Like (ECL) Cell Effects

In 39 patients treated with oral pantoprazole 40 mg to 240 mg daily (majority receiving 40 mg to 80 mg) for up to 5 years, there was a moderate increase in ECL-cell density starting after the first year of use which appeared to plateau after 4 years.

In a nonclinical study in Sprague-Dawley rats, lifetime exposure (24 months) to pantoprazole at doses of 0.5 to 200 mg/kg/day resulted in dose-related increases in gastric ECL-cell proliferation and gastric neuroendocrine (NE)-cell tumors. Gastric NE-cell tumors in rats may result from chronic elevation of serum gastrin concentrations. The high density of ECL cells in the rat stomach makes this species highly susceptible to the proliferative effects of elevated gastrin concentrations produced by proton pump inhibitors. However, there were no observed elevations in serum gastrin following the administration of pantoprazole at a dose of 0.5 mg/kg/day. In a separate study, a gastric NE-cell tumor without concomitant ECL-cell proliferative changes was observed in 1 female rat following 12 months of dosing with pantoprazole at 5 mg/kg/day and a 9 month off-dose recovery. (See **PRECAUTIONS**, Carcinogenesis, Mutagenesis, Impairment of Fertility).

Other Effects

No clinically relevant effects of pantoprazole on cardiovascular, respiratory, ophthalmic, or central nervous system function have been detected. In a clinical pharmacology study, pantoprazole 40 mg given once daily for 2 weeks had no effect on the levels of the following hormones: cortisol, testosterone, triiodothyronine (T3), thyroxine (T4), thyroid-stimulating hormone (TSH), thyronine-binding protein, parathyroid hormone, insulin, glucagon, renin, aldosterone, follicle-stimulating hormone, luteinizing hormone, prolactin and growth hormone.

In a 1-year study of GERD patients treated with pantoprazole 40 mg or 20 mg, there were no changes from baseline in overall levels of T3, T4, and TSH.

Clinical Studies

PROTONIX Delayed-Release Tablets were used in all clinical trials.

Erosive Esophagitis (EE) Associated with Gastroesophageal Reflux Disease (GERD)

A U.S. multicenter double-blind, placebo-controlled study of PROTONIX 10 mg, 20 mg, or 40 mg once daily was conducted in 603 patients with reflux symptoms and endoscopically diagnosed EE of grade 2 or above (Hetzel-Dent scale). In this study, approximately 25% of enrolled patients had severe EE of grade 3 and 10% had grade 4. The percentages of patients healed (per protocol, n=541) in this study were as follows:

[See second table above]

Erosive Esophagitis Healing Rates (per protocol)

Week	PROTONIX 10 mg QD (n = 153)	PROTONIX 20 mg QD (n = 158)	PROTONIX 40 mg QD (n = 162)	Placebo (n = 68)
4	45.6%+	58.4%+#	75.0%+*	14.3%
8	66.0%+	83.5%+#	92.6%+*	39.7%

+($p < 0.001$) PROTONIX versus placebo.
*($p < 0.05$) versus 10 mg, or 20 mg PROTONIX
#($p < 0.05$) versus 10 mg PROTONIX

In this study, all PROTONIX treatment groups had significantly greater healing rates than the placebo group. This was true regardless of *H. pylori* status for the 40-mg and 20-mg PROTONIX treatment groups. The 40-mg dose of PROTONIX resulted in healing rates significantly greater than those found with either the 20- or 10-mg dose.

A significantly greater proportion of patients taking PROTONIX 40 mg experienced complete relief of daytime and nighttime heartburn and the absence of regurgitation starting from the first day of treatment compared with placebo. Patients taking PROTONIX consumed significantly fewer antacid tablets per day than those taking placebo.

PROTONIX 40 mg and 20 mg once daily were also compared with nizatidine 150 mg twice daily in a U.S. multicenter, double-blind study of 243 patients with reflux symptoms and endoscopically diagnosed EE of grade 2 or above. The percentages of patients healed (per protocol, n=212) were as follows:

[See first table at top of next page]

Once daily treatment with PROTONIX 40 or 20 mg resulted in significantly superior rates of healing at both 4 and 8 weeks compared with twice daily treatment with 150 mg of nizatidine. For the 40 mg treatment group, significantly greater healing rates compared to nizatidine were achieved regardless of the *H. pylori* status.

A significantly greater proportion of the patients in the PROTONIX treatment groups experienced complete relief of nighttime heartburn and regurgitation starting on the first day and of daytime heartburn on the second day compared with those taking nizatidine 150 mg twice daily. Patients taking PROTONIX consumed significantly fewer antacid tablets per day than those taking nizatidine.

Long-Term Maintenance of Healing of Erosive Esophagitis

Two independent, multicenter, randomized, double-blind, comparator-controlled trials of identical design were conducted in GERD patients with endoscopically-confirmed healed erosive esophagitis to demonstrate efficacy of PROTONIX in long-term maintenance of healing. The two U.S. studies enrolled 386 and 404 patients, respectively, to receive either 10 mg, 20 mg, or 40 mg of PROTONIX (pantoprazole sodium) Delayed-Release Tablets once daily or 150 mg of ranitidine twice daily. As demonstrated in the table below, PROTONIX 40 mg and 20 mg were significantly superior to ranitidine at every time point with respect to the maintenance of healing. In addition, PROTONIX 40 mg was superior to all other treatments studied.

[See second table above]

PROTONIX 40 mg was superior to ranitidine in reducing the number of daytime and nighttime heartburn episodes from the first through the twelfth month of treatment. PROTONIX 20 mg, administered once daily, was also effective in reducing episodes of daytime and nighttime heartburn in one trial.

[See third table above]

Erosive Esophagitis Healing Rates (per protocol)

Week	PROTONIX 20 mg QD (n = 72)	PROTONIX 40 mg QD (n = 70)	Nizatidine 150 mg BID (n = 70)
4	61.4%+	64.0%+	22.2%
8	79.2%+	82.9%+	41.4%

+(p < 0.001) PROTONIX versus nizatidine.

Long-Term Maintenance of Healing of Erosive Gastroesophageal Reflux Disease (GERD Maintenance): Percentage of Patients Who Remained Healed

	PROTONIX 20 mg QD	PROTONIX 40 mg QD	Ranitidine 150 mg BID
Study 1	n = 75	n = 74	n = 75
Month 1	91*	99*	68
Month 3	82*	93*#	54
Month 6	76*	90*#	44
Month 12	70*	86*#	35
Study 2	n = 74	n = 88	n = 84
Month 1	89*	92*#	62
Month 3	78*	91*#	47
Month 6	72*	88*#	39
Month 12	72*	83*	37

* (p < 0.05 vs ranitidine), #(p <0.05 vs PROTONIX 20 mg)

Note: PROTONIX 10 mg was superior (p < 0.05) to ranitidine in study 2 but not study 1.

Number of Episodes of Heartburn (mean ± SD)

		PROTONIX 40 mg QD	Ranitidine 150 mg BID
Month 1	Daytime	5.1 ± 1.6*	18.3 ± 1.6
	Nighttime	3.9 ± 1.1*	11.9 ± 1.1
Month 12	Daytime	2.9 ± 1.5*	17.5 ± 1.5
	Nighttime	2.5 ± 1.2*	13.8 ± 1.3

* (p < 0.001 vs ranitidine, combined data from the 2 U.S. studies)

Most Frequent Adverse Events Reported as Drug Related in Short-term Domestic Trials

	% Incidence			
	Study 300-US		Study 301-US	
Study Event	PROTONIX (n = 521)	Placebo (n = 82)	PROTONIX (n = 161)	Nizatidine (n = 82)
Headache	6	6	9	13
Diarrhea	4	1	6	6
Flatulence	2	2	4	0
Abdominal pain	1	2	4	4
Rash	<1	0	2	0
Eructation	1	1	0	0
Insomnia	<1	2	1	1
Hyperglycemia	1	0	<1	0

Note: Only adverse events with an incidence greater than or equal to the comparators are shown.

INDICATIONS AND USAGE

Short-Term Treatment of Erosive Esophagitis Associated With Gastroesophageal Reflux Disease (GERD)

PROTONIX® (pantoprazole sodium) Delayed-Release Tablets are indicated for the short-term treatment (up to 8 weeks) in the healing and symptomatic relief of erosive esophagitis. For those patients who have not healed after 8 weeks of treatment, an additional 8 week course of PROTONIX may be considered.

Maintenance of Healing of Erosive Esophagitis

PROTONIX Delayed-Release Tablets are indicated for maintenance of healing of erosive esophagitis and reduction in relapse rates of daytime and nighttime heartburn symptoms in patients with gastroesophageal reflux disease (GERD). Controlled studies did not extend beyond 12 months.

CONTRAINDICATIONS

PROTONIX Delayed-Release Tablets are contraindicated in patients with known hypersensitivity to any component of the formulation.

PRECAUTIONS

General

Symptomatic response to therapy with pantoprazole does not preclude the presence of gastric malignancy.

Owing to the chronic nature of erosive esophagitis, there may be a potential for prolonged administration of pantoprazole. In long-term rodent studies, pantoprazole was carcinogenic and caused rare types of gastrointestinal tumors. The relevance of these findings to tumor development in humans is unknown.

Information for Patients

Patients should be cautioned that PROTONIX Delayed-Release Tablets should not be split, crushed or chewed. The tablets should be swallowed whole, with or without food in the stomach. Concomitant administration of antacids does not affect the absorption of pantoprazole.

Drug Interactions

Pantoprazole is metabolized through the cytochrome P450 system, primarily the CYP2C19 and CYP3A4 isozymes, and subsequently undergoes Phase II conjugation. Based on studies evaluating possible interactions of pantoprazole with other drugs, no dosage adjustment is needed with concomitant use of the following: theophylline, antipyrine, caffeine, carbamazepine, diazepam, diclofenac, digoxin, ethanol, glyburide, an oral contraceptive (levonorgestrel/ethinyl estradiol), metoprolol, nifedipine, phenytoin, warfarin, midazolam, clarithromycin, metronidazole, or amoxicillin. Clinically relevant interactions of pantoprazole with other drugs with the same metabolic pathways are not expected. Therefore, when co-administered with pantoprazole, adjustment of the dosage of pantoprazole or of such drugs may not be necessary. There was also no interaction with concomitantly administered antacids.

Because of profound and long lasting inhibition of gastric acid secretion, it is theoretically possible that pantoprazole may interfere with absorption of drugs where gastric pH is an important determinant of their bioavailability (e.g., ketoconazole, ampicillin esters, and iron salts).

Carcinogenesis, Mutagenesis, Impairment of Fertility

In a 24-month carcinogenicity study, Sprague-Dawley rats were treated orally with doses of 0.5 to 200 mg/kg/day, about 0.1 to 40 times the exposure on a body surface area basis, of a 50-kg person dosed at 40 mg/day. In the gastric fundus, treatment at 0.5 to 200 mg/kg/day produced enterochromaffin-like (ECL) cell hyperplasia and benign and malignant neuroendocrine cell tumors in a dose-related manner. In the forestomach, treatment at 50 and 200 mg/kg/day (about 10 and 40 times the recommended human dose on a body surface area basis) produced benign squamous cell papillomas and malignant squamous cell carcinomas. Rare gastrointestinal tumors associated with pantoprazole treatment included an adenocarcinoma of the duodenum at 50 mg/kg/day, and benign polyps and adenocarcinomas of the gastric fundus at 200 mg/kg/day. In the liver, treatment at 0.5 to 200 mg/kg/day produced dose-related increases in the incidences of hepatocellular adenomas and carcinomas. In the thyroid gland, treatment at 200 mg/kg/day produced increased incidences of follicular cell adenomas and carcinomas for both male and female rats.

Sporadic occurrences of hepatocellular adenomas and a hepatocellular carcinoma were observed in Sprague-Dawley rats exposed to pantoprazole in 6-month and 12-month toxicity studies.

In a 24-month carcinogenicity study, Fischer 344 rats were treated orally with doses of 5 to 50 mg/kg/day, approximately 1 to 10 times the recommended human dose based on body surface area. In the gastric fundus, treatment at 5 to 50 mg/kg/day produced enterochromaffin-like (ECL) cell hyperplasia and benign and malignant neuroendocrine cell tumors. Dose selection for this study may not have been adequate to comprehensively evaluate the carcinogenic potential of pantoprazole.

In a 24-month carcinogenicity study, B6C3F1 mice were treated orally with doses of 5 to 150 mg/kg/day, 0.5 to 15 times the recommended human dose based on body surface area. In the liver, treatment at 150 mg/kg/day produced increased incidences of hepatocellular adenomas and carcinomas in female mice. Treatment at 5 to 150 mg/kg/day also produced gastric fundic ECL cell hyperplasia.

A 26-week p53 +/− transgenic mouse carcinogenicity study was not positive.

Pantoprazole was positive in the *in vitro* human lymphocyte chromosomal aberration assays, in one of two mouse micronucleus tests for clastogenic effects, and in the *in vitro* Chinese hamster ovarian cell/HGPRT forward mutation assay for mutagenic effects. Equivocal results were observed in the *in vivo* rat liver DNA covalent binding assay. Pantoprazole was negative in the *in vitro* Ames mutation assay, the *in vitro* unscheduled DNA synthesis (UDS) assay with rat hepatocytes, the *in vitro* AS52/GPT mammalian cell-forward gene mutation assay, the *in vitro* thymidine kinase mutation test with mouse lymphoma L5178Y cells, and the in vivo rat bone marrow cell chromosomal aberration assay.

Pantoprazole at oral doses up to 500 mg/kg/day in male rats (98 times the recommended human dose based on body surface area) and 450 mg/kg/day in female rats (88 times the recommended human dose based on body surface area) was found to have no effect on fertility and reproductive performance.

Pregnancy

Teratogenic Effects

Pregnancy Category B

Teratology studies have been performed in rats at oral doses up to 450 mg/kg/day (88 times the recommended human dose based on body surface area) and rabbits at oral doses up to 40 mg/kg/day (16 times the recommended human dose based on body surface area) and have revealed no evidence of impaired fertility or harm to the fetus due to pantoprazole. There are, however, no adequate and well-controlled studies in pregnant women. Because animal reproduction studies are not always predictive of human response, this drug should be used during pregnancy only if clearly needed.

Nursing Mothers

Pantoprazole and its metabolites are excreted in the milk of rats. It is not known whether pantoprazole is excreted in human milk. Many drugs which are excreted in human milk have a potential for serious adverse reactions in nursing infants. Based on the potential for tumorigenicity shown for pantoprazole in rodent carcinogenicity studies, a decision should be made whether to discontinue nursing or to discontinue the drug, taking into account the benefit of the drug to the mother.

Pediatric Use

Safety and effectiveness in pediatric patients have not been established.

Use in Women

Erosive esophagitis healing rates in the 221 women treated with PROTONIX (pantoprazole sodium) Delayed-Release

Continued on next page

Protonix—Cont.

Tablets in U.S. clinical trials were similar to those found in men. In the 122 women treated long-term with PROTONIX 40 mg or 20 mg, healing was maintained at a rate similar to that in men. The incidence rates of adverse events were also similar for men and women.

Use in Elderly

In short-term U.S. clinical trials, erosive esophagitis healing rates in the 107 elderly patients (≥65 years old) treated with PROTONIX were similar to those found in patients under the age of 65. The incidence rates of adverse events and laboratory abnormalities in patients aged 65 years and older were similar to those associated with patients younger than 65 years of age.

ADVERSE REACTIONS

Worldwide, more than 11,100 patients have been treated with pantoprazole in clinical trials involving various dosages and duration of treatment. In general, pantoprazole has been well tolerated in both short-term and long-term trials.

In two U.S. controlled clinical trials involving PROTONIX 10-, 20-, or 40-mg doses for up to 8 weeks, there were no dose-related effects on the incidence of adverse events. The following adverse events considered by investigators to be possibly, probably or definitely related to drug occurred in 1% or more in the individual studies of GERD patients on therapy with PROTONIX.

[See fourth table at top of previous page]

In international short-term double-blind or open-label, clinical trials involving 20 to 80 mg per day, the following adverse events were reported to occur in 1% or more of 2805 GERD patients receiving pantoprazole for up to 8 weeks.

[See table below]

In two U.S. controlled clinical trials involving PROTONIX 10-, 20-, or 40-mg doses for up to 12 months, the following adverse events considered by investigators to be possibly, probably or definitely related to drug occurred in 1% or more of GERD patients on long-term therapy.

Most Frequent Adverse Events Reported as Drug Related in Long-term Domestic Trials

	% Incidence	
Study Event	PROTONIX (n = 536)	Ranitidine (n = 185)
Headache	5	2
Abdominal pain	3	1
Liver function tests abnormal	2	<1
Nausea	2	2
Vomiting	2	2

Note: Only adverse events with an incidence greater than or equal to the comparators are shown.

In addition, in these short- and long-term domestic and international trials, the following treatment-emergent events, regardless of causality, occurred at a rate of ≥ 1% in pantoprazole-treated patients: anxiety, arthralgia, asthenia, back pain, bronchitis, chest pain, constipation, cough increased, dizziness, dyspepsia, dyspnea, flu syndrome, gastroenteritis, gastrointestinal disorder, hyperlipemia, hypertonia, infection, liver function tests abnormal, migraine, nausea, neck pain, pain, pharyngitis, rectal disorder, rhinitis, SGPT increased, sinusitis, upper respiratory tract infection, urinary frequency, urinary tract infection, and vomiting.

Additional treatment-emergent adverse experiences occurring in <1% of pantoprazole-treated patients from these trials are listed below by body system. In most instances the relationship to pantoprazole was unclear.

BODY AS A WHOLE: abscess, allergic reaction, chills, cyst, face edema, fever, generalized edema, heat stroke, hernia, laboratory test abnormal, malaise, moniliasis, neoplasm, non-specified drug reaction, photosensitivity reaction.

CARDIOVASCULAR SYSTEM: abnormal electrocardiogram, angina pectoris, arrhythmia, atrial fibrillation/flutter, cardiovascular disorder, chest pain substernal, congestive heart failure, hemorrhage, hypertension, hypotension, myocardial infarction, myocardial ischemia, palpitation, retinal vascular disorder, syncope, tachycardia, thrombophlebitis, thrombosis, vasodilatation.

DIGESTIVE SYSTEM: anorexia, aphthous stomatitis, cardiospasm, colitis, dry mouth, duodenitis, dysphagia, enteritis, esophageal hemorrhage, esophagitis, gastrointestinal carcinoma, gastrointestinal hemorrhage, gastrointestinal moniliasis, gingivitis, glossitis, halitosis, hematemesis, increased appetite, melena, mouth ulceration, oral moniliasis, periodontal abscess, periodontitis, rectal hemorrhage, stomach ulcer, stomatitis, stools abnormal, tongue discoloration, ulcerative colitis.

ENDOCRINE SYSTEM: diabetes mellitus, glycosuria, goiter.

HEPATO-BILIARY SYSTEM: biliary pain, hyperbilirubinemia, cholecystitis, cholelithiasis, cholestatic jaundice, hepatitis, alkaline phosphatase increased, gamma glutamyl transpeptidase increased, SGOT increased.

HEMIC AND LYMPHATIC SYSTEM: anemia, ecchymosis, eosinophilia, hypochromic anemia, iron deficiency anemia, leukocytosis, leukopenia, thrombocytopenia.

METABOLIC AND NUTRITIONAL: dehydration, edema, gout, peripheral edema, thirst, weight gain, weight loss.

MUSCULOSKELETAL SYSTEM: arthritis, arthrosis, bone disorder, bone pain, bursitis, joint disorder, leg cramps, neck rigidity, myalgia, tenosynovitis.

NERVOUS SYSTEM: abnormal dreams, confusion, convulsion, depression, dry mouth, dysarthria, emotional lability, hallucinations, hyperkinesia, hypesthesia, libido decreased, nervousness, neuralgia, neuritis, neuropathy, paresthesia, reflexes decreased, sleep disorder, somnolence, thinking abnormal, tremor, vertigo.

RESPIRATORY SYSTEM: asthma, epistaxis, hiccup, laryngitis, lung disorder, pneumonia, voice alteration.

SKIN AND APPENDAGES: acne, alopecia, contact dermatitis, dry skin, eczema, fungal dermatitis, hemorrhage, herpes simplex, herpes zoster, lichenoid dermatitis, maculopapular rash, pruritus, skin disorder, skin ulcer, sweating, urticaria.

SPECIAL SENSES: abnormal vision, amblyopia, cataract specified, deafness, diplopia, ear pain, extraocular palsy, glaucoma, otitis externa, taste perversion, tinnitus.

UROGENITAL SYSTEM: albuminuria, balanitis, breast pain, cystitis, dysmenorrhea, dysuria, epididymitis, hematuria, impotence, kidney calculus, kidney pain, nocturia, prostatic disorder, pyelonephritis, scrotal edema, urethral pain, urethritis, urinary tract disorder, urination impaired, vaginitis.

Postmarketing Reports

There have been spontaneous reports of adverse events with the post-marketing use of pantoprazole. These reports include anaphylaxis (including anaphylactic shock); angioedema (Quincke's edema); anterior ischemic optic neuropathy; severe dermatologic reactions, including erythema multiforme, Stevens-Johnson syndrome, and toxic epidermal necrolysis (TEN, some fatal); hepatocellular damage leading to jaundice and hepatic failure; pancreatitis; and rhabdomyolysis. In addition, also observed have been confusion, hypokinesia, speech disorder, increased salivation, vertigo, nausea, tinnitus, and blurred vision.

Laboratory Values

In two U.S. controlled, short-term trials, 0.4% of the patients on PROTONIX 40 mg experienced SGPT elevations of greater than three times the upper limit of normal at the final treatment visit. In two U.S. controlled, long-term trials, none of 178 patients (0%) on PROTONIX 40 mg and two of 181 patients (1.1%) on PROTONIX 20 mg, experienced significant transaminase elevations at 12 months (or earlier if a patient discontinued prematurely). Significant elevations of SGOT or SGPT were defined as values at least three times the upper limit of normal that were non-sporadic and had no clear alternative explanation. The following changes in laboratory parameters were reported as adverse events: creatinine increased, hypercholesterolemia, and hyperuricemia.

OVERDOSAGE

Some reports of overdosage with pantoprazole have been received. A spontaneous report of a suicide involving an overdosage of pantoprazole (560 mg) has been received; however, the death was more reasonably attributed to the unknown doses of chloroquine and zopiclone which were also taken since two other reported cases of pantoprazole overdosage involved similar amounts of pantoprazole (400 and 600 mg) with no adverse effects observed. One patient tolerated a dose of 320 mg per day for 3 months. Doses of up to 240 mg per day, given intravenously for seven days, have been administered to healthy subjects and have been well tolerated.

Pantoprazole is not removed by hemodialysis.

Single oral doses of pantoprazole at 709 mg/kg, 798 mg/kg and 887 mg/kg were lethal to mice, rats and dogs, respectively. The symptoms of acute toxicity were hypoactivity, ataxia, hunched sitting, limb-splay, lateral position, segregation, absence of ear reflex, and tremor.

DOSAGE AND ADMINISTRATION

Treatment of Erosive Esophagitis

The recommended adult oral dose is 40 mg given once daily for up to 8 weeks. For those patients who have not healed after 8 weeks of treatment, an additional 8-week course of PROTONIX may be considered. (See **INDICATIONS AND USAGE.**)

Maintenance of Healing of Erosive Esophagitis

The recommended adult oral dose is one PROTONIX 40 mg Delayed-Release Tablet, taken daily. (See **Clinical Studies.**)

Adverse Events in GERD Patients in Short-term International Trials

	% Incidence			
Study Event	Pantoprazole Total (n=2805)	Ranitidine 300 mg (n=594)	Omeprazole 20 mg (n=474)	Famotidine 40 mg (n=239)
Headache	2	3	2	1
Diarrhea	2	2	2	<1
Abdominal pain	1	1	<1	<1

No dosage adjustment is necessary in patients with renal impairment, hepatic impairment, or for elderly patients. No dosage adjustment is necessary in patients undergoing hemodialysis.

PROTONIX Delayed-Release Tablets should be swallowed whole, with or without food in the stomach. If patients are unable to swallow a 40 mg tablet, two 20 mg tablets may be taken. Concomitant administration of antacids does not affect the absorption of PROTONIX.

Patients should be cautioned that PROTONIX Delayed-Release Tablets should not be split, chewed or crushed.

HOW SUPPLIED

PROTONIX® (pantoprazole sodium) Delayed-Release Tablets is supplied as 40 mg yellow oval biconvex delayed-release tablets imprinted with PROTONIX (brown ink) on one side.

They are available as follows:

NDC 0008-0841-10 bottles of 100
NDC 0008-0841-81 bottles of 90
NDC 0008-0841-91 bottles of 1000
NDC 0008-0841-99 carton of 10 Redipak® blister strips of 10 tablets each

PROTONIX is supplied as 20 mg yellow oval biconvex delayed-release tablets imprinted with P20 (brown ink) on one side.

They are available as follows:

NDC 0008-0843-81 bottles of 90
NDC 0008-0843-99 carton of 10 Redipak® blister strips of 10 tablets each

Storage

Store PROTONIX® Delayed-Release Tablets at 20°–25°C (68°–77°F); excursions permitted to 15°–30°C (59°–86°F). [See USP Controlled Room Temperature].

Rx only

U.S. Patent No. 4,758,579
Manufactured for Wyeth Laboratories
A Wyeth-Ayerst Company
Philadelphia, PA 19101
under license from
Byk Gulden Pharmaceuticals
D78467 Konstanz, Germany
CI 7482-2 Revised August 22, 2001

RAPAMUNE® ℞

Oral Solution and Tablets
[*răp'-a'mūn*]
(sirolimus)

Prescribing information for this product, which appears on pages 3584–3589 of the 2002 PDR, has been completely revised as follows. Please write "See Supplement A" next to the product heading.

> **WARNING:**
> Increased susceptibility to infection and the possible development of lymphoma may result from immunosuppression. Only physicians experienced in immunosuppressive therapy and management of renal transplant patients should use Rapamune®. Patients receiving the drug should be managed in facilities equipped and staffed with adequate laboratory and supportive medical resources. The physician responsible for maintenance therapy should have complete information requisite for the follow-up of the patient.

DESCRIPTION

Rapamune® (sirolimus) is an immunosuppressive agent. Sirolimus is a macrocyclic lactone produced by *Streptomyces hygroscopicus*. The chemical name of sirolimus (also known as rapamycin) is (3*S*,6*R*,7*E*,9*R*,10*R*,12*R*,14*S*,15*E*,17*E*,19*E*,21*S*,23*S*,26*R*,27*R*,34a*S*) - 9,10,12,13,14,21,22,23,24,25,26,27,32,33,34,34a-hexadecahydro-9,27-dihydroxy-3-[(1*R*)-2-[(1S,3*R*,4*R*)-4-hydroxy - 3 - methoxycyclohexyl]-1-methylethyl]-10,21-dimethoxy-6,8,12,14,20,26-hexamethyl-23,27-epoxy- 3*H*-pyrido[2,1-*c*][1,4] oxaazacyclohentriacontine-1,5,11,28,29 (4*H*,6*H*,31*H*)-pentone. Its molecular formula is $C_{51}H_{79}NO_{13}$ and its molecular weight is 914.2. The structural formula of sirolimus is shown below.

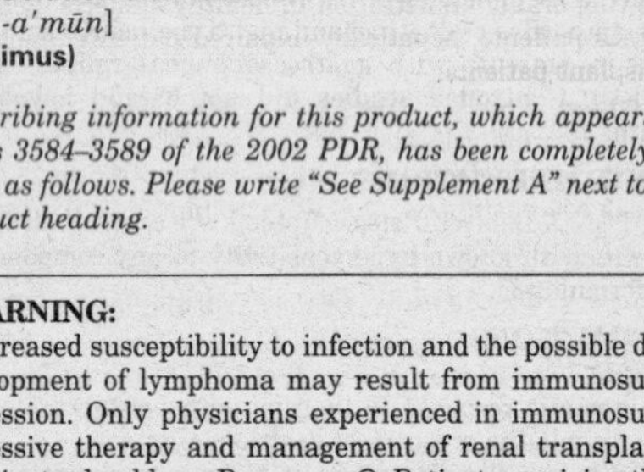

Sirolimus is a white to off-white powder and is insoluble in water, but freely soluble in benzyl alcohol, chloroform, acetone, and acetonitrile.

Rapamune® is available for administration as an oral solution containing 1 mg/mL sirolimus and as a white, triangular-shaped tablet containing 1 mg sirolimus.

The inactive ingredients in Rapamune® Oral Solution are Phosal 50 PG® (phosphatidylcholine, propylene glycol, mono- and di-glycerides, ethanol, soy fatty acids, and ascorbyl palmitate) and polysorbate 80. Rapamune Oral Solution contains 1.5% - 2.5% ethanol.

The inactive ingredients in Rapamune® Tablets include sucrose, lactose, polyethylene glycol 8000, calcium sulfate, microcrystalline cellulose, pharmaceutical glaze, talc, titanium dioxide, magnesium stearate, povidone, poloxamer 188, polyethylene glycol 20,000, glyceryl monooleate, carnauba wax, and other ingredients.

CLINICAL PHARMACOLOGY

Mechanism of Action

Sirolimus inhibits T lymphocyte activation and proliferation that occurs in response to antigenic and cytokine (Interleukin [IL]-2, IL-4, and IL-15) stimulation by a mechanism that is distinct from that of other immunosuppressants. Sirolimus also inhibits antibody production. In cells, sirolimus binds to the immunophilin, FK Binding Protein-12 (FKBP-12), to generate an immunosuppressive complex. The sirolimus:FKBP-12 complex has no effect on calcineurin activity. This complex binds to and inhibits the activation of the mammalian Target Of Rapamycin (mTOR), a key regulatory kinase. This inhibition suppresses cytokine-driven T-cell proliferation, inhibiting the progression from the G_1 to the S phase of the cell cycle.

Studies in experimental models show that sirolimus prolongs allograft (kidney, heart, skin, islet, small bowel, pancreatico-duodenal, and bone marrow) survival in mice, rats, pigs, and/or primates. Sirolimus reverses acute rejection of heart and kidney allografts in rats and prolonged the graft survival in presensitized rats. In some studies, the immunosuppressive effect of sirolimus lasted up to 6 months after discontinuation of therapy. This tolerization effect is alloantigen specific.

In rodent models of autoimmune disease, sirolimus suppresses immune-mediated events associated with systemic lupus erythematosus, collagen-induced arthritis, autoimmune type I diabetes, autoimmune myocarditis, experimental allergic encephalomyelitis, graft-versus-host disease, and autoimmune uveoretinitis.

Pharmacokinetics

Sirolimus pharmacokinetic activity has been determined following oral administration in healthy subjects, pediatric dialysis patients, hepatically-impaired patients, and renal transplant patients.

Absorption

Following administration of Rapamune® (sirolimus) Oral Solution, sirolimus is rapidly absorbed, with a mean time-to-peak concentration (t_{max}) of approximately 1 hour after a single dose in healthy subjects and approximately 2 hours after multiple oral doses in renal transplant recipients. The systemic availability of sirolimus was estimated to be approximately 14% after the administration of Rapamune Oral Solution. The mean bioavailability of sirolimus after administration of the tablet is about 27% higher relative to the oral solution. Sirolimus oral tablets are not bioequivalent to the oral solution; however, clinical equivalence has been demonstrated at the 2-mg dose level. (See **CLINICAL STUDIES** and **DOSAGE AND ADMINISTRATION**).

Sirolimus concentrations, following the administration of Rapamune Oral Solution to stable renal transplant patients, are dose proportional between 3 and 12 mg/m^2.

Food effects: In 22 healthy volunteers receiving Rapamune Oral Solution, a high-fat meal (861.8 kcal, 54.9% kcal from fat) altered the bioavailability characteristics of sirolimus. Compared to fasting, a 34% decrease in the peak blood sirolimus concentration (C_{max}), a 3.5-fold increase in the time-to-peak concentration (t_{max}), and a 35% increase in total exposure (AUC) was observed. After administration of Rapamune Tablets and a high-fat meal in 24 healthy volunteers, C_{max}, t_{max}, and AUC showed increases of 65%, 32%, and 23%, respectively. To minimize variability, both Rapamune Oral Solution and Tablets should be taken consistently with or without food (See **DOSAGE AND ADMINISTRATION**).

Distribution

The mean (±SD) blood-to-plasma ratio of sirolimus was 36 (± 17.9) in stable renal allograft recipients, indicating that sirolimus is extensively partitioned into formed blood elements. The mean volume of distribution (V_{ss}/F) of sirolimus is 12 ± 7.52 L/kg. Sirolimus is extensively bound (approximately 92%) to human plasma proteins. In man, the binding of sirolimus was shown mainly to be associated with serum albumin (97%), α_1-acid glycoprotein, and lipoproteins.

Metabolism

Sirolimus is a substrate for both cytochrome P450 IIIA4 (CYP3A4) and P-glycoprotein. Sirolimus is extensively metabolized by O-demethylation and/or hydroxylation. Seven (7) major metabolites, including hydroxy, demethyl, and hydroxydemethyl, are identifiable in whole blood. Some of these metabolites are also detectable in plasma, fecal, and urine samples. Glucuronide and sulfate conjugates are not present in any of the biologic matrices. Sirolimus is the major component in human whole blood and contributes to more than 90% of the immunosuppressive activity.

Excretion

After a single dose of [^{14}C]sirolimus in healthy volunteers, the majority (91%) of radioactivity was recovered from the feces, and only a minor amount (2.2%) was excreted in urine.

SIROLIMUS PHARMACOKINETIC PARAMETERS (MEAN ± SD) IN RENAL TRANSPLANT PATIENTS (MULTIPLE DOSE ORAL SOLUTION)[a,b]

n	Dose	$C_{max,ss}$[c] (ng/mL)	$t_{max,ss}$ (h)	$AUC_{\tau,ss}$[c] (ng•h/mL)	CL/F/WT[d] (mL/h/kg)
19	2 mg	12.2 ± 6.2	3.01 ± 2.40	158 ± 70	182 ± 72
23	5 mg	37.4 ± 21	1.84 ± 1.30	396 ± 193	221 ± 143

a: Sirolimus administered four hours after cyclosporine oral solution (MODIFIED) (e.g., Neoral® Oral Solution) and/or cyclosporine capsules (MODIFIED) (e.g., Neoral® Soft Gelatin Capsules).
b: As measured by the Liquid Chromatographic/Tandem Mass Spectrometric Method (LC/MS/MS).
c: These parameters were dose normalized prior to the statistical comparison.
d: CL/F/WT = oral dose clearance.

SIROLIMUS PHARMACOKINETIC PARAMETERS (MEAN ± SD) IN RENAL TRANSPLANT PATIENTS (MULTIPLE DOSE TABLETS)[a,b]

n	Dose (2 mg/day)	$C_{max,ss}$[c] (ng/mL)	$t_{max,ss}$ (h)	$AUC_{\tau,ss}$[c] (ng•h/mL)	CL/F/WT[d] (mL/h/kg)
17	Oral solution	14.4 ± 5.3	2.12 ± 0.84	194 ± 78	173 ± 50
13	Tablets	15.0 ± 4.9	3.46 ± 2.40	230 ± 67	139 ± 63

a: Sirolimus administered four hours after cyclosporine oral solution (MODIFIED) (e.g., Neoral® Oral Solution) and/or cyclosporine capsules (MODIFIED) (e.g., Neoral® Soft Gelatin Capsules).
b: As measured by the Liquid Chromatographic/Tandem Mass Spectrometric Method (LC/MS/MS).
c: These parameters were dose normalized prior to the statistical comparison.
d: CL/F/WT = oral dose clearance.

SIROLIMUS PHARMACOKINETIC PARAMETERS (MEAN ± SD) IN 18 HEALTHY SUBJECTS AND 18 PATIENTS WITH HEPATIC IMPAIRMENT (15 MG SINGLE DOSE - ORAL SOLUTION)

Population	$C_{max,ss}$[a] (ng/mL)	t_{max} (h)	$AUC_{0-\infty}$ (ng•h/mL)	CL/F/WT (mL/h/kg)
Healthy subjects	78.2 ± 18.3	0.82 ± 0.17	970 ± 272	215 ± 76
Hepatic impairment	77.9 ± 23.1	0.84 ± 0.17	1567 ± 616	144 ± 62

a: As measured by LC/MS/MS

SIROLIMUS PHARMACOKINETIC PARAMETERS (MEAN ± SD) IN PEDIATRIC PATIENTS WITH STABLE CHRONIC RENAL FAILURE MAINTAINED ON HEMODIALYSIS OR PERITONEAL DIALYSIS (1, 3, 9, 15 MG/M^2 SINGLE DOSE)

Age Group (y)	n	t_{max} (h)	$t_{1/2}$ (h)	CL/F/WT (mL/h/kg)
5 - 11	9	1.1 ± 0.5	71 ± 40	580 ± 450
12 - 18	11	0.79 ± 0.17	55 ± 18	450 ± 232

Pharmacokinetics in renal transplant patients

Rapamune Oral Solution: Pharmacokinetic parameters for sirolimus oral solution given daily in combination with cyclosporine and corticosteroids in renal transplant patients are summarized below based on data collected at months 1, 3, and 6 after transplantation. There were no significant differences in any of these parameters with respect to treatment group or month.

[See first table above]

Whole blood sirolimus trough concentrations (mean ± SD), as measured by immunoassay, for the 2 mg/day and 5 mg/day dose groups were 8.59 ± 4.01 ng/mL (n = 226) and 17.3 ± 7.4 ng/mL (n = 219), respectively. Whole blood trough sirolimus concentrations, as measured by LC/MS/MS, were significantly correlated (r^2 = 0.96) with $AUC_{\tau,ss}$. Upon repeated twice daily administration without an initial loading dose in a multiple-dose study, the average trough concentration of sirolimus increases approximately 2 to 3-fold over the initial 6 days of therapy at which time steady state is reached. A loading dose of 3 times the maintenance dose will provide near steady-state concentrations within 1 day in most patients. The mean ± SD terminal elimination half life ($t_{1/2}$) of sirolimus after multiple dosing in stable renal transplant patients was estimated to be about 62 ± 16 hours.

Rapamune Tablets: Pharmacokinetic parameters for sirolimus tablets administered daily in combination with cyclosporine and corticosteroids in renal transplant patients are summarized below based on data collected at months 1 and 3 after transplantation.

[See second table above]

Whole blood sirolimus trough concentrations (mean ± SD), as measured by immunoassay, for the 2 mg oral solution and 2 mg tablets over 6 months, were 8.94 ± 4.36 ng/mL (n = 172) and 9.48 ± 3.85 ng/mL (n = 179), respectively. Whole blood trough sirolimus concentrations, as measured by LC/MS/MS, were significantly correlated (r^2 = 0.85) with $AUC_{\tau,ss}$. Mean whole blood sirolimus trough concentrations in patients receiving either Rapamune Oral Solution or Rapamune Tablets with a loading dose of three times the maintenance dose achieved steady-state concentrations within 24 hours after the start of dose administration.

Special Populations

Hepatic impairment: Sirolimus (15 mg) was administered as a single oral dose to 18 subjects with normal hepatic function and to 18 patients with Child-Pugh classification A or B hepatic impairment, in which hepatic impairment was primary and not related to an underlying systemic disease. Shown below are the mean ± SD pharmacokinetic parameters following the administration of sirolimus oral solution.

[See third table above]

Compared with the values in the normal hepatic group, the hepatic impairment group had higher mean values for sirolimus AUC (61%) and $t_{1/2}$ (43%) and had lower mean values for sirolimus CL/F/WT (33%). The mean $t_{1/2}$ increased from 79 ± 12 hours in subjects with normal hepatic function to 113 ± 41 hours in patients with impaired hepatic function. The rate of absorption of sirolimus was not altered by hepatic disease, as evidenced by C_{max} and t_{max} values. However, hepatic diseases with varying etiologies may show different effects and the pharmacokinetics of sirolimus in patients with severe hepatic dysfunction is unknown. Dosage adjustment is recommended for patients with mild to moderate hepatic impairment (see **DOSAGE AND ADMINISTRATION**).

Renal impairment: The effect of renal impairment on the pharmacokinetics of sirolimus is not known. However, there is minimal (2.2%) renal excretion of the drug or its metabolites.

Pediatric: Limited pharmacokinetic data are available in pediatric patients. The table below summarizes pharmacokinetic data obtained in pediatric dialysis patients with chronically impaired renal function.

[See fourth table above]

Geriatric: Clinical studies of Rapamune did not include a sufficient number of patients > 65 years of age to determine whether they will respond differently than younger patients. After the administration of Rapamune Oral Solution, sirolimus trough concentration data in 35 renal transplant patients > 65 years of age were similar to those in the adult population (n = 822) 18 to 65 years of age. Similar results were obtained after the administration of Rapamune Tablets to 12 renal transplant patients > 65 years of age compared with adults (n = 167) 18 to 65 years of age.

Gender: After the administration of Rapamune Oral Solution, sirolimus oral dose clearance in males was 12% lower than that in females; male subjects had a significantly longer $t_{1/2}$ than did female subjects (72.3 hours versus 61.3 hours). A similar trend in the effect of gender on sirolimus oral dose clearance and $t_{1/2}$ was observed after the administration of Rapamune Tablets. Dose adjustments based on gender are not recommended.

Race: In large phase III trials using Rapamune Oral Solution and cyclosporine oral solution (MODIFIED) (e.g., Neoral® Oral Solution) and/or cyclosporine capsules (MODIFIED) (e.g., Neoral® Soft Gelatin Capsules), there were no significant differences in mean trough sirolimus concentrations over time between black (n = 139) and non-black (n = 724) patients during the first 6 months after transplantation at sirolimus doses of 2 mg/day and 5 mg/day. Similarly, after administration of Rapamune Tablets (2 mg/day) in a phase III trial, mean sirolimus trough concentrations over 6 months were not significantly different among black (n = 51) and non-black (n = 128) patients.

CLINICAL STUDIES

Rapamune® (sirolimus) Oral Solution: The safety and efficacy of Rapamune® Oral Solution for the prevention of or-

Continued on next page

Rapamune—Cont.

gan rejection following renal transplantation were assessed in two randomized, double-blind, multicenter, controlled trials. These studies compared two dose levels of Rapamune Oral Solution (2 mg and 5 mg, once daily) with azathioprine (Study 1) or placebo (Study 2) when administered in combination with cyclosporine and corticosteroids. Study 1 was conducted in the United States at 38 sites. Seven hundred nineteen (719) patients were enrolled in this trial and randomized following transplantation; 284 were randomized to receive Rapamune Oral Solution 2 mg/day, 274 were randomized to receive Rapamune Oral Solution 5 mg/day, and 161 to receive azathioprine 2-3 mg/kg/day. Study 2 was conducted in Australia, Canada, Europe, and the United States, at a total of 34 sites. Five hundred seventy-six (576) patients were enrolled in this trial and randomized before transplantation; 227 were randomized to receive Rapamune Oral Solution 2 mg/day, 219 were randomized to receive Rapamune Oral Solution 5 mg/day, and 130 to receive placebo. In both studies, the use of antilymphocyte antibody induction therapy was prohibited. In both studies, the primary efficacy endpoint was the rate of efficacy failure in the first 6 months after transplantation. Efficacy failure was defined as the first occurrence of an acute rejection episode (confirmed by biopsy), graft loss, or death.

The tables below summarize the results of the primary efficacy analyses from these trials. Rapamune Oral Solution, at doses of 2 mg/day and 5 mg/day, significantly reduced the incidence of efficacy failure (statistically significant at the <0.025 level; nominal significance level adjusted for multiple [2] dose comparisons) at 6 months following transplantation compared to both azathioprine and placebo.

[See first table above]
[See second table above]

INCIDENCE (%) OF THE PRIMARY ENDPOINT AT 6 MONTHS: STUDY 1[a]

Parameter	Rapamune® Oral Solution 2 mg/day (n = 284)	Rapamune® Oral Solution 5 mg/day (n = 274)	Azathioprine 2-3 mg/kg/day (n = 161)
Efficacy failure at 6 months	18.7	16.8	32.3
Components of efficacy failure			
Biopsy-proven acute rejection	16.5	11.3	29.2
Graft loss	1.1	2.9	2.5
Death	0.7	1.8	0
Lost to follow-up	0.4	0.7	0.6

a: Patients received cyclosporine and corticosteroids.

INCIDENCE (%) OF THE PRIMARY ENDPOINT AT 6 MONTHS: STUDY 2[a]

Parameter	Rapamune® Oral Solution 2 mg/day (n = 227)	Rapamune® Oral Solution 5 mg/day (n = 219)	Placebo (n = 130)
Efficacy failure at 6 months	30.0	25.6	47.7
Components of efficacy failure			
Biopsy-proven acute rejection	24.7	19.2	41.5
Graft loss	3.1	3.7	3.9
Death	2.2	2.7	2.3
Lost to follow-up	0	0	0

a: Patients received cyclosporine and corticosteroids.

Patient and graft survival at 1 year were co-primary endpoints. The table below shows graft and patient survival at 1 year in Study 1 and Study 2. The graft and patient survival rates at 1 year were similar in the Rapamune- and comparator-treated patients.

[See third table above]

1-YEAR GRAFT AND PATIENT SURVIVAL (%)[a]

Parameter	Rapamune® Oral Solution 2 mg/day	Rapamune® Oral Solution 5 mg/day	Azathioprine 2-3 mg/kg/day	Placebo
Study 1	(n = 284)	(n = 274)	(n = 161)	
Graft survival	94.7	92.7	93.8	
Patient survival	97.2	96.0	98.1	
Study 2	(n = 227)	(n = 219)		(n = 130)
Graft survival	89.9	90.9		87.7
Patient survival	96.5	95.0		94.6

a: Patients received cyclosporine and corticosteroids.

The reduction in the incidence of first biopsy-confirmed acute rejection episodes in Rapamune-treated patients compared to the control groups included a reduction in all grades of rejection.

[See fourth table above]

In Study 1, which was prospectively stratified by race within center, efficacy failure was similar for Rapamune Oral Solution 2 mg/day and lower for Rapamune Oral Solution 5 mg/day compared to azathioprine in black patients. In Study 2, which was not prospectively stratified by race, efficacy failure was similar for both Rapamune Oral Solution doses compared to placebo in black patients. The decision to use the higher dose of Rapamune Oral Solution in black patients must be weighed against the increased risk of dose-dependent adverse events that were observed with the Rapamune Oral Solution 5 mg dose (see **ADVERSE REACTIONS**).

[See fifth table above]

PERCENTAGE OF EFFICACY FAILURE BY RACE AT 6 MONTHS

Parameter	Rapamune® Oral Solution 2 mg/day	Rapamune® Oral Solution 5 mg/day	Azathioprine 2-3 mg/kg/day	Placebo
Study 1				
Black (n = 166)	34.9 (n = 63)	18.0 (n = 61)	33.3 (n = 42)	
Non-black (n = 553)	14.0 (n = 221)	16.4 (n = 213)	31.9 (n = 119)	
Study 2				
Black (n = 66)	30.8 (n = 26)	33.7 (n = 27)		38.5 (n = 13)
Non-black (n = 510)	29.9 (n = 201)	24.5 (n = 192)		48.7 (n = 117)

Mean glomerular filtration rates (GFR) at one year post transplant were calculated by using the Nankivell equation for all subjects in Studies 1 and 2 who had serum creatinine measured at 12 months. In Studies 1 and 2 mean GFR, at 12 months, were lower in patients treated with cyclosporine and Rapamune Oral Solution compared to those treated with cyclosporine and the respective azathioprine or placebo control.

Within each treatment group in Studies 1 and 2, mean GFR at one year post transplant was lower in patients who experienced at least 1 episode of biopsy-proven acute rejection, compared to those who did not.

Renal function should be monitored and appropriate adjustment of the immunosuppression regimen should be considered in patients with elevated serum creatinine levels (see **PRECAUTIONS**).

OVERALL CALCULATED GLOMERULAR FILTRATION RATES (CC/MIN) BY NANKIVELL EQUATION AT 12 MONTHS POST TRANSPLANT

Parameter	Rapamune® Oral Solution 2 mg/day	Rapamune® Oral Solution 5 mg/day	Azathioprine 2-3 mg/kg/day	Placebo
Study 1	(n = 233)	(n = 226)	(n = 127)	
Mean (SE)	57.4 (1.28)	55.1 (1.28)	65.9 (1.69)	
Study 2	(n = 190)	(n = 175)		(n = 101)
Mean (SE)	54.9 (1.26)	52.9 (1.46)		61.7 (1.81)

Rapamune® Tablets: The safety and efficacy of Rapamune Oral Solution and Rapamune Tablets for the prevention of organ rejection following renal transplantation were compared in a randomized multicenter controlled trial (Study 3). This study compared a single dose level (2 mg, once daily) of Rapamune Oral Solution and Rapamune Tablets when administered in combination with cyclosporine and corticosteroids. The study was conducted at 30 centers in Australia, Canada, and the United States. Four hundred seventy-seven (477) patients were enrolled in this study and randomized before transplantation; 238 patients were randomized to receive Rapamune Oral Solution 2 mg/day and 239 patients were randomized to receive Rapamune Tablets 2 mg/day. In this study, the use of antilymphocyte antibody induction therapy was prohibited. The primary efficacy endpoint was the rate of efficacy failure in the first 3 months after transplantation. Efficacy failure was defined as the first occurrence of an acute rejection episode (confirmed by biopsy), graft loss, or death.

The table below summarizes the result of the primary efficacy analysis at 3 months from this trial. The overall rate of efficacy failure in the tablet treatment group was equivalent to the rate in the oral solution treatment group.

[See first table at top of next page]

The table below summarizes the results of the primary efficacy analysis at 6 months after transplantation.

[See second table at top of next page]

Graft and patient survival at 12 months were co-primary efficacy endpoints. There was no significant difference between the oral solution and tablet formulations for both graft and patient survival. Graft survival was 92.0% and 88.7% for the oral solution and tablet treatment groups, respectively. The patient survival rates in the oral solution and tablet treatment groups were 95.8% and 96.2%, respectively.

The mean GFR at 12 months, calculated by the Nankivell equation, were not significantly different for the oral solution group and for the tablet group.

The table below summarizes the mean GFR at one-year post-transplantation for all subjects in Study 3 who had serum creatinine measured at 12 months.

OVERALL CALCULATED GLOMERULAR FILTRATION RATES (CC/MIN) BY NANKIVELL EQUATION AT 12 MONTHS POST TRANSPLANT: STUDY 3

	Rapamune® Oral Solution	Rapamune® Tablets
Mean (SE)	58.3 (1.64) n = 166	58.5 (1.44) n = 162

INDICATIONS AND USAGE

Rapamune is indicated for the prophylaxis of organ rejection in patients receiving renal transplants. It is recommended that Rapamune be used in a regimen with cyclosporine and corticosteroids.

CONTRAINDICATIONS

Rapamune is contraindicated in patients with a hypersensitivity to sirolimus or its derivatives or any component of the drug product.

WARNINGS

Increased susceptibility to infection and the possible development of lymphoma and other malignancies, particularly of the skin, may result from immunosuppression (see **ADVERSE REACTIONS**). Oversuppression of the immune system can also increase susceptibility to infection including opportunistic infections, fatal infections, and sepsis. Only physicians experienced in immunosuppressive therapy and management of organ transplant patients should use Rapamune. Patients receiving the drug should be managed in facilities equipped and staffed with adequate laboratory and supportive medical resources. The physician responsible for maintenance therapy should have complete information requisite for the follow-up of the patient.

As usual for patients with increased risk for skin cancer, exposure to sunlight and UV light should be limited by wearing protective clothing and using a sunscreen with a high protection factor.

Increased serum cholesterol and triglycerides, that may require treatment, occurred more frequently in patients treated with Rapamune compared to azathioprine or placebo controls (see **PRECAUTIONS**).

In phase III studies, mean serum creatinine was increased and mean glomerular filtration rate was decreased in patients treated with Rapamune and cyclosporine compared to those treated with cyclosporine and placebo or azathioprine controls (see **CLINICAL STUDIES**). Renal function should be monitored during the administration of maintenance immunosuppression regimens including Rapamune in combination with cyclosporine, and appropriate adjustment of the immunosuppression regimen should be considered in patients with elevated serum creatinine levels. Caution should be exercised when using agents which are known to impair renal function (see **PRECAUTIONS**).

In clinical trials, Rapamune has been administered concurrently with corticosteroids and with the following formulations of cyclosporine:

- Sandimmune® Injection (cyclosporine injection)
- Sandimmune® Oral Solution (cyclosporine oral solution)
- Sandimmune® Soft Gelatin Capsules (cyclosporine capsules)
- Neoral® Soft Gelatin Capsules (cyclosporine capsules [MODIFIED])
- Neoral® Oral Solution (cyclosporine oral solution [MODIFIED])

The efficacy and safety of the use of Rapamune in combination with other immunosuppressive agents has not been determined.

Hepatic Artery Thrombosis: In two multicenter, randomized, controlled studies in de novo liver transplant recipients, the use of sirolimus in combination with cyclosporine or tacrolimus was associated with an increase in hepatic artery thrombosis. Most cases occurred within 30 days post-transplantation and most led to graft loss or death. The safety and efficacy of Rapamune® (sirolimus) as immunosuppressive therapy have not been established in liver transplant patients, and therefore, such use is not recommended.

PRECAUTIONS

General

Rapamune is intended for oral administration only.

Lymphocele, a known surgical complication of renal transplantation, occurred significantly more often in a dose-related fashion in Rapamune-treated patients. Appropriate post-operative measures should be considered to minimize this complication.

Lipids

The use of Rapamune® (sirolimus) in renal transplant patients was associated with increased serum cholesterol and triglycerides that may require treatment.

In phase III clinical trials, in *de novo* renal transplant recipients who began the study with normal, fasting, total serum cholesterol (fasting serum cholesterol < 200 mg/dL), there was an increased incidence of hypercholesterolemia (fasting serum cholesterol > 240 mg/dL) in patients receiving both Rapamune® 2 mg and Rapamune® 5 mg compared to azathioprine and placebo controls. In phase III clinical trials, in *de novo* renal transplant recipients who began the study with normal, fasting, total serum triglycerides (fasting serum triglycerides < 200 mg/dL), there was an increased incidence of hypertriglyceridemia (fasting serum triglycerides > 500 mg/dL) in patients receiving Rapamune® 2 mg and Rapamune® 5 mg compared to azathioprine and placebo controls.

Treatment of new-onset hypercholesterolemia with lipid-lowering agents was required in 42 - 52% of patients enrolled in the Rapamune arms of the study compared to 16% of patients in the placebo arm and 22% of patients in the azathioprine arm.

Renal transplant patients have a higher prevalence of clinically significant hyperlipidemia. Accordingly, the risk/benefit should be carefully considered in patients with established hyperlipidemia before initiating an immunosuppressive regimen including Rapamune.

Any patient who is administered Rapamune should be monitored for hyperlipidemia using laboratory tests and if hyperlipidemia is detected, subsequent interventions such as diet, exercise, and lipid-lowering agents, as outlined by the National Cholesterol Education Program guidelines, should be initiated.

In clinical trials, the concomitant administration of Rapamune and HMG-CoA reductase inhibitors and/or fibrates appeared to be well tolerated.

During Rapamune therapy with cyclosporine, patients administered an HMG-CoA reductase inhibitor and/or fibrate should be monitored for the possible development of rhabdomyolysis and other adverse effects as described in the respective labeling for these agents.

Renal Function

Patients treated with cyclosporine and Rapamune were noted to have higher serum creatinine levels and lower glomerular filtration rates compared with patients treated with cyclosporine and placebo or azathioprine controls. Renal function should be monitored during the administration of maintenance immunosuppression regimens including Rapamune in combination with cyclosporine, and appropriate adjustment of the immunosuppression regimen should be considered in patients with elevated serum creatinine levels. Caution should be exercised when using agents (e.g., aminoglycosides, and amphotericin B) that are known to have a deleterious effect on renal function.

Antimicrobial Prophylaxis

Cases of *Pneumocystis carinii* pneumonia have been reported in patients not receiving antimicrobial prophylaxis. Therefore, antimicrobial prophylaxis for *Pneumocystis carinii* pneumonia should be administered for 1 year following transplantation.

Cytomegalovirus (CMV) prophylaxis is recommended for 3 months after transplantation, particularly for patients at increased risk for CMV disease.

Information for Patients

Patients should be given complete dosage instructions (see **Patient Instructions**). Women of childbearing potential should be informed of the potential risks during pregnancy and that they should use effective contraception prior to initiation of Rapamune therapy, during Rapamune therapy and for 12 weeks after Rapamune therapy has been stopped (see **PRECAUTIONS: Pregnancy**).

Patients should be told that exposure to sunlight and UV light should be limited by wearing protective clothing and using a sunscreen with a high protection factor because of the increased risk for skin cancer (see **WARNINGS**).

Laboratory Tests

It is prudent to monitor blood sirolimus levels in patients likely to have altered drug metabolism, in patients ≥13 years who weigh less than 40 kg, in patients with hepatic impairment, and during concurrent administration of potent CYP3A4 inducers and inhibitors (see **PRECAUTIONS: Drug Interactions**).

Drug Interactions

Sirolimus is known to be a substrate for both cytochrome CYP3A4 and P-glycoprotein. The pharmacokinetic interaction between sirolimus and concomitantly administered drugs is discussed below. Drug interaction studies have not been conducted with drugs other than those described below.

Cyclosporine capsules MODIFIED:

Rapamune Oral Solution: In a single dose drug-drug interaction study, 24 healthy volunteers were administered 10 mg sirolimus either simultaneously or 4 hours after a 300 mg dose of Neoral® Soft Gelatin Capsules (cyclosporine capsules [MODIFIED]). For simultaneous administration, the mean C_{max} and AUC of sirolimus were increased by 116% and 230%, respectively, relative to administration of sirolimus alone. However, when given 4 hours after Neoral® Soft Gelatin Capsules (cyclosporine capsules [MODIFIED]) administration, sirolimus C_{max} and AUC were increased by 37% and 80%, respectively, compared to administration of sirolimus alone.

Mean cyclosporine C_{max} and AUC were not significantly affected when sirolimus was given simultaneously or when administered 4 hours after Neoral® Soft Gelatin Capsules (cyclosporine capsules [MODIFIED]). However, after multiple-dose administration of sirolimus given 4 hours after Neoral® in renal post-transplant patients over 6 months, cyclosporine oral-dose clearance was reduced, and lower doses of Neoral® Soft Gelatin Capsules (cyclosporine capsules [MODIFIED]) were needed to maintain target cyclosporine concentration.

Rapamune (sirolimus) Tablets: In a single-dose drug-drug interaction study, 24 healthy volunteers were administered 10 mg sirolimus (Rapamune Tablets) either simultaneously or 4 hours after a 300 mg dose of Neoral® Soft Gelatin Capsules (cyclosporine capsules [MODIFIED]). For simultaneous administration, mean C_{max} and AUC were increased by 512% and 148%, respectively, relative to administration of sirolimus alone. However, when given 4 hours after cyclosporine administration, sirolimus C_{max} and AUC were both increased by only 33% compared with administration of sirolimus alone.

Because of the effect of cyclosporine capsules (MODIFIED), it is recommended that sirolimus should be taken 4 hours after administration of cyclosporine oral solution (MODIFIED) and/or cyclosporine capsules (MODIFIED), (see DOSAGE AND ADMINISTRATION).

INCIDENCE (%) OF THE PRIMARY ENDPOINT AT 3 MONTHS: STUDY 3[a]

	Rapamune® Oral Solution (n = 238)	Rapamune® Tablets (n = 239)
Efficacy Failure at 3 months	23.5	24.7
Components of efficacy failure		
Biopsy-proven acute rejection	18.9	17.6
Graft loss	3.4	6.3
Death	1.3	0.8

a: Patients received cyclosporine and corticosteroids.

INCIDENCE (%) OF THE PRIMARY ENDPOINT AT 6 MONTHS: STUDY 3[a]

	Rapamune® Oral Solution (n = 238)	Rapamune® Tablets (n = 239)
Efficacy Failure at 6 months	26.1	27.2
Components of efficacy failure		
Biopsy-proven acute rejection	21.0	19.2
Graft loss	3.4	6.3
Death	1.7	1.7

a: Patients received cyclosporine and corticosteroids.

Cyclosporine oral solution: In a multiple-dose study in 150 psoriasis patients, sirolimus 0.5, 1.5, and 3 mg/m²/day was administered simultaneously with Sandimmune® Oral Solution (cyclosporine Oral Solution) 1.25 mg/kg/day. The increase in average sirolimus trough concentrations ranged between 67% to 86% relative to when sirolimus was administered without cyclosporine. The intersubject variability (%CV) for sirolimus trough concentrations ranged from 39.7% to 68.7%. There was no significant effect of multiple-dose sirolimus on cyclosporine trough concentrations following Sandimmune® Oral Solution (cyclosporine oral solution) administration. However, the %CV was higher (range 85.9% - 165%) than those from previous studies.

Sandimmune® Oral Solution (cyclosporine oral solution) is not bioequivalent to Neoral® Oral Solution (cyclosporine oral solution MODIFIED), and should not be used interchangeably. Although there is no published data comparing Sandimmune® Oral Solution (cyclosporine oral solution) to SangCya® Oral Solution (cyclosporine oral solution [MODIFIED]), they should not be used interchangeably. Likewise, Sandimmune® Soft Gelatin Capsules (cyclosporine capsules) are not bioequivalent to Neoral® Soft Gelatin Capsules (cyclosporine capsules [MODIFIED]) and should not be used interchangeably.

Diltiazem: The simultaneous oral administration of 10 mg of sirolimus oral solution and 120 mg of diltiazem to 18 healthy volunteers significantly affected the bioavailability of sirolimus. Sirolimus C_{max}, t_{max}, and AUC were increased 1.4-, 1.3-, and 1.6-fold, respectively. Sirolimus did not affect the pharmacokinetics of either diltiazem or its metabolites desacetyldiltiazem and desmethyldiltiazem. If diltiazem is administered, sirolimus should be monitored and a dose adjustment may be necessary.

Ketoconazole: Multiple-dose ketoconazole administration significantly affected the rate and extent of absorption and sirolimus exposure after administration of Rapamune Oral Solution, as reflected by increases in sirolimus C_{max}, t_{max}, and AUC of 4.3-fold, 38%, and 10.9-fold, respectively. However, the terminal $t_{1/2}$ of sirolimus was not changed. Single-dose sirolimus did not affect steady-state 12-hour plasma ketoconazole concentrations. It is recommended that sirolimus oral solution and oral tablets should not be administered with ketoconazole.

Rifampin: Pretreatment of 14 healthy volunteers with multiple doses of rifampin, 600 mg daily for 14 days, followed by a single 20 mg-dose of sirolimus, greatly increased sirolimus oral-dose clearance by 5.5-fold (range = 2.8 to 10), which represents mean decreases in AUC and C_{max} of about 82% and 71%, respectively. In patients where rifampin is indicated, alternative therapeutic agents with less enzyme induction potential should be considered.

Drugs which may be coadministered without dose adjustment

Clinically significant pharmacokinetic drug-drug interactions were not observed in studies of drugs listed below. A synopsis of the type of study performed for each drug is provided. Sirolimus and these drugs may be coadministered without dose adjustments.

Acyclovir: Acyclovir, 200 mg, was administered once daily for 3 days followed by a single 10-mg dose of sirolimus oral solution on day 3 in 20 adult healthy volunteers.

Digoxin: Digoxin, 0.25 mg, was administered daily for 8 days and a single 10-mg dose of sirolimus oral solution was given on day 8 to 24 healthy volunteers.

Glyburide: A single 5-mg dose of glyburide and a single 10-mg dose of sirolimus oral solution were administered to 24 healthy volunteers. Sirolimus did not affect the hypoglycemic action of glyburide.

Nifedipine: A single 60-mg dose of nifedipine and a single 10-mg dose of sirolimus oral solution were administered to 24 healthy volunteers.

Norgestrel/ethinyl estradiol (Lo/Ovral®): Sirolimus oral solution, 2 mg, was given daily for 7 days to 21 healthy female volunteers on norgestrel/ethinyl estradiol.

Continued on next page

Rapamune—Cont.

Prednisolone: Pharmacokinetic information was obtained from 42 stable renal transplant patients receiving daily doses of prednisone (5–20 mg/day) and either single or multiple doses of sirolimus oral solution (0.5-5 mg/m^2 q 12h).

Sulfamethoxazole/trimethoprim (Bactrim®): A single oral dose of sulfamethoxazole (400 mg)/trimethoprim (80 mg) was given to 15 renal transplant patients receiving daily oral doses of sirolimus (8 to 25 mg/m^2).

Other drug interactions

Sirolimus is extensively metabolized by the CYP3A4 isoenzyme in the gut wall and liver. Therefore, absorption and the subsequent elimination of systemically absorbed sirolimus may be influenced by drugs that affect this isoenzyme. Inhibitors of CYP3A4 may decrease the metabolism of sirolimus and increase sirolimus levels, while inducers of CYP3A4 may increase the metabolism of sirolimus and decrease sirolimus levels.

Drugs that may increase sirolimus blood concentrations include:

Calcium channel blockers: nicardipine, verapamil.

Antifungal agents: clotrimazole, fluconazole, itraconazole.

Macrolide antibiotics: clarithromycin, erythromycin, troleandomycin.

Gastrointestinal prokinetic agents: cisapride, metoclopramide.

Other drugs: bromocriptine, cimetidine, danazol, HIV-protease inhibitors (e.g., ritonavir, indinavir).

Drugs that may decrease sirolimus levels include:

Anticonvulsants: carbamazepine, phenobarbital, phenytoin.

Antibiotics: rifabutin, rifapentine.

This list is not all inclusive.

Care should be exercised when drugs or other substances that are metabolized by CYP3A4 are administered concomitantly with Rapamune. Grapefruit juice reduces CYP3A4-mediated metabolism of Rapamune and must not be used for dilution (see **DOSAGE AND ADMINISTRATION**).

Herbal Preparations

St John's Wort *(hypericum perforatum)* induces CYP3A4 and P-glycoprotein. Since sirolimus is a substrate for both cytochrome CYP3A4 and P-glycoprotein, there is the potential that the use of St. John's Wort in patients receiving Rapamune could result in reduced sirolimus levels.

Vaccination

Immunosuppressants may affect response to vaccination. Therefore, during treatment with Rapamune, vaccination may be less effective. The use of live vaccines should be avoided; live vaccines may include, but are not limited to measles, mumps, rubella, oral polio, BCG, yellow fever, varicella, and TY21a typhoid.

Drug-Laboratory Test Interactions

There are no studies on the interactions of sirolimus in commonly employed clinical laboratory tests.

Carcinogenesis, Mutagenesis, and Impairment of Fertility

Sirolimus was not genotoxic in the *in vitro* bacterial reverse mutation assay, the Chinese hamster ovary cell chromosomal aberration assay, the mouse lymphoma cell forward mutation assay, or the *in vivo* mouse micronucleus assay.

Carcinogenicity studies were conducted in mice and rats. In an 86-week female mouse study at dosages of 0, 12.5, 25 and 50/6 (dosage lowered from 50 to 6 mg/kg/day at week 31 due to infection secondary to immunosuppression) there was a statistically significant increase in malignant lymphoma at all dose levels (approximately 16 to 135 times the clinical doses adjusted for body surface area) compared to controls. In a second mouse study at dosages of 0, 1, 3 and 6 mg/kg (approximately 3 to 16 times the clinical dose adjusted for body surface area), hepatocellular adenoma and carcinoma (males), were considered Rapamune related. In the 104-week rat study at dosages of 0, 0.05, 0.1, and 0.2 mg/kg/day (approximately 0.4 to 1 times the clinical dose adjusted for body surface area), there was a statistically significant increased incidence of testicular adenoma in the 0.2 mg/kg/day group.

There was no effect on fertility in female rats following the administration of sirolimus at dosages up to 0.5 mg/kg (approximately 1 to 3 times the clinical doses adjusted for body surface area). In male rats, there was no significant difference in fertility rate compared to controls at a dosage of 2 mg/kg (approximately 4 to 11 times the clinical doses adjusted for body surface area). Reductions in testicular weights and/or histological lesions (e.g., tubular atrophy and tubular giant cells) were observed in rats following dosages of 0.65 mg/kg (approximately 1 to 3 times the clinical doses adjusted for body surface area) and above and in a monkey study at 0.1 mg/kg (approximately 0.4 to 1 times the clinical doses adjusted for body surface area) and above. Sperm counts were reduced in male rats following the administration of sirolimus for 13 weeks at a dosage of 6 mg/kg (approximately 12 to 32 times the clinical doses adjusted for body surface area), but showed improvement by 3 months after dosing was stopped.

Pregnancy

Pregnancy Category C: Sirolimus was embryo/feto toxic in rats at dosages of 0.1 mg/kg and above (approximately 0.2 to 0.5 the clinical doses adjusted for body surface area). Embryo/feto toxicity was manifested as mortality and reduced fetal weights (with associated delays in skeletal ossification). However, no teratogenesis was evident. In combination with cyclosporine, rats had increased embryo/feto mortality compared to Rapamune alone. There were no effects on rabbit development at the maternally toxic dosage of 0.05 mg/kg (approximately 0.3 to 0.8 times the clinical doses adjusted for body surface area). There are no adequate and well controlled studies in pregnant women. Effective contraception must be initiated before Rapamune therapy, during Rapamune therapy, and for 12 weeks after Rapamune therapy has been stopped. Rapamune should be used during pregnancy only if the potential benefit outweighs the potential risk to the embryo/fetus.

ADVERSE EVENTS OCCURRING AT A FREQUENCY OF ≥ 20% IN ANY TREATMENT GROUP IN PREVENTION OF ACUTE RENAL REJECTION TRIALS (%)[a] AT ≥ 12 MONTHS POST-TRANSPLANTATION FOR STUDIES 1 AND 2

Body System Adverse Event	Rapamune® Oral Solution —2 mg/day— Study 1 (n = 281)	Rapamune® Oral Solution —2 mg/day— Study 2 (n = 218)	Rapamune® Oral Solution —5 mg/day— Study 1 (n = 269)	Rapamune® Oral Solution —5 mg/day— Study 2 (n = 208)	Azathioprine 2-3 mg/kg/day Study 1 (n = 160)	Placebo Study 2 (n = 124)
Body As A Whole						
Abdominal pain	28	29	30	36	29	30
Asthenia	38	22	40	28	37	28
Back pain	16	23	26	22	23	20
Chest pain	16	18	19	24	16	19
Fever	27	23	33	34	33	35
Headache	23	34	27	34	21	31
Pain	24	33	29	29	30	25
Cardiovascular System						
Hypertension	43	45	39	49	29	48
Digestive System						
Constipation	28	36	34	38	37	31
Diarrhea	32	25	42	35	28	27
Dyspepsia	17	23	23	25	24	34
Nausea	31	25	36	31	39	29
Vomiting	21	19	25	25	31	21
Hemic And Lymphatic System						
Anemia	27	23	37	33	29	21
Leukopenia	9	9	15	13	20	8
Thrombocytopenia	13	14	20	30	9	9
Metabolic And Nutritional						
Creatinine increased	35	39	37	40	28	38
Edema	24	20	16	18	23	15
Hypercholesteremia (See **WARNINGS** and **PRECAUTIONS**)	38	43	42	46	33	23
Hyperkalemia	15	17	12	14	24	27
Hyperlipemia (See **WARNINGS** and **PRECAUTIONS**)	38	45	44	57	28	23
Hypokalemia	17	11	21	17	11	9
Hypophosphatemia	20	15	23	19	20	19
Peripheral edema	60	54	64	58	58	48
Weight gain	21	11	15	8	19	15
Musculoskeletal System						
Arthralgia	25	25	27	31	21	18
Nervous System						
Insomnia	14	13	22	14	18	8
Tremor	31	21	30	22	28	19
Respiratory System						
Dyspnea	22	24	28	30	23	30
Pharyngitis	17	16	16	21	17	22
Upper respiratory infection	20	26	24	23	13	23
Skin And Appendages						
Acne	31	22	20	22	17	19
Rash	12	10	13	20	6	6
Urogenital System						
Urinary tract infection	20	26	23	33	31	26

a: Patients received cyclosporine and corticosteroids.

Use during lactation

Sirolimus is excreted in trace amounts in milk of lactating rats. It is not known whether sirolimus is excreted in human milk. The pharmacokinetic and safety profiles of sirolimus in infants are not known. Because many drugs are excreted in human milk and because of the potential for adverse reactions in nursing infants from sirolimus, a decision should be made whether to discontinue nursing or to discontinue the drug, taking into account the importance of the drug to the mother.

Pediatric use

The safety and efficacy of Rapamune in pediatric patients below the age of 13 years have not been established.

Geriatric use

Clinical studies of Rapamune Oral Solution or Tablets did not include sufficient numbers of patients aged 65 years and over to determine whether safety and efficacy differ in this population from younger patients. Data pertaining to sirolimus trough concentrations suggest that dose adjustments based upon age in geriatric renal patients are not necessary.

ADVERSE REACTIONS

Rapamune® Oral Solution: The incidence of adverse reactions was determined in two randomized, double-blind, multicenter controlled trials in which 499 renal transplant patients received Rapamune Oral Solution 2 mg/day, 477 received Rapamune Oral Solution 5 mg/day, 160 received azathioprine, and 124 received placebo. All patients were treated with cyclosporine and corticosteroids. Data (≥ 12 months post-transplant) presented in the table below show the adverse reactions that occurred in any treatment group with an incidence of ≥ 20%.

Specific adverse reactions associated with the administration of Rapamune (sirolimus) Oral Solution occurred at a significantly higher frequency than in the respective control group. For both Rapamune Oral Solution 2 mg/day and 5 mg/day these include hypercholesterolemia, hyperlipemia, hypertension, and rash; for Rapamune Oral Solution 2 mg/day acne; and for Rapamune Oral Solution 5 mg/day anemia, arthralgia, diarrhea, hypokalemia, and thrombocytopenia. The elevations of triglycerides and cholesterol and decreases in platelets and hemoglobin occurred in a dose-related manner in patients receiving Rapamune.

Patients maintained on Rapamune Oral Solution 5 mg/day, when compared to patients on Rapamune Oral Solution 2 mg/day, demonstrated an increased incidence of the following adverse events: anemia, leukopenia, thrombocytopenia, hypokalemia, hyperlipemia, fever, and diarrhea.

In general, adverse events related to the administration of Rapamune were dependent on dose/concentration.

[See table above]

At 12 months, there were no significant differences in incidence rates for clinically important opportunistic or common transplant-related infections across treatment groups, with the exception of mucosal infections with *Herpes simplex*, which occurred at a significantly greater rate in patients treated with Rapamune (sirolimus) 5 mg/day than in both of the comparator groups.

The table below summarizes the incidence of malignancies in the two controlled trials for the prevention of acute rejection. At 12 months following transplantation, there was a very low incidence of malignancies and there were no significant differences among treatment groups.

[See table at top of next page]

Among the adverse events that were reported at a rate of ≥3% and <20%, the following were more prominent in patients maintained on Rapamune 5 mg/day, when compared to patients on Rapamune 2 mg/day: epistaxis, lymphocele, insomnia, thrombotic thrombocytopenic purpura (hemolytic-uremic syndrome), skin ulcer, increased LDH, hypotension, facial edema.

The following adverse events were reported with ≥3% and <20% incidence in patients in any Rapamune treatment group in the two controlled trials for the prevention of acute rejection, BODY AS A WHOLE: abdomen enlarged, abscess, ascites, cellulitis, chills, face edema, flu syndrome, generalized edema, hernia, *Herpes zoster* infection, lymphocele, malaise, pelvic pain, peritonitis, sepsis; CARDIOVASCULAR SYSTEM: atrial fibrillation, congestive heart failure, hemorrhage, hypervolemia, hypotension, palpitation, peripheral vascular disorder, postural hypotension, syncope, tachycardia, thrombophlebitis, thrombosis, vasodilatation; DIGESTIVE SYSTEM: anorexia, dysphagia, eructation, esophagitis, flatulence, gastritis, gastroenteritis, gingivitis, gum hyperplasia, ileus, liver function tests abnormal, mouth ulceration, oral moniliasis, stomatitis; ENDOCRINE SYSTEM: Cushing's syndrome, diabetes mellitus, glycosuria; HEMIC AND LYMPHATIC SYSTEM: ecchymosis, leukocytosis, lymphadenopathy, polycythemia, thrombotic thrombocytopenic purpura (hemolytic-uremic syndrome); METABOLIC AND NUTRITIONAL: acidosis, alkaline phosphatase increased, BUN increased, creatine phosphokinase increased, dehydration, healing abnormal, hypercalcemia, hyperglycemia, hyperphosphatemia, hypocalcemia, hypoglycemia, hypomagnesemia, hyponatremia, lactic dehydrogenase increased, SGOT increased, SGPT increased, weight loss; MUSCULOSKELETAL SYSTEM: arthrosis, bone necrosis, leg cramps, myalgia, osteoporosis, tetany; NERVOUS SYSTEM: anxiety, confusion, depression, dizziness, emotional lability, hypertonia, hypesthesia, hypotonia, insomnia, neuropathy, paresthesia, somnolence; RESPIRATORY SYSTEM: asthma, atelectasis, bronchitis, cough increased, epistaxis, hypoxia, lung edema, pleural effusion, pneumonia, rhinitis, sinusitis; SKIN AND APPENDAGES: fungal dermatitis, hirsutism, pruritus, skin hypertrophy, skin ulcer, sweating; SPECIAL SENSES: abnormal vision, cataract, conjunctivitis, deafness, ear pain, otitis media, tinnitus; UROGENITAL SYSTEM: albuminuria, bladder pain, dysuria, hematuria, hydronephrosis, impotence, kidney pain, kidney tubular necrosis, nocturia, oliguria, pyelonephritis, pyuria, scrotal edema, testis disorder, toxic nephropathy, urinary frequency, urinary incontinence, urinary retention.

Less frequently occurring adverse events included: mycobacterial infections, Epstein-Barr virus infections, and pancreatitis.

Rapamune® Tablets: The safety profile of the tablet did not differ from that of the oral solution formulation. The incidence of adverse reactions up to 12 months was determined in a randomized, multicenter controlled trial (Study 3) in which 229 renal transplant patients received Rapamune Oral Solution 2 mg once daily and 228 patients received Rapamune Tablets 2 mg once daily. All patients were treated with cyclosporine and corticosteroids. The adverse reactions that occurred in either treatment group with an incidence of ≥20% in Study 3 are similar to those reported for Studies 1 & 2. There was no notable difference in the incidence of these adverse events between treatment groups (oral solution versus tablets) in Study 3, with the exception of acne, which occurred more frequently in the oral solution group, and tremor which occurred more frequently in the tablet group, particularly in Black patients. The adverse events that occurred in patients with an incidence of ≥3% and <20% in either treatment group in Study 3 were similar to those reported in Studies 1 & 2. There was no notable difference in the incidence of these adverse events between treatment groups (oral solution versus tablets) in Study 3, with the exception of hypertonia, which occurred more frequently in the oral solution group and diabetes mellitus which occurred more frequently in the tablet group. Hispanic patients in the tablet group experienced hyperglycemia more frequently than Hispanic patients in the oral solution group. In Study 3 alone, menorrhagia, metrorrhagia, and polyuria occurred with an incidence of ≥3% and <20%.

The clinically important opportunistic or common transplant-related infections were identical in all three studies and the incidences of these infections were similar in Study 3 compared with Studies 1 & 2. The incidence rates of these infections were not significantly different between the oral solution and tablet treatment groups in Study 3.

In Study 3 (at 12 months), there were two cases of lymphoma/lymphoproliferative disorder in the oral solution treatment group (0.8%) and two reported cases of lymphoma/lymphoproliferative disorder in the tablet treatment group (0.8%). These differences were not statistically significant and were similar to the incidences observed in Studies 1 & 2.

Other clinical experience: Cases of interstitial lung disease [including pneumonitis, and infrequently bronchiolitis obliterans organizing pneumonia (BOOP) and pulmonary fibrosis], some fatal, with no identified infectious etiology have occurred in patients receiving immunosuppressive regimens including Rapamune. In some cases, the interstitial lung disease has resolved upon discontinuation or dose reduction of Rapamune. The risk may be increased as the trough Rapamune level increases.

There have been rare reports of pancytopenia.

Hepatotoxicity has been reported, including fatal hepatic necrosis with elevated sirolimus trough levels.

Abnormal healing following transplant surgery has been reported, including fascial dehiscence and anastomatic disruption (e.g., wound, vascular, airway, ureteral, biliary).

OVERDOSAGE

There is minimal experience with overdose. During clinical trials, there were two accidental Rapamune ingestions, of 120 mg and 150 mg. One patient, receiving 150 mg, experienced an episode of transient atrial fibrillation. The other patient experienced no adverse effects. In general, the adverse effects of overdose are consistent with those listed in the **ADVERSE REACTIONS** section (see **ADVERSE REACTIONS**).

General supportive measures should be followed in all cases of overdose. Based on the poor aqueous solubility and high erythrocyte and plasma protein binding of Rapamune, it is anticipated that Rapamune is not dialyzable to any significant extent. In mice and rats, the acute oral lethal dose was greater than 800 mg/kg.

INCIDENCE (%) OF MALIGNANCIES IN PREVENTION OF ACUTE RENAL REJECTION TRIALS: AT 12 MONTHS POST-TRANSPLANT[a]

Malignancy	Rapamune® Oral Solution 2 mg/day (n = 511)	Rapamune® Oral Solution 5 mg/day (n = 493)	Azathioprine 2-3 mg/kg/day (n = 161)	Placebo (n = 130)
Lymphoma/lymphoproliferative disease	0.4	1.4	0.6	0
Non-melanoma skin carcinoma	0.4	1.4	1.2	3.1
Other malignancy	0.6	0.6	0	0

a: Patients received cyclosporine and corticosteroids.

DOSAGE AND ADMINISTRATION

It is recommended that Rapamune Oral Solution and Tablets be used in a regimen with cyclosporine and corticosteroids. Two-mg Rapamune oral solution has been demonstrated to be clinically equivalent to 2-mg Rapamune oral tablets; hence, are interchangeable on a mg to mg basis. However, it is not known if higher doses of Rapamune oral solution are clinically equivalent to higher doses of tablets on a mg to mg basis. (See **CLINICAL PHARMACOLOGY: Absorption**). Rapamune is to be administered orally once daily. The initial dose of Rapamune should be administered as soon as possible after transplantation. For *de novo* transplant recipients, a loading dose of Rapamune of 3 times the maintenance dose should be given. A daily maintenance dose of 2 mg is recommended for use in renal transplant patients, with a loading dose of 6 mg. Although a daily maintenance dose of 5 mg, with a loading dose of 15 mg was used in clinical trials of the oral solution and was shown to be safe and effective, no efficacy advantage over the 2 mg dose could be established for renal transplant patients. Patients receiving 2 mg of Rapamune Oral Solution per day demonstrated an overall better safety profile than did patients receiving 5 mg of Rapamune Oral Solution per day.

To minimize the variability of exposure to Rapamune, this drug should be taken consistently with or without food. Grapefruit juice reduces CYP3A4-mediated metabolism of Rapamune and must not be administered with Rapamune or used for dilution.

It is recommended that sirolimus be taken 4 hours after administration of cyclosporine oral solution (MODIFIED) and/or cyclosporine capsules (MODIFIED).

Dosage Adjustments

The initial dosage in patients ≥13 years who weigh less than 40 kg should be adjusted, based on body surface area, to 1 mg/m^2/day. The loading dose should be 3 mg/m^2.

It is recommended that the maintenance dose of Rapamune be reduced by approximately one third in patients with hepatic impairment. It is not necessary to modify the Rapamune loading dose. Dosage need not be adjusted because of impaired renal function.

Blood Concentration Monitoring

Routine therapeutic drug level monitoring is not required in most patients. Blood sirolimus levels should be monitored in pediatric patients, in patients with hepatic impairment, during concurrent administration of strong CYP3A4 inducers and inhibitors, and/or if cyclosporine dosing is markedly reduced or discontinued. In controlled clinical trials with concomitant cyclosporine, mean sirolimus whole blood trough levels, as measured by immunoassay, were 9 ng/mL (range 4.5 – 14 ng/mL [10th to 90th percentile]) for the 2 mg/day treatment group, and 17 ng/mL (range 10 - 28 ng/mL [10th to 90th percentile]) for the 5 mg/day dose.

Results from other assays may differ from those with an immunoassay. On average, chromatographic methods (HPLC UV or LC/MS/MS) yield results that are approximately 20% lower than the immunoassay for whole blood concentration determinations. Adjustments to the targeted range should be made according to the assay utilized to determine sirolimus trough concentrations. Therefore, comparison between concentrations in the published literature and an individual patient concentration using current assays must be made with detailed knowledge of the assay methods employed. A discussion of the different assay methods is contained in *Clinical Therapeutics*, Volume 22, Supplement B, April 2000.

Instructions for Dilution and Administration of Rapamune® Oral Solution

Bottles

The amber oral dose syringe should be used to withdraw the prescribed amount of Rapamune® Oral Solution from the bottle. Empty the correct amount of Rapamune from the syringe into only a glass or plastic container holding at least two (2) ounces (1/4 cup, 60 mL) of water or orange juice. No other liquids, including grapefruit juice, should be used for dilution. Stir vigorously and drink at once. Refill the container with an additional volume (minimum of four [4] ounces (1/2 cup, 120 mL)) of water or orange juice, stir vigorously, and drink at once.

Pouches

When using the pouch, squeeze the entire contents of the pouch into only a glass or plastic container holding at least two (2) ounces (1/4 cup, 60 mL) of water or orange juice. No other liquids, including grapefruit juice, should be used for dilution. Stir vigorously and drink at once. Refill the container with an additional volume (minimum of four [4] ounces (1/2 cup, 120 mL)) of water or orange juice, stir vigorously, and drink at once.

Handling and Disposal

Since Rapamune is not absorbed through the skin, there are no special precautions. However, if direct contact with the skin or mucous membranes occurs, wash thoroughly with soap and water; rinse eyes with plain water.

HOW SUPPLIED

Rapamune® Oral Solution is supplied at a concentration of 1 mg/mL in:

1. Cartons:
   NDC # 0008-1030-06, containing a 2 oz (60 mL fill) amber glass bottle.
   NDC # 0008-1030-15, containing a 5 oz (150 mL fill) amber glass bottle.

In addition to the bottles, each carton is supplied with an oral syringe adapter for fitting into the neck of the bottle, sufficient disposable amber oral syringes and caps for daily dosing, and a carrying case.

2. Cartons:
   NDC # 0008-1030-03, containing 30 unit-of-use laminated aluminum pouches of 1 mL.
   NDC # 0008-1030-07, containing 30 unit-of-use laminated aluminum pouches of 2 mL.
   NDC # 0008-1030-08, containing 30 unit-of-use laminated aluminum pouches of 5 mL.

Rapamune® Tablets are available as follows: 1 mg, white, triangular-shaped tablets marked "RAPAMUNE 1 mg" on one side.

NDC # 0008-1031-05, bottle of 100 tablets.
NDC # 0008-1031-10, Redipak® cartons of 100 tablets (10 blister cards of 10 tablets each).

Storage

Rapamune® Oral Solution bottles and pouches should be stored protected from light and refrigerated at 2°C to 8°C (36°F to 46°F). Once the bottle is opened, the contents should be used within one month. If necessary, the patient may store both the pouches and the bottles at room temperatures up to 25°C (77°F) for a short period of time (e.g., up to 24 hours for the pouches and not more than 15 days for the bottles).

An amber syringe and cap are provided for dosing and the product may be kept in the syringe for a maximum of 24 hours at room temperatures up to 25°C (77°F) or refrigerated at 2°C to 8°C (36°F to 46°F). The syringe should be discarded after one use. After dilution, the preparation should be used immediately.

Rapamune Oral Solution provided in bottles may develop a slight haze when refrigerated. If such a haze occurs allow the product to stand at room temperature and shake gently until the haze disappears. The presence of this haze does not affect the quality of the product.

Rapamune® Tablets should be stored at 20° to 25°C (USP Controlled Room Temperature) (68° - 77°F). Use cartons to protect blister cards and strips from light. Dispense in a tight, light-resistant container as defined in the USP.

℞ only

US Pat. Nos.: 5,100,899; 5,212,155; 5,308,847; 5,403,833; 5,536,729.

PATIENT INSTRUCTIONS FOR RAPAMUNE® (SIROLIMUS) ORAL SOLUTION ADMINISTRATION

Bottles

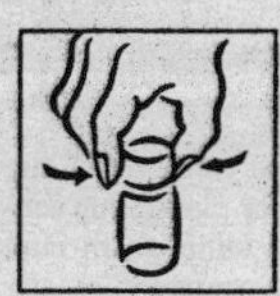

1. Open the solution bottle. Remove the safety cap by squeezing the tabs on the cap and twisting counterclockwise.

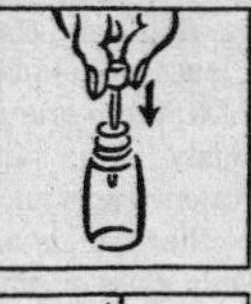

2. On first use, insert the adapter assembly (plastic tube with stopper) tightly into the bottle until it is even with the top of the bottle. Do not remove the adapter assembly from the bottle once inserted.

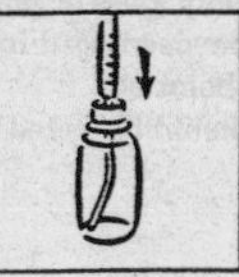

3. For each use, tightly insert one of the amber syringes with the plunger fully depressed into the opening in the adapter.

Continued on next page

Rapamune—Cont.

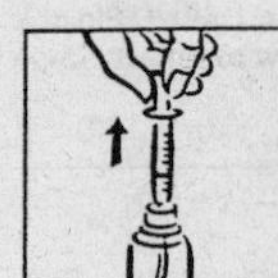

4. Withdraw the prescribed amount of Rapamune® (sirolimus) Oral Solution by gently pulling out the plunger of the syringe until the bottom of the black line of the plunger is even with the appropriate mark on the syringe. Always keep the bottle in an upright position. If bubbles form in the syringe, empty the syringe into the bottle and repeat the procedure.

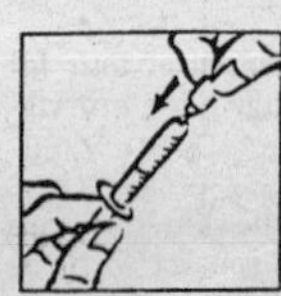

5. You may have been instructed to carry your medication with you. If it is necessary to carry the filled syringe, place a cap securely on the syringe—the cap should snap into place.

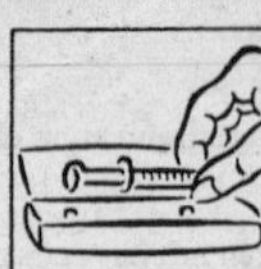

6. Then place the capped syringe in the enclosed carrying case. Once in the syringe, the medication may be kept at room temperature or refrigerated and should be used within 24 hours. Extreme temperatures (below 36°F and above 86°F) should be avoided. Remember to keep this medication out of the reach of children.

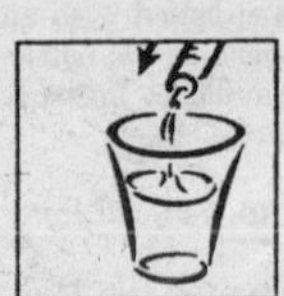

7. Empty the syringe into a glass or plastic cup containing at least 2 ounces (1/4 cup; 60 mL) of water or orange juice, stir vigorously for one (1) minute and drink immediately. Refill the container with at least 4 ounces (1/2 cup; 120 mL) of water or orange juice, stir vigorously again and drink the rinse solution. Apple juice, grapefruit juice, or other liquids are NOT to be used. Only glass or plastic cups should be used to dilute Rapamune® Oral Solution. The syringe and cap should be used once and then discarded.

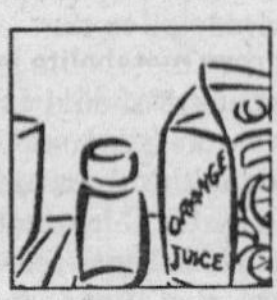

8. Always store the bottles of medication in the refrigerator. When refrigerated, a slight haze may develop in the solution. The presence of a haze does not affect the quality of the product. If this happens, bring the Rapamune® Oral Solution to room temperature and shake until the haze disappears. If it is necessary to wipe clean the mouth of the bottle before returning the product to the refrigerator, wipe with a dry cloth to avoid introducing water, or any other liquid, into the bottle.

PATIENT INSTRUCTIONS FOR RAPAMUNE® (SIROLIMUS) ORAL SOLUTION ADMINISTRATION

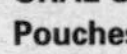

Pouches

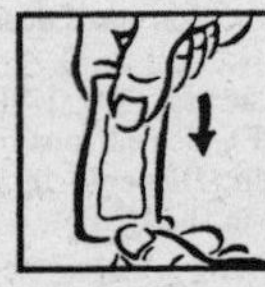

1. Before opening the pouch, squeeze the pouch from the neck area to push the contents into the lower part of the pouch.

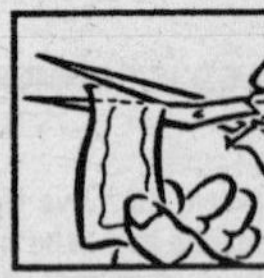

2. Carefully open the pouch by folding the marked area and then cutting with a scissors along the marked line near the top of the pouch.

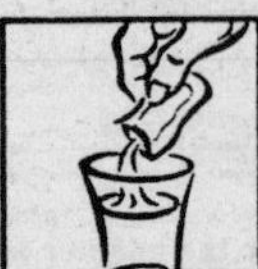

3. Squeeze the entire contents of the pouch into a glass or plastic cup containing at least 2 ounces (1/4 cup; 60 mL) of water or orange juice, stir vigorously for one (1) minute and drink immediately. Refill the container with at least 4 ounces (1/2 cup, 120 mL) of water or orange juice, stir vigorously again and drink the rinse solution. Apple juice, grapefruit juice or other liquids are NOT to be used. Only glass or plastic cups should be used to dilute Rapamune® Oral Solution.
4. Unused pouches should be stored in the refrigerator.

Wyeth Laboratories
Division of Wyeth-Ayerst Pharmaceuticals Inc.
Philadelphia PA 19101
CI 7713-1 Revised April 8, 2002

SONATA® ℂ ℞

[sō' nă-tă]
(zaleplon)
Capsules

Prescribing information for this product, which appears on pages 3591–3595 of the 2002 PDR, has been revised as follows. Please write "See Supplement A" next to the product heading.

In the third sentence of the paragraph under the subheading ***Metabolism*** *in the* **CLINICAL PHARMACOLOGY** *section,* "CYP3A4" *should be deleted and replaced with* "cytochrome P_{450} (CYP)3A4."

The paragraph following the subheading ***"Controlled Trials Supporting Effectiveness"*** *under* **Clinical Trials** *in the* **CLINICAL PHARMACOLOGY** *section should be deleted and replaced with the following paragraph:*

Sonata (typically administered in doses of 5 mg, 10 mg, or 20 mg) has been studied in patients with chronic insomnia (n = 3,435) in 12 placebo- and active-drug-controlled trials. Three of the trials were in elderly patients (n = 1,019). It has also been studied in transient insomnia (n = 264). Because of its very short half-life, studies focused on decreasing sleep latency, with less attention to duration of sleep and number of awakenings, for which consistent differences from placebo were not demonstrated. Studies were also carried out to examine the time course of effects on memory and psychomotor function, and to examine withdrawal phenomena.

The second paragraph of the subsection "Non-elderly patients:" *following the subheading* ***Chronic Insomnia*** *under* **Clinical Trials** *in the* **CLINICAL PHARMACOLOGY** *section should be deleted and replaced with the following paragraph:*

Adult outpatients with chronic insomnia were evaluated in six double-blind, parallel-group sleep laboratory studies that varied in duration from a single night up to 35 nights. Overall, these studies demonstrated a superiority of Sonata 10 mg and 20 mg over placebo in reducing LPS on the first 2 nights of treatment. At later time points in 5-, 14-, and 28-night studies, a reduction in LPS from baseline was observed for all treatment groups, including the placebo group, and thus, a significant difference between Sonata and placebo was not seen beyond 2 nights. In a 35-night study, Sonata 10 mg was significantly more effective than placebo in reducing LPS at the primary efficacy endpoint on nights 29 and 30.

The second and third paragraphs following the subheading ***Withdrawal Emergent Anxiety and Insomnia*** *under* ***Studies Pertinent to Safety Concerns for Sedative/Hypnotic Drugs*** *under* **Clinical Trials** *in the* **CLINICAL PHARMACOLOGY** *section should be deleted and replaced with the following:*

Zaleplon has a short half-life and no active metabolites. At the primary efficacy endpoint (nights 29 and 30) in a 35-night sleep laboratory study, polysomnographic recordings showed that wakefulness was not significantly longer with Sonata than with placebo during the last quarter of the night. No increase in the signs of daytime anxiety was observed in clinical trials with Sonata. In two sleep laboratory studies involving 14- and 28-nightly doses of Sonata (5 mg and 10 mg in one study and 10 mg and 20 mg in the second) and structured assessments of daytime anxiety, no increases in daytime anxiety was detected. Similarly, in a pooled analysis (all the parallel-group, placebo-controlled studies) of spontaneously reported daytime anxiety, no difference was observed between Sonata and placebo.

Rebound insomnia, defined as a dose-dependent temporary worsening in sleep parameters (latency, total sleep time, and number of awakenings) compared to baseline following discontinuation of treatment, is observed with short- and intermediate-acting hypnotics. Rebound insomnia following discontinuation of Sonata relative to baseline was examined at both nights 1 and 2 following discontinuation in three sleep laboratory studies (14, 28, and 35 nights) and five outpatient studies utilizing patient diaries (14 and 28 nights). Overall, the data suggest that rebound insomnia may be dose dependent. At 20 mg, there appeared to be both objective (polysomnographic) and subjective (diary) evidence of rebound insomnia on the first night after discontinuation of treatment with Sonata. At 5 mg and 10 mg, there was no objective and minimal subjective evidence of rebound insomnia on the first night after discontinuation of treatment with Sonata. At all doses, the rebound effect appeared to resolve by the second night following withdrawal. In the 35-night study, there was a worsening in sleep on the first night off for both the 10-mg and 20-mg groups compared to placebo, but not to baseline. This discontinuation-emergent effect was mild, had the characteristics of the return of the symptoms of chronic insomnia, and appeared to resolve by the second night after zaleplon discontinuation.

The paragraph following the subheading ***Other Withdrawal-Emergent Phenomena*** *under* ***Studies Pertinent to Safety Concerns for Sedative/Hypnotic Drugs*** *under* **Clinical Trials** *in the* **CLINICAL PHARMACOLOGY** *section should be deleted and replaced with the following:*

The potential for other withdrawal phenomena was also assessed for in 14- to 28-night studies, including both the sleep laboratory studies and the outpatient studies, and in open-label studies of 6- and 12-month durations. The Benzodiazepine Withdrawal Symptom Questionnaire was used in several of these studies, both at baseline and then during days 1 and 2 following discontinuation. Withdrawal was operationally defined as the emergence of 3 or more new symptoms after discontinuation. Sonata was not distinguishable from placebo at doses of 5 mg, 10 mg, or 20 mg on this measure, nor was Sonata distinguishable from placebo on spontaneously reported withdrawal-emergent adverse events. There were no instances of withdrawal delirium, withdrawal associated hallucinations, or any other manifestations of severe sedative/hypnotic withdrawal.

The following paragraph should be added to the end of the subsection following the subheading "Use in patients with depression" under **General** *in the* **PRECAUTIONS** *section:*

This product contains FD&C Yellow No. 5 (tartrazine) which may cause allergic-type reactions (including bronchial asthma) in certain susceptible persons. Although the overall incidence of FD&C Yellow No. 5 (tartrazine) sensitivity in the general population is low, it is frequently seen in patients with aspirin hypersensitivity.

The entire **ADVERSE REACTIONS** *section should be deleted and replaced with the following:*

ADVERSE REACTIONS

The premarketing development program for Sonata included zaleplon exposures in patients and/or normal subjects from 2 different groups of studies: approximately 900 normal subjects in clinical pharmacology/pharmacokinetic studies; and approximately 2,900 exposures from patients in placebo-controlled clinical effectiveness studies, corresponding to approximately 450 patient exposure years. The conditions and duration of treatment with Sonata varied greatly and included (in overlapping categories) open-label and double-blind phases of studies, inpatients and outpatients, and short-term or longer-term exposure. Adverse reactions were assessed by collecting adverse events, results of physical examinations, vital signs, weights, laboratory analyses, and ECGs.

Adverse events during exposure were obtained primarily by general inquiry and recorded by clinical investigators using terminology of their own choosing. Consequently, it is not possible to provide a meaningful estimate of the proportion of individuals experiencing adverse events without first grouping similar types of events into a smaller number of standardized event categories. In the tables and tabulations that follow, COSTART terminology has been used to classify reported adverse events.

The stated frequencies of adverse events represent the proportion of individuals who experienced, at least once, a treatment-emergent adverse event of the type listed. An event was considered treatment emergent if it occurred for the first time or worsened while receiving therapy following baseline evaluation.

Adverse Findings Observed in Short-Term, Placebo-Controlled Trials

Adverse Events Associated With Discontinuation of Treatment

In premarketing placebo-controlled, parallel-group phase 2 and phase 3 clinical trials, 3.1% of 744 patients who received placebo and 3.7% of 2,149 patients who received Sonata discontinued treatment because of an adverse clinical event. This difference was not statistically significant. No event that resulted in discontinuation occurred at a rate of ≥1%.

Adverse Events Occurring at an Incidence of 1% or More Among Sonata 20 mg-Treated Patients

Table 1 enumerates the incidence of treatment-emergent adverse events for a pool of three 28-night and one 35-night placebo-controlled studies of Sonata at doses of 5 mg or 10 mg and 20 mg. The table includes only those events that occurred in 1% or more of patients treated with Sonata 20 mg and that had a higher incidence in patients treated with Sonata 20 mg than in placebo-treated patients.

The prescriber should be aware that these figures cannot be used to predict the incidence of adverse events in the course of usual medical practice where patient characteristics and other factors differ from those which prevailed in the clinical trials. Similarly, the cited frequencies cannot be compared with figures obtained from other clinical investigations involving different treatments, uses, and investigators. The cited figures, however, do provide the prescribing physician with some basis for estimating the relative contribution of drug and non-drug factors to the adverse event incidence rate in the population studied.

Table 1
Incidence (%) of Treatment-Emergent Adverse Events in Long-Term (28 and 35 Nights) Placebo-Controlled Clinical Trials of Sonata[1]

Body System Preferred Term	Placebo (n = 344)	Sonata 5 mg or 10 mg (n = 569)	Sonata 20 mg (n = 297)
Body as a whole			
Abdominal pain	3	6	6
Asthenia	5	5	7
Headache	35	30	42
Malaise	<1	<1	2
Photosensitivity reaction	<1	<1	1
Digestive system			
Anorexia	<1	<1	2
Colitis	0	0	1
Nausea	7	6	8
Metabolic and nutritional			
Peripheral edema	<1	<1	1

Nervous system			
Amnesia	1	2	4
Confusion	<1	<1	1
Depersonalization	<1	<1	2
Dizziness	7	7	9
Hallucinations	<1	<1	1
Hypertonia	<1	1	1
Hypesthesia	<1	<1	2
Paresthesia	1	3	3
Somnolence	4	5	6
Tremor	1	2	2
Vertigo	<1	<1	1
Respiratory system			
Epistaxis	<1	<1	1
Special senses			
Abnormal vision	<1	<1	2
Ear pain	0	<1	1
Eye pain	2	4	3
Hyperacusis	<1	1	2
Parosmia	<1	<1	2
Urogenital system			
Dysmenorrhea	2	3	4

1: Events for which the incidence for Sonata 20 mg-treated patients was at least 1% and greater than the incidence among placebo-treated patients. Incidence greater than 1% has been rounded to the nearest whole number.

Other Adverse Events Observed During the Premarketing Evaluation of Sonata

Listed below are COSTART terms that reflect treatment-emergent adverse events as defined in the introduction to the **ADVERSE REACTIONS** section. These events were reported by patients treated with Sonata (zaleplon) at doses in a range of 5 mg/day to 20 mg/day during premarketing phase 2 and phase 3 clinical trials throughout the United States, Canada, and Europe including approximately 2,900 patients. All reported events are included except those already listed in Table 1 or elsewhere in labeling, those events for which a drug cause was remote, and those event terms that were so general as to be uninformative. It is important to emphasize that although the events reported occurred during treatment with Sonata, they were not necessarily caused by it.

Events are further categorized by body system and listed in order of decreasing frequency according to the following definitions: **frequent** adverse events are those occurring on one or more occasions in at least 1/100 patients; **infrequent** adverse events are those occurring in less than 1/100 patients but at least 1/1,000 patients; **rare** events are those occurring in fewer than 1/1,000 patients.

Body as a whole—**Frequent:** back pain, chest pain, fever; **Infrequent:** chest pain substernal, chills, face edema, generalized edema, hangover effect, neck rigidity.

Cardiovascular system—**Frequent:** migraine; **Infrequent:** angina pectoris, bundle branch block, hypertension, hypotension, palpitation, syncope, tachycardia, vasodilatation, ventricular extrasystoles; **Rare:** bigeminy, cerebral ischemia, cyanosis, pericardial effusion, postural hypotension, pulmonary embolus, sinus bradycardia, thrombophlebitis, ventricular tachycardia.

Digestive system—**Frequent:** constipation, dry mouth, dyspepsia; **Infrequent:** eructation, esophagitis, flatulence, gastritis, gastroenteritis, gingivitis, glossitis, increased appetite, melena, mouth ulceration, rectal hemorrhage, stomatitis; **Rare:** aphthous stomatitis, biliary pain, bruxism, cardiospasm, cheilitis, cholelithiasis, duodenal ulcer, dysphagia, enteritis, gum hemorrhage, increased salivation, intestinal obstruction, abnormal liver function tests, peptic ulcer, tongue discoloration, tongue edema, ulcerative stomatitis.

Endocrine system—**Rare:** diabetes mellitus, goiter, hypothyroidism.

Hemic and lymphatic system—**Infrequent:** anemia, ecchymosis, lymphadenopathy; **Rare:** eosinophilia, leukocytosis, lymphocytosis, purpura.

Metabolic and nutritional—**Infrequent:** edema, gout, hypercholesteremia, thirst, weight gain; **Rare:** bilirubinemia, hyperglycemia, hyperuricemia, hypoglycemia, hypoglycemic reaction, ketosis, lactose intolerance, AST (SGOT) increased, ALT (SGPT) increased, weight loss.

Musculoskeletal system—**Frequent:** arthralgia, arthritis, myalgia; **Infrequent:** arthrosis, bursitis, joint disorder (mainly swelling, stiffness, and pain), myasthenia, tenosynovitis; **Rare:** myositis, osteoporosis.

Nervous system—**Frequent:** anxiety, depression, nervousness, thinking abnormal (mainly difficulty concentrating); **Infrequent:** abnormal gait, agitation, apathy, ataxia, circumoral paresthesia, emotional lability, euphoria, hyperesthesia, hyperkinesia, hypotonia, incoordination, insomnia, libido decreased, neuralgia, nystagmus; **Rare:** CNS stimulation, delusions, dysarthria, dystonia, facial paralysis, hostility, hypokinesia, myoclonus, neuropathy, psychomotor retardation, ptosis, reflexes decreased, reflexes increased, sleep talking, sleep walking, slurred speech, stupor, trismus.

Respiratory system—**Frequent:** bronchitis; **Infrequent:** asthma, dyspnea, laryngitis, pneumonia, snoring, voice alteration; **Rare:** apnea, hiccup, hyperventilation, pleural effusion, sputum increased.

Skin and appendages—**Frequent:** pruritus, rash; **Infrequent:** acne, alopecia, contact dermatitis, dry skin, eczema, maculopapular rash, skin hypertrophy, sweating, urticaria, vesiculobullous rash; **Rare:** melanosis, psoriasis, pustular rash, skin discoloration.

Special senses—**Frequent:** conjunctivitis, taste perversion; **Infrequent:** diplopia, dry eyes, photophobia, tinnitus, watery eyes; **Rare:** abnormality of accommodation, blepharitis, cataract specified, corneal erosion, deafness, eye hemorrhage, glaucoma, labyrinthitis, retinal detachment, taste loss, visual field defect.

Urogenital system—**Infrequent:** bladder pain, breast pain, cystitis, decreased urine stream, dysuria, hematuria, impotence, kidney calculus, kidney pain, menorrhagia, metrorrhagia, urinary frequency, urinary incontinence, urinary urgency, vaginitis; **Rare:** albuminuria, delayed menstrual period, leukorrhea, menopause, urethritis, urinary retention, vaginal hemorrhage.

The first paragraph under the subheading "Dependence" under **Abuse, Dependence, and Tolerance** *in the* **DRUG ABUSE AND DEPENDENCE** *section should be deleted and replaced with the following paragraph:*

Dependence

The potential for developing physical dependence on Sonata and a subsequent withdrawal syndrome was assessed in controlled studies of 14-, 28-, and 35-night durations and in open-label studies of 6- and 12-month durations by examining for the emergence of rebound insomnia following drug discontinuation. Some patients (mostly those treated with 20 mg) experienced a mild rebound insomnia on the first night following withdrawal that appeared to be resolved by the second night. The use of Benzodiazepine Withdrawal Symptom Questionnaire and examination of any other withdrawal emergent events did not detect any other evidence for a withdrawal syndrome following abrupt discontinuation of Sonata therapy in pre-marketing studies.

The paragraph under the subheading "Tolerance" under **Abuse, Dependence, and Tolerance** *in the* **DRUG ABUSE AND DEPENDENCE** *section should be deleted and replaced with the following paragraph:*

Tolerance

Possible tolerance to the hypnotic effects of Sonata 10 mg and 20 mg was assessed by evaluating time to sleep onset for Sonata compared with placebo in two 28-night placebo-controlled studies and latency to persistent sleep in one 35-night placebo-controlled study where tolerance was evaluated on nights 29 and 30. No development of tolerance to Sonata was observed for time to sleep onset over 4 weeks.

CI 6001-3 Revised November 26, 2001

TRIPHASIL®-21 ℞

[*trī-fă 'sĭl*]

Tablets

(levonorgestrel and ethinyl estradiol tablets—triphasic regimen)

Prescribing information for this product, which appears on pages 3600–3605 of the 2002 PDR, has been revised as follows. Please write "See Supplement A" next to the product heading.

The paragraph that is the entire **CLINICAL PHARMACOLOGY** *section should be deleted and replaced with the following:*

Combination oral contraceptives primarily act by suppression of gonadotropins. Although the primary mechanism of this action is inhibition of ovulation, other alterations include changes in the cervical mucus (which increase the difficulty of sperm entry into the uterus) and the endometrium (which reduce the likelihood of implantation).

PHARMACOKINETICS

Absorption

Levonorgestrel is rapidly and completely absorbed after oral administration (bioavailability about 100%). Levonorgestrel is not subject to first-pass metabolism or enterohepatic circulation and therefore does not undergo variations in absorption after oral administration. Ethinyl estradiol is rapidly and almost completely absorbed from the gastrointestinal tract but, due to first-pass metabolism in gut mucosa and liver, the bioavailability of ethinyl estradiol is between 38% and 48%.

There have been no formal multiple-dose studies conducted using Triphasil. However, a multiple-dose study was done in 22 women using a monophasic, low dose combination of 0.10 mg levonorgestrel and 0.02 mg ethinyl estradiol. Maximum serum concentrations of levonorgestrel were found to be 2.8 ± 0.9 ng/mL (mean ± SD) at 1.6 ± 0.9 hours after a single dose, reaching a steady state at day 19. Observed levonorgestrel concentrations increased from day 1 to days 6 and 21 by 34% and 96%, respectively. Unbound levonorgestrel concentrations subsequently increased from day 1 to days 6 and 21 by 25% and 83%, respectively, however, the accumulation of unbound levonoregestrel was approximately 14% less than total levonorgestrel accumulation. The kinetics of total levonorgestrel were non-linear due to an increase in binding of levonoregestrel to SHBG, which is attributed to increased SHBG levels that are induced by the daily administration of ethinyl estradiol. Ethinyl estradiol reached maximum serum concentrations of 62 ± 21 pg/mL at 1.5 ± 0.5 hours after a single dose, reaching steady state at day 6. Ethinyl estradiol concentrations increased by 19% from days 1 to 21 consistent with an elimination half-life of 18 hours.

Single-dose studies with Triphasil have been conducted with the following data reported below in Table I. Plasma concentrations have been corrected below to reflect single tablet dosing/day.

TABLE I: MEAN (SE) PHARMACOKINETIC PARAMETERS OF TRIPHASIL IN SINGLE-DOSE STUDIES

Levonorgestrel

Dose LNG/EE µg	C_{max} ng/mL	t_{max} h	$t_{1/2}$ h	AUC ng•h/mL
50/30	1.7 (0.1)	1.3 (0.1)	23 (2.2)	17 (1.5)
75/40	2.1 (0.2)	1.5 (0.2)	15 (1.2)	21 (2.0)
125/30	2.5 (0.2)	1.6 (0.1)	23 (1.4)	34 (3.0)

Ethinyl Estradiol

Dose LNG/EE µg	C_{max} pg/mL	t_{max} h	$t_{1/2}$ h	AUC pg•h/mL
50/30	141 (9)	1.4 (0.1)	8.1 (1.0)	1126 (113)
75/40	179 (13)	1.6 (0.2)	14 (1.7)	2177 (244)
125/30	115 (10)	1.5 (0.1)	8.8 (1.6)	1072 (170)

Distribution

Levonorgestrel is bound to SHBG and albumin. Levonorgestrel has high binding affinity for SHBG that is 60% of that of testosterone. Ethinyl estradiol is about 97% bound to plasma albumin. Ethinyl estradiol does not bind to SHBG, but will induce SHBG synthesis.

Metabolism

Levonorgestrel: The most important metabolic pathway occurs in the reduction of the Δ4-3-oxo group and hydroxylation at positions 2α, 1β, and 16β, followed by conjugation. Most of the metabolites that circulate in the blood are sulfates of 3α,5β-tetrahydro-levonorgestrel, while excretion occurs predominately in the form of glucuronides. Some of the parent levonorgestrel also circulates as 17β-sulfate. Metabolic clearance rates may differ among individuals by several-fold, and this may account in part for the wide variation observed in levonorgestrel concentrations among users.

Ethinyl estradiol: Cytochrome P450 enzymes (CYP3A4) in the liver are responsible for the 2-hydroxylation that is the major oxidative reaction. The 2-hydroxy metabolite is further transformed by methylation and glucuronidation prior to urinary and fecal excretion. Levels of Cytochrome P450 (CYP3A) vary widely among individuals and can explain the variation in rates of ethinyl estradiol 2-hydroxylation. Ethinyl estradiol is excreted in the urine and feces as glucuronide and sulfate conjugates, and undergoes enterohepatic circulation.

Excretion

The elimination half-life for levonorgestrel is approximately 36 ± 13 hours at steady state. Levonorgestrel and its metabolites are primarily excreted in the urine (40% to 68%) and about 16% to 48% are excreted in the feces. The elimination half-life of ethinyl estradiol is 18 ± 4.7 hours at steady state.

SPECIAL POPULATIONS

Hepatic Insufficiency

No formal studies have evaluated the effect of hepatic disease on the disposition of Triphasil. However, steroid hormones may be poorly metabolized in patients with impaired liver function.

Renal Insufficiency

No formal studies have evaluated the effect of renal disease on the disposition of Triphasil.

Drug-Drug Interactions

Interactions between ethinyl estradiol and other drugs have been reported in the literature.

- *Interactions with Absorption:* Diarrhea may increase gastrointestinal motility and reduce hormone absorption. Similarly, any drug which reduces gut transit time may reduce hormone concentrations in the blood.
- *Interactions with Metabolism:*
  Gastrointestinal wall: Sulfation of ethinyl estradiol has been shown to occur in the gastrointestinal (GI) wall. Therefore, drugs which act as competitive inhibitors for sulfation in the GI wall may increase ethinyl estradiol bioavailability (e.g., ascorbic acid).
  Hepatic metabolism: Interactions can occur with drugs that induce microsomal enzymes which can decrease ethinyl estradiol concentrations (e.g., rifampin, barbiturates, phenylbutazone, phenytoin, griseofulvin).
- *Interference with Enterohepatic Circulation:* Some clinical reports suggest that enterohepatic circulation of estrogens may decrease when certain antibiotic agents are given, which may reduce ethinyl estradiol concentrations (e.g., ampicillin, tetracycline).
- *Interference in the Metabolism of Other Drugs:* Ethinyl estradiol may interfere with the metabolism of other drugs by inhibiting hepatic microsomal enzymes or by inducing hepatic drug conjugation, particularly glucuronidation. Accordingly, plasma and tissue concentrations may either be increased or decreased, respectively (e.g., cyclosporine, theophylline).

CI 7461-1 Issued May 2, 2001

Key to Controlled Substances Categories

Products listed with the symbols shown below are subject to the Controlled Substances Act of 1970. These drugs are categorized according to their potential for abuse. The greater the potential, the more severe the limitations on their prescription.

CATEGORY	INTERPRETATION
CII	**HIGH POTENTIAL FOR ABUSE.** Use may lead to severe physical or psychological dependence. Prescriptions must be written in ink, or typewritten and signed by the practitioner. Verbal prescriptions must be confirmed in writing within 72 hours, and may be given only in a genuine emergency. No renewals are permitted.
CIII	**SOME POTENTIAL FOR ABUSE.** Use may lead to low-to-moderate physical dependence or high psychological dependence. Prescriptions may be oral or written. Up to 5 renewals are permitted within 6 months.
CIV	**LOW POTENTIAL FOR ABUSE.** Use may lead to limited physical or psychological dependence. Prescriptions may be oral or written. Up to 5 renewals are permitted within 6 months.
CV	**SUBJECT TO STATE AND LOCAL REGULATION.** Abuse potential is low; a prescription may not be required.

Key to FDA Use-in-Pregnancy Ratings

The U.S. Food and Drug Administration's use-in-pregnancy rating system weighs the degree to which available information has ruled out risk to the fetus against the drug's potential benefit to the patient. The ratings, and their interpretation, are as follows:

CATEGORY	INTERPRETATION
A	**CONTROLLED STUDIES SHOW NO RISK.** Adequate, well-controlled studies in pregnant women have failed to demonstrate a risk to the fetus in any trimester of pregnancy.
B	**NO EVIDENCE OF RISK IN HUMANS.** Adequate, well-controlled studies in pregnant women have not shown increased risk of fetal abnormalities despite adverse findings in animals, or, in the absence of adequate human studies, animal studies show no fetal risk. The chance of fetal harm is remote, but remains a possibility.
C	**RISK CANNOT BE RULED OUT.** Adequate, well-controlled human studies are lacking, and animal studies have shown a risk to the fetus or are lacking as well. There is a chance of fetal harm if the drug is administered during pregnancy; but the potential benefits may outweigh the potential risk.
D	**POSITIVE EVIDENCE OF RISK.** Studies in humans, or investigational or post-marketing data, have demonstrated fetal risk. Nevertheless, potential benefits from the use of the drug may outweigh the potential risk. For example, the drug may be acceptable if needed in a life-threatening situation or serious disease for which safer drugs cannot be used or are ineffective.
X	**CONTRAINDICATED IN PREGNANCY.** Studies in animals or humans, or investigational or post-marketing reports, have demonstrated positive evidence of fetal abnormalities or risk which clearly outweighs any possible benefit to the patient.